SRB's

Volume 1

Surgical Operations

Text and Atlas

Volume 1

SRB's Surgical Operations

Text and Atlas

Third Edition

Sriram Bhat M MS (General Surgery) FRCS (Glasgow)
Professor and Unit Head
Department of Surgery
Kasturba Medical College
Mangaluru, Karnataka, India

Honorary Medical Officer
Government District Wenlock Hospital, Mangaluru
Dakshina Kannada, Karnataka, India
e-mail: meera_sriram2003@yahoo.com

Forewords

K Ganesh Pai
Ashok Pandit

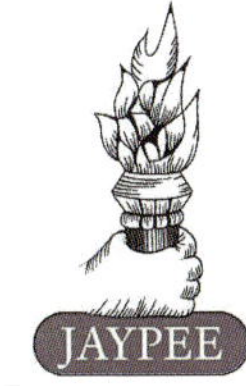

JAYPEE BROTHERS MEDICAL PUBLISHERS
The Health Sciences Publisher
New Delhi | London

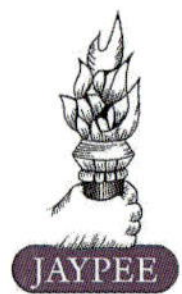

Jaypee Brothers Medical Publishers (P) Ltd

Headquarters
Jaypee Brothers Medical Publishers (P) Ltd
EMCA House, 23/23-B
Ansari Road, Daryaganj
New Delhi 110 002, India
Landline: +91-11-23272143, +91-11-23272703
+91-11-23282021, +91-11-23245672
Email: jaypee@jaypeebrothers.com

Corporate Office
Jaypee Brothers Medical Publishers (P) Ltd
4838/24, Ansari Road, Daryaganj
New Delhi 110 002, India
Phone: +91-11-43574357
Fax: +91-11-43574314
Email: jaypee@jaypeebrothers.com

Overseas Office
JP Medical Ltd.
83, Victoria Street, London
SW1H 0HW (UK)
Phone: +44 20 3170 8910
Fax: +44 (0)20 3008 6180
Email: info@jpmedpub.com

Website: www.jaypeebrothers.com
Website: www.jaypeedigital.com

SRB's Surgical Operations: Text and Atlas (2 Volumes)

First Edition: 2014
Second Edition: 2018
Revised Reprint: 2024
Third Edition: **2025**

ISBN: 978-93-5696-956-8

Printed at: Samrat Offset Pvt. Ltd.

This book is dedicated to
My beloved father

***Late* Mr Krishna Bhat Muguli**

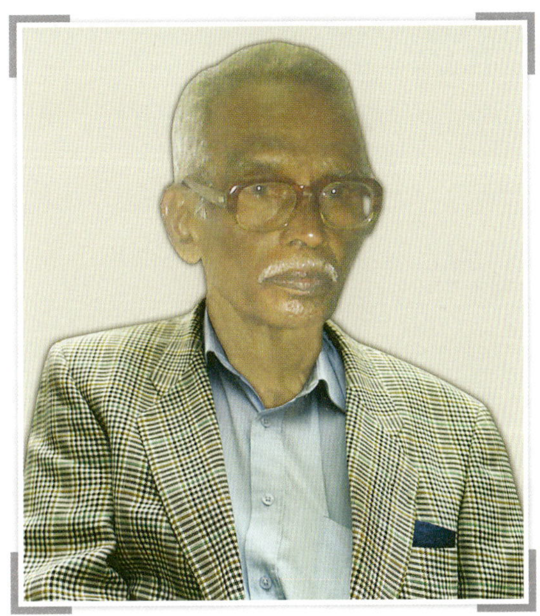

from whom I have learnt *simplicity, contentment, humility and dedication*

and

Mangala Hospital and Mangala Kidney Foundation, Mangaluru, India

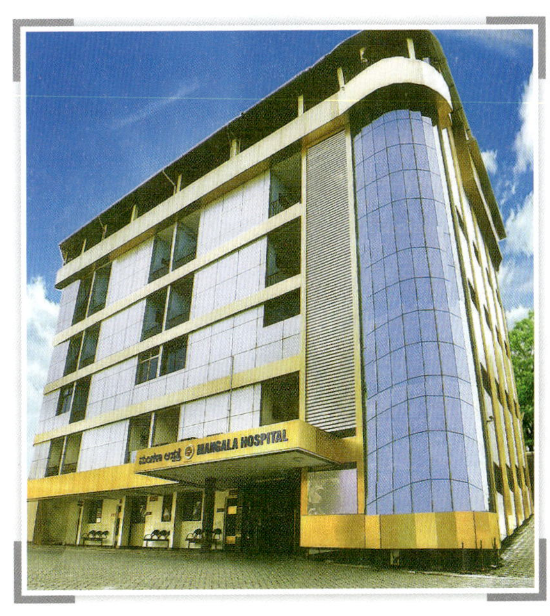

Contributors

Amit Jain MS
Consultant and Head
Amit Jain's Institute of Diabetic Foot and Wound Care
Brindhavvan Areion Hospital
Bengaluru, Karnataka, India

Arunkumar MS MCh (Surgical Gastroenterology)
Consultant Surgical Gastroenterologist
Kochi, Kerala, India
Contributed to chapters on Surgeries of Liver and Gallbladder, and Surgeries of Pancreas

Ashok Pandit MS MCh (Urology)
Urologist
Yenepoya Hospital
Kodialbail, Mangaluru, Karnataka, India
Contributed to chapter on Urologic Surgeries

Ashok Shetty MS MCh (Cardiothoracic)
Cardiothoracic Surgeon
Mangaluru, Karnataka, India
Contributed to chapter on Surgeries in Arterial Diseases

CS Rajan MS FRCS
Professor
Mallya Hospital
Consultant Surgeon
Annaswamy Mudaliar General Hospital
Bengaluru, Karnataka, India
Ex-Head
Department of Surgery
St. Martha's Hospital, Bengaluru (2003–2013)
Contributed on topic Intercostal Tube Drainage in chapter of Principles of Surgical Management in Trauma

Keshavprasad MS
Associate Professor
Department of Surgery
Kasturba Medical College
Mangaluru, Karnataka, India
Contributed to chapters on Basics in Laparotomy and Laparoscopy; Surgeries of Liver and Gallbladder, and Surgeries of Pancreas

Meera Karanth P MD (Obs & Gynae)
Consultant Gynaecologist
Mangaluru, Karnataka, India
Wrote the chapter on Surgeries in Obstetrics and Gynaecology

Venkatesh Udupa MS (Surgical Gastroenterology)
Department of HPB Surgery and Liver Transplantation
St. Vincent's University Hospital
Dublin, Ireland
Contributed to chapter on Surgeries of Liver and Gallbladder

Foreword

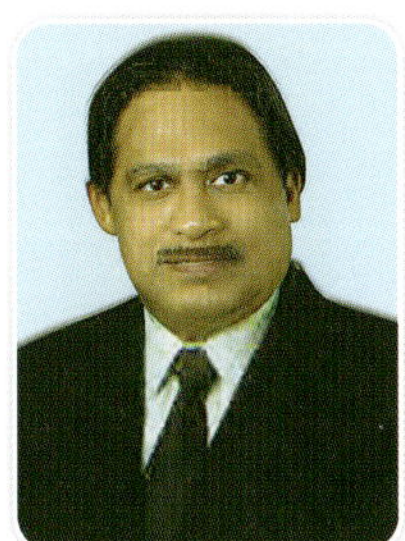

It is my pleasure to write a foreword for *SRB's Surgical Operations: Text and Atlas*, third edition. Let me, at the outset, congratulate Dr Sriram Bhat M for launching this fantastic book. Dr Bhat belongs to a rare breed of surgeons, who has not only mastered the art of excellence in teaching but also bestowed with superb skill in surgery and documentation. This facet has been put on record by bagging Good Teacher Award twice from Kasturba Medical College, Mangaluru, Karnataka, India, a constituent college of the prestigious university, Manipal Academy of Higher Education (MAHE), Manipal and churning out about half a dozen textbooks related to surgery. These books have been well received and sold like cakes within India and abroad.

I have gone through the contents of this book and it is quite fascinating. It has about 1,450 pages containing coloured illustrations of operative procedures spread across fields of general surgery, gastrointestinal tract surgery, urology, vascular surgery, and basic laparoscopy. A study of this book, at the very least, stimulates surgeons to think about their own technique. It is unlikely that a surgeon who is expert in a particular operation will turn to this book for advice about that operation, but it is to be expected that the same surgeon will obtain useful information from this book when called upon to operate in a less familiar field. I sincerely appreciate and applaud with deep admiration the efforts put in by Dr Bhat (fondly referred as SRB by his students and colleagues) devoting his valuable time at the cost of his family and professional life towards this aesthetic collection which, in a nutshell, is extremely par excellent.

I, therefore, wholeheartedly support this book and recommend its use by undergraduate and postgraduate students, general surgeons, and all those who need guidance in the field of operative surgery and basic laparoscopy.

K Ganesh Pai MS MCh (Paediatric Surgery)
Senior Paediatric Surgeon and Paediatric Urologist
Emeritus Professor of Paediatric Surgery
Kasturba Medical College
Mangaluru, Karnataka, India

Foreword

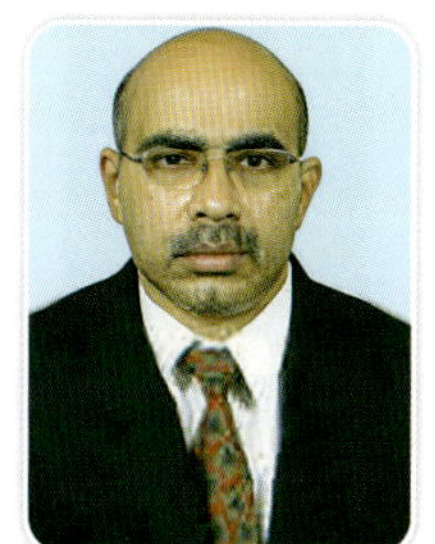

No matter how well read and proficient in clinical skills, the ultimate test of a surgeon is the operation theatre. Although a mastery of operative surgery does require a lifetime's practice, having a good teacher/mentor and access to a thorough text on operative surgery, will shorten the learning curve. This textbook with its exhaustive coverage of practically all surgical procedures (common and otherwise) will definitely be useful to both undergraduate and postgraduate students of surgery as well as practitioners of the art. The plentiful illustrations are simple and enhance the understanding.

It is my distinct privilege to have been associated with Dr Sriram Bhat M since his time as a postgraduate in surgery and has a great love for teaching. The large number of students who flock his weekly bedside clinics in Government District Wenlock Hospital, Mangaluru, Dakshina Kannada, Karnataka, India, ever since he joined the faculty of general surgery, is a testament to his ability to impart knowledge. Having worked with him for over 30 years, I have seen him growing in stature and knowledge as a surgeon. He picks up new skills like laparoscopy through sheer hard work. Dr Bhat also has prodigious literary output. He has written more than five books in relation to surgery for medical, dental and nursing graduates. His *SRB's Manual of Surgery* has proved hugely popular among undergraduates in India and abroad. Having seen his labour day and night at documenting the various surgical procedures and, of course, the laborious collating, writing and proofreading often into the wee hours of the morning reminded me of Duke Elder (of the classic ophthalmic text) who reputedly made with barely an hour's sleep! I thank Dr Bhat for giving me this unique honour of writing the foreword for this operative book which I am certain will also prove equally popular and useful.

Ashok Pandit MS MCh (Urology)
Consultant Urologist
Mangaluru, Karnataka, India

Preface to the Third Edition

It is a great pleasure to bring this third edition of *SRB's Surgical Operations: Text and Atlas*, almost 6 years after the release of the second edition in 2018. The first edition was released in 2014, and both editions were very well appreciated by the postgraduate students and fellow colleagues and on their insistence, I intend to bring out the third edition. The main aim of this book is to reach out to all students, the basic principles involved in the art of surgery by bringing out in a lucid way the steps involved in various procedures, from the simplest of the procedures to the most complex radical surgeries. There were few shortcomings in the first and second editions. They are addressed adequately along with correction of mistakes in the text and diagram. Few current concepts are updated in most of the chapters. I deeply indebt all those who supported me to bring out this edition. Diabetic foot management is changing in approach which is added in specific by none other than our country's renowned surgeon, Dr Amit Jain from Bengaluru, Karnataka, India. I thank Professor K Ganesh Pai, a renowned paediatric surgeon from Mangaluru, and my dear friend, colleague, and renowned urologist, Dr Ashok Pandit in Mangaluru for writing Forewords to this edition also. I acknowledge all contributors in helping me directly or indirectly in bringing out this third edition.

My special thanks go to our beloved Group Chairman Shri Jitendar P Vij of M/s Jaypee Brothers Medical Publishers (P) Ltd, New Delhi, India, for his constant encouragement for all my works.

I always remember all my patients from whom I have taken different photographs for the book. I wish and pray for their health and recovery.

I accept any criticism and comments about this edition from readers and followers of this book. I hope this edition will be immensely helpful to all surgical postgraduates and all practicing surgeons of this country and abroad in treating different conditions surgically.

Sriram Bhat M
e-mail: meera_sriram2003@yahoo.com

Preface to the First Edition

It was my long dream after writing *SRB's Manual of Surgery* to pen in relations to operative technique in detail from simplest procedure to essential advanced major procedures needed to general surgeons and surgical postgraduates. I took nearly 4 years to make my dream near true in the form of *SRB's Surgical Operations: Text and Atlas*. I have included umpteen numbers of illustrations and photographs. Basic principles and techniques of suturing and dissection are also dealt with in detail. It will be useful to all categories of students and consultants to learn the basics. Gastrointestinal surgery is discussed in detail with illustrations. Urology mainly open methods are discussed adequately if not extensively. Basic laparoscopy and usual laparoscopy surgeries are discussed with highlighting the robotic surgeries, liposuction and so on. It differs from other operative surgery books by its unique presentations in detail with surgical anatomy and operative photographs of most of the procedures. I presume students and consultants will enjoy its reading. I am always grateful to Shri Jitendar P Vij (Group Chairman) of M/s Jaypee Brothers Medical Publishers (P) Ltd, New Delhi, India, for his support and encouragement towards me to bring out this book. Any comments and healthy criticisms are well accepted.

Sriram Bhat M
e-mail: meera_sriram2003@yahoo.com

Acknowledgements

I am happy to bring out the third edition of the book *SRB's Surgical Operations: Text and Atlas*. This is due to constant help and support of many.

- I thank our Chancellor Dr Ramdas M Pai, Pro-Chancellor, Vice-Chancellor, Pro-Vice-Chancellor of Manipal Academy of Higher Education, and Dean, Kasturba Medical College (KMC), Mangaluru and Manipal, Karnataka, India.
- I thank the Head, Department of Surgery, KMC, and Professor Ashfaque Mohammad, for his constant encouragement in academic work and progress.
- I always remember my senior teachers, Professor CR Ballal, Professor Suresh Kamath, Professor K Prakash Rao, *Late* Professor Subramanya Bhat, Professor Bhaskar Shetty, and Professor Ramachandra Pai, for their constant help.
- I thank Professor K Ganesh Pai, Paediatric Surgeon, for his encouragement and for writing foreword to this book. He was my thesis guide and is a renowned paediatric surgeon.
- I thank by beloved friend, popular urologist, Dr Ashok Pandit, Mangaluru, who has been helping me in my entire surgical career. He happily agreed to write foreword to this book.
- My special thanks go to Dr Jayaram Shenoy, Dr Jayaprakash Rao, and Professor Thangam Verghese, for their affection and support.
- Surgical unit heads in our college Drs Manohar Pai, Poornachandra, Shivaprasad Rai, Yogishkumar, Sunil Kumar Shetty, Rajesh Ballal, Rahul Bhat, and Shivananda Prabhu have always been supportive of my work and are worth to be remembered always.
- I am grateful to all my teachers and colleagues in the surgery department, who directly or indirectly helped me to bring out this edition.
- I appreciate District Medical Officer and Resident Medical Officer of Government District Wenlock Hospital, Mangaluru, for their kind help.
- I will never forget my close associate Dr Ganapathy, Mangala Hospital, Kadri, Mangaluru, and Dr Anitha Bhat, Anaesthetist, for their affectionate help and encouragement in all my endeavours. They always stood with me in my difficulties.
- My special thanks go to Professor Sribatsa Kumar Mohapathra, Veer Surendra Sai Medical College (VSSMC), Burla, Sambalpur, Odisha, India, and Dr Arunkumar, Surgical Gastroenterologist, Kochi, Kerala, India.
- I sincerely thank all earlier and recent contributors to this edition.
- I sincerely thank Professor Navinchandra Shetty, Head, Department of Radiology, KMC, Mangaluru and also other faculty of the department, for their help in providing and guiding me in X-rays, CT scans, and imaging methods.
- I thank Drs Shibu Mohan, Keshavaprasad, Ahris, Rupa, and Sadhan and all faculties in the surgery department.
- I sincerely appreciate Drs Raghavendra Bhat and Ravichandra, Consultants, Department of Radiology, Yenepoya Medical College, Mangaluru, for their contribution and affectionate help.
- I thank Dr Suresh Pai, *Late* Dr Ashok Shetty (Cardiothoracic Surgeon), Dr Muralidhar Pai (Neurosurgeon), *Late* Dr Vivekanand Prabhu (Paediatric Surgeon), Dr Sadashiva Rao (Paediatric Surgeon), Dr Narayana Bhat (Paediatric Surgeon), and Dr Prashanth Mallya (Anaesthetist), for their help and contributions.
- I thank my friend Dr Jagadish for his contributions to X-ray and opinion on dental and faciomaxillary topics.
- My wife, Dr Meera Karanth P helped me day and night in revising this edition and without her help this would not have been possible. My beloved daughter Ananya helped me in drawing new diagrams artistically. I enjoy her love and affection toward me.
- I remember my students Dr Ravi CR (Chitradurga), Dr Ashwini Polnaya (Mangaluru), Dr Ishwara Keerthi, Dr Sudesh, Dr Narasimha Murthy, Dr Nithin, Dr Ashish Singh, and Dr Aromal, for their special contributions.
- I thank all staff in the operation theatre and others in Mangala Hospital and Government District Wenlock Hospital, Mangaluru, for their help in taking photographs of different surgeries regularly.
- I thank all my students, especially postgraduates of surgery department, who were helping regularly in bringing out this edition.
- Words are not sufficient to remember all my patients, who are the main material for the book. I pray for their good health always.
- I appreciate Shri Jitendar P Vij (Group Chairman), Mr Ankit Vij (Managing Director), Ms Sunita Katla (PA to Group Chairman and Publishing Manager), and the whole team of M/s Jaypee Brothers Medical Publishers (P) Ltd, New Delhi, India, for doing appreciable work in their respective field of printing and publishing.
- I also extend my appreciation to the working team of M/s Jaypee Brothers Medical Publishers (Bengaluru branch), for their timely help.

Contents

VOLUME 1

VOLUME 2

1

CHAPTER

Introduction and Principles in Operative Surgery

Surgery is an *art,* but it is not just an art; it is an art with principles, dedication, determination, gentleness, and tissue respect. It is an *irreversible art* work which if improperly done can be counterproductive. Doing surgery without principle is like an operator doing job without knowing the outcome.

It is often wrongly considered that quicker the surgeon, better he is. *Fast surgery* is probably a *glamour* than an essentiality. *Speed* of the operator is only a *short-term* impression. Rapid operator concept itself is a *myth.* It is the *accuracy and delicacy* of the procedure which is more important. Speed comes eventually by practice, experience, skill and knowledge. One should not force the speed; it should be spontaneous. It is the *precision* which is more important than speed. *However,* quickness is needed in surgical emergencies especially in trauma and torrential bleeding situations. It again does not mean that one can violate the principles. *Art of surgery* means knowing proper surgical anatomy, surgical pathology, tissue respect and handling technique, gentleness, proper haemostasis, asepsis, good knowledge of different instruments and skill. *A surgeon* should be artistic, innovator, teacher, principled and superb operator.

Every surgical condition may not require surgery. Individual patient is assessed and planned for surgery accordingly. *Planning, thinking, skill, execution* are the assets of proper surgery. Doing wrong procedure in wrong time, with *wrong need* even through a brilliant technical execution will give a poor result. He may be considered as a *good operator* but a *poor surgeon.*

Often there are many surgical procedures as therapy for a single disease. *Merits and demerits* of each and which is ideal to that particular situation should be analysed prior to deciding the procedure. The so called '*decision making*' is very important since olden days.

Adequate length of incision; proper retraction; *minimum touch* technique (means dissection is done with instruments mainly and with fingers when needed and avoid unnecessary rough tissue handling); haemostasis; tissue respect; gentleness; patience; tolerance; avoiding restlessness; adequate exposure; safety methods; proper knowledge of different techniques; anticipation of problems; so prevention of problems; tackling ability of on table complications; taking help of additional/senior/experienced surgeons when needed without any ego—are the basic essentials of a *quality* surgeon.

Five essential qualities to be a good surgeon

1. *Lady's finger* (should be gentle in handling patients and tissues).
2. *Lion's heart* (being brave to take decisions).
3. *Eagle's eye* (carefully watching changes occurring in the patient during treatment).
4. *Horse's leg* (immense stamina to withstand long hours of surgery).
5. *Camel's belly* (ability to carry on without food for hours).

Clinician is the one who listens patiently; who sees carefully; who feels evidentially; who hears silently.

A clinician should show *'empathy'* towards patient (ability to understand what the patient is undergoing through; have self-confidence/positive attitude thereby can impart confidence in the patient; should be honest while treating the patient.

Safe surgery needs—clear surgical anatomy; right anaesthesia; haemostasis; asepsis; skill with patience; learning attitude; dedication and determination.

Surgery should not be a glamour; but it should be a dedicated profession.

POSITION OF THE SURGEON

Surgeon has to spend large amount of time continuously in the operation theatre. So, he needs both physical as well as mental strength for this. He should be comfortable, and relaxed. Posture is important while doing surgery. Otherwise, surgeon may develop back/neck pain or other postural abnormalities. Many procedures like surgeries of hand and brain are often comfortably done in sitting position. It is good practice to make assistant and scrub nurse also to sit during such procedures as assistants also should be comfortable while doing the procedure. Shoulder should be relaxed and elbow should be relaxed and flexed at 90°.

Suturing involves using of biceps muscle to move hand from a pronated to a supinated position in a natural rolling motion and is called as *forehand suturing.* So right-hand surgeon assumes his body and foot for greatest efficiency. Suturing is done from right side with needle position aiming towards surgeons left foot. Both feet are placed perpendicular to the table; both parallel to each other.

Backhand manoeuvre is done by moving hand from supinated position to roll backward to reach pronated position. Position of feet and body of the surgeon should be reversed or altered depending on the convenient of technique like backhand suturing. Often both feet may be required to be placed parallel to the table. Scalpel blade is usually used in backhand movement. Suturing is preferred in *forehand* movement. Scissor is pointed towards left of the right-hand surgeon. Electrocautery cutting is directed towards right foot like scalpel blade.

Position *of right-hand* surgeon and *left-hand* surgeon even though vary; it is better every surgeon to have a fair skill of using both hands effectively. Which side of the patient surgeon should stand even though is a matter of convenience; but in usual practice, surgeon stands on right side of the patient if he is a right-hand surgeon or left-hand surgeon. But surgeon should be flexible enough to *change the side* as required or as when difficulty arises during the procedure. There should not be prejudiced or have a prefixed idea about these things as *comfort of the surgeon* is the priority.

There are *separate instruments* manufactured for left-hand surgeons. But due to limited availability and cost factor and because of less number of left-hand surgeons overall (even though exact ratio is not known, probably left-hand surgeons are less than 1%) makes left-hand surgeons compulsorily use right-hand instruments successfully.

Even though, it is often categorised as minor and major operations, it should be considered that *all surgeries are major*. By experience and knowledge surgeon may feel that surgery is minor. Practically if one looks in patient's angle; for each patient whatever procedure he/she is undergoing is important and is always for the first time. For surgeon again it is imperative to execute enough care and skill whether the procedure/surgery are small or big. So optimum care is mandatory for all procedures, without any shortcomings.

HISTORY OF SURGERY

It is interesting to know little bit of the history in relation to surgery. Its evolvement was gradual, slow with lot of trial and errors. Acceptance, criticism were the problems in developing the newer avenues. There are so many contributors for development and progress of surgery since many centuries **(Figs. 1-1 to 1-26)**.

Wound closure had originated as early as 17th century BC.

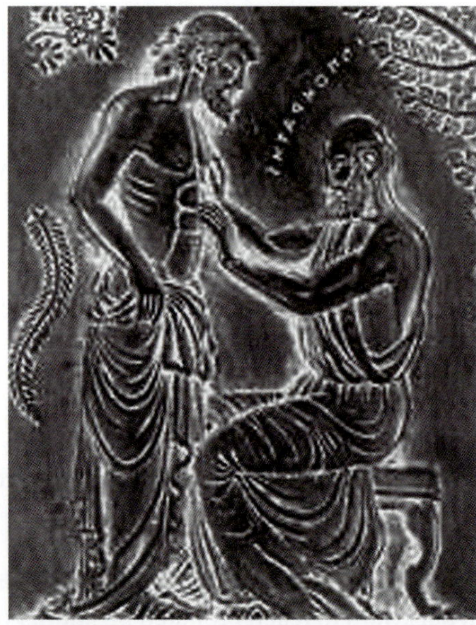

Fig. 1-1: Hippocrates (400 BC). He described umbilical hernia, acute abdomen, terminal ill patient in peritonitis, and his famous oath.

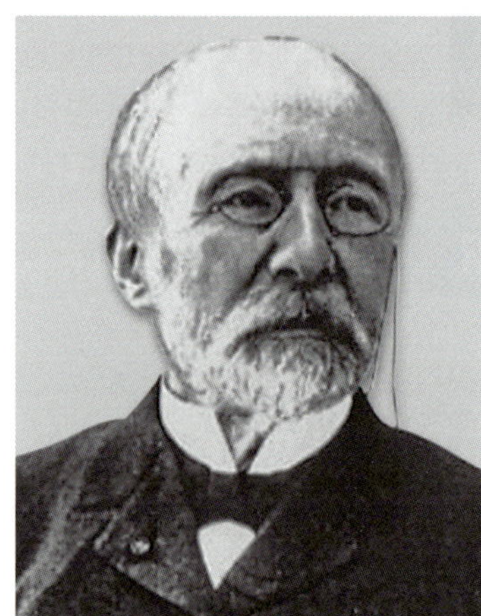

Fig. 1-2: Courvoisier. He did extensive work on biliary surgery. He originated his famous Courvoisier's law.

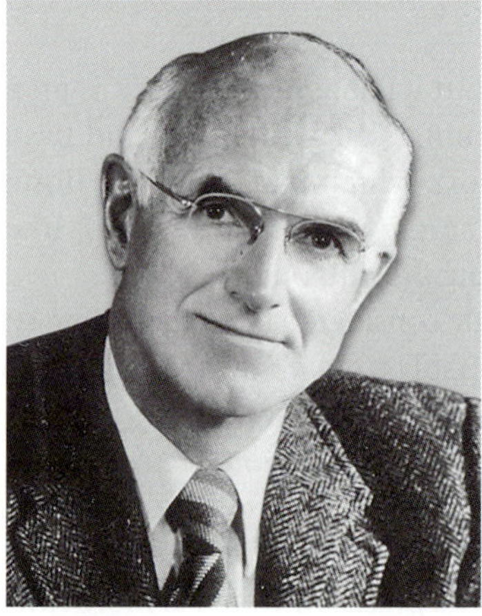

Fig. 1-3: Joseph E Murray. He got Nobel Prize in 1990 for organ and cell transplantation along with E Donnall Thomas. He did first successful human kidney transplantation between identical twins in December 23, 1954 on a patient Richard Herric who lived and married recovery room nurse.

Sushruta in ancient India gave the concept of nasal reconstruction after loss of nose following punishment in 600 BC. He repaired intestine perforation using ant heads–natural stapling. It was called as 'Sushruta era' **(Fig. 1-4)**. *Sushruta Samhita* is premedieval period treatise in surgery. Book had five sections.

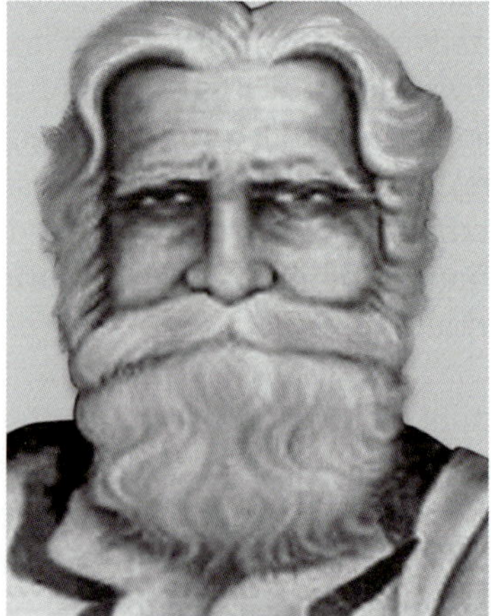

Fig. 1-4: Sushruta.

Abu Kassim (1000 BC) used suture materials prepared from animal intestine to close the bowel. In 12th century silk became a suture material.

Successful human skin graft was done by **Sir Astley Cooper** in 1817.

Andreas Vesalius from Padua, Italy (1514–1564) gave the importance of human anatomy in surgery **(Fig. 1-5)**. He gave concept of human dissection in learning anatomy and surgery. He wrote anatomy book 'De Humani Coporis Fabrica Libri'.

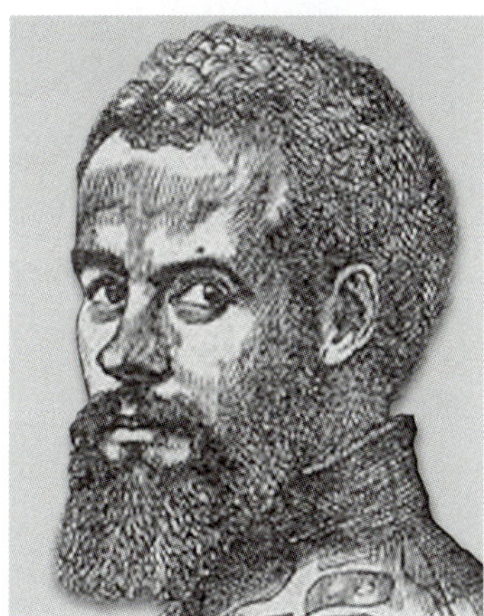

Fig. 1-5: Andreas Vesalius.

Chester B McVay worked as Chief of Surgery at the Yankton Clinic and Sacred Heart Hospital in Yankton; USA from 1946 to 1980. He received numerous awards and had his chapters in four medical books. He did extensive work on inguinal and femoral hernias and related surgeries.

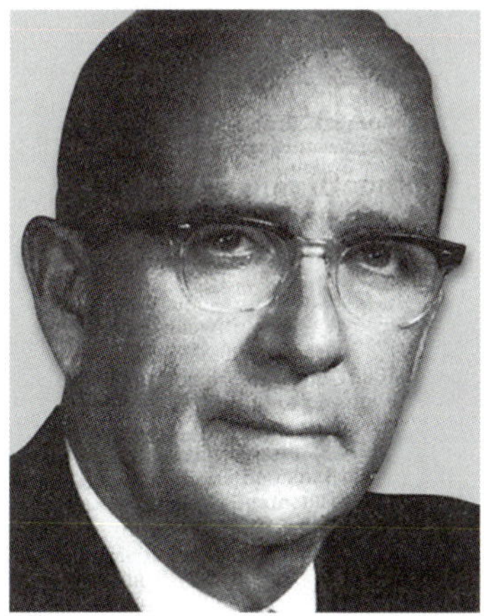

Fig. 1-6: Chester B McVay. He did extensive work on hernia surgery.

Ambroise Pare (Paris; 1510–1590) did revolution in surgery by practicing ligation of individual vessels doubly especially in amputation **(Fig. 1-7)**. He said, "I treated him; God cured him". He started concept of controlled experimentation.

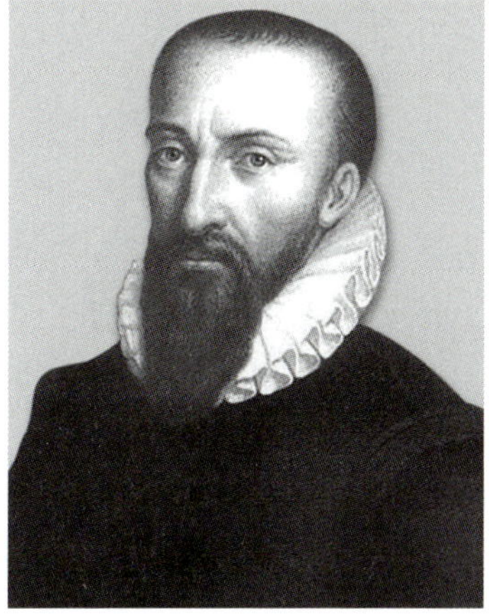

Fig. 1-7: Ambroise Pare.

Albucasis, Moorish clinician (AD 952, Arab) did first successful thyroidectomy; was bold, venturesome operator. He wrote that time famous medical book '*al-Tasrif*'. He also used catgut, cotton sutures. He also used to do small bowel anastomosis.

John Hunter (Glasgow, England; 1728–1793) an excellent surgeon **(Fig. 1-8)** of that time wrote many books on surgery, war wounds. He had outstanding collections of 13,000 specimens which were present in the Museum of Royal College of Surgeons which was destroyed during World War II by Nazi bombing. He described aneurysms and, its treatment, shock, phlebitis, nasogastric feeding, and respiratory assisting. He died of inoculation of syphilis and gonorrhoea by mistake. He thought of transplantation and angiogenesis and did experiments on it. He gave the importance of experimental surgery, study of anatomy and natural history in surgery.

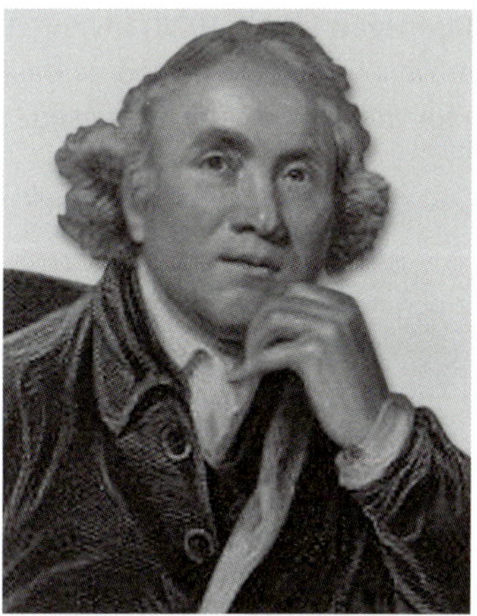

Fig. 1-8: John Hunter.

Joseph Lister (Scotland/England; 1827–1912) evoluted the concept of asepsis and antisepsis. He started chemical antisepsis using carbolic acid. He originated proper cleaning of the wound and area prior to surgery to improve the results and reduce the sepsis. He started the use of sterile sutures in surgery. His era is called as *Listerism*. He invented Lister's sinus forceps, pointed scissors, catgut ligature. He is rightly known as the father of modern surgery **(Fig. 1-9)**.

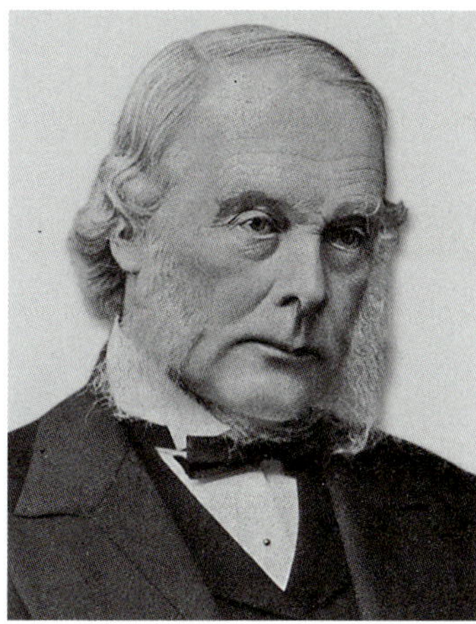

Fig. 1-9: Joseph Lister.

William TG Morton, a Boston dentist, on October 16th in 1846, gave ether anaesthesia for the first time successfully to a patient Gilbert Abbott who was operated by John Collins Warren to remove jaw tumour **(Fig. 1-10)**.

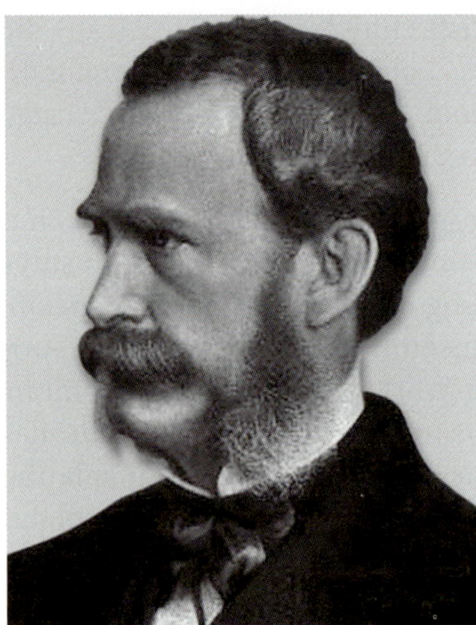

Fig. 1-10: William TG Morton.

Wilhelm Conrad Roentgen (1845–1923) invented X-rays (1895) also called as Roentgen rays which was used as basic diagnostic tool. He got Nobel Prize for the same which was used **(Fig. 1-11)**.

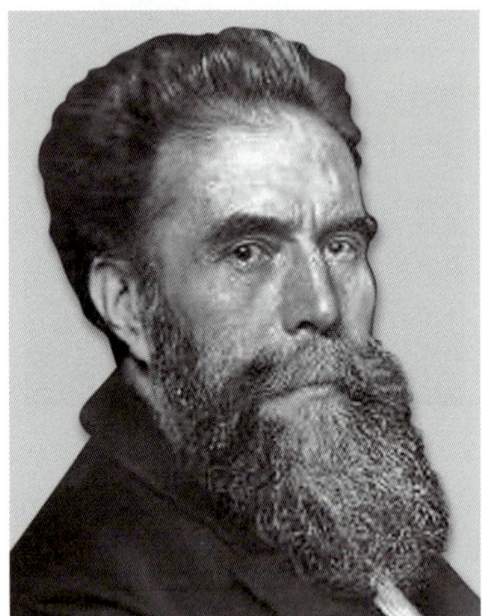

Fig. 1-11: Wilhelm Conrad Roentgen.

Rudolph Matas (America; 1860–1957) **(Fig. 1-12)** was a pioneer in vascular surgery; started endoaneurysmorrhaphy.

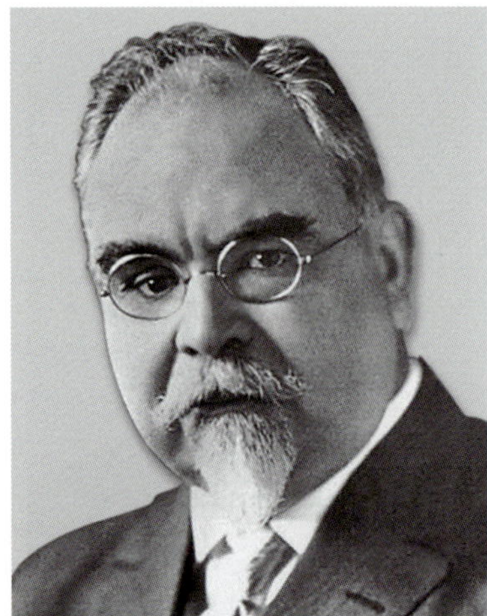

Fig. 1-12: Rudolph Matas.

William S Halsted (America; 1852–1922) **(Fig. 1-13)** did extensive work on surgeries of breast and hernia. Halsted concept in carcinoma of breast and Halsted's radical mastectomy has ruled surgical era for a century until concept has changed from 1980 onwards. He started the use of gloves during surgery. He also started residency training in United States. He did work on hernia surgery also.

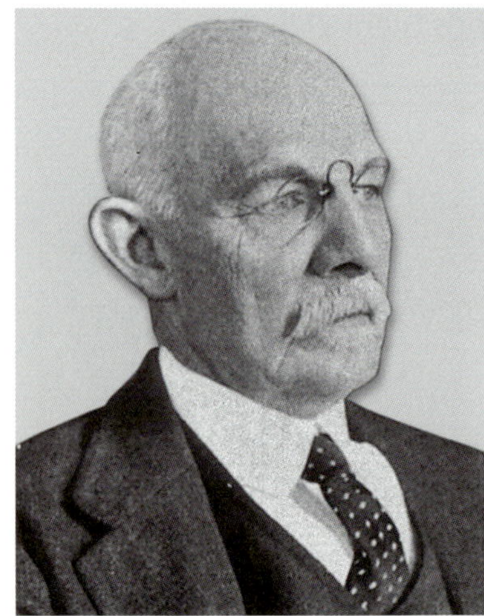

Fig. 1-13: William S Halsted.

Bernard von Langenbeck (German; 1810–1887) **(Fig. 1-14)** did lots of contributions to surgery in technique, precision and instruments. He did first successful cholecystectomy in 1882.

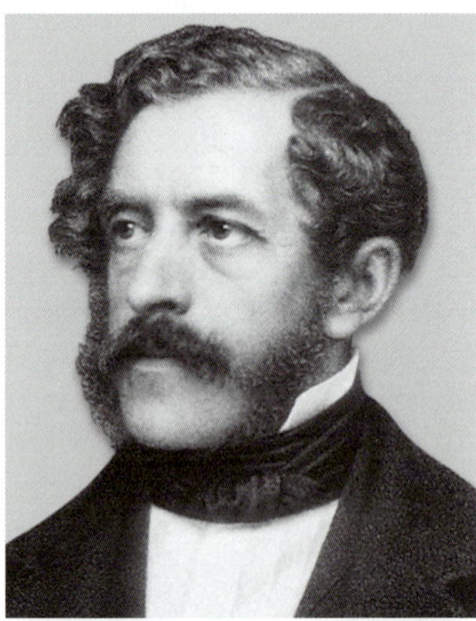

Fig. 1-14: Bernard von Langenbeck.

Theodor Billroth (Vienna; 1829–1894) **(Fig. 1-15)** did extensive work in abdominal surgery. Billroth anastomosis after gastrectomy is good old popular method.

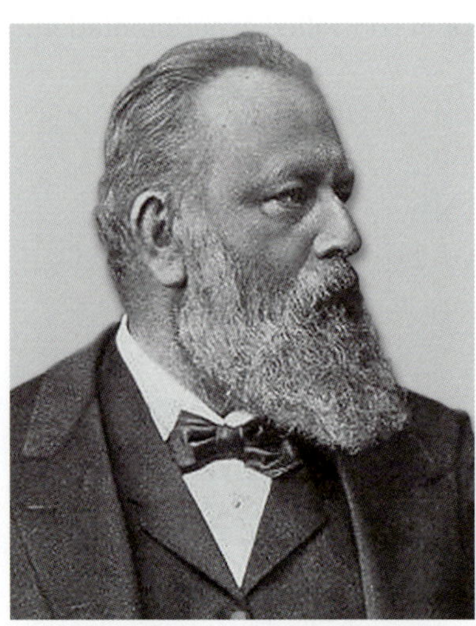

Fig. 1-15: Theodor Billroth.

Schlatter first did successful total gastrectomy in 1897.

Senn did successful appendicectomy in 1889.

Lester Dragstedt did vagotomy for peptic ulcer.

Allen Oldfather Whipple (1881–1963) **(Fig. 1-16)** did successful pancreaticoduodenectomy for pancreatic cancer in 1935.

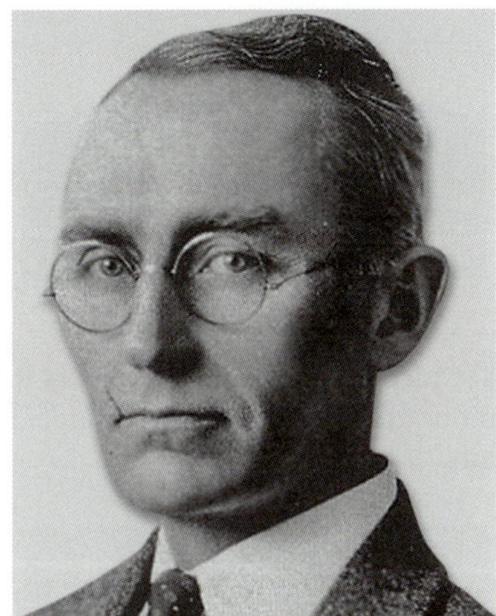

Fig. 1-16: Allen Oldfather Whipple.

Franke in 1900 did total pancreatectomy.

Wendell did first successful hepatic resection in 1911.

Lembert (1826, France) started inverting seromuscular sutures.

Edoardo Bassini (1844–1924) started classical Bassini's repair for inguinal hernia in 1884 as tissue repair which dominated hernia treatment for nearly a century; but now becoming a surgical legacy **(Fig. 1-17)**.

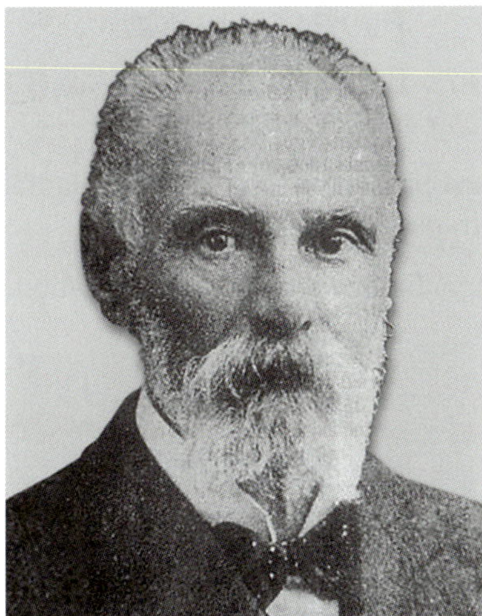

Fig. 1-17: Edoardo Bassini. He did lot of work in hernia surgery. Tissue repair for inguinal hernias under his name ruled the system for a century and now slowly becoming surgical legacy.

Theodor Kocher (Berne; Switzerland, August 25, 1841–1917) was the *first surgeon to get Nobel Prize* (1909) **(Fig. 1-18)**.

He did extensive work on thyroid surgeries and designed present technique of thyroid surgeries. He was from Switzerland. He was the first to do excision of thyroid in 1876. By 1912 he did thousands of thyroidectomies with eventual mortality rate as 0.18%.

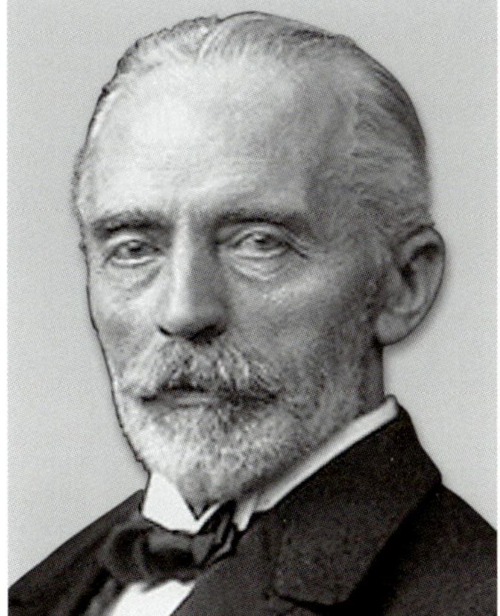

Fig. 1-18: Theodor Kocher.

He has written Kocher's Textbook of Operative Surgery in 1892. Many surgical avenues are after his name—Kocher's vein; Kocher's forceps (has got tooth in the tip); Kocherisation (duodenal mobilisation); Kocher's incision (right subcostal for open cholecystectomy); Kocher's thyroidectomy incision; Kocher's test; Kocher's method for reduction of shoulder dislocation; Kocher's arched incision for opening the knee joint; Kocher's method of fixation of uterus; Kocher's invagination technique for inguinal hernia; Kocher's eye sign of thyrotoxicosis (on starring accentuation of lid retraction); Kocher-Debre Semelaigne syndrome (myxoedema, generalised muscle hypertrophy, cretinism, short stature); Kocher Lorenz elbow fracture (osteochondral fracture of capitellum). He did experimental works on gunshot injuries. Theodor Kocher Institute, Kochergasse, Kocher Park, are his memories in the city of Berne.

Harvey Cushing, Halsted's resident, started the practice of experimental surgery. He was interested in the field of neurosurgery. He started and showed the essentiality of electrocoagulation in neurosurgery.

John H Gibbon (1903–1973) **(Fig. 1-19)** developed extracorporeal circulation for cardiac surgery.

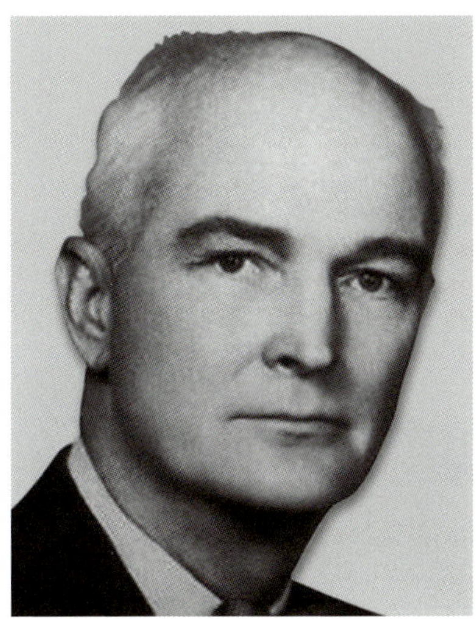

Fig. 1-19: John H Gibbon.

Alfred Blalock (1889–1964) **(Fig. 1-20)** was a pioneer in cardiac surgery. He discovered successful surgical therapy for Fallot's tetralogy.

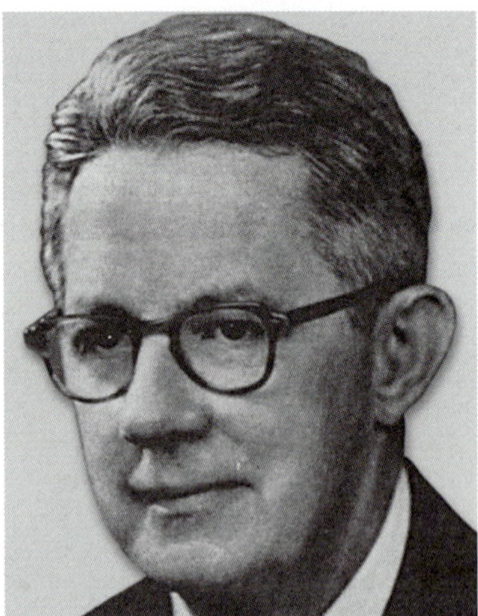

Fig. 1-20: Alfred Blalock.

Owen H Wangensteen, a very popular surgical teacher pioneered in colonic surgery **(Fig. 1-21)**.

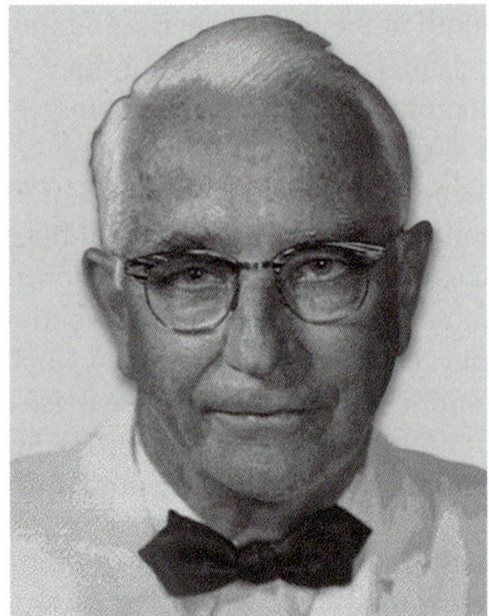

Fig. 1-21: Owen H Wangensteen.

Francis D Moore (Fig. 1-22) gave importance of metabolism in surgery.

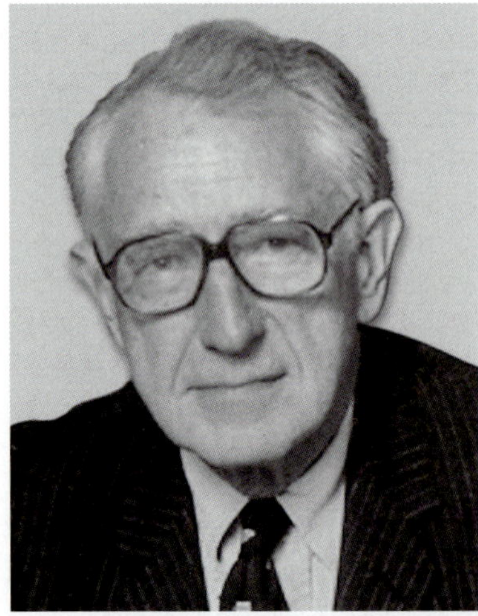

Fig. 1-22: Francis D Moore.

Jonathan Rhoads (Fig. 1-23) did extensive work on surgical nutrition and surgical oncology.

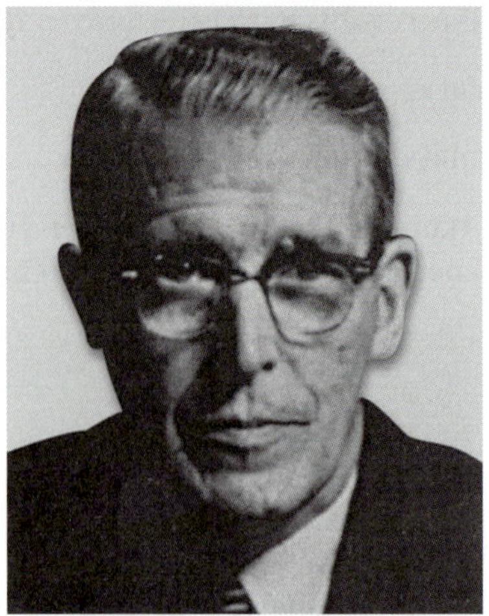

Fig. 1-23: Jonathan Rhoads.

Charles Huggins (Chicago) **(Fig. 1-24)** got Nobel Prize for effects of hormones on tumour growth and use of orchidectomy in advanced carcinoma prostate.

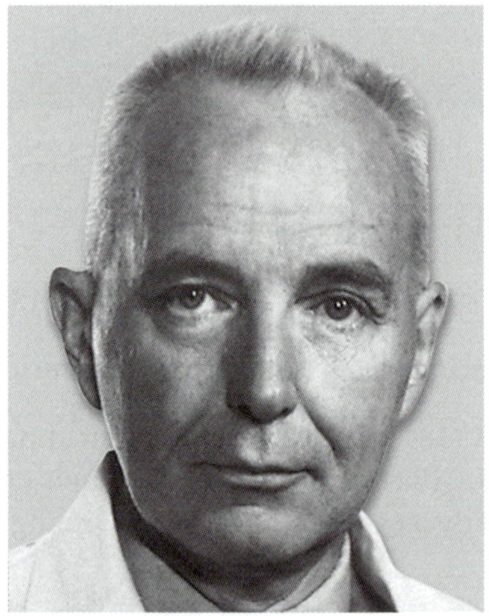

Fig. 1-24: Charles Huggins.

Alexis Carrel (1873–1944) **(Fig. 1-25)** got Nobel Prize in 1912 for his work on vascular anastomosis.

Christian Bernard pioneered in heart transplantation. He did first successful heart transplantation in 1967.

Ullmann in Vienna did first kidney transplantation (1902).

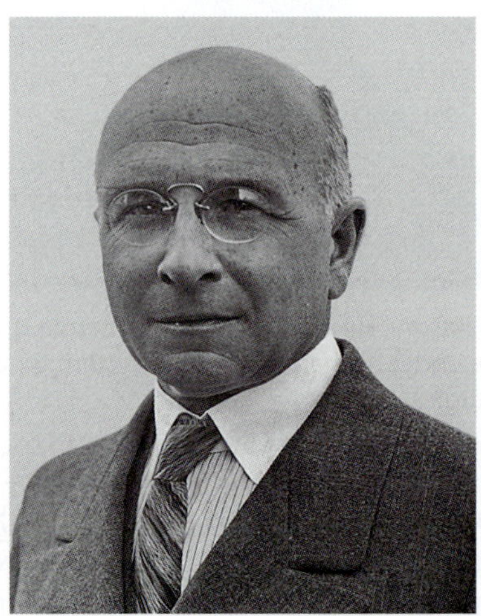

Fig. 1-25: Alexis Carrel.

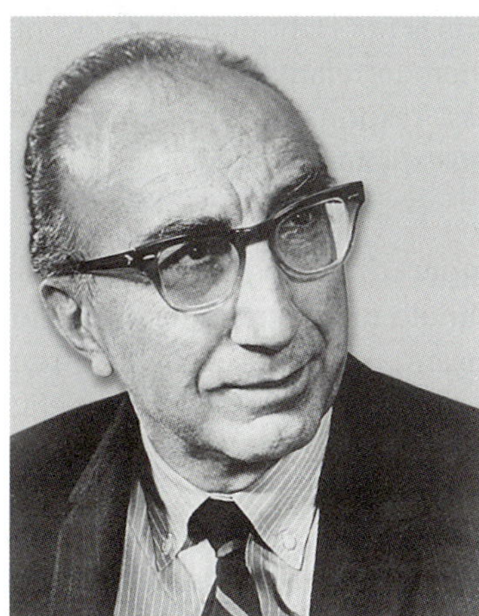

Fig. 1-26: Michael D Bakey. He did extensive work on vascular surgery and aneurysms.

George Kelling (Dresdon, 1901) did first laparoscopy using cystoscope in dog and called as celioscopy. Hans Christian started it in humans. Zollikofer (1924) brought CO_2 for pneumoperitoneum. *Kalk* is father of laparoscopy surgery. Janos Verres (Hungary, 1938) used spring needle to create pneumoperitoneum. Fourestier, Gladu and Valmiere used cold light fiberglass illumination (France, 1952). Kurt Semm (German, 1977) used automatic insufflation device.

Semm in 1983 did first successful *laparoscopic appendicectomy.*

Mouret P did first *laparoscopic cholecystectomy* in France in 1987.

Surgeons who won Nobel prize are Theodor Kocher (1909); Alexis Carrel (for his work on vascular anastomosis, 1912), Charles Huggins (urologist and oncologist for management of carcinoma prostate and hormone therapy, 1966); Joseph Murray (organ transplantation, 1990).

ETHICS IN SURGERY

Ethical principles are very important in surgical field. Finalising the accurate diagnosis or possibilities, recommending the treatment, explaining the merits and demerits of different procedures or recommended procedure, risks, complications should be explained to the patient.

Community values, its basic knowledge is essential to a surgeon in influencing the patient about the illness. In many countries, states and communities, close relatives of a patient do not want the patient to be informed about the major disease he is suffering like cancer or life-threatening illness. Here decision making is done by close relative of the patient like son/father/mother/brother/sister. The so called *truth telling* to the patient is purposely avoided to maintain the will power of the patient or details about the illness is informed to the patient gradually so that the patient is made to understand and accept the reality of the situation. It is always better to explain the patient that in many diseases, it is only possible to *give adequate care* but not complete cure.

Resources; individual identity of the patient; education of the patient; help of relatives; patient's ability to understand; planning are the important factors needed. Often it is better to reveal the details of the disease in presence of two attendees/relatives/caregivers. In the court of law/*legally* it is better to take signature of the witness for informed consent with date. Surgeon should have a registered *legally permissible recognised degree* certificate to perform different operations.

Behaviour of the surgeon with the patient, relatives of the patient, hospital staff, theatre staff, residents, students and colleagues should be proper. Shouting, abusing, manhandling should be avoided as much as possible even under stress.

Avoid negligence like retaining of mops during surgery, not giving adequate postoperative care, etc. Negligence is not accepted in court of law. In difficult situations surgeons should not hesitate to take the help of another surgeon. Reasonable care is essential. Act of omission or act of commission both are considered in negligence.

Documenting in detail about the surgery in case sheets, daily follow-up notes, progress notes with timings, informed consent are important. It is better every surgeon should have a clear idea about legal aspects of his practice. It is also better to have a legal advisor to clarify the doubts whenever needed.

It should always be remembered that surgeon is basically a part of the *public life*. He should respect the dignity of patient and caregivers; psychological, social and spiritual aspect of the patient should be considered; refrain from committing crimes; competence, compassion should be present; should educate the patient and community; teach the *future learners* of surgical profession with love and interest. One should *never* bring cast, community, religion, race during practice. *Only human life* and humanity should be the goal.

Oaths used in medical field are Hippocratic oath; Sushruta and Charaka oath of India; declaration of Geneva.

Medical Ethics

Medical ethics is a system of principles governing medical conduct. (1) Doctor-patient relationship is moral trust between two. Doctor is considered as one who is near to God in India. (2) Professional confidence and secret about the patient is important. (3) Ethical practice is a must from the surgeon. Unethical practices are—advertising; selling medications; accepting gifts, commissions, bonus, etc; unnecessary criticising professional colleagues; conflicts of interests. (4) In dealing with medical insurance. (5) In undertaking newer innovative techniques. (6) Ethics in blood transfusions: Permission should be sought before blood transfusions. Jehovah's witnesses are people with special faith as they never accept blood transfusions which is said to be against their eternal life. Care should be used in managing critical patient of such faiths. (7) Doctor should not refuse treatment and care based on certain diseases like—HIV infection. (8) Risk and benefits of surgery should be weighed before deciding the procedure. (9) Following proper legal backgrounds in organ transplantation—the Transplantation of Human Organ Act, 1994. (10) Information about need for use of ventilator, duration, chances, risks, when to discontinue the ventilator need should be discussed with patient's close relative properly with informed consent. (11) Avoiding **medical negligence**—one should remember that anything that goes wrong is not negligence. *Reasonable standard of care and skill* is needed in treating the patient. Breach of duty by the doctor/surgeon to achieve standard care and skill is called as negligence. If there is damage, then only patient is allowed to claim the negligence. Without damage, patient cannot claim the negligence. General and special damages can be claimed by the patient as financial compensation. Act of commission or act of omission—both are considered in negligence. Surgeon is responsible for negligence of nurses, assistants, theatre staffs or technicians.

Res Ipsa Loquitur is obvious negligence—'thing speaks for itself' like retaining mop/gauze. Contributory negligence is due to act of omission.

Usually, **section 304A** is filed which is a bailable warrant in court of law with summons to the surgeon as accused. Expert witnesses and other documents like case sheets, medicine bills, and certificates are used in examination and cross examination.

Consumer Protection Act (1986) deals with medical negligence cases. It is basically based on documents and affidavits provided by the patient and the doctors.

Often surgeons can be called as **expert witness** in the court of law. He should act fair and accurate without siding anybody. He should have enough proofs and evidences of standard books or journals about what he is telling and documenting in the court. He should be prepared prior about his witness role.

Consent

Permission granted by the patient to the surgeon to make a diagnostic or therapeutic intervention or to have therapy is called as **consent.**

Informed consent is more valid. All relevant information should be provided about benefits, risks of the procedure, present condition in acute cases, need for repeat procedures, intensive care, approximate expenses, probable period of hospital stay, etc. Abiding patient from taking the decision is not correct. *Prevailing silence* between doctors and patients is not right in present day of modern practice. During rounds patient or relative of the patient should be informed about the progress, response or any complications every time. It is always better to explain the patient about the illness in patient's own language.

Valid consent—operating surgeon himself should obtain the consent; patient should understand the discussion/details given to give informed consent; patient must be free from coercion to give consent; details about the procedure, risks, benefits, complications of the procedure; patient should be allowed to query his/her doubts or to clarify his/her suspicions. Person giving consent should be above 18 years, conscious and mentally alert. Parents should give consent if patient is below 18 years. In handicapped or mentally retarded patients, parents or guardians can give consent. In an *emergency condition or in unconscious patient*, procedure and treatment can be done without consent even in the absence of any relative, but after informing and taking written permission from the hospital authority.

Patient presenting himself in surgeon's clinic itself is consent for examining—**implied consent**. When patient cannot give consent, consent taken from close relative is called as **substituted consent**. Consent taken for one procedure can be considered as consent for additional inevitable essential procedure (decided during initial procedure) and is called as *extension doctrine.*

2 CHAPTER

Preoperative Preparation, Operation Room and Postoperative Care

Operations may be *elective* wherein patient is properly prepared with all investigations and precautions or *emergency* wherein immediate surgery is required to save the life of the patient like in perforation of bowel, haemorrhage and trauma.

Patient is admitted prior to date of the elective surgery. In young individual it is sufficient to admit the patient on the day of surgery, provided evaluation is done earlier on outpatient basis. If patient is elderly or asthmatic or with other systemic comorbidities, it is better to admit him earlier and manage the systemic problems with the help of a physician, cardiologist and anaesthetist. Patient is evaluated with essential investigations like haemogram, urine analysis, renal function and liver function test, ECG, blood electrolytes, chest X-ray, echocardiography. Physician and Cardiologist's opinion taken and required treatment given. If patient is markedly anaemic prior to surgery, blood transfusion is required. Asthma and other respiratory diseases, diabetes has to be managed properly prior to surgery. Electrolyte supplement prior to surgery is required in certain conditions.

Prior to shifting the patient to operation theatre following rules should be followed:

- Correct identification of the patient—identification tag is a must.
- Informed consent of the patient for the surgery should be taken. If patient is less than 18 years then consent of parent or guardian is taken.
- Preparation of the patient according to the requirement is done. Present concept is preparation should be done just before surgery on the operation theatre table, even though what usually followed is preparation in the ward often on previous night which is convenient rather than a right way.
- Nothing should be given orally 6–8 hours before surgery.
- Bladder should be empty before sending the patient to the theatre. If required the patient is catheterised.
- Enema, as per instruction should be given.
- Ornaments, dentures, nail polish, hearing aids, contact lenses should be removed before shifting the patient.
- The patient must wear head cover, feet covers, theatre dress.
- Pre-medication, as per instruction should be given.
- Ward nurse should accompany the patient to theatre and should hand over the patient to theatre nurse.

PREOPERATIVE ASSESSMENT

History

1. Chronic cough, smoking, alcohol, drug intake, drug allergy.
2. Any previous diseases like hypertension, diabetes mellitus, epilepsy, bronchial asthma, tuberculosis, hepatitis, cardiac diseases, bleeding disorders and renal diseases.
3. Drug therapy: Steroids, antihypertensives, sedatives, antibiotics, antiepileptics, aspirin.
4. History relevant to different systems—cardiovascular; renal; hepatic; thyroid disease; endocrinal like adrenal; metabolic; nutritional.
5. History suggestive of fluid loss like diarrhoea, vomiting; intestinal obstruction; burns; haemorrhage; trauma.
6. Past history of surgery, its detail and if possible one should collect the old medical records.
7. History suggestive of coagulation disorders like haemophilia, anticoagulant therapy.

Patient with history of recent myocardial infarction should avoid surgery for 6 months unless it is an emergency. Patients with valvular heart disease/on prosthesis need prophylactic antibiotic. Patient with coagulative diseases need specific corrections as needed prior to surgery.

Examination

General: Posture, teeth, mouth opening, dilated veins, neck movements, tremor, airway, anaemia, oedema, jaundice and cyanosis.

Respiratory system: To look for asthma, tuberculosis, emphysema, chronic obstructive pulmonary disease (COPD).

Airway: Mouth opening, Malampatti scoring, tyromental distance, temporomandibular joint assessment.

Cardiovascular system: Hypertension, ischaemic heart disease, arrhythmias, cardiac failure, valvular diseases.

Spine: Curvature, intervertebral space, skin over the back for any infection.

Other systems: Abdomen, skeletal system.

Preoperative Investigations

Haematocrit, blood sugar, blood urea, serum creatinine, electrolytes, chest-X ray, electrocardiography (ECG), blood grouping, blood-gas analysis, cardiac assessment.

Prothrombin time, bleeding time, clotting time, platelet count, liver function tests, pulmonary function tests, arterial blood gas assessment, serum calcium, T3, T4, thyroid stimulating hormone (TSH)—in specific surgical diseases.

Different imaging methods for confirming the diagnosis.

Preoperative Care and Treatment

Control of respiratory and cardiac diseases taking special care from cardiologists, chest therapists, and respiratory physiotherapist. Smoking should be stopped (at least 15 days prior to surgery, but ideally one month prior to elective surgery); prophylactic antibiotics; bronchodilators; steroid inhalers are given. Asthmatic patients are often on steroid therapy and may need intravenous hydrocortisone prior to surgery.

- Renal assessment with blood urea, serum creatinine, urine analysis (albumin, specific gravity) and serum electrolytes is done. In compromised kidney function, nephrologist's opinion and therapy is asked for. Adequate hydration, catheterisation in major surgery for hourly urine output monitoring, avoidance of nephrotoxic drugs in patients with renal failure are the steps to be remembered.
- Improvement of haemoglobin status is required, if anaemia is present. Minimum haemoglobin *ideally* needed for elective surgery is 10 g% (*Safer zone* for anaesthesia tolerance is 7 g% haemoglobin). Nutrition should be adequate. Proper protein diet in elective surgery is good. In emergency situation, parenteral nutrition is given.
- Preoperative antibiotics are given as per instructions of the surgeon. It is used only if there is existing infection like abscess, skin infection or in peritonitis. In elective cases perioperative antibiotics are given like in inguinal hernia mesh repair.
- Blood should be kept ready for major surgeries for transfusion.
- Control of diabetes mellitus and cardiac diseases is important. It is better to take physician's help/cardiologist's opinion prior to surgery. An echocardiography or treadmill test is better for cardiac evaluation. On the day of surgery (two hours prior to surgery) fasting sugar should be checked. Urine sugar, urine *ketone bodies* and *serum potassium* estimation are essential in diabetic patients. It is better to start on insulin therapy if the patient is on oral hypoglycaemic drugs prior to surgery. Often intravenous infusion of 5 units plain insulin in 5% dextrose and 5 mEq of potassium chloride at rate of 50 mL/hour are needed. Hourly blood sugar and serum potassium estimation is needed to maintain blood sugar level at 100–180 mg% and potassium level at 4–5 mEq/mL.
- **All smokers should be asked to stop smoking ideally** *four weeks prior to surgery* in elective surgeries even though patient may not follow the instruction.
- Any preoperative fluid deficits should be corrected with proper monitoring. Monitoring is done using estimation of *hourly urine output*, electrolyte estimation. Usually normal saline or Ringer lactate is used.
- Purgatives/enema are given prior to surgery as sphincter relaxation occurs during general anaesthesia or spinal anaesthesia.
- Skin preparation is done by shaving the area, or by using depilation creams. Ideally it should be done just prior to surgery *in the operation theatre* using clippers. Patient should take proper bath prior to surgery.
- Patient should be kept nil oral for 8 hours (In children up to 4 hours prior liquid can be given for short duration procedures). Fasting prior to surgery is essential to prevent life-threatening aspiration. In emergency surgical situations (like in trauma), nasogastric tube is passed to remove the gastric content; prokinetic drugs are given to rapid the gastric emptying; drugs which decrease the pH of the stomach and to decrease the gastric secretions are given.
- *Prophylactic antibiotics* are given in cardiac surgeries, prosthetic surgeries, trauma, gastrointestinal surgeries, gynaecological surgeries, and oral cavity surgeries. Overuse of antibiotics should be avoided due to development of resistance. Based on their features, wounds should be classified as clean, clean contaminated, contaminated and dirty infected. Clean wound has got less than 2% infection rate whereas dirty infected wound has got 30% infection rate. Common bacteria contaminating the surgical wounds are *Staphylococcus aureus, Staphylococcus epidermidis* and Gram-negative organisms. Prophylactic antibiotics are given on the operation theatre table at the time of induction of anaesthesia. Further doses may be given during surgical procedure if operation time is more than 4 hours. Usually low toxic antibiotics like 2nd generation cephalosporins and metronidazole are given. Concept of antibiotics in contaminated dirty wounds, severe cellulitis, abscess, sepsis, peritonitis is different where patient is prone for septicaemia and its life-threatening problems. Therefore, higher dose of higher generation antibiotics should be used without any hesitation. Sepsis is more common in AIDS or immunosuppressed patient.
- Hyper/hypothyroidism both are equally dangerous for any surgery. Both should be corrected prior to surgery. Toxicity is controlled by proper antithyroid drugs. Hypothyroidism is corrected by oral L thyroxin once a day daily morning. Toxicity if not controlled may precipitate toxic crisis which has got very high mortality.
- Patients with long-term steroid therapy for any cause should have injection hydrocortisone intravenously 100 mg 6th hourly prior to surgery, at the time of induction of anaesthesia and later continued 6th hourly for 2 days of postoperative period which later is gradually reduced and withdrawn.
- Special preparations for gastric/colonic or biliary surgeries should be done.
  - *Colonic preparation:* Low residue diet for 72 hours; bowel wash with saline; gut irrigation using oral polyethylene glycol with electrolytes taken in two litres of water in 2 hours to clear the entire bowel. It acts by osmotic hygroscopic action. It is also achieved by oral intake of mannitol for 2–3 days. Bowel antiseptics like neomycin 1 gram three times/day prior to surgery is given. *Total gut irrigation* is done by passing nasogastric tube through which normal saline is infused. It is infused (8 litres of saline) until clear saline is passed per anum. [*On-table colonic lavage* can be done by passing a tube through performed appendicectomy opening (purse string suture is placed) and another opening in distal colon just proximal to obstruction and saline is irrigated from first to second tube continuously to achieve proper cleaning of the colon].
  - *Gastric preparation in gastric outlet obstruction:* Here patient is having hypokalaemia, hyponatraemia, hypomagnesaemia, hypochloraemia, hypocalcaemia with metabolic alkalosis and *paradoxical aciduria*. Correction of dehydration, electrolytes, anaemia (blood), hypoproteinaemia (amino acids, total parenteral nutrition), hypocalcaemia (intravenous calcium gluconate) and alkalosis is essential in these patients. Gastric lavage is done for 5 days prior to surgery by passing stomach (Ewald's) tube using normal saline to remove residual food, to decrease mucosal oedema, and to maintain gastric tone.
  - *In obstructive jaundice:* Specific problems are altered prothrombin time (bleeding tendency), hypoalbuminaemia and malnutrition, sepsis, anaemia, dehydration and diminished carbohydrate reserve. *Hepatorenal syndrome* is specific problem postoperatively—due to endotoxaemia, acute tubular

necrosis due to toxins, sludging of bile salts in the renal tubules, hypovolaemia. Management is by—adequate fluid infusion (*hydration*), fresh frozen plasma; mannitol infusion; antibiotics; injection vitamin K 10 mg intramuscular once a day for 5 days; intravenous dextrose to improve the carbohydrate reserve. Albumin infusion is usually *not needed* in these patients.

Note:
Informed consent is absolute need.

OPERATIVE RISK ASSESSMENT

It is important in children, old age; obesity; liver, renal, respiratory and cardiac dysfunctions; sepsis; chronic illness and malignancy. If patient is undergoing surgery for disease like hernia which may be elective, the *risk here due to concomitant disease* like of cardiac or respiratory or renal problems is important.

If patient is undergoing surgery for surgical problem like perforated appendicitis or acute gallbladder disease like empyema gallbladder or peritonitis, *here risk is of primary disease* (appendicitis/empyema gallbladder) due to sepsis.

Premedication

It is given one hour before surgery.

For sedation and relief of anxiety: Pethidine 50 mg/morphine 10 mg/diazepam 10 mg. Midazolam 1–2.5 mg.

To suppress vagal activity: Atropine 0.6 mg IM.

To reduce vomiting: Promethazine (phenergan) 12.5 mg.

ASA (American Association of Anesthesiologists) grading of the patient for surgery

1. Normal individual.
2. Mild–moderate one systemic disease under control—diabetes and hypertension under control; mild obesity, alcohol intake, smoking.
3. Severe systemic disease/multiple systemic diseases—uncontrolled diabetes and hypertension; activity limited due to disease.
4. Incapacitating systemic disease—high risk.
5. Moribund status—imminent risk of life—surgery as life saving procedure.
6. Brain dead patient.

Class 'E' is added to each type if it is an emergency surgery.

DISINFECTION AND STERILISATION

Concept of asepsis is started in 19th century. Ignaz Semmelweis showed reduction of the puerperal fever by washing hands prior to delivery. Lister used carbolic acid as an antiseptic to reduce surgical infection. Lawson Tait introduced principles of asepsis.

Asepsis

Asepsis means organisms are prevented to access the patient or individual. It is a state of being free from disease causing contaminants or preventing contact with microorganisms. Term is used to those methods to promote or to induce asepsis in an operative field to prevent infection to make the surgical field "sterile"; means it is free of all biological contaminants; but it is difficult to achieve; and so elimination of infection is the goal of asepsis, not sterility. There are two types of asepsis—medical and surgical (Ayliffe et al. 2000). Medical or clean asepsis reduces the number and prevents the spread of organisms; surgical or sterile asepsis eliminates microorganisms from surgical area.

The practice of surgical asepsis begins with cleaning the object in question using the principles of medical asepsis followed by a sterilisation process creating an environment in a surgical suite or special procedure room, to avoid any possible infection to the patient also with proper attire (scrubs, cap, mask, gloves, shoe covers).

Antisepsis

It means prevention of infection by inhibiting the growth and multiplication of microorganisms so that making the field free of microorganisms.

Disinfection (Table 2-1)

It is the killing of as many micoorganisms as possible from a surface by physical or chemical means. Articles or surfaces that cannot be sterilised in the operation theatre or special procedure room must be disinfected. Disinfectant may be with or without tuberculocidal activity. It eliminates many or all pathogenic microorganisms, except bacterial spores (usually) *on inanimate objects.*

TABLE 2-1: The Centre of Disease Control (CDC) and Prevention has given three levels of disinfection.

	High	*Intermediate*	*Low*
Vegetative bacteria	+	+	+
Tubercle	+	+	–
Spores	+	+/–	–
Fungi	+	+	
Lipid and medium-sized viruses	+	+	+/–
Non-lipid and small-sized viruses	+	+/–	–

Sterilisation

It is freeing of an article from pathogens by killing or removing all bacteria, spores, fungi and viruses.

- **Bioburden:** The number and types of viable organisms with which an object is contaminated.
- **Decontamination:** The process by which contaminated items are rendered safe for personnel without protective attire to handle or render item safe for reuse. Objects are made safe to handle or use or discard by eliminating all pathogens.
- **Cleaning** is removal of organic and inorganic material from objects and surfaces; done manually or mechanically using water with detergents or enzymatic products.
- **Biological indicator:** It is sterilisation process monitoring device consisting of a standardised viable population of microorganisms of high resistance to mode of sterilisation being monitored.
- **Chemical indicator:** It is sterilisation process monitoring device designed to respond with a characteristic chemical change to one or more parameters of sterilisation cycle.
- **Chemosterilisers:** A chemical used for destroying all forms of microbiological life including spores.
- **Terminal sterilisation:** Sterilisation process carried out after final packaging of the item.
- **Sterility assurance level (SAL):** The probability of survival of microorganisms after a terminal sterilisation process and is predictor of efficacy of the process. A SAL of 10^{-6} indicates non-sterile item.

Contd...

Contd...

- **H Spaulding classification of sterilising materials:** (1) Critical items—Objects that enter sterile tissue or the vascular system must be sterile as high risk of contamination with microorganisms. They include surgical instruments, cardiac and urinary catheters, implants and ultrasound probes used in sterile body cavities, etc. (2) Semi-critical items—They contact with mucous membranes or non-intact skin like respiratory therapy and anaesthesia equipment, endoscopes, laryngoscope blades, oesophageal manometry probes, anorectal manometry catheters, etc. (3) Non-critical items—They come in contact with intact skin but not mucous membrane. As intact skin acts as an effective barrier to most pathogens, the sterility of objects coming in contact with intact skin is not critical. They are—bedpans, blood pressure cuffs, crutches and hospital computers, etc.

METHODS OF STERILISATION AND DISINFECTION

Methods of sterilisation

1. **Physical Method**
   - Thermal (heat) methods
     - Dry heat: Red heat, flaming, incineration, hot air oven, infrared.
     - Moist heat: Below 100°C, at 100°C, above 100°C
   - Radiation method: non-ionising; ionizing—electromagnetic, particulate.
   - Filtration method: Earthenware, asbestos, sintered glass, membrane.
   - Sunlight.
2. **Chemical Method**
   - Liquids: Alcohols, aldehydes, phenolics, halogens, heavy metals, surface active agents, dyes.
   - Gaseous: Formaldehyde, ethylene oxide, plasma.

Physical Methods

Heat Sterilisation

Heat sterilisation involves destruction of enzymes and other essential cell constituents is the most widely used and reliable method of sterilisation. It is more effective in hydrated state where under conditions of high humidity, hydrolysis and denaturation occur, thus lower heat input is required.

In dry state, oxidative changes occur, and so high heat input is needed. This method is used only to the thermostable products, but it is also used for moisture-sensitive materials for which dry heat (160–180°C) sterilisation, and for moisture-resistant materials for which moist heat (121–134°C) sterilisation is used. The degree of heat, the exposure time and the presence of water decides the efficiency of heat sterilisation. Lethal chemical events take place mediated through water and oxygen; presence of water lower exposure time is sufficient to achieve sterilisation.

Incineration, flaming, red heat and hot air oven are examples of dry heat sterilisation. Autoclave, boiling water are examples of moist heat sterilisation.

In dry heat, higher temperature is used (160–180°C) with exposure time up to 2 hours, depending upon the temperature employed. Dry heat shows good penetrability and non-corrosive nature which is useful in sterilising glass and metal surgical instruments, non-aqueous thermostable liquids and thermostable powders. Dry heat destroys bacterial endotoxins/pyrogens and so sterilised glass bottles can be filled aseptically; which are difficult to sterilise by other means.

Hot Air Oven (Dry Heat)

Articles are packed in special craft papers and then placed in a thermostatically controlled dry heat steriliser **(Fig. 2-1)**. Here temperature is raised and lowered slowly to prevent breakage by uneven expansion. It is mainly suitable for ophthalmic instruments and glass items but not plastics or rubber. It is useful for sterilisation of powders, grease, oil and glass syringes. Depending on the holding temperature timing of keeping instruments varies: 150°C – 150 minutes; 160°C – 120 minutes; 170°C – 60 minutes; 180°C – 30 minutes; 190° C – 6–12 minutes.

An insulated chamber surrounded by an outer case containing electric heaters; a fan; shelves; thermocouples; temperature sensor; door locking controls. Articles are first wrapped in containers of cardboard, paper or aluminium; the materials are arranged to ensure uninterrupted air flow; the oven may be pre-heated for materials with poor heat conductivity; the temperature is allowed to fall to 40°C, before collecting the sterilised material.

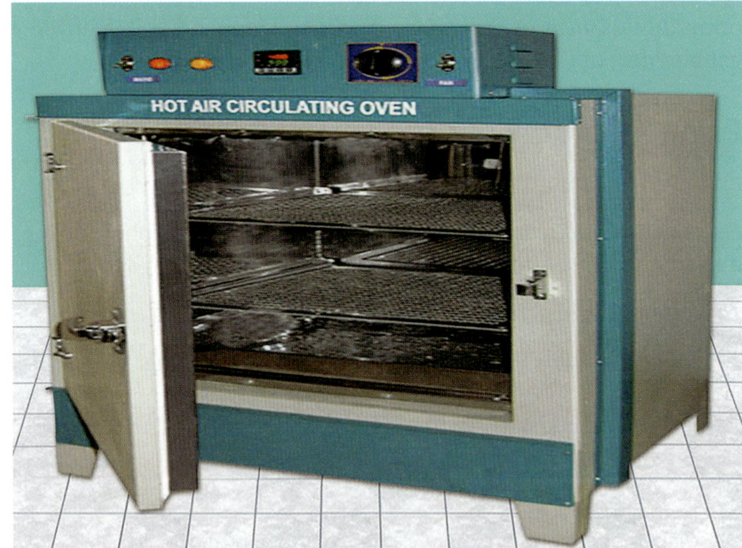

Fig. 2-1: Hot air oven.

Flaming

It is done using Bunsen burner. It is used for small glass objects or metals.

Burning or Incineration

It is used to disinfect contaminated articles like dressings. It is used to sterilise medical and other biohazardous wastes; it burns the material into ashes. Incinerator is a mini furnace wherein wastes are placed and burnt.

Glass Bead Sterilisation

Glass beads are heated to 425°C to 475°C; then instruments are doused into the glass beads to sterilise them. It practiced in dental procedures but it is not approved by FDA and CDC.

Boiling

Boiling kills bacteria but not spores. Boiling may be used as a means of disinfection if no other method is available; however, many spores are able to resist the heat of boiling (212°F or 99°C) for many hours.

To increase the effectiveness of boiling, sodium carbonate may be added to the water in quantity to make a 2% solution. If an object is to be disinfected by boiling and sodium carbonate is added to the water, it should be boiled for 15 minutes. If sodium carbonate is not added, boiling time should be 30 minutes. Boiling is used to disinfect syringes, utensils; but not used for gloves, rubber materials **(Fig. 2-2)**.

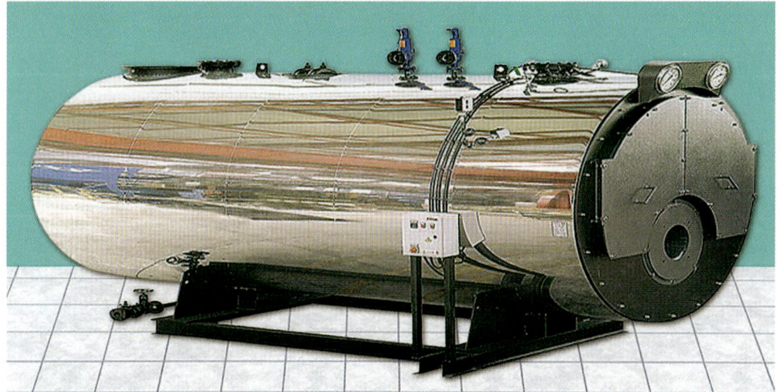

Fig. 2-2: Boiler as steriliser.

Tyndalisation (John Tyndall)

It is boiling for 20 minutes in atmospheric pressure then cooling and incubating for a day then again boiling which is repeated for 4 times. It allows the spores to germinate which will be killed in further boiling. It is a lengthy procedure and prions are not killed. It is presently an obsolete method.

Autoclave

It is *moist heat [steam (dry saturated steam)]* sterilisation (converter, steam steriliser). Saturated steam under pressure is used to sterilise the instruments—121°C with pressure of 15 pounds/sq. inch (2 kg/sq cm; 100 KPa) for 15–20 minutes. Autoclave contains a chamber where packed instruments are kept; through the chamber steam is passed at a set point of time, pressure and temperature. *Jacket* is the portion surrounding the chamber maintains the temperature of chamber. The equipment are first cleaned thoroughly (scrub, sonication, ultrasound, pulsed air, etc.), dried and then packed in muslin, linen or papers which are easily penetrated by steam to place in the chamber. After sterilisation, it is depressurised and cooled slowly and gradually to avoid boiling while releasing pressure. Autoclave kills all bacteria, spores, fungi, viruses but not prions. For prions 121°C for 60 minutes or 134°C for 18 minutes is needed; even then most virulent CJD and BSE strains cannot be sterilised **(Table 2-2)**.

TABLE 2-2: Temperature, pressure and time relations in autoclave.

Temperature in °C	*Pressure lb/inch^2*	*Time in minutes*
121	20	10
126	20	10
134	30	3.5
150	50	Few seconds

Jacket is the portion surrounding the chamber maintains the temperature of chamber. The equipment are first cleaned thoroughly, dried and then packed in muslin, linen or papers which are easily penetrated by steam to place in the chamber. Autoclave has got meter and charts which display temperature and pressure. Indicator tape is placed over the packed box/tray which change its colour once sterilisation is complete.

A cylindrical or rectangular chamber, with capacities ranging from 400 to 800 litres; water heating system or steam generating system; steam outlet and inlet valves; single or double doors with locking mechanism; thermometer or temperature gauge; pressure gauges. For porous loads (dressings) sterilisers are generally operated at a minimum temperature of 134°C for one hour, and for bottled fluid, sterilisers employing a minimum temperature of 121°C are used. One should confirm that there should be sufficient water in the autoclave to produce the steam. The stages of autoclaving technique are—air removal, steam admission and sterilisation cycle with heating up, holding/exposure, and cooling stages.

Autoclave uses pressurised steam to destroy microorganisms; for efficient heat transfer, steam must flush the air out of the autoclave chamber. The drain screen at the bottom of the chamber should be checked and cleaned if blocked. If there is block with debris, a layer of air may form at the bottom of the autoclave, interfering efficient operation. Autoclave functioning should be tested periodically with biological indicators like spores of *Geobacillus stearothermophilus*. Autoclave is very useful for most of the items to sterilise but is not acceptable for rubber, plastics, and equipment that would be damaged by high temperature **(Figs. 2-3A to E)**.

Conditioning/heat up phase: Air should be evacuated before sterilisation, from the chamber as it reduces the amount of steam entering the autoclave and so also the temperature achieved.

Exposure/sterilisation phase: As the steam enters the load, it gives Latent heat to materials rapidly on contact.

Postexposure/exhaust phase: At the end the steam should be exhausted from the autoclave to avoid condensation of water on the load when cool air is admitted.

Note:

Flash sterilisation—refers to steam sterilisation of items for immediate use. Autoclave can also be carried out at low temperature and low pressure steam **(LTS)** at 37 kPa with 74°C, but it would not kill spores. The addition of vapour of formaldehyde to this is called as low pressure steam and formaldehyde **(LTSF)** which can kill many if not all spores. Ordinarily rubber goods, linens and metals are autoclaved.

Principle: Water boils when its vapour pressure equals that of surrounding atmosphere; when water is boiled in closed chamber with increased pressure, the temperature at which it boils and that of steam which is formed will exceed 100°C. When steam comes in contact with cooler surface condenses to water giving its latent heat to that surface. Thus 1,600 mL of steam at 100°C and at atmospheric pressure condenses into 1 mL of water at 100°C and releases 518 calories of heat. Moist heat causes destruction of microorganisms by denaturation of macromolecules, primarily proteins. This method is a faster process than dry heat sterilisation.

Characteristics of steam: It should be optimum, otherwise efficacy will be decreased. It should be free from air, liquid or solid particles; for this, filters can be installed.

Advantages of autoclave: It can kill all bacteria, spores and viruses. Rapid sterilisation, ease of use, good penetration, economical,

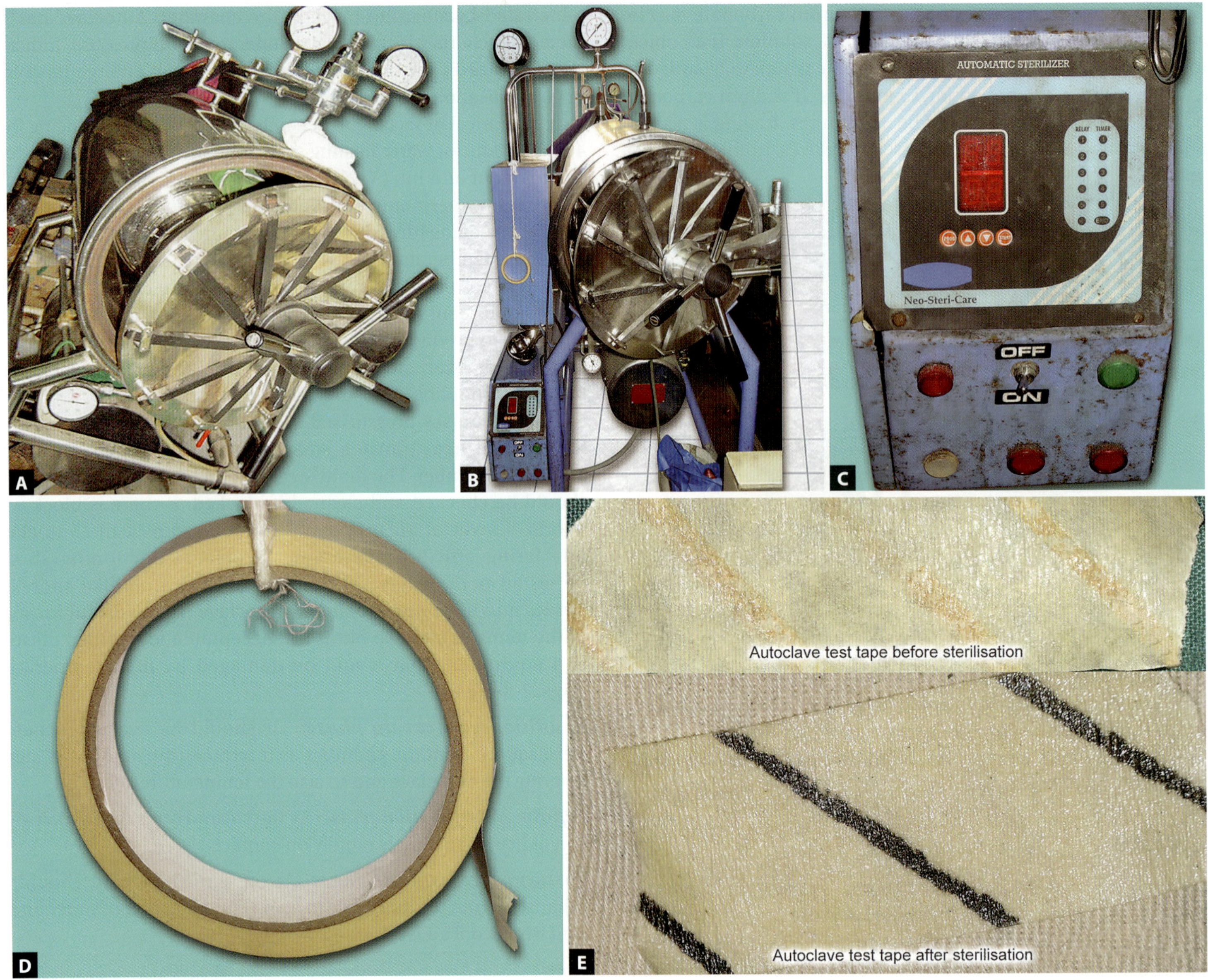

Figs. 2-3A to E: Autoclave machine. It is commonly used method of sterilisation in operation theatre. Autoclave test tape is used to confirm the adequacy and completion of the sterilisation; colour changes to black once autoclave is complete.

absence of toxic products/residues and materials can be prepackaged and kept sterile until use.

Disadvantages: Heat sensitive materials are damaged like plastic and rubber goods. It causes blunting of cutting edges, crossing of metal surfaces. Oil, grease, powders are not sterilised because of lack of penetration. It causes shortening of life of electronic components.

Problems with the steam: Steam quality should be greater than 97%. Water, if present, results in wet steam. If the pressure is too high, it will cause the steam to rain and packs will become wet. If the pressure is too low, the steam will be superheated which is less able to transfer heat to items and it will be difficult to attain uniform temperature.

Autoclave performance: It is confirmed independently by biological indicator. Commonly used are—spores of heat resistant bacteria *Geobacillus stearothermophilus* (*Bacillus stearothermophilus*). These spores are kept in glass vials or strips which are placed inside the autoclave chamber in difficult places where stream to reach.

Six classes of indicators are available

Class 1: These are internal and external process indicator; these inform that item has been exposed to sterilisation process; e.g. external process indicator—autoclave tape. Green coloured stick turns black if autoclave is complete. It contains special protein which gets denatured only in specified temperature and pressure; any alteration or fluctuation will not cause denaturation and strip will remain same colour.

Class 2: Bowie-Dick test for vacuum steam steriliser. They only access vacuum pump efficiency and detect the presence of air leaks and gases in steam.

Class 3: Temperature tube; contains chemicals that melts and sometimes changes colour when the appropriate temp is attained.

Class 4: Respond to one or more sterilisation parameters. It contains ink that changes colour when exposed to correct combination of sterilisation parameters.

Class 5: It is known as integrating indicators or integrators; it respond to all parameters of sterilisation over a specified range of temperatures.

Class 6: These are emulating indicators; these are designed to react to all critical parameters over a specified range of sterilisation cycles for which the stated values are based on the settings of the selected sterilisation cycles.

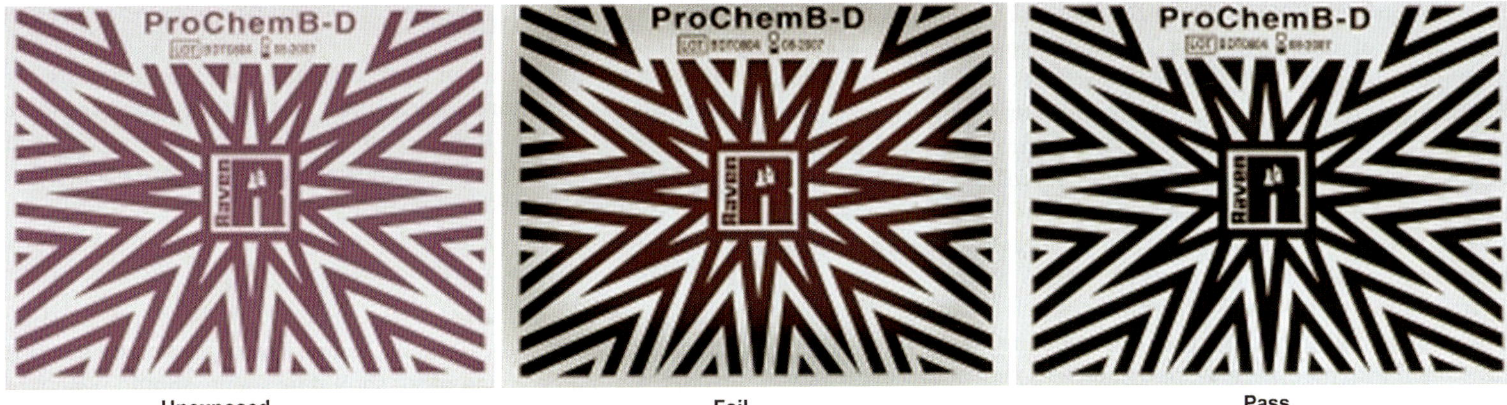

Fig. 2-4: Bowei Dick test for sterilisation completion.

D-value is the decimal reduction time, is the expression of the degree of sterilisation. It denotes the time needed to reduce the initial number to one tenth (1/10) of the initial number. It varies with the microorganism, temperature, water activity and pH. For medical devices and injections, a sterility assurance level of at least 10^{-6} is need. In autoclave, 121°C with a pressure 100 KPa with a sterility assurance level of 10^{-4} for a product with a bioburden 10^{6} and a D value of 2 minutes. Prions are not eliminated with this. 131°C for 60 minutes or 134°C for 18 minutes is required for sterilisation for prions.

Bowie Dick test pack: Bowie Dick test pack is a series of air removal and steam penetration barriers; chemical indicator is located in the centre; the test pack is placed directly into an empty steam steriliser chamber; during sterilisation, steam should displace the air through the barrier material within the pack. A uniform change from yellow to blue/purple on the indicator sheet indicates that all the air was removed and replaced by steam. It is manufactured in the absence of lead or other heavy metals. It is done after a warm up cycle at the beginning; it verifies that steriliser effectively removes air **(Fig. 2-4)**.

Pasteurisation

It is a high level disinfectant. The equipment is immersed in water at an elevated temperature of usually 80°C for 10 minutes or 70°C for 30 minutes. It cannot kill all spores and viruses. So it is recommended for situations where absolute sterility is not required—breathing tubes, endotracheal tubes, reservoir bags, face masks, laryngoscope blades and any rubber goods **(Fig. 2-5)**.

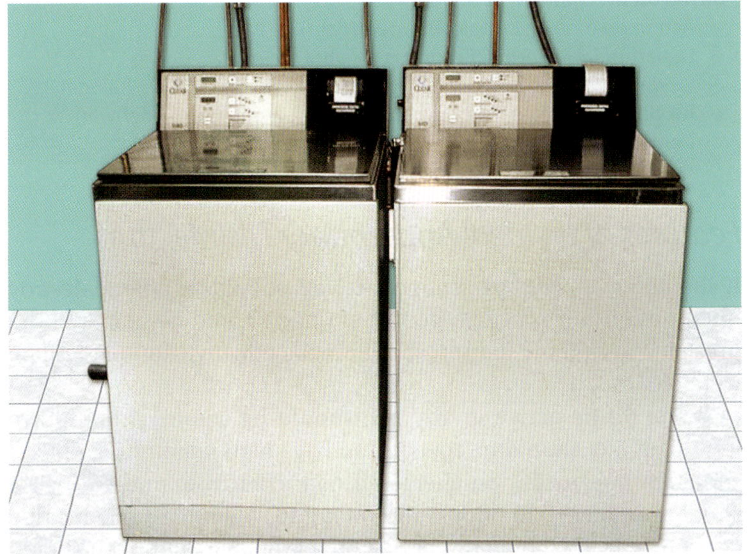

Fig. 2-5: Pasteurisation.

Advantages: It is simple, inexpensive and reliable. It does not emit toxic fumes; it is less damaging to instruments as low temperature is required.

Disadvantages: Items will be wet and must be dried. Prepackaging is not possible. Plastic and rubber articles lose their shape and antistatic properties because of repeated exposure to high temperatures.

Radiation

Sterilisation can be achieved using electromagnetic radiation such as electron beams, X-rays, gamma rays or irradiation by subatomic particles. Electromagnetic or particulate radiation can be adequately energetic to ionise atoms or molecules (ionising radiation) or less energetic (non-ionising radiation).

Ionising Type of Radiation

Atomic gamma radiation is used for commercial purpose to sterilise suture materials, disposable materials in packets. It is viable, safe and cheaper. All disposable materials like gloves, tubes are sterilised by this method. Gamma radiation is very penetrating; commonly used for sterilisation of disposable medical equipment, such as syringes, needles, cannulas and intravenous sets, and food. It is emitted by a radioisotope, usually Cobalt-60(^{60}Co) or caesium-137(^{137}Cs). Cobalt-60 gamma photons have about twice the energy of caesium-137 radiation, and so greater penetrating range.

Gamma radiation: It is very penetrating; commonly used for sterilisation of disposable medical equipment, such as syringes, needles, cannulas and intravenous sets, and food. It is emitted by a radioisotope, usually Cobalt-60(^{60}Co) or caesium-137(^{137}Cs). Cobalt-60 gamma photons have about twice the energy of caesium-137 radiation, and so greater penetrating range. Sterilisation by irradiation with gamma rays may affect material properties sometimes.

Electron beam processing: It is also commonly used for sterilisation. Electron beams use an on-off technology and provide a much higher dosing rate than gamma or X-rays; so less exposure time is needed reducing thereby any potential degradation to polymers. But electron beams are less penetrating than either gamma or X-rays. Proper concrete shields to protect workers and the environment from radiation exposure are essential.

X-rays: High-energy X-rays causes irradiation of large packages and pallet loads of medical devices. They sufficiently penetrate to treat multiple pallet loads of low-density packages with very good dose uniformity ratios. X-ray sterilisation does not require chemical or radioactive material: high-energy X-rays are generated at high intensity by an X-ray generator that does not require shielding when not in use. X-rays are generated by bombarding a dense material such as tantalum or tungsten with high energy electrons in a process known as bremsstrahlung conversion.

Irradiation with X-rays or gamma rays, electromagnetic radiation rather than particles, does not make materials radioactive. Irradiation with particles may make materials radioactive, depending upon the type of particles and their energy and the type of target material. Neutrons and very high-energy particles make materials radioactive; but have good penetration; lower energy particles (other than neutrons) cannot make materials radioactive but have poorer penetration.

Non-ionising Radiation

It is either infrared radiation or ultraviolet radiation used to reduce the bacteria in air, water. Bacteria and virus are vulnerable to ultraviolet rays below 3000A°. Exposure to eyes and skin can cause burn injury. Ultraviolet (UV) light irradiation from a germicidal lamp is useful for sterilisation of surfaces and transparent objects. Materials that are transparent to visible light absorb UV. UV irradiation is used to sterilise the interiors of biological safety cabinets between uses, but is ineffective in shaded areas, including areas under dirt. It may damage some plastics such as polystyrene foam when exposed for prolonged time.

Filtration Sterilisation

Filtration process removes the microorganisms but does not destroy. It prevents the passage of both viable and non-viable particles. Sieving, adsorption and trapping within the matrix of the filter material are different methods. Sterilising grade filters are used in heat sensitive injections, ophthalmic solutions, biological products and air and other gases for supply to aseptic areas. It is also used as part of the venting systems on fermentors, centrifuges, autoclaves and freeze driers. Membrane filters are used for sterility testing.

Two types of filters are used in filtration sterilisation:

Depth filters: They are made up of diatomaceous earth, unglazed porcelain filter, sintered glass or asbestos. Here fibrous or granular materials are so packed as to form twisted channels of minute dimensions.

Membrane filters: These are made of cellulose acetate, cellulose nitrate, polycarbonate, and polyvinylidenefluoride with porous membrane about 0.1 mm thick. The membranes are supported on a frame and fluids are made to transverse membranes by positive or negative pressure or by centrifugation.

High efficiency particulate air (HEPA): It can remove up to 99.97% of particles >0.3 µm in diameter. Air is first passed through prefilters to remove larger particles and then passed through HEPA filters. **Filtration for sterilisation of liquids:** Membrane filters of 0.22 µm pore diameter are used; sintered filters are used for corrosive liquids, viscous fluids and organic solvents. Titre reduction value, the depth of the membrane, its charge and the tortuosity of the channels are the deciding factors in filtration.

Chemical Agents

Chemicals are used when heat sterilisation is inappropriate for materials like electronic, fibreoptics, plastics, etc. (heat sensitive instruments). Gas or liquid chemicals are used. Chemicals used should be compatible when such sterilised articles are being used. It is performed by soaking item in the solution. It kills the organisms by coagulation/alkylation of proteins and also by enzymatic degradation and lysis of cell membranes.

The criteria to be satisfied in the chemical methods are: Must be capable of killing spores; should be non-corrosive; should be non-irritant; should be economical; should be stable; should penetrate grease and fibres; should be non-toxic.

Factors Influencing chemical sterilisation: (1) **Concentration of the chemical:** Rate of killing of bacteria varies directly with the concentration of the disinfectant. (2) **Temperature:** It should be designed to be used at room temperature. (3) **Evaporation and light deactivation:** Volatile agents evaporate easily like—chlorine products. Exposure to light adversely affects the disinfectant. (4) **pH:** Alcohols work best in alkaline PH while aldehydes work best in acidic pH. (5) **Bioburden:** The effectiveness of the disinfectant depends on the nature and number of contaminating microorganisms. (6) **Characteristics of the item to be sterilised:** A disinfectant solution will be effective only if it can contact all the surfaces on the item. (7) **Time:** Time required for different chemical agents to function effectively varies from seconds to hours. (8) **Use pattern:** It refers to how many times the solution can be used. (9) **Use and storage life:** Use life indicates limited period of time during which activated solution can be used. Storage life is the time period after which the unused or inactivated product is no longer deemed effective.

Classification of disinfectants

Based on consistency
- Liquid (alcohols, phenols).
- Gaseous (formaldehyde vapour).

Based on spectrum of activity
- High level.
- Intermediate level.
- Low level.

Based on mechanism of action
- Action on membrane (alcohol, detergent).
- Denaturation of cellular proteins (alcohol, phenol).
- Oxidation of essential sulphydryl groups of enzymes (H_2O_2, halogens).
- Alkylation of amino, carboxyl and hydroxyl group (formaldehyde).
- Damage to nucleic acids (formaldehyde).

Features of an Ideal Antiseptic or Disinfectant

It should have wide spectrum of activity; should be able to destroy microbes within practical period of time; should be active in the presence of organic matter; should make effective contact and be wettable.

It should be active in any pH; should be stable; should have long shelf life; should be speedy and have high penetrating power; should be non-toxic, non-allergenic, non-irritative or non-corrosive; should not have bad odour; should not leave non-volatile residue or stain; efficacy should not be lost on reasonable dilution; it should be cheaper and easily available.

Detergents

They are surface active agents. They contain fat-soluble long chain hydrocarbons and water-soluble ions which concentrate between cell membrane and surrounding medium causing membrane disruption. Detergents can be anionic or cationic. Negatively charged long chain hydrocarbons are anionic detergents. Cationic detergents are fat soluble with positive charges and combine with quaternary nitrogen atom and are called as quaternary ammonium compounds (quats). Cetrimide and bezalkonium compounds are quats. 2% detergent solutions are used. They are active against vegetative cells, mycobacteria and enveloped viruses.

Quaternary Ammonium Compounds

They are low level disinfectants, e.g. benzalkonium chloride. They are bactericidal, fungicidal and viricidal but not sporicidal. They are effective against gram-positive than gram-negative and marginally effective against *Pseudomonas*. They inactivate HIV but not hepatitis virus. They are inactivated by organic materials. Side effects are allergic reactions and contact dermatitis. Quats are biocides that also kill algae. Newer analogues are more effective with short contact time and effective against bacteria, viruses, fungi and mycobacteria.

Dyes

Acridine and aniline dyes are used as antiseptics and disinfectants. They interact with bacterial nucleic acids and so microbicidal. Aniline dyes such as crystal violet, malachite green and brilliant green; Acridine dyes such as acriflavine and aminacrine are commonly used dyes. Acriflavine is a mixture of proflavine and euflavine; only euflavine has effective antimicrobial properties. They are more effective against gram-positive bacteria. They may be used topically as antiseptics to treat mild burns. They are used as paint on the skin to treat bacterial skin infections. *Melachite green* is used in Lowenstein Jenson medium for growth of *Mycobacterium tuberculosis*.

Phenolic Compounds

They are used as standard to compare the efficacy of other agents. They are intermediate to low level disinfectants. It is derived from carbolic acid (phenol), one of the oldest germicides. It is the oldest known disinfectant used by Lister. Phenol (5%) is prepared from coal tar. They are bactericidal, fungicidal and viricidal but not sporicidal. They are active in the presence of organic matter. They are irritant to skin and mucous membranes, have bad odour. They are absorbed by rubber and residual disinfectant may cause tissue irritation. ***Cresol*** is more powerful and non-toxic. 5% solution is used. ***Lysol*** is emulsified cresol with soap. 2% solution is effective. Hexachlorophene, thymol [derived from herb thyme (intermediate level disinfectant)], amylmetacresol (is present in strepsils), α phenylphenol, chloroxylenol, triclosan are other phenolic products. *Triclosan* is organic phenyl ether which acts against gram-positive bacteria and to some extent against many gram-negative bacteria. It also acts on fungi and viruses.

They are bactericidal, fungicidal, mycobactericidal but are inactive against spores and most viruses. They are not inactivated by organic matter. The corrosive phenolics are used for disinfection of ward floors, in discarding jars in laboratories and disinfection of bedpans.

Phenol is considered as standard and measurement of effectiveness of other compounds is assessed as *"phenol coefficient"*. Disinfectant is compared with phenol using *Salmonella typhi* and *Staphylococcus aureus*. Disinfectants which are more effective than phenol has got phenol coefficient >1; and less effective one has got coefficient <1.

Disadvantages: Phenols are often toxic and irritant.

Halogens

They oxidise essential **sulphydryl** group enzymes thus killing microbes. But they are rapidly inactivated in the presence of organic matter. Iodine is corrosive and staining. Bleach solution is corrosive and will corrode stainless steel surfaces.

Iodophors

It is a combination of iodine and carrier with a resulting complex providing sustained release reservoir of iodine. They are bactericidal, viricidal and tuberculocidal but not sporicidal. These are intermediate to low level disinfectants. They corrode the metallic items and non-metallic items may be stained or discoloured. They are non-irritant and do not stain skin. *Povidone-iodine* is a good example, which is commonly used. *Tincture iodine* is 2% iodine in 70% alcohol. Iodine when combined with neutral carrier polymers like polyvinylpyrrolidone forms iodophors. Povidone-iodine is a good example. Iodophores allow slow release and so minimise the irritation. For handwashing iodophores are diluted in 50% alcohol. 10% povidone iodine is used undiluted in pre- and postoperative skin disinfection **(Fig. 2-6)**.

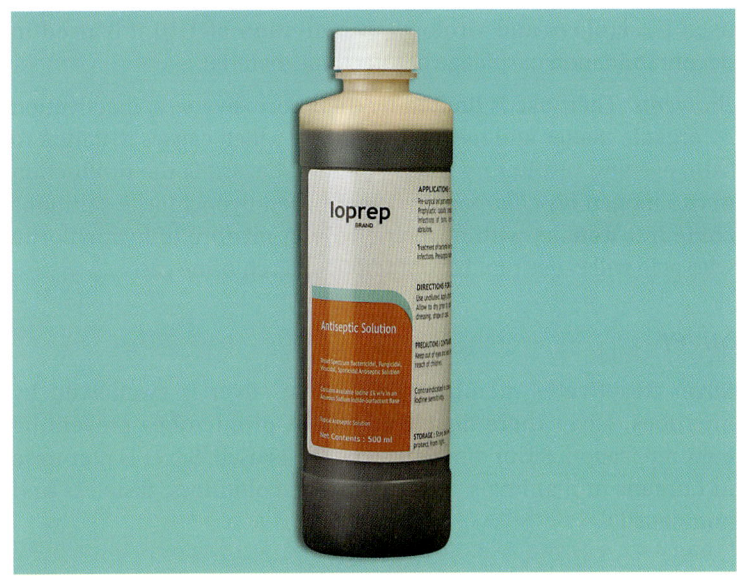

Fig. 2-6: Iodophors as antiseptic and disinfectant.

Chlorine and Chlorine Compounds

They are intermediate level disinfectants. They are active against bacteria and viruses but not spores. They are available both in liquid (sodium hypochlorite) and solid (calcium hypochlorite, bleaching powder) forms. They are most widely used, inexpensive and fast acting. *EUSOL: Edinburgh University Solution* **(Figs. 2-7A and B)** contains sodium hypochlorite, boric acid and calcium hydroxide. *Eusol bath* is dipping the ulcer bearing part in dilute eusol solution for 30 minutes 2–3 times a day. It is highly effective against HIV. Household bleach is an inexpensive and excellent source of sodium hypochlorite. A *1:100 to 1:1000* dilutions is effective against HIV. *1:5 to 1:10* dilution is effective against hepatitis. It also inactivates Cruetz Feldt Jakob disease with an exposure time of *1 hour*.

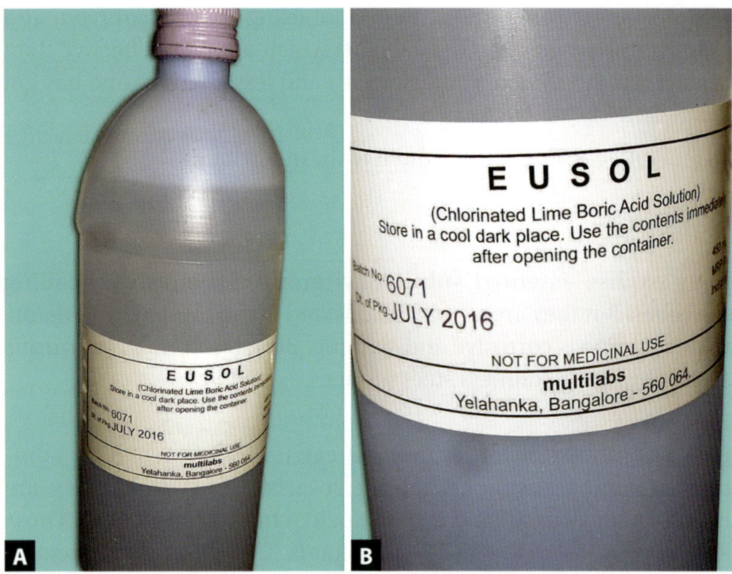

Figs. 2-7A and B: Eusol—Edinburgh university solution.

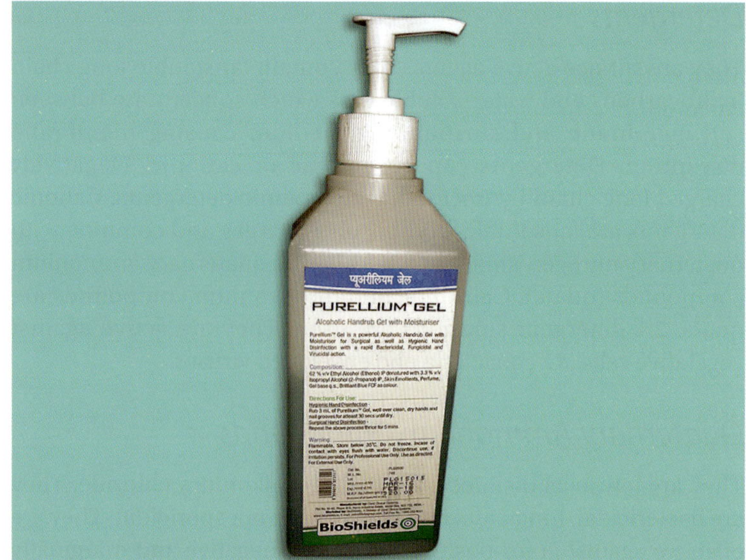

Fig. 2-8: Alcohol used as disinfectant and antiseptic.

Sodium hydroxide is also added to hypochlorite so as to stabilise it to prevent it from decomposing into chlorine. But such solution becomes strongly basic. Chloramines, chloramines T are also used as disinfectant. Chlorine oxide which is derived from precursor sodium chlorite and sodium and potassium chlorate is also commonly used.

Chlorine gas is used to bleach water. Household bleach is used to disinfect floors in dilution of 1:10. In higher concentrations chlorine is used to disinfect swimming pools. 0.5% sodium hypochlorite is used in serology and virology; at a dilution of 1:10 it is used in decontamination of spillage of infectious material.

Problems: Their use is limited by their corrosiveness, inactivation by organic matter and may leave residue which causes irritation to skin, eye and respiratory tract. Potential hazard is the production of carcinogen *bis-chloromethyl ether*, when hypochlorite solutions come into contact with formaldehyde. A mixture of hypochlorite with acid will cause rapid evolution of toxic chlorine gas.

Silver

Silver deactivates membrane proteins; silver is swallowed by microbes; silver there deactivates DNA of microbes preventing their replication. Silver dihydrogen citrate is used. Silver is non-toxic to humans and animals. It is odourless, colourless, tasteless and non-caustic.

Copper Alloy

It helps in reducing 99% bacterial contamination with 2 hours of exposure. It kills gram -ve and +ve bacteria after exposure for 2 hours. It also shows continuous antibacterial activity even after repeated contamination.

Alcohols

Alcohol dehydrates cells, disrupts membrane and causes coagulation of proteins. Ethyl or isopropyl alcohols (ethanol or isopropanol) are used. It is intermediate level disinfectants. Ethyl alcohol is bactericidal in 60–90% concentration and isopropyl alcohol in 60% concentration. 70% ethyl alcohol (spirit) is better. They kill bacteria but not spores, action against viruses is variable. Recommendation is—exposure to 70% ethanol for *15 minutes* to inactivate the hepatitis virus but *1 minute for HIV*. Their effectiveness is limited because of rapid evaporation, lack of ability to penetrate organic matter. They are used mainly to disinfect external surfaces of equipment like thermometers, stethoscopes, ventilators, fibreoptic cables. They can damage mounting of lensed instruments and tend to swell and harden rubber. Methyl alcohol kills fungal spores **(Fig. 2-8)**.

Alcohols are basically antiseptics rather than disinfectant as it is used mainly on living tissue surfaces. They are non-corrosive, but due to limited contact time as it gets evaporated rapidly their effects get reduced unless surface is submerged into the liquid. They are more effective when combined with distilled water which facilitates the diffusion through cell membrane. 70% ethanol diluted in water is effective against many bacteria. 80% ethanol and 5% isopropanol is effective to deactivate viruses like HIV, hepatitis B and C. Alcohol efficacy is enhanced by adding wetting agent dodecanoic acid (coconut soap) which is also effective against *Clostridium difficile*.

Aldehydes

Aldehydes act through alkalisation of amino, carboxy and hydroxyl groups damaging nucleic acids. They kill all microorganisms including spores.

Formaldehyde

It is useful to disinfect the rooms like operation theatre. It is effective at a high temperature and humidity of 80–90%. It is commonly used to fumigate the room. 500 mL of formalin with one litre of water is boiled to get formaldehyde vapour. Adding potassium permanganate to the same solution can create formaldehyde vapour. Room is kept closed for 12 hours. It is less expensive and has got longer half life. Paraformaldehyde is used to get the vapour formaldehyde. It is used principally in water-based solution called formalin. Vapour can be generated from paraformaldehyde tablets which contain 95% formaldehyde in a polymerised form. 40% formaldehyde (formalin) is used for surface disinfection and fumigation of rooms, chambers, operation theatres, wards, sick rooms. Fumigation is achieved by boiling formalin, heating paraformaldehyde or treating formalin with potassium permanganate. It also sterilises bedding, furniture and books. 10% formalin with 0.5% tetraborate sterilises clean metal instruments. It is a high level disinfectant. It is non-corrosive and is not inactivated by organic matter. It is widely used for sterilisation of endoscopic equipment, catheters, etc. For better effect it needs relative humidity of 60–80% and temperature of 37°C. Residual formaldehyde may affect the skin, but it can be neutralised by ammonia. Its use is limited by its pungent odour and fumes. It should be handled as a potent sensitiser and probable carcinogen.

Methanol is added to increase its half life.

Glutarldehyde (cidex 2%)

It is used to sterilise sharp instruments. Instruments should be dipped for 22 hours to achieve complete sterilisation. It is potent bactericide, sporicide, fungicide and viricide. The presence of solid materials and block of tissues need still longer time as it will take more time to penetrate these tissues. It is volatile and toxic to skin and also on inhalation. Its half life is short—less than 2 weeks **(Figs. 2-9A and B)**.

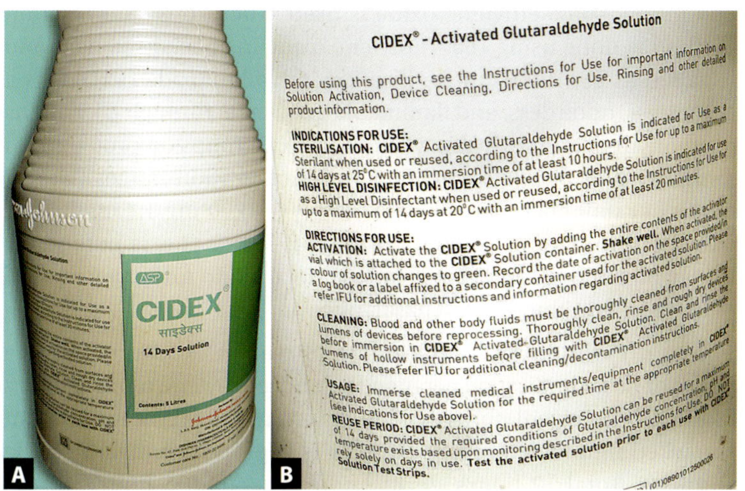

Figs. 2-9A and B: Cidex—glutaraldehyde solution 2%.

It is a saturated dialdehyde. It is used in 1.0% concentration (but highly effective in 2% concentration). It is *high level disinfectant*. It kills spores within 12 hours and viruses within 10 minutes. It is widely used because of their excellent biocidal properties, activity in the presence of organic matter, non-corrosiveness and non-coagulation of proteinaceous material. 2% glutaraldehyde is used to sterilise thermometers, cystoscopes, bronchoscopes, centrifuges, anasethetic equipment. An exposure of at least 3 hours at alkaline pH is required for action by glutaraldehyde. 2% formaldehyde at 40°C for 20 minutes is used to disinfect wool and 0.25% at 60°C for 6 hours to disinfect animal hair and bristles. Glutaraldehyde requires alkaline pH and only those articles that are wettable can be sterilised.

Disadvantages: It is noxious and irritating to tissues and hence thorough rinsing of all exposed materials is mandatory. Prepackaging is not possible and equipment will be wet. Pseudomembranous laryngitis has been linked to disinfection of tracheal tubes with glutaraldehyde.

Hydrogen Peroxide (H_2O_2)

It is used as topical oxygen therapy. Because of its effervescence and release of nascent oxygen it removes the tissue debris. It is used to clean wounds, cavities, ulcers and as mouthwash, as ear drops to clear ear wax.

H_2O_2, being a strong oxidant is used to sterilise rigid scopes and heat sensitive articles. Its cycle time is less (30 minutes). It is available as both liquid and vaporised form. It is an effective bactericidal, fungicidal, viricidal and sporicidal. It is commercially available as 3% solution but can be used up to 25% concentration. It is non-corrosive and not inactivated by organic matter but irritant to skin and eyes. Vapor can be used to sterilise/disinfect the rooms/aircrafts. It gets decomposed in light; proteinaceous organic materials reduce its activity. 3% should be used for skin, ulcers and wounds. 6% is used to decontaminate the instruments **(Fig. 2-10)**.

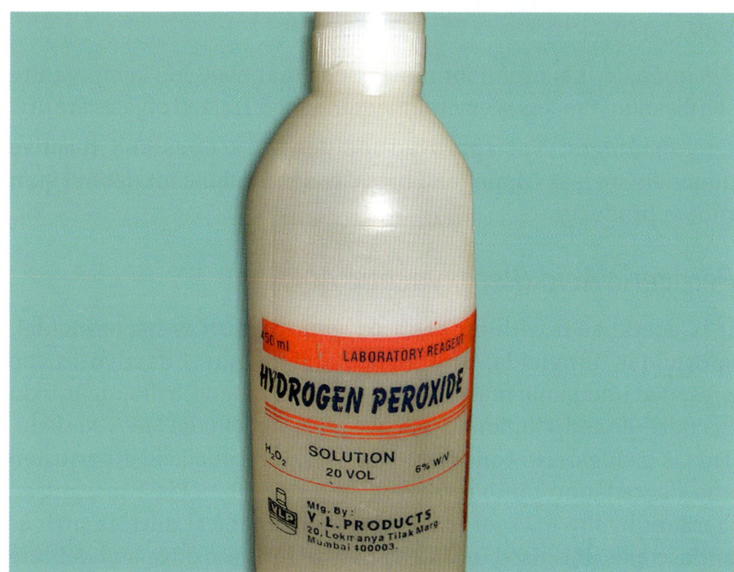

Fig. 2-10: Hydrogen peroxide topical agent.

Problems of H_2O_2: It has low penetration capacity and not compatible with cellulose products like paper. Suture materials or nylon materials will become brittle with this. It is irritant to skin and eyes. It is toxic when used with a concentration of more than 10%. Vapor is hazardous to lungs.

Hydrogen peroxide vacuum chamber sterilisation: Hydrogen peroxide solution in a vacuum chamber is dispersed to create a plasma cloud. There will be oxidisation of key cellular components, which inactivates the microorganisms. The plasma cloud exists only while the energy source is turned on; when it is turned off, water vapor and oxygen are formed, resulting in no toxic residues and harmful emissions. The temperature is maintained in the 40–50°C range, which makes it suitable for use with heat and moisture sensitive devices. The instruments are wrapped prior to sterilisation and can either be stored or used immediately. ***Phases***—a *vacuum phase* to create vacuum in the chamber and to drop the pressure to less than one pound per square inch (for 20 minutes). In the *injection phase*, rise in pressure is created by introducing the aqueous hydrogen peroxide into the vacuum chamber which vaporises into a gas. In *diffusion phase* the hydrogen peroxide vapor spreads throughout the chamber raising the pressure which drives the sterilant into the packs with instruments killing the microorganisms. In *plasma phase* the radiofrequency energy is applied to remove the electrons from some of the molecules to create low temperature plasma cloud. This leads into the activated compounds to lose their high energy and recombine to form oxygen and water. In *venting phase*, filtered air is introduced into the chamber to allow the chamber to return to atmospheric pressure to facilitate opening of the door which lasts for one minute.

Ozone

Ozone sterilisers use O_2, water and electricity to produce ozone. It is a gas used for disinfecting water, laundry, foods, air, and surfaces.

It destroys many organic compounds, resulting in rapid decolourisation and deodorisation in addition to disinfection. It decomposes relatively quickly; it is used to remove the bulk of oxidisable matter from the water, which would produce small amounts of organochloride if treated with chlorine only. Ozone has a very wide range of applications from municipal to industrial water treatment due to its powerful reactivity. Hydrogen peroxide is sometimes mixed with colloidal silver.

Advantages: It is useful for most goods that need low temperature sterilisation. Process is environment friendly. Treated objects are dry.

Disadvantages: Not approved for flexible scopes and reactive materials such as copper and brass. It is unsuitable for natural gum rubber products.

Peracetic Acid (Peroxyacetic Acid)

It is acetic acid with an extra oxygen atom. It is bacteriocidal, sporicidal, fungicidal and viricidal. They are effective in the presence of organic matter. But it is corrosive and irritating to skin in concentrated solution. It is active ingredient in the *Steris* sterilant. This is a single use concentrate of 35% peracetic acid + corrosion and degradation inhibitors. Peracetic acid (0.2%) is a recognised sterilant by the FDA for use in sterilising medical devices such as endoscopes. It is used in wide variety of heat sensitive and delicate instruments. It is used on wet or dry items and there is no personnel exposure. It can be situated in the operating room suite. It is useful only for totally immercible objects and only small number instruments can be processed in a cycle. Peracetic acid is a disinfectant produced by reacting hydrogen peroxide with acetic acid. It is effective against many microorganisms and is not deactivated by catalase and peroxidase, the enzymes that break down hydrogen peroxide. It also breaks down to acetic acid and hydrogen peroxide which are safer end products. It can be used under wide temperature range (0–40°C), wide pH range (3.0–7.5), in clean or hard water conditions, and is not affected by protein residues. It needs precleaning, leak testing, appropriate tray to immerse objects. Sterilant is provided in a sealed single use container and premixing or dilution is not done. Devices should tolerate 55°C temperature.

Performic Acid

It is the simplest and powerful perorganic acid. It is formed by the reaction of hydrogen peroxide and formic acid, it shows more rapid action than peracetic acid; later breaks down into water and carbon dioxide.

Potassium Permanganate ($KMnO_4$)

It is a purplish-black crystalline powder that colours everything it touches, through a strong oxidising action. It stains "stainless" steel, which somehow limits its use and makes it necessary to use plastic or glass containers. It is used to disinfect aquariums and is used in community swimming pools to disinfect ones feet before entering the pool. It is widely used to disinfect community water ponds and wells in tropical countries, as well as to disinfect the mouth before pulling out teeth. It can be applied to wounds in dilute solution.

Potassium peroxymonosulfate is another disinfectant; used as a 1% solution in water, and keeps for one week once it is made up. It kills bacteria, viruses, and fungi; it is expensive, very effective, its pink colour fades as it is used up. It is the principal ingredient in *Virkon*, is a wide-spectrum disinfectant used in laboratories.

GASEOUS STERILISATION

Ethylene Oxide Sterilisation

Ethylene oxide (ETO) is used for 70% of sterilisations and 50% of medical devices. It is done with a temperature of 30–60°C with more than 30% humidity and gas concentrations of 200–800 mg/L. Ethylene oxide penetrates well through paper, plastics, clothes, etc. It kills bacteria, spores, viruses, fungi and is highly effective and compatible. But it is inflammable, toxic and can be carcinogenic and may affect the reproductive system. ETO steriliser needs biological validation after installation, repair and failure. Gas chamber and micro-dose methods—are two methods used. Ethylene oxide is delivered into a chamber containing ethylene oxide and diluents gases like carbon dioxide and halogenated hydrocarbon. Now commonly 100% ethylene oxide is used. Micro-dose sterilisation method is done using 100% ethylene oxide in specialised bags and is called as gas diffusion sterilisation. Ethylene oxide $(CH_2)_2O$ is a colourless, odourless, and flammable gas. It acts through alkylations of sulphydryl, amino, hydroxyl and carboxyl groups on proteins and amino groups of nucleic acids. The concentration ranges (weight of gas per unit chamber volume) from 800–1200 mg/L for ethylene oxide with operating temperatures of 45–63°C. Gas is potentially mutagenic and carcinogenic; can produce acute toxicity; irritation of the skin, conjunctiva and nasal mucosa.

Phases are—initial preconditioning phase, an exposure phase, a phase of post-sterilisation aeration to remove ethylene oxide residues like ethylene glycol and ethylene chlorohydrin. Here instrument is packed in a sealed plastic cover. It is kept in the ethylene oxide steriliser. Total 12 hours sterilisation is needed; 6 hours for gas sterilisation and another 6 hours for gas to come out. It is good way of sterilisation. Once instrument is sterilised, it can be kept and used for 6 months. Problem is cost factor, time duration needed (minimum 12 hours) for sterilisation **(Figs. 2-11A to D)**.

Formaldehyde (HCHO): It is similar to ethylene oxide with similar action from a range of 15–100 mg/L with a temperature of 70–75°C.

Low temperature steam formaldehyde (LTSF) steriliser: It operates with sub atmospheric pressure steam; air is removed by evacuation and steam is admitted to the chamber.

Others

Chlorhexidine (hibitane) is useful antiseptic. It is a non-detergent chemical disinfectant usually used in the concentration of 0.5% in 70% alcohol for skin. Tubes, masks, etc. are sterilised by keeping for 20 min in 0.1% aqueous solution. Chlorhexidine can be used in an isopropanol solution for skin disinfection, or as an aqueous solution for wound irrigation. It is also used as an antiseptic handwash. 20% chlorhexidine gluconate solution is used for preoperative hand and skin preparation. Chlorhexidine gluconate is also mixed with quaternary ammonium compounds like cetrimide to get better antimicrobial effects (savlon). Chlorhexidine is inactivated by soap water.

Cetrimide is cationic surfactant (cetavlon). 2% solution is used. *Savlon* is combination of cetrimide and hibitane (chlorhexidine). It is very commonly used antiseptic in operation theatres and wards **(Fig. 2-12)**.

Hexachlorophene (cinthol): It is not used in infants and children because it can get absorbed through intact skin in this age group causing severe neurotoxicity. Hexachlorophene is chlorinated diphenyl and is less irritant. It has marked effect over gram-positive bacteria but not over gram-negative bacteria, mycobacteria, fungi and viruses.

Dettol (chloroxylenol)—5% solution is used. Chloroxylenol is less irritant and is used for topical purposes; is more effective against gram-positive bacteria than gram-negative bacteria. Chloroxylenol is inactivated by hard water **(Fig. 2-13)**.

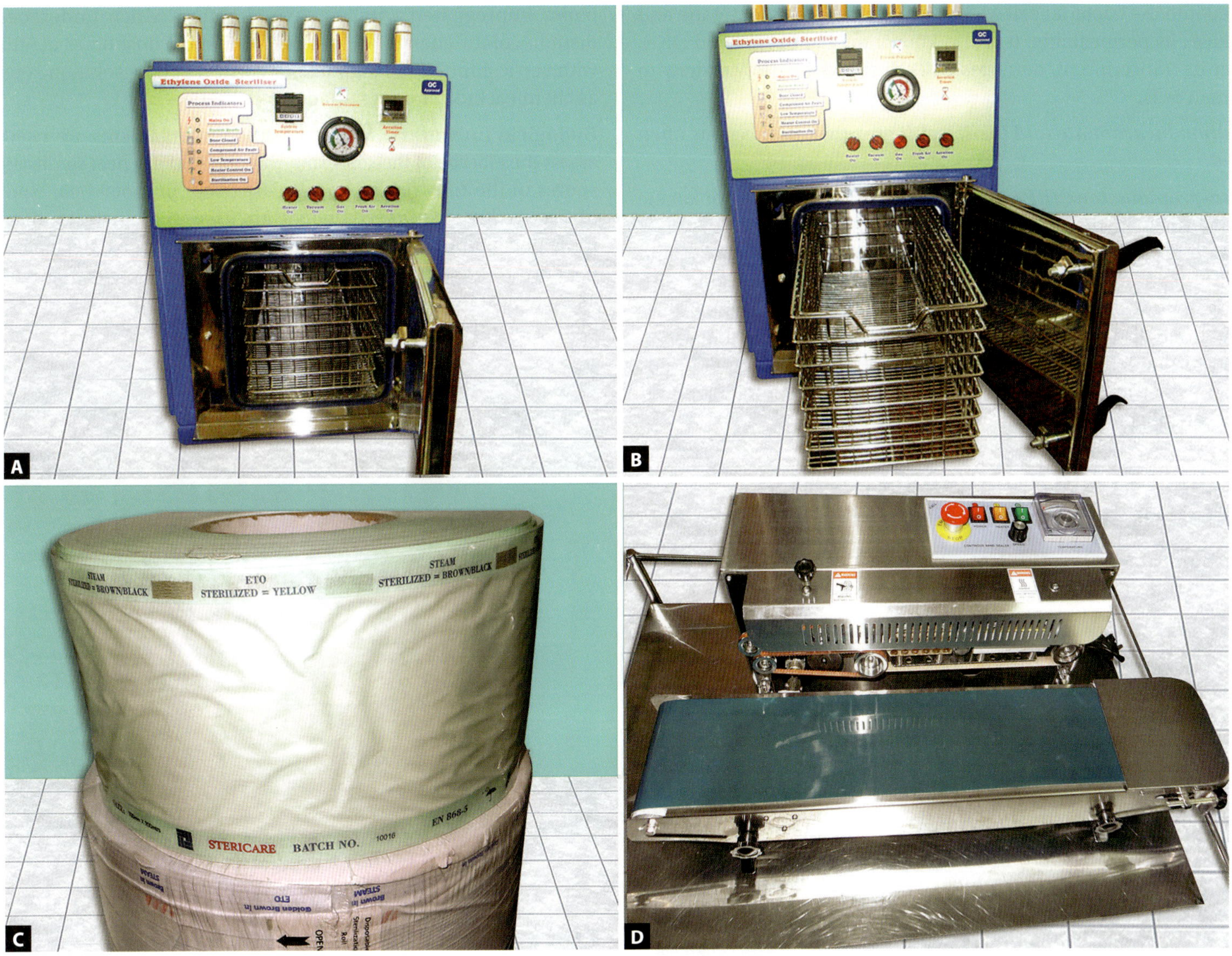

Figs. 2-11A to D: Ethylene oxide steriliser.

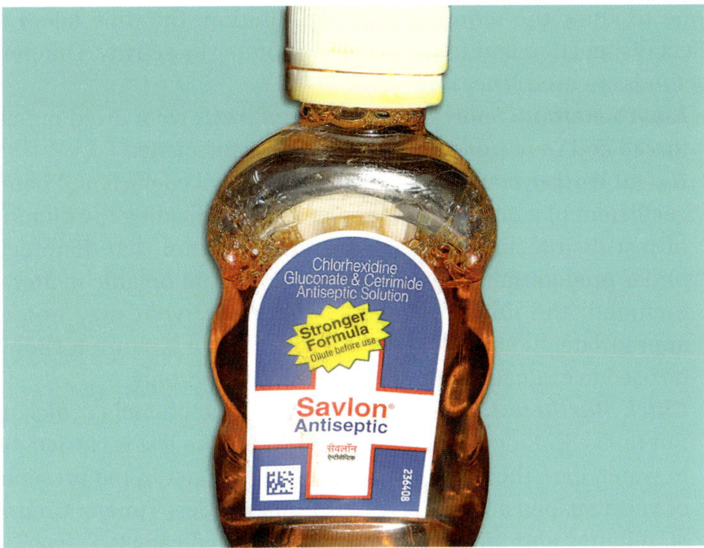

Fig. 2-12: Savlon—cetrimide with chlorhexidine.

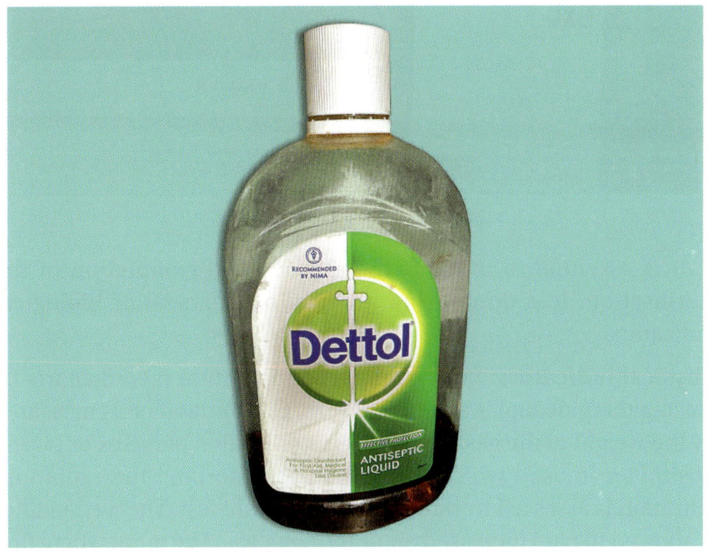

Fig. 2-13: Dettol—chloroxylenol.

Acriflavine and proflavine are orange-red coloured dyes used as antiseptics. It is effective against gram-positive and few gram-negative organisms. It retains its activity in pus and body fluids.

The polymer of polyaminopropyl biguanide is bactericidal at very low concentrations (10 mg/L). The polymer strands are incorporated into the bacterial cell wall, which disrupts the membrane and reduces its permeability. It is also known to bind to bacterial DNA, alter its transcription, damages DNA. It shows very low toxicity to human cells.

Sodium bicarbonate and lactic acids are other disinfectants often used.

Beta-propiolactone (BPL): It is a condensation product of ketane with formaldehyde.

It is an alkylating agent which by alkylation of carboxyl and hydroxyl groups becomes microcidal. It is a colourless liquid with pungent to sweetish smell. It is an effective sporicidal agent. 0.2% is used to sterilise biological products. It is more efficient in fumigation than formaldehyde. It is used to sterilise vaccines, tissue grafts, surgical instruments and enzymes. But its poor penetrating power and carcinogenicity limits its use.

Evaluation and Monitoring Process of Different Sterilisation Methods

Mechanical monitor (indicator) (Fig. 2-14): It is the device that records time, temperature and pressure precisely.

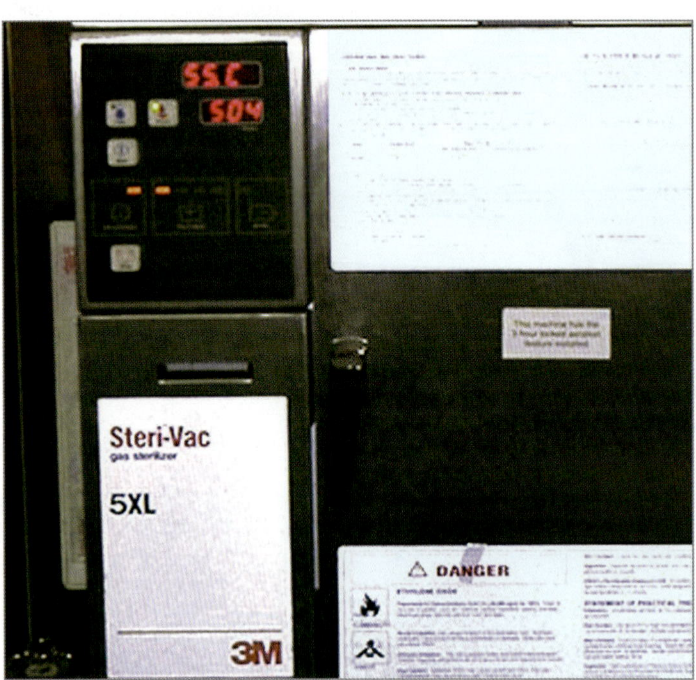

Fig. 2-14: Mechanical indicator.

It is essential to monitor the efficacy and completion of the sterilisation. It is done using physical or chemical or biological indicators.

Physical indicators: It is usually by temperature record charts by placing thermocouples at different sites. Gas sterilisation is measured by the weight of the gas. In radiation sterilisation persplex or plastic dosimeter is used which darkens after absorbing the radiation. Filtration is assessed by bubble point pressure test. The wetted filter is allowed to pass increased air or nitrogen gas. The point where first gas bubble comes is the maximum pore size. Gas or air pressure is further raised to allow generalised bubble formation; pressure difference here if it is below the expected then filter is at fault.

Chemical indicators: Coloured strips or tapes are placed in the chamber; change in the colour indicates the completion of the sterilisation. In gas sterilisation, Royach Sacket, the indicator paper impregnated with reactive chemical which undergoes a distinct colour change on reaction. Chemical dosimeter acidified with cerric ammonium sulphate or cerric sulphate solution is used as chemical indicator for radiation sterilisation.

Biological indicators: Spores of different organisms are used to assess the efficacy of the sterilising chambers. In dry heat sterilisation, spores of the *Clostridium* species are used. In moist heat, spores of *Geobacillus stearothermophilus* are used as biological indicator in sealed ampoules of the culture media. In gas sterilisation, *Bacillus subtilis var:niger* and *Bacillus subtilis var.golbigii* are used as biological indicator. *S. marcesence and B. diminuta* are used as biological indicators for filtration sterilisation **(Fig. 2-15)**.

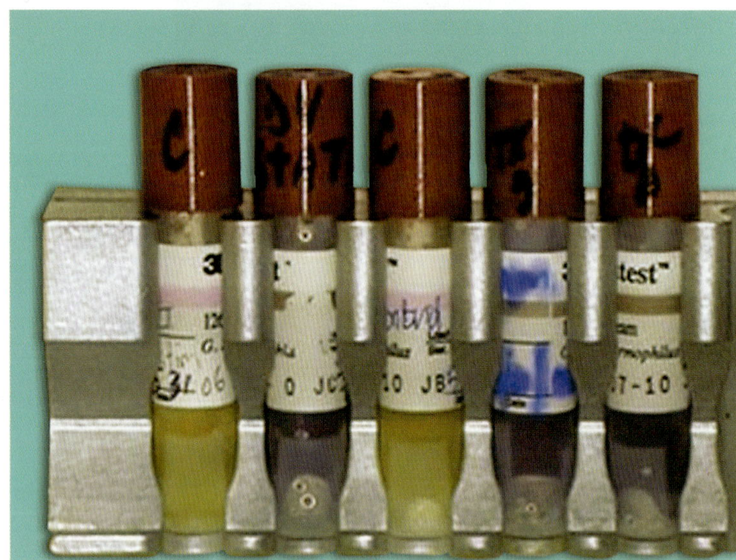

Fig. 2-15: Biological indicator is very good method of assessing the efficacy of the sterilisation.

Efficacy Tests for Disinfectant

As disinfectants lose their activity on standing and in the presence of organic matter, their activity must be periodically tested. It is done to know the required effective dilution, the time taken to effect disinfection and to periodically monitor its activity. Different methods are used. *They are:*

- ***Koch's method:*** Spores of *Bacillus anthracis* were dried on silk thread and were subjected to action of disinfectants.
- ***Rideal Walker method:*** It is based on phenol coefficient. Phenol coefficient of a disinfectant is calculated by dividing the dilution of test disinfectant by the dilution of phenol that disinfects under predetermined conditions. But here no organic matter is included; the microorganism *Salmonella typhi* may not be appropriate; the time allowed for disinfection is short; it should be used to evaluate phenolic type disinfectants only.
- ***Chick Martin test:*** This test is also similar to phenol coefficient. But unlike in Rideal Walker method where the test is carried out in water, here the disinfectants are made to act in the presence of yeast suspension or 3% dried human feces. Time is fixed at 30 minutes and the organism used to test efficacy is *S. typhi* as well as *S. aureus*.

- ***Capacity use dilution test (Kelsey-Sykes test):*** The capacity test determines the appropriate dilution use of the disinfectants. The stability test (Maurer) determines the stability and long-term effectiveness of disinfectant dilution. The capacity and stability test help to find out the ideal and the choice of a disinfectant.
- ***In-use test (Kelsey and Maurer):*** This test estimates the number of living organisms in a vessel of disinfectant in actual use. The disinfectant that is already in use is diluted 1 in 10 by mixing 1 mL of the disinfectant with 9 mL of sterile nutrient broth. Ten drops of the diluted disinfectant is placed on two nutrient agar plates. One plate is incubated at 37°C for 3 days; other is kept at room temperature for 7 days. The number of drops that yielded growth is counted after incubation. If their growth in more than five drops on either plate, it represents failure of disinfectant.

OPERATION THEATRE ROOM (OPERATION THEATRE COMPLEX)

History of Operation Theatre (OT)

In 1893, Henry Burdett noted "in many large hospitals two and sometimes three, operation rooms (ORs) are provided, one being arranged in the form of a theatre, and provided with accommodation for a considerable number of students" with viewing galleries. Probably word "*operation theatre*" usage has come for this reason **(Figs. 2-16A and B)**.

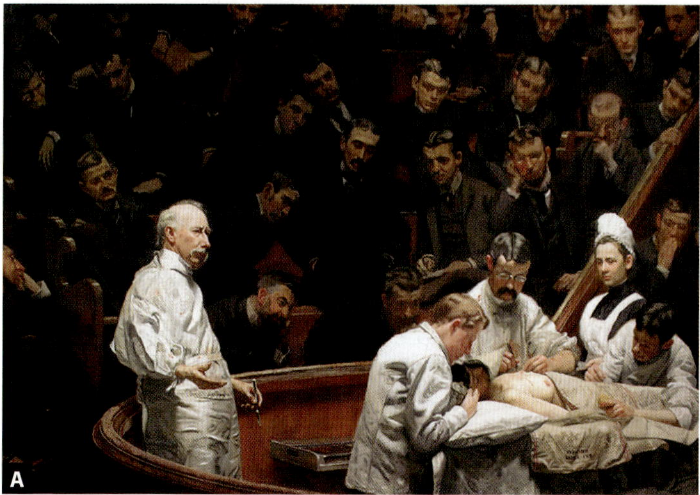

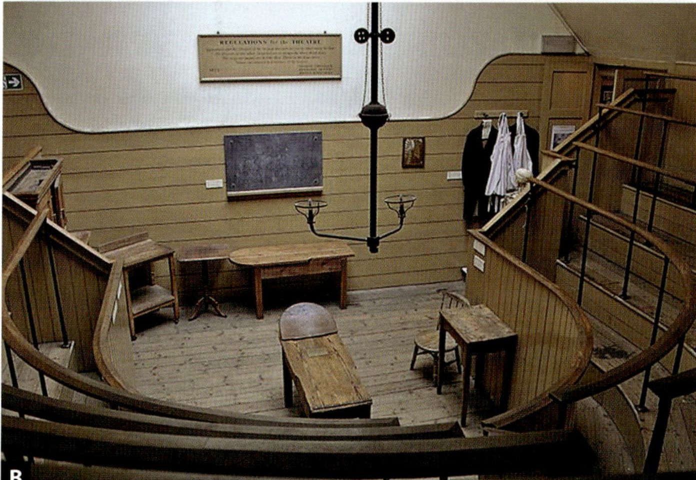

Figs. 2-16A and B: Operation being conducted before the 18th century—historical and Operation Theatre in the 18th century with gallery.

In 1867, Lister's antisepsis methods are getting popular. ORs/theatres are designed to eliminate infection. OTs are made at a convenient access to wards but severed from aerial contact with wards. Changing clothes while entering the OT has become standard instead of their regular clothes started as practice. Washing hands prior to surgery, wearing rubber gloves (1878) became standard. In 1886, von Bergmann started steam sterilisation. Face masks and caps started in the 20th century. In 1884, a German surgeon Gustav Neuber implemented set of restrictions to ensure sterilisation and aseptic operating condition through use of gowns, caps, and shoe covers. He invented autoclave. He also introduced separate OT for infected and uninfected cases. In 1890, standard surgical gloves were introduced by William Halsted and made it mandatory.

In 1962, the principles of theatre suite design were adopted in the surgical departments. The theatre sterile supply unit (TSSU) prepared instrument packs as part of the theatre suite with theatre staff supervision. But the linen and swabs were sterilised in the central sterile supply department (CSSD). Sterile packs containing general sets of instruments, and packs for particular operations are stored in the previously occupied by the steriliser room. The clean and dirty traffic flow separation in the theatre suite is planned to have asepsis rather than antisepsis.

General Considerations

Operation theatre is like a temple to all surgeons. It is complex area with proper principles, protocols, guidelines, and rules which are essential for safety of the patients who are undergoing the surgical procedures.

Every operation theatre should have a waiting area, entrance, surgeon's changing and relaxing room, separate changing room and relaxing room for nurses, autoclave and sterilisation room, OT scrub area, all sets of instruments, instruments for anaesthesia, adequate number of racks, toilets, air-conditioned ventilator, OT tables, trolleys to shift patients, OT laundry, good light, ultrasound machine, C-Arm image intensifier.

Operation theatre should have an adjoining postoperative ward. This ward should be close to the OT, easily accessible (surgeon and anaesthetist should be able to rush to the postoperative ward in a short period without changing their OT dress).

In many theatres light music is played to calm the patient just before inducing anaesthesia.

OT complex and theatre should be easy to clean floor, roof and walls. An individual unit for instrument cleaning, washing, and arranging should be present where the instruments are kept ready, packed and autoclaved as directed.

A separate room for pathologists with facilities for frozen section and relaxing should be present.

OR will be specifically designed and reserved for respective fields depending on workloads and turn over, such as, orthopaedic surgeries, spine surgeries, replacement surgeries, cardiac surgeries, neurosurgeries, ophthalmology surgeries, and laparoscopic surgeries.

Computers, preparation areas, staff areas, and instrument areas should be strategically placed to improve the efficiency. Clean work area, soiled work area, restricted area, and unrestricted areas should be strategically arranged to have safe, smooth uninterrupted OR work.

A microbiologically "ultra clean air system" wherein clean air directed centrally low downward and rapidly outward to minimise

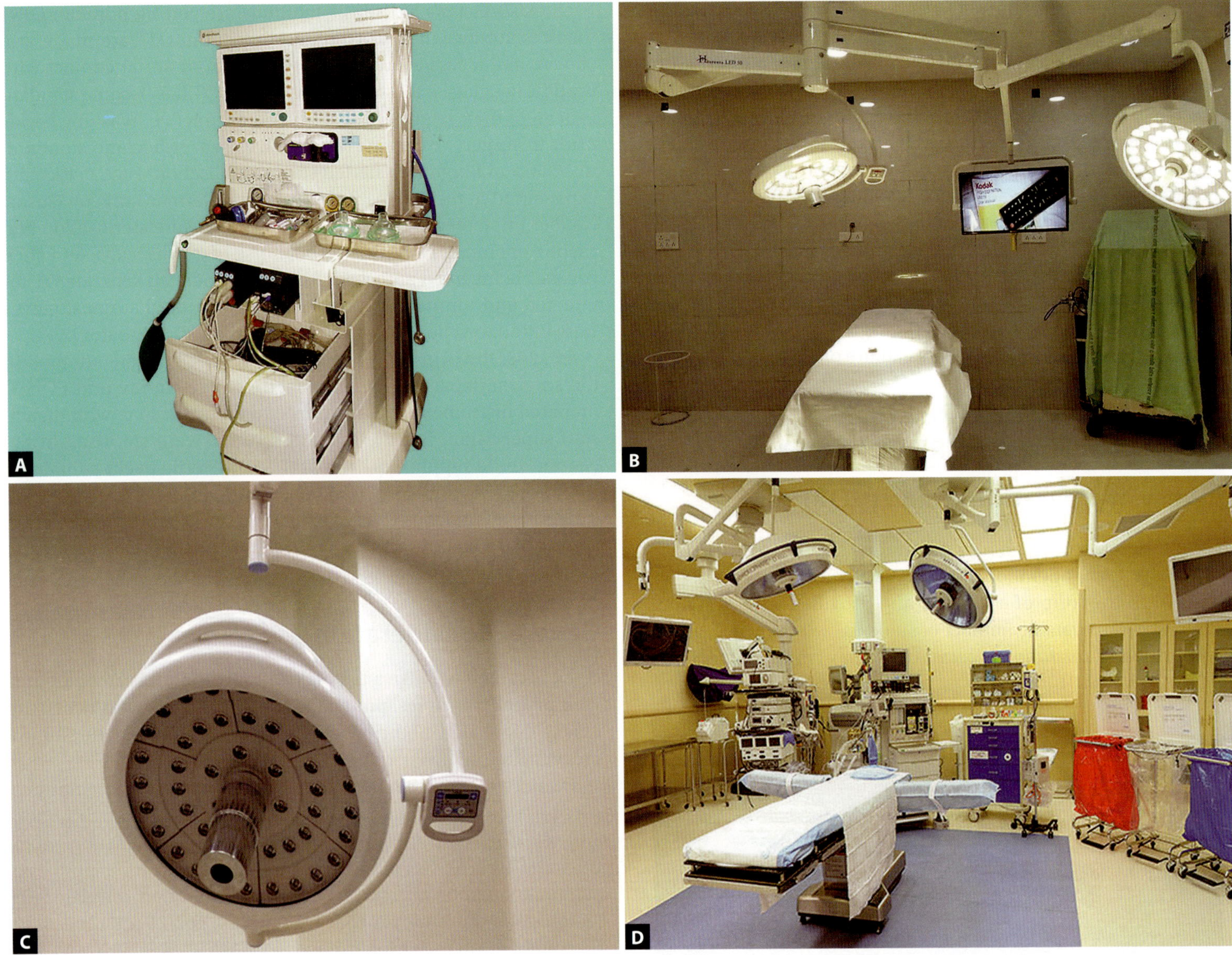

Figs. 2-17A to D: Essential needs of operation theatre (OT). High-tech operation system in OT complex. Anaesthesia machine is also seen.

infection and sepsis over surgical field. Many theaters now have "scavenger" extraction systems to remove anaesthetic gases from the atmosphere.

The adaptive layout for operating theatre **(ALOT)** in hospitals is used to have the "most efficient" layout placement for operating facilities, corridors, and elevators in a designated area with a set of professional standards. Such standards include regulations on hygiene, safety, and security of doctors, medical staff, patients, and visitors; movements of technologies; and specifications of operating rooms. *Two types of operation theatre complex are used—(1) Conventional and Non-integraed, (2) Hybrid, integrated and digital.*

Hybrid, Integrated, Digital OR: In Hybrid OR, specialised imaging devices are brought to and installed in the OR like MRI, CT, ultrasound, Doppler, intraoperative imaging devices, vascular imaging devices, etc. In integrated type, patient information, audio, video, surgical and room lights, building automation, and specialised equipment, including imaging devices, could all communicate with one another; often all these can be commanded from a central console by one operator **(Figs. 2-17 and 2-18)**.

Types of operation theatre

- **Based on sterility:**
  - Ultrasterile OT [cardiothoracic and vascular surgery (CTVS) and transplant OT]
  - Sterile OT
  - Septic OT
- **Based on construction:**
  - Modular OT
  - Non-modular OT
- **Based on timing of surgery:**
  - Routine OT
  - Emergency OT

Principles of an Operation Theatre

- An air-conditioning is a must to have a filtered continuous flow of air.
- Doors and windows should be kept closed as much as possible.
- Ward nurse should hand over the patient to theatre nurse with all details, case sheets, tag, side of surgery, blood to be transfused, and pre-medication details. While shifting the patient ward nurse

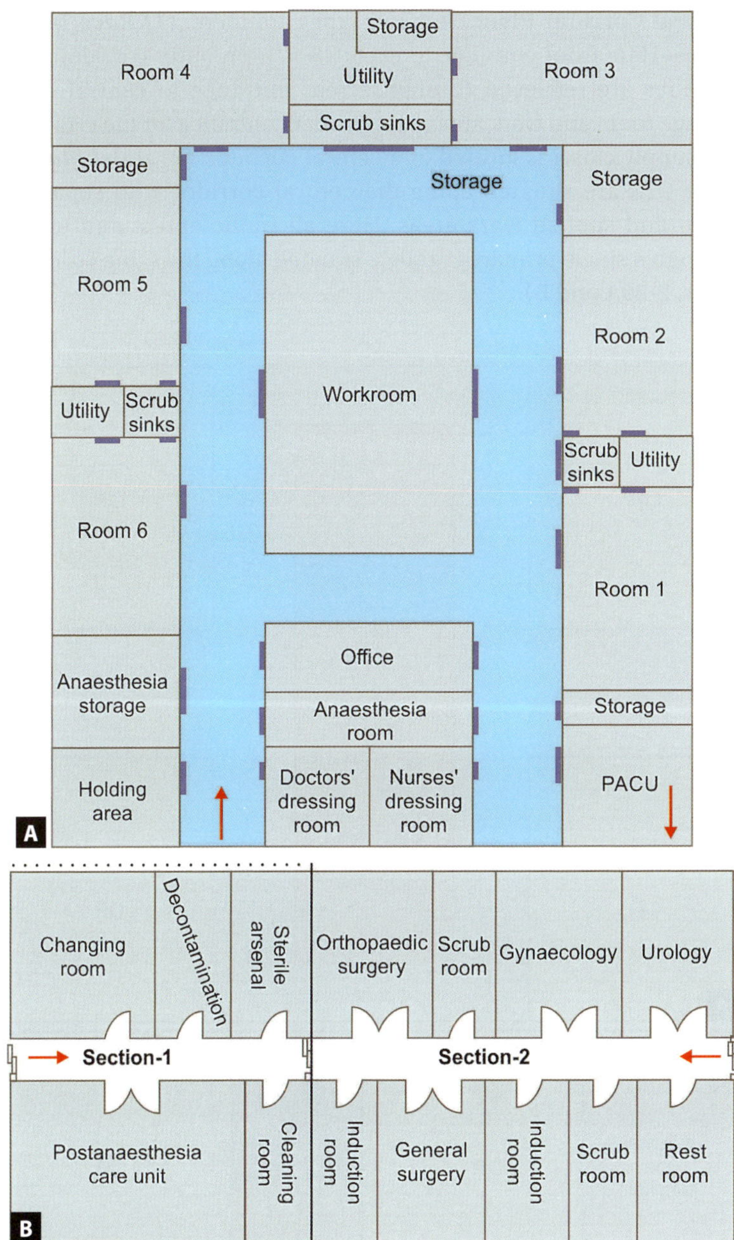

Figs. 2-18A and B: (A) Two section operation theater (OT) complex design; (B) Provisional plan for OT work area. (PACU: postanaesthesia care unit)

must take care of the airway and IV line of the patient, must keep tongue depressor, swabs, airway in the trolley.

- Patient should be shifted to theatre always in a trolley. Patient should remove all ornaments and wear theatre gowns, cap, and feet covers.
- Patient must be transferred from ward trolley to theatre trolley, which should have modern accessories like oxygen, side guards, drip stand, oxygen masks, pulse oximeter placing area, tiltable couch.
- Patient's trolley and ward blankets should not be taken inside the operation theatre.
- Initially patient should be kept in preoperative room and later should be shifted to theatre. Anaesthetist and surgeon and also theatre nurse should accompany the patient.
- Theatre nurse should confirm the consent form, case sheets, site and side of the surgery, etc.
- Separate theatre shoes should be worn by surgeons, anaesthetists, theatre nurses and assistants.
- Unnecessary movements, speaking loudly, laughing, should be avoided as patient inside the theatre may be awake especially when under spinal anaesthesia.
- All persons entering the theatre should wear theatre dress (pant and shirt), cap, mask, footwear or shoes (shoes are ideal). Material for dress should be smooth, non-woven fabric, which is easily boilable. Cap should cover and conceal hair fully.
- Clothes, dresses should be washed, daily cleaned, ironed and kept ready. Fresh, clean cotton blanket should be used for the patient in theatre.
- Ideally all mobile phones should be switched off inside the theatre.
- Any public person or relative of the patient should not be allowed inside the theatre. Selected people may be allowed only by prior permission from medical director of the hospital and from operating surgeon.
- One ***senior nurse*** is made in-charge of all activities in the theatre like shifting patients, arranging theatre tables, autoclave and other sterilisation methods, cleaning the instruments, packing the instruments for autoclave. She decides the duties of her junior nurses and makes a list of nurses for that day surgical scrubbing.

  Operation theatre assistant and technicians are also under her supervision and should follow her instructions strictly. She should be answerable for any default and problems in the theatre occurred or created by her fellow nurses and theatre boys.
- ***Scrub nurse*** is the one, who washes to assist the surgeon, arranges the instrument table and gives instruments to surgeon during procedure. She should be well aware of the steps of surgery and instruments required. She should be alert, quick, and understandable.
- One nurse in each theatre works as a ***circulating nurse*** who provides additional instruments required during surgical procedure. She also takes care of the counting of the surgical mops and swabs used. Used mops or swabs should be kept hanging in mop rack or swab rack which should be visible to the operating team. Name, procedure and number of mops collected and used should be written on a blackboard. Scrub nurse and circulating nurse are fully in-charge and responsible for swab counts. *She also will be legally questioned and penalised along with the surgeon if there is negligence in mop count.*
- Theatre nurse and OT assistant should accompany the patient while handing over to postoperative nurse from OT.
- Patient should be shifted outside the OT once anaesthetist confirms the fitness for shift. It is the anaesthetist who decides when to shift, how to shift and how long the patient should be in postoperative ward.

Modes of infection and sepsis in OT

- Patient's skin.
- Surgeon, nurses and OT technicians, by unclean hands, nostrils, throat, skin.
- Contamination of OT floor and wall.
- Improper sterilisation.
- Poor handling of instruments.
- Poor packing and poor storage of instruments.
- Theatre clothes, footwear and shoes.
- Not disinfecting the OT properly and adequately after using the OT for infected cases.

Occupational Safety and Health Administration (OSHA) Protocols

- Shoes must be comfortable with closed heel and toe and not cloth covered. Cloth-covered shoes may allow blood, body fluids, and other liquids to permeate. Cloth-covered shoes will not protect the feet should a heavy object fall on them.
- Personal hygiene must be meticulous. A shower should be taken shortly before beginning a workday in the operating theatre.
- Jewellery, long or artificial fingernails, and nail polish are prohibited as they harbour microorganisms. Piercing jewellery must be removed as it may become loose and fall onto the sterile field.
- All persons who expect to proceed from the unrestricted zone into the semi-restricted zone must go to the dressing area, wear a scrub suit and tuck the blouse of the suit into the pants.
- All hairs, beards, or mustaches must be covered with a surgical cap and mask. Hair must be confined as it sheds microorganisms with movement.
- Shoe covers must be placed over shoes to reduce contamination and to protect shoes from coming in contact with blood and body fluids.
- Before proceeding into Zone 3, all persons must scrub hands and arms for medical asepsis. It is believed that bare skin may shed microorganisms. In many institutions, all who are not scrubbed for the surgical procedure must wear a scrub jacket to cover bare arms.
- Before entering a room where a surgical procedure is in progress, a mask must be worn. The masks worn in the theatre room must be single and high-filtration type.

Operation Theatre Design

Operation theatre design principles revolve around traffic control, environmental control, prevention of surgical site infection (SSI), absolute sterility, adequate space, and quick and easy reachability. There will be clear separation of clean and soiled areas, strategic design of entire area to have adequate space for different needs with the help and suggestions of engineers and technical experts. Different designs and plans are used for OT complex **(Fig. 2-19)**.

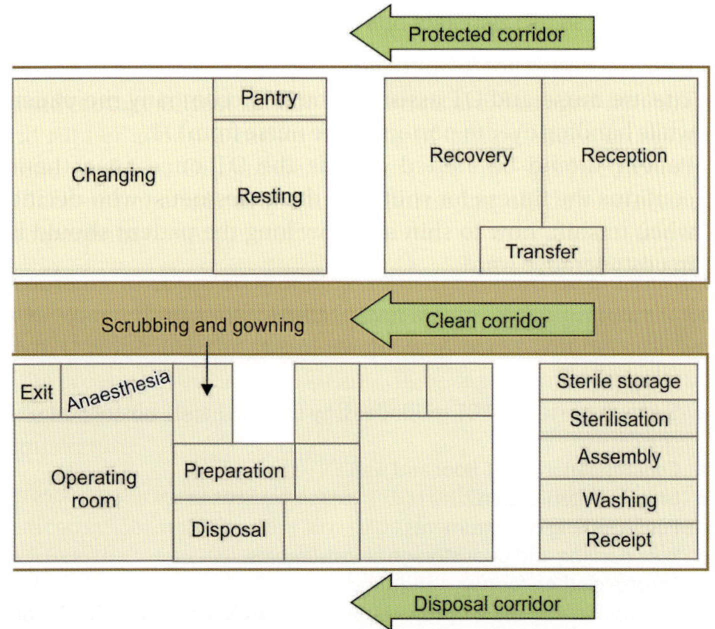

Fig. 2-19: Basic design of operation theatre (OT) complex.

Central Corridor Plan: Here two types are there. ***(1) Race Track Plan***—Here front entrance to each OR is from outer corridor and supplies are retrieved through a rear entrance to central core storage room and work areas. The primary entrance for the OTs and the supply closet is located in a central corridor. ***(2) Hotel Plan***—Here ORs are situated along the central corridor with separate clean and spoiled work areas. Here all traffic enters and exists through a single primary entrance situated along the same corridor **(Figs. 2-20A and B)**.

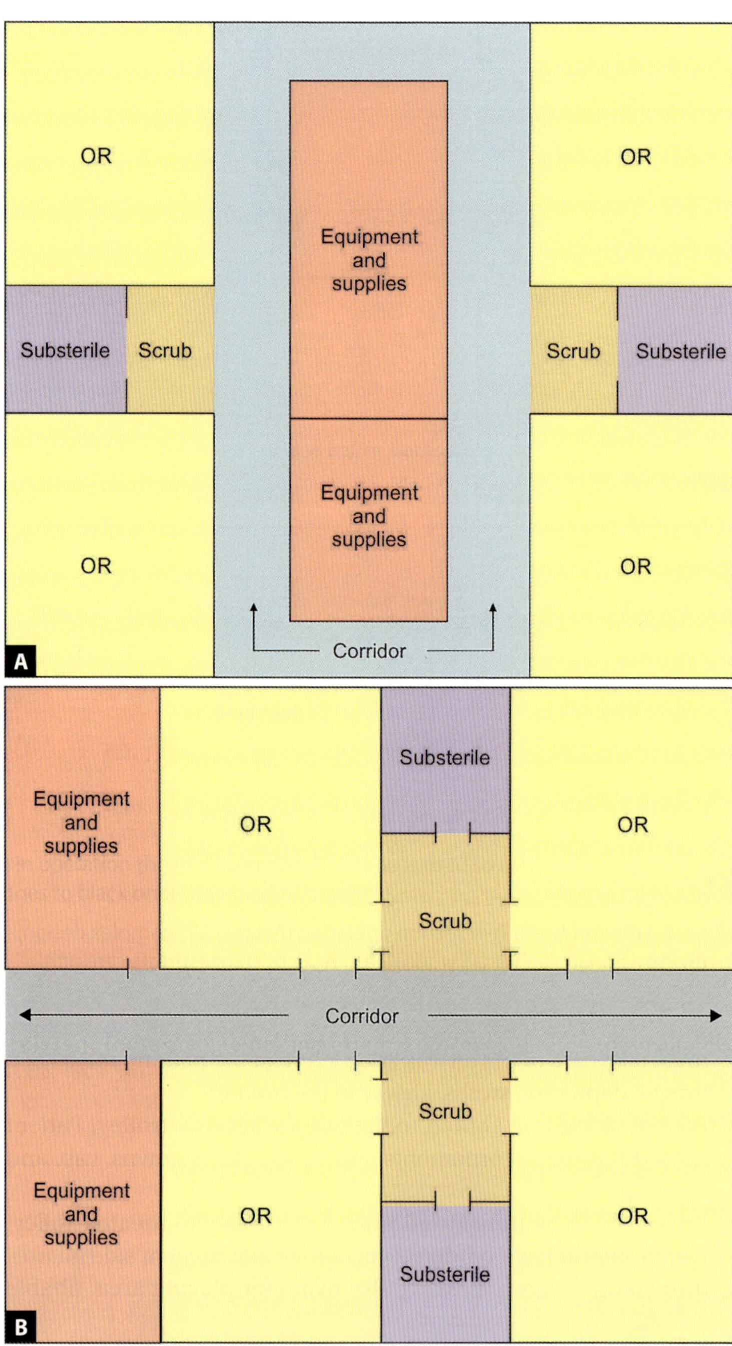

Figs. 2-20A and B: (A) Typical race track plan of central corridor; (B) Typical hotel room type corridor. (OR: operation room)

Peripheral Corridor Plan: Here front entrance to each OR is from the peripheral corridor and supplies are retrieved through a rear entrance from the OR to the central storage and work areas. *Note:* Grouping or cluster plan with peripheral and central corridor: It is combination of both.

Different Zones in Operation Theatre Complex

For effective traffic control, to reduce bacterial load, and to avoid SSI different zones are created in OT complex:

- Protective/outer zone/unrestricted zone
- Semi-restricted zone/sub-sterile area/clean zone
- Restricted zone/sterile area
- Disposable zone/disposable area

Protective Zone/Unrestricted Zone: Here hospital persons, patient, and patient attendants can move with street clothes. It also connects to store room, cleaner room, and equipment store room. It contains maintenance workshop, kitchen/pantry, firefighting device, emergency exit, service room, and closed-circuit TV control area.

Semi-restricted Area/Clean Zone: Here street clothes are changed and OT clothes (OT gowns), OT slippers (*chappals*), cap, and mask as OT attire are cleaned as per guidelines. Here street clothes are not allowed. Only OT-related personnel and staffs are allowed from this zone onward. It has changing rooms for medical or paramedical staffs, rest rooms, toilets, OT administrative room, stores, records, computers, pre- and postoperative rooms, intensive care unit (ICU), postanaesthesia care unit (PACU), and sterile zones.

Restricted Zone/Sterile Area: This is the sterile main OT and OR area. Here patient is in OT gowns and covers, only essential persons will enter this area. Unnecessary inside and outside movements should be restricted. Overcrowding in OR should be avoided. Keeping this area calm and silence is also important. OR is considered as a sanctity place by surgeons and is a serious work area.

Disposable Zone or Area: It contains disposable corridor and utility area (dirty). But OT attire is mandatory here. Often there is a transition zone wherein patient and his personnel enter the semi-restricted area through this wearing a cover gown or jumpsuit, cap, and shoe covers.

Sub-areas: Sub-areas are also important. They are—Nurse's station/counter; Preoperative Check/Reception Area; Holding Area; Induction Room; Postanaesthetic Care Unit; Staff Rooms; Offices for Nurses and Anaesthetists; Laboratory; Seminar/Conference Room; Radiology Services; Store Room; Housekeeping Storage Areas; Sterile Supply Room; Scrub Room; Waiting Room; Visitor's Gallery; Housekeeping Storage Areas; Sterile Supply Room; Utility Room; Disposal or Sluice Room.

Operating Room (OR)

The standard OR should be square or rectangular in shape with adequate space for free movements of personnel, trolleys, wheel chairs, C-Arm, monitors, electrosurgical nits, laparoscopic trolleys, etc. It should be 20 × 20 × 10 feet with a floor space of 400 square feet. Cardiothoracic and neurosurgery ORs should be bigger with 30 × 20 × 10 feet dimensions of 600 square feet space. OR for minor surgery or endoscopy rooms can be of 18 × 18 × 10 feet dimensions with 324 square feet space **(Figs. 2-21A and B)**.

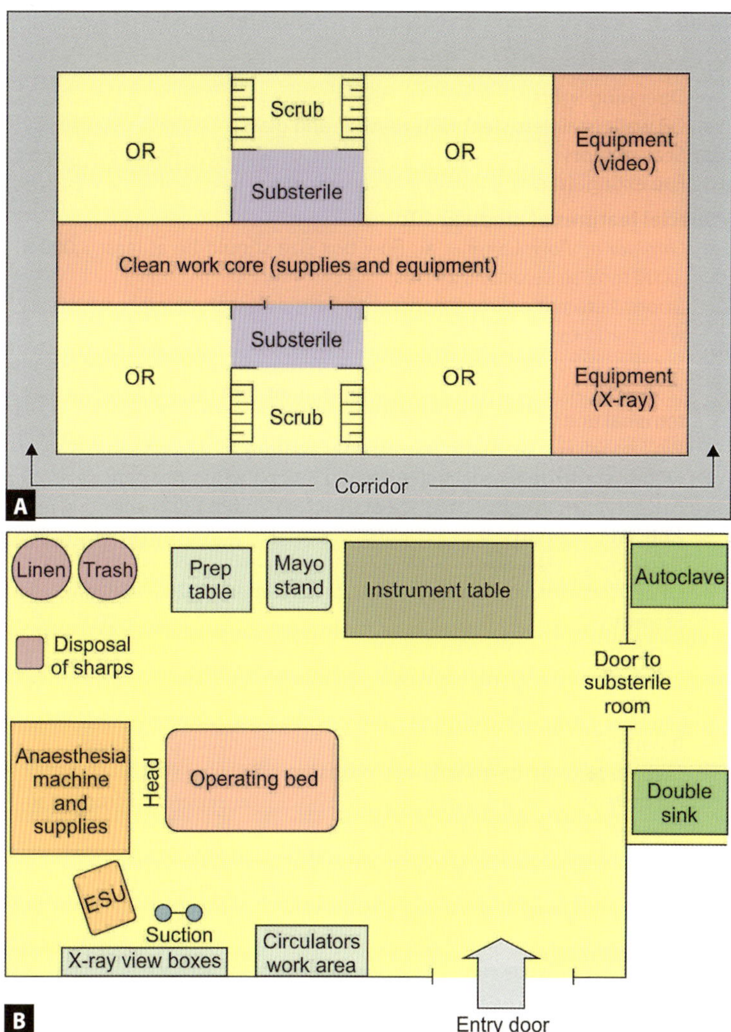

Figs. 2-21A and B: Arrangements in the operation room. (ESU: electrosurgical unit)

Operation room:

- ***Procedure room:*** 150 square feet floor area with 12 ft minimum clear dimensions at the head, sides, and foot of the OR bed. Local anaesthesia used here
- ***General OR:*** 250–400 square feet floor area with 15–18 ft minimum clear dimensions at the head, sides, and foot of the OR bed. Local, general, and regional anaesthesia used here
- ***Other ORs:*** Range in size from 600 to 650 square feet with a 24- to 25-foot width and accommodate multiple ceiling-mounted booms, monitors, and high-technology equipment such as robotics and controlling consoles

OR requirements:

- *Ventilation:* Air conditioning—recirculating and non-recirculating; 20–30 air exchanges/hour; Laminar air flow; Positive pressure system in operation theatre (OT); Temperature between 20 and 24°C
- *Piped gases in OT:* Outlets for O_2, suction, and N_2O are minimum
- *Electricity:* Power line of 230 V; Suspended ceiling outlets should have locking plugs to avoid accidental disconnection; Wall outlets should be 1.5 m above the ground; Emergency generators
- *Lighting:* Minimum of 2,000 lux light is required in OT room;
- General OT room lighting to surgical site should not exceed 1:5; Lights should be freely mobile horizontally and vertically
- Anaesthesia equipment
- Communicating devices

Contd...

Contd...

- Operating table
- Operating lights
- OR walls (stainless steel, HPL, drywall, and glass)
- Sealed doors
- Fire extinguisher

Special features of modular OT:
- *Laminar air flow:* Laminar air flow box size should be at least 3,000 × 3,000 mm; air velocity 0.24 m/s
- *Doors:* Automatic sliding doors with hermetic seal; stainless steel door with thickness not <1.5 mm; dimension of 2,100 × 1,500 mm
- *Surgical pendant:* Should contain a minimum of –10 socket outlet (230 V, 13 A); 2 oxygen terminal units; 2 air terminal units; 2 vacuum terminal units; 1 CO_2 terminal unit
- *Wall panel:* Fire resistant; pre-powder coating of walls; stainless steel with silicone rubber seal between two wall panels to hermetic seal
- *False ceiling* galvanised steel sheet of at least 1 mm thickness
- Antistatic flooring
- X-ray/image view box
- *OT LED light:* Intensity—160,000 lux; field diameter—200–420 mm
- Storage unit
- Scrub station
- OT information board

Septic OT:
- It is a place where surgeries with risk of infections are performed
- *Location:* Should be away from main aseptic OT
- All instruments and clothing used should be separated from main theatre
- Separate clothing room and scrub room
- Separate sterilisation room with flash autoclave machine

Precautions in Operation Room

Operation room checklist should be followed strictly. Unnecessary opening of doors, personnel entry should be avoided. Fire safety measures should be arranged. Prevention of radiation exposure and lead shielding should be followed **(Fig. 2-22)**.

Hazards in Operation Room

Physical hazards; Chemical hazards; Fire hazards; Electrical hazards; Biological hazards; Reproductive hazards should be considered and taken care off.

Fire Hazards

It is most important and most dangerous hazards in OT complex. Operation room is highly susceptible area for major fires and explosion as it is oxygen and gases enriched area with high-electric power generator and lines.

Fire triangle with fuel, oxygen, and ignition source as the components will make OR more susceptible. A flammable gas, vapor or liquid [e.g., ethylene oxide (EO), alcohol, ether, and methane from the bowel], and dry sponges are flammable. During skin preparation, alcohol-based solutions can ignite if not permitted to dry before draping. Laser, electrosurgical units, cords, and power cables are ignition agents. Pure oxygen or air with >21% oxygen combusts to get fire. Highly flammable anaesthetic agents (e.g., cyclopropane and ether) are changed to in favour of halogenated agents.

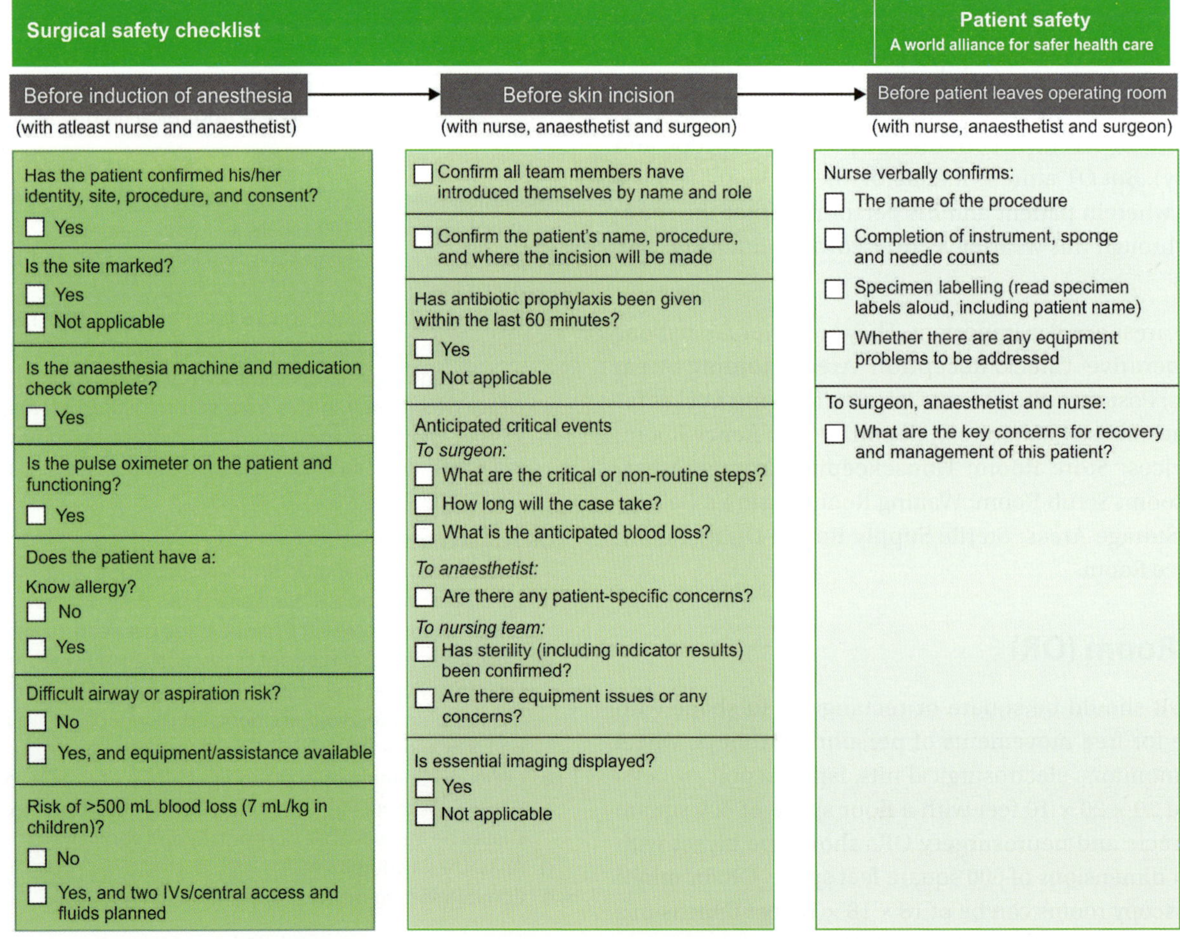
Surgical safety checklist

Patient safety
A world alliance for safer health care

Before induction of anesthesia
(with atleast nurse and anaesthetist)

Has the patient confirmed his/her identity, site, procedure, and consent?
☐ Yes

Is the site marked?
☐ Yes
☐ Not applicable

Is the anaesthesia machine and medication check complete?
☐ Yes

Is the pulse oximeter on the patient and functioning?
☐ Yes

Does the patient have a:
Know allergy?
☐ No
☐ Yes

Difficult airway or aspiration risk?
☐ No
☐ Yes, and equipment/assistance available

Risk of >500 mL blood loss (7 mL/kg in children)?
☐ No
☐ Yes, and two IVs/central access and fluids planned

Before skin incision
(with nurse, anaesthetist and surgeon)

☐ Confirm all team members have introduced themselves by name and role

☐ Confirm the patient's name, procedure, and where the incision will be made

Has antibiotic prophylaxis been given within the last 60 minutes?
☐ Yes
☐ Not applicable

Anticipated critical events
To surgeon:
☐ What are the critical or non-routine steps?
☐ How long will the case take?
☐ What is the anticipated blood loss?
To anaesthetist:
☐ Are there any patient-specific concerns?
To nursing team:
☐ Has sterility (including indicator results) been confirmed?
☐ Are there equipment issues or any concerns?

Is essential imaging displayed?
☐ Yes
☐ Not applicable

Before patient leaves operating room
(with nurse, anaesthetist and surgeon)

Nurse verbally confirms:
☐ The name of the procedure
☐ Completion of instrument, sponge and needle counts
☐ Specimen labelling (read specimen labels aloud, including patient name)
☐ Whether there are any equipment problems to be addressed

To surgeon, anaesthetist and nurse:
☐ What are the key concerns for recovery and management of this patient?

Fig. 2-22: Surgical safety checklist—an essential component of safe surgery.
Source: World Health Organization

These non-combustible agents are mixed with medical air, oxygen, or nitrous oxide **(Fig. 2-23)**.

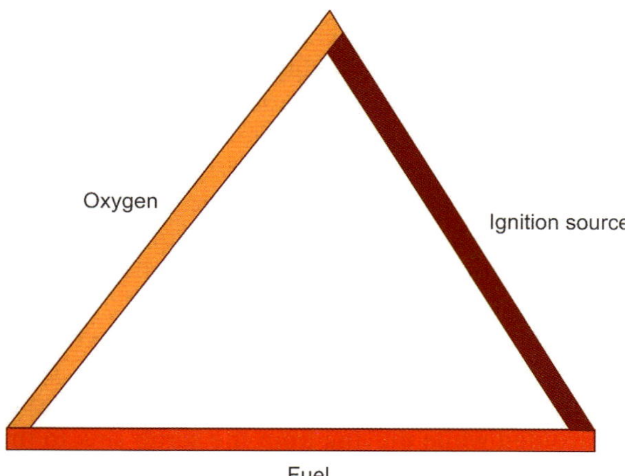

Fig. 2-23: Fire triangle in Operation Room.

Safety measures: Keeping flammable agents away from the igniting agents; explosion proof electric plugs; friction less bags; blankets with less static electricity (avoid woollen or synthetic blankets); antistatic buckets; and gaps between the equipment are some safety measures. Adequate knowledge of fire safety, fire alarm, and fire extinguishers should be there to all OT workers. *Three types of fire extinguishers are present—Class A:* Pressurised water for combustible materials such as paper and wood; *Class B:* Carbon dioxide or dry chemicals to control flammable agents like oil, gas, or liquids; and *Class C:* Halon bromochlorodifluoromethane (halon) halogenated compressed gas to control electrical or laser fire. **Types of Safety measures: (1) PASS method: P**ull the safety ring out of the handle; **A**im the nozzle; **S**queeze the handle; **S**weep the spray over the base of the fire. **(2) RACE method: R**escue anyone who is in immediate danger; **A**ctivate the fire alarm; **C**ontain the fire, if possible; **E**vacuate the area.

Operation Room Design

Designing operation theatre complex and Operation Room (OR) should be done properly keeping in mind with adequate space, power system, modular arrangements, waste disposal, sterility, laminar airflow, adequate water supply, drainage system, etc. It should be designed with planning in consultation with experienced consultants, engineers, technical people.

Operation room (OR) design principles

- *Infection control:* Physical separation—consider these—clean areas; contaminated areas; containment; confinement; *Environmental*—standards for—electrical circuits; gases; lighting
- *Efficiency*—physical effort; materials; time plan; space plan
- *Floor plan*—central core; transitional area
- *Traffic patterns*—unrestricted (transitional area, attire, lounge, toilet, and rest room); semirestricted [patient holding area, check in point, surgical offices, communication central; corridors; scrub sink areas; equipment and supply rooms/storage; utility work room, central processing decontamination area; clean processing room with assembly and sterilisation; anaesthesia work room; postanaesthesia care unit (PACU), postoperative recovery room]; sterile/restricted (cleanest area monitored strictly)
- *Equipment*—(1) Operation table/bed—adjustable, padded, with removable arm boards and leg holders, kidney bridge, should have cassette attachment for X-ray/image taking; should able move in different directions with remote control or through pedals. (2) Back table

Contd...

Contd...

covered with sterile drape to keep sterile surgical instruments (mayo stand—adjustable stand with supports, attached to OR table, should be covered with sterile drape. (3) Kick buckets, single ring stand, double ring stand to hold basins. (4) Preparation table, step stools, blanket warmers, clocks, stopwatch. (5) X-ray view box, computers, intercom, telephones, supply cabinets, in room supply storage
- *Airflow in OR*—air pressure, air exchanges, high-efficiency particulate air (HEPA) filters, laminar airflow
- *Humidity* control (50–60%); temperature (68–73°F); electricity care
- Inline gas and suction; lighting to OR and OT table (over head)
- *Special procedure rooms*; integrated OR system to provide centralised control of equipment
- *Other working areas*—offices, patient holding areas, scrub areas, substerile area, sterile instrument room; equipment storage area, utility work room; decontamination area; clean processing area; anaesthesia work room; PACU; surgery waiting area; family conversation/counselling room
- *Team approach*—radiology, pathology, infection control team, surgeon, nurses, technicians, biomedical engineering, material management, central supply, pharmacy, blood bank system; risk management, switch boards and other delicate systems, medical records, maintenance services
- *Administration and policies*; accreditation—process, reimbursement, audit, meeting; healthcare policies
- *Structure and management*—directors (decision making); administration (responsibilities); medical staff (patient services)
- *Chain of command*—vertical and horizontal alignment

Risk Management in Operation Theatre Complex

- Protocol and guidelines should be strictly followed.
- Protective attire and safety equipment should be made available to employees, as appropriate.
- Monitoring devices should be used in all hazardous locations as recommended by regulatory agencies.
- Regular programmes should be conducted to keep employees informed about hazards and safeguards; should be taught how to use and care for new equipment; employees must know the location and use of emergency equipment, such as fire extinguishers and shutoff valves; employees must wear protective attire; and regular maintenance of all potentially hazardous equipment.
- Faulty or malfunctioning equipment should be taken out of service; injury and unsafe conditions should be reported; and early response whenever problem or risk arises.
- Regular health check-up and documentation of all OT complex healthcare personnel is a must. If any injury or disease/illness occurs to OT personnel, early notification and assessment should be done.

Most common causes of contamination	The surgical team
• The use of contaminated instruments • Contaminated gloves • Wet or damp sterile field • Microorganisms blown onto a surgical site	• Surgeon • Surgical assistant • Nurses—scrub nurse; circulating nurse • Physician assistant • Anaesthesiologist • Nurse anaesthetist • Operation theatre technician • Radiology technician

Contd...

Contd...

Precautions	Surgical technician
• Ventilation ducts must have special filters • Airflow in the theatre room should be unidirectional • Air pressure in the theatre room should be greater than in the outside corridors • Humidity is to be controlled to prevent static electricity • Theatre room doors should remain closed as much as possible	• His duty is always to maintain a clean and sterile environment for the surgical team to perform needed surgeries properly • He will be in-charge of scrubbing in and keeping instruments sterile and organised. He may be asked to assist by handing instruments • He will have to have knowledge of surgical machines, all instruments and sterilisation procedure • He will be in-charge of shifting the patient before and after surgery. Surgical technician play a very important role in the operating room

Operation Theatre Nurse

The operating room nurse's jobs and duties consists of education, preparation and coordination of patient care. OR or perioperative registered nurses are responsible for maintaining the sterile conditions in the operating room and monitoring patients during the operation. They are also responsible for continued care during and after the procedure.

Skin Preparation and Draping for Sterile Procedures

Skin preparation: The purpose of skin preparation is to remove as many microorganisms as possible by mechanical and chemical means to reduce the potential chance of infection. There are two aspects to skin preparation for a sterile procedure: (1) *Mechanical* and (2) *Chemical*

Chemical method of skin preparation: The area to be penetrated should be cleaned with an antiseptic solution. Once you start to clean the area of interest, do this in a circular motion beginning in the center and working outward. One should not cross anything over the area that has been prepared. *Draping for sterile procedure*: After the skin has been prepared, sterile drapes are prepared around the area of interest. It must be handled as little as possible; disposable sterile cloth towel are mainly used, however, a fenestrated drape may be used. It should be placed so that they are within the limits of the area prepared. They are folded so that they overlap and the folds face the operative site.

Scrubbing and Wearing OT Gown and Glove

Both hands, forearms up to elbow joints should be rinsed with running water and soap. Any ring, jewellery, wristwatch should be removed prior to the scrub. Prescrub wash should be done up to both elbow joints. Nails should to cut short; nail polish ideally should be avoided. Using brush and soap, finger nails, hands on both sides are cleaned. Then forearm is brushed and washed. Procedure is repeated three times (presently whether need to brush the hands are *controversial*). Two types of scrubbing methods are present. One is *timed scrub method*—scrubbing is done part by part for certain minutes properly. Other is *counter stroke method*—fingers, hands, forearms are scrubbed with counted number of strokes: 15 strokes for finger nails, 10 strokes for palm, thumb and fingers of each hand, 10 strokes for back of each hand, 10 strokes for each forearm. Flow of water rinse should be from finger and hands towards elbow, i.e. from clean area towards unclean area. For that folded hands should be raised upwards to allow proper flow of water from clean towards unclean area. After thorough rinsing the hands by running water, hands are washed with antiseptic solution and then with warm water.

Presently brushless scrub technique is equally effective and is popular. 90% alcohol with chlorhexidine gluconate is commonly used. Initial prescrub wash is done using water. Hands should be dried before using alcohol based rub to make it more effective. Fingers, hands, forearms, and 5 cm above the elbow should be scrubbed using antiseptic solution.

Once fully scrubbed, he/she should not touch with hands any objects or his/her own face or parts of body. Once the surgical hand scrub is complete, contamination of the hands and forearms should be avoided while moving from the scrub sink to the sterile table by keeping the hands in front of the body and above the waist. If there is potential for contact with the door, it is necessary to back through the door. She should keep her hands and fingers tucked with each other with forearm and hands outstretched. Using a sterile towel, forearm and hands are dried up. Both hands are inserted into the armholes of the sterile gown. The gown is not touched or pulled but both arms are kept outstretched. Circulating nurse will pull back the tapes of the gown and ties it over the back.

A back wrap gown has got two tapes to tie on the front aspect. After wearing gloves, one tape is given to the scrubbed scrub nurse/surgeon who is already with gown and gloves. She/he will encircle the gown round and bring it in front and give to the surgeon to be tied it with other tape.

Techniques of Wearing the Surgical Gloves

There are three methods of wearing the surgical gloves—*closed gloving technique*; the *open gloving technique* and *assisted gloving technique*.

Closed glove technique: Here after wearing sterile surgical gown, hands are kept inside the sleeves of the sterile gown. Folded part of the glove (cuff) is held through the gown sleeve without bringing the hand and fingers outside the sleeve. Glove is held with one hand and is inverted on to the opposite sleeve and hand and over the wrist of the opposite hand; fingers and hand are moved towards the glove across the cuff correspondingly. Gloved hand and fingers will hold the folded another glove over its cuff and is again inverted over the sleeve of the opposite hand covered with gown sleeve; and by repeated finger forward movements fingers are covered with glove. Final adjustment is done by clasping the fingers and sleeves and gown cuff can be adjusted at the end properly. It is ideal method as it is entirely sterile method; but it is often difficult to slide fingers into the appropriate corresponding glove fingers and often time consuming **(Figs. 2-24A and B)**.

Open Gloving technique: Ideally it should be done when procedures are done using only gloves without gown, but this technique is commonly practiced even after wearing sterile gown. Glove packet is opened; folded cuff of the glove is held with fingers of opposite hand; fingers of ipsilateral hand are slid into the glove towards corresponding finger part of the glove; once all fingers are slid into the glove properly, using this gloved fingers opposite glove is held by insinuating under the folded cuff of the opposite glove. Opposite fingers and hand are slid into the glove; held cuff is everted over the wrist or the gown sleeve; final adjustment is done by apposing the fingers **(Figs. 2-25A and D)**.

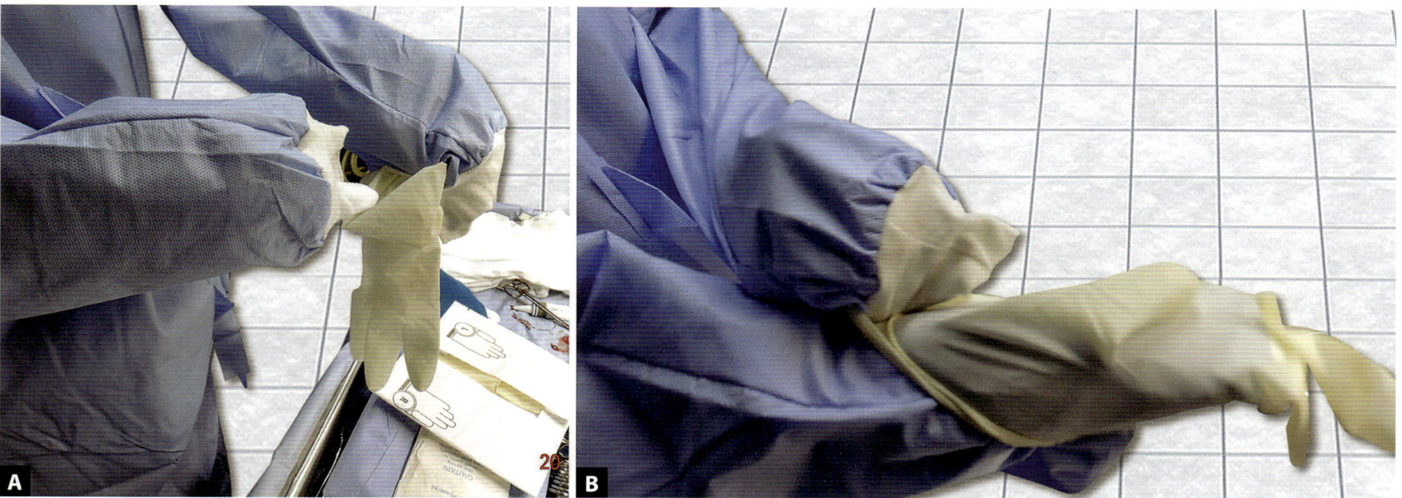

Figs. 2-24A and B: Wearing glove closed method.

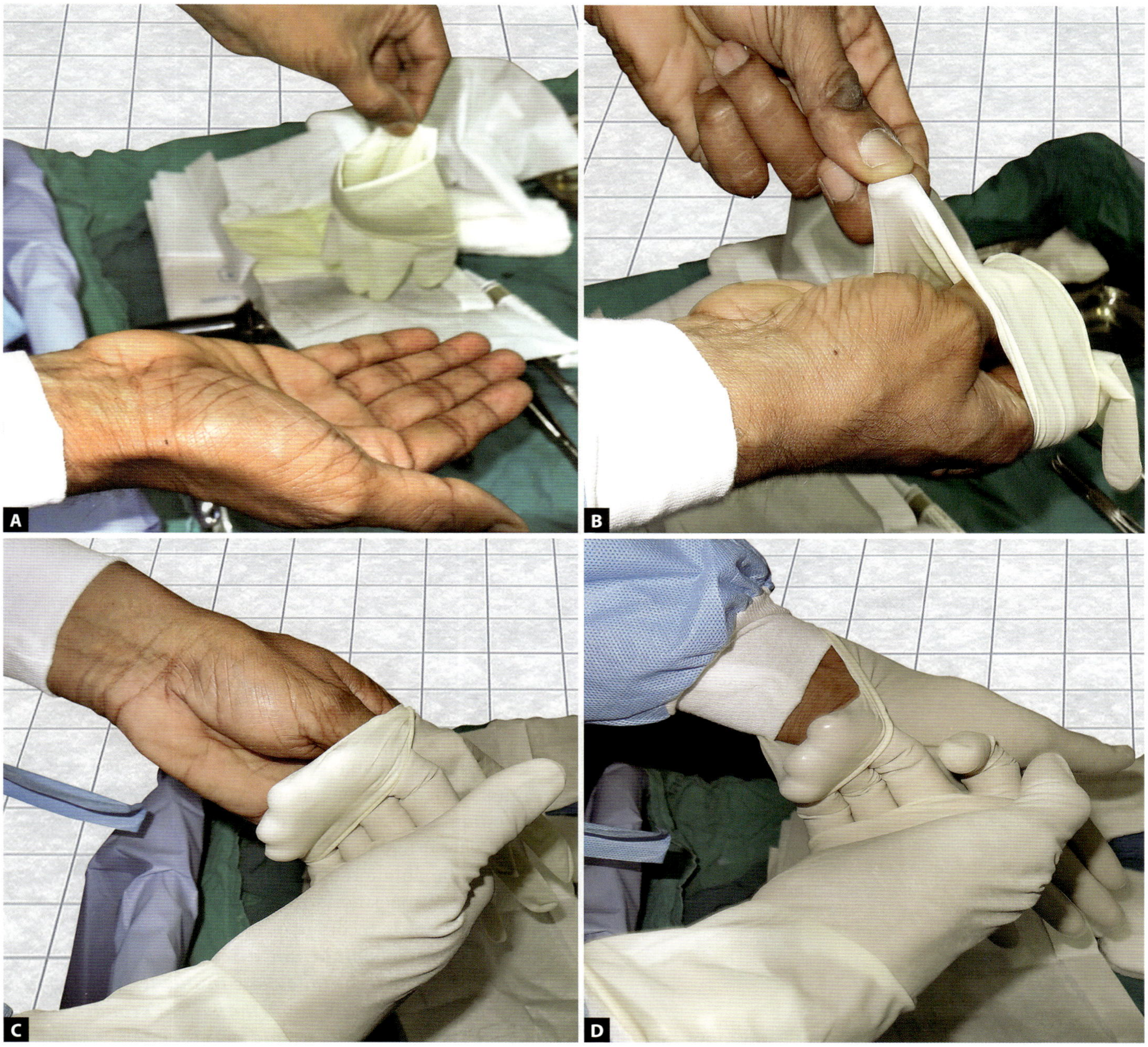

Figs. 2-25A to D: Wearing glove open method.

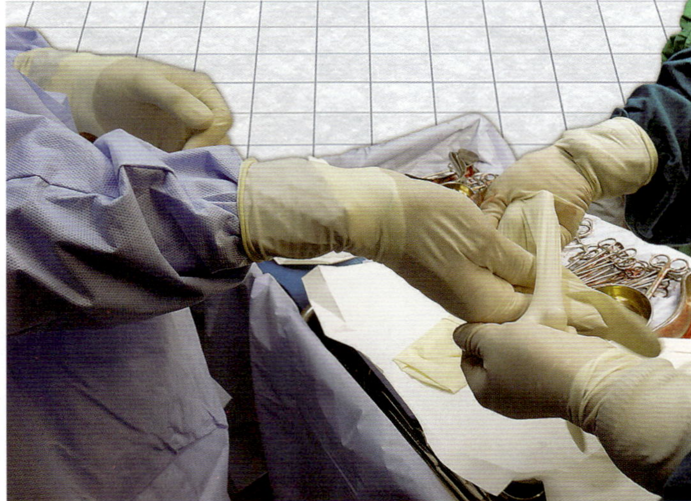

Fig. 2-26: Wearing glove by assisted method.

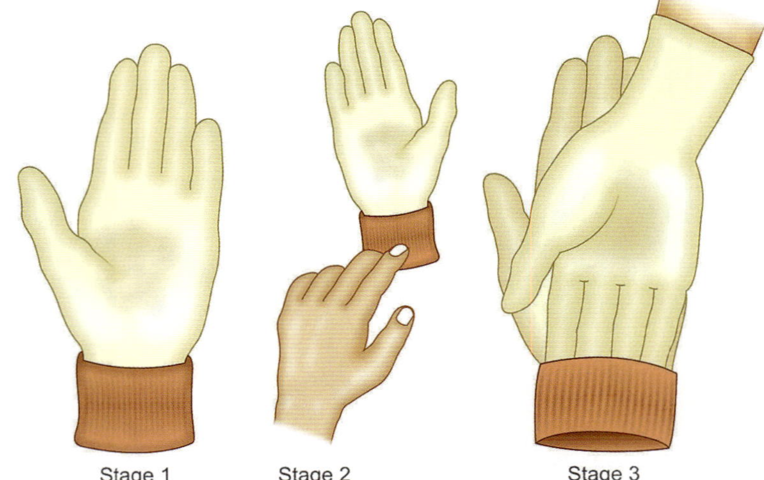

Fig. 2-27: Correct method of wearing gloves.

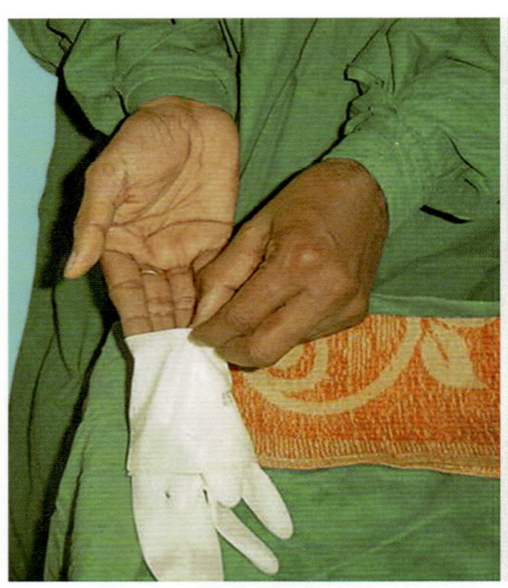

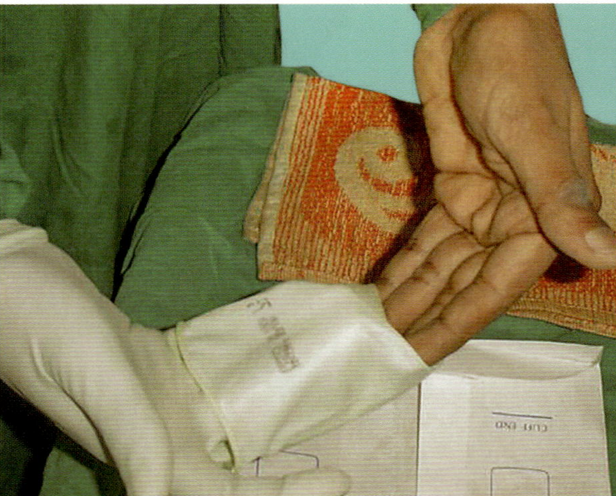

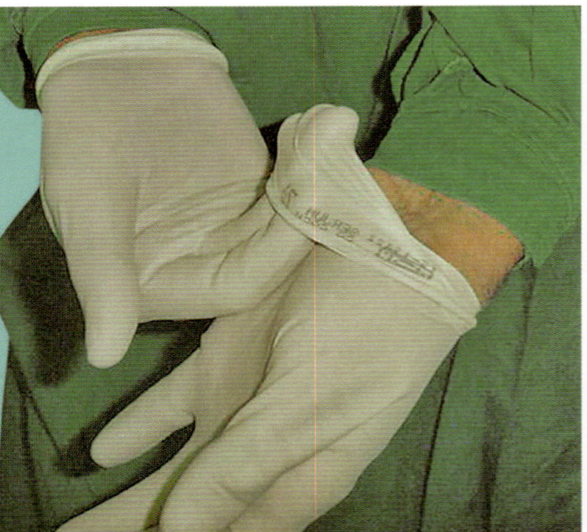

Fig. 2-28: Method of wearing glove.

Assisted gloving technique: Here assistant or scrub nurse helps the surgeon to wear the glove. He/she picks up the glove from the glove cover using his sterile gloved fingers; glove cuff is partly inverted and held widely using both hands of the assistant/scrub nurse; surgeon slides his fingers and hand into the glove; assistant takes the opposite glove again similarly to allow the surgeon to pass his hand into glove; final adjustment and everting of the glove cuff over the sleeves of the gown is done to complete the sterile method of wearing the gloves **(Figs. 2-26 to 2-28)**.

Theatre technique of wearing gloves

- After using glove powder, with the bare hand inner aspect of the cuff of the glove is held. It is pulled over the hand. It should not be wrapped over the wrist cuff of the gown at this stage.
- Fingers of this gloved hand should hold the cuff of the other glove from outside and it is slided over the fingers and hand.
- Now cuff of the glove is pulled proximally over the wrist of the gown using other gloved fingers.

Circulating Nurse

One who supplies all additional instruments and mops. She also keeps the mop counts.

Duties of Circulating Nurse

- Keeping counts of instruments, and mops given to scrub nurse. Instruments are kept in bundles of five, ten and so on. So counting will be easier.
- Taking care of swab rack, collecting the used mops from scrub nurse and hanging the mops in groups of five. Mops presently used in many theatres are having radio-opaque threads and so can be easily identified when needed by taking X-ray or through a C-Arm.
- Collection of specimens, pus, fluids and labelling with name, unit, number. It may be for culture, cytology or for histopathology.
- Keeping account of the disposable instruments and suture materials, drugs and fluids used in each procedure.
- Noting the duration of the surgery, quantity of blood transfused and type of anaesthesia given.
- Documenting in record book or theatre computer.

Theatre nurse should not discuss outside or reveal about the procedure or technique done in theatre with anybody. It is surgeon's duty to explain about the patient's condition, procedure done and problems. She should never comment about anything that happen in theatre (Figs. 2-29 and 2-30).

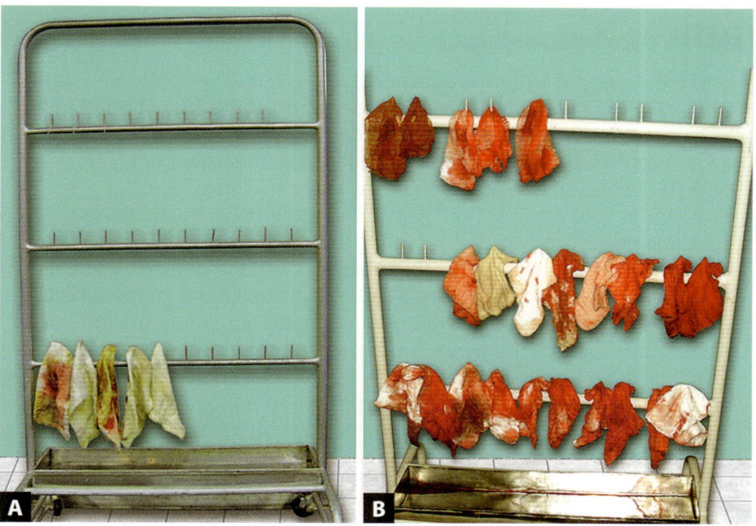

Figs. 2-29A and B: OT mop rack to keep used mops during surgery.

Septic Operation Theatre

- All infected cases like abscess drainage, amputation for gangrene, slough excision, dressing of large ulcers should be done in a separate OT. Otherwise clean surgeries may get infected. It is especially important when orthopaedic surgeries are going on.
- Entrance to septic OT must be separate from that of main OT.
- Staffs working in septic OT should not enter main OT.
- Instruments for septic OT should be kept separately.
- Drapes, towels, mops should be placed in a plastic bag after use and sent to laundry immediately. It should be labelled as *infected.*
- Circulating nurse should wear gloves while working in a septic OT.
- Disinfection of shoes is essential once it is used in septic OT.
- Daily disinfection of OT is essential.
- Swab culture of the OT materials at regular intervals is needed.
- Separate Boyle's apparatus is used in septic OT.
- Dress is changed when one comes out of septic OT and enters the main OT.

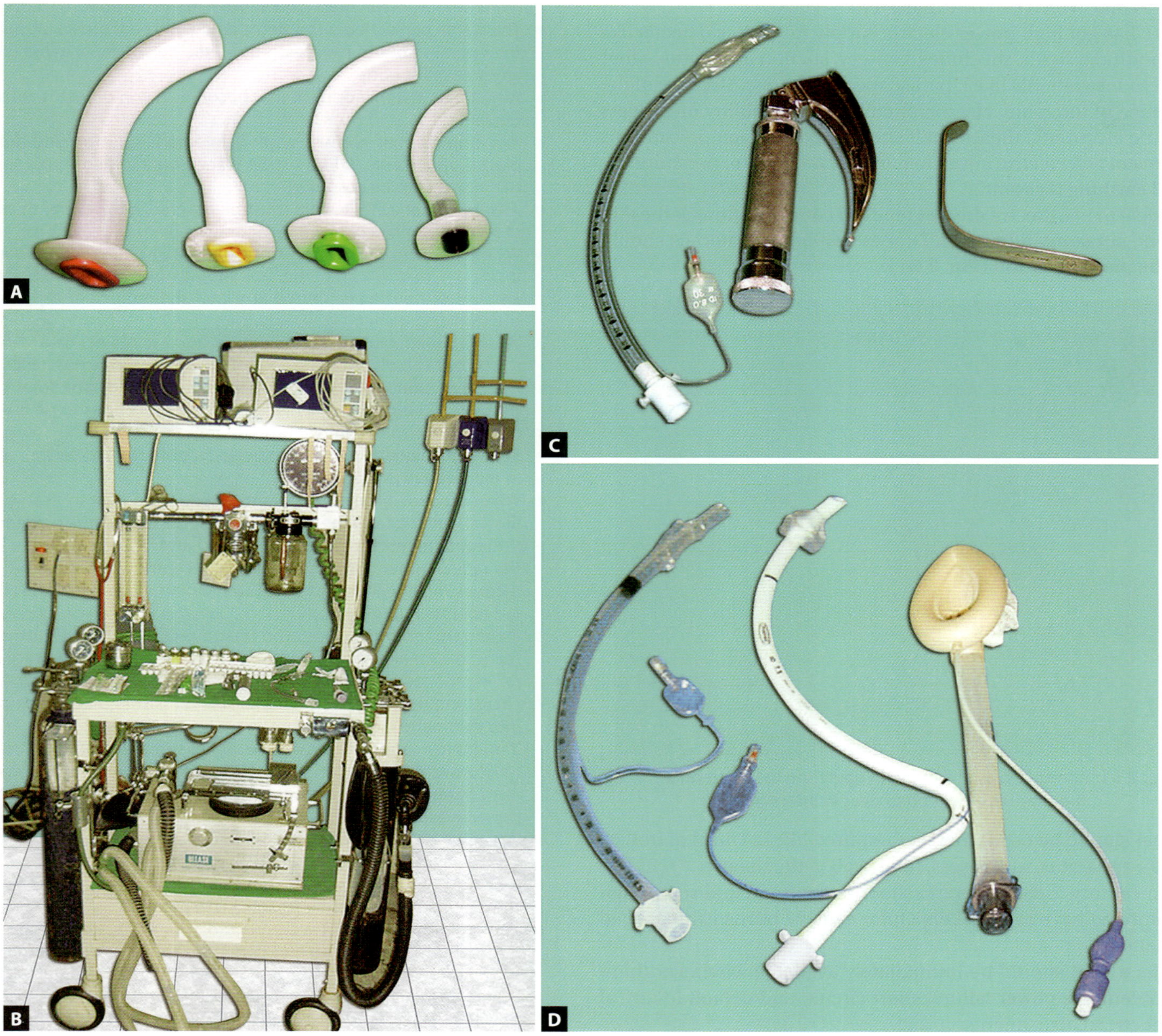

Figs. 2-30A to D: Different materials required to give anaesthesia: (A) Airway; (B) Boyle's apparatus; (C) Direct laryngoscope; (D) Laryngeal mask airway (LMA)—a special device tube to give anaesthesia.

Prevention of infection

- Cleaning of the patient's skin where incision is placed by povidone iodine, cetrimide, spirit.
- Isolation of surgical area by proper draping with green towels.
- Transparent sheeting of the skin through which skin incision is placed.
- Adhesive films to the skin.
- Use of on table parenteral antibiotic in major cases.
- Always clean cases are done first and then infected cases.
- Proper sterilisation.
- Double autoclaving for orthopaedic and ophthalmology cases.

Precautions in an Operation Theatre

- In the absence of proper safety measures and precautions, OT is a place where one is prone for accidental trauma and injuries, which may be danger to patient as well as to theatre personnel.
- Main danger exists in some anaesthetic agents, which may cause life-threatening explosions. It may cause burns, loss of vision, hearing loss, damage to OT, may also sometimes cause death. Ether is one, which can be explosive.
- An OT has got high power electric supply for its basic needs like air condition, lights, machines, cautery, suction apparatus, other modern instruments like laparoscope, C-Arm, etc. Because of the presence of too many electric circuits and possibility of dangers of static electricity, theatre staff should take enough precautions to prevent any electric injury to patients and theatre personnel.
- Good earthing is essential.
- It is ideal to use theatre dresses made of cotton (cotton clothes) to patient, surgeon and nurses. Drapes and other materials should also be made of cotton **(Fig. 2-31)**.

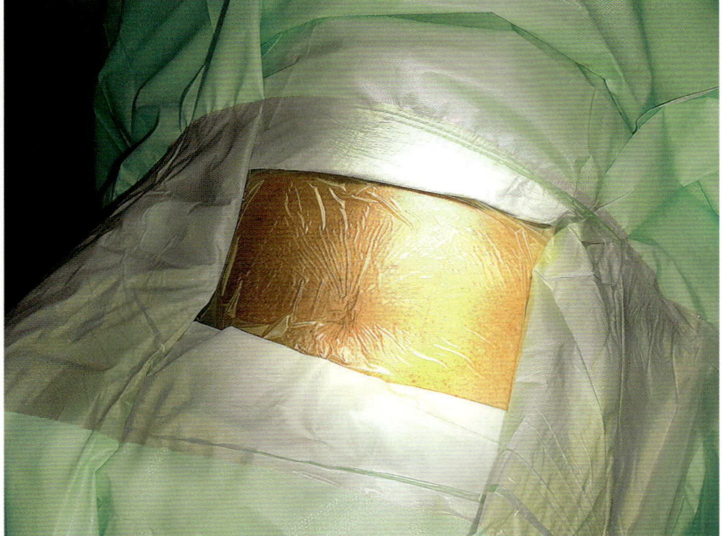

Fig. 2-31: Adhesive plastic draping in operation theatre reduces the chances of wound or deeper infection.

- Rubber should be used wherever required like in wheel of trolley, Boyle's apparatus, mattresses, floor, wall of the theatre.
- When cautery is used, electric shock is common and so enough precautions have to be taken. Often cautery burns can occur to the patient.
- An electrician should be immediately available whenever there is problem like power failure, short circuit, and default in any of the electrical instruments.

Beware of possible anaesthetic explosions and electrical injuries in OT.

Rules in sterile area in operation theatre

- If the sterility of an item is questionable, it is not to be considered sterile.
- Once a sterile field has been prepared, it must not be left unattended as it may become contaminated and presumed to be sterile.
- An unsterile person does not reach across a sterile field.
- A sterile person does not lean over an unsterile area.
- A sterile field ends at the level of the tabletop or at the waist of the sterile person's gown.
- Anything that drops below the tabletop or sterile person's waistline is no longer sterile and may not be brought up to the sterile tabletop. The only parts of the sterile gown considered sterile are the areas from the waist to the shoulders in front and the sleeves from 2 inches above the elbow to the cuffs.
- The cuffs of the sterile gown are considered non-sterile because they collect moisture. Cuffs must always be covered by sterile gloves.
- The edges of a sterile wrapper are not considered sterile and must not touch a sterile object.
- Sterile drapes are placed by a sterile person. The sterile person places the drapes on the area closest to him first to protect his sterile gown.
- A sterile person must remain within the sterile area. He must not lean on tables or against the wall.
- If one sterile person must pass another, they must pass back-to-back.
- The sterile person faces the sterile field and keeps sterile gloves above the waist in front of his chest. The sterile person must avoid touching any area of his body.
- Any sterile material or pack that becomes damp or wet is considered unsterile.
- Any objects that are wet with disinfectant solution and are to be placed on a sterile field must be placed on a folded sterile towel for the moisture to be absorbed.
- A wet area on a sterile field must be covered with several thicknesses of sterile towelling or an impervious drape.
- When pouring sterile solution, the lid should face upward and inside the lid or the lip of the flask should not be touched. First a small amount of solution is poured and later the remainder is poured into the sterile container.
- When a sterile solution is to be poured into a container on a sterile field, the container is placed at the edge of the sterile field by the sterile person.
- Overhead units must be cleaned with a disinfectant solution, and portable radiographic machines and image receptors to be used must be cleaned with a disinfectant solution.
- Sterile technique must be maintained for all items and persons involved in the invasive procedure.
- When needed image receptors should be placed prior to cleaning; scout films should be taken before draping the patient for the procedure.
- If the image receptors must be placed after the procedure is begun, the radiographer may pass the image receptor to the scrub nurse who receives the image receptor in a sterile plastic bag and places it at the radiographer's direction.
- If the radiographer places the image receptor himself, the surgical team must make room for him. He may place the image receptor by raising the sterile drapes touching only the inside of the drape, or the circulating nurse may lift the drapes and assist in placing the cassette into the image receptor holder.
- If multiple images are to be taken, all personnel who are not scrubbed must leave the operation theatre. The scrubbed members of the team must wear protective radiation apparel. They may also step behind protective lead-lined screens.
- When hands are directly exposed to radiation, leaded sterile gloves as well as all other protective equipment must be worn.
- Pregnant female personnel should not be present in the operation theatre when radiographic imaging is in progress.
- The radiographer must wear his radiation detection badge on the outside of the lead apron and under the sterile gown during imaging procedures. The badge must be checked at prescribed intervals.
- During imaging, all unnecessary instruments must be removed from the operative field and a sterile drape must be placed over the open incision.
- All dressings must be treated as if they are contaminated, because drainage from wounds may harbour pathogenic microorganisms.

Most important people in OT

- First and foremost is the ***patient***.
- Next are surgeon and anaesthetist.
- Essential are theatre nurses and theatre assistant.
- Surgery is a team work. All are important.

POSTOPERATIVE CARE

In all major prolonged surgeries, patient is kept in postoperative ward. Postoperative set up should be clean, air conditioned, well equipped set up with restricted entries. Rules followed in operation theatre should be followed here also. Postoperative ward should be adjacent to the main operation theatre. It should be equipped with all essential life-saving drugs, tubes, ventilators, oxygen supply line, suction devices, and monitors to each bed. One nurse should exclusively attend one patient. An anaesthetist should be in-charge of the postoperative ward. Nurse should be well trained, quick, and observant and should able to manage emergency situation. Defibrillator and needful things to manage cardiac arrest should be available in postoperative ward **(Figs. 2-32 and 2-33)**.

Following care should be taken:

- Use of dry bed sheets, clean beds and clothing, waterbeds/air mattresses, change of position, leg exercises, needed positioning depending on obesity, respiratory reserve, and type of surgery the patient underwent should be taken care of. Oxygen is given through mask or cannula.
- *Proper monitoring* with oxygen saturation, pulse, blood pressure, respiration, and urine output is needed. Central venous pressure (CVP) line is often required for major cases.
- *Drains, tubes* (nasogastric tube, urinary catheters) should be observed for quantity and colour of the contents. Intercostal tubes, abdominal drains, tubes like T tube, stenting tubes should be taken care of **(Figs. 2-34A and B)**. Often if patient is having many tubes in postoperative period it is better to label each tube for better nursing purpose. Nasogastric tube is placed in most of the abdominal surgeries to decompress stomach, so as to prevent aspiration, and as a therapy for ileus. It is usually kept connected to a bag/bottle allowing continuous flow. Intermittent suction also should be added to clear the stomach at 4th hourly interval. Tube is removed once bowel sounds are heard, patient passes flatus or stool and once total aspiration becomes less than 200 mL per day.
- Surgical cases done under spinal anaesthesia or in case of small procedures, patient can be kept for 3 hours in recovery room for observations before sending to bed. But it is surgeon's discretion to decide how long to keep the patient in postoperative ward. For example, patient who underwent transurethral resection of prostate (TURP) under spinal anaesthesia is usually kept in post-operative ward for minimum of 12 hours to watch for irrigation and bleeding.

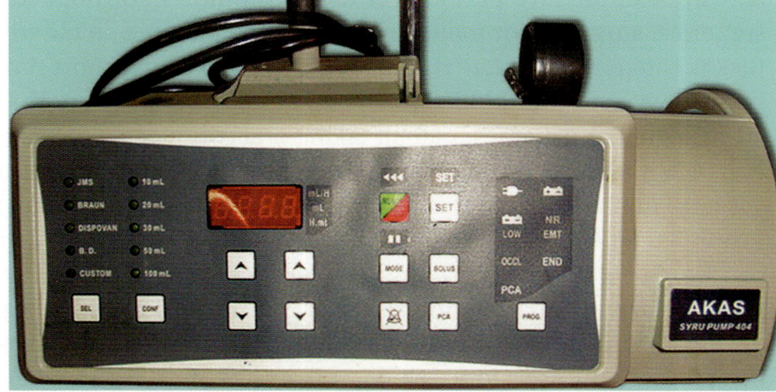

Fig. 2-32: Infusion pump is used in postoperative period to have a proper control about the infusion of fluids, drugs, etc.

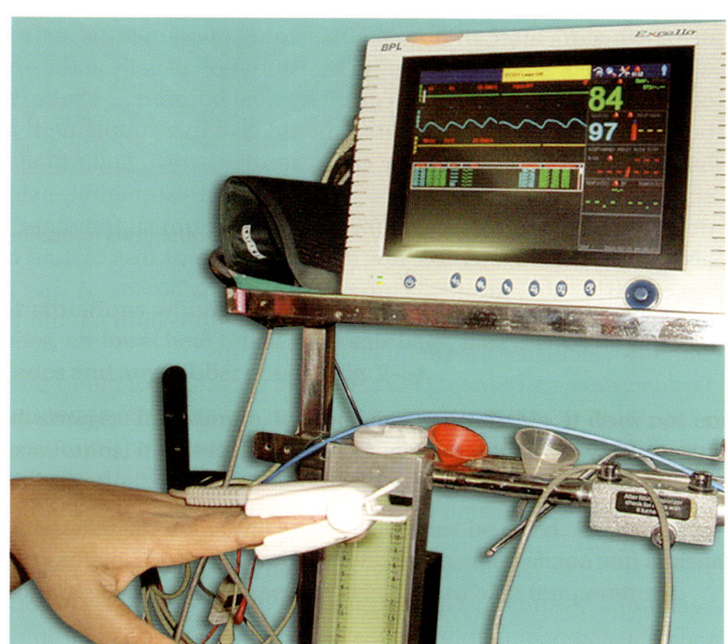

Fig. 2-33: Pulse oximeter. It is usually portable. Different types may be available. One showing just O2 saturation and pulse rate to cardiac waves is available. It is non-invasive, continuous real time device. Amount of light absorbed by a solution is directly proportional to the amount of solute in it. It contains two light emitting diodes—660 nm (for reduced haemoglobin absorption) and 940 nm (for oxyhaemoglobin absorption). Ratio of absorption of these two wavelengths is oxygen saturation. Normal saturation is 98–100%. It is monitored in fingers, toes. Limitations are patient movements, electrical interference, and vasoconstriction, presence of carboxyhaemoglobin or methaemoglobin.

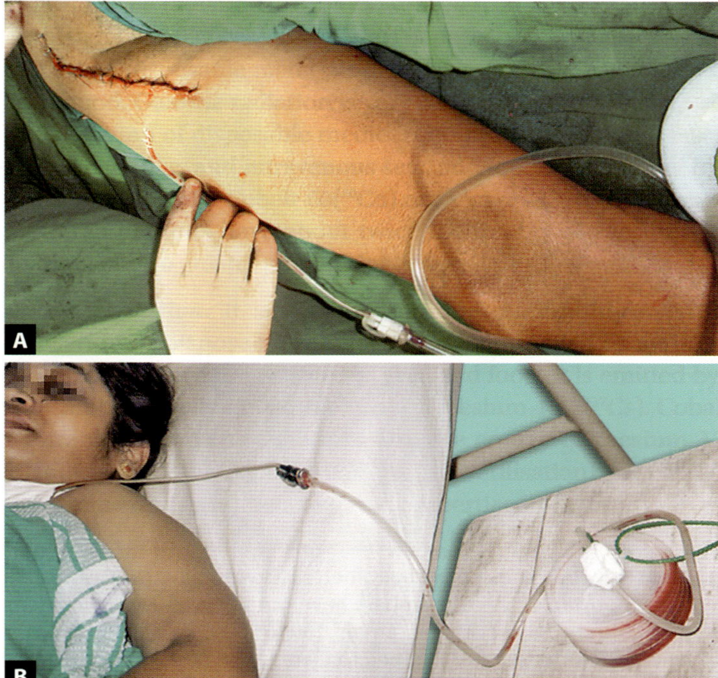

Figs. 2-34A and B: Postoperative drain should be taken care of.

- *Postoperative fluid management* should be proper and adequate. It is decided on individual patient depending on type of surgery, on table complications, duration of recovery, respiratory reserve, electrolyte status, etc. Fluid need is monitored by hourly urine output and CVP measurement. *Extracellular fluid loss and third space fluid loss* occurs in first postoperative period. *Commonest electrolyte deficit* in postoperative period is *potassium* which usually occurs after 48 hours. Potassium supplement is started when needed, after confirmation by estimation usually at the end of 2nd postoperative day. It is given by *slow infusion* as 1 mEq/kg body weight. Experienced nurse should give this supplement as bolus push of potassium may cause cardiac arrest. Sodium also commonly gets deranged. It is corrected after estimation, using double strength saline. Calcium and magnesium supplement is also often needed. *Sensible loss of fluid* is obvious loss of fluid by nasogastric tube, drains, urine output; *insensible loss* is due to metabolism, temperature, and hyperventilation. Both should be carefully calculated for adequate fluid therapy.
- *Postoperative assessment chart*—regular recording of blood pressure, pulse, respiration, urine, drain, etc. is a must. Postoperative examination of respiratory system for crepitations (pulmonary oedema), of legs for deep vein thrombosis (DVT) (pain, swelling and tenderness in calf), cardiovascular system and of abdomen is done daily.
- *Postoperative respiratory physiotherapy* is given to remove secretions. Respiratory distress may be due to cough, secretions, pain causing poor diaphragmatic movements, drugs like atropine. Proper pain relief; coughing, removal of secretions, breathing exercises using balloons or spirometer, steam inhalation, saline nebulisation, bronchodilators, mobilisation are encouraged **(Fig. 2-35)**. To prevent deep vein thrombosis (DVT) leg exercises and early mobilisation are done. It is better to take the help of a physiotherapist for the same.

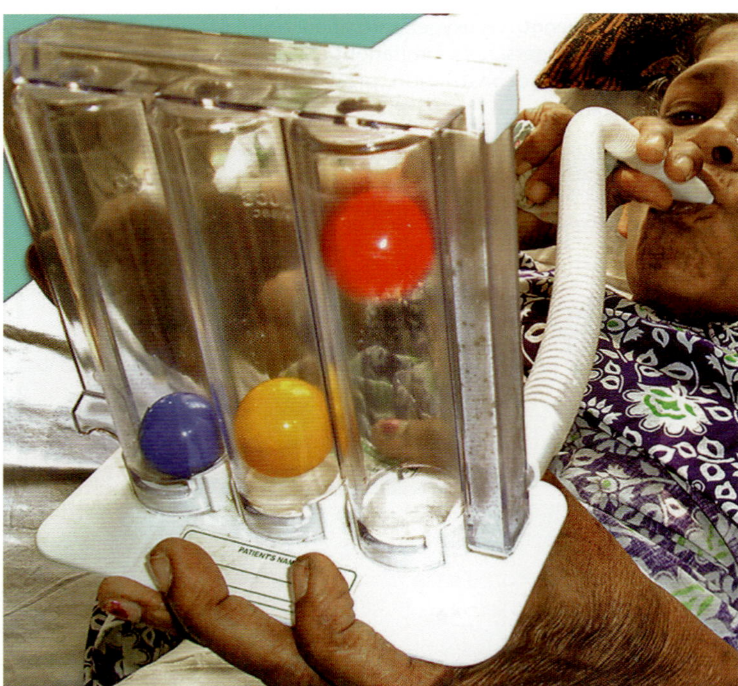

Fig. 2-35: Flow-based incentive spirometer is commonly used as it is light weight and portable. Three chambers have got three balls one in each of different colours. Each registers an air flow of 600/900/1200 cc/second respectively. Volume inspired can be calculated. Rise of the ball in chamber indicates the extent of flow of air. It is used in postoperative lung expansion. It is also used to prevent atelectasis, preoperative improvement of respiratory reserve. Larger device indicating inhaled air volume also in use.

- Postoperative investigations are done as and when needed based on clinical and monitoring grounds. Haemoglobin %, total count, serum electrolytes, serum creatinine, serum bilirubin are commonly done. In critical patients arterial blood gas analysis, haematocrit, platelet count, prothrombin time are done at regular intervals. Chest X-ray should be done if pneumonia, effusion or ARDS is suspected postoperatively. ECG should be taken when needed.
- *Antibiotics* are continued for 48 hours and stopped. It is continued in infective/septic cases or in septicaemia.
- Diabetes should be managed depending on blood sugar level using insulin. Later it can be changed to oral hypoglycaemic drugs after consultation with physician in charge.
- *Postoperative nutrition*—In usual surgeries oral feeding is started in 6–8 hours once patient is conscious and without any nausea. Initially started with 50 mL/hour liquid, later semisolid and finally solid normal diet is used. It takes 2 days to have normal diet in surgeries other than gastrointestinal. In abdominal surgery it is delayed until, bowel sounds appear, patient passes flatus and nasogastric tube aspiration becomes less than 200 mL per day. Early oral feeding in abdominal surgery is under trial at present. In gastrointestinal surgery, it takes usually 5 days to start oral feeding. In major gastrointestinal surgeries, intestinal fistulas, total parenteral nutrition (TPN) is a must with all essential elements, otherwise sepsis, wound dehiscence, anastomotic leak can occur.
- *Postoperative pain* relief is essential. If pain is not relieved it leads to tachypnoea, tachycardia, pneumonia, atelectasis, hypertension, and aggravate cardiac problems. Pain units are present in hospitals to manage pain by analgesics like non-steroidal anti-inflammatory drugs (NSAIDs) and tramadol, sedation like morphine and pethidine, epidural analgesia. Often *continuous intravenous infusion* of analgesics is needed. *Patient controlled analgesia* is training patient to self-administer the drug using triggering button which delivers the controlled dose of analgesics. Opioids can cause nausea and vomiting and so antiemetic should be given. NSAIDs can be nephrotoxic especially in elderly and gastric irritant and so patient should be monitored. Antihistamine injection like ranitidine (50 mg intravenously) or injection of proton pump inhibitors should be given along with NSAIDs. Pain reduces in intensity in 48 hours after surgery. If pain persists after 48 hours, it should be evaluated for sepsis, haematoma, ileus, collection, nerve irritation, pneumonia, DVT, etc.
- *Prevention of postoperative DVT* is important. Risk of DVT is 30% in postoperative period. It is more common in orthopaedic surgeries, surgeries for malignancy, in obese patients, in elderly. Risk is categorised as *low risk* (age less than 40 years; short time surgery without immobilisation); *moderate risk* (age more than 40 years; major surgeries; patient taking oral contraceptives); *high risk* (age above 40 years, cardiac illness, major operation, pelvic surgery, malignancy, prolonged postoperative immobilisation). Prophylactic low dose heparin/low molecular weight heparin can be given on the day of surgery and continued for 5 days postoperatively. Early mobilisation, compression stockings to legs during surgery and postoperative period, leg exercises, pneumatic compression devices are other modalities used. Patient should stop oral contraceptives 4 weeks prior to major surgery.

- *Postoperative fever* is the one surgeon is really worried about. Fever in 24 hours may be due to intravenous fluid, inflammatory response, atelectasis, DVT, inflammation at the site of intravenous cannula, urinary infection. Up to 5 days it may be due to pneumonia, catheter-induced infection, cellulitis at infusion site, thrombophlebitis, DVT. After 5 days it may be due to collection at operative site, bacteraemia, septicaemia, pneumonia. Total count, liver function tests, urine analysis, chest X-ray, blood culture, ultrasound of the site like abdomen, occasionally CT scan is needed for proper evaluation to identify the cause of fever. Higher generation antibiotics are needed. Proper monitoring is needed. Anastomotic leak, subphrenic abscess, pelvic abscess has to be thought of. Empyema, late DVT has to be ruled out. Doppler scan of both limbs should be done if suspected. Drainage of pus, re-surgery has to be considered.
- *Surgical wound management* is also important. Clean surgical wound is inspected only after 48 hours. Infected wound should be inspected in 24 hours. Timing of suture removal depends on type of surgery, site of surgery. It is removed usually in 4–5 days in face, in 7–10 days in the abdomen, back, limbs. There may be danger of wound dehiscence in early removal of sutures. Very late removal may cause wound infection. Timing is decided by surgeon on individual basis. Suture is removed with all aseptic precautions. It is removed from deeper part of the knot which is pulled towards the line of incision **(Figs. 2-36A and B)**.

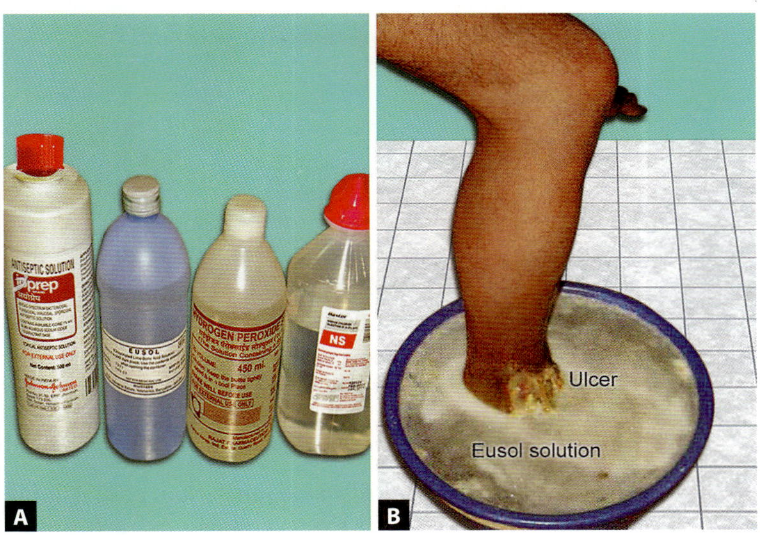

Figs. 2-36A and B: Dressing solutions used in different dressings. Patient dipping his ulcer leg in dilute eusol solution—Eusol bath (Edinburgh University Solution—boric acid, sodium hypochlorite, calcium hydroxide).

SURGICAL COMPLICATIONS

It is said that complications tend to occur in spite of adequate precaution and care in surgical practice. If any surgeon tells that he had zero percent of complications then it is logic that he has not operated at all. But complications can be reduced; often can be prevented by proper preoperative care and preparation. One has to remember that complication is not negligence. Complications during postoperative period is categorised as respiratory, cardiac, renal, hepatic, gastrointestinal, generalised, postoperative fever, deep venous thrombosis and so on.

It is usually classified as: (1) ***Intraoperative*** complications. (2) ***Immediate postoperative*** complications. (3) ***Late postoperative*** complications.

Respiratory Complications

It is the *most common* postoperative complication. Precipitating factors are old age, obesity, smoking, asthma, bronchitis, associated cardiac illness, postoperative pain, aspiration. 25% of postoperative deaths are due to respiratory infection.

Atelectasis

Atelectasis is collapse of basal lung alveoli which can be prevented by respiratory physiotherapy, control of pain, effective coughing. It is the most common postoperative respiratory complication. Narcotics, anaesthetic agents, abdominal/thoracic wound pain cause pulmonary shunt development that eventually leads into atelectasis, pneumonia, respiratory failure, etc. It is common in smokers, and obese individuals. Pneumonia can develop eventually in these patients. Deep breathing, proper coughing, usage of spirometer, respiratory physiotherapy are the important ways to treat and prevent it.

Aspiration

Aspiration is common in postoperative period causing collapse of lung, bronchopneumonia—***Mendelson's syndrome***. Large quantity of aspiration can cause complete blockage of airway and instant death. Often it is due to chemical (acid) induced severe laryngeal spasm. Immediate ventilation using intubation and ventilator; suction and clearing of airway, bronchoscopy and clearing are the measures needed. Prevention of aspiration is important. For this keeping the patient nil oral in postoperative period for 12 hours is beneficial. Sideward positioning of the patient; prokinetics, passing nasogastric tube are often needed. Once aspirated sudden laryngeal spasm, sepsis, bronchospasm, respiratory failure may develop. It is treated with antibiotics, immediate bronchoscopy, bronchodilators, and ventilator support. Role of steroid support is *not well* accepted even though commonly practiced. *Postoperative pneumonia* is commonly due to nosocomial infection by *Pseudomonas*, *Klebsiella* and *Enterobacter*. Both lung pneumonia/atelectasis may be life threatening and an emergency situation.

Pulmonary Oedema

Pulmonary oedema with accumulation of fluid in the alveoli causing hypoxaemia is a common postoperative complication. It is due to fluid overload, cardiac cause and acute lung injury due to toxins, sepsis. Pulmonary capillary wedge pressure (PCWP) is ideal to identify it with abnormal chest X-ray. It is treated with restricted fluid, diuresis, and oxygen supplement often with ventilator support.

Acute/Adult Respiratory Distress Syndrome

Acute/adult respiratory distress syndrome (***ARDS***) is a form of respiratory failure with fluid accumulation in the alveoli, widened/thickened alveoli-capillary space, diffuse inflammatory response in both lungs with PaO_2/FIO_2 ratio less than 200 and PCWP less than 18 mmHg. It is critical entity leading into respiratory failure and death. Patient develops tachypnoea, tachycardia, dyspnoea, cyanosis with coarse crepitations all over the lungs on both sides. Patient will be in respiratory failure with reversal of arterial PaO_2 and $PaCO_2$. *Management:* Patient needs ventilator support with initial FIO_2 at 100%; positive end expiratory pressure (PEEP); tidal volume

6–8 mL/kg; peak pressure at 35 cm of water; $PaCO_2$ is maintained at 40 mmHg; inspiratory/expiratory ratio is at 1:2. Later FIO_2 is weaned to 60%. ARDS is now classified as classical type III respiratory failure. Chest X-ray is a useful tool to diagnose. Monitoring of pulmonary capillary wedge pressure is needed. Fluid restriction and diuretics are part of the therapy. Complications of ventilator have to be watched for—dependency, sepsis with resistant bacteria, endotracheal tube blockage. Tracheostomy if needed is *always* better. TPN, enteral nutrition, prevention of thrombocytopenia and bleeding by transfusing FFP or platelets whenever needed is essential. Development of uraemia should also be watched for by assessing the renal functions repeatedly.

Criteria for weaning from ventilator are—respiratory rate less than 25/minute; PaO_2 more than 70 mmHg; $PaCO_2$ less than 45 mmHg; minute ventilation 8 litre/minute; tidal volume 6 mL/kg; negative inspiratory force is minus 25 cm of H_2O.

Acute lung injury is similar but here PaO_2/FIO_2 ratio is less than 300 and PCWP is less than 18 mmHg. It is little less severe than ARDS.

Respiratory Failure

Respiratory failure is defined as a status with arterial partial pressure of oxygen less than 60 mmHg; arterial partial pressure of CO_2 more than 60 mmHg. Aspiration, pneumonia, sepsis, lung injury, transfusion, ARDS, acute lung injury, fat embolism are common causes. There is diminished diffusion across alveolar membrane causing cyanosis and hypoxia. *Type I respiratory failure* is *hypoxic condition* with reduced PaO_2 but normal $PaCO_2$. There is hypoventilation, AV shunts, ventilation perfusion mismatch, and low venous oxygen. *Type II hypercapnic respiratory failure* is reduced PaO_2 with increased $PaCO_2$. There is also increased CO_2 production with widened dead space. *Type III respiratory failure is typical ARDS* with development of hyaline membrane; reduced diffusion; decrease in surfactant; raise in pulmonary arterial pressure; progressive atelectasis; respiratory arrest. Management is similar to ARDS. Monitoring at regular intervals is essential. Tracheostomy may be a life-saving need **(Figs. 2-37 to 2-39)**.

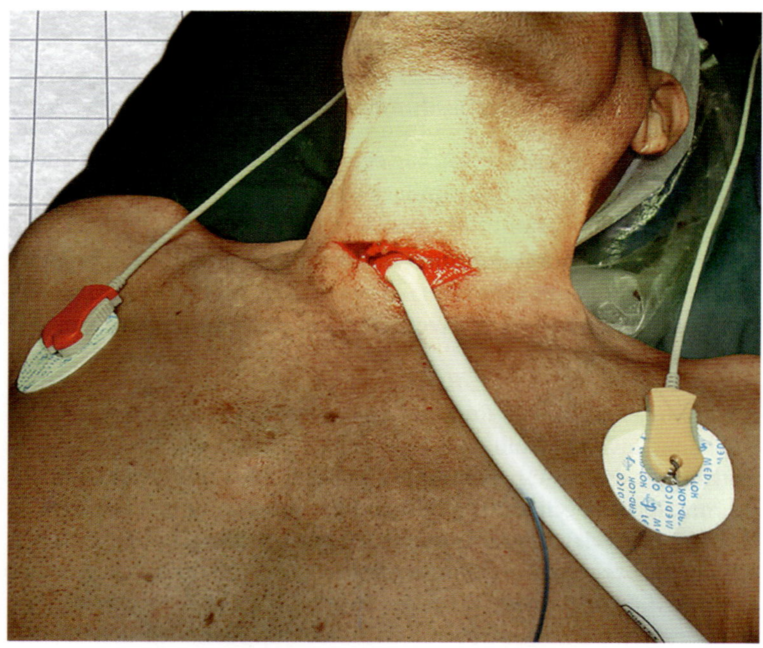

Fig. 2-37: On table tracheostomy tube placement.

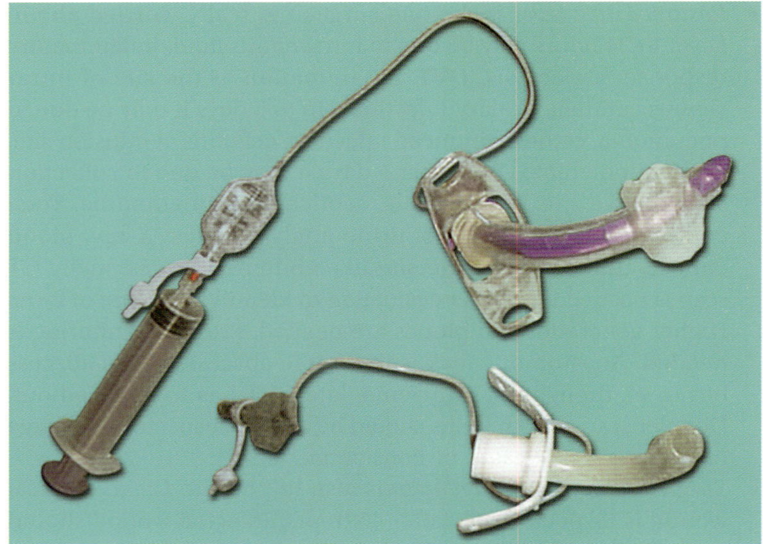

Fig. 2-38: Synthetic tracheostomy tube—PVC.

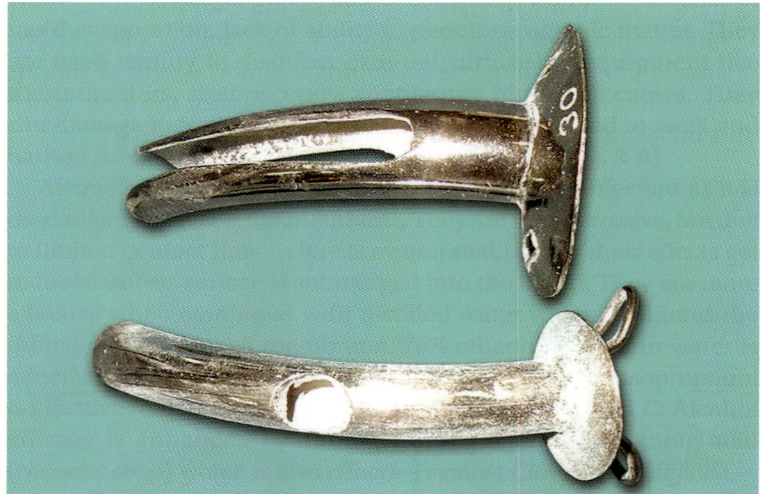

Fig. 2-39: Fuller's biflanged tracheostomy tube having outer tube and inner tube. Inner tube is having an opening on the convex surface. Inner tube is longer than outer tube.

Other than above measures, nitric oxide inhalation; partial liquid ventilation; fluorocarbon assisted gas exchange; extracorporeal membrane oxygenators are used.

Fat Embolism (Ernst Von Bergmann, in 1873)

About 90% major trauma especially with fractures develop fat embolism from aggregation fat globules and chylomicrons derived from bone marrow. Fat globules release fatty acids which act as toxins. It is common in fracture long bones, multiple fractures. It is observed after intramedullary nailing, liposuction, joint reconstruction, parenteral lipid infusion, cardiopulmonary bypass, pathological fractures. Only 5–10% will develop ***fat embolism syndrome (FES)***. FES shows respiratory distress (ARDS), skin manifestations. Approximately 20–30% of the population have a patent foramen ovale; fat emboli pass through the pulmonary circulation causing the systemic manifestations of FES, particularly involving the brain and kidneys. As a result of the occluded cerebral vasculature, patients exhibit encephalopathy, localised cerebral oedema. FES has got 20% mortality **(Table 2-3)**.

TABLE 2-3: Gurd and Wilson criteria for FES.

Major criteria	*Minor criteria*
♦ Symptoms and radiologic evidence of respiratory insufficiency ♦ Cerebral sequelae unrelated to head injury or other conditions ♦ Petechial rash–over upper body, axillae	♦ Tachycardia (heart rate >110/min) ♦ Pyrexia (>38.5°C) ♦ Retinal changes or petechiae ♦ Renal dysfunction ♦ Jaundice ♦ Acute drop in haemoglobin level ♦ Sudden thrombocytopenia ♦ Elevated erythrocyte sedimentation rate ♦ Fat microglobulinemia

Features:

Pulmonary: Cyanosis, tachypnoea, right heart failure, froth in mouth and nostrils, fat droplets in sputum, eventually respiratory failure. *Cutaneous*: Petechial haemorrhages in the skin. *Cerebral*: Drowsy, restlessness, disorientation, constricted pupils, pyrexia and coma. *Retinal artery emboli* is the earliest sign to appear, causing *striae haemorrhages, fluffy exudates* confirmed on fundoscopic examination. *Kidney*: Blockage in renal arterioles results in fat droplets in urine.

Differential diagnosis: Pulmonary embolism, thrombotic thrombocytopenic purpura.

Investigations: Presence of fat lobules in the blood obtained by pulmonary capillary wedging is diagnostic; haemoglobin estimation, platelet count and total WBC count; chest X-ray shows snow storm appearance; CT chest is useful; CT head is done to rule of causes of intracranial injuries; transoesophageal echocardiography (TEE) may be of use in evaluating the intraoperative release of marrow contents into the bloodstream during intramedullary reaming and nailing; bronchoalveolar lavage with staining for fat will show lipid inclusions.

Treatment: Adequate oxygenation with ventilator support (ICU care); hydration, nutrition, achieving haemodynamic stability, prevention of DVT, avoiding volume overload with proper fluid therapy; methylprednisolone may be useful; but use of heparin, low molecular dextran and other steroids are controversial even though commonly used; albumin transfusion may be helpful as it binds with fatty acids to reduce the lung injury; early fixation of the fractures; placement of IVC filters will prevent the chances of fat embolism or emboli reaching into the lungs.

Air/Gas Embolism

Causes: Through venous access like intravenous (IV) cannula, most common cause; during artificial pneumothorax; during surgeries of neck and axilla; traumatic opening of major veins sucking air inside, causing embolism; during fallopian tube insufflation; laparoscopic surgeries; during illegal abortion.

Features: It causes respiratory distress, haemoptysis, convulsions, unconsciousness, visual and hearing disturbances, fatigue and numbness, paralysis, haemodynamic instability and coma.

- Amount of air required causing ***venous air/gas embolism*** is 15 mL. *To precipitate symptoms in venous embolism 100 mL of air required. 100 mL of air at a rate more than 100 mL/second is fatal.*
- When the air enters the right atrium, it gets churned up forming foam which enters the right ventricle and blocks the pulmonary artery.

Contd...

Contd...

- ***Mill-Wheel murmur (machinery)*** heard over the precordium through a stethoscope is diagnostic.
- During open heart surgery/therapeutic pneumothorax, by accidental pulmonary vein puncture or in atrial septal defect (ASD) air may enter left side of the heart (*paradoxical air embolism*) causing coronary block or cerebral air embolism.
- ***Arterial gas embolism*** is more dangerous and often early fatal. *2 mL of gas/air is fatal in cerebral circulation; and 0.5 mL is fatal in coronary arteries.*
- Through paravertebral veins also air embolism can occur to brain.

Treatment: Patient is placed in *Trendelenburg left lateral decubitus position*. The Trendelenburg position keeps left ventricular air bubble away from the coronary artery ostia (which are near the aortic valve) so that air bubbles do not enter and occlude the coronary arteries. Left lateral decubitus positioning helps to trap air in the non-dependent segment of the right ventricle (where it is more likely to remain instead of progressing into the pulmonary artery and occluding it). The left lateral decubitus position also prevents the air from passing through a potentially patent foramen ovale (present in as many as 30% of adults) and entering the left ventricle, from which it could then embolise to distal arteries. Hyperbaric oxygen is useful in both venous and arterial gas/air embolism as it reduces the ischaemia, reduces the bubble size; in arterial gas embolism it removes the nitrogen from the bubble so that it improves perfusion and oxygenation. By passing a needle, the air has to be aspirated from the right ventricle. Often requires life-saving open thoracotomy to aspirate the excess air causing the block.

Pulmonary Embolism

Pulmonary embolism is often life-threatening complication in postoperative period. Its incidence is 30% with death rate 10%. Endothelial damage, stasis, hypercoagulable status are the *risk factors*. Trauma, fractures, major surgery, obesity, old age, postpartum period, pregnancy, malignancy, venous catheters, neurologic causes, varicose veins, inherited thrombophilia are the *main causes.* Commonest origin is deep venous thrombosis (DVT) in *iliofemoral* region. Pulmonary embolism may be *massive* in 10% of cases blocking pulmonary artery leading to instant death. *Medium and small emboli* block the lung capillaries at periphery causing infarction. *Presentations are*—pain, swelling, tenderness in the leg; pleuritic chest pain; sudden onset dyspnoea; tachycardia; haemoptysis; inspiratory crackles; loud second heart sound; audible fourth heart sound; tachypnoea. *ECG* shows right bundle branch block, right axis deviation, P wave pulmonale. Chest X-ray may show infarction in lung (*wedge shaped*). Change in arterial blood gas is obvious. Venous duplex US shows evidence of DVT in legs. *Pulmonary CT angiography* even though is *gold standard*, and ideal most sensitive investigation; it is not commonly done as it is invasive, not available, needs expertise to do it. *Echocardiography* is non-invasive, can be done bed side, available in most of the centers. It shows hypokinesia and dilatation of right ventricle, paradoxical motion, pulmonary hypertension; but it is not as sensitive as pulmonary angiography. *D-dimer* assay is typical as negative result excludes pulmonary embolism; but positive result will not confirm the diagnosis. D-dimer is degraded product of a cross-linked fibrin blood clot. *Helical CT angiogram* is technically easier, commonly done CT than CT pulmonary angiogram. *V/Q lung scan* is the initial test of choice but it is not available. Echocardiography, helical CT angiogram scan, venous Doppler scan, D-dimer assay are commonly practiced evaluatory methods. *Treatment*—heparin; LMWH; fondaparinux (synthetic pentasaccharide anticoagulant which inhibits factor Xa) *Ultrafractionated heparin* is very useful as a bolus 70 units/kg followed by 1000 units/hour intravenously with maintaining partial thromboplastin time two times the control. Warfarin, oral anticoagulant 5–10 mg daily is started as an *overlap therapy* with heparin for 2 days before stopping heparin. *Thrombolytic agents* like streptokinase, urokinase, and recombinant tissue plasminogen activator that dissolves the clot rapidly is useful in massive pulmonary embolism. Transcatheter thrombolysis and embolectomy is also useful. IVC filter placement is better method to prevent embolism in high-risk groups.

Cardiac Complications

Elective operation in a patient who had myocardial infarction recently should be ideally deferred for 6 months. In an emergency situation such rule cannot be applied.

Myocardial Infarction

Myocardial infarction (MI) can develop on table preoperatively which has got high mortality; or in postoperative period. Old age, obesity, patient already with history earlier of ischaemic attacks are more prone to develop MI. In suspected cases repeated cardiac isoenzymes—CPK MB should be done. ECG and echocardiography, immediate call for cardiologist is a must. Often MI is precipitated by surgical stress, shock, haemorrhage, hypovolaemia, hypoxia, electrolyte imbalance and prolonged anaesthesia. Measures taken are—pain relief, oxygen, nebulisation, CVP monitor, avoiding fluid overload, vasopressors, emergency angiogram and angioplasty by balloon or stent.

Postoperative Hypertension

Postoperative hypertension may be due to pain, hypoxia, hypothermia, fluid overload, trauma (head), internal bleeding, and crisis of certain disease like pheochromocytoma. *Hypertensive crisis* in postoperative period is dangerous. There is severe raise in blood pressure (diastolic >110 mmHg); organ dysfunction; cerebral and subarachnoid haemorrhage; stroke; acute cardiac problems; bleeding from surgical wound site. Sodium nitroprusside, nitroglycerin, labetalol, esmolol, enalaprilat, nicardipine are the different drugs tried. At time 25% of blood pressure is controlled, which then is gradually allowed to become normal. Rapid control may lead into stroke, organ hypoperfusion.

Cardiac Arrest

It is the cessation of the heart. Heart stops contracting. Causes: All causes for shock. Structural causes like coronary artery diseases, myocardial hypertrophy, carditis, cardiomyopathy; conduction problems; valvular heart diseases; hypoperfusion status due to shock of any cause; metabolic causes; sudden reduction in cardiac output due to tension pneumothorax, pulmonary embolism, anaphylaxis, acute blood loss; toxins; drugs. There will be finally *ventricular fibrillation* before leading into cardiac arrest. Profound circulatory failure develops causing typical features.

Features of cardiac arrest:
- No palpable pulse—radial/femoral/carotid.
- Heart sounds not heard.
- Cessation of respiration, apnoea—cyanosis occurs.
- Development of unconsciousness with convulsions.
- Pupils start dilating.
- Cessation of bleeding.
- ECG shows asystole/ventricular fibrillation.

Critical period—once heart and lungs stop, brain death occurs in 3 minutes.

Immediate measures—cardiopulmonary resuscitation (CPR)

- **Airway** open by head tilt—chin lift; jaw thrust manoeuvre; clean the airway by finger or Heimlich method.
- **Breathing**—spontaneous/mouth to mouth/bag and mask.
- **Cardiac** compression.
- **Drugs** and **defibrillator**.
- **ECG, endotracheal** tube and monitor.

Basic life measures:
- **External cardiac compression (massage):** Patient is laid flat on a *hard surface (never on soft surface)*. Manual compression is exerted over the lower sternum, using both hands one over other without bending the elbow at a rate of 60–70 per minute. Rib cage damage during procedure can very well be ignored (Heel of right hand is placed over the sternum 5–8 cm above xiphoid process and left hand is placed over it) **(Fig. 2-40)**.
- At the same time, another person should give *mouth to mouth breathing* at a rate of 10-20 per minute after clearing the airway by removing froth, and dentures if present **(Fig. 2-41)**. A bag with mask can be used to ventilate using air or oxygen.
- Endotracheal intubation and ventilator support.

Observations to be made are:

- Groin pulse.
- Respiration and breath sounds.
- Blood pressure.
- Pupillary reaction.
- ECG activity.

Once patient recovers, the cause and sequelae has to be managed properly.

Sequelae are due to hypoxia and circulatory collapse

- Cerebral oedema and permanent brain damage.
- Acute/adult respiratory distress syndrome (ARDS).
- Renal failure.

Advanced life support:
- Intubation, 100% oxygen support.
- Proper venous line ideally central or peripheral as an emergency should be assessed.
- Endotracheal intubation and administration of epinephrine/atropine/lignocaine in 10 mL saline is given twice as intravenous dose. Intracardiac drugs are *not used* now.
- **Internal open cardiac massage:** This method is used when cardiac arrest occurs in the operation theatre during surgery, acute tamponade, and acute bilateral pneumothorax. Left side thorax is opened through a *rapid lengthy* incision along 4th or 5th intercostals space. Initially heart with intact pericardium is

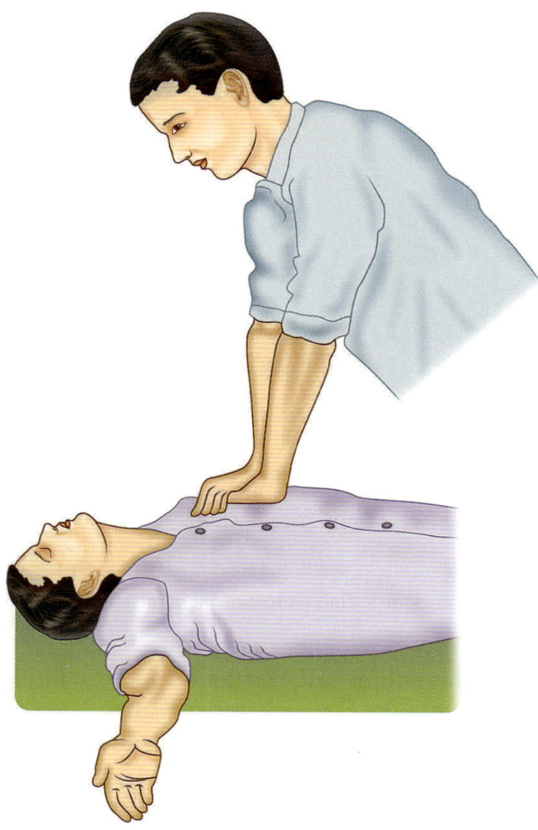

Fig. 2-40: Technique of cardiac massage.

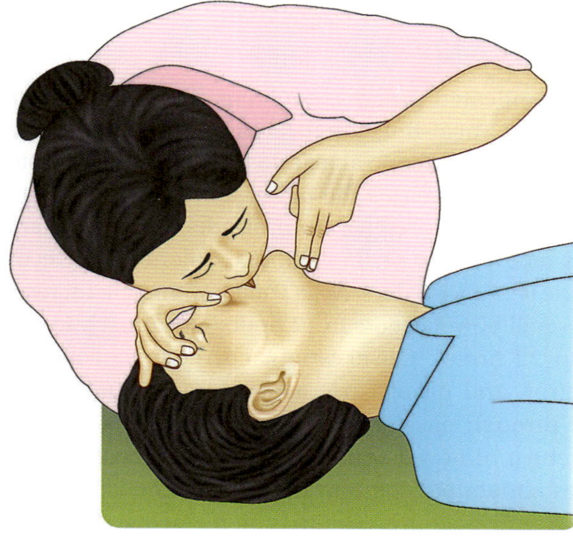

Fig. 2-41: Technique of mouth-to-mouth respiration. Note patient's nose should be held closed with right hand of the doctor/assistant and with left hand lower jaw should be pushed forward.

rhythmically compressed and relaxed using left hand against sternum. Mean time costal cartilages above and below are cut with a knife to have a better exposure. Pericardium is opened in front of the phrenic nerve. Direct cardiac massage is undertaken until heart regains its function and later shifted to ventilatory support and critical care **(Fig. 2-42)**.

- **Defibrillation technique:** Jelly is applied to the site of electrodes. One electrode is placed at the base of heart to the right of the sternum, other over the estimated area of the apex of the heart **(Fig. 2-43)**. ***Ensure that nobody is in contact with the patient.***

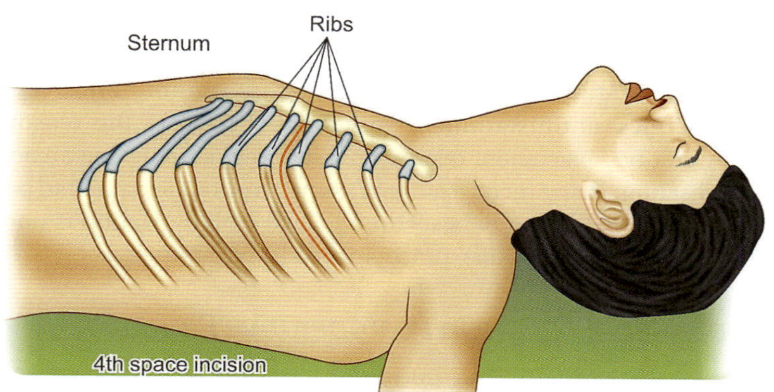

Fig. 2-42: Left thoracotomy for open internal cardiac massage.

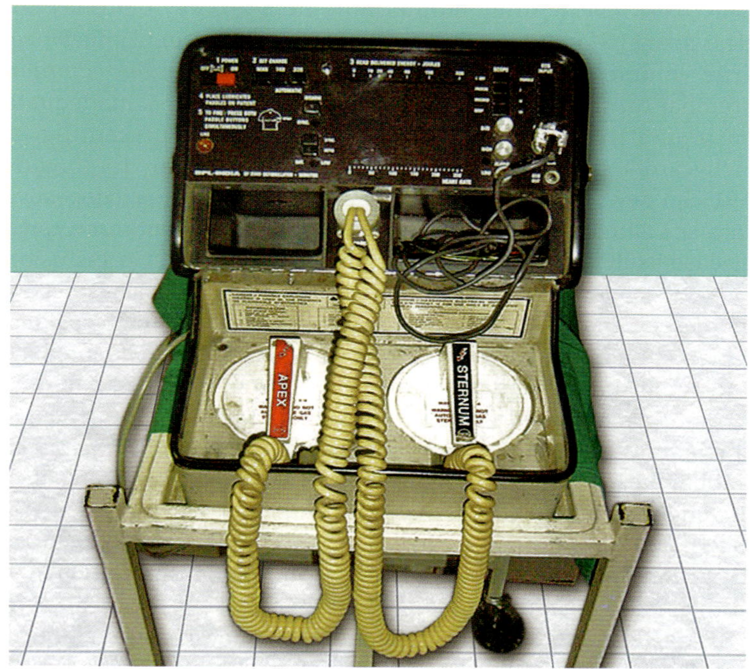

Fig. 2-43: Defibrillator is used in case of cardiac arrest.

The defibrillator is activated. Ventilation and ECG monitoring is resumed immediately. Defibrillation up to 3 times (200; 300 and 360 Joules) is done.

- Injection of 1:10,000 adrenaline (1 mg IV) and 10% calcium chloride intravenously. It is repeated every 3 minutes. Lignocaine 1.5 mg/kg IV; repeated every 3 minutes. Procainamide 30 mg/minute up to a total dose of 17 mg/kg; atropine 1 mg intravenously.
- Correction of hypoxia, acidosis, hypothermia, hypotension, hypovolaemia, potassium imbalance.
- Sodium bicarbonate 8.4% injection, hydrocortisone injection.
- Analysis of blood gas (PCO_2 and PO_2), and assessment of serum electrolytes at repeated intervals.
- Urinary catheterisation, Ryle's tube insertion.
- Monitoring the patient with BP, pulse, respiration, and temperature chart—critical care in ICU.

Renal/Urinary Complications

Postoperative Retention of Urine

About 20% of postoperative patients develop retention of urine. Perineal, gynaecological, pelvic surgeries are common causes.

Surgery done under spinal anaesthesia is also common cause. Wound pain, difficulty in straining, pre-existing prostate enlargement, stricture urethra, phimosis, drugs (sympathomimetics, anti-cholinergics, antihistamines) and constipation are the reasons. Hot water bag placement over hypogastric region, relieving anxiety, mobilisation, doing rectal examination may make the patient to pass urine. If still retention persists then Foley's catheterisation is done. Alpha adrenergic blockers, prazocin are also used often.

Acute Renal Failure in Postoperative Period

Acute renal failure in postoperative period is common and often it is real challenge to manage. It is increase in serum creatinine level—relative increase of 50% or absolute increase by 1 mg%. It can be oliguric ARF (output less than 480 mL/day) or non-oliguric ARF (isosthenuric urine output more than 2 L/day but does not clear toxins). Both cause electrolyte and haemodynamic imbalance. True volume depletion in postoperative period is the *common* prerenal *cause*. It may be due to vomiting, diarrhoea, inadequate postoperative fluid replacement, haemorrhage presenting as tachycardia, hypotension, low jugular venous pulse, dry tongue. ARF can develop due to associated pulmonary oedema, congestive cardiac failure, as hepatorenal syndrome, nephritic syndrome, renal disease itself. It can be also immunologic, idiopathic, transfusion induced; *septicaemia induced* (decreased peripheral vasoconstriction, increased renal vasoconstriction, toxins) also. Aminoglycosides, *NSAIDs* (inhibits glomerular afferent vasodilatation) are nephrotoxic and renal parameters have to be monitored in these patients. Haemolysis or rhabdomyolysis can cause renal failure. It needs adequate fluid therapy, mannitol therapy—25 gram intravenous, sodium bicarbonate intravenous to keep urine pH more than 6.5 so that pigment haem gets dissolved. *Investigations:* **Prerenal ARF** is identified by low urinary sodium (less than 20 mEq/L), less than 1% of fractional excretion of sodium, high serum sodium, and blood urea nitrogen and creatinine ratio is more than 20:1. In **renal cause of ARF**, fractional excretion of sodium is higher than 1% due to tubular damage. Urinary sodium level is more than 50 mEq/L. Creatinine clearance test is ideal. *Treatment:* Haemodynamic management; *fluid challenge* using 500 mL normal saline infusion in 30 minutes; frusemide 100–400 mg intravenously; 20% mannitol; *dopamine* infusion at a rate of 3 μg/kg/minute; haemodialysis until kidney regains its function adequately. During haemodialysis, fluid intake should be monitored properly by taking help of a nephrologist; twice a day monitoring of serum electrolytes; *sudden hyperkalaemia* more than 5.5 mEq/dL is a risk for cardiac arrest and so potassium supplement should be avoided and IV calcium, DNS with insulin should be started. Adequate calorie is essential and is supplemented orally or parenterally **(Fig. 2-44)**.

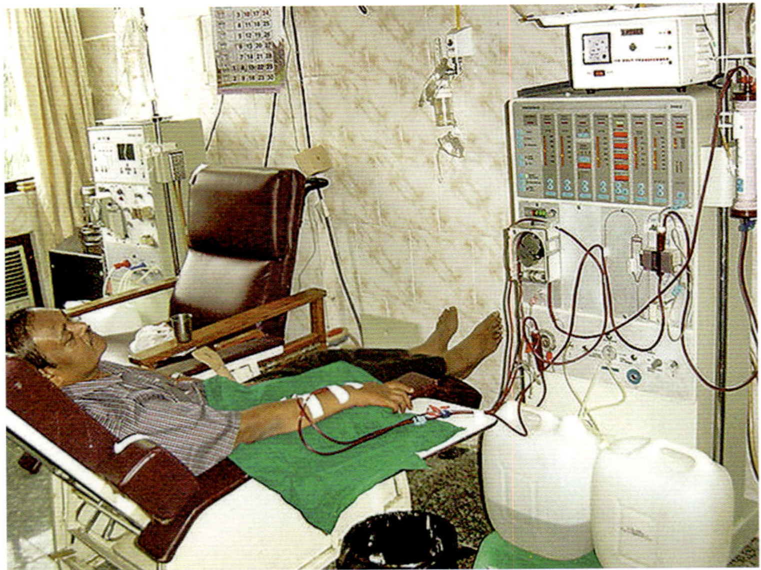

Fig. 2-44: Haemodialysis to a renal failure patient.

Gastrointestinal Complications

Acute Erosive Gastritis

It is seen in critically ill patients; ICU patients; in severe trauma and burns *(Curling's ulcer);* head injury and intracranial diseases (Cushing's ulcer); drugs like aspirin, NSAIDs. It is due to gastric mucosal disruption, ischaemia, decreased gastric epithelial turnover, and reduced prostaglandin production (PG increases epithelial turnover, bicarbonate, mucus, mucosal blood flow). Gastroduodenoscopy confirms the diagnosis. It is treated by nasogastric aspiration, saline wash, proton pump inhibitors or H2 blockers. Sucralfate is an aluminium salt of sulfated sucrose binds only to ulcer bed but not to normal gastric mucosa, which increases the prostaglandin level, binds pepsin and bile acids, blocks the back diffusion of hydrogen ions, and protects stomach from colonisation by bacteria. Vasopressin, misoprostol (it is PGE1 used in NSAIDs-induced gastritis), laser coagulation using gastroscope are other methods. Vagotomy, total gastrectomy to control postoperative bleeding is rarely needed nowadays.

Postoperative Ileus

Ileus is a complicated process involving altered gastrointestinal nervous system, local hormonal factors, inflammatory factors, bowel handling and narcotic analgesia. Resection and anastomosis of bowel temporarily ceases the bowel activity due to inability to transmit the peristaltic waves from duodenal pacemaker. Small bowel ileus recovers usually in 48 hours. Colonic ileus recovers in 4 days, gastric ileus in 4–5 days. *Note:* Patient without ileus, recovery of motility of small bowel occurs in 12 hours; of stomach in 48 hours; of colon in 72 hours. Observation, correction of electrolytes, sepsis control, and nasogastric aspiration is usually sufficient. Aspiration through nasogastric tube less than 200 mL; passing of flatus, return of bowel sounds are signs of recovery. Rarely if ileus causes abdominal compartment syndrome laparotomy may be required and decompression is done using decompressor. *Bowel obstruction* occurring within 30 days after surgery is called as *early postoperative* bowel obstruction. It can be due *to primary ileus* without any precipitating factors or *secondary ileus* with precipitating factors or *mechanical bowel obstruction* commonly due to adhesions (90%). *Ileus* is a complicated process involving altered gastrointestinal nervous system, local hormonal factors, inflammatory factors, bowel handling, and narcotic analgesia. Resection and anastomosis of bowel temporarily ceases the bowel activity due to inability to transmit the peristaltic waves from duodenal pacemaker. *CT abdomen* is ideal to diagnose type of bowel obstruction, complications, peritonitis and also to decide whether surgical intervention is needed. *Treatment* is initially conservative—fluids, correction of electrolytes, sepsis. But if needed re-exploration is done to correct the mechanical obstruction of the bowel.

Acute Abdominal Compartment Syndrome

It is increased intra-abdominal pressure more than 12 mmHg (normal pressure is about 5 mmHg) with hypoxia, increasing peak airway pressure, poor ventilation, oliguria. *Causes:* Ascites, pancreatitis, bowel wall oedema, fluid collection, major abdominal procedures, liver transplantation, contents of large long-standing hernias once reduced into the peritoneal cavity, non-compliant abdominal wall when closed with tension, trauma, packing abdomen, paralytic ileus, coagulopathies. Diaphragm gets displaced upwards causing hypoxia, hypercapnia, and acidosis. Pressure more than 25 mmHg causes compression of IVC and portal vein leading into reduced venous return to heart and increased peripheral resistance. Right atrial and pulmonary arterial occlusion pressure decreases. Kidneys get compressed directly leading into decreased GFR and urine output. Mesenteric vein compression → decreased perfusion → intramucosal acidosis, bowel wall oedema. Increased CVP reduces the cerebral blood outflow and increases the intracranial pressure. *Features:* Difficulty in breathing, oliguria, tense distended abdomen, reduced cardiac output, deterioration in level of consciousness, acidosis and respiratory failure. *Investigations:* Measurement of pressure using a transducer through a urinary bladder Foley's catheter; measurement through gastric catheter; abdominal perfusion pressure measurement; assessment of renal infiltration gradient; CT abdomen. Pressure is graded as Grade I—10–15 cm H_2O; Grade II—15–25 cm H_2O; Grade III—26–35 cm H_2O; Grade IV—>35 cm H_2O. *Treatment:* Emergency surgery and decompression, drainage of the abdominal fluid, muscle relaxant, ventilator, laparostomy, mesh/biomesh/sterile bag cover, vacuum-assisted closure are methods available.

Postoperative Gastrointestinal Bleeding

It may be upper gastrointestinal (GI) or lower gastrointestinal bleeding. Upper GI bleed may be due to peptic ulcer, stress gastritis, variceal bleed, Mallory Weiss bleeding, arteriovenous (AV) malformations and anastomotic bleed. Bleeding stress ulcers can occur, when gastric pH is less than 4.0. Lower GI bleed may be due to diverticulosis, colitis, bowel ischaemia, AV malformations. Precipitating factors are trauma, burns, head injury, coagulopathies, sepsis, disseminated intravascular coagulation (DIC), drugs. Tarry coloured stool/melaena and haematemesis or blood in the nasogastric tube is the feature of upper GI bleed. Haematochezia, loose stool are the features of lower GI bleed. Rapid bleed can cause hypotension, tachycardia and shock. Gastroscopy or colonoscopy confirms the diagnosis. *Treatment:* Blood transfusion; conservative therapy by saline wash, intravenous H2 blockers (Ranitidine 50 mg/ Famotidine), proton pump inhibitors, sucralfate, monitoring and maintaining the clotting factors, antibiotics, maintaining the INR using injection vitamin K or fresh frozen plasma, platelet transfusion; endoscopic control of bleeding by tamponade, epinephrine, laser, clips, banding, heater probe; angiographic embolisation using gel foam, clot, coils through superior or inferior mesenteric arteries. Occasionally surgical intervention is needed especially when there is refractile anastomotic leak. Re-anastomosis or subtotal gastrectomy, vagotomy are the procedures used.

Stomal Complications

It can be early or late. Early can be retraction, necrosis, abscess formation, high output systemic failure, and leak. Late can be prolapse, stenosis, parastomal hernia, fistula, excoriations, and bowel obstruction.

Anastomotic Leak

It is a common complication in gastrointestinal surgery often dreadful and life threatening. It may be intestinal or pancreatic or biliary fistulas/leak.

Factors: Poor blood supply, sepsis, emergency resections, malignancy, old age, obesity, smoking, immunocompromised patients, fluid collection or abscess formation, steroid therapy (steroid prevents collagen formation and healing), hypotension and hypoxia on table and in immediate postoperative period, presence of drains, shock, malnutrition, deficiencies, stapler-related factors, specific diseases like carcinoma, tuberculosis, Crohn's disease, diverticulitis. Uncontrolled leak, abscess formation, electrolyte imbalance, anaemia, malnutrition, sepsis are the effects. Renal failure, multiorgan failure and death can occur if not controlled. Fistula should be *classified as low output or high output* depending on the quantity of fluid effluent in the fistula. If it is less than 500 mL it is called as low output fistula; if more than 500 mL it is high output fistula. Often it is *also* classified as *low* (below 200 mL/ 24 hours); *moderate* (between 200–500 mL); *high* (more than 500/day). In pancreatic fistula if less than 200 mL it is classified as low or more than 200 mL it is high. *Skin excoriation* (effluent dermatitis) initially allergic later with skin infection is common presenting as pain, ulcers, intractable itching. In proximal fistula electrolyte imbalance, fluid loss, malabsorption is severe whereas in distal fistula (colonic) it is less severe.

Investigations: CT abdomen, CT fistulogram, contrast GI studies, enteroclysis, endoscopies, cystoscopy to see enterovesical fistula.

Treatment: Total parenteral nutrition (TPN); evaluation of site of leak as whether it is end/lateral/low/high fistula; antibiotics; skin care with zinc oxide cream, adhesives, barriers, sealants, pouches; blood transfusion; rest to bowel by keeping the patient nil orally so that luminal secretions are reduced. If there is abscess, bleeding, peritonitis, bowel ischaemia re laparotomy is done. Timing of re exploration is in 24–48 hours once patient is stabilised. Thorough peritoneal wash with warm saline is given. Site of leak is identified. Ileostomy, colostomy or internal by pass procedures are done depending on individual patients and site of pathology. *Spontaneous closure* of fistula is expected in 60% of patients. *Favourable factors for spontaneous closure of fistula are*—tract more than 2 cm, single straight tract, lateral type, non-epithelialised tract, without sepsis or abscess or foreign body, defect in the bowel wall less than 1 cm, without distal obstruction and absence of specific diseases, adequate nutrition. In 40% cases *surgical intervention* and correction is needed. *Unfavorable factors are*—short tract less than 2 cm, multiple tracts, associated internal tracts, end fistula, epithelialisation, presence of infection or abscess, and bowel wall defect more than 1 cm, presence of specific diseases, foreign body, and malnutrition. Somatostatin and its analogues help in reducing the GI secretions thereby reduce the fistula output. Enteral nutrition can very well be used in low proximal fistulas or in colonic fistulas. *Fistuloclysis* is a newer method of infusing the nutrient fluid directly through the fistula into the GI tract.

Bile Leak

Bile leak is related to biliary surgery. It is 0.2% in open cholecystectomy and 0.7% in laparoscopic surgery.

Causes may be—leak from cystic duct stump, leak from accessory duct, injury to common bile duct or hepatic duct, biliary anomalies, thermal injury to CBD, late disruption and leak. Complete transection of CBD or hepatic ducts, avulsion of cystic duct, complex injuries with laceration of CBD can occur. *MRCP is diagnostic.* ERCP and CT abdomen is also done to assess proper pathology, site of disruption and to plan the proposed therapy. Pathology may be bilioma formation, biliary peritonitis, biliary fistula through drain site or through the wound, formation of abscess **(Fig. 2-45)**.

Presentations are—initially asymptomatic but later jaundice, cholangitis, abdomen pain and tenderness, features of sepsis.

Treatment: ERCP and stenting, aspiration of bilioma, in partial injury T tube insertion with repair by open method, in complete transection choledochoenterostomy should be done. It needs proper care, skill, patience and meticulous dissection. Drains must be placed at the site.

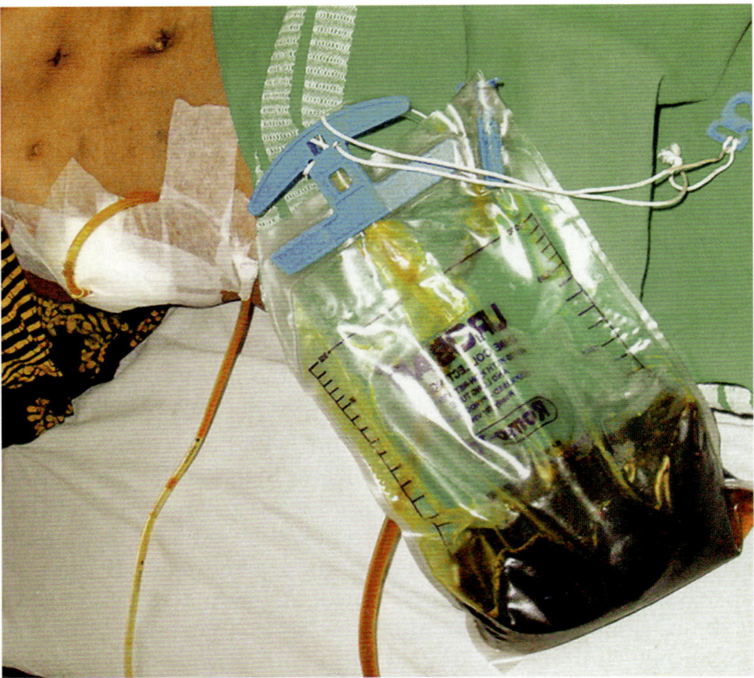

Fig. 2-45: Biliary fistula in a difficult postoperative laparoscopic cholecystectomy patient. It needs ERCP and stenting.

Clostridium Difficile Colitis

Clostridium difficile is a gram-positive spore bearing anaerobic bacillus. Spores exist in the environment and GI tract as a dormant status. *Antibiotic use* disturbs the microflora of the colon allowing this organism to get released from germinated spores. Bacteria release toxins—toxin A (enterotoxin) and toxin B (cytotoxin) cause various effects. *Effects are*—asymptomatic, mild colitis; *Pseudomembranous colitis*; fulminant colitis; toxic megacolon. Its incidence is increased by over use of antibiotics. Its mortality is also increased now (15%). It is common in general surgery, vascular surgery, old age, patients in ICU, HIV, patients on chemotherapy. Patients with long duration or multiple antibiotic therapies are more prone to its infection. Even single dose antibiotic therapy is known to cause *Clostridium difficile* sepsis. *Features:* Pain abdomen, foul smelling loose stool, fever, distension of abdomen, septic shock, dehydration, toxaemia are the features. *Treatment:* Careful use of antibiotics, aseptic precautions are important to prevent the infection. It is treated with vancomycin (orally/enema/IV) or metronidazole or rifampicin. Use of *Lactobacillus acidophilus and Saccharomyces cerevisiae* is also helpful. Occasionally surgical intervention with total colectomy and ileostomy may be needed as a life-saving measure.

Postoperative Psychosis

Acute postoperative psychosis is often seen. Presentations are either depression or mania or like schizophrenia with delusions. It is often difficult to differentiate the condition from electrolyte imbalance and other metabolic derangements. Proper evaluation and then help of a psychiatrist is needed. Usually patient becomes alright once he recovers from the actual illness and postoperative period, but needs counselling and drug therapy.

Postoperative Fever (See above)

It is the common problem in postoperative period. ***Malignant hyperthermia*** is rapidly increased metabolic crisis during/after exposure to anaesthesia which is often life threatening (10% mortality). It is usually inherited as *autosomal dominant* disease where there is increased calcium efflux in skeletal muscle from sarcoplasmic reticulum to myoplasm. *Triggering anaesthetic agents* (halothane, enflurane, isoflurane, desflurane) and depolarising muscled relaxants like succinyl choline causes increased calcium concentration in *Mycoplasma*. It leads into uncontrolled hypermetabolism in muscles leading into hypoxia, lactic acidosis, hypercapnia, breaking of ATP (adenosine triphosphate), excessive heat generation, hyperkalaemia, myoglobulinuria, DIC, systemic ischaemia and failure. Commonly susceptibility runs in family, with earlier or family history of recurrent myalgia, pain and fever after exercise, and often caffeine intolerance. Muscle biopsy (creatine kinase assay), halothane/caffeine contraction tests are useful. Such susceptible patients should have trigger-free anaesthesia like barbiturates, benzodiazepines, propofol, ketamine, nitrous oxide, non-depolarising neuromuscular blockers). *Manifestations* usually develop *immediately* after administering the triggering drugs like tachycardia, arrhythmias, temperature, and muscle rigidity, inability to open the mouth with masseter spasm, tachypnoea, hypotension, and hyperthermia. *Treatment strategies* are—discontinuation of the surgery, stop and use alternate anaesthetic agent, dantrolene intravenously 2.5 mg/kg bolus and repeated once in 5 minutes until recovery, hyperventilation, surface cooling by different methods like tepid sponging of entire body, coolant usage, cool parenteral fluids, correction of acidosis, beta blockers, lignocaine injection, correction of hyperkalaemia, hypercalcaemia, hypercapnia, dialysis if needed, ICU care.

Postoperative Hypothermia

A 2°C drop in the core temperature causes hypothermia with metabolic derangements.

Causes of hypothermia are prolonged surgical procedure, transfusion, intravenous fluids, low room temperature (air condition), anaesthesia (propofol), and vascular phenomenon.

Effects of hypothermia—vasoconstriction, poor organ perfusion, arrhythmias, decreased coagulation function (risk of bleeding), altered macrophage action and sepsis, reduced oxygenation of tissues, poor healing, neurological disturbances, acid-base imbalance, poor cardiac and respiratory effort, bradycardia, coma. A temperature *below 35°C* is critical. Shivering with coldness is the initial presentation. Core temperature is *monitored* in pulmonary artery blood, tympanic membrane, oesophagus, pharynx, rectum and urinary bladder. Warm intravenous fluids, warmed clothes, humidifier/warmer, usage of warming device, covering of the head, humidifying inhalation gases, warm saline wash in surgical fields, rewarming infusion devices, rarely cardiopulmonary bypass are the *treatment plans.* Single dose hydrocortisone may be helpful.

Surgical Wound Complications

Seroma Formation

A seroma is a collection of liquefied fat, serum, lymph fluid in a closed surgical wound under the skin in subcutaneous plane and is clear, yellow and viscous. It is often seen after skin grafting, mastectomy, surgery in inguinal region, after lymph node dissections, after mesh placing surgery. Suction drains prevent seroma formation. Once seroma is formed, it is aspirated. If there is failure even after two times of aspiration, then open drainage is done. Often seroma can get infected when it should be drained and fluid should be sent for culture. When mesh is present underneath, it need not to be removed in every patient. Mesh should be removed only when there is resistant infection.

Flap Necrosis

Flap necrosis is common in surgeries like mastectomy, amputations, and different plastic surgeries **(Figs. 2-46A and B)**. Viable part should be allowed to separate from non-viable part so as to facilitate eventual debridement of the non-viable necrosed area. Further coverage of the area is done based on the extent of the flap necrosis and anatomical location. Additional flap reconstruction or skin grafting is used as options.

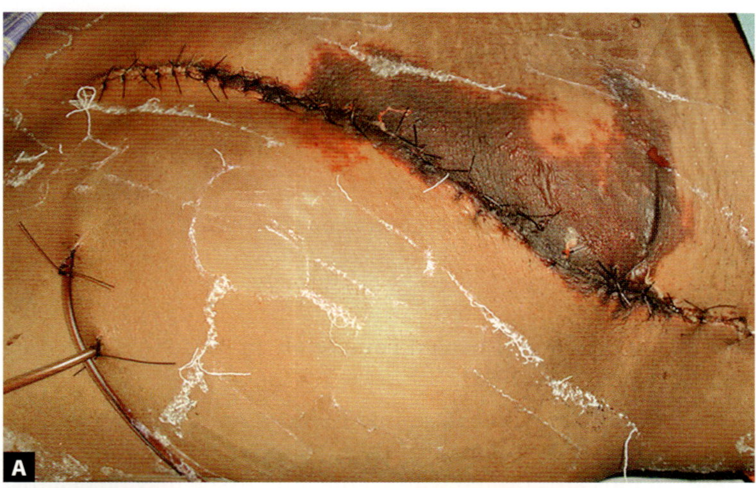

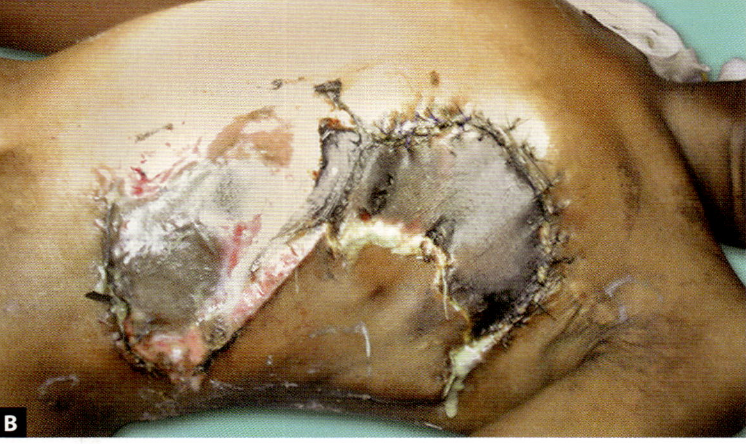

Figs. 2-46A and B: Postoperative flap necrosis.

Haematoma Formation

It is an abnormal collection of blood either under the wound (traumatic or surgical) or in a potential space developed pathologically or after surgery. It can occur in subcutaneous plane, in the muscle, deep to muscle or in cavities like in the abdomen, thorax or intracranially **(Fig. 2-47)**.

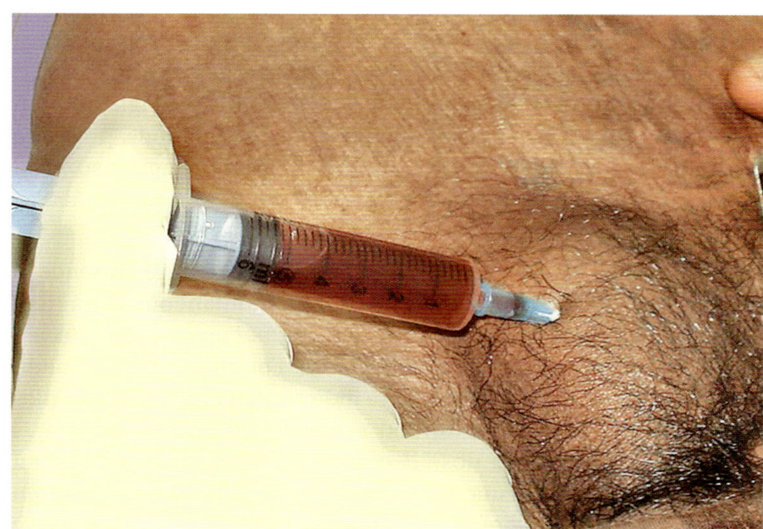

Fig. 2-47: Postoperative haematoma formation.

Causes: Inadequate haemostasis during surgery, slipping of ligatures, drug-induced (anticoagulants, aspirin, clopidogrel), depleted clotting factors.

Presentations: Pain, localised bluish or purple swelling, skin discolouration, tenderness often fluctuant. Large haematoma at different locations can cause different problems like airway obstruction in neck; paralytic ileus in the abdomen, features of raised intracranial tension in brain; respiratory distress in thorax, etc. Anaemia, DIC, sepsis are other problems. Often bleeding may not get controlled and may be life threatening especially in the cavities. It can get infected also.

Investigations: Haematoma is confirmed by ultrasound, aspiration or CT scan (inside cavities). Prothrombin time, partial thromboplastin time, platelet counts, haemoglobin estimation, are other needed evaluation methods.

Treatment: It should be treated by surgical drainage, correction of clotting factors. Patients on heparin therapy should stop the heparin 3 hours before surgery; low molecular weight heparin (LMWH) 15 hours before surgery; warfarin therapy 3 days before surgery; clopidogrel 6 days before surgery. International normalised ratio *(INR)* should be *less than 1.5* before surgery.

Surgical Site Infection

It may be (superficial) in skin and subcutaneous tissue; (deep) in fascia and muscles; internal cavities at the site of operation (organ space*). Superficial wound infection* will show purulent discharge with erythema, pain and oedema involving skin and subcutaneous infection in less than 30 days. *Deep wound infection* is purulent discharge from deeper plane, with clinical or sonological or radiological evidence of deeper abscess, fever, pain, tenderness or wound dehiscence through deeper plane in less than 30 days. *Organ space infection* is purulent discharge from a drain placed at organ space, bacteria cultured from fluid from organ space, confirmed abscess in organ space clinically or by evaluation methods with infection in less than 30 days without an implant or with infection less than one year with an implant. *Commonest bacteria* are group D *Enterococcus, Staphylococcus aureus,* and *Escherichia coli. Commonest time* of postoperative infection is 5–6 days postoperatively. 80% of infections occur within 30 days. *Factors related to surgical wound infection (Patient factors)*—old age, obesity, smoking, alcohol intake, ischaemia, poor blood supply, diabetes mellitus, anaemia, malnutrition, immunosuppression, steroid therapy, associated malignancy, hypoxia, hyperlipidaemia, radiotherapy site; *(Treatment/hospital factors)*—foreign body in the wound, improper sterilisation, poor asepsis methods, presence of drains, emergency surgery, surgery in sepsis, lengthy surgical procedure, nosocomial infection. Surgical wounds are classified as clean, clean contaminated and dirty **(Table 2-4)**.

Management of infection: Features of *infected wound* are presence of pus/infected fluid in the main wound, pus spontaneously draining from disrupted wound, fluid culture positive for bacteria. For infected wounds *therapeutic antibiotics* are given. For clean contaminated wounds preoperative antibiotics are indicated. It is given 30 minutes before surgery and is continued every 4 hours until surgery is over and later standard dose is continued. Only in certain clean surgical cases like mastectomy *prophylactic antibiotics* are given preoperatively; but it should be stopped in immediate postoperative period (usually antibiotics are not necessary in clean cases except in certain occasions) **(Figs. 2-48 to 2-51)**. Wound sutures are opened. Fluid/pus are drained. Fluid is sent for culture study (controversial). Open wound debridement is done and thorough warm saline wash is given. Wound is packed and dressed. Regular dressing is done until wound granulates well. Wound may close spontaneously by epithelialisation or scarring or may need secondary suturing or skin grafting if wound area is wide. Wound vacuum dressings are very useful in large, deep wounds **(Fig. 2-52)**. Use of drain in surgical wound is controversial. Closed suction drains in deep spaces are advised. In usual surgical wounds drain is not necessary.

TABLE 2-4: Surgical wounds—classification

Clean wound	*Clean contaminated*	*Contaminated*	*Dirty wound*
Primary closure of the wound	Primary closure of the wound	Open/traumatic wound	Open—suppurative wound
No hollow viscus injury	Controlled hollow viscus injury	Evidence of inflammation is present	Evidence of severe inflammation
No evidence of inflammation	No evidence of inflammation	Spillage of viscus is present—uncontrolled	Untreated, uncontrolled spillage of the content
Proper aseptic methods used	Mechanical drain usage	Infection rate—25%	Pus in the surgical field
Elective surgery	Infection rate—<8%		Infection rate—40%
Infection rate—<3%			

Prevention of surgical wound infections

- Proper aseptic care.
- Proper meticulous dissection, haemostasis, preservation of blood supply, gentle tissue handling.
- Proper wash, irrigation using warm saline.
- Avoiding foreign body in the wound, maintaining normal temperature.

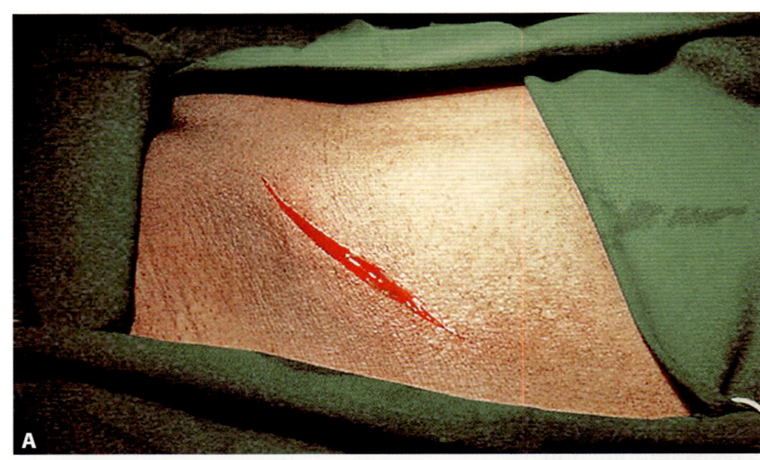

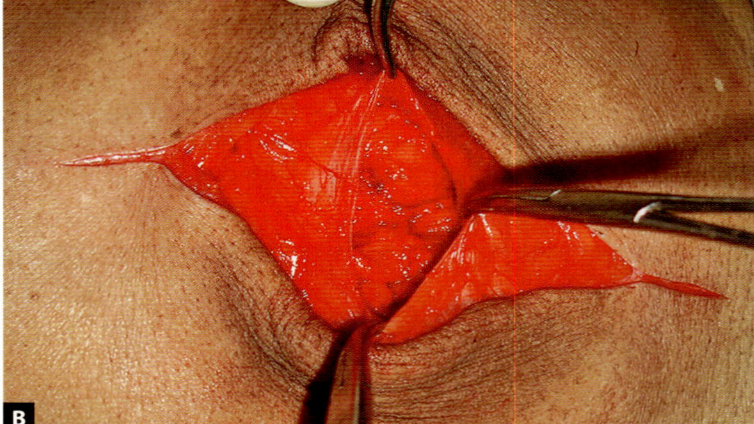

Figs. 2-48A and B: Clean wound (see Table 2-4).

Chronic Wound

A wound which is not healed completely in 30 days is called as chronic wound **(Fig. 2-53)**.

Causes: Debilitating illness, steroid therapy, immunosuppression, poorly nourished patients, obesity, malignancy, radiotherapy. These wounds are covered with granulation tissue may be healthy, unhealthy or exuberant. Once granulation tissue becomes healthy with clear discharge skin grafting is done to cover the defect. Often if area is not wide, then secondary suturing is done.

Wound Dehiscence

It is *acute wound failure* in postoperative period with separation of wound edges including *all layers.* For all practical purposes it is observed in abdominal wound and so it is synonymous with *burst abdomen/abdominal wound dehiscence* **(Fig. 2-54)**. It is sudden, rapid all layer wound giving way precipitated by severe cough or vomiting causing salmon coloured serosanguinous discharge. Intra-abdominal anastomotic leak has to be considered other than usual causes of wound sepsis. Under anaesthesia, thorough exploration of the contents is done. After warm saline wash, wound is closed

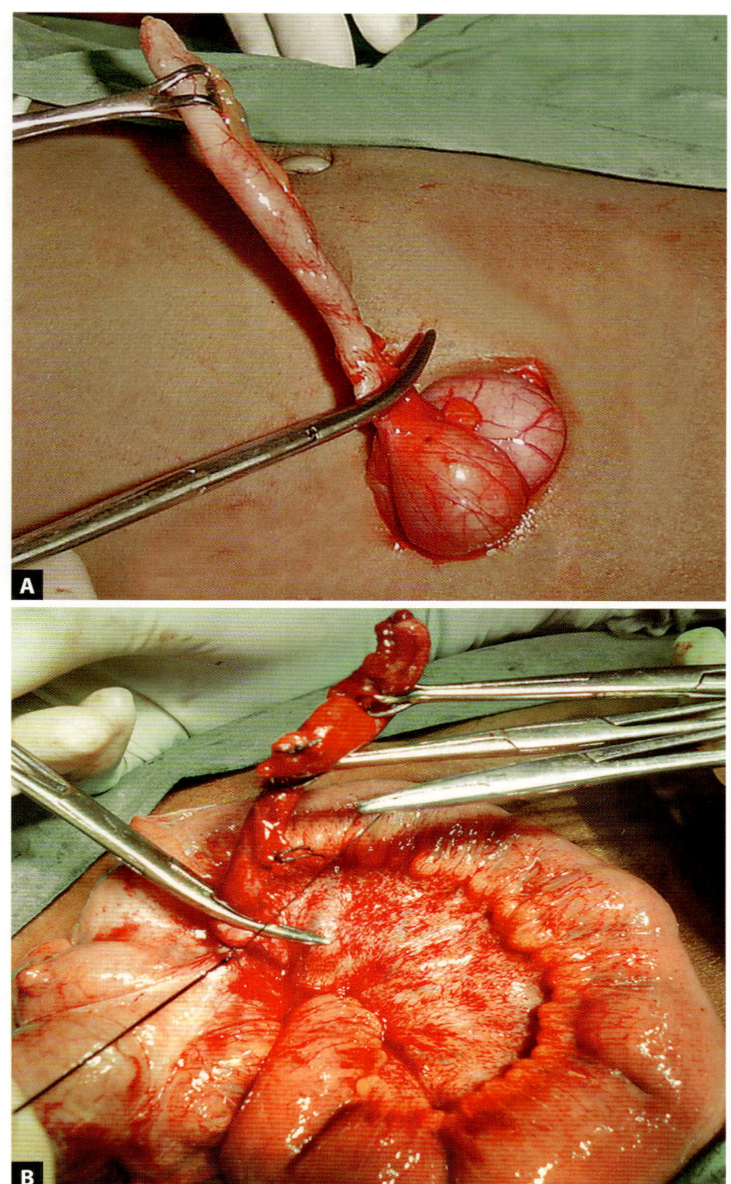

Figs. 2-49A and B: Clean contaminated wound (see Table 2-4).

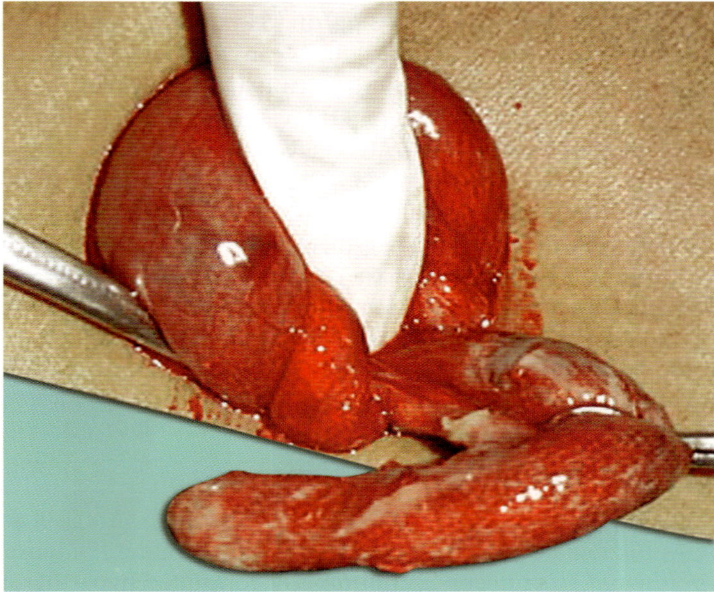

Fig. 2-50: Contaminated wound (see Table 2-4).

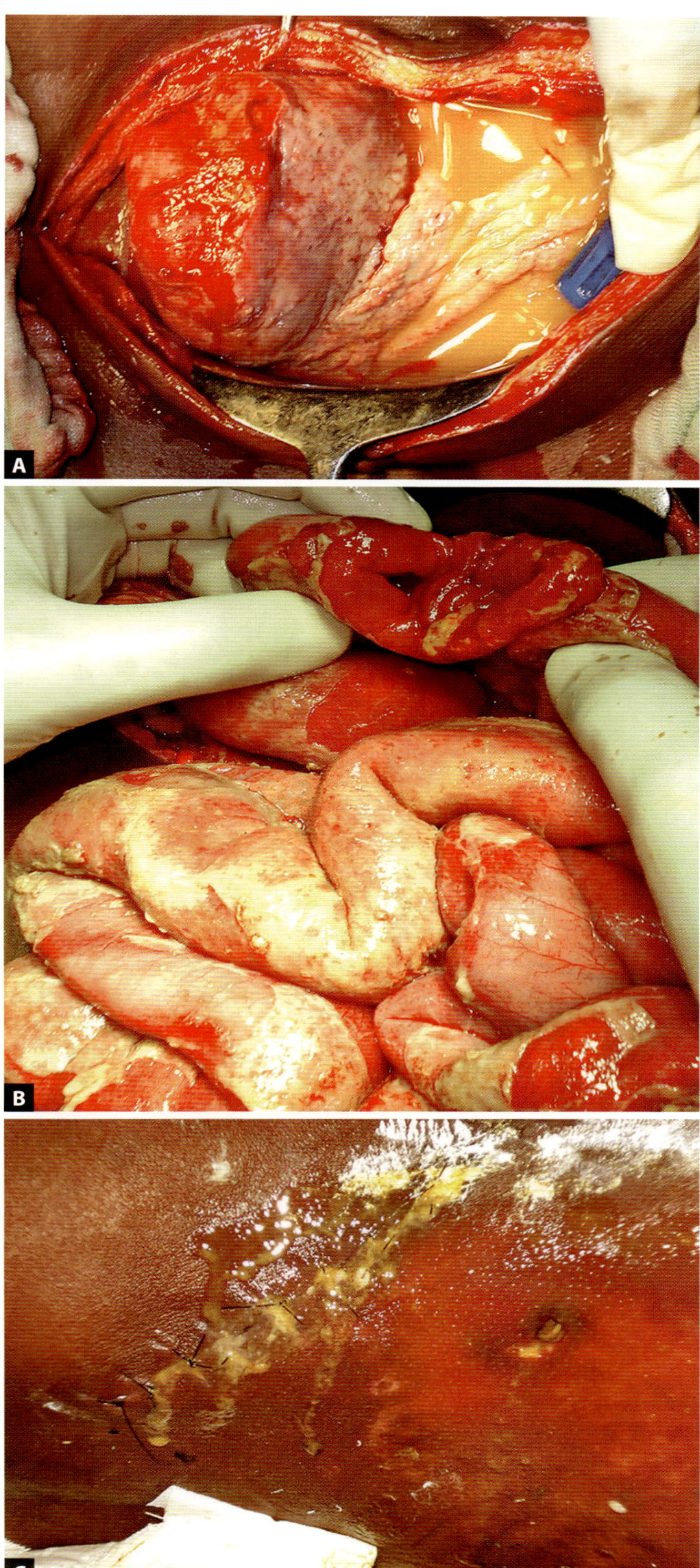

Figs. 2-51A to C: Dirty wound (see Table 2-4).

primarily with interrupted non-absorbable monofilament sutures or using absorbable mesh or biologic prosthesis (decellularised porcine submucosa/dermis or human cadaveric dermis). Wound vacuum system using cell foam, semiocclusive drape and suction over the wound can be very useful. It gives immediate cover to the contents;

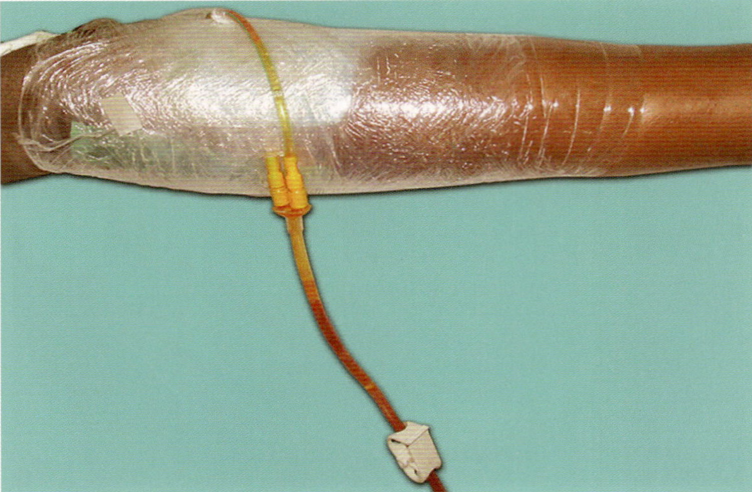

Fig. 2-52: Vacuum dressing.

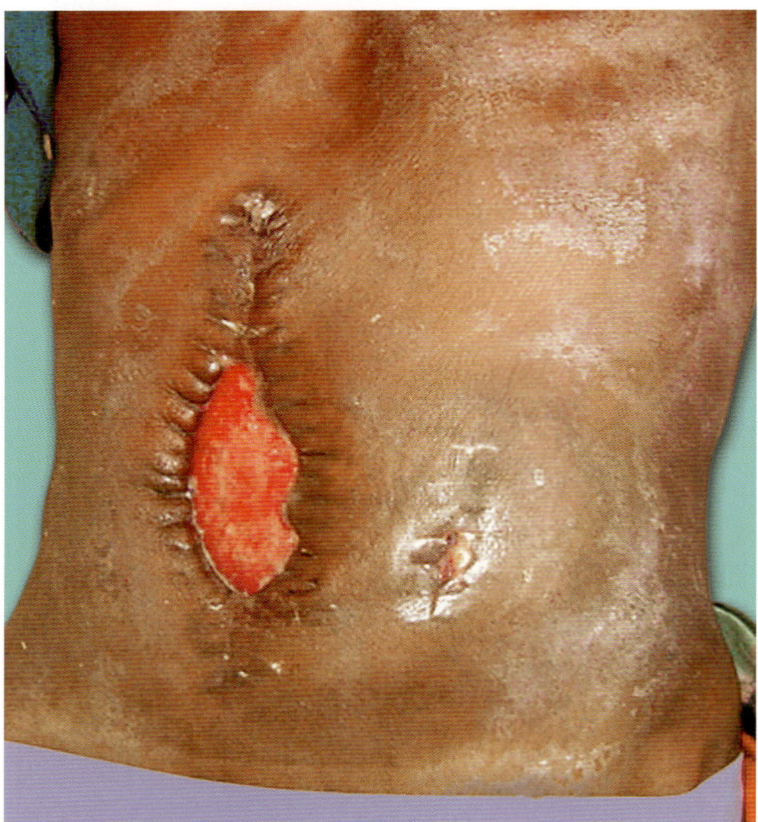

Fig. 2-53: Chronic wound.

removes the interstitial fluid, reduces the bowel oedema; increases the perfusion and healing; lessens the bacterial contamination. Intestinal fistulas, late hernia formation are the problems.

Adrenal Insufficiency

Acute Adrenal Insufficiency

Acute adrenal insufficiency in postoperative period may be due to destruction of gland by haemorrhage, necrosis, thrombosis which is secondary to sepsis, toxins, antiphospholipid syndrome or postpartum necrosis; critically ill patients; abrupt stopping of long-term steroid therapy; surgical adrenalectomy. Acute adrenal insufficiency is *difficult to diagnose* in a critically ill patients. Unexplained hypotension,

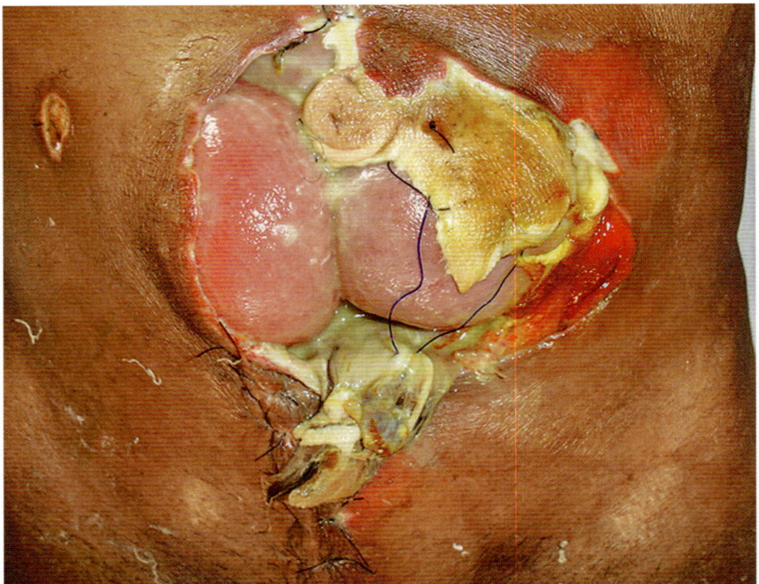

Fig. 2-54: Burst abdomen/acute wound failure/abdominal wound dehiscence.

haemodynamic instability, hyponatraemia not responding to normal saline, hypoglycaemia and uraemia persistent inflammation are the features. *Treatment* is high dose intravenous hydrocortisone or methylprednisolone, volume correction, correction of hyponatraemia. Sodium level *below* 120 mmol/L is dangerous.

Chronic Adrenal Insufficiency

Chronic adrenal insufficiency may be primary or secondary. *Primary* is due to primary adrenal gland destruction by autoimmune disease (Addison's disease). *Secondary* is due to diseases of hypothalamous or anterior pituitary or due to chronic use of steroids causing suppression of hypothalamo-pituitary-adrenal axis inducing adrenal atrophy. *Features*: Fatigue, weakness, anorexia, weight loss, diarrhoea, decreased libido, depression, dizziness hyponatraemia, hypoglycaemia, hyperkalaemia, acidosis. *Primary type* shows increased pigmentation of skin and mucous membrane due to elevated ACTH. *Secondary type* shows headache, visual disturbances, hypoadrenalism, and decreased ACTH level, loss of hair, pallor, hypothyroidism, oligomenorrhoea, and diabetes insipidus. Morning plasma cortisol level less than 3 μg/dL (83 mmol/L) is diagnostic (Normal is more than 19 μg/dL); between 3–19 is equivocal but suspicious of adrenal insufficiency; above 19 μg/dL rules out adrenal insufficiency. In primary type ACTH level in plasma is more than 100 pg/mL. In secondary type ACTH level is less. Aldosterone level in plasma may be reduced. *Rapid ACTH stimulation test* is useful. 250 μg cosynthropin is injected IV/IM and serum cortisol is measured in 60 minutes which will be 20 μg/dL or more in normal individual. If cortisol secretion is not increased then it is adrenal insufficiency. *Metyrapone test*: After oral administration of metyrapone, if there is insufficient increase in plasma 11-deoxycortisol and low plasma cortisol level (<8 μg/dL) then it is secondary adrenal insufficiency. Condition is treated by IV hydrocortisone and fludrocortisone.

Other Complications

Hyperthyroid Crisis or Hypothyroidism

Hyperthyroid crisis occurs in improperly controlled hyperthyroid patient undergoing surgery of thyroid or other surgery. It causes dehydration, shock, hyperthermia, hypotension, cardiac arrhythmias. It is treated in critical care unit with beta blockers, antithyroid drugs, hydrocortisone, tepid sponging, antipyretics, Lugol's iodine, digitoxin, fluid therapy, heparin, plasmapheresis, proper monitoring. *Hypothyroidism* is not rare and is equally dangerous in anaesthetised patient. It should be confirmed by assessing T3, T4 and TSH levels. It is treated with l thyroxin therapy.

Syndrome of Inappropriate ADH (SIADH) Secretion

It causes chronic normovolemic hyponatraemia (serum sodium less than 135 mmol/L). *ADH* is arginine vasopressin synthesised in hypothalamus transported to and stored in posterior pituitary; secretes into blood to regulate water excretion. ADH is secreted by thirst, nausea, hypoglycaemia, hypovolemia and drugs like ACE inhibitors, dopamine, NSAIDs. SIADH is caused by trauma, stroke, ADH producing tumour, drugs. *Features* are anorexia, lethargy, convulsions, hyponatraemia, hypotonic plasma, urine osmolality in excess of plasma osmolality, increased urinary sodium excretion, absence of oedema, normal kidney function. *Treatment:* Fluid restriction is the main therapy, IV normal saline in significant symptomatic SIADH (not to every patient), or acute SIADH of less than 3 days duration. Slow gradual correction is the principle as rapid correction of sodium level causes permanent neurological damage. Frusemide occasionally can be used.

Postoperative Convulsions

It could be *primary* related primary intracranial diseases like tumour/trauma/haemorrhage in the brain. It could be *secondary* due to electrolyte imbalance, metabolic derangements, sepsis, systemic diseases, MODS, hypoxia, hypoglycaemia, hypomagnesaemia, drugs. Intravenous diazepam or phenytoin sodium is used. In refractory cases gabapentin is used. Later patient is assessed with CT head and electroencephalogram.

Postoperative Stroke

It is due to either ischaemia (common) or haemorrhage. Ischaemia is due to hypotension, thrombosis or emboli from heart. Haemorrhagic stroke (less common) is due to bleeding disorders, hypertension and anticoagulants. Patient is evaluated with CT head, echocardiography and cardiac evaluation, blood analysis (bleeding time, clotting time, prothrombin time and platelet count), carotid angiogram (CT angiogram). It is managed with the help of cardiologists and neurologists using mannitol, dexamethasone, anticonvulsants, cardiac management, thrombolytics.

Postoperative Epistaxis

It may be due to blood dyscrasias, anticoagulants, hypertension and trauma during intubation (nasal) or during insertion of nasogastric tube. *Anterior epistaxis* is due to septum and turbinates and is commonly due to tubes. It is controlled by pressure using thumb and fingers or packing using gauze. Posterior nasal bleeding (*posterior epistaxis*) is more dangerous and is torrential; difficult to manage. It needs posterior nasal packing; Foley's catheter insertion per nostril and inflating balloon with 30 mL distilled water to cause tamponade for 3–5 days; blood transfusions; occasionally ligation of sphenopalatine and ethmoidal arteries is needed.

Postoperative Sinusitis

Postoperative sinusitis commonly involving the maxillary sinus is of nosocomial origin mainly due to *Staphylococcus aureus* and *Pseudomonas* bacteria. It is also common in patients with ventilator. It is often dangerous as it may lead into life-threatening postoperative pneumonia or brain abscess. Purulent nasal discharge, facial pain (if patient is awake), fever are the features. CT sinus and discharge study confirms the diagnosis. Proper antibiotics, often sinus drainage are the treatment needed.

Postoperative Parotitis

Postoperative parotitis is not an uncommon entity especially in elderly postoperative patients in diabetic and in immunosuppressed patients. Pain, tenderness, diffuse swelling, trismus, stridor due to airway obstruction, oedema of floor of the mouth, dysphagia are the features. Often it can cause toxaemia and septicaemia. Once abscess forms it needs proper incision and drainage through proper incision under general anaesthesia. Tracheostomy is often a need.

Intensive Care in Surgery

A critically ill patient is one who has life-threatening illness or injury with one or more failing organs, essentially needing intensive care support **(Figs. 2-55A and B)**.

Mortality is 50% if there are two organ failures; 85% if there are three organ failures; near 100% if there are four organ failures.

Monitoring

Arterial Blood Pressure

Non-invasive measurement of blood pressure is commonly done using either manual cuff or automated device. Measurement by invasive direct intra-arterial blood pressure is done by placing a cannula into the artery (radial artery) and connecting to a pressure transducer to record every beat accurate blood pressure. Intra-arterial cannulation can cause complications like haematoma, thrombosis of artery, infection, bleeding, arteriovenous fistula and pseudoaneurysm.

Monitoring Heart Rate, Respiratory Rate and Temperature

Heart rate and respiratory rate are assessed through monitor in the intensive care unit (ICU). Temperature is assessed by placing the thermometer in the axilla. Special temperature monitoring devices are also available. Continuous ECG monitoring gives heart rate (above 100 is tachycardia; below 60 is bradycardia). Lead II is used to assess P wave. Chest leads are used to assess infarction and dysrhythmias.

Central Venous Pressure

It is a method to measure the right atrial pressure by placing a venous catheter (20 cm) into the superior vena cava (SVC). Commonly for central venous pressure (CVP) monitoring, a venous catheter is passed through right internal jugular vein or infraclavicular subclavian vein to the SVC (used for TPN purpose). Or occasionally a long catheter (60 cm) can be passed through basilic vein (not commonly done). Under radiological guidance, initially a needle

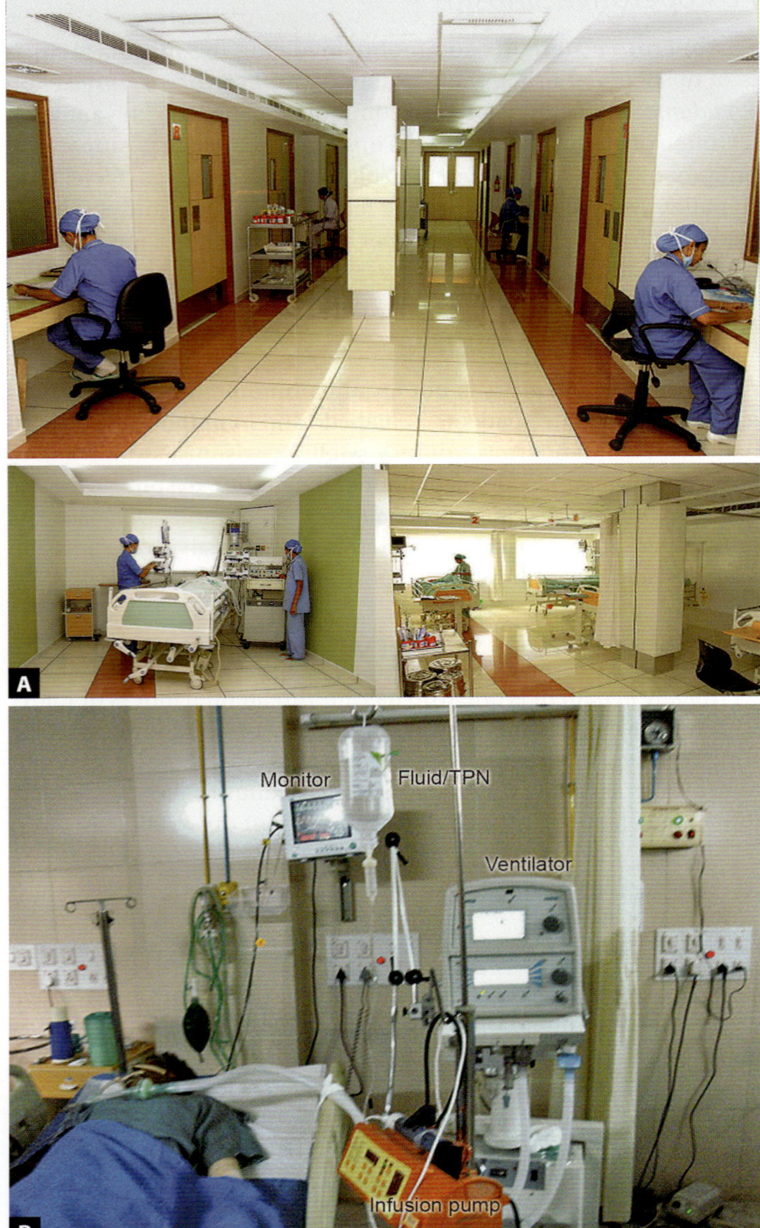

Figs. 2-55A and B: Intensive care unit showing ICU bed with facilities. *Courtesy:* Unity health complex, Mangaluru.

is passed 3 cm above the medial end of the clavicle, in the hollow between the two heads of sternomastoid muscles, directing towards the suprasternal notch into the right internal jugular vein. Then through a guidewire, a venous catheter is passed into the SVC through right internal jugular vein, which can also be confirmed by changes in flow during inspiration and expiration. Catheter is connected to saline manometer, taking manubriosternal angle (*angle of Louis*) as zero point. Normal value is 2–10 cm of water/ 0–4 mmHg. CVP has got a, c and v upwards waves; x and y downwards waves. *'a'* is atrial contraction (absent in atrial fibrillation); *'c'* is tricuspid valve bulging during ventricular contraction; *'x'* is atrial relaxation; *'v'* is atrial filling; *'y'* is tricuspid valve opening and ventricular filling. If less than 2 cm, more fluid is infused. If more than 10 cm, fluid infusion should be restricted. Right atrial pressure is directly related to ventricular end-diastolic pressure, i.e. filling pressure of right ventricle which is directly related to ventricular end

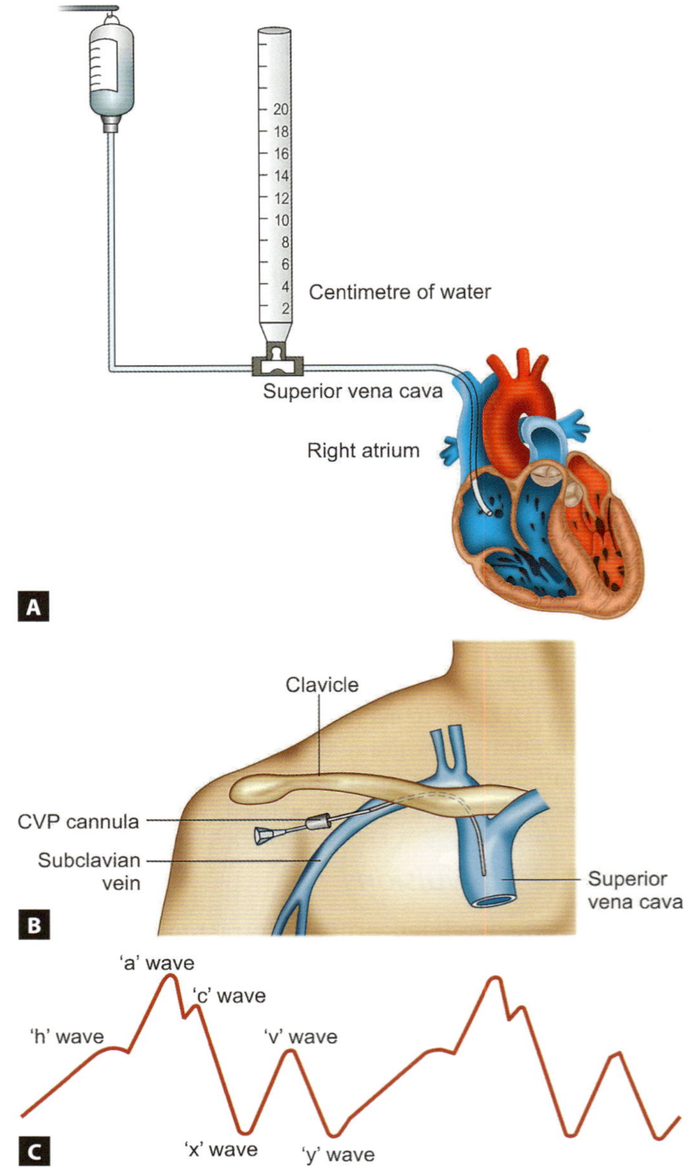

Figs. 2-56A to C: Central venous pressure (CVP) is used to monitor the patient. Note the location of the central venous catheter. Note the CVP wave pattern.

diastolic volume, i. e. evidence of overall volume of fluid in the body. *CVP monitoring is used* for fluid resuscitation in shock, patients with hypotension of any cause; for multiple drug therapy; for TPN. CVP is a useful indicator of cardiac filling if both right and left ventricles are functioning equally well. In ischaemic heart disease, cardiomyopathies, cardiac valvular disease left ventricular function is affected. In pulmonary hypertension right ventricular function is affected. Response to bolus of 500 mL fluid administration shows transient rise with a fall of central venous pressure which suggests low circulating volume **(Figs. 2-56A to C)**.

Complications of CVP: Pneumothorax; haemothorax; injury to brachial plexus and vessels; bleeding; sepsis; air embolism; catheter erosion into bronchus, right atrium; catheter displacement.

Pulmonary Capillary Wedge Pressure

It is a better indicator of circulating blood volume and left ventricular function. Catheter used *is Swan Ganz* triple channel pulmonary artery balloon catheter. It is used to differentiate right and left ventricular failure, pulmonary embolus and septic shock; to measure cardiac output, to monitor fluid therapy, inotropic agents and vasodilators. **Procedure:** Under strict aseptic precaution, using cannula and guidewire, catheter is passed through internal jugular vein, into the right atrium. Balloon is inflated by 1.5 mL of air and then negotiated into pulmonary artery, until it reaches a small branch and wedges it. Pressure at this point is called as *pulmonary capillary wedge pressure (PCWP). PCWP* normally is 8–12 mmHg, considering midaxillary point as zero reference point. After that balloon is deflated to get pulmonary artery pressure which is normally 25 mmHg systolic and 10 mm Hg diastolic. PCWP catheter can be kept *in situ* only for 72 hours. PCWP gives left atrial pressure and filling pressure of left ventricle. Present pulmonary artery floatation catheter (PAFC) has got a lumen at superior vena cava or right atrium to give CVP also **(Fig. 2-57)**.

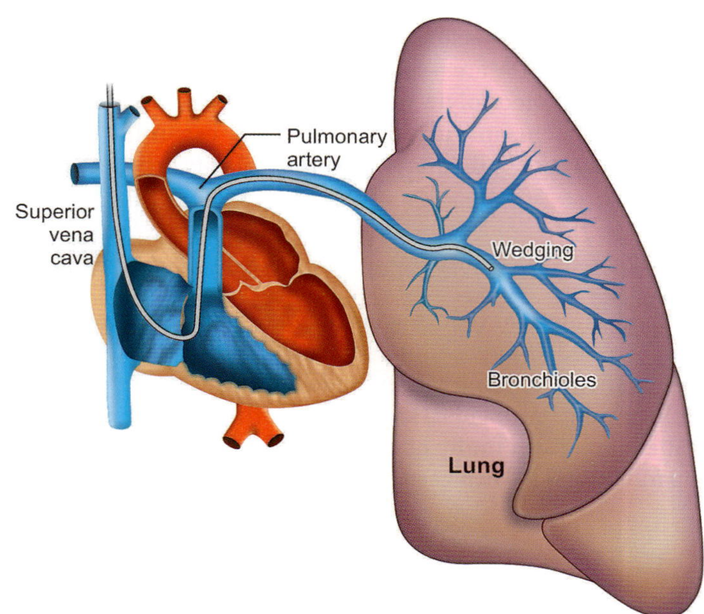

Fig. 2-57: Pulmonary capillary wedge pressure (PCWP) is better index of shock. But it is technically difficult and cannot be kept for more than 72 hours. It cannot be used for perfusion purpose unlike CVP line.

Complications of PCWP: Arrhythmias; heart block; pulmonary artery thrombosis; pulmonary artery rupture; balloon rupture; pulmonary infarction; pneumothorax; haemothorax; bleeding; sepsis; thrombosis.

Arterial Oxygen Saturation Measurement

Pulse oximeter gives continuous reading of the oxygen saturation which is placed on the pulp of the finger. It is by using diode light probe having two wavelengths—red band of 660 nm for reduced haemoglobin; infrared band of 940 nm for oxygenated haemoglobin. Difference in absorbance of both gives saturation. It is easier rapid way of assessing the oxygen saturation. *Limitations of pulse oximeter* are—it is not accurate once saturation is below 70%; vasoconstriction, hypovolaemia, hypothermia, drugs, carboxyhaemoglobin, shivering, improper positioning will give false values.

Arterial Blood Gas Analysis

It is ideal way of assessing the metabolic or hypoxic or oxygenation status. It includes pH (7.30–7.44); PCO_2 (35–45 mmHg); PaO_2 (75–100 mmHg); PAO_2 (alveolar partial pressure of oxygen); CO_2 concentration (TCO_2 24–28 mmHg); bicarbonate estimation (22–26 mmol/L); O_2 saturation (95%) and temperature. Normal capnograph shows initial steep upstroke (sudden increase in CO_2 in expired gas); slow raising plateau (suggests alveolar emptying); a rapid fall (during inspiration). 6th hourly ABG analysis is needed in critical patient.

Core Temperature Assessment

Core temperature is measured by placing thermometer in oesophagus or rectum or at tympanic membrane. Rectal temperature is 0.5°C more than oesophageal temperature. Temperature below 35°C cannot be measured with standard thermometers but needs low reading thermometers.

Urine Output Measurement

Hourly urine output should be measured. It should be more than 1.0 mL/kg/hour which indicates good cardiac output. Urine output less than 0.5 mL/kg/hour indicates poor cardiac output.

Cardiac Monitoring

Continuous cardiac monitoring is essential. It indicates rhythm changes, rate, wave forms, etc.

Other Assessments

Assessment of blood urea, serum creatinine, serum electrolytes, urinary electrolytes, urinary urea and creatinine. In *prerenal failure* urinary sodium is less than 10 mmol/L. Urinary urea and serum urea ratio is 10:1. It is more than this when there is inability to concentrate urine. Assessment of liver function, *coagulation profiles* (bleeding time—BT, clotting time—CT, prothrombin time—PT, activated partial thromboplastin time—APTT, thrombin time—TT, fibrin degradation products—FDP, D dimer assay, platelet count) are also important. Total count may be increased in sepsis but it is a poor indicator as it may not be raised in cold septic shock. Neutrophil count is more reliable. Intracranial pressure monitoring (ICP) is ideal in patient with head injury, with encephalopathy using invasive ICP bolts. Acidosis/alkalosis should be assessed.

Scoring of Illness

Therapeutic intervention scoring system *(TISS)* is used. Scoring is between 1–4. More the score means more intervention is needed and worse outcome. Acute physiology assessment and chronic health evaluation (APACHE) is another scoring system used in places. APACHE 3 is the present version used. Acute physiology score (APS) is also used with 34 parameters and each having 0–4 grading.

ICU Management

Fluid Management

Initially it is with crystalloids like normal saline or Ringer lactate; later by colloids, blood. It is decided at regular intervals in individual patients in individual diseases.

Inotropic Agents

Inotropic agents like dopamine, dobutamine, adrenaline, noradrenaline or isoprenaline are used in hypotension and altered cardiac status. *Dopamine* is given as 2 to 5 μg/kg/minute (low dose) in oliguria to improve urine output as it causes renal and splanchnic *vasodilatation*. Moderate dose of 5–10 μg/kg/minute is *inotropic* through β1 receptors of the heart. High dose of more than 10 μg/kg/minute causes peripheral *vasoconstriction* through α1 receptors. Dopamine is mainly used in septic shock. *Dobutamine* has mainly inotropic effect on heart without vasodilatation or vasoconstriction effects. Dobutamine is mainly used in cardiogenic shock.

Management of Respiration

It is the second most important aspect in ICU. Respiration should be assessed for existing problems. Endotracheal intubation, tracheostomy, management of ARDS, placement of intercostals tube when needed, assessment of respiratory failure, antibiotic therapies are important. Laryngoscopes, endotracheal tubes, Magill's forceps, fibreoptic intubation set, CO_2 detector should be available in ICU. If initial oxygen therapy is not adequate, then artificial ventilation is started using endotracheal intubation. Tracheostomy *is ideal* if prolonged ventilation is needed (more than 7 days). Problems with these tubes are—infection, bleeding, blockage and causing crisis, disconnection, acute gastric dilatation.

Management of renal failure, hyperkalaemia, acidosis, electrolyte derangements as required. Often haemodialysis may be needed.

Nutritional Support

Polymeric diet (proteins, glucose, triglycerides) or elemental diet (free amino acids, glucose, fat-soluble medium and long chain fatty acids) or disease specific diet are given. Patients on ventilator are given low carbohydrates, proteins and high fat diet. Patients with hepatic encephalopathy are given more branched chain amino acids with less aromatic amino acids. Enteral nutrition *is ideal* either orally or through nasogastric tube or through gastrostomy or jejunostomy. *Total parenteral nutrition (TPN)* is used *when needed*—poor GI absorption; acute pancreatitis; severely malnourished and catabolic patients; when oral food/enteral nutrition cannot be given for 10 days; GI fistulas. TPN is given through central vein like subclavian or internal jugular vein. ***Harris Benedict equation*** is used to calculate the required calorie [For men = 66 + (113.7 × weight in kg) + (5 × height in cm) – (6.8 × age in years). For women = 655 + (9.6 × weight in kg) + (1.8 × height in cm) – (4.7 × age in years)]. 60% of total calorie needed is provided from glucose and 40% of calorie is from fat. Protein is given to maintain the nitrogen to calorie ratio as 1:150. TPN fluids contain 20% dextrose, 20% fat in emulsion; 20% amino acids, electrolytes, vitamins, trace elements. *Complications of TPN* are—catheter displacement, sepsis, bleeding, pneumothorax, electrolyte imbalance, trace element deficiency (zinc, copper, chromium and selenium), essential fatty acid deficiency, biotin deficiency, hyperosmolarity, catheter block, cholestasis.

Other Supportive Methods

Often neuromuscular blocking agents may be required to paralyse the patient. Sedation is commonly used to reduce anxiety, reduce oxygen demand, to improve ventilation. Analgesics are often given to reduce pain. Antacids/H2 blockers/proton pump inhibitors/sucralfate are given orally or parenteral (H2 blockers and proton pump inhibitors) to keep gastric pH above 4.

3

CHAPTER

Basic Principles of Incision, Dissection, Suturing and Haemostasis

PRINCIPLES OF INCISION

Holding the Instruments

Surgical instruments are essential armamentarium for proper surgery. Instruments are held in two ways. *Better method* is by *fingertip pressure* wherein thumb and ring fingers are placed in finger bows of the instrument. Precise fine relaxed movements are essential for proper work up of the instruments. Bizarre hurried movements will not give precision. *Second method* of holding the instruments is tight *vise like grip* using fist of the hand. It gives a good grip but precision may not be adequate. Surgical trainee to begin with prefers this method as he thinks that grip is essential part in holding the instrument. Even though this method may be useful in some situations, it is ideal to use the method of fingertip pressure and practice it for eventual smooth precise work **(Figs. 3-1A and B)**. Middle finger of the surgeon is kept behind the handle and index finger is extended along the length of the handle. It is said that slow, definitive, precise and non-repetitive movements actually gives faster surgery than haphazard, frenzied, rapid movements (Please refer Chapter 5—Instruments for details about each instruments).

Surgeon should be like *an artist* (creative/innovative worker) *not just an artisan* (skilled worker).

One should remember that surgeon *risks the lives* of others daily and so optimum *efficiency* is needed in him. Both sin of commission or sin of omission should be avoided as much as possible.

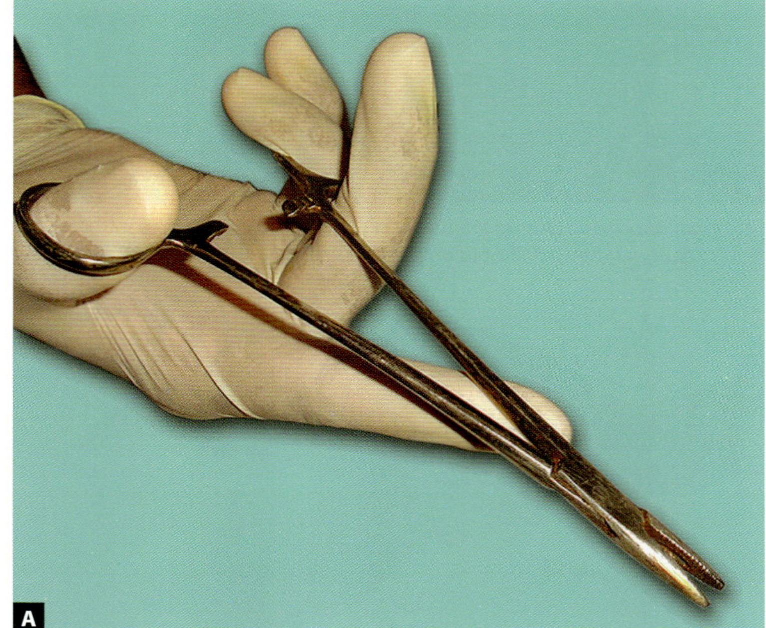

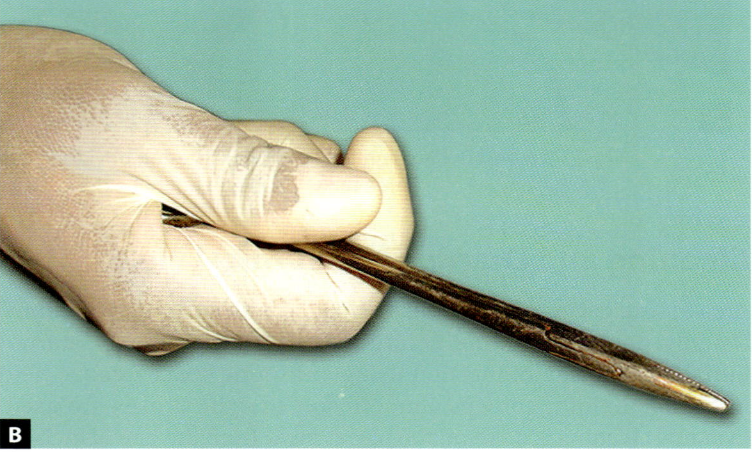

Figs. 3-1A and B: Holding needle holder by fingertip pressure (ideal) and also by tight vise grip (acceptable method).

Anaesthesia and Positioning of the Patient

Surgeon or assistant should be present beside the patient while giving anaesthesia even though it is commonly not followed. Once anaesthesia is given, proper positioning of the patient depending on the surgery which he does should be done by surgeon itself. For example, proper positioning for thyroidectomy, nephrectomy, sympathectomy, laparoscopic surgeries should be done and confirmed by the surgeon himself as it is important to have a proper position while operating **(Figs. 3-2A to C)**. Surgeon should be physically and mentally comfortable while operating.

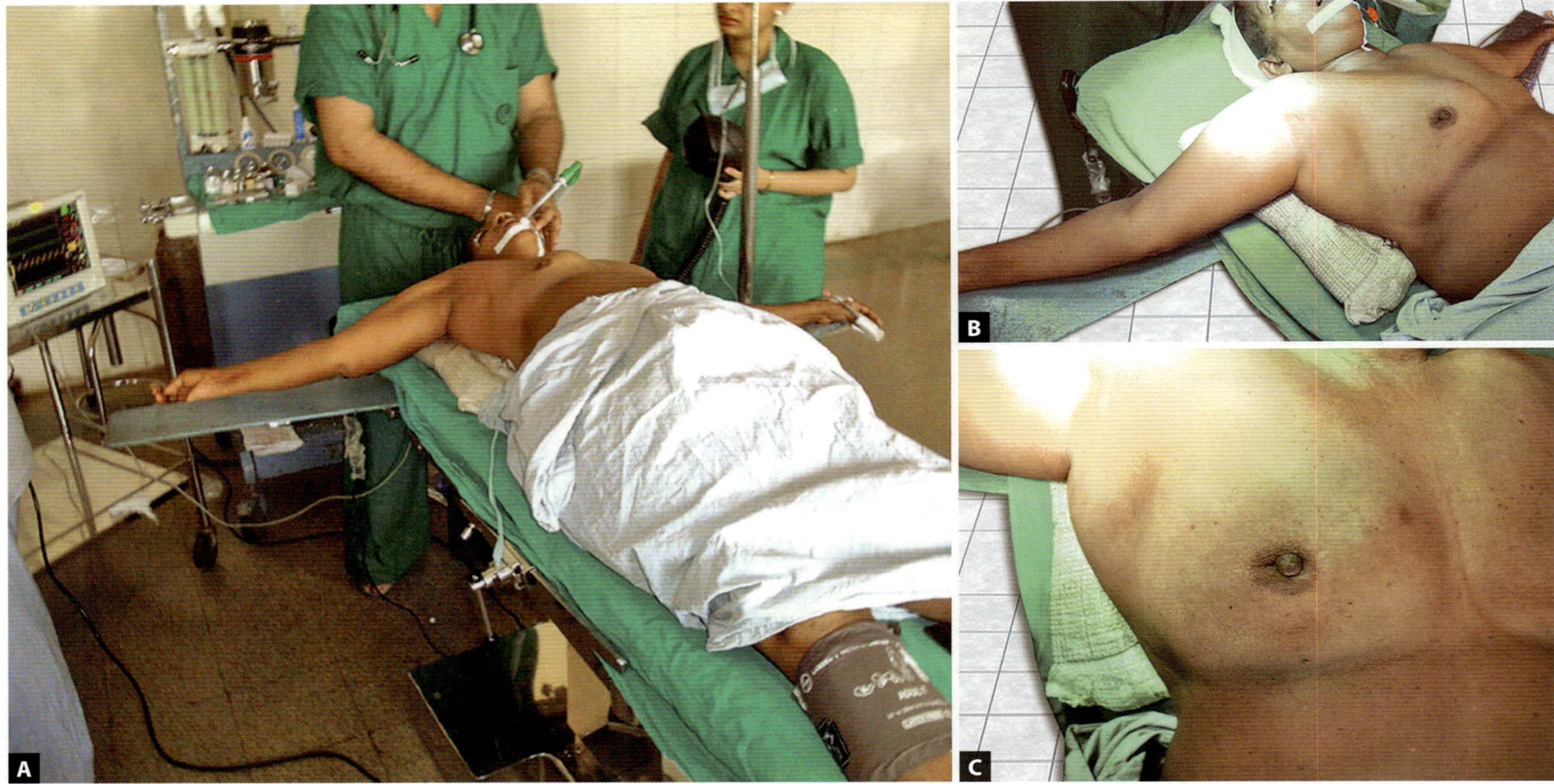

Figs. 3-2A to C: During anaesthesia surgeon should be present beside the patient. After anaesthetist gives permission positioning of the patient done. Surgeon himself should do the positioning. He should be fully satisfied with the position of the patient. Proper positioning makes surgery easier.

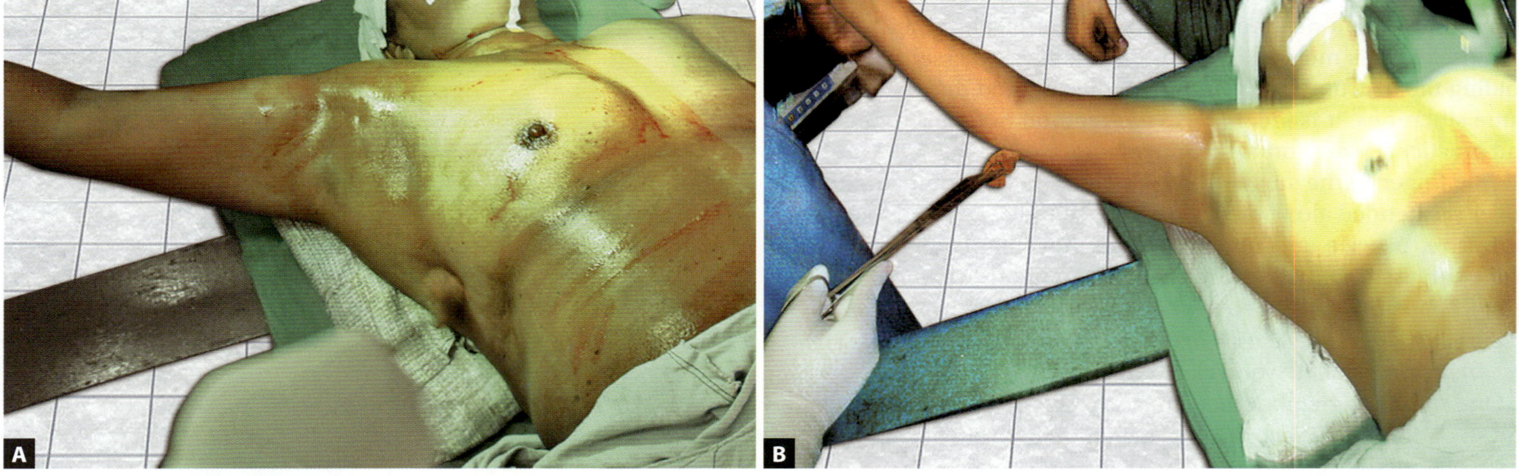

Figs. 3-3A and B: Cleaning the surgical field using povidone iodine. It is cleaned first at the site of incision; later outer area of the field. Three times cleaning should be done. Last one is used to clean mainly at the site of incision.

Cleaning and Draping the Surgical Field

Area of surgical incision should be cleaned with antiseptic solutions. Usually povidone iodine solution is used. Cleaning is started initially at the site of incision using antiseptic soaked gauze held in sponge holding forceps. Smooth soft straight strokes are used. Eventual cleaning is done on the places away from the line of incision on either side. Adequate wider area should be cleaned. Usually cleaning is done two times. Often two separate antiseptics are used each time like povidone iodine first and surgical spirit next **(Figs. 3-3A and B)**. It is matter of surgeon's choice than any standard. Care should be taken while cleaning crevices like umbilicus or skin folds. After cleaning, draping is done using sterile surgical towels. Towels of different colours are used—green/blue/violet, etc. Green is the commonly preferred colour. Sterile disposable plastic sticking sheets (*adhesive plastic drapes*) are also used in deeper part of the towel. Often incising area is covered with such sterile sticking plastic sheets and incision is made through this plastic **(Figs. 3-4A to C)**. All these different methods are used to prevent sepsis. Towel clips are used in the corners to hold the drapes.

Making the Incision

Ideally incision should be marked using sterile marking ink. Its length, type, placing should be decided depending on the proposed surgical technique **(Fig. 3-5)**. Scalpel is used to make the incision. Depth control is better when belly of the scalpel is used.

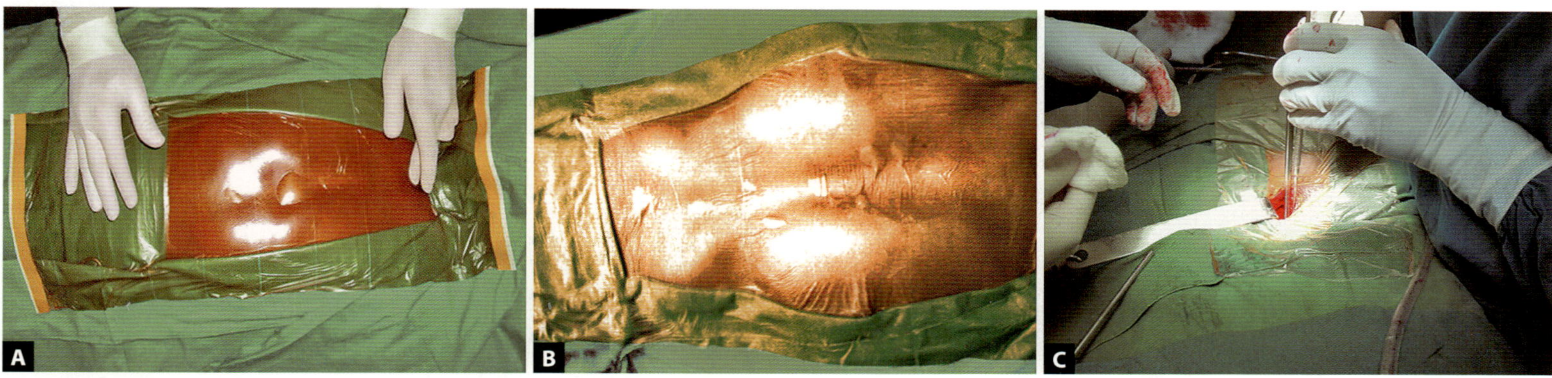

Figs. 3-4A to C: Draping is important to reduce infection. Adhesive plastic drapes are ideal. Incision is made through it. Photographs show draping at abdomen, thorax, and back (spine).

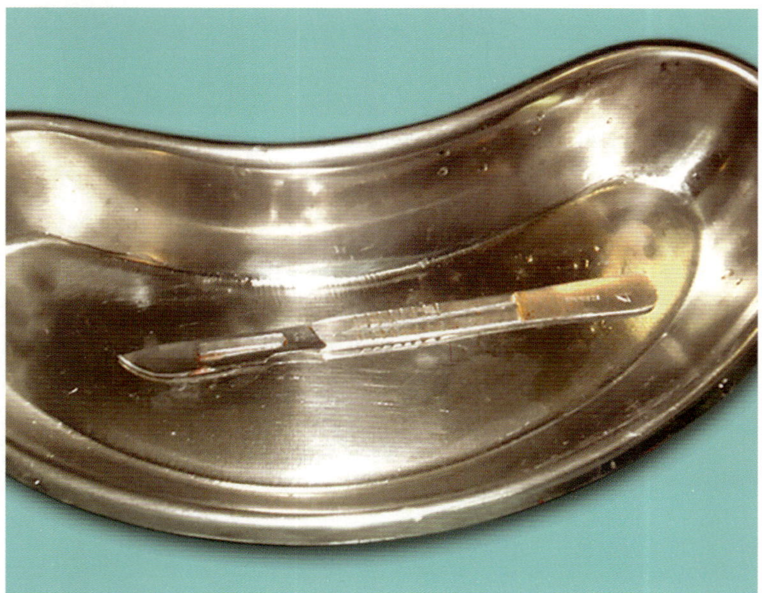

Fig. 3-5: Knife with blade should be given to the surgeon in a kidney tray. Same should be returned to scrub nurse. It should not be kept over the patient. It should be kept only in a kidney tray on an instrument trolley.

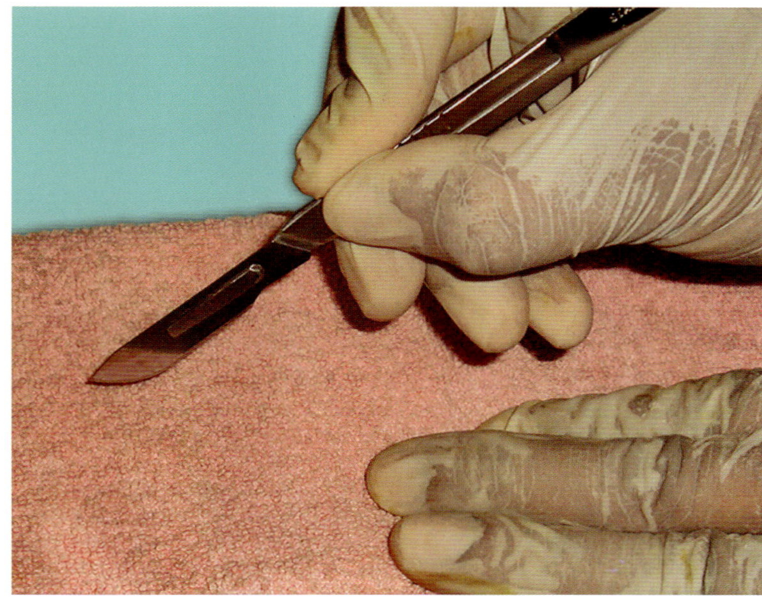

Fig. 3-7: Pen holding position.

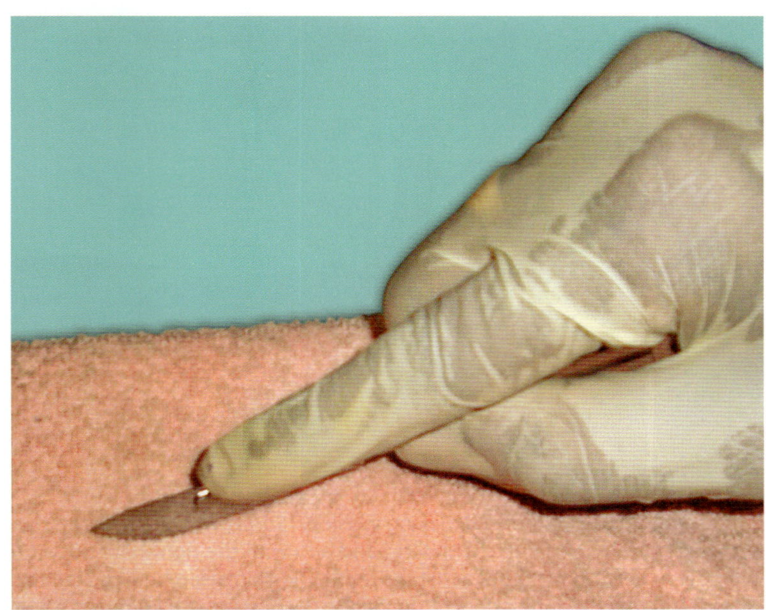

Fig. 3-6: Dinner knife position.

- *Dinner knife position* is used while making lengthy incision. Sustained pressure by the index finger over the knife with depth control is the technique **(Fig. 3-6)**.
- *Pen holding/writing position* is used to make incision over the vessels/nerves/tumours. Skin flap or tissues without natural plane can be dissected using this method **(Fig. 3-7)**.
- *Fiddle bow position* is used to make incisions with less pressure on delicate tissues. It is with least pressure, fine dissection is done with firm grip **(Figs. 3-8A and B)**.
- *Stab position of the knife* is used in draining an abscess or making an incision to pass drains. No. 11 blade is usually used **(Fig. 3-9)**.
- *Grasping position* is used to make long sweeping cuts.

Incision should be in a single stroke cutting both skin and subcutaneous tissues. Repeated superficial flimsy strokes should be avoided. Once adequate incision is made small bleeders in the cut edges of the incision is cauterised using coagulation current. Many bleeding points stop spontaneously by pressure. Further incision is carried out with scalpel or cutting cautery. Cutting cautery transects the fat and tissues precisely but only partially haemostatic

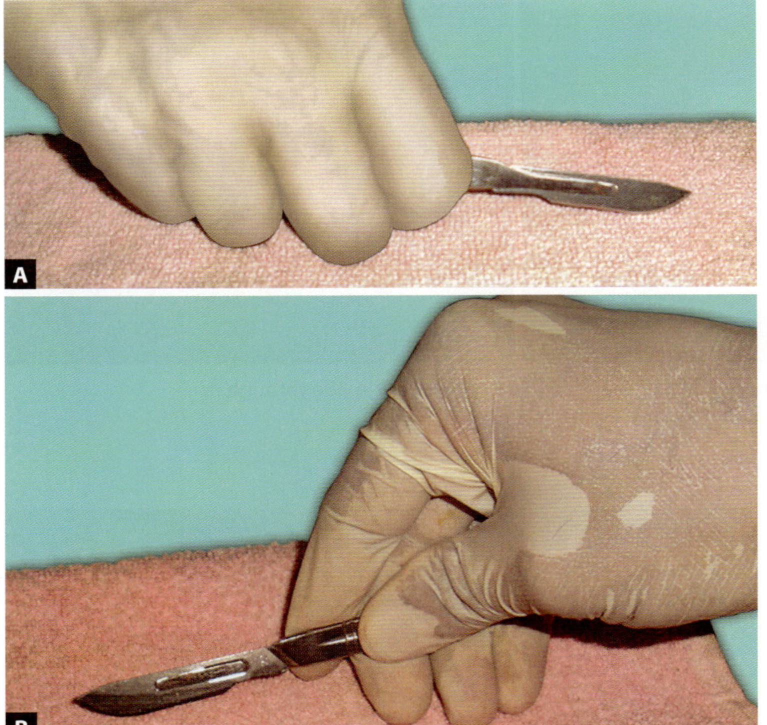

Figs. 3-8A and B: Fiddle bow position.

Fig. 3-9: Stab position of knife for drainage of an abscess.

Principles in making incision (Figs. 3-10A and B)

- Incision should be planned well prior to surgery for adequacy, for possible need for extension during course of the surgery, and indeed be cosmetically acceptable. Ideally incision site should be marked using sterile marker or methylene blue.
- Incision is done to access the deeper structure. It should be done parallel to crease lines. It should not cross across flexor aspects of the joints.
- It should be planned in such a way that scars are cosmetically accepted.
- Clean single stroke firm incision should be made with required depth. Repeated strokes and movements should be avoided. Blade should be at right angle to the surface.
- Knife should be perpendicular to skin to begin with blade pointing perpendicular to skin. But later blade should be parallel with curvature/belly of the blade on the site of the incision.
- While making lengthy incision like in abdomen, incision area should be stretched between thumb and index fingers of the other hand of surgeon.
- Another method is—using the fingers of left hand with the gauze, one lateral part of the marked incision line is held with traction; opposite side is similarly held by the assistant; deep stroke incision is placed using belly of the scalpel (22), cutting full thickness of skin and subcutaneous tissue, extending into the entire proposed length of the line of incision. It is commonly used in the abdomen.
- While making incisions care should be taken to avoid injuries to deeper structures like muscle/nerves/vessels/bowel.
- Patient should be symmetrically lying down on the operating table.
- In the abdomen with a previous laparotomy scar, present incision should be at a newer site. If skin is incised over the same scar, often excision of scar is needed. Dissection in the deeper plane and opening of the peritoneum should be started at fresh site so as to prevent injuries to deeper contents like bowel.
- Length of the incision should be adequate. There is no point in struggling in small holed blind surgeries.
- During surgery, if need arises, one should not hesitate to extend the incision.
- Use of diathermy in skin incision is controversial although cutting diathermy is used for this purpose. Thermal injury of the skin may result in poor scar.
- Incision should be parallel to natural lines/Langer lines/hair lines/eyebrow.

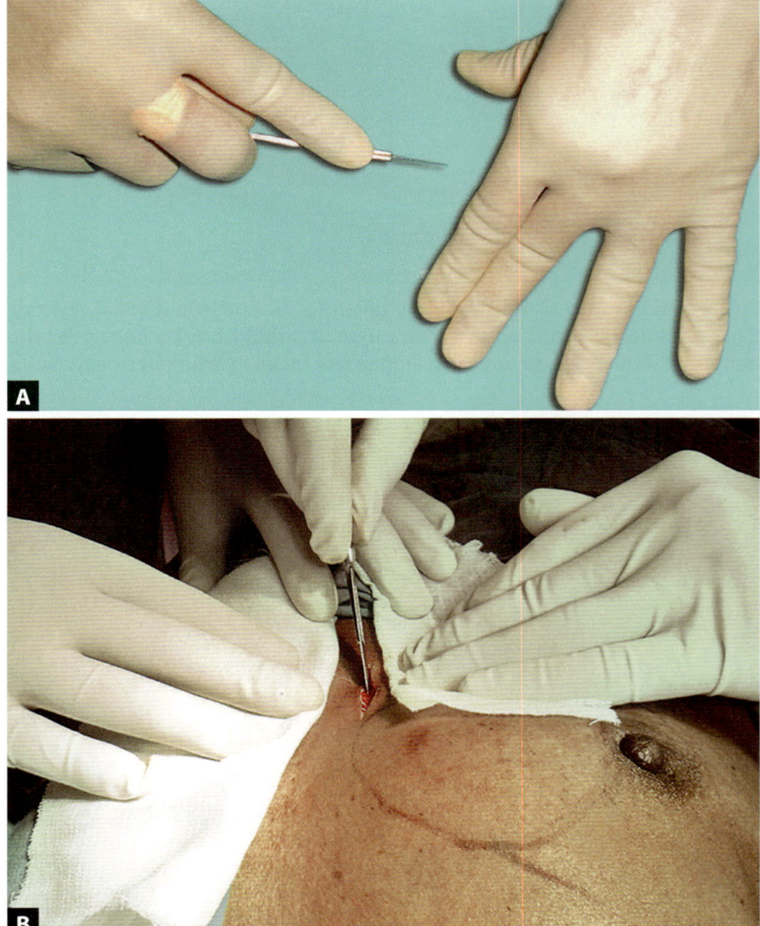

Figs. 3-10A and B: Methods of making incisions. Surgeon can stretch the skin between thumb and fingers with left hand and with the right-hand incision is made. In second method, assistant holds the skin stretched by traction on each side by placing fingers of the hands over gauze and surgeon makes incision.

with least tissue trauma. Many surgeons prefer to use coagulation current to transect fat and fascial layers. It is good haemostatic but causes more tissue damage, oedema, infection. Blended cautery is ideal in such situation rather than coagulation cautery. Blended cautery cuts well with adequate haemostasis but with lesser tissue damage. Cautery is used for dissection in most places even in depth and all laparoscopic procedures. Good quality cautery, proper settings and earthing (in monopolar), precaution to avoid inadvertent injury of important adjacent structures are most important while using the cautery.

In the abdomen *upper midline incision* is commonly used extending below across *left of the umbilicus* **(Figs. 3-11A and B)**. Linea alba is cut using scalpel or cutting cautery. Peritoneum is held between two artery forceps. It is felt with fingers to confirm that no abdominal contents are grasped. Peritoneum is cut using scalpel blade holding obliquely. Cut edges on either side are held using artery forceps. Long curved scissor (Metzenbaum) with closed blades is passed under the entire length of the incision to confirm that there no adhesions. Blades are opened and peritoneum is cut in the line of incision. Peritoneum is opened on left of the falciform ligament because this area is vascular.5 mm wide of linea alba should be left attached to the umbilicus so that while closing proper bites are taken at this point to prevent incisional hernia at this site **(Figs. 3-12A to C)**.

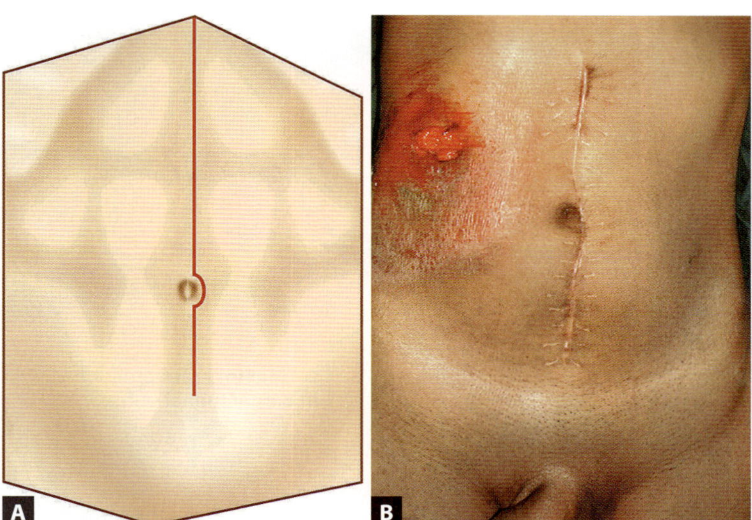

Figs. 3-11A and B: Midline incision is universally used in the abdomen. Adequate incision is a must. Extension below is done from left of the umbilicus.

In the *lower midline incision,* lower part of the incision should be done carefully. Rectus sheath should be opened up to the pubis bone beyond the pyramidalis muscle. Preperitoneal fat is adherent to the peritoneum and urinary bladder in the lower most part. This part is vascular and thickened. This part of the peritoneum need not be incised as it will not improve the exposure further instead it will cause unnecessary troublesome bleeding.

Holding the Skin and Tissues

Skin is held using toothed dissecting forceps. *Fine Adson's toothed forceps* are available. Tough structures are also held using toothed forceps. Structures like subcutaneous tissue, fascia, bowel wall, vessel wall are held using non-toothed forceps. Holding pressure and grip should be optimum in such a way that after releasing it should not show the imprint of the forceps tip. Forceps is held over the serrations on the outer surface like as a pen holding fashion. It is the *fine grip* which holds the tissue rather than force. Haemostat (artery forceps) is also used often to hold fascia, peritoneum, aponeurosis, etc. Tissues should be held using instruments as much as possible to avoid unnecessary tissue trauma. But fingers must be used when you need '*tissue touch/tissue feel*', to confirm the surgical anatomy/to confirm the operability or extent of the pathology/to confirm the relation. *Finger dissection* is a well-accepted surgical method but unnecessary usage should be avoided. Artery forceps should not be used to hold skin, bowel or delicate structures. Allis tissue forceps is used to hold skin flaps and tough structures. It is not used to hold bowel and delicate structures.

Retraction

Retraction of tissues in the depth is essential while doing surgery. Langenbeck retractor is used to retract skin and subcutaneous tissues. Different retractors are available to use in the deeper plane. Non-self retaining retractor (manual) when used needs the constant help of assistant. When self-retaining retractor is used,

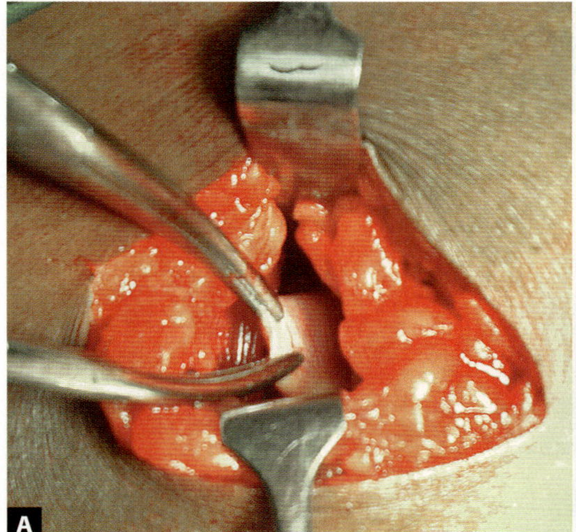

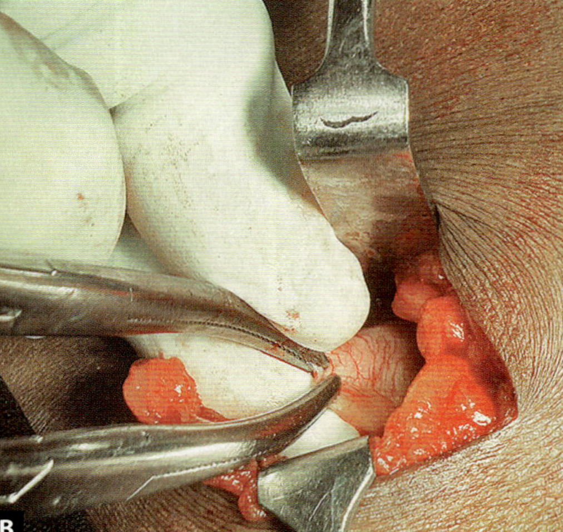

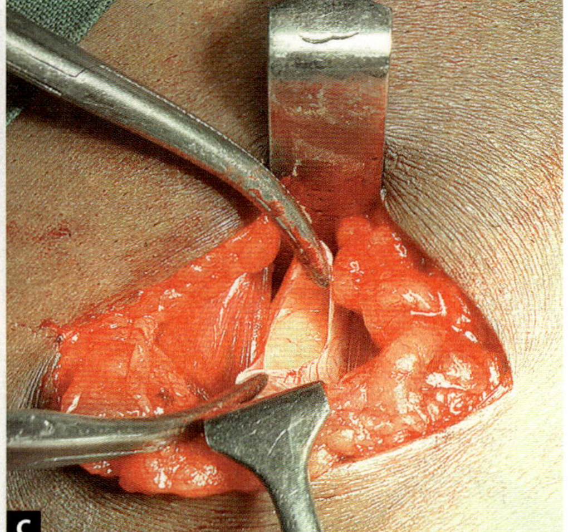

Figs. 3-12A to C: Opening the peritoneum using knife or scissor after confirming on intra-abdominal contents are held with artery forceps.

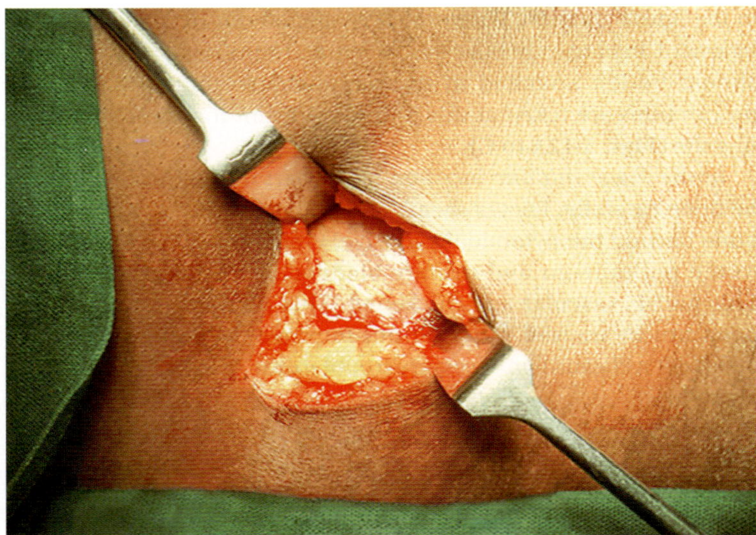

Fig. 3-13: After draping proper retraction is needed to continue with surgery. Assistant holds the retractors. Two hands of the surgeon should be free for dissection and proceeding with surgery.

assistant's hands are free to help surgeon during surgery. Surgeon's both hands should be free to do the procedure. Often many general surgeons do surgery with one hand while retracting the tissues with other hand. This should be avoided as much as possible. But when traction to the tissue is needed then surgeon should hold or retract the tissues with traction to undertake further steps of the dissection **(Figs. 3-13 and 3-14)**. Adequate incision of *sufficient length* and proper *stable exposure* are *the two basic essentials* of good surgical practice.

Exposure and Isolation of the Surgical Dissecting Area of Interest

Adequate exposure is done using proper incision, proper positioning, good retraction, by assistants, proper packing and keeping away other adjacent organs/tissues/structures. For example, in open method of cholecystectomy with Kocher's subcostal incision, mops are placed medially over the stomach and below over the colon and above the liver to expose the field adequately.

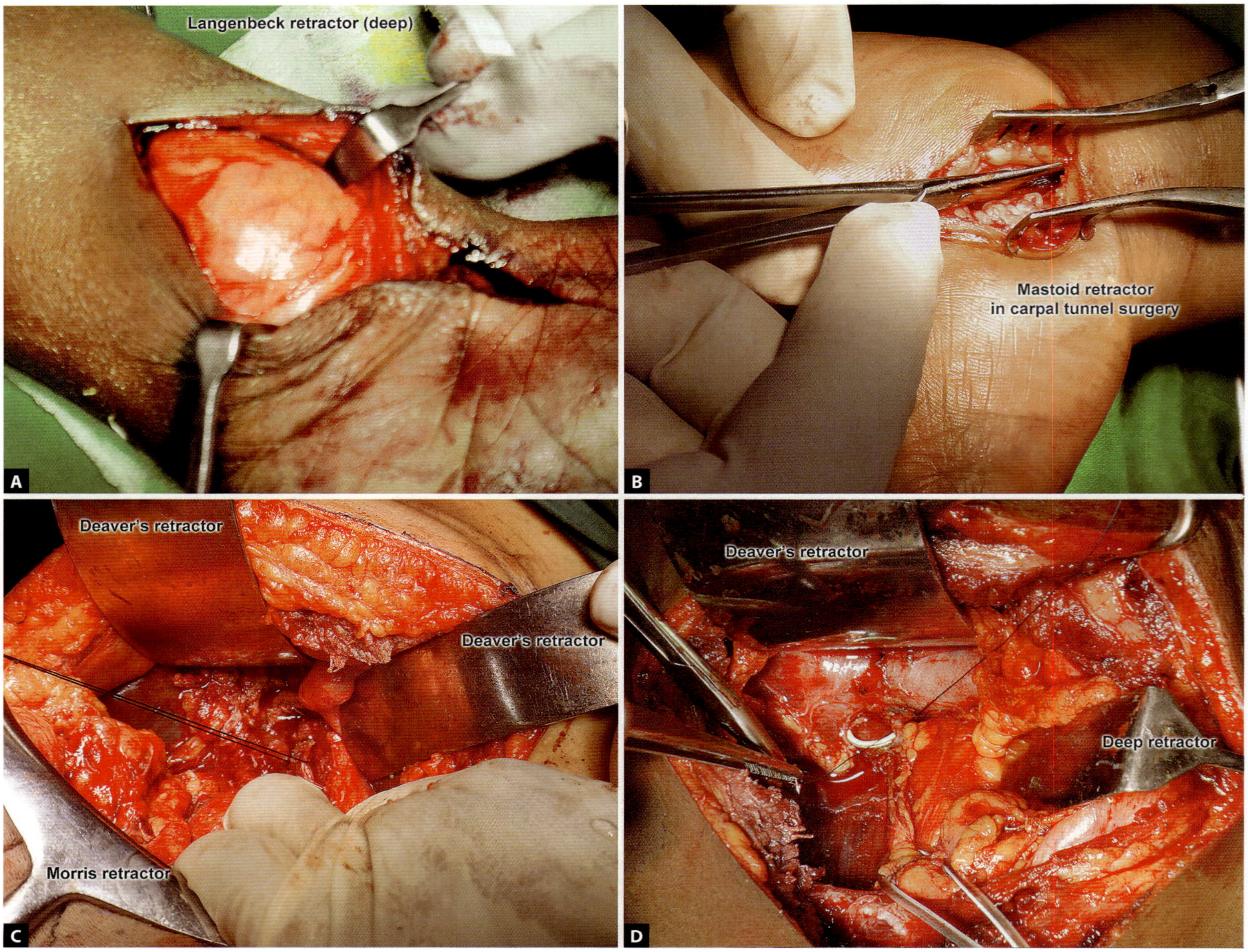

A: Langenbeck retractor (deep)

B: Mastoid retractor in carpal tunnel surgery

C: Deaver's retractor; Deaver's retractor; Morris retractor

D: Deaver's retractor; Deep retractor

Figs. 3-14A to D

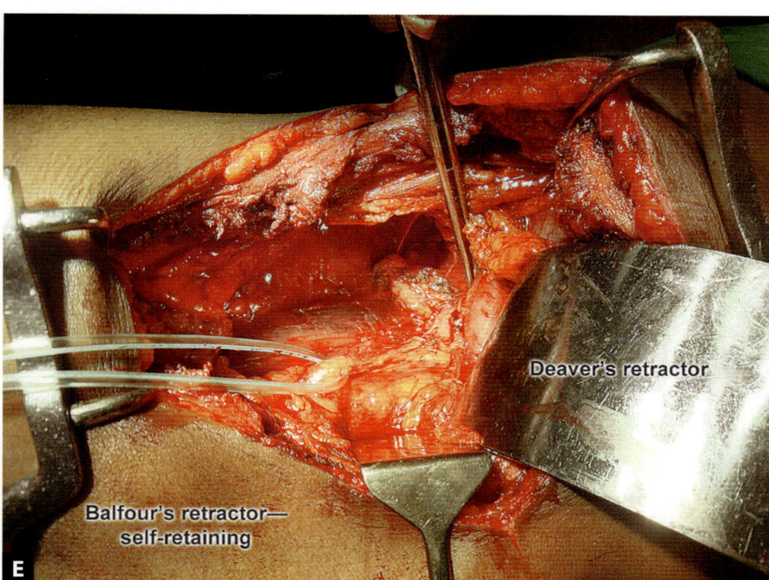

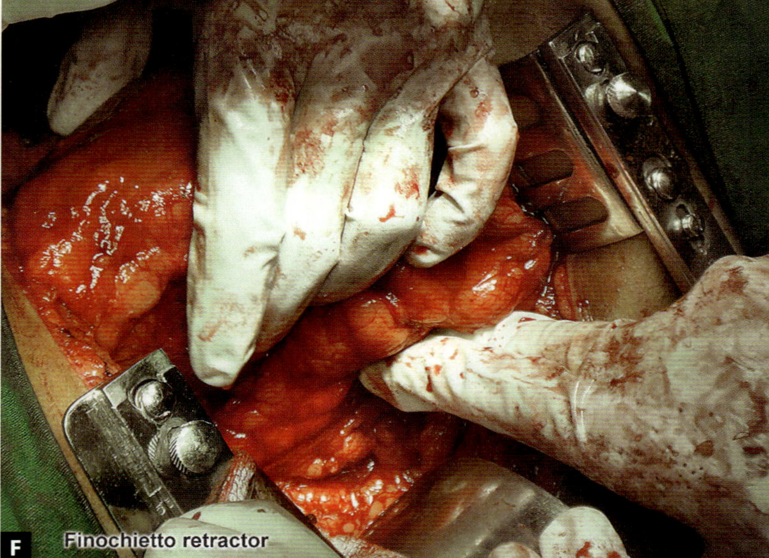

Figs. 3-14E and F

Figs. 3-14A to F: Different retractors are used at different places to retract tissues so has to expose the surgical field clearly.

DISSECTION

Dissection means identifying and separating the anatomical planes. Delineating right plane in right way is a real surgical craft. It comes by constant repetitive work, dedication and thinking. A beginner becomes a master once he masters this basic asset of surgical handicraft. Dissection should be least traumatic and with least blood loss.

Different methods available are:

Finger dissection: Left index finger is used for finger dissection. Gentle smooth finger strokes or sweeps are good way of dissection especially in the abdomen during Kocherisation, gastrectomy, adhesion removal, vagotomy, hiatus hernia surgery, pelvic surgery. However, when there are adhesions blind finger dissections close to the vessels and forcible finger dissections are to be avoided **(Fig. 3-15)**.

Scalpel dissection: It is ideal one to create a plane which is not natural. Scalpel is held in 45° angle to the line of incision. It is used to raise skin flaps in mastectomy, thyroidectomy. It is useful in dissecting dense scar tissue, tough structures. Scalpel is also used (No. 15) in cutting the bowel during resection **(Figs. 3-16A and B)**.

Peanut dissection (Kutner): It is very popular method of dissection in many places like dissection of Calot's triangle in cholecystectomy, urinary bladder dissection, to dissect the planes in pedicles during thyroidectomy, to skeletonise the lymphatics, to dissect the loose areolar tissue to achieve proper plane **(Figs. 3-17A and B)**. It is small 1.5 cm wet gauze held firmly in a long artery forceps.

Large folded wet gauze (10 × 10 cm) in a sponge holding forceps is used for dissection to push avascular loose areolar tissue while separating urinary bladder from uterine cervix; to elevate the peritoneum during lumbar sympathectomy, to separate stomach from pancreas posteriorly **(Fig. 3-18)**.

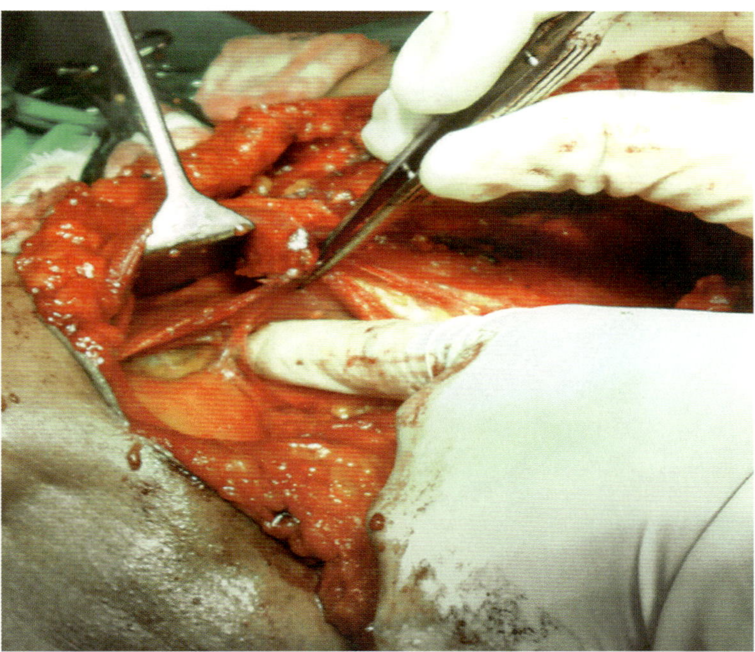

Fig. 3-15: Finger dissection is one of the methods of dissection. It gives anatomical feel (tissue feel); depth can be assessed; extent of the pathology can be assessed; blunt dissection can be carried out. It should be gentle, careful dissection. Rough usage of finger should be avoided as it may injure adjacent tissues often causing unpleasant bleeding.

Scissor dissection: Closed blades of scissor is commonly used to dissect the tissues which also give proprioception feel of the tissues. Dense tissues are dissected and cut with scissors. Gentle precise controlled movements are necessary. It achieves a clean sharp dissection **(Figs. 3-19A to D)**.

Cautery dissection: It is presently commonly used method of dissection. Cutting cautery is used for dissection. Coagulation is used in between as and when needed to control bleeding.

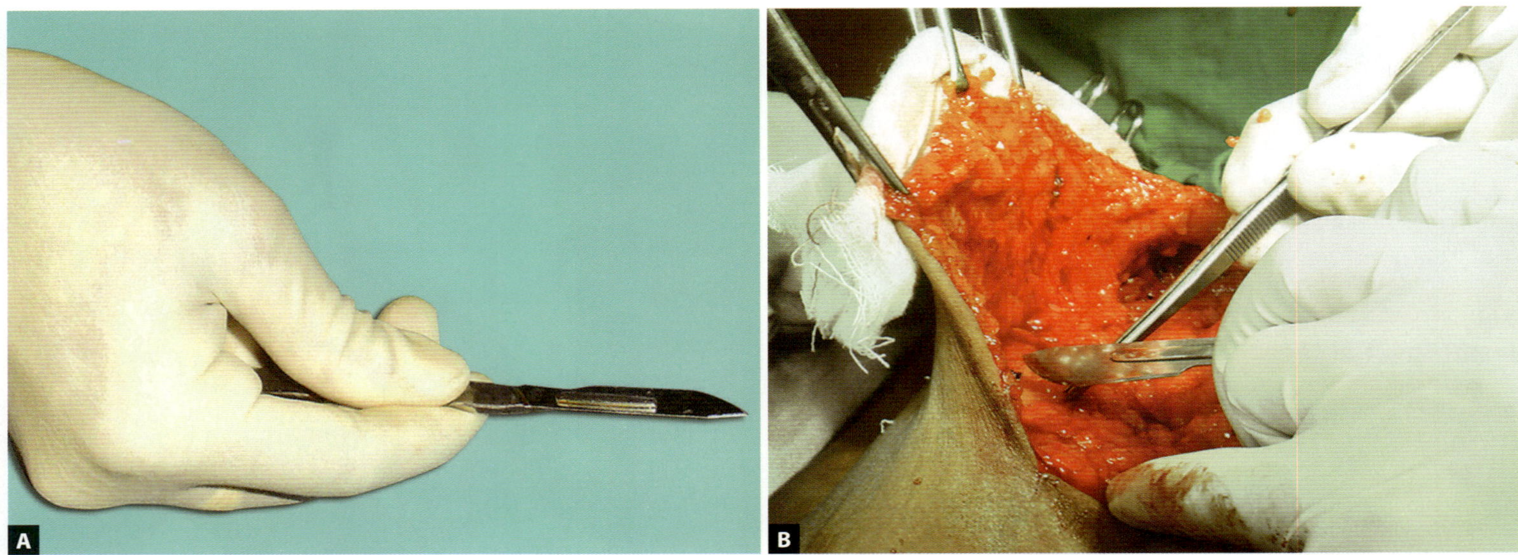

Figs. 3-16A and B: Scalpel dissection is used commonly when there is no natural plane.

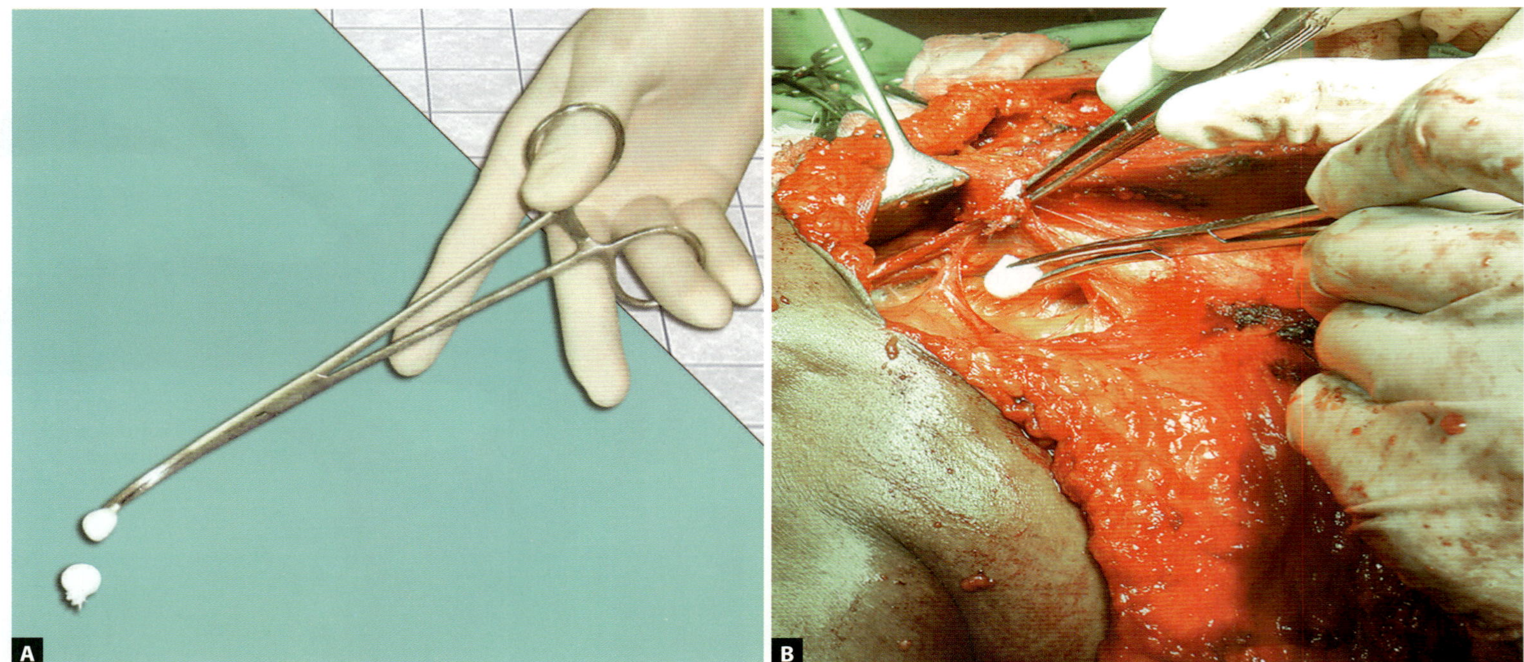

Figs. 3-17A and B: Peanut dissection is commonly used to dissect loose areolar tissue.

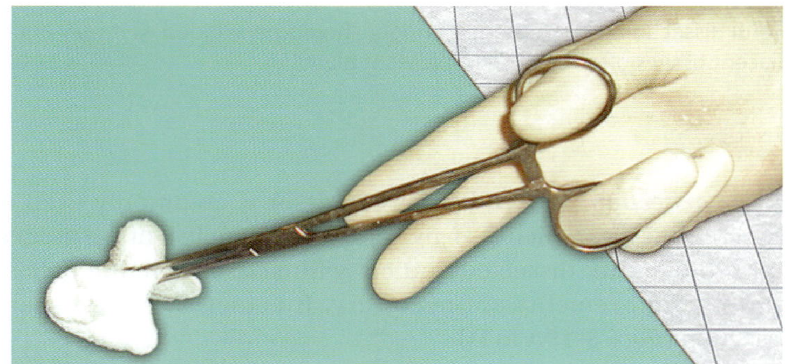

Fig. 3-18: Gauze dissection is used along loose areolar tissues; to separate urinary bladder from uterine cervix during hysterectomy, etc. it is used with gentle sweep movements over the tissues.

It is not advisable to use coagulation current for dissection as it causes too much charring and tissue destruction. So, infection and flap necrosis will be higher. Many surgeons are habituated to use coagulation current for dissection as it is easier and bloodless **(Figs. 3-20A and B)**.

Note

Proper anaesthesia; good exposure; adequate retraction; meticulous dissection; patience; decision making skill on the operation table; skilled assistant; taking help of another surgeon without any ego are—the need for *successful surgery* and to become *successful surgeon*. ***'SEE AND CUT and CUT AND SEE'***

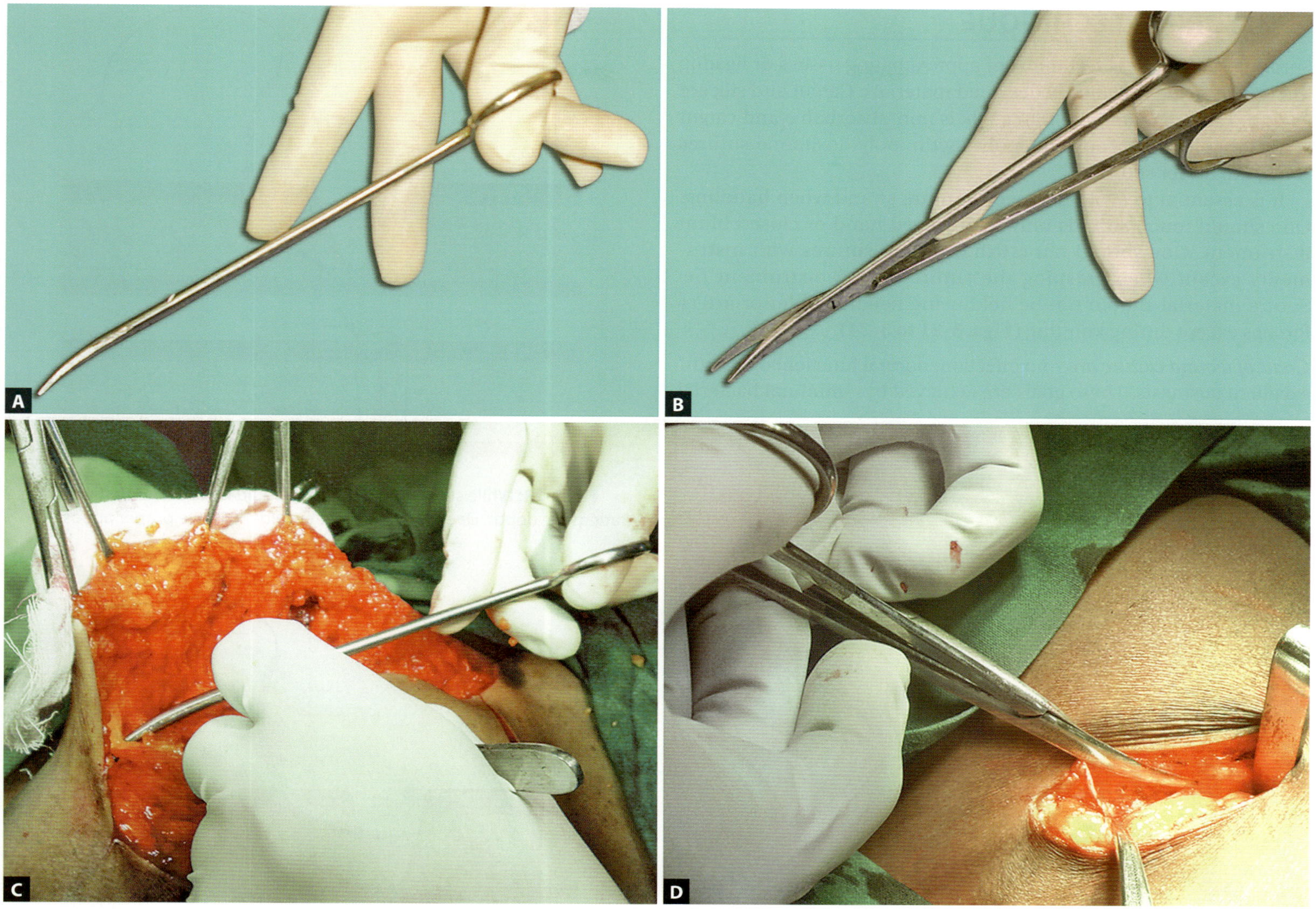

Figs. 3-19A to D: Various methods of holding and using scissor during dissection. Scissor dissection is one of the good controlled methods of dissection.

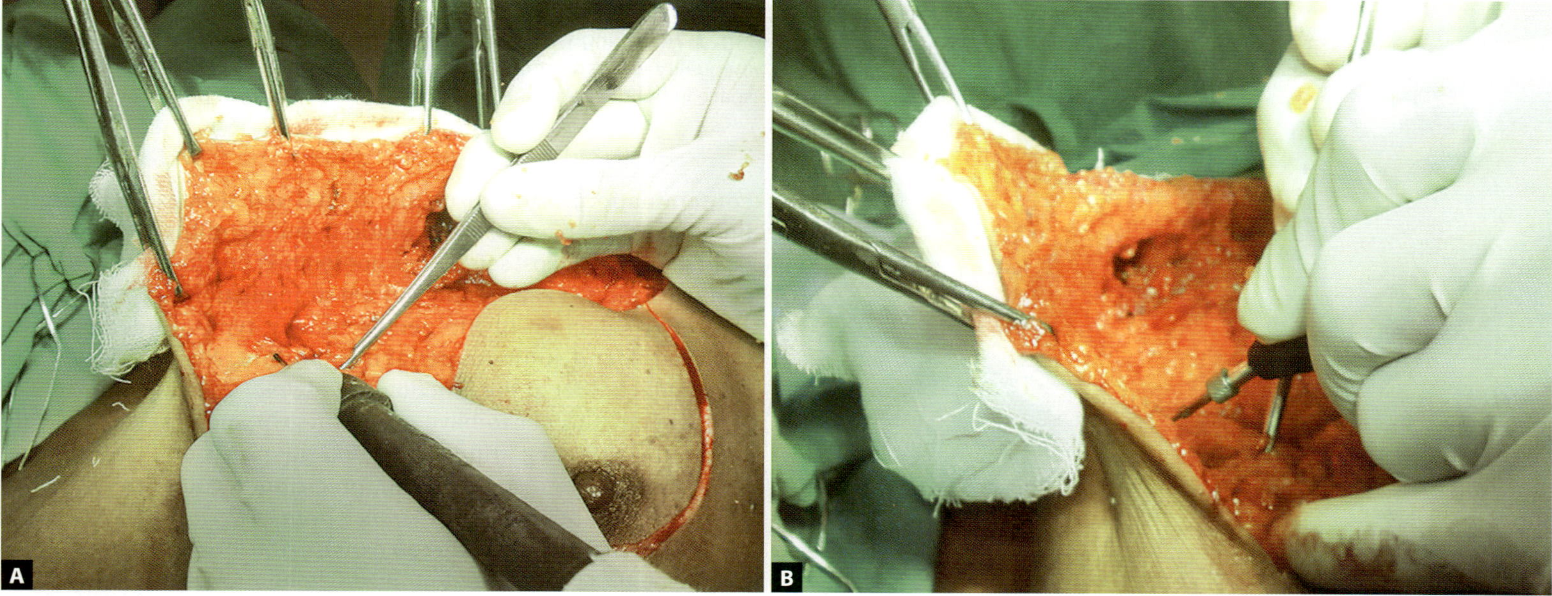

Figs. 3-20A and B: Cutting cautery is used for dissection. Coagulation current may cause charring. Coagulation is used to control bleeding. Cautery dissection here used to raise skin flaps in mastectomy.

SUTURING TECHNIQUE

Suturing is an art. It is technique of approximating tissues or ligating the vessels using specifically designed materials. Catgut and silk are good old suture materials (1887). Silk is non-absorbable and catgut is absorbable. Polypropylene, polyglactin, polydioxanone sutures (PDS) are newer sutures.

It is essential to avoid damage to suture strand when handling. One should touch strands only with gloved hand or closed blunt instrument. One should not crush or crimp sutures with instruments except when grasping the suture during instrument tie. Suture material should not be held using needle holder or artery forceps except during knotting **(Figs. 3-21 to 3-24)**.

Goals of wound closure are—no infection; normal function; optimum/excellent cosmesis. These goals are achieved by—minimal bacterial contamination; removal of the devitalised tissues with foreign bodies; proper haemostasis; gentle tissue handling using forceps (skin toothed forceps, soft tissues nontoothed fine forceps); optimum approximation of tissues only but not strangulation.

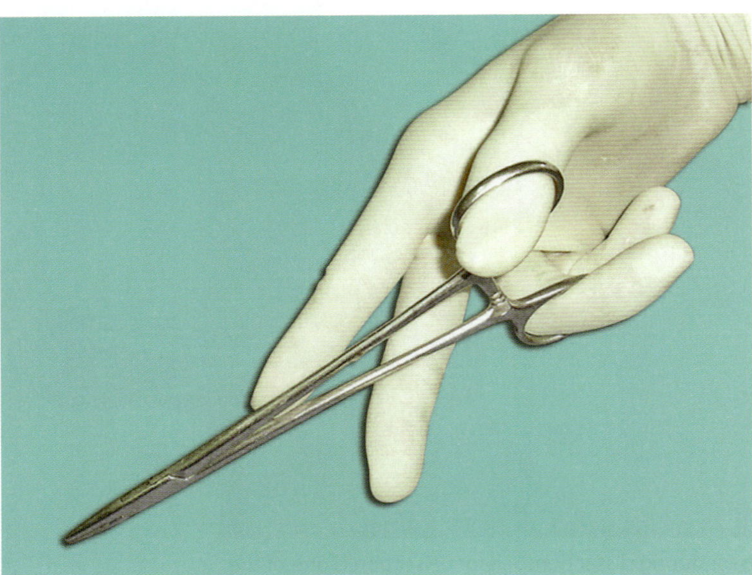

Fig. 3-21: Holding the needle holder properly and knowing its movement in rotational axis is important for proper suturing and knotting. It is the precise gentle rotation which is essential; not pushing flimsy movement.

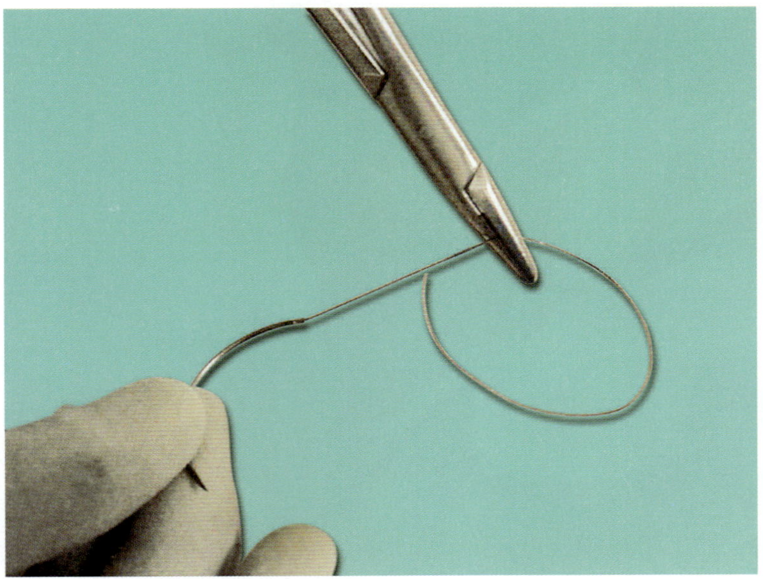

Fig. 3-22: Holding the suture material using needle holder unnecessarily should be avoided.

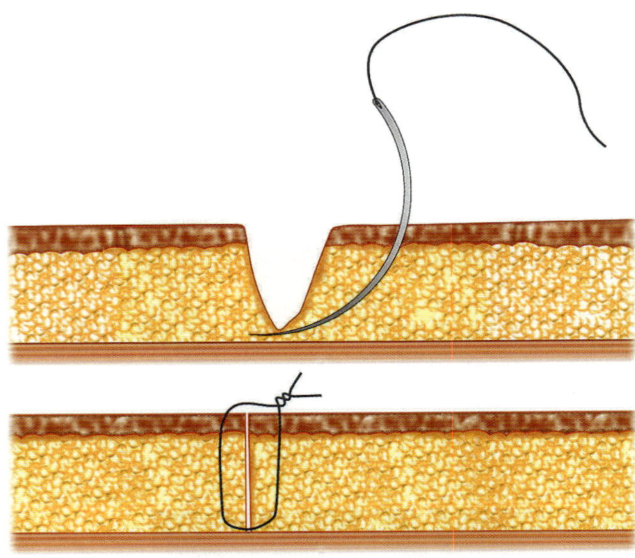

Fig. 3-23: While suturing needle bite should be taken correctly with adequate depth. Deeper part should be wider to have proper apposition.

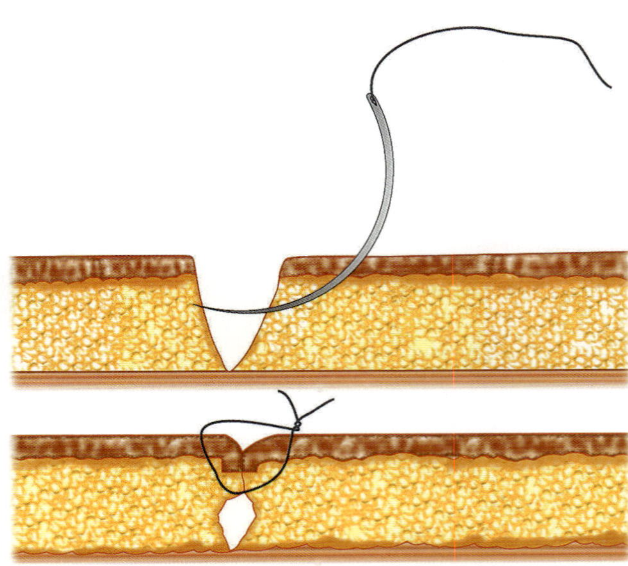

Fig. 3-24: Taking wrong bite of needle with inadequate depth, width and inequality will cause poor apposition and alignment and also creating dead space in the deeper plane causing seroma formation or poor scar later.

Proper selection of the needle holder, type of needles (size, curve, etc), and suture material is important. Needle is placed in the needle holder at the junction of *proximal 2/3rds to distal 1/3rd* of the needle holder to have optimum grip and precision. If held more proximal, then grip will be good but precision is inadequate. If needle is more distally placed, precision is good but with poor grip. Needle is held *half the distance from swaged end.* Grasping of the needle should be neither too tight nor too loose. Optimum *grasp* should be there. Alignment of needle holder jaw should be proper. Needle should not rotate during grasping. Needle and needle holder should function as a *single unit* **(Figs. 3-25A and B)**.

Features of needle holder/needle driver should be

- Appropriate sized needle holder for the respective needle should be used
- Needle should be grasped 1/2 to 2/3rds distance from swaged area
- Tips of the jaws should meet
- Needle should stay firm and stable within the jaw while using
- Needle should be placed securely
- Needle holder should be locked while using, but should not be overclosed
- Needle holder should always be directed by surgeon's thumb
- Rotation movement should be used
- Optimum grip and optimum control are needed for precision work
- Stability and dexterity are important

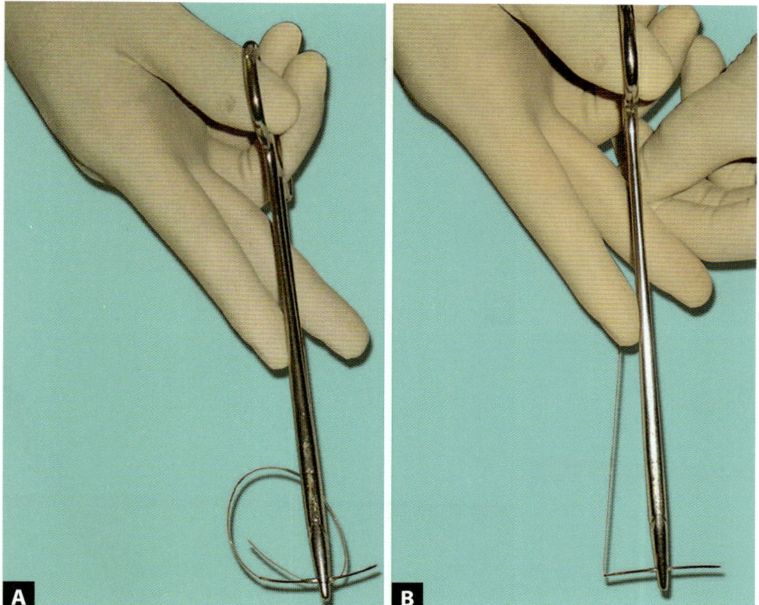

Figs. 3-25A and B: Holding the needle with a needle holder.

Correct placement of the needle is essential to have proper easy penetration of the tissue at desired angle. Usually needle holder (driver) is held using thumb and fourth fingers and index finger rests on the fulcrum of the needle holder to create stability. Often needle holder can be held in the palm to increase the dexterity.

Tissue to be penetrated by needle should be held using dissecting forceps. For skin and tough structures toothed forceps are used; for bowel, soft tissues, muscles, vessels, peritoneum, etc. are held using nontoothed forceps. Often finer forceps like Adson's forceps are used. Undue traction on the tissue should not be done as it may traumatise or tear the tissues. If tissues are in depth or bulky instead of taking bites together from the wound edges, it is preferable to take bites one after other from each edge of the wound so that precision in taking the adequate tissue bite with alignment becomes perfect.

Needle should enter the tissue/skin perpendicular to the surface at 90° allowing smooth entry without any tissue damage; similarly needle should exit out through exit tissue also perpendicularly in 90°. Width, depth at entry point and exit points should become near mirror image of each other. While bringing out of the exit tissue, needle tip should be held using forceps ideally even though it is done using needle holder especially in deeper tissues. Coordinated use of forceps and needle driver with alternating pronating and supinating hand actions with needle holder is important to achieve effective efficient least traumatic suture placement creating a rectangular suture path.

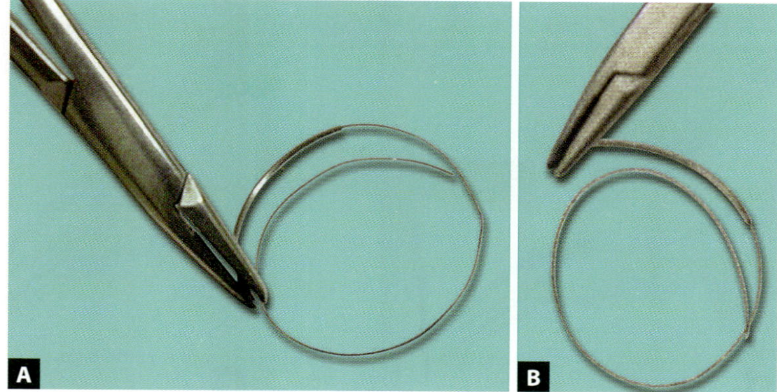

Figs. 3-26A and B: Holding the needle tip with needle holder should be avoided. It is held only during knotting process.

Needle is passed through smaller thickness of the tissue. Excess tissue bite should be avoided. It is the smooth, rotation movement than the movement with force which is important. Proper sized needle should be taken depending on the thickness and texture of tissue/tissue resistance which is to be apposed. *Rotation force* should be in the direction of the curvature of needle. Twisting or bending needle tip should be avoided. Holding the needle tip with instrument will cause blunting or breaking of the tip and if such broken tip is entangled in the tissue it is very difficult to identify it **(Figs. 3-26A and B)**.

Cutting needles are used for skin, tough structures, mucoperiosteum. *Round bodied needles* are used for smooth tissues like fat, peritoneum, muscle, bowel, vessel anastomosis, etc. Usual *width of the tissue* taken is 5 mm. But finally, it depends on the thickness, tissue strength and condition to which patient is getting operated upon. In retention sutures of abdomen or Smead-Jones closure width taken is 3 cm. Distance between each bite is important. It should not be too closer or too far. In the skin 1 cm gap sutures are sufficient. In the bowel 5 mm gap sutures are needed to have complete sealing of the bowel edge and also haemostasis. Tissue should be handled carefully. Only required tissue should be grasped. Bulk grasping should be avoided. Smaller sized suture is better **(Figs. 3-27 and 3-28)**.

While suturing after taking the proper needle bite through one edge of the wound (skin or tissues), needle holder is released but forceps should hold the tissue/skin edge until needle holder is completely released and adequate length of the needle tip is visible; then forceps is released from the tissue and needle is grasped using forceps to place it in the needle holder again. Needle is again similarly pierced from inside outside to complete the suturing; again here also needle tip should pierce and visible to hold the needle tip with forceps; entire act of suturing requires proper fine pronation and supination of the wrist. Bites from the both edges of the wound can be taken together without releasing the needle from the needle holder but forceps is released from first edge to second edge while taking respective needle bites. It is done in surface wounds; but while suturing in the depth it is ideal to take bites from each edge separately so that proper bite is ensured. Needle should pierce 5 mm from the wound edge in general but perpendicular to the tissue, i.e. equidistant from the both cut edges **(Figs. 3-29A to M)**.

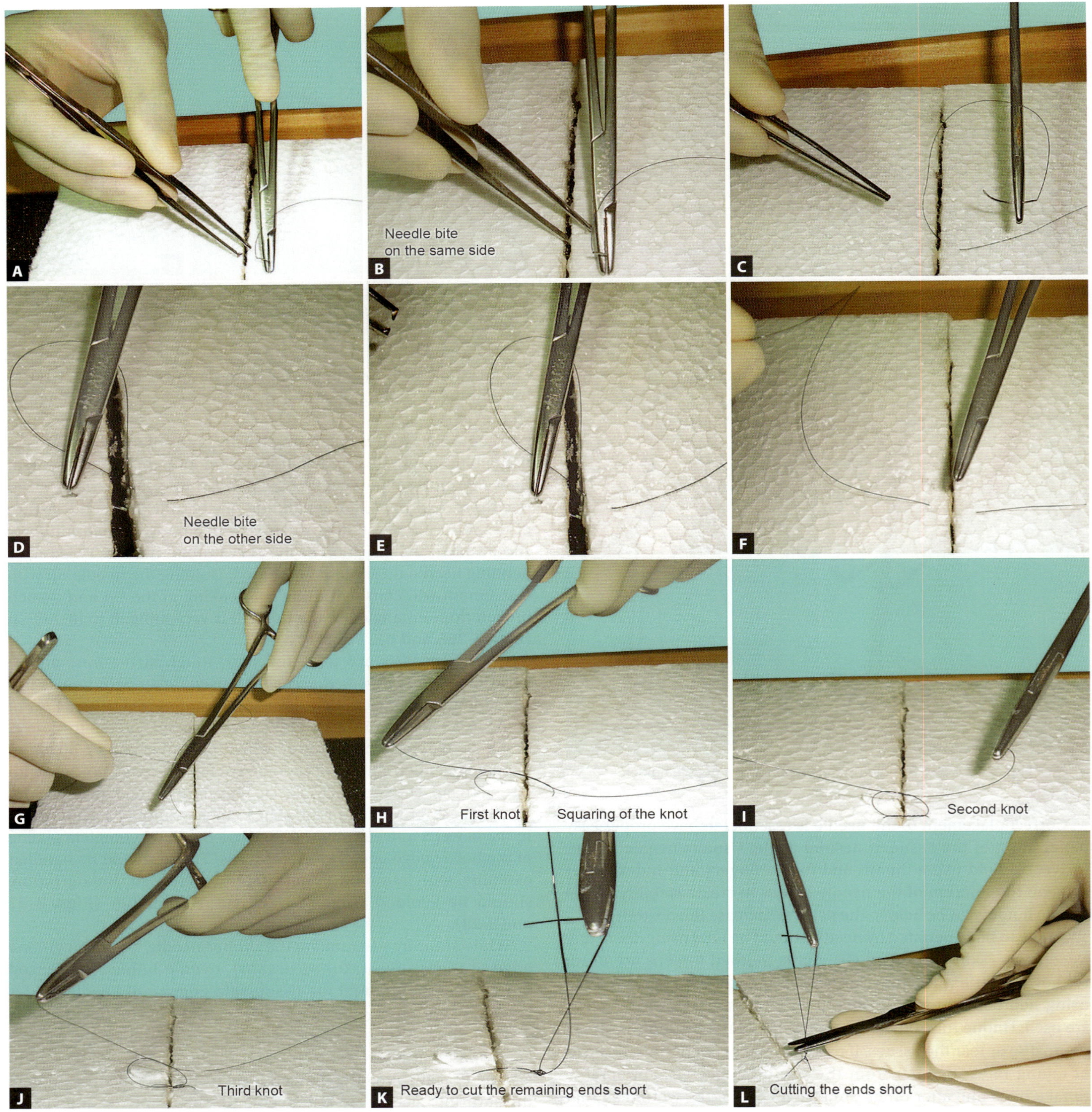

Figs. 3-27A to L: Instrument suturing and knotting—simple suture.

Size of the suture material is decided in relation to the strength of the tissues. Usually 3-zero is used. Thicker tissues may need 2-zero sutures. Abdominal wall closure needs 1 or zero or 1-zero suture material.

Ideally interrupted sutures are better. It holds and apposes well. It maintains the blood supply of the tissue edge. But in many places like gastrojejunostomy continuous sutures can be used.

It is better to take bite from each edge of the tissue *separately* even though it looks more time consuming. When both edges are held together and needle is forced through them, there are chances of having lateral movements which can cause tear at the first point of entry of the needle resulting in poor apposition of the tissue. It can be used safely if the edges are close enough without tension and if one can avoid lateral movements while taking bite of second edge **(Fig. 3-30)**.

Learner *should practice* holding the tissues with instruments than hand. It is common that beginner prefers to use hands than instruments as it is easier, but holding tissues with instruments is better. In certain occasions hand is used to hold the tissues; otherwise by enlarge instruments are used.

Type of suture material used depends on the tissue and condition for which suturing is done. Once wound attains maximum strength sutures are no longer required. Slow healing wounds need non-absorbable sutures. Rapidly healing wound need absorbable sutures. Rapid healing, least irritation is achieved by smaller sized,

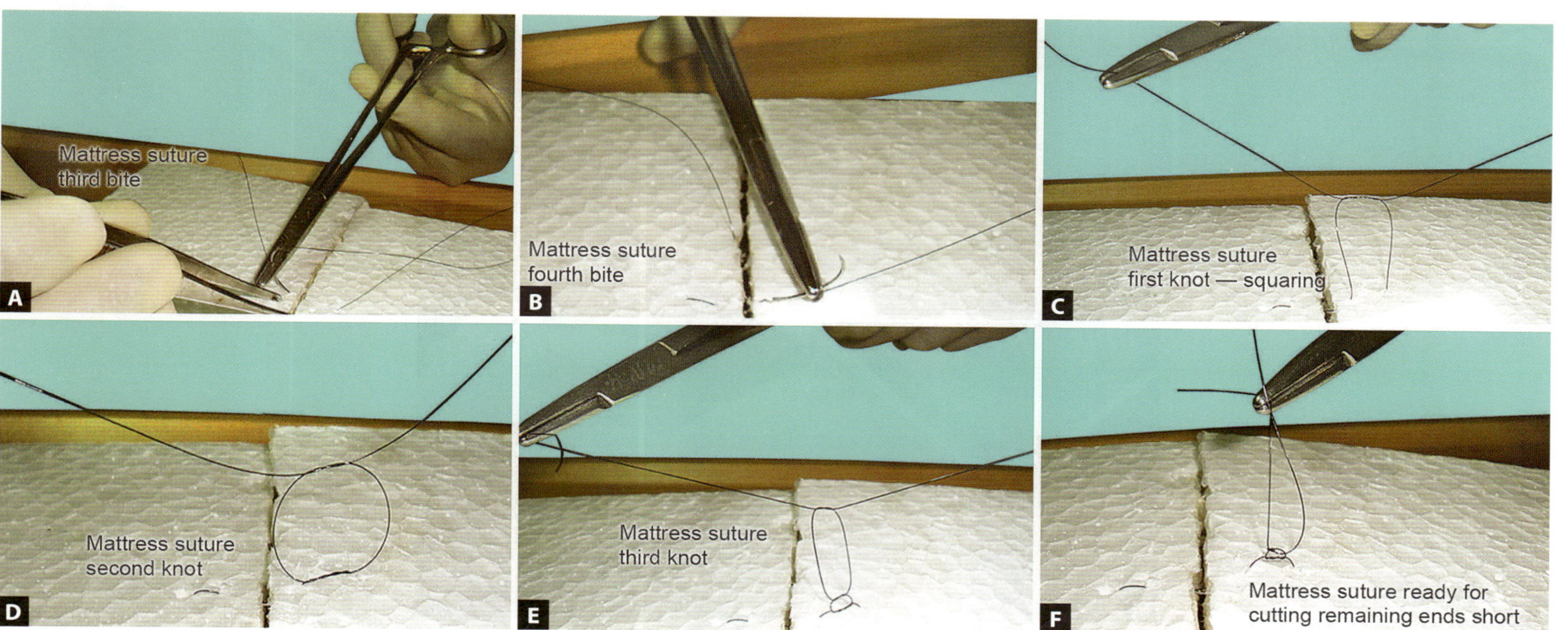

Figs. 3-28A to F: Method of placing mattress sutures and knotting with squaring.

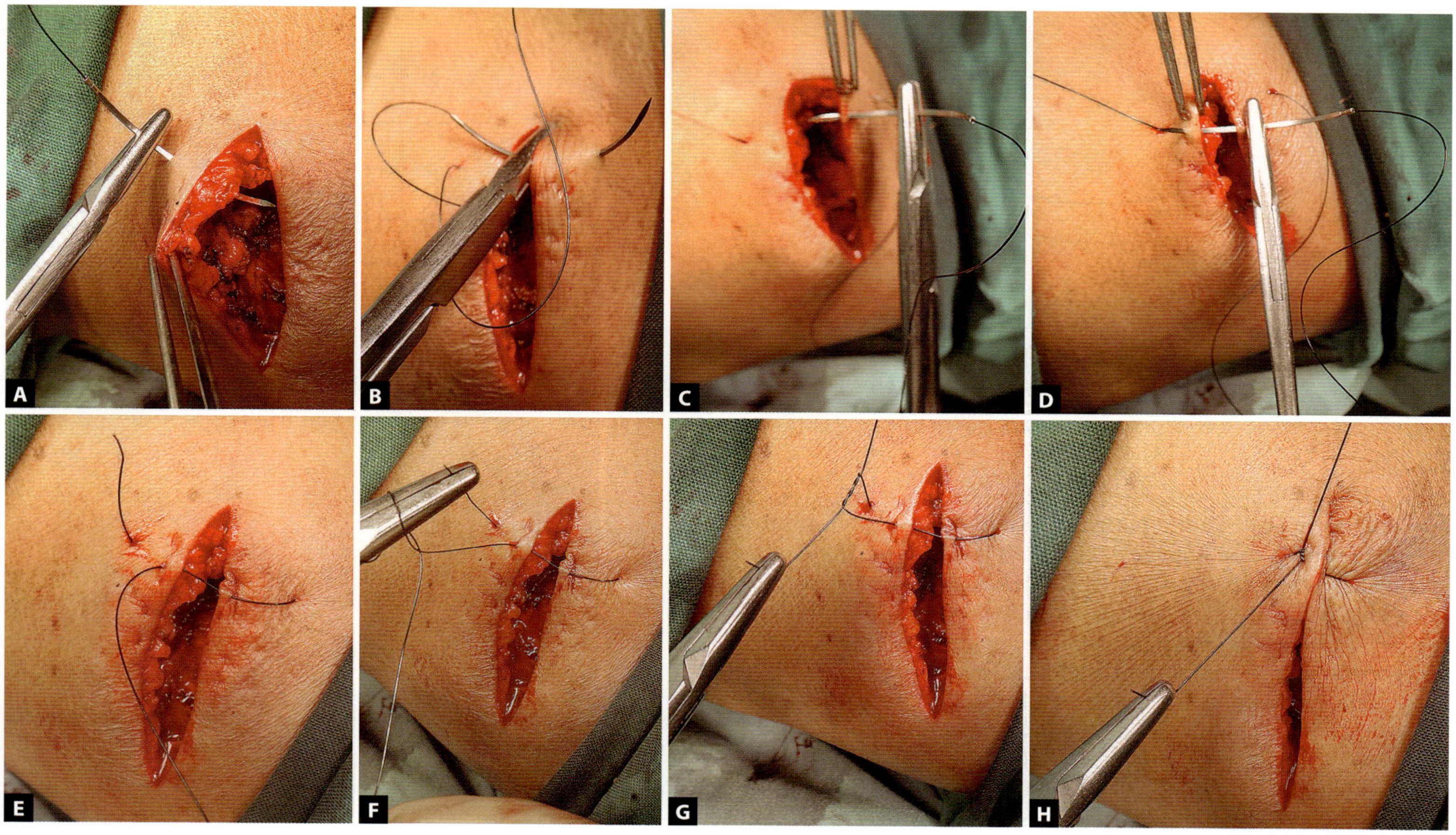

Figs. 3-29A to H

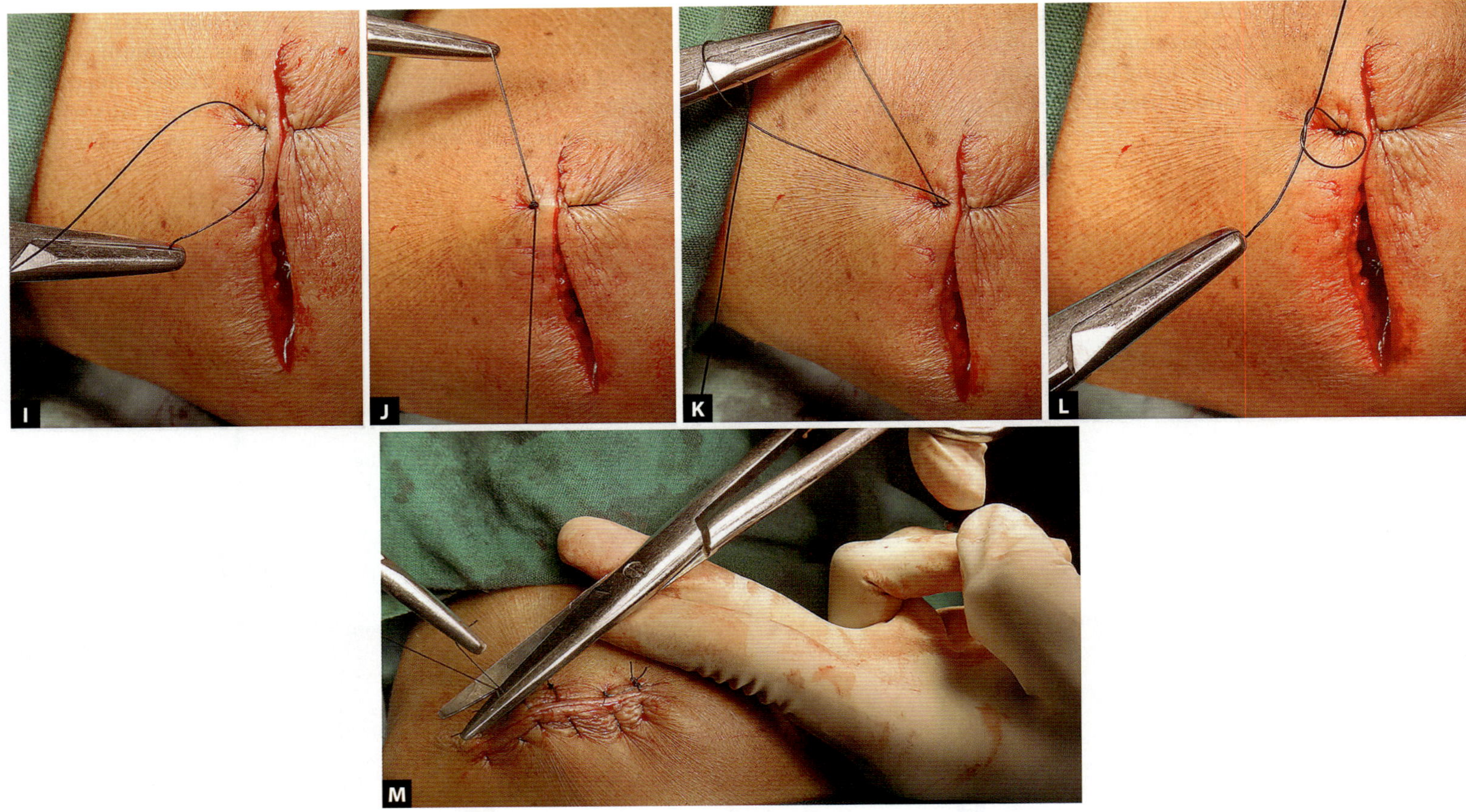

Figs. 3-29I to M

Figs. 3-29A to M: Technique of taking bites in vertical mattress suture and placing the knot securely. It is one of the commonest suture methods used.

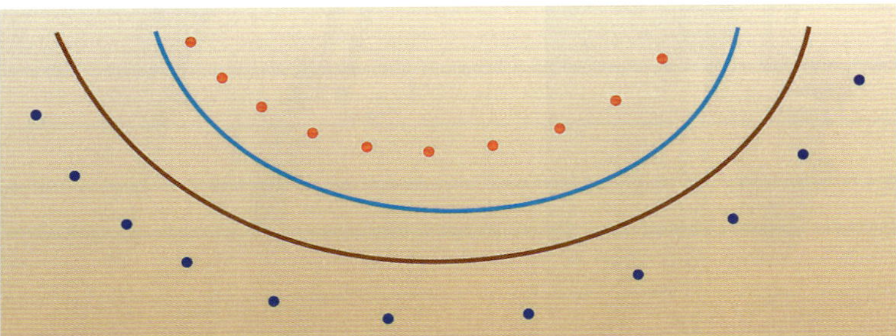

Fig. 3-30: By marking the corresponding points of each edge of the wound before suturing, makes it easier to take bites at proper anatomical level to achieve good wound alignment and apposition without causing disparity.

monofilament, inert suture material. In bowel absorbable suture material used—3-zero is ideal; often 2-zero is also used. Silk is also used in many centres. Interrupted sutures are better especially in oesophagus, colorectum, and contaminated field. Continuous sutures are used in stomach and jejunum. Single layer is well accepted; it gives wider lumen; maintains blood supply. Double layer using silk/linen for outer seromuscular; full thickness Connell/Gambee sutures for inner layer using absorbable sutures like 3-zero Vicryl is also equally good. It is time consuming, may lessen the luminal diameter. But it is more secure. In biliary tree and urinary system rapidly absorbing sutures like 3-zero Vicryl are used. Patient age, nutrition, immunosuppression, malignancy, sepsis, acute nature are other factors which decide the type of suture material used **(Fig. 3-31)**.

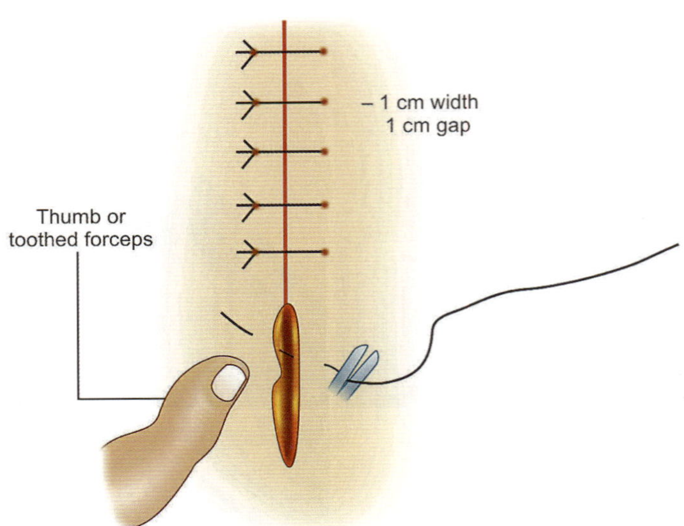

Fig. 3-31: Equidistant, proper correct bite, counter pressure using thumb or toothed forceps on the opposite edge, rotation precise gentle movements are the basic principles of suturing.

Note:

After suturing needle should be returned to scrub nurse with needle holder.

Suture material selection and usage

- ***The choice of type and size of the suture material*** for a particular procedure is based on the known physical and biologic characteristics of the suture material and the healing properties of the sutured tissues. It also depends on condition of the disrupted tissues and the condition of the patient and post-operative status. In potentially contaminated tissues, monofilament sutures are better (like polypropylene). When cosmetic result is anticipated, fine inert monofilament sutures are used.
- *In vascular suturing*, monofilament polypropylene is used which is inert, least infective, least reactive, high tensile strength and thrombus formation is least. Size selection depends on the size of the vessel and situation where it is being used – 4-zero to 7-zero – are used. Polyester is preferred for suturing artificial heart valves, myocardium and vascular prosthesis.
- *In irradiated field*, not only the normal healing process is delayed but the tolerance to the trauma of irradiated tissue is markedly reduced. So with extremely careful and gentle surgical technique with avoidance of tension and mattress sutures as they further increase the degree of ischemia is needed. Non-absorbable polypropylene or polyglactin absorbable can be used. Intermittent sutures are ideal than continuous one.
- *In microsurgical procedure*, polyamide or polypropylene 10-zero is used.
- When a wound has reached maximal strength, sutures are no longer needed. Tissues that ordinarily heal slowly such as skin, fascia and tendons should be sutured with non-absorbable sutures. Tissues that heal rapidly such as peritoneum, liver, small intestine, muscles, stomach, colon and bladder are sutured with absorbable sutures; but in gastrointestinal tract non-absorbable sutures are also used. Suture should be stronger than the sutured tissues. It is not good to use more suture material than necessarily needed to avoid adverse problems like crumpling and tissue strangulation.
- The selection of the suture material is based on (1) The condition of the wound; (2) The tissues to be repaired; (3) The tensile strength of the suture material; (4) Knot holding characteristics of the suture material; (5) The reaction of the surrounding tissues to the suture materials.
- Forward wrist movement (*fluid movement of the wrist*) and backhand movement are important movements in suturing. Mainly wrist and partly elbow movements are used as combined. Shoulder movements should be restricted as much as possible. Height of the table and stance of the surgeon and changing stance as per need are equally important for effective suturing.
- *Correct placement of the needle* (*Needle arming*) is essential to have proper easy penetration of the tissue at desired angle. Needle should be held in the middle of the needle in the needle body at needle proximal 1/3rd using needle holder; distal jaw of the needle holder at distal 1/3rd to proximal 1/3rd part needle should be placed; needle holder should be locked adequately. Usually needle holder (driver) is held using thumb and fourth fingers and index finger rests on the fulcrum of the needle holder to create stability. Often needle holder can be held in the palm to increase the dexterity.
- Tissue to be penetrated by needle should be held using dissecting forceps. For skin and tough structures toothed forceps are used; for bowel, soft tissues, muscles, vessels, peritoneum etc. are held using nontoothed forceps. Often finer forceps like Adson's forceps are used. Undue traction on the tissue should not be done as it may traumatise or tear the tissues. If tissues are in depth or bulky instead of taking bites together from the wound edges, it is preferable to take bites one after other from each edge of the wound so that precision in taking the adequate tissue bite with alignment becomes perfect.
- Needle should enter the tissue/skin *perpendicular to the surface at 90° allowing smooth entry* without any tissue damage; similarly needle should exit out through exit tissue also perpendicularly in 900. Width, depth at entry point and exit points should become near mirror image of each other. *While bringing out of the exit tissue, needle (body) proximal to the tip should be held using forceps ideally even though it is done using needle holder especially in deeper tissues. Needle tip should not be held as repetitive friction will blunt or dull the needle tip or tip may rarely break also.* Coordinated use of forceps and needle driver with alternating pronating and supinating hand actions with needle holder is important to achieve effective efficient least traumatic suture placement creating a rectangular suture path.
- Needle is passed through smaller thickness of the tissue. Excess tissue bite should be avoided. It is the smooth, rotation movement than the movement with force which is important. Proper sized needle should be taken depending on the thickness and texture of tissue/tissue resistance which is to be apposed. *Rotation force* should be in the direction of the curvature of needle.

Different Types of Suturing

Simple everting suture: It is used in skin. Bites at deeper plane should be wider than superficial plane. Edges should be everted once this stitch is placed **(Fig. 3-32)**.

Simple interrupted fascial suture: It is used in abdominal wall like in closure of *McBurney* incision by taking about 5–8 mm of tissue bite **(Figs. 3-33A and B)**.

Vertical mattress suture (Stewart): Deep bite is taken from one edge; passed through deeper part of opposite edge and brought out on the opposite edge surface; again close to the superficial margin of opposite side bite is taken and is passed through similar edge of same side to bring out as mattress suture **(Figs. 3-34 to 3-36)**.

Horizontal mattress suture: It is not commonly used in skin. It is often used in retention sutures (tension sutures), fascial closure, and ventral hernia repair, to achieve haemostasis. Here bite is taken like a square with two-time bites on each side one below the other **(Fig. 3-37)**.

Haemostatic figure of eight suture: It is basically used for haemostasis. It is used in circumcision to ligate frenular artery, bleeders withdrawn into the soft tissues. Vicryl or polypropylene (2-zero/3-zero) is used.

Continuous over and over simple suture: It is continuous suture used in peritoneum, fascia, aponeurosis. Vicryl is used usually.

Subcuticular suture: It is used in skin closure. Needle bite is taken initially at one corner; it is continued by taking bites at the white dermis each side alternatively to reach the other end of the wound; which is then brought out through the corner of the wound. Usually absorbable polyglycolic acid is used (3-zero) using curved cutting needle **(Figs. 3-38 and 3-39)**. It is difficult to place subcuticular sutures using round body needle. Absorbable suture is not removed. Nonabsorbable monofilament suture can also be used. Its ends are left long or tied loosely over gauze. It is removed in 10 days. Often there may be difficulty in pulling out the sutures. Subcuticular suture gives cosmetically better scar. But if sutures thicker than 3-zero is used it will cause inflammatory reaction in the apposed wound causing no cosmetic benefit. Subcuticular sutures should not be used in trauma, infective areas, and emergency surgeries. There is controversy whether it has got advantage over interrupted sutures using fine material except in avoiding (in absorbable subcuticular)/easier (non-absorbable subcuticular) suture removal.

Skin staplers: It is stainless steel staplers applied using specialised disposable devices to the skin. It is quicker and apposes well. It is used in major surgeries. It saves time compared to suture closure

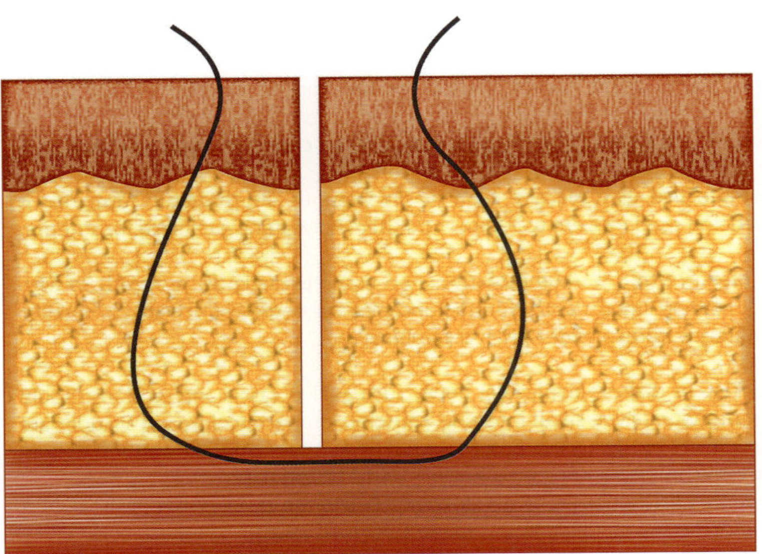

Fig. 3-32: Bite should be equidistant on both edges of the wound to achieve eversion of the wound edges. Inversion of the edge should be avoided.

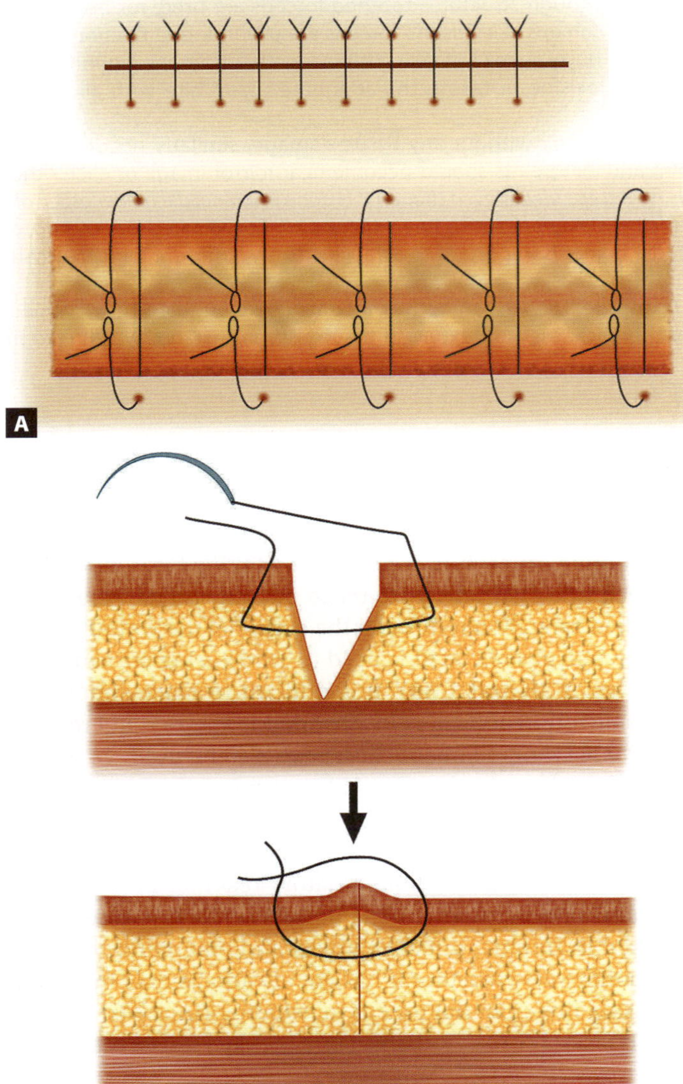

Figs. 3-33A and B: Simple interrupted suture.

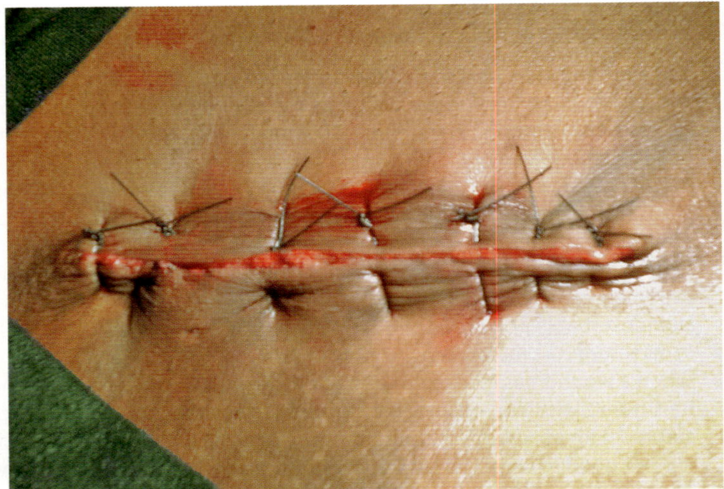

Fig. 3-34: Vertical mattress sutures.

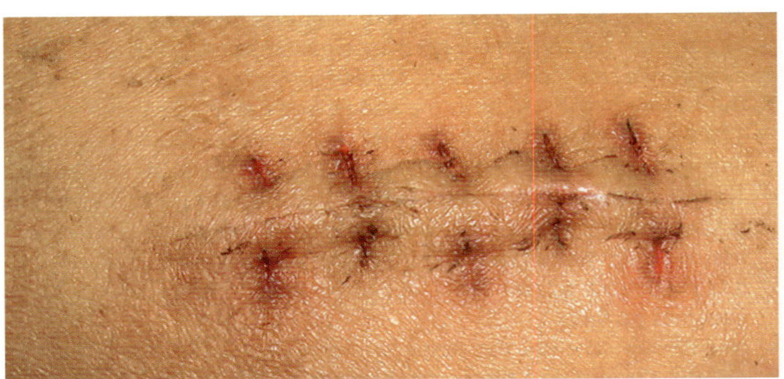

Fig. 3-35: Scar of interrupted sutures—vertical mattress sutures.

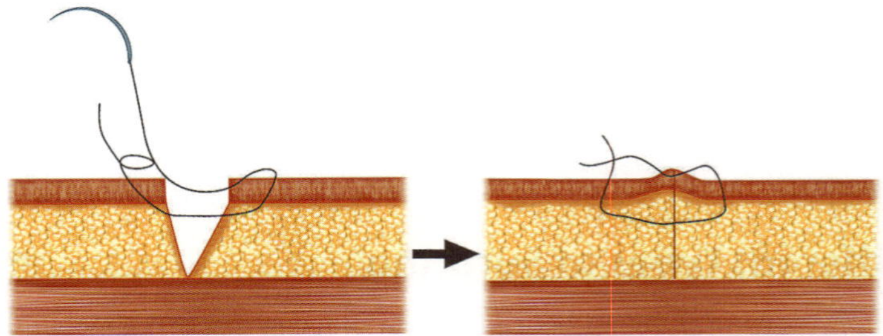

Fig. 3-36: Vertical mattress suture (Stewart).

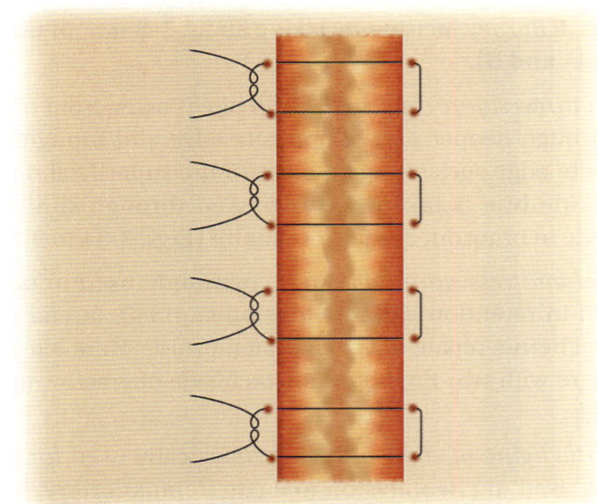

Fig. 3-37: Horizontal mattress sutures.

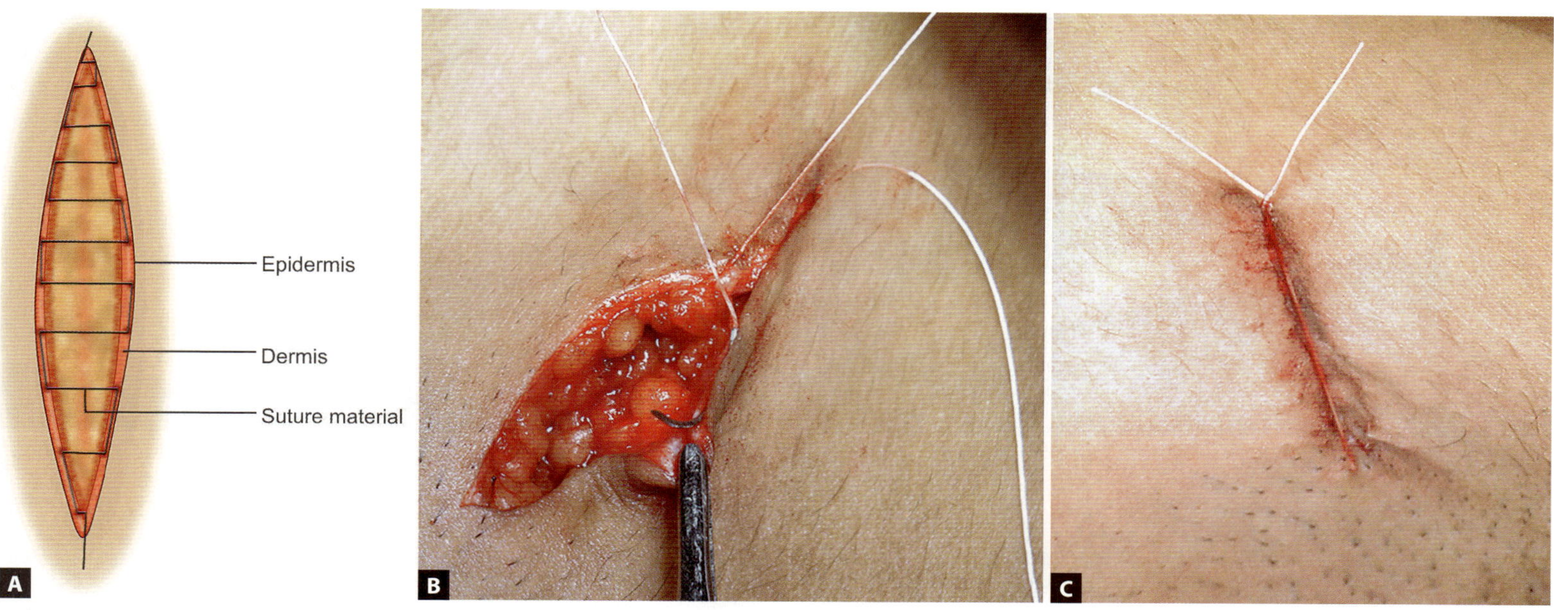

Figs. 3-38A to C: Technique of subcuticular suture placing.

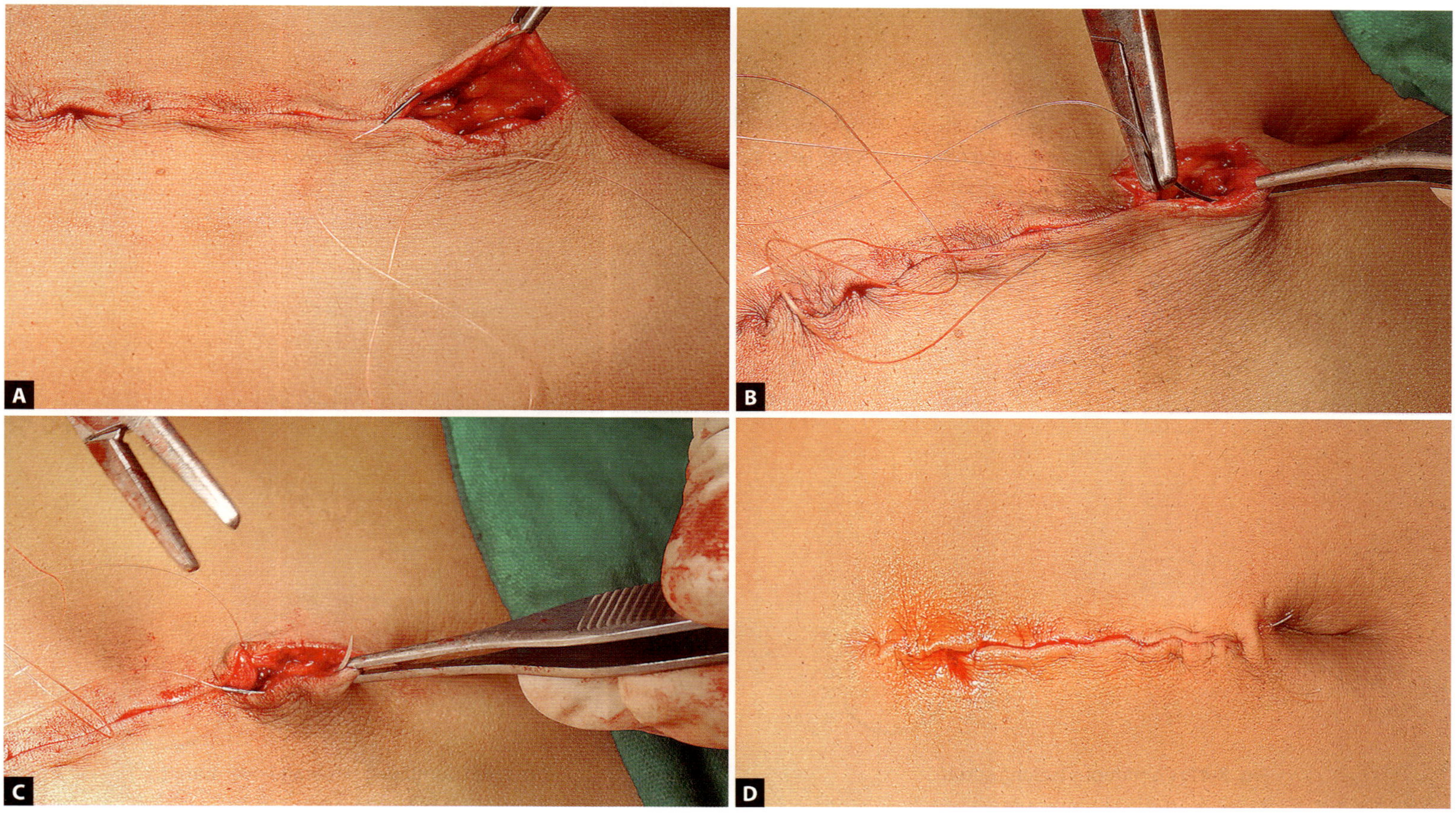

Figs. 3-39A to D: Subcuticular suturing using absorbable suture—poliglecaprone (monocryl) suture material.

of the skin. Two wound edges should be held in proper alignment before applying skin staplers. Removal needs special instrument. It gives good cosmetic result **(Figs. 3-40A to D)**.

Continuous locking sutures (Continuous blanket sutures): It is not commonly used in skin. It is used in closure of fascial layer. It holds well and is haemostatic. It is commonly used in closure of rectus sheath. Nonabsorbable suture material is usually used. It does not cause bunching of the wound **(Fig. 3-41)**.

Continuous over and over suture: It is continuous sutures taken at equidistant. It should not be very tight as more tightening may cause strangulation of the wound edge; it may cause bunching of the wound; but it saves time **(Fig. 3-42)**.

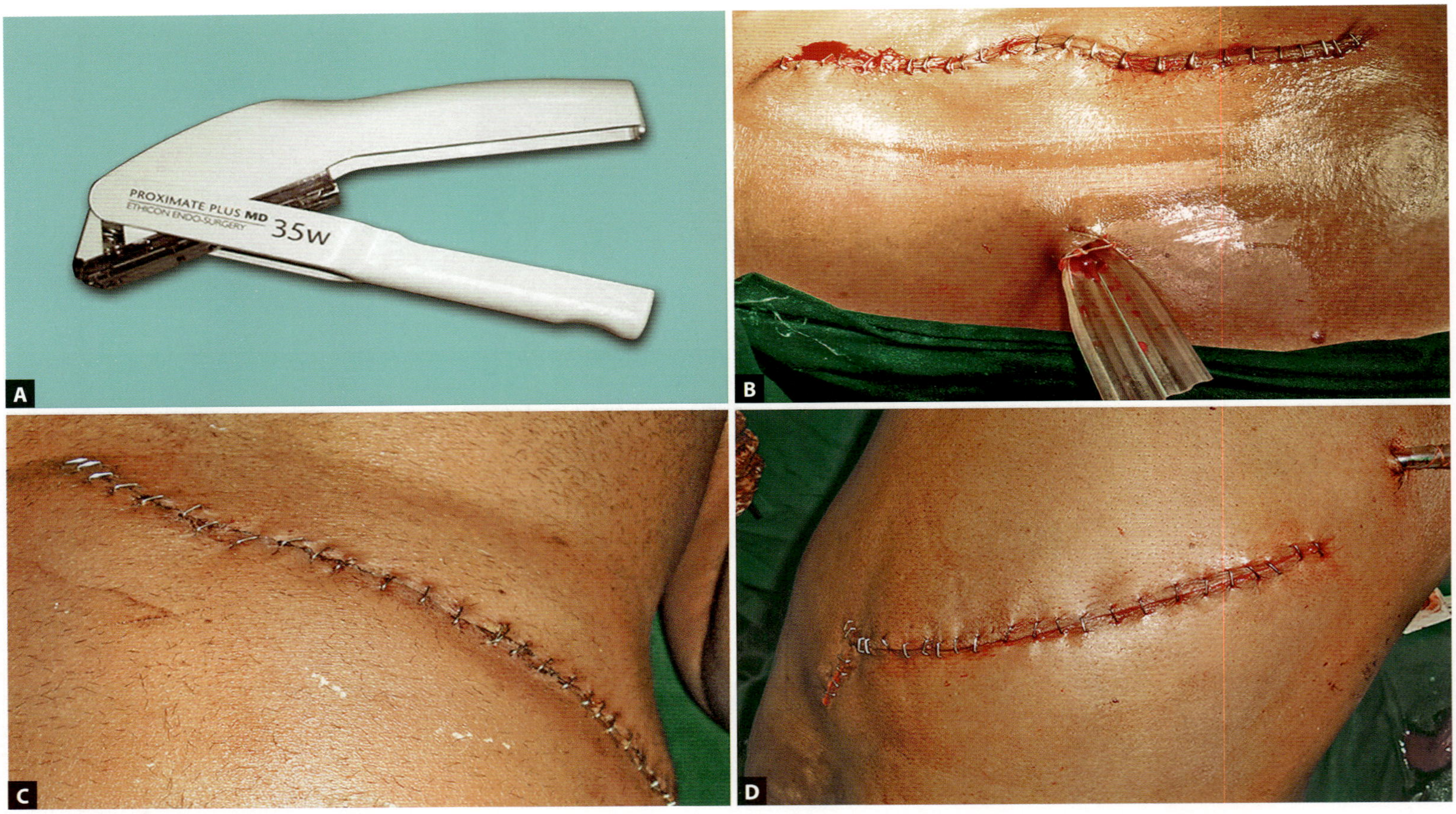

Figs. 3-40A to D: Skin stapler is used to close large surgical skin incision. It is faster and cosmetically accepted.

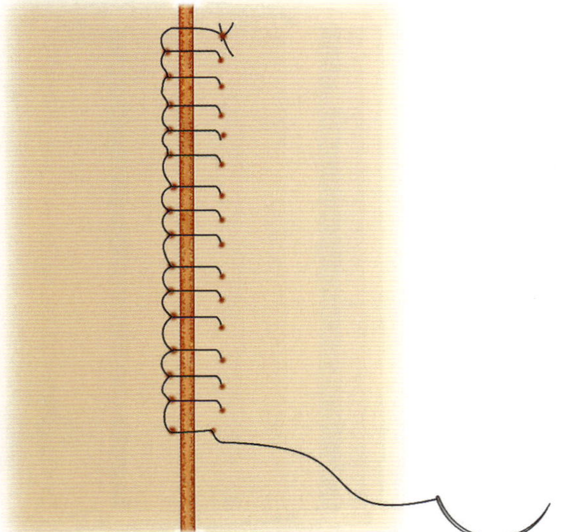

Fig. 3-41: Continuous locking suture.

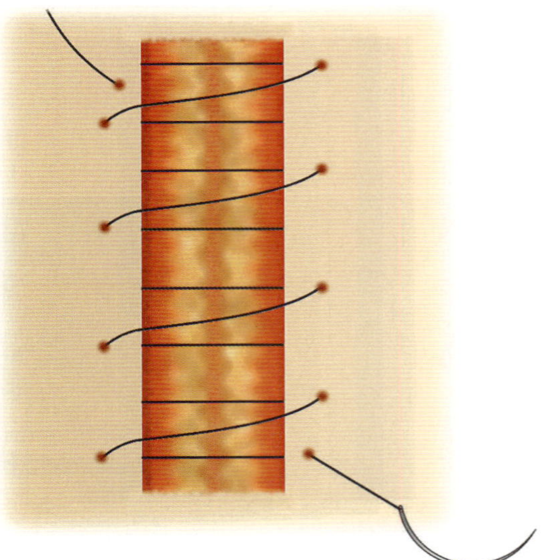

Fig. 3-42: Continuous over and over suture.

Continuous 'mass closure' using one or zero monofilament non-absorbable suture material commonly used in closure of abdominal incisions especially midline. Bites are taken at 1 cm width from wound edge; with each bite at 1 cm interval. Single strand or loop suture material can be used for this. This method is commonly used **(Fig. 3-43)**.

Note:

Jenkin's rule—suture length to wound length ratio should be at least 4:1 often may be even 6:1 as skin and soft tissues lengthen significantly under strain; to accommodate this lengthening lengthier suture material is needed.

The three point suture: It is used in suturing triangular flap/flaps to have correct apposition. Dermal bites should be at the same levels on both edges **(Fig. 3-44)**.

Retention sutures (Tension sutures): It is even though practiced in many centres, ideally it should be avoided. It is used during closure of laparotomies done for acute conditions like peritonitis, obstruction wherein patient's general condition is not good; layer by

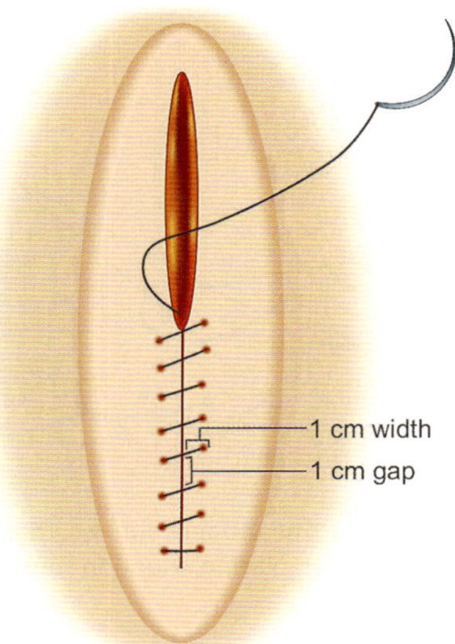

Fig. 3-43: Continuous mass closure of the abdomen.

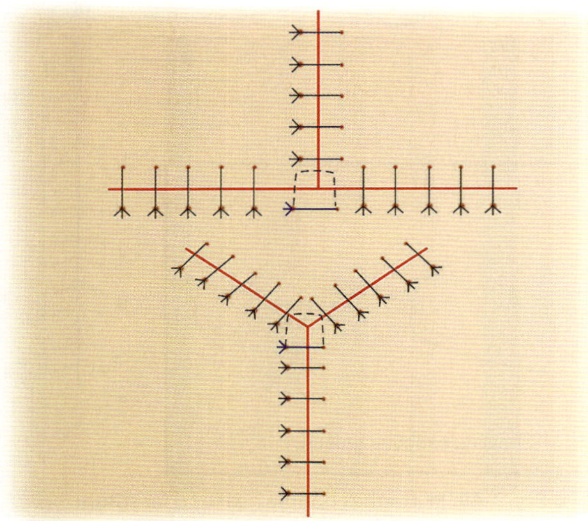

Fig. 3-44: Three-point suturing is used in apposing junction of the triangular flaps.

layer closure may cause acute wound failure with burst abdomen; when quick closure is a need of the day. Its use is getting replaced by *Smead-Jones* sutures or interrupted single layer deeper sutures. Retention sutures are taken as full thickness sutures placed 3–5 cm away from the wound. Large curved cutting needle is used. Number zero or one monofilament suture material like polyethylene is used. First bite is taken away from the wound from skin to peritoneum into the peritoneal cavity; needle is then brought back 3–5 cm away from the opposite edge of the wound; suture material is passed through a supportive sterile tube (cut drip set tube) of 2–3 cm length; near the edge of the skin of the existing side needle and suture material is passed; similar bite is taken on the same side of skin edge; suture is passed through one more sterile tube of 2–3 cm size and is kept ready for knotting after completion of placing all sutures. Each suture is placed with a gap of 1.5–2 cm. Knotting is started from one corner; but if closure is difficult then central knots is put first. While knotting in deeper plane, bowel and omentum should be guarded with finger or placing mop or using a special curved bow-like instrument (*Sergeant Instrument*) so as to prevent entangling or injuring these structures.

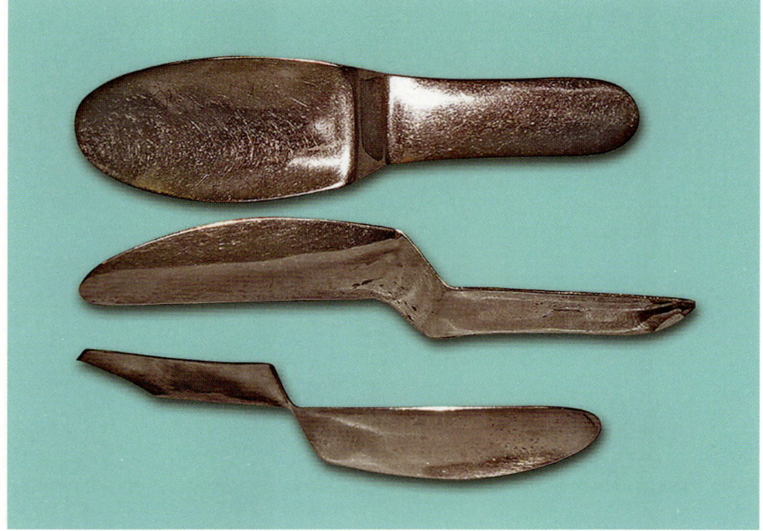

Fig. 3-45: Sergeant retractor used during closure of the abdomen to prevent abdominal content coming out.

Sutures are cut once all knots are tied on one side of the wound. Skin may be apposed using separate sutures **(Fig. 3-45)**.

In *vertical mattress retention sutures,* tubes cross the wound. *In horizontal mattress retention sutures*, bites are taken like a square and sterile tubes are placed parallel to the wound (not crossing). In this type, number of sutures needed is less than vertical type. Distinct advantages of horizontal mattress retention suture type are not clear but it is said that it is stronger than vertical mattress retention suture. But chances of bowel or omentum getting trapped are higher in this **(Figs. 3-46 and 3-47)**.

Modified Smead-Jones closure: It is interrupted specialised suture used in the closure of abdomen as single layer excluding the skin. Linea alba is held with Allis' forceps. *Number one* polyethylene or PDS suture material is used. First bite on one side taken 3 cm away (width) from the margin from outside to inside; it is then passed through the corresponding opposite edge with 3 cm width from inside to outside; later again one small loop of 5 mm width from the edges of each side of the wound from first bite site to second bite site is taken; suture is knotted on the free edge of the first bite side. Full thickness bite holds the suture and maintains the tension in the wound. Smaller loop keeps the linea alba in apposed place. Large curved *Ferguson needle* is better to place these sutures. Each suture is placed at 2 cm interval. This is the type of suturing used at present in acute abdominal conditions instead of the retention sutures. Here also it is better to place all sutures under proper vision and knotting is done at the end **(Fig. 3-48)**. At least four knots should be placed. Excessive tension should be avoided. In upper abdomen peritoneum need not be included in the bite; but in lower abdomen as linea alba is indistinct, peritoneum is included in this.

LE Hughes double near and far suture: It is similar with same indications as Smead-Jones, with double near and far sutures placed to have a strong loop with knot on one side **(Fig. 3-49)**.

Single layer seromucosal suture of bowel: It is now well-practiced method of suturing of the bowel. Interrupted seromucosal sutures using 3-zero/2-zero Vicryl or PDS takes up well. Nonabsorbable silk or linen also can be used. These nonabsorbable sutures are good old suture materials which are even now well accepted. Only drawback presumed is formation of suture granuloma at the anastomotic site **(Fig. 3-50)**.

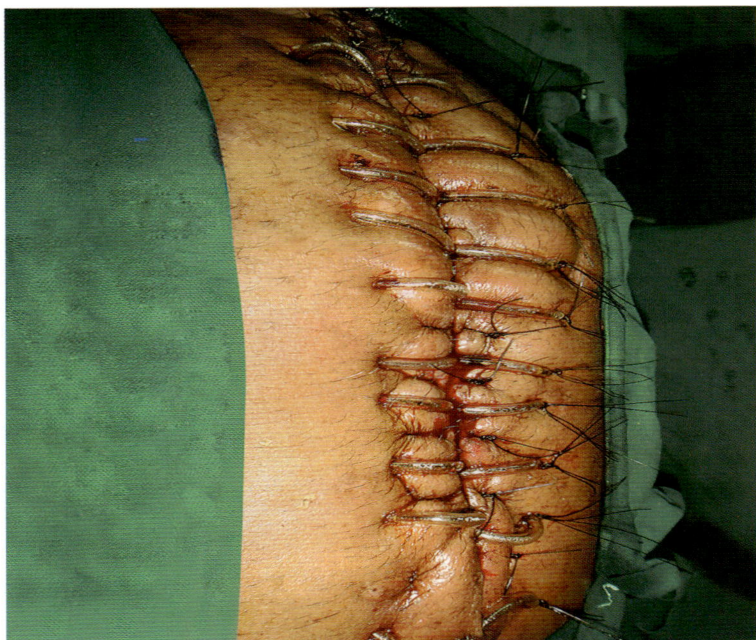

Fig. 3-46: Vertical mattress retention sutures. It is full thickness single layer suture.

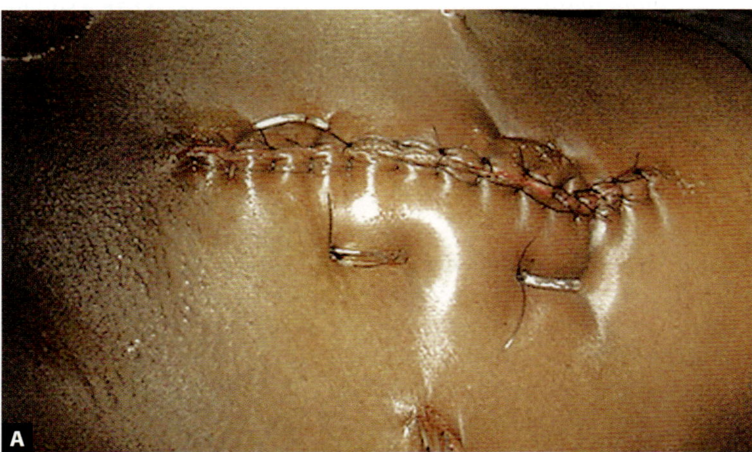

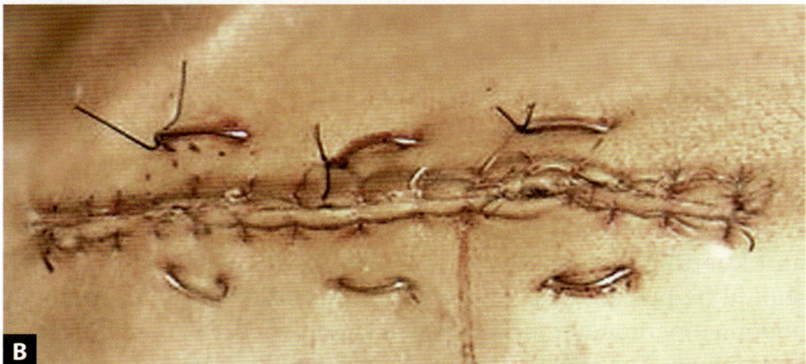

Figs. 3-47A and B: Horizontal mattress suture.

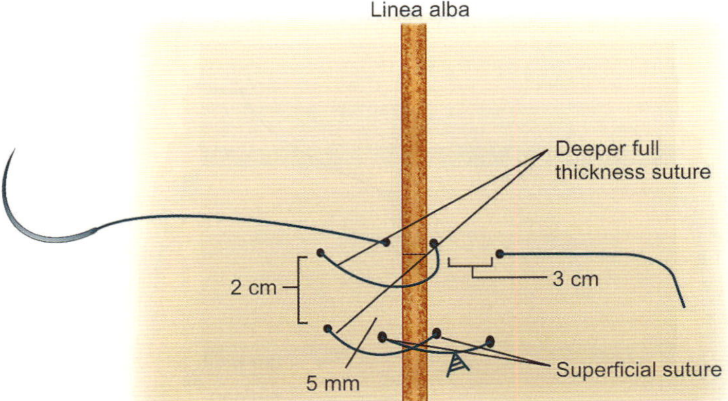

Fig. 3-48: Modified Smead-Jones sutures. These sutures are better than placing retention sutures.

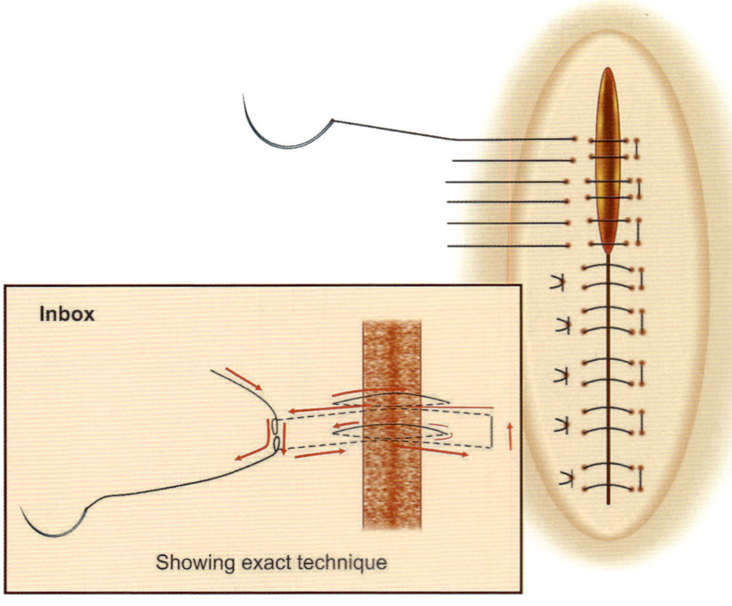

Fig. 3-49: LE Hughes double near and far suture.

Gambee single layer full thickness (all layers) sutures using Vicryl are also used in bowel anastomosis. It can also be used as continuous sutures especially during gastrojejunostomy. *Continuous suturing* is quicker; alternate bites should be locked to prevent purse string effect; anterior layer is closed with inverting sutures. *Interrupted suture* is more stable and stronger with less chances of anastomotic disruption. It also maintains the blood supply better than continuous sutures. Width of suture bite taken should be less over mucosal part than seromuscular part. Bites are taken 3 mm from the cut edge of the serosa; each bite is taken in a 5 mm gap **(Fig. 3-51)**.

Lembert suture: It is the commonly used seromuscular suture. Silk 3-zero or Vicryl 3-zero is used. Deep seromuscular suture including submucosal layer is taken at a point 5 mm from the cut edge of the serosa; this bite emerges at same line closure at 2 mm from the cut edge of serosa; bite is taken on the opposite part of the bowel at 2 mm from the serosal cut edge as seromuscular which emerges at 5 mm point away in the same longitudinal line and knot is placed. It can be used as continuous suture also **(Fig. 3-52)**.

Cushing suture: It is similar to Lembert suture wherein seromuscular bites are taken parallel to the cut edge of the serosa (at 2 mm from the cut edge). Thickness of tissue taken is 5 mm. Both interrupted and continuous sutures can be taken **(Fig. 3-53)**.

Halsted suture: It is actually seromuscular horizontal mattress suture. Care must be taken to avoid excessive tension over the suture line as this may lead into ischaemia of the anastomotic site **(Fig. 3-54)**.

Connell suture: Here suture material passes through all the layers of the intestine from serosa to mucosa; again brought out through all layers of the intestine on the same side from mucosa to serosa;

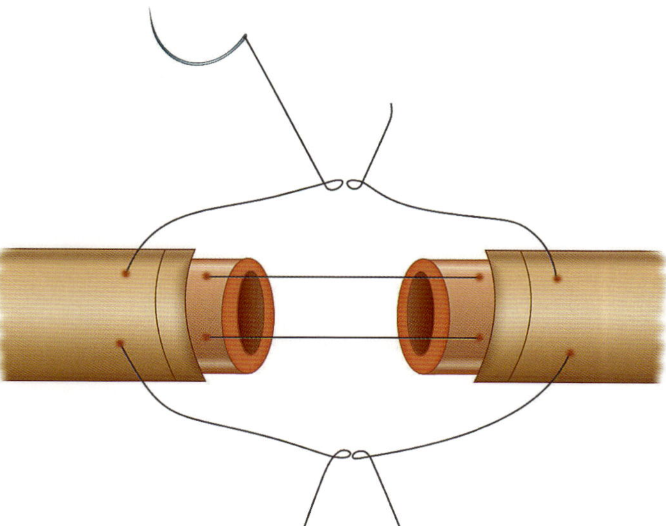

Fig. 3-50: Single layer seromucosal layer suturing of the bowel.

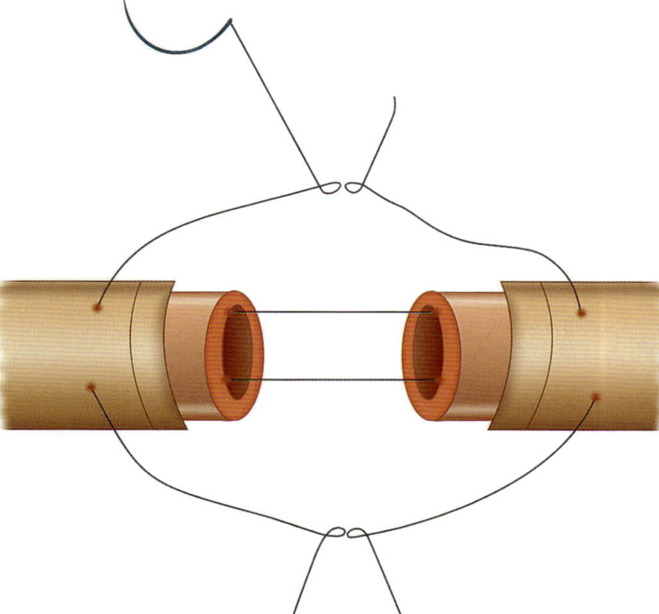

Fig. 3-51: Gambee suture.

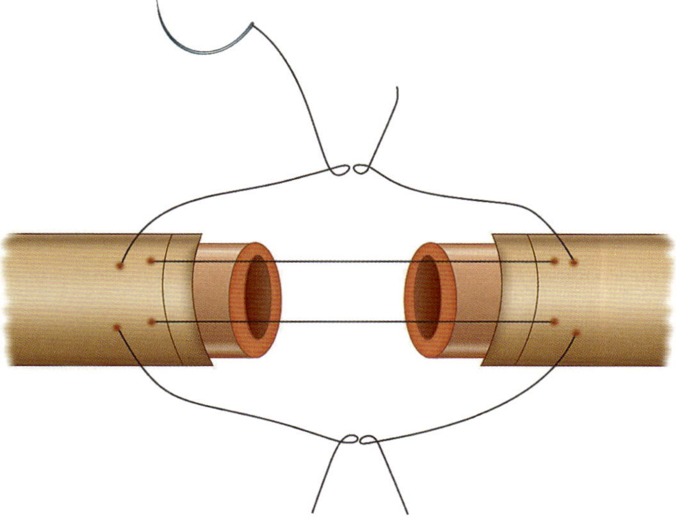

Fig. 3-52: Lembert suture.

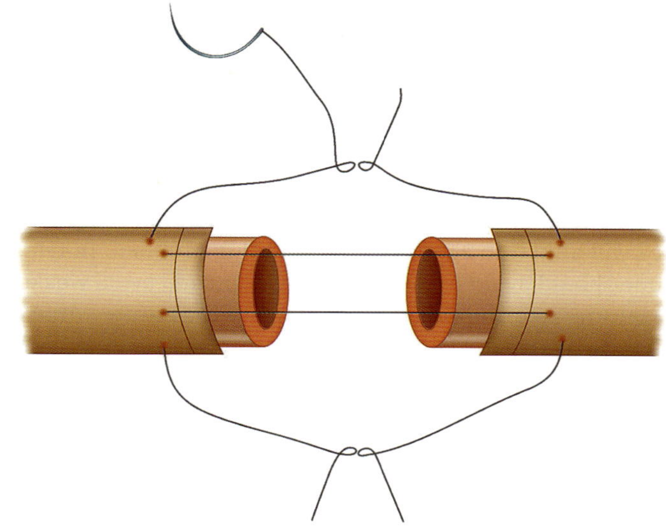

Fig. 3-53: Cushing suture.

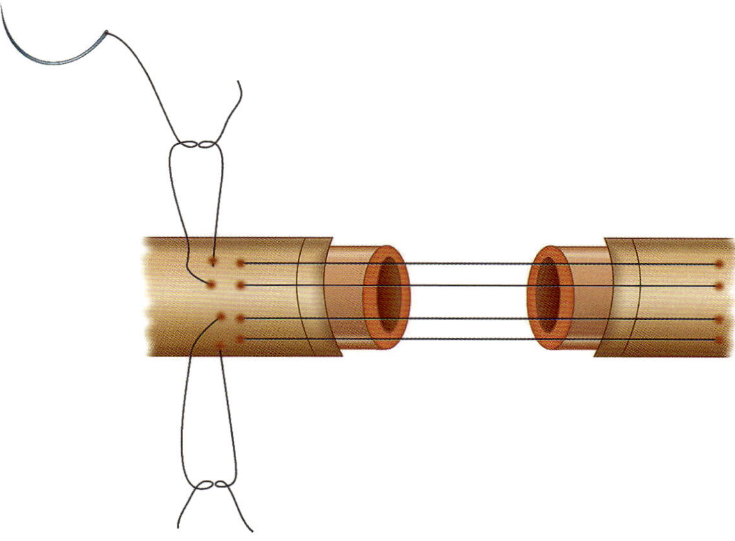

Fig. 3-54: Halsted suture.

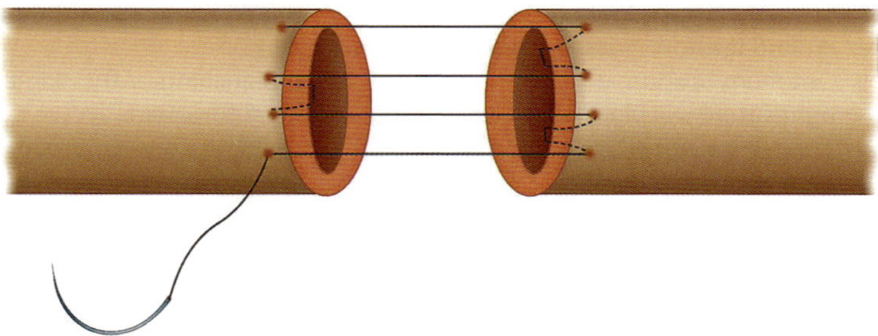

Fig. 3-55: Connell suture for bowel anastomosis.

passed over opposite segment of the bowel; passing from serosa to lumen/mucosa and from mucosa to outside towards serosa; again coming towards same side to repeat the technique. It is very good technique to invert the mucosal part of the anterior layer. It is commonly used in double layer anastomosis but can be used in single layer anastomosis **(Fig. 3-55)**. Connell suture apposes well; achieves good mucosal inversion. But it is *not adequately haemostatic* and so bleeders on the cut edge of the bowel should be ligated or cauterised individually.

KNOT TYING TECHNIQUE

Principles

The knot must be simple, firmly tied and should not slip. Knots must be as small as possible and ends should be cut as short as possible in the tissues. Skin sutures which are to be removed should be kept around 1 cm length so that removal is easier. But keeping too long sutures will abut into adjacent knots causing problem. In tying the knot one should avoid friction between strands to avoid weakening of the suture; one should avoid damage to the suture while tying knot. Excessive tension while tying knot will lead to suture breakage or tissue damage. Strength should be optimum; neither too tight nor too loose. Beginners tend to put too tight knots. Too tight sutures may cause tissue strangulation. After tying the first loop tension should be maintained on the strand to avoid loosening of knot. Final throw should be as nearly horizontal as possible. The surgeon should not hesitate to change stance or position in order to place secure flat knot. Usually three knots are sufficient. First knot is the best knot. In retention sutures or if polypropylene is used as suture material, then maximum 4/5 knots have to be placed. Any additional knots will not help in stability of knot or do not add to the strength of a securely tied square knot.

First throw/knot should be gently pushed and guided using index finger **(Fig. 3-56)**.

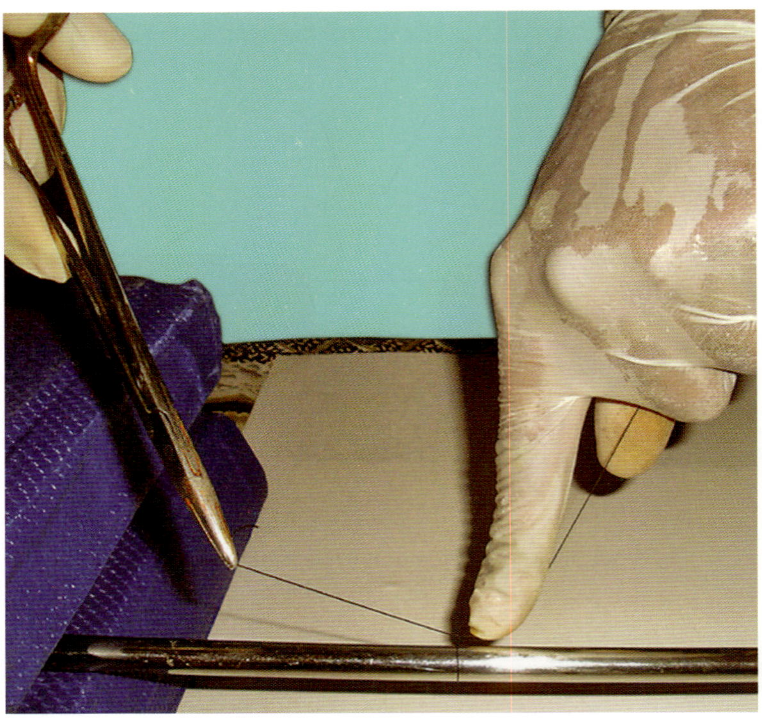

Fig. 3-56: First throw/knot should be gently pushed and guided using index finger.

Remember about suturing

- Width of the bite of suture on each side of the wound edge should be equal—*coarse* adjustment.
- Gap between the sutures should be equal. It may be 1 cm gap in skin; 3–5 mm gap in bowel; 1–2 mm gap in vessel.
- Slight eversion of the wound edge causes proper apposition. Scar will be cosmetically acceptable.
- Deeper bite in the tissue by the needle should be wider than superficial to achieve adequate eversion.
- Inversion of edges may cause overlapping, delayed healing, delayed wound gap and poor scarring.
- Knots should be on one side of the bites on the corner of the optimal side which is the wound edge which is on lower level—gives *fine* adjustment.
- Bites should be adequate and deep enough; superficial unequal bites will cause improper apposition.
- Thumb can be used to push the skin against the needle bite from opposite side.
- Suturing is done from more mobile edge of the wound towards relatively immobile side.
- Flap of the tissue/skin when sutured, knot should be on the opposite side of the edge of the flap.
- Vertical mattress sutures give a good eversion.
- Improper alignment of the wound edges in a curved or lengthy wounds can be prevented by placing the key sutures at salient points which are identified by holding the edges taut using skin hooks or marking corresponding points on each edge to have proper adjustment and to prevent distortion.
- Wound tension should be distributed equally.
- Optimum tension at suture line will not cause blanching of the skin and will only leave thin/least suture mark whereas more tension with abnormally tight suture will blanch the skin causing obvious suture mark.
- Apposition, not strangulation of the tissues should be done. Optimum tension and number of stitches should be used. Excessive stitches are also should be avoided.
- Matching and alignment of wound edges are important. Dog ear should be avoided. In lengthy wound, first suture is placed centrally; next one is between end of the wound and the first suture; this will allow proper apposition and avoids dog ear formation.
- Curve of the needle should be followed; levering causes damage.
- Least tissue trauma, atraumatic handling, optimum precision are the need.
- Suturing and knotting is an art; a craft; is a fine work.
- Slow, precise, first bite should be careful and best bite; rapid, clumsy bite is not a good bite; one should avoid repetition.
- Matching landmarks on either sides of the wound should be identified properly.
- Suturing is easier with multifilament suture material like silk than monofilament suture material. Silk has got best handling ability, knot holding property, least memory. Suture insertion and passage through tissues is easier with silk.
- Tissues should be handled gently; heavy retraction of the tissues should be avoided.
- Proper selection of sutures and needles is important.
- Layers should be approximated properly but as tension free (layer by layer).
- Dead space should be obliterated.
- Skin and tough structures like periosteum needs cutting needles; atraumatic eyeless needle with sutures. are ideal.
- Interrupted sutures are better whenever there is oedema, infection/inflammation or in secondary suturing. Non-absorbable monofilament sutures are advisable here.
- Subcuticular or absorbable sutures are used in clean wounds.

Different Knot Tying Techniques

Hand Knot Tying

Two hands and single hand techniques are used. Two hands technique is ideal. *Aberdeen hand knot* is also used to end the continuous suture.

Two hands technique is commonly used. It is done using left hand in right hander; end of the thread/suture material is held between thumb and index finger of left hand; this part of the thread will pass behind the little finger of left hand, encircling it, and coming forward towards between thumb and index finger. Opposite end of the thread which is held in right hand is looped in front across middle finger; middle finger stretching and holding this right-hand loop will be flexed at the distal interphalangeal joint and looped around the left-hand thread end to create first knot which is held between apposed middle and ring fingers. These two fingers with the thread are pulled towards left to release the knot; knot is squared by directing the left hand towards the opposite side; knot is tightened by gentle push using pulp of left index finger. Further two knots are also placed similarly **(Figs. 3-57 and 3-58)**.

Single hand technique is done using left hand index finger. Thread is held similarly but between left thumb and left middle finger; looping is done using left index finger. This method is used whenever thread is small or there is less space in the area. It is little cumbersome to do compared to two hands technique **(Figs. 3-59A to H)**.

Two hand technique and single hand is also done in another method: With the left hand between thumb and index finger one end of the thread is held (held proximal to the pulp these two fingers) with loop coming in front from below; other end of the thread holding in right hand is passed across index finger of left hand coming from behind up and forward close to the other end of the thread in left hand; apposed pulps of the thumb and index finger is looped around it

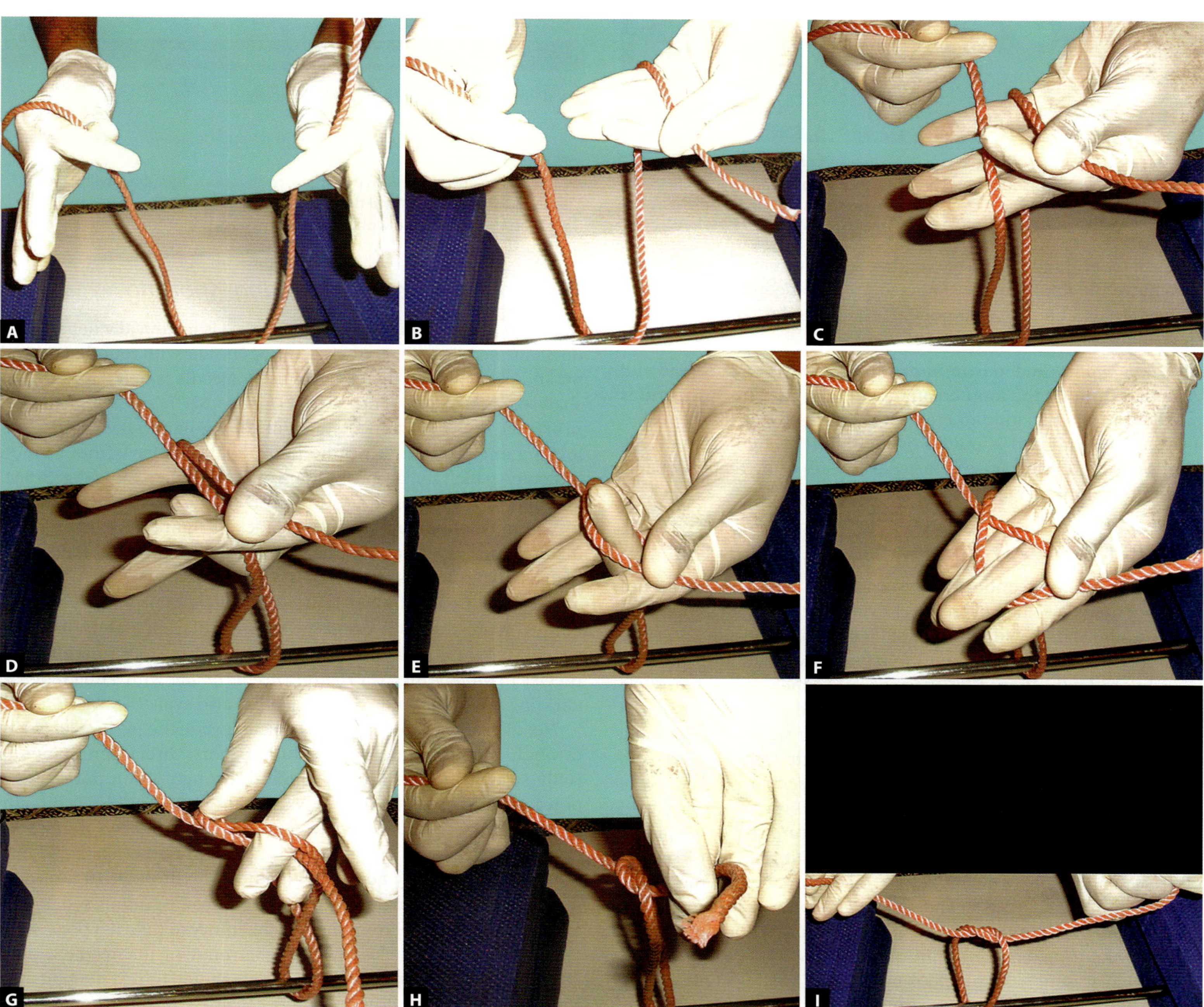

Figs. 3-57A to I: Hand knotting using two hands technique.

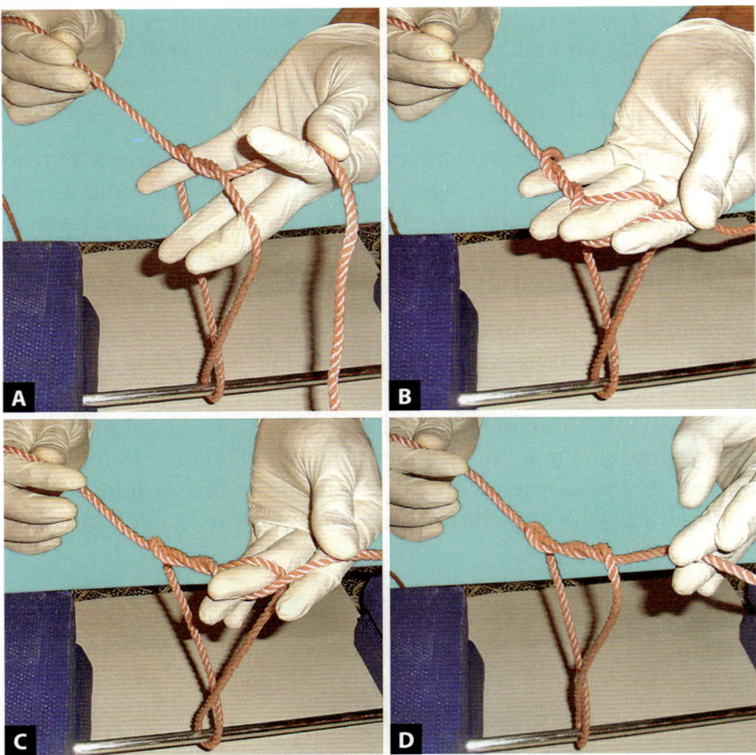

Figs. 3-58A to D: Two hands technique use and placing surgeon's knot with two loops/throws in the knot with squaring.

and left-hand thread tip is passed between these two finger pulps to achieve the knot. Further knots are repeated similarly. Surgical knots can also be placed. Knots can be placed in similar way by single hand technique **(Figs. 3-60A to S)**.

Aberdeen knot is used in continuous sutures at the end. Thread end is passed through the loop created in earlier last bite/turn; end is passed through this loop to create a new loop; once it is repeated 4–5 times thread end is pulled firmly tightly to tighten the knot. It is used while closing linea alba/rectus sheath using nonabsorbable continuous sutures **(Figs. 3-61A to M)**.

Instrument Knot Tying

This is the basic essentiality for surgery. Different types of knot tying are there. Needle holder is held with one hand; long limb side of the suture is held with other hand; instrument (needle holder) is looped (throws) around the suture usually twice for surgical knot (first knot ideally should be *surgical knot*—means two loops are taken); instrument is crossed to opposite side to square the knot and gently knot is tightened; tightening of the knot should be adequate enough means neither too tight to strangulate the tissue nor too loose so as to create a gap; this first knot is *essentially the best knot* in knotting; gentle traction should be held to the strand to avoid loosening of the first knot; two ends of the suture should be pulled in opposite direction with equal gentle traction. Second knot is taken as a single loop which is usually taken from behind the suture material (opposite direction and squared in opposite direction) and is tightened; third knot is again single loop (or often double loop like surgeon's knot) taken from front of the suture material (alike first knot single or double loop) and is tightened. One has to remember that usually three firm proper knots are sufficient. It is always considered that even though first knot is the holding knot total two knots (only one additional knot) are *insufficient* and *so three knots* are a must **(Figs. 3-62A to K)**.

Only in suture material like polypropylene which has highest *memory* (recoiling tendency and so poor knot holding ability) five knots are put. Any further knots put will not help in strengthening the knot further; so it is waste of energy by the surgeon and unnecessary creating bunch in the knot. After placing first knot it is always better to fix the knot with surgeon's index finger to confirm the adequacy of tightness of the knot **(Figs. 3-63A to H)**.

Instrumental knotting is more precise than hand knotting; as it creates optimum regulated tension at the suture line; and knot guidance and placement is better with instrument.

Laparoscopic Knot Tying

Problems with laparoscopic suturing are—lack of tissue perception, depth; limitation of movement of the instruments; difficulty in suturing and knotting inside; restricted space of working; need for high skill level by the laparoscopic surgeon.

Prerequisites for laparoscopic suturing

- Perfect health—mentally and physically.
- Hand-eye coordination.
- Visual perception, ability to concentrate and dedication, determination.
- Precision, proper camera operator.
- Learning curve, repetitive training, motivation, discipline, willpower.
- Proper instruments and their usage.
- Triangulation of two working instruments is important.

Types of Laparoscopic Suturing/Knotting

A. *Intracorporeal suturing and knotting:* It is technically demanding one. Fine needle with suture is used. *Ski needle* with rounded curved tip and triangular straight shaft is used. Needle is held at triangular shaft so that needle will not swivel. *Dundee 'Ski' needle* with flattened proximal cross section instead of triangular makes improved locking and fixation of needle into needle holder without much difficulty, which makes positioning of the needle easier **(Fig. 3-64)**. Standard curved needles are also commonly used but with swiveling problem. Polyfilament, coloured (black or fluorescent white), and 3-zero suture materials are ideal. Polyfilament material holds well with easy knotting ability.

Excellent needle holder is an asset for intracorporeal knotting. Semm, Wolf, Ethicon, Cook, MBG are different needle holders available. Szabo and Berci needle holder gives 360° rotation with precise manoeuvring. *Self-righting needle holder* with a notch inside allowing self-positioning of the needle is also available.

Needle with suture material is placed inside the peritoneal cavity through—5 mm reducer cross 10 mm port; direct percutaneous (only straight needle); Reich method through 5 mm port (5 mm port is removed, gently needle with 5 mm needle holder is directly pushed along the track of the removed port into the peritoneal cavity under laparoscope guidance and 5 mm port is again slid into the abdominal cavity across needle holder); through 10 mm port directly. Needle entangling in the tissues, needle cutting, separation of the suture material from the needle, injury to the vital organs are the problems which may occur while introducing the needle.

Entrance bite and exit bite in the tissue should be taken separately. Knot is formed by either through 'C' loop or 'O' loop. *Square knot, square slip knot* (square knot untumbled to form slip knot),

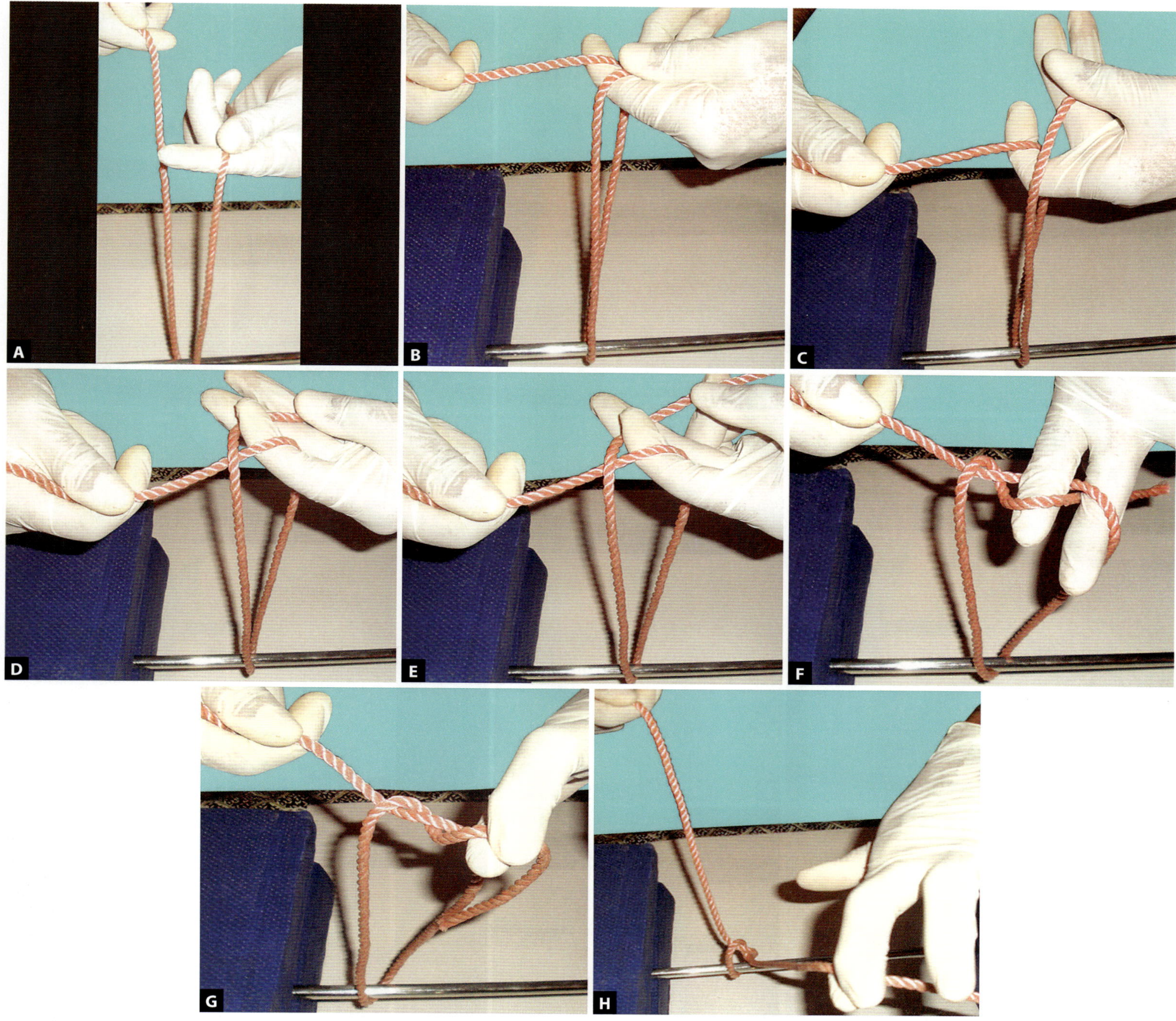

Figs. 3-59A to H: Making knot with single hand technique. Even though surgeon should learn this technique as it is used when suture ends are short. It is not necessary to use this technique for fascination purpose. It is always better to use two hands technique which is more comfortable.

ligature slip knot, surgeon's knot are placed. Jamming slip knot, Aberdeen knot (terminal knot) are other knots which can be placed. *Intracorporeal twist technique* is another method used in laparoscopic suturing. One end of the suture is rotated over the needle holder with suture tip holding for three loops; other grasper/needle holder holding other end of the suture is released to hold tip of the looped suture material; needle holder of the looped suture releases the tip of the looped suture and is allowed to hold and create a loop of the free other end of the suture which after releasing the loop across this loop forms a knot; further pull releases the loop achieving a firm knot **(Figs. 3-65 to 3-66)**.

Jamming slip knot is a starter knot used in continuous suturing. After double looping through needle holder, little away from the end, the suture is grasped to form a loop to which knot is slipped and further knots tighten it. This knot near the end of the suture material acts as a first knot of the continuous suture which avoids intracorporeal knotting and hastens the suturing **(Fig. 3-67)**.

B. *Extracorporeal knotting:* It is commonly advocated in laparoscopy as it is convenient, safe and effective. Long 90 cm suture is used; needle with suture may be passed through tissue inside under laparoscopic vision and brought out through the 5 mm/10 mm port. Similarly ligature also can be looped around the specific structure and ends of the suture are brought out for knotting. After placing extracorporeal knotting, it is pushed to the required site through a knot pusher. Additional knots similarly can be placed. Different types of extracorporeal knots are:

1. *Roeder's knot* (By Roeder used for tonsillectomy in 1918): Semm used this in laparoscopy. Catgut is commonly used.

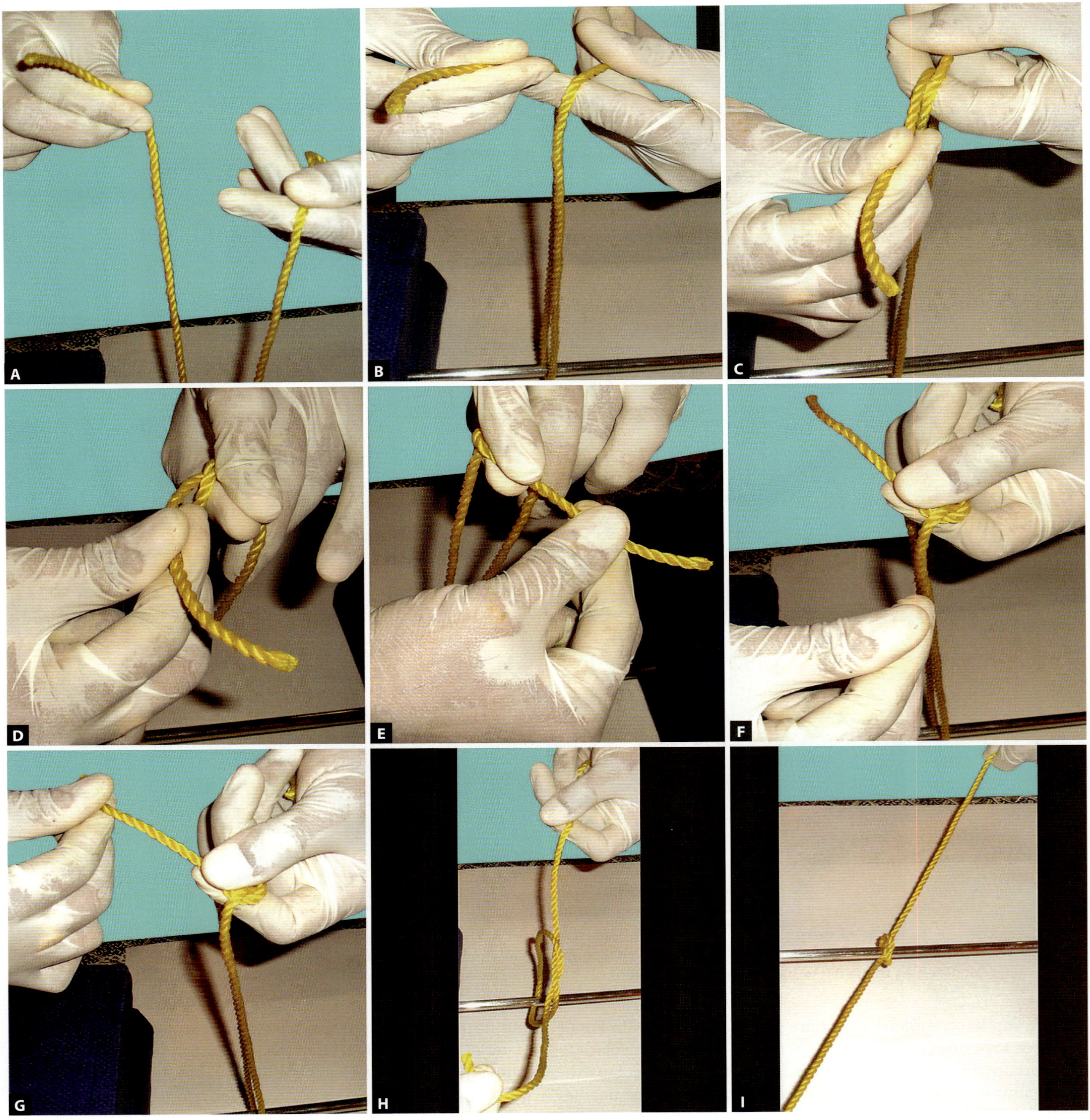

Figs. 3-60A to I

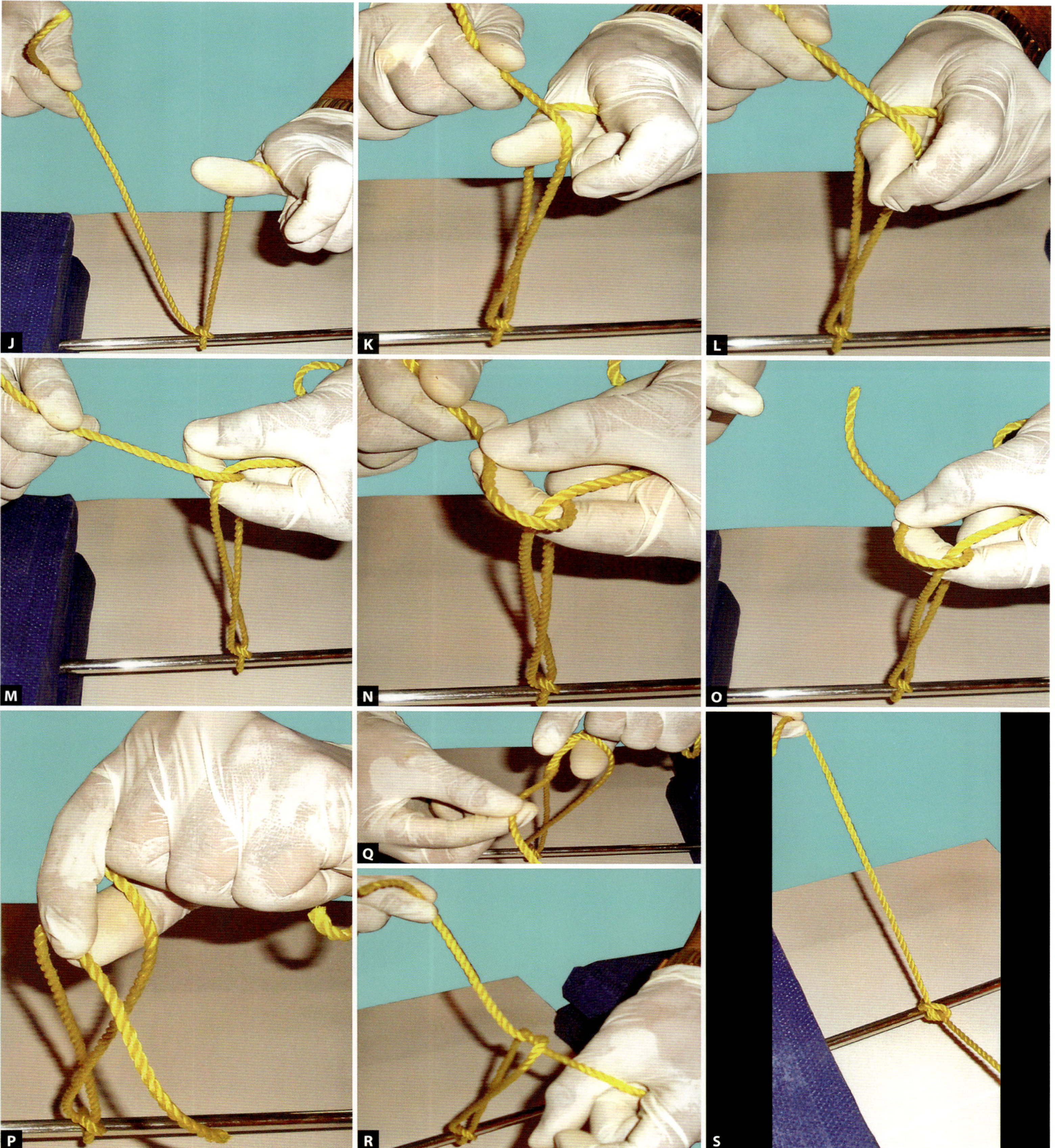

Figs. 3-60J to S

Figs. 3-60A to S: Two hands technique hands knotting using mainly thumb and index finger; here apposed thumb and index fingers move across loop to create knot.

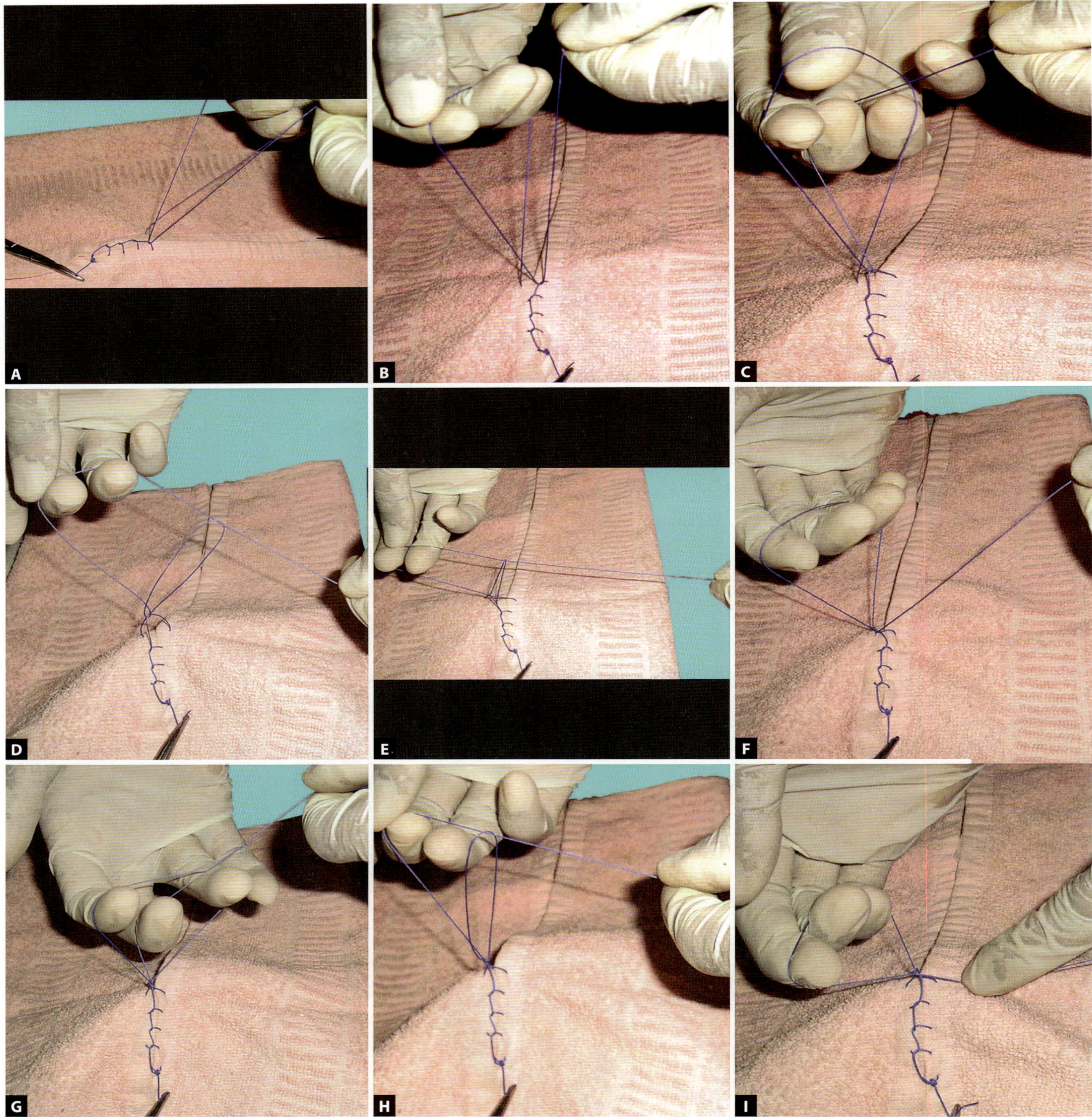

Figs. 3-61A to I

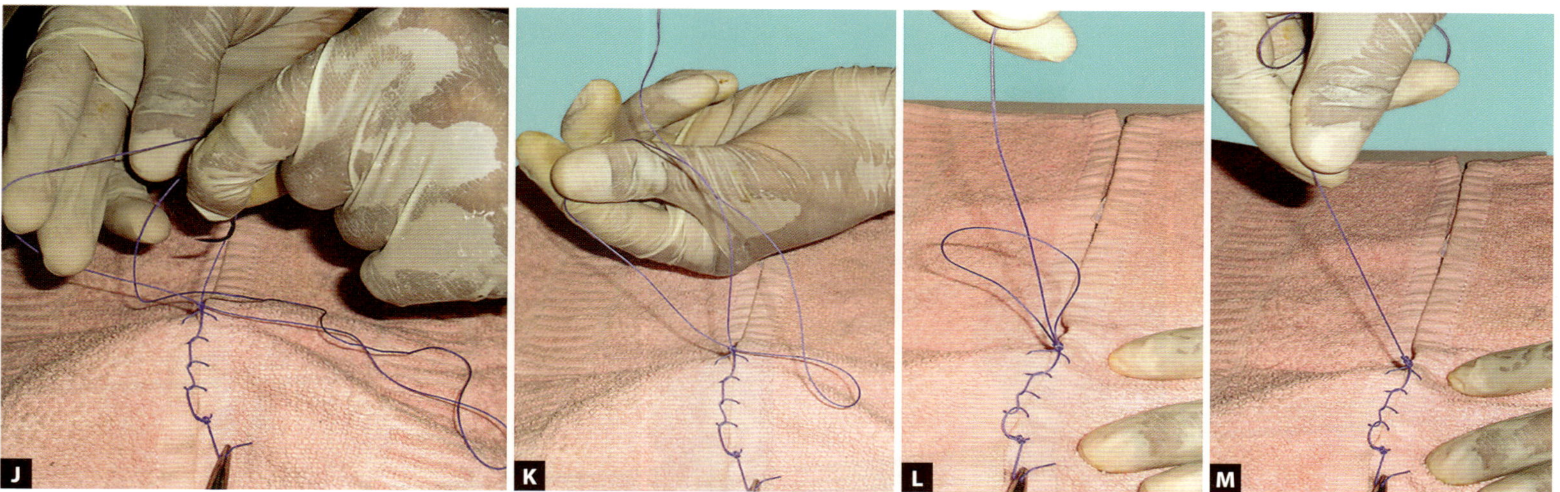

Figs. 3-61J to M

Figs. 3-61A to M: Photographs showing how exactly Aberdeen knot is placed. Usually used at the end of linea alba suturing.

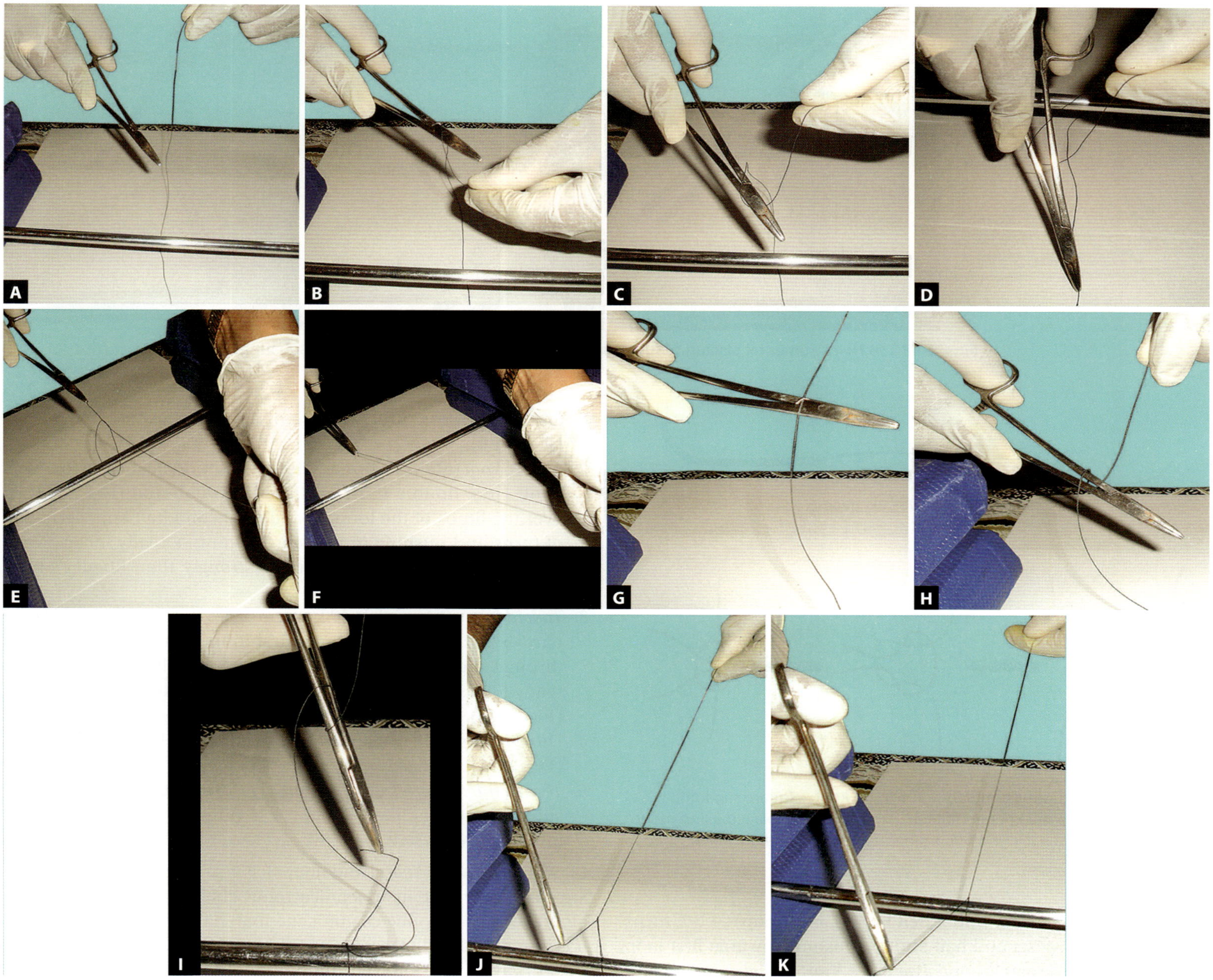

Figs. 3-62A to K: Placing reef knot using needle holder instrument. Knot should be squared for proper secure knot to get.

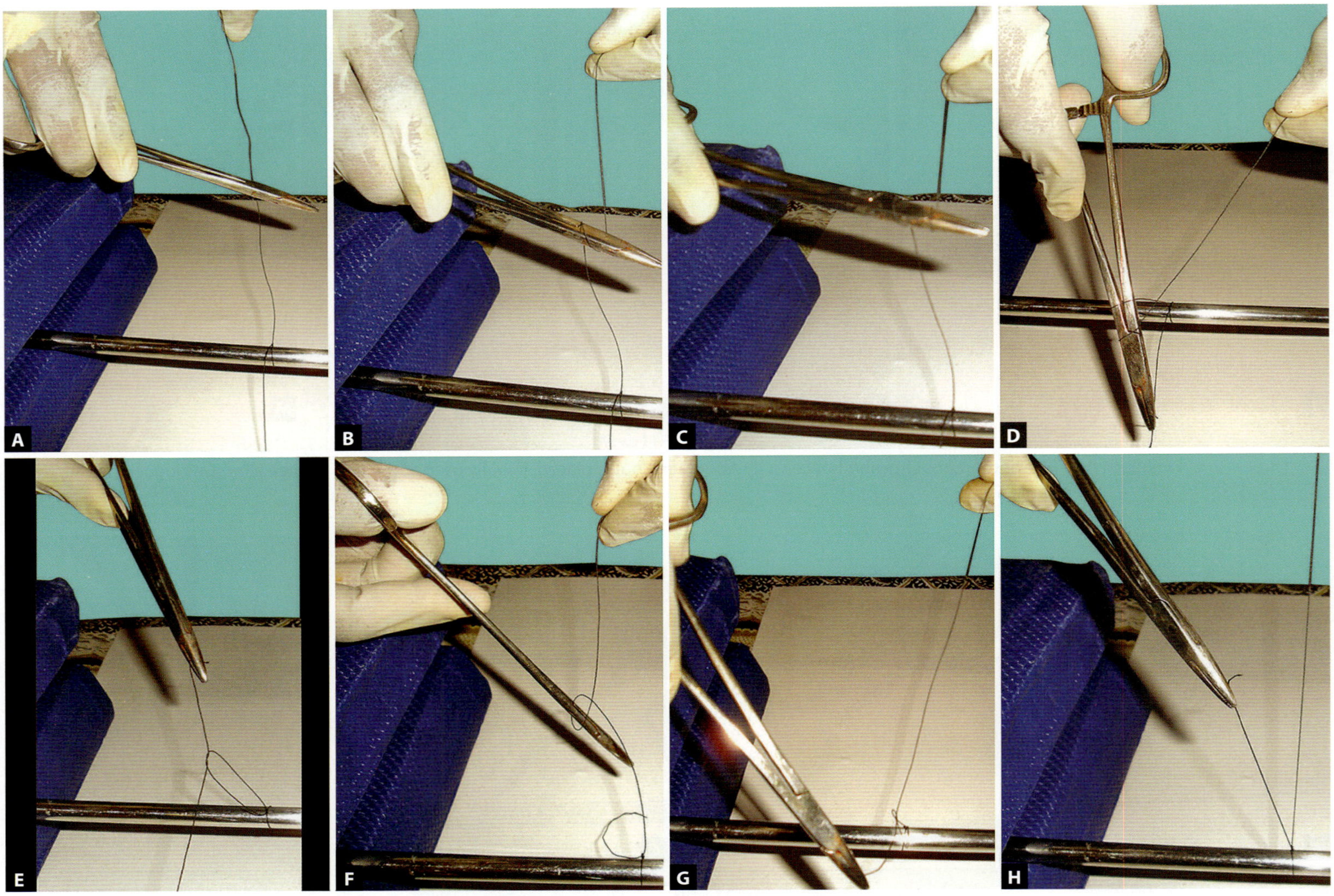

Figs. 3-63A to H: Instrumental placing of surgeon's knot (double throw of first loop with squaring)

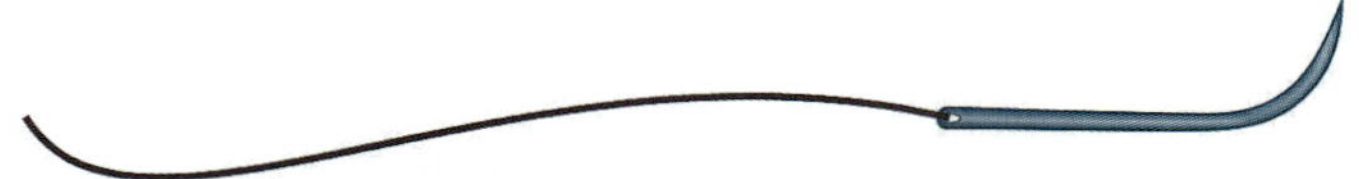

Fig. 3-64: Dundee Ski needle.

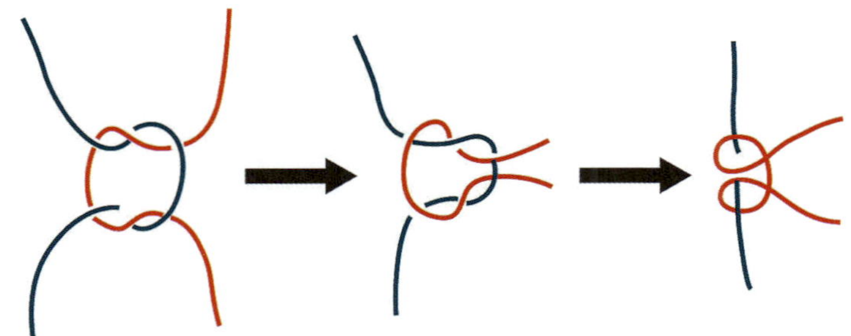

Fig. 3-65: Square knot untumbled to form slip knot—square slip knot. It has got ability to secure the knot in difficult places. It can be placed using monofilament suture material. It maintains adequate tissue tension. It is pushed in place by sliding.

Silk also can be used. Initial half knot (single loop) → 3½ turns over the loop → second half knot → pushing towards first loop → tightening creates good Roeder's knot which can be slid over the suture material easily → pushed after loop is passed around the structure like base of appendix using knot pusher **(Fig. 3-68)**.

2. *Melzer knot* (Melzer Germany 1991): It is modification of Roeder's knot. Here double initial half knot (double loop) → 3½ turn over the limbs of the loop → double second half knot → taking of turns and pushing to tighten the knot → ready for use with a loop. It is used with PDS and is *stronger* than Roeder's knot **(Fig. 3-69)**.
3. *Tayside knot:* Initial half knot → 4½ turn loop on standing part → tail is passed through first loop → tail is again passed through the first loop → tail is pulled to tighten the knot and ready for use. It is modified Fisherman's utility knot (Scotland) **(Fig. 3-70)**.
4. *Duncan slip knot:* Half hitch is added to the loop after 3½ turn **(Fig. 3-71)**.
5. *Texas Endosurgery Institute Knot (TEI Knot):* It is useful for many suture materials like PDS but it is difficult to do and several methods are present.

C. *Pre-formed slip knots* (Endoloops): It is pre-looped sutures which are commonly used in appendicectomy, cholecystectomy or ligating blood vessels. Chromic catgut is the material commonly used here. It is introduced and placed using 5 mm endoloop pusher. Disposable pushers with pre-knotted endoloops are available. Metal knot pusher is not disposable (reusable) with a Roeder's knot.

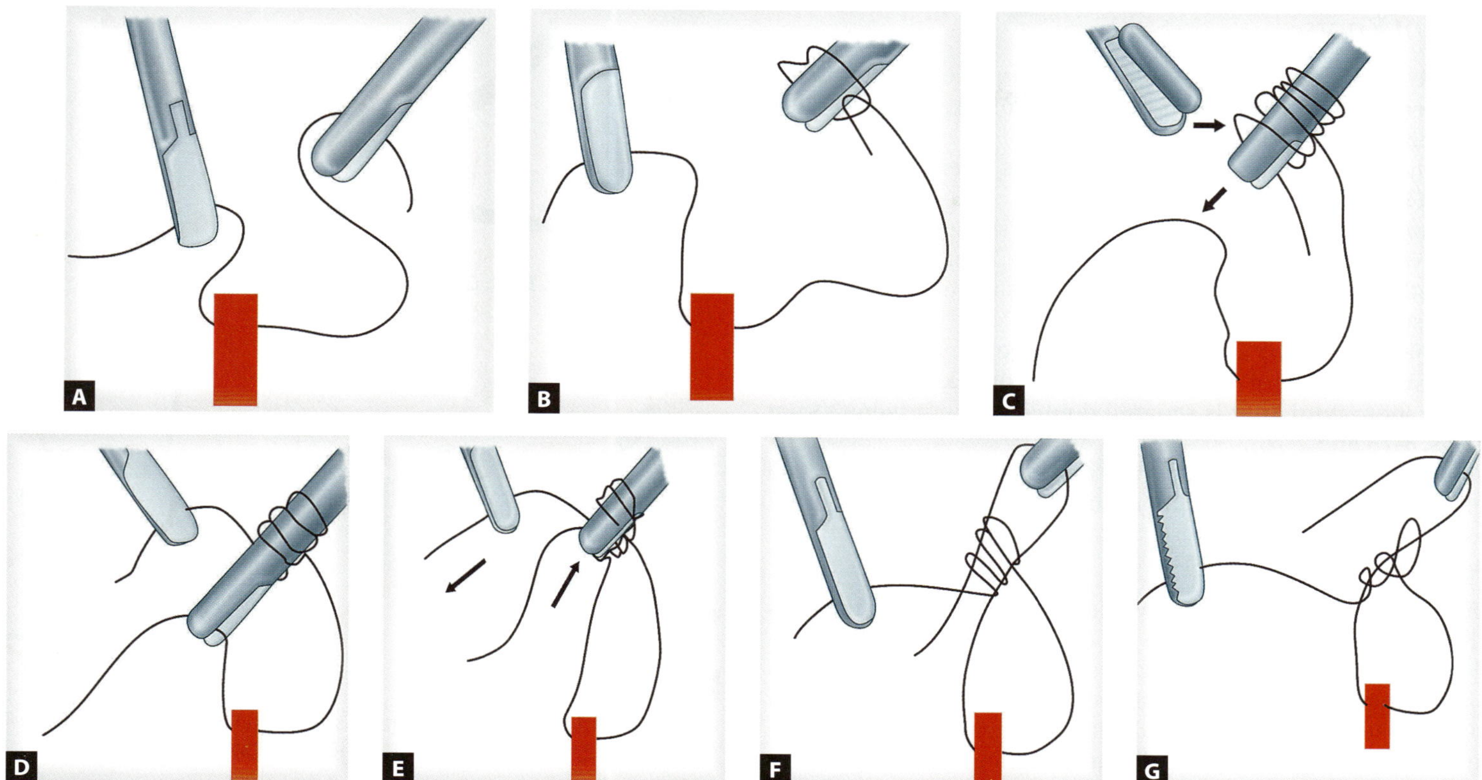

Figs. 3-66A to G: Intracorporeal twist knotting.

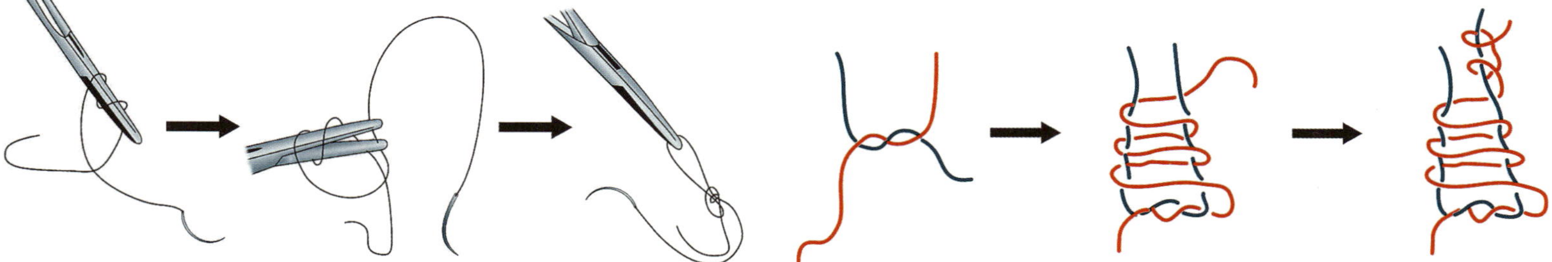

Fig. 3-67: Jamming slip knot.

Fig. 3-70: Melzer knot.

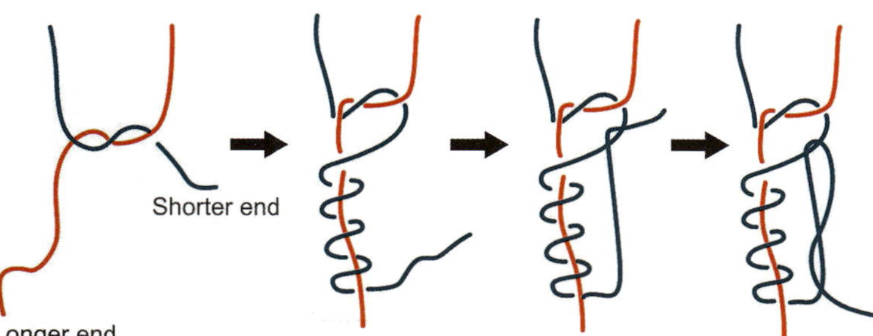

Fig. 3-68: Tayside knot.

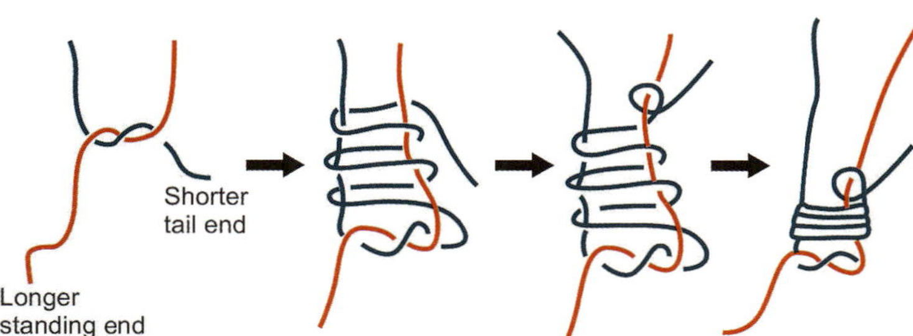

Fig. 3-69: Roeder's knot.

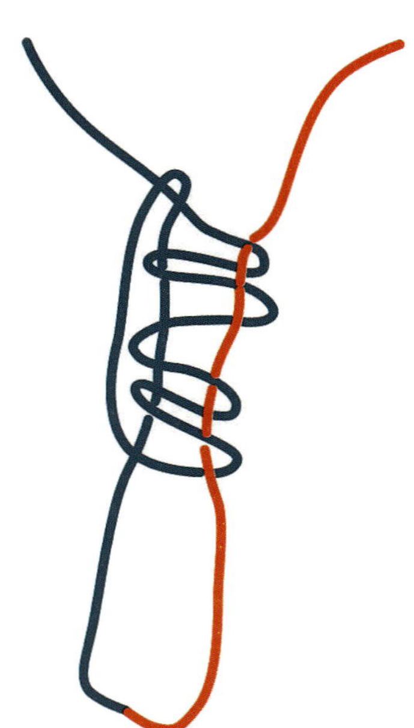

Fig. 3-71: Duncan slip knot.

Different Knots

1. *Reef knot* with squaring is ideal knot and commonly used. Correct squaring is essential. If it is not done knot gets spoiled and loosened **(Fig. 3-72)**.
2. *Granny knot* is not safe when second loop is taken from the same side **(Fig. 3-73)**.
3. *Surgeon's knot* with one extra loop in the first knot with squaring. It prevents loosening and slipping of the knot and maintains strength and tension required with the tissue and so becomes a more secure knot **(Figs. 3-74A and B)**.
4. *Modified fisherman's knot:* First knot has got three loops/throws with surgeon's knot with squaring; second knot is squared single loop; third knot is squared double throw surgeon's knot **(Figs. 3-75 and 3-76)**.
5. *Triple modified reef knot:* It is the reef with three knots instead of two. It is actually the commonly used knot **(Fig. 3-77)**.

Dog-Ear

After excision of a circular lesion while closing the wound, the ends of the wound gets elevated like pronouncement called as 'dog-ear'. If this is sutured as it is, it causes a prominence resulting in unsatisfactory cosmetic scar. Such wound is sutured until dog ear is formed; later dog-ear is excised with lengthening of the wound; suturing continued to create lengthier clean sutured wound eventually leading into a linear scar **(Fig. 3-78)**.

Principles in knotting

- Optimum grip; optimum control; optimum precision—is essential.
- Hold the suture with needle holder only during knotting (not in other time).
- Knot must be as small as possible.
- In skin, after knotting ends of interrupted sutures are cut neither too short nor too long; usually 1 cm of length is kept which is equivalent to gap between sutures. In deeper plane it should be kept short.
- One should avoid friction between strands while knotting. This can be minimised by holding sutures loosely; not tightly like a string. If so it will cause sawing effect and reduces the strength of the suture.
- Holding the suture with excessive tension will break the suture and traumatise the tissues. Folding with minimum tension allows free movement of the suture for finer suturing.
- First knot is the important knot; after placing first knot gentle traction to the strand is needed to avoid loosening of the first knot. Two ends of the suture should be pulled in opposite direction with equal gentle traction.
- Knotting is for proper apposition and approximation of the tissues; not for strangulation; so too tight suture should be avoided. Optimum tension should be used. It comes to a surgeon by repeated practice and experience. Surgeon should adjust his stance and position to place the knot properly.
- All knots ideally should be squared for stability by pulling in opposite direction.
- Friable edges of the wound cause poor knot holding and placement.

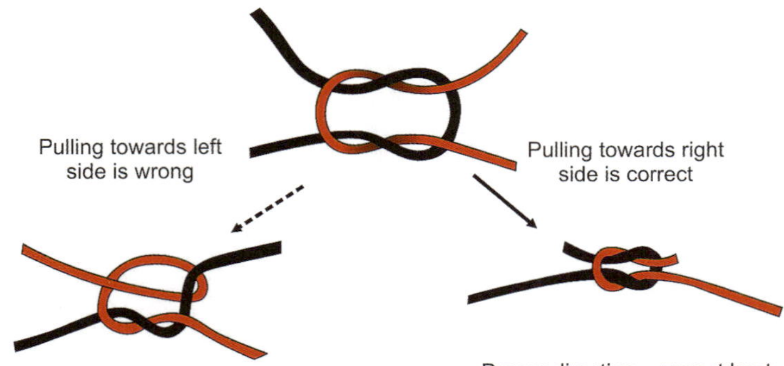

Fig. 3-72: Reef knot.

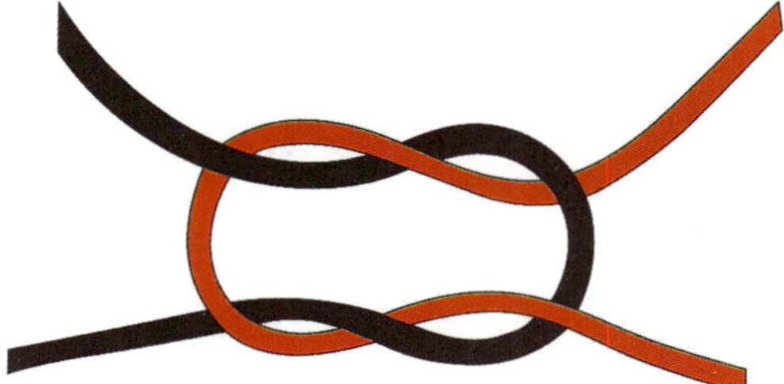

Fig. 3-73: Granny knot. It is not commonly used.

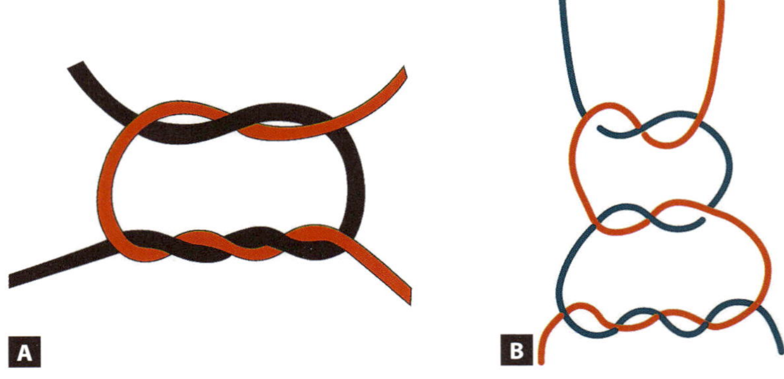

Figs. 3-74A and B: Typical surgeon's knot is taking two loops/throws in first knot with squaring. It holds well without slippage.

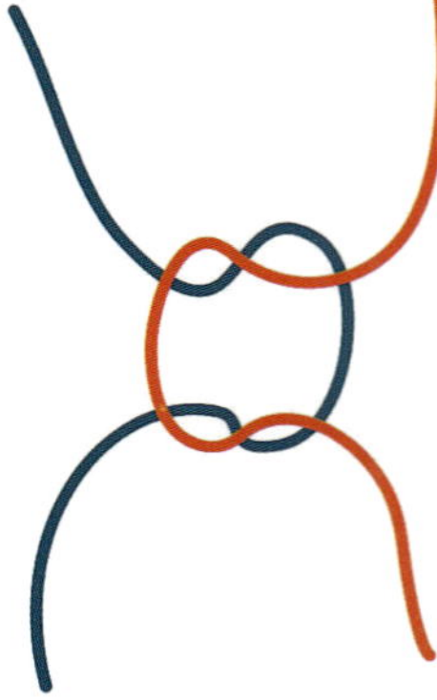

Fig. 3-75: Squaring of knot should be done to make it secure, especially first throw/knot should be squared.

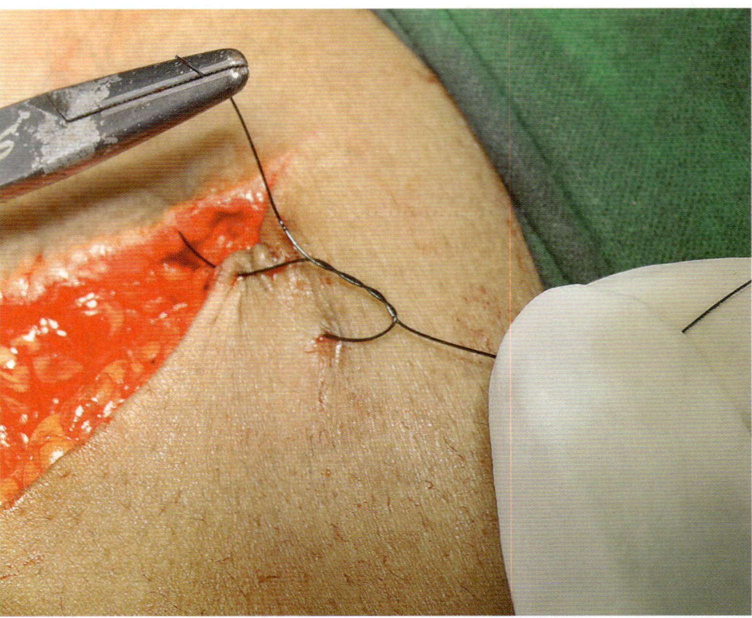

Figs. 3-76: Squaring is important to achieve a safe and secure knot.

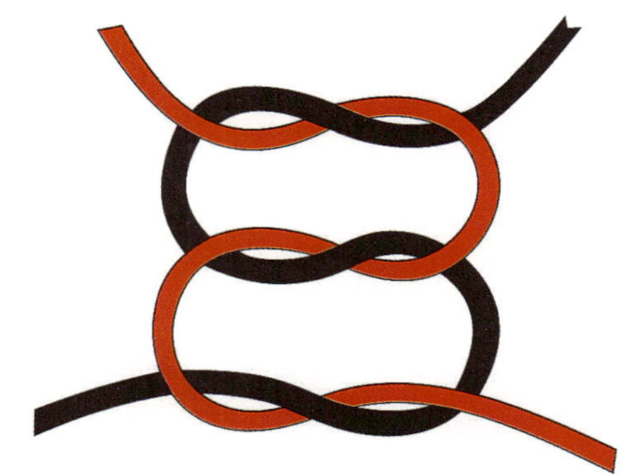

Fig. 3-77: Reef with three knots is used here which is more secure.

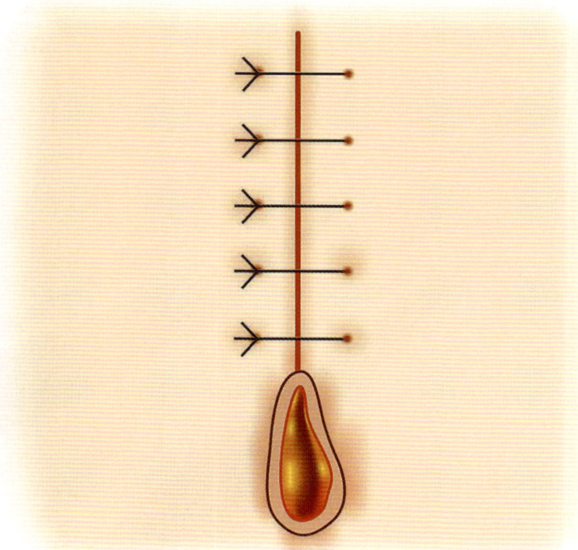

Fig. 3-78: Dog-ear often develops at the end of the wound. It is rectified by cutting excess skin and suturing creating a lengthy scar.

SUTURE REMOVAL

Suture cutting scissor is used with sharp tips. Suture is cut on one side deep to the knot; it is pulled using forceps *towards the wound line* so that to prevent entering the exposed part of the suture to get into the deeper part of suture line during removal and also to prevent wound dehiscence. Cut suture if pulled away from the wound line, chances of wound dehiscence is likely. Surgeon should use wrist and finger movements. B P handle with *11 number pointed sharp blade* also can be used. Patient should be always in lying down position. Suture removal is also an art **(Figs. 3-79A to E)**.

HAEMOSTASIS

Control of bleeding is essential part of the surgical technique. Small oozing gets controlled on its own by natural haemostatic methods. All other bleeding either from small or large vessel needs proper secure control before further proceeding with surgery. There are many methods to control bleeding.

Gauze/Mop Pack

Wet gauze packed over a diffuse area with pressure over it controls the diffuse bleeding. Size of the gauze needed is decided based on the area of ooze. Small gauze/large gauze/mop/mops can be used. Small saline wet gauze is used in small area like raising in thyroid flap. Large gauze may be used in wider area with fat disposition like raising flaps in mastectomy. Mops are used in the abdomen and in brisk torrential bleeding like in liver injury. Often mops are kept in place to develop adequate tamponade and haemostasis and are removed in 24–48 hours once patient is well stabilised. During surgery when sudden bleeding occurs by inadvertent cutting of the vessel, hurried applying of the haemostat should be avoided as it is blind application. Instead it is better to pack the area with mop with firm pressure, after few minutes mop is removed gently to identify the point of bleeder which is held using a haemostat **(Fig. 3-80)**. Suction device should be used to keep field clean and clear to identify the severity and point of bleeding. *Note:* Mopping is the essential part of the surgery. *Rubbing* over the tissues using mop *should not* be done.

Use of Haemostat

Usually medium sized curved haemostat is used. In the depth large sized artery forceps can be used. Occasionally right-angle forceps also is used. Mosquito forceps is also used for small bleeders like in head, face and neck surgery. Commonly bleeder should be identified precisely and caught with the artery forceps like a point. When identification becomes difficult due to retraction or presence of fat, convex part of the artery forceps is used to hold the tissue with the bleeder. Again unnecessary holding of extra tissues should be avoided in this method as it may lead into deeper tissue destruction. After applying the haemostat it should be confirmed that bleeding has stopped by mopping and suction. While placing the ligature around the haemostat tip of the haemostat should be pointing forward (assistant should hold the haemostat gently and carefully and surgeon will place the ligature). Always make sure that haemostat is not catching the vital adjacent structure which may be incorporated in ligature **(Figs. 3-81A to F)**.

In scalp bleeding or scalp incision galea should be held with straight or curved artery forceps/haemostat at many points and turned back over the skin to stop bleeding.

Bleeding area can be lifted with non-toothed forceps and underneath tissue can be cross clamped with haemostat.

Use of Ligature

Ligation of bleeding vessel is essential in many places. Small vessel are cauterised after holding with haemostat. Wider vessel should be ligated. Polyglycolic acid 2-zero or 3-zero can be used. Silk also can be used as it holds well with good strength. Once surgeon places the first knot, assistant *gently* releases the haemostat and removes it. Haemostat should not be released suddenly.

Mounted tie is used for small or medium vein ligation. Here two ligatures are placed with 0.5 or 1 cm gap around the vein using two haemostats and tied securely. Vein in between is cut safely. If it is artery two ligatures are placed proximally and one ligature distally before cutting in between. Larger vein ligation also needs double ligation proximally **(Fig. 3-82)**.

Ligating the larger vessel like left gastric artery, branches of mesenteric vessel and superior thyroid artery needs additional care as slippage in reality is a definitive risk. In such occasions ideal method could be to dissect the vessel from adjacent tissue and

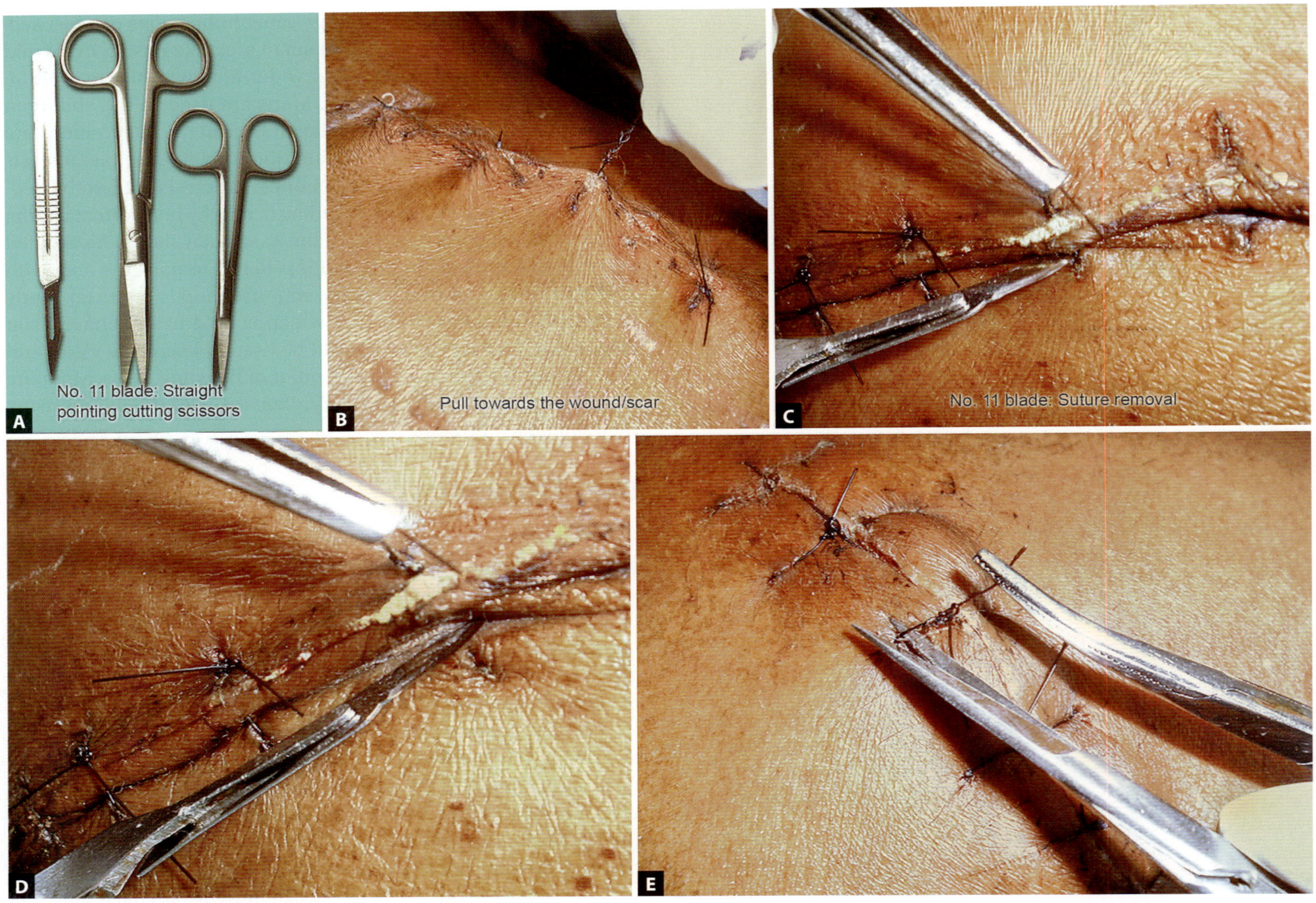

Figs. 3-79A to E: Suture removal is an art. It is done with all aseptic precautions. Suture is cut behind the knot and suture is held at the knot using dissecting forceps or haemostat, and pulled towards the wound so that wound dehiscence will not occur and outer part of the suture material is not dragged inside the track during removal to reduce the possible chances of infection along the track.

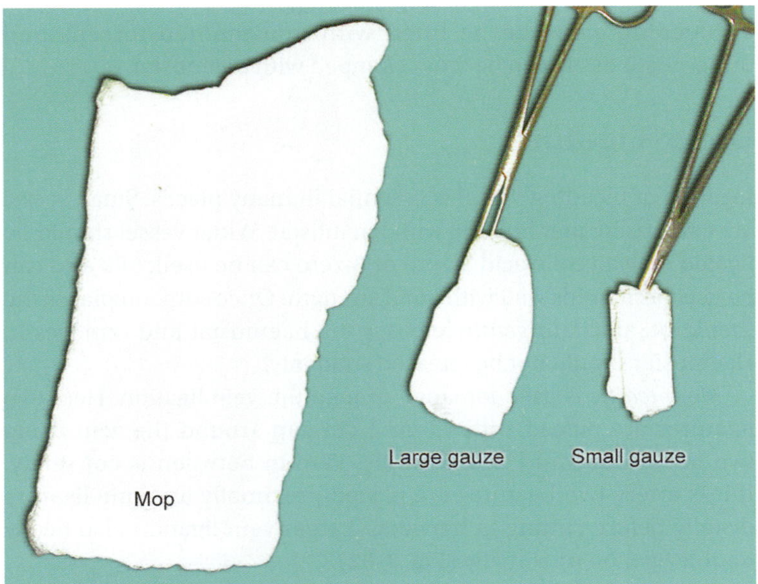

Fig. 3-80: Packing is common method to control bleeding temporarily. Small gauze, large gauze or mop/mops are used depends on the area, depth and severity of bleed.

fat for 1.5 cm (*skeletonisation of the vessel*) length and ligating it. Ligation of such vessel needs special care. Initially vessel is cross clamped using *Mixter/Miegster* clamp. Using long haemostat lengthy ligature (silk or polyglycolic acid) is passed around the Mixter clamp and tied using hand knot. One more ligature is placed again 2 mm proximal to earlier ligature. Stump of the vessel should be around 1 cm beyond the distal ligature **(Fig. 3-83)**.

Often in resection of the tissue like gastrectomy, mastectomy, colectomy, intestinal resection, main vessel (gastric artery/gastro-epiploic artery/mesenteric vessel branch) is isolated and dissected for about 2 cm length and ligature is passed using Mixter clamp as a feeding ligature and tied. Proximal two ligatures are placed at 2 mm apart. Distal ligature is placed away at 1.5 cm gap. Vessel is cut using curved scissor or with no. 15 blade (part behind the vessel should be guarded by placing flat surface of the dissecting forceps or any other instrument) leaving 1 cm vessel proximally and 0.5 cm vessel distally. Two firm proper proximal ligatures are sufficient even though many surgeons have got the habit of placing 3 or more proximal ligatures. Only one proximal ligature is technically sufficient but is not advisable; so two proximal ligatures are probably ideal **(Fig. 3-84)**.

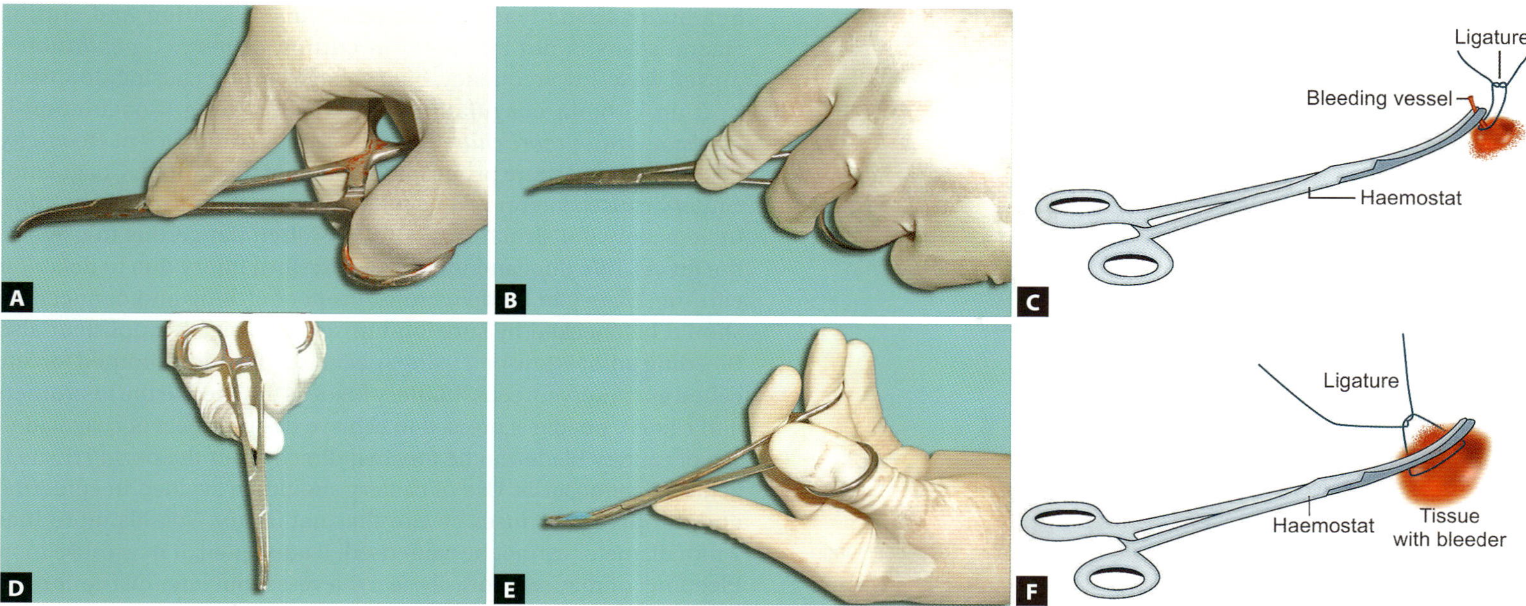

Figs. 3-81A to F: Haemostat is used in two ways. Holding is done on the tip when bleeder point is visualised and is ligated. If tissue is bleeding, tissue is held with the convex part of the haemostat and ligated.

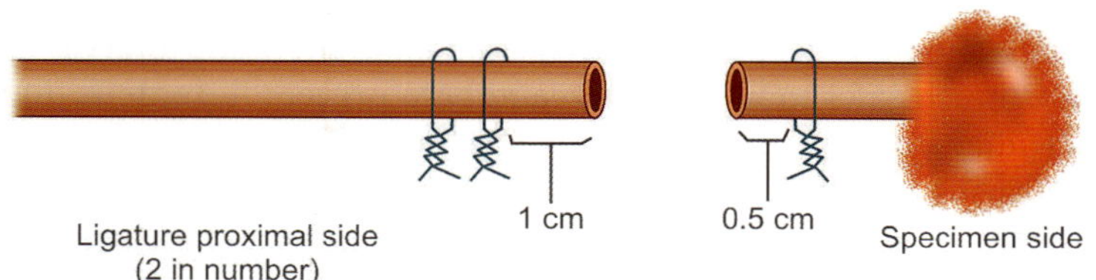

Fig. 3-82: Vessel is cut between knots with adequate gap in between to prevent knot slippage. Ideally proximal two ligations and distal one ligation are needed.

Transfixation Ligature

Transfixation prevents the slippage of the suture. It is used in big vessel ligation or when oozing tissues are held and ligated. Gastric vessels, mesenteric branches, in obese patients where ligature may not hold, in vessels in the depth-are the indications. It is better to use transfixation suture whenever surgeon feels that just ligature may not be sufficient to secure.

Needle with the suture is passed underneath the haemostat over middle of the grasped tissue, first knot encircles half of the tissue on one side; then suture is looped around the opposite side of the grasped tissue and knot is placed. Once such *figure of eight stitch* is completed then only haemostat is released by the assistant. Further knots are placed over it. Safety of the ligature can be achieved by passing the needle *second time* underneath the tissue again before knotting **(Fig. 3-85)**.

Underrunning of the Tissue

It is not possible to catch the area and control the bleeding if bleeding point is not identified and is not pointed. Any blind struggle to hold the area with haemostat will aggravate the bleeding without achieving any thing. In such occasion it is wiser to place continuous locking sutures in tissue bed where bleeding occurs using 3-zero polyglycolic acid/silk/polypropylene sutures. Repeated mopping and suction of the area is essential. However, surgeon should take care and be aware of presence of some major vessels and vital structures in that deeper plane. Depth control in these sutures is

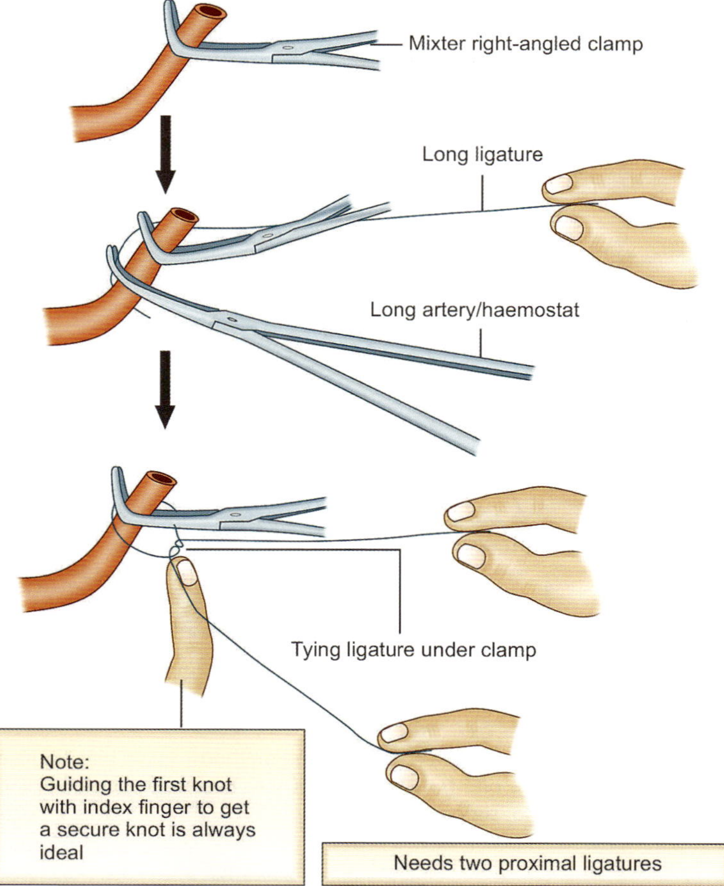

Fig. 3-83: In the depth vessel should be dissected first properly. Mixter/Miegster clamp is applied. Ligature is passed underneath using long haemostat. Ligature is placed by firm knot which is directed using index finger.

also important. Usually bleeding stops by placing few locking sutures. Locked loops should be held by the surgeon himself so that tearing through the tissues by the suture material is avoided and gentle traction to lift the tissue to facilitate further bites is achieved.

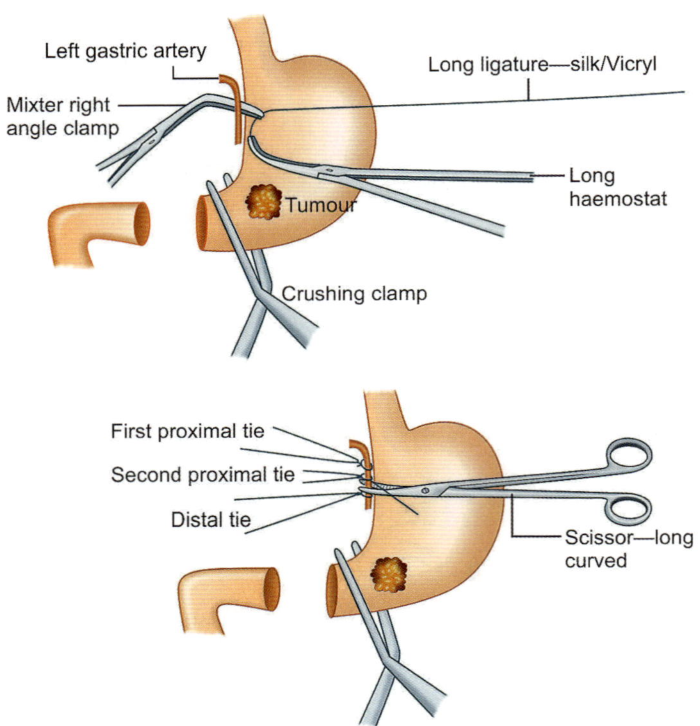

Fig. 3-84: Once adequate length of the vessel is dissected properly from surrounding tissues, using Mixter clamp ligatures are placed—two proximally; one distally. Vessel is cut between proximal and distal ligatures.

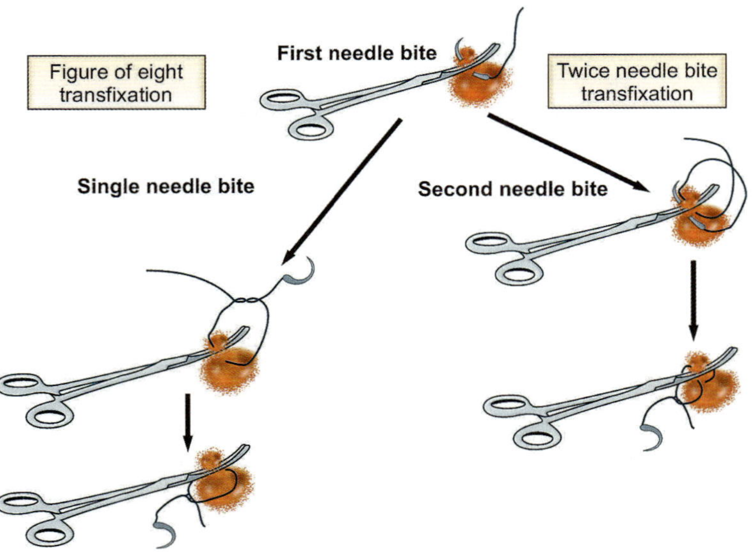

Fig. 3-85: Transfixation suture. it is done by two methods. Single bite, figure of eight suture or double bite transfixation is used. Both hold knots in place with minimal chance for slippage.

Diathermy

Diathermy is most commonly used tool for haemostasis at present. Monopolar cautery or bipolar cautery is used for haemostasis. It is high density current which is made to pass into the tissue in need (target tissue) to cut or control bleeding (coagulate).

In monopolar cautery current passes through a grounding electrode kept behind thigh/buttock of the patient. Monopolar device delivers two types of current—cutting and coagulation. *Cutting* is continuous, high frequency low voltage current causing rapid heating of tissue leading into tissue disintegration and cutting. Haemostasis is not adequate in cutting cautery. *Coagulation* is pulsed wave, low frequency, high voltage current causing slow tissue heating, protein coagulation and vessel sealing. Coagulation in *fat tissue causes more charring* as fat is poor conductor of electricity, destruction and more prone for infection of the wound. Coagulation cautery causes lateral heat significant enough to cause heat injury to adjacent vital structure/tissue. It is often dangerous to use near the bowel, bile duct and major vessels. Burn injury due to default in earthing plate can be dangerous. Proper earthing and connections should be checked by surgeon himself. It is legally important also. Bleeding point is grasped using specialised fine non-toothed forceps called as cautery forceps. Cautery blade is touched to the instrument and cautery peddle is pressed to achieve desired effect of coagulation. Tip of cautery blade can be touched directly over the oozing tissue to achieve haemostasis. Use of cautery should be avoided in epidermis and dermis as it causes severe thermal injury. Vessels more than 2 mm diameter cannot be cauterised. If attempted, it may cause more bleeding; or may temporarily seal the vessel but later disruption can occur to cause re bleeding in postoperative period.

In bipolar cautery, current passes from one blade of the bipolar forceps across the grasped tissue in between towards other blade directly without earthing. It causes heating only in between blades of the bipolar forceps. Lateral heat and adjacent tissue injury is less. It is much safer to use bipolar cautery to prevent hazardous injury to adjacent vital structures (bowel, CBD, IVC, major artery/vein). It causes coaptive coagulation. It is not used for cutting. It is very useful in laparoscopic surgery. Earthing plate is not needed in bipolar cautery. Bipolar coagulation is slower compared to monopolar coagulation. It often checks the surgeon's patience.

Ligasure/Ligaseal/Ultrasonic Shears/Laser/Harmonic Scalpel (Focus)

These are the different energy sources presently available to control bleeding which coagulate and seal wider vessels even up to 5–7 mm diameter. It is very useful in hysterectomy, colectomy, gastrectomy, resections, pancreatic surgery, thyroidectomy and in advanced laparoscopic surgeries.

Haemostatic Clips

Haemoclips are applied directly over the vessel circumferentially. It is useful in thyroidectomy, gastrectomy, colectomy, oesophagectomy, etc. It should not be applied blindly without visualising the vessel/bleeding vessel. Improper application may cause uncontrolled bleeding. Before applying it direction of the clip, structure underneath should be assessed properly. It may injure adjacent structures, or lacerate the vessel clipped if not placed properly. Precise gentle placement assures the haemostasis and speeds the surgery. Haemoclips are used in open as well as laparoscopic surgery.

Tourniquets

Tourniquet is a device which compresses or constricts the part specifically limb by applying around the limb circumferentially and raising the pressure. It temporarily occludes the vessels completely so that bleeding will not occur distal to its application. Tourniquet means to turn (Greek). It is used to cut off the blood supply to a limb temporarily so that a bloodless field is created while performing the surgery.

Historically primitive tourniquet like rope and stick wherein rope is twisted around the limb using a stick was in practice **(Fig. 3-86)**. Jean Louise Petit, a French surgeon devised metallic tourniquet in 1718 **(Fig. 3-87)**. Joseph Lister in 1864 advocated exsanguinations of blood prior to tourniquet application to achieve proper bloodless field. In 1873, Friedrich von Esmarch developed his famous *Esmarch's rubber tourniquet* which is more effective and safer than metallic one. In 1904, Harvey Cushing invented *pneumatic tourniquet*. This is better than Esmarch's rubber tourniquet in relation to its quickness to inflate and deflate and lesser chances of nerve paralysis. In 1908, August Bier introduced two tourniquets to give segmental or regional anaesthesia; presently it is popular as intravenous regional anaesthesia (IVRA/*Bier's block*). In 1980, James McEven from Canada invented microprocessor controlled tourniquet; these modern automatic tourniquets are self-controlled, self-calibrated safety devices. In 2000, Dr Nome Gavriely, invented silicone ring or elastic ring tourniquet which contains elastic silicone ring, stockinet, pull straps made up off ribbon to encircle the limb. Silicone ring while rolling along the limb will exsanguinate the limb and once in place desired occlusion is created to act like tourniquet.

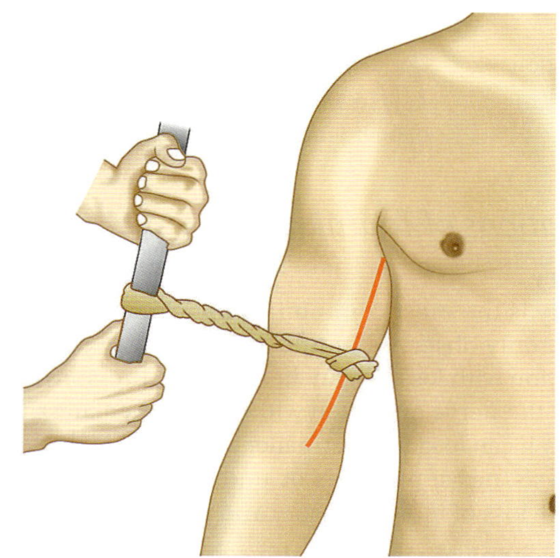

Fig. 3-86: Historical primitive tourniquet with rope and stick.

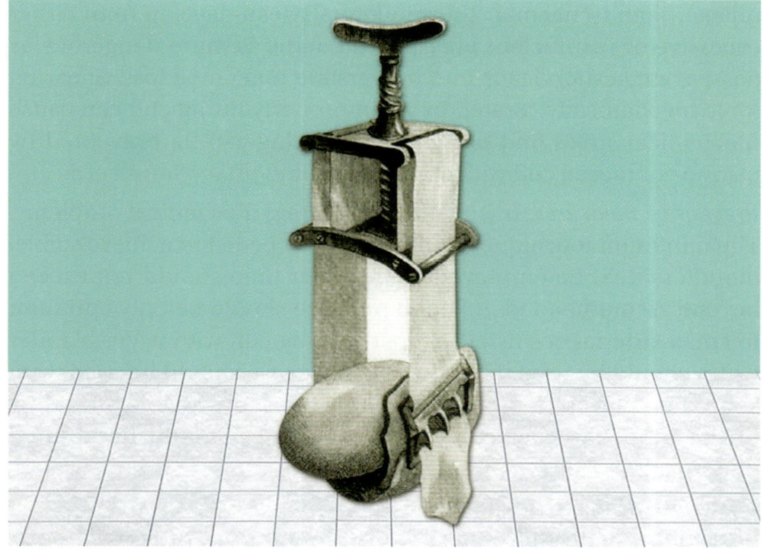

Fig. 3-87: Petit metallic tourniquet (1718).

As it is narrow tourniquet it gives wider surgical field to operate and device is sterile too.

Limb should be exsanguinated before applying/inflating the tourniquet. It is done using a bandage or pressurised Rhys-Davis exsanguinator. A tourniquet is applied in mid-thigh and above the elbow in upper limb. It should not be closer to joints. It is not applied over the forearm or leg. It is applied over layers of gauze/cotton, but not over bare skin. Guidelines for tourniquet pressure in adult are—50 mmHg above the systolic blood pressure in upper limb; 100 mmHg above the systolic blood pressure in lower limb. If bleeding is still observed then additional 25 mmHg pressure is increased. Tourniquet time is 60 minutes for upper limb; 90 minutes for lower limbs. If further tourniquet is needed it should be deflated completely for 15 minutes and again reinflated again for additional standard time period. It is very important to keep tubing, connectors, gauges, pressure source should be clean and in working condition. Limb occlusion pressure (LOP/minimum tourniquet pressure needed) should be found out by gradually increasing the tourniquet pressure until distal arterial pulse ceases which is confirmed by Doppler stethoscope. Cuff pressure should be monitored continuously and alarming system should be used.

Uses: To attain blood less field in limb surgeries of upper and lower limbs, orthopaedic surgeries, soft tissue tumours, amputations. It is used (rubber tourniquet) to get access to veins for IV injections and IV sampling. Tourniquet is used in diagnostic tests for varicose veins, purpura (ITP), etc. It is used as a first aid in bleeding conditions of limbs, snake bite (it is controversial). Tourniquets are also often used for small procedures in fingers and toes. In trauma it is very useful to stop bleeding temporarily from the limb.

Types: (1) *Rubber tourniquet:* Simple red rubber catheter is used for drawing blood, to have access to veins **(Fig. 3-88)**. (2) *Pneumatic tourniquet.* Used in limbs, will give the arterial pressure and also acts as a tourniquet [Sphygmomanometer cuff **(Fig. 3-89)** is simpler and easily available type]. (3) Esmarch rubber *elastic bandage tourniquet.* (4) Specialised sophisticated tourniquets are available which gauge pressure, timing accurately **(Figs. 3-90A and B)**. (a) Contoured and wide cuff tourniquet has more surface area with the limb dispersing cuff force and pressure. (b) Silicone ring autotransfusion tourniquet device exsanguinates the blood from the limb and occlude the limb very fast. It is simple to use and self-contained. (c) Automatic tourniquet systems are self-monitored automatic one and is less complicated and more precise. (d) Combat self-applied tourniquets are useful in war fields to apply to wounded soldiers quickly to prevent blood loss.

Contraindications: In all peripheral vascular diseases and atherosclerosis; infection; DVT; crush injuries; sickle cell disease.

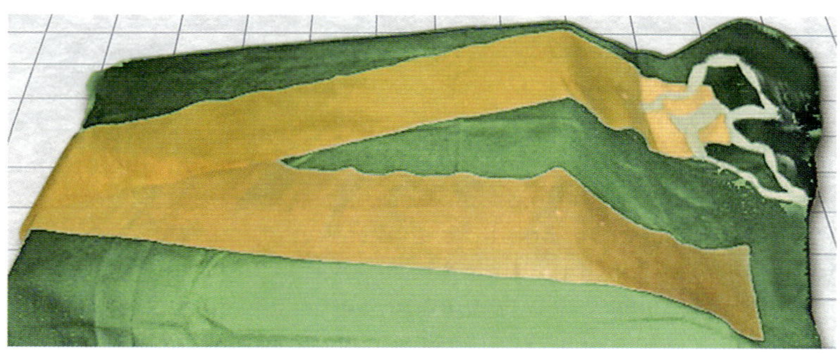

Fig. 3-88: Esmarch rubber tourniqient.

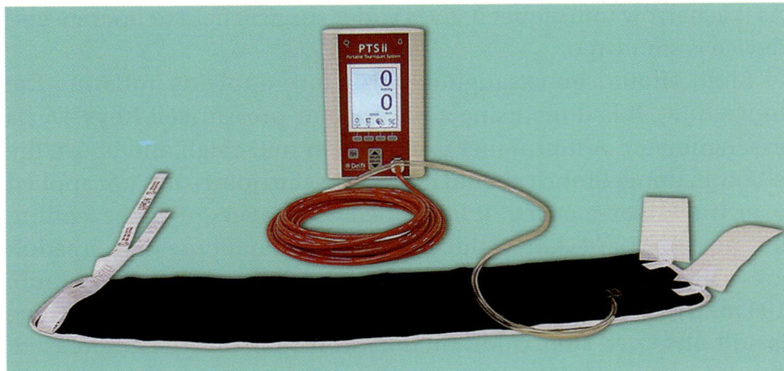

Fig. 3-89: Wide cuff tourniquet.

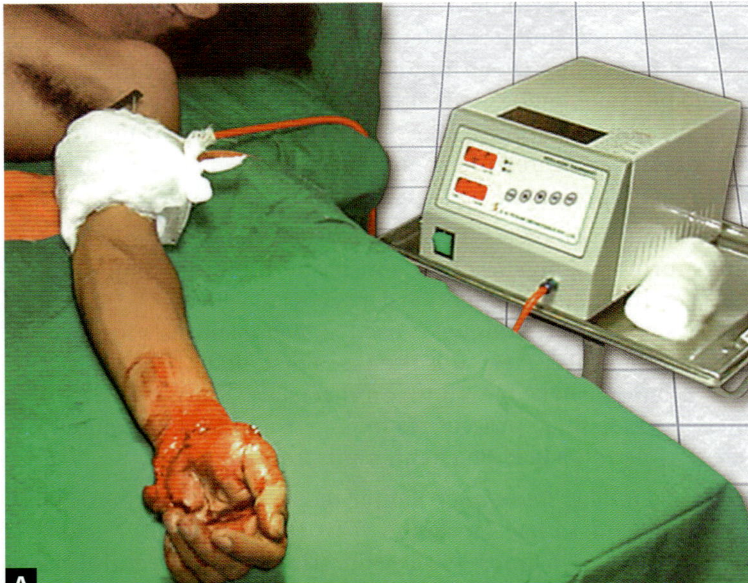

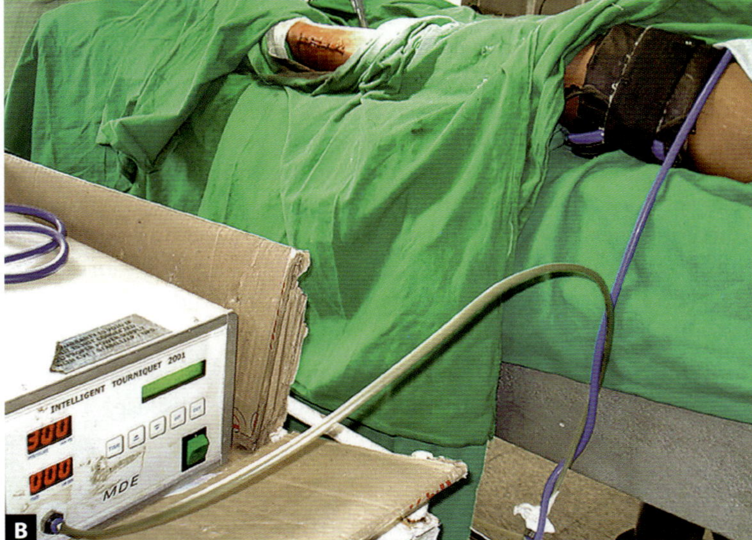

Figs. 3-90A and B: Automatic gauged pressure tourniquet.

Complications: It may crushing effect on muscles in thigh which may lead on to crush syndrome; tourniquet palsy (radial nerve) in upper limb; infection; improper application of tourniquet will lead to more bleeding; forgetting the removal of tourniquet or using more time to release may compromise the blood supply of the limb leading to severe ischaemia and gangrene. Tourniquet pain can occur with hyperaemia, hyperthermia and pain following reperfusion. Skin changes like blistering, ischaemic necrosis, post-tourniquet syndrome with pain, numbness, paresis, stiffness and pallor can develop **(Table 3-1)**.

Note:
Tourniquet time for upper limb is one hour and for lower limb is one and half to two hours.

TABLE 3-1: Bruner's rules of ten for the safe use of tourniquet (Modified by Barithwaite and Klenerman).

Size of the tourniquet	Arm 10 cm; thigh 15 cm or wider
Application	Apply only to a healthy limb or with proper caution to unhealthy limb
Site of application	Upper arm or middle/upper thigh
Padding	At least two layers of orthopaedic wool
Skin preparation	Occlude to prevent soakage of wool
Pressure	50–100 mmHg above the systolic pressure in arm; double systolic pressure for thigh; or 250–350 mmHg for lower limb
Time	2 hours for lower limb; 1 hour for upper limb; maximum time 3 hours only
Temperature	Avoid heating like very hot lights; cool if feasible to keep tissues moist
Documentation	Duration and pressure
Calibration and maintenance	At least weekly against mercury manometer or teat gauge; 3 monthly maintenance

Complications of Tourniquets

Nerve Injury

Nerve injury is the most common complication of tourniquet. It is more commonly observed in upper limb. It may be mild transient loss of function with loss of pain, heat, cold or pressure along the distribution of the nerve and often with muscle weakness temporarily. Occasionally it can lead into permanent, irreversible damage. It causes limb paralysis/nerve paralysis or tourniquet paralysis syndrome. There will be loss of motor, sensory and proprioceptive functions.

Causes: Mechanical stress on the nerves under the cuff at the edges (proximal edge commonly) and ischaemia of nerves under or distal to the cuff are the causes of nerve injury. Mechanical pressure directly under the cuff leads to irreversible nerve damage quicker than ischaemia. Tourniquet palsy can develop from either excessive or insufficient pressure; the latter is more dangerous as passive congestion leads into irreversible functional loss. Shearing force mechanically created by an improperly fitting cuff can cause mechanical stress and palsy. This shearing can be prevented by using a contoured cuff with appropriate limb protection sleeve.

Preventive measures: It is mainly preventing mechanical problems. The minimum tourniquet pressure that is needed to achieve stable, bloodless field be employed. Tourniquet time should not exceed beyond recommended. Inflation pressure should be only optimum to create arterial occlusion. Properly fitting cuff with wider bladder width should be used. Limb protection sleeve should be used. Cuff should be placed at proper location. One should avoid wrinkling of the tube. Two layered tubular stockings should be applied underneath.

Post-tourniquet Syndrome

Post-tourniquet syndrome (PTS) is pronounced, prolonged post-operative post-tourniquet swelling of the limb. In 50% of cases cause is hyperemia after release of tourniquet. Another 50% is due to postischaemic reactive hyperemia as a response to clean the limb of the metabolic products due to anoxia. Other causes are—oedema or a postoperative haematoma or prolonged bleeding from the surgical wound. Features of PTS are—oedema, stiffness, pallor, weakness without paralysis and subjective numbness without objective anaesthesia. PTS is mainly due to prolonged ischaemia rather than mechanical compression. This occurs due to application of tourniquet for prolonged time and inappropriate cuff pressures causing venous outflow block with inadequate arterial flow block. Calcified vessels in elderly and in patients who are on long-term steroid therapy and prolonged clotting time of different causes can lead into PTS.

Intraoperative Bleeding

It is due to underinflation of the cuff leading into venous pooling; inadequate initial exsanguination; improper cuff; excessive padding. Re-application of appropriate cuff scientifically corrects this problem.

Compartment Pressure Syndrome

The compartment is the area between the two tough fascia layers of a muscle group. Only extremely small amount of fluid in this space exists normally allowing contraction and relaxation of the muscles within the covering fascia. Pain which is severe and cannot be controlled by any analgesics; muscle weakness, paraesthesia, decreased or absent pulses, tense skin over the limb, occasionally irreversible paralysis—are the features. Causes—external compression with an increase in compartment contents due to trauma or surgery is the cause. It is due to prolonged tourniquet ischemia time. Previous history of compartment syndrome; McArdle's disease (a muscle phosphorylase deficiency disease exhibit compartment-like syndromes after about 20 minutes of vigorous exercise); patients who had a cast placed on the limb prior to tourniquet release are more prone for compartment syndrome after tourniquet. So ideally solid cast should be placed after the release of the tourniquet.

Pressure Sores and Chemical Burns

Pressure sores and skin blisters are due to skin breakdown, friction, or soft tissue folding under the tourniquet. Pressure necrosis or shearing is due to inadequate padding or faulty cuff application in patients with loose or thin skin, obese or elderly patients, compromised circulation like in elderly or diabetic. Chemical burns are caused by skin preparation solutions seeping under the tourniquet cuff. When the cuff is inflated, the solution is held tightly against the patient's skin. Adhesive tape should be used between the distal edge of the cuff and surgical site. Cuff should be positioned high in the limb away from the joints. Proper use of limb protection sleeve is essential. Readjusting the cuff should be avoided once inflated as it will cause shearing trauma to the skin underneath.

Digital Necrosis

Digital necrosis is common when tourniquet is applied over the fingers or toes. It is common while using a Penrose drain, rubber band, or a rolled finger of the surgical glove as a tourniquet. It is more common when used in patients with vascular diseases and diabetes.

Toxic Reactions

It is due to sudden release of tourniquet especially occurs during intravenous regional anaesthesia (IVRA). It may cause drowsiness, convulsions, respiratory depression and cardiac arrest.

The major cause of adverse effects of IVRA and/or failure of the technique is technical error. A toxic reaction may result from:

Thrombosis

Deep venous thrombosis (DVT) and the associated risk of pulmonary embolism are a major problems especially in orthopaedic surgery of lower extremities; deep venous thrombosis is considered to be as the source of pulmonary embolism in several cases of tourniquet-related cardiac arrest.

Tourniquet Pain

Tourniquet pain (most common) is dull, aching pain throughout the limb may develop during and following tourniquet use. The initial sensation of pressure at the tourniquet site progresses often to numbness and paralysis, progressing to complete paralysis. A severe, aching sensation at the site of the tourniquet or distal extremity progressively develops.

Thermal Damage

Tourniquet prevents heat dissipation from the limb which may precipitate thermal damage from heat generated by surgical lights or powered surgical instruments. Frequent irrigation, special draping and low-power surgical lights are recommended.

Hyperthermia

Tourniquets use is associated with a progressive increase in central body temperature especially in paediatric patients so may lead into hyperthermia. So aggressive warming of the child should be avoided.

Rhabdomyolysis

Rhabdomyolysis is due to the release of the cellular contents after damage to skeletal muscle; presents as—fever and tachycardia, pain, tenderness, oedema, dark urine, and oliguria.

Metabolic Changes

Metabolic changes occur in the ischaemic limb after applying tourniquet like increased $PaCO_2$, lactic acid and potassium and decreased levels of PaO_2 and pH leading into hypoxia, hypercarbia, and acidosis of the tissue. Deflation should be done slowly to prevent sudden release of these metabolites and their effects to respiratory, cardiac and cerebral tissues.

Control of Sudden Severe Bleeding during Surgery

It is often encountered problem in major surgery like pancreatic surgery, nephrectomy, splenectomy, oesophagectomy, biliary surgeries, surgeries in neck, and surgeries for malignancies. Methods used to control haemorrhage temporarily are—(1) *Finger pressure* and packing: Applying pressure directly over the site is the ideal method as immediate pressure instead of struggling to catch the bleeder using haemostat. *Pringle manoeuvre* by holding the foramen Winslow between thumb and fingers is one of the methods to control bleeding in liver. Iced sterile saline pack can be used in kidneys to reduce the metabolic activity and so to increase the compression period. (2) Usage of clamps carefully with proper suctioning: Satinsky clamp and other vascular clamps are soft and stable which can be applied effectively across a bleeding major vessel like portal vein/inferior vena cava (IVC)/major artery. (3) Proximal and distal control using vascular clamps or umbilical tapes in major vessels like aorta. (4) Extend the incision to expose the area adequately. Visualisation, suction should be optimised. Adequate number of blood should be arranged for transfusion. Needed assistants may be increased. If needed surgeon should not hesitate to call another experienced surgeon for help. (5) Permanent control of bleeding by vascular suturing using fine 4-zero polypropylene sutures or other definitive procedures. (6) Monitoring the patient for disseminated intravascular coagulation (DIC), coagulation changes, further bleeding, sepsis, cardiac arrest, acute respiratory distress syndrome (ARDS), respiratory problems, metabolic consequences.

Other Methods

Topical agents: They are collagen or cellulose matrix which stimulates clot formation over the oozing surface. They also prevent disruption of clot already formed. *Microfibrillar collagen powder* (Avitene) can be sprinkled over bleeding surface through forceps. It is used when oozing surface is irregular. But it is costly. *Oxidised cellulose* (surgicel) is placed over the bleeding area **(Fig. 3-91)**. *Gelatin* sponge, topical thrombin, gelatin matrices (floseal), topical cryoprecipitate, topical EACA (Epsilon amino caproic acid), alginate materials, temporalis muscle patch (neurosurgery) are other materials used. *Bone wax* is bees wax with almond oil; it is used in bleeding bone marrow.

Endoscopic control of haemorrhage using laser, sclerotherapy, clips, etc. are tried. Angiogram and therapeutic embolisation using coils, gel foam, clot is used in bleeding duodenal ulcer, colonic bleeding **(Figs. 3-92 to 3-95)**.

Endostaplers and endoclips are used in laparoscopic surgery safely.

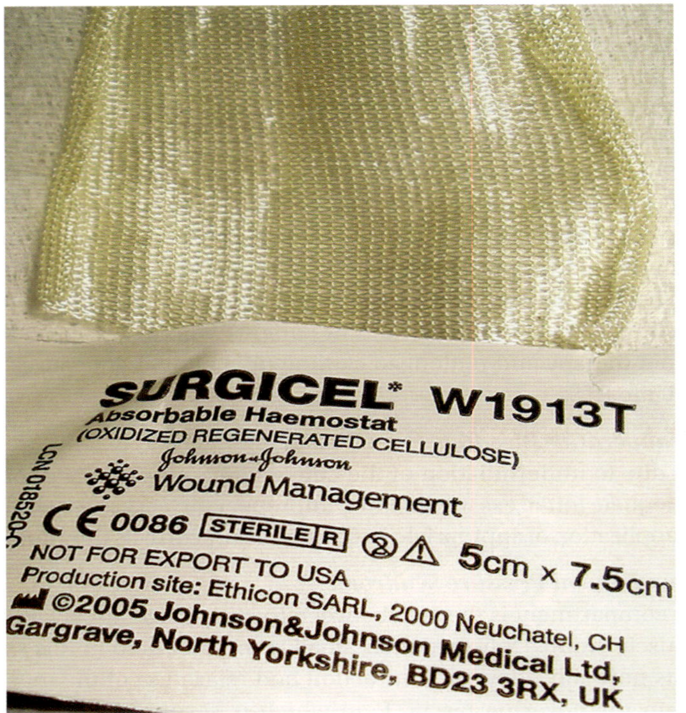

Fig. 3-91: Surgicel.

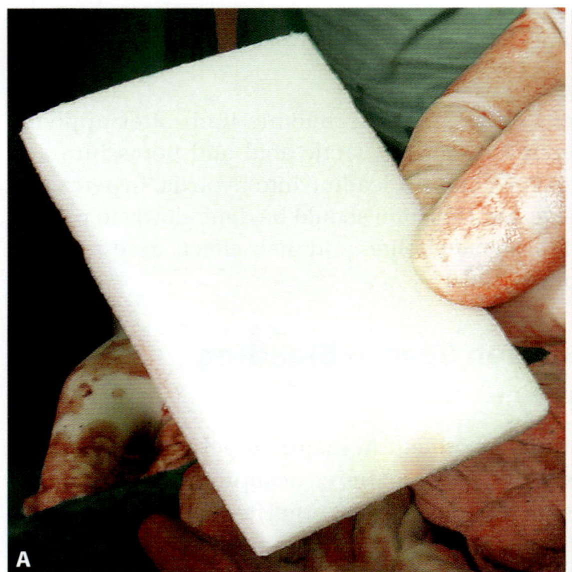

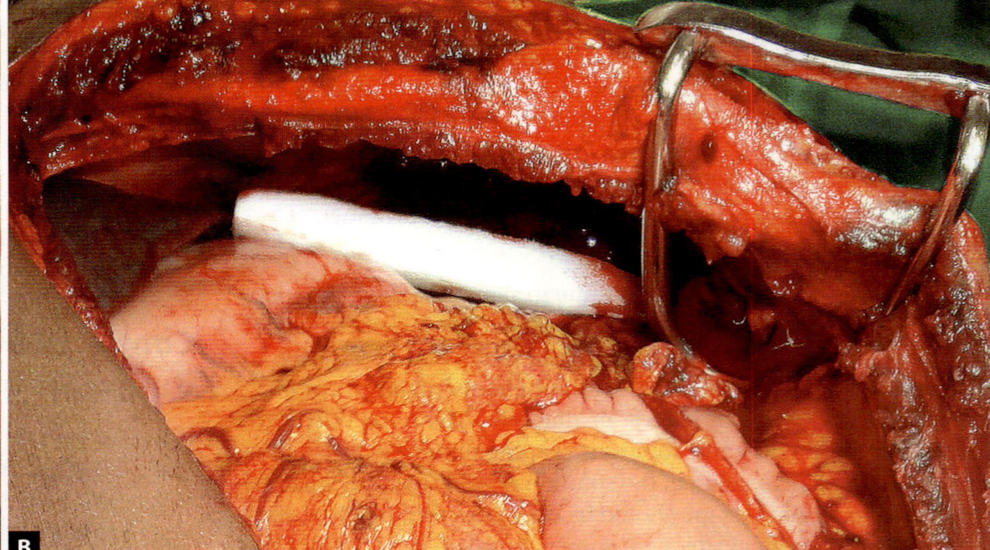

Figs. 3-92A and B: Gel foam.

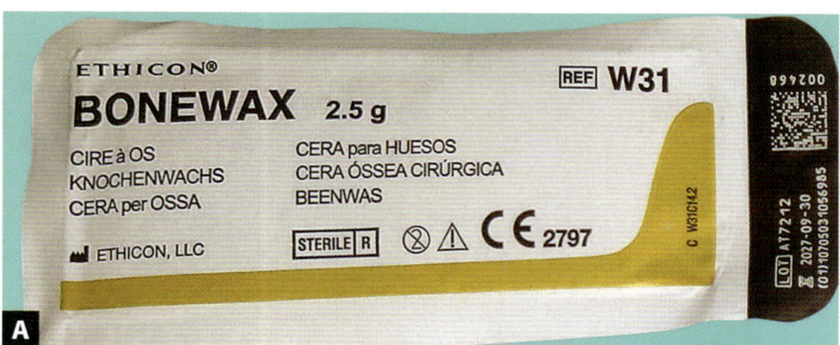

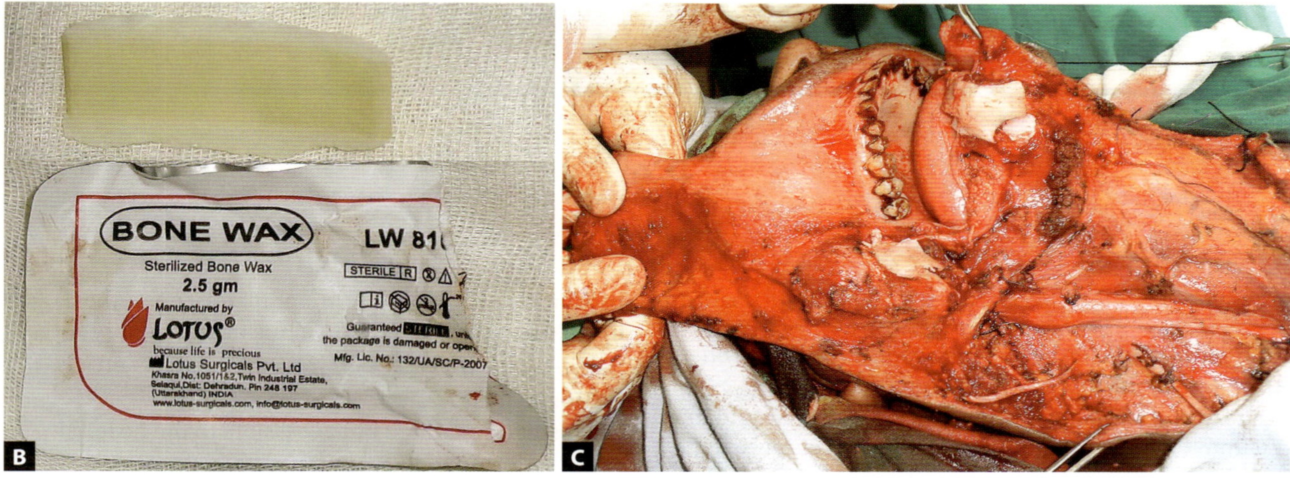

Figs. 3-93A to C: Bonewax is bees wax in almond oil; used to control bleeding from cut end of bones.

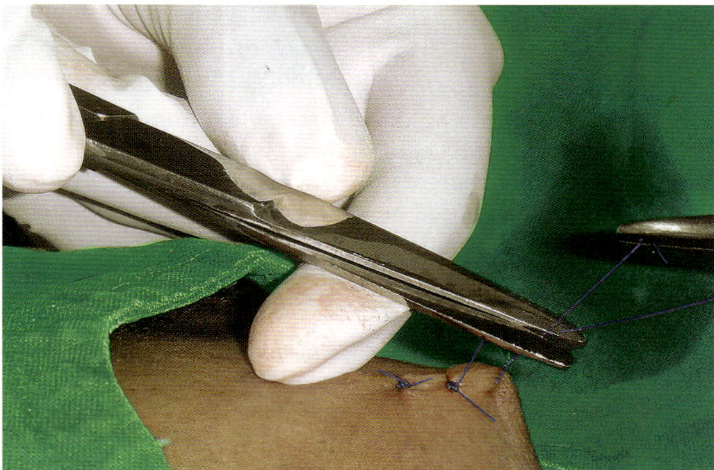

Fig. 3-94: Cutting the end of the knot.

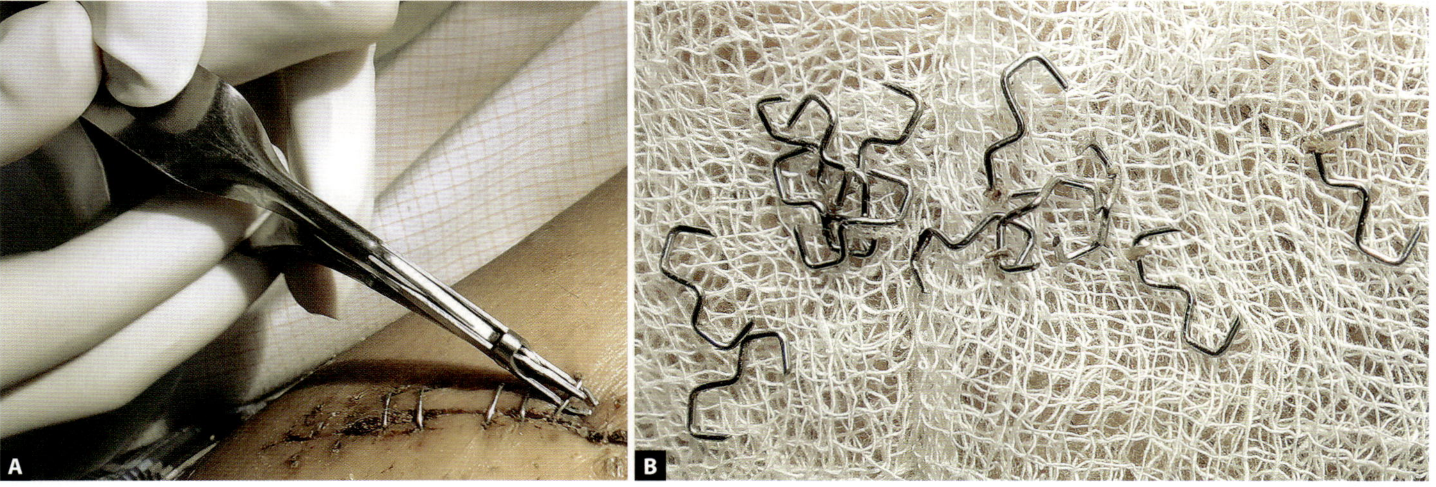

Figs. 3-95A and B: Clip removal in skin stapling.

4

CHAPTER

Day Care Surgery, Ambulatory Surgery and Outpatient Surgery

DEFINITION

It is a confusing entity with so many words with difficult understanding. It is fast developing and so equally important.

Day care surgery or ambulatory surgery is said wherein patient is discharged within 23 hours of admission (USA); or surgery done without night stay (UK). It is often also called as *ambulatory surgery/ minimal stay surgery.*

Even though all are similar, technical meanings are little different.

Day care surgery means patient is fit to return home in 23 hours usually with overnight stay. *Ambulatory surgery means* patient recovers after surgery and returns home in the same evening. *Office surgery means* patient recovers from surgery and returns home in few hours. *Outpatient surgery* is different from day care surgery in that, patient is not previously fully assessed in outpatient surgery. Only minor procedures are done in this. Patient is not admitted in outpatient surgery. In day care and ambulatory surgery patient is admitted in the hospital.

Day care surgery has been defined by *the Royal College of Surgeons* as when the surgical day care patient is admitted for investigation or operation on a planned non-resident basis and who nonetheless requires facilities for recovery. This definition excludes upper and lower gastrointestinal (GI) endoscopies, outpatient procedures such as flexible cystoscopy, and minor superficial surgery under local anaesthesia, none of which require full day case facilities for recovery.

It is a *unique upcoming field* in surgery wherein surgeon, general practitioner, nurse at care centre, anaesthetist work in hand so that hospital stay and cost is reduced. Patient who has been prepared prior by all evaluation methods comes to the hospital, undergoes surgery/procedure, gets discharged at evening.

The cases are usually carried out under local, regional or general anaesthesia (monitored anaesthesia). Facilities and standards of care in the day care surgical unit must be alike to those provided for inpatient. The patient is to be formally admitted to day care unit, full work up and documentation is done and there should be facilities to observe the patient for 12 hours.

INTRODUCTION

In 19th century (1903) Glasgow surgeon James Nicoll did many day care surgeries in children. Dr RM Waters of Sioux City of Iowa in 1918 did first day care surgery under general anaesthesia. Dudley Street ambulatory surgical centre started in Providence Rhode Island in 1968 by Charles Hill. Society for ambulatory anaesthesia has established in 1984 for safety and undertaking of ambulatory surgery.

Ambulatory surgical set up may be:

- Hospital integrated.
- Hospital separated but accessible to the hospital.
- Satellite ambulatory unit.
- Free standing unit—totally independent.
- Office based unit—mainly in USA (20% surgeries) but are said to be inadequately equipped.

Levels of ambulatory surgery are:
Minor (LA); major (GA/epidural); inpatient ambulatory surgery.

Assessment done prior to surgery are by*—pre-anaesthetic clinics* with system evaluations; *health questionnaire* by surgeon and physician; *telephonic interviews.*

Patient selection, patient information, patient acceptance are important parts in day care surgery.

Types of day care centres

Hospital Integrated Unit: This unit provides a designated area to which patients are admitted and from which they are discharged home and in which pre-operative evaluation and preparation are carried out. The hospital operating rooms and recovery rooms are used for both inpatients and day care surgery patients.

Hospital Autonomous Unit: This totally self-sufficient unit is located within the hospital but operates totally independent of other portions of the hospital.

Hospital Satellite Unit: This is an autonomous facility which is operated by the hospital personnel but located away from the hospital campus.

Free Standing Unit: This is an autonomous unit which is not part of any other healthcare facility.

Procedures done in day care surgery set up are:
Excision of deep swellings; lymph node excision biopsy; therapeutic endoscopies; all procedures for haemorrhoids; hydrocele surgery; circumcision; hernia surgery; gynaecologic procedures. Minor amputations; orthopaedic procedures like reduction, minor plating and screwing of bones, arthroscopies, surgeries of peripheral joints, surgeries for carpal tunnel syndrome, ear surgeries, small laryngeal and nasal surgeries, many ophthalmic surgeries like cataract surgeries, laser, etc.

Inguinal hernia, femoral hernia, small umbilical hernia, excision of skin tumours, many plastic surgeries are done as day care surgery.

Basic requirements are—in-house anaesthesiologist; recovery room; theatre and recovery room/ward nurse; all essential surgical set up including monitor, ventilator.

The procedures that can be undertaken as day care surgical procedures are as per the BADS (British Association of Day Surgery) or Audit Commission of UK which came up with 'Basket of 20' surgical procedures to provide a more consistent measure of performance. The 25 procedures included as found updated in the report of the Audit Commission of UK, 2000 are as follows (Updated report, 2001): (1) Orchidopexy. (2) Circumcision. (3) Inguinal hernia repair. (4) Excision of breast lump. (5) Anal fissure dilatation or excision. (6) Haemorrhoidectomy. (7) Laparoscopic cholecystectomy. (8) Varicose vein stripping or ligation. (9) Transurethral resection of bladder tumour. (10) Excision of Dupuytren's contracture. (11) Carpal tunnel decompression. (12) Excision of ganglion. (13) Arthroscopy. (14) Bunion operations. (15) Removal of metalware. (16) Extraction of cataract with/without implant. (17) Correction of squint. (18) Myringotomy. (19) Tonsillectomy. (20) Submucous resection. (21) Reduction of nasal fracture. (22) Operation for bat ears. (23) Dilatation and curettage/hysteroscopy. (24) Laparoscopy. (25) Termination of Pregnancy. *The BADS* has recommended inclusion of another fifty procedures under the name of Trolley of procedures.

Selection criteria are:

American Society of Anesthesiologists (ASA) category I and II patients can be taken up for day care surgery. ASA III/or beyond are contraindicated for day care surgery.

ASA (American Society of Anesthesiologists) grading of the patient for surgery

1. Normal individual.
2. Mild–moderate systemic disease—diabetes and hypertension under control.
3. Severe systemic disease—uncontrolled diabetes and hypertension.
4. Incpacitating systemic disease.
5. Moribund status.

Class E – Emergency surgery.

Exclusion criteria for day care surgery

- ASA grade beyond III or more.
- Obesity (BMT >35). Hypertension—not controlled.
- Surgery requiring more than one hour.
- Surgery with anticipation of major fluid/blood loss or needs post-operative critical care.
- Pre-term babies and infants less than 3 month's age.
- Patient living in far and not easily reachable or able to transport easily.
- Unstable psychiatric illness.
- If proper caregiver is not available.
- Uncontrolled diabetes, alcohol abuse, COPD, severe asthma, epilepsy.
- Pregnancy.

Final evaluation is done just prior to the date of surgical procedure. Patient should be assessed by surgeon, anaesthesiologist, and a physician. Once evaluation is done surgery should be undertaken ideally within 2 weeks.

Haematocrit, ECG, renal function tests—blood urea and serum creatinine, blood sugar level, chest X-ray are to be taken. Other relevant investigations are done depending on specific disease patient is having or suspected like cardiac (echocardiography, cardiologist opinion), respiratory diseases.

Patient should be asked to stop smoking at least 2 weeks prior to surgery.

Type of anaesthesia should be decided by surgeon and in-house anaesthesiologist. Local anaesthesia is commonly used at present for small procedure like tapping, excisions, circumcision and hydrocele. Open inguinal or femoral hernia surgery is commonly done at present under local anaesthesia unless hernia is irreducible/large or patient is contraindicated for local anaesthesia. Laryngeal mask airway (LMA) or combined oropharyngeal airway are commonly used. Minimal or no premedication is the usual practice in day care surgery.

Laparoscopic hernia repair (TEP/TAPP) also can be done under day care surgery but under general anaesthesia.

Proper written consent for anaesthesia, procedure, day care surgery with consent for possible needed admission if at all due to some complications should be taken.

Spinal or epidural anaesthesia also can be used in many procedures.

List of day care surgery for the day should be decided previous day after collecting clear information from the patient about him being coming for surgery without fail. Some inadvertent reason if patient fails to turn up, then person on waiting list can be called upon for surgery if he is prepared and ready to do so.

TECHNIQUE

Technique is same as like any theatres. There is no deviation in principles and methodology of the procedure.

Sutures can be interrupted or absorbable subcuticular. Dressings are placed. Patient is asked to remove dressing in 3 days and is allowed to take bath normally in 3 days.

Ward nurse will monitor the patient properly about the recovery and should document it. Once she is sure of proper recovery then patient is discharged with proper intimation about oral drugs, diet, and rest in the house, to call and attend immediately in dire problems. Usually patient is discharged in 6 hours if procedure is done under local anaesthesia; in 8–12 hours if procedure is done under general/epidural/spinal anaesthesia. Clear cut discharge criteria should be followed and should be decided by anaesthesiologists and surgeons. *Aldrete scoring system* is used for fitness for discharge and safe transfer of the patient to the house.

Aldrete score sheet/table

Definition

Aldrete score is a medical scoring system for the measurement of recovery after anaesthesia (post-anaesthesia) which includes activity, respiration, consciousness, blood circulation and colour.

Activity	Score
Able to move 4 extremities voluntarily or on command	2
Able to move 2 extremities voluntarily or on command	1
Able to move 0 extremities voluntarily or on command	0
Respiration	
Able to breathe deeply and cough freely	2
Dyspnoea or limited breathing	1
Apneic	0
Consciousness	
Fully awake	2
Arousable on calling	1
Not responding	0
Circulation	
B/P ± 20% of pre-anaesthetic level	2
B/P ± 20% to 50% of pre-anaesthetic level	1
B/P ± 50% of pre-anaesthetic level	0
Colour	
Normal	2
Pale, dusky, blotchy, jaundiced	1
Cyanotic	0

Advantages of Day Care Surgery

Reduction in hospital cost as admission and more days stay in the hospital and reduced nursing care is possible.

Large numbers of surgeries are done and so waiting period is reduced. Operation theatre getting blocked by emergency procedures is prevented.

Hospital will have less administrative and nursing works.

Reduced risk of infections is achieved by day care surgery.

Early mobilisation, less interference of domestic works, better personal care by family members including food.

Psychologically patient will be better once he reaches home.

Disadvantages of Day Care Surgery

Patient care taker becomes more responsible in taking care of the patient.

Complications if develop, may not be identified properly like—pain, giddiness, bleeding, vomiting.

Patients from very far places may not be suitable candidates as in case of emergency it may not be possible to reach back to the hospital at the earliest.

Contraindications

Old age, all exclusion criteria mentioned above in the table, psychological (stressed or psychosis patients), social problems in taking care of the patient or need for travelling (poor transport) back very far.

Care Once at Home

This is equally important as patient has undergone surgery just few hours back. It is mainly the patient, family members.

Patient should take rest that date (night) once he reaches home; diet should be initially liquid and later normal diet. Patient should be informed about one or two episodes of possible development of vomiting post-operatively due to anaesthesia which usually subsides eventually.

Informed caregiver mostly one of the close family member is essential part of the day care surgery.

All instructions should be given in *a written form* clearly in understanding simple way.

Driving, decisive works, exercises should be avoided for 24 hours.

Any additional instructions should be taken as when needed over the phone by the patient.

Follow up by telephone in 12 hours, 24 hours and 48 hours should be done by the day care centre (by nurse or anaesthetist or surgeon) as a mandatory.

Patient should be called for suture removal and if needed post-operative evaluation depending on the condition to which patient undergoes surgery.

General practitioner/family physician of the family/patient should aware of the patient undergoing surgery; he should visit give care to the patient. Extra responsibility comes to general practitioner.

Present Trend for Day Care Surgery

It is rapidly emerging field in surgery—in different specialties also. It *reduces cost*, mental agony to patient and family members. *Minimal hospital stay* makes it acceptable to the patient. 30% (in USA)—40% (in UK) cost savings occur by day care surgery.

70% surgeries in USA and 60% surgeries in UK are done by day care surgery. 20% surgeries in India.

Home diet given with care and feeling of away from hospital makes better and faster recovery.

Infection rate comes down drastically in day care surgery because of avoidance of hospital acquired resistant infection.

Day care surgery probably reduces the disability.

Post-operative nausea and vomiting (50%); post-operative pain and post-operative drowsiness/dizziness (50%) are the *common complications* in day care anaesthesia.

But proper selection, proper follow up, immediate reaching facility to the hospital in case of emergency mainly *post-operative bleeding*, often vomiting, dehydration due to poor intake, severe pain, discomfort and sedation—are prerequisite care.

It is developing field which needs modern anaesthetic and surgical set up with outstanding team and set up.

Alertness; ambulation; analgesia and alimentation—*basis for* day care of surgery.

Advantages of day care surgery	**Factors relevant for success of day care surgery**
♦ Cost containment ♦ Decompression of busy hospital beds ♦ Patient care at home with family members ♦ Stress to patient is reduced ♦ To contain administrative and nursing workload in hospitals ♦ Early mobilisation ♦ Home diet is better acceptable by the patient	♦ Patient acceptability ♦ Patient selection ♦ Feasibility for day care ♦ Patient information and facilities for quick communication ♦ Post-operative care ♦ Identification of complications once discharged and facilities to reach hospital quickly if need arises ♦ Audit
Disadvantages ♦ Family members should give adequate post-operative care who are not trained or experienced ♦ Complications if arises often find difficult to take decisions ♦ Inability to communicate and reach back to operated hospital if needed	**Contraindications** ♦ Old age, ASA grade > III ♦ Obesity, hypertension, uncontrolled diabetes mellitus, alcohol abuse, COPD, asthma, epilepsy, pregnancy ♦ If proper care giver is not available at home ♦ Major surgeries—more than 1 hour, fluid and blood loss, severe sepsis related, infants less than 3 months

5

CHAPTER

Instruments

Surgical instruments are essential for any surgery, whether minor or major. All instruments should be sterilised prior to use to prevent infection.

Parts of an instrument (Fig. 5-1)

- Two finger bows for holding.
- A ratchet or lock.
- A pair of shaft or body.
- Joint either box type (with a slot) or pivot (attached by a screw).
- Pair of blades at terminal part.

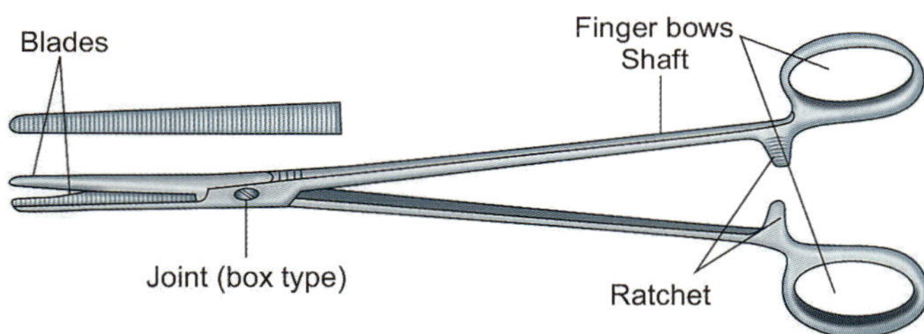

Fig. 5-1: Parts of an instrument.

CHEATLE'S FORCEPS

It is used to pick sterilised articles like instruments and drapes so to avoid touching the instruments while transferring them from one tray/table to other. It is kept dipped in antiseptic solutions like savlon/cidex. It does not have lock. It is heavy metallic forceps with curved blades with serrations. One blade of the proximal handle has got rounded ring for inserting finger and other blade may be having ring or often has got free hook to have proper grip **(Figs. 5-2A to C)**.

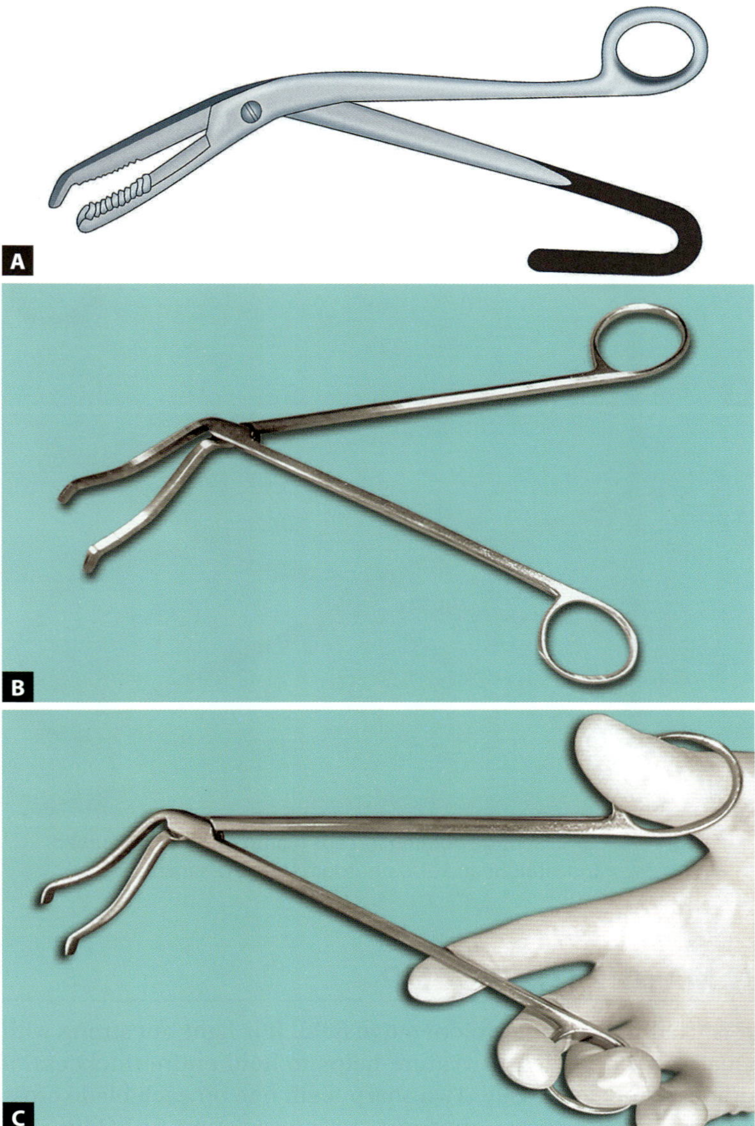

Figs. 5-2A to C: Cheatle's forceps.

SPONGE HOLDING FORCEPS (RAMPLEY'S)

It has got fenestrated, serrated flat round distal end. It is 22.5 cm long; has a ratchet and two long blades **(Figs. 5-3A to C)**.

It is used to clean the operative field. Because of the length, the surgeon's hand will not get contaminated while cleaning the patient, it is also used to swab the cavities, to mop the oozing area, to hold gallbladder or cervix or tongue or bowel or stomach during surgeries, for blunt dissections or as ovum forceps. It can also be used to dry the operative field using gauze. It can be used for blunt dissection with a wet firm swab held on the tip in vagotomy, sympathectomy. It can be used as haemostatic with a large gauze at the tip. It is used to hold Hartmann's pouch in open cholecystectomy. It is used to clean the vaginal cavities.

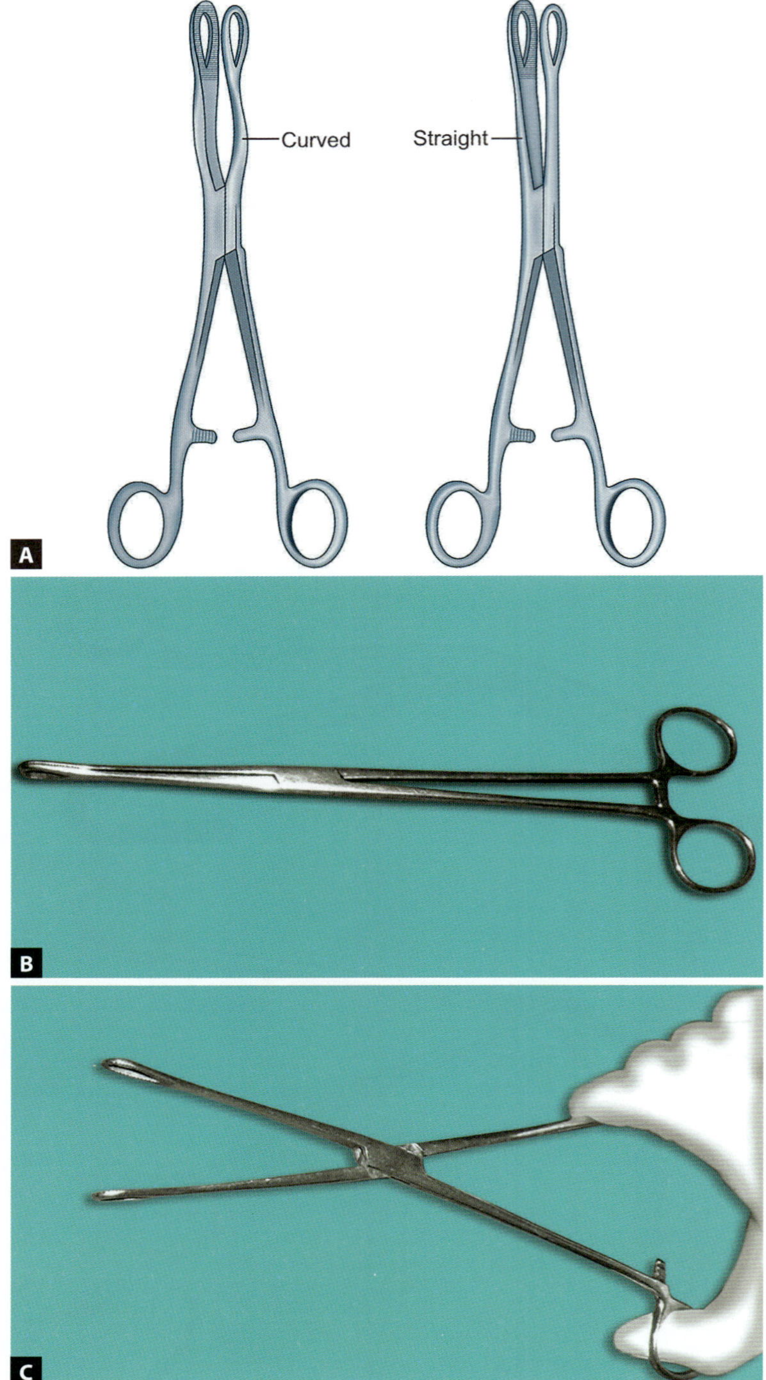

Figs. 5-3A to C: Sponge holding forceps (Rampley's)—both curved and straight and also photograph of the same.

MAYO'S TOWEL CLIP

It is used to fix drapes in operative field. It is light but strong with small curved blades. Curvature helps to hold entire thickness of drapes firmly and easily. Two sharp teeth one on each blade cross each other but do not approximate (cross action tip) **(Figs. 5-4 and 5-5)**.

It is used to fix suction tubes, diathermy wires and laparoscopic cables on operative table. It is used to fix ribs in flail chest. It can be used to hold cord in hernia or to hold tongue if specific instruments are not available. It can be used to hold dental wiring; patella during patellectomy; in faciomaxillary fractures.

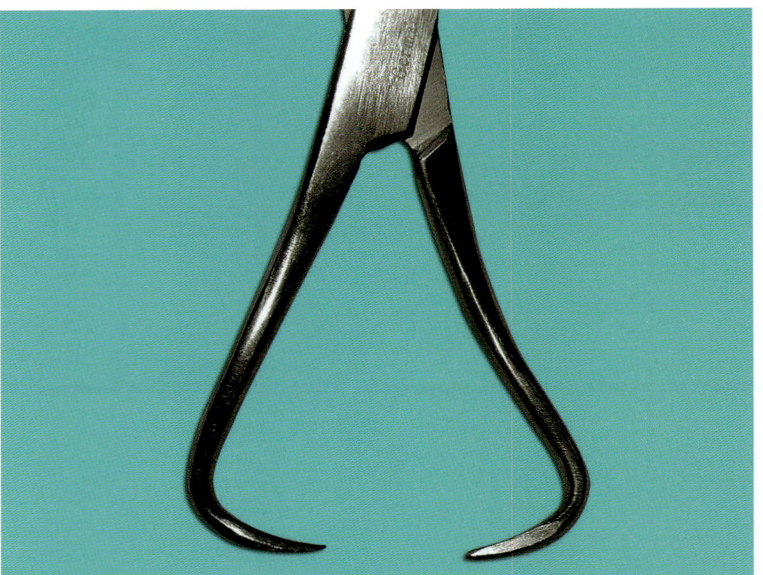

Fig. 5-4: Towel clip with cross action tip.

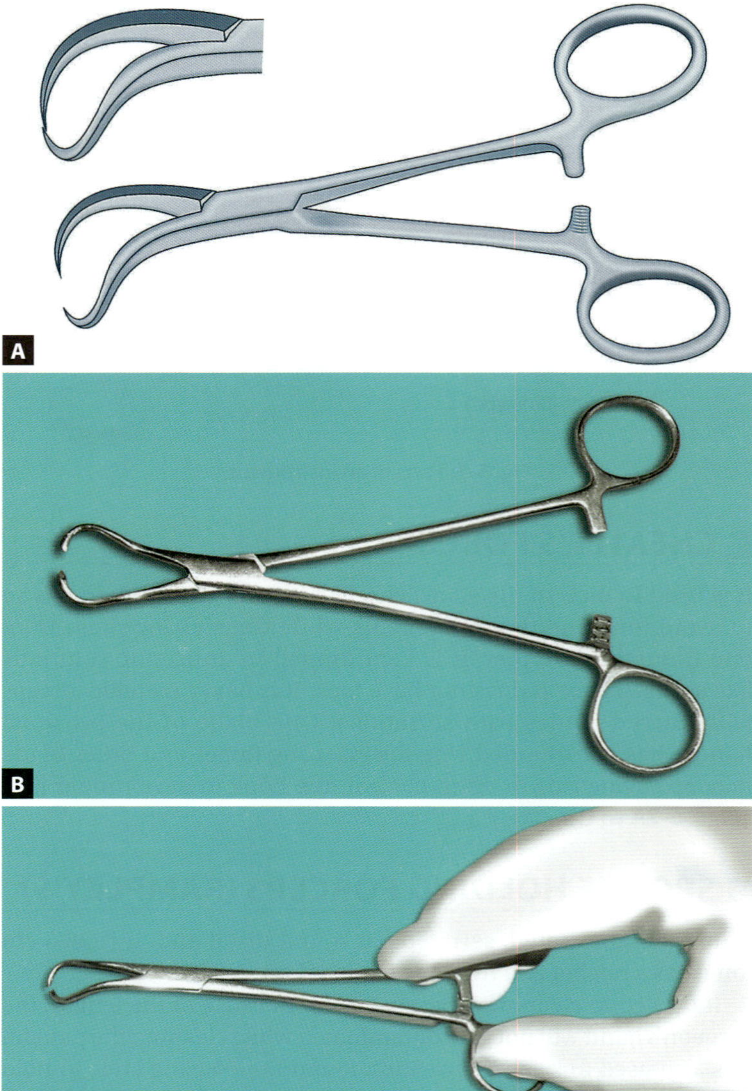

Figs. 5-5A to C

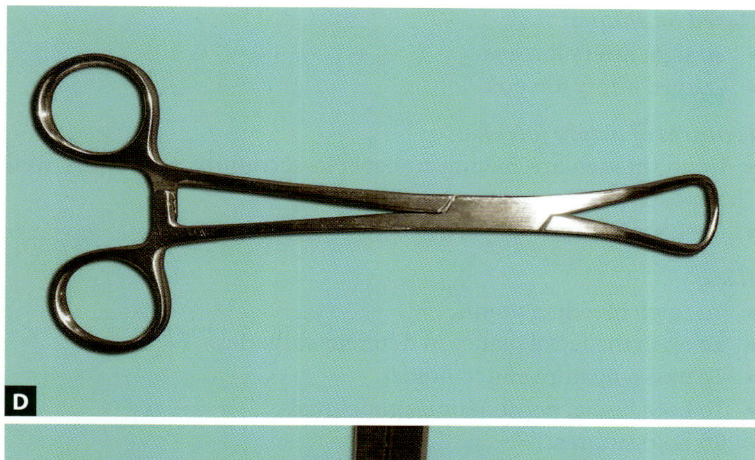

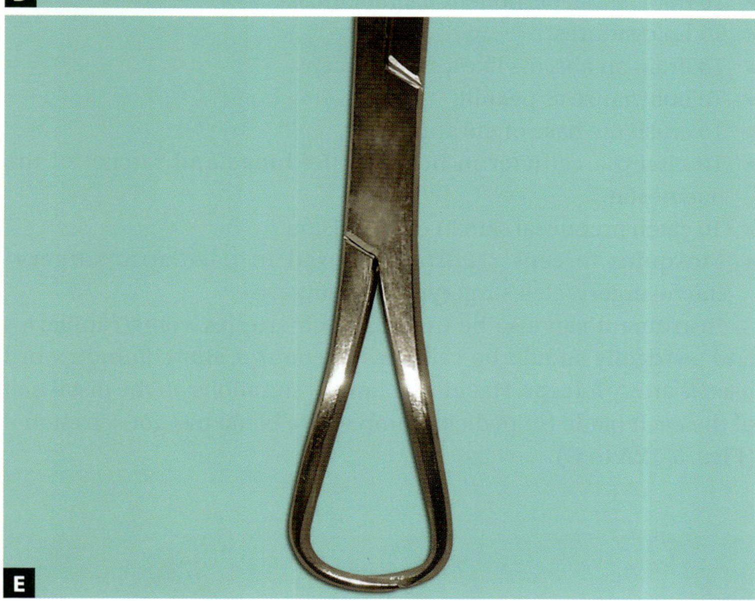

Figs. 5-5D and E
Figs. 5-5A to E: Mayo's towel clip.

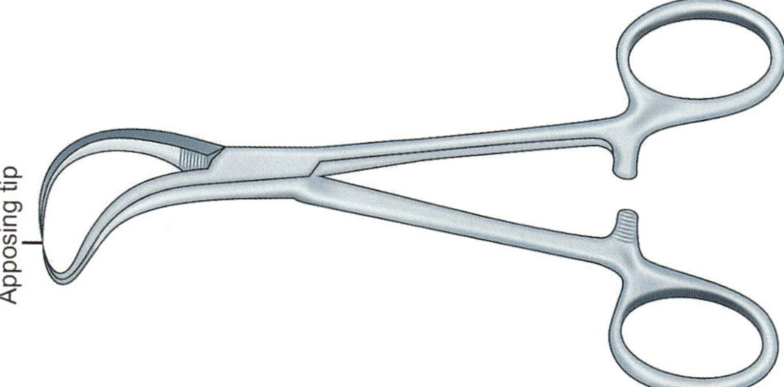

Fig. 5-6: Backhaus' towel clip.

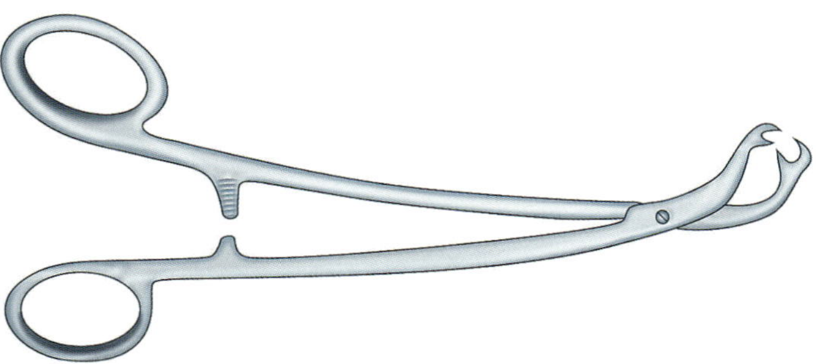

Fig. 5-7: Moynihan's tetra towel clip—it is with long blades with a curvature with two teeth in each blade (total four).

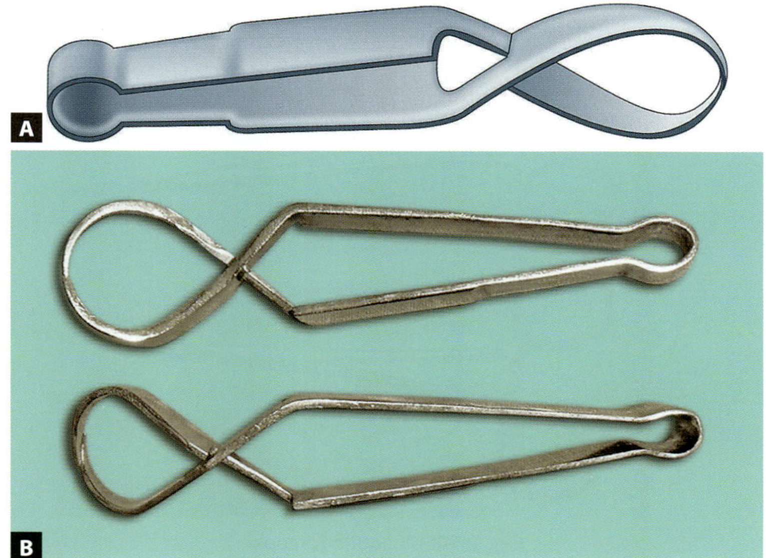

Figs. 5-8A and B: Doyen's towel clips.

BACKHAUS' TOWEL CLIP

It has got a ratchet catch, curved sharp ends which approximate each other, but do not cross each other (approximating tip, but no cross action in tip) **(Fig. 5-6)**.

MOYNIHAN'S TETRA TOWEL CLIP/FORCEPS

It is used to hold the cut edges of the skin incision to the four corners of the draped tetra towels so as to isolate the operative field. Isolation also can be achieved by suturing the drape margins to the subcutaneous tissue at different points or using adhesive plastic drape to skin through which the drape skin incision is made **(Fig. 5-7)**.

DOYEN'S TOWEL CLIP

It is a short instrument with curved ends with sharp points. Handles join at proximal ends. When handles are pressed tips open, when handles are released tips close and firmly grip the towel **(Figs. 5-8A and B)**. It has got cross action tip.

Towel clips

- Mayo's—cross action tip; no approximation.
- Backhaus'—approximating tip; no cross action.
- Doyen's—tension blades open when pressed and vice versa.
- Moynihan's tetra forceps/towel clip to isolate cut edge of the skin incision for isolation; has got two teeth on each blades.
- Bull dog towel clip—has got cross section action with tapering points
- Gray's towel clips—not used now.

ARTERY FORCEPS (HAEMOSTAT)

Types (Figs. 5-9 to 5-11)

Based on size:

- Small or mosquito artery forceps: *Mosquito forceps* is so called because of its fine tip which can even catch the proboscis of a mosquito—Halsted haemostat.
- Medium-sized artery forceps.
- Large artery forceps.

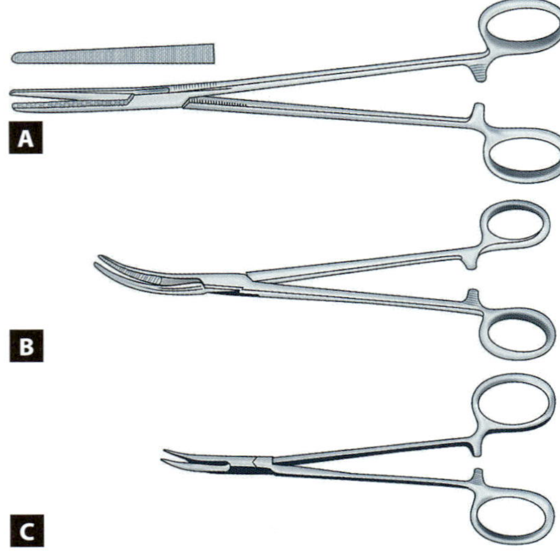

Figs. 5-9A to C: Artery forceps: (A) Straight; (B) Curved; (C) Mosquito (Halsted).

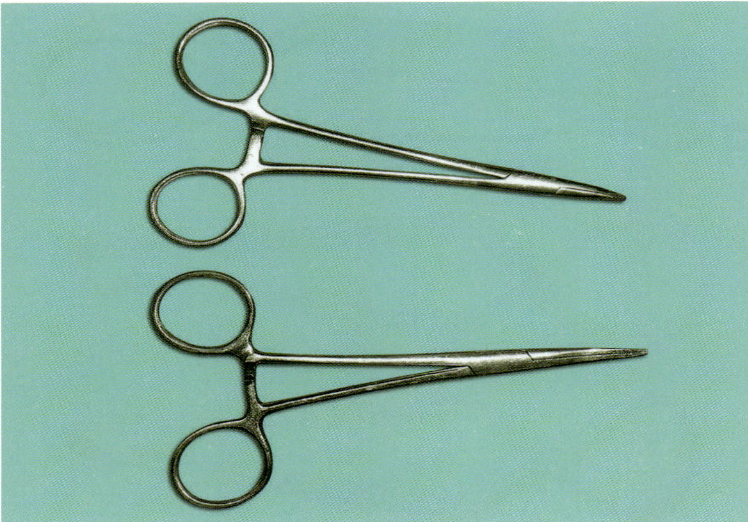

Fig. 5-10: Mosquito forceps.

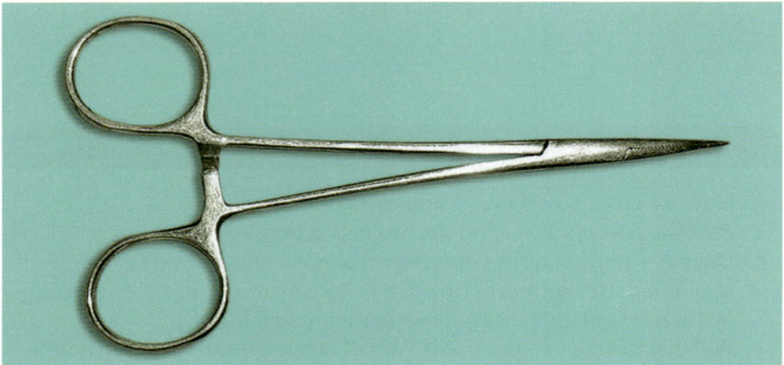

Fig. 5-11: Small-sized curved Halsted haemostat—mosquito artery forceps.

Based on shape:

- Straight artery forceps.
- Curved artery forceps.

Features of artery forceps:

- Distal blades are having transverse serrations which are well apposed.
- Lock in the proximal part.

Uses:

- To catch bleeding points.
- To open the facial planes in different surgeries.
- To pass a ligature and to hold it.
- To hold fascia, peritoneum, aponeurosis.
- To hold sutures.
- To drain an abscess like a sinus forceps.
- To hold gauze as peanut.
- To crush the base of the appendix.
- To clamp a catheter in between the hinge and ratchet of the haemostat.
- To catch prepuceal skin in circumcision.
- Mosquito forceps *(Halsted)* is used in paediatric surgery/microsurgery/cleft surgery/plastic surgery.

Instrument can also be used to catch arteries/veins/capillaries and so ideally should be called as *haemostat*. But common word used is artery forceps. Haemostat has got serrations on the distal half of the each blade (in pedicle clamp entire blade has got serrations) **(Figs. 5-12A to C)**.

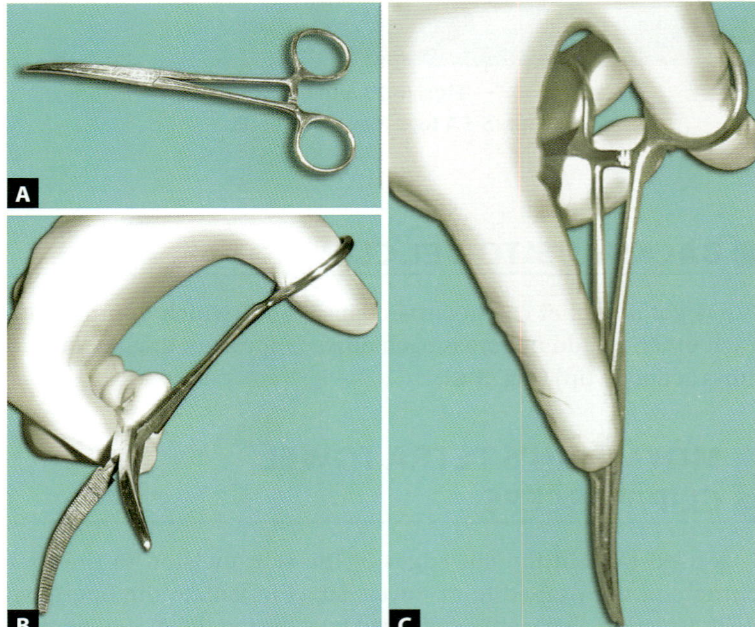

Figs. 5-12A to C: Artery forceps showing its inner aspect with transverse serrations–Spencer-Wells haemostat/pedicle clamp. It is better called as haemostat. Many named artery forceps/haemostats are available with little different in features. More or less all serve similar functions. Serrations in entire length of the distal blades is traditionally a stout haemostat or pedicle clamp (Spencer-Wells) whereas traditional artery forceps has got serrations only near the tip/distal half of the inner blade. There is no need to remember such confusing entities even though these are facts.

Medium sized, curved half serrated haemostat, called as *Kelly's artery forceps* **(Figs. 5-13 and 5-14)**.

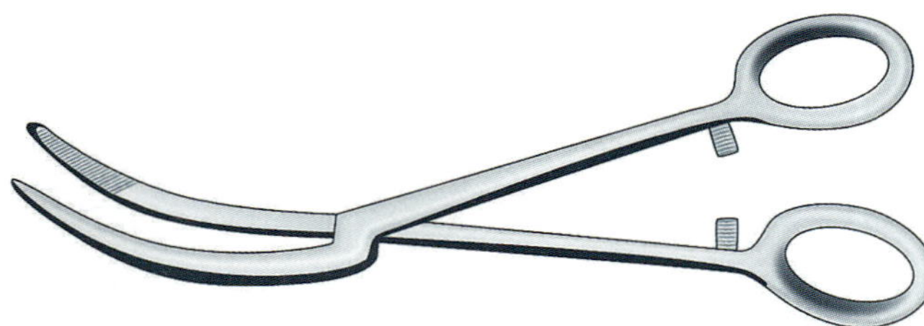

Fig. 5-13: Kelly's artery forceps—commonly used haemostat.

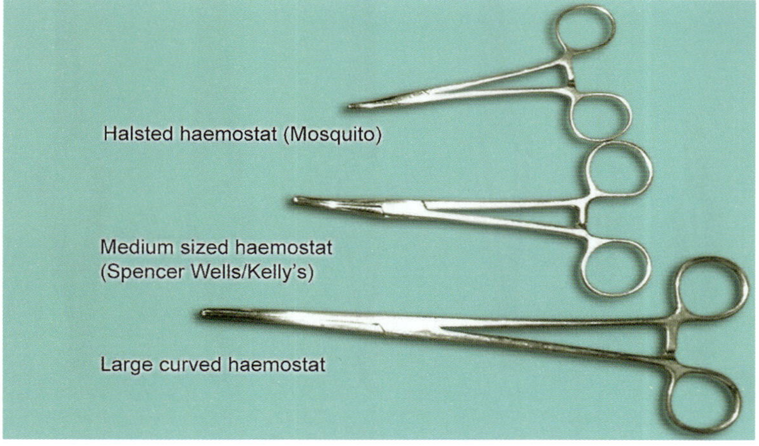

Fig. 5-14: Different sized curved haemostats.

NEGUS ARTERY FORCEPS

It is stout long jawed instrument (forceps) with distal part of the jaws bent like a hook with transverse serrations. It is used to catch bleeding part of the tissues prior to ligation. Initially bleeding area is clamped with haemostat, later Negus artery forceps is clamped underneath and artery is released. It facilitates easier passage of the ligature across the bleeding vessels or tissues **(Figs. 5-15 and 5-16)**.

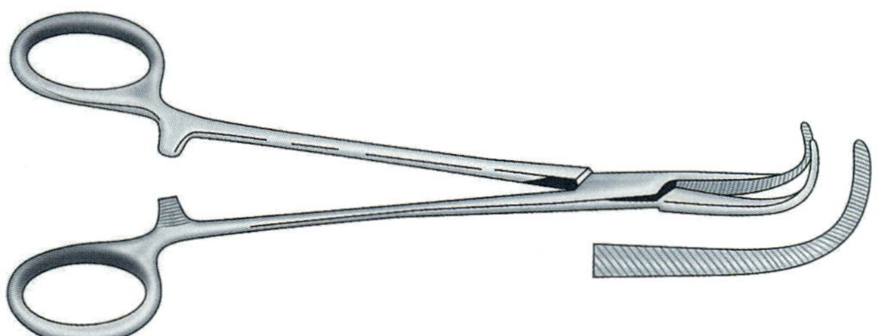

Fig. 5-15: Negus artery forceps.

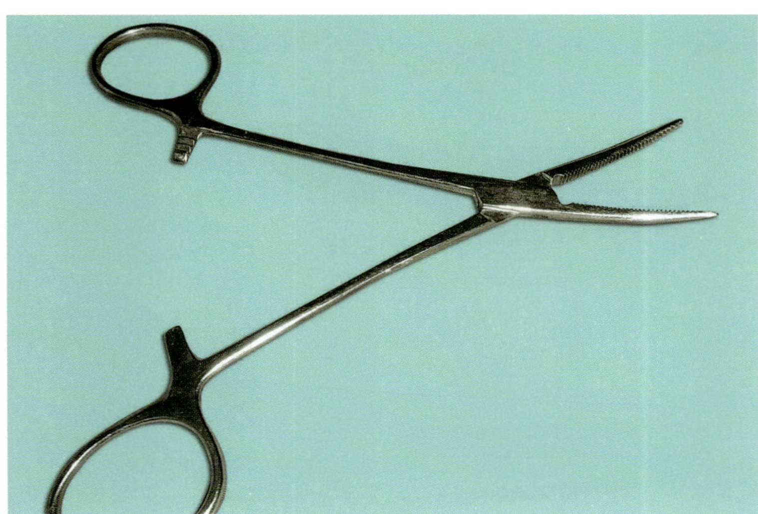

Fig. 5-16A

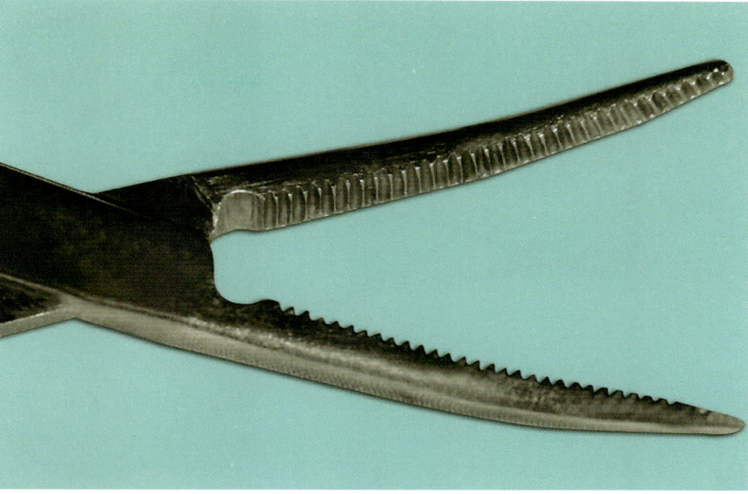

Fig. 5-16B

Figs. 5-16A and B: Artery forceps: Haemostat—typical look.

RIGHT ANGLE FORCEPS—MEISTER'S/LAHEY'S/MIXTER'S

It has got 90° curves in terminal 1 cm part of the blades. Blades are *longitudinally* serrated. It has got a ratchet. Tip is blunt. It is used to dissect pedicles and to pass ligatures, to dissect the vagus and ligate in vagotomy, to hold bleeding vessels in depth, to dissect major vessels, to dissect and pass ligatures to cystic duct and cystic artery in cholecystectomy and in thyroid, biliary, splenic, gastric, renal and pelvic surgeries **(Figs. 5-17A to D)**.

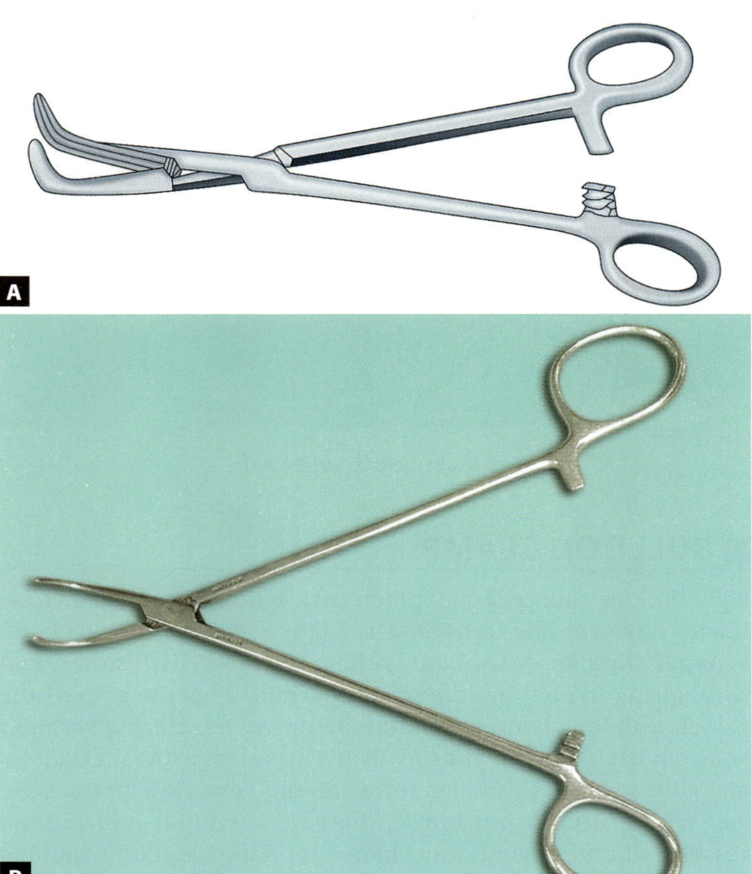

Figs. 5-17A and B

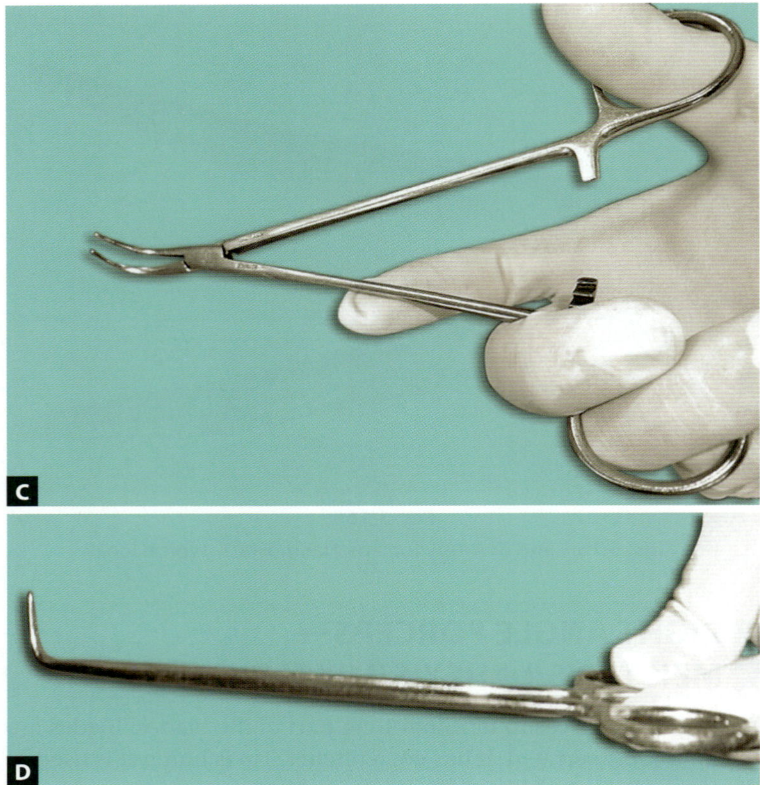

Figs. 5-17C and D

Figs. 5-17A to D: Meigster right angle forceps.

WELLS' ARTERIAL CLAMP

It has got doubly right-angled distal blades with longitudinal serrations in the jaw. It is used to clamp pedicles like in nephrectomy or splenectomy **(Fig. 5-18)**.

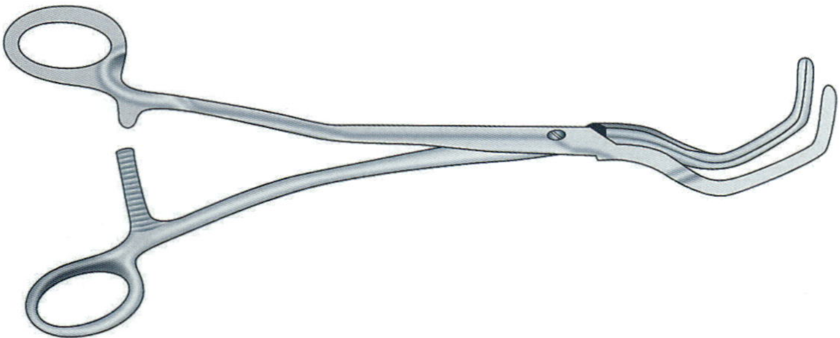

Fig. 5-18: Wells' arterial clamp.

BULLDOG CLAMP

Light bulldog clamp has got pinch cock action to open and close. Blades have got fine transverse serrations. Pott's bulldog clamp is paper clip like instrument with strong jaws (with serrations) with spring loaded handle which permits a secure grip of the vessel. Bulldog clamp is used to clamp vessels during vascular anastomosis like for creating AV fistula in patient with renal failure; major vessel surgeries as for aorta, inferior vena cava, portal vein, etc. With a firm grip it blocks the vessel without injuring the vessel wall and without any chance for slippage. Pott's bulldog clamp is used for large vessels like aorta, vena cava **(Figs. 5-19 and 5-20)**.

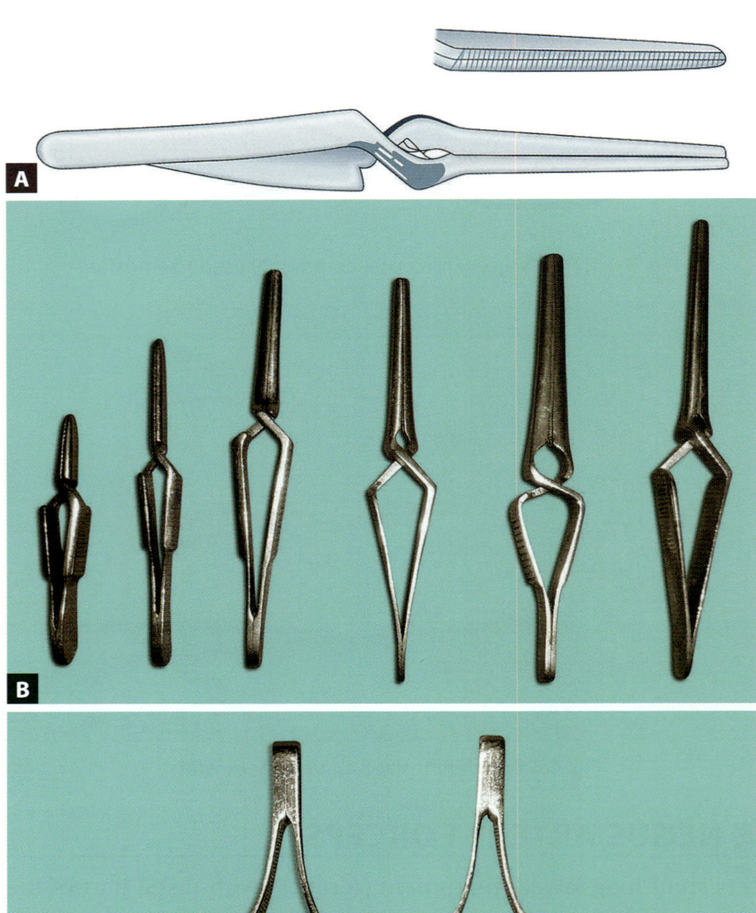

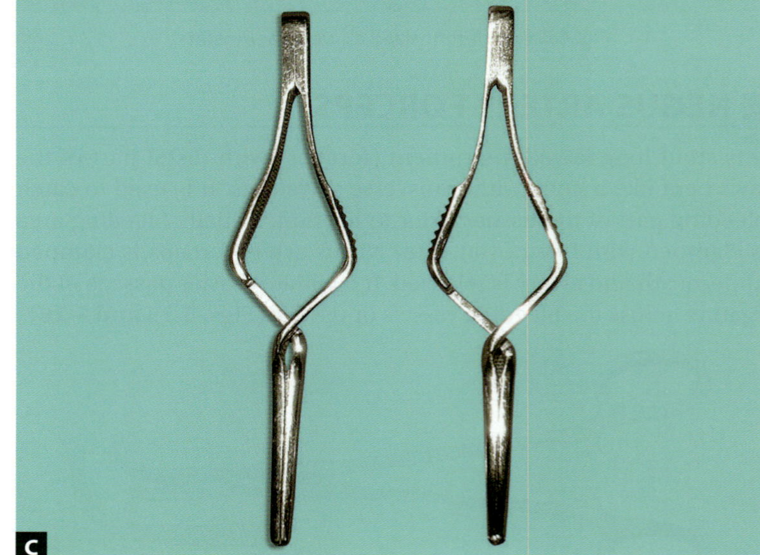

Figs. 5-19A to C: Bulldog clamp used to clamp vascular system—artery or veins. Different sizes are available.

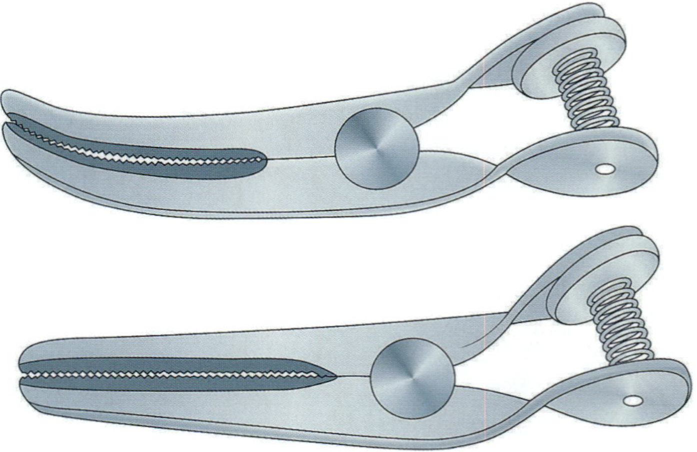

Fig. 5-20: Pott's bulldog clamp.

SATINSKY VASCULAR CLAMP

It is light atraumatic long instrument with C shaped distal blades which has got fine teeth within. It has got a ratchet. It can be applied to part of the circumference of the vessel in portal vein, iliac veins, inferior vena cava while removing tumor thrombus in renal cell carcinoma, in pancreatectomy, major vessel surgeries. Vascular anastomosis can be done using it **(Figs. 5-21A to C)**.

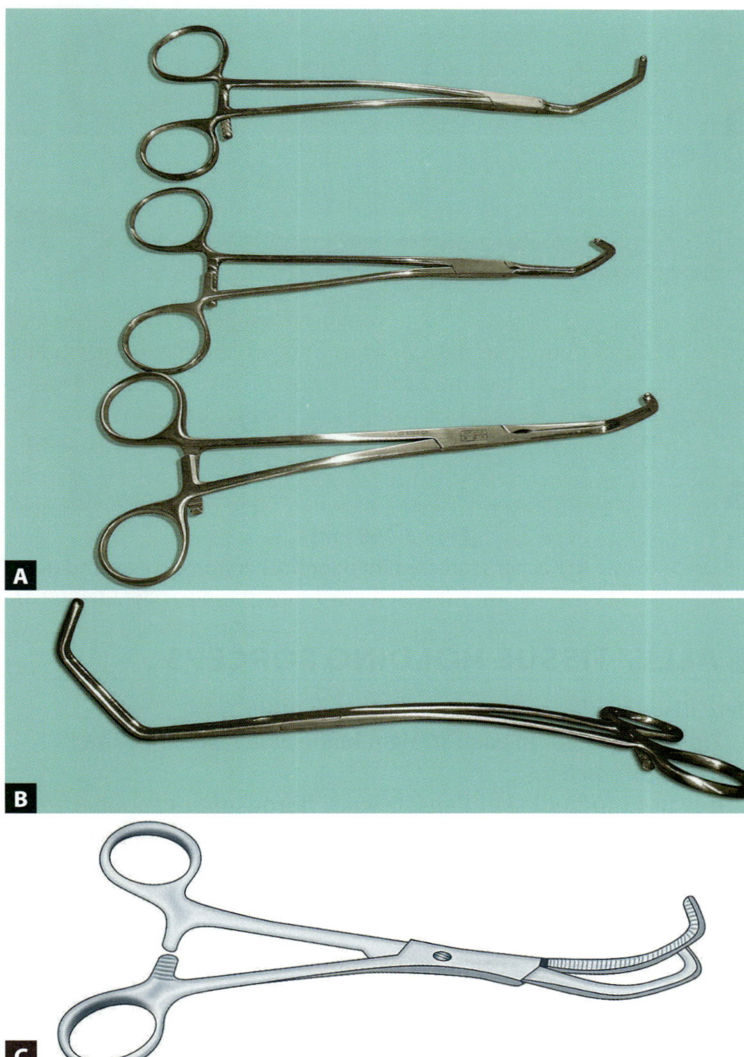

Figs. 5-21A to C: Satinsky vascular clamp.

DE BAKEY'S VASCULAR CLAMP

Its blades are long and well angulated so that it can be used to clamp vessels/bleeders in the depth with good grip without damaging the vessel wall **(Figs. 5-22A to C)**.

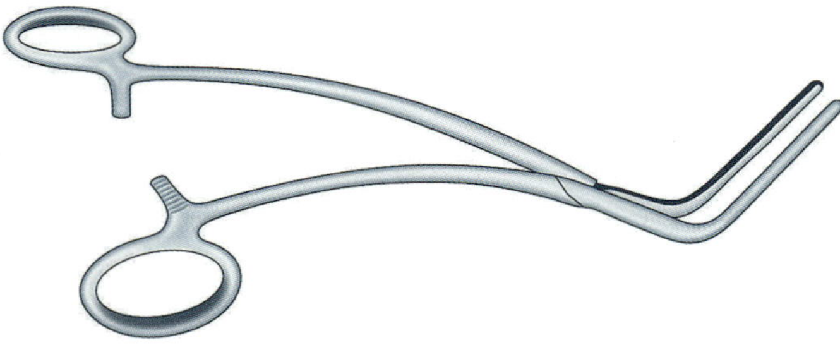

Fig. 5-22A

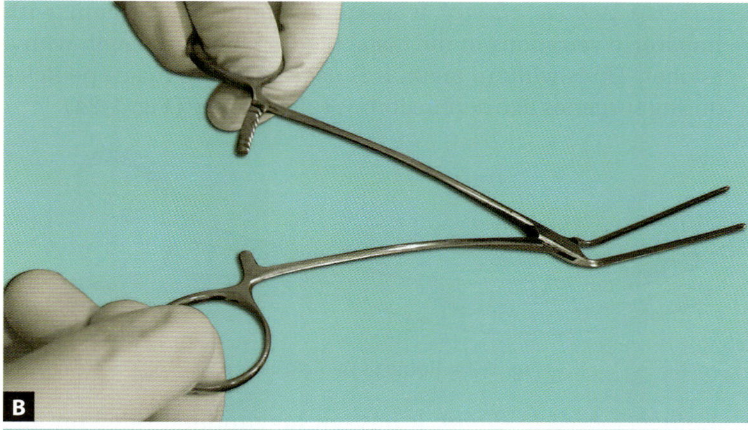

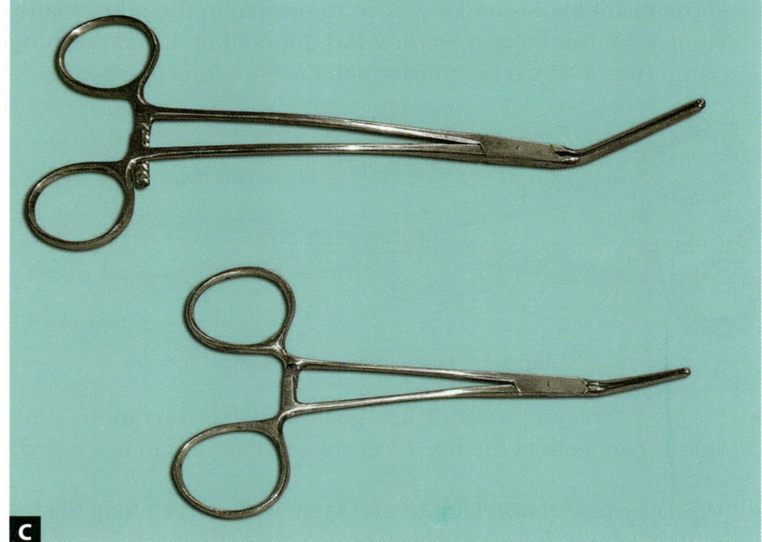

Figs. 5-22B and C

Figs. 5-22A to C: De Bakey's vascular clamp.

PEDICLE CLAMPS

A pedicle clamp is a stout haemostat with straight or curved blades with a ratchet. Entire blades are serrated here. It can be with or without teeth.

- *Spencer-Wells pedicle clamp/artery forceps:* It has blunt tip without teeth. It can be straight or curved. Its blades are entirely serrated. It can be small/straight/large **(Fig. 5-23)**.

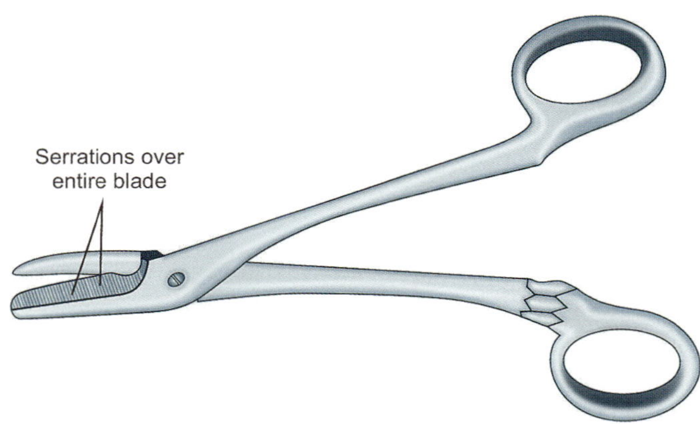

Fig. 5-23: Spencer-Wells' clamp/artery forceps.

- *Robert's pedicle clamp:* It is stout curved instrument with transverse serrations in the distal blades on entire length with a ratchet. Tip is without teeth. It is used to clamp major pedicles during surgeries like nephrectomy/splenectomy **(Fig. 5-24)**.

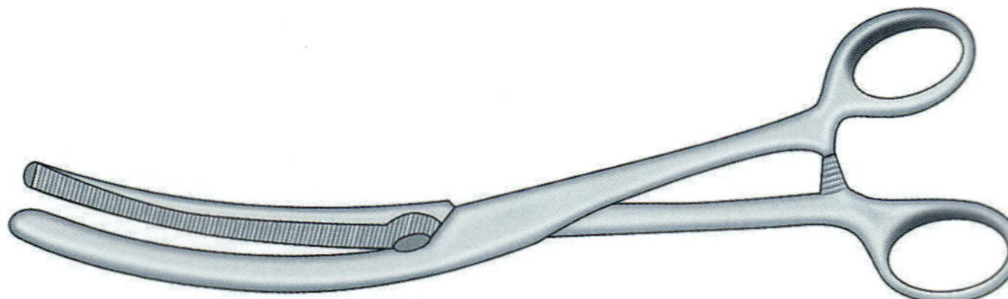

Fig. 5-24: Robert's pedicle clamp.

- *Maingot's pedicle clamp:* It has got longitudinal ridge on one of the distal blades and a groove to receive in the other blade. Tip has got one-in-two teeth. It has got ratchet. It is a crushing clamp **(Fig. 5-25)**. It is stronger than Kocher's forceps/clamp.

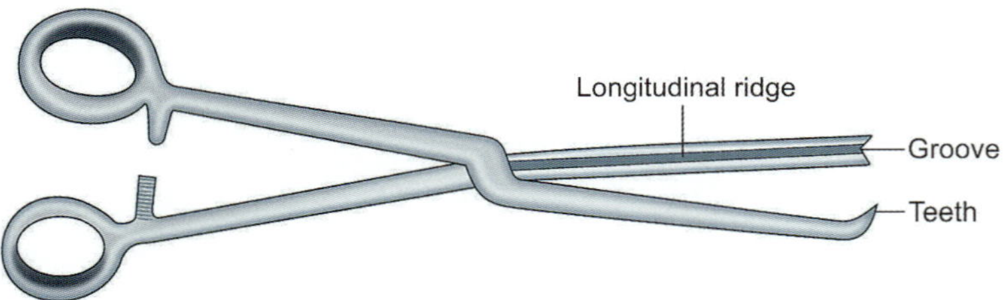

Fig. 5-25: Maingot's pedicle clamp.

- *Kocher's forceps/clamp:* It has got transverse serrations with one-in-two teeth at the tip. It has got a ratchet. It can be curved/straight.
- *Mayo's pedicle clamp* is stout and large with curved long blades with serrations. It is useful in clamping major pedicles.

KOCHER'S FORCEPS

It has got serrations in the distal blades and apposing tooth in the tip. It holds the tissues/pedicle well and prevents slippage of the tissues and retraction of the vessels/bleeders. It can be straight or curved; small/medium or large type **(Figs. 5-26A to C)**.

It is used to hold pedicles, tough structures, cut ends of the muscles like—in thyroidectomy/haemorrhoidectomy/mastectomy/polypectomy/hysterectomy.

It is used to hold tough/fibrous structures like in palms/soles/scalp to prevent retraction of vessels during surgery.

It is used to hold peanuts (gauze pellets of 3–4 mm sized used in blunt dissection).

It is used to hold gauze for blunt dissection; to hold resected bowel; to hold ribs during rib resection.

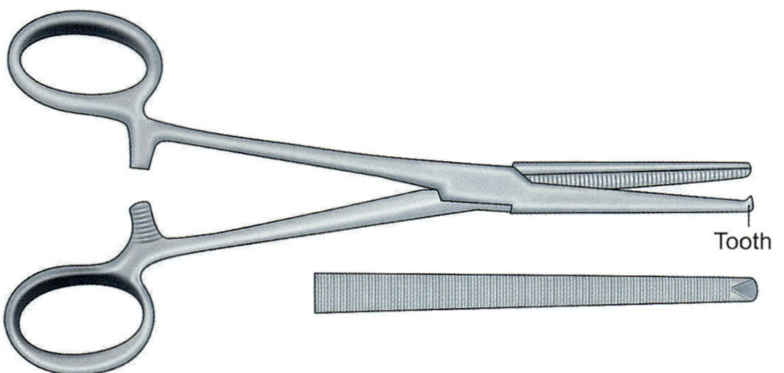

Fig. 5-26A

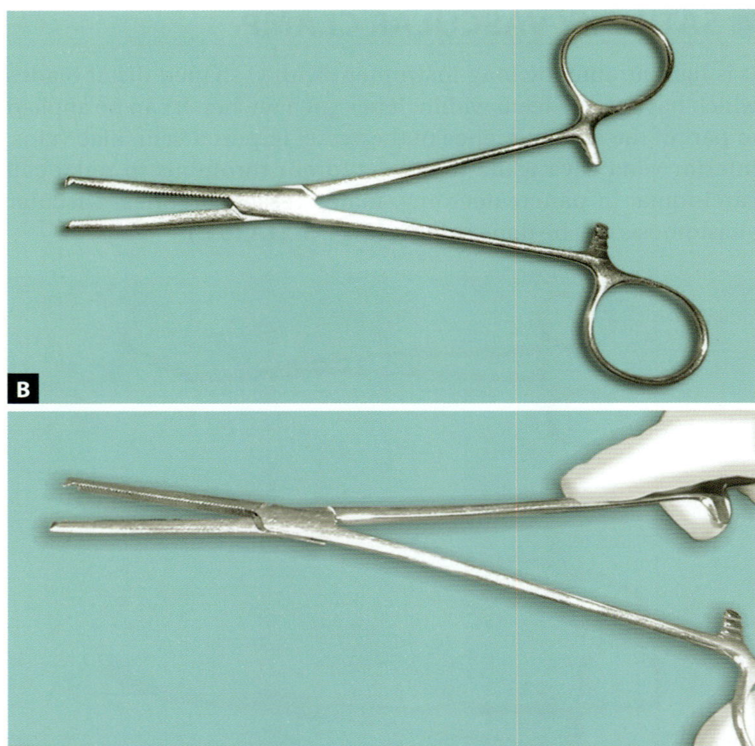

Figs. 5-26B and C

Figs. 5-26A to C: Kocher's forceps (Theodor Kocher from Switzerland got Nobel prize for his extensive work on thyroid surgery—also refer Chapter 1).

ALLIS' TISSUE HOLDING FORCEPS

Here distal blades are not apposing each other.

Tip has got teeth in each straight blade which are apposing.

It has got *ratchet*.

It is used to hold skin flaps, fascias, fibrous tissue, aponeurosis, galea (in craniotomy) and bladder wall **(Figs. 5-27A to C)**. It is essential instrument in any surgery whether major or minor. It can be small/medium/large. Large Allis is used in hysterectomy to hold vaginal wall and tough structures. It is better not to use this instrument to hold delicate structures like bowel/vessel wall.

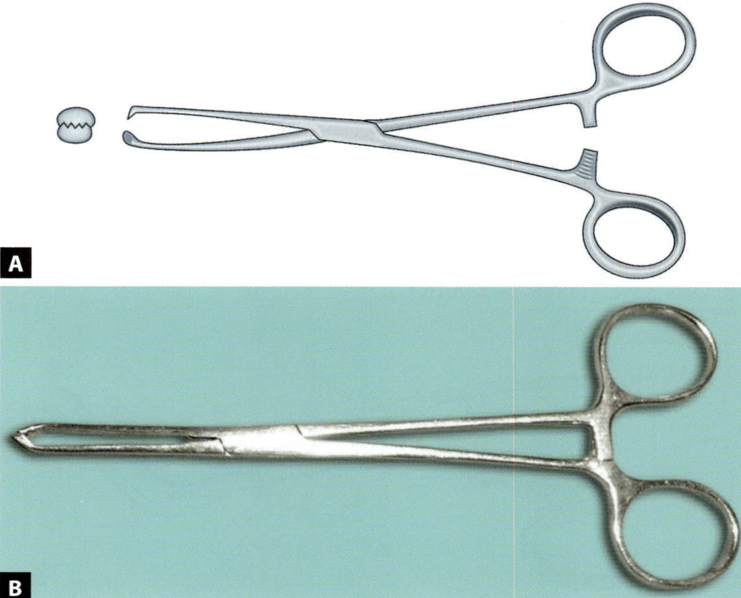

Figs. 5-27A and B

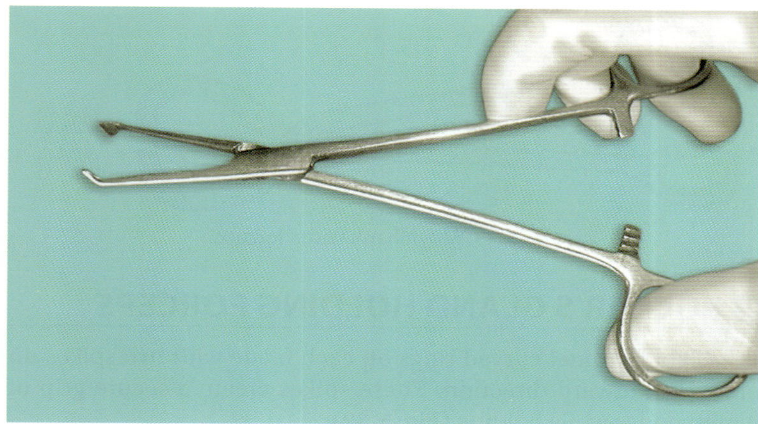

Fig. 5-27C

Figs. 5-27A to C: Allis' tissue holding forceps.

BABCOCK'S FORCEPS

The distal parts of distal blades are curved with triangular fenestra in it which allows soft tissues to bulge out. Tip is non-traumatic with transverse serrations/ridges on it. It has got a ratchet.

It is used to hold any part of the bowel, Fallopian tubes, appendix, urinary bladder, ureter, spermatic cord, lymph node **(Figs. 5-28A to C)**.

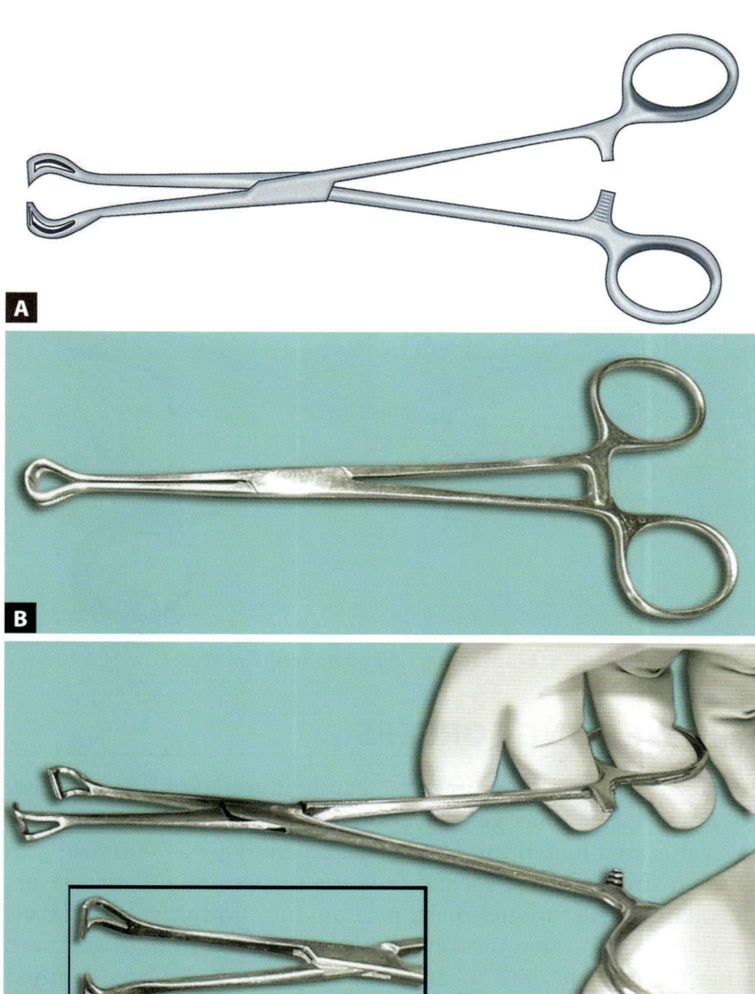

Figs. 5-28A to C: Babcock's forceps.

LANE'S TISSUE HOLDING FORCEPS

It has got thick, stout distal blades with oval fenestra in each blade with a broad expanded curvature at the end. It has got apposing tooth (one in two) at the tip and a ratchet **(Figs. 5-29A to C)**.

It is used to hold bulky and tough structures (like to hold breast during mastectomy; to hold salivary glands while excising); to hold lymph nodes; to hold tumour tissue. It is also used as towel clip and sponge holding forceps. It is used to hold linea alba and aponeurosis.

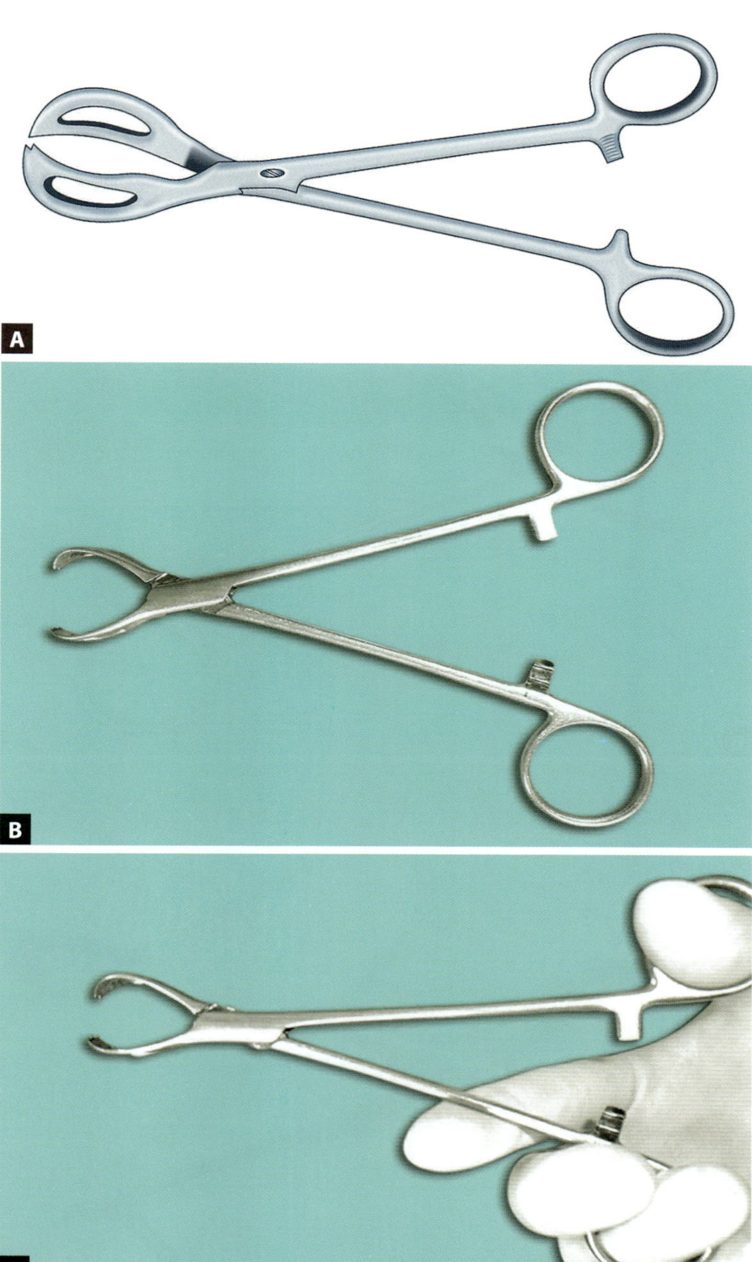

Figs. 5-29A to C: Lane's tissue holding forceps.

MORRANT-BAKER'S APPENDIX HOLDING FORCEPS

It is like Lane's forceps but with apposing serrations proximal to the tooth. These serrations give a good grip on mesoappendix while holding appendix in appendicectomy. Its use is replaced by Babcock's forceps **(Figs. 5-30A to C)**.

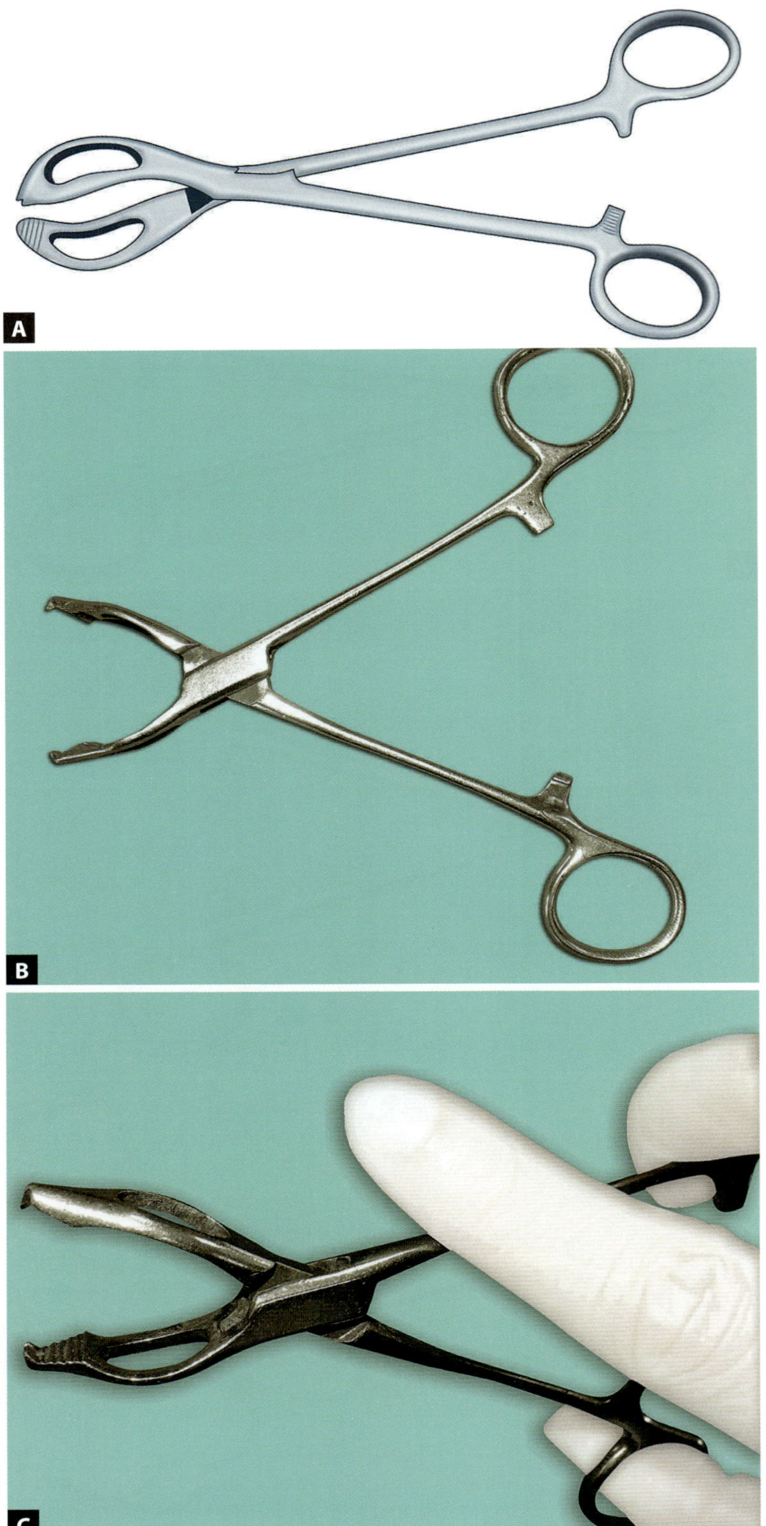

Figs. 5-30A to C: Morrant-Baker's tissue holding forceps.

MOYNIHAN'S TISSUE FORCEPS

It is the tissue holding forceps with thinner and curved blades. Its uses are like Allis' forceps **(Fig. 5-31)**.

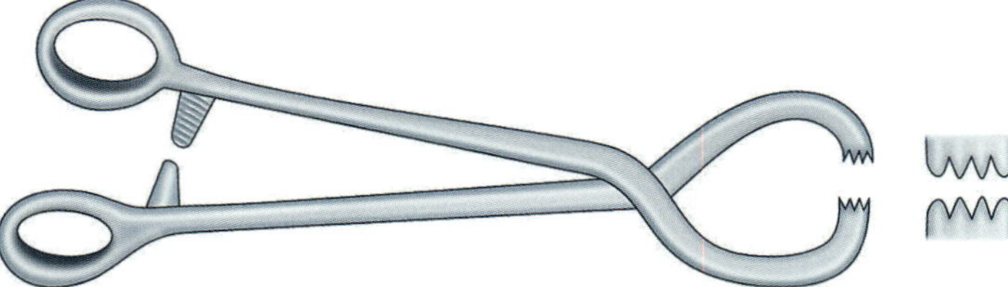

Fig. 5-31: Moynihan's tissue forceps.

KOCHER'S GLAND HOLDING FORCEPS

It has got terminal curved rings on each blade with two spikes on each with inward direction. These spikes create a secure grip of lymph nodes while holding **(Fig. 5-32)**.

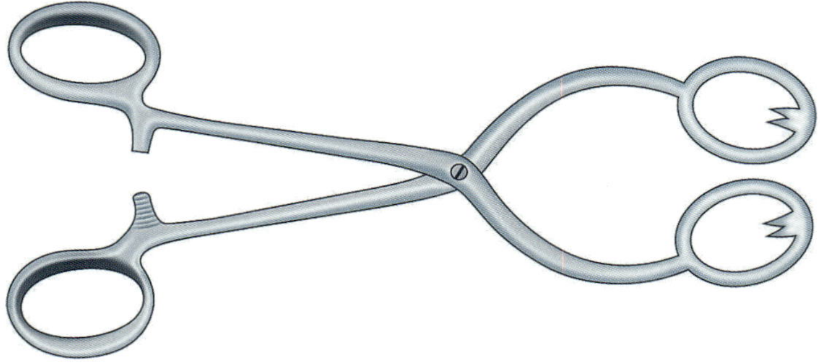

Fig. 5-32: Kocher's gland holding forceps.

YOUNG'S GLAND FORCEPS

It has got long blades with each blade having rounded flat end with a fenestra without any serrations on its inner aspect. It is atraumatic. It has got ratchet. It is used to hold lymph nodes, cyst wall during surgical excision **(Fig. 5-33)**.

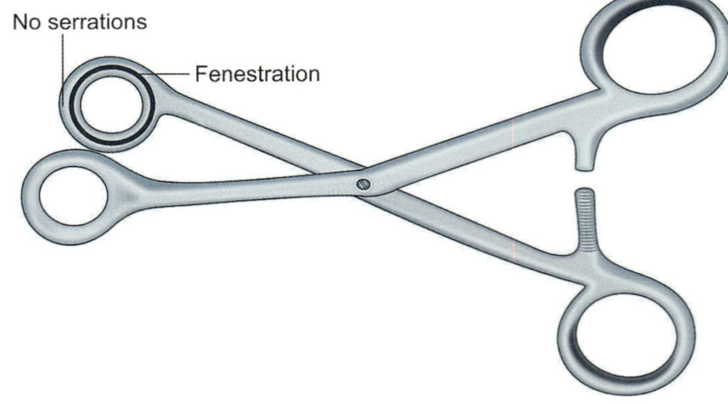

Fig. 5-33: Young's gland holding forceps.

DISSECTING FORCEPS

It is basic essential instrument. It can be toothed or non-toothed. Its outer surface has got serrations/grooves in the middle part. Over this area fingers are placed like a pen to get a good firm grip of the instrument. It is used to hold the tissues and different layers like skin, fascia, aponeurosis, peritoneum, bowel, vessel, nerve, muscle, etc. Toothed dissecting forceps is used to hold skin and other tough structures. It can be one in two/two in three toothed forceps. It is also used for suture removal **(Figs. 5-34 to 5-36)**.

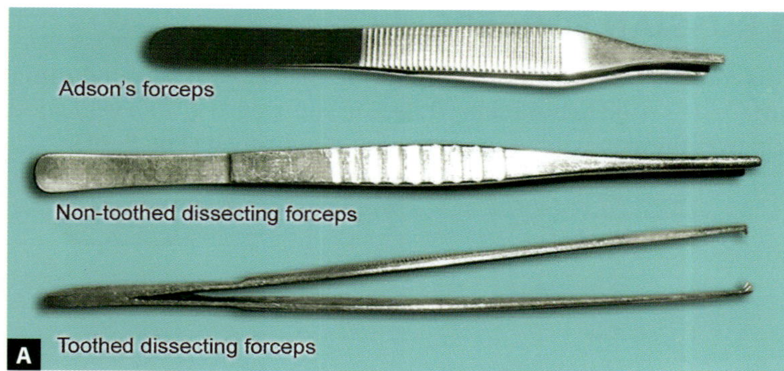

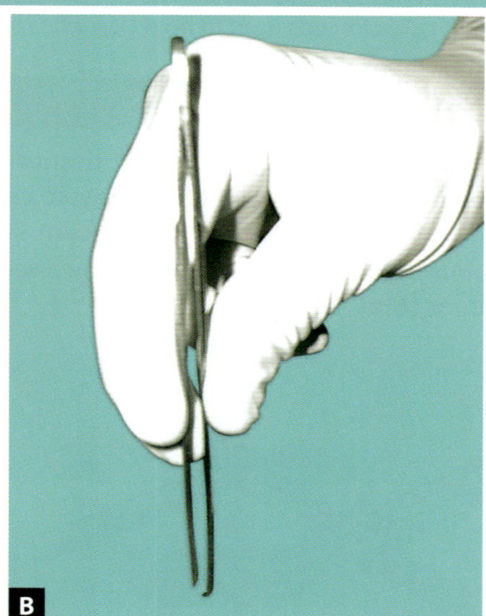

Figs. 5-34A and B: Different types of dissecting forceps. Photograph showing how to hold dissecting forceps.

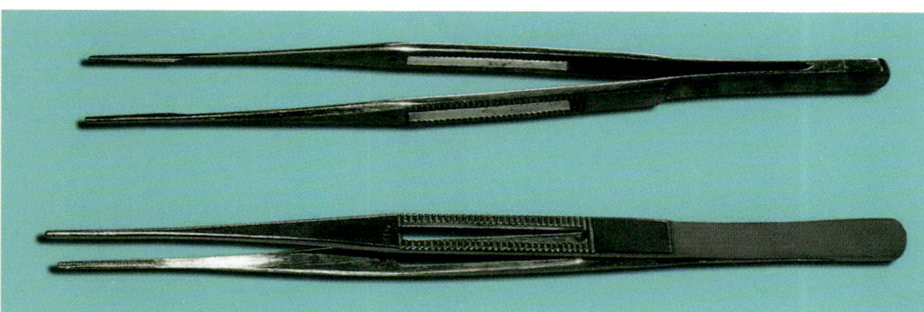

Fig. 5-35: Fine forceps.

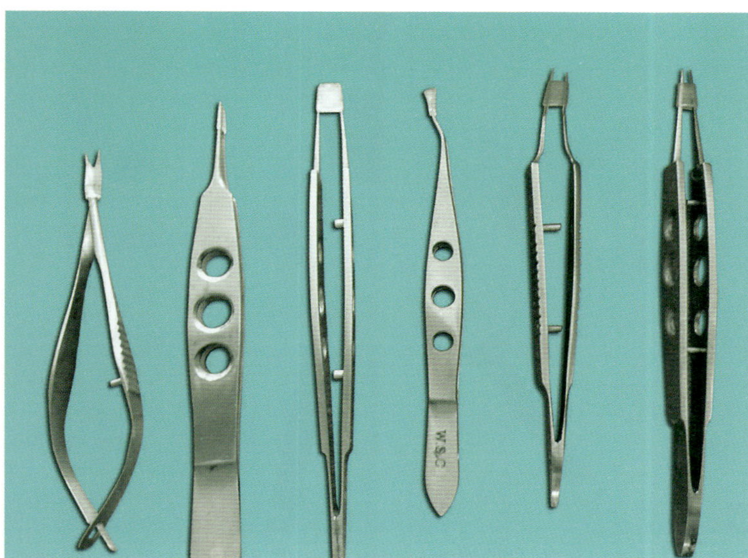

Fig. 5-36: Vascular forceps.

Plain Non-toothed Dissecting Forceps

It is used to hold delicate soft, friable structures like peritoneum, vessels, bowel, nerves, and tendons. It cannot be used to hold skin or tough structures. During surgical dissection it is used to hold/fix/steady/stretch the structures as needed. It is also used to hold and cauterise small bleeding vessels **(Figs. 5-37A to F)**.

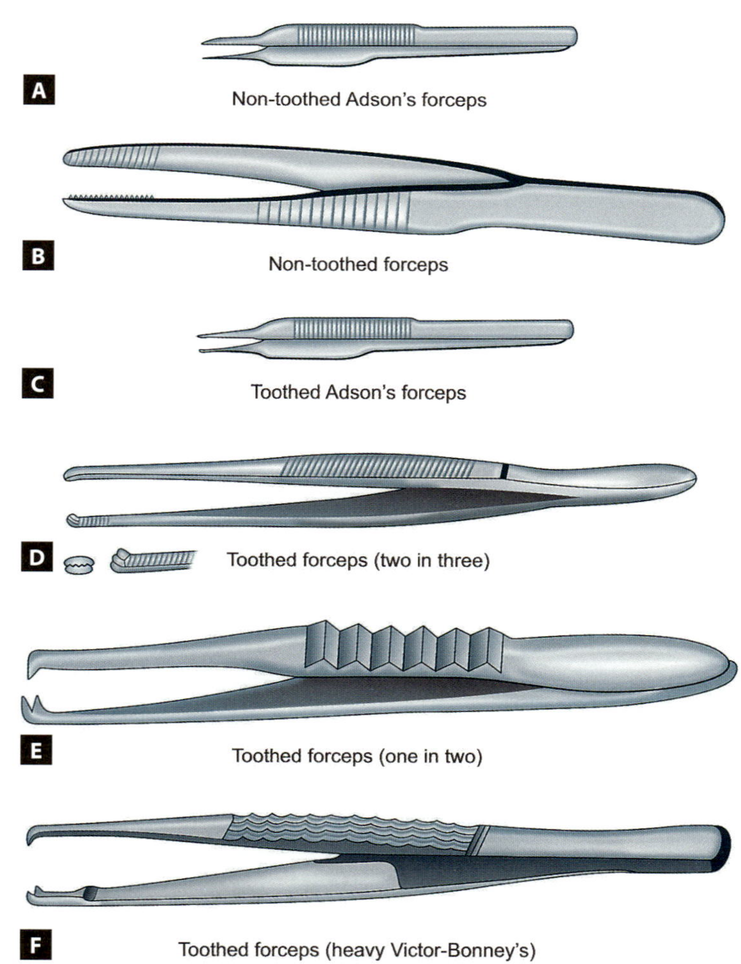

Figs. 5-37A to F: Dissecting forceps: (A) Non-toothed Adson's fine forceps; (B) Non-toothed forceps; (C) Toothed Adson's fine forceps; (D) Toothed forceps–two in three type; (E) Toothed forceps-one in two type; (F) Toothed forceps—heavy Victor-Bonney's type.

Toothed-dissecting Forceps

It is used to hold skin and tough structures like fascia, aponeurosis; to remove sutures. It is not used to hold delicate structures like bowel/vessel/nerve. It can have one in two teeth or two in three teeth. Small, fine forceps used for fine works is called as Adson's forceps. *Adson's forceps* can be toothed or non-toothed. *Victor-Bonney's* forceps is heavy toothed dissecting forceps.

KOCHER'S THYROID DISSECTOR

It has got a curved blade with vertical grooves on it. There is an eye on its tip. It is used to dissect the upper pole of thyroid in thyroidectomy and to place as a surface while cutting the superior pedicle. Through eye ligature can be passed **(Fig. 5-38)**.

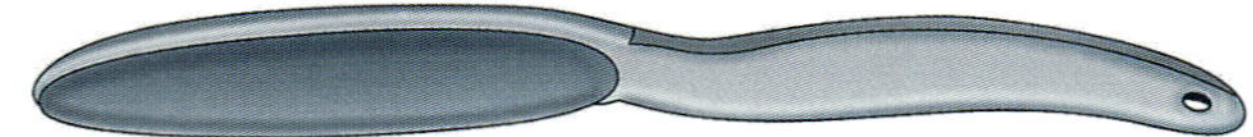

Fig. 5-38: Kocher's thyroid dissector.

SINUS FORCEPS (LISTER'S)

It has got straight, long blades with serrations in the tip. It does not have ratchet. Serrations allow it hold and break the loculi or wall of the abscess cavity. It is a blunt instrument and so least traumatic and so adjacent neurovascular bundle will not get damaged **(Figs. 5-39A to D)**.

It is used to drain pus from abscess cavity (*Hilton's method)*. It is called as sinus forceps because it is initially originated to pack the sinus cavities. It is also used to pack nasal cavity and ear. It is less traumatic.

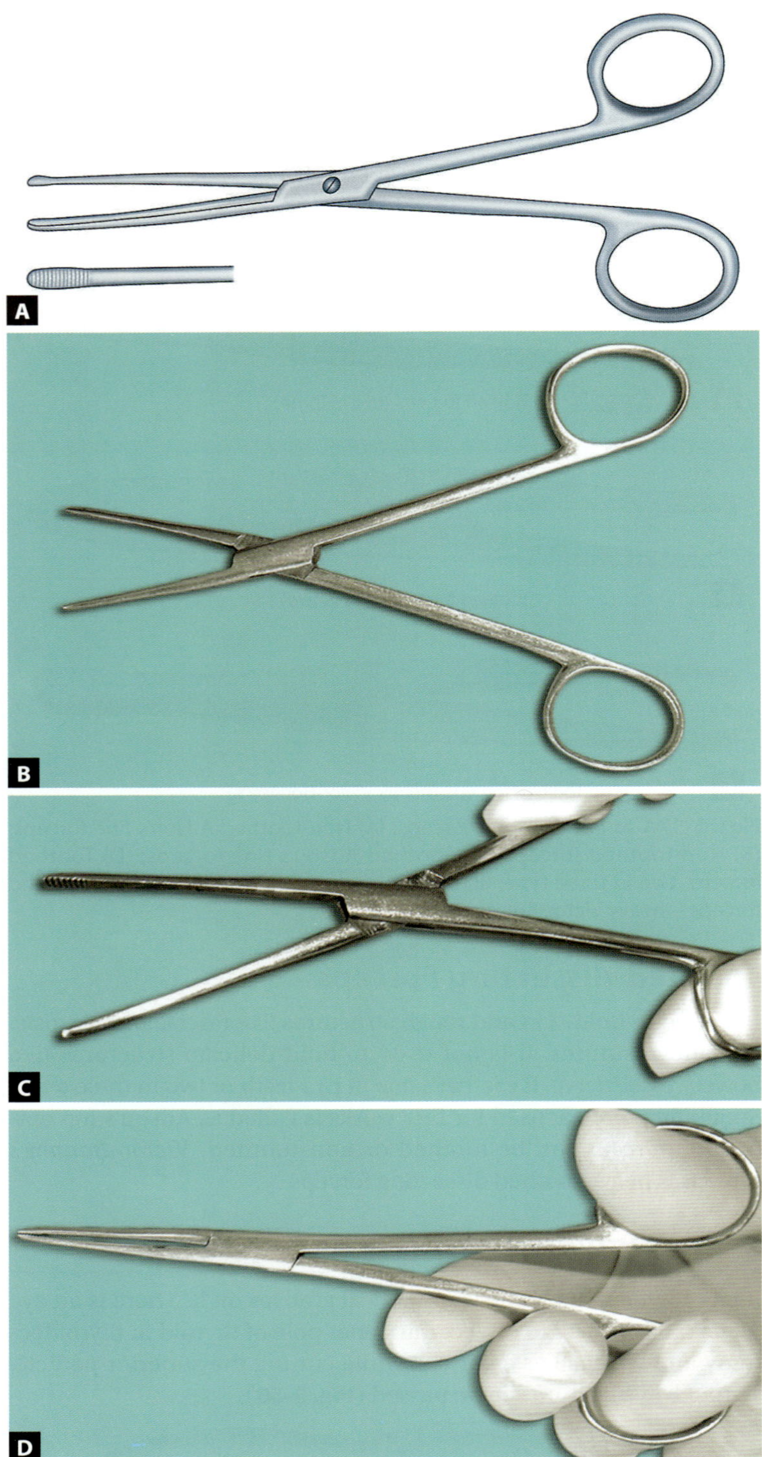

Figs. 5-39A to D: Lister's sinus forceps. It does not have lock. It has got serrations on the inner aspect of the distal blades.

RUSSIAN FORCEPS

This forceps has got clubbed tip in the blades with serrated inner surface. It is used to hold skin while skin suturing. It gives a very good grip over the skin while suturing without injuring it **(Fig. 5-40)**.

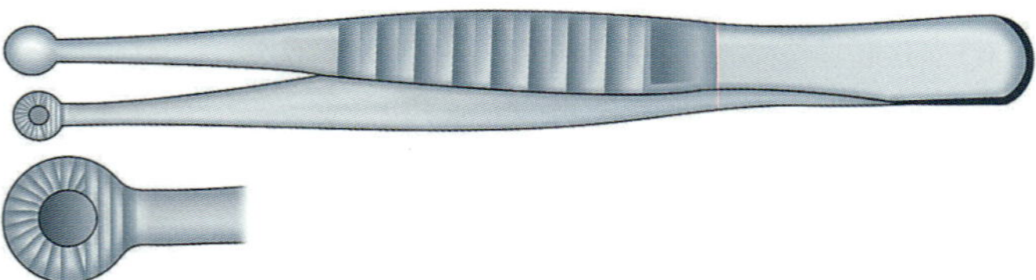

Fig. 5-40: Russian forceps used to hold skin while suturing.

RETRACTORS

A retractor is an instrument used to retract tissues away from the operating field; to expose surgical field properly; to carry out surgery precisely and also to prevent damage to adjacent structures while conducting operation. It also prevents the unnecessary handling of the adjacent tissues **(Figs. 5-41 and 5-42)**.

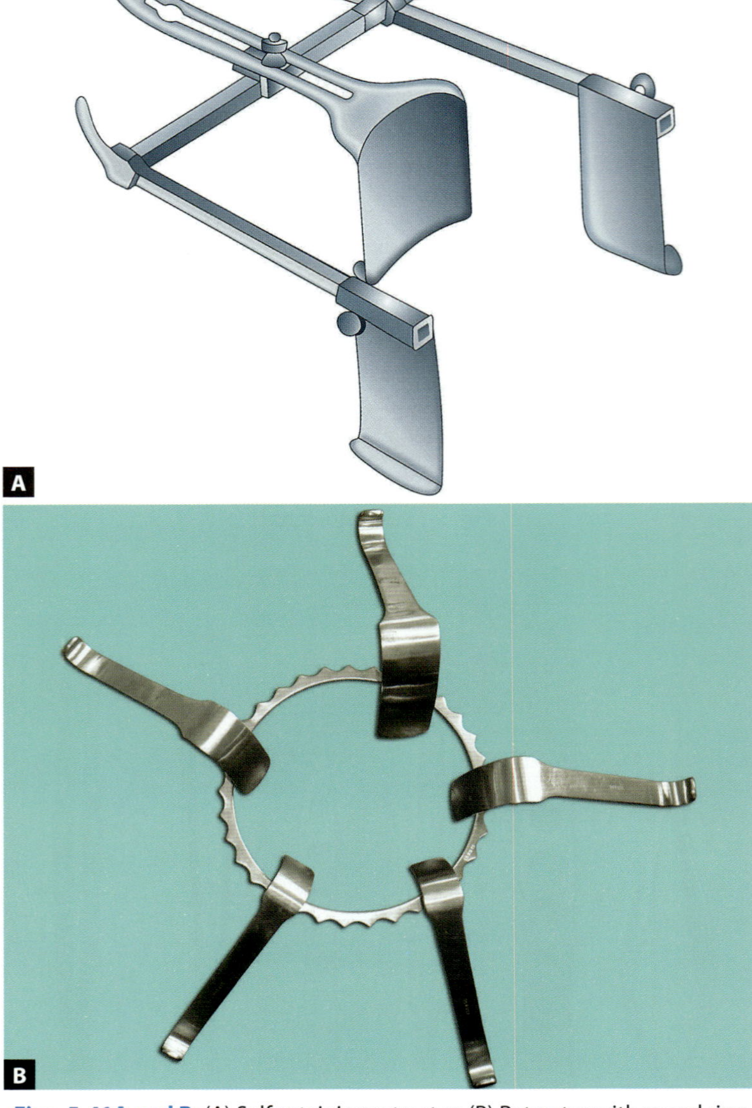

Figs. 5-41A and B: (A) Self-retaining retractor; (B) Retractor with round ring and flanges on it.

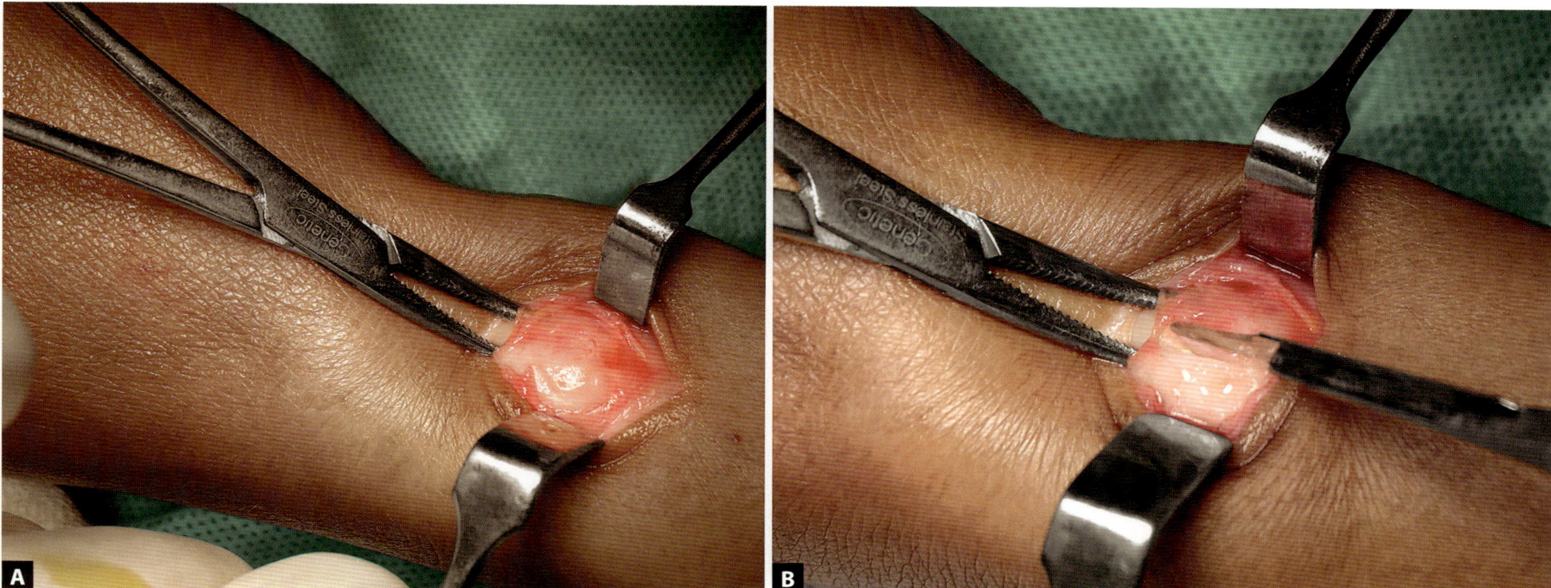

Figs. 5-42A and B: Retractors are used for safe dissection and cutting. It exposes the field well and delineates the anatomy also better.

Types of retractors:

- *Light retractor* is used to retract vessels, nerves, tendons or any delicate structures.
- *Heavy, stout retractors* are used to retract abdominal wall, ribs, sternum, etc.
- *Broad, flat retractors* are used to retract at curved different angles like for liver, spleen, kidney, bowels, etc.
- *Hook retractors* are used to retract soft tissues.

Retractor may be *plain/non-self-retaining/manual* (which is held by an assistant and its position is adjustable time to time) or *self-retaining* (fixed retraction and continuous non-altered/mechanical). Retractor can also be self-illuminating also with a power lamp at the corner of the blade. Drawback of the manual retraction is that assistant can get fatigue by continuous retraction. Over retraction and injury is possible here.

Self-retaining retractor will not allow regular relaxation of tissues and non-adjustable. It is also bulky. But it maintains fixed in position and assistant hands are free for additional work. It may inflict tissue trauma underneath. Placing mops under these instruments will reduce such adverse effect. Fixed deep blades may injure deeper structures like bowel in abdomen. These fixed retractors can be of different types. Chain retractor is cheap good retractor used to retract costal margins in abdomen with blade placing under the costal margin/lower sternum. Its proximal end is connected to an ordinary chain which is fixed to upper end of the table through a stirrup. It is used for surgeries for hiatus hernia, achalasia cardia and lower oesophagus; surgeries of spleen, biliary systems. Upper hand retractors, Omni retractors are different complex retractors used with ends attached to both sides of the operating table. These retractors provide stable exposure of the surgical field to operating surgeon.

Remember: Retraction should be gentle and adequate. Over retraction can cause injury to the retracted organ/tissues and often bleeding.

Uses of retractors

- Retraction of cut edges of the incision.
- To hold important structures like liver/spleen, etc. away from surgical field.
- To steady the tissues.
- To control bleeding.
- To avoid inadvertent trauma to adjacent structures.

SINGLE HOOK RETRACTOR

It is used to retract the skin. It is used in excision of swellings like cyst, lipoma and neurofibroma. It is used to hold skin flaps while raising the flaps **(Figs. 5-43A to C)**.

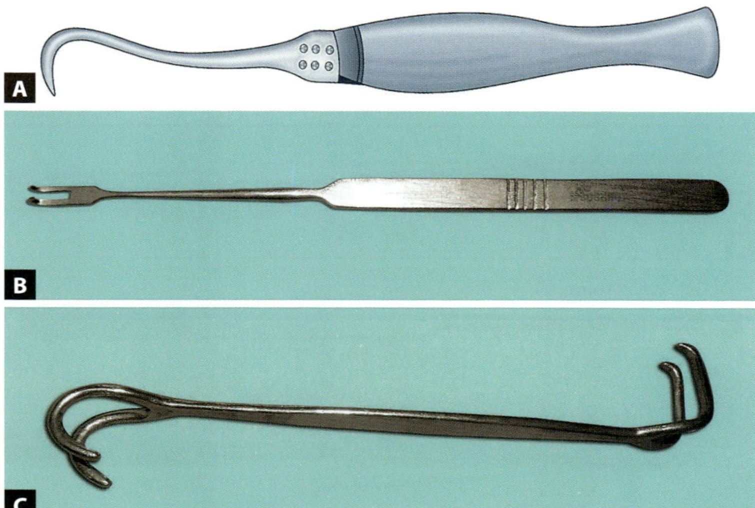

Figs. 5-43A to C: (A) Single hook retractor; (B) Double hook retractor; (C) Double biflanged retractor.

VOLKMANN'S RETRACTOR/CAT'S PAW

It is used to retract fascias in soles and palms. There are multiple hooks with pointed edges. Uses are same as single hook retractor. Handle has got serrations. It cannot be used to retract delicate tissues due to presence of sharp teeth at the retracting end **(Figs. 5-44 and 5-45)**.

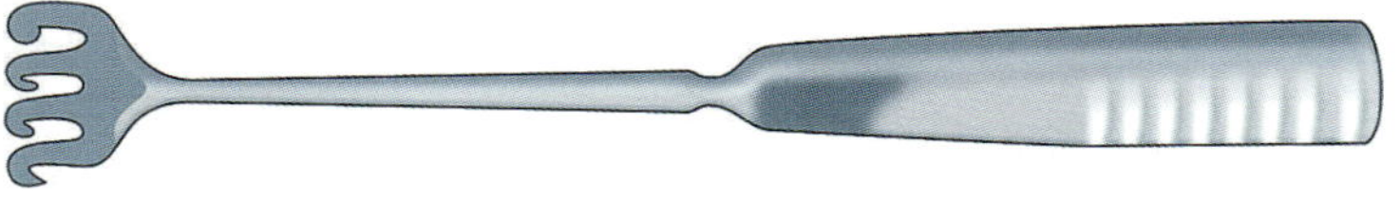

Fig. 5-44: Volkmann's retractor.

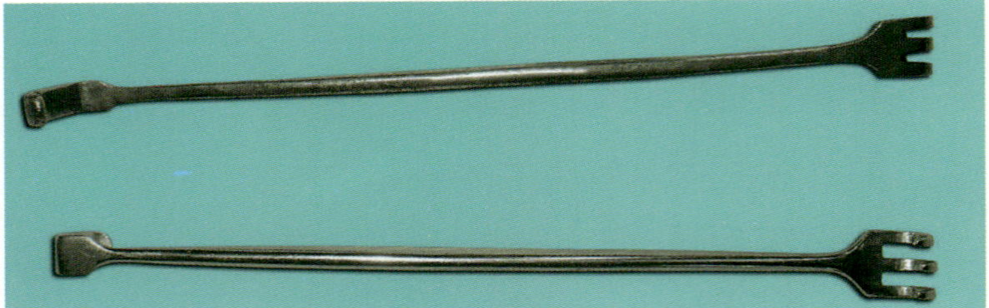

Fig. 5-45: One side double hook and other side usual retracting retractor.

FISCH NERVE HOOK

It is a fine delicate blunt nerve hook used to retract nerves during surgery. Examples: Spinal accessory nerve and hypoglossal nerve retraction in block dissection; ilioinguinal nerve in hernia surgery; lingual and hypoglossal nerves in submandibular surgeries; facial nerve in parotidectomy **(Fig. 5-46)**.

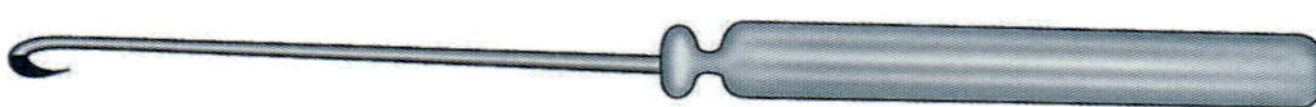

Fig. 5-46: Fisch nerve hook.

SKIN HOOK

It has got sharp curved tip to hold skin with a single puncture. It is used to hold skin flaps during its raise. It is essential instrument in plastic surgery **(Figs. 5-47A to C)**.

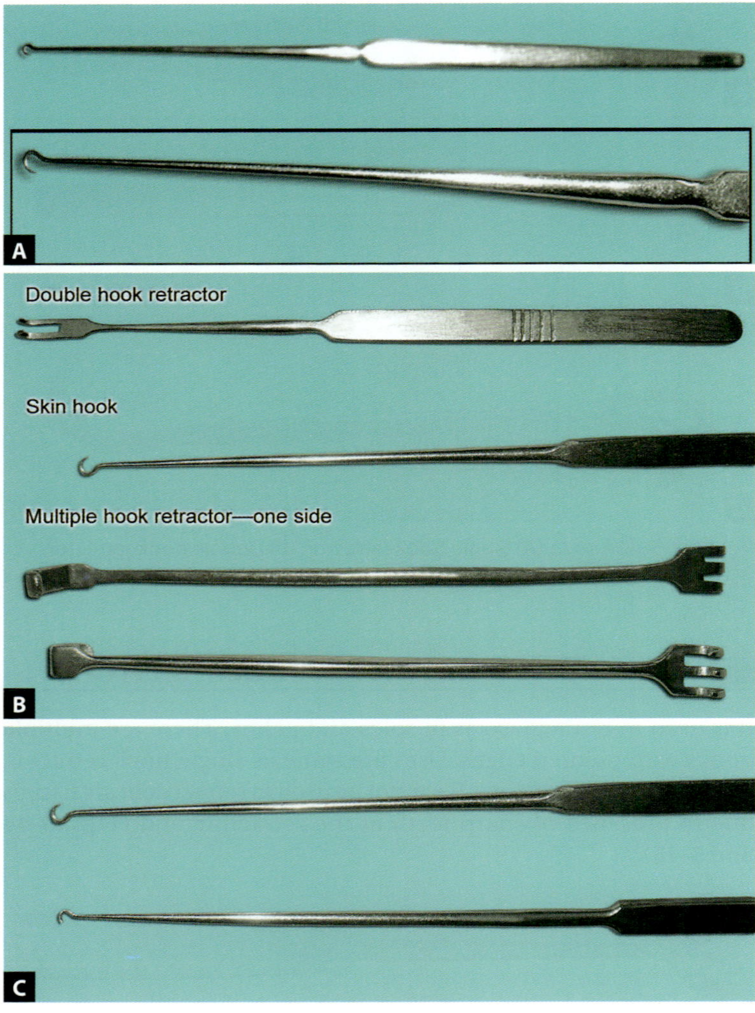

Figs. 5-47A to C: Skin hook retractors of different types.

LANGENBECK'S RETRACTOR

It has got a long handle and a small solid blade. It is used in hernia surgery or any superficial surgeries to retract skin, fascia and aponeurosis, etc. It can be single bladed or double bladed. It is a superficial retractor. It is used to retract structures like skin, fascia or muscle **(Figs. 5-48A and B)**.

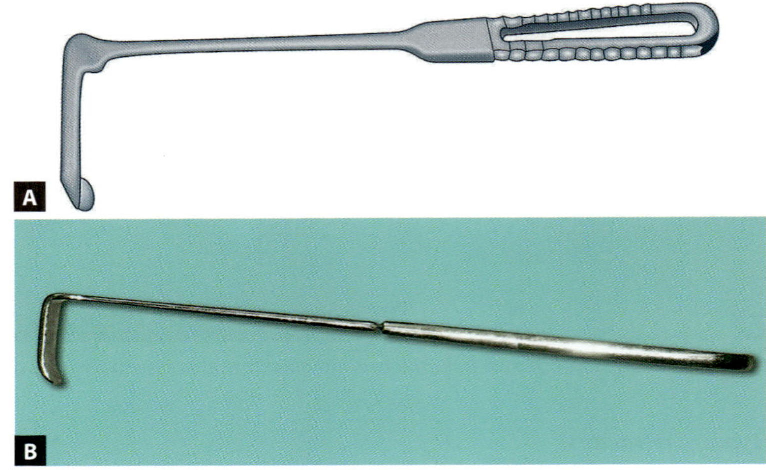

Figs. 5-48A and B: Langenbeck's retractor.

CZERNY'S RETRACTOR (HERNIA RETRACTOR)

This retractor has got thick and small blade on one side and biflanged hook on the other side in opposite directions. It is used in surgeries like hernia, laparotomy especially during closure. Bleeders in the edge can be identified and cauterised easily. It is a superficial retractor. Biflanged end facilitates placing the terminal stitch on the end of the wound during closure **(Figs. 5-49A and B)**.

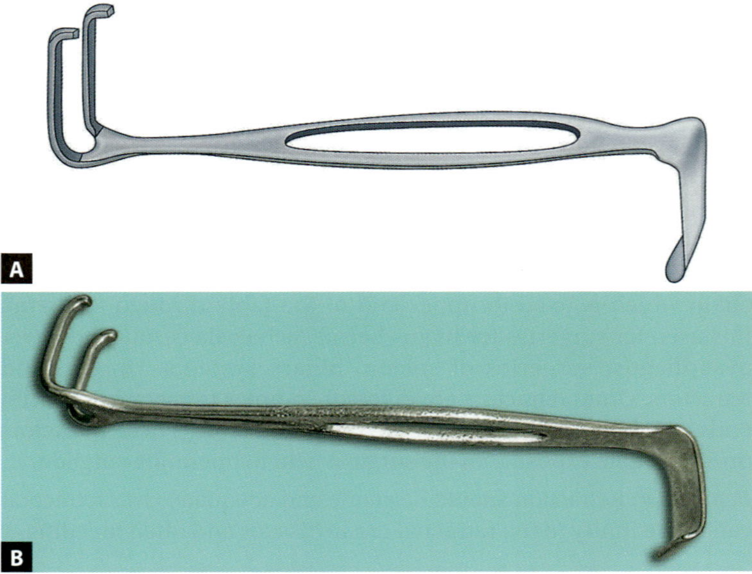

Figs. 5-49A and B: Czerny's retractor.

RIGHT ANGLE RETRACTOR

Here handle and blade are at right angle to each other **(Figs. 5-50A and B)**.

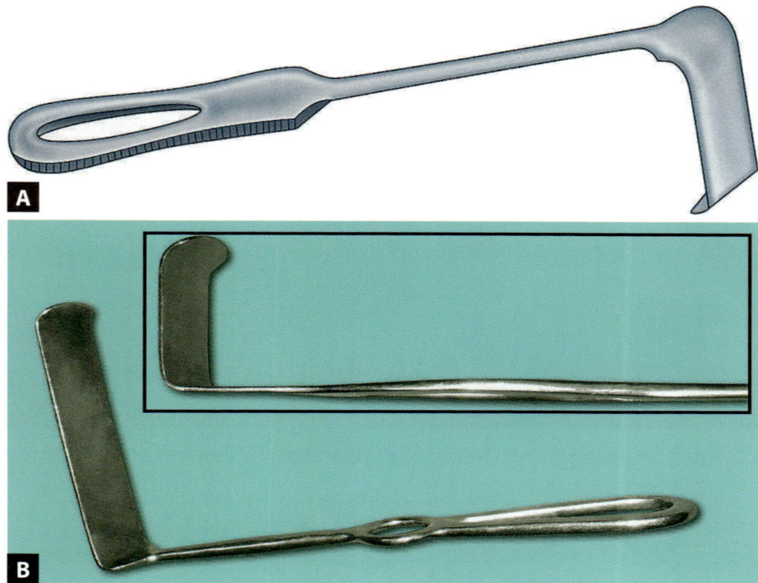

Figs. 5-50A and B: Right angle retractor.

MORRIS' RETRACTOR

It may be single blade type or double blade type. It has flat transversely curved blade. There is a blunt projecting ridge with backward projection to have a better hold.

It is used to retract abdominal wall incisions/loin incisions/subcostal wounds/any wounds in depth. Beak end of the retractor end prevents it from slipping from depth of the wound and holds well to wound. It needs an assistant to retract as it is manual retractor. Its use in many places is replaced by self-retaining retractor **(Figs. 5-51A and B)**.

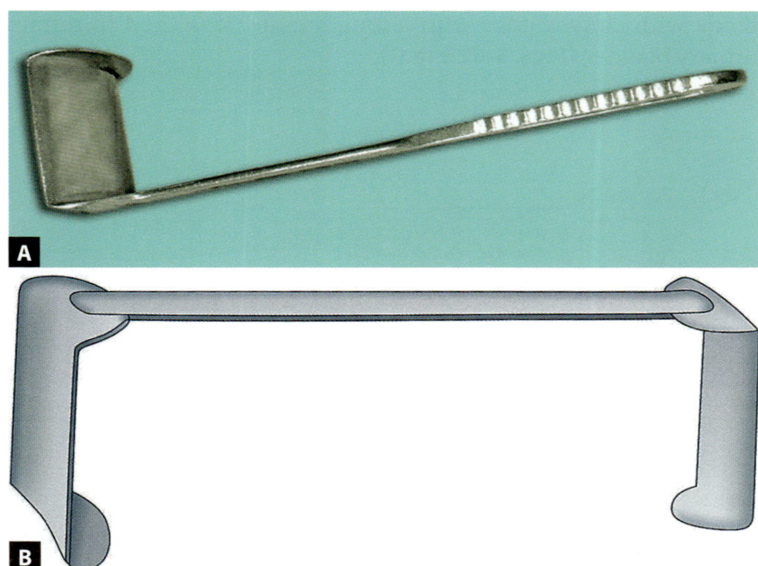

Figs. 5-51A and B: Morris retractors—(A) Single blade (one sided) and (B) Double blade (both sided).

'C' SHAPED RETRACTOR—ROUX

It is C shaped with curve at both ends. It is used to retract wounds like in hernia, appendicectomy, wide excisions, oral surgery, etc. C shape gives a proper grip **(Figs. 5-52A and B)**.

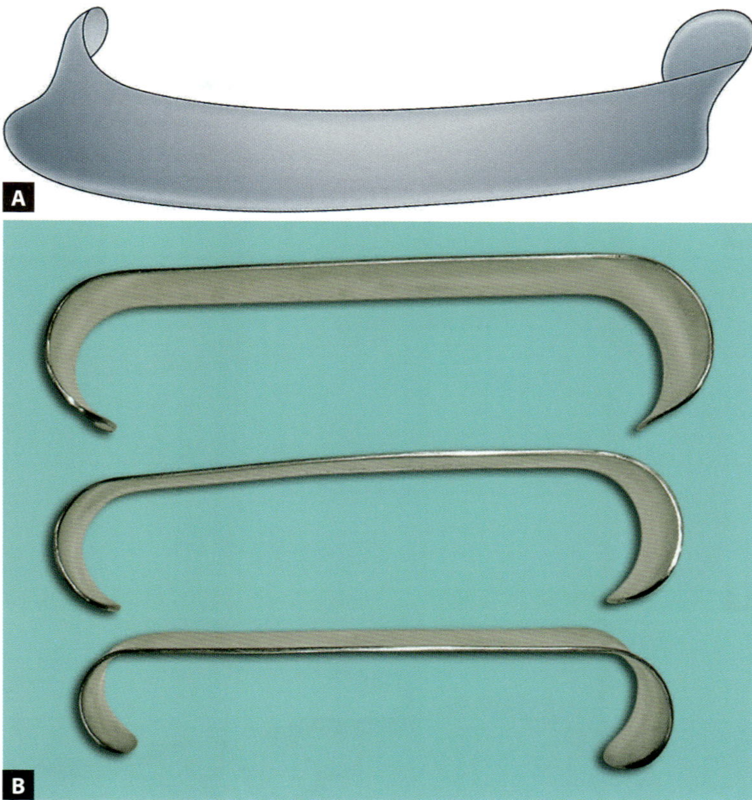

Figs. 5-52A and B: 'C' shaped retractor.

'S' SHAPED RETRACTOR

Here blunt curves on each end are in opposite directions. Uses are like C shaped retractor **(Fig. 5-53)**.

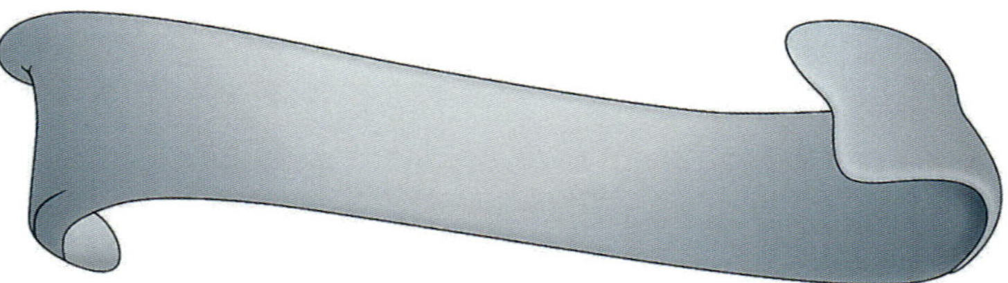

Fig. 5-53: 'S' shaped retractor.

DEAVER'S RETRACTOR

It is an instrument in shape of question mark (?). It is stout but atraumatic. Its action is *levering* of the tissues not by push or pull or traction. Moist mops should be kept underneath prior to placing this retractor. It is a retractor with a broad, gently curved long blade. It has got strong handle **(Figs. 5-54 and 5-55)**.

It is used to retract the abdominal wall. It is used to retract liver, spleen and other abdominal viscera. It is atraumatic and gives adequate exposure of the surgical field. All major abdominal surgeries like vagotomy, cholecystectomy, gastrectomy, pancreatic surgeries, colonic surgeries, kidney surgeries, anterior resection/abdomino-perineal resection, bladder surgeries, lumbar sympathectomy need this instrument.

KEYLAND'S RETRACTOR

It has got flat wide blade with a right angle handle. It is manual retractor. It is used like Deaver's retractor **(Fig. 5-56)**.

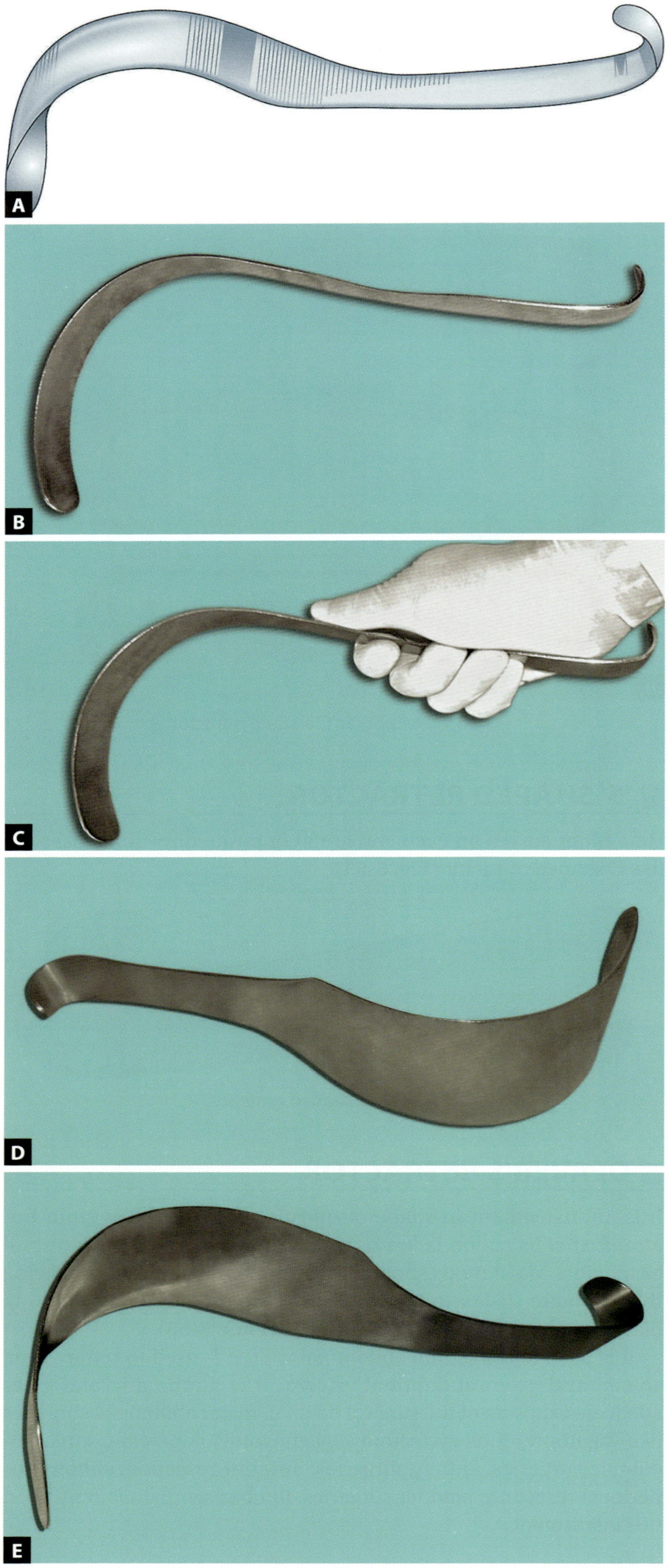

Figs. 5-54A to E: Deaver's retractor (manual)/Deaver liver retractor—used to retract liver, spleen, soft tissues, bowel.

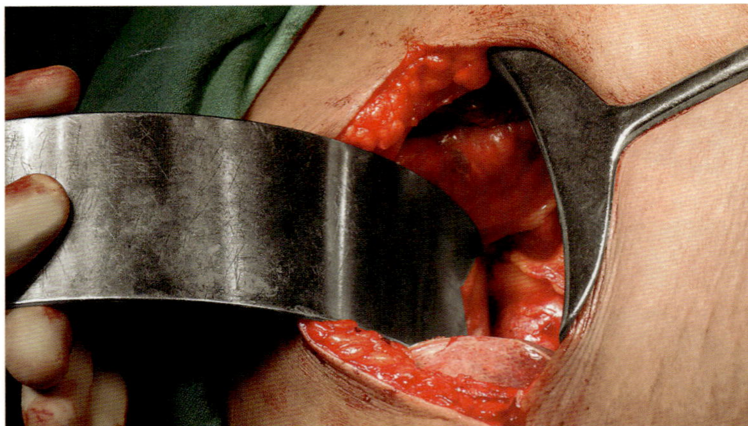

Fig. 5-55: Manual retractors used in laparotomy—Deaver's and Morris.

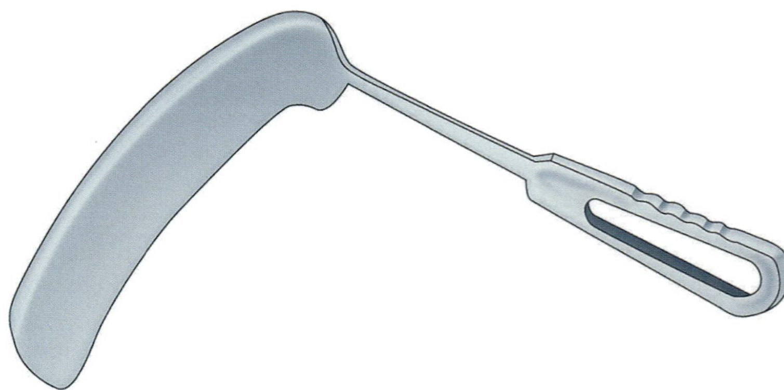

Fig. 5-56: Keyland's retractor (manual).

DOYEN'S RETRACTOR

It is used in pelvic surgeries and in laparotomies. It has a curved blade with convex edge with a long handle. It is used to retract urinary bladder **(Figs. 5-57A to C)**.

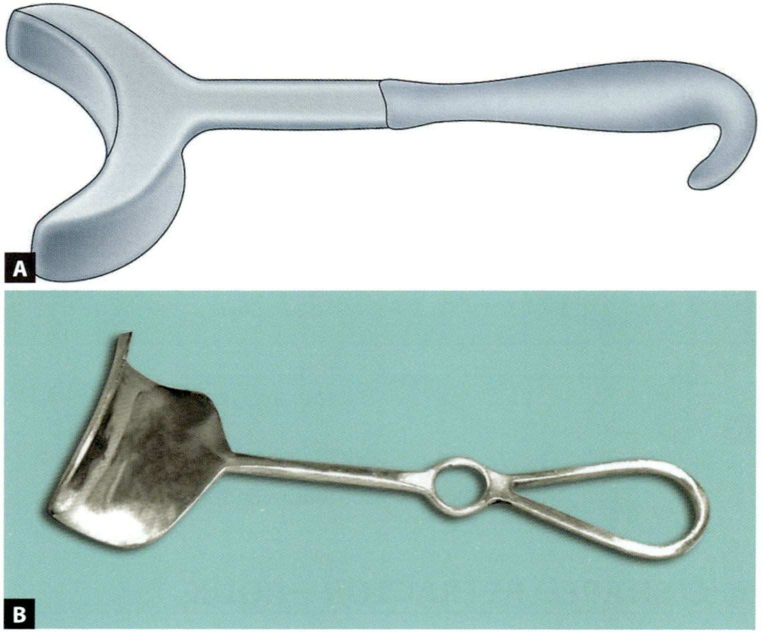

Figs. 5-57A and B

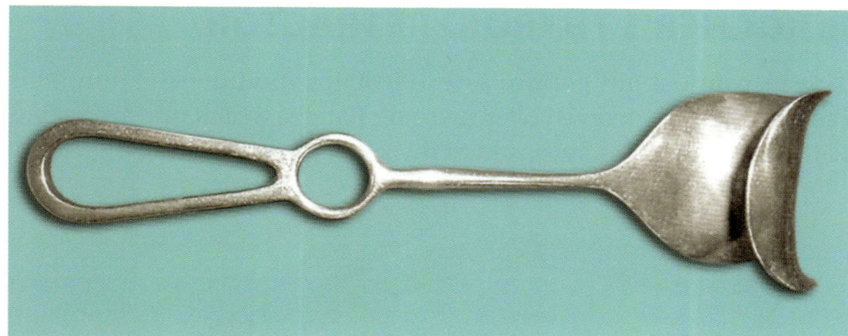

Fig. 5-57C

Figs. 5-57A to C: Doyen's retractor.

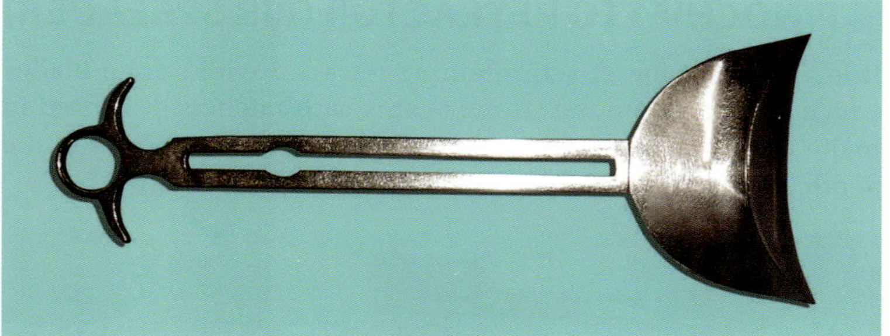

Fig. 5-58C

Figs. 5-58A to C: Balfour's self-retaining retractors.

BALFOUR'S SELF-RETAINING RETRACTOR

It has got different adjustable blades so as to retract abdominal wall and tissues during surgery. It has got quadrangular metal frame. Two side heavy blades are hook shaped to fit into the wound sides **(Figs. 5-58A to C)**. There is a detachable third blade to retract the viscera. One of the side blades has got screw to adjust the width of the retraction by side blades. Detachable blade is also fixed through an adjustable screw with a slot. Closed instrument is inserted into the wound and adequately widened as required to have its use. Tissues/bowel/organs should not be trapped while widening and adjusting.

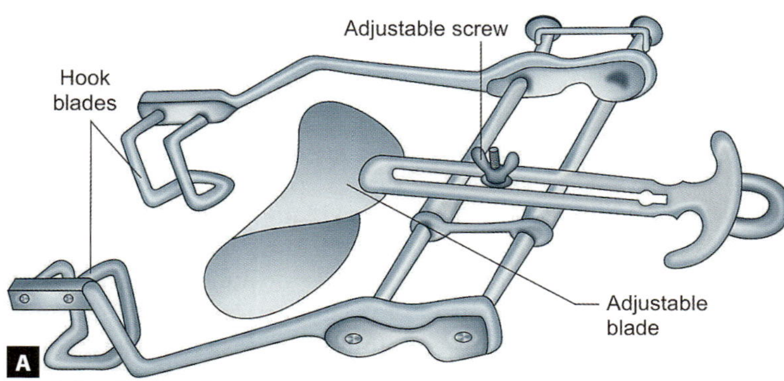

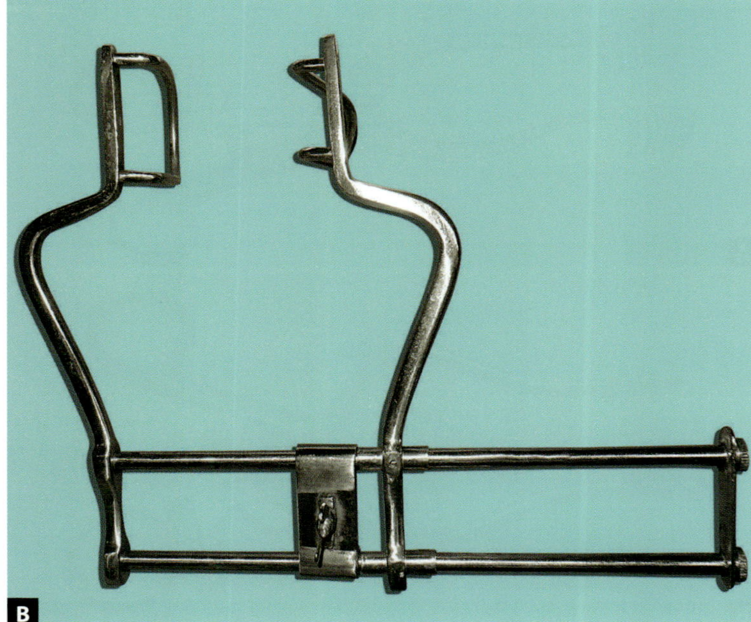

Figs. 5-58A and B

MILLIN'S SELF-RETAINING RETRACTOR

It has got three-sided triangular metal frame with two flat side blades and one long S shaped adjustable blade which has got two curves to retract urinary bladder or lower abdominal wall by each as needed. It is used in Millin's open prostatectomy and other pelvic surgeries **(Fig. 5-59)**.

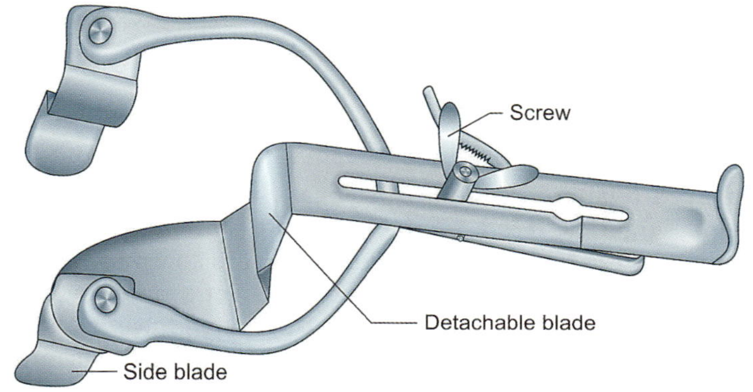

Fig. 5-59: Millin's self-retaining retractor.

ALM RETRACTOR

It is a small self-retaining retractor with broad beam which has got blades; ends of the blades have got hooks to retract; blades are widened after placing under the skin edges or tissue edges; using screw in the beam blades are widened to achieve effective retraction. Adjustment joint proximally also facilitates the proper stability and placement of the retractor **(Fig. 5-60)**.

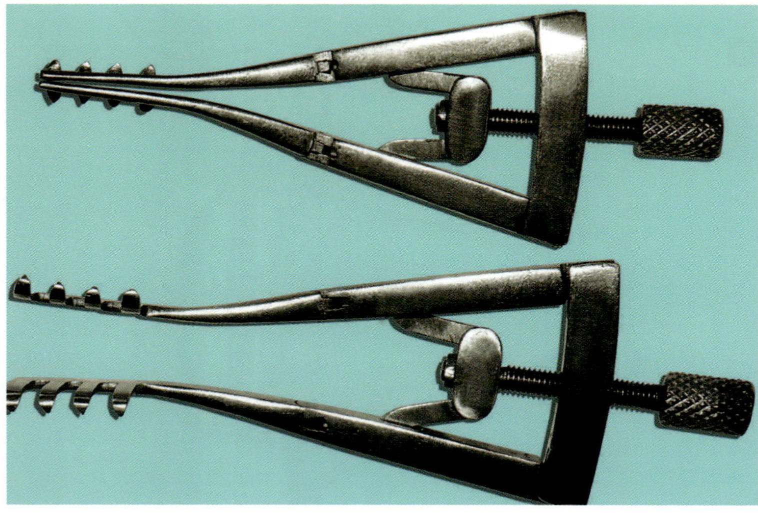

Fig. 5-60: ALM retractor. It is used in small surface surgery as self-retaining retractor.

FINOCHIETTO RETRACTOR (RIB SPREADER)

It is a special type of self-retaining retractor with strong blades which are placed on the strong beams with ratchets. It is used in major surgeries like nephrectomy, laparotomies, surgeries in the depth. It is used as a rib spreader in thoracotomy **(Fig. 5-61)**.

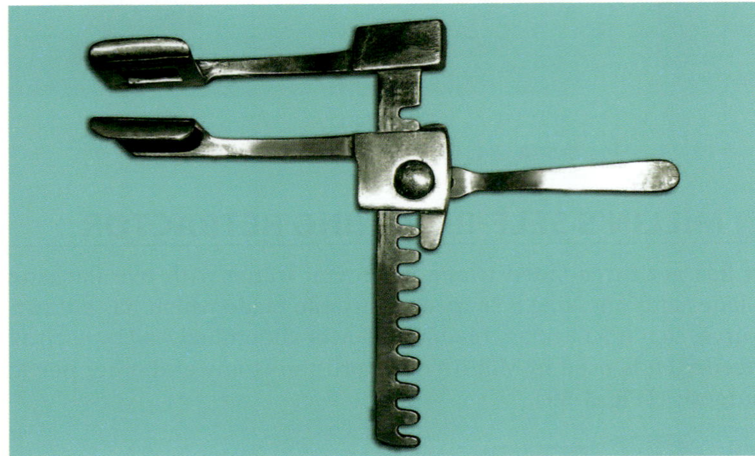

Fig. 5-61: Finochietto retractor.

JOLL'S THYROID RETRACTOR

It is a self-retaining retractor specifically used for thyroid/parathyroid surgeries. It is a semicircular retractor with two blades attached with a handle. End of the blades are sharp like a towel clip with a catch/ratchet on it. Handle has got a screw by which instrument can be opened or closed. Upper and lower skin flaps can be retracted well in thyroid surgery using this instrument **(Figs. 5-62A and B)**.

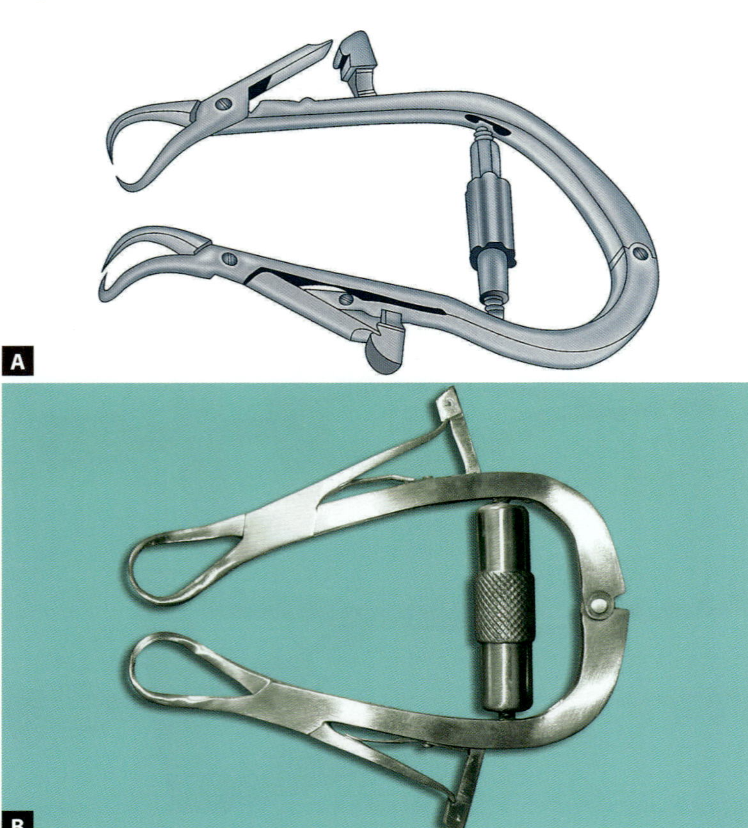

Figs. 5-62A and B: Joll's thyroid retractor.

KOCHER'S THYROID RETRACTOR

This instrument has got two side adjustable multihooked terminals (adjustable with screws) over two side flanges which are connected with a lockable joint. It is used in thyroidectomy **(Fig. 5-63)**.

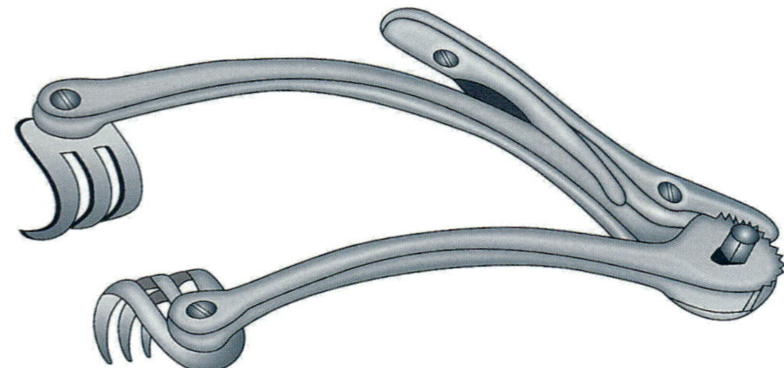

Fig. 5-63: Kocher's thyroid retractor.

MACINTOSH DEPRESSOR (RETRACTOR)

Macintosh depressor (retractor) is used as a guard while dissecting tissues over delicate vital structures like nerve, vessels. It safeguards the delicate structures underneath. Example—It is used in carpal tunnel release to guard the underlying median nerve while cutting the flexor retinaculum **(Fig. 5-64)**.

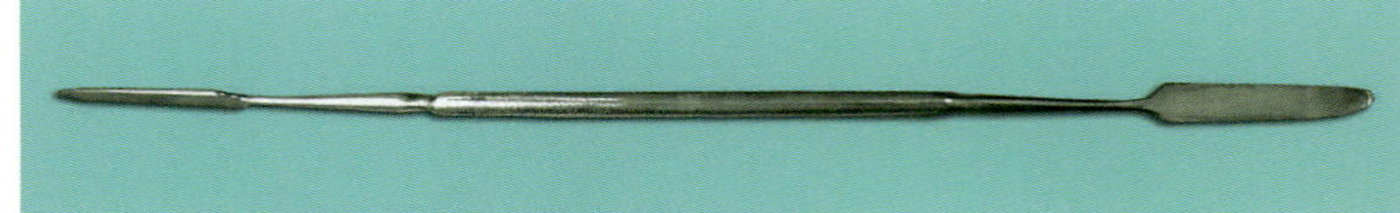

Fig. 5-64: Macintosh depressor (retractor) is used as a guard while dissecting tissues over delicate vital structures like nerve, vessels.

MOLLISON'S MASTOID RETRACTOR

It is stout instrument with curved long blades which has got sharp outward curved teeth to retract tissues. Proximal shaft has got ratchet with finger bows. It is self-retaining, haemostatic and gives wide exposure of the field. It is used in mastoid surgery, laminectomy, to retract scalp in neurosurgery, limb surgeries, etc. When shafts are approximated blades will open **(Figs. 5-65A to C)**.

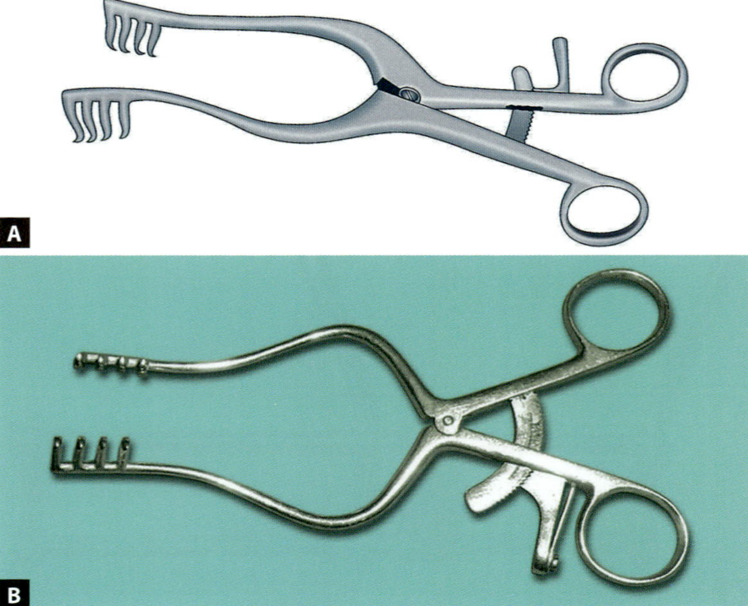

Figs. 5-65A and B

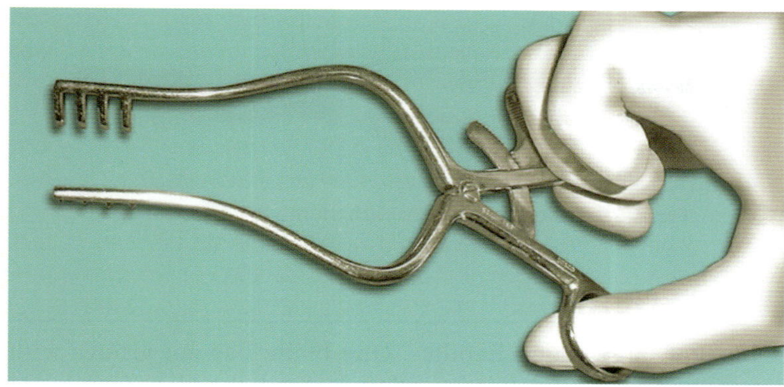

Fig. 5-65C
Figs. 5-65A to C: Mollison's mastoid retractor.

BLADDER NECK RETRACTOR

It is thin, long instrument with two thin long distal blades. Proximal thin shafts have got a ratchet. When ratchet closes, the blades will open. It is used in retracting bladder neck in bladder surgeries **(Fig. 5-66)**.

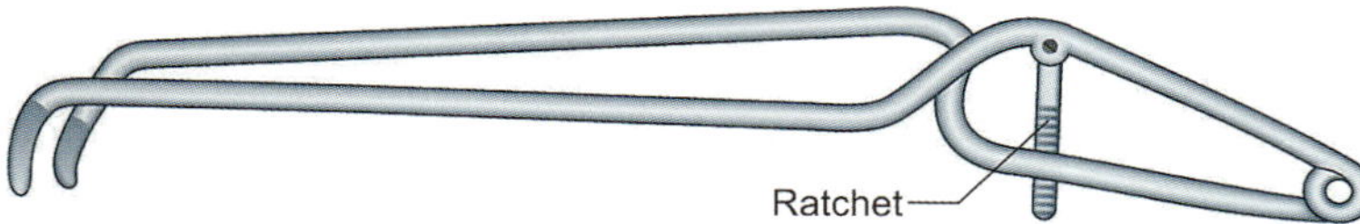

Fig. 5-66: Bladder neck retractor.

CHEEK RETRACTOR

It is single piece instrument with acutely angled blade with inward curled round margin. It is used to retract cheek to inspect the oral cavity as well as to take biopsy of a lesion for diagnosis; dental extractions; interdental wiring; excision of lesions in jaw, gums and oral cavity (epulis, papillomas, mucous cysts, etc.) **(Fig. 5-67)**.

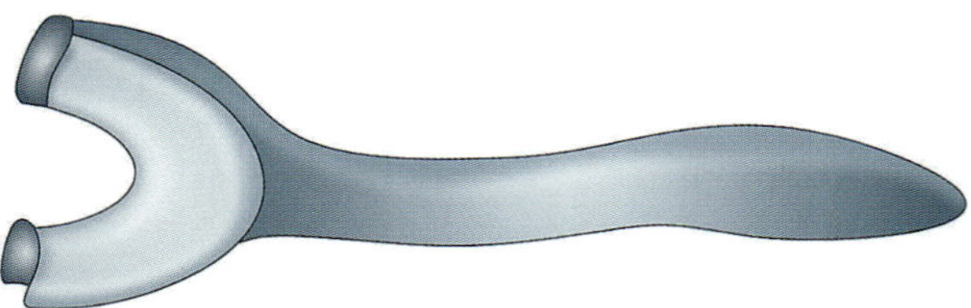

Fig. 5-67: Cheek retractor.

SCAPULA RETRACTOR

It has got a long stout handle with broad right-angled blade with serrations. It is used to retract scapula during thoracotomy **(Fig. 5-68)**.

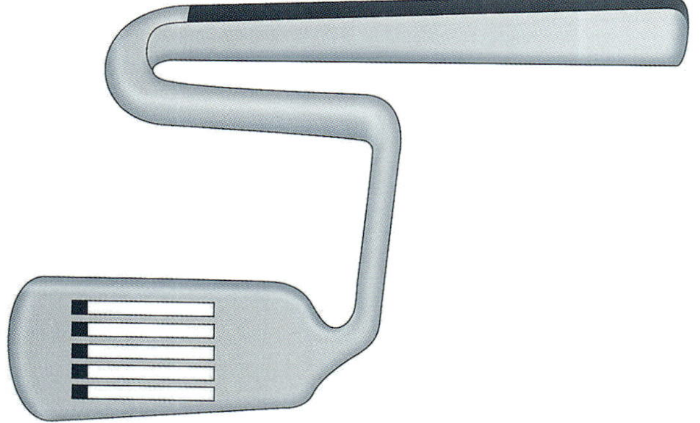

Fig. 5-68: Scapula retractor.

KIDNEY HILUM RETRACTOR

It has got curved C shaped small blade with a long malleable shaft which is slightly curved. It is used in extended pyelolithotomy (Gilvernet's) to retract renal hilar tissues so as to reach the pelvis. Intrarenal pelvis is approached by this manner to remove the stone **(Fig. 5-69)**.

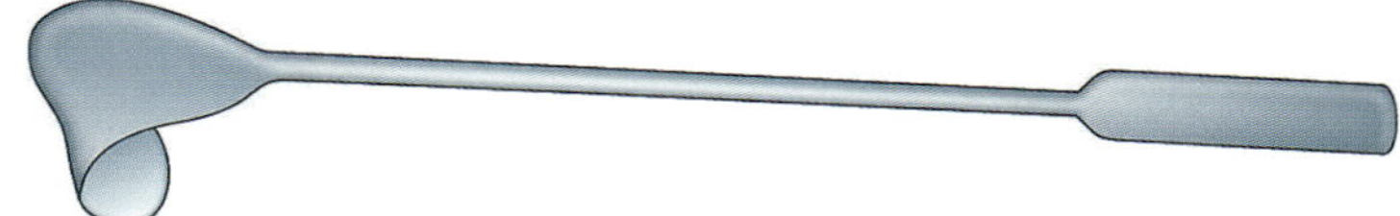

Fig. 5-69: Kidney hilum retractor.

MORRIS KIDNEY RETRACTOR

It has got blade of 6.5 × 5 cm in size with a curve. There is a blunt projecting ridge directed inwards. It is used in renal surgeries like nephrolithotomy, pyelolithotomy, pyeloplasty and nephrectomy **(Fig. 5-70)**.

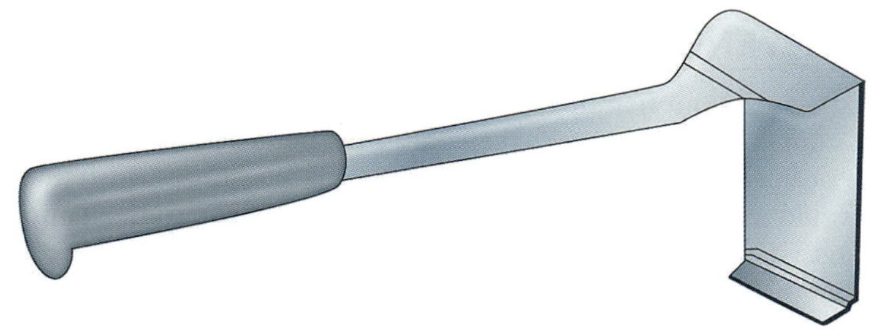

Fig. 5-70: Morris kidney retractor.

ALLISON'S LUNG RETRACTOR

It has got long handle with light blade. Blade is made up of wires. Blade is at right angle to the handle. It is used to retract lungs. Lung can expand between wires of the blade. It is atraumatic. It is used in oesophageal surgery, thoracic sympathectomy, mediastinal surgery **(Figs. 5-71A and B)**.

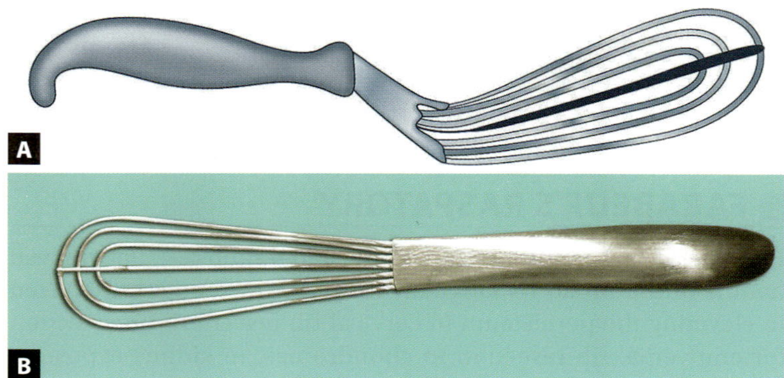

Figs. 5-71A and B: Allison's lung retractor.

RIB RETRACTOR (TUFFIER'S)

There is a strong short shaft with blades attached to it at right angles. One blade is fixed whereas other one is adjustable which can be fixed with a screw at required width. Blades are deep with outer flanges so as to hold with a proper grip. It is used in thoracotomy in lung/oesophageal and cardiac surgeries (trauma, tumours, mitral valvotomy, mediastinal tumours, diaphragmatic hernia, oesophagectomy, etc.). It is a self-retaining retractor **(Fig. 5-72)**. Other rib retractor used is Quervain's rib retractor which is stronger with wing-like blades, fixed with a screw.

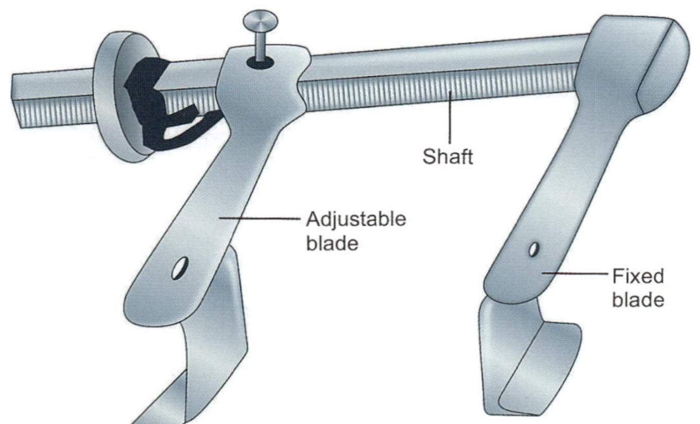

Fig. 5-72: Self-retaining rib retractor.

DOYEN'S RIB RASPATORY

It has got a stout handle with a curved semicircular distal blade to pass under the rib surface for separating the periosteum after incising the periosteum of the rib. Using periosteal elevator periosteum is elevated and raspatory is passed under the periosteum from upper margin of the rib to prevent injury to intercostal vessels. There are separate instruments for right side and left side. Handle is held with blade facing forward and upward to determine the side **(Figs. 5-73A and B)**.

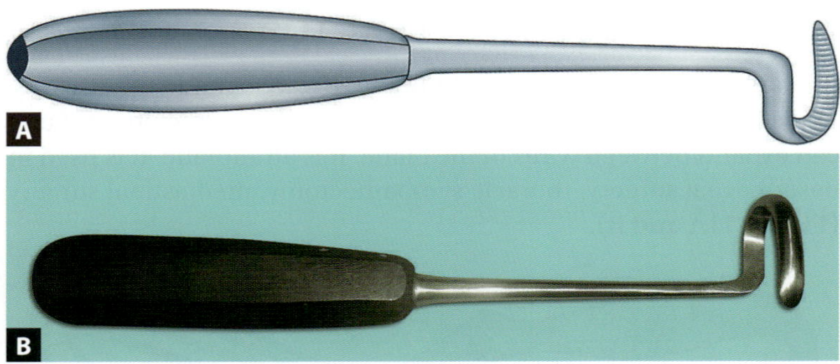

Figs. 5-73A and B: Doyen's rib raspatory.

FARABEUF'S RASPATORY

It is a periosteal elevator with a corrugated thumb rest, flat grooved handle and a broad rectangular blade (beveled edge). It is used in elevating the periosteum in cervical rib resection, rib resection for empyema, rib resection in chondromas, in kidney exposure, in osteomyelitis of ribs. Periosteum is retained so that regeneration and remodeling can occur; intercostal vessels and nerves are protected. It is not used to elevate the inner surface of the ribs where Doyen's raspatory is used **(Figs. 5-74 and 5-75)**.

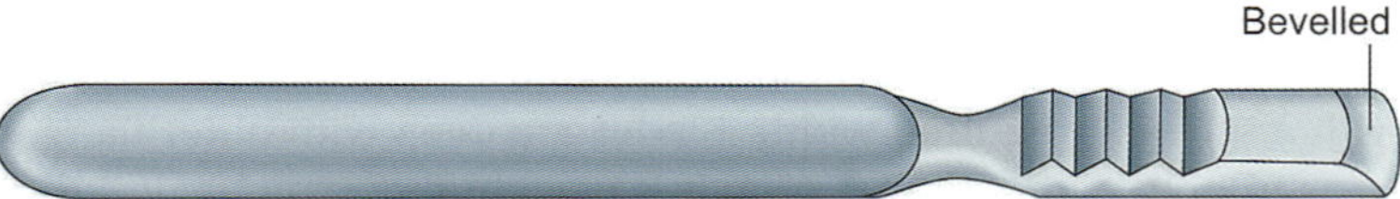

Fig. 5-74: Farabeuf's raspatory with thumb rest.

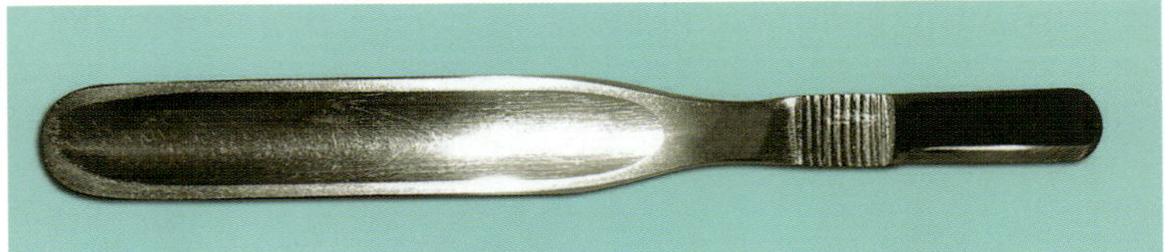

Fig. 5-75: Periosteal elevator with thumb rest (Farabeuf's).

RIB SHEAR

It has got large rough handles. One blade has got groove with serrations and is blunt. It is passed underneath the rib as a protector to the adjacent tissues. Other blade is cutting one which apposes over the groove of first blade. It cuts the rib from front. Instrument is used for rib resection **(Figs. 5-76A to D)**.

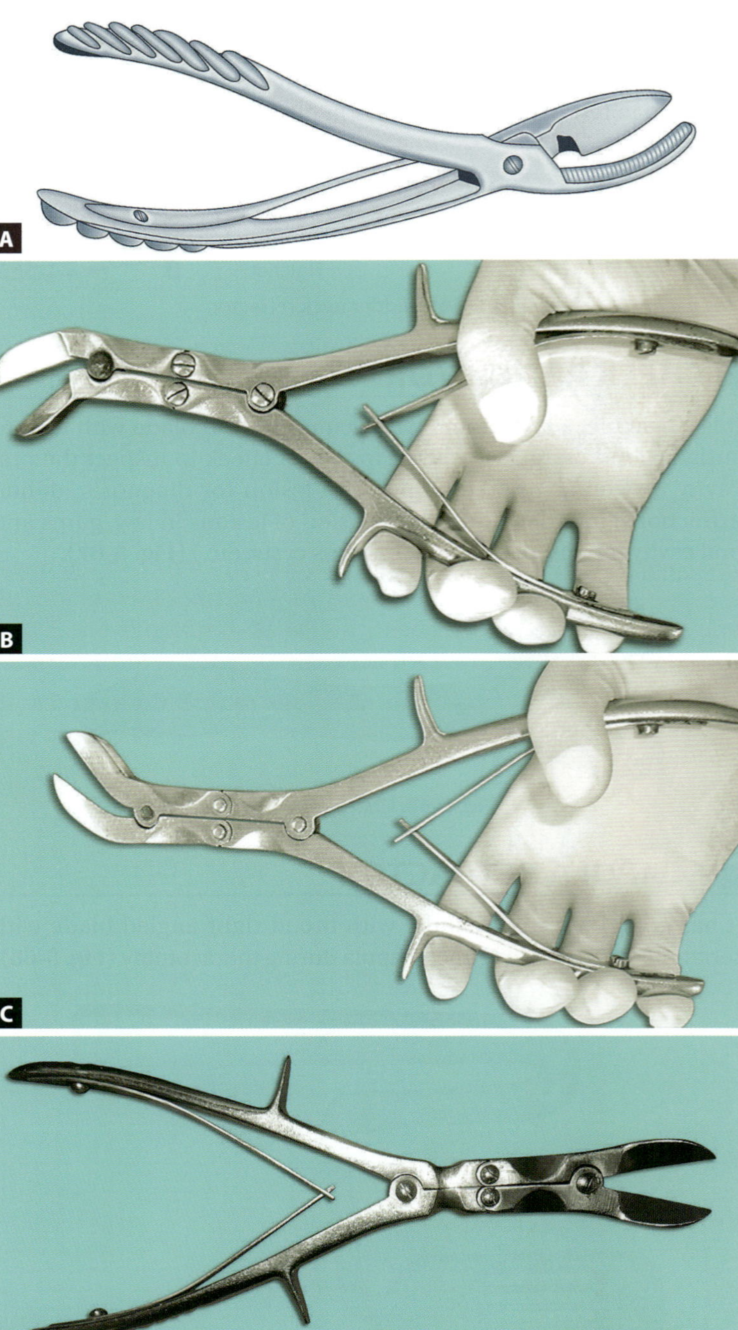

Figs. 5-76A to D: Rib shear used to cut the ribs.

RIB APPROXIMATOR

It has two strong curved blades with teeth; proximal blade is mobile but can be fixed by a screw whereas distal blade is fixed. It is used to approximate the ribs during closure of thoracotomy. Two blades are placed adjacent to ribs and proximal blade is apposed adequately and fixed with screw. Thoracotomy wound is closed in layers. Screw is loosened to remove the rib approximator **(Figs. 5-77A and B)**.

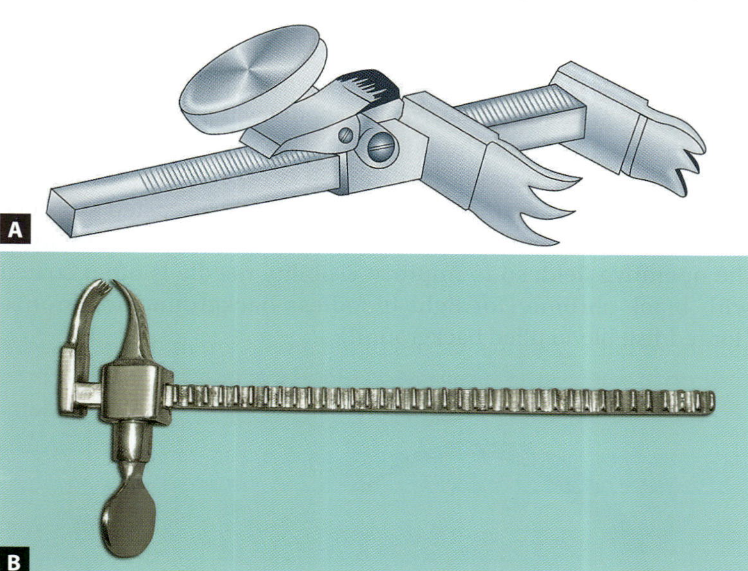

Figs. 5-77A and B: Rib approximator is used in closure of thoracotomy wound.

BONE SAW AND BONE FILE

Bone saw is used to cut the bone during amputation; according to the need direction can be achieved but it is hand held and so needs firm grip and stamina to use it; often it get blunted making job more difficult. Its use is replaced by electric saw or Gigli saw **(Fig. 5-78)**.

Bone file is used to smoothen the cut edge of the amputated stump to eliminate the sharp areas **(Fig. 5-79)**.

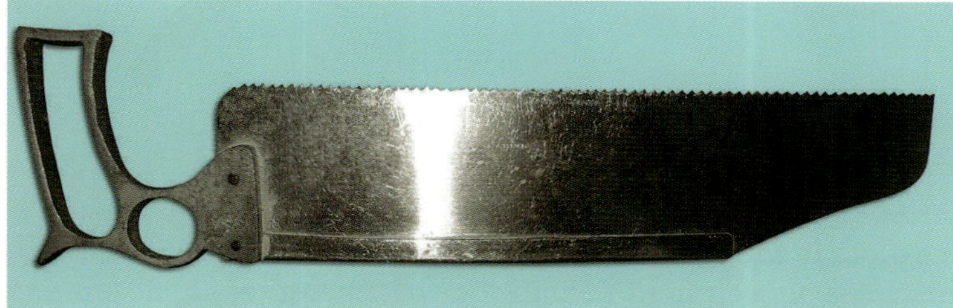

Fig. 5-78: Bone saw—it is used to cut the bone in amputation. Now electric saw or Gigli saws are commonly used.

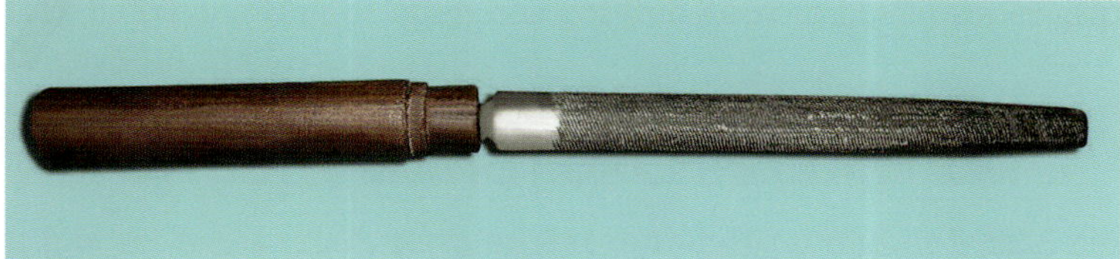

Fig. 5-79: Bone file—it is used to smoothen the cut bones to eliminate sharp areas.

DUVAL'S LUNG HOLDING FORCEPS

Its distal blades have triangular aperture with its inner surface being finely serrated to have firm grip on the lungs without any trauma. Blades are gently curved which imparts a smooth action. It is used to hold the lung during lobectomy/pneumonectomy **(Figs. 5-80A to C)**.

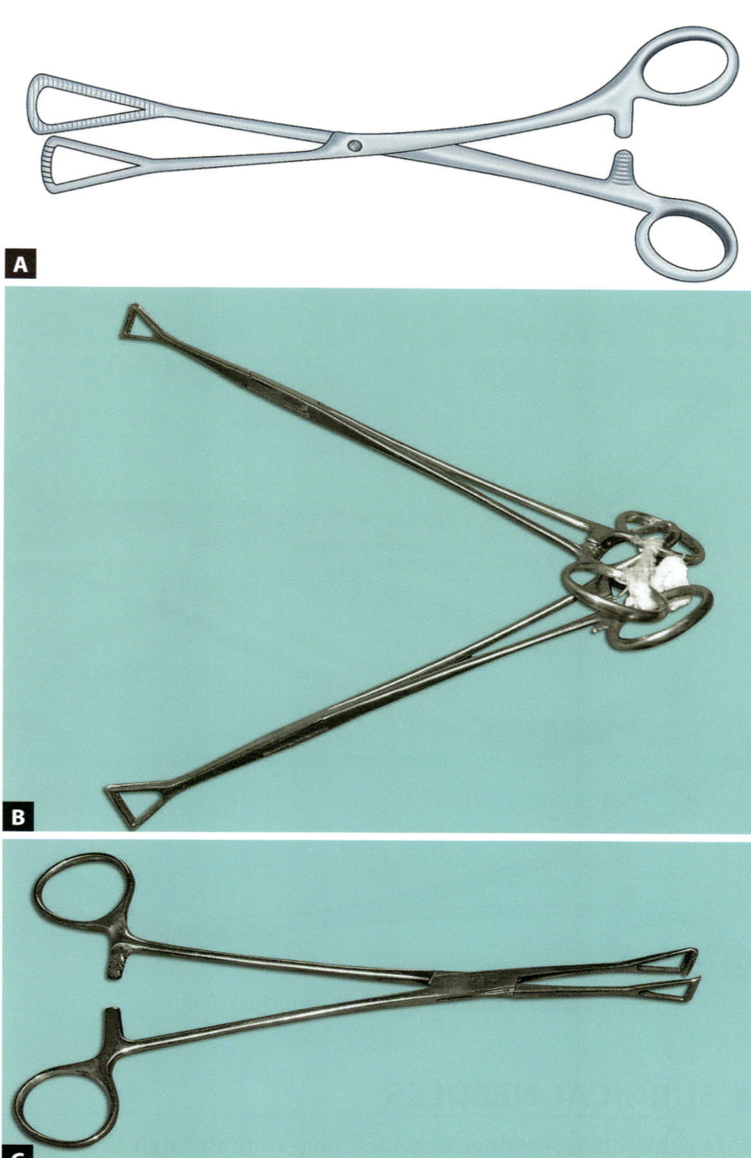

Figs. 5-80A to C: Duval's lung holding forceps.

FRIEDRICH'S LUNG HOLDING FORCEPS

It has got four pronged blades. Each prong is having sigmoid curve with a ball at the tip. It is atraumatic because of smooth ball. It is used to hold wider area of lung tissue **(Fig. 5-81)**.

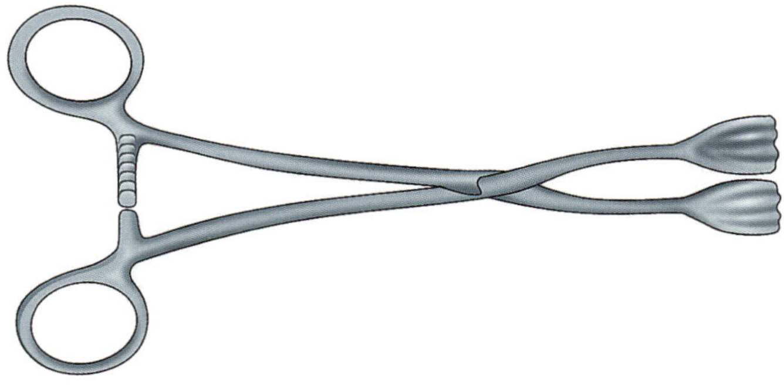

Fig. 5-81: Friedrich's lung holding forceps.

BICKFORD'S BRONCHIAL CLAMP

It has got long distal blade which has got two bends with longitudinal serrations and spikes on the inner surface. It is used to clamp the bronchus as it holds the cartilaginous part firmly **(Figs. 5-82A to C)**.

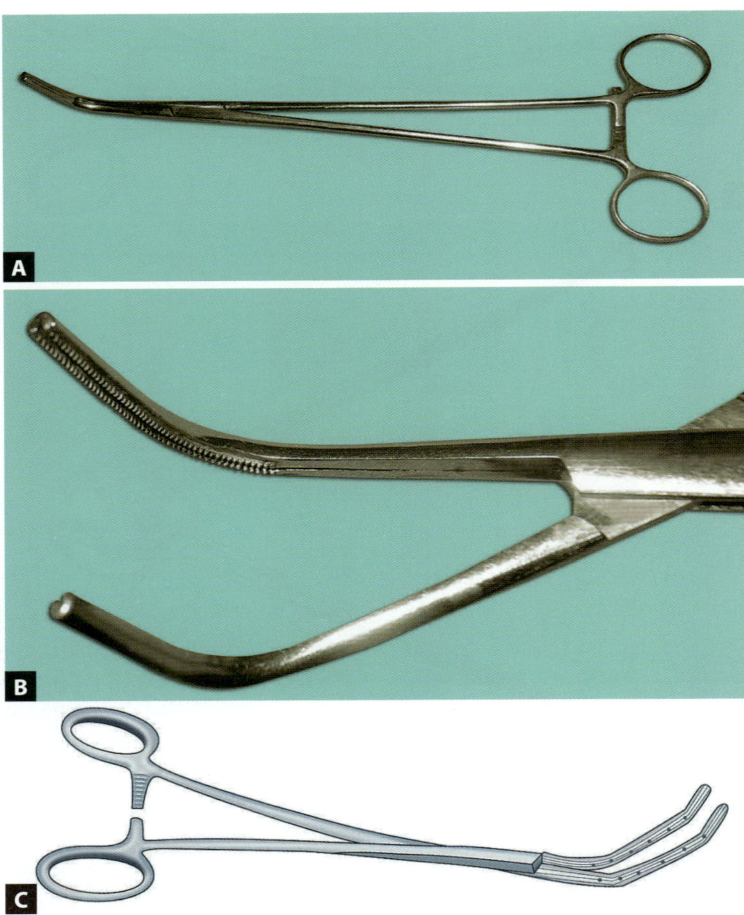

Figs. 5-82A to C: Bickford's bronchial clamp.

SURGICAL NEEDLES

Surgical needles are devices which penetrate through the tissues to pass sutures across the wounds which are to be approximated. So needle creates a channel or track to pass the needed suture material with less tissue disruption, with minimum risk of bleeding without compromising the wound blood supply.

Historically thorns, ivory and bone were used as needles and horse hairs were used as sutures. Plant fibres and animal tissues were used as ligatures and sutures in historical days. Later copper and bronze needles were used for suturing. Metal needles became popular in 14th century. Cistercian Monks started eyed needles. Glovemakers straight needle, sailmakers curved needle, handled distal eyelet needle (from gimlet of leather workers) which was used by Pare in 1564 as crooked needles were different needles used in olden days **(Fig. 5-83)**.

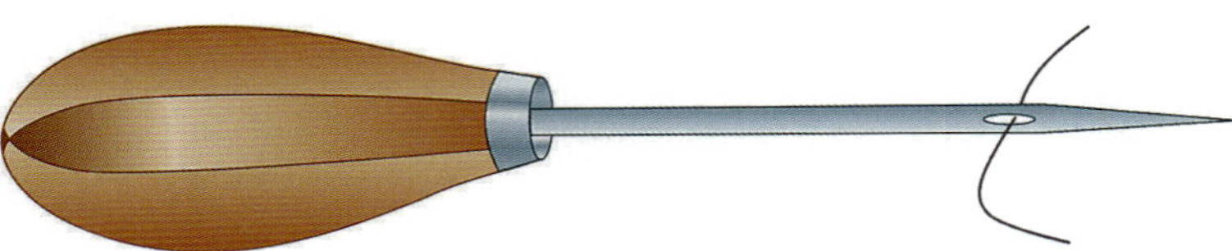

Fig. 5-83: Crooked Pare needle.

In 1275, Salicet found triangular cutting needle which showed better penetrating property. Mondeville in 1320 started scooping the needle near the eye to accommodate the bulk of the suture material. In 1774, Petit introduced the eyeless concept of the needle where suture material placed in a slot in the needle hub to act like a pincer **(Fig. 5-84)**. In 1874, Gaillard from San Francisco invented atraumatic needle with its hub end being drilled to place catgut suture which was called as *Eureka needle* **(Fig. 5-85)**.

Integral flanged needle **(Fig. 5-86)** has come in 1921 by Ovington (Davis and Geck Company). Now, high quality stainless steel is used to manufacture needle. Strength and rigidity are the two important features of a suitable needle. Needle should withstand the optimum force; it may bend but should not break with great force. Needle should have very smooth finish which is created by polishing to clear all burrs on the surface. Needle also should be coated to reduce tissue resistance. But needle often glare to reduce the visibility at the operative field; so to improve visibility needle is often coated with black chrome (for light bloodless background) or bronze (for reddish blood filled background).

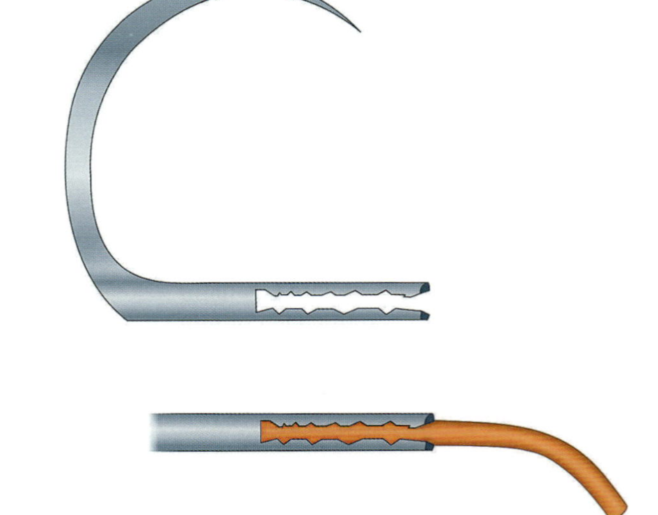

Fig. 5-84: Petit eyeless concept of a needle.

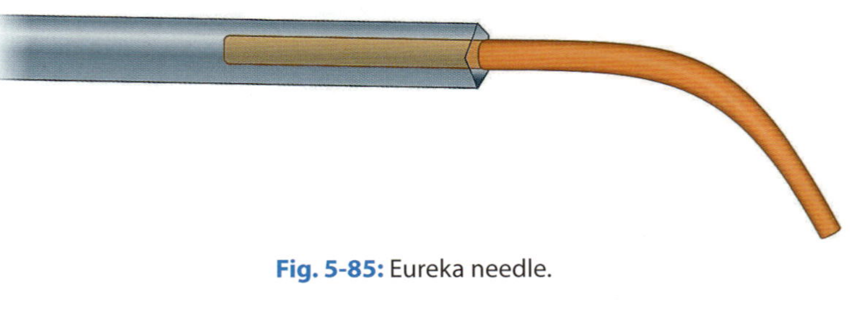

Fig. 5-85: Eureka needle.

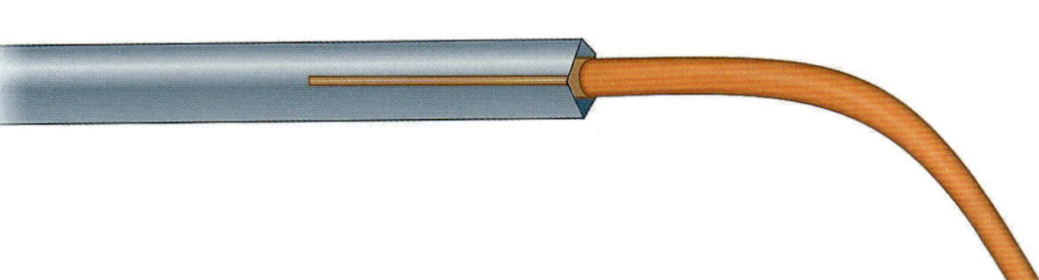

Fig. 5-86: Integral flanged head needle.

Features of Surgical Needle

Needle Integrity

Needle should be strong and should stay firmly in the needle holder (driver) when it is grasped; it should not bend or break during passage through the tissues. Needle rear and tip ends are weak and prone for bend or break. Broken needle may get lost in the tissues or cavities and often carries real difficult to identify and remove it; in such situation C-arm imaging may be needed to pinpoint the location of the lost broken needle part. Needle should be rotated along the line and through the tissues needed. It should not be twisted or forced by push. Usually centre of the needle is placed at the junction of proximal 2/3rd and distal 1/3rd of the jaw of the needle driver. Integrity and stability of the needle holder should be maintained by the manufacturer.

Size of the Needle

While selecting the size, both length and diameter of the needle, are important for particular suturing. Length is selected depending on the bulk of the tissue being sutured. Diameter of the needle is selected depending on the resistance of the target tissues. Tough structure like ligaments are sutured using wider stronger cutting needle; smooth tissues like bowel is sutured using thinner round body needle.

Length of the Needle

It is essential to select the ideal length of the needle to approximate the given particular tissues. It is selected by assessing the distance between entrance and exit bite points. Wider the distance lengthier the needle needed. But it is difficult to pass lengthier needle through the tissues as it may get deflected in the needle holder. Withdrawal of the needle is also difficult after holding near its tip.

Diameter (Gauge) of the Needle

Diameter of the needle is equally important in proper suturing technique. Ratio between diameters of needle and suture material is 2:1 for larger suture and 3:1 for smaller suture even though ideal ratio being 1:1 which is not possible to achieve.

Types

Based on the Edge

- *Round body needle:* It is round and smooth on cross section. It is used to suture muscles/intestines/soft tissues/vessels/nerves/tendons/peritoneum.
- *Taper round needle:* Round bodied needle tapering smoothly towards the tip.
- *Conventional cutting needle:* Here needle is triangular on cross section with apex facing inward. It is used to suture skin/aponeurosis/tough structures. Cutting edge is inside the curve.
- *Reverse cutting needle:* Here needle is triangular (reverse) on cross section with apex facing outward. It increases the strength and is less likely to bend while suturing. Here cutting edge is outside the curve.
- *Taper cut needle:* Here tip of the needle is cutting or reverse cutting in section but eventually tapers into the body as round in section. It improves the penetration of needle but minimises the trauma.
- Blunt pointed needles are used to suture friable organs like liver/spleen/kidneys.
- *Spatulated side cutting needle* (saber lock): It is like a spatula with two lateral side cutting edges.
- *Micropoint needles*, either round bodied or reverse cutting or spatulated, are used in ophthalmic surgery and microsurgery. It has got an extra honing process.
- *Trocar point needle* is stout strong cutting end with a robust round body. It is used in obstetrics and gynaecology.
- *Tru taper needle* is one with tip angle of needle is at 22 degrees (unlike conventional angle is 32 degrees). It is used in vascular surgery.
- *Visiblack needles:* Needles coated with black so that they are visible better in red background. It also prevents the glare from the focus lights by the needles.
- *Dolphin nose needle* is specially designed needle used for surgeries in patients with hepatitis and AIDS which minimises the risk of puncturing the gloves and fingers of the surgeon.
- *JB needle* (Juergen-Breunner needle): Oval round bodied needle with a steep curve at the distal half to have easy passage of the needle through bowel in gastrointestinal surgeries.
- *Port closure needle* in laparoscopic surgeries.
- *Ski needle* with a ski shaped curvature in the distal part so as to have easy passage through the port for laparoscopic intracorporeal suturing.

Based on Curvature

- *Straight needle:* It was once commonly used needle (*Keith needle for skin and Bunnel needle for GIT*). It can be cutting or round bodied. It too can be with eyelet or atraumatic. Atraumatic straight round body needle with chromic catgut suture were popular in olden days while doing bowel anastomosis. Straight needle is still often used in skin suturing especially by beginners; it is quiet useful in laparoscopic surgery also.
- *Curved needle:* ¼, ½, ⅜, and ⅝ circle etc. ½ and ⅜ are commonly used. It is the wrist movement which rotates the needle through tissues. Surgeons often reconfigure the needle to their personal preference. While bending the needle to needed movement, needle at the point of bent gets weakened and may break. Needle holder should not be used to reshape the needle as carbide jaw of the needle holder may burr the surface of the needle making it more traumatic.
- *Compound needles:* Here configurations at the tip and body are different. J-shaped needle, fishhook needle **(Fig. 5-87B)**, compound curved needles are different types which are self explanatory. They are used in depth to have controlled penetration of the needle during suturing—suturing in depth in the pelvis, in ophthalmology suturing.
- *Endoski needle:* This needle is specially devised for laparoscopic surgery **(Fig. 5-87A)** Here proximal straight component of the needle with distal dynamic part is curved as half of a half circle; straight component is one and half trims of the curved one. The shaft is either triangular or rhomboid. Triangular type avoids both swivel and deflection of the needle. Rhomboid type resists swivel.

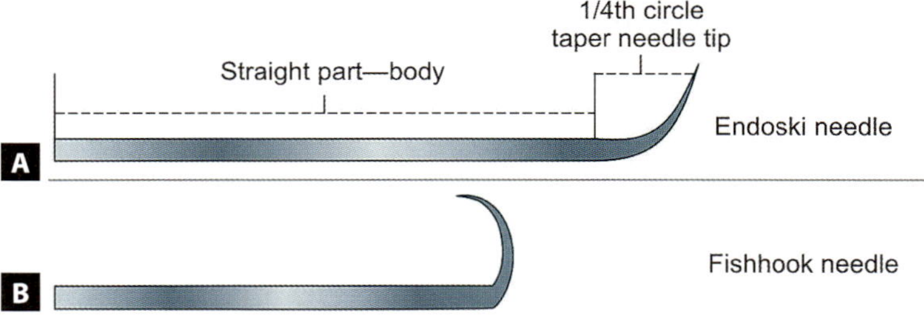

Figs. 5-87A and B: (A) Endoski needle used in laparoscopy commonly; (B) Fishhook needle used in depth.

Curved part is tapered. Needle can be passed through 5 mm port easily into the peritoneal cavity. Needle is held using laparoscopic needle holder along the straight component. But while driving the needle direction of the dynamic end needle tip is difficult to make out so that any deflection if occurs cannot be identified easily.

Based on Existence of the Eye

- *Atraumatic needle* is eyeless. Here suture material is attached to the needle by *swaging* (Mr Merson of England). Size of the suture material and that of needle is same or less and so tissue trauma is less. It is single stranded. Needle once used is disposed (Not reusable). It is available as sterilised pack. These needles can be round body or cutting. As it is single use needle, patient develops a new guaranteed sharp sterile needle. Accidental unthreading is not present. High quality efficacy of the needle is present, so suturing is easier, quicker and better.
- *Traumatic needle:* It is eyed needle (French eyelet—14th century). Needle in the eye area is wider than the body of the needle and so tissue trauma is more. These needles are reusable. It should be sterilised prior to reuse. Accidental fall of thread or needle may be problematic here **(Figs. 5-88 and 5-89)**.
- *Half curved needles at both ends of a straight part (Canoe needle).*

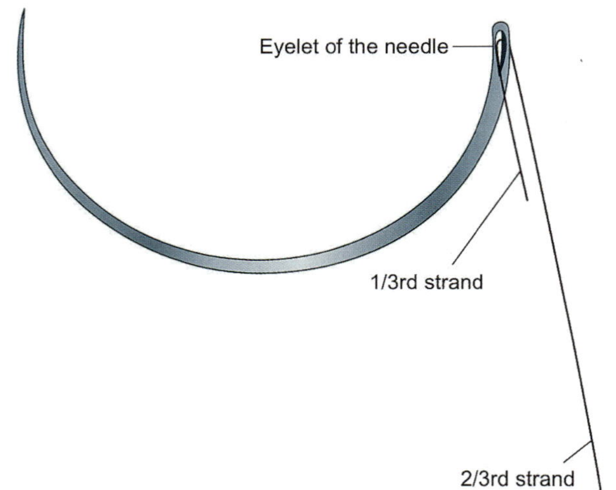

Fig. 5-88: Eyelet needle—suture material here is double stranded.

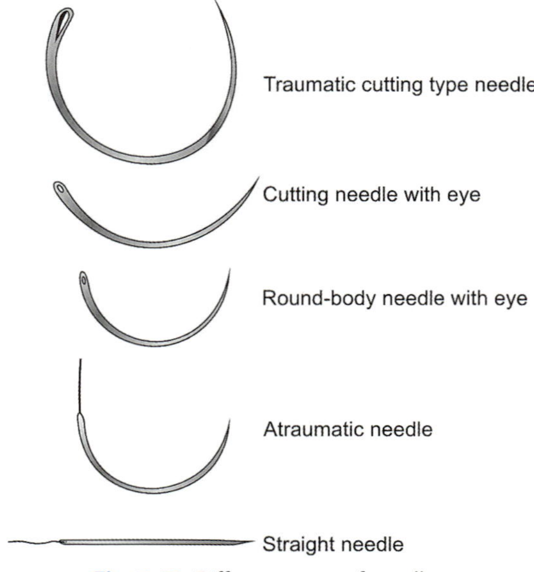

Fig. 5-89: Different types of needles.

Parts of a Surgical Needle

It is important to know the different parts of the surgical needle. Types, profiles, different configurations decide the selection of the needle in different suturing. Operating surgeon should have reasonable idea about the configurations of different types of needles. Important parts are—needle tip, body and swage end **(Figs. 5-90A and B)**.

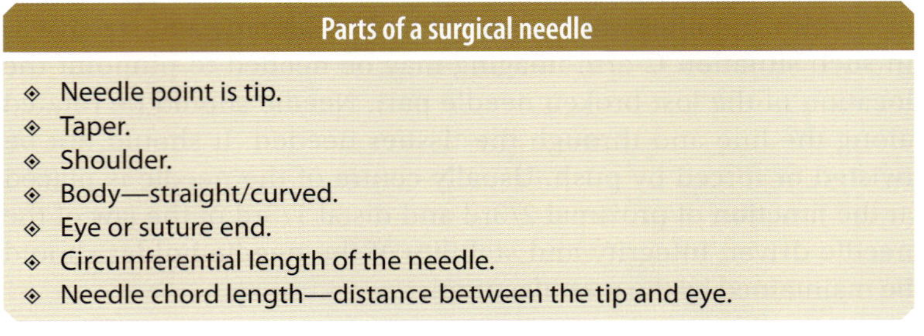

Parts of a surgical needle

- Needle point is tip.
- Taper.
- Shoulder.
- Body—straight/curved.
- Eye or suture end.
- Circumferential length of the needle.
- Needle chord length—distance between the tip and eye.

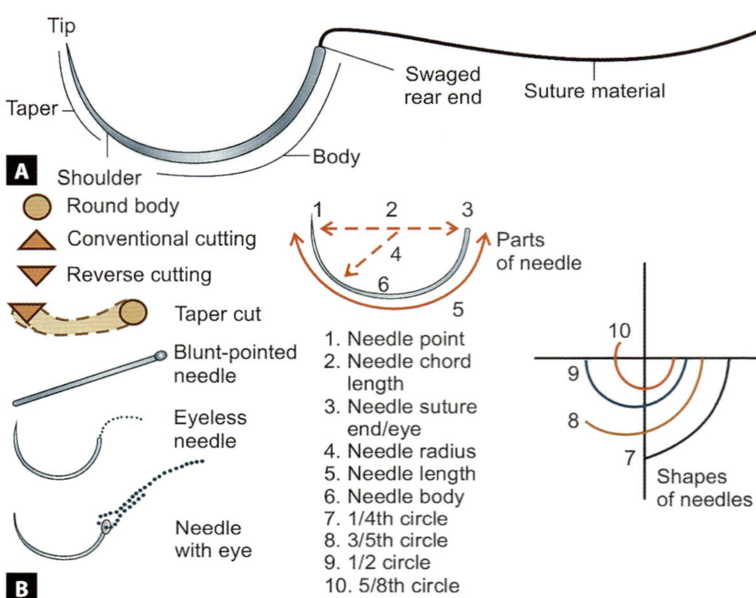

Figs. 5-90A and B: Different parts of the needle. Different types of needles. Diagram also shows the eyeless/eyed needles and gives the meanings of 1/4th, 1/2, 3/8th and 5/8th circle needles.

Needle Tip

Distal most part of the needle is needle tip. It is the one which allows the penetration of the needle through the tissues efficiently. Tip is sharp enough to penetrate the tissues. Easy penetration depends on tapering ratio, cross section of the needle. Blunt tip needle is used in infected cases to avoid possible injury to the operating team.

Tapering of the Needle

Needle tapers up to the shoulder of the needle but tapering distance varies. Tapering ratio is the ratio between distance between the needle point and shoulder of the needle and diameter at body of the needle. If tapering length is 8 mm and diameter at body is 2 mm then tapering ratio is 4:1. Usually 3:1 tapering ratio is commonly used. More the tapering the ratio better the penetration capacity; but needle is prone for bending and loss of strength. Tapering tip may be cutting or round bodied (non-cutting). Round bodied taper tip is used in vascular and bowel anastomosis to achieve minimum trauma it the tissue track. Cutting tip is used for skin and tough structures. Cutting tip may be conventional triangular (Δ) or reverse cutting (∇). Spatulated tip is also useful in tough structures like cornea, periosteum and ligaments. Here tip (apex) is triangular or reverse and proximally taper up to the shoulder of the needle as rhomboid spatulated again either as conventional or inverse spatula **(Figs. 5-91 and 5-92)**.

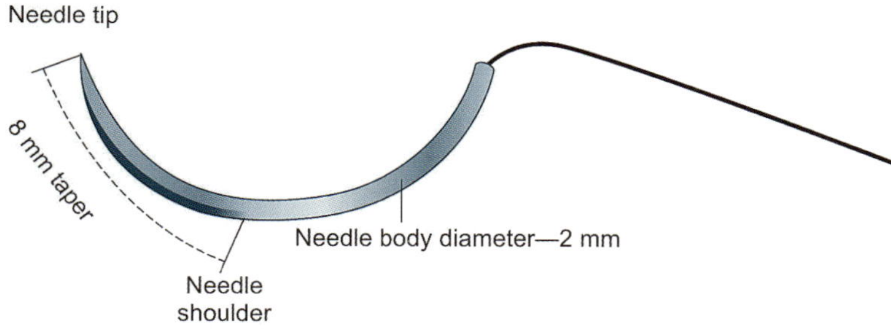

Fig. 5-91: Tapering ratio of the needle is the ratio between distance between the needle point and shoulder of the needle and diameter at body of the needle.

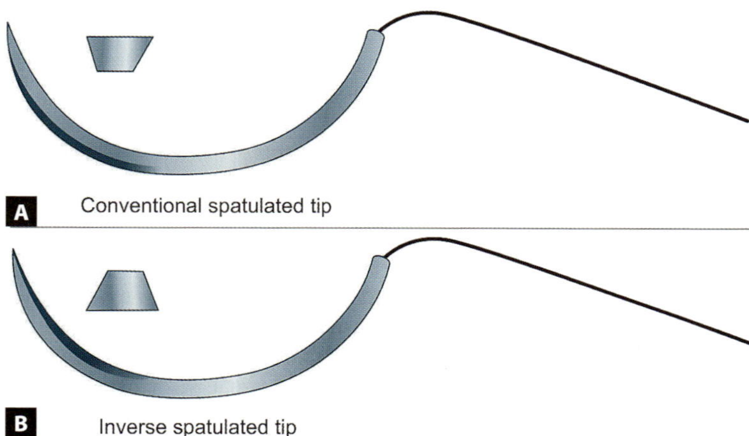

Figs. 5-92A and B: Spatulated needle tips: (A) Conventional spatulated; (B) Inverse spatulated.

Shoulder of the Needle

It is the junction of the body and taper of a needle. Configurations will be different on either sides of the shoulder. Needle driver (holder) is placed in the body just proximal to the shoulder.

Needle Body

Body of the needle is the part proximal to the shoulder or proximal to taper. Body extends up to the rear end that is swage. It may be rounded or oval (currently popular) or triangular or reverse cut or flattened hexagonal or rhomboid or diamond shaped on cross section. Body may be having grooves or ribs on the inner and outer surfaces of the body. Body may be straight or curved **(Fig. 5-93)**.

Curved needle is commonly used. This curve used with a dynamic driving force using needle driver to penetrate through the tissues effectively and efficiently. Shape, size, dimension of the curvature, strength, stability of needle are important to have an optimum safe and efficient needle. Needle should be grasped properly by the needle holder; this grasp efficiency prevents the needle from deflecting and moving in the jaws of the needle holder. Needle should be strong enough to pass through the tissues required without bending or breaking. It should be easily penetrable and should withstand the force used to pass the needle.

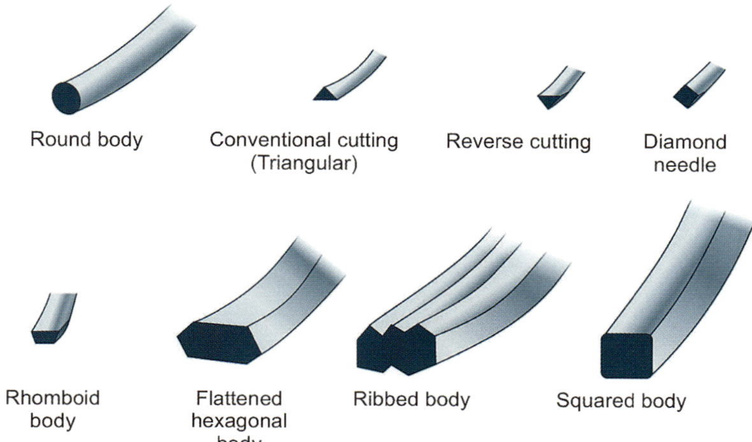

Fig. 5-93: Different types of the body of the needle.

Features of an ideal surgical needle

- It is made up of high quality stainless needle.
- It should be stable to be grasped by the jaws of the needle driver.
- It should be adequately sharp enough to penetrate the required tissue.
- It should be sterile and corrosive resistant.
- Smaller diameter is ideal to minimise the tissue trauma.
- *Strength* (resistance to deformation during passage through tissues); *ductility* (resistance to breakage after bending); *sharpness* (ability to penetrate the tissues easily); *clamping moment* (stability of the needle in a needle driver) are different qualities/characteristics decides the needle performance.

Different Techniques to Attach the Needle to Suture Material in Atraumatic Eyeless Needle

Attached suture material should be secure and strong; should not get detached from the needle. Eyeless needle with sutures are easy to use; less traumatic to tissues as it is single stranded. Eyed needle (French eyelet) has got oval eyelet opening to pass the suture material; suture is pulled back to create a double strands (double back). One end is kept shorter than the other by one-third of longer one. Single suture is used for tying. But track will be wider as it has to pass wider eyelet of the needle and two strands of the suture initially. In atraumatic needle, track will be same as of the needle and suture material.

Swaging

Rear end of the needle is first flattened; it is folded to create a U-shaped channel; the suture is kept in his groove and metal is folded around the channel to grip the suture end using a precise force to achieve security. Diameter is reconstituted and burrs are eliminated. Here double strands of a suture material are eliminated. It also allows the placement of needle on both ends of a suture material to create a *double armed suture*. One should remember the *swaging junction is the weakest point* of a suture material **(Figs. 5-94 and 5-95)**.

Crimping

Using mechanical device or laser, a tunnel is drilled at the rear end of the needle. End of the suture material is inserted into the tunnel. It is crimped in place securely using optimum force. Crimping is used for a larger diameter suture **(Fig. 5-96)**.

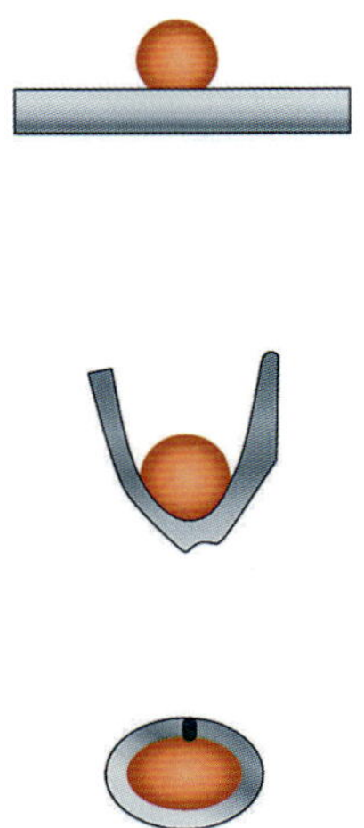

Fig. 5-94: Swaging of the needle to the suture material—rear end is flattened; then folded to create a U; suture is placed into the groove of created U and arms of the U is folded to create strong 'O' with suture material end captured inside.

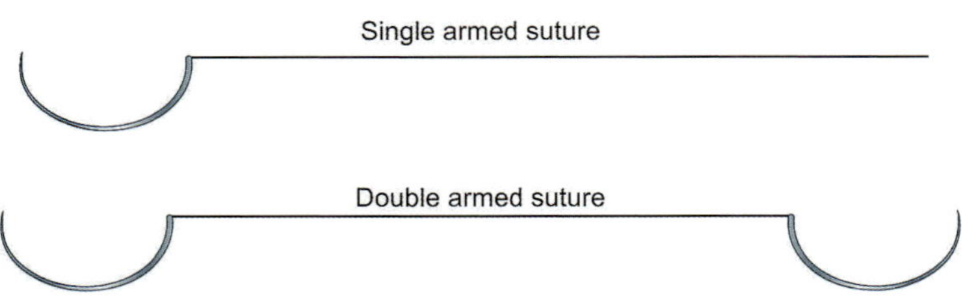

Fig. 5-95: Single armed and double armed sutures.

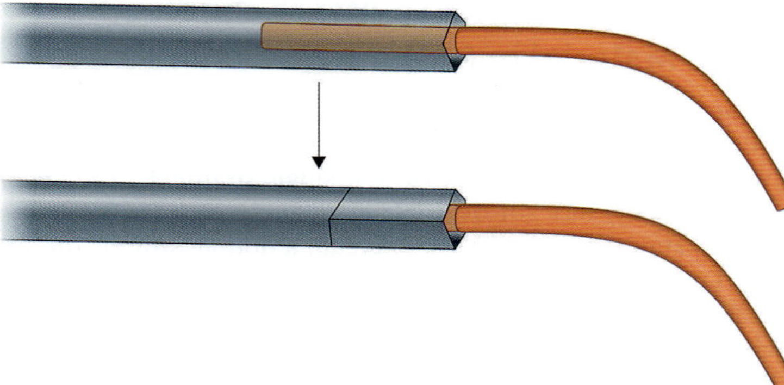

Fig. 5-96: Crimping method.

Metalised Suture

It is done to eliminate weak point created either by swaging or crimping. Electroplating and dipping was tried to attach the suture. But it is not in common usage.

Usually suture is attached to the *end of the needle*. Often in *middle attachment needle (shuttle needle)* suture material is attached to middle of a straight needle. It is useful in laparoscopic surgery but otherwise causes double track in the tissue passage. *Detachable suture* material is often used where purposefully suture material is attached to needle with a low force so that after passage through the tissue needle can be detached from the suture material with reasonable distraction force on the suture and needle in opposite directions. It is useful in some open surgeries but should not be used in laparoscopic surgeries. Chances of needle getting lost in the surgical field are higher when such needles are used **(Figs. 5-97 and 5-98)**.

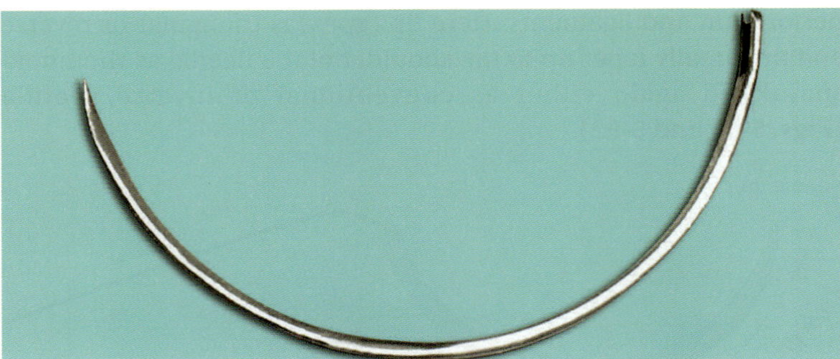

Fig. 5-97: Surgical needle.

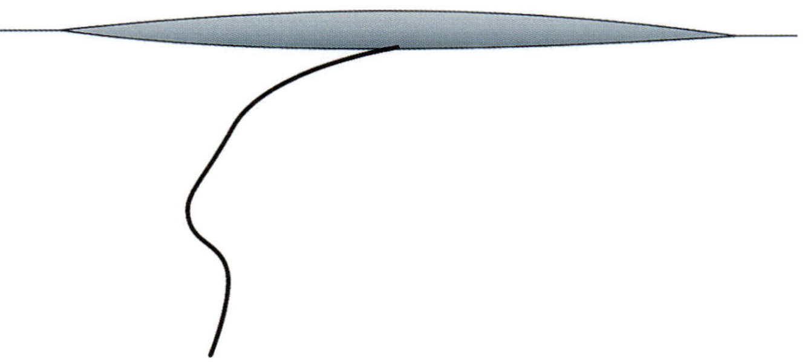

Fig. 5-98: Shuttle needle.

Note

- Weakest part of the needle is part near the eye.
- Needle is sterilised in cidex/Lysol. It should not be autoclaved as tip gets blunt.
- The needle is held at its centre by placing it at the junction of the proximal 2/3rd and distal 1/3rd to have optimal grip, control and precision.
- Needles can be ¼ circle, ½ circle, ⅜ circle or ⅝ circle at their curvatures **(refer Figs. 5-90A and B)**. Needles of different curvature are used at different places depending on the depth of the suturing.
- Needles are made up of stainless steel.
- Atraumatic needles are available as sterilised packs. They are sterilised by ethylene oxide or gamma sterilisation along with the sutures which they coexist.
- *Gallie's needle* is large eyed needle which was earlier used in hernias to suture the defect using fascia lata strips.
- *Lane's needle* is half circle cutting needle with a large eye.
- *Mayo needle* is obstetric needle with a large square eye and is strong.
- *Hagedorn reverse flattened point fish hook needle* used for suturing inaccessible sites.
- *Symonds round bodied fish hook needles.*
- *Bonney Reverdin needle* is a special needle with an eye which is open to one side with small slender shutter which can slid and closed after passing the suture material.
- *Kous Netzoff aluminium needle is* used to suture the liver tear.

NEEDLE HOLDER

Smaller distal blades with criss-cross serrations often with a groove in the middle are the features of a needle holder. Often there is a longitudinal groove in the middle of the distal blade between serrations. Ratio of length of handle to blades is 4:1.

It may be straight or curved. It may be available in different sizes. While holding a needle in a needle holder one should get a good control and good grip. This is achieved by placing the needle at junction of proximal 2/3rd and distal 1/3rd of the blade. Needle holder should be held between thumb and ring finger. Curved needle holders are available to hold the needles and work at the depth like in pelvis/thoracic cavity for better manoeuvrability and visualisation. Needle holder is sterilised by autoclave **(Figs. 5-99A to C)**. *Tungsten-carbide inner surface coated needle holder* is available which has got longer duration of life due to reduced wear and tear of the instrument because of tungsten coating.

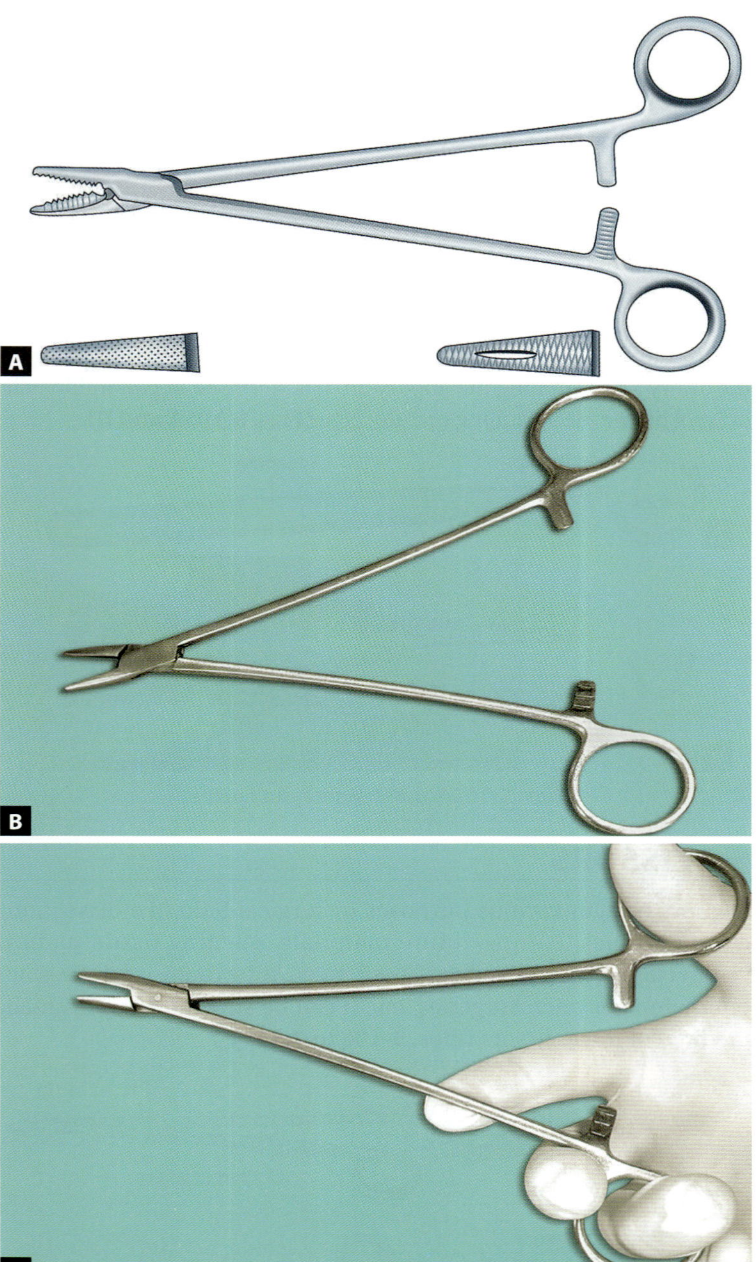

Figs. 5-99A to C: Needle holder.

BARD-PARKER'S HANDLE (BP HANDLE)

Bard-Parker's handle is a flat stainless steel instrument with a slot on narrower side on both surfaces to attach scalpel blade. 3, 4, 5 and 7 numbered blades are available. Number 4 handle is wider. Scalpel blades 10, 11, 12, and 15 fit into Bard-Parker handle numbers 3, 5 and 7. Scalpel blades 18, 19, 20, 21, 22, 23 and 24 fit into slot of Bard-Parker's blade number 4. New blade is used into the slot of the handle for each patient and so sharpness of the blade is maintained. BP handle is sterilised by autoclave **(Figs. 5-100 and 5-101)**.

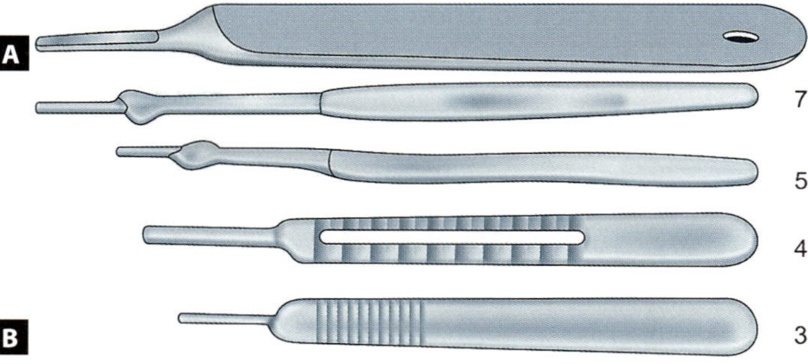

Figs. 5-100A and B: Bard-Parker's handles—3, 4, 5 and 7.

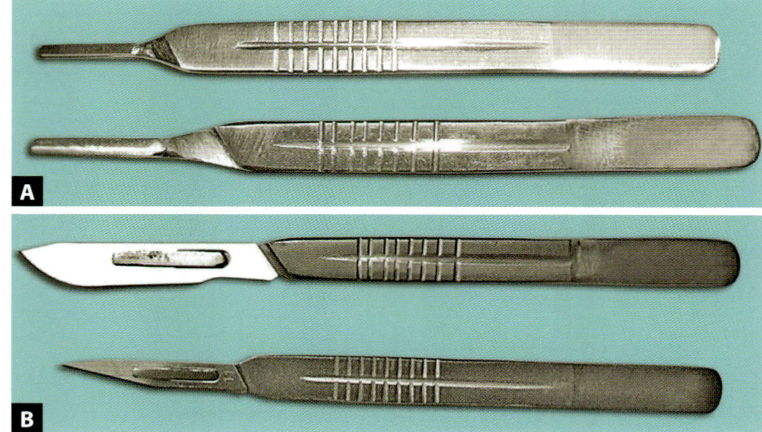

Figs. 5-101A and B: (A) Bard-Parker handles number 3 and 4; (B) Blades used are no. 2 and no. 1.

SURGICAL BLADES

They are detachable blades. Number 11 blade is stab knife blade which is used in incision and drainage of an abscess and also in making small incision like for drains. Number 12 blade is curved one, used for tonsillectomy. Here cutting edge faces surgeon. Number 15 is used in plastic surgery, head and neck surgery, face surgeries. Numbers 20, 22 and 24 used in skin incisions of major surgeries like laparotomy, thoracotomy, craniotomy, incisions in limb. Blades are sterilised by gamma radiation with aluminum foil packing. Commonly blades are used only once and then disposed. If sterilisation is needed it is done using cetrimide/lysol immersion (not autoclave or boiling). Scalpel is also used for dissections of fascial planes, raising skin flaps, hernial sac, etc. Fine lateral oblique strokes are used for such dissections. One should have a control over the depth of dissection. When scalpel is used in the abdomen like while cutting the bowel, it should be used in such a way that sharp edge of the blade should face forward so that to avoid inadvertent injury to deeper vital structures. Bowel is cut from mesenteric margin towards anti-mesenteric surface **(Figs. 5-102 and 5-103)**.

Different Ways of Placing Incisions

- *Dinner knife position* is used while making a lengthy incision.
- *Pen holding/writing position* is used to make incision over the vessels/nerves/tumours.
- *Fiddle-bow position* is used to make incisions with less pressure on delicate tissues.
- *Grasping position* is used to make long sweeping cuts.

- *Stab position* is used to drain an abscess using no. 11 blade with no. 3 BP handle. It is also used to make an incision to pass a drain corrugated or tube.

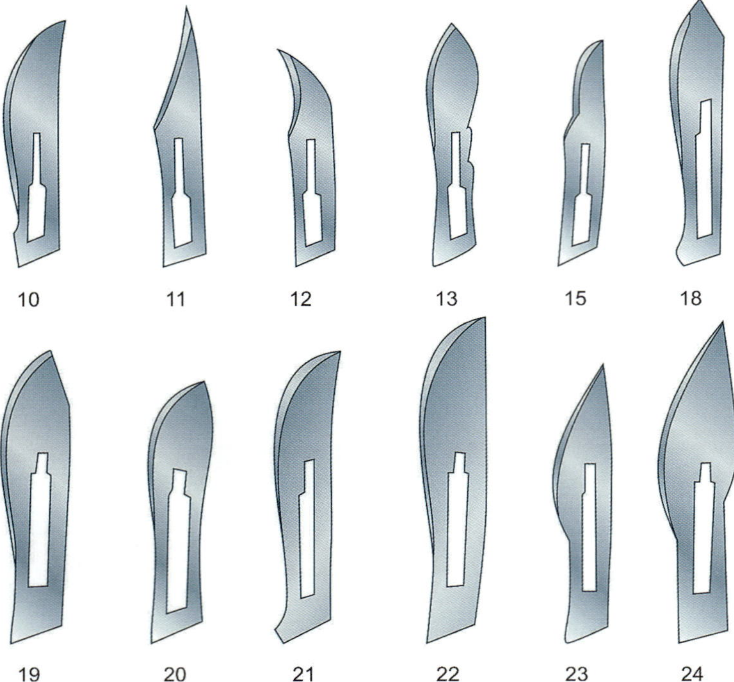

Fig. 5-102: Surgical blades of different numbers. Blades are detachable and used only once.

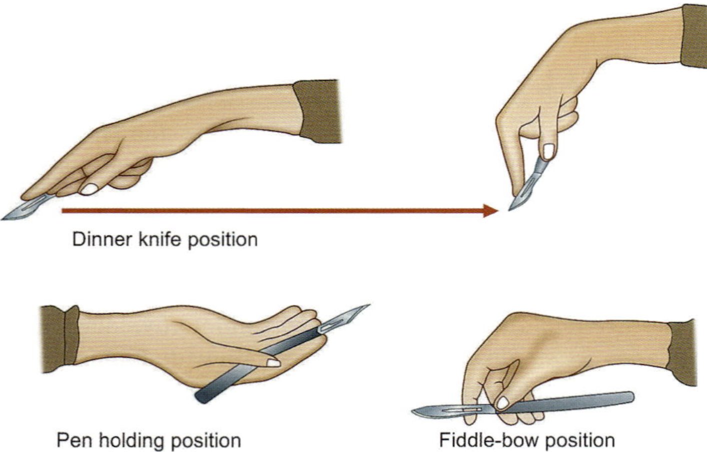

Fig. 5-103: Different positions/methods used to hold knife while making incisions or doing dissections in different surgeries.

Principles in making incision

- Incision should be planned well prior to surgery for adequacy, for possible need for extension during course of the surgery, and indeed be cosmetically acceptable. Ideally incision site should be marked using sterile marker or methylene blue.
- Clean single stroke firm incision should be made with required depth. Repeated strokes and movements should be avoided.
- Knife should be perpendicular to skin to begin with blade pointing perpendicular to skin. But later blade should be parallel with curvature/belly of the blade on the site of the incision.
- While making lengthy incision like in abdomen, incision area should be stretched between thumb and index fingers of other hand of the surgeon.
- Care should be taken to avoid injuries to deeper structures like muscle/nerves/vessels/bowel while making incisions.

TENOTOMY KNIFE

Tenotomy knife straight/curved with a short cutting edge with a fixed handle is used in congenital torticollis to cut sternomastoid muscle, congenital talipes equinovarus, adductor tenotomy and lateral sphincterotomy for fissure in ano **(Fig. 5-104)**.

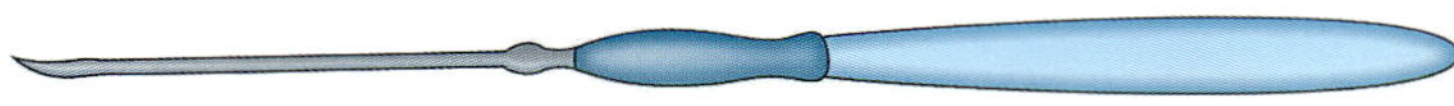

Fig. 5-104: Tenotomy knife.

ANEURYSM NEEDLE

Aneurysm needle is stout instrument with a deep hook in one end with an eye opening in the blunt tip. Eye proceeds as a deep groove in the needle proximally which allows the ligature to stay firmly. This facilitates the passage of the ligatures across the deeper plane around the blood vessels; to ligate the vessel in continuity; in venesection; to pass the ligature around any tubular structures. Earlier it was used to ligate the artery while treating the aneurysm. It is sterilised in glutaraldehyde or lysol but never by boiling or autoclave **(Figs. 5-105A and B)**.

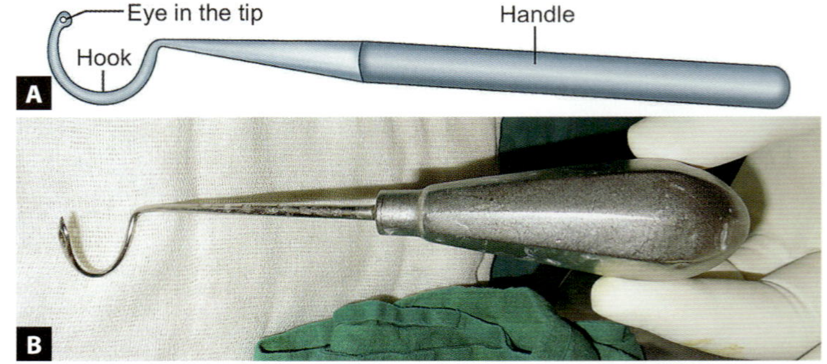

Figs. 5-105A and B: Aneurysm needle.

SCISSORS

Scissors has got various purposes in surgical field like dissection, cutting tissues, cutting suture materials, opening tissue planes, venesection, cutting bandages, corrugated/tube drains and dressing, ophthalmic or microsurgeries, etc. It can be straight, curved, small, medium or long scissors **(Figs. 5-106 to 5-111)**.

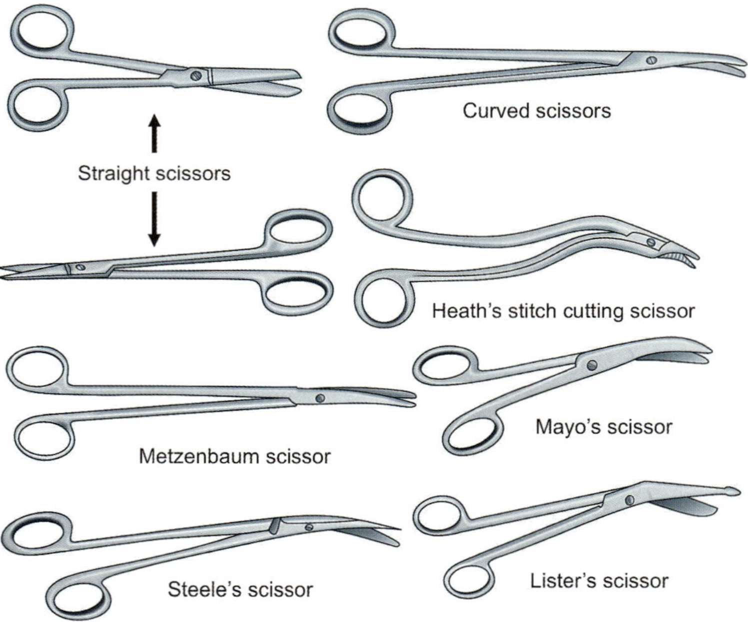

Fig. 5-106: Different scissors used in surgical practice.

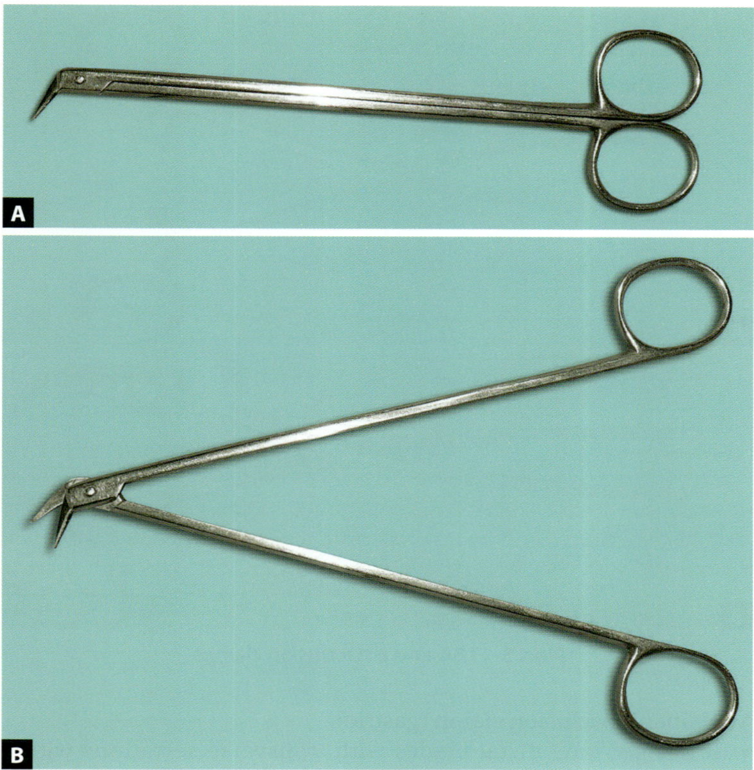

Figs. 5-107A and B: Potts-Smith scissor.

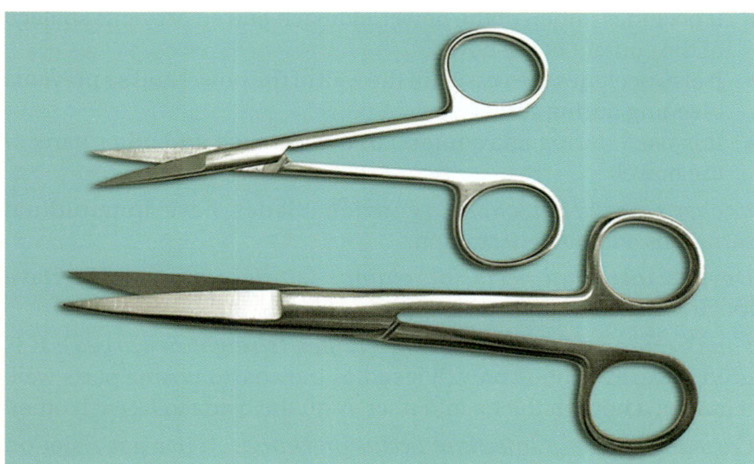

Fig. 5-108: Straight scissors used for suture cutting.

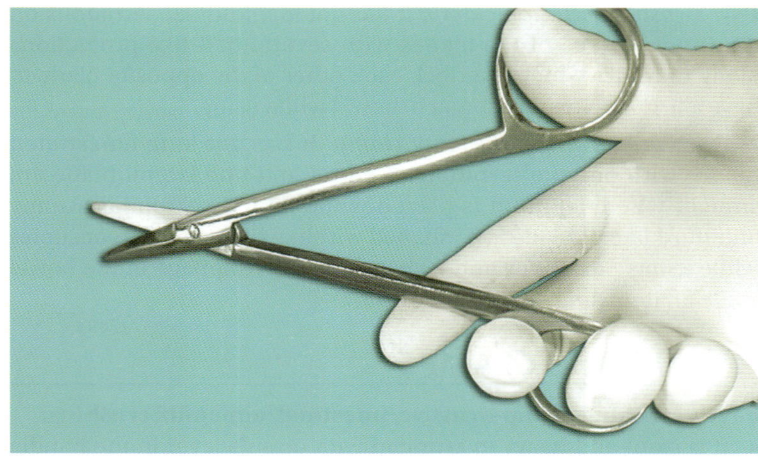

Fig. 5-109: Scissor showing method of holding it.

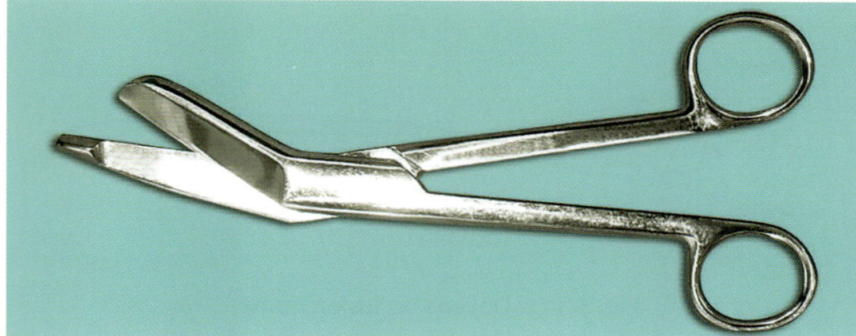

Fig. 5-110: Lister's bandage cutting scissor. Distal blades are bent at angle so that it is passed easily under the bandage. Lower blade has got flat blunt atraumatic tip. This part is passed under the bandage as it is atraumatic. Scissors are sterilised by chemical method using lysol or glutaraldehyde. Scissors are not autoclaved; not boiled.

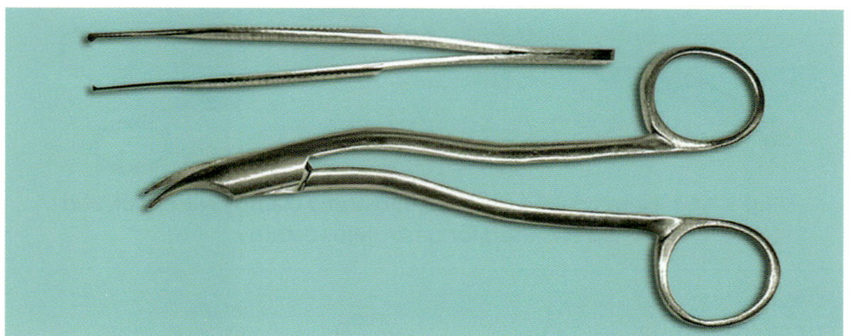

Fig. 5-111: Heath's suture cutting scissor with toothed forceps.

Different scissors are:

Mayo's scissors—are long and stout scissors. It can be blunt tipped/ pointed tip/straight or curved.

Mc Indoe scissor—is having fine small blade. It is used mainly for dissection and in cutting delicate structures.

Metzenbaum scissor—has got long blades in comparison to shaft. It is used in depth dissection like vagotomy, cholecystectomy, pelvic surgeries, etc.

Heath suture cutting scissor—has got long shaft, small curves angled blades with tip is having fine serrations which ensures the proper grip of the suture material to be cut. Suture is held with dissecting forceps and is cut using Heath's scissor between knot and skin where suture enters.

Steele's scissor is like Metzenbaum scissor with similar use.

Lister's bandage/dressing cutting scissor has got flat lower blade to avoid damage to skin. Lower blade has got a knob at the terminal.

BOWEL OCCLUSION CLAMPS

Different types of occlusion clamps are discussed as follows **(Figs. 5-112 to 5-118):**

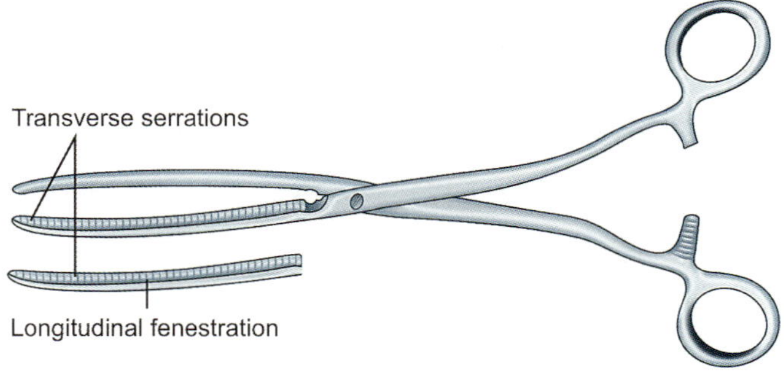

Fig. 5-112: Moynihan's occlusion clamp.

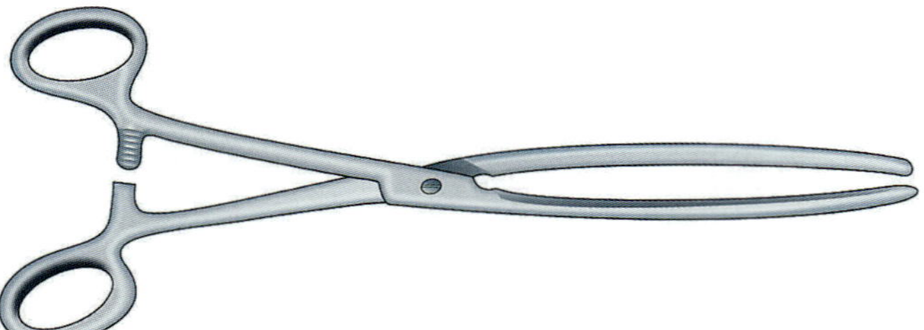

Fig. 5-113: Doyen's occlusion clamp.

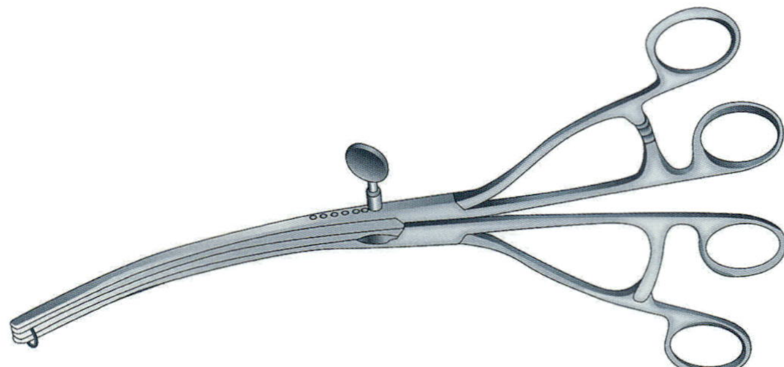

Fig. 5-114: Lane's paired gastrojejunostomy clamps with hook and screws used for gastrojejunostomy.

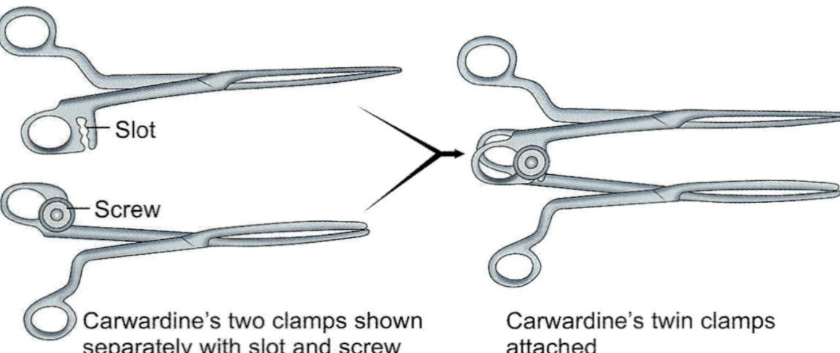

Fig. 5-115: Carwardine's twin intestinal occlusion clamp with screw and slot to fix. It is used to have easier intestinal anastomosis.

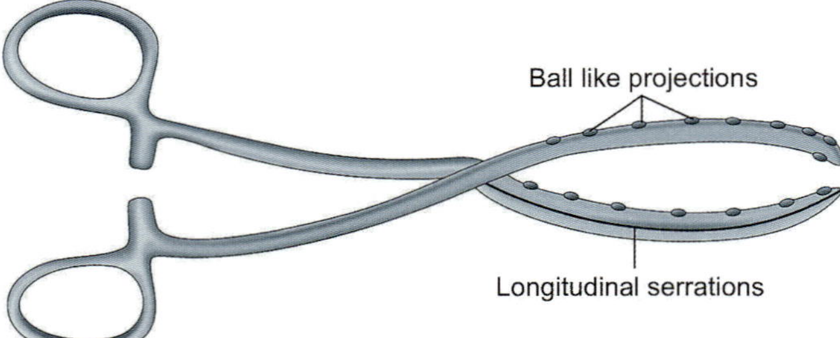

Fig. 5-116: Payr's gastric occlusion clamp.

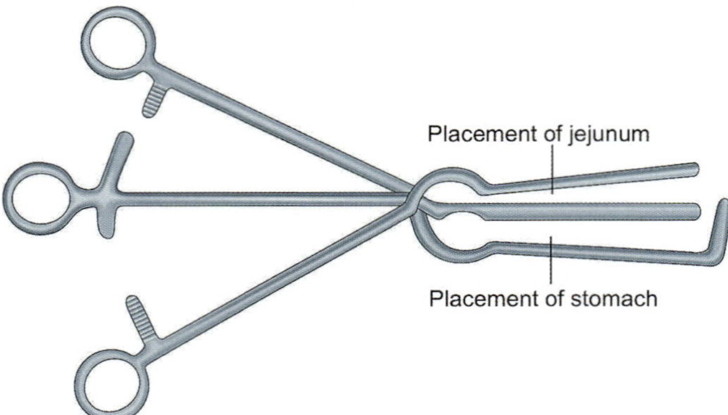

Fig. 5-117: Moynihan's gastrojejunostomy clamp.

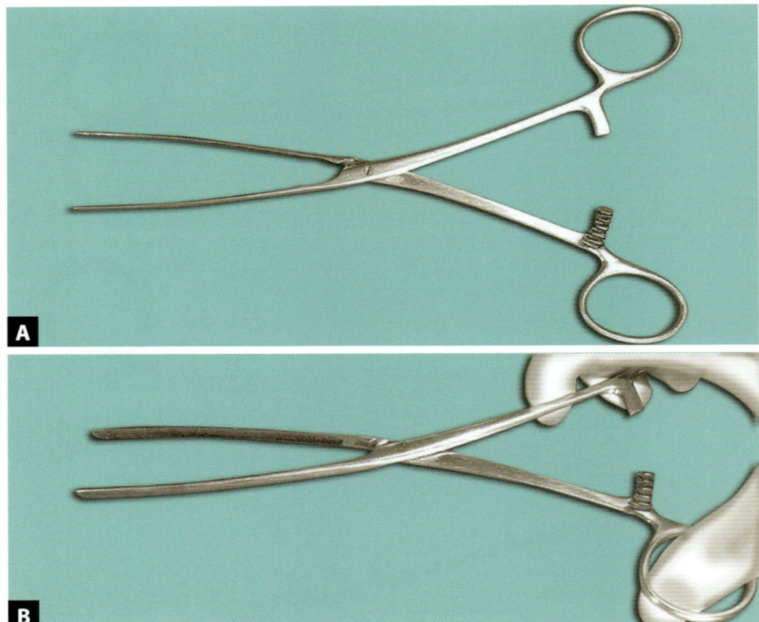

Figs. 5-118A and B: Occlusion clamps.

Moynihan's occlusion clamp (gastric)

- It has got long distal blades with transverse serrations with a longitudinal fenestration one on each blade.
- It may be straight or curved.
- It is non-traumatic, non-crushing type.
- It occludes lumen of the bowel/stomach and so prevents spillage of the content of the bowel.
- It also occludes the vessels in the wall of the bowel and so prevents bleeding during surgery.
- It is used during anastomosis of the stomach and other parts of the bowel.

Kocher's occlusion clamp (gastric): Blades have longitudinal serrations without fenestration.

Doyen's intestinal occlusion clamps (straight or curved): Have longitudinal serrations with apposing blades.

Lane's paired gastrojejunostomy clamps (straight or curved): It is used in gastrojejunostomy. It steadies the anastomosing parts well. It has got a hook at the tip and a screw on the blade to fix each other.

Carwardine's twin intestinal occlusion clamps: It has got a slot on one part shaft and a corresponding screw on the other part shaft. These slot and screw fits into each other to facilitate proper intestinal anastomosis.

Payr's gastric occlusion clamp: It has got longitudinal serrations on the inner surface of the blades with several ball-like projections along the sides which interlock each other of the opposite blade to have a firm grip on the stomach/bowel while using.

Moynihan's gastrojejunostomy clamp: It has got long fenestrated blades with oblique serrations. Central and one lateral blade are straight where jejunum is placed while doing gastrojejunostomy and third lateral blade is 'L' shaped within which stomach occupies while using. Serrations and L shape prevents slippage of the bowel while anatomising.

CRUSHING CLAMPS

Payr's crushing clamp—gastric/intestinal/appendix crushing:

- It is stout and heavy instrument with double lever in the handle with longitudinal serrations.

- Once applied it crushes the bowel. So before applying it, line of resection of stomach/bowel should be assessed properly. It is applied to the part which has to be removed. Viability of the bowel is lost once it is applied.
- It is used in gastrectomy, resection and anastomosis of the bowel.
- It can be gastric crushing or intestinal crushing or appendix crushing clamp. All are similar; only size of the blades is smaller in intestinal and appendix crushing clamps **(Figs. 5-119 and 5-120)**.

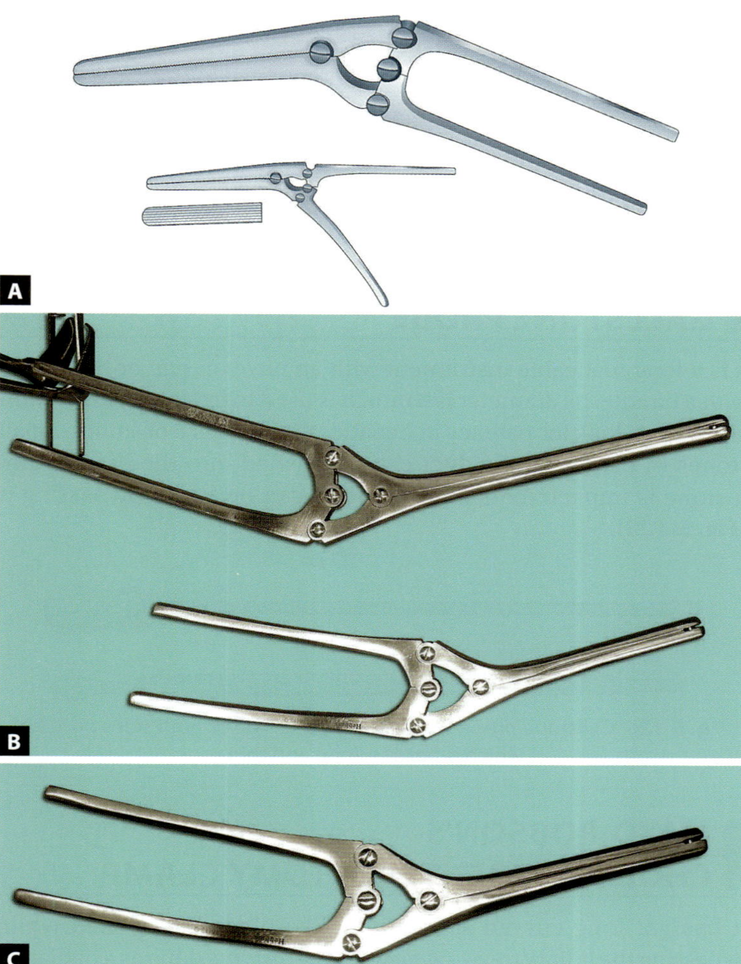

Figs. 5-119A to C: Payr's (gastric) crushing clamp.

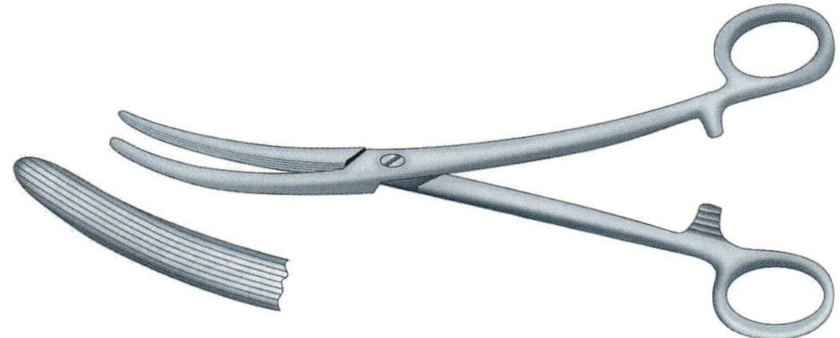

Fig. 5-120: Parker-Kerr crushing clamp.

Parker-Kerr crushing clamp: It is a stout and heavy crushing clamp with longitudinal serrations.

DESJARDIN'S CHOLEDOCHOLITHOTOMY FORCEPS

It has got long distal blades with smooth serrations and fenestra in the tip. It does not have lock and so accidental damage to CBD mucosa or crushing of the CBD stone are avoided.

It is used for choledocholithotomy (removal of CBD stones). Length and curve facilitate the stone extraction better. In laparoscopic cholecystectomy, it can be used to remove stones from gallbladder by passing through the 10 mm port so that makes delivery of the gallbladder easier. Disadvantage is that instrument may dilate the CBD significantly while manipulating **(Figs. 5-121A to D)**.

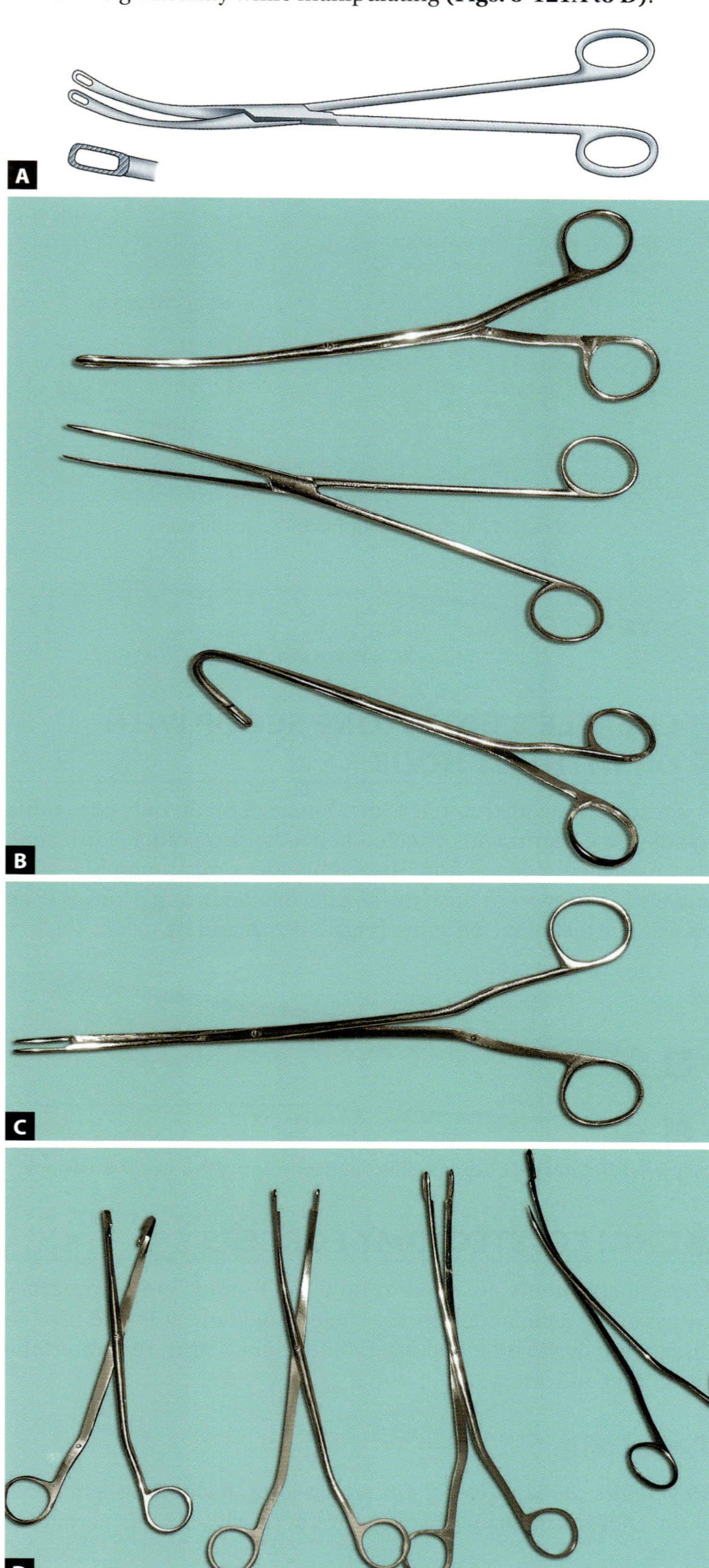

Figs. 5-121A to D: Desjardin's choledocholithotomy forceps.

Lawson-Tait choledocholithotomy forceps/Alligator forceps is used which has got alligator jaws that facilitate passage through a narrow duct with lesser chances of dilating the duct.

BAKES DILATOR

It is long malleable metallic instrument with club at the terminal end. It is available in different sizes **(Fig. 5-122)**.

It is used to assess the CBD, duodenal papilla for patency or block. Dilator is passed through the choledochotomy opening downwards to reach the metal tip (olive blunt tip) to duodenum. It signifies the patency. It is called as *steel sign*. Dilators are passed gradually from lesser diameter to higher diameter size **(Fig. 5-123)**.

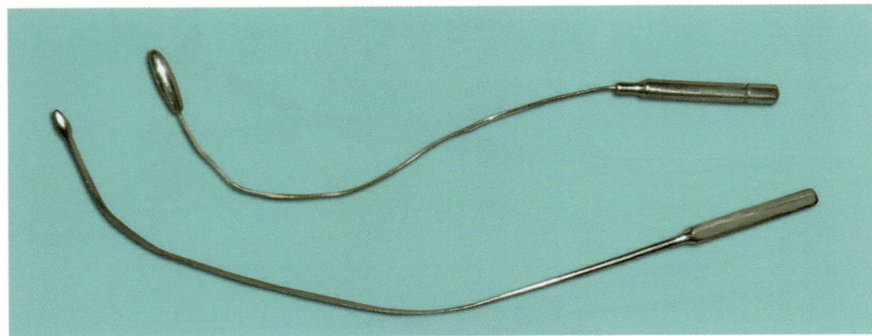

Fig. 5-122: Bakes common bile duct dilator.

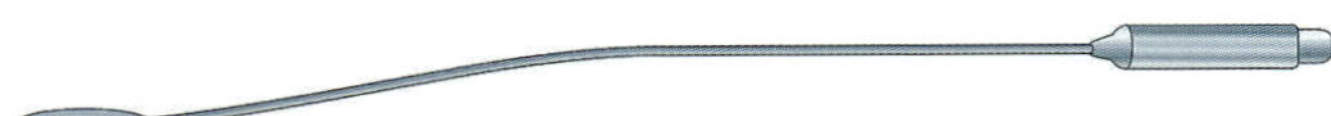

Fig. 5-123: Bakes dilator.

CHEATLE'S GALLSTONE SCOOP WITH OR WITHOUT HOOK

It is flexible long instrument with a blunt scoop on one side with a handle. Few instruments often contain a hook on other side. Scoop is to remove the debris from the gallbladder or common bile duct; and also to support or push the stone while removing. Hook is used to dislodge the impacted stone **(Figs. 5-124A and B)**.

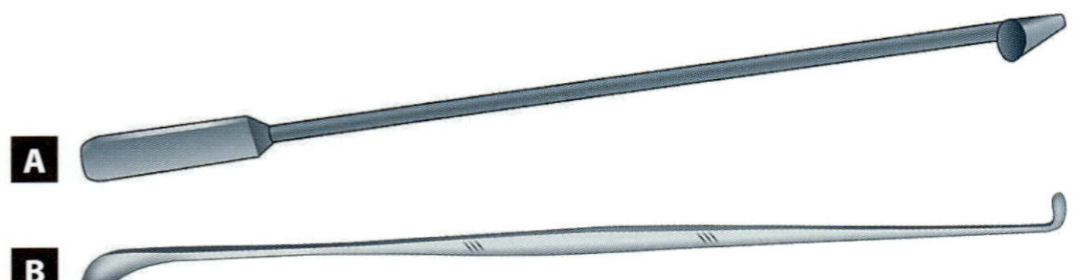

Figs. 5-124A and B: Cheatle's gallstone scoop and also scoop with a hook.

CHOLECYSTECTOMY FORCEPS

These instruments are used to hold the fundus and Hartmann's pouch of the gallbladder during cholecystectomy. It is also used to dissect the cystic duct and artery and to pass ligature around the cystic duct and artery.

Types (Fig. 5-125)

Moynihan's cholecystectomy forceps has long shafts with slight curve at the short distal blades like a parrot beak with oblique serrations inside.

Henry-Gray's cholecystectomy forceps is similar but has right-angled blades with transverse serrations.

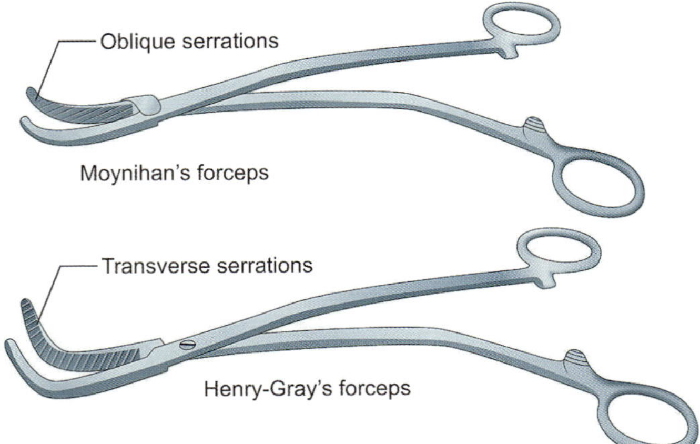

Fig. 5-125: Cholecystectomy forceps—two types: Moynihan's parrot beak curved. Henry Gray's right angled.

GALLSTONE PROBE

It is a long malleable instrument with an olive on one or both ends with a handle. Its diameter is 6 mm. It is used to explore the common bile duct to look for patency in hepatic, and presence of stones. Small stones in common bile duct can be pushed into the duodenum. If stone is impacted, its exact location can be found by passing it **(Fig. 5-126)**.

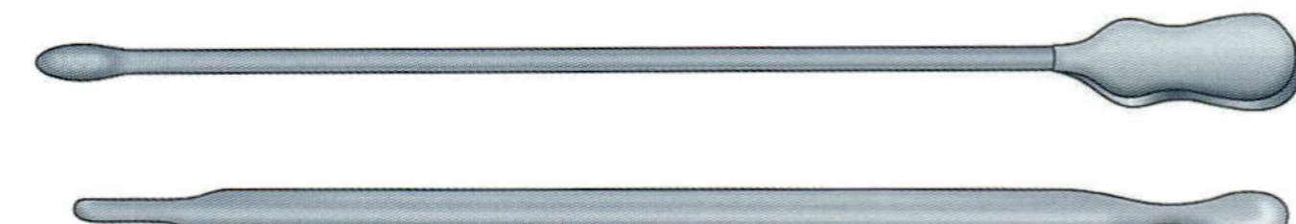

Fig. 5-126: Gallstone probe is available as one side or both sides olive tip which is flexible, long and thin.

MAYO-ROBSON'S CHOLECYSTOENTEROSTOMY CLAMP

It has got long curved semicircle—like blades. It is used while bypassing the biliary tree—*cholecystoenterostomy* done as a palliative procedure in obstructive jaundice (in carcinoma head of the pancreas or periampullary or carcinoma distal common bile duct) **(Fig. 5-127)**. This clamp is used to clamp the gallbladder to keep in position while doing cholecystojejunostomy. But choledochojejunostomy Roux-en-Y is a better palliative bypass procedure because narrow cystic duct may get blocked later causing re-obstruction of the biliary tree. Cystic duct may end into the common bile duct lower down and its junction may get involved by the tumour invasion causing re-block and so failure of the palliative procedure.

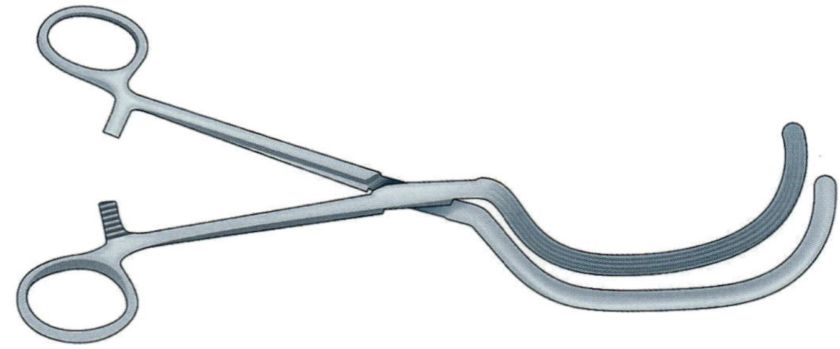

Fig. 5-127: Mayo-Robson's cholecystoenterostomy clamp.

KEHR'S 'T' TUBE

- It is used after opening of CBD (choledochotomy). CBD is closed with 'T' tube in situ.
- It is made up of latex or red rubber. 'T' tube has got horizontal part which is kept in the CBD and vertical part which is allowed to come out to drain bile **(Figs. 5-128A to C)**. Amount of bile draining is measured daily.
  Before removal of 'T' tube, patency of CBD should be confirmed.

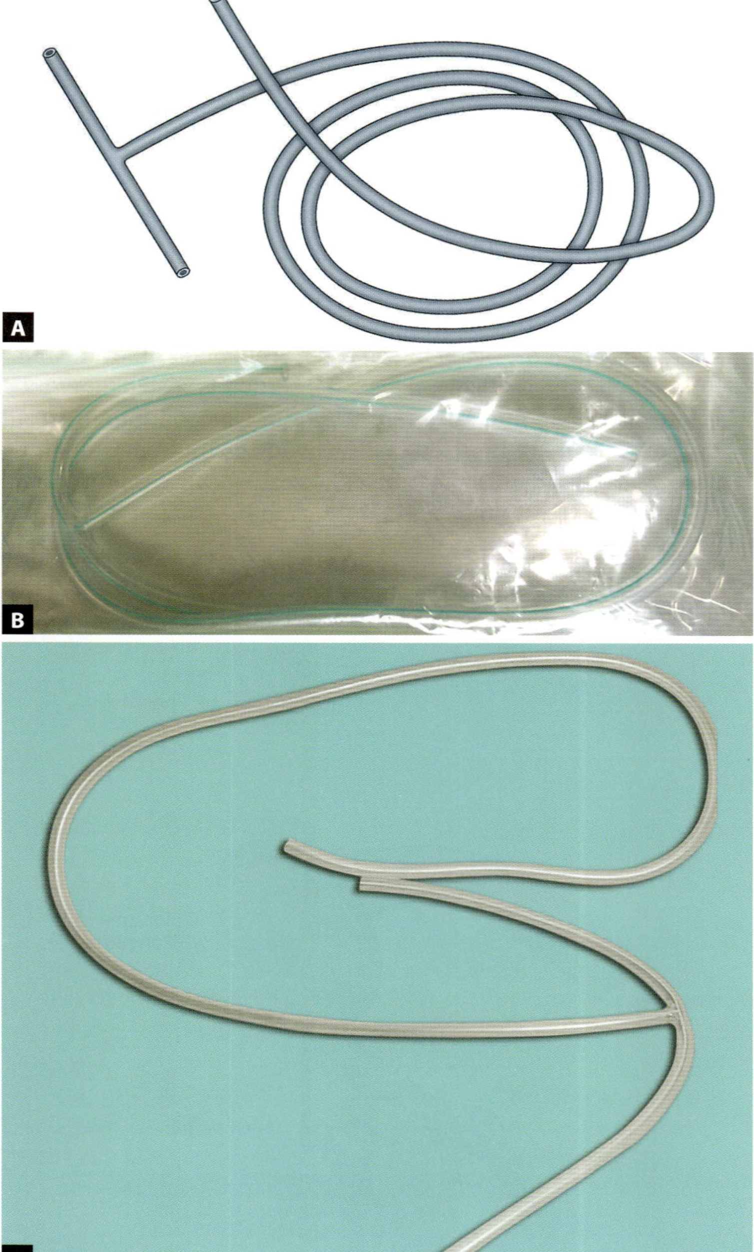

Figs. 5-128A to C: Kehr's 'T' tubes.

It is done by following methods:

- The vertical limb (done in 10–14 days) is clamped and observed for development of pain, fever and jaundice in 24 hours. If normal then one can presume that there is no obstruction in the CBD.
- Water-soluble iodine dye is injected through the tube to visualise biliary tree and free flow of dye into the duodenum (post-operative 'T' tube cholangiogram). It is done in 14 days which is the time required to develop fibrous track. Once there is free flow tube is removed and track gets closed on its own.

Complications/problems of T tube

- Kinking/block/break in T tube
- Displacement/slipping of T tube out of common bile duct may cause biliary peritonitis
- Improper pancreatic duct drainage due to tube
- Impaired enterohepatic circulation
- Biliary infection, secondary haemorrhage, bile leak and peritonitis, foreign body reaction
- Difficulty in removal even after adequate pressure is managed by gradual continuous pressure and occasionally exploration may be needed.

Note:

Montgomery T tube is used as a specialised combined device acts like a tracheal stent and airway both; used in laryngotracheal surgeries in specialised centres.

SUCTION INSTRUMENTS

These are essential instruments needed in all surgeries to suck out blood from the surgical field, pus, infected fluid, fluid in peritoneal/thoracic/cranial cavities. It has got a *suction tip* of varying types, *suction tube* which connects tip to the *suction apparatus* and suction creating system, either central suction system *or* power suction system with two suction glass bottles connected to each other *or* manual suction apparatus (now not used). Suction tip has got a long bent tube with openings at one end to suck the fluid, with a stout handle which has got a proximal ridged part at the other end to which suction tube (rubber or plastic) is attached, which in turn is connected to suction apparatus. Suction tip and suction tubes should be sterile. They are sterilised by autoclave **(Fig. 5-129)**.

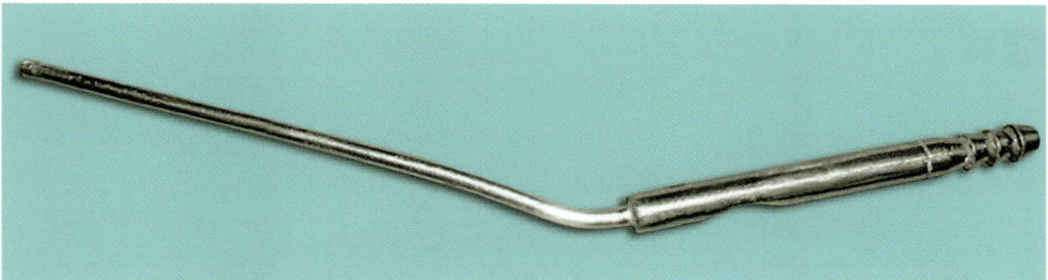

Fig. 5-129: Suction tip.

Types of suction tips:

- *Adson's fine suction tip*: It is angled with a vent/thumb rest to control the suction as needed. It is a fine suction tip which is used in meticulous surgeries like plastic, vascular and reconstructive surgeries. It cannot be used when large quantity of blood/pus/fluid/clot needs to be sucked out **(Figs. 5-130A to C)**.

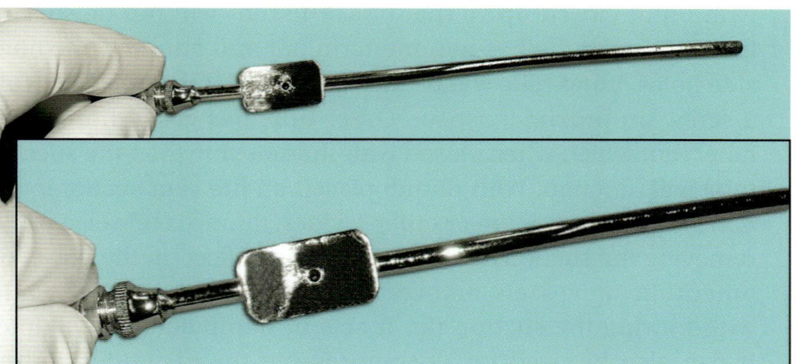

Fig. 5-130A

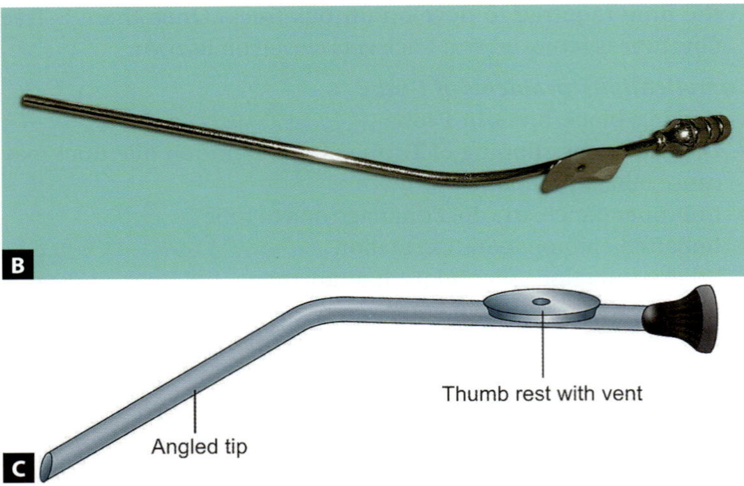

Figs. 5-130B and C

Figs. 5-130A to C: Adson's suction cannula is used for fine suctioning and alone the delicate structures.

- *Yankauer suction tip:* It is large suction tip used mainly in peritoneal cavity after lavage; in haemoperitoneum; in peritonitis; in pelvis; in thoracotomy; etc. It has got central hole with outer small multiple holes. It creates strong suction and so may suck omentum; bowel wall, etc. So with one hand bowel and omentum should be pushed aside while sucking the fluid. Often its tip is supported by a rubber tube. When it is present, care is taken to see that it is not left inside the peritoneal cavity by inadvertent slippage **(Figs. 5-131A and B)**.

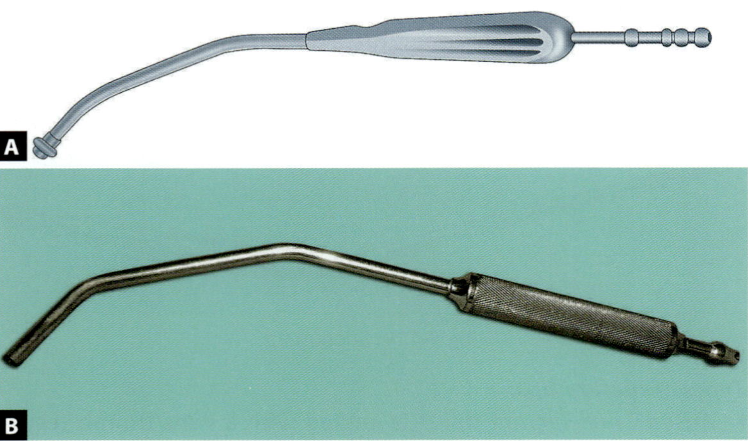

Figs. 5-131A and B: Yankauer's suction tube.

- *Poole's multiperforated suction tip:* It has got outer and inner tubes—one inside the other. Outer tube has got multiple holes with blunt closed tip so that bowel/tissues will not be sucked inside. Inner tube has got one terminal and another proximal side holes. Inner tube will be inside the outer tube attached with a screw on proximal aspect. Outer tube has got a thumb rest hole/vent which when closed with thumb, only then the suction tube will function. With thumb placed on the vent suctioning is done in the peritoneum or other cavities, thumb is released while removing the suction tube so that sucking effect on the bowel or omentum or vessels or over the stoma is prevented while withdrawing the suction tip. It acts by sump action principle. It can also be used for decompressing the distended bowel **(Figs. 5-132A and B)**.

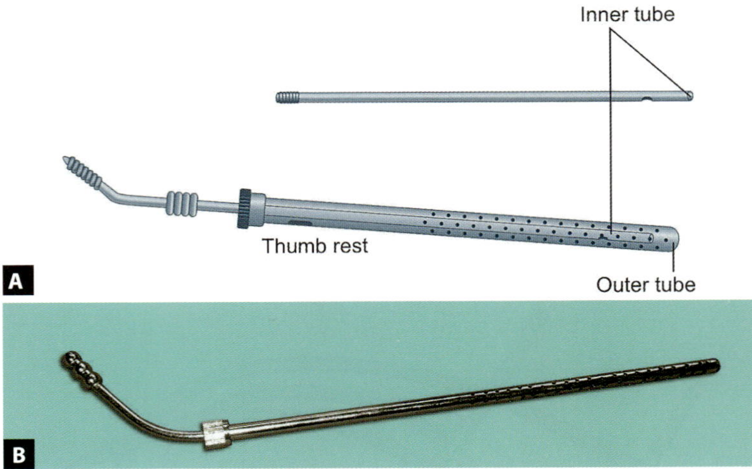

Figs. 5-132A and B: Poole's suction tip (device).

TRACHEOSTOMY TUBE

Types (Figs. 5-133 to 5-136)

1. *Fuller's bivalved tracheostomy tube:* It has got outer tube and inner tube. Outer tube is biflanged and so insertion is easier. Inner tube is longer with an opening on its posterior aspect. Inner tube can be removed and re-inserted easily whenever required. Outer tube flanges are weak and sharp and can break or cause trauma to the tracheal wall. It cannot be used during radiotherapy.

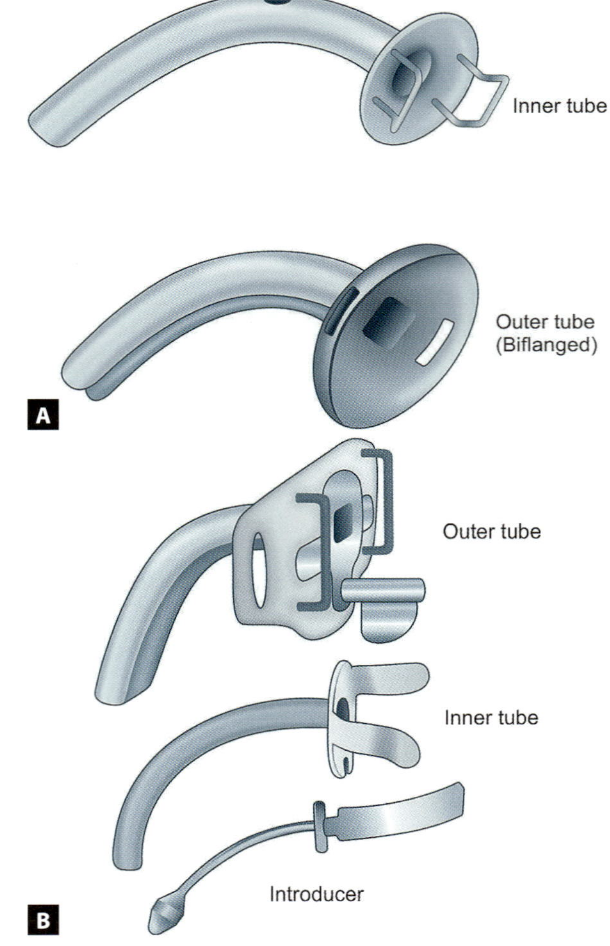

Figs. 5-133A and B: Tracheostomy tubes: (A) Fuller's tube; (B) Jackson's tube.

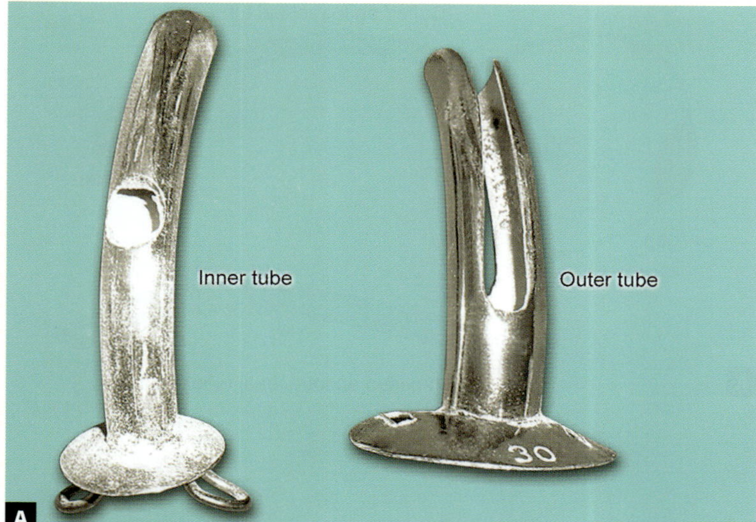

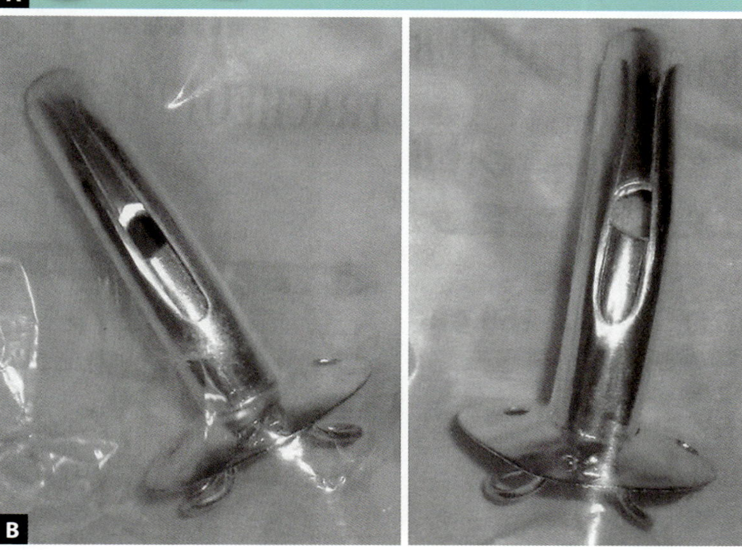

Figs. 5-134A and B: Fuller's biflanged tracheostomy tube. It is made up of German silver. Outer biflanged tube is compressible and so acts like a tracheal dilator. Inner tube is longer than outer tube with opening on the convex part which allows phonation and re-education during decannulation. Inner tube can be removed out cleaned properly and can be replaced again with ease. Tracheostomy opening in the neck when blocked with finger, patency of airway and phonation can be checked.

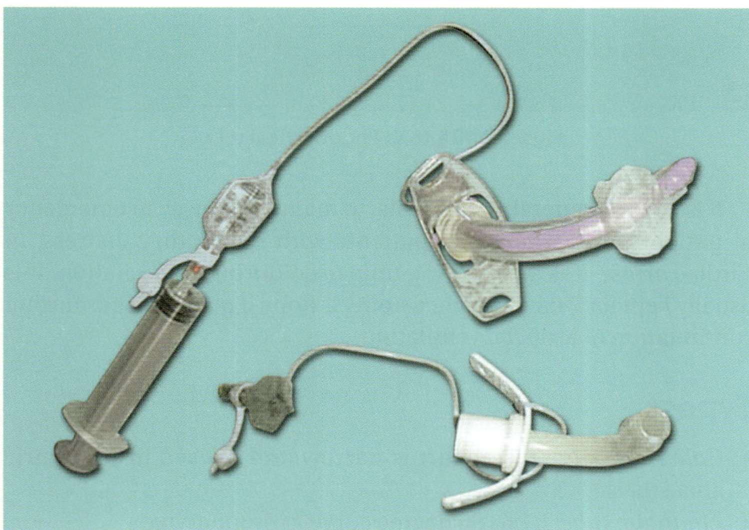

Fig. 5-135: Synthetic disposable tracheostomy tube. Usually number 8.0 or 8.5 is used.

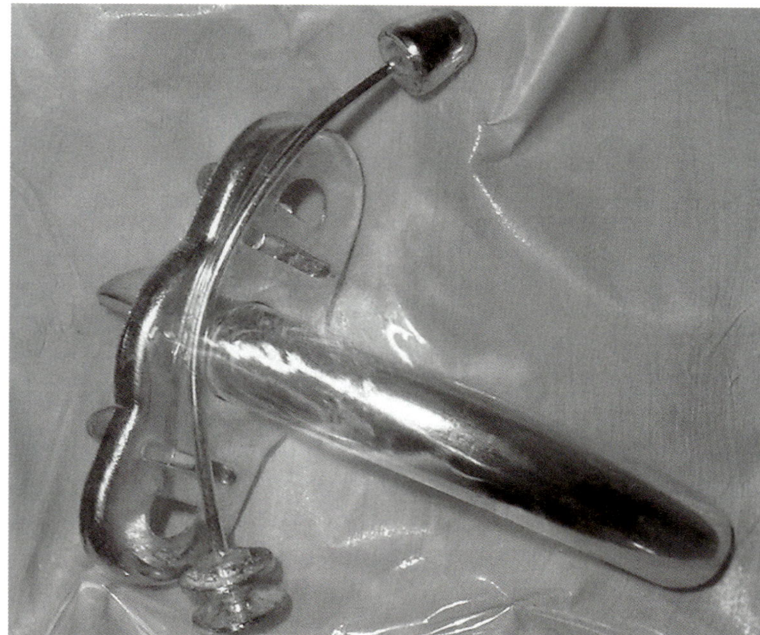

Fig. 5-136: Chevalier Jackson's tracheostomy tube.

2. *Jackson's tracheostomy tube:* It has got outer tube, inner tube and an obturator. Outer tube has got lock mechanism for inner tube with holes on either side for straps and shield for protection. Inner tube is longer than outer tube. Obturator guides insertion of tube. It is not used in radiotherapy. With tube in place patient cannot speak.
3. *Red-rubber tracheostomy tube.*
4. *PVC tracheostomy tube.*

Modern tracheostomy tubes are made of plastic. They are soft, least irritant and disposable. They have inflatable cuff which makes it easier to give assisted ventilation. Cuff should be deflated at regular intervals to prevent pressure necrosis of trachea (For assisted ventilation endotracheal tube can be kept for 7 days. Beyond that period patient needs tracheostomy for further ventilation).

Indications for tracheostomy:

- In head, neck and facial injuries.
- Tetanus.
- Tracheomalacia after thyroidectomy.
- Laryngeal oedema/spasm.
- Major head and neck surgeries like commando's operation, block dissection, etc.

TRACHEAL DILATOR (TROUSSEAU'S)

Here blades open up while approximating the handle. Blades have got club shaped blunt tip. It is used to dilate the tracheal opening during tracheostomy and to keep it open while introducing the tracheal dilator (**Figs. 5-137A and B**).

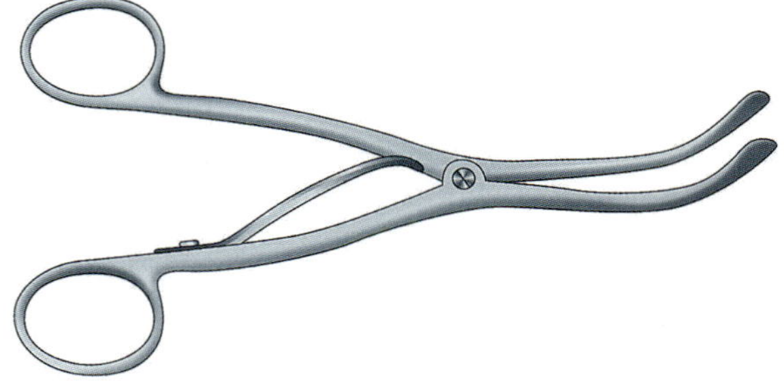

Fig. 5-137A

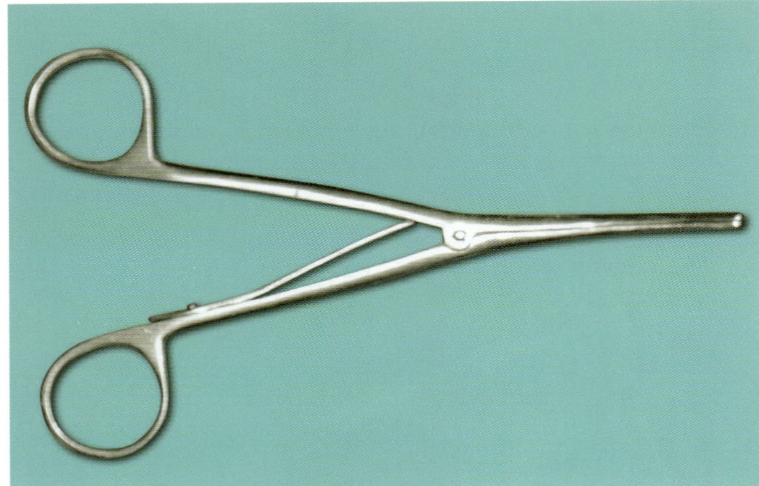

Fig. 5-137B

Figs. 5-137A and B: Tracheal dilator.

TRACHEAL HOOK

It is single blunt hook/sharp hook with a handle which is used to stabilise the trachea, retract strap muscles and isthmus during tracheostomy by placing under the cricoid to pull it upwards. Sharp hook is used to stabilise the trachea. Blunt hook is used to retract strap muscles **(Fig. 5-138)**.

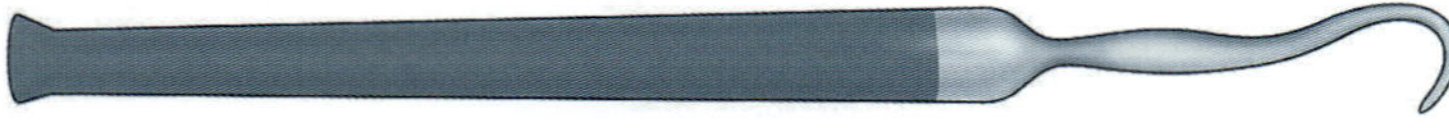

Fig. 5-138: Tracheal hook.

CRICOID HOOK

It has got thin shaft and two curved prongs at the end of the blade with a handle. It is used to retract the isthmus during tracheostomy **(Fig. 5-139)**.

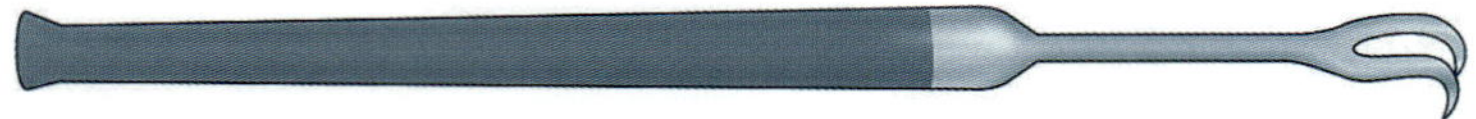

Fig. 5-139: Cricoid hook.

ENDOTRACHEAL TUBE

It is a gently curved tube used to pass into the trachea via the nasal/oral route. It is made up of India rubber or portex. It may be cuffed or non-cuffed (plain). Cuff is present on the distal part of the tube which is inflated using air through a fine tube present on the body of the endotracheal tube. Small pilot balloon on the proximal part is present to check the tension of the cuff. Cuff prevents aspiration and air leak. Capacity of the cuff is 4 ml and often tip is radiopaque. When non-cuffed tube is used, ribbon gauze should be packed around it to protect airway from aspiration. Its distal end is beveled—38 degrees towards left as tube is passed from the right angle of the mouth of the patient. It has got a thick black mark which should pass just beyond the vocal cords. Cuff should be 3 cm beyond vocal cords in adult and 1 cm beyond vocal cords in infants. Different sized tubes are available depending on age of the patient. Number 6.5 to 8.0 in females and 8.0 to 9.5 in males are used. Styllet is often used while passing the endotracheal tube for easy intubation **(Figs. 5-140A to C)**.

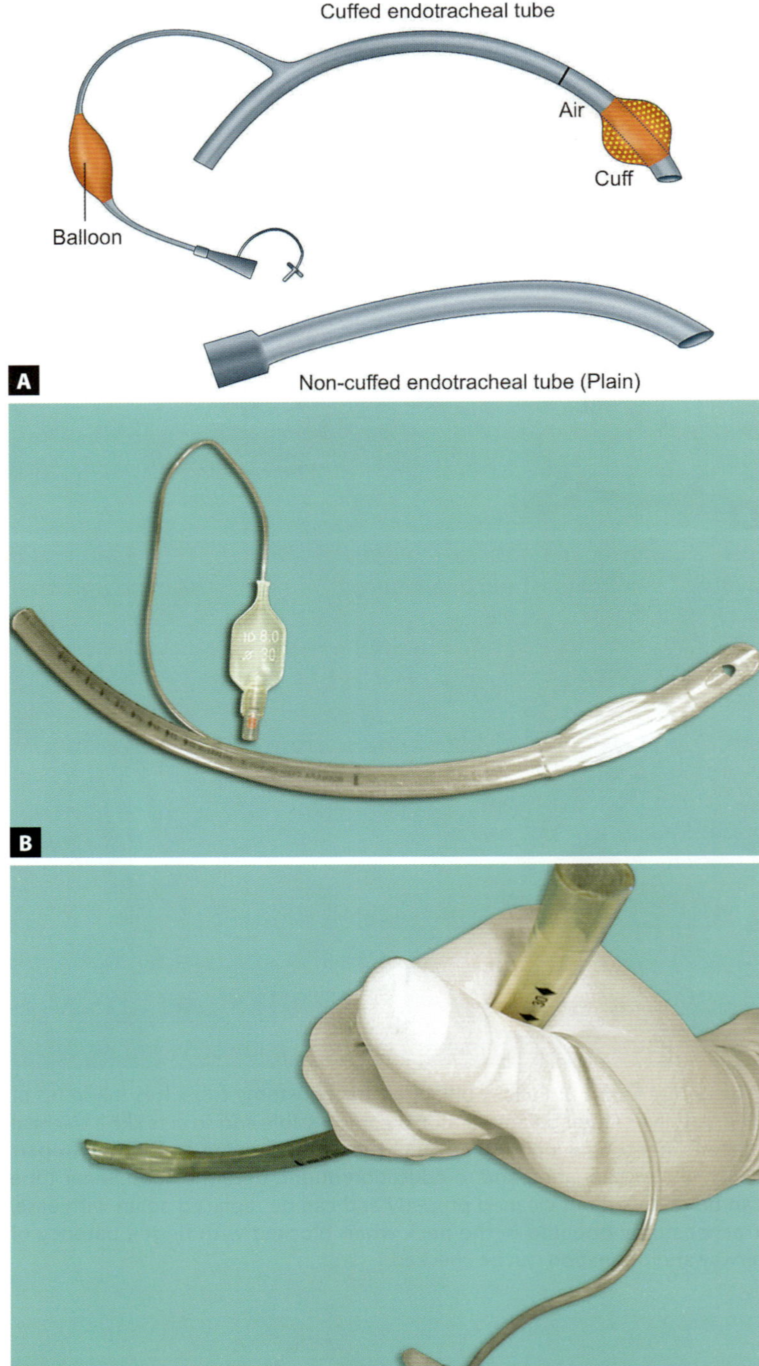

Figs. 5-140A to C: Endotracheal tube.

It is used in general anaesthesia, to maintain airway in emergency in patients with trauma, in patients with respiratory distress, in cardiac arrest. It is a life-saving tube used during resuscitation. It is usually kept for 7 days. Tracheostomy is done if patient needs further continuation of artificial ventilation.

Types

- *Cole tube:* Here distal part is narrow and is used in paediatric anaesthesia.
- *Lindholm tube:* It has 90 degree curve at oropharynx.
- *Rae preformed tracheal tube:* There is bending in the part of the tube that remains outside. It can be oral or nasal bends.

- *Spiral embedded/armoured/reinforced*: Middle segment of the tube is spirally embedded with nylon/metal filaments to make it resistant for kinking and tolerable in high pressure.
- *Endotrol tube* has got cable like mechanism to have a control over the tip.
- *Hi-low jet three*—lumen tracheal tube with main lumen for ventilation, second for jet ventilation, suctioning, oxygenation and bronchoscopy, third one for irrigation and sampling from trachea.
- *Laser shield endotracheal tube* which is made up of silicon with impregnation of metal particles.
- *Oxford endotracheal tube*: Here 2 cm of nasal end of the tube is bent at 90 degrees and is used in cleft lip and cleft palate surgeries.

Complications of Endotracheal Tube

- Oesophageal intubation—most dangerous and should be identified by ventilation, auscultation, absence of vapour in the proximal part of the tube. It should be removed and reintroduced immediately.
- Trauma to oral/nasal/pharynx/larynx.
- Right sided intubation as right bronchus is shorter, wider than left and it is in line with tracheal lumen. Left side will not get ventilated in this situation.
- Bronchial obstruction/aspiration.
- Infection—bronchopneumonia, septicaemia.
- Kinking, blocking of the tube.
- Tracheal dilatation/erosion.
- Inadvertent extubation/difficult extubation.
- Laryngeal/pharyngeal oedema, laryngitis.
- Vocal cord dysfunction/laryngeal or tracheal narrowing.

DIRECT LARYNGOSCOPE

It is to visualise larynx; consists of a handle and blade. Handle contains batteries as light source. Blade can be straight or curved and detachable. It contains an illuminating bulb at the tip. Light gets on only when blade is straightened when ready for use when it comes in contact with handle.

Macintosh blade is commonly used which is curved with a flange to push the tongue to opposite side. Blade is designed for right hander to push the tongue towards left. For left hander separate laryngoscope with blades are used. Bulb at the blade comes in contact with handle once blade is opened right angle to cause illumination. Fibreoptic laryngoscope is brighter with bulb in the handle so that bulb falling into oropharynx or larynx is prevented. Tip of the blade is used to press vallecula so that epiglottis gets lifted to view the glottis. Blades may be small, medium, large or extra large **(Figs. 5-141A and B)**.

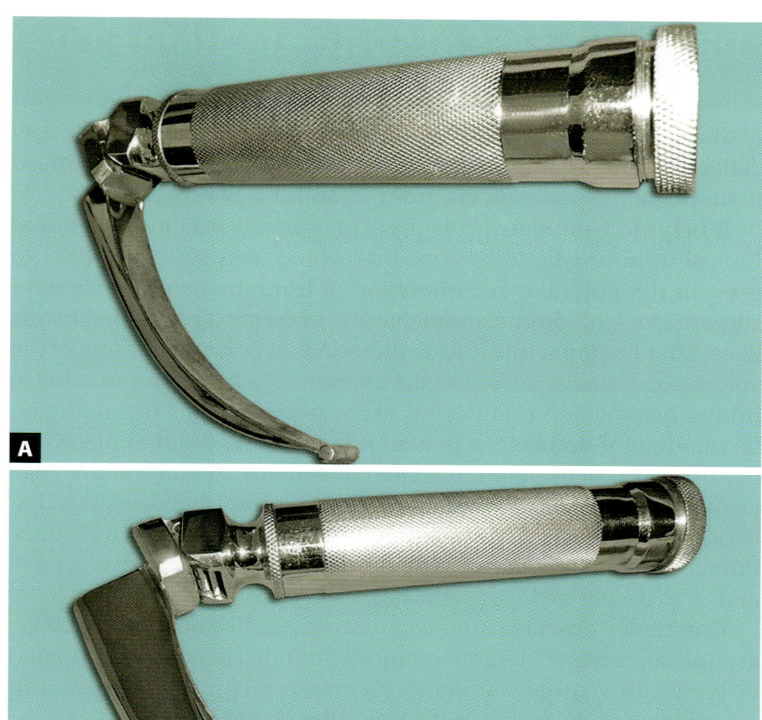

Figs. 5-141A and B: Macintosh laryngoscope.

Miller blade: It consists of straight blade which is used in children and in difficult cases with tip passing behind the epiglottis to view glottis. Miller blades are available as 0, 1, 2, 3 and 4.

Problems: Trauma to oropharynx, tachycardia, hypertension, arrhythmias. Inadvertent loosening of the bulb and falling into oropharynx or larynx is real risk.

MAGILL'S FORCEPS

It is long, sidewise angulated with fenestrated blades with rings in the handle without ratchets. Angulation helps while using in proper vision of oropharynx. It is used to assist in endotracheal intubation, nasotracheal intubation, removal of dentures, teeth, foreign body from the oropharynx in anaesthetised patient. It is used to pass nasogastric tube under vision in anaesthetised patient. Oropharyngeal packing is done under vision using Magill's forceps **(Figs. 5-142A and B)**.

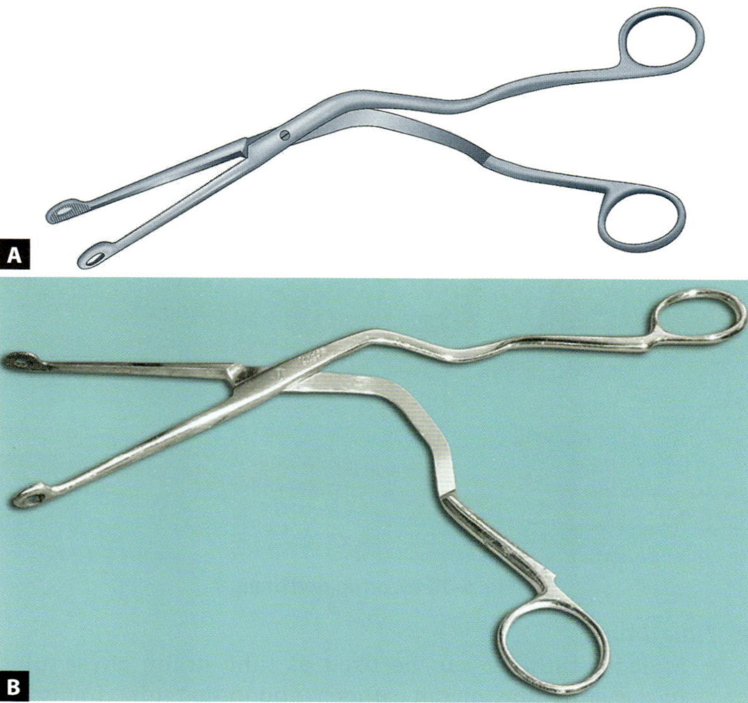

Figs. 5-142A and B: Magill's forceps.

DRAINS (PLEASE ALSO REFER CHAPTER 18, PAGE NO. 594)

A drain is a device which creates a channel which allows any collected fluid to come out after closure of the main wound. It is used to drain fluid, blood, pus, etc. from wounds or cavities.

It helps to eliminate dead space; to evacuate existing accumulation of fluid or gas; to remove pus, blood, serous, chyle, bile; to prevent the potential accumulation of fluid or gas probably after surgery like laparotomy, thoracotomy; to create a controlled fistula like—after common bile duct exploration. Accurate recording of the volume of drainage as well as the contents are important to achieve proper healing and monitor for excessive bleeding. Depending on the amount of drainage, a patient may have the drain in place one day to weeks. Signs of new infection or copious amounts of drainage are a warning sign. Open drains will have protective dressings that need to be changed daily or as required. Red rubber drains induce immense tissue reaction and often may be helpful to create a track and so to isolate cavities (peritoneal cavity in biliary drainage).

Criteria for drainage are—septic surgeries like abscess drainage, aseptic surgeries with large quantity fluid discharge is anticipated or wider area surgery is done; to create a controlled fistula; in anticipation of the anastomotic leak **(Figs. 5-143A to C)**.

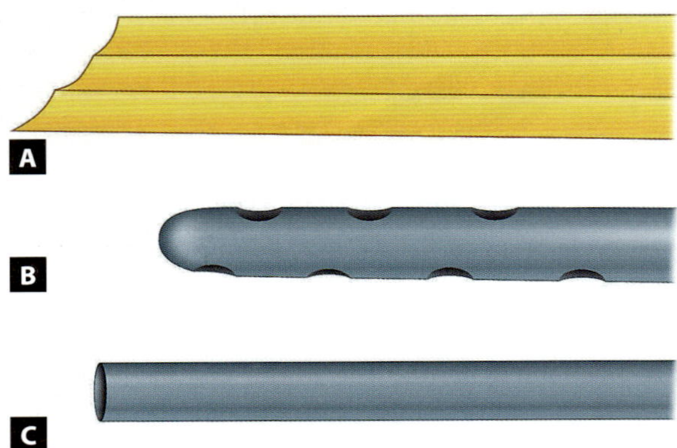

Figs. 5-143A to C: Drains: (A) Corrugated rubber drains; (B) Multiple perforated drains; (C) Tube drain.

Types

1. *Corrugated rubber drain:* It drains by capillary action and gravity. It is cheaper and technically easier. But it allows soakage of dressings and causes discomfort to the patient **(Fig. 5-144)**.

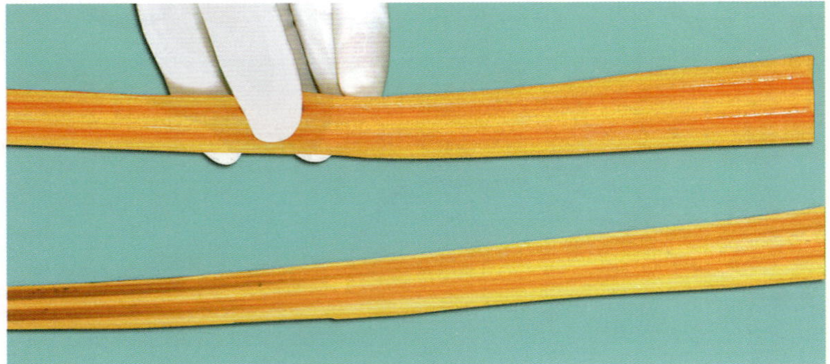

Fig. 5-144: Corrugated drain.

2. *Tube drains:*
   - Malecot catheter can be used as tube drain; chest tube, nasogastric tube, pigtail catheter, abdominal tube drains are other examples.
   - Penrose soft latex rubber tube **(Fig. 5-145)**
   - Multiple perforated tubes
3. *Closed suction tube drain system*—JP drain, Redivac drain.
4. *Glove drain-* glove finger is used as a drain.
5. *Wick drain* is a gauze drain to drain pus, discharge, etc.

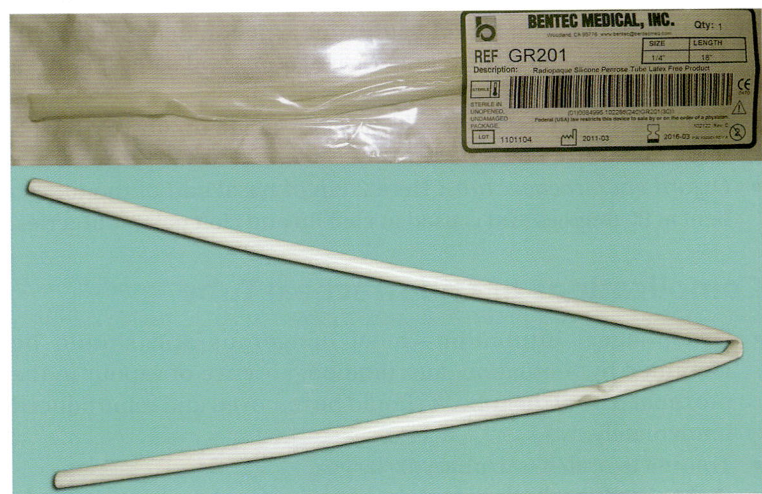

Fig. 5-145: Penrose drain—a tube drain.

Advantages of tube drains

- Quantity of fluid like bile, pus can be measured.
- It can be kept for longer time.
- Skin excoriation will not occur.
- Patient will be more comfortable.
- Infection rate is less.
- Removal is easier.
- Dye can be injected and cavity or communication can be assessed using 'C-arm'.

Classification of Drain System

- *Open (static) drains:* Corrugated drain, Penrose drain (soft latex rubber tubing). Infection rate is higher.
- *Closed siphon drains:* Here drain is connected to a sterile bag with or without one-way valve. It reduces the infection.
- *Closed suction drain:* Here negative pressure of –100 to –500 mmHg is used to create vacuum to drain the secretions.
- *Sump suction drain:* Here negative suction with a parallel air-vent is used to prevent the adjacent soft tissues being sucked into the lumen of the drain.
- *Under water seal drain* to drain pleural space.

Drains may be open or closed: Corrugated drains are open types. They drain by gravity and capillary action. It may cause entry of infection into the inside cavity. Blockage, improper drainage may be problem. Closed drains are tube drains—different tube drains are available with different size and texture. Usually 24 number tube is used in cavities. But finally selection is done depending on the anatomical location, type of surgery, cavities and anticipation of the drainage.

Drain may be active or passive: Active drains are connected to a suction system. It drains fluid completely; it prevents entry of infection; it promotes healing faster; it eliminates the dead space. But it may injure the tissues adjacent which may get sucked in. Passive drains are equally effective but are gravity dependent (like intercostal and abdominal tube drains) and so may get blocked/clogged.

Different drains are:

Jackson-Pratt drain (JP drain, brain drain, 1972) is a closed suction device consists of a perforated round or flat tube connected to a negative pressure collection device which is a bulb with a drainage port which can be opened to remove fluid or air. After compressing the bulb to remove fluid or air, negative pressure is created as the bulb returns to its normal shape. It is used in surgeries of abdomen, breast, brain, joints, etc. **(Figs. 5-146A to C)**.

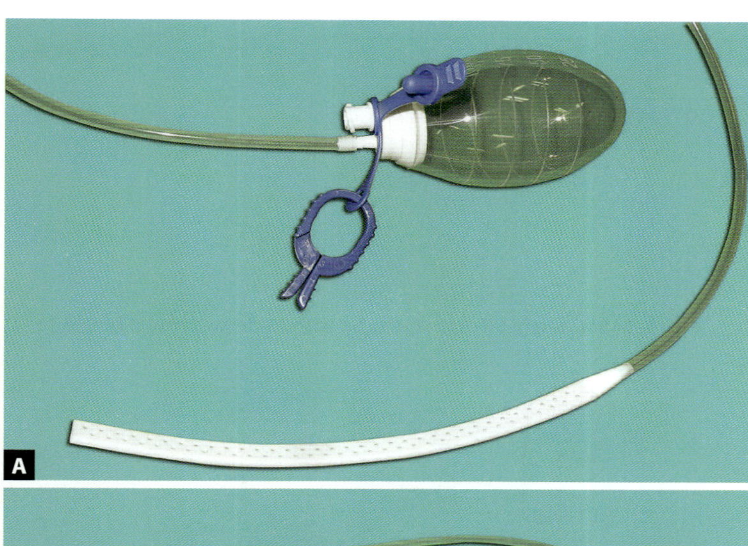

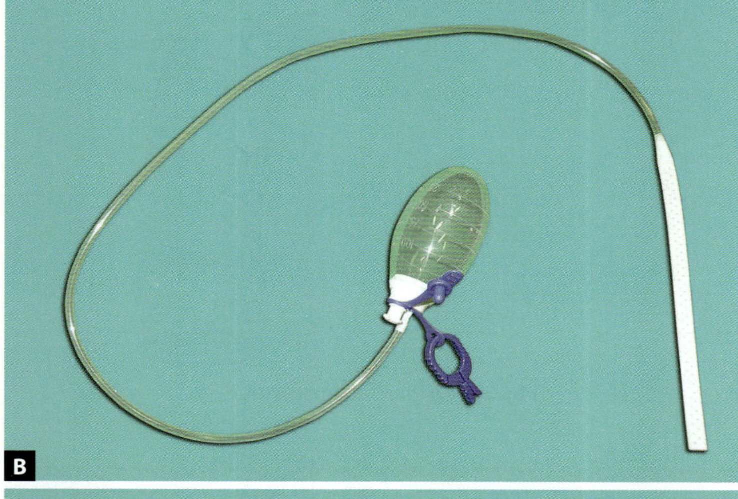

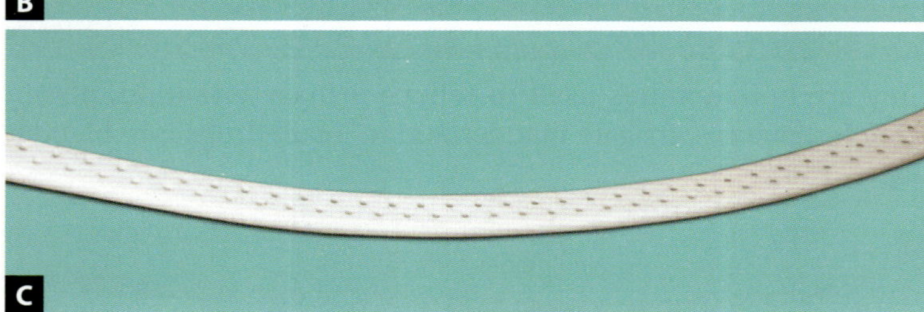

Figs. 5-146A to C: Jackson-Pratt suction drain.

Blake drain: It is a round silicone tube with channels to carry fluid to a negative pressure collecting system. Drainage is achieved by capillary action, allowing fluid to travel through the open grooves into a closed cross section, which contains the fluid and allows it to be suctioned. *Vacuum therapy:* It is a negative pressure suction wound therapy which creates a closed system using foam and through which a tube is made to pass outside which is connected to suction device. It is used in open wounds, large ulcers. Suctioning is done initially continuously and later intermittently; after 4–6 days. Wound dressing and foam is removed to inspect the area. This method allows rapid formation of the granulation tissues.

Pigtail drain tube (pigtail): It is a type of catheter that removes unwanted body fluids from an organ, duct or cavities. Pigtail drains are inserted under strict radiological guidance to ensure correct positioning. A pigtail is a sterile, thin, long, universal catheter with a locking tip that once inserted and adjusted by the radiologist forms a pigtail shape. A guide wire is also part of the sterile insertion kit. The tip of the pigtail has several holes to facilitate the drainage. The open end of the catheter has an outlet, which is compatible with an intravenous (IV) Luer lock. Pigtails are inserted percutaneously under guidance (USG or CT usually by a radiologist). It is used in nephrostomy, draining fluid or abscess from organs like liver, draining pus or fluid from cavities like in postoperative situation or from biliary system, etc.

Davol drain: It is a soft, supple silicone with X-ray opaque strip. It minimises the trauma and blockage. Drains have a triple lumen configuration; large center lumen for maximum removal; filtered air vent helps reduce risk of infection; third lumen allows irrigation and instillation of medication. 0.3 micron antibacterial filter removes virtually all bacteria from incoming air. Suture cuff helps fasten drain.

Redivac drain: Redivac drain is a close system drain with many holes at the end of a fine tube(s); it is connected to an evacuated glass bottle providing suction. It is used to drain blood beneath the skin, e.g. after mastectomy or thyroidectomy, or from deep spaces, e.g. around a vascular anastomosis **(Figs. 5-147A and B)**.

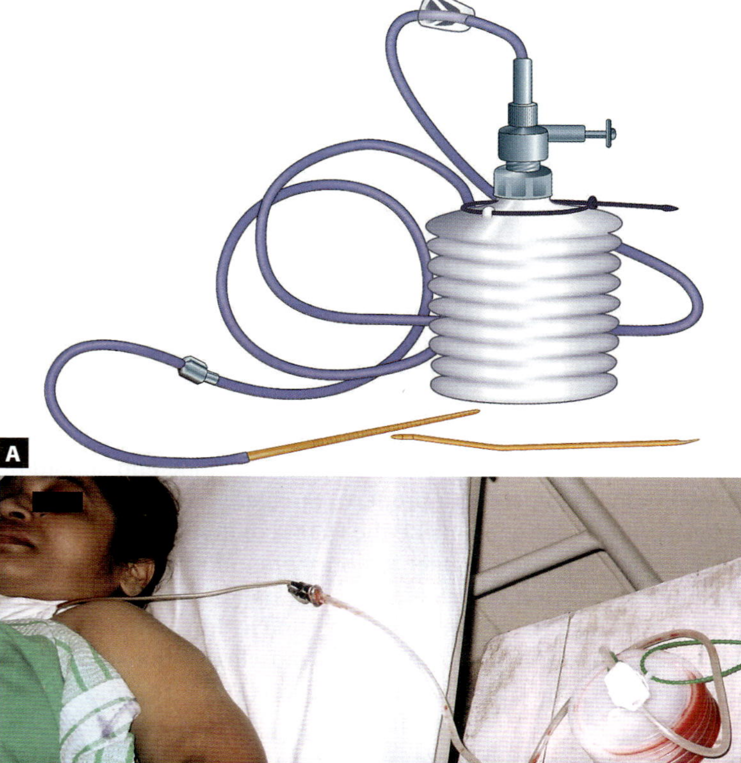

Figs. 5-147A and B: Romovac suction drain. Here suction is created by pressing the suction corrugation. There is a sharp metallic introducer to pass the tube into the required area after puncturing the skin. It is used for thyroidectomy, mastectomy, radical dissection, wide excisions, flap surgeries, etc.

Indications for Drains

- In drainage of an abscess.
- In bleeding surgical conditions like trauma, per-operative bleed.
- In haemothorax, pyothorax or pneumothorax.
- In acute abdominal conditions like peritonitis, haemoperitoneum.
- In major abdominal surgeries like of pancreas, biliary tree, stomach etc.
- In thyroid surgery.
- In hydrocele surgery.

Problems in Drains

- Infection through the drain.
- Displacement, discomfort, pain.
- It may not drain adequately and can give false information—failure of functioning.
- It may interfere with healing process inside.

Presently keeping a drain itself is a question of debate and controversy all over. Older dictum was 'when in doubt keep a drain and the surgeon can sleep happily'—is questioned at present.

Drains if not used properly may be counterproductive.

Note:

- A drain should be placed always in most dependent position and should be brought out through shortest straight route with a separate stab incision. It should be anchored to skin securely. Corrugated drain should be kept with adequate length otherwise it may get into the abdominal cavity during phases of respiration.
- Drain is removed once amount of drain output becomes minimal or less than 25 mL. Drain is removed by gentle pull after cutting the anchoring suture. After thyroidectomy it is kept for 24 hours; after mastectomy it is kept for 5 days; T tube is removed in 10–14 days. Abdominal drains are removed in 5–7 days. It may be kept for longer time in pancreatic and biliary surgeries probably to create a safe fistula. Drain can be shortened and removed; usually it is cut 2 cm daily.

INTERCOSTAL DRAINAGE TUBE

It is made up of portex with proximal end having multiple holes which is inserted into the pleural space. Other end is connected to a glass tube the tip of which is dipped inside the under water bottle which allows the expulsion of air outside. This tube end should be dipped in the water column properly. Smaller glass tube often bent in between is not dipped inside the water column which allows the air to go out. It is used in haemothorax/pneumothorax/empyema/after thoracic/oesophageal surgeries. In haemothorax/empyema, chest tube is inserted in the midaxillary line in 6th intercostal space. It is easier to pass the tube in this line as muscles are thin and patient will be comfortable if tube is in this position **(Fig. 5-148)**.

PAUL'S DRAINAGE TUBE

It is a bent glass tube with two ends. Edge with two collars is passed through the enterotomy into the intestine and fixed with a purse string suture. End with a single collar is attached to a rubber tube to remove the bowel contents from distended bowel. It is not used now **(Fig. 5-149)**.

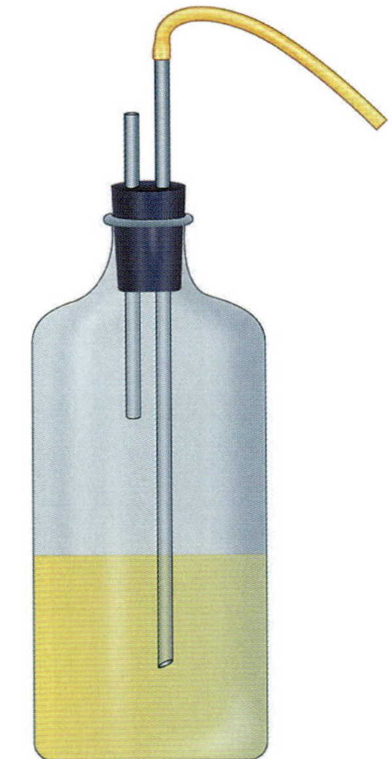

Fig. 5-148: Intercostal drainage tube with underwater seal bottle.

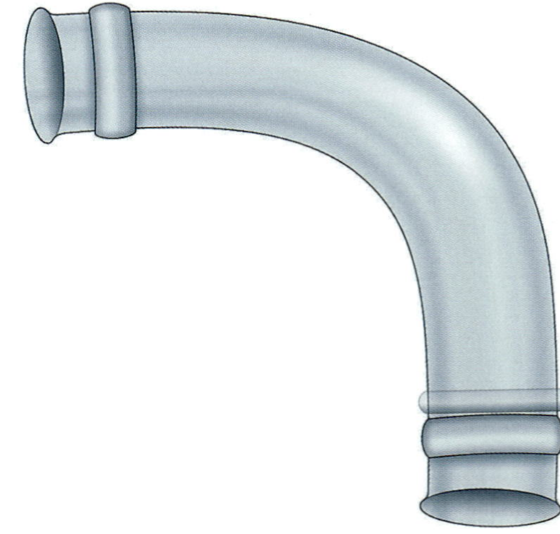

Fig. 5-149: Paul's drainage tube.

CATHETERS

They are hollow tubes used to relieve urinary retention, obtain urine for analysis, irrigate bladder and to instill drugs into bladder **(Fig. 5-150)**.

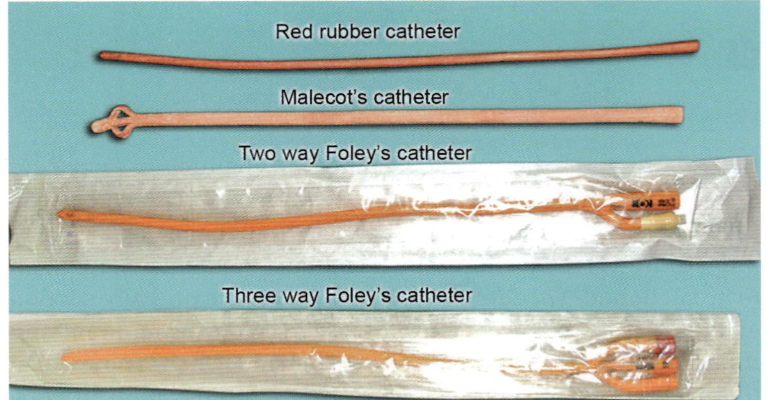

Fig. 5-150: Different urinary catheters—non-self-retaining red rubber catheter; self-retaining Malecot's catheter; self-retaining Foley's catheter.

India rubber catheter	Latex rubber	Metal catheters	Polyethylene catheters
◈ Red in color contains high sulphur ◈ Heat resistant ◈ Causes more irritation	◈ Softer, smooth, less irritant ◈ Can be kept for long time ◈ Sterilised by boiling, autoclave or gamma radiation	◈ Female and male catheters are different ◈ Used in difficult catheterisation ◈ To empty bladder prior to vaginal hysterectomy	◈ Transparent and stiffer **Gum elastic catheters** ◈ From gum resins with cotton/silk impregnated ◈ Formalin vapor sterilisation ◈ Boiling or autoclave cannot be done ◈ Not used now

Uses

- To pass per urethrally in retention of urine of any cause [BPH, stricture, trauma).
- To measure the urine output in renal failure, postoperative patients and terminally ill patients, and patients under critical care.
- After prostatectomy or TURP—three way catheter is used for irrigation also. Here it is also used as haemostatic by inflating more distilled water into the balloon and giving traction causing tamponade effect.
- Paraplegia/neurogenic bladder—initially Foley's catheter is used later condom drainage is better.
- To give bladder wash in haematuria, infection, etc.
- Percutaneous suprapubic cystostomy.
- Cholecystostomy.
- To drain fistulas.
- To control bleeding from nostrils/post-haemorrhoidectomy secondary haemorrhage.
- In children to give enema or to do barium/contrast enema X-rays.
- In obstructed labour, during caesarean section surgery, prior to abdominal hysterectomy (for 1 day), at the end of vaginal hysterectomy (for 5 days), post-partum haemorrhage, during abortion often.
- To check cervical incompetence 8 F Foley's catheter is used.
- After vesicovaginal fistula repair it is kept for 14–21 days.
- After Wertheim's operation it is kept for 14 days.
- After bladder injury repair it is kept for 10–14 days.

Types

- *Nonself-retaining catheter:* Simple red rubber catheter.
- *Self-retaining catheter:* Foley's catheter, Malecot's catheter, Gibbon's catheter, De-Pezzer catheter.

Types of Catheterisation

a. *Indwelling catheterisation:* When a catheter is left behind in bladder and remains so it is called an indwelling catheter.
   It is achieved by:
   - Balloon tip of catheter
   - Foley's catheter
   - Flower tip of catheter
   - Malecot's catheter, De-Pezzers
   - Strapping catheter externally
   - Gibbon's catheter.

b. *Intermittent catheterisation:* A sterile catheter is introduced intermittently by the patient or by others.

FOLEY'S CATHETER (FREDRICK EUGENE BASIL FOLEY, AMERICAN UROLOGIST)

It is a *self-retaining* urinary catheter made up of *latex*. It has got a balloon near the tip into which distilled water is infused to make it *self-retainable*. Usually Foley's catheter is kept for 7 days. It is *sterilised* by radiation **(Fig. 5-151).**

Size:	Adults	16 F.
	Children	8 F or 10 F.

(**F**—*French unit, Charriere unit, where each unit equals 0.33 mm).* 16 F means circumference of the catheter is 16 mm. Diameter is on-third of circumference).

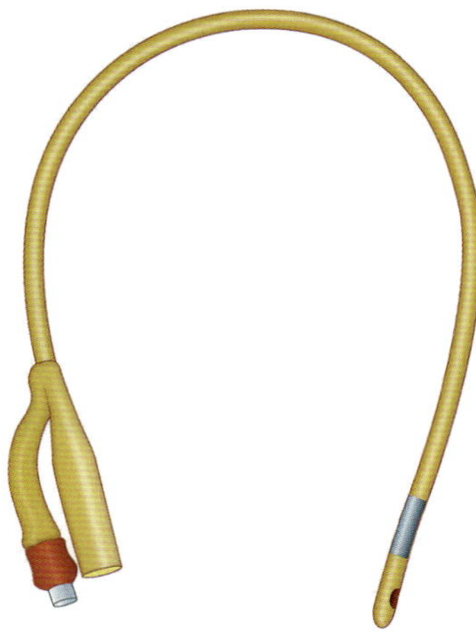

Fig. 5-151: Foley's catheter.

Types

1. Two-way Foley's **(Fig. 5-152A).**
2. Three-way Foley's: To give bladder irrigation, e.g. following TURP **(Fig. 5-152B).**
3. Silicon coated Foley's: To reduce reaction and so as to keep for longer period (3 months).

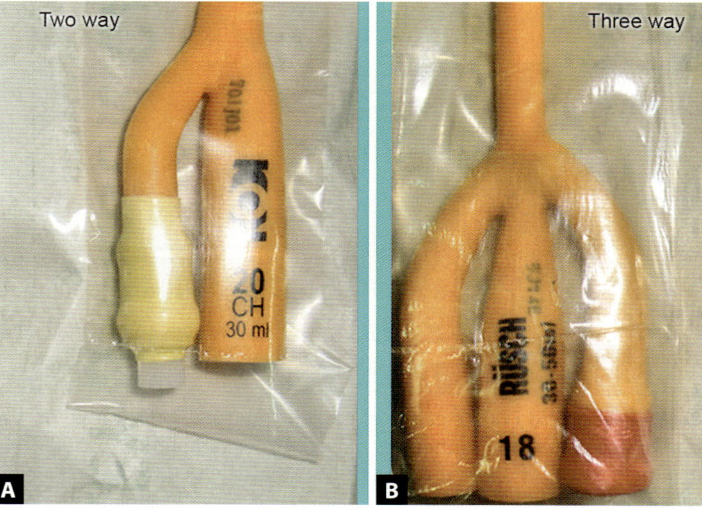

Figs. 5-152A and B: (A) Two-way Foley' and (B) Three-way Foley's catheters.

Procedure

After cleaning under strict asepsis, lignocaine gel is lubricated into the urethral meatus. Catheter is passed into the urethra. Sometimes *Maryfield introducer* is used to pass Foley's catheter. Once catheter is in the bladder, urine will flow out. It is now connected to an *urosac bag* **(Fig. 5-153)**. Balloon is inflated with 20–30 mL (amount is written on the catheter) of distilled water to make it self-retainable. During removal of the catheter same amount of water should be removed from the balloon before pulling out the catheter. After passing catheter, prepucial skin should be placed backwards otherwise iatrogenic paraphimosis can develop **(Figs. 5-153 to 5-155)**.

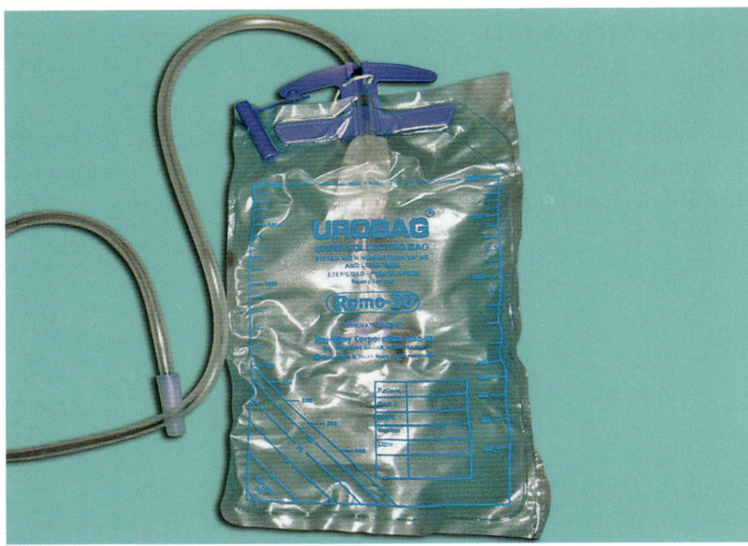

Fig. 5-153: Urosac bag.

Complications

- Infection.
- Encrustation.
- Bleeding.
- Stone formation.
- Blockage, false passage.
- Stricture.
- Difficulty in removal of the catheter due to blockage of the balloon channel. Here bulb of Foley's can be punctured from above under ultrasound guidance or ether can be injected into the balloon so as to burst it but it may cause chemical cystitis or a stilette (ureteric catheter stilette) can be passed into the channel.

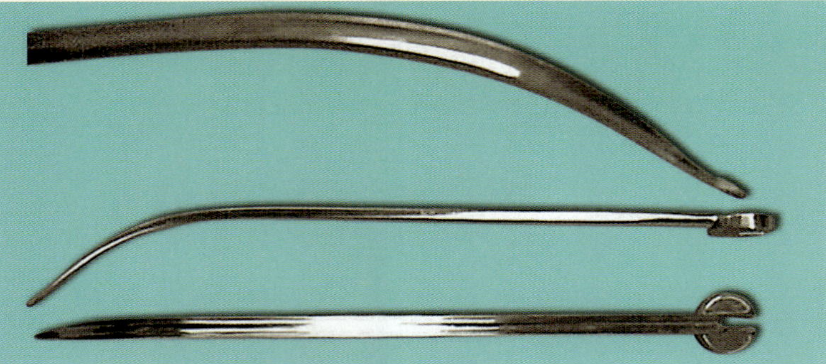

Fig. 5-154: Maryfield Foley's catheter introducer. It has got groove on the convex surface over which catheter is placed. Tip of catheter is hooked on to projection on the tip of the introducer. Once catheter with introducer is inside, introducer is released and removed retaining the catheter which is inflated adequately.

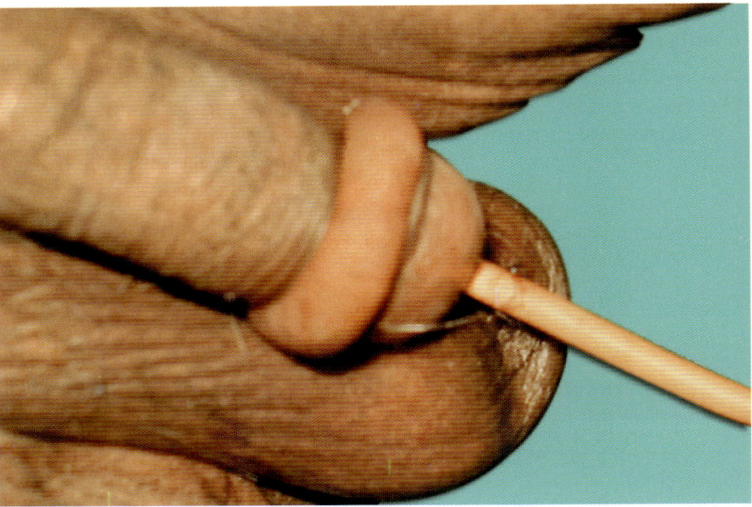

Fig. 5-155: Iatrogenic paraphimosis developed after Foley's catheterisation due to failure to place back the prepucial skin.

MALECOT'S CATHETER

It is self-retaining urinary catheter with an umbrella or flower at the tip. It is made of red rubber, contains sulphur and so it is radiopaque **(Fig. 5-156)**.

It is never introduced per urethrally. It is sterilised by boiling.

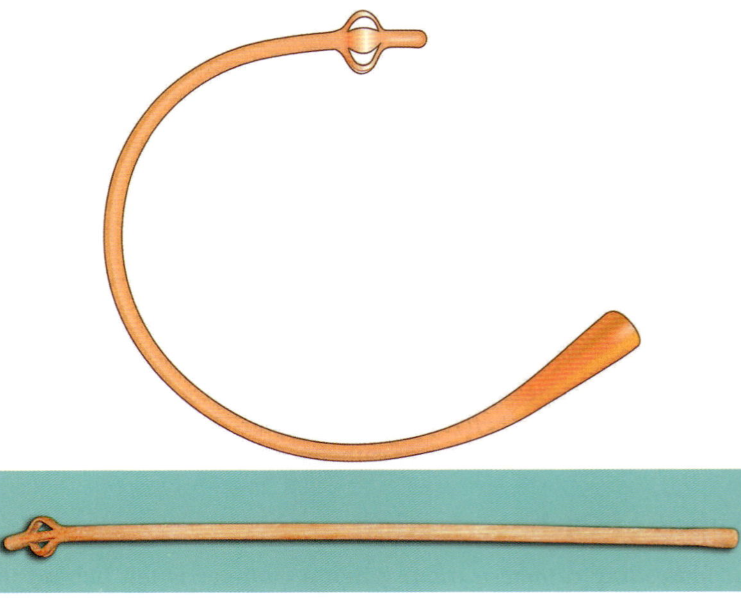

Fig. 5-156: Malecot's catheters.

Uses

- Suprapubic cystostomy (SPC):
  - In case of urinary retention when Foley's catheterisation fails (after two trials).
  - For diversion of urine following bladder, prostate or urethral surgeries.
- For continuous drainage of abscess cavities:
  - Perinephric abscess.
  - Pyonephrosis.
  - Subphrenic abscess.
  - Amoebic liver abscess.
- Cabot's nephrostomy.
- Cholecystostomy.
- Infected pseudocyst of the pancreas.
- Gastrostomy, caecostomy (tube type).

Advantages

- Malecot's catheter can be kept for a long period of time (3 months).
- It drains fluid adequately.
- Less infection rate.
- Removal is easier.

Disadvantage

Surgery (open method) is required to insert the catheter.

Suprapubic Cystostomy

It is placing of Malecot catheter into the bladder above the pubis by open method, or percutaneously under guidance using Foley's catheter. It is a temporary opening through the abdomen into the bladder.

Prerequisite: Bladder must be full and is confirmed by dullness below the umbilicus or by ultrasound.

Indication: Retention of urine when urethral catheterisation fails.

Procedure: Under local anaesthesia (Xylocaine 2% above the pubis, in the midline) or general anaesthesia, a vertical midline incision of 3 cm in length is placed through linea alba. Skin, fascia, anterior rectus sheath are incised. Recti are retracted. In extraperitoneal space, peritoneum with pad of fat is reflected upward. Bladder is identified by the pattern of detrusor muscle and vesical venous plexus and is confirmed by aspirating urine through a syringe. The bladder is opened near the fundus. Urine is aspirated. Bladder wall is inspected for any pathology. Malecot catheter is straightened using artery forceps and placed in the bladder. Sutures are placed around the Malecot catheter. Wound is closed in layers.

In percutaneous suprapubic cystostomy (SPC), Foley's catheter is passed into the bladder using trocar and cannula.

Complications

- Injury to bowel, peritoneum.
- Infection.

SIMPLE RED RUBBER CATHETER

It is a non self-retaining urinary catheter. It is stiffer than Foley's catheter. Its tip is rounded and blunt. Opening is only on the side wall (In flatus tube opening is present on both sides and also at the tip).

Here *English unit* to number: Diameter = $\frac{1 + \text{Catheter number}}{2}$ is used to **(Figs. 5-157A and B)**.

Uses:

- Used to drain urine from the bladder temporarily in retention of urine.
- To find out residual urine. After passing urine, catheter is introduced into the bladder. The amount of retained urine is measured. If it is more than 30–50 mL it signifies obstruction. It often increases more than 200 mL in conditions like BPH and indicates significant obstruction that needs surgical intervention like TURP.
- While doing cystography to infuse dilute iodine dye into the bladder.
- Single gentle passage of the red rubber catheter is tried as a diagnostic method to identify the urethral/bladder/renal injuries.

Haematuria signifies urinary tract injury. Measured normal saline is infused into the bladder and return volume is collected; if it is less, then it indicates injury to bladder.

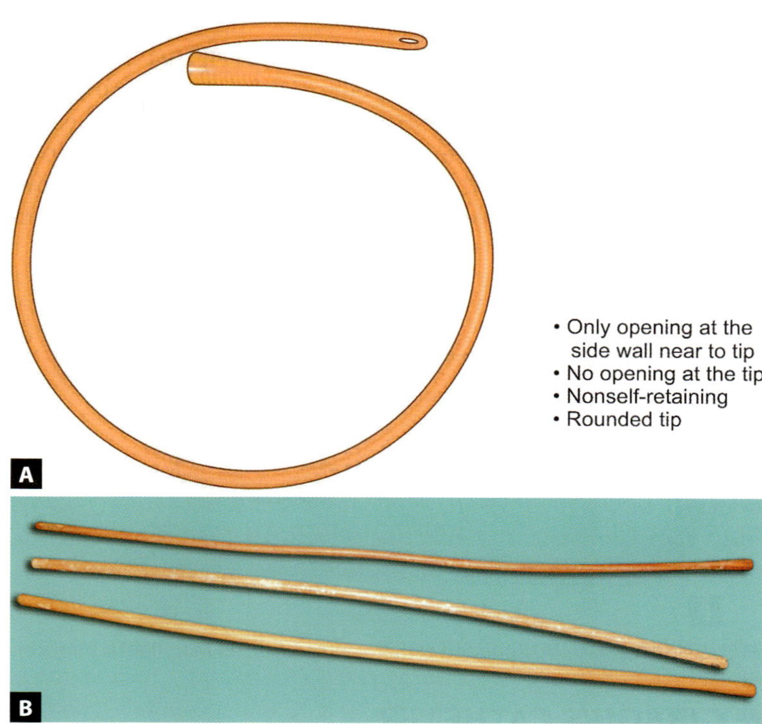

Figs. 5-157A and B: Simple nonself-retaining red rubber catheter.

- For administration of intravesical chemotherapy or therapeutic BCG infusion into the bladder per urethral in bladder carcinoma.
- To collect urine from the bladder for culture and sensitivity.
- To identify the urethra in perineal surgery/urethral surgery/penectomy.
- To dislodge and push back the calculus impacted in the urinary meatus or in the urethra.
- To administer nasal oxygen.
- For suction of throat/endotracheal tube/tracheostomy tube.
- As a tourniquet for venesection and surgeries of fingers and toes.
- Used as a sling in many places like to hold cord, to hold vagus, to hold pedicles, to hold oesophagus/bowel/ureter.
- To irrigate and clear the pus after opening the abscess cavity/or any other cavities in depth.
- To irrigate common bile duct after choledochotomy; to irrigate ureter/renal pelvis after stone removal.
- In pregnancy, labour, puerperium.
- Just prior to vaginal hysterectomy after draping to empty the bladder red rubber or female metal catheter is used.
- Often to diagnose tracheo-oesophageal fistula.

DEPEZZER'S CATHETER

It is a self-retaining catheter with a bulb at the end which makes it self-retaining. Its uses are like Malecot's catheter. It cannot be passed per urethral. Usually 24 French size is used **(Fig. 5-158)**.

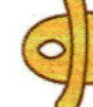

Fig. 5-158: Depezzer's catheter.

CATHETER INTRODUCER

It is used to negotiate the catheter into the urethra or in other places wherever it is used.

Two types:

- Long slender metallic type with rounded tip **(Fig. 5-159A)**.
- Maryfield introducer–it is long curved flat metallic introducer with a longitudinal groove over its convex surface over its entire length which ends at the tip as a blunt projection. This projection helps in hooking the catheter tip (Foley's catheter) and the groove accommodates the body of the catheter and prevents it from slipping away **(Fig. 5-159B)**.

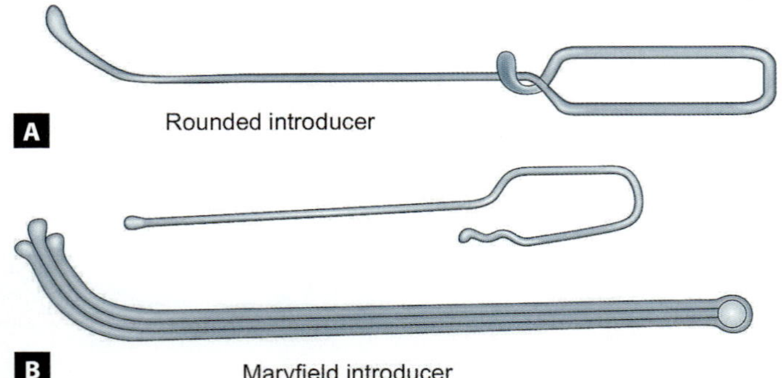

Figs. 5-159A and B: (A) Rounded catheter introducer; (B) Maryfield introducer.

GIBBON'S CATHETER

It is a self-retaining catheter made up of plastic with a stilette in it which makes its passage easier through urethra. There are different sizes for males and females because of the difference in length of the urethra in male and female. Catheter has two ribbons attached which can be used to fix to the genitalia by adhesive plaster. Gibbon's catheter is least irritant to urethra **(Fig. 5-160)**.

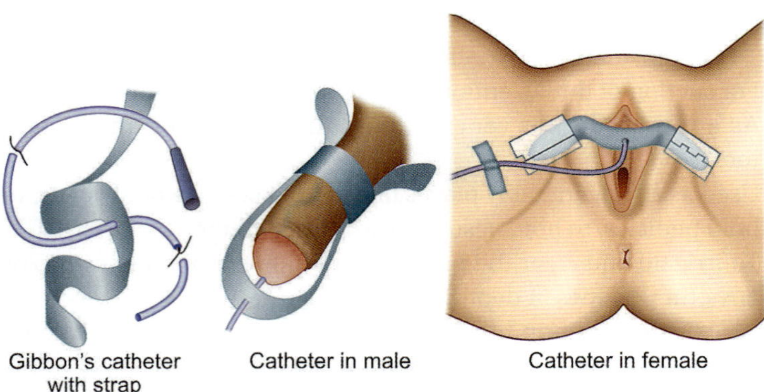

Fig. 5-160: Gibbon's catheter. Note the look and method of fixing in male and female.

TIEMANN CATHETER (FIG. 5-161)

It is made up of PVC with beaked, stiff tip. Different colour codes are used on the beaked tip for different numbers of the catheter. Side holes are located proximal to the colour codes.

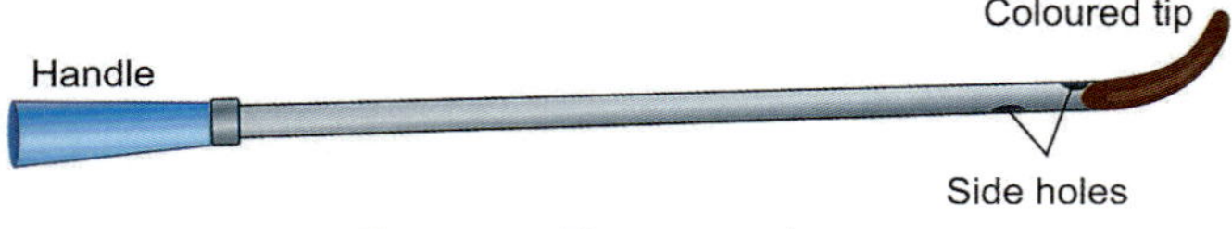

Fig. 5-161: Tiemann catheter.

No. 12—White
No. 14—Green
No. 16—Vermilon
No. 18—Red
No. 20—Yellow
No. 22—Maroon
No. 24—Blue

METAL CATHETERS

They are metal catheters which are stiff and can be passed into the urethra even if other catheters fail.

Two Types

a. *Male metal catheter:*
It is long tube with a curve at the tip. Tip is rounded and blunt with side holes. Two rings near the base help in holding the catheter. It is used to empty the bladder in retention of urine when other types of catheter fail. With prior lubrication of urethra using adequate quantity of lignocaine jelly, it is passed like a dilator with all aseptic precautions. Catheter is passed through the external meatus into the urethra. Once it reaches the bulbar urethra a resistance is felt, then handle is rotated across the inguinal ligament, groin towards the midline over to the abdomen. Sudden release of resistance is felt as catheter enters the bladder. Urine will come out of the catheter easily. Catheter will stay there firmly only if entered properly **(Fig. 5-162)**.

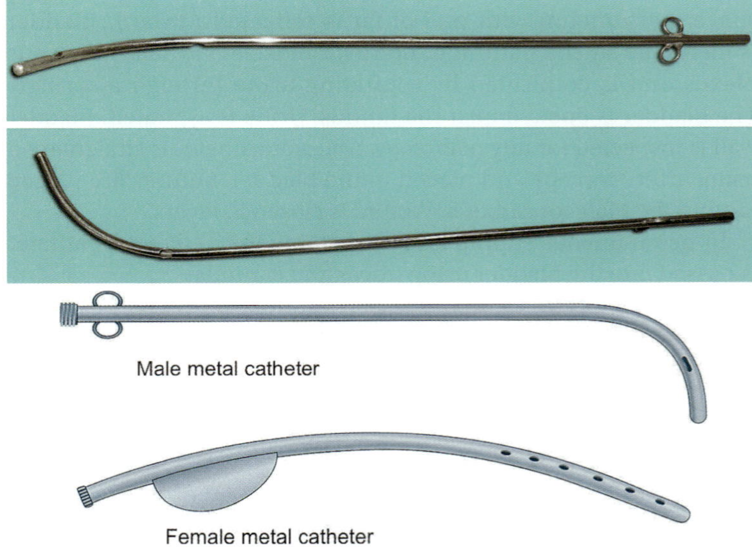

Fig. 5-162: Diagram showing male and female metal catheters.

b. *Female metal catheter:*
It is short metallic catheter. Tip is rounded with multiple side holes. It has got one flat curved handle. It is used to empty the bladder in pelvic surgeries like vaginal hysterectomy **(Fig. 5-163)**.

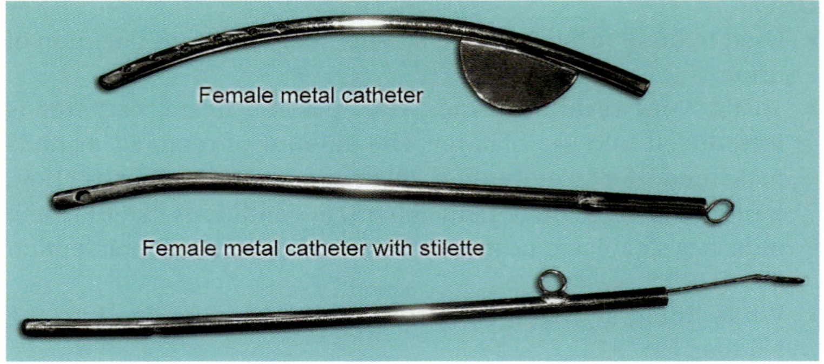

Fig. 5-163: Female metal catheter—two types are there. One can observe the stilette.

URETERIC CATHETER

It is thin slender flexible radiopaque tube of 70 cm length with a black mark at every 5 cm junction. French unit is used. 3-8 French (F) are available. Initially cystoscope is passed and under visualisation ureteric catheter is passed through ureteric orifice with a stilette. Stilette maintains the stiffness and patency of the catheter. It can be olive tipped; whistle; coude'; or open ended. It is used while doing retrograde pyelography (RGP); to collect selective urine sampling in tuberculosis; to assess and relieve the ureteric obstruction; as an ureteric stent **(Figs. 5-164A and B)**.

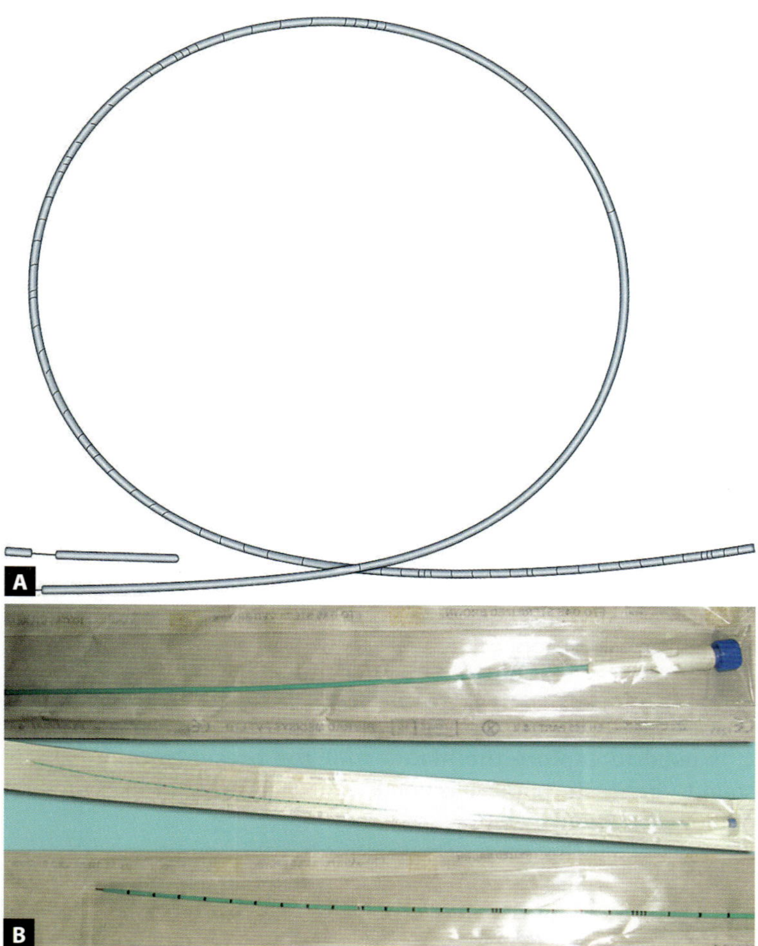

Figs. 5-164A and B: Ureteric catheters.

URETHRAL DILATORS

- Lister's dilator.
- Clutton's dilator.
- Filiform bougies.
- Gum elastic bougies.
- Olive tip bougies.
- Whip bougies.

LISTER'S URETHRAL DILATOR

It has got olive tip with a rounded handle. Handle is rounded with numbers marked. Denominator is circumference in mm at the base of the Lister's dilator **(Figs. 5-165A and B)**. Numerator signifies circumference just proximal to the olive tip (narrowest point). Difference between denominator and numerator is 3 mm. So each dilator is narrowed for 3 mm from base to proximal end of olive tip. Circumference of olive tip is equal to circumference in the base. Numbering is based on English scale (diameter in mm) = Number/2 + 1. It is used to dilate stricture urethra; to pass catheter by open rail road technique in rupture urethra.

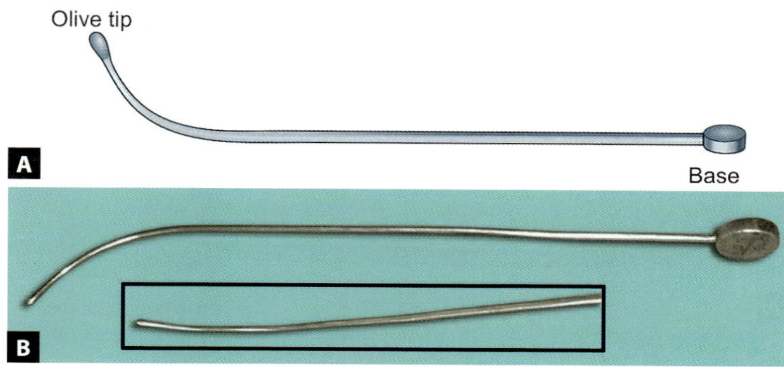

Figs. 5-165A and B: Lister's urethral dilator.

With all aseptic precautions urethral dilatation is done (proper cleaning and draping). It is done under local lignocaine jelly application or under general anaesthesia. Dilator is passed up to the bulb when a resistance is felt. Then handle is gently curved over the inguinal ligament, groin and over the abdomen towards midline. A feel of entry into the bladder is felt while entering the bladder. Once left like that dilator stays there firmly with free side-to-side movement otherwise it will fall back **(Figs. 5-166A and B)**.

Persistent pain; severe resistance and bleeding per urethra are the features to consider failure of the dilator entering into the bladder.

False passage; bleeding; infection and fistula formation are the complications of urethral dilatation.

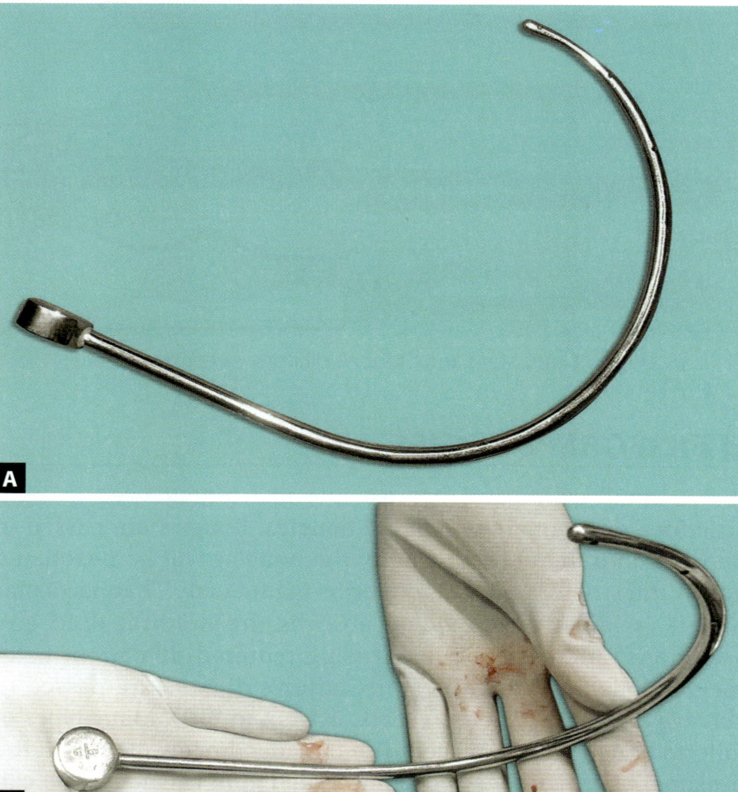

Figs. 5-166A and B: Curved urethral negotiator.

CLUTTON'S DILATOR

It is a long metallic instrument with a curve and blunt tip at the end. Handle is violin shaped. It is numbered in English units. Denominator of the part signifies the circumference in the base and numerator suggests the circumference in the tip **(Figs. 5-167 and 5-168)**. Difference between denominator and numerator is 4. Numbers are like 6/10; 8/12; 10/14—so on. Set 12 of dilators are available.

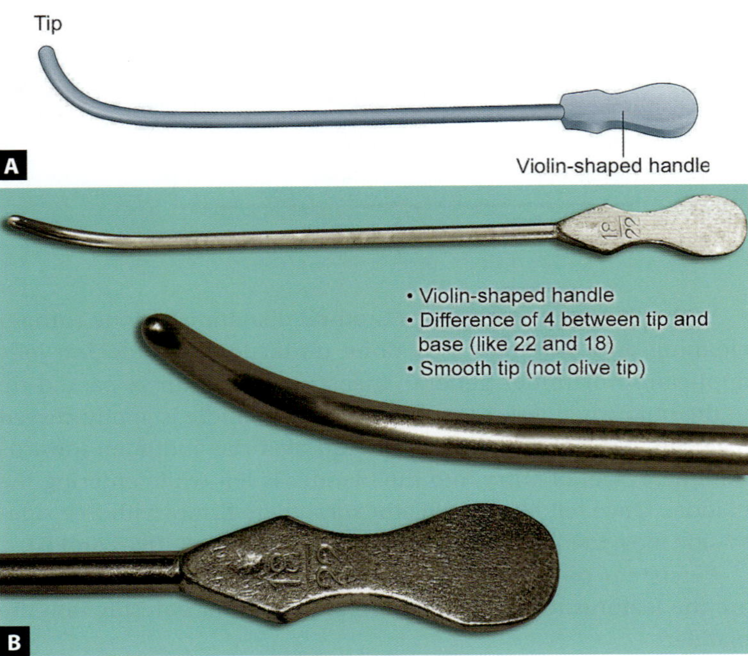

Figs. 5-167A and B: Clutton's dilator—it has violin-shaped handle.

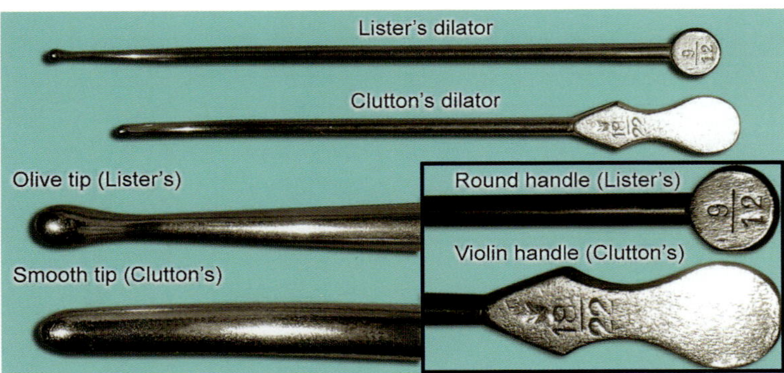

Fig. 5-168: Lister's and Clutton's dilators—a comparison.

FILIFORM BOUGIES

It is a small cylindrical hygroscopic instrument used in tight strictures to negotiate one of the bougies. Bougies are passed in bunches into the urethra. One of the bougies will be negotiated across the stricture by trial and error manoeuvre. That particular bougie is left in place which absorbs the urethral fluid and secretions; and gets swollen causing required dilatation. Later metallic dilators like Lister's or Clutton's dilators are passed to achieve adequate dilatation **(Figs. 5-169A and B)**. Many types of filiform bougies are furnished with threaded hollow mounts at the proximal ends. Larger sized screw ended gum elastic bougie can be attached to the filiform follower thread to do the subsequent dilatation.

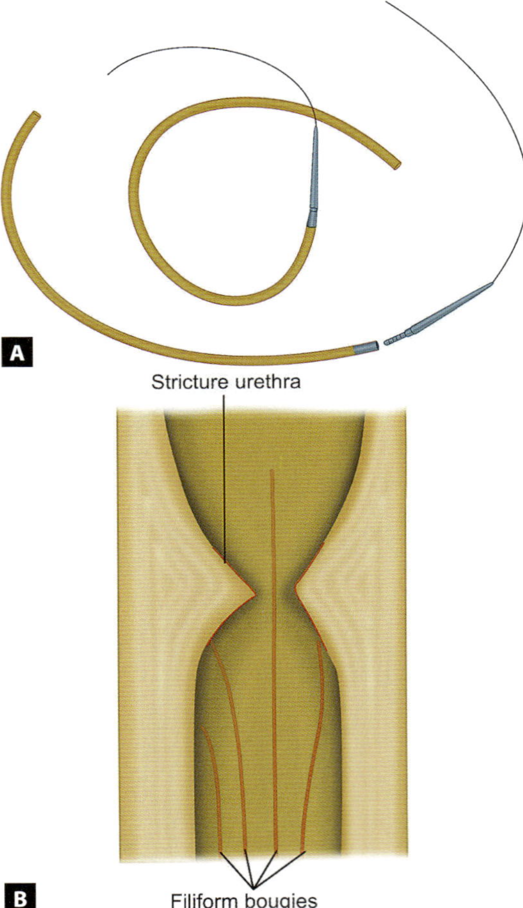

Figs. 5-169A and B: Filiform bougie with followers. One of the bougie can be negotiated through the tight strictures and which helps in further dilatation through metallic dilators.

BLADDER SOUND

It is used to explore the bladder for the presence of stones by sound—hence the name. It is not used now. It can be used as urethral dilator **(Fig. 5-170)**.

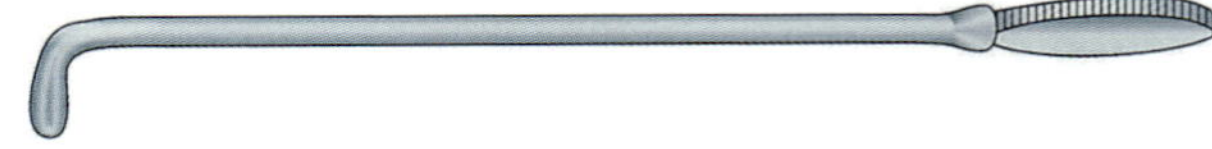

Fig. 5-170: Bladder sound.

THOMPSON-WALKER'S SUPRAPUBIC CYSTOLITHOTOMY FORCEPS

It has got a spoon shaped elongated concave blades with spikes on the inner surface which gives secure grip of the stone from the bladder. It has no ratchet. Shaft has got a ring for placement of thumb and another is curved open to place four fingers. It is used to hold and remove stones from the urinary bladder in suprapubic cystolithotomy **(Fig. 5-171)**.

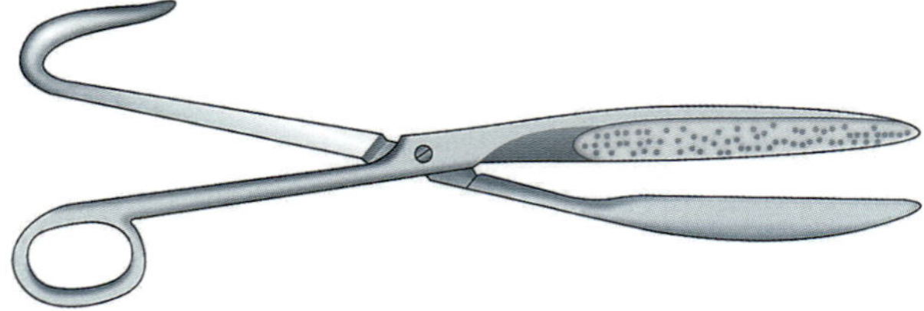

Fig. 5-171: Thompson-Walker's suprapubic cystolithotomy forceps.

BOOMERANG NEEDLE

It is sharply curved needle attached to a special holder with a spring within it. Needle has got sharp point and a slot. Suture material is passed through the slot to pass deep into the tissues. When handle is compressed through spring, needle rotates inwards passing through the tissues in front. It is used in suturing prostatic capsule in open prostatectomy **(Fig. 5-172)**.

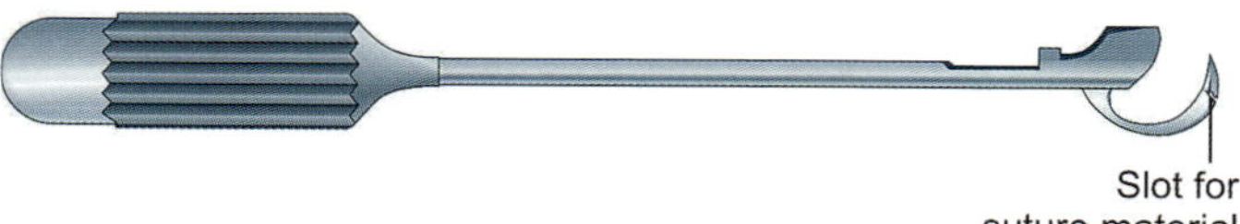

Fig. 5-172: Boomerang needle used to suture prostatic capsule in open prostatectomy.

NASOGASTRIC TUBE/RYLE'S TUBE

It is one meter long which is made up of red rubber or plastic. Original Ryle's tube was made up of moulded red rubber **(Figs. 5-173A and B)**. Presently used nasogastric tubes are made up of polyethylene or portex. Tip is blunt without opening. Subterminal multiple openings are present on all the sides. It is sterilised by gamma rays.

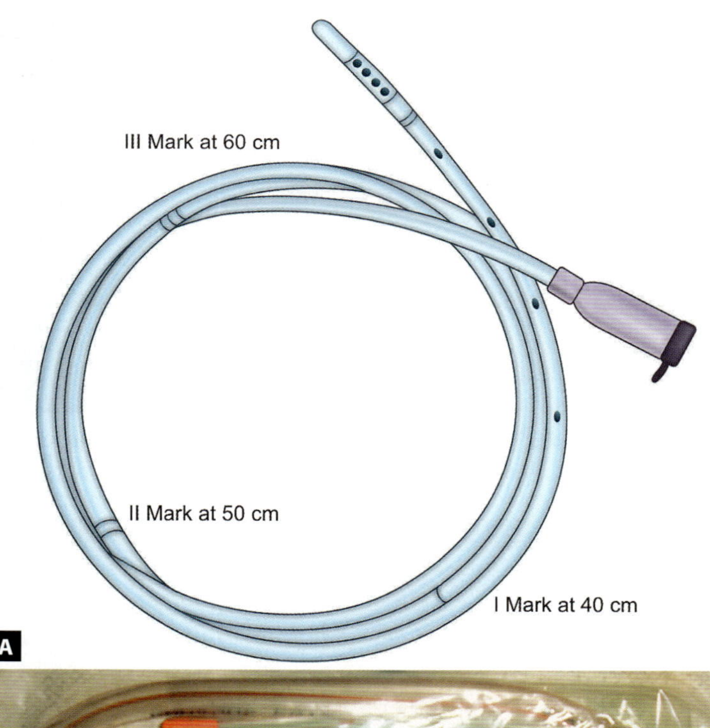

Figs. 5-173A and B: Ryle's tube.

It has got three lead shots in the tip which makes it radiopaque. It also facilitates easy passage of the tube through the oesophagus. Once tube is inside the stomach, bile/gastric juice will come out of the proximal end, often confirmed by aspiration. Stethoscope is placed over the stomach; syringe with air is pushed into the tube; if tip of the tube is in the stomach air entering into the stomach can be heard through the stethoscope.

It is passed through one of the nostrils using xylocaine 2% jelly. Under anaesthesia it is passed using Magill's forceps. It should be fixed securely to the nostrils otherwise it may get displaced or come out. It should be replaced with new tube in 2 weeks. Intermittent suction or continuous open drainage can be done depending on requirement. In postoperative period it is removed once patient passes flatus; or adequate bowel sounds are heard; and content in the tube is reduced to less than 50 mL.

It has got markings at different levels:

- At 40 cm distance, indicates the level of gastro-oesophageal junction.
- At 50 cm distance, indicates the level of body of the stomach.
- At 60 cm distance, indicates the level of the pylorus.
- At 65 cm distance, indicates the level of the duodenum.

Indications

Diagnostic:

- For gastric function tests. To assess free acid and total acid—in gastric/duodenal ulcers; pyloric obstruction/carcinoma stomach (exfoliative cytology); achylia; Zollinger-Ellison syndrome; pernicious anaemia; saline load test to confirm gastric motility and outlet obstruction; small bowel enema.
- Hollander's test for completion of vagotomy.
- To diagnose tracheo-oesophageal fistula.
- Baid test for pseudocyst of the pancreas.

Therapeutic:

- In acute abdominal conditions like peritonitis/obstruction, etc.
- In abdominal trauma.
- After abdominal surgeries.
- In pyloric stenosis.
- In upper GIT bleeding.
- In paralytic ileus, gastric dilatation to decompress the bowel.
- For feeding purpose in comatose patients, faciomaxillary injuries, major head and neck surgeries, head injuries, pharyngolaryngeal surgeries; surgeries for cleft palate.

Ryle's tube is British type, made up of red rubber, usually 75 cm in length, with lead shot in the tip. It is available as different sizes from 8 French to 18 French units.

Levin's tube is American tube made up of portex, 125 cm in length. *Now it is commonly used tube.*

Complications

- Injury to nostrils and bleeding.
- Pharyngitis/rhinitis.
- Discomfort/unacceptancy.
- Ulceration in the pharynx/oesophagus.
- Aspiration pneumonia as lower sphincter is kept open—dangerous complication—may cause death also.
- Perforation of oesophagus.

Nasogastric tube is contraindicated in corrosive oesophageal burns in initial phases for 2 weeks.

INFANT FEEDING TUBE

It does not have lead shots and no markings. It is used in children and infants similar to Ryle's tube **(Fig. 5-174)**. Length: 52 cm

Sizes: FG 5, 6, 7, 8, 9, 10, 11, 12, 13, 14, 15, 16, 17, 18

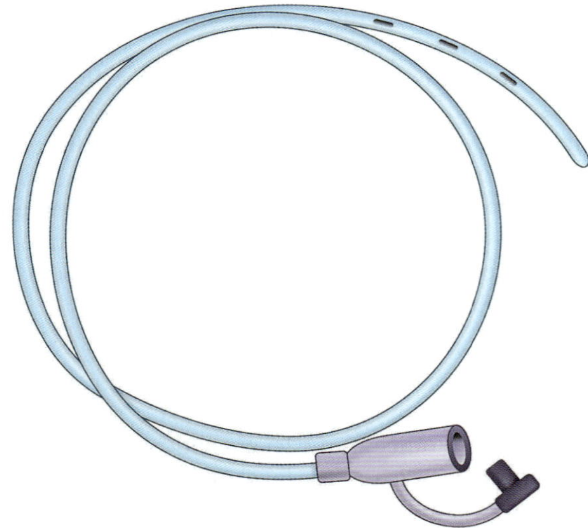

Fig. 5-174: Infant feeding tube.

FLATUS TUBE

It is made up of India rubber, 45 cm in length. There is one opening in the tip and another on the side proximal to the tip (Urinary catheter like red rubber catheter has no opening on the tip, only side opening is present) **(Fig. 5-175)**. It is used in sigmoid volvulus to decompress and derotate; in paralytic ileus; in subacute intestinal obstruction. It is passed per anal into the rectosigmoid area. Proximal end is connected to water container to observe the quantity of air bubble which signifies the amount of gas getting deflated.

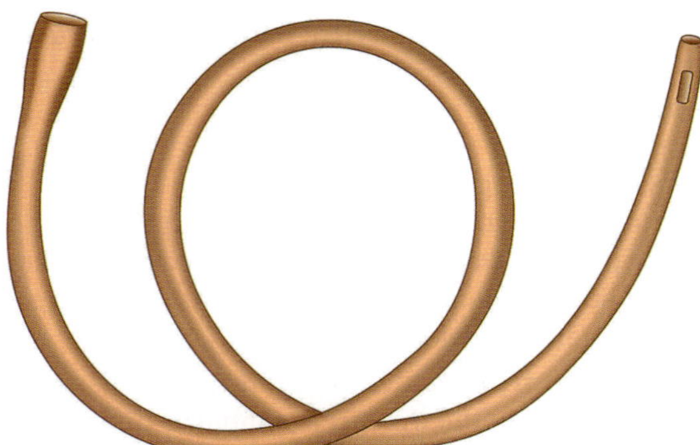

Fig. 5-175: Flatus tube.

HERNIA BISTOURY

It has got a handle and a flat blade with a small cutting edge on one side near the tip. Tip is blunt. Instrument is used to divide constriction band in strangulated hernia, to cut lacunar ligament in femoral hernia. It helps to protect adjacent structures while cutting the band **(Fig. 5-176)**.

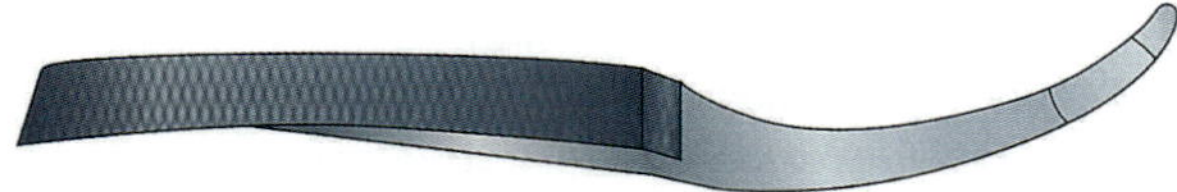

Fig. 5-176: Hernia bistoury.

COLLINGWOOD STEWART'S RING-SHAPED BLADE HERNIA FORCEPS

It has got semicircular tips which when approximated forms as ring. It has got a ratchet to have a proper grip. It is used to hold cord structures during inguinal hernia surgery so that hernioplasty/herniorrhaphy can be done effectively **(Figs. 5-177 and 5-178)**.

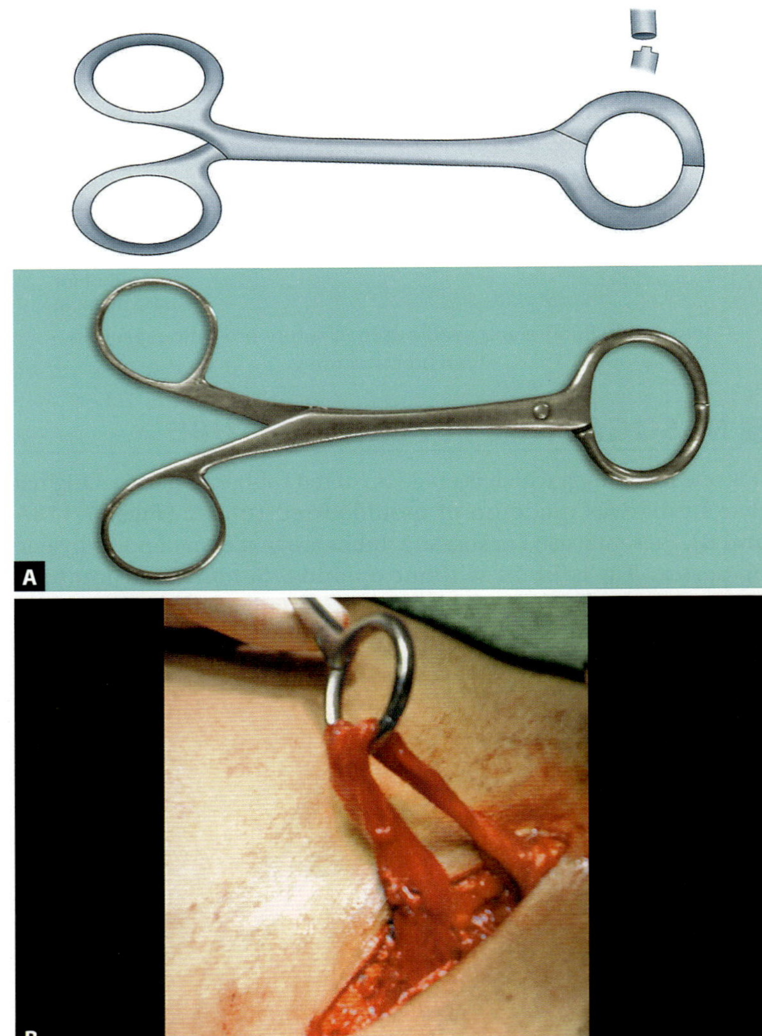

Figs. 5-177A and B: Cord holding forceps/ring forceps used to hold cord structures in inguinal hernia surgery.

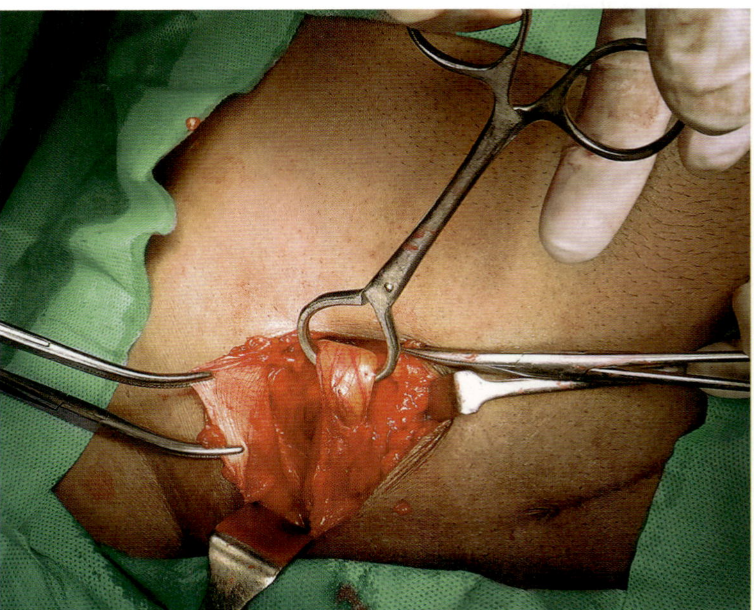

Fig. 5-178: Collingwood Stewart cord holding forceps used in open inguinal hernia surgery.

POLYPROPYLENE MESH

It is polypropylene white coloured monofilament, nonabsorbable, inert, malleable, strong, synthetic mesh used for hernioplasty. Presently prosthetic mesh repair is standard except probably Shouldice repair. Mesh is fixed using polypropylene suture material which is blue in colour **(Figs. 5-179A and B)**.

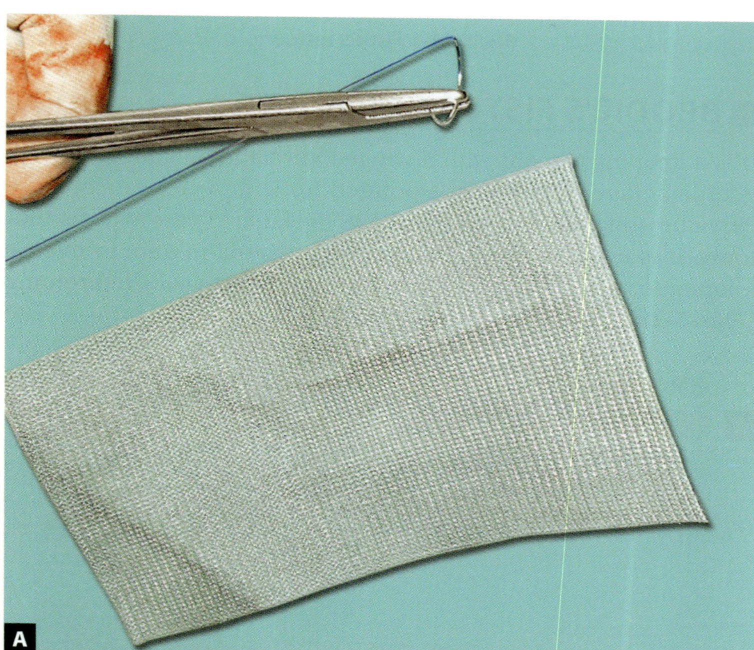

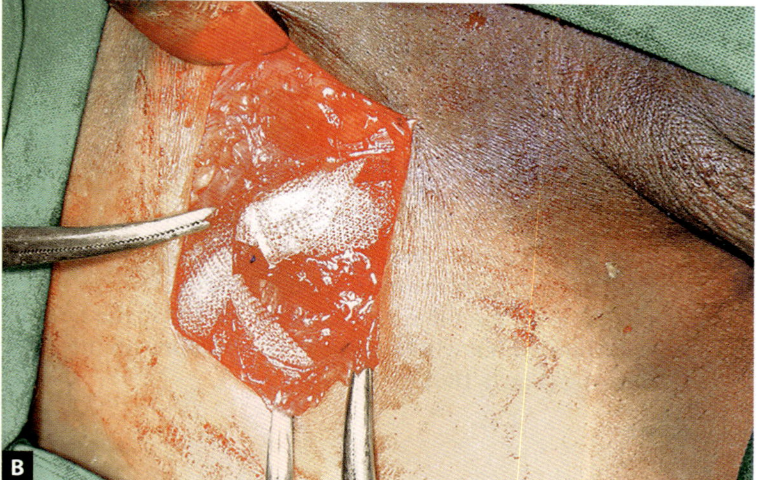

Figs. 5-179A and B: Polypropylene mesh used for hernioplasty.

TROCAR AND CANNULA

Trocar has got stout handle with a sharp pointed distal end. Trocar passes through the cannula of different sizes and snugly fits into proximal end of cannula. Trocar with sheath is punctured into the needed place and trocar is removed. Through sheath fluid is evacuated. Through the sheath Foley's catheter can also be passed to keep in place. It is used in per cutaneous cystostomy, draining hydrocele fluid, draining pus from gallbladder, pleural cavity, maxillary antrum, etc. **(Figs. 5-180A and B)**.

HERNIA DIRECTOR

Hernia director is used to protect the bowel in strangulated/obstructed hernia while releasing the narrow constricting band.

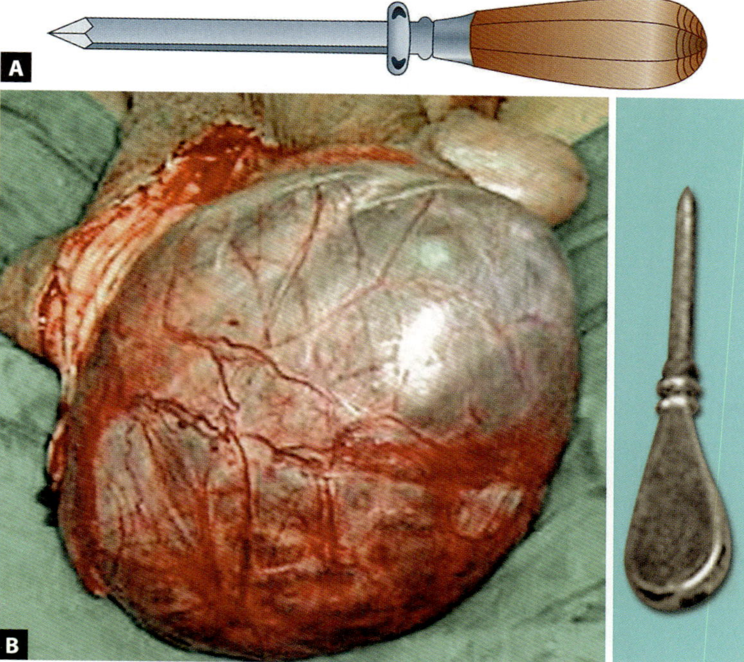

Figs. 5-180A and B: Trocar and cannula.

Key's hernia director has got grooved gently curved long blade with ridged stout handle. Childe's hernia director has two wings on sides of the blades as a guard with a handle. Constriction ring is cut using hernia bistoury **(Fig. 5-181)**.

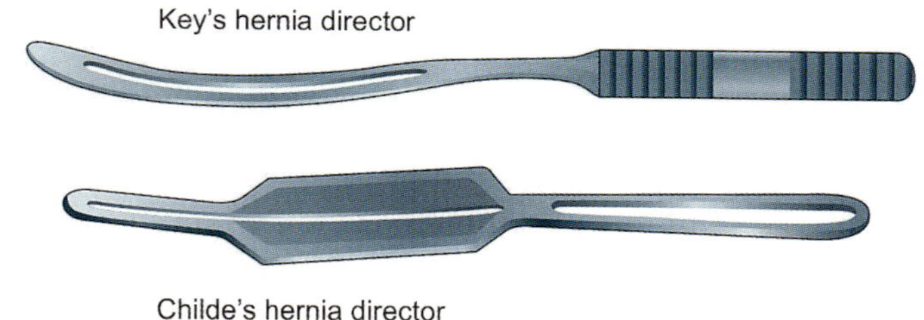

Fig. 5-181: Key's and Childe's hernia directors.

PROCTOSCOPE (KELLY'S)

Indications

- *Diagnostic:* Piles, fissure in ano, polyps, stricture, to see internal opening in fistula, carcinoma or any rectal bleeding
- *Therapeutic:* Injection therapy for partial prolapse or piles, cryotherapy for piles, banding for piles, polypectomy, biopsy for carcinoma rectum or anorectum.

Types

- *Illuminating* with a bulb at the distal part.
- *Non-illuminating.*

Parts

Proctoscope is conical shape, with proximal diameter more than the distal, so as to illuminate the light at the required site properly. *Obturator* is the inner part which allows the easy insertion of the proctoscope. Usual medium sized proctoscope is 10 cm in length with proximal diameter of 3.5 cm and distal diameter of 2.5 cm—tapering. This tapering allows light to reflect and pass distally. Proximal funnel-shaped flange is 5 cm in diameter **(Figs. 5-182A and B)**.

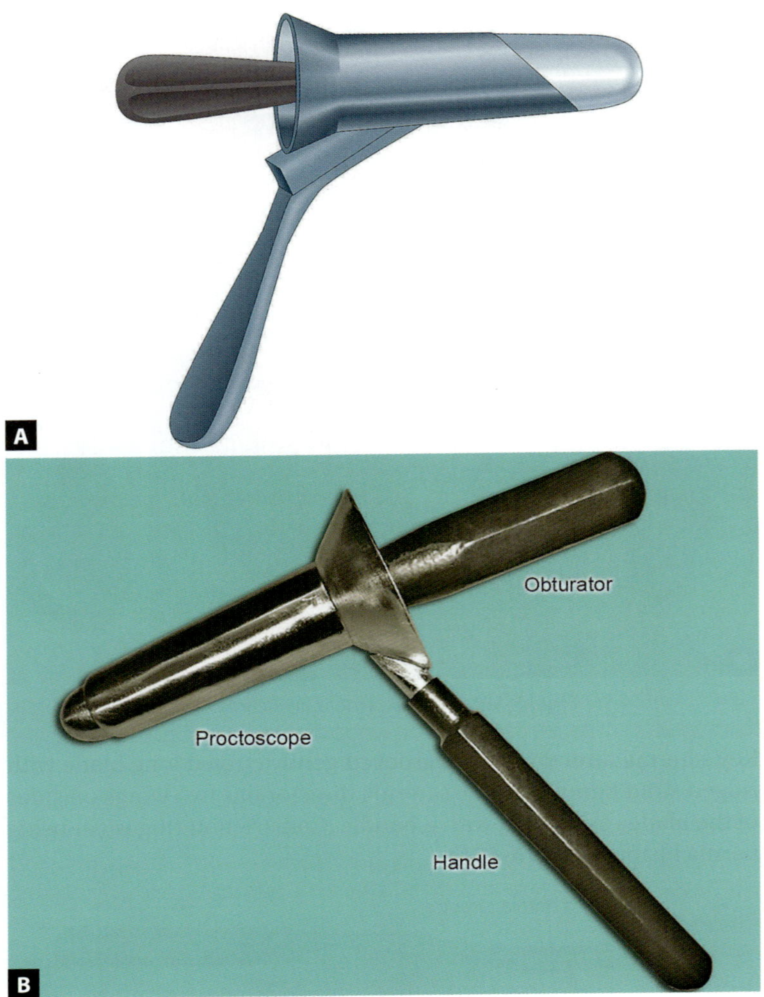

Figs. 5-182A and B: Proctoscope.

Positions for Proctoscopy

- Left lateral position (common).
- Right lateral.
- Lithotomy.
- Knee-elbow position.

Technique of proctoscopy

After doing digital examination, proctoscope with the obturator is introduced inside; through the anal canal in the direction towards the umbilicus. The obturator is removed. Proctoscope is withdrawn and during the course of withdrawal, any pathology has to be looked for.

Acute anal fissure is contraindication for proctoscopy.

SAINT MARK'S ANAL DILATOR

It is hollow conical instrument with both ends closed. Distal end is tapered, smooth and rounded. It is available in three different sizes. It is used for anal dilatation in post-anorectal surgeries and in anal stenosis. Xylocaine jelly is applied to the blunt tip and is gently passed through the anal canal to achieve dilatation **(Fig. 5-183)**.

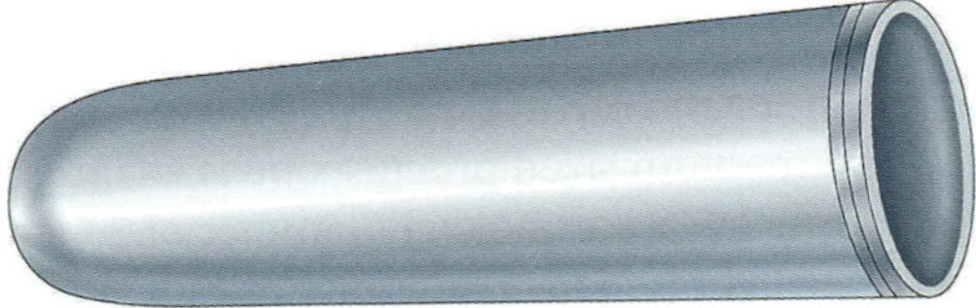

Fig. 5-183: Saint Mark's anal dilator.

FISTULA BISTOURY

It is a long blade with solid knife with a cutting edge. It is used to lay open the fistula in ano along with Brodie's fistula probe **(Fig. 5-184)**.

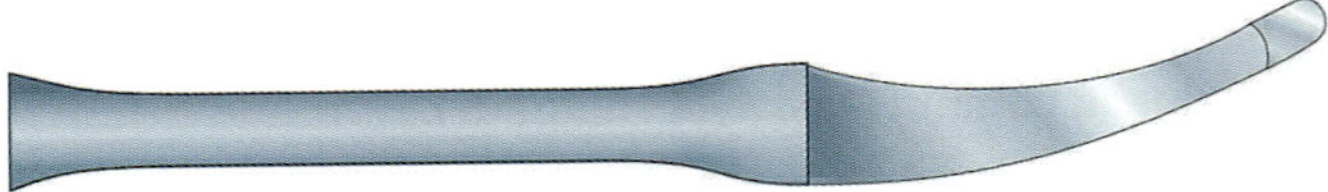

Fig. 5-184: Fistula bistoury.

BRODIE'S FISTULA DIRECTOR

It is a long instrument with a winged flat handle. Shaft is curved, gradually tapering to form a pointed tip with a groove along the curvature longitudinally which allows the knife to pass to do fistulotomy. It is used in probing and treating fistula in ano; to release tongue tie as a guide and protector and in external urethrotomy **(Figs. 5-185A and B)**.

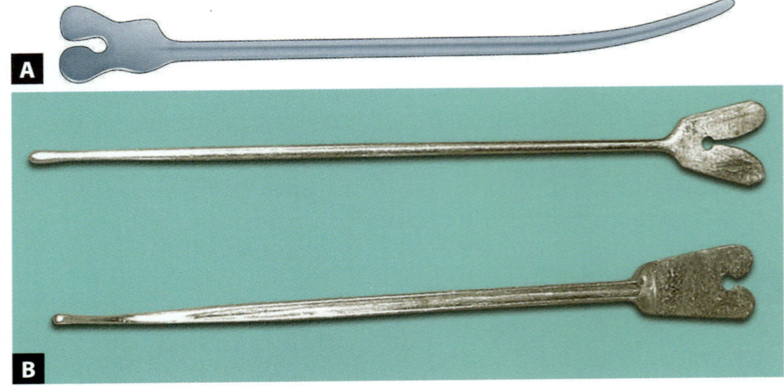

Figs. 5-185A and B: Brodie's fistula director.

PILE HOLDING FORCEPS

It has got long distal blades ending as a ring. Each has got fenestra with a groove on its inner surface. It is used to hold pile mass during haemorrhoidectomy. It differs from sponge holding forceps which has got serrations on the inner aspect of the ring. Tongue holding forceps is also similar but without groove or serrations on the inner aspect of the ring **(Fig. 5-186)**.

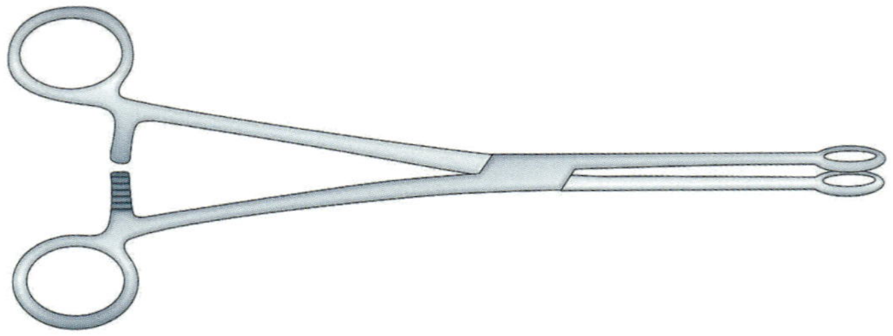

Fig. 5-186: Pile holding forceps has got groove on the inner aspect of the rings in the distal blades.

YEOMAN'S PUNCH BIOPSY FORCEPS

It has got two short stout jaws on the tip. Upper jaw is rectangular, mobile and cutting. Lower jaw is fixed and is having a cup. Through a handle (without ratchet) jaws can be closed and opened. Mobile jaw takes punch biopsy from the rectal lesion whereas fixed jaw accommodates the biopsy tissue in the cup **(Fig. 5-187)**. It is used to take biopsy from rectal lesions like carcinoma, ulcers, polyps, etc.

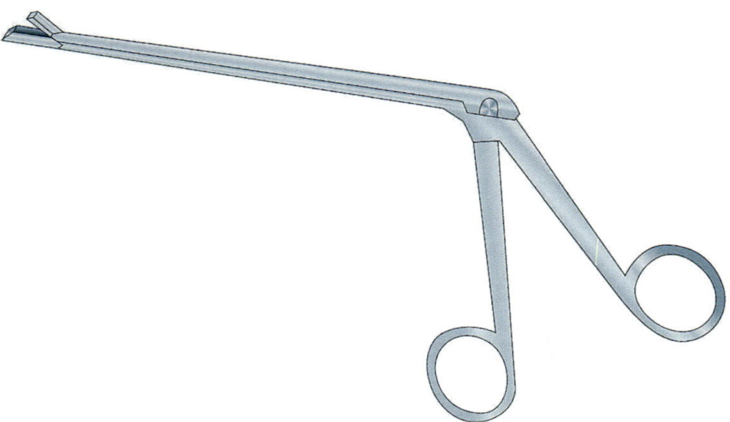

Fig. 5-187: Yeoman's punch biopsy forceps.

MOYNIHAN'S GLASS TUBE

This glass tube of 20 cm in length with a beveled one end and other end connected to a rubber tube with a two circular ridges to facilitate the holding of the purse string suture around the tube. It is used to decompress the proximal bowel in intestinal obstruction without contaminating the peritoneal cavity **(Fig. 5-188)**.

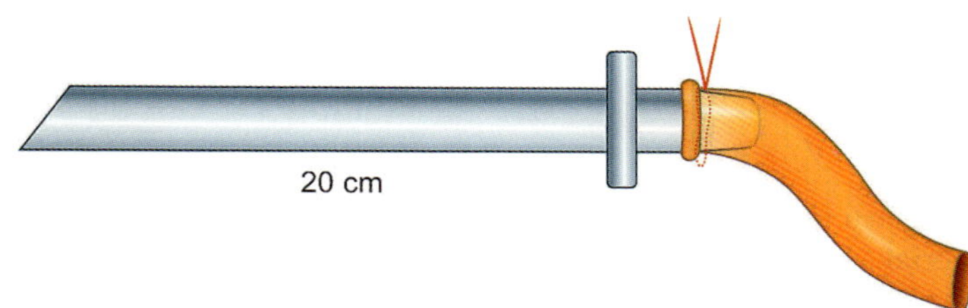

Fig. 5-188: Moynihan's glass tube to decompress bowel in intestinal obstruction.

DUPUYTREN'S ENTEROTOME

It has a stout distal blade with longitudinal serrations. It has got butterfly nut and screw on the proximal end which when tightened causes crushing effect on the structure between the blades. It is specifically used in *colostomy closure extraperitoneally* by placing this instrument over the spur of the colostomy. It is kept in place for 5–7 days and if needed further tightening can be done using screw. Spur gets necrosed and colostomy closes gradually on its own or by placing few sutures in front **(Fig. 5-189)**. Presently colostomy closure is done intraperitoneally by formally suturing bowel wall either single layer or two layers.

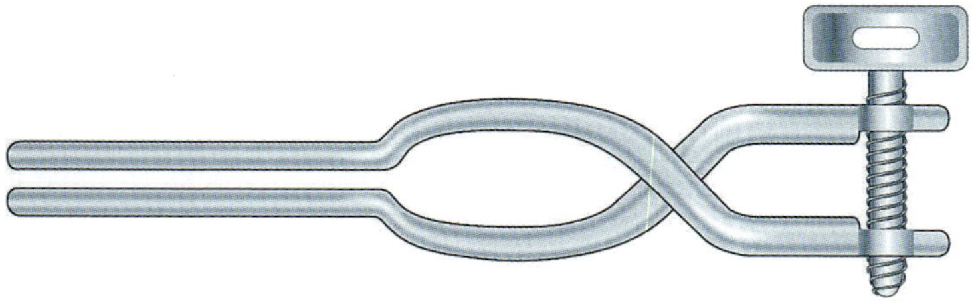

Fig. 5-189: Dupuytren's enterotome used for extra peritoneal closure of the colostomy by crushing the spur.

SPIGOT

It is a glass rod of 10 cm length, with one end narrow and blunt. In colostomy, once a loop of the colon is delivered through the abdominal wound it is used to pass through the mesocolon. It stabilises the loop of colon in position and prevents it from slipping into the peritoneal cavity **(Fig. 5-190)**. It is rarely used now.

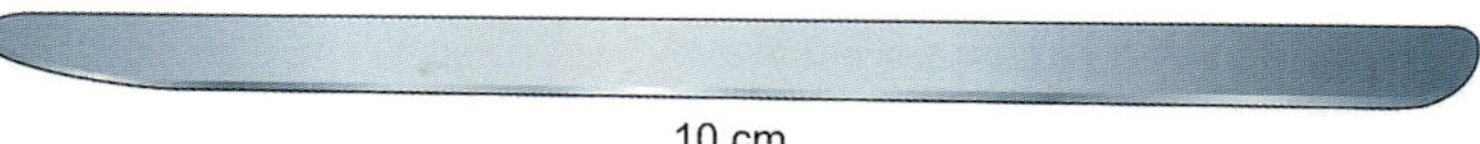

Fig. 5-190: Spigot used in as colostomy glass rod to prevent the slipping of the colon into the peritoneal cavity.

HUDSON BRACE WITH PERFORATOR AND BURR

Hudson's brace is used to do burr holes in skull bone. Using brace initially perforator is used to reach and open the inner table. Perforator should be carefully used to avoid injury to deeper structures. Later burr is used to widen the hole made by perforator **(Fig. 5-191)**.

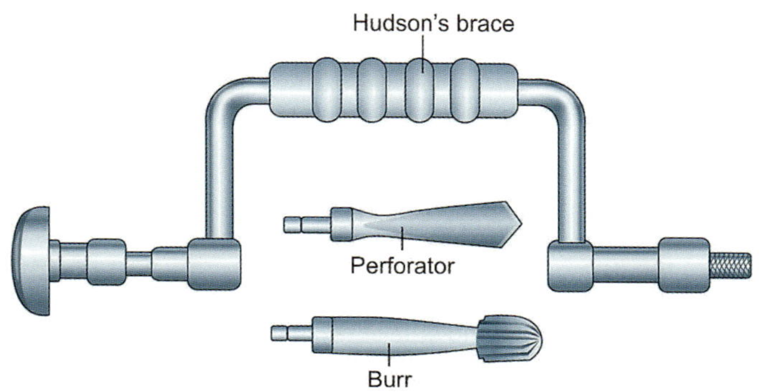

Fig. 5-191: Hudson's brace perforator and burr.

SUTURE MATERIALS

Classification

Suture material is classified based on its origin, absorption and structure.

Absorbable

- *Natural*—monofilament: Catgut (natural amino acid polymer).
- *Synthetic*
  - Monofilament: Poliglecaprone (monocryl); polyglyconate (Maxon); polydioxanone suture (PDS).
  - Multifilament: Coated polyglycolic acid (Dexon); polyglactin 910; lactomer copolymer (polysorb).

Nonabsorbable

- *Natural*
  - Monofilament
  - Multifilament: Surgical silk (natural amino acid polymer), surgical linen (natural cellulose polymer), cotton
- *Metallic:* Stainless steel—monofilament; stainless steel—multifilament.
- *Synthetic*
  - Monofilament: Polypropylene, polyethylene, polyamide, polyester monofilament.
  - Multifilament: Polyamide braided, polyester braided.

Based on coating:
- ***Coated***
- ***Uncoated***

Based on filaments:
- **Monofilament:** Catgut, poligrecaprone, polyglyconate, PDS, polypropylene, polyamide, polyethylene
- **Multifilament:**
  - *Braided:* Silk, polyamide braided, Polyglactin 910, Dexon.
  - *Twisted:* Cotton, linen.

Monofilament suture materials are smooth, strong and least reactive which will not allow bacteria to harbour. But handling and knot handling properties are poor. Polypropylene shows good memory. Recoiling tendency of the suture material is called as *memory* of the suture material. Higher the memory difficult is the handling and knotting. Lesser the memory means better the handling quality.

Multifilament sutures are easier to handle with less memory. But they may harbour bacteria easily and in infected field they are not suitable. They cause more reaction to tissues.

Features of ideal suture material

- It should be least reactive, should not allow harbouring of the bacteria.
- It should be nonelectrolytic, noncapillary, nonallergenic, noncarcinogenic.
- It should have good/high tensile strength.
- It should have proper knot holding property with easy handling ability.
- It should have good BSR (Breaking strength retention).
- It should have low modulus of elasticity.
- It should have less memory. Memory is inherent capacity of the suture material to return to or maintain its original gross shape which is related to plasticity, pliability and diameter.
- It should be amenable for proper sterilisation.
- It should be easily available and cheaper.

Properties of the Suture Material

Mechanical properties are assessed using tensiometer (Instrom machine) by recording stress strain curve evaluating the yield stress, breaking stress and modulus of the elasticity.

Biological properties are biodegradability, tissue reaction, tissue incorporation, infection rate, material deposition like calcium on to the placed suture material. It depends on the chemical nature of the suture material, type of material (mono or multifilament), surface charge on the suture material.

Surgical properties are—handling, tissue sliding, tensile strength, knot run down and knot holding (knot security).

Biology of Suture Materials

As suture material is a foreign body, both cellular response and enzymatic activity occur together. Tissue reaction is more to natural absorbable suture material than synthetic absorbable suture material. Plain catgut shows more tissue reaction than chromic catgut. Tissue reaction is more towards silk, linen or cotton compared to polyamide, polyester or polypropylene (least).

Suture Tensile Strength

It is breaking strength of the suture material, which is important in holding tissues in approximated position during stages of wound healing. Inadequate tensile strength or rapid loss of tensile strength may result in disruption of the suture line. As apposed tissue needs at least initial 7 days to regain its tensile strength, at least for 7 days tissues should be kept in apposition by suture material.

Tensile strength is the one which holds the tissues in approximation until tissue wound heals strongly. So adequate tensile strength is very essential component of a suture material. Breaking strength of a suture material is expressed either in grams per denier (weight of a fibre 9,000 metre long) or newtons per tex (weight of a fibre 1,000 metre length). It is also related to the size and diameter of the suture material.

Breaking Strength Retention

Breaking strength retention (BSR) is related to the rate and extent of the biodegradability of the suture. It is studied by immersing the suture in fluids as in vitro BSR or putting into animal tissues as in vivo BSR. It reflects the duration of the tensile strength maintained in the tissue.

Elasticity of the Suture Material

It is the ability to deform or stretch when suture is subjected to a progressive distraction force and inability to reach back to its original dimension even after force is removed beyond yield point. It is the measure of the ability of the suture material to regain its original form and length after deformation.

Capillarity

It is the extent to which absorbed fluid is transferred along the suture material.

Fluid absorption: It is the ability of the suture material to take up fluid after immersion.

Knot-pull Tensile Strength

It is the breaking strength of knotted suture material (10–40% weaker after deformation by knot placement); knot strength: It is the amount of force necessary to cause a knot to slip. *Straight pull tensile strength:* It is the linear breaking strength of suture material.

Plasticity

It is the measure of the ability to deform without breaking and to maintain a new form after relief of the deforming force. *Pliability*: It is the ease of handling of suture material so that knot tension can be adjusted and secure knots can be placed comfortably.

Absorption Time

It is not equal to tensile strength period. Absorption of suture material may be rapid or delayed or slow. Ideally tensile strength and absorption time should last for at least 3 weeks to have an efficient tissue apposition. Catgut gets absorbed by cellular response and phagocytosis; synthetic absorbable suture gets absorbed by hydrolysis using tissue fluids.

Absorbable Sutures

Natural Absorbable Suture

Plain and chromic catgut, collagen sutures, Cargile membrane, fascia lata, kangaroo tendon are different natural absorbable sutures.

Only catgut is used now. Collagen suture is derived from tendo-Achilles of cattle containing 100% collagen; its action its similar like catgut but it is more stiff; it is no longer used. Cargile membrane is derived from submucosa of caecum of ox. It was once practiced to cover removed pleura or peritoneum or to prevent adhesions after abdominal surgery. It is also no longer used. Fascia lata is derived from same individual's thigh or from cattle. It was once used in hernia repair, in correction of drooping of the upper eyelid and in facial palsy. Kangaroo tendon is derived from the tendons of the tail of the kangaroos. It shows high tensile strength but is no more in use.

Catgut

It is monofilament natural absorbable suture material. It is derived from submucosa of jejunum of sheep or serosa of cattle intestine. It contains 99% collagen—protein by nature. It gets absorbed by enzymatic degradation by proteolytic enzymes derived from macrophages. It can be plain or chromic catgut (treated with chromic acid). Heat treated fast absorbing gut is also available. Fast absorbing gut is used often in transepidermal suturing wherein suture removal is not necessary and impractical. Fast absorbing gut should only be used for skin not in deeper tissues. Plain catgut causes more reaction but for shorter period compared to chromic catgut. Plain catgut loses its tensile strength completely in 15 days; chromic catgut in 30 days. Tissue reaction is early and rapid in plain and slower in chromic catgut. Handling and knot holding property is good in catgut. Plain catgut is straw coloured and chromic is brown coloured. Plain catgut is wet whereas chromic catgut is dry (so it is smooth). Plain catgut is used in apposition of the subcutaneous tissue, ligating bleeders in the subcutaneous tissue and often in circumcision. Chromic catgut is used in obstetric and gynaecological surgeries like caesarean or legation of pedicles in hysterectomy. Catgut is ideal for surgical slip knots due to its rough texture which imparts an intrinsic resistance for reverse slipping. So it is commonly used as endoloops in laparoscopic surgeries as in laparoscopic appendicectomy. Sterile dry packed chromic catgut is suitable for slip knot. Alcohol packed chromic catgut once unpacked can be made dry if left for 15 minutes. It is used also in suturing the muscle, ligating pedicles in infected field, etc. Once atraumatic straight needled chromic catgut was popular in bowel anastomosis is no longer advocated. Many of catgut uses are replaced by other synthetic absorbable sutures.

It is manufactured by—after washing, intestine is slit longitudinally into four strands; muscle and fat are removed using water spry—*sliming*. Chemical bath saponification is also used to remove fat. Strands are spun together, dried with tension and electronically polished. It is absorbed by inflammatory reaction and phagocytosis.

Chromic catgut is catgut with chromic acid salt. The catgut is treated with 20% chromium salt in water with 5 parts of glycerine. It is brown in colour. Its absorption time is 21 days. It is used in suturing muscle, fascia, external oblique aponeurosis, ligating pedicles, etc. Atraumatic sutures are manufactured either by swaging or by entangling the suture material into the grooved proximal part of the needle by mechanical pressure. Wound suture material in a support card is packed in a foil envelope with isopropyl alcohol. It is sterilised by gamma radiation.

Synthetic Absorbable Sutures

They are polymers and carbohydrate by nature, absorbed by hydrolysis. They can be monofilament or multifilament—braided. Braiding may be either looping or in multiplicity. They maintain higher tensile strength and so keep the approximation stronger for longer period. They are usually pliable, smooth, glides along the tissues smoothly. They are biodegradable by hydrolysis and less reactive with easy handling property with less memory. They can be monofilament or multifilament suture materials. Polydioxanone (PDS), polyglyconate (Maxon), poliglecaprone (Monocryl), biosyn and Caprosyn are monofilament types of synthetic absorbable sutures. Coated polyglycolic acid (Dexon), polyglactin (polyglycolide co-lactide; polyglactin 910), lactomer copolymer (polysorb) are multifilament absorbable suture materials.

Polyglyconate (Maxon, Davis and Geck)

It is *monofilament absorbable* synthetic suture material which is absorbed by hydrolysis releasing glycolic acid and hydrogen ion which lowers the pH in the tissue and so least infection rate. It is a copolymer of glycolic acid and trimethylene carbonate. It lasts longer period taking around 6 months to get absorbed. It shows good handling features in both open surgery and laparoscopy. Its dyed colour is visible and stains under the skin. It shows excellent tensile strength, knot holding property and minimum memory.

Glycomer 631 (Biosyn, Covidien)

It is *monofilament absorbable* synthetic suture material showing good handling features and tensile strength. Its absorption is slow taking 4 months to get absorbed.

Polyglytone 621 (Caprosyn)

It is *fast absorbing monofilament* synthetic suture material which is absorbed in 8 weeks and its tensile strength lasts for 10 days only. So it is used in suturing low tension approximations. It contains glycolide, caprolactone, trimethylene carbonate and lactide.

Poliglecaprone 25 (Monocryl, Ethicon)

It is *monofilament absorbable* synthetic suture material with excellent handling features with smooth surface, pliable (less stiff and less hard), adequate knot holding property causing minimal tissue reaction. This suture material is very easy to bend and to stretch. Gliding and passage through tissues is smooth and less dragging and so minimises the trauma to tissues. It is copolymer of 75% glycolide and 25% caprolactone. It shows high tensile strength for 3 weeks and absorbed by hydrolysis in 90 days. It does not have package memory and so recoiling and inadvertent knotting is not present. Proper tissue sliding, adequate elasticity, ideal handling, visible transparent colour makes it as ideal absorbable monofilament suture material. It is sterilised by ethylene oxide.

Polydioxanone Suture Material (PDS)

It is the *strongest monofilament absorbable* suture material which lasts longer period maintaining its tensile strength in the wound. It is nonreactive, absorbable, synthetic suture material. It contains polymerised para dioxanone 97%; 3% copolymerised lactide. It is absorbed by hydrolysis. PDS II is improvised version of the PDS I in relation to handling property. PDS glides through tissues well but can cause crinkling. It is absorbed by hydrolysis. It is very good for open surgery but not suitable for endoscopic surgery. *V Loc* is the barbed suture which is self-anchoring and no knots are required; it contains 0 number polydioxanone suture material with axially barbed segments.

Polyglactin 910 (Vicryl, Ethicon)

It is *braided, multifilament*, synthetic, coated, *absorbable* suture material which is a polymer made up of glycolic acid with lactide component. Ratio is 9 of polyglycolic acid to 1 lactide. Lactide being hydrophobic reduces the water molecule ingress into the copolymer preventing the breakdown of the linkage of the glycolic acid copolymer chain thereby increasing the longevity of the suture material and its tensile strength. Lactide reduces the regularity and crystallinity of the copolymer making it to have greater pliability. Polyglactin shows more tensile strength and handling character than many other suture materials. Coated polyglactin suture material contains 50% polyglactin (polyglactin coat component contains 35% polyglycolide and 65% lactide) and 50% calcium stearate (it is an absorbable fatty acid lubricant). This coating reduces the surface friction of the braided suture material without altering the quality of the suture material like absorption, reaction, tensile strength. It is absorbed by hydrolysis (not protein degradation) and so least reactive. It gets absorbed in 90 days; maintains tensile strength for 30 days.

Polyglactin 910 (Vicryl) is most commonly used suture material in all open surgeries and in laparoscopic surgeries. It is not used in cardiovascular and neural suturing. Rapidly absorbing type (Vicryl rapid; velosorb fast) is also available which gets absorbed in 2 weeks. Antibacterial polyglactin (Vicryl plus) suture material is also often used. *Triclosan* is nontoxic, noncarcinogenic, antibacterial agent (not antibiotic) which is safe and effective and is used to protect the suture material from bacterial colonisation (Vicryl plus).

It is sterilised by ethylene oxide. It is stored in an optimum temperature below 25°C. Life of packed material is 5 years.

Coated Polyglycolic Acid (Dexon II, Davis and Geck)

It is polyglycolic acid with bioabsorbable copolymer of polyoxypropylene and polyoxyethylene coated with polycaprolate multifilament suture material. Its features are almost similar to polyglactin.

Lactomer Copolymer—Polysorb

It is *braided, multifilament*, synthetic *absorbable* suture material consists of glycolide and lactide (93.5:6.5). It is coated with glycolide and caprolactone. It is suitable for both open and laparoscopic and for both interrupted and continuous suturing. It has got good tensile strength, tissue glide, knot holding capacity, easy handling properties. It gets absorbed in 3 months. But being purple in colour it shows poor visibility. It is very useful for laparoscopic suturing and extracorporeal slip knot placement.

Uses of absorbable suture materials

- In bowel anastomosis like gastrojejunostomy, resection and anastomosis—Vicryl (2 zero) is used.
- In cholecystojejunostomy (CCJ), choledochojejunostomy (CDJ), pancreaticojejunostomy—Vicryl is used.
- In suturing muscle, fascia, peritoneum, subcutaneous tissue, mucosa.
- In ligating pedicles, e.g. ligation of pedicles during hysterectomy. 1-zero chromic catgut or Vicryl are used.
- In circumcision usually 3-zero plain or chromic catgut or Vicryl rapid are used.

Absorbable suture materials should not be used in suturing tendon, nerves, vessels (vascular anastomosis) or in hernia surgery where tissue approximation under stress is needed.

Nonabsorbable Suture Materials

Natural

Silk

Silk is *natural, nonabsorbable, multifilament, braided* suture material. Silk is derived from cocoon of the silkworm larvae. Silk is protein by nature. It is coated with a wax which reduces the capillary action. It causes cellular tissue reaction; it shows very high tensile strength which is lost in 2 years. It has got very good handling and knot holding property. It is sterilised by gamma irradiation.

It is available as atraumatic eyeless needled sutures, precut (sutupak) sutures, with micropoint needles for ophthalmologic surgeries.

Linen

It is *natural, nonabsorbable, multifilament, twisted* suture material. Linen is a cellulose material derived from the flax. *Flax* is blue flowered plant that is grown for its seed and textile fibres; textile fibre is made from the stalk of this tree used as a twisted multifilament suture material. It has got very good handling and knot holding property. Its tensile strength increases by 100% when it is wet. It is commonly used for ligatures, to tie pedicles.

Cotton

It is *natural, nonabsorbable, multifilament twisted* suture material derived from the hairs of the seed of the cotton plant.

Synthetic

Synthetic nonabsorbable suture materials are hydrocarbon polymers derived from oil and coal. They are biocompatible usually non-biodegradable or slowly biodegradable and do not swell in the tissues. They show high flexibility and tensile strength, inertness, resistance to creep, and low melting point. But they have got poor knot retaining ability and knot may spill after placing. Usually they are monofilament but multifilament materials are available like of polyester; multifilament is created by braiding from a multiplicity of monofilaments or by looping of a single filament.

Nylon (New York, London)

It is ***polyamide*** usually monofilament, synthetic, nonabsorbable suture material. It has got good tensile strength with minimal tissue reaction. But it shows high memory and so recoiling tendency and knot holding difficulty is common and so needs 4–5 throws to place the knot. It is slowly biodegradable. Polyamide suture (Ethilon, Ethicon; Dermalon, Davis and Geck) is available as atraumatic sutures and as sutupak sutures. Polyamide multifilament sutures are also available.

Dacron and Terylene/Polyesters

They are ***polyester*** synthetic, nonabsorbable, multifilament, braided sutures with high tensile strength with least reaction. But it has got a tendency to cut through; so Teflon or PTFE coating is provided.

Ethibond is polyester sutures coated with polybutylate which prevents increase in diameter of the suture material and avoids flake in the tissues. Ethibond has got 8 carrier molecules. Newer version, *ethibond excel* has got 16 carrier molecules which is smoother and better. It is used in cardiovascular and neurological surgeries. It is available in white and green colours to facilitate suturing in valve surgeries. It is very useful for slip knots in extracorporeal slip knot in laparoscopic surgeries.

Polypropylene

It is monofilament, nonabsorbable, synthetic suture material. It has got high tensile strength with least reaction. It slides down through tissues easily but has got high memory with recoiling tendency and needs minimum 5 throws to have a secure knot. It is less thrombogenic and inert. It is elastic and can fracture by undue grasping with forceps.

It is commonly used in all repairs like hernia, vascular and neural anastomosis, tendon suturing.

Polyethylene

It is not commonly used as it is not as strong as other synthetic suture materials. It is a polymer by nature. It stretches and has got poor knot holding property.

Expanded PTFE

It is a nonabsorbable suture material with least reaction, better handling, with porous microstructure. It is good suture material but is not commonly used.

Polybutester—Novafil

It is monofilament, blue coloured, synthetic suture material which has got adequate flexibility, suppleness and strength. Polybutester suture is a monofilament containing copolymer containing butylene terephthalate and polytetramethylene ether glycol. It with low forces yield greater elongation and the elasticity is superior allowing the suture to return to its original length once the load is removed.

Stainless Steel Metallic Non-toxic Suture/Wire (Steel, Tantalum, Silver)

They are useful in approximating bones and tough structures, in orthopaedic and thoracic surgeries (sternotomy or thoracotomy), in reconstructive surgeries, surgeries of skull base or head and neck, sinus surgeries, in dental surgeries. It is iron chromium nickel molybdenum alloy. Monofilament is called as steel suture/metallic suture. Multifilament is called as metallic/steel wire which can be twisted or braided. Metallic sutures/wires are difficult to handle and to use, may cause injury to surgeons but they are very high tensile strength and low reactivity. Kinking is another problem.

Barbed Suture

It is knotless surgical suture which has got barbs on its surface which once penetrates the tissue lock the suture preventing from getting loosened. It is often used in cosmetic surgery. It is now more popular in key hole and laparoscopic surgery.

Uses of Nonabsorbable Suture Materials

For repair in herniorrhaphy; for closure of abdomen after laparotomy; for vascular anastomosis (6-zero), nerve suturing, tendon suturing; in tuboplasty, vasovasostomy —8-zero to 10-zero are used; in ophthalmic surgeries; for tension suturing in the abdomen; for suturing the skin **(Figs. 5-192A and B)**.

Numbering of suture material

2—Thick. For pedicle ligation.
1—
1—zero.
2—zero. For bowel suturing.
3—zero.
4—zero.
5—zero. For vascular anastomosis.
6—zero.
7—zero.
8—zero.
9—zero. For ophthalmic surgery. Requires microscopy

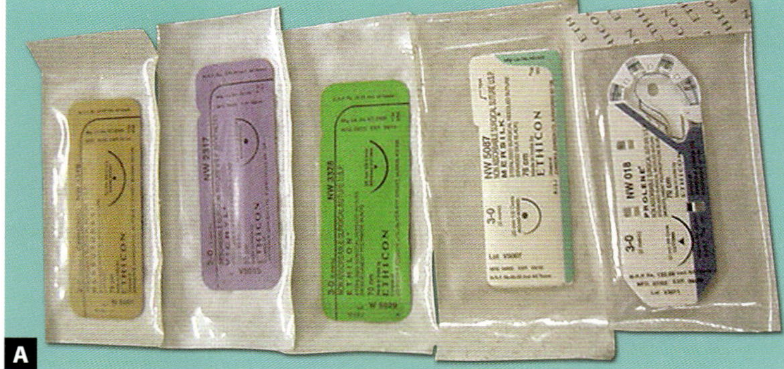

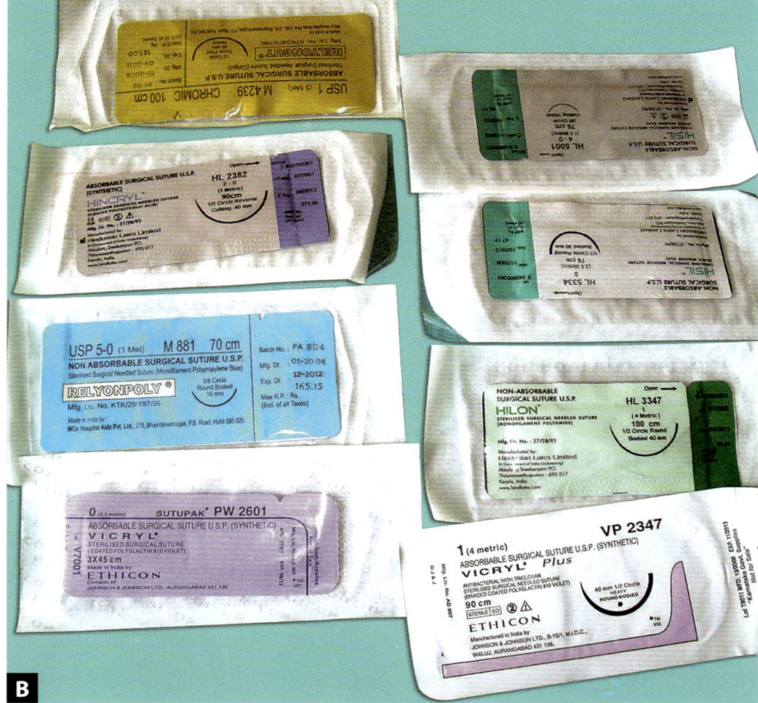

Figs. 5-192A and B: Different types of suture materials (with pack).

Note:

- Length of the suture material is written on the packs. It can be 45 cm; 76 cm; 90 cm or 152 cm so on.
- Company code for a particular suture material is important to identify it in detail.
- Lot number, batch number, needle description, needle curvature, needle size are mentioned on the packs.
- Name of manufacturing company, license number, manufacture date and expiry dates are mentioned on the pack.

Types of Suturing (Fig. 5-193)

1. Continuous suturing.
2. Interrupted simple suturing.
3. Interrupted mattress suturing.
4. Subcuticular suturing.
5. Horizontal tension suturing.
6. Vertical tension suturing.

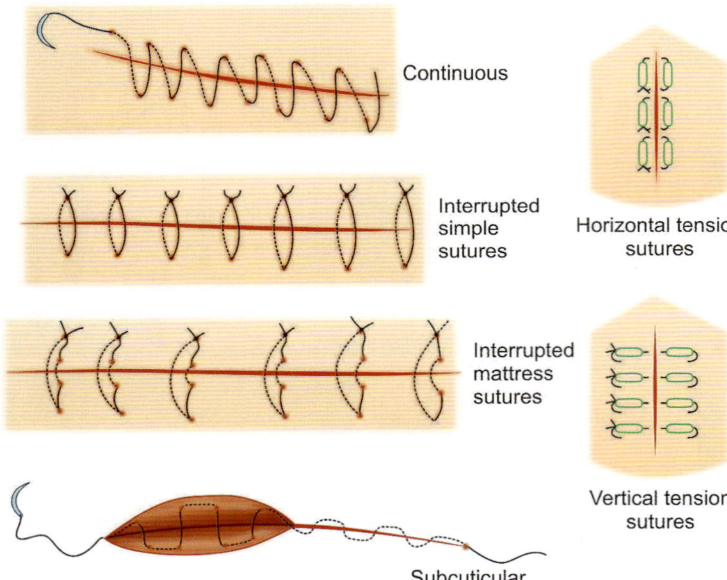

Fig. 5-193: Types of suturing.

Types of Knots (Fig. 5-194)

1. Reef knot.
2. Granny knot.
3. Surgeon's knot.

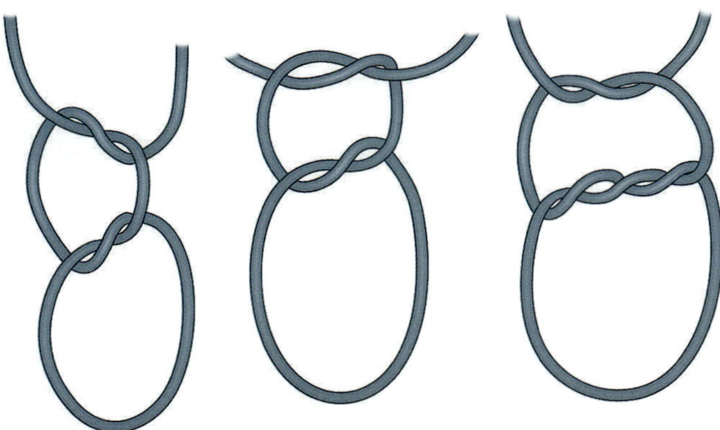

Fig. 5-194: Types of knots

MITCHEL'S CLIP DEVICE

- *Mitchel's metal clip:* It has got two sharp points on their teeth to grip the edges of the skin wound when applied.
- *Mitchel's clip applicator:* It has got a groove on the inner surface of each blade with a tooth on the ends of the blades to apply the clips to the edges of skin wound.
- *Mitchel's clip extractor:* It has got short distal blades, one blade has a hood which comes in front of the clip while another blade is flat which comes under the clip, with pressure on the finger rings clip is extracted. It does not have ratchet.
- *Mitchel's clip magazine:* Here clips are arranged in a row and other end with teeth is used to hold the skin margins together like a toothed forceps **(Fig. 5-195)**.

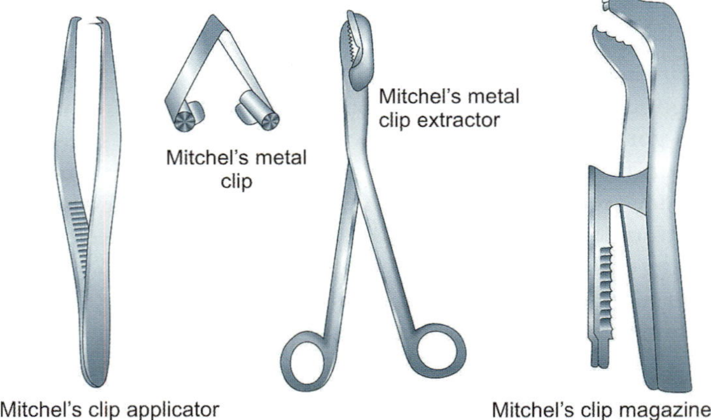

Fig. 5-195: Mitchel's clip devices with clip, applicator, extractor and clip magazine.

TOUHY EPIDURAL CATHETER

It is used in epidural catheterisation while giving epidural anaesthesia, for pain relief. Its tip is bent to direct towards the epidural space; it has got stilette also **(Figs. 5-196A and B)**.

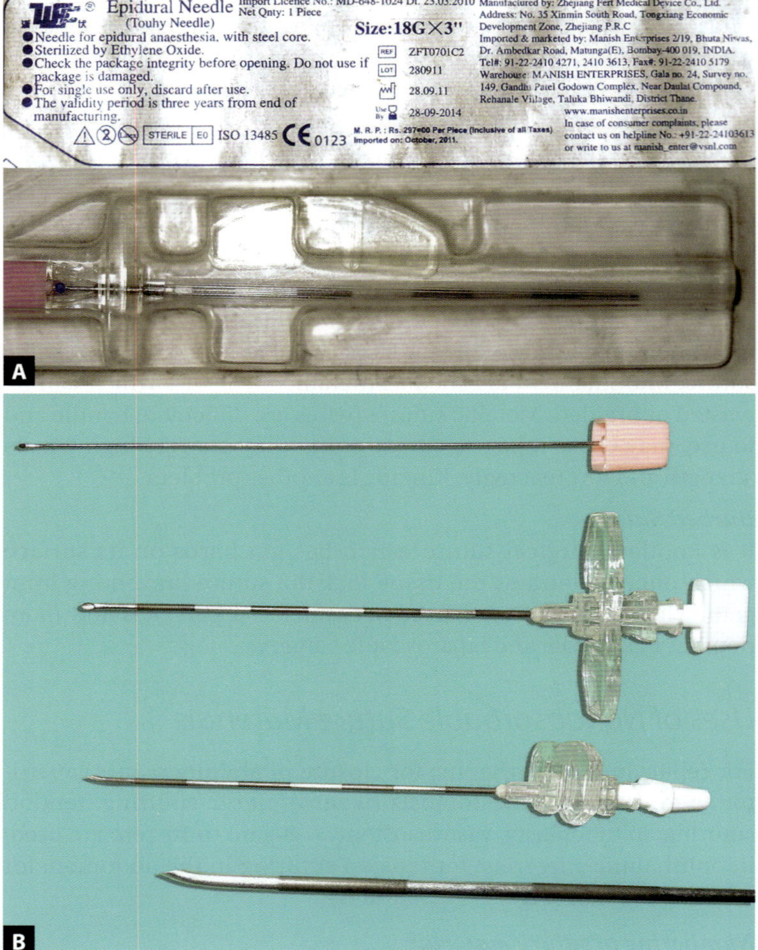

Figs. 5-196A and B: Touhy epidural catheter.

SYRINGES

It is basic instrument in medical practice used to give injections through any route, aspirate fluids, to give wash over surface or deeper places.

Types

Bectin Dickenson syringe (BD syringe): It is a glass syringe with a glass piston and barrel having a nozzle at the end to fit into the BD needle. Proximal end of the barrel has got a rim with one side being flat that prevents from rolling and breakage. It is sterilised by boiling. Disposable plastic BD syringes are commonly used now which is sterilised by gamma radiation. BD injection syringes are available as 2 mL, 3 mL, 5 mL, 10 mL, 20 mL, 50 mL and 100 mL capacity. 1 mL tuberculin/insulin syringes, Luer-lock BD syringes (needle can be locked near the nozzle to prevent slipping of the needle) are other modifications **(Fig. 5-197)**.

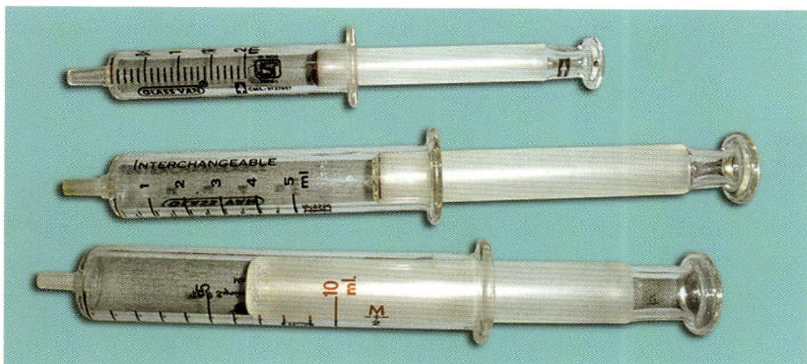

Fig. 5-197: Bectin Dickenson syringe (BD syringe).

Record syringes: It is like BD syringe with a metallic screw at the proximal end of the barrel which can fix the barrel of the syringe so that piston will not come out.

Gabriel syringe: It is used for injection sclerotherapy for internal piles using 5% phenol in almond/olive oil (almond/vegetable oil acts as a vehicle which holds phenol for long period of action). It is a stainless steel syringe with two metallic finger brims near the proximal end. One more metallic finger brim is present on the proximal end of the piston to place thumb while injecting. Special needle which may be straight or curved and sharply pointed is used for injection of haemorrhoids. Patient is placed in left lateral position. Using proctoscope pedicle/upper part of the piles is identified. Sclerosant is injected into the submucosal plane only which is confirmed by pale bleb with thin vessels over it. If it turns as white patch it means it is more superficial and needle is withdrawn and replaced in submucosal plane. 4 ml at each site with two piles in one sitting is done and further injections are given if needed with a 3 weeks gap until complete sclerosis and obliteration of piles occurs **(Fig. 5-198)**.

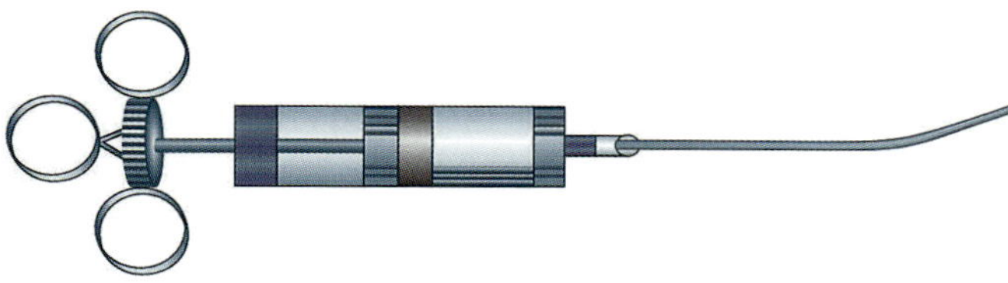

Fig. 5-198: Gabriel syringe.

Indications for sclerotherapy in piles	Contraindications for sclerotherapy
◈ 1st and early 2nd degree piles	◈ Infection at the site
◈ Piles in pregnancy and old individuals	◈ Secondary piles
	◈ Association of fissure in ano or fistula in ano

Asepto Syringe/Dakin's Syringe

It is made up of glass with broad flanged proximal end to which a rubber bulb can be fitted into it. It has got a tapered tip through which tubes/catheters can be fit to give wash, to suck the contents. It is used to give bladder wash in infection, in post-prostatectomy period, to give wash in different cavities and in depth, to instill methylene blue into the bladder to find out any fistula, to remove clots from prostate or other cavities during surgery **(Fig. 5-199)**.

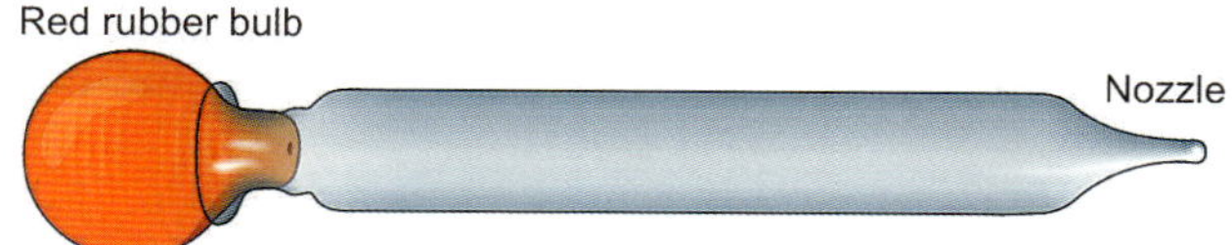

Fig. 5-199: Asepto syringe used for bladder wash.

Toomy Syringe

It is used to give bladder wash through cystoscope while doing transurethral resection of prostate (TURP). It has got a metallic nozzle which fits well into the cystoscopic sheath. It creates a strong suction force to suck the irrigated fluid **(Fig. 5-200)**.

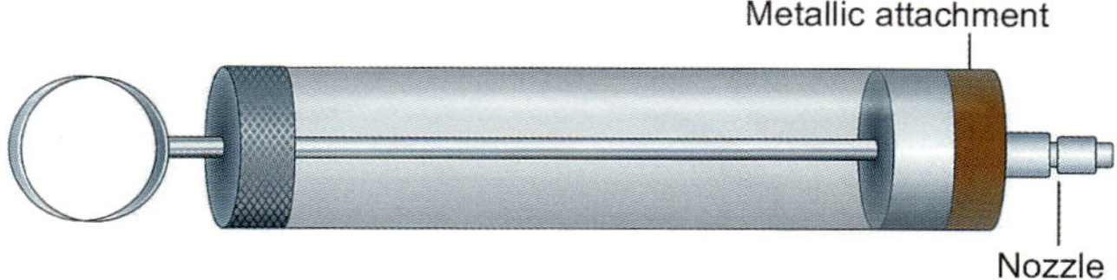

Fig. 5-200: Toomy syringe.

DOYEN'S MOUTH GAG

It has got flat, broad, strong, curved distal blades which has got serrations on the outer aspect so as to have proper grip over teeth. Blades are covered with rubber tubes to prevent injury to enamel. It is used for biopsies in oral cavity, dental extraction, tonsillectomy, excisions of small oral cavity lesions **(Figs. 5-201A to C)**.

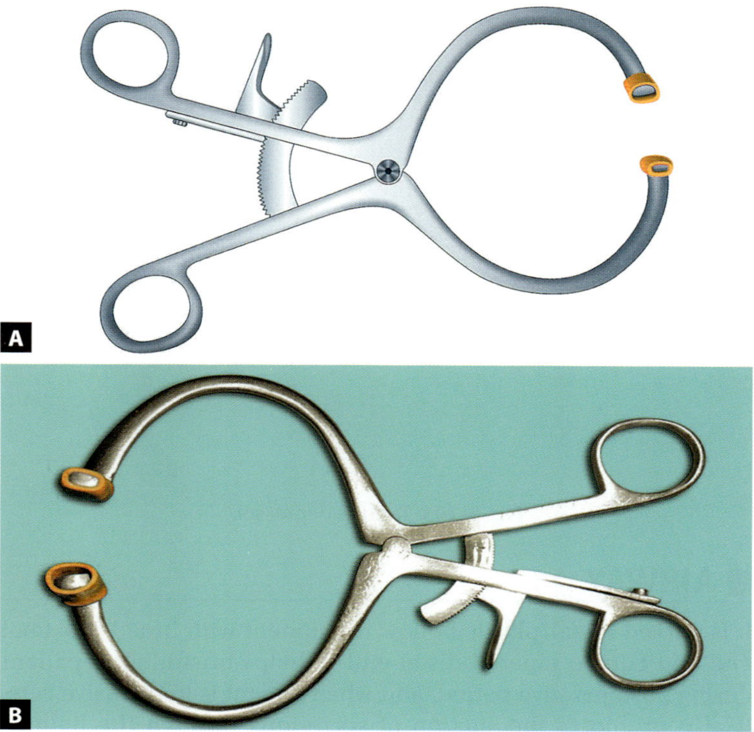

Figs. 5-201A and B

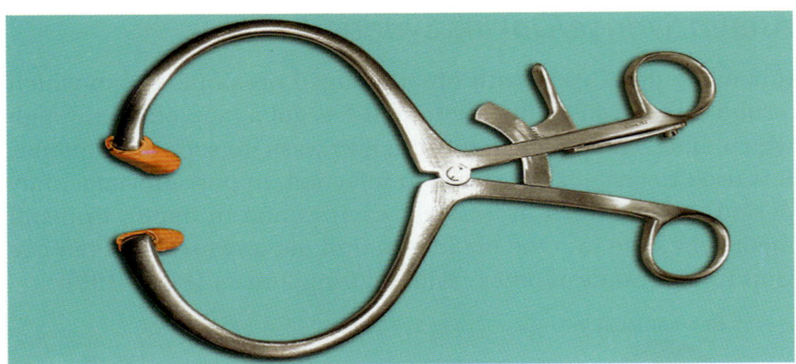

Fig. 5-201C

Figs. 5-201A to C: Doyen's mouth gag.

JENNINGS MOUTH GAG

It is a self-retaining mouth gag with a thin rim and ratchet. Blades fit into the alveolar margins not on the teeth. So it is useful in edentulous patients. It has got a gap to pass endotracheal tube **(Fig. 5-202)**.

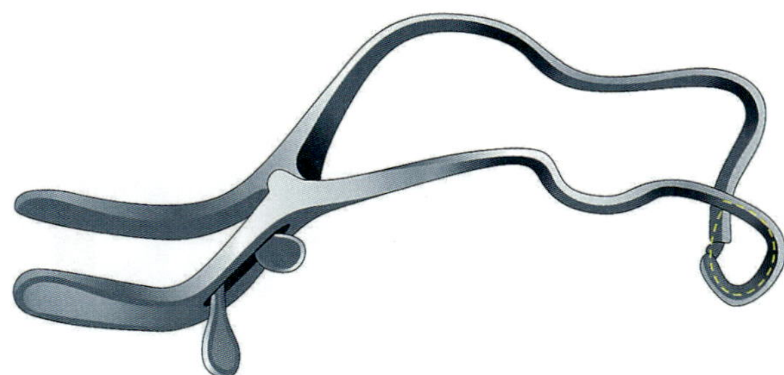

Fig. 5-202: Jening's mouth gag.

TONGUE DEPRESSOR

It is a flat steel atraumatic plate with a 90 degree angle at the centre. Ends are rounded with smooth edge. It is used to inspect posterior third of tongue, oral cavity, tonsils, to take biopsy, etc. Anterior two-third of the tongue is depressed gently with tongue depressor **(Fig. 5-203)**.

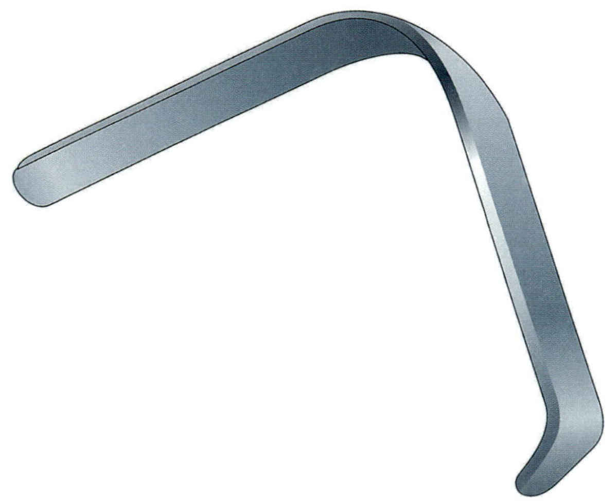

Fig. 5-203: Tongue depressor.

AIRWAY

It is curved metal/plastic hollow instrument with broad proximal end and curved tapered distal end. It helps breathing to patient during postoperative period, and when patient is in intensive care. It also promotes the suction of secretions through the hollow. It prevents fall back of tongue in unconscious patient, in patient with head injury and during induction of general anaesthesia. In a patient with epilepsy it is used to prevent falling back of tongue during convulsion **(Figs. 5-204A and B)**.

It is oropharyngeal airway. It has got a flange (prevents swallowing of airway and keeps it in place), bite block (prevents biting and kinking) and curved body. *Guidel disposable airway* is available in different sizes. *Ovassapian airway* is modified with round channel to facilitate easy passage of fibreoptic bronchoscope. Airway which is cuffed is another modification of airway which can be connected to breathing circuits.

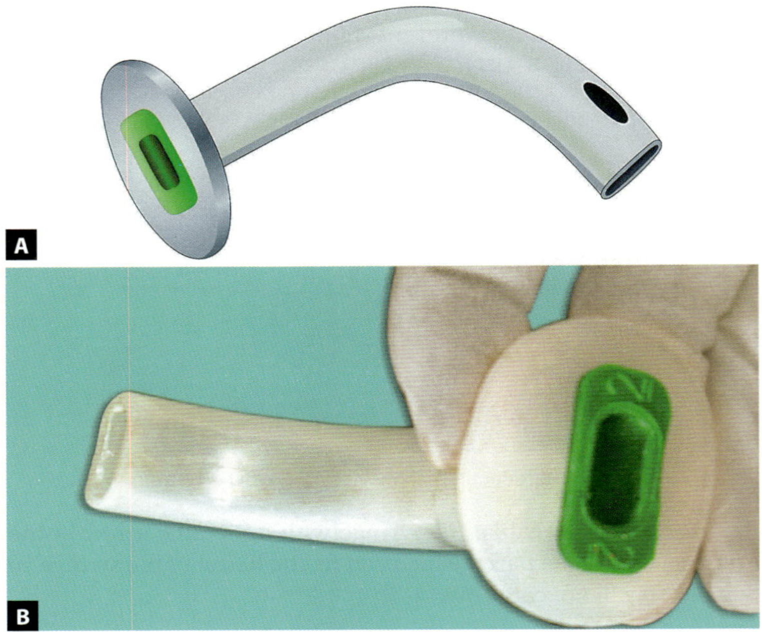

Figs. 5-204A and B: Airway.

HUMBY'S KNIFE

It is used to take split skin graft from donor site. Usually graft is taken from thigh. Often it can also be taken from arm, leg, and forearm. Humby's knife has got stout handle, two flat leaves in blade, one of which is fixed and other can be rotated **(Figs. 5-205A and B)**. Disposable skin grafting blade is passed between the rods into the flat leave which has got three knobs which fits exactly into the openings of the blade. Front leaf has got slots which when pushed gets fixed over the blade. Using firm constant pressure with sawing action split skin is harvested from the thigh. Punctuate bleeding over the donor area confirms the proper skin harvesting. Donor graft is placed over the sterile wooden board. Multiple small window cuts are made to prevent formation of seroma. Skin is placed over the recipient bed and fixed using polypropylene sutures or skin staples. Dressing is placed and part is immobilised. Graft is inspected on 5th day for take up. Donor area is inspected after 10 days and kept open without dressing. Stages of graft intake are—stage of plasmatic imbibition, stage of revascularisation and stage of circulation.

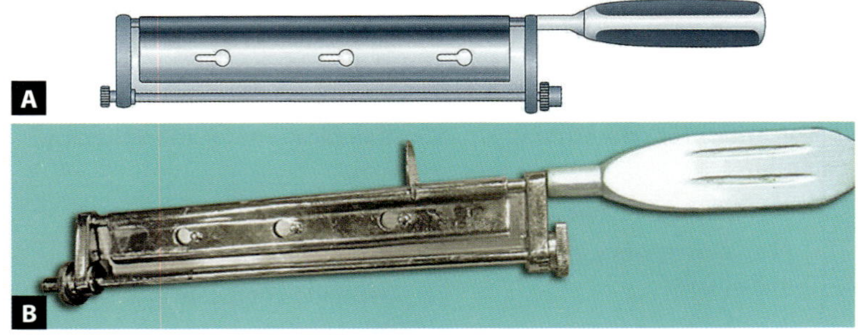

Figs. 5-205A and B: Humby's knife to harvest skin graft.

Other knives used for harvesting skin graft are (Figs. 5-206A to E):

- Braithwaite's skin grafting knife—disposable blade.
- Watson's skin grafting knife—disposable blade.
- Thiersch's skin grafting knife—it has got knife with permanent blade.
- Electrical dermatome.

MYER'S VEIN STRIPPER

It is used strip off varicose vein usually long saphenous vein. It is passed from above just below the saphenofemoral junction. Usually stripping is done up to the middle of the leg. Saphenous neuralgia is a rare complication **(Fig. 5-207)**.

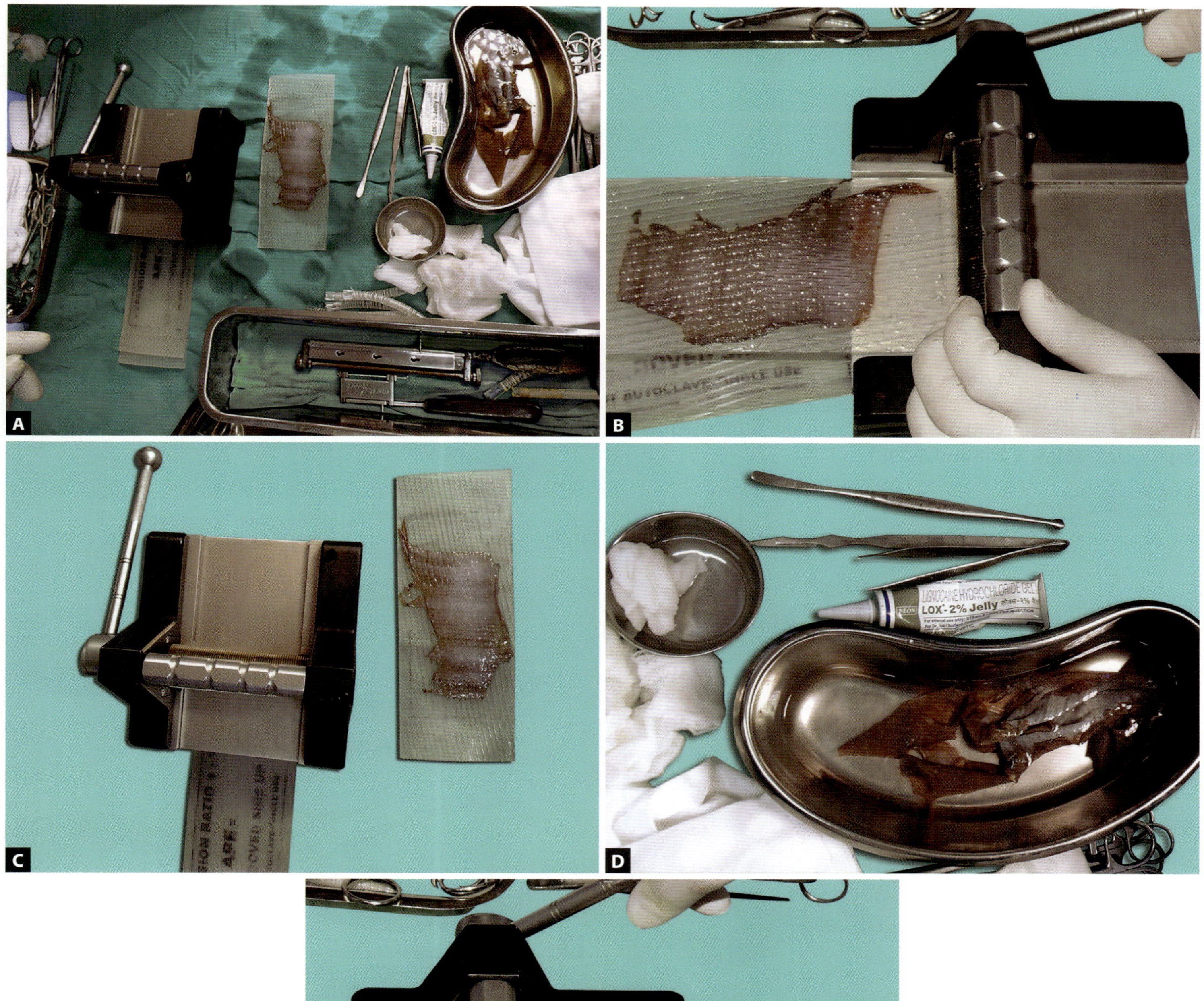

Figs. 5-206A to E: Mesher used for skin grafting in wider recipient area.

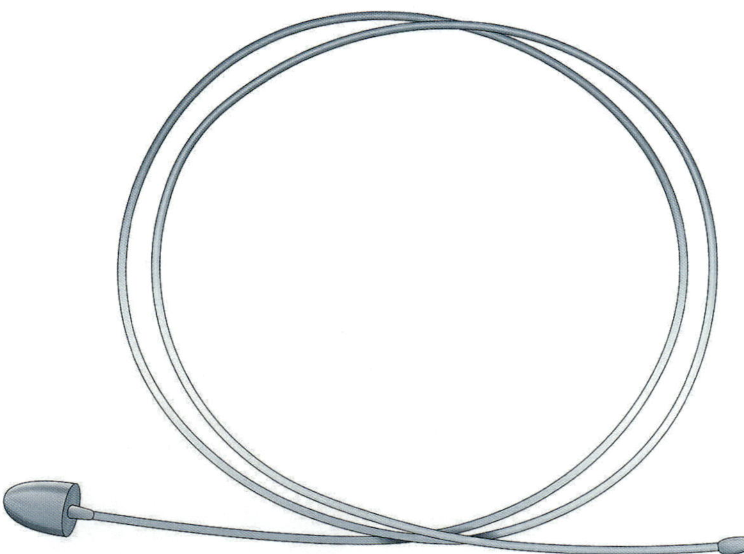

Fig. 5-207: Myer's vein stripper.

BONE CUTTING FORCEPS

It has got short blades with sharp firm cutting edges to cut bones; with a stout handle with ridges. It gives optimum mechanical force to cut bones/bone spurs. Some instruments are supported with leverage system **(Figs. 5-208 and 5-209)**.

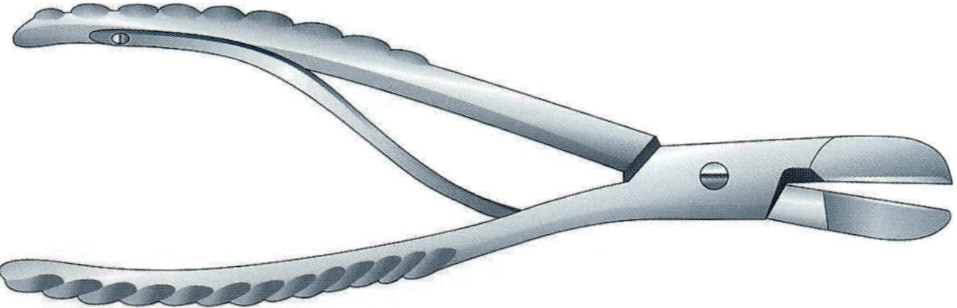

Fig. 5-208: Bone cutting forceps.

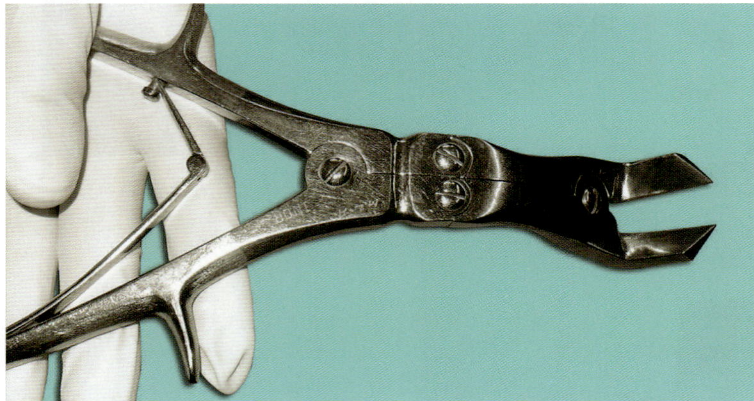

Fig. 5-209: Bone cutter in amputation of small bones, in cutting ribs, etc. It is strong and stout instrument.

BONE ELEVATOR/BONE LEVER

It has got curved blade with blunt edge and serrations on concave surface. Proximal long shaft has got ring for grip. Some bone lever has got proximal knife-like handle instead of ring. It is used in manipulating the fracture segments in open reduction and so to isolate fracture ends from surrounding soft tissues. It is also used to elevate the fracture segments/bone from the depth for placement of nails/fixation **(Fig. 5-210)**.

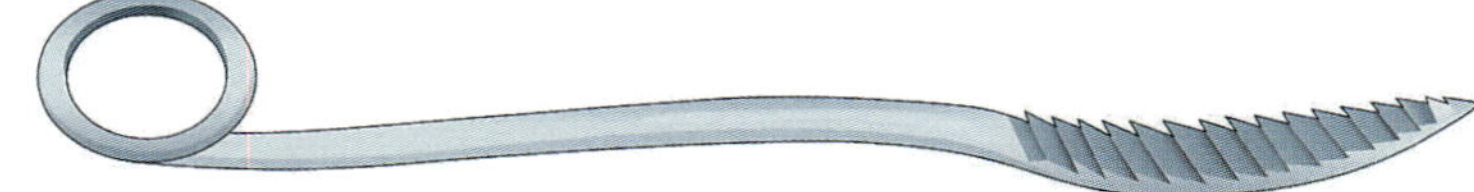

Fig. 5-210: Bone elevator/bone lever.

BONE NIBBLER

It has got sharp edges in the tip with blades being concave. It may be having single action/double action joint. It is used to nibble the bone in pieces like in craniectomy, rib resection, amputations of small bones, etc. **(Figs. 5-211 and 5-212)**.

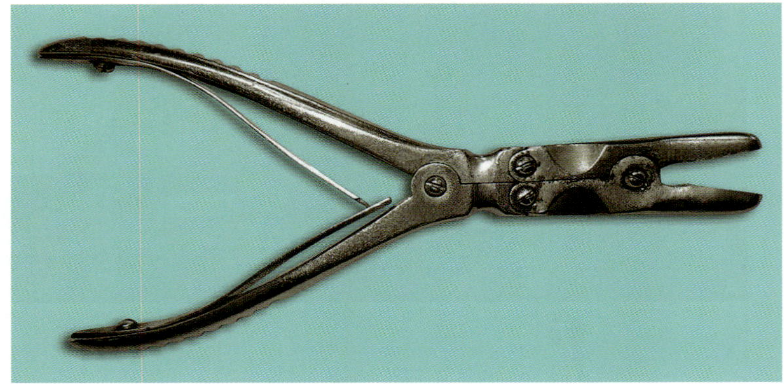

Fig. 5-211: Double action bone nibbler.

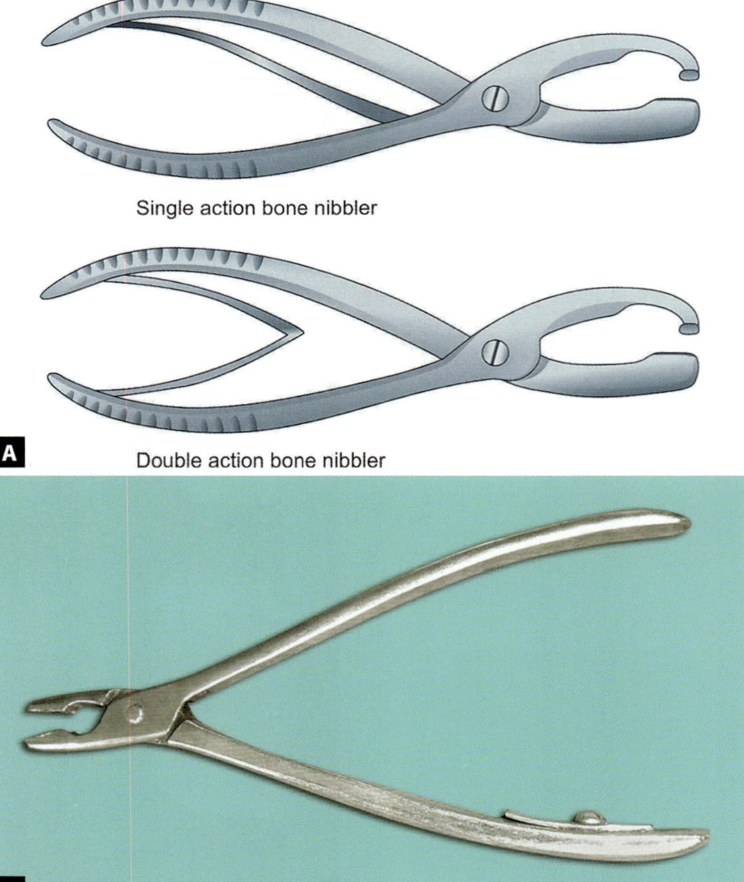

Figs. 5-212A and B: Bone nibbling forceps/bone nibbler.

SEQUESTRECTOMY FORCEPS/ SEQUESTRUM HOLDING FORCEPS

It has a stout blade with thick transverse serrations with a groove in the middle without a ratchet. It is used to remove sequestrum in osteomyelitis. Sequestrum should be formed before removal X-ray should show clear radiolucency around dense dead bone—a sign of complete separation of the sequestrum **(Fig. 5-213)**.

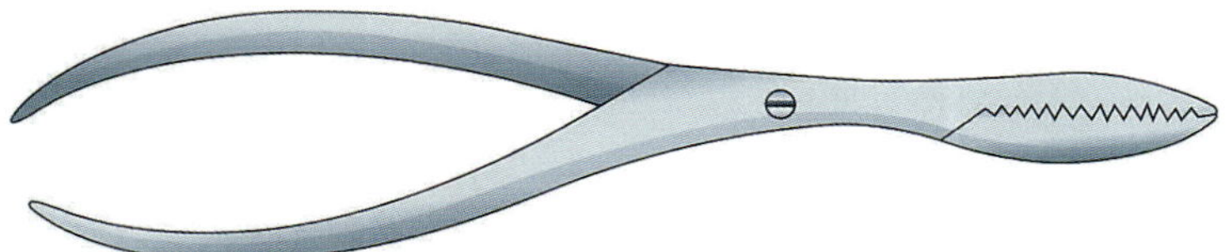

Fig. 5-213: Sequestrectomy forceps/sequestrum holding forceps.

FERGUSSON'S BONE HOLDING FORCEPS/LION FORCEPS

It has got curved blade with stout blunt teeth, looks like jaw of a lion. Bone is held in the gap between the jaws. It is used to hold bones in open reduction of fractures, maxilla in maxillectomy, and mandible in mandibular fixation **(Fig. 5-214)**.

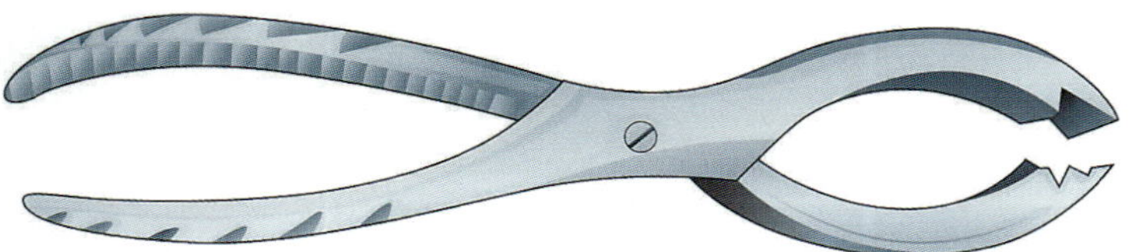

Fig. 5-214: Fergusson's bone holding forceps/lion forceps.

CHISEL

Chisel has got proximal rounded flat head which receives the blows of a mallet. Handle is stout, 10 cm in length. Shaft is of equal size of handle which ends as one side bevelled only (abrupt beveling). It is used to chip the bone using mallet blow. It is also used in bone grafting, sequestrectomy, etc. (**Figs. 5-215A and B**).

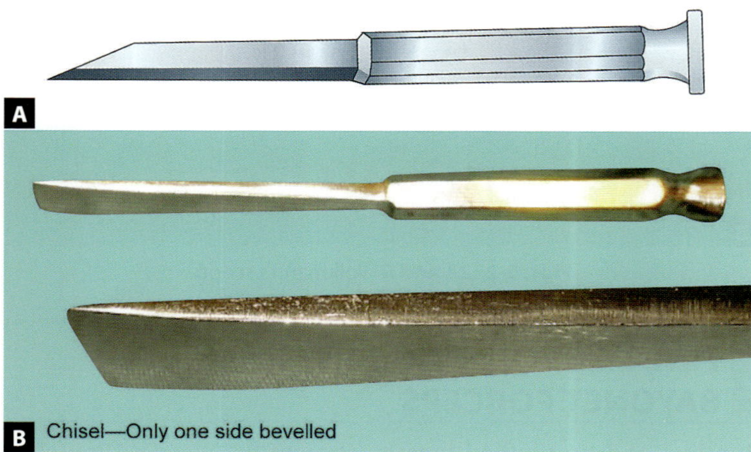

Figs. 5-215A and B: Chisel.

OSTEOTOME

It is similar to chisel but both sides is bevelled and beveling is gradual. Shaft has got the marks to find out the length of the osteotome inside the wound. It is used for all osteotomies in different congenital and acquired conditions **(Figs. 5-216A and B)**.

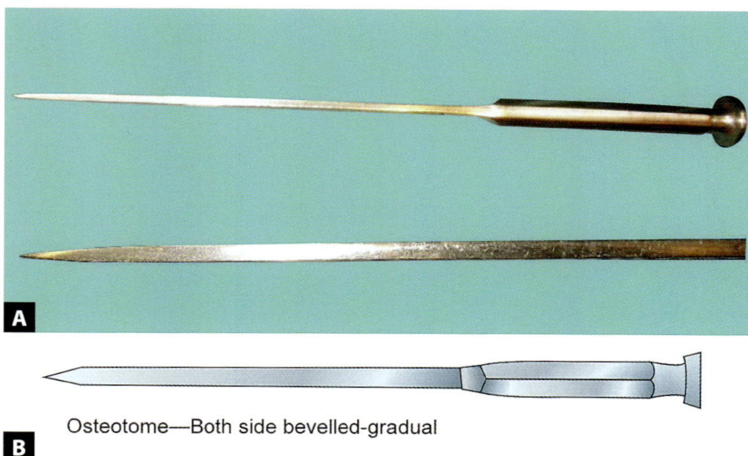

Figs. 5-216A and B: Osteotome.

MALLET

Mallet is a hammer made up of stainless steel or lead. It is lighter than conventional hammer. It is used to give repeated blows on the flat surface over the head of chisel or osteotome. Blow should be flat without rebound **(Fig. 5-217)**.

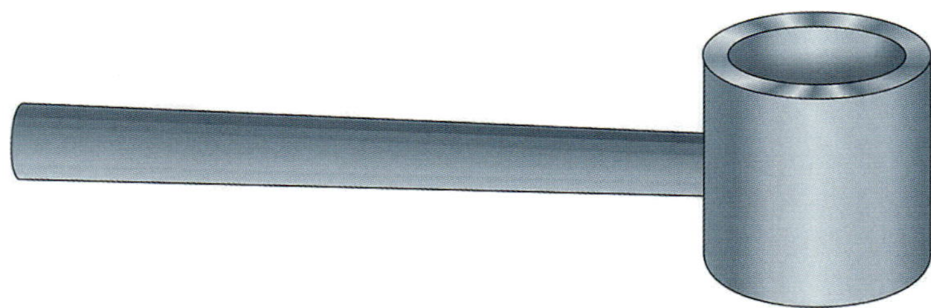

Fig. 5-217: Mallet.

GIGLI'S SAW

It is 14 inches long with four flexible metal wires braided together with rough sharp surface. It has got loops on either ends to hook the handles on it which is essential while cutting the bone. It is used to cut the bones like mandible, maxilla, amputation of femur/tibia, skull bones between the trephine holes. It is originally used to cut the pubic bone in narrow pelvis **(Figs. 5-218A and B)**.

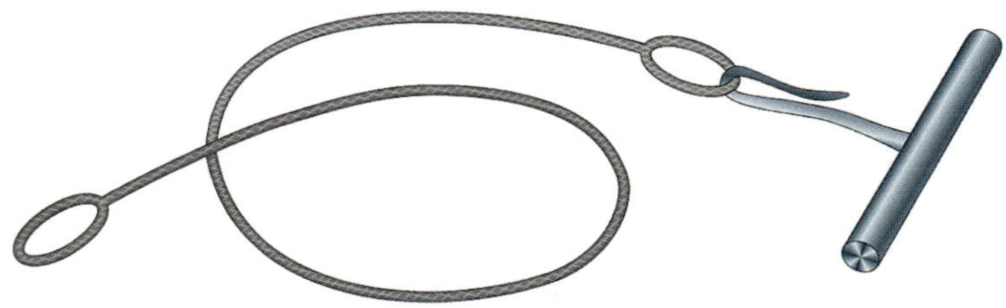

Fig. 5-218A

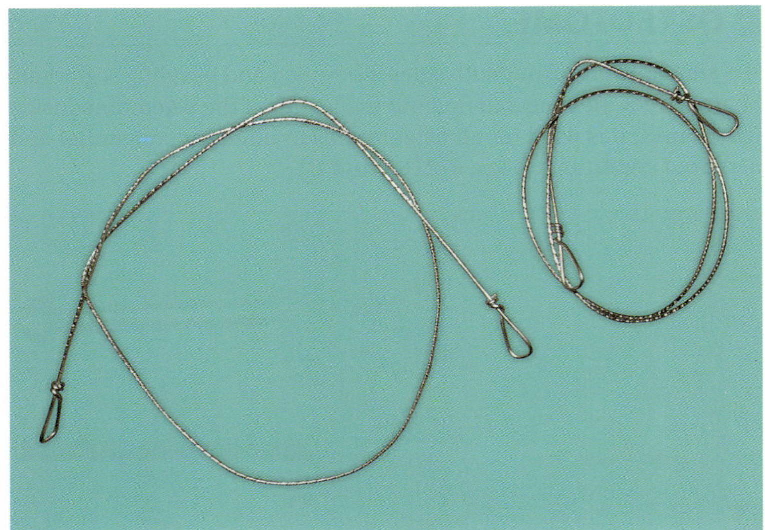

Fig. 5-218B

Figs. 5-218A and B: Gigli's saw/Gigli's wire saw.

KIDNEY TRAY

It is the tray which is kidney shaped. It is used to collect material like fluid, clots, pus, foreign body, gauze, to keep BP handle with blade, to collect daughter cysts in hydatid cyst surgery, in necrosectomy of pancreas, etc. It is sterilised and kept in instrument trolley **(Fig. 5-219)**.

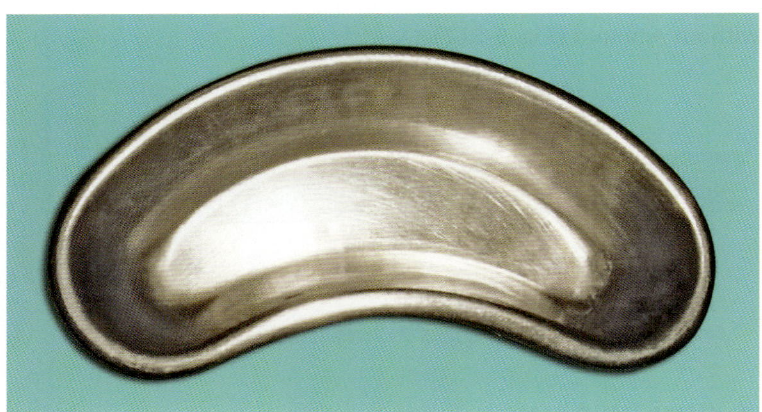

Fig. 5-219: Kidney tray.

GALLIE CUP

It is used as a sterilised cup in the instrument trolley to provide antiseptic cleaning solution like povidone iodine, surgical spirit; to keep needles, gauze in the trolley, to collect material, to keep saline needed during surgery. It is essential instrument in all surgery **(Fig. 5-220)**.

MAYO'S TABLE

It is the table which is fixed to the side of the operating table and it crosses across the OT table so that draping is done over it to keep instruments over it. Instruments will not fall down if surgeon uses it. It is used when position of the patient is in such a way that it is difficult to place instruments over direct draping. Examples are surgeries in kidney position, lateral position, head and neck surgeries **(Fig. 5-221)**.

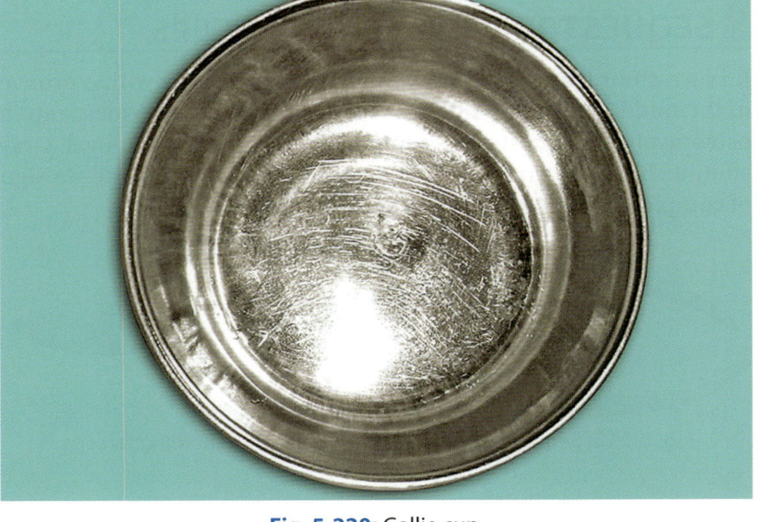

Fig. 5-220: Gallie cup.

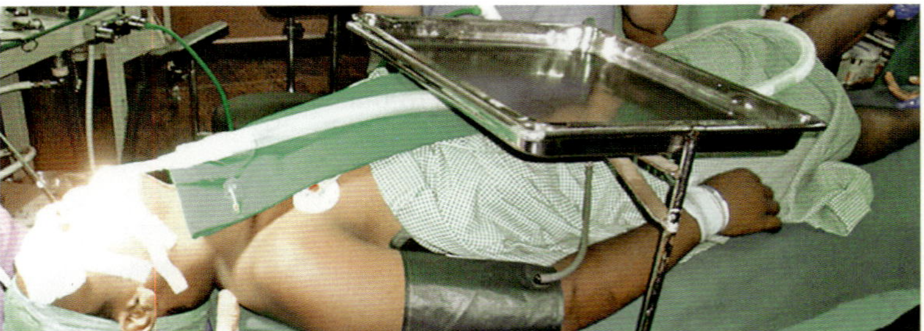

Fig. 5-221: Mayo's table.

VOLKMANN'S SCOOP

It is spoon shaped strong stout instrument with serrations in the middle part. Ends are spoon shaped with cups. Spoons on the ends are of different sizes. It is used to scoop granulation tissue, ulcer bed, before skin grafting, to collect tissues, scoop sinus cavities, clearing necrotic materials from abscess cavities, curette cavities and sinus track in chronic osteomyelitis **(Figs. 5-222A and B)**.

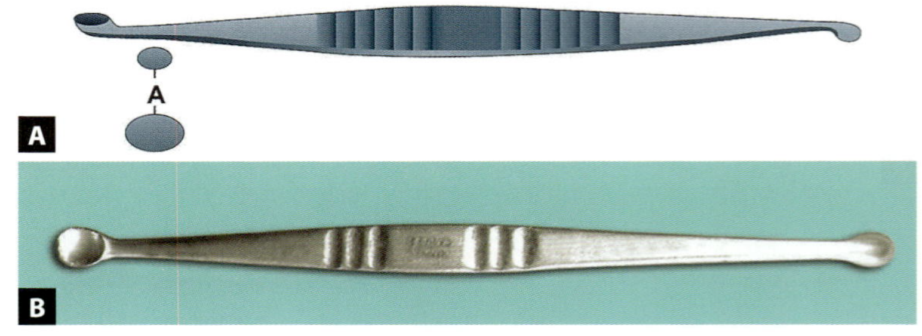

Figs. 5-222A and B: Volkmann's scoop.

FINE LENGTHY STRAIGHT AND BAYONET FORCEPS

Toothed and no toothed lengthy straight or *bayonet* (French—dagger/long blade of rifle) forceps are used in fine dissection and holding tissues and cauterising tissues. Many cautery instruments are fine and often with bayonet. Bayonet shape gives proper vision in depth to proceed with procedure or cautery **(Fig. 5-223)**.

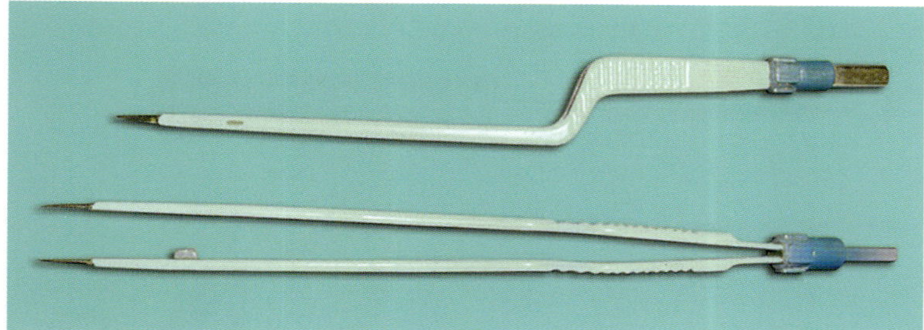

Fig. 5-223: Straight lengthy and bayonet forceps.

CYSTOSCOPE

It is the instrument used by urologists, to visualise urinary bladder, for removal of urinary bladder stones, for TURP, for stricturotomy in urethral stricture, for taking biopsy **(Fig. 5-224)**.

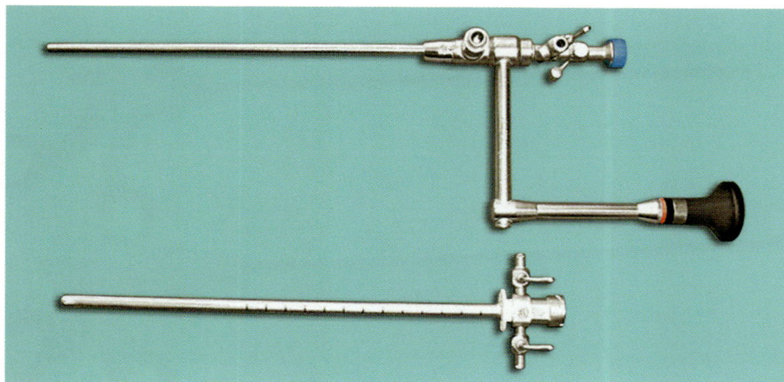

Fig. 5-224: Cystoscope.

AMBU BAG

It is a manual resuscitator with self-inflating bag, bag inlet and non-rebreathing valve. Self-inflating bag returns back into its original shape after compression. During compression air/oxygen enters the patient through non-breathing valve. When compression is released air enters through unidirectional valve to return the bag to its original shape. Exhaled air of the patient returns to atmosphere through non-breathing valve. It is *assisted manual breathing unit*. It can be connected to oxygen reservoir or to atmosphere air. It is used in cardiopulmonary resuscitation, during transporting critically ill patients **(Fig. 5-225)**.

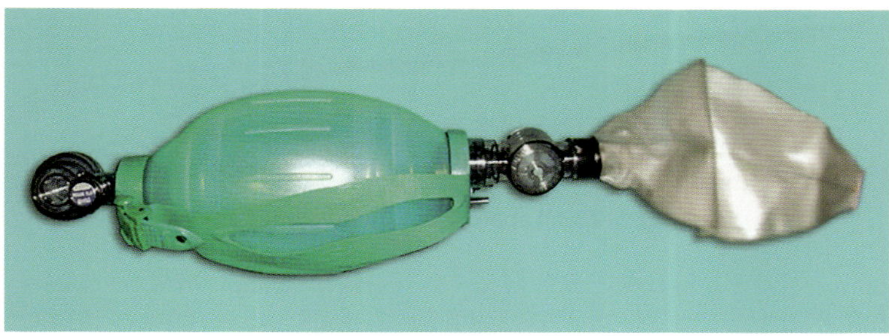

Fig. 5-225: Ambu bag.

LAPAROSCOPIC INSTRUMENTS

There is separate set of laparoscopic instruments with 3 chip camera, telescope light source, CO_2 insufflator, various instruments, harmonic scalpel, etc. Details about that are discussed in appropriate places **(Figs. 5-226 to 5-239)**.

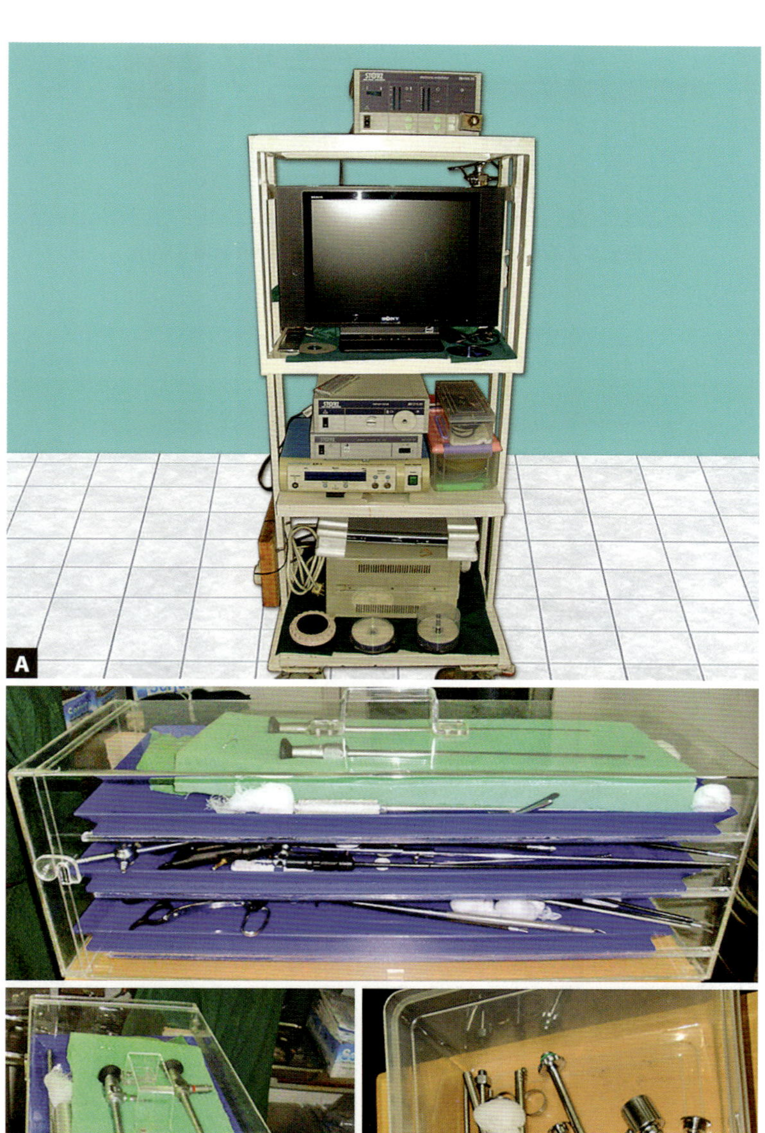

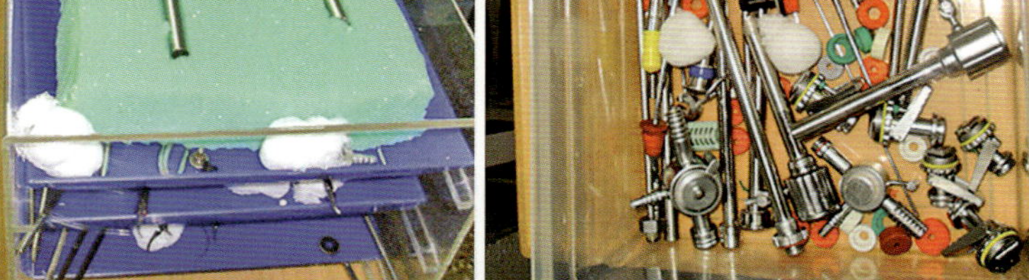

Figs. 5-226A and B: Laparoscopic instrument trolley and set.

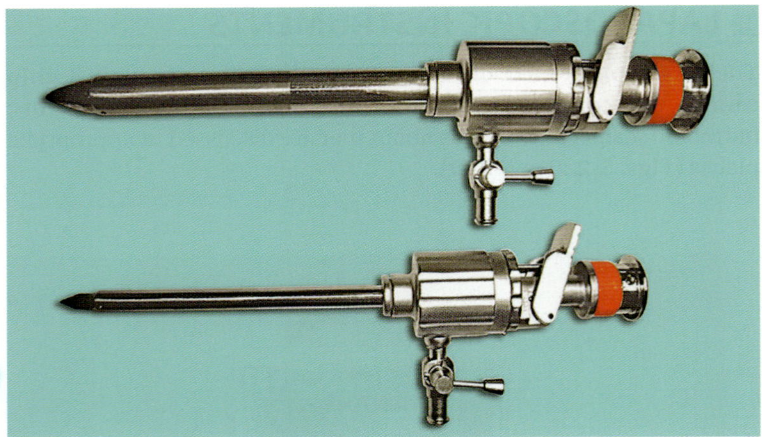

Fig. 5-227: Laparoscopic trocars—10 mm and 5 mm.

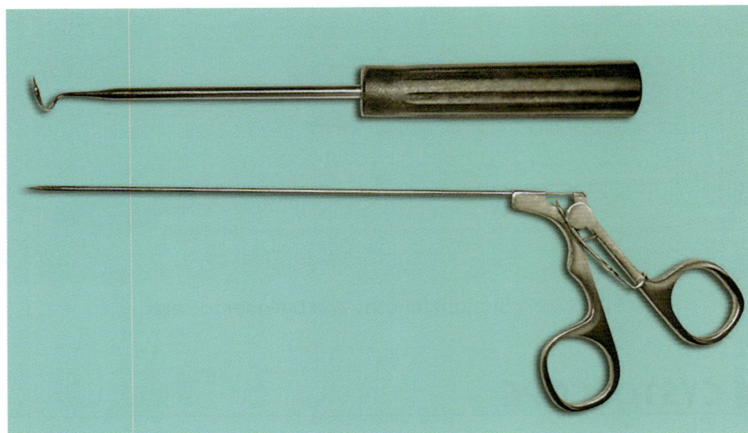

Fig. 5-230: Laparoscopic port closure needle. First one is curved needle; second one is standard laparoscopic closure needle.

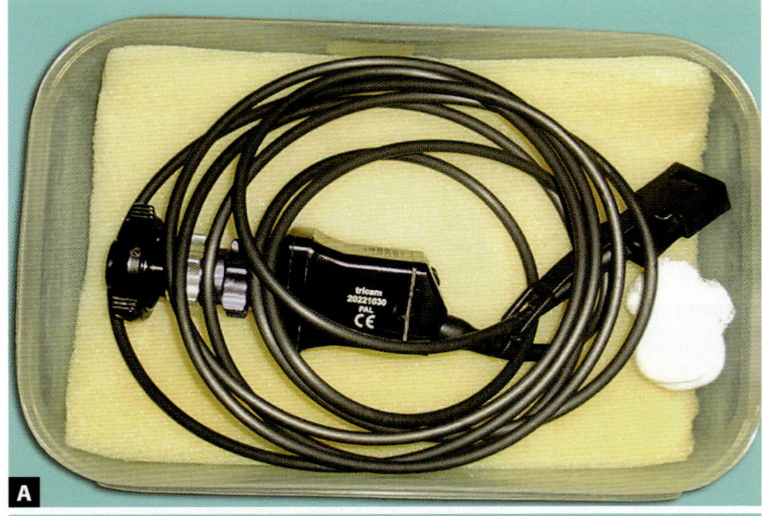

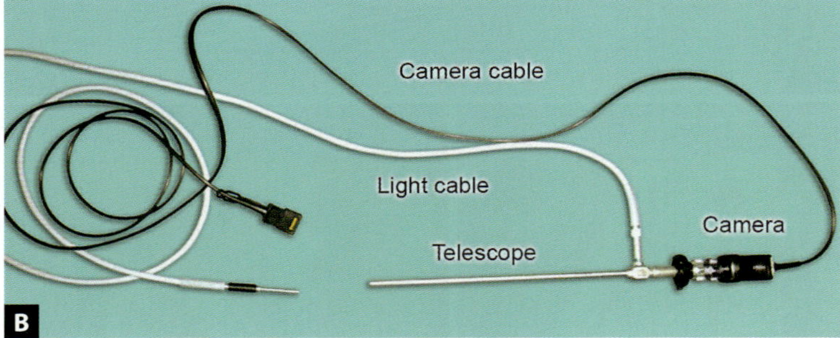

Figs. 5-228A and B: Laparoscopic camera, light cable, camera cable and telescope.

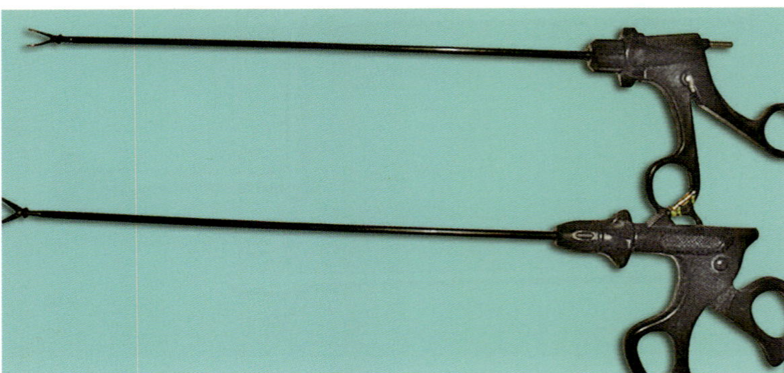

Fig. 5-231: Laparoscopic instruments. They are long fine rotating instruments—scissor, Maryland dissector, grasper, Babcocks forceps, toothed grasper, right-angled dissector, etc.

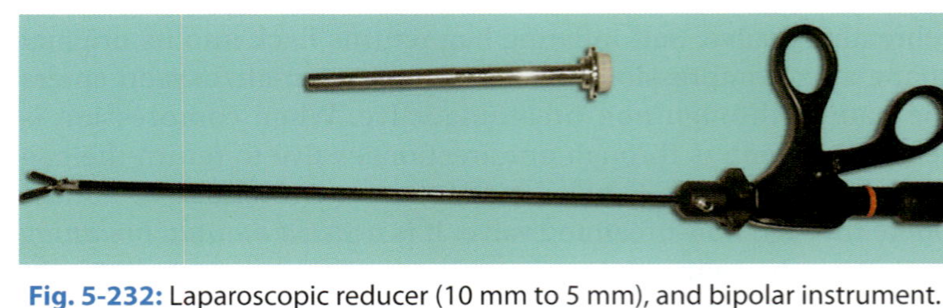

Fig. 5-232: Laparoscopic reducer (10 mm to 5 mm), and bipolar instrument.

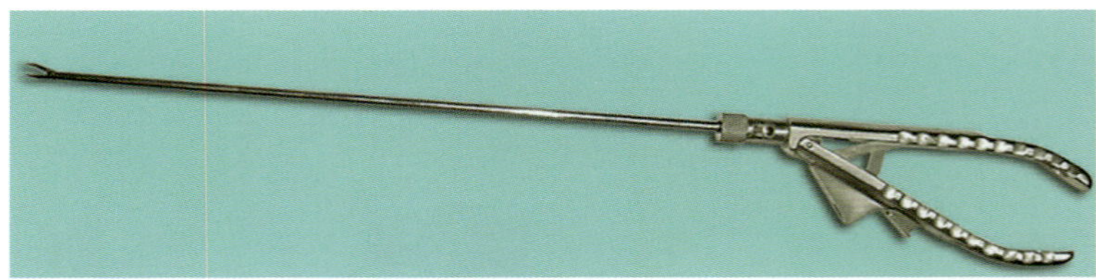

Fig. 5-233: Laparoscopic needle holder.

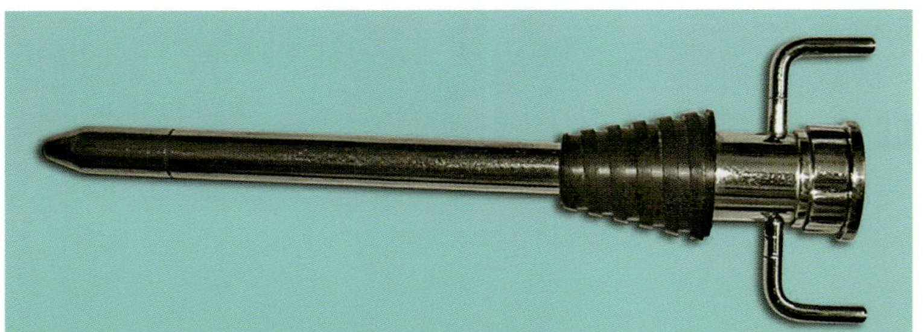

Fig. 5-229: Laparoscopic Hassan's cannula.

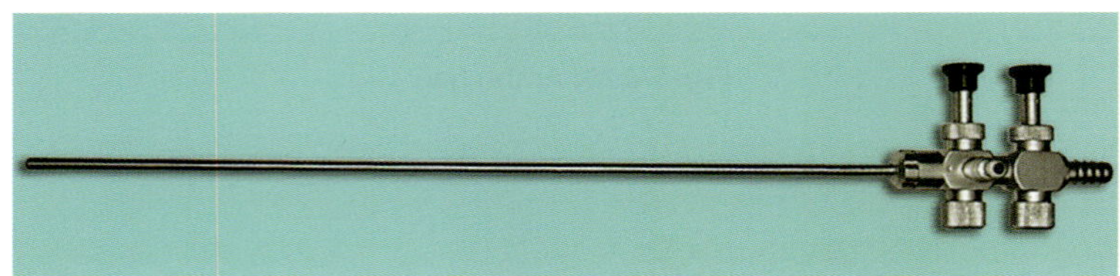

Fig. 5-234: Laparoscopic suction device.

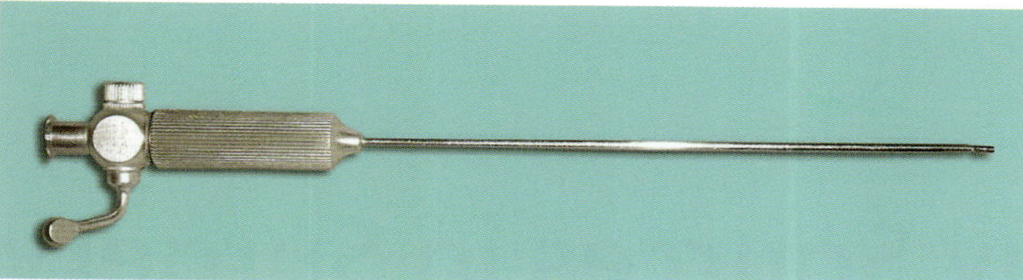
Fig. 5-235: Veress needle.

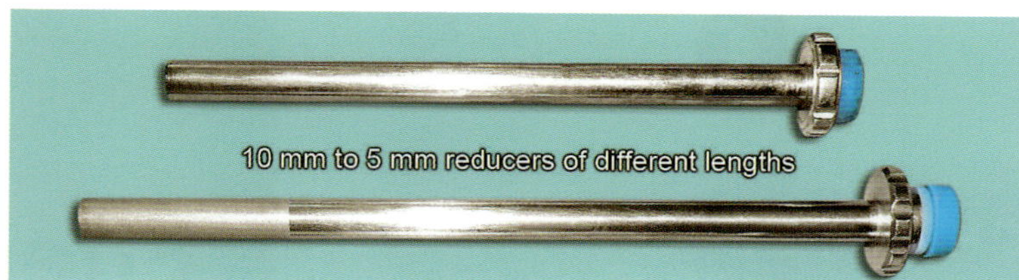

Fig. 5-238: Reducer.

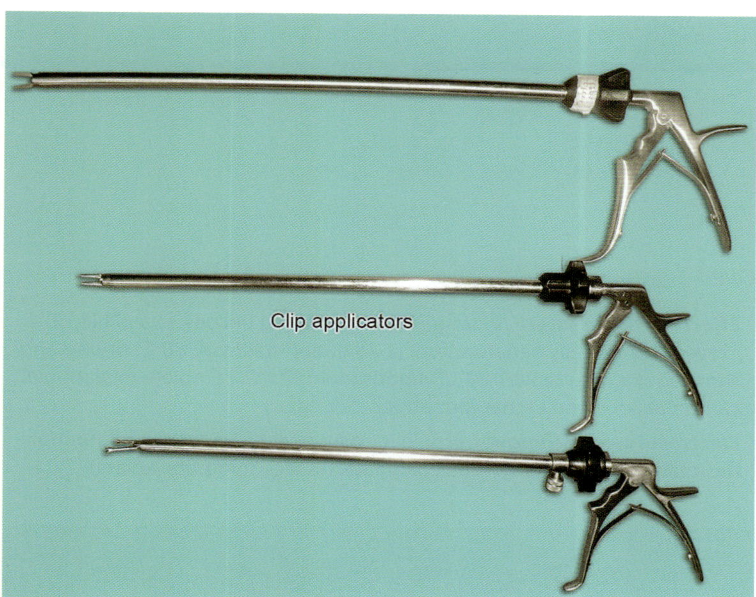

Fig. 5-236: Clip applicators.

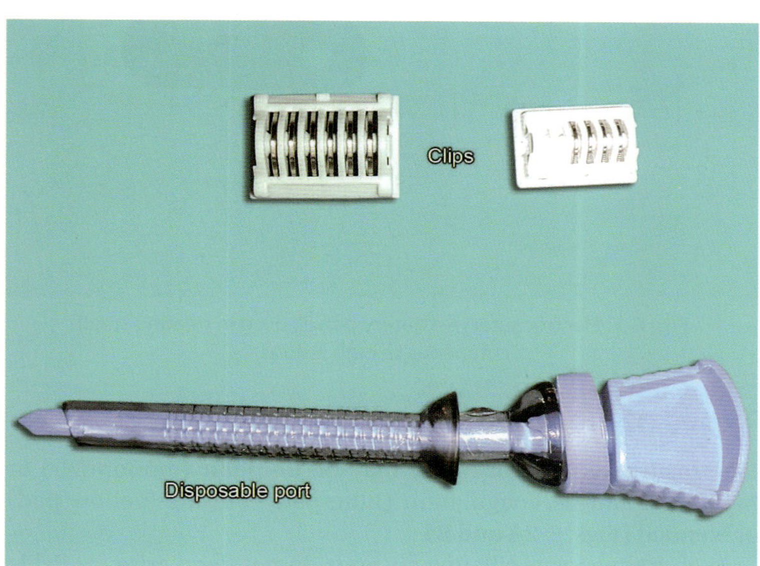

Fig. 5-237: Disposable port.

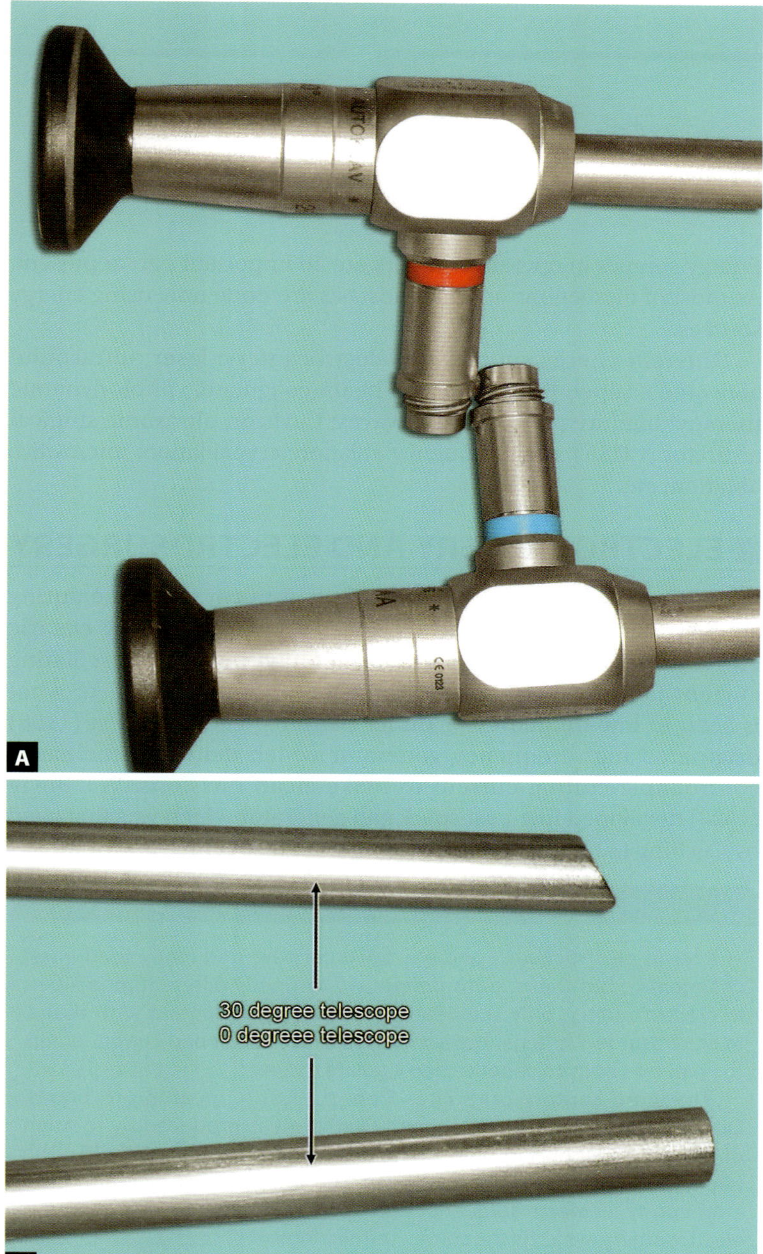

Figs. 5-239A and B: Telescope.

6

CHAPTER

Energy Sources in Surgery

Energy sources in operative surgery are an important part at present. As most of dissections and haemostasis are done now using energy sources.

Different energy sources are electrocautery; laser; ultrasound activated scalpel; ligasure; argon beam coagulator; photodynamic therapy; high frequency sound waves; Cavitron ultrasonic surgical aspirator (CUSA); radiofrequency ablation; cryoablation; microwave ablation, etc.

ELECTROCAUTERY AND ELECTROSURGERY

It is a method to achieve haemostasis and to cut the tissue during surgery using intrinsic thermal effect of high frequency electric current. In 1890 D'Arsonval found that high frequency oscillating current is not capable of neuromuscular stimulation like what is seen in low frequency or direct currents. Lee de Forest (1908) originated high frequency generator which delivered the easily controllable cutting current to make clean incisions. WT Bovie (1928) developed low-cost spark gap generator which was first used by Cushing in neurosurgical procedures **(Fig. 6-1)**.

Note

The terms electrocautery and electrosurgery are frequently used interchangeably; but these terms define two distinctly different modalities. In electrocautery, only the heated wire comes in contact with tissue. In electrosurgery, the patient is included in the circuit and current enters the patient's body to vaporise or coagulate tissue.

The word cautery originates from the Latin, meaning to brand. Diathermy means 'dielectrical heat'. Diathermy is produced by rotation of molecular dipoles in high frequency alternating electric field—the effect produced by a microwave oven. The word Diathermy is also used erroneously for electrosurgery device. In operation theatre device used is electrosurgery, which is the correct terminology.

In electrocautery, current does not pass through the patient. DC or AC is passed through a resistant metal wire electrode, generating heat. The heated electrode is then applied to living tissue to achieve haemostasis or tissue destruction. It is used in dermatology, ophthalmology, plastic surgery, etc. It is safe in patients with pacemakers, defibrillators, deep brain stimulators. It is safer but burns and risk of explosion is there when come in contact with alcohol or oxygen. Risk of human papilloma virus (HPV) and hepatitis B and *Staphylococcus aureus* infection is present while using. Electrocautery devices can be in the form of disposable battery-powered pens or line-powered thermal cautery units.

Contd...

Contd...

Effects of temperature on tissues: 45°C: collagen uncoils, reversible; 60°C: irreversible protein denaturation, coagulation necrosis; 80°C: drying and shrinkage of tissues; 90–100°C: vaporisation; 125°C: complete oxidation of carbon residue and eschar formation.

Electrosurgery techniques are: Electrosurgical coagulation; fulguration; desiccation; electrotomy. (Cut; coagulate; dissect; fulgurate; ablate).

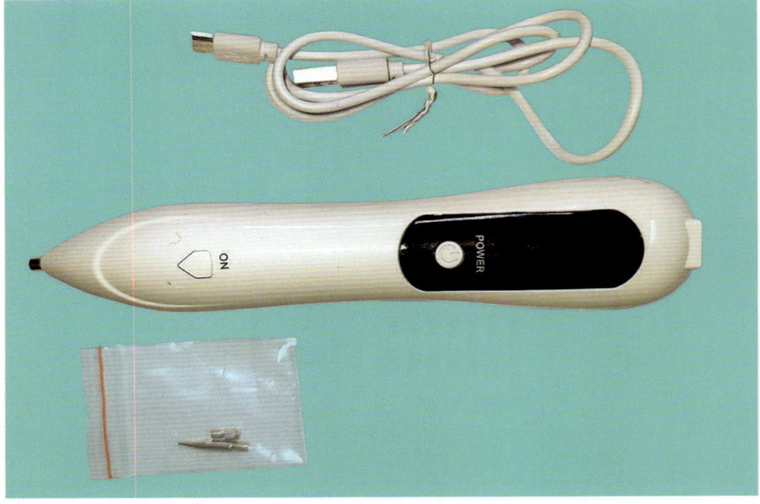

Fig. 6-1: Electrocautery—cautery pencil; used in treating small cutaneous benign lesions.

Types of Electrosurgery/Electrocautery

Electrosurgery/electrocautery may be unipolar (monopolar) or bipolar. It can be coagulation (blue pad), cutting (yellow pad) or blended **(Figs. 6-2A and B)**.

High frequency oscillating currents do not depolarise excitable membranes; current greater than 10,000 Hz do not cause muscle contractions and nerve stimulation.

Electrosurgical units (*ESU, Diathermy*) used in operating rooms convert standard electrical frequencies from the wall outlet, which are 50 to 60 Hz, to much higher frequencies, 500,000 to 3,000,000 Hz. This is important to minimise nerve and muscle stimulation, which occurs at electrical currents below 10,000 Hz. High frequency (3 lakh to 6 lakh Hz) current, is allowed to pass through the tissue to create conduction heat achieving haemostasis. High frequency

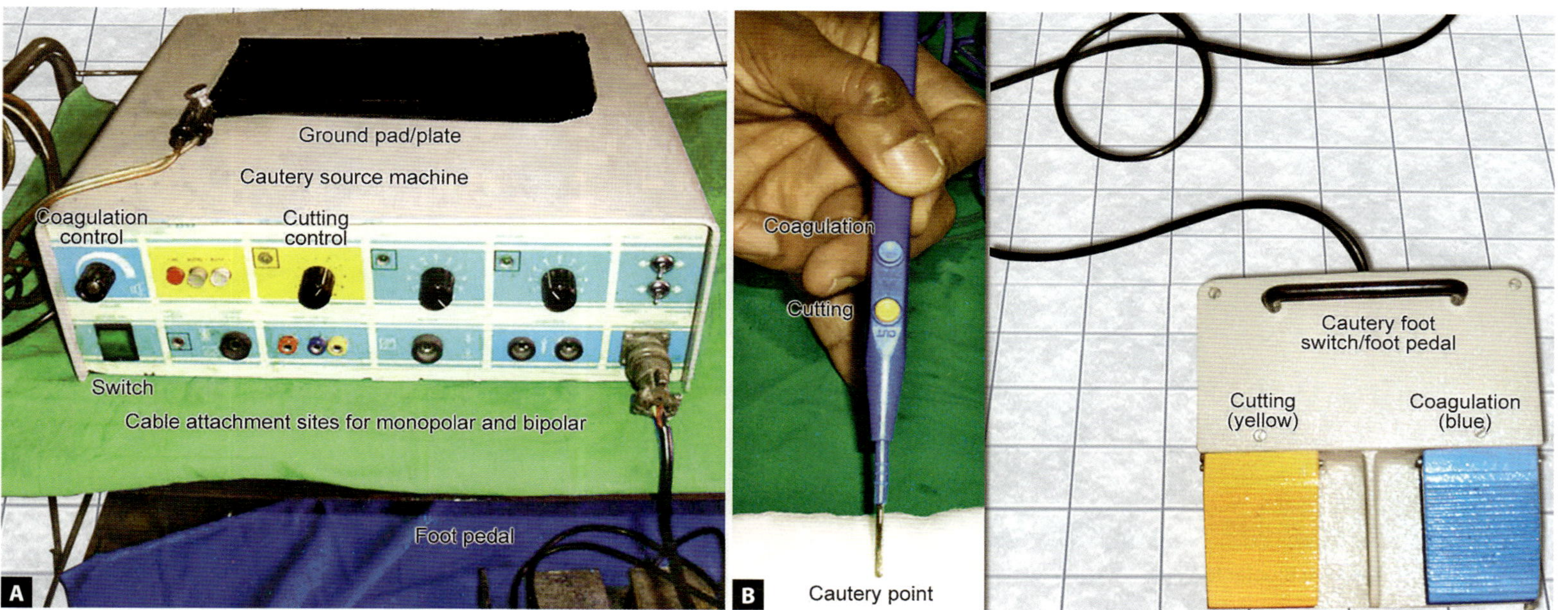

Figs. 6-2A and B: Cautery machine and its components.

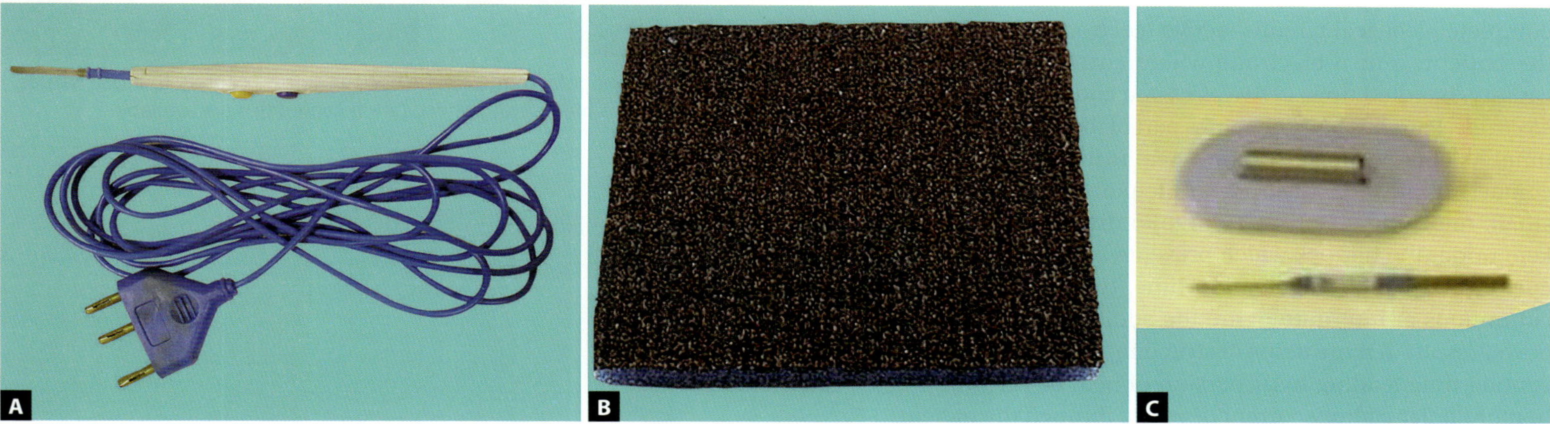

Figs. 6-3A to C: (A) Monopolar cautery pencil with (B) Bovie scratch pad for non-Teflon tip; (C) Teflon tip with Bovie cleaner for it is also shown.

>100 kHz alternate current will no longer stimulate the nerve or muscle. This electrosurgical current causes dehydration, coagulation and vaporisation of tissues.

In monopolar type, current flows from generator to patient through active electrode and returns back through the return electrode to the generator. It is *pulsed wave, low frequency and high voltage* current for *coagulation cautery.*

It is *continuous wave, high frequency and low voltage in cutting* type of monopolar cautery. Active electrode passes through a fine probe to the needed tissue area; whereas return electrode is with 22 square inches of surface area (minimum 10 square inch); flat plate placed under muscular surface with gel conductive coating. Active electrode contacts in less area than return electrode. Current gets concentrated in less area of active electrode to achieve needed effects. Effects may be coagulation or cutting. Coagulation is achieved by protein denaturation and coagulation necrosis. Cutting is due to rapid focal tissue heating causing tissue disintegration without any coagulation necrosis. So, cutting cannot cause coagulation. Coagulation at the tip of probe can cause cutting but with more charring.

In monopolar diathermy, the patient forms part of the electrical circuit, only one side of the generator output is connected to the active electrode; the other side is connected to a return plate under the patient; the plate provides a wider safe path for the current to pass back to the diathermy **(Figs. 6-3A to C)**.

In bipolar diathermy, the current flows between the tips of the forceps, one tip acting as an active electrode and the other as a return; the patient's tissue acts as the conducting medium, through which the current will flow. Cutting current is not produced here; only coagulation current is produced and the field of coagulation is limited to the contact area between the tips of forceps. Surrounding tissues are safer and no earthling (ground plate) is needed. Usually only foot switch is used in bipolar not hand switch **(Fig. 6-4)**.

Electric circuit: It contains (1) *Hot wire*—that connects to the switch; (2) *Neutral wire*—serves as pathway for electrons to return to energy source completing the circuit; (3) *Ground wire*—separate wire that safely conveys leaking electrons to ground avoiding electric shock and injury to patient and OT personnel. Direct current (DC) flows in one direction from negative pole to positive pole. In alternate current (AC) flow of current reverses periodically; one complete cycle occurs when current moves in one direction and then reverses its course; one AC cycle is called as Hertz (Hz).

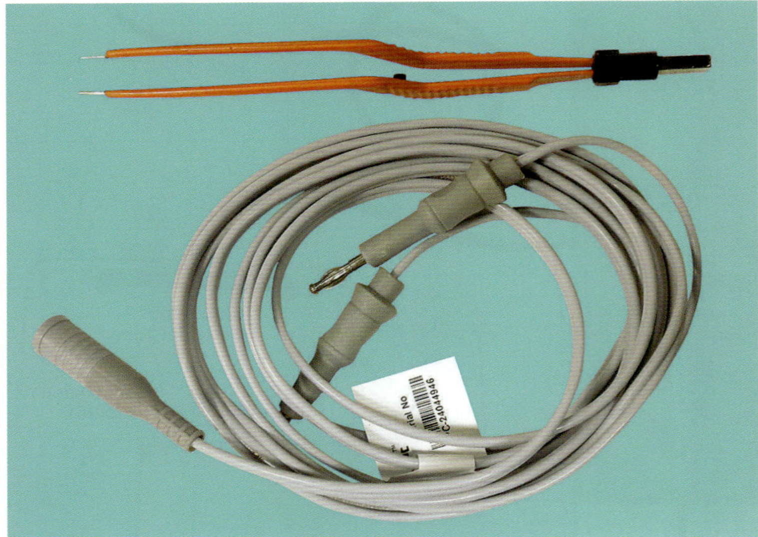

Fig. 6-4: Bipolar forceps—non-sticky type.

Monopolar Cautery

Electrosurgical unit consist of: (1) The electrical generator. (2) To complete electrical circuit—active electrode where current enters the patient; return electrode where current exits. In monopolar cautery, handled tip is *active electrode* and grounding pad is *return electrode*. Patient's body becomes part of the circuit during activation time. As energy conversion into heat is inversely related to area of contact, application electrode at the point in the surgeon's hand is small, returning electrode is large to disperse energy at the plate kept under the buttock which prevents burn injury. Power settings, current frequencies, activation time, type of waveforms whether continuous or intermittent are the additional factors related. High power results in more tissue destruction; low power needs prolonged contact time leading to dispersion of heat to surrounding tissues. In monopolar cautery current *disperses* through the patient.

In monopolar cautery, *continuous waveform* gives cutting current to incise the tissues; *intermittent waveform* gives coagulation current.

In cutting mode, more heat is generated rapidly over the target tissue with less lateral thermal heat—pure cutting effect with sinusoidal waveform with high frequency current (temperature at the tissue contact point is >600°C causing instant vaporisation and cutting).

Cutting cautery allows accurate, precise incisions in the tissues whether curved/circular/in different directions. It is good in relatively avascular area; for fine dissection. Here only tip of the cutting electrode should come in contact with tissues without any resistance and pressure. This active electrode should be clean and should have adequate high power. Epidermis and dermis should never be cut by cutting cautery (even though many surgeons advocate); deep dermis can be cut with his. But then it is preferable to make entire length of the incision by selected scalpel blade and from subcutaneous plane onward to proceed with cautery dissection **(Fig. 6-5)**. Cutting mode can be—low; pure; blend. ***Blend*** (*Blended waveform)* is not a mixture of coagulation and cutting but produces cutting effect with haemostasis with modified duty cycle. It is a blend of pure sinusoidal cutting current with periodic dampened coagulation current. Tissue is heated and water in the cell dries out. It can be used as cutting or coagulation current by contact with tissue. As we go from Blend 1 to Blend 3 the duty cycle is progressively reduced. A lower duty cycle produces less heat. Blend 1 is able to vaporise tissue with minimal haemostasis; Blend 3 is less effective at cutting but has maximum haemostasis **(Figs. 6-6A and B)**.

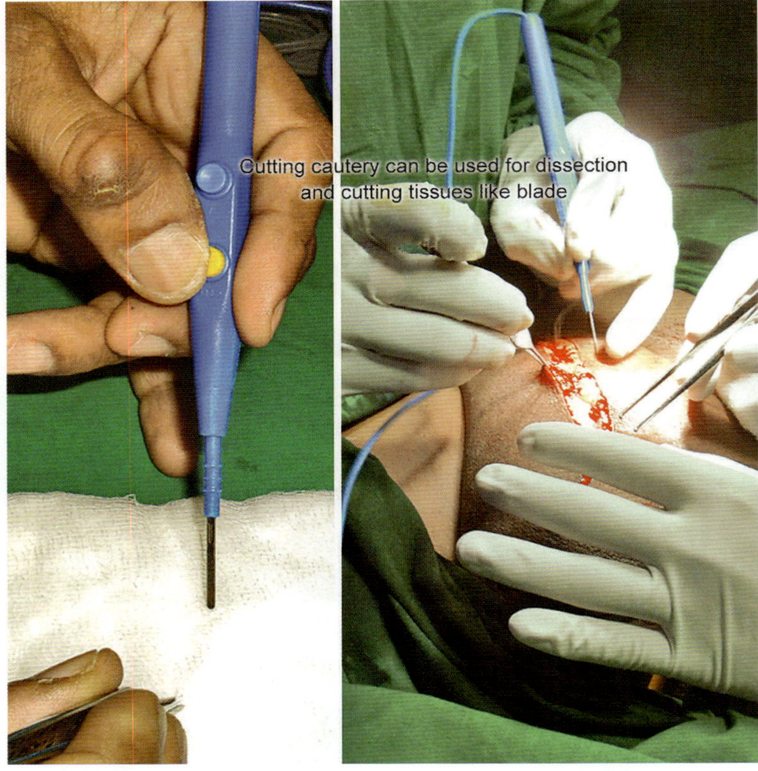

Fig. 6-5: Monopolar mode can be used as cutting cautery to incise tissues like a blade. Long, short, Teflon coated tips are available.

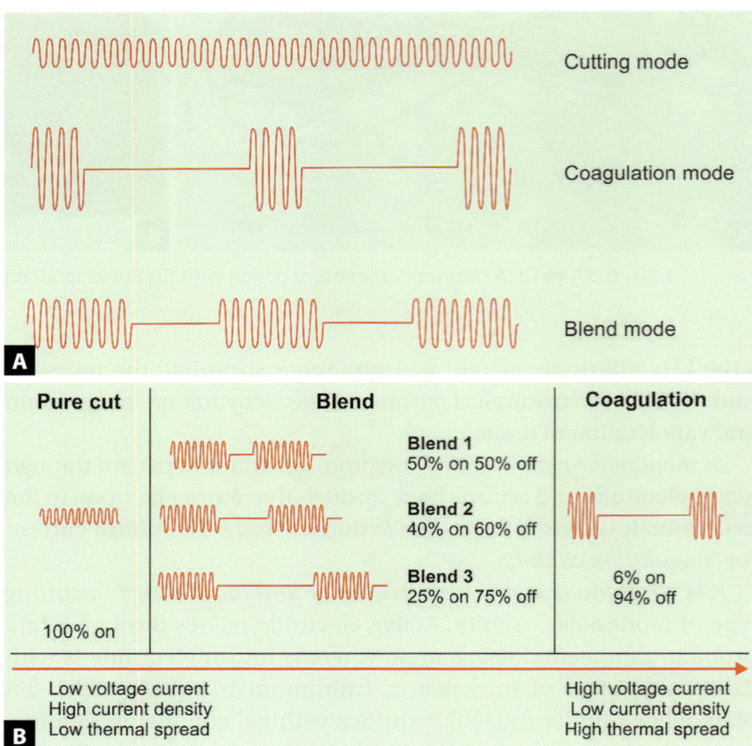

Figs. 6-6A and B: Waveforms in cutting, coagulation and blend types of monopolar electrosurgical unit.

In coagulation mode less heat with slow frequency is generated causing tissue dehydration, vessel thrombosis with more lateral thermal injury (series of dampened sinusoidal waves with rapid bursts leading into desiccation, coagulation, thrombosis, destruction). Coagulation current is used for haemostasis by two methods: (1) *Obliterative coagulation* is achieved by direct contact between active electrode and bleeding points which is suitable for bleeders less than 0.5 mm in size. (2) *Co-aptive coagulation* is achieved by holding the edges of the vessel or bleeding tissue with a haemostat or forceps and applying current to the instrument which is suitable for larger vessels between 0.5 and 1.5 mm in size. Desiccation of coagulation current is used like a cutting device but by proper tension and counter tension in the tissue. Excessive tension is essential in such situation. Control switch is either in a hand piece or in the foot pedal (blue coagulation; yellow cutting) **(Figs. 6-7 to 6-9)**. Coagulation mode can be—desiccate 1,2,3; fulgurate; LCF fulgurate; Spray.

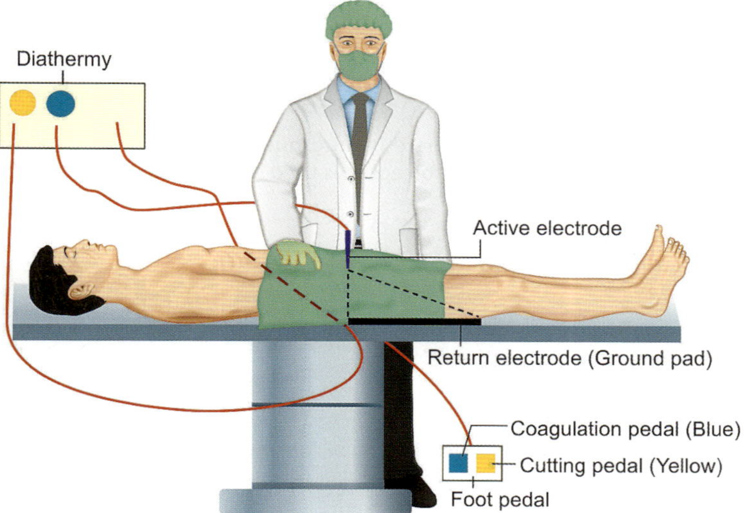

Fig. 6-7: Monopolar cautery. It requires ground pad as return electrode. It can be used both for cutting and coagulation effects of the cautery.

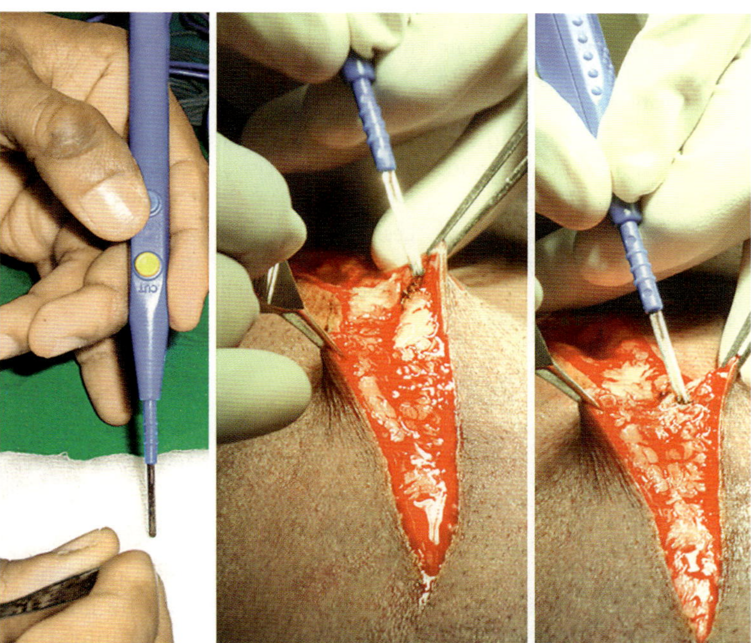

Fig. 6-8: Obliterative coagulation is used for tiny bleeders to control.

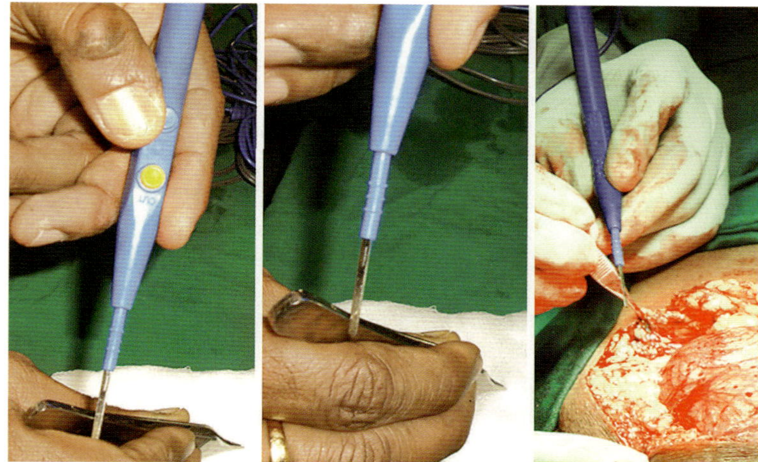

Fig. 6-9: Co-aptive coagulation is used for little larger vessels. Here bleeding vessel is held with specific cautery forceps or usual forceps and cautery point is touched to the cautery forceps to coagulate the vessel.

Earthling ground plate (return pad, diathermy pad, dispersive pad): *Types of patient plates used are*—reusable and disposable; disposable is ideal but reusable is economical. Disposable plates are—conductive adhesive plates which are generally thin, lightweight and flexible with its conductive adhesive which works like gel having continuous adhesive border. Plates should not be placed near scars, implant sites or ECG electrodes; a muscular well-vascularised area is most suitable like buttocks, thigh, calf, upper arm, back, etc. **(Fig. 6-10)**.

Removable Energy Management system (REM system) continuously monitors the heat buildup in the ground plate; it is connected to the patient and to generator. Indicator illuminates green when system is proper; any changes it illuminated red as a warning sign. Newer instant response technology which recognises the changes in the tissues 200 times per second is also available which provides the instrument high power efficiency rating **(Figs. 6-11A and B)**.

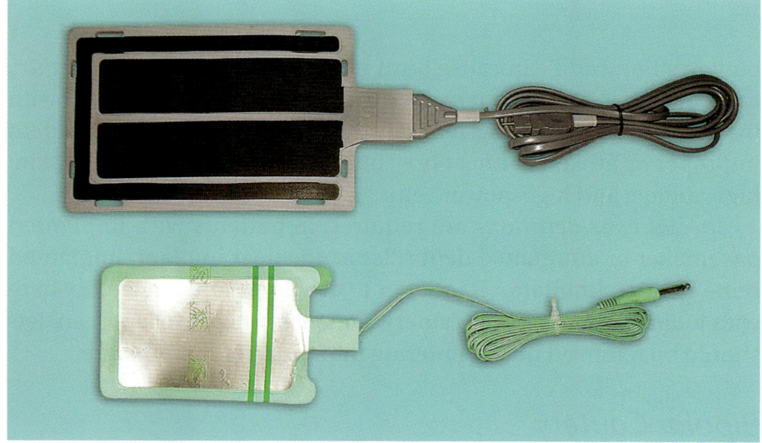

Fig. 6-10: Return pad used in monopolar cautery. It can be reusable or disposable.

Plate site must be clean, dry and shaved; skin integrity should be protected; patient should not rest on dispersive plate clamp; settings should be determined by the surgeon; all connections, contact points should be checked for safety; fluid should not be allowed to pool adjacent to the ground plate. Patient should not be in contact with any metal (earthed objects like drip stand, OT table edge) as much as possible. Active electrode should be kept safely when it is not in use as tip of the active electrode may come in contact with the

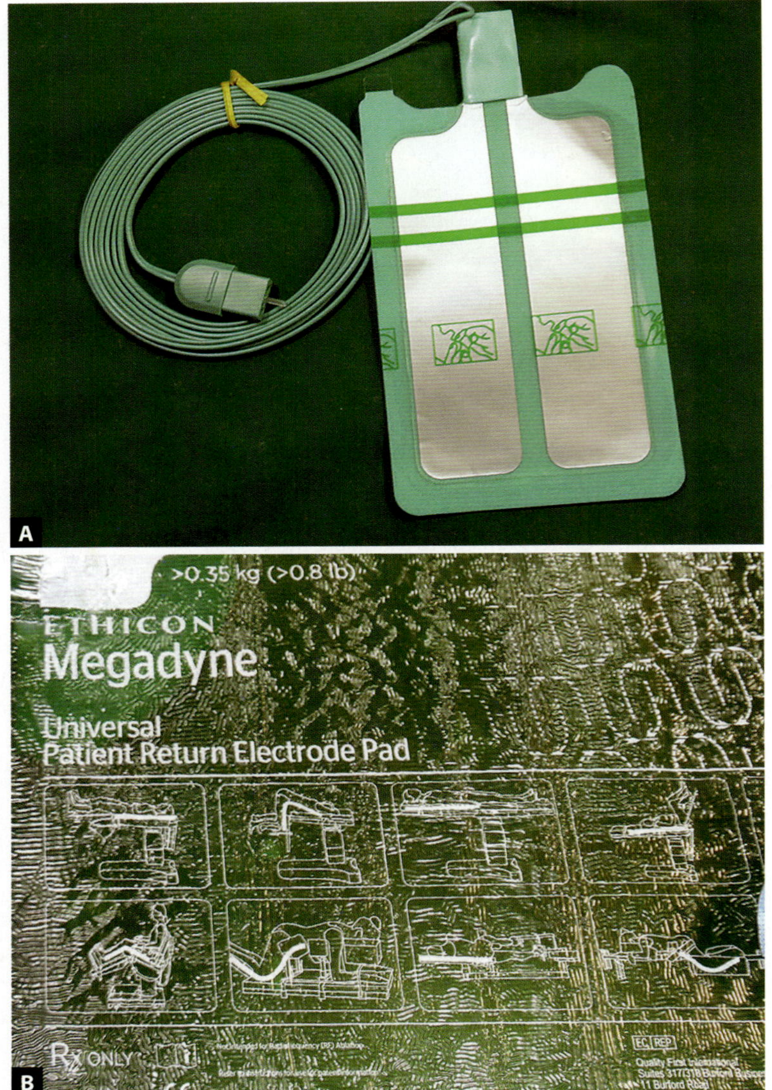

Figs. 6-11A and B: Different dispersive electrode/pads (Earthling pads).

patient's body and can cause burn injury inadvertently. *Burn injury* can develop if plate is not properly in contact with the patient with inadequate surface area; hairs in the return electrode plate area; improper or broken connections; inflammable material on the skin; high voltage and high-power setting.

Special considerations are required in patients with implanted pacemaker or automated defibrillator, cochlear implant, implanted bone growth stimulator; it is better to avoid monopolar cautery here with judicial use of bipolar cautery. Patient's body jewelleries, anklets should be removed before entering into the operation theatre.

Bipolar Cautery

Here one tip of bipolar forceps acts as active electrode and another tip as return electrode with the tips of the forceps with grasped tissue in between completing the circuit. *Grounding pad is not required in this.* It gives precise thermal coagulation. There is no chance of lateral thermal injury. Electrical energy is concentrated between the two electrodes. Current is *not dispersed* through the patient. It causes co-aptive obliteration. It is meant only for coagulation. It causes self-limiting coagulation of tissues in between tips of two electrodes in which after tissue desiccation prevents further flow of current. If tips of bipolar forceps come in contact with each other without any tissue in between, this may create a short circuit which should be avoided. Bipolar is not used for cutting. Bipolar cautery can seal a vessel up to 7 mm in size **(Figs. 6-12 to 6-14)**. Bipolar can have three types of working operations—precise; standard; macro.

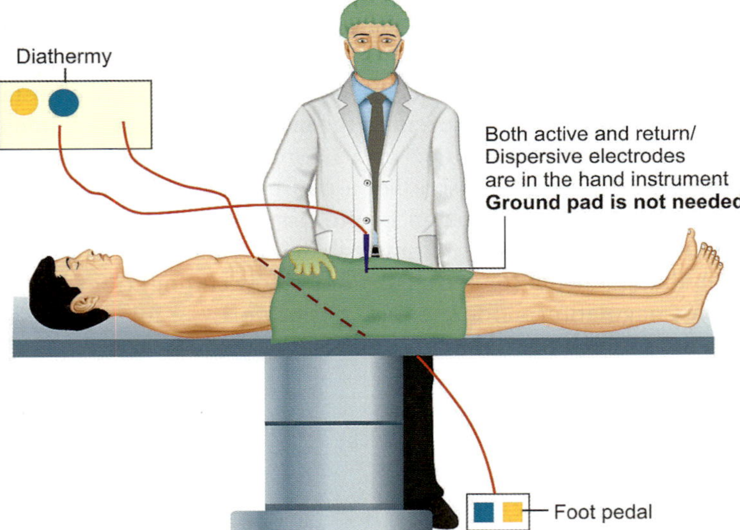

Fig. 6-12: Bipolar cautery. There is no ground pad. Active and return electrodes are in the tip of the forceps. It is used only for coagulation not for cutting.

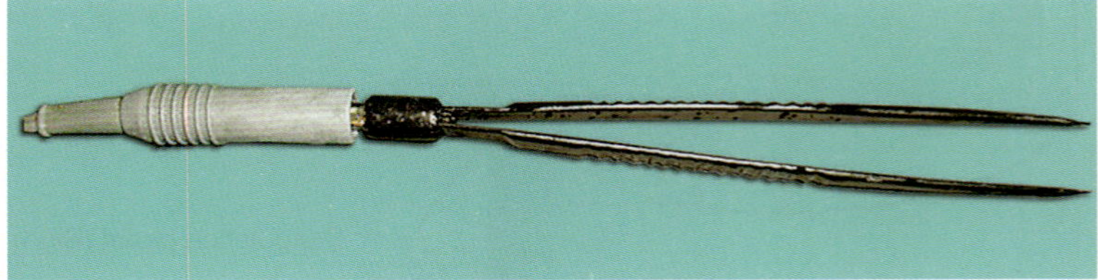

Fig. 6-13: Bipolar cautery forceps.

Monopolar cautery	*Bipolar cautery*
Active electrode in the hand instrument; return electrode in the grounding pad—plate kept under leg/thigh/buttock of the patient	Both active and return electrodes are in hand instrument tips. Grounding pad is not needed
Achieves both cutting and coagulation effect depends on need	Achieves only coagulation effect (co-aptive) but precise and accurate. Not used for cutting tissues or dissection purpose
Chances of large tissue injury, lateral thermal heat problems, can interfere with pacemakers; can cause deep burn injury	Less tissue injury; no lateral thermal heat problems; safe with pacemakers; less chance of burn injury

Tates rule: Only the surgeon holding the hand piece cautery should control the foot pedal (never allow a sister or assistant) to prevent miscommunication and risk of inappropriate current application and injury to patient.

Precautions while using electrosurgical device

Machine should be inspected periodically for default. Connections and wires should be checked. Wet area should not be allowed. Alcohol containing solutions when used for preparation, it should be allowed to dry up properly. Power settings should be

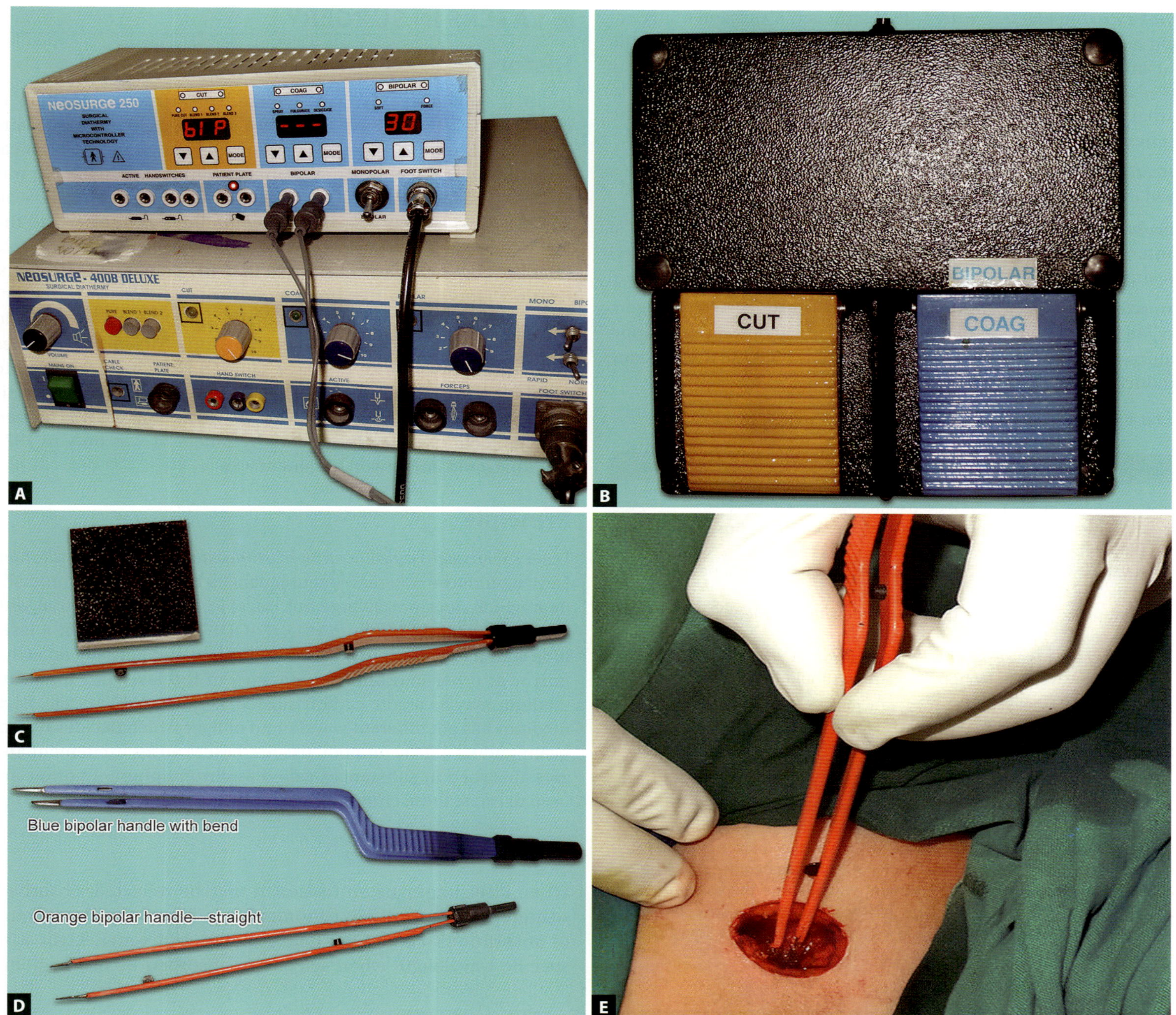

Figs. 6-14A to E: Bipolar cautery system—source, forceps, different type tips, foot pedal, functioning in tissues.

only optimum not very high. Active electrode pencil when not in use should be kept away from wet surface of the drape and should not come in contact with patient's body. Grounded metal objects should not touch patient's body. Dispersive electrode should be placed in proper dry place with surface area adequate contact.

Problems with Cautery

Active electrode injuries: It is accidental activation of the electrode. It is prevented by storing hand electrode device in a plastic cover when not in use. Adhesive plastic drape prevents accidental touch of adjacent skin. It is better to have proper activation sound tone (different for cutting and cautery). One should avoid unnecessary touching of the adjacent tissues with active electrode.

Return electrode injury: If contact between grounding pad and skin is not proper or inadequate, it will lead into high resistance and impedance causing burn injury. It is usually deep wide area burn. It amounts for negligence legally. Often return electrode monitoring alarm device is used which if contact between grounding pads and skin is insufficient, will give alarm and automatically shuts down.

Coupled current diversion: Here active electrodes come in contact with a conductor of electricity—staples, clips or guidewires. It is important in laparoscopic surgery.

Uncoupled current diversion: It occurs in monopolar co-aptive coagulation. It may be due to perspiration inside the glove. Hole (glove tear) in the glove may or may not be there. It is unintended diversion of current across thin insulators/capacitor. Double glove or changing the glove will prevent this.

Flame injuries: It may be due to flammable anaesthetics, flammable solvents, high oxygen tension, ether, etc. Cautery should never be used in close association with inflammable items.

Smoke during electrocautery: It obstructs the surgeon's surgical field especially in laparoscopic surgery. It is bacterial mutagenic causing increased chances of sepsis. Cautery of condyloma may cause aerosolisation of the virus particles. In laparoscopic surgery, partial opening of the knob of the port to release smoke during the cautery procedure reduces the field obstruction due to smoke.

Infection and cautery: Charred tissue/cauterised tissue may be a good media for bacterial colonisation.

Pacemaker interference: Monopolar cautery may cause electrical contact between active electrode and pacemaker unit (cardiac) causing its block.

Intestinal gas explosions: It is due to presence of hydrogen, oxygen and methane in the bowel. Mechanical bowel preparation reduces such gas load. Mannitol/sorbitol may increase the methane production in the bowel.

Burn injury: To surgeon/assistant/scrub nurse.

About electrocautery

- It is the commonest device used for haemostasis.
- It causes tissue dehydration and vessel thrombosis or tissue disintegration.
- Always proper electrical connections and ground pad fitting should be confirmed.
- Monopolar cautery should be avoided in a patient with cardiac pacemaker.
- Igniting agents like alcohol (excess usage of surgical spirit), ether should be avoided. Monopolar cautery should be avoided in testis/cord/during circumcision.
- Tip of the cautery point should be insulated with quiver when not in use.
- Only using surgeon should activate the diathermy—*Tates rule*.
- Insulation of the laparoscopic instrument should be 100% otherwise it causes burn of adjacent tissue or port site. Instrument to instrument *direct coupling* and tissue damage can occur. If insulation is improper between trocar port and plastic sleeve of the instrument it leads into *capacitance coupling* and damage. *Retained heat* from the tip of the laparoscopic cautery instrument will damage the tissue if tip is made to rest on any vital tissues (like *spatula or hook* instrument after use if touches diaphragm, liver or colon may cause heat injury of the respective organs.

LASERS IN SURGERY

History

In 1960, Theodore Maiman invented the ruby laser which is considered to be the first successful optical or light laser. Many historians claim that Theodore Maiman invented the first optical laser; however, there is some controversy that Gordon Gould was the first. The first gas laser (helium neon) was invented by Ali Javan in 1960. The gas laser was the first continuous-light laser and the first to operate "on the principle of converting electrical energy to a laser light output." It has been used in many practical applications. Gordon Gould was the first person to use the word ***"laser"***. Many believe that Gordon Gould made the first light laser. Gould was a doctoral student at Columbia University under Charles Townes, the inventor of the laser. Gordon Gould was inspired to build his optical laser in 1958. He failed to file for a patent for his invention until 1959. As a result, Gordon Gould's patent was refused and his technology was exploited by others. It was only in 1977 Gordon Gould finally won his patent war.

Principle

Laser means *light amplification by stimulated emission of radiation*. Device produces coherent, intense, parallel beam of monochromatic light which does not diverge but travel in the same direction with same wavelength. Medium (CO_2/DIODE) is contained in a laser tube with a fully reflective mirror at one end and partially reflective mirror at other end allowing passage of the laser beam. Lasing medium may be argon, carbon dioxide, krypton, Nd:YAG, etc. Each medium has got different wavelength of light which decides type of beam and its effects on body tissues. Laser causes excitement and gets absorbed in substances called as chromophore. Photons are used to excite these chromophore molecules **(Figs. 6-15A and B)**.

Effects of Laser

When laser impinges on tissues, it may be reflected, absorbed, scattered or transmitted. Chromophores determine the amount of absorption—commonly haemoglobin and water. Light with specific wavelength when selectively absorbed by haemoglobin

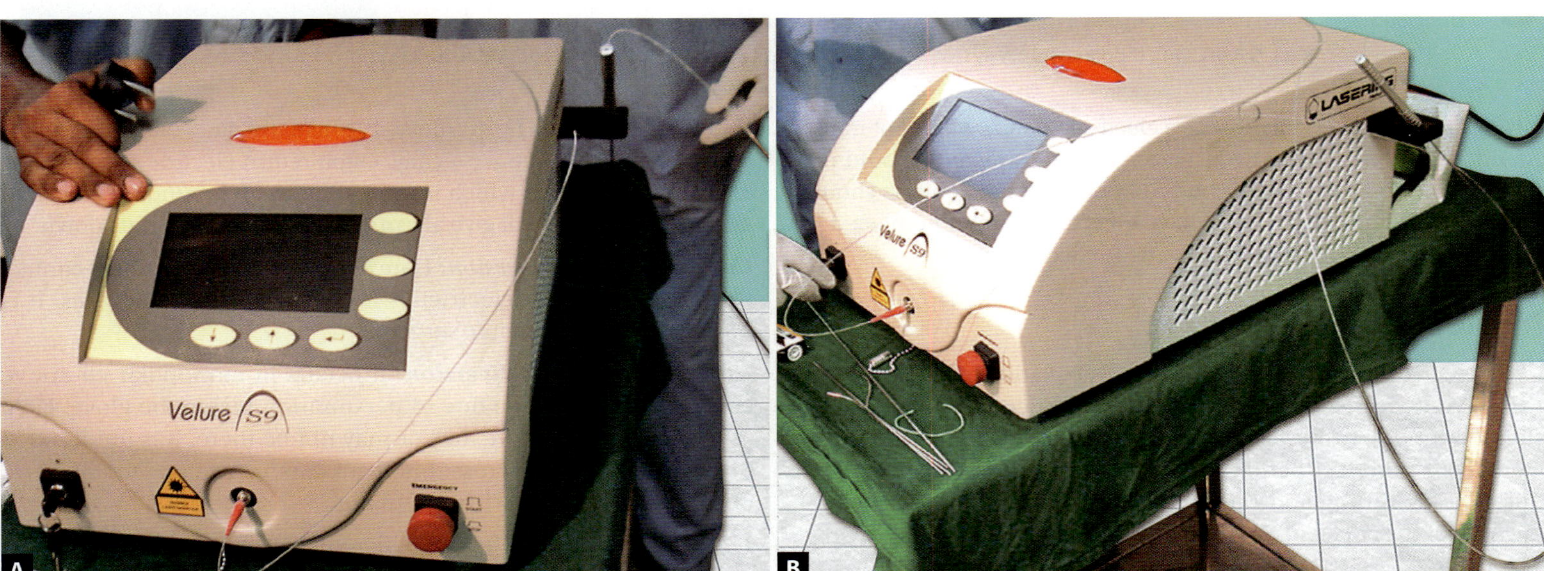

Figs. 6-15A and B: Typical laser instrument with laser fibre.

causes vessel sclerosis with least changes in surrounding tissue (like blue green light of argon laser). When absorbed by water cells are vaporised to steam with minimum charring and least damage to surrounding cells (like infrared light of CO_2 laser). Effects of laser depends on total energy, wavelength, target tissue optical characters, spot size, etc. Total energy is product of power and exposure duration. Thermal tissue destruction leads into oedema, protein denaturation, tissue contraction, cell water boiling. Entire effects cause haemostasis, tissue dissection, etc. There is less collateral damage. It can be applied to surface of target tissue or interstitially using a probe under image guidance. Photosensitising agents enhance laser effect. Energy penetration is least with argon laser, moderate with CO_2 laser, maximum in Nd: YAG laser.

Different Lasers Used

Argon laser: It is used mainly for coagulation, partly for tissue removal. It produces blue green coherent light (absorption by pigments and haemoglobin). It also passes through clear colourless structure without absorption. It can be targeted to lesions through clear normal structures. It can be used to vessel precisely without spread of energy beyond. It is used in port-wine stain, vascular lesions, and skin tumours.

Neodymium: Yttrium-Aluminum-Garnet (Nd:YAG) laser: It is a laser whose active medium is a crystal of yttrium, aluminum, and garnet doped with neodymium ions, and whose beam is in the near infrared spectrum of 1060 nm wavelength. It is equally effective for blood vessel coagulation and tissue removal. It produces infrared coherent light which is deeply absorbed in tissues without any colour specificity. As it causes perivascular tissue contraction and fibrosis, it can be used to control larger vessel bleeding than argon laser. Thermal damage to adjacent tissues is possible. It is very useful in endoscopic laser surgery in tracheobronchial tree, upper and lower gastrointestinal tract and urinary system.

Carbon dioxide laser: It is used mainly in haemorrhoids and perianal surgery. CO_2 laser is one of the earliest gas laser invented (by Kumar Patel Bell Labs in 1964). It is the highest power continuous wave laser with wavelength of 9.4–10.6 μm producing infrared light beam. It is used in skin resurfacing (laser facelifts), dermabrasion, naevus sebaceous, rhinophyma, haemorrhoidal surgery, cervical dysplasia (cervical intraepithelial neoplasia/CIN) surgery, vocal cord tumours, blepharoplasties, etc. **(Figs. 6-16A to D)**.

Neon laser: It is used in combination with CO_2 laser or other lasers (Holmium/Nd: YAG). Use is similar like CO_2 laser.

Holmium laser: It is used in prostate surgery, urinary bladder surgery, etc. It is used commonly in urology. Holmium lithotripsy in 2100 nm wavelength is useful to fragment the stone. It can be used safely endoscopically. Pulsed laser is safer to prevent injury to basket or ureter. Holmium YAG/pulsed dye laser is used usually. It fragments or vapourises the stone well; can be used through ureteroscope; highly efficacious; does not require any manipulation of stone. Drawback is it is time consuming.

Dye laser is a laser with organic dye as the active medium, whose beam is in the visible light spectrum. Pulsed dye laser: It is a type of laser used in cosmetic procedures.

Pulsed dye lasers are non-ablative, which means that they target tissue in the deeper layers of skin, leaving the top-most layers uninjured. Pulsed dye lasers are typically used to address cosmetic skin problems such as unsightly veins and pigmentation problems, fine lines around the eyes, and stretch marks.

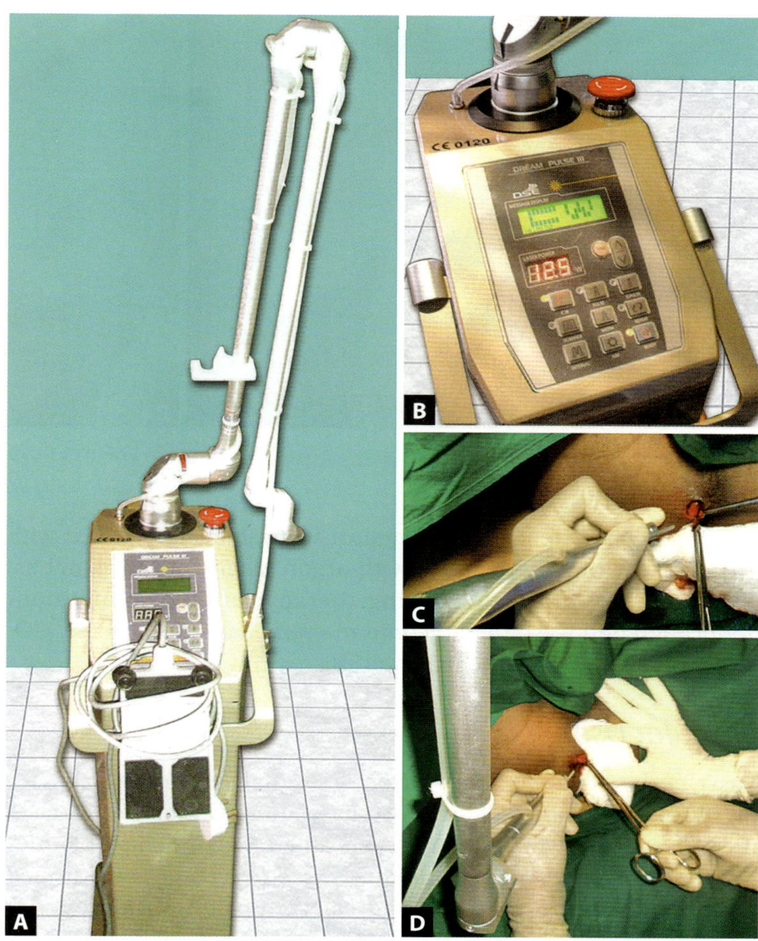

Figs. 6-16A to D: Carbon dioxide laser used for haemorrhoidectomy.

Excimer laser is a laser with rare gas halides as the active medium, whose beam is in the ultraviolet spectrum and penetrates tissues only a short distance; used in ophthalmological procedures and laser angioplasty.

Helium-neon laser is a laser with a mixture of ionised helium and neon gases as the active medium, whose beam is in the red visible light spectrum; used as a guiding beam for lasers operating at non-visible wavelengths.

Krypton laser is a laser with krypton ionised by electric current as the active medium, whose beam is in the yellow-red visible light spectrum; used for photocoagulation.

KTP laser is one in which a beam generated by a neodymium:YAG laser is directed through a potassium titanyl phosphate crystal to produce a beam in the green visible spectrum; used for photoablation and photocoagulation.

Uses of Laser

Cutaneous Use

Laser in general surgery is used to cut tissues during surgery; destroy or remove tissues; to cauterise the bleeding vessels; to seal lymphatics in malignancy to reduce spread; to remove naevus, warts; to reduce skin wrinkles **(Figs. 6-17A to C)**.

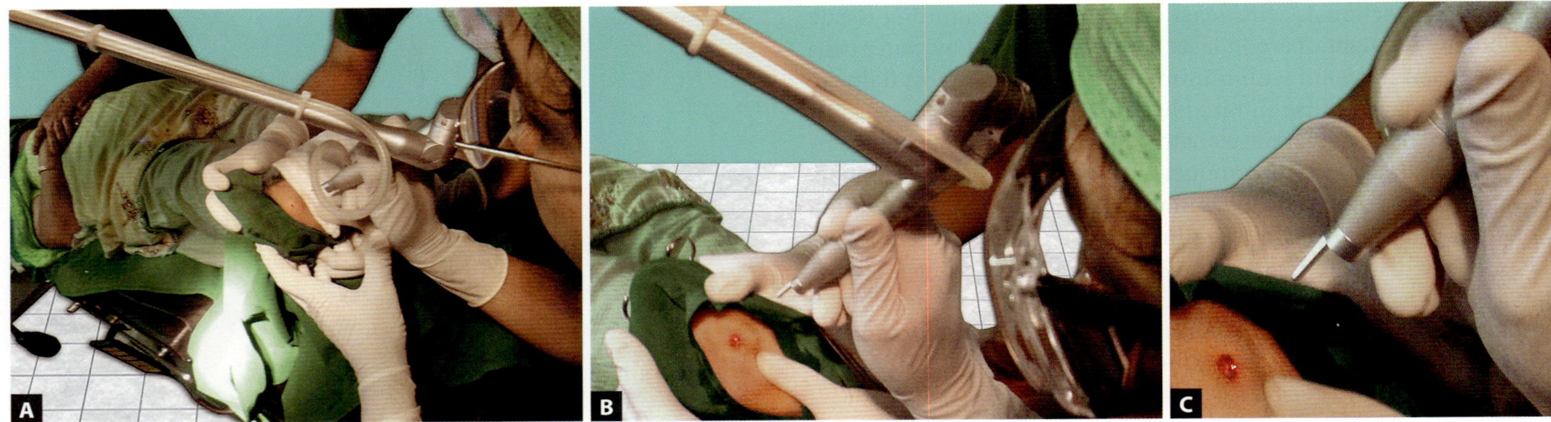
Figs. 6-17A to C: Use of laser in surface surgery.

Superficial dermal lesions like port-wine stains are treated with argon laser. Initially painting with argon laser until it blanches; ice is applied prior and during therapy; antibiotic ointment application and wash therapy until re-epithelialisation occurs. CO_2 laser is used for many facelift surgeries.

Vascular Use

Laser endarterectomy, laser arterial recanalisation, laser angioplasty, laser assisted balloon angioplasty are different arterial laser therapies. CO_2, argon, Nd:YAG lasers ablate only calcified plaques but high risk of vessel perforation. *Pulsed laser* causes controlled removal of both calcified and non-calcified plaques with less risk of vessel wall perforation. Newer *smart lasers* are available in which fluorescent spectra signals are used to direct when to fire laser and when not to. It identifies the normal vessel wall from plaques and stops firing once normal vessel wall reaches.

Laser-assisted vascular anastomosis (LAVA) is more precise, with high patency rate and reduced surgical time. It is under trial. Argon laser/diode laser is used for medium and large vessels; CO_2 laser is used for small vessels. Aneurysm formation is the major drawback in this technique. However, it is a promising future non-suture anastomosis method for vessels.

Endovenous laser ablation (EVLA): Laser heat produced steam bubbles causes endothelial thermal damage, occlusion of vein and fibrosis preventing neovascularisation. Diode laser is used commonly. Great saphenous vein just below knee level; small saphenous vein at mid-calf level is cannulated; guidewire is passed; 5 French catheter is passed; 0.1% xylocaine (Tumescent anaesthetic agent—500 mL normal saline + 8.4% sodium bicarbonate + 30 mL 1% xylocaine with adrenaline—causes compression, anaesthesia, absorption of heat) is injected around the vein on its entire length; laser fibre is inserted beyond the tip of the catheter; laser is fired (12 watts in thigh, 10 watts in leg) stepwise with withdrawal; compression bandage is applied for one week; later patient is advised to wear stockings for 6 months. External manual pressure is applied over the vein. It is done on outpatient basis/day care surgery. It is scarless, can be done under local anaesthesia; shows good recovery. It can cause bruising, phlebitis, sepsis **(Fig. 6-18)**.

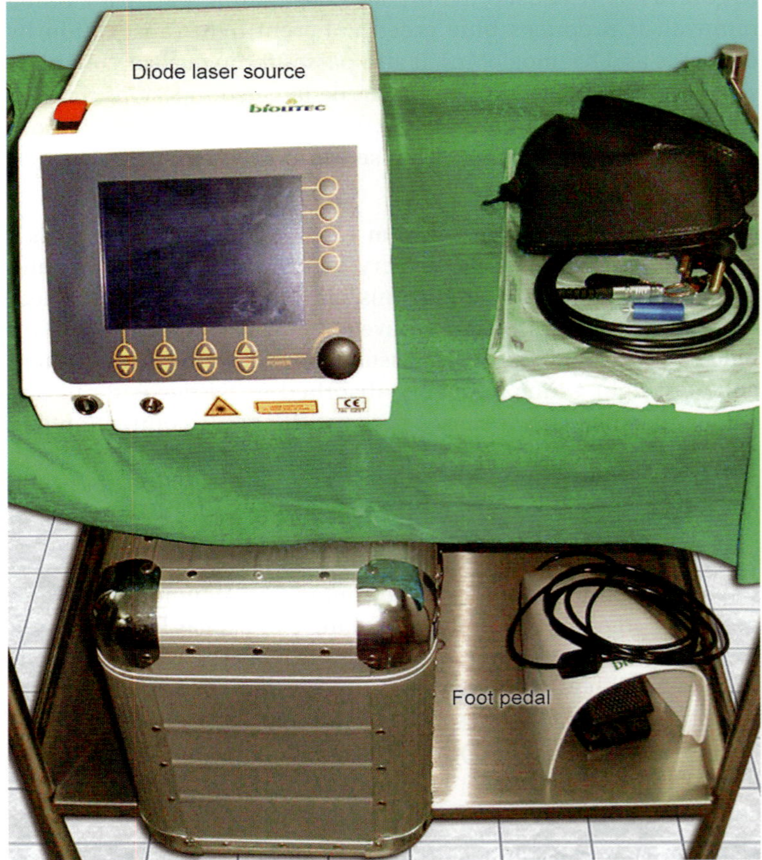

Fig. 6-18: Diode laser—commonly used for varicose vein.

Laser in Gastrointestinal Diseases

Gastrointestinal vascular malformations are very well treated with laser. Argon laser is ideal for small lesions as chances of perforation are less. Nd:YAG laser is used for wider lesions. Laser is done usually from periphery to centre of the lesion.

Laser is useful in early gastric cancer with protruded lesions or depressed lesions less than 1 cm in size without any ulceration. It is either done by high energy output photothermal destruction using helium neon laser or by low energy output photochemical destruction using argon dye laser, 72 hours after intravenous injection of a porphyrin derivative to sensitise the tumour tissue. Low energy output laser is not useful in bleeding or stenosed tumour.

Nd:YAG laser photocoagulation is used for bleeding peptic ulcers and oesophageal varices. But it has not become popular.

Laser photocoagulation is used for palliation of inoperable oesophageal and oesophagogastric carcinomas to relieve dysphagia. Advantages are—easier, simpler, avoids major surgery, immediately effective, can be repeated as needed. In non-obstructing tumour approach is from distal part of the tumour to proximal part using Nd:YAG laser. Endocavitory radiotherapy using endoscopically delivered iridium 192 immediately after laser ablation prolongs the dysphagia free intervals.

In colorectal carcinoma with obstruction or bleeding, laser is used to relieve the obstruction by coring the tumour tissue. In advanced malignancy, repeated laser may be needed. In early carcinoma with obstruction initial decompression prior to definitive surgery can be done using Nd:YAG laser.

In liver it is used for surface laser coagulation and for liver resection. In liver resection segmental vessel ligation, skeletonisation of large vessel, cone resection of the metastatic liver nodule and haemostasis is achieved using laser. Single unit CO_2 and Nd:YAG laser is used.

Biliary laser lithotripsy is done using Nd:YAG laser wherein laser fibre is passed through endoscopy/percutaneous transhepatic/ tube tract approach. Stone is fragmented and extracted. Calcified or large cholesterol stones may be difficult to retrieve by laser method. Thermal damage of the biliary mucosa which is dangerous can be minimised by using coumarin flash lamp pulsed dye laser.

CO_2 laser is used for haemorrhoidectomy wherein anoderm, mucosa are excised. CO_2 laser is superficial, controlled and precise. Sloughing, secondary haemorrhage, abscess formation are the complications **(Fig. 6-19)**.

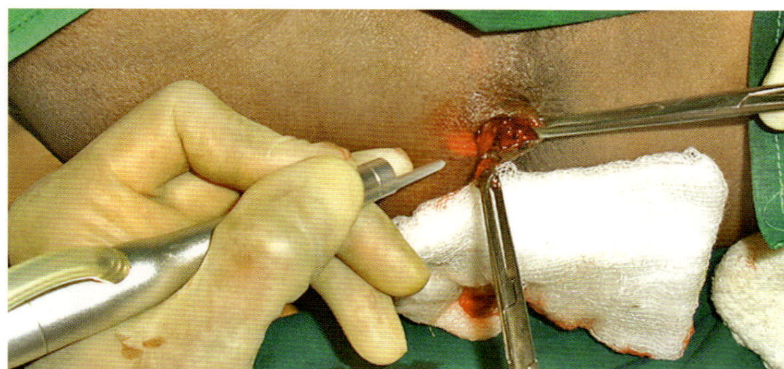

Fig. 6-19: Laser haemorrhoidectomy.

Uses in Urology

CO_2 laser is useful in removal of lesions over external genitalia like condyloma acuminata, haemangiomas, palliation in penile carcinoma in case of refusal for penile amputation, malignant melanoma and other lesions on genitalia.

Holmium YAG laser is used in urinary bladder tumour, prostatectomy, stone fragmentation, during partial nephrectomy, etc.

Other Uses

Laser is extensively used in vocal cord diseases, carcinoma larynx and oropharynx.

Laser is very common tool used in various procedures in ophthalmic diseases—retinal detachment, iridotomy, dacryocystitis, capsulotomy, lens liquefaction, glaucoma.

Advantages of Laser in Surgery

It is precise with minimal damage to adjacent tissue. It creates bloodless field. It reduces the postoperative pain. It often can be done under local anaesthesia. It is faster especially in removing small lesions.

Precautions

All reflecting instruments should be avoided as reflection through these instruments may target into normal tissue causing its destruction. Coated non-reflective instruments are better to be used.

Everyone in theatre should wear protective spectacles.

Normal tissues should be protected using wet towels.

In oropharyngeal laser surgery jet ventilation technique is used for anaesthesia to prevent possible ignition **(Figs. 6-20 and 6-21)**.

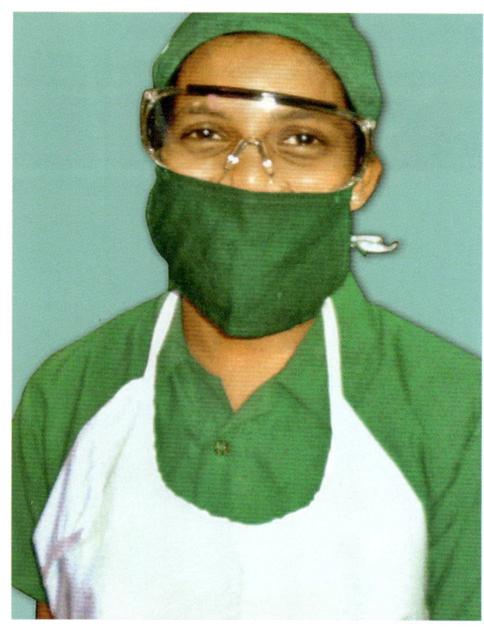

Fig. 6-20: Operation theatre staff should wear special goggles to protect eyes during laser surgery.

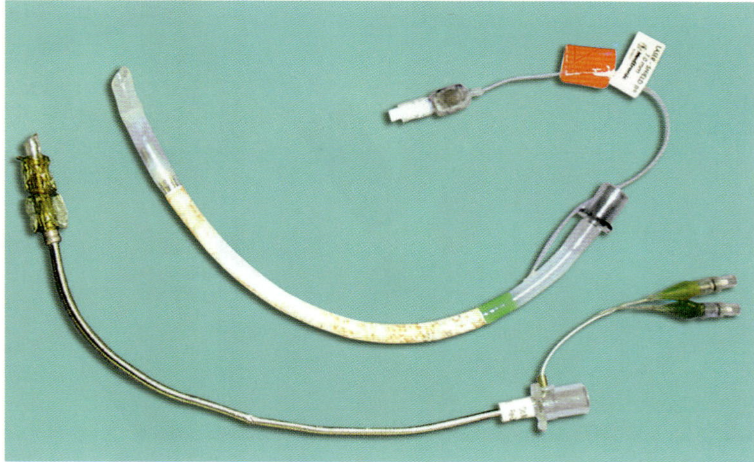

Fig. 6-21: Special endotracheal tubes are used to give anaesthesia when laser is used in the oral/pharyngeal/laryngeal area.

Problems with Laser

Smoke and fine particles can deposit in alveoli causing reduced mucociliary clearance, bronchiolitis, and emphysema. It is better to use high efficiency masks or smoke evacuator.

Injury to major vessel or bowel due to misdirection of the laser can occur. Bowel necrosis and perforation may become evident after few days.

Venous gas embolism is common during laparoscopic or hysteroscopic laser surgery.

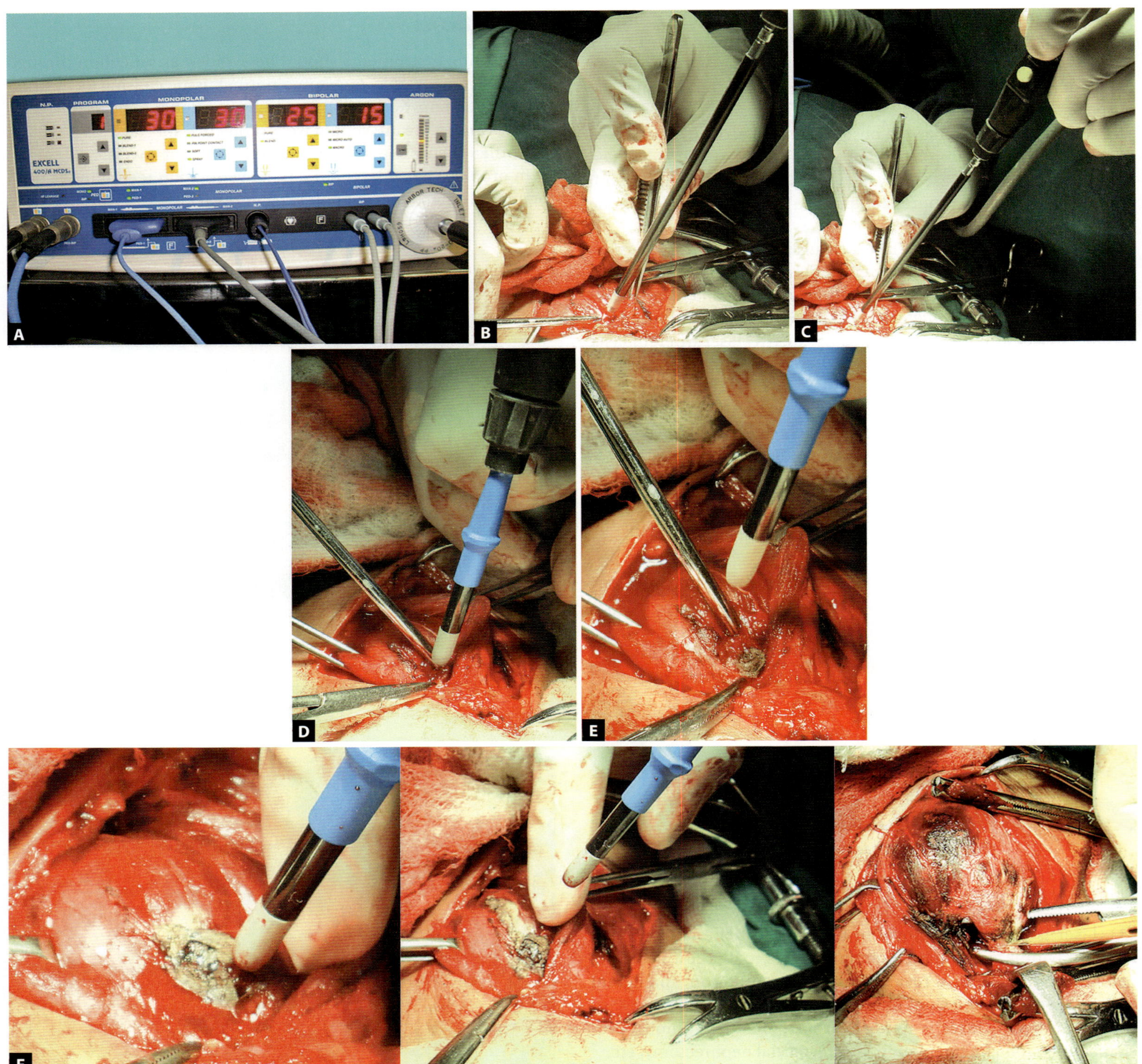

Figs. 6-22A to F: Argon beam coagulator used for surface thermal coagulation.

Fire of drapes, burns to theatre personnel can occur if it is used inappropriately without enough care.

Cost, availability and expertise availability are the further drawbacks.

ARGON BEAM COAGULATOR

Here steady flow of electrons is established through electrically activated and ionised argon gas causing monopolar electric circuit between hand-held probe and target tissue. It leads into thermal coagulation of the tissue to a depth up to 6 mm maximum. Regular Bovie hand held probe is used. It is commonly used in surface bleeding in an organ like liver, spleen, kidney, thyroid, etc. **(Figs. 6-22A to F)**.

LOW AND HIGH FREQUENCY SOUND WAVE ENERGY

Low frequency sound waves are used for diagnosis. High frequency ultrasound is used for dissection, coagulation and cutting tissues.

Extracorporeal Shock Wave Lithotripsy

Extracorporeal shock wave lithotripsy (ESWL) is acoustic shock waves used to fragment renal stones commonly and gallstones occasionally. High energy shock waves are passed through a water tissue interface and focused under C-Arm guidance over the stone to fragment it. This energy is generated using piezoelectric or electromagnetic method **(Fig. 6-23)**.

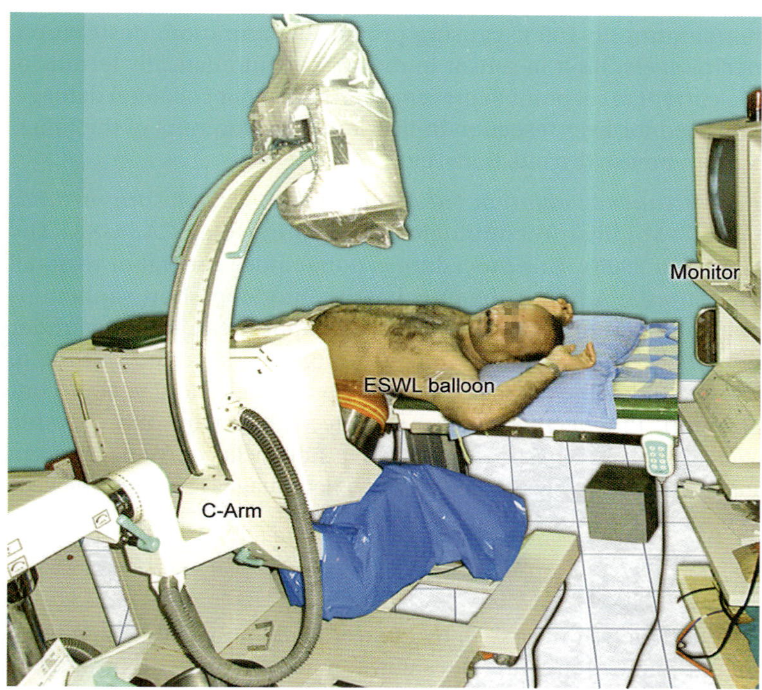

Fig. 6-23: Extracorporeal shock wave lithotripsy (ESWL).

Harmonic Scalpel

It is bipolar ultrasound energy of high frequency (of 55,000 vibrations/second—5.55 kHtz) used to dissect tissues by creation of stress and friction in the tissues, heat and denaturation of the protein. It is actually ***ultrasound activated scalpel*** with high energy mechanical vibrations leading to transfer of energy causing dissection. It coagulates the vessel, cuts the tissue facilitating the dissection. Surrounding tissues are not affected. It is now used in open procedure (FOCUS) as well as in laparoscopic surgeries. It can seal vessel up to 5 mm. Instrument contains one movable blade and one stationary. Stationary blade is ultrasonically activated **(Fig. 6-24)**. It is not dependent on current energy and so current diversion or ground pad injury is not there. Tissue should come in contact with active blade. It causes less smoke and steam but smoke created should be removed by constant suction to reduce the infection rate. Temperature is just 50–100°C (unlike in diathermy which is 150–400°C). It develops bloodless safe dissection with least damage to adjacent structures. Disadvantage is cost factor.

Harmonic scalpel (HS) is high power system working at a frequency of 55.5 kHz or 55,500 vibrations/sec. It is ultrasonic dissection (Ultracision). Hand piece contains US transducer with piezoelectric crystal sandwiched under pressure among metal cylinders. The US generator converts ultrasonic energy into mechanical energy. Denatured protein coagulum develops due to tamponade and coaptation. Harmonic scalpel has three compatible probes that are the shear, blade and a hook. The shear has opposite silicon padding which is absent in blade and hook. The shear can coagulate vessels

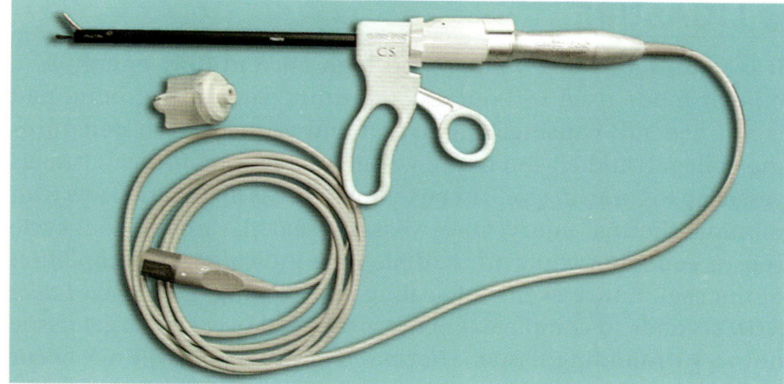

Fig. 6-24: Harmonic scalpel.

up to 5 mm, whereas the hook and blade only 2 mm in diameter. The harmonic scalpel probes reach the temperature of 8°C; on prolonged use also temperature remains below 250°C which is far less than other electrosurgical sources resulting in reduced lateral thermal spread and charring. Vibration of the active probe prevents sticking of coagulated tissues over it; but mist production could affect the visibility. Smoke formation is less in harmonic scalpel. It uses slow energy with lowest mean burst pressure with lateral thermal damage is less than 1 mm. it causes mist production and may impair the visibility but smoke formation is minimal.

CAVITRON ULTRASONIC SURGICAL ASPIRATOR (CUSA)

It contains a knife which has got ultrafrequency oscillating tip (23000 cps) which fractures, fragments and dissects the solid tissue with preservation of nerves and vessels. Soft tissues are fragmented, washed and aspirated with the same instrument. Lower frequency ultrasound energy is used to dissect the solid organ tissues with low fibre, high water content. It is used in dissection of liver, pancreas, brain, spinal cord. It causes less blood loss and clarity dissection. It allows individual ligation or clipping of vessels and biliary ductules in liver resection. It is useful in non-cirrhotic liver tumours. In pancreas it is useful in endocrine pancreatic tumours. It is used also in partial nephrectomy, partial splenectomy and many gynaecological procedures **(Fig. 6-25)**.

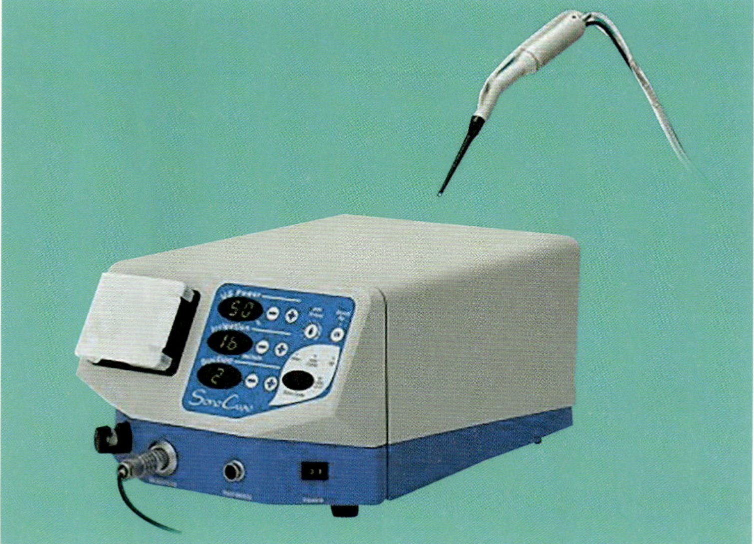

Fig. 6-25: Cavitron ultrasonic surgical aspirator (CUSA) device.

LIGASURE

It is continuous low voltage and high current flow energy in a bipolar mode used without any returning electrode (ground pad is not needed) causing coagulation and vessel seal. It denatures the collagen and elastin of the vessel wall causing its seal. It seals vessel up to 7 mm in size. Tissue temperature is maintained low with minimal thermal injury. Once vessel is sealed, through cool cycle sensor generator shuts off. Audible tone indicates the completion of the seal. Entire events of sealing and cooling (cool cycle) take 5–10 seconds to complete. Energy is targeted over the target tissue not to surrounding tissue. Thermal energy spread will not occur beyond 1.5 mm of surrounding tissue. Ligasure is very useful in laparoscopic surgeries as well as in open surgeries like hysterectomy, thyroidectomy, haemorrhoidectomy, liver surgery, splenectomy, colectomy, etc. It minimises blood loss and avoids blood transfusion **(Figs. 6-26A to F)**.

Ligasure vessel sealing system (LVSS) seals tissue by administration of high current and low voltage that of 180 V as compared electrocautery. LVSS uses high co-aptive pressure creating tissue temperature under 1000°C causing rupture of hydrogen cross-links resulting in a vascular seal with high tensile strength. Melted collagen and elastin in the vessels form a permanent seal; secure seal of blood vessels up to 7 mm diameter is achieved. Smoke formation causes problem in visibility and so delays the procedure. In LVSS, there is a feedback from the tissue that controls the energy delivery and automatically discontinues it, when the seal cycle completes eliminating the guesswork of operating surgeon for completion of the seal. It seals vessel permanently. But lateral thermal damage of approximately 2 mm is observed but much less than electrocautery units. LVSS produces smoke which affect visibility. Sticking is less. LVSS has got moderate mean burst pressure with slower energy with lateral thermal damage is about 2 mm.

Problems with ligasure are—its size (large); dissection is not possible; sticking of the instrument and tissue avulsion while removing the instrument; availability.

Advantages are—bloodless; obviates blood transfusion; presence of feedback controlled safety system; being bipolar adjacent tissue safety is ensured; ground pad return electrode is not needed; reduces the surgical time as it reduces the need of number of suture ligatures for the vessel; major vessels can also be well sealed.

RADIOFREQUENCY ABLATION

Radiofrequency ablation is used for curative or palliative procedures for tumours; for neuralgia, bone pain, arrhythmias. High frequency alternating current is transmitted through the electrode to the tissues (350–500 kHz) to release kinetic energy elevating the tissue temperature to 100°C causing protein denaturation, desiccation, necrosis, etc. Built in sensor in the system automatically terminate the current at set point to prevent over-heating or collateral damage. It is used for liver resection in liver tumours, tumours of the lungs, kidney, breast, thyroid, bone, etc.

Radiofrequency ablation (RFA) method (VNUS closure method) (VNUS Medical Technologies Inc; Sunnyvale, CA, USA) (by Goldman 2000): This procedure is done under general or regional anaesthesia. A RFA catheter is passed into long/short saphenous vein near saphenofemoral or saphenopopliteal junction under guidance. 85°C temperature is used for longer period of time to cause endothelial damage, collagen denaturation and venous constriction. Phlebectomy is done while withdrawing the catheter. Wall of the vein is destroyed through its full thickness. Vein transform into a cord, which gets dissolved by macrophages and immune cells **(Figs. 6-27A to C)**.

CRYOTHERAPY

It is destruction of tissues by controlled cooling. Cryoprobe with an automatic defrosting device is connected to liquid nitrogen or nitrous oxide or CO_2 container. Nitrous oxide produces temperature of minus 98°C; CO_2—minus 60°C; liquid nitrogen—minus 180°C; Freon—minus 190°C. Nitrous oxide is used in many procedures like cryotherapy for piles, surface lesions. Nitrous oxide is easily available, cheaper, achieves optimum temperature. Cryoablation for liver tumour is achieved using liquid nitrogen or argon cryosystem. It induces intracellular crystallisation, dehydration, denaturation of protein and obliteration of microcirculation. Even though it is haemostatic often freezing and defrosting is inadequate causing haemorrhage **(Fig. 6-28)**.

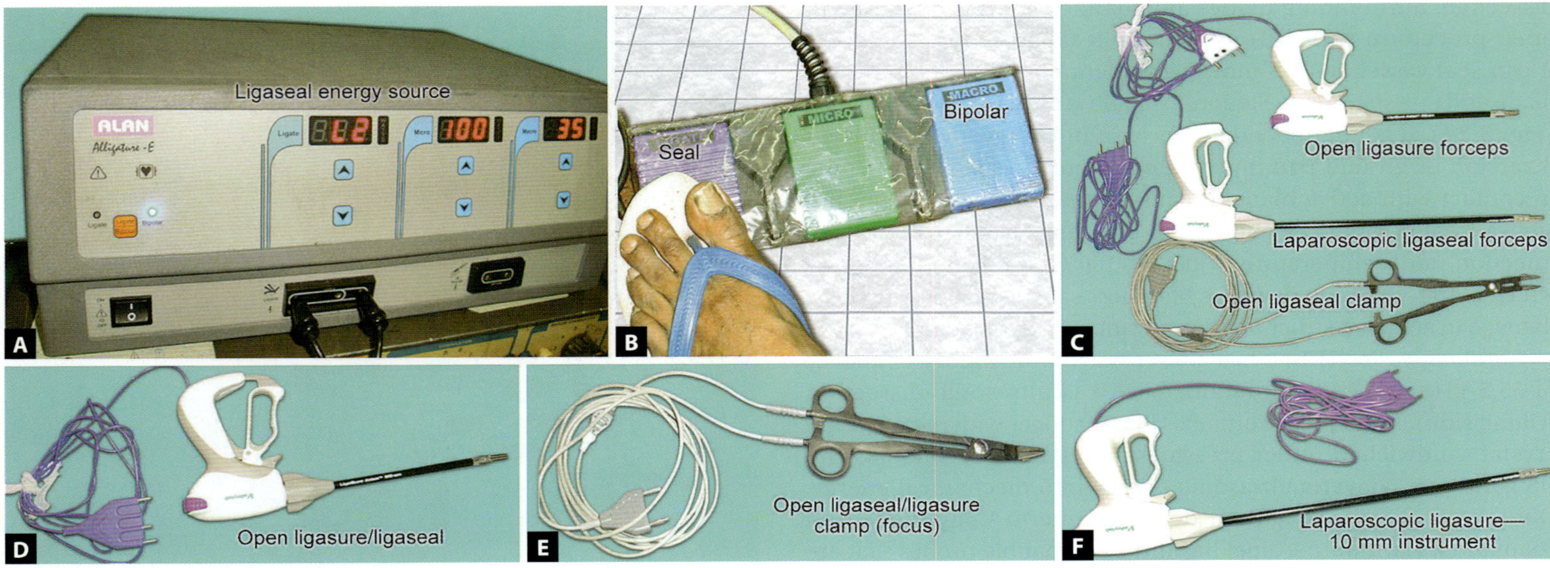

Figs. 6-26A to F: Ligasure/ligaseal set and instruments. It can be used in laparoscopy or open surgery. For open surgery ligaseal instrument or clamp (focus) can be used. For laparoscopic procedures 5 mm or 10 mm ligaseals are available. Dissection is not possible with these instruments.

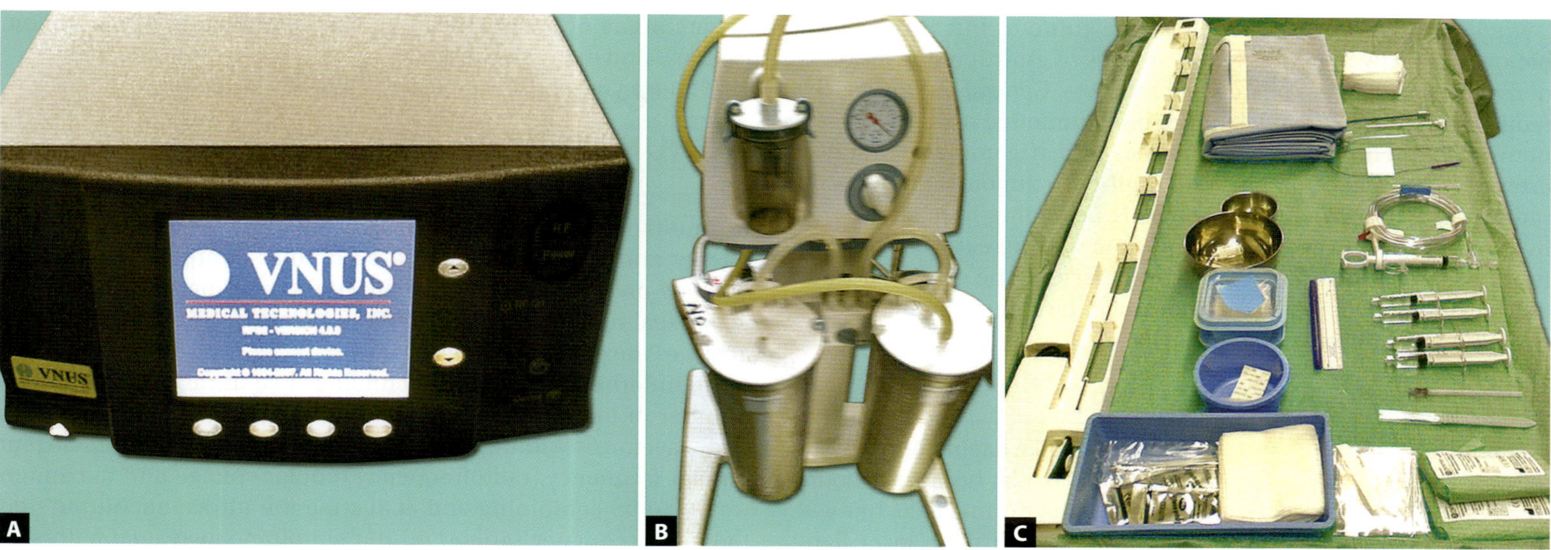

Figs. 6-27A to C: Radiofrequency ablation device system.

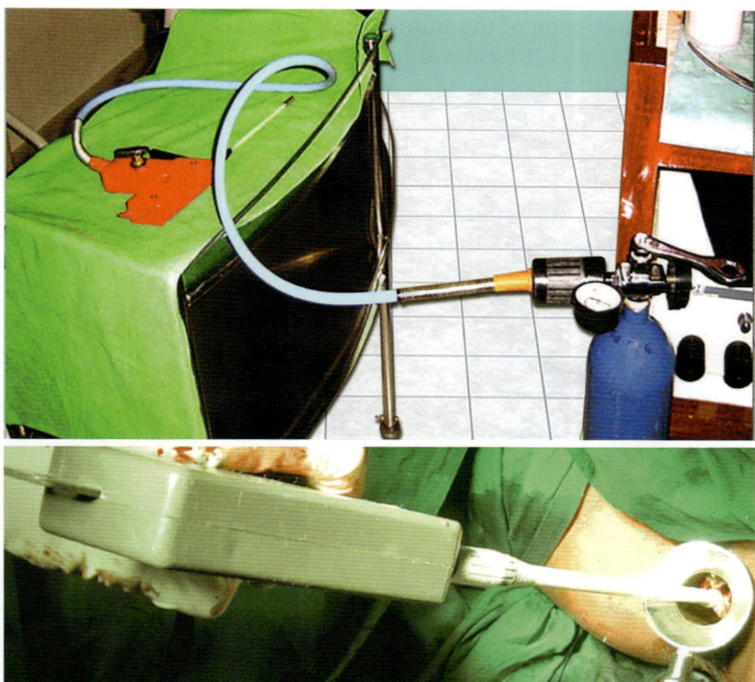

Fig. 6-28: Cryosurgery instrument and its use in treating haemorrhoids.

MICROWAVE ABLATION

Under image guidance microwave energy probe is placed over the target tissue to create a rapidly alternating electrical field releasing energy in the form of heat causing coagulation necrosis. It is used in liver tumour ablation, cardiac arrhythmias, benign prostatic hyperplasia, endometrial diseases, partial nephrectomy.

RADIOSURGERY

Radiosurgery was first developed at the Karolinska Institute of Stockholm, Sweden in 1949 using proton. In 1968 gamma knife is used and standardised.

High energy gamma radiation is used as an energy source through a gamma knife to target tissue in a circular fashion on a specific point without injuring adjacent normal brain tissue. It is used to treat epilepsy, arteriovenous malformations and brain tumours. It is also called as stereotactic radiotherapy. It operates by directing highly focused beams of ionising radiation with high precision. It is a relatively recent technique (1951) which is used to ablate, by means of a precise dosage of radiation, intracranial and extracranial tumours and other lesions that could be otherwise inaccessible or inadequate for open surgery. The *Gamma Knife*, is a new device exclusively for radiosurgery, consists of radioactive sources of Cobalt-60 placed in a kind of helmet with central channels for irradiation, using ***gamma rays***. In the latest version of this device, 192 sources of radioactive cobalt direct gamma radiation to the centre of a helmet, where the patient's head is inserted. This is called the *Leksell Gamma Knife Perfexion*.

Patients can be treated within five days as an outpatient. The average hospital stay for a craniotomy (conventional neurosurgery, requiring the opening of the skull) is about 15 days. Radiosurgery costs less than conventional surgery, and with much less morbidity, e.g. mortality, pain and post-surgical complications, such as haemorrhage and infection. The period of recovery is minimal, and the patient may return to his or her normal lifestyle, without any discomfort. Radiosurgery still has got limitations and disadvantages. It is difficult and dangerous to treat masses larger than 3 cm because it will require very high doses of radiation. Fractionated radiotherapy may be a better option ideally combined with surgical debulking. The duration of time required to achieve the desired effects is much longer than surgery; it can take up to 2 years for arteriovenous malformations. During that time, the patient remains at risk for a rebleed. For treatment of tumours, radiosurgery does not physically remove the tumour, rather stops it from growing larger. Therefore, it is not a good option when the tumour presents with significant mass effect on vital structures of the brain or spinal cord and when it causes increased intracranial pressure. Open surgery is needed to relieve pressure, remove the tumour totally or debulk it to make it a better target for radiosurgery. Open surgery and radiosurgery are often used in conjunction for many types of brain tumours. Stereotactic radiosurgery can successfully treat many different types of tumours, both benign and malignant. The malignant brain tumours treated most often are the brain metastases. Radiosurgery is particularly a good option for patients who are with poor surgical risks due to other medical causes.

Radiosurgery does not remove the tumour, but results in a biological inactivation of the tumour, lack of growth of the lesion is normally considered to be treatment success. General indications for radiosurgery include many kinds of brain tumours, such as acoustic neuromas, meningiomas, metastases and trigeminal neuralgia, arteriovenous malformations and skull-base tumours. Stereotactic radiotherapy to extracranial lesions is becoming popular like for liver metastases, liver cancer, lung cancer, pancreatic cancer, etc. It has been demonstrated that radiosurgery can be a very safe and efficient method for the management of many difficult brain lesions, while it avoids the loss in quality of life.

PHOTODYNAMIC THERAPY

Systemic injection of photosensitising agent like haematoporphyrin derivative will bind selectively to tumour or vascular beds. In 48 hours this photosensitiser gets cleared off from the normal cells but will be retained in tumours even after 48 hours. Through laser light applied over the tumour, *photosensitiser* is activated. It causes thermal reaction → fluorescence effect → ***single oxygen formation*** → selective tumour destruction. Singlet oxygen is a very aggressive chemical and will very rapidly react with any nearby biomolecules. These destructive reactions will kill cells through apoptosis or necrosis. Technique was initially used in recurrent carcinoma of breast with skin metastases. It is also used in diagnosis and treatment of tracheobronchial carcinoma and oesophageal carcinoma.

Other uses are—in non-small cell lung cancer; pancreatic cancers; squamous cell carcinoma of skin; basal cell carcinoma; recurrent superficial bladder cancer; recurrence and chest wall involvement in carcinoma of breast. It can be used for macular degeneration, psoriasis and many skin lesions.

Photosensitiser used at present clinically is *photofrin*.

THUNDERBEAT

It is integrated form of surgical energy from a single instrument. It simultaneously delivers ultrasonically generated frictional heat energy and electrically generated bipolar energy. It has higher bursting pressure and highly reduced thermal speed than Ligasure vessel sealing system (LVSS) and the harmonic scalpel (HS). It can achieve 7 mm vessel sealing.

Thunderbeat has similar technology like ultrasonic energy like number of instrument sockets, footswitch options, output levels and waveforms without any much difference in the input current bipolar frequency, radiofrequency bipolar voltage and maximum watts. So by combining and activating the ultrasonic output and the high frequency bipolar output simultaneously enable to seal and cut vessels and to cut and coagulate soft tissue. Bipolar output enables vessels sealing and haemostasis. The ultrasonic output enables to seal and cut vessels and to cut and coagulate soft tissues. The handpiece plug of the thunderbeat transducer which converts drive current into ultrasonic output is connected to the thunderbeat socket of the USG 400. The high frequency bipolar current and drive current are supplied to the transducer via a cable eliminating the need to connect a cord of the ESG-400. There is minimum lateral thermal damage. It has got high mean burst pressure and fastest in cutting without any visibility impairment with least mist and smoke production **(Figs. 6-29A to G)**.

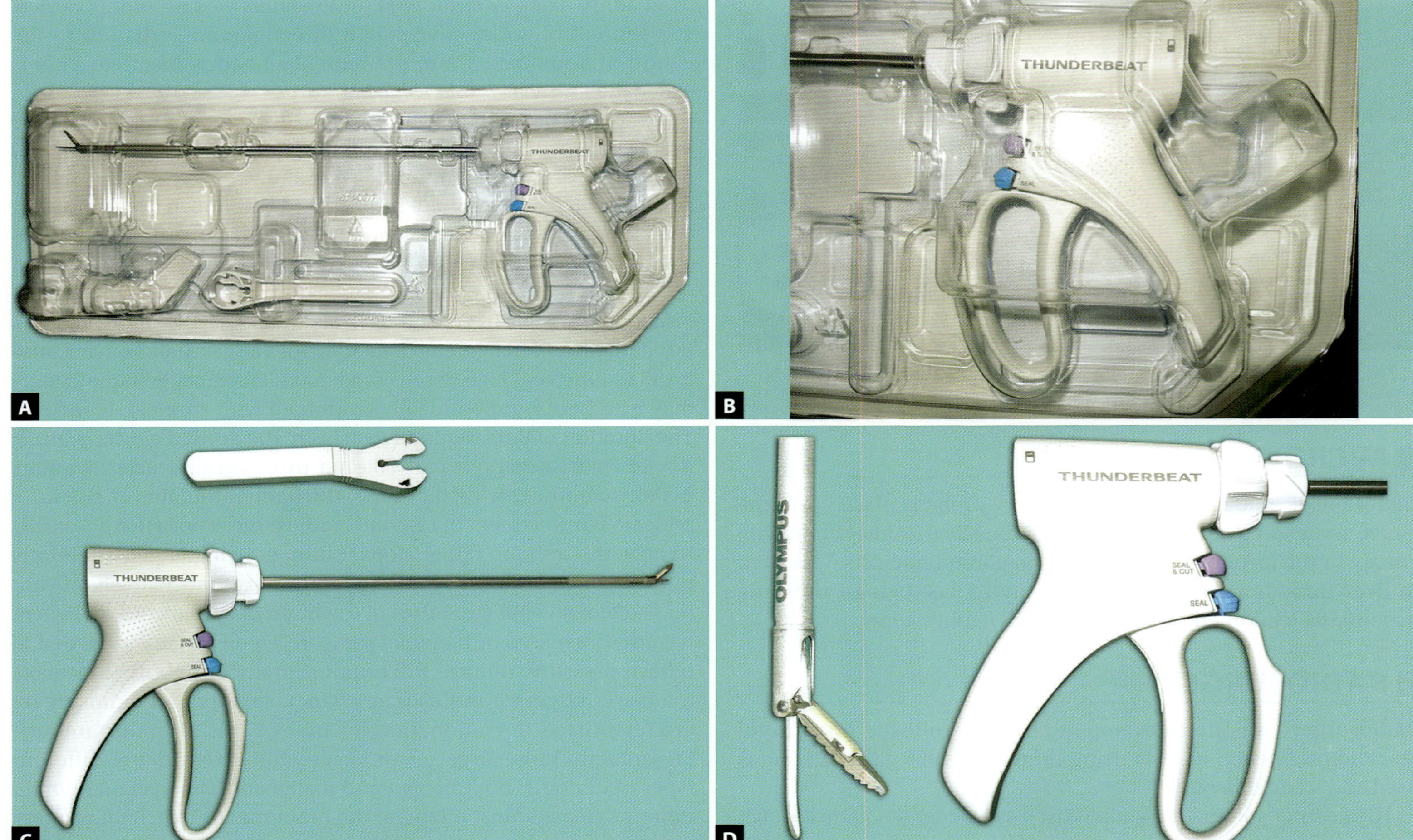

Figs. 6-29A to D

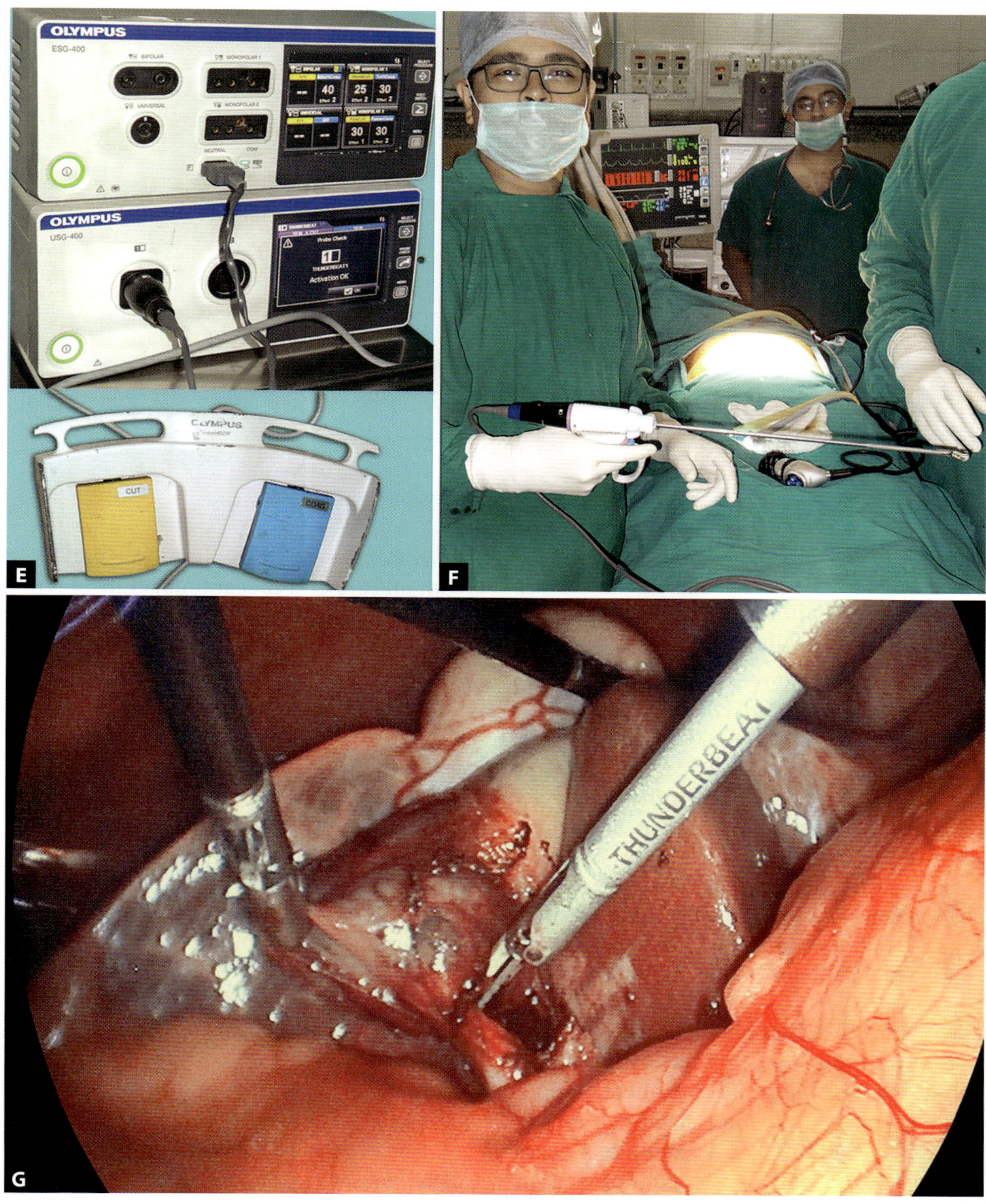

Figs. 6-29E to G

Figs. 6-29A to G: Thunderbeat—an integrated energy device.

7

CHAPTER

Basic Surgical Procedures

URINARY CATHETERISATION

Catheters used: Simple non-self-retaining red rubber catheter, Foley's self-retaining catheter, Gibbon's catheter, metal catheter.

Urethral catheters may be indwelling (self-retaining) or short-term (non-self-retaining) or *intermittent or external catheters.* Indwelling catheters may be urethral or suprapubic (open SPC or trocar SPC). External catheters are *condom catheters* (Texas catheter) which enclose penis firmly and through its tip catheter tube continues towards external collecting bag. It is used in bedridden, comatose, stroke, old age patients. It reduces the chances of urosepsis and prevents bed wetting, smell and social problems but it is often difficult to maintain. It needs to be changed daily or more times a day. Simple non-self-retaining red rubber catheter, Foley's self-retaining catheter, Gibbon's catheter, metal catheter (male and female)—are different catheters used.

Catheters can be made up of rubber, peripheral venous catheter (PVC), silicone or latex. Robinson catheter is not having balloon in the tip and is used for short-term or intermittent catheterisation. In adult 16–18 F is used. In children, smaller sized catheter is used (child age divided by 2 and adding 8; for example, 4 years old child requires—4/2 = 2 + 8 = 10 F catheter. Straight tip is used usually; Coude tip with a curve at the tip is used in patients with BPH; haematuria catheter and 3-way catheters are used in patients with haematuria and post-bladder or prostate surgeries **(Figs. 7-1 to 7-5)**.

Indications: Retention of urine due to BPH, stricture urethra, trauma (with all care and precaution gently one trial is done); in all major surgeries in post-operative period; in patients with acute conditions and patients in shock to measure the hourly urine output.

Causes of retention of urine

Bladder outlet obstruction

- Benign prostatic hyperplasia (BPH), carcinoma prostate.
- Prostatitis, prostatic abscess.
- Bladder carcinoma close to bladder neck.
- Bladder stone obstructing bladder neck.
- Hypertrophy of bladder neck muscle.
- Stricture at bladder neck.

Causes at urethral level

- Urethral stricture—may be due to trauma or inflammatory (gonococcal/non-specific) or neoplastic or after catheterisation/cystoscopy or after surgery (TURP/urethral surgery/perineal urethrostomy).
- Urethral stone.
- Tumours.
- Posterior urethral valve.
- Urethral trauma.
- Meatal stenosis.
- Pinhole meatus/phimosis.

Other causes

- Post-operative period.
- Post-surgery—after haemorrhoidectomy/fissurectomy/fistulectomy.
- Spinal injury/spinal surgery/spinal anaesthesia.
- Drugs like anti-cholinergics, anti-depressants or anti-hypertensives.

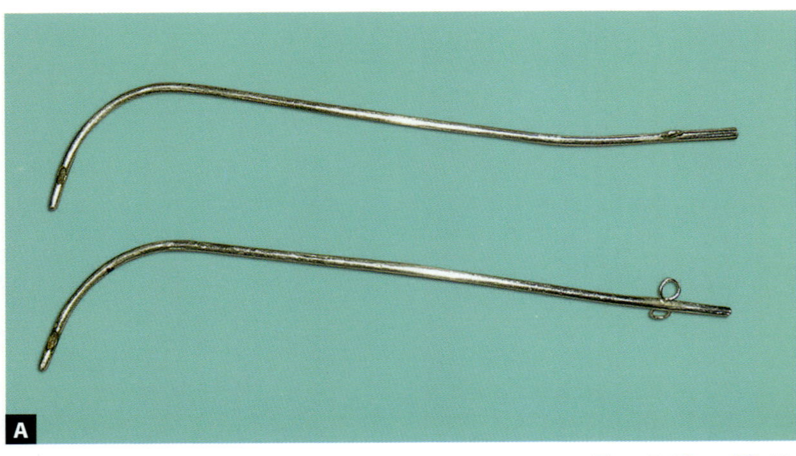

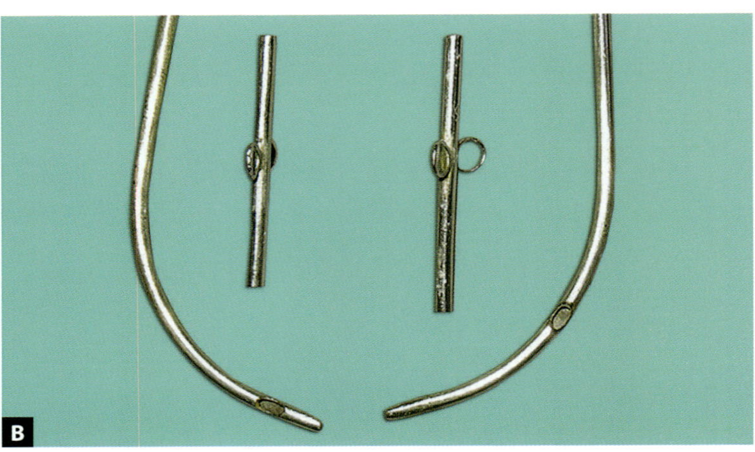

Figs. 7-1A and B: Male metal catheter.

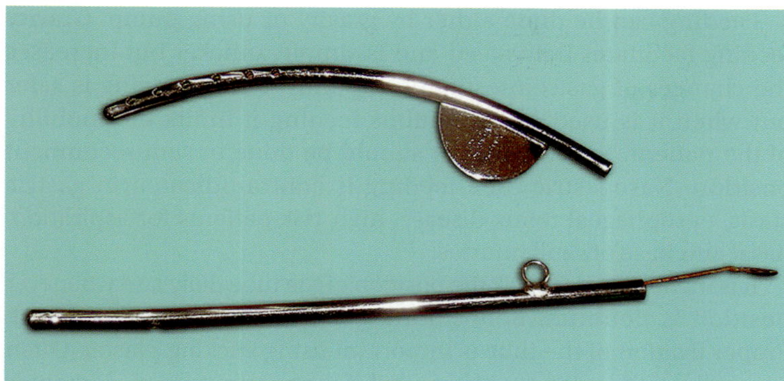

Fig. 7-2: Female metal catheter.

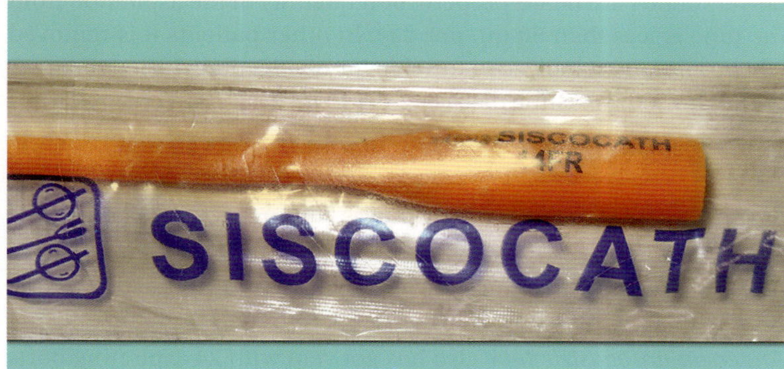

Fig. 7-3: Catheter used for intermittent catheterisation.

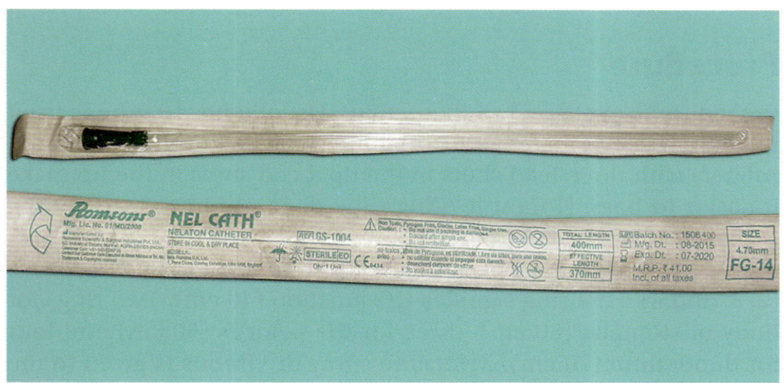

Fig. 7-4: Stiff single use non-self-retaining urinary catheter.

Foley's catheter is commonly used. Urosac bag, gloves, sterile towel, 2% xylocaine jelly and distilled water are needed.

Procedure

The patient is explained about the procedure. Sterile gloves are worn after handwash. Patient will be in supine position with legs apart. Genitalia are cleaned with povidone iodine solution. Draping is done using sterile towel. Prepuce is retracted and glans is cleaned again. 20 mL of 2% xylocaine is taken in a syringe and pushed into the urethra through the external meatus. After 5 minutes, penis is held vertically (so that urethra gets straightened to make easier passage of the catheter) and Foley's catheter tip is lubricated with jelly and is gently passed into the urinary bladder. Urine flow through the catheter confirms that it is inside the bladder. It is advanced further more and balloon near the tip is inflated *using distilled water*. Air is not used for this purpose. Normal saline may get crystallised and so ideal is distilled water. (Note: in endotracheal tube only air is used to inflate the balloon. Water should never be used because if balloon bursts aspiration can occur). Quantity inflated should be noted in the case sheet. Usually 20 mL is used. It is actually written in the Foley's catheter. After inflation catheter is pulled out to confirm that balloon is inflated properly. Catheter is connected to urosac bag. Prepuce is placed in normal position otherwise paraphimosis (iatrogenic) can develop.

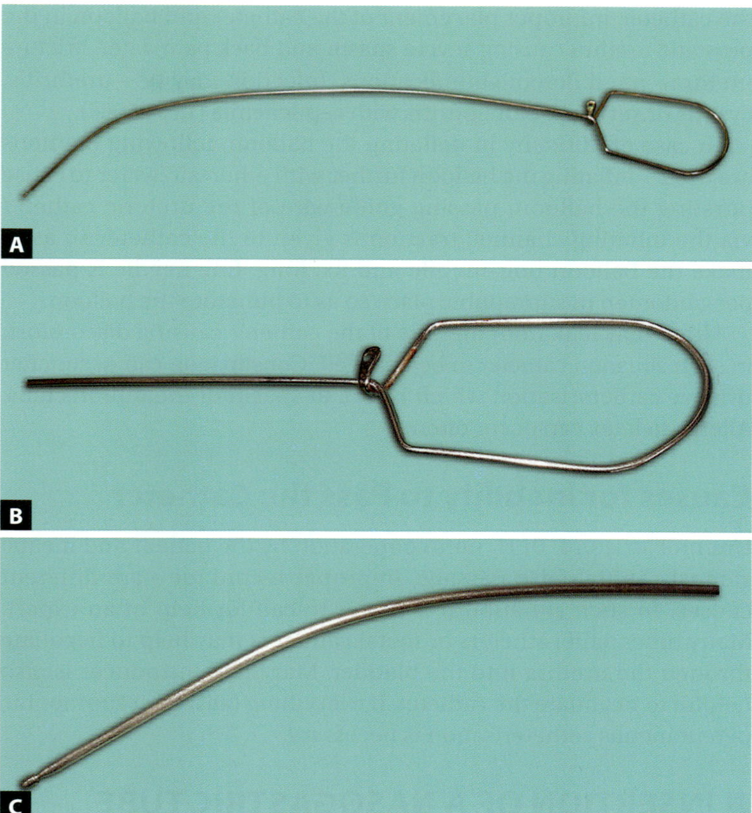

Figs. 7-5A to C: Foley's catheter introducer.

In adult 16 F catheter is used. F-French unit—16 mm circumference (Charriere unit). Often Foley's catheter is kept for 7–10 days. If there is a need to keep catheter for more than 10 days then silicon coated Foley's catheter is used as it is least reactive. Foley's catheter is made up of latex. In children 10 F or 8 F is used.

Three-way Foley's catheter is used to irrigate the bladder with normal saline/glycine solution continuously in post-TURP (transurethral resection of prostate) or after bladder surgery or after bladder trauma.

Foley's catheter often is reinforced with tension wires to prevent block and is called as haematuric Foley's catheter.

Maryfield introducer is used often to pass the Foley's catheter into the bladder. It has got a curve with a groove over the convex part to accommodate the catheter.

Balloon should be *deflated completely* before removal of the catheter otherwise urethral injury and haematuria can occur.

In females, labia majora are retracted apart to identify the urethral orifice to pass the catheter.

Complications of Catheterisation

Infection, false passage, bleeding (haematuria), inability to deflate the balloon while removing the catheter, allergic reactions, bladder/urethral spasm, clouding of the urine, urethral pain, urine leak by the side of the catheter tube, bladder stone formation, blockage of the catheter, improper placement of the catheter and balloon in the prostatic urethra causing severe spasm and back pain, later stricture urethra—are different complications. Infection may be—urethritis, cystitis or severe pyelonephritis with septicaemia (urosepsis).

In case of difficulty in deflating the balloon, following methods are used—inflating the balloon further with ether/air/water to cause bursting the balloon; passing guide wire of the ureteric catheter via the inflating channel; traction is given to the catheter so as to make the balloon non-mobile and fix, long, fine needle is passed per-abdomen in suprapubic place so as to puncture the balloon.

Urine may leak from the side of the catheter causing discomfort; in such situation catheter to be changed. Constipation can occur after urinary catheterisation which is due to spasm of the puborectalis. Allergy to latex can occur often.

Causes for Inability to Pass the Catheter

Urethral stricture, BPH, non-cooperation by the patient and meatal stenosis, initial false passage, improper technique—are different causes. In such situation it is better to call for help of an expert. Many times, stiff catheters or metal catheters may help to negotiate through the urethra into the bladder. Maryfield introducer is also helpful to negotiate the catheter. If everything fails, then suprapubic percutaneous catheterisation is necessary.

INSERTION OF A NASOGASTRIC TUBE

Indications

For decompressing stomach in intestinal obstruction, after abdominal surgery. It prevents aspiration and distension of intestines.

For gastric function tests: In gastric outlet obstruction to decompress the stomach and also to give stomach wash. Stomach tube is better (Ewald's tube) for this.

For feeding purpose: In post-operative patients, bedridden patients who cannot swallow, in comatose patients, in patients with major head and neck surgeries like laryngectomy, pharyngectomy in post-operative period.

Baid test: Passed Ryle's tube will be palpable per abdomen in pseudocyst of pancreas as stomach is stretched forward. Ryle's tube will not enter the stomach in Boerhaave's syndrome, gastric volvulus.

Often nasogastric tube is helpful in guarding the oesophagus in major neck surgeries. It is used in all oesophageal and gastric surgeries, often as a tube drain whenever needed either in open or laparoscopic surgeries.

Indications may be diagnostic or therapeutic: Diagnostic indications are—upper gastrointestinal (GI) problems, gastric function tests, for contrast study of gastrointestinal tract (GIT), Baid test, etc. Therapeutic indications are—in intestinal obstruction to decompress the bowel, in gastric dilatation, for feeding purpose, in toxic ingestion for irrigation, for total gut irrigation, in post-operative period GI surgeries.

Note:

Relative contraindications are—bleeding oesophageal varices, alkali ingestion, coagulation disorders, patient not accepting the tube.

Usually, nasogastric tube can be kept for few weeks; polyurethane and silicone tubes can be kept for longer period of 6–8 weeks which are unaffected by gastric juice. PVC tube is kept only for 2–3 weeks. Any further need of tubing requires gastrostomy (PEG).

Feeding can be done either by gravity or using pump. Gravity feeding facilitates bolus feed and is simple, quicker but increases the chances of gastrointestinal symptoms. Pump feeding is safer but when it is used as continuous feeding it limits the mobility of the patient. Feeding ideally should be done in semirecumbent position. Nasogastric tube feeding is contraindicated in gastric stasis, oesophageal reflux disease, high-risk patients for aspiration, nasal and base of skull injuries.

It is mandatory to check the position of the tube daily and whenever position is doubtful. Repositioning is needed if it is displaced. Proper fixation of the tube is important using sticking plaster. Often suture fixation is done to the nostril if long-term tube placement is required; but it is painful and causes more discomfort to the patient.

Nasogastric tube is removed when the patient passes flatus or bowel sounds are heard properly or if quantity of the aspiration from the tube is less than 50 mL per day. In other patients it is removed whenever patient looks comfortable for oral feeding during recovery period from the existing disease.

Types

Single lumen Levin's nasogastric tube is commonly used.

Salem Sump double lumen catheter in which one is for aspiration, other is for venting to reduce the negative pressure and so preventing the gastric mucosa being drawn into the catheter.

Anderson nasogastric tube also has got vent with 24 aspirating ports which also prevent clogging.

Dobhoff nasogastric tube has got a weight at the end which pulls the tube downwards while inserting into the oesophagus.

Procedure

Procedure is explained to the patient. Usually no. 16 tube is used in adult. It is one meter (100 cm) long usually of plastic (earlier red rubber) with three lead shots in the tip. Lead shots in the tip make it easier to pass. (Infant feeding tube does not have lead shots). In children, size is determined by—age + 16 divided by 2 (if age is 6, then 6 + 16 = 22/2 = 11). It has got different marking ring/rings (2, 3, and 4). First ring signifies OG junction (40 cm). Two rings for body of stomach (50 cm), three for the pylorus (60 cm) and four for duodenum (70 cm). Xylocaine spray or viscous is given to the patient. Nasal xylocaine spray or instillation of the xylocaine viscous into the nostril is also done. Length is assessed by nose to ear to xiphisternum (NEX) or by nose to umbilicus of the patient. Position is sitting upright with neck flexed position.

Xylocaine jelly 2% is lubricated to the tube. It is passed one of the nostrils (wider one) horizontally until it reaches the posterior pharyngeal wall. Patient is asked to swallow if needed with the help of cup of water. Tube passes through the relaxed cricopharyngeus and then into oesophagus. Afterwards it is easier to pass into the oesophagus. Once it is in the oesophagus adequately tube is fixed to nostril. 'No swallow' technique is better wherein patient is asked to take deep breath and hold while passing the tube across the pharynx which closes the glottis with epiglottis so that keeps cricopharynx open **(Figs. 7-6 and 7-7)**.

In difficult situation lifting the oropharynx upwards using two fingers will facilitate the tube insertion. One can use direct laryngoscope to guide the tube towards the oesophagus using Magill forceps. Lifting the thyroid cartilage upwards and in front will also help in facilitating the tube downwards. Freezing the nasogastric tube will stiffen the tube which makes passing the tube easier. Ureteric guide wire as stylet also can be used in difficult situation.

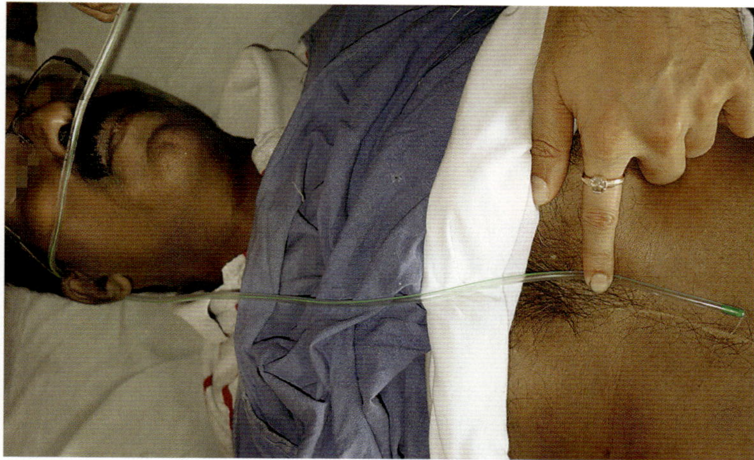

Fig. 7-6: NEX (nose to ear to xiphisternum) measurement for nasogastric tube.

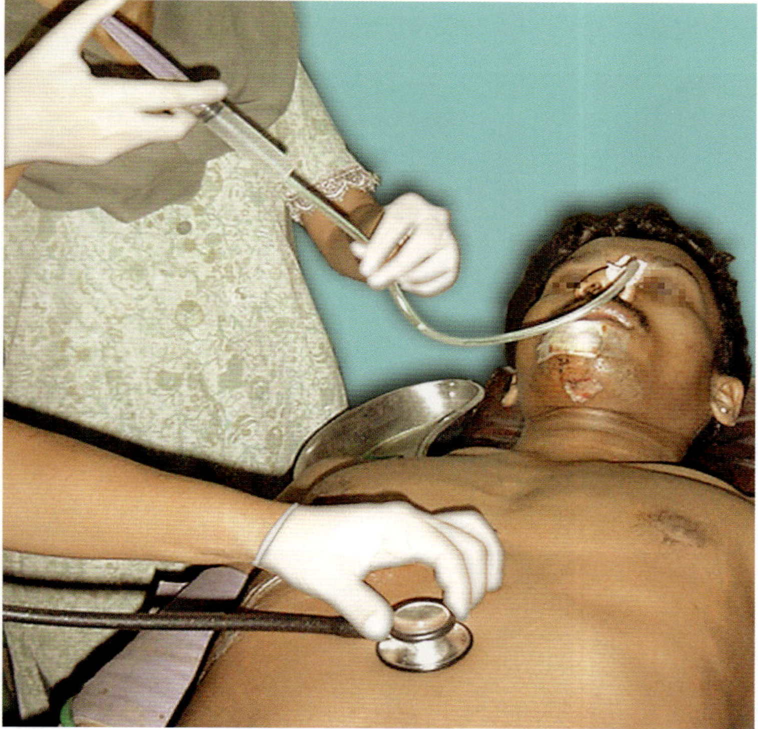

Fig. 7-7: After passing the Ryle's tube to the stomach, air from the syringe should be infused through the tube and when auscultated gush of air into the stomach can be heard which confirms that tube tip is in the stomach.

Confirmation of the tube in the stomach is done by aspirating the bile and also by injecting 30 mL of air into the stomach through the tube which can be heard in the epigastrium with a stethoscope as a gurgling sound. Taking an X-ray and confirming is a better method. *Colorimetric capnography* may be better way to confirm the position of the tube. If patient is able to speak properly then tube is not in the trachea. Checking the pH of the gastric aspirate is ideal but it is technically difficult.

Problems and Complications

Often tube gets coiled in the pharynx and becomes difficult to negotiate to oesophagus. Bleeding from nostril is not uncommon after the insertion. Aspiration can occur theoretically as it keeps OG junction patent. Oesophageal perforation, anastomotic dehiscence, tracheal intubation, pneumonia, proximal displacement, blockage of the tube, discomfort are all possible other complications which can occur.

ABSCESS DRAINAGE

Abscess is a localised collection of pus lined by granulation tissue covered by pyogenic membrane. It contains pus in loculi **(Fig. 7-8)**.

Bacteria causing abscess: Staphylococcus aureus, Streptococcus pyogenes, Gram-negative bacteria (*E. coli, Pseudomonas, Klebsiella*), and anaerobes.

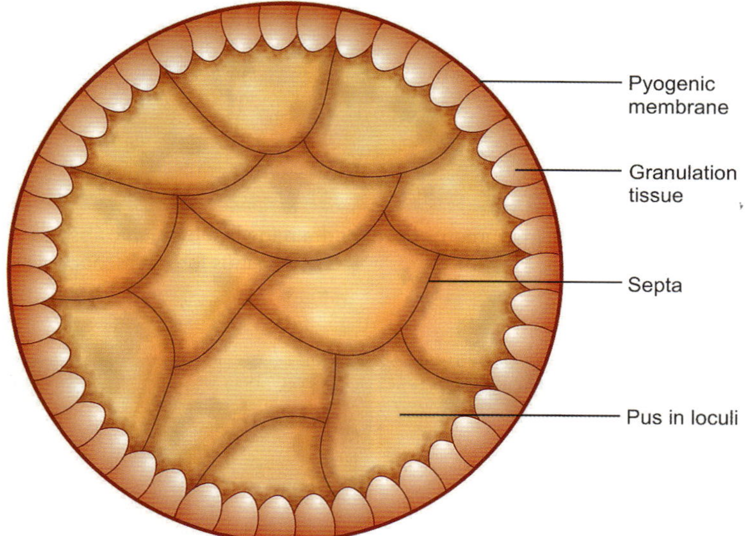

Fig. 7-8: Pyogenic abscess—parts.

Factors precipitating abscess formation: General condition of the patient: Nutrition, anaemia, age of the patient; Associated diseases: Diabetes, HIV, immunosuppression; Type and virulence of the organisms; Trauma, haematoma, and road traffic accidents.

Abscess should be drained once it is formed only under the cover of antibiotics.

Features of formed abscess

- Pointing tenderness
- Visible pus
- Excruciating pain
- Localised swelling
- Induration (brawny induration).

Abscess is Drained by Hilton's Method

Under general or regional anaesthesia, after cleaning and draping, using needle with syringe pus is confirmed by aspiration. Adequate incision is made over the skin longitudinal along the line of neurovascular bundle. Pyogenic membrane is opened using sinus forceps. Pus is collected for culture and sensitivity. All loculi should be broken. Wound is washed with saline or povidone iodine. Gauze drain or corrugated drain is placed in the wound. Antibiotics are continued. Wound is allowed to granulate and heal **(Figs. 7-9 to 7-11)**.

Incision and loop drainage (I and LD): It is incising the abscess and placing silicone tubes or drains/loops in the cavity to have continuous drainage of the abscess. After incision and drainage through a small incision, second small incision is made at the outer edge, a vessel loop is passed through incisions and tied loosely (air knot). This is left in pace for a several days until the cavity heals and free of discharge. This avoids repeated packing of the cavity at regular dressings. If the abscess is more than 5 cm, loop drainage technique is better.

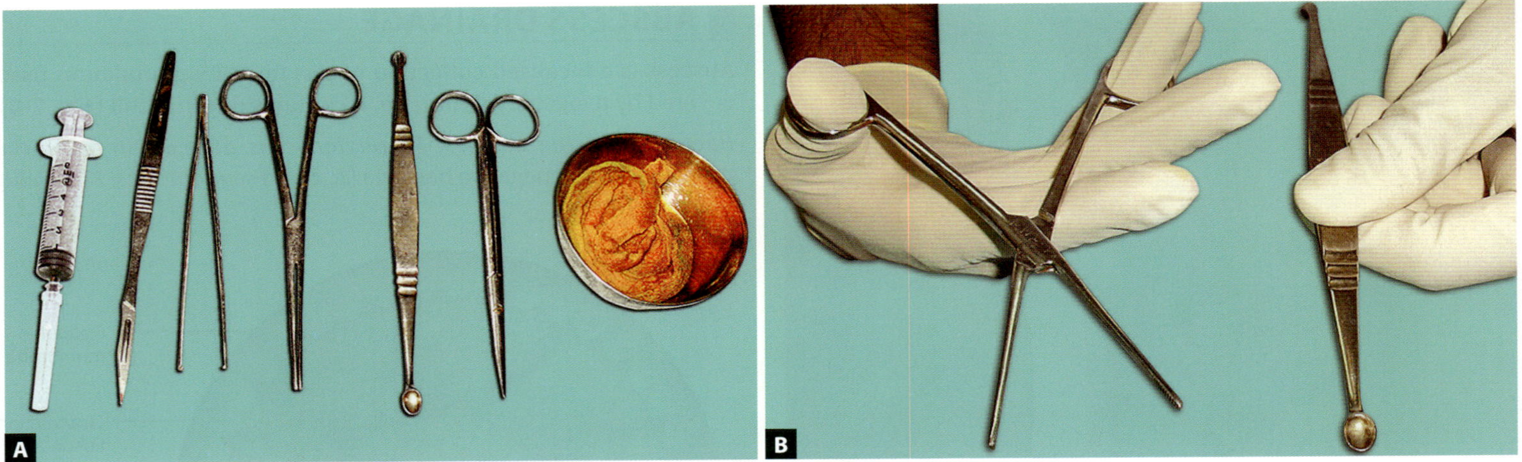

Figs. 7-9A and B: Instruments used for drainage of a pyogenic abscess—syringe with needle for aspiration; 11 number blade; toothed dissecting forceps; Lister's sinus forceps; scoop; scissor; roller pack soaked in povidone iodine.

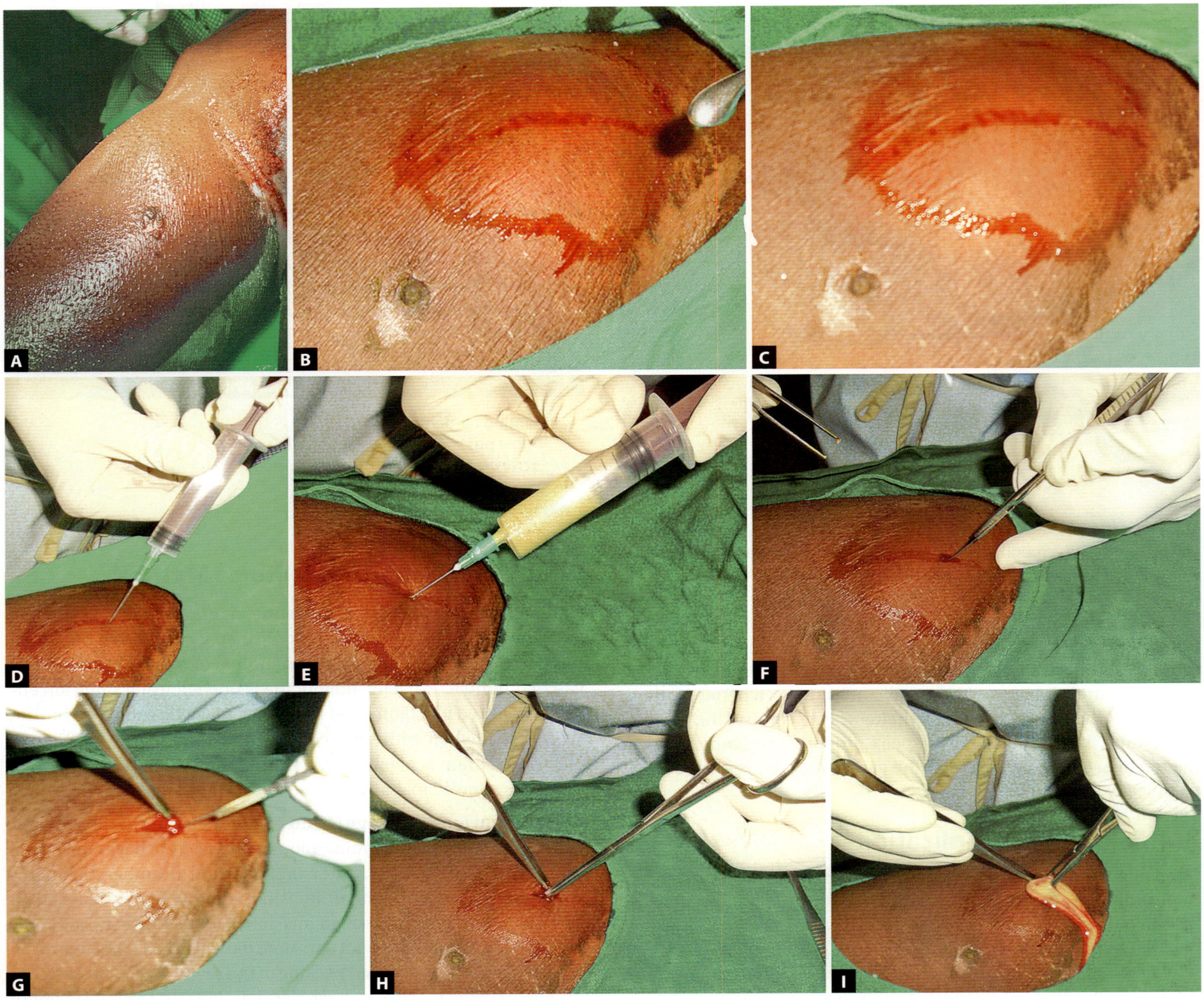

Figs. 7-10A to I

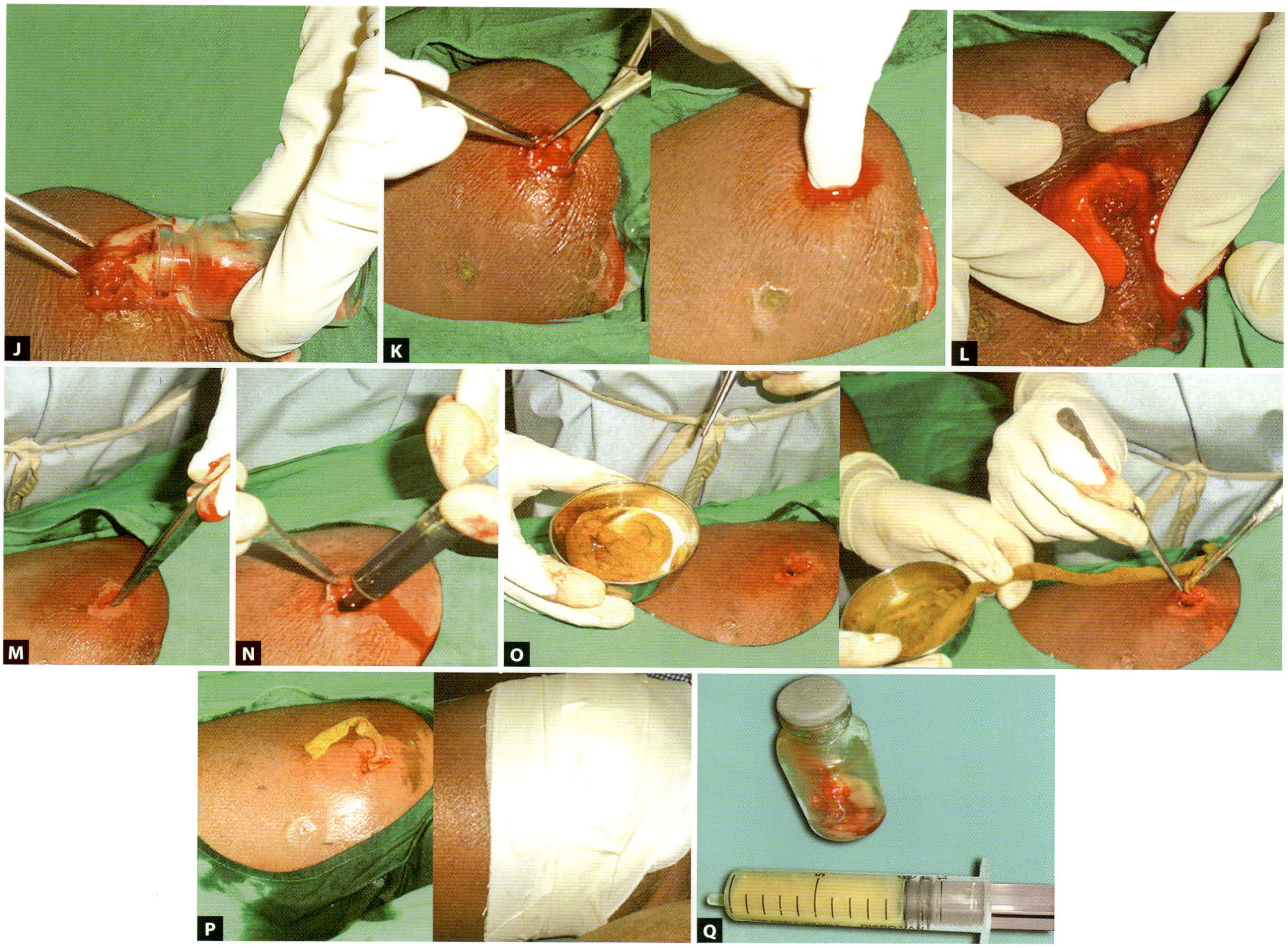

Figs. 7-10J to Q

Figs. 7-10A to Q: Technique of draining pyogenic abscess. 11 number blade is used to make incision. Lister's sinus forceps is used to drain abscess. Often scoop is used gently to remove unhealthy tissues from the wall of the abscess cavity. Cavity is packed with gauze. Dressing placed. Pus sent for culture.

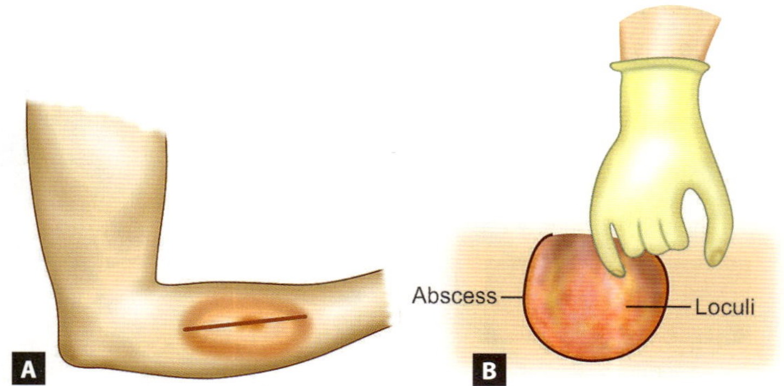

Figs. 7-11A and B: Incision should be longitudinal along the line of neurovascular bundle. Loculi should be broken using little finger or blades of sinus forceps.

Incisions should be of 5 mm sized small only, multiple incisions can be made to place many loops not more than 4 cm away from the main centre/summit incision. Most crucial is surgeon must be diligent in breaking all loculi and through a warm saline wash using a 20 cc syringe **(Figs. 7-12A to C)**.

Local anaesthesia may not act as pus is acidic in nature and xylocaine will not be effective in this acidic media.

Complications: Improper drainage and residual abscess; septicaemia; sinus formation; if abscess is located near major vessels, sloughing of the vessel wall leading to torrential haemorrhage occasionally.

Sarcoma and aneurysms may mimic pyogenic abscess especially when it is deep seated and so necessary investigations like CT scan and aspiration of the content should be done before incision and drainage **(Figs. 7-13 and 7-14)**.

Abscess in special locations may not show features of formed abscess. In those locations abscess should be drained without waiting for features of formed abscess—pointing, fluctuation. They are—parotid abscess; breast abscess; Ludwig's angina—it is actually a cellulitis not an abscess but needs exploration and decompression; thigh abscess; ischiorectal abscess.

Parotid Abscess

Parotid abscess presents as severe pain and tender swelling in the parotid region in front of the tragus. Often patient will be toxic,

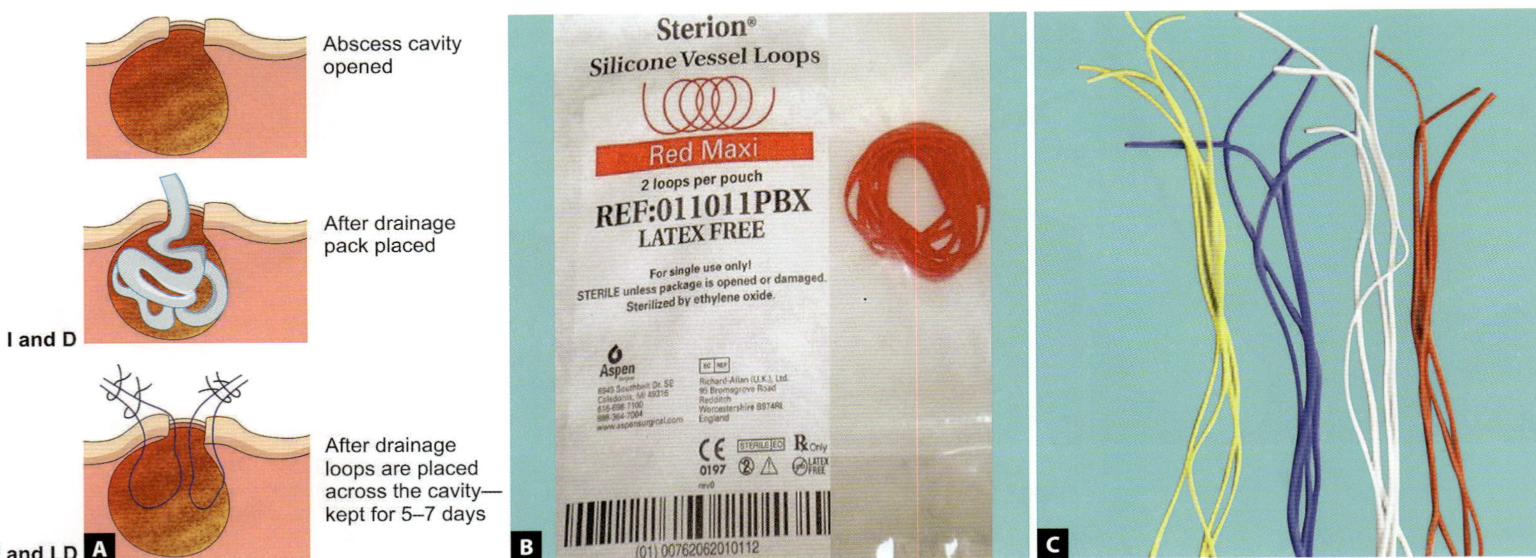

Figs. 7-12A to C: Incision (I) and drainage (D) and incision and loop drainage (LD) with silicone vessel loops.

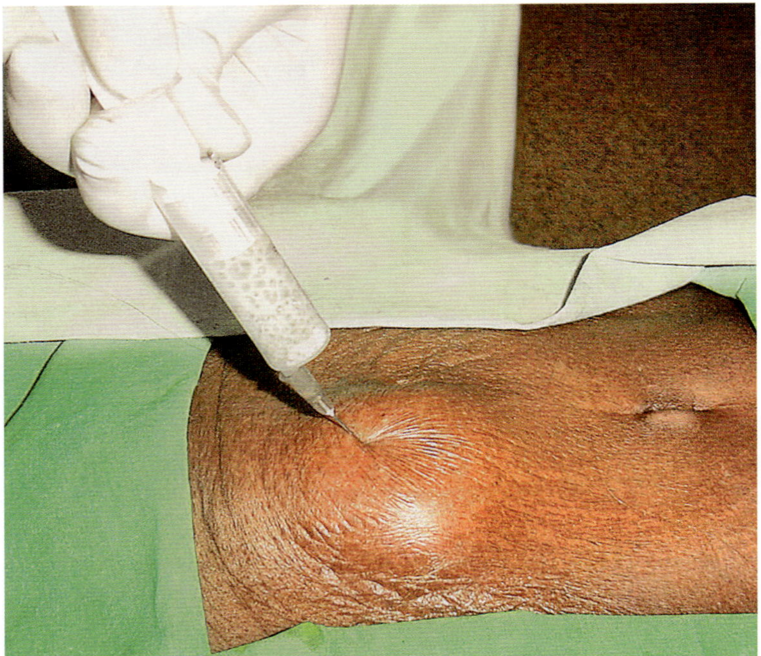

Fig. 7-13: Aspiration of abdominal wall abscess. Aspiration of abscess prior to making incision is absolute need.

dehydrated with trismus. Parotid abscess is drained under general anaesthesia with endotracheal tube in place. *Blair's* vertical incision is placed in front of the tragus. Abscess cavity is opened using sinus forceps with multiple horizontal incisions in deeper plane. Care should be taken not to traumatise the facial nerve. After draining pus and proper saline wash drain is placed into the wound. Loose sutures in the skin may be placed. Facial nerve injury, septicaemia, laryngeal oedema and local spread of sepsis are the complications. Infection when spreads to pharynx/larynx/parapharyngeal space needs tracheostomy **(Fig. 7-15)**.

Note:

Lilienthal (1917) originally described this concept. He started 'S' incision (vertical running incision in front of the tragus downwards curving under the ear and extending into the neck in front of the sternocleidomastoid muscle along the skin crease). Anterior skin flap is raised; then multiple horizontal incisions are made along the parotid sheath to break all septae underneath to archive proper drainage of the pus. Later in 1923, Blair and Padgett popularised the technique and also proposed and practiced the essentiality of the early drainage of the parotid abscess to avoid complications like extensive necrosis, septicaemia even though their proposal of early intervention is opposed initially by many. That is why technique is

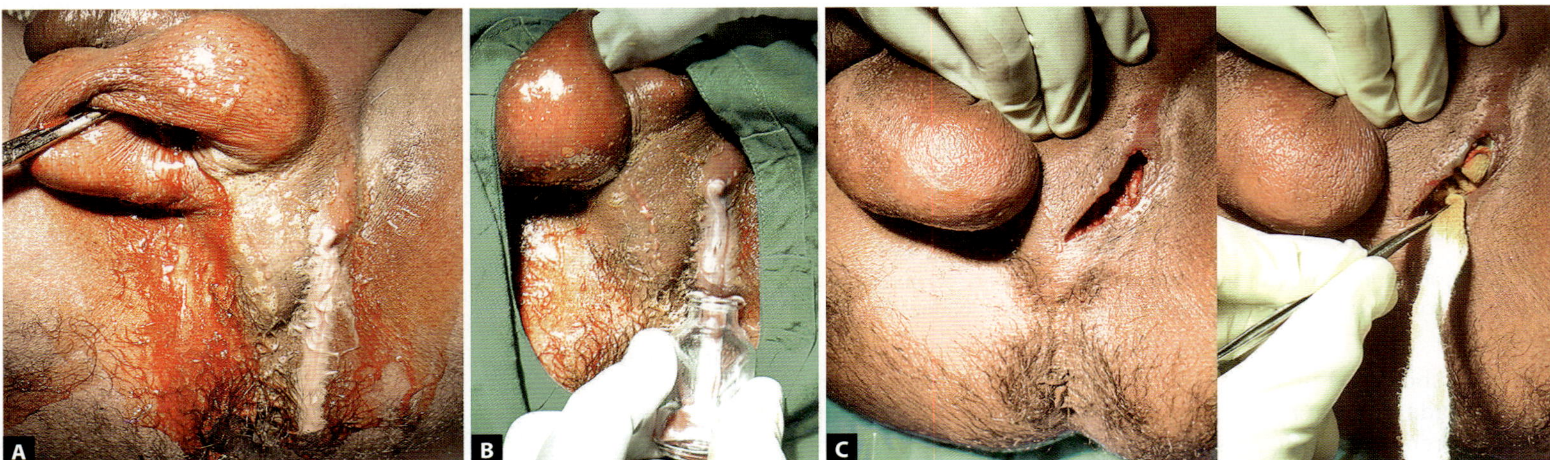

Figs. 7-14A to C: Abscess in the perineum which is drained and packed.

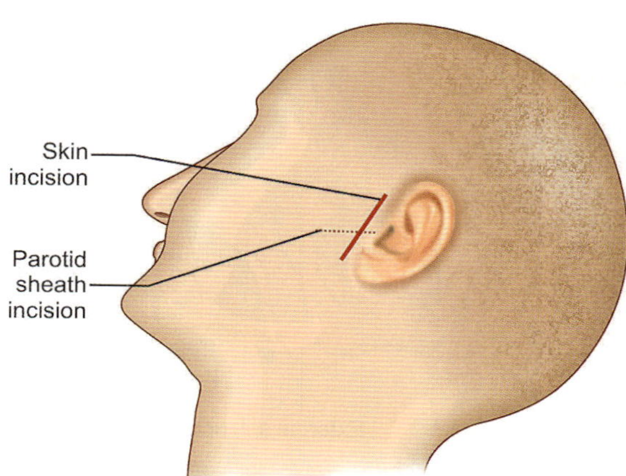

Fig. 7-15: Blair incision used to drain the parotid abscess.

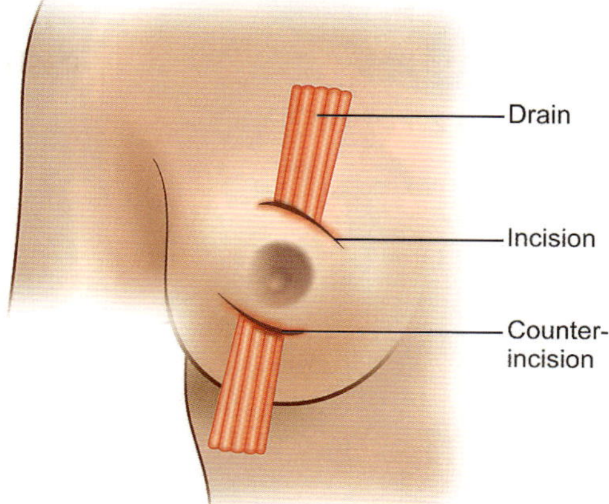

Fig. 7-16: Incision and counter-incision for breast abscess.

often called as Blair's method of drainage. Possible complications of surgery are—facial nerve injury, sinus/fistula formation.

Early drainage reduces the oedema, trismus, toxaemia, septicaemia and improves the perfusion making antibiotics to act better.

Breast Abscess

Breast abscess is commonly due to *Staphylococcus aureus*. It is common in lactating women. It should always be drained under general anaesthesia. There will not be any localisation. Diffuse swelling and tenderness all over the breast is common. Occasionally tender axillary lymph nodes may be palpable. After cleaning and draping, pus is aspirated and confirmed initially. Either circum-areolar or submammary incision is done. After draining pus and breaking loculi, a counter-incision is made on the upper aspect. After proper saline wash of the wound, drain is placed across the *incision and counter-incision*. If patient is lactating, suppression of lactation is done using Bromocryptine 2.5 mg. Regular expression of milk either manually or using breast pump should be done. Otherwise recurrent infection or fistula can occur.

Acute breast abscess may mimic mastitis carcinomatosis/ inflammatory carcinoma of breast.

Breast abscess which is not drained but treated with antibiotics may form organised, hard, non-tender swelling in the breast called as *Antibioma* which mimics carcinoma breast. Antibioma contains thick walled fibrous tissue with sterile pus as flaques inside. It needs excision **(Figs. 7-16 to 7-19)**.

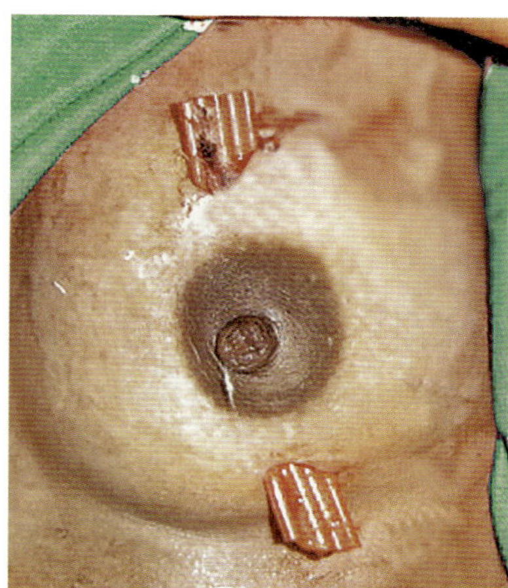

Fig. 7-17: Photograph showing placement of drain in breast abscess.

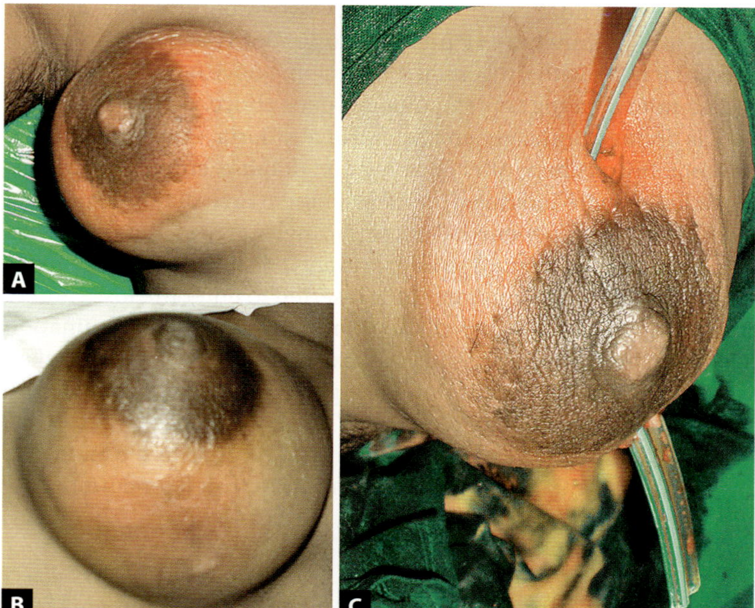

Figs. 7-18A to C: Typical breast abscess showing features of acute inflammation. Drain should be placed after incision and drainage in such abscesses. Often gauze drain can be used.

Axillary Abscess

Axillary abscess is drained under general anaesthesia with axilla in hyperextended position and a sandbag under the shoulder. A 5 cm incision is made under the anterior axillary fold longitudinally. Skin and superficial fascia is incised. Using sinus forceps deep fascia is opened parallel to the line of the axillary vessels. Care is taken not to injure axillary vessels (vein). After draining pus and saline wash, gauze/corrugated drain is placed. Antibiotics are continued. Complications are sinus formation, bleeding, shoulder stiffness.

Ischiorectal Abscess

Ischiorectal fossa (pyramidal shape 5 cm depth and 2 cm width) lies between anal skin and levator ani. Right and left communicates with each other. Laterally, it is related to fascia covering obturator internus and ischial tuberosity; medially to levator ani and external sphincter; posteriorly sacrotuberous ligament and gluteus maximus; anteriorly urogenital diaphragm; below, the floor by skin. Above it is related to

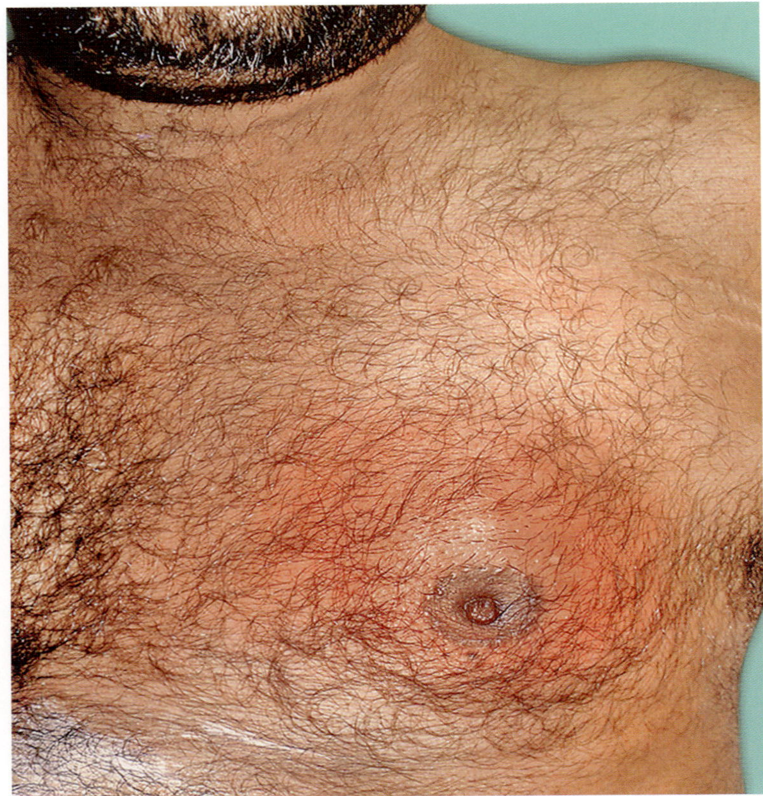

Fig. 7-19: Breast abscess in a male patient. Breast abscess even though is uncommon in male, it can occur during puberty.

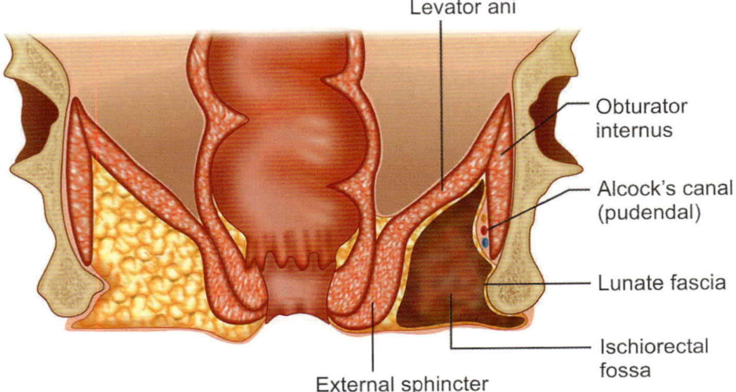

Fig. 7-20: Anatomy of ischiorectal fossa. Note the boundaries and Alcock's canal.

lunate fascia and pudendal neurovascular bundle in pudendal canal (*Alcock's canal*). There is no deep fascia under the skin in ischiorectal fossa. *Fascia lunata* (semilunar shaped hence the name) covers fascia on the levator ani medially, covers fascia on the obturator internus laterally (pudendal canal is located between obturator fascia and fascia lunata transmitting internal pudendal vessels and nerves); in front it fuses with urogenital diaphragm; above fascia is arched as tegmentum creating suprategmental space above.

It is drained under general/spinal anaesthesia. Procedure is done in lithotomy position. After cleaning and draping, cruciate incision is placed over more indurated/more prominent area of the ischiorectal fossa. Incision is deepened. Parts of the angles of the flaps are excised (diamond-shaped wound) so as to prevent it to close to form recurrent abscess formation. Sinus forceps is inserted to enter the fossa and to drain the pus. Using finger all loculi are broken. Rectal examination is done to find out the possibility of existing fistula. Cavity is packed with gauze and dressing is done using 'T' bandage. Antibiotics and regular dressings are required **(Figs. 7-20 to 7-22)**.

Digital examination of the rectum should be done to see for fistula. If fistula is present, fistulectomy is done at same or later period.

Ludwig's Angina

It is an inflammatory oedema of submandibular region and floor of the mouth, commonly due to streptococcal infection. There is bilateral brawny cellulitis of sublingual and submandibular region. It is common in severely ill and in advanced malignancy, causing *trismus, laryngeal oedema*. Extension of infection into *parapharyngeal space* may lead to dreaded internal *jugular vein thrombosis*. As the infection is deep to the deep fascia in a closed fascial plane; it spreads very fast causing dangerous complications.

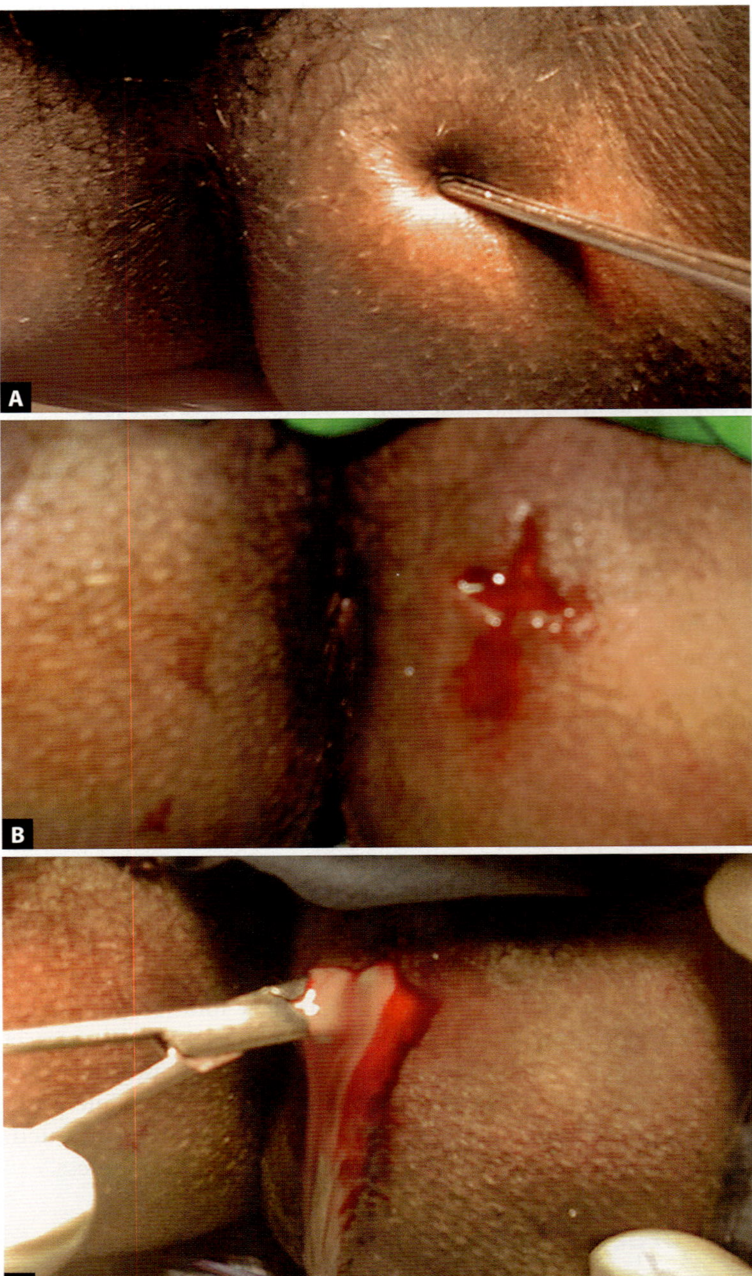

Figs. 7-21A to C: Ischiorectal abscess drainage under general anaesthesia. Note the cruciate incision placed and pus is gushing out.

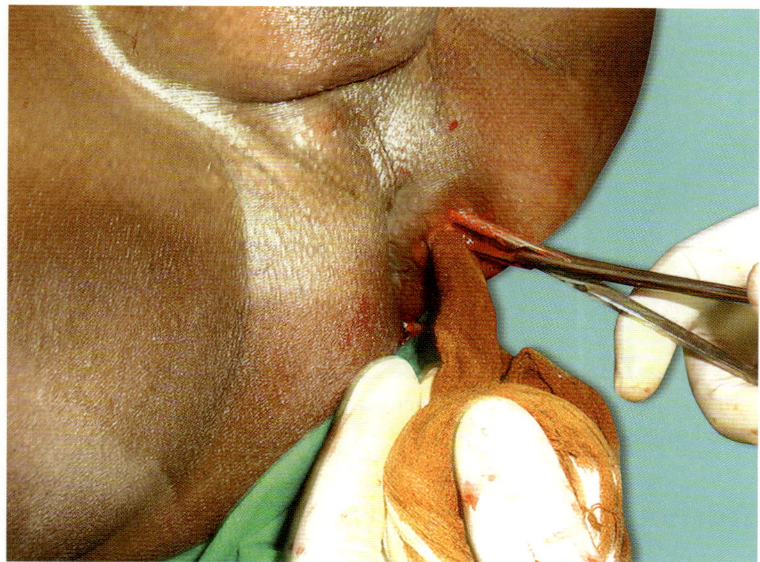

Fig. 7-22: Ischiorectal abscess cavity packed after drainage. Cruciate incision and creation of diamond-shaped wound is essential.

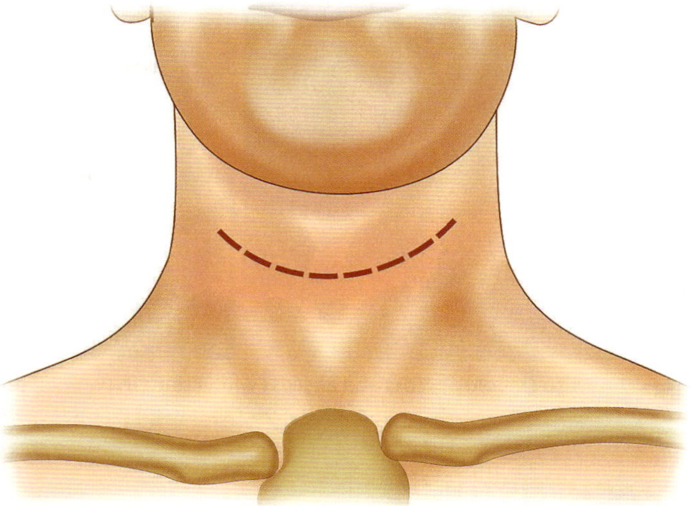

Fig. 7-23: Incision for draining Ludwig's angina.

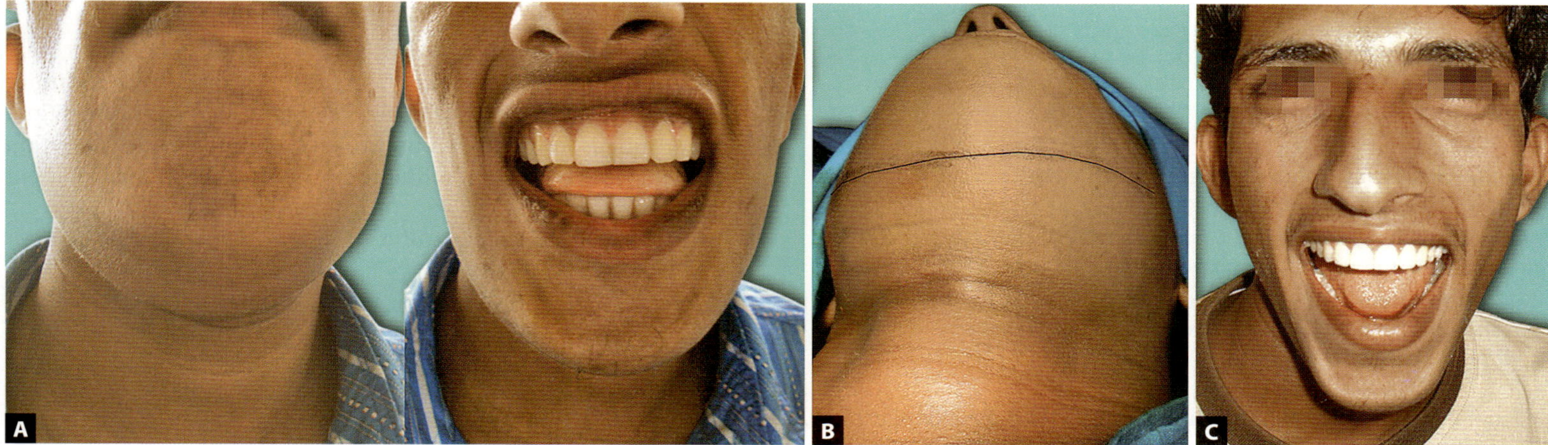

Figs. 7-24A to C: Ludwig's angina is drained by decompression incision in the submandibular region with cutting of both mylohyoid muscles. Patient after recovery could open the mouth.

Clinical features: Fever, toxicity, diffuse swelling, dysphagia, dyspnoea, and trismus.

Treatment: Antibiotics-penicillins (high dose 20 lac 4th–6th hourly), cefoperazone, sulbactam, metronidazole-anti-microbial; IV fluids for adequate hydration **(Figs. 7-23 and 7-24)**.

Decompression of the submandibular region is done, by making a deep incision extending into the deep fascia and also *cutting both the mylohyoid muscles*. Either it is left open or *delayed suturing is done,* (better option) or it is loosely sutured with a drain in situ.

Complications: Laryngeal oedema and respiratory distress may require tracheostomy; septicaemia; Extension of infection into parapharyngeal space.

Cold Abscess

It is due to caseation necrosis and localisation in a tuberculous infection. There will not be any signs of inflammation. It is well localised, soft, cystic, non-tender swelling without any warmness. It is commonly due to tuberculous lymphadenitis, but can occur in tuberculosis of spine, kidney or other areas. Fine needle aspiration cytology (FNAC) shows caseation necrosis, macrophages and typical epithelioid cells. Cold abscess is drained using *non-dependent incision*. After drainage wound is sutured without placing a drain **(Figs. 7-25A to D)**.

Treatment of cold abscess: When there is cold abscess; initially it has to be aspirated. [Needle is introduced into the cold abscess in a non-dependent site along a *'Z' track* (in zigzag pathway) so as to prevent sinus formation]. But if it recurs, then it should be drained. Drainage is done through a *non-dependent incision*. After draining the caseating material, *wound is closed without placing a drain.* *Surgical removal of tuberculous lymph nodes*: It is done by raising skin flaps and removing all caseating material and lymph nodes. Care should be taken not to injure major structures.

Indications for surgical removal of tubercular lymph nodes

- There is no local response to chemotherapy.
- When sinus persists.

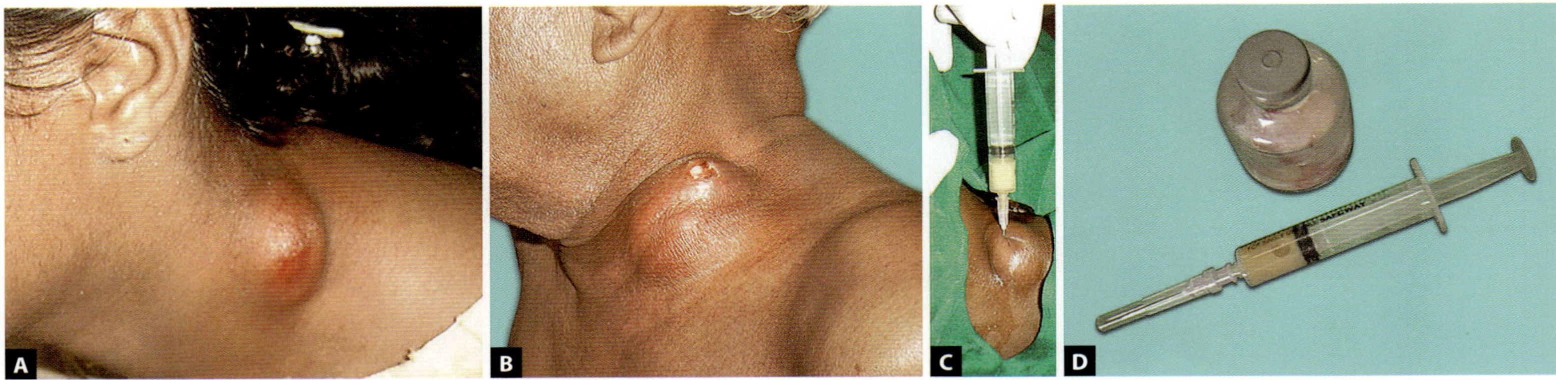

Figs. 7-25A to D: Cold abscess and abscess with a sinus in two different patients. It is aspirated in a zigzag track manner. Open drainage is done through non-dependent incision; wound later closed without placing any drain.

TRACHEOSTOMY

Tracheostomy is making an opening in the anterior wall of trachea and converting it into a stoma on the skin surface. It is done for airway maintenance. It is a life-saving procedure.

Types

- Emergency tracheostomy.
- Elective tracheostomy.
- Permanent tracheostomy.

High tracheostomy—above the level of isthmus. It can cause tracheal stenosis. It is above 2nd tracheal ring.

Mid-tracheostomy—ideal and commonly used. It through 2nd and 3rd rings behind isthmus. It is approached by dividing thyroid isthmus.

Low-tracheostomy—below the isthmus level. It is deep and impinges the suprasternal notch. It can cause torrential bleed which is difficult to control.

Tracheostomy tube has got outer cannula with neck flange/plate, inner cannula which can be removed when cleaning is needed; and obturator which is used to facilitate smooth insertion of the tracheostomy tube. It can be metallic or non-metallic. Cuffed or non-cuffed. Cuffed tube may be with disposable or reusable inner cannula. Fenestrated cuffed or non-cuffed tracheostomy tubes are also available.

Tracheostomy can be classical or bedside percutaneous dilatational tracheostomy **(Fig. 7-26)**.

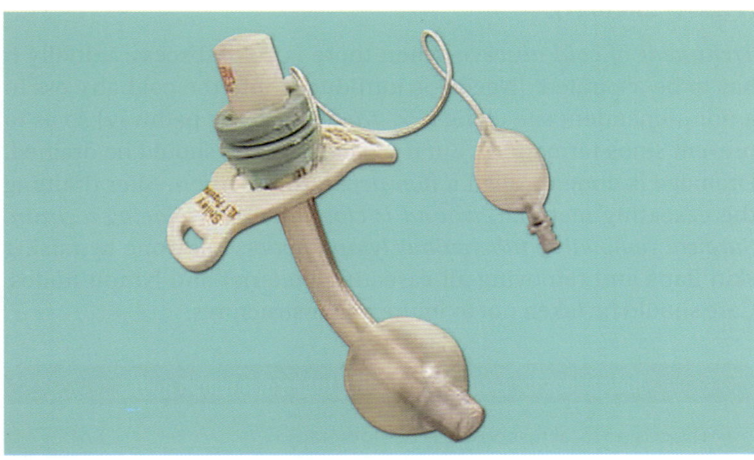

Fig. 7-26: Sheily tracheostomy tube.

Tracheostomy Tubes

1. ***Fuller's bivalved tracheostomy tube:*** It has got a outer tube and an inner tube. Outer tube is biflanged and so insertion is easier. Inner tube is longer with an opening on its posterior aspect. Inner tube can be removed and re-inserted easily whenever required. Using inner tube patient can speak. It is not used in radiotherapy.
2. ***Jackson's tracheostomy tube:*** It has got outer tube, inner tube and an obturator. Outer tube has got lock mechanism for inner tube with holes on either side for straps and shield for protection. Inner tube is longer than outer tube. Obturator guides insertion of tube. It is not used in radiotherapy. With tube in place patient cannot speak.
3. Red-rubber tracheostomy tube.
4. ***PVC tracheostomy tube***.

Tubes can be cuffed or non-cuffed. It can be fenestrated or non-fenestrated. It can be metal or polyvinyl chloride. Metal tubes are commonly used for permanent tracheostomies. Inner tube can be removed for cleaning purpose. They do not prevent patient from developing aspiration. It is not used for mechanical ventilation purpose.

Shiley's fenestrated tube has got inner and outer tube. Outer cannula has got cuff which can be inflated if mechanical ventilation is needed. Inner tube is changeable and can be non-fenestrated or fenestrated. Non-fenestrated tube is used when mechanical ventilation is needed (outer tube cuff should be inflated). Fenestrated inner tube is used when needs to speak (with deflated outer tube). One way speaking valve may be used along with this to allow air to enter from atmosphere but air exits through fenestra into upper airway. Oxygen can be attached to this speaking valve **(Figs. 7-27 to 7-30)**.

Modern tracheostomy tubes are made of plastic. They are soft, least irritant and disposable. They have inflatable cuff which makes it easier to give assisted ventilation. Cuff should be deflated at regular intervals to prevent tracheal pressure necrosis. For assisted ventilation, endotracheal tube can be kept for 10–14 days. Beyond that period patient needs tracheostomy for further ventilation as endotracheal tube *in situ* beyond this period may cause damage to trachea, larynx and also precipitate life-threatening sepsis.

Indications for Tracheostomy

In head, neck and facial injuries; tetanus; tracheomalacia after thyroidectomy or bilateral recurrent laryngeal nerve palsy;

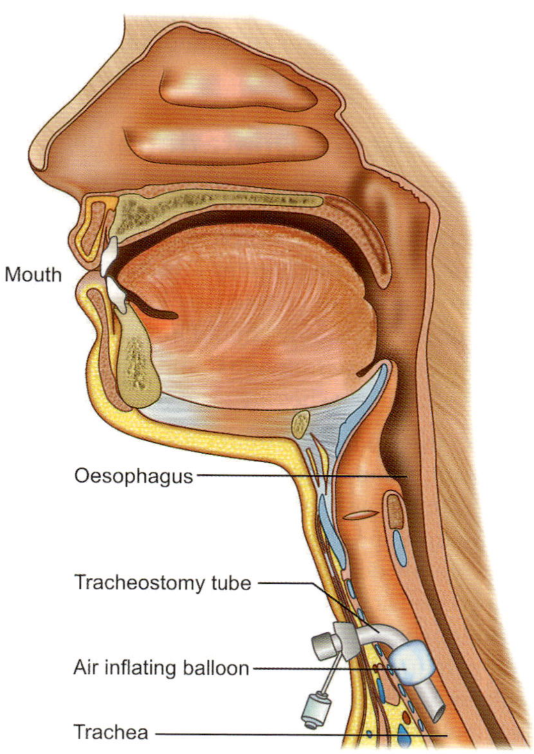

Fig. 7-27: Position of tracheostomy tube.

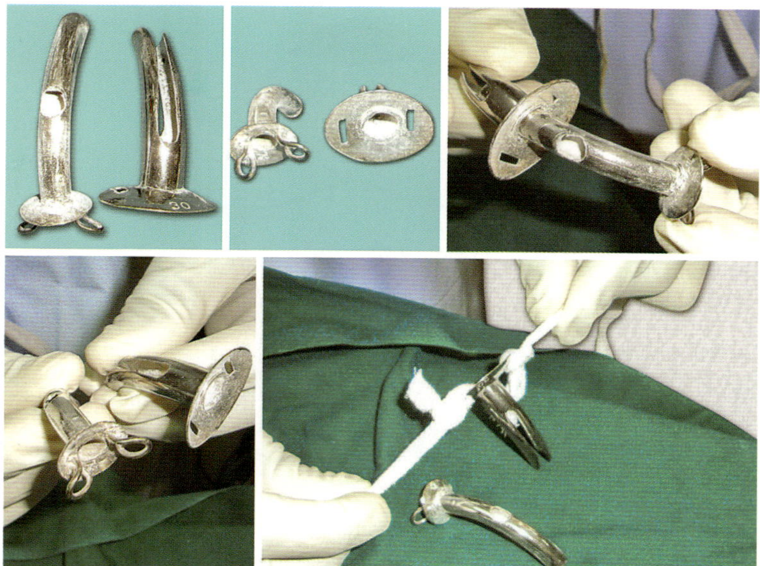

Fig. 7-29: Fuller's biflanged tracheostomy tube.

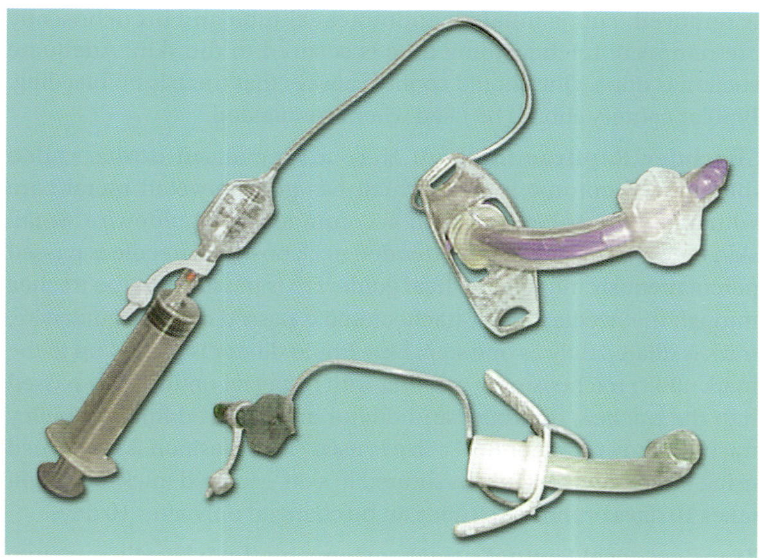

Fig. 7-28: Tracheostomy tube with inflation part and syringe (inflated with air)—polyvinyl chloride.

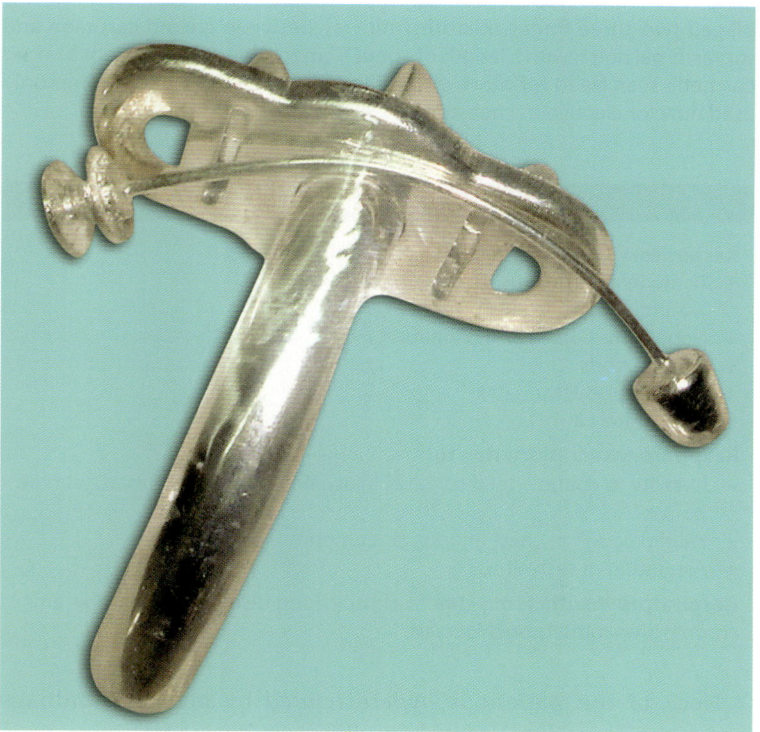

Fig. 7-30: Chevalier Jackson's tracheostomy tube.

laryngeal oedema/spasm; major head and neck surgeries like Commando's operation, block dissection; acute laryngitis as in diphtheria; carcinoma larynx, foreign body larynx, burns mouth, pharynx, larynx; respiratory paralysis like bulbar palsy; respiratory failure due to asthma, acute respiratory distress syndrome (ARDS).

Technique of Tracheostomy

Approaches—(1) *Vertical midline* incision: It extends from cricoid cartilage to sternal notch. It is used in emergency and often in elective tracheostomy. Tracheal stenosis less likely in this incision and also spontaneous closure is much rapid when compared to horizontal incision. It gives rapid access with less dissection but gives a poor scar. (2) *Horizontal* incision: It can be used in elective tracheostomy. It is placed two—three finger breadths/midway between cricoid cartilage and suprasternal notch with a length of about 5 cm transversely. It has got a better cosmetic scar. Need for more dissection is the drawback but is commonly used now for elective tracheostomy. (3) *Percutaneous approach* using a needle, cannula, guidewire, and serial plastic dilators followed by tracheostomy tube insertion **(Fig. 7-31)**.

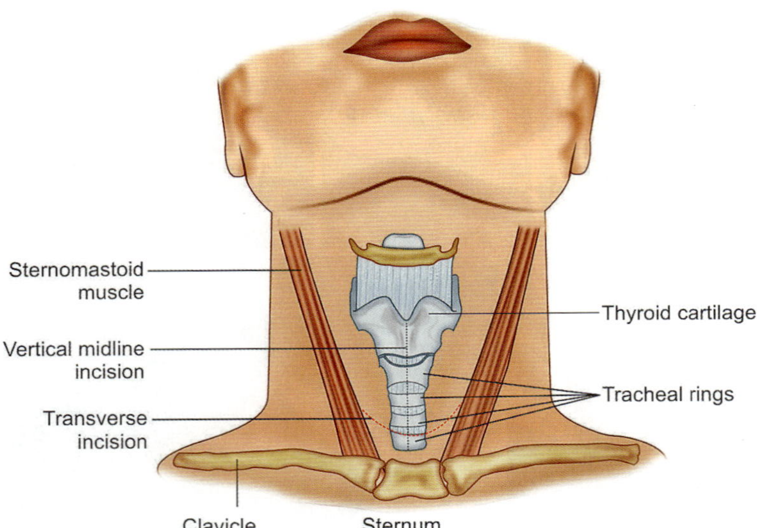

Fig. 7-31: Vertical midline or transverse incisions are used for tracheostomy. ***Vertical midline*** extends from cricoid cartilage to sternal notch. It is used in emergency and often in elective tracheostomy. Tracheal stenosis less likely in this incision and spontaneous closure is much rapid in this compared to horizontal incision. It gives rapid access with less dissection but leads into poor scar. ***Transverse incision*** can be used in elective tracheostomy. It is placed two-three finger breadths/midway between cricoid cartilage and suprasternal notch with a length of about 5 cm transversely. It has got a better cosmetic scar. Need for more dissection is the drawback but is commonly used now for elective tracheostomy.

Indications for tracheostomy

Respiratory obstruction due to:
- Acute infections causing oedema larynx.
- Trauma.
- Neoplasms—benign/malignant.
- Foreign body.
- Bilateral abductor palsy.
- Congenital causes.

Respiratory secretions due to:
- Inability to cough—tetanus, head injury, neurological causes, strychnine poison.
- Painful cough in chest injuries, pneumonia.
- Aspiration of secretions.

Respiratory insufficiency due to chronic lung diseases like emphysema, chronic bronchitis, bronchiectasis.

Neck of the patient is *hyperextended* by placing sandbags under the shoulder. Vertical (midline) or horizontal incision is made. eep fascia is opened. Strap muscles are retracted laterally. Isthmus is divided or retracted *upwards*. Inferior thyroid veins may cause bleeding and needs careful ligation. A few drops of lignocaine are instilled into the trachea to suppress the cough reflex. Trachea is fixed with tracheal hook. 2nd and 3rd or 3rd and 4th tracheal rings are opened and circular opening is made or a tracheal flap (*B'jork flap*—flap sutured to inferior margin of the incision) with base downwards is made. In elderly with calcified stiff trachea, cartilage rings are excised otherwise flap is commonly used. Tracheostomy tube is placed. It is tied around the neck. Usually 8.0 or 8.5 sized tracheostomy tubes are used. If the patient is having endotracheal tube as it is common in many situations, anaesthetist will remove the endotracheal tube and tracheostomy tube is inserted and connected to ventilator immediately. Proper suctioning of the trachea prior to insertion of the tube is better. Skin incision is sutured or packed to prevent formation of subcutaneous emphysema **(Figs. 7-32A to I)**.

Bedside Percutaneous Dilatational Tracheostomy

It is done instead of open method as percutaneous one. One should able to extend the neck of the patient adequately and distance between suprasternal notch to cricoid cartilage should be at least 1 cm. Percutaneous tracheostomy should not be done in children younger than 12 years, obese individual and with coagulopathies. Different methods and approaches are used **(Figs. 7-33A to I)**.

Cigalia (Hopkins) method: Here under general anaesthesia with neck extension cleaning and draping is done. Larynx is stabilised and pulled cephalad. Skin is incised for 2 cm vertical or horizontal; blunt dissection is done up to pre-tracheal fascia; existing endotracheal tube is withdrawn after deflating the cuff gently up to the glottis; bronchoscopy is passed across the glottis (through the endotracheal tube) to illuminate the skin incision. Needle is passed into the tracheal lumen percutaneously through the skin incision directed caudally. Needle tip is seen and confirmed by bronchoscopy already placed; needle should never puncture the posterior wall of the trachea (most important); guidewire is passed into the trachea through the needle or its cannula (if needle is cannulated one); needle is removed; serial dilators are passed to dilate the track; once adequately dilated, tracheostomy tube is put across the dilator into the trachea; dilator is removed; cuff is inflated; endotracheal tube and bronchoscopy are removed; tracheostomy tube is secured to the skin. Adequate suction is done. One should confirm always that there is no bleeding. Bipolar cautery should be used whenever needed.

Shachner Rapitrac method: Here a specialised device called dilator tracheotome is used which has got a beveled metal core with a hole in its centre which accommodates a guidewire. Small skin incision is placed with extended neck position; needle is passed percutaneously into the trachea; guidewire is passed into the trachea through the needle; dilator tracheotome is passed over the guidewire; track is dilated fully as one step; blue Rhino dilator is passed up to the mark 40 Fr; tracheostomy cannula with a special obturator is passed into the trachea; obturator and dilator are removed finally. Sheiley tracheostomy tube 8 or 8.5 Fr size is used. Tube position is confirmed using bronchoscope. Tube is sutured to skin. Matured track formation takes 10 days or more; so tube can be changed only after 10 days.

Translaryngeal Fantoni's tracheostomy method: Needle puncture into the trachea is done with cranial direction under bronchoscopic visualisation; tracheal cannula is inserted with a pull-through technique in retrograde direction along the orotracheal route. Cannula should be rotated downward at the end to achieve final pointing.

Note:
- First tracheal ring should never be used to do tracheostomy as perichondritis of cricoid cartilage with stenosis can occur—subglottic stenosis.
- Skin should not be sutured or loosely sutured to prevent development of subcutaneous emphysema.
- Cautery should be used during tracheostomy as much as possible to prevent oozing/bleeding from places like muscles and tracheal cut edge. Often torrential haemorrhage known to occur which may need a reexploration to control bleeding.

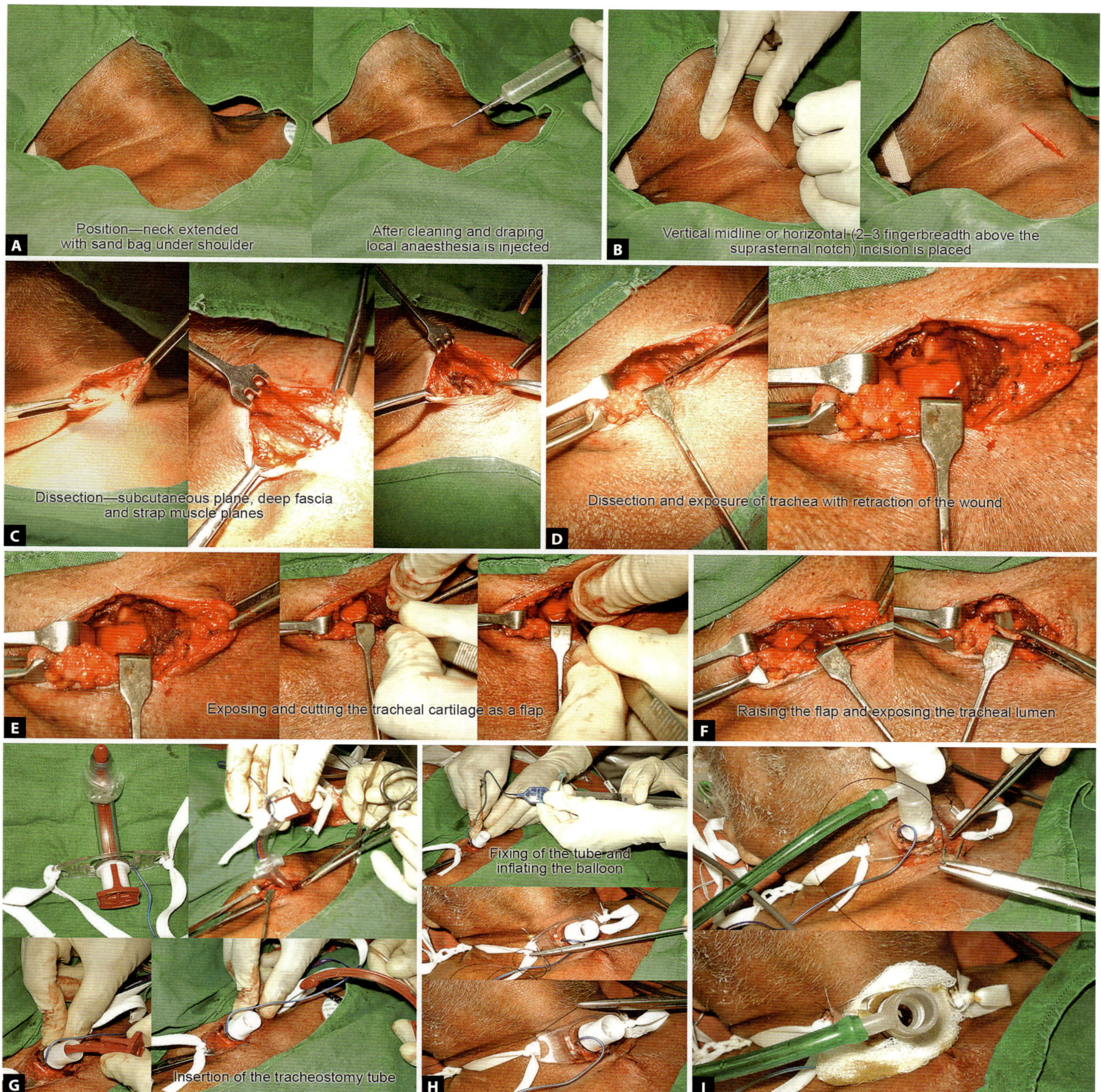

Figs. 7-32A to I: Steps in tracheostomy.

- In children trachea is soft and compressible and may get displaced easily and dissection may injure recurrent laryngeal nerve or carotid. Procedure is done under general anaesthesia with endotracheal tube in place or after insertion of bronchoscopy. Neck extension in children may cause innominate vein, thymus and pleura to be pulled upward allowing their possible injury. Silk sutures should be placed on the trachea prior to incising it. Trachea should not be excised in children; only it should be incised. Tracheostomy tube size should be carefully selected. Too lengthy tube will impinge on carina. Only portex tube should be used. Metallic tube is not advisable in children.

Tracheostomy Care

Regular suctioning and cleaning of the tube is needed. Humidification of the inspired air is done using normal saline/Ringer lactate.

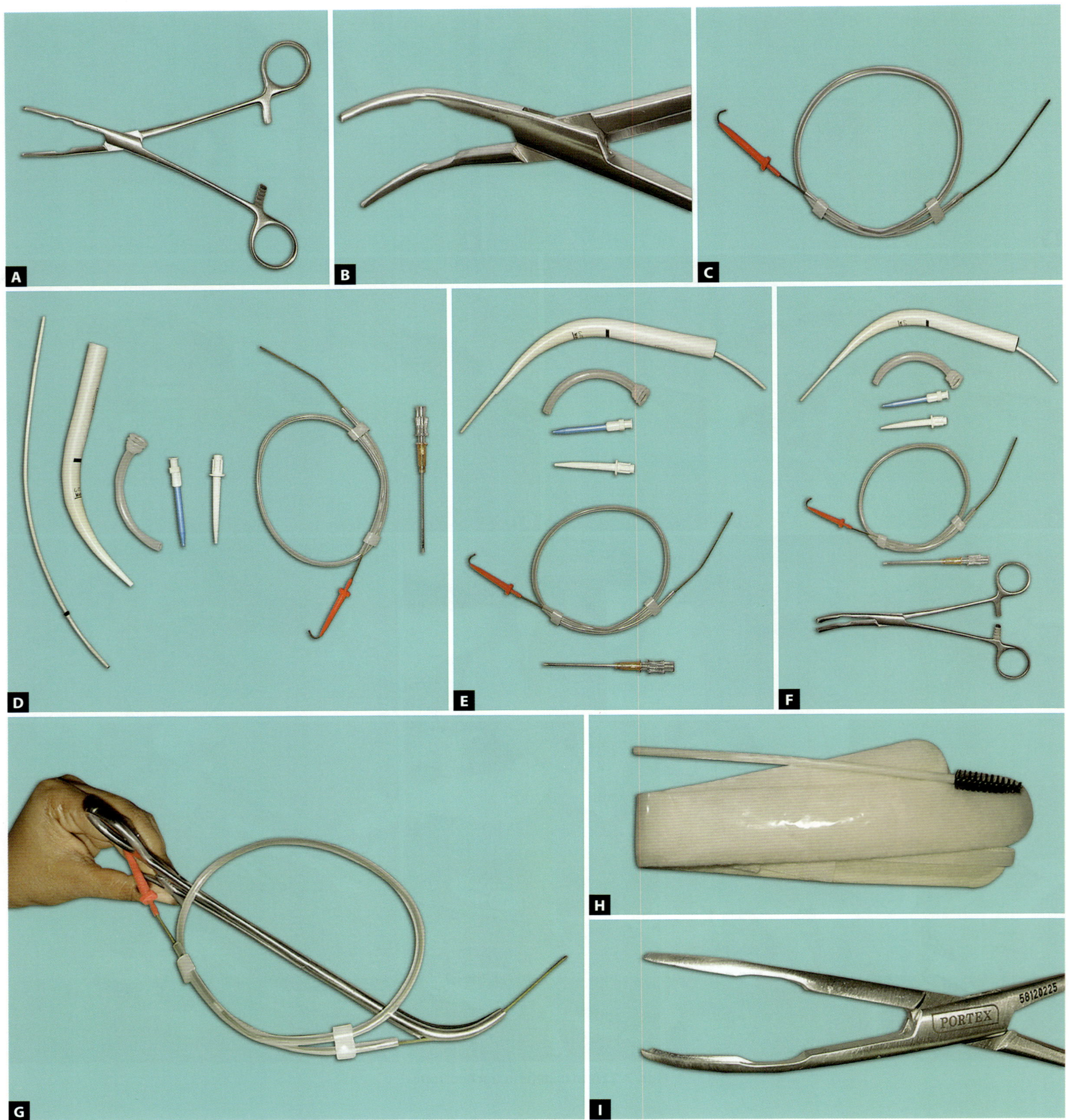

Figs. 7-33A to I: Percutaneous tracheostomy set.

Acetylcysteine, mucolytic agent is used to liquefy secretions or crusts so as to prevent blockage. Constant observation of the patient for block, bleeding, and periodic deflation of the cuff of the tube for short period to prevent pressure necrosis of tracheal mucosa, prevention of infection are the other care required.

Decannulation of tracheostomy should be done with care especially in children as sudden respiratory distress can occur and in such occasion emergency re-insertion of the tube should be done. Cuff deflation and decannulation is done when patient is able to maintain airway and regains adequate swallowing reflex.

Initially it can be changed to metal tracheostomy tube. Once patient breathes well properly, regains normal cough reflex tracheostomy tube is entirely removed and wound is sealed with dressing. Opening closes spontaneously in few days on its own. Tracheostomy set is kept ready at bedside for emergency insertion in case if patient finds difficult to breathe again. Post-decannulation respiratory distress may be due to sustenance of existing pathology; tracheal obstruction due to granulation tissue, oedema, subglottic stenosis, tracheomalacia, tracheostomy dependency.

Flexible bronchoscopy may be needed to clear the lower airway through the tracheostomy tube **(Figs. 7-34 to 7-37)**.

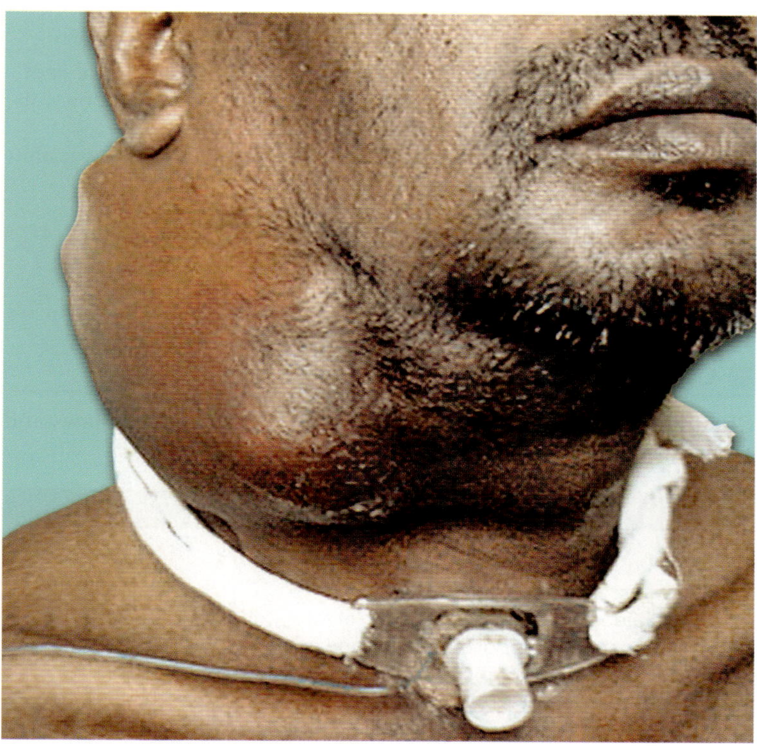

Fig. 7-34: Advanced secondaries in neck with tracheostomy tube to control respiratory stridor.

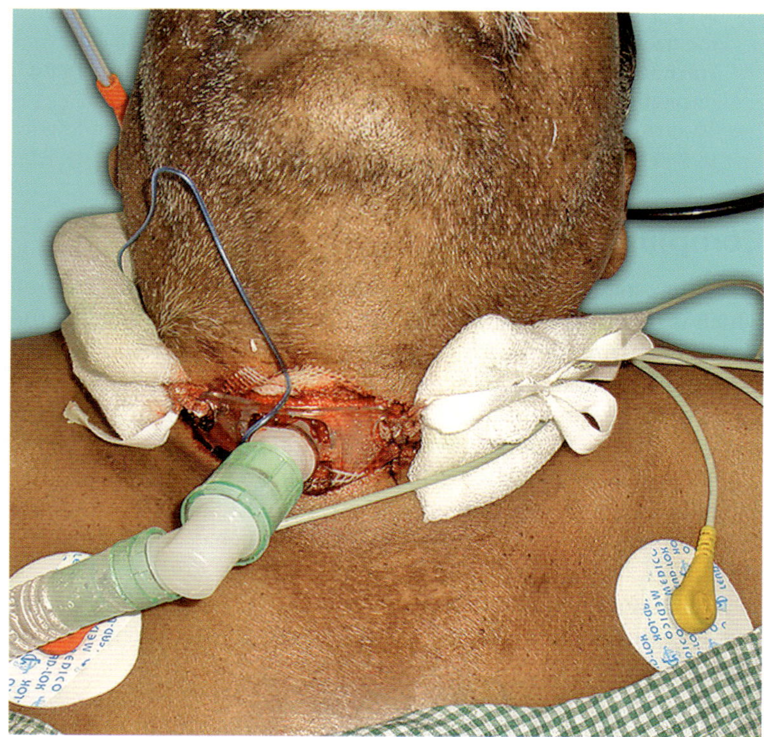

Fig. 7-36: Tracheostomy in position connected to ventilator.

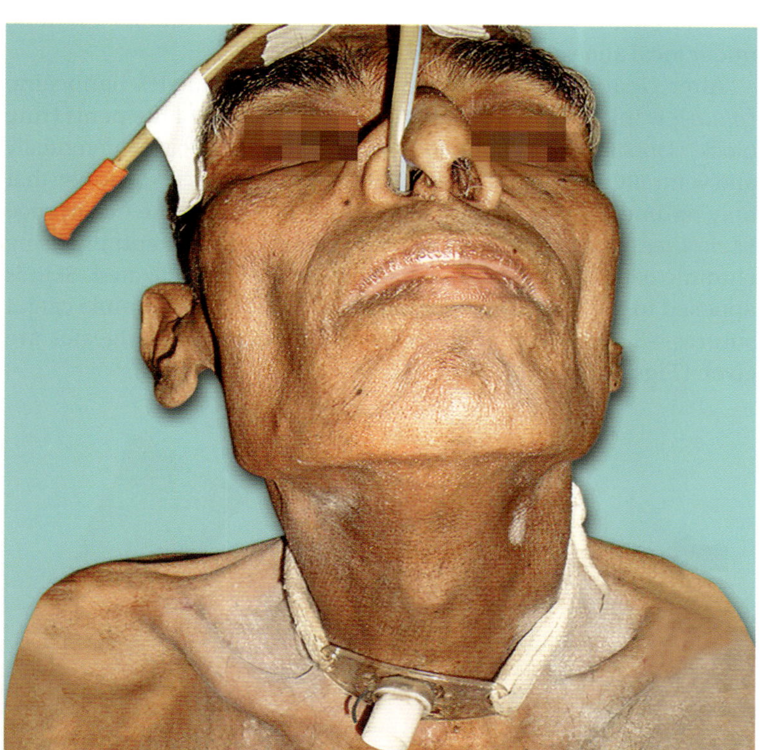

Fig. 7-35: Permanent tracheostomy is done in a patient who underwent total laryngopharyngectomy for carcinoma larynx. Patient is on nasogastric tube for feeding purpose.

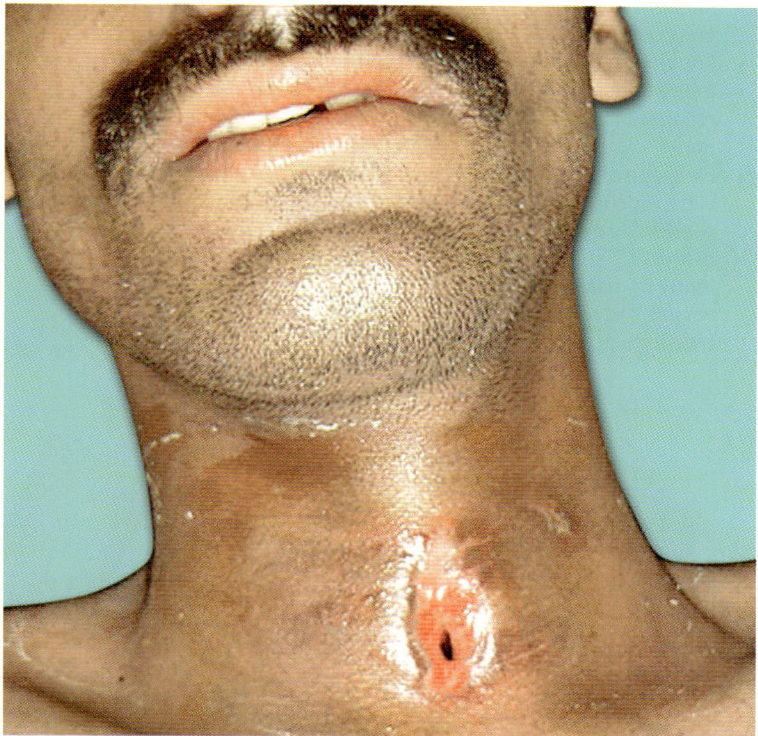

Fig. 7-37: Tracheostomy track without tube in situ.

Functions of the tracheostomy

- Alternate pathway for respiration bypassing the upper airway.
- It decreases the dead space by 50% and reduces the resistance to airflow so as to improve the ventilation.
- It prevents aspiration in bulbar palsy, coma, and haemorrhage from larynx/pharynx.
- In injuries of head, chest, abdomen, in respiratory paralysis lower airway is kept clean and patent by doing suction of the secretions through the tracheostomy tube.
- Tracheostomy is better and ideal for intermittent positive pressure respiration (IPPR).
- To give general anaesthesia when endotracheal intubation is not possible.

Complications of Tracheostomy

Bleeding, aspiration of blood and secretions, sudden apnoea which is due to sudden washing out of CO_2 (sudden removal of the respiratory stimulant). 5% CO_2 in oxygen is administered in such situation, pneumothorax, surgical emphysema in the neck, mediastinal emphysema, injury to adjacent structures like oesophagus, recurrent laryngeal nerve, thyroid gland, tracheal stenosis, laryngeal stenosis due to perichondritis of cricoid cartilage, tracheitis/tracheobronchitis, displacement/blockage of the tube or erosion of the tube into major vessels, tracheo-oesophageal, tracheoarterial fistula.

In children thymus and innominate vein may be in the lower neck crossing the trachea which may be injured during tracheostomy **(Table 7-1)**.

TABLE 7-1: Complications of tracheostomy.

Early	*Late*	*Delayed*
• Bleeding • Pneumothorax • Subcutaneous emphysema • Pneumomediastinum • Injury to oesophagus, recurrent laryngeal nerve • Blockage of tube by clots, mucus, sputum causing respiratory distress • Injury to major vessels and torrential bleeding	• Sepsis • Accidental decannulation • Damage to the tube/ balloon and so aspiration or improper functioning • Late haemorrhage	• Tracheal erosion • Tracheomalacia • Tracheo-oesophageal fistula • Tracheal stricture • Formation of unhealthy granulation tissue in the track • Recurrent infection

Nursing care

- Consent should be taken
- Materials like tracheostomy tubes (8.5 size), sterile gown, drapes, gloves, cap, mask, tracheostomy sterile set, gauze, local anaesthetic agent, suction apparatus and tubes, connecting tubes to ventilator, sterile syringes should be kept ready.
- During procedure the patient is monitored for vital signs.
- Proper nursing care of the tracheostomy tube is done like, humidifying, cleaning, suction, care of the wound, checking of cuff pressure.
- Tracheal dilator and additional tracheostomy tube should be kept ready at bedside in case of blockage of existing tube/balloon not getting inflated to replace with a new one.
- Absolute asepsis like scrubbing hands, using sterile equipment are essential.
- Sterile suction tubes should be used.
- Care of inner tube is essential in case of metal tracheostomy tube.
- Regular dressing of the wound is needed. Antibiotics are required to prevent pulmonary sepsis.

CIRCUMCISION

Circumcision is the surgical removal of penile foreskin. In Jews and Muslims it is done as religious ceremony.

Indications

- Religious.
- Phimosis.
- Paraphimosis after doing initial dorsal slit.
- Balanitis and balanoposthitis (common in diabetics).
- Early carcinoma of prepuce or glans penis—both diagnostic as well as therapeutic purpose.
- Certain sexually transmitted diseases, e.g. herpes infection.

Procedure

In children it is done under general anaesthesia. In adults it is done under local anaesthesia.

After cleaning and draping, local anaesthesia [1% lignocaine *(plain)*] is injected circumferentially near the root of the penis (ring block). Dorsal skin is cut up to the corona and later circumferentially and ventrally. The skin is cut with inner layer. Care is taken to see that only optimum (less) skin is cut ventrally to prevent the occurrence *of chordee*. Frenular artery is transfixed and ligated ventrally using chromic catgut (2-0 or 3-0). Small bleeders are also ligated. Skin is apposed to the cut edge of corona using interrupted chromic catgut sutures—3 zero. Post-operatively, antibiotics and analgesics are given **(Figs. 7-38 and 7-39)**.

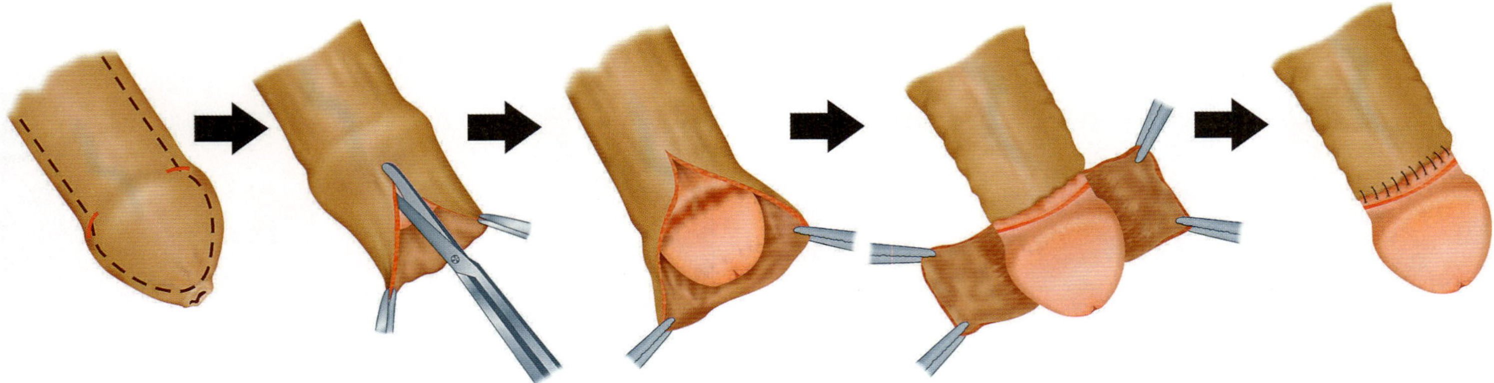

Fig. 7-38: Circumcision technique.

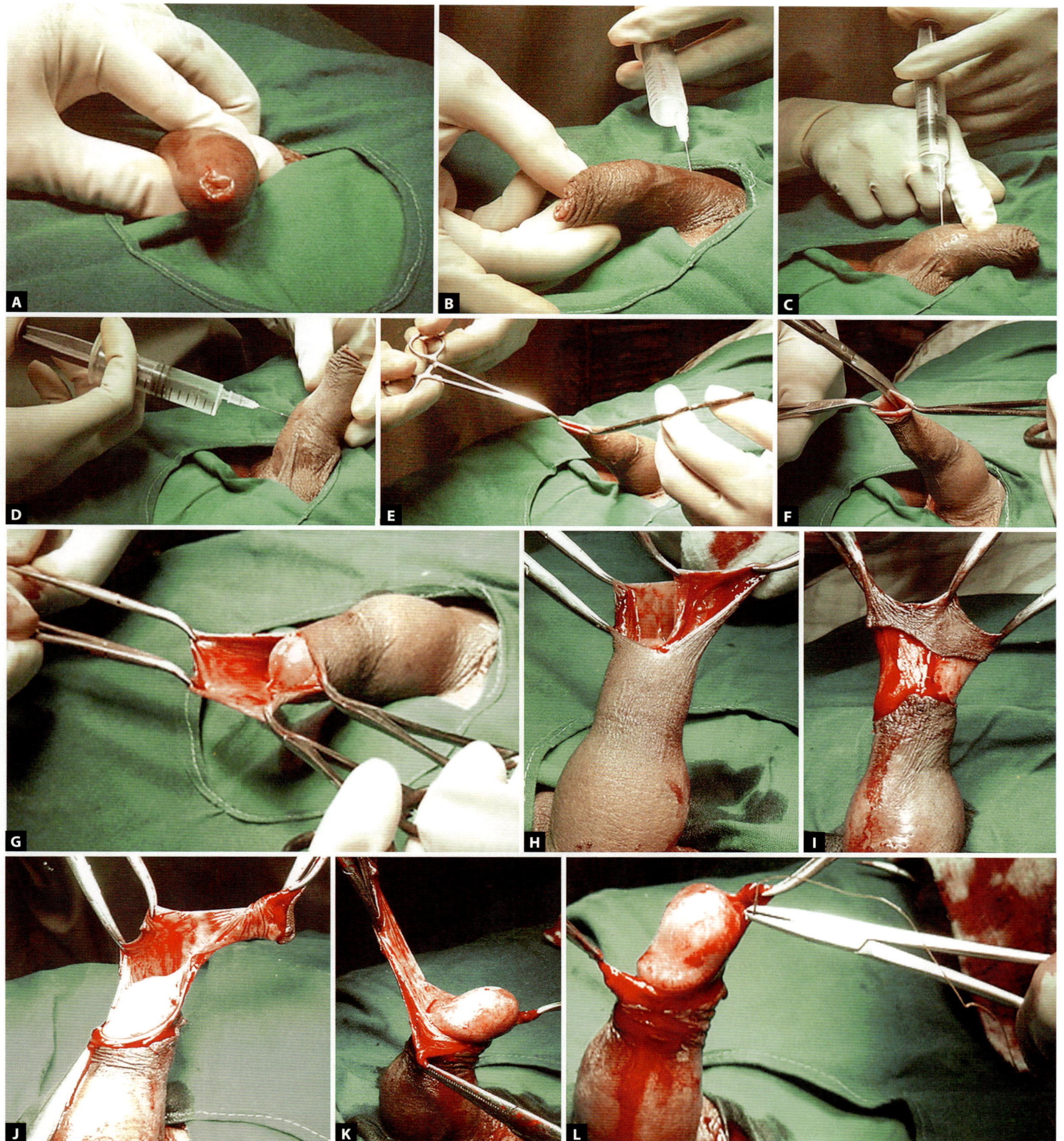

Figs. 7-39A to L

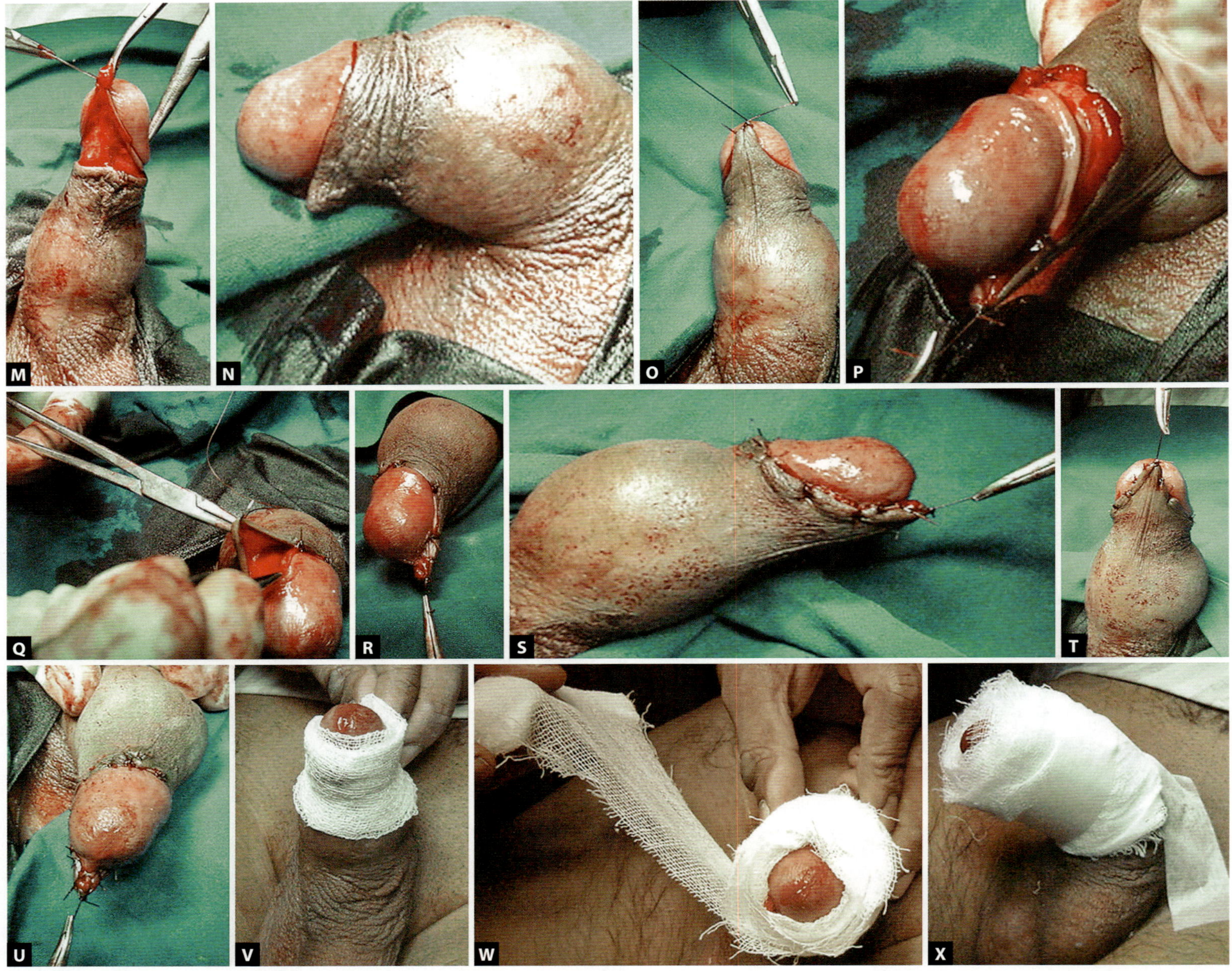

Figs. 7-39M to X

Figs. 7-39A to X: Operative steps of circumcision.

Note:

The word circumcision is from Latin *circumcidere*, meaning "to cut around".

Advantages of circumcision: It reduces the risks of penile cancer, urinary infection, sexually transmitted diseases and maintains the better hygiene.

- One should not use xylocaine with adrenaline as local anaesthetic for circumcision.
- One should avoid using monopolar cautery; judicial bipolar cautery usage is admitted. Monopolar cautery may precipitate gangrene of the glans.
- One should cut less skin on the ventral aspect to prevent formation of chordee.
- Always should use absorbable sutures (3-0 or 4-0 chromic catgut or rapid Vicryl).
- Interrupted sutures are better than continuous sutures.

Plastic Cap—Hollister Bell Cap Technique

This cap is fitted over the glans penis and prepuce is rolled over it. A tight ligature is tied over it near base of the prepuce. In 7 days, skin and prepuce sloughs off sheds with the cap. Bleeding will not occur due to thrombosis of prepuceal vessels. Technique can be used for religious circumcision/balanoposthitis without phimosis. It is contraindicated in phimosis and paraphimosis.

Complications

(1) Reactionary haemorrhage due to slipping of ligature from frenular artery or dorsal vein—Here patient presents with pain, swelling, dressing soaked with blood. Vitals are normal. Wound reopened under local anaesthesia; bleeder is identified after removal of the clot; it is securely ligated and wound closed again. (2) Infection. (3) Stricture urethra near the external meatus in children. (4) Chordee due to removal of excess skin on the ventral aspect. (5) Rarely priapism can occur.

DORSAL SLIT OF PREPUCE

Indications

Paraphimosis; to do biopsy from a growth underneath the prepuce either in the glans or in prepuce itself.

After cleaning and draping, xylocaine plain (1%) is injected into the root of the penis circumferentially. Using two mosquito forceps oedematous prepuceal skin is held. Dorsally skin in midline is cut. Fibrous ring/constriction ring proximally is identified and is cut. Once released properly skin will move freely. 'V' shaped cut edge is sutured with continuous plain/chromic catgut. Dressing is placed over the wound. Patient needs formal circumcision at a later period (after 3 weeks) once oedema subsides **(Figs. 7-40 and 7-41)**.

EXCISION OF THE SWELLING

Swellings like sebaceous cyst, lipoma, pyogenic granuloma, papilloma are excised usually under local anaesthesia. Dermoid cyst which is extending into the deeper plane should be excised under general anaesthesia.

After cleaning and draping, xylocaine 1% injection is infiltrated around the swelling and underneath the swelling by lifting the swelling.

Incision

The following incisions are indicated in different situations **(Figs. 7-42 to 7-45):**

- In sebaceous cyst *elliptical incision* is placed encroaching the punctum.
- In swellings like lipoma/ganglion *linear incision* is placed.
- In swelling like papilloma/pyogenic granuloma *circumferential elliptical incision* covering the entire lesion is placed.
- *Circular or oval incision* is used whenever wide excision is needed or skin grafting is planned over it like excision of basal cell carcinoma lesion, etc. Such excision once done it is often difficult to close the defect primarily but needs skin grafting or flap locally.

Procedure

Skin flaps on either side are raised adequately until edge of the swelling is clearly seen. Using scissor sharp dissection is done to

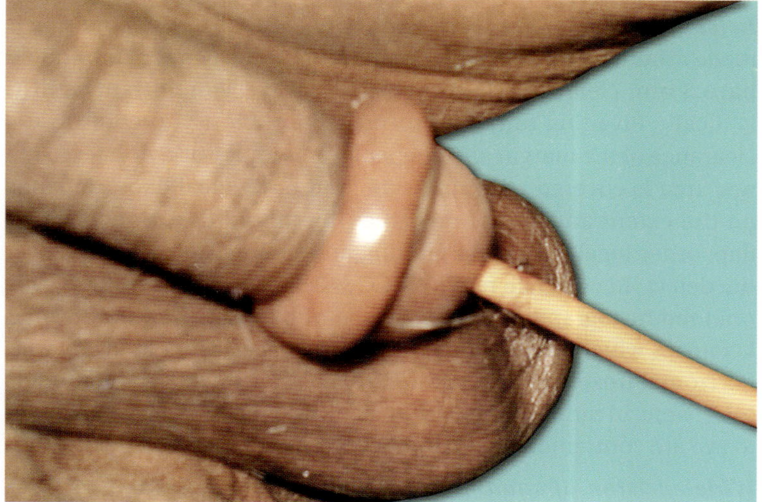

Fig. 7-40: Paraphimosis developed after urethral catheterisation. It needs manual reduction using lignocaine jelly or dorsal slit to release it by cutting the constriction band on the dorsum of the penis.

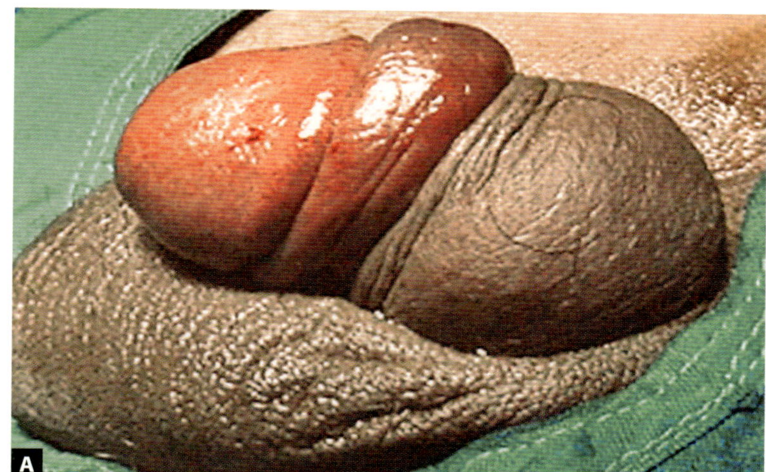

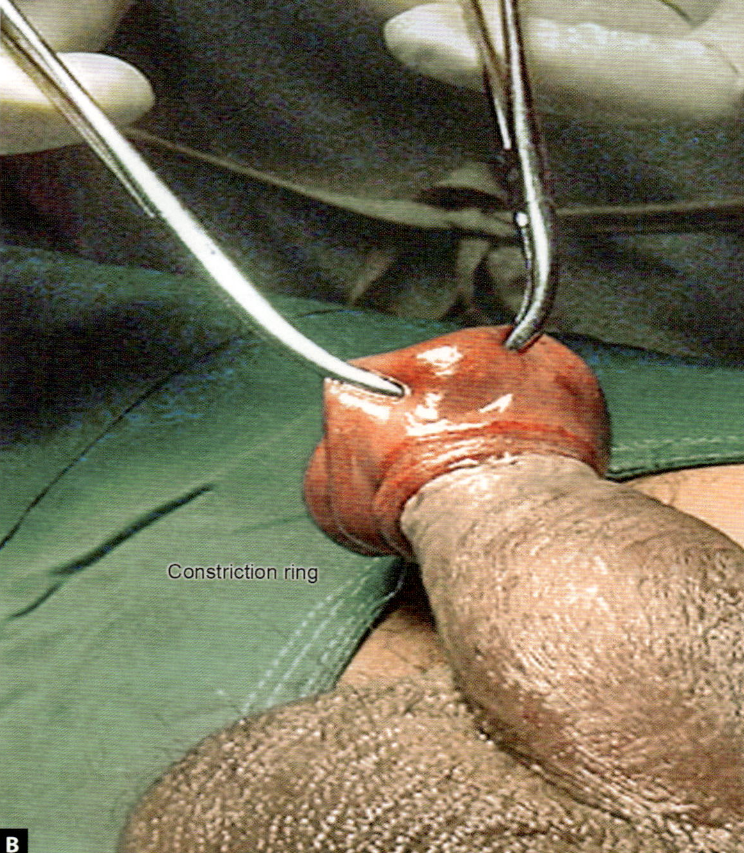

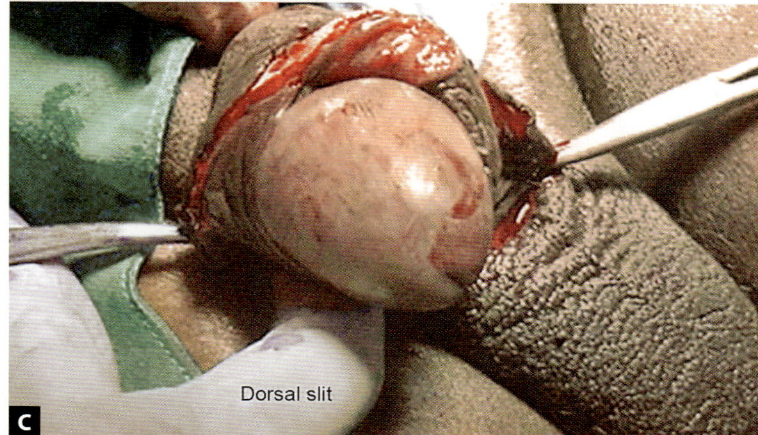

Figs. 7-41A to C: Paraphimosis showing constriction ring and dorsal slit over the ring.

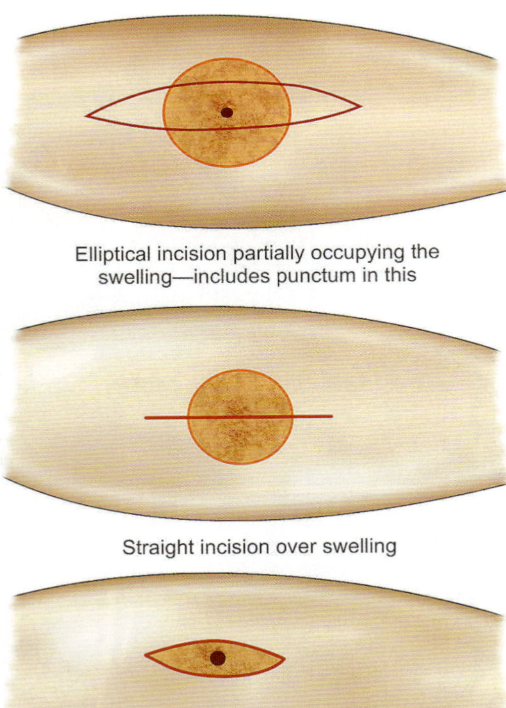

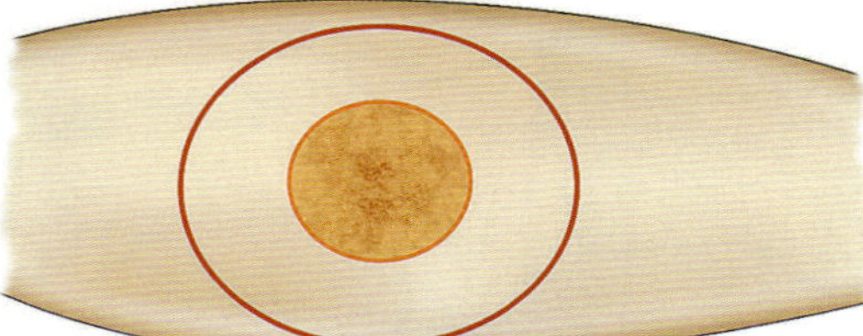

Fig. 7-42: Different incisions used as surgical approaches to remove swelling.

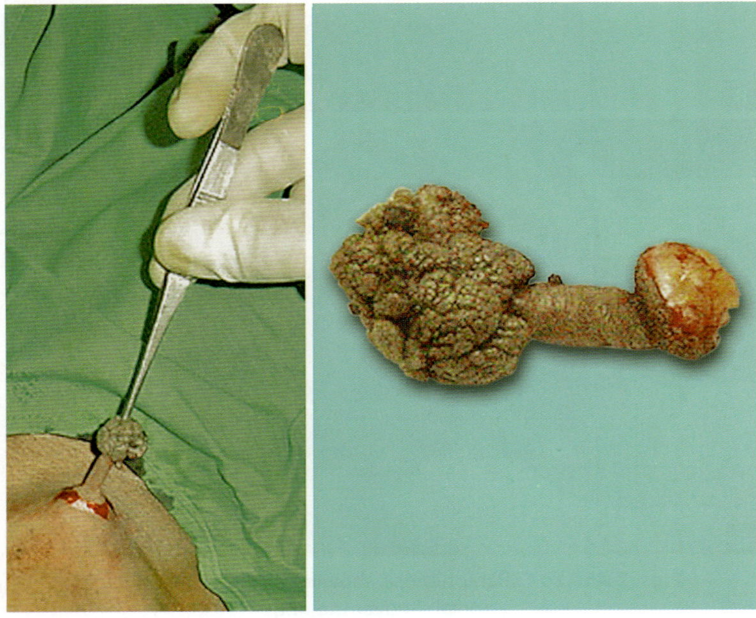

Fig. 7-43: Excision of papilloma with circumferential incision.

remove the entire swelling. Bleeding points are cauterised/ligated. Skin is closed using non-absorbable monofilament polypropylene/ polyethylene 3-zero sutures.

In a ***sebaceous cyst***, capsule should be removed completely otherwise recurrence can occur. Often avulsion of the capsule also is done to complete the procedure. Punctum should be in the centre of the elliptical incision; length of the ellipse should be equal to the diameter of the cyst. Width of the incision varies, depends on the achievement of proper skin apposition during closure. Stretched skin over the cyst (scalp, face) allows wider ellipse; whereas in unstretched skin like in back, narrow ellipse is made. It is easier to begin the dissection at the ends of the elliptical incision than on the summit. Natural plane should be reached by sharp dissection and later blunt dissection can be used over the surface of the capsule. Sharp dissection is done using cautery or scissor or no 15 blade. Artery forceps or mosquito forceps (Halsted) are used to create the plane. Skin hook, fine retractors are needed. If cyst punctures, cyst wall is held up for traction to visualise the plane for dissection. Often cyst is deliberately punctured on the summit and traction is given to the cyst wall to proceed with dissection. If there is more inflammation, wound is left open to granulate and heal. In infected sebaceous cyst, excision is not done. Only incision and drainage is done as it is difficult to identify the cyst capsule and results in poor scarring if any attempt is made. Often it is observed that cyst wall lining gets destroyed completely causing no recurrence; so only drainage in severely infected cyst **(Figs. 7-46 and 7-47)**.

In lipoma linear incision is deepened until capsule of the lipoma is reached. Colour of lipoma is different from surrounding fat and lobules are larger. Squeezing out or winkling of lipoma through the incision can be done using finger which minimises the length of the incision. Retraction, counter traction, sharp and blunt dissection is needed for excision. Large lipoma also can be easily excised under local anaesthesia. Diffuse lipoma needs general or regional anaesthesia for excision. Lipoma in certain locations like back is often adherent to muscles or has extension into muscle plane. In such occasion, muscle should be spilt and small vessels should be ligated or cauterised for proper complete excision (general anaesthesia is needed). In a large swelling like of large lipoma drainage tube must be kept for 48 hours. Dressing is placed. Antibiotics and analgesics are given. Suture removed in 5–8 days. Liposuction for removal of lipoma is not ideal.

In wide excision of basal cell carcinoma (BCC), circular incision is made around the lesion with 5 mm clearance. Deeper plane should have 3 mm clearance. Depth clearance is very important as BCC is locally invading tumour. Frozen section biopsy to confirm the clearance of the margin and deeper layer is important. After excision raw area is covered with split skin graft or by local flaps, depends on the extent and site of raw area. Rhomboid flap, transposition flap, other local flaps, skin grafting are the methods used to cover the defect. Recurrence rate for BCC is 2%. *MOHS*—Microscopically oriented histographic surgery is used often in BCC, SCC and solar keratoses which is described by MOHS. It is excision in layers with horizontal frozen section control. BCC is sensitive for radiotherapy but lesions in pinna, lacrimal canaliculi and those in close proximity to eye are contraindicated for radiotherapy **(Figs. 7-48A to I)**.

Wide excision of squamous cell carcinoma is similar to BCC. Clearance margin kept is 1 cm. Frozen section biopsy for confirmation of clearance from margin and depth is essential. Defect is closed by transposition/rotation flap/skin grafting depending on

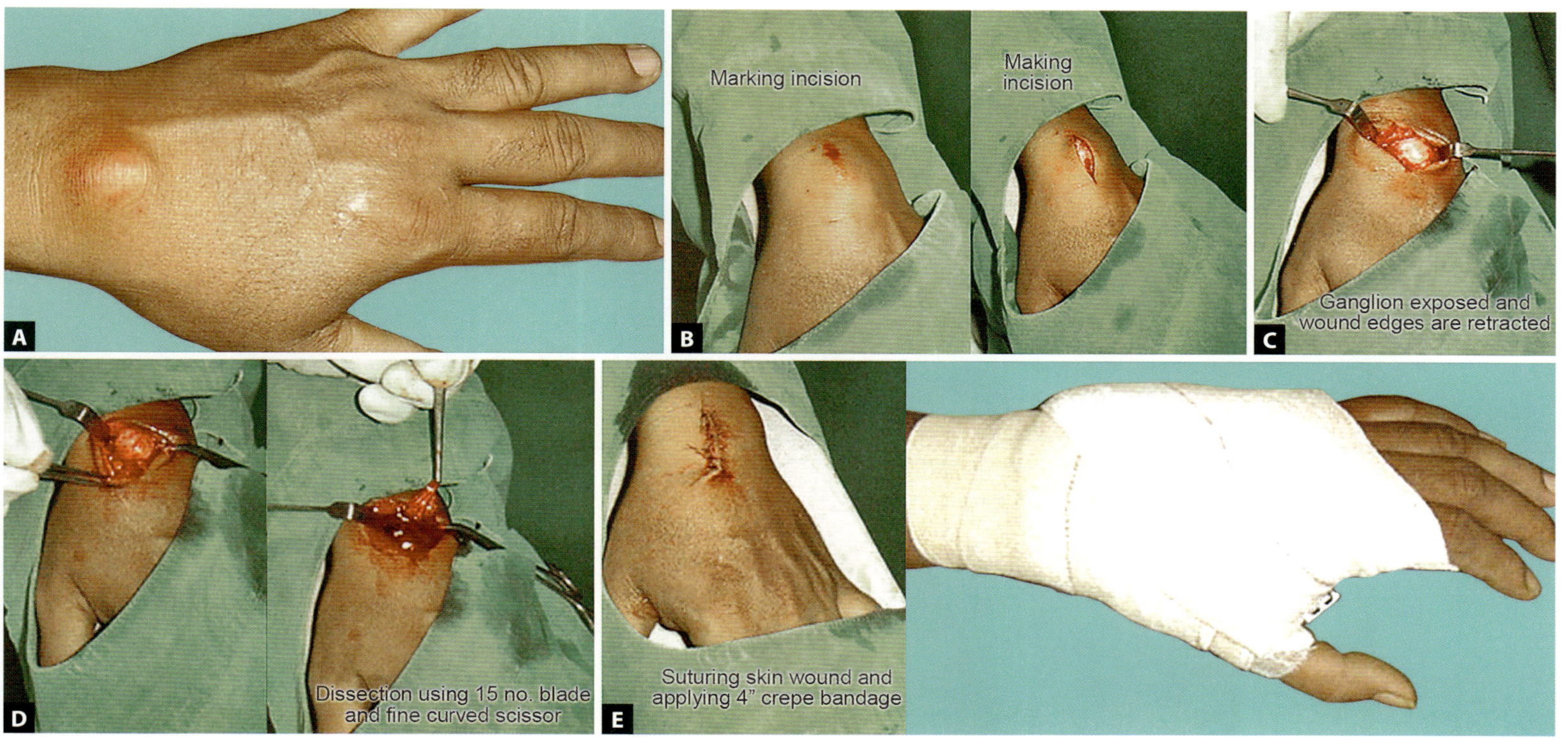

Figs. 7-44A to E: Steps in excision of ganglion.

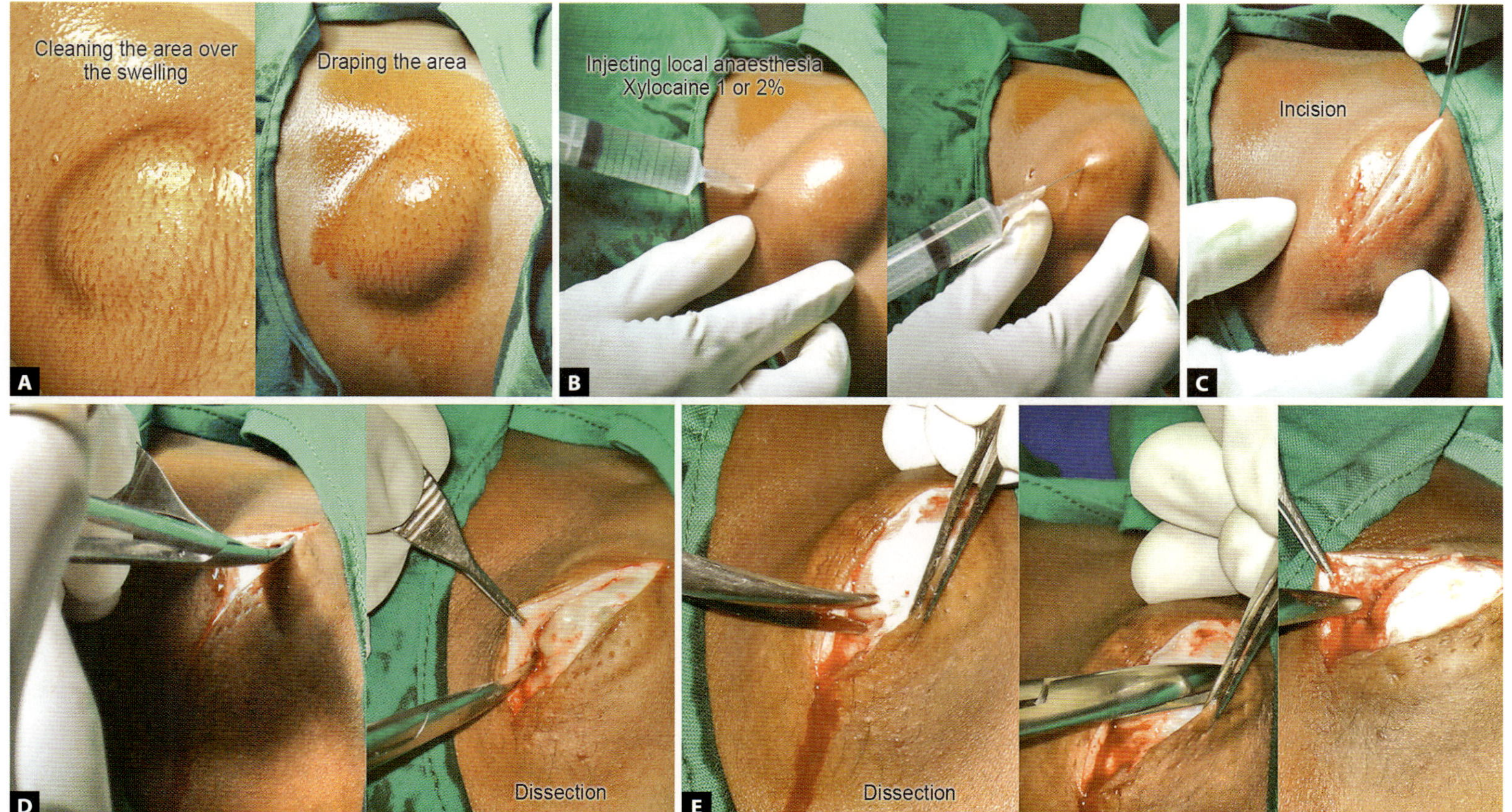

Figs. 7-45A to E

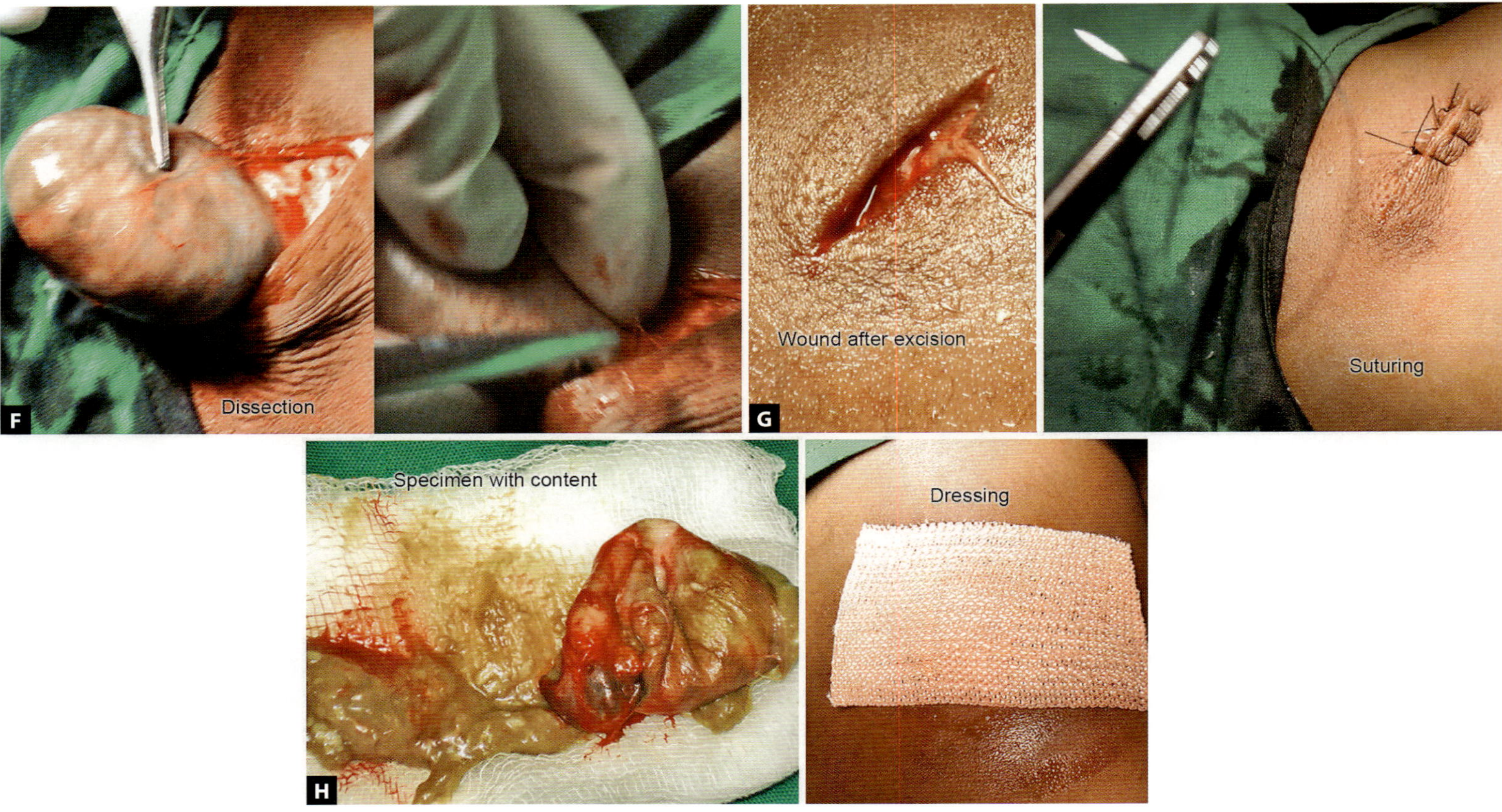

Figs. 7-45F to H

Figs. 7-45A to H: Excision of cyst—steps. Often it is necessary to place elliptical incision around the punctum in case of excision of sebaceous cyst with punctum.

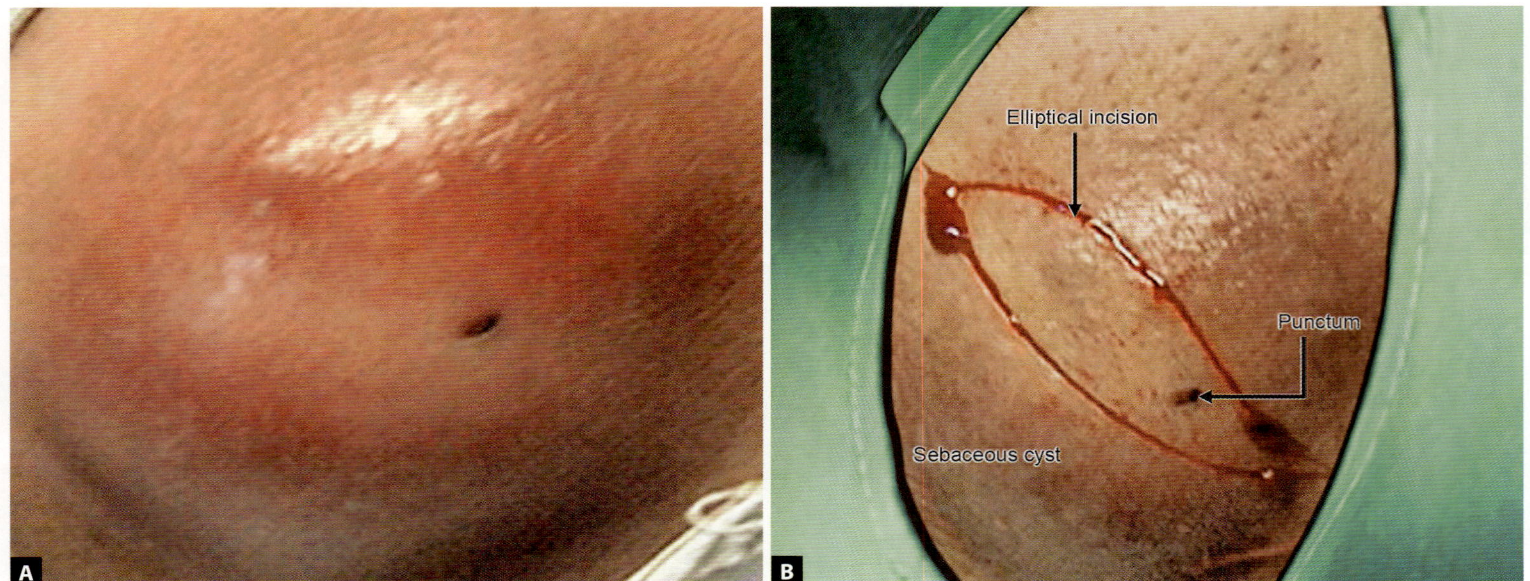

Figs. 7-46A and B: Sebaceous cyst with elliptical incision encroaching the punctum.

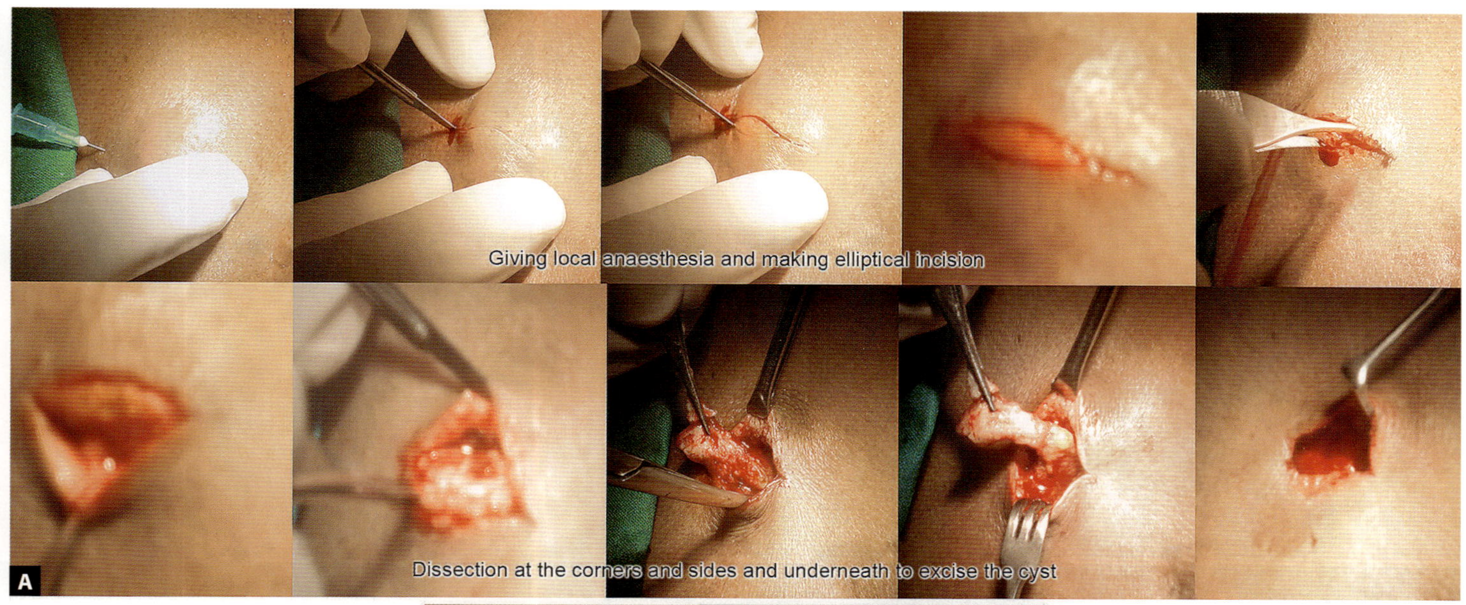

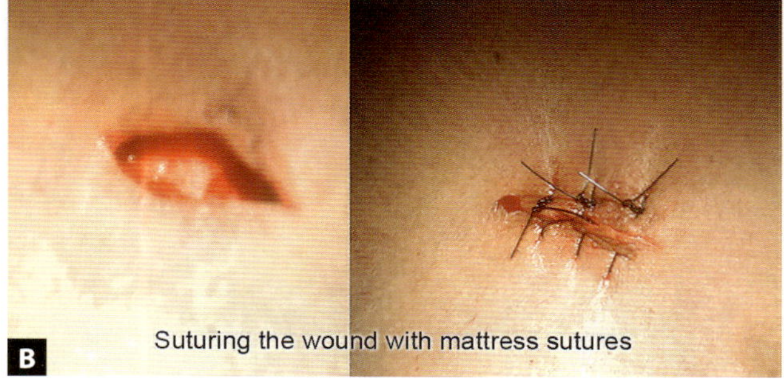

Figs. 7-47A and B: Steps in sebaceous cyst excision.

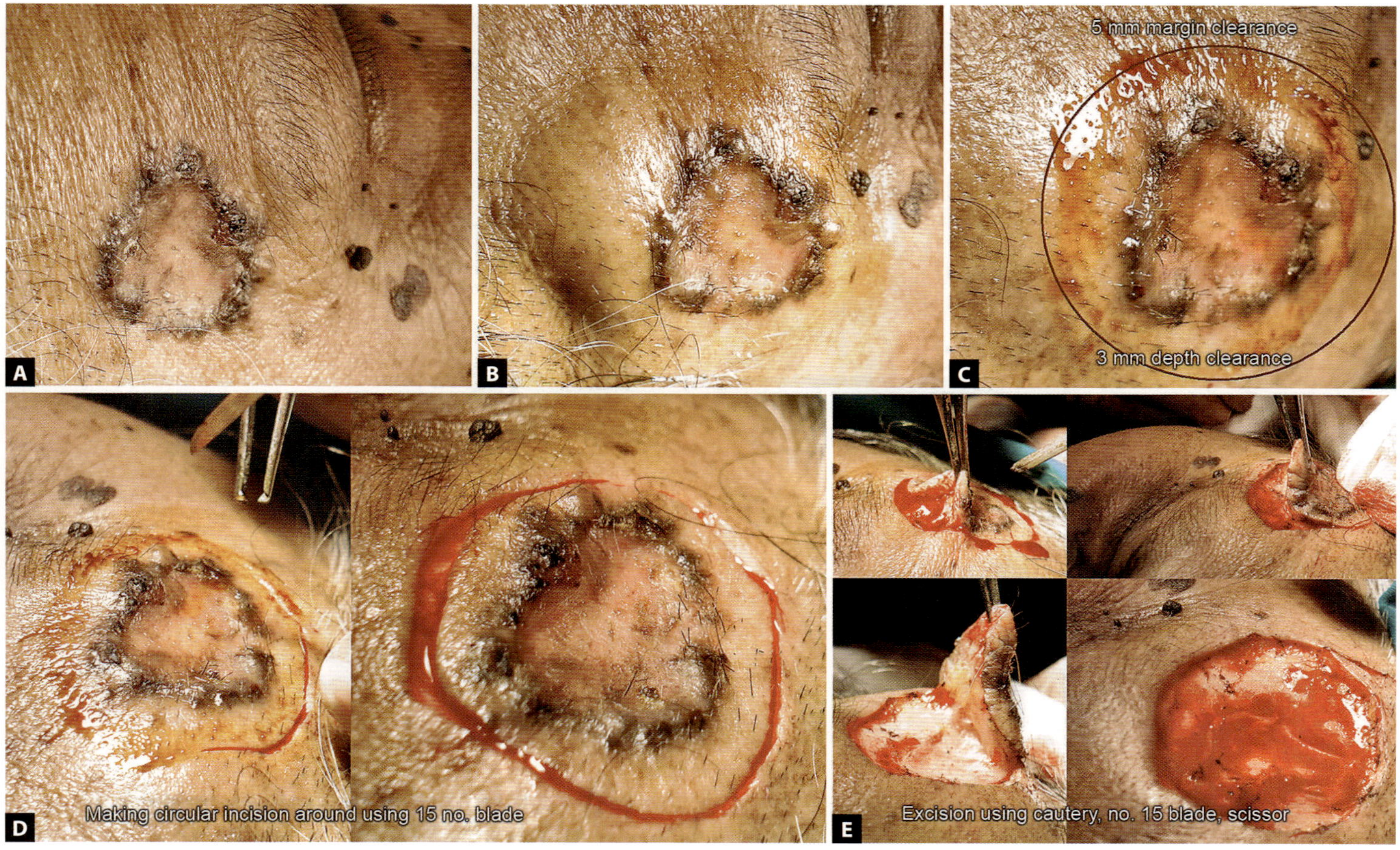

Figs. 7-48A to E

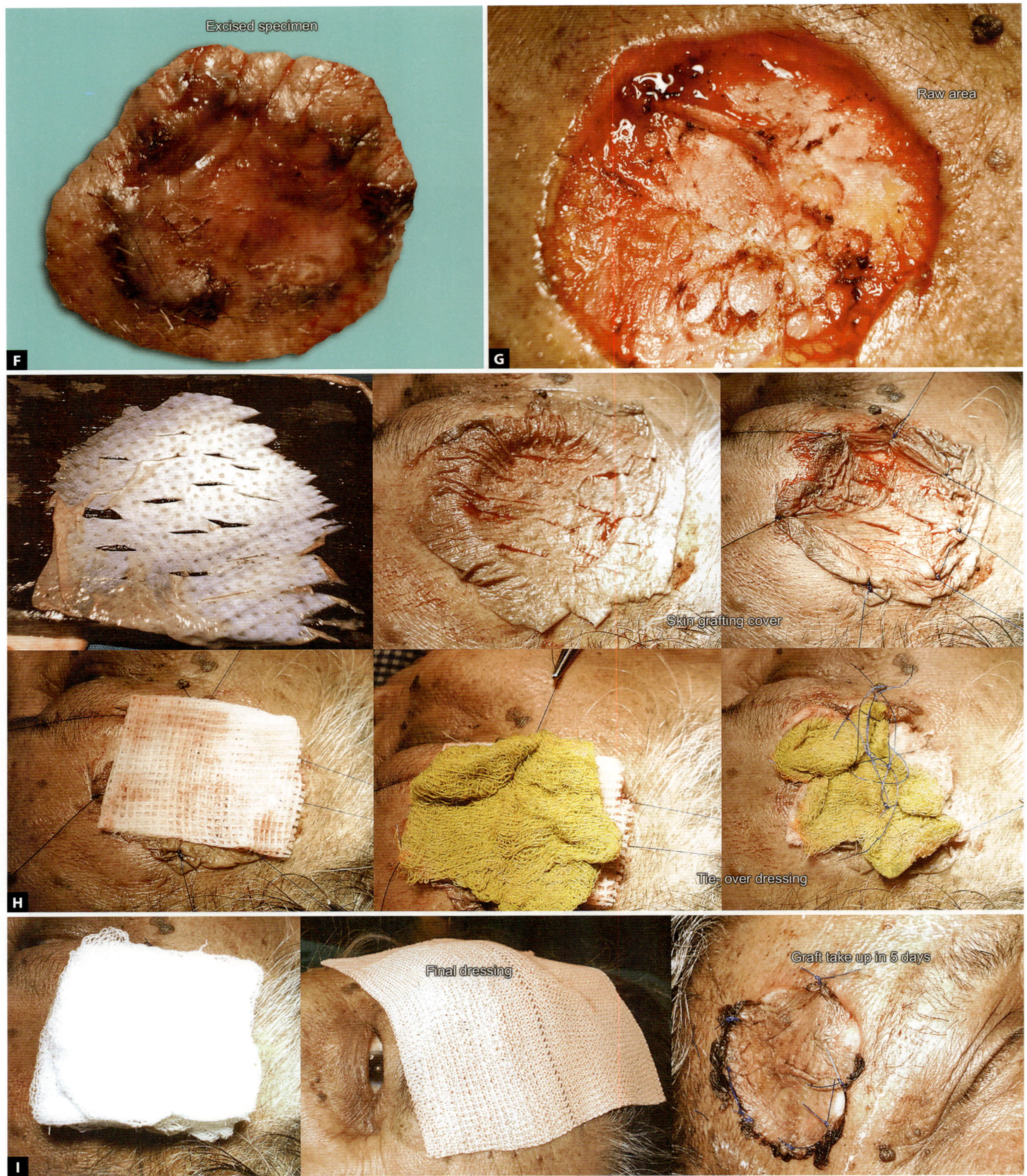

Figs. 7-48F to I

Figs. 7-48A to I: Wide excision of BCC and split skin grafting over it with tie over dressing. Graft has taken up well when seen after 5 days.

location of the carcinoma. Disarticulation of the toe/ray amputation/ forefoot amputation/below knee amputations are done for recurrent or wider or deeper or aggressive disease. Regional lymph node block dissection is done (ilioinguinal/axillary/neck) if nodes are positive by FNAC. It is usually/ideally done in same sitting now; but may be postponed for 3 weeks. Radiotherapy/cryosurgery/laser are other methods used for primary disease. Chemotherapy using 5 fluorouracil/adriamycin/vincristine/cisplatin are also added **(Figs. 7-49A to D)**.

MOHS surgery, also known as **chemosurgery**, originated by a general surgeon, ***Dr Frederic E Mohs***, is microscopically controlled surgery (*Microscopically oriented histographic surgery*) used to treat common types of skin cancer. Complete *circumferential peripheral and deep margin* assessment is the key feature. *Mohs micrographic surgery* is an advanced treatment process for *non-melanotic skin cancer* (basal cell cancer, squamous cell cancer, sebaceous carcinoma, extramammary Paget's disease, dermatofibrosarcoma protuberans, etc.) that offers the highest possible cure rate for many skin cancers and simultaneously minimises the sacrifice of normal tissue. Mohs section should include 100% of the epidermal margin, but greater than 95% is often accepted. Ideally 100% of the epithelial margin should be available to be reviewed on serial sectioning of the Mohs specimen. The team consists of the Mohs surgeon, histotechnician, pathologist and the reconstructive surgeon. The *Mohs surgeon* identifies the cancer and its margin, often with the aid of dermatoscopy. He removes the cancer under local anaesthesia

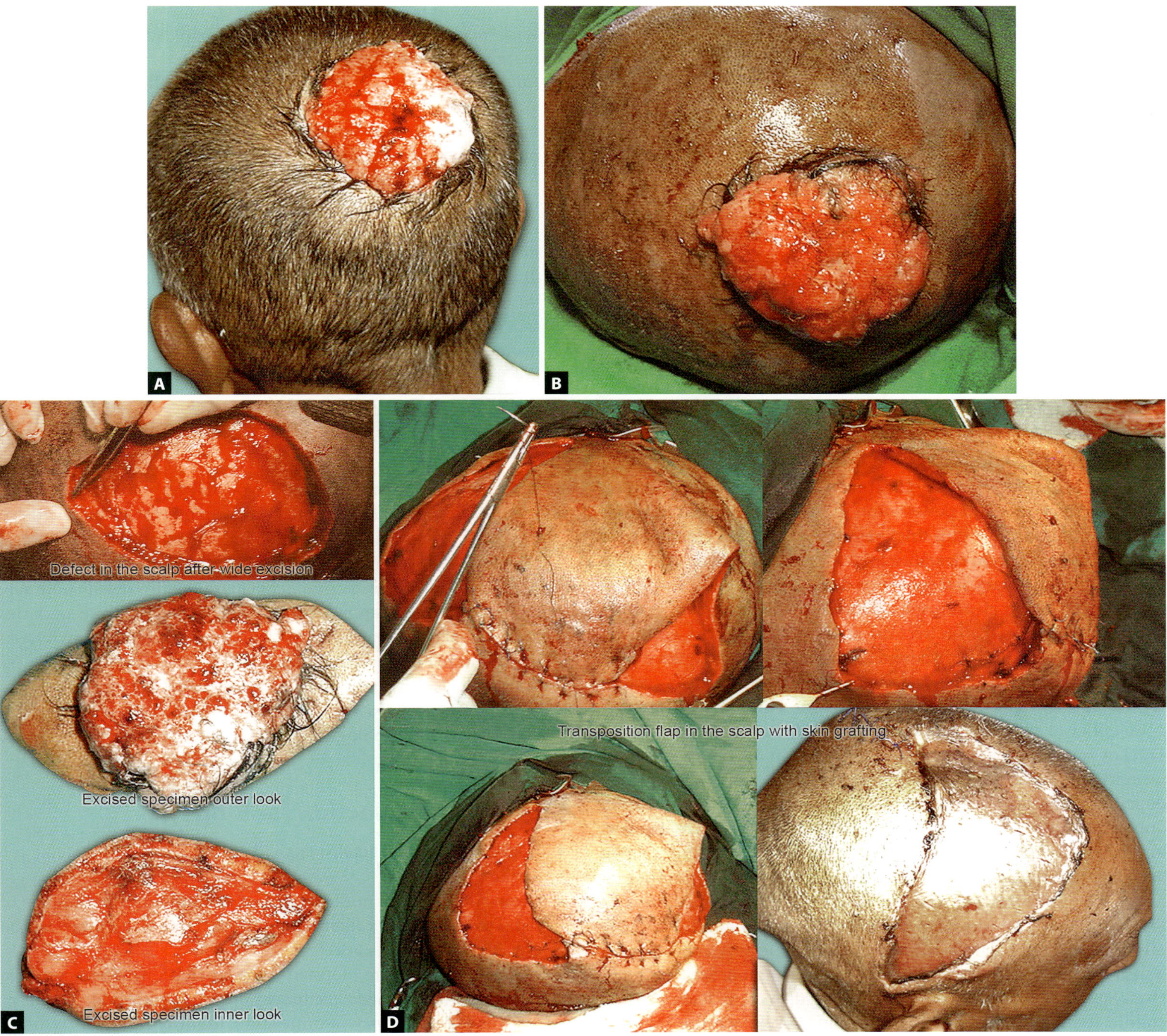

Figs. 7-49A to D: Squamous cell carcinoma scalp. Wide excision is done. Transposition flap is done to cover the defect. Flap donor area is covered with split skin graft.

and prepares it for histology processing. This is accomplished by cutting the specimen (if required), staining the specimen for orientation, and sending it to the laboratory. The *histotechnician* prepares the tissue for Mohs processing by flattening the surgical margin on a flat surface initially. Then the flat surgical surface is mounted on a cryostat to be sectioned and prepared for glass slides to be read by the pathologist. The *pathologist* examines the slide for residual tumours, and marks the location of the tumour on the pathology report and sends it back to the Mohs surgeon. Completion of surgery with margin clearance is informed to Mohs surgeon by the pathologist. Defect is covered by a reconstructive/*plastic surgeon.*

Mohs surgery is performed *in four* levels—(1) Surgical removal of tissue (Surgical Oncology). (2) Mapping the piece of tissue, freezing and cutting the tissue between 5 and 10 micrometers using a cryostat, and staining with hematoxylin and eosin (H&E) or other stains (including T. Blue). (3) Interpretation of microscope slides (Pathology). (4) Reconstruction of the surgical defect (Reconstructive Surgery). The procedure is usually performed under local anaesthesia, can be done as day care surgery. A small scalpel is utilised to cut around the visible tumour. A very small surgical margin is utilised, usually with 1 to 1.5 mm of free margin or uninvolved skin. The amount of free margin removed is much less than the usual 4–6 mm required for the standard excision of skin cancers. After each surgical removal of tissue, the specimen is processed, cut on the cryostat and placed on slides, stained with H and E and then read by the Mohs surgeon/pathologist who examines the sections for cancerous cells. If cancer is found, its location is marked on the map (drawing of the tissue) and the surgeon removes the indicated cancerous tissue from the patient. This procedure is repeated until no further cancer is found. Anti-coagulants are commonly used along with Mohs surgery.

Mohs procedure is very useful for BCC (98–100% cure rate). It is also useful in SCC (90–94% cure rate).

In excision of melanoma—clearance needed is more than BCC/SCC as it is more aggressive. Clearance to be achieved is decided based on thickness and penetration of the lesion. 1 cm clearance is done for less than 1 mm thickness lesion; 1–2 cm clearance for 1–2 mm thickness; 2 cm clearance for 2–4 mm thick lesion. As incision biopsy of the primary lesion is not done, in clinically suspected lesion initial 2 mm clearance excision of suspected lesion is done with immediate *paraffin section* study. Once report confirms the diagnosis with depth/thickness accurately in mm, definitive wide excision and reconstruction is done at a later period. Frozen section is of no use for depth/thickness assessment. Paraffin section study is essential to plan the final clearance and predict the prognosis. Thickness in mm is the most essential factor in melanoma as far as primary is considered. Reconstruction may be by flap or skin grafting depending on the location of the lesion. Donor area should be from opposite limb, as lesions in the limb may cause secondary deposits in the denuded donor raw area if taken from same side limb. Digital amputation/disarticulation are needed for digital melanoma. Amputation of proximal phalanx may be sufficient if lesion is in the subungual site otherwise disarticulation is needed. Presently prophylactic regional node dissection is not done as systemic spread is also the deciding factor in prognosis of melanoma. Sentinel node biopsy is better and ideal to decide for block dissection. Radiolabelled colloid is injected to the lesion around day before the surgery. Pre-operative scintigraphy is done or node is identified using hand-held gamma camera. Radiolabelled colloid slowly reaches the node but stays there long time. It is often done in combination with injection of blue dye intraoperatively which reaches the node rapidly in 10 minutes but disappears from the node early. Positive sentinel node biopsy indicates regional block dissection. Melanoma is not radiosensitive and so it is used only in intracranial and spinal secondaries. Chemotherapy has also got fewer roles but is commonly used post-operatively using melphalan and DTIC. Isolated limb perfusion even though practiced in many centres, its benefits are not proved. Laser, MOHS, cryosurgery is not commonly used in melanoma **(Figs. 7-50 and 7-51)**.

Note:

- *Enucleation* is removal of the swelling within the tissue of origin with normal part of tissue of origin being retained. For example—enucleation of prostate in benign prostatic hyperplasia (BPH).
- *Excision* is removal of tissue/tumour entirely with its capsule.
- *Wide excision* is removal of tumour with surrounding tissue margin adequately for clearance.
- *Compartment excision* is removal of tumour/diseased tissue with all adjacent soft tissues in one compartment except neurovascular bundle. It is done in limbs for soft tissue sarcoma as a curative but limb saving procedure.
- *Radical excision/radical block dissection* is removal of tumour widely with adjacent soft tissues with lymph node dissection.
- *Retraction, traction/counter traction, sharp* and *blunt* dissection is needed for excision. In inflammatory area or adherent area sharp dissection is done using diathermy or scissor or no. 15 blade. When there is proper plane with loose areolar tissue, blunt dissection is done using finger or peanut. Blind dissection should be avoided.

LYMPH NODE BIOPSY

Indications

- Lymphoma to find out the grade, type of lymphoma.
- Secondaries in the lymph node only when FNAC is inconclusive but clinically node is significant. Significant node is one which is based on size (variable in different locations and type of primary but hard node >1 cm is significant) and texture (hard) probably harbouring tumour spread. FNAC is the first choice in secondaries as biopsy of node may block the lymphatics and may allow spread of tumour to next level of nodes.
- Tuberculosis of lymph node, Catscratch disease.
- Rare lymphatic diseases.
- Sarcoidosis, immunological diseases, infectious mononucleosis, SLE.

Site of Node Selection for Biopsy

- Neck nodes—superficial/deep.
- Axillary node.
- Groin node—these nodes can often be non-specific because of repeated recurrent inflammation. Hard, large sized node can be considered as significant.
- Abdominal nodes are biopsied using laparoscopy. Thoracoscopic biopsy or mediastinoscopic biopsy of lymph node is also done.
- Sentinel node biopsy is done after identifying the first node using markers; commonly done in carcinoma of breast/penis/melanoma.

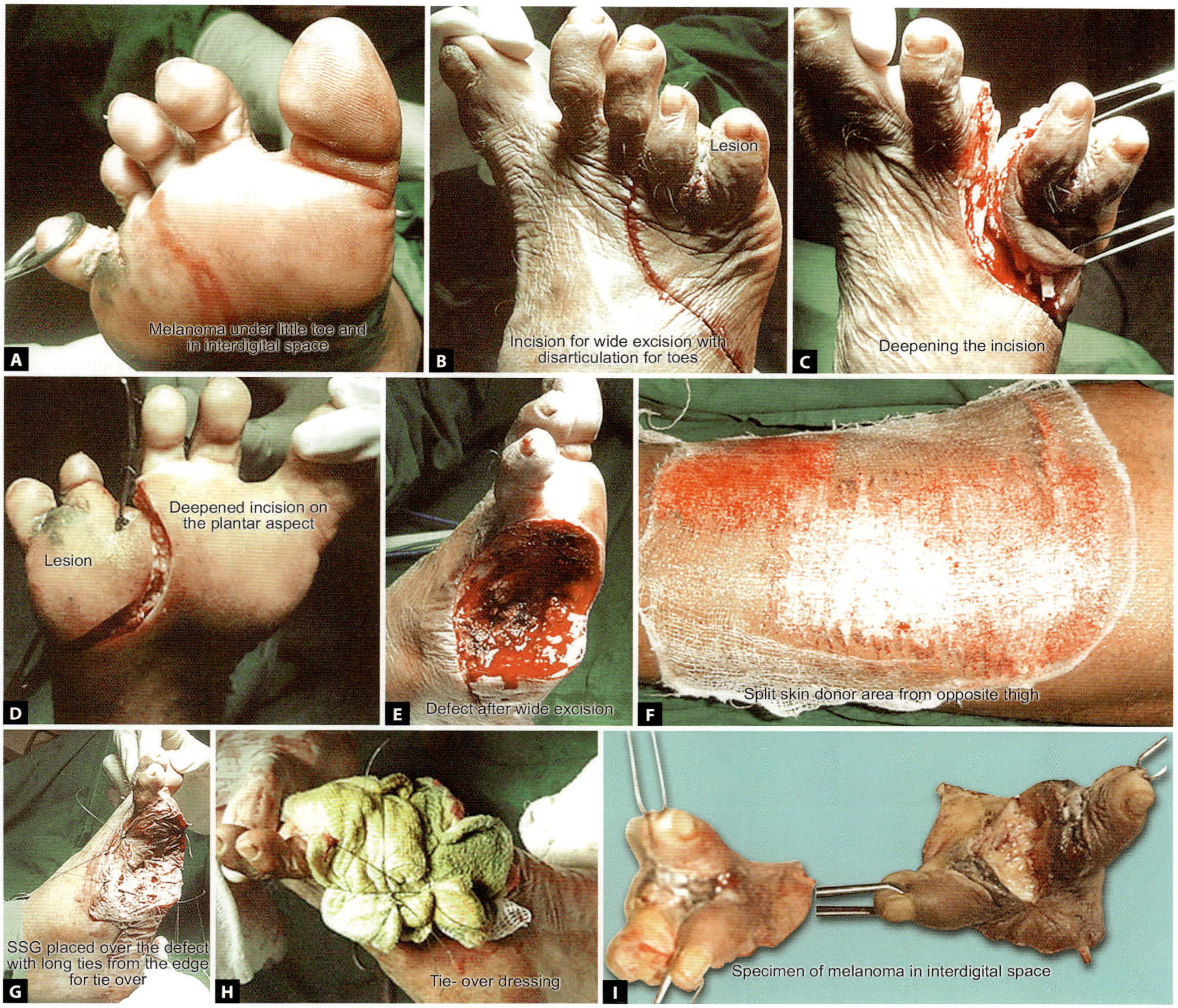

Figs. 7-50A to I: Wide local excision of melanoma with disarticulation of toes. Skin grating is done to cover the defect. Flap is ideal in many places like plantar aspect of the foot but technically difficult.

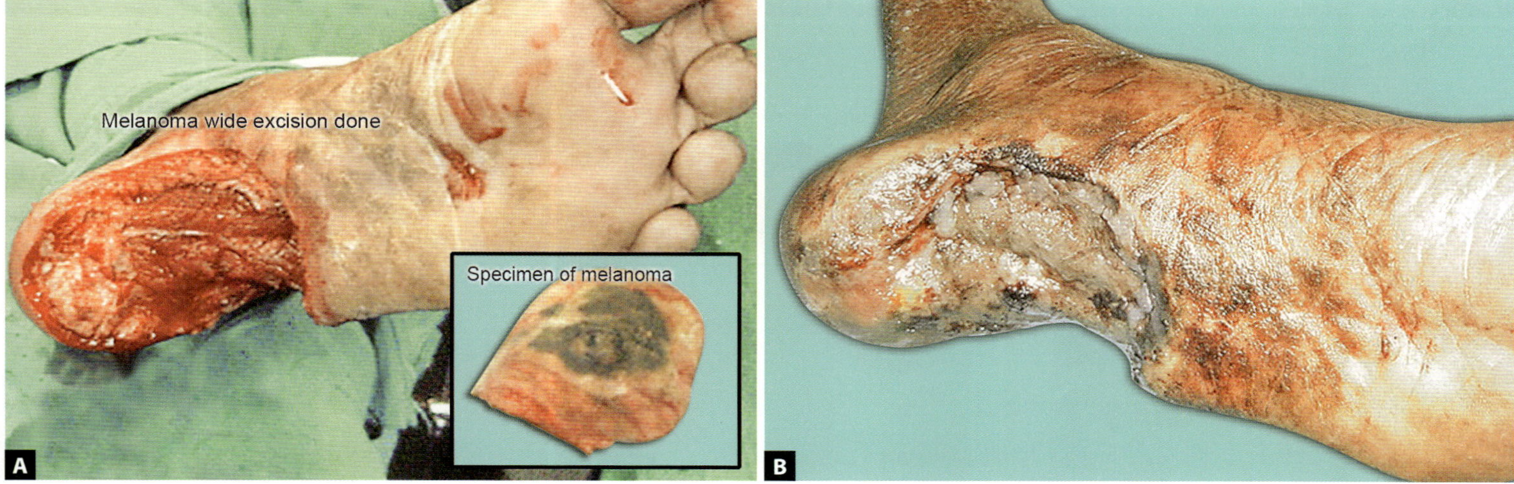

Figs. 7-51A and B: Wide excision of a melanoma in sole with split skin grafting.

Procedure

Lymph node biopsy *ideally* should be done under *general anaesthesia.* Superficial nodes/nodes in upper posterior triangle may be removed under local anaesthesia—xylocaine 1%.

After cleaning and draping, incision is placed. Incision is decided depending on the site of the lymph node. It is usually horizontal in the neck over the lymph node. It is better to mark the incision line using marking ink. Adequate incision is essential otherwise technique will be difficult. After skin incision, fascia is incised. Lymph node is identified based on shape, colour and texture. Node is separated from adjacent structures. Node is held using Lane's tissue holding forceps. One should avoid breaching the capsule as much as possible to retain the lymph node architecture. After removal haemostasis is maintained. Diathermy or ligation using fine absorbable sutures (polyglactic acid) is used. (Earlier surgeon used to cut the node to see the inner texture and to get imprint cytology over a slide; but now pathologists prefer to send the node without cutting). It is fleshy in Hodgkin's lymphoma. It is yellowish caseating in tuberculosis and dark, haemorrhagic in secondaries. Skin is closed with interrupted sutures using monofilament non-absorbable sutures or absorbable subcuticular sutures. Sutures removed in 7 days.

Ideally entire one node with its intact capsule should be removed especially in lymphomas. Often excision it may be difficult because of fibrosis and adherent lymph nodes **(Figs. 7-52A to F)**.

Lymph node can be studied as histology slides, culture, AFB staining, AFB culture or other special staining for fungal infection. Immunohistochemistry has got major role in lymphoma.

Often when result is inconclusive repeat biopsy may be needed.

Complications and Difficulties

Bleeding is due to injury to small or major vessels (jugular veins in neck; femorals in groin; axillary vein or branches in axilla). Adjacent nerves also may get injured (accessory, intercostobrachial, femoral). Sepsis, haematoma formation, lymph ooze, fungation may be other problems.

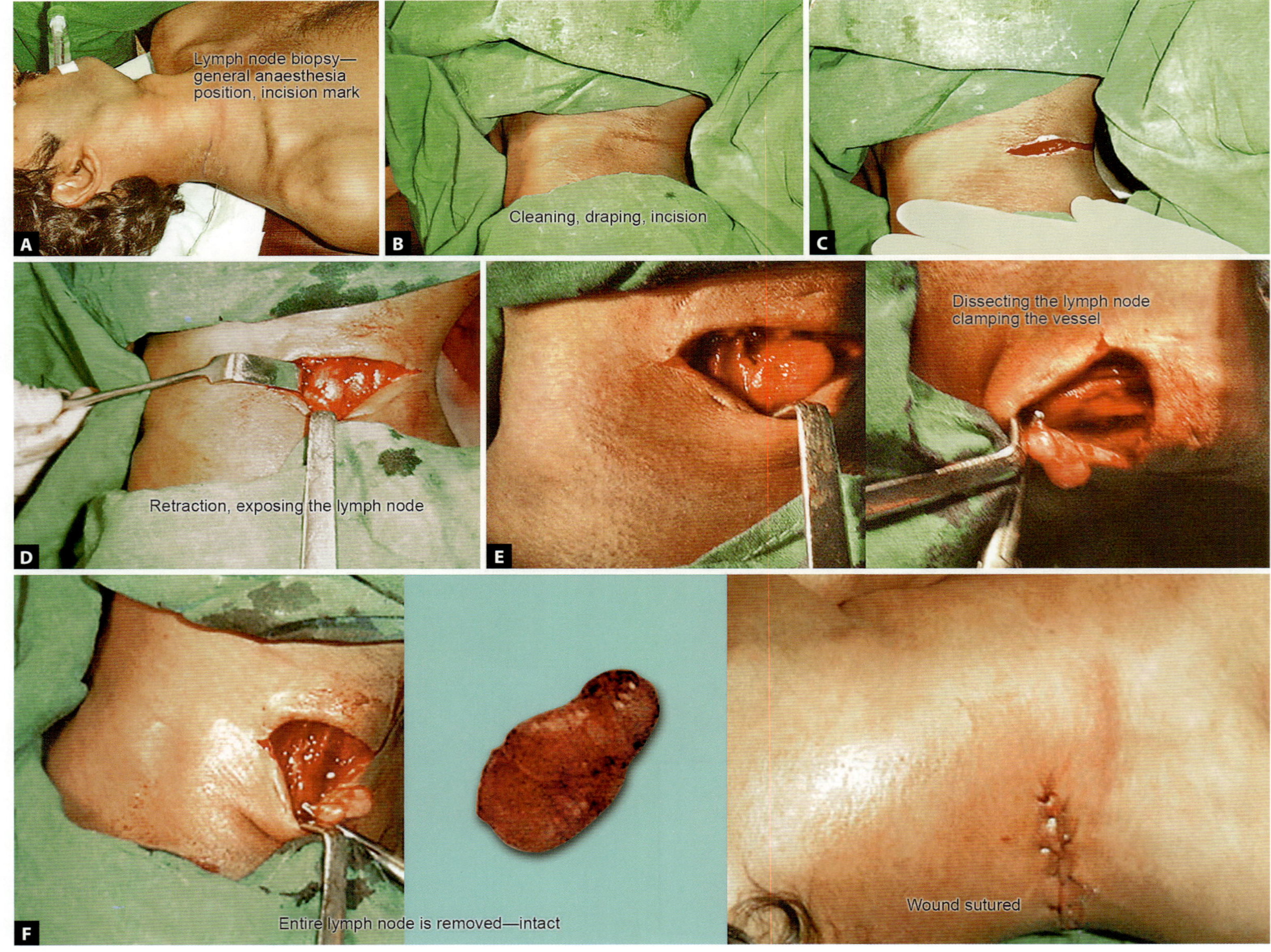

Figs. 7-52A to F: Technique of lymph node biopsy.

LIVER BIOPSY

It is removal of bit of the liver tissue percutaneously for histological purpose.

Paul Ehrlich started liver aspiration in 1883; percutaneous liver biopsy first started in 1920. Presently it is done as percutaneous/transvenous (jugular)/laparoscopic/open abdominal surgery. Percutaneous liver biopsy is done presently always under USG/CT guidance. Tissue is assessed for cytology, immunohistochemistry, copper, tuberculosis, fibrosis, markers, etc. Hepatitis, primary biliary cirrhosis, sclerosing cholangitis, cirrhosis, haemochromatosis, metabolic liver diseases, biliary atresia, to check response for therapy—are different current indications. It is done only selectively in hepatocellular carcinoma in advanced inoperable cases to begin palliative therapy. In liver secondaries biopsy of liver is not advocated usually as a prime confirmative method; only if all evaluation and confirmation methods through primary sites fail, then biopsy of liver is done.

Percutaneous needle liver biopsy is commonly done. Vim Silverman, Menghini, Jamshidi and Klatskin needles are different liver biopsy needles. Transjugular liver biopsy is done in case of ascites or if patient is having uncontrolled bleeding problems or if there is a need to assess pressure gradient.

Prerequisites

Prothrombin time (PT) should be normal before doing liver biopsy, otherwise severe bleeding can occur. Normal value of prothrombin time is 12–16 seconds (it is compared to control and difference should be less than 4 sec between test and control) (or normal PT INR). It is corrected by giving injection vitamin K 10 mg IM for 5 days. Even after that if PT remains still high then fresh blood transfusion (FFP) is done to correct it.

If ascites is present, tapping should be done prior to liver biopsy.

Blood grouping and cross matching should be done.

History of taking anti-coagulants like warfarin, aspirin, clopidogrel should be asked; if patient is taking these drugs they should be stopped for 5 days to avoid possible chances of haemorrhage.

Indications

(1) Cirrhosis, chronic hepatitis, haemochromatosis, Wilson's disease. (2) Hepatoma in inoperable stage to confirm as hepatocellular carcinoma (HCC) to give palliative therapy. In secondaries liver biopsy is usually not done as it may precipitate failure or ascites. (3) Granulomatous liver diseases, metabolic and storage diseases, familial diseases. (4) Unexplained long-term fever wherein all other usual investigations are normal. (5) Chronic hepatitis, biliary atresias.

Ishak fibrosis score progression is assessed by liver biopsy sequentially at regular intervals; normal is <22. The fibrosis score is defined as follows: F0—no fibrosis; F1—portal fibrosis without septa; F2—portal fibrosis with rare septa; F3—numerous septa without cirrhosis; F4—cirrhosis. ***METAVIR scoring system*** is also used in hepatitis C infection mainly to see fibrosis and necroinflammatory activity (A0—no; A1—mild; A2—moderate; A3—severe).

Contraindications

Bleeding diathesis, platelet count below 60,000, widened prothrombin time (if PT INR is >1.5), Hydatid disease, wherein it will precipitate anaphylaxis, haemangiomas, ascites, infection in close proximity—lung/diaphragm/peritoneum and liver congestion.

Procedure

Patient should be kept nil oral for 6 hours. Injection atropine 0.6 mg should be given intramuscularly. Patient will be lying on his back very close to the edge. Often 30° propped up position is used. After cleaning and draping, 9th intercostal space in the midaxillary line is marked. Xylocaine 1% is injected into the skin, subcutaneous tissue, deeper tissues up to liver capsule. He or she is then asked to lie on the back with the right elbow to the side and the right hand under the head. The patient is instructed to lie as still as possible during the procedure. He or she is warned to expect a sensation resembling a punch in the right shoulder, but to hold still in spite of the momentary feeling. Needle used is either *Vim-Silverman needle or Menghini needle* (better option).

Using Vim Silverman's needle: It has got three parts—trocar, cannula and split (biflanged) needle **(Fig. 7-53)**. Trocar snugly fits properly into the cannula. Trocar with cannula is passed into the liver tissue when patient holds the breath in deep inspiration. Trocar entering the liver tissue can be felt. Patient is asked to relax and breath comfortably. Trocar is removed. Split needle is much longer than cannula. It is held in the hand to keep ready for penetration into the liver. Patient is again asked to hold the breath properly. Split needle is passed fully to core the liver tissue beyond the existing cannula; cannula is pushed further over the split needle to include the cut liver tissue; cannula with split needle is rotated 180°; cannula with needle is removed entirely. Split needle is removed carefully and opened to collect the cut liver tissue for biopsy. Patient is asked to breath normally afterwards. Procedure can be repeated once again. Further repetitive procedure to get more tissue in the same sitting is not advisable due to high risk of liver injury and bleeding. Tissue is often collected in *Bouin's solution* which contains 75% picric acid.

Presently guided liver biopsy is commonly recommended and popular, i.e. ultrasound (US) guided, CT guided, laparoscopy guided.

Menghini needle method: Percutaneous liver biopsy is done with a special hollow needle, called as Menghini needle, attached to a suction syringe. 3 mL sterile saline is taken into the syringe with specific Menghini needle **(Fig. 7-54)**. Once needle is inside the intercostal space after injecting local anaesthesia, 2 mL of saline is injected to clear the skin fragments in it. Aspiration vacuum is created in the syringe, kept like that and needle is moved forward into the liver. Meantime patient should hold his breath completely in expiration. Needle is connected to the syringe with already created vacuum and withdrawn immediately. It will contain sucked liver tissue which is carefully collected on a glass receptacle containing saline. This method is safer and reliable.

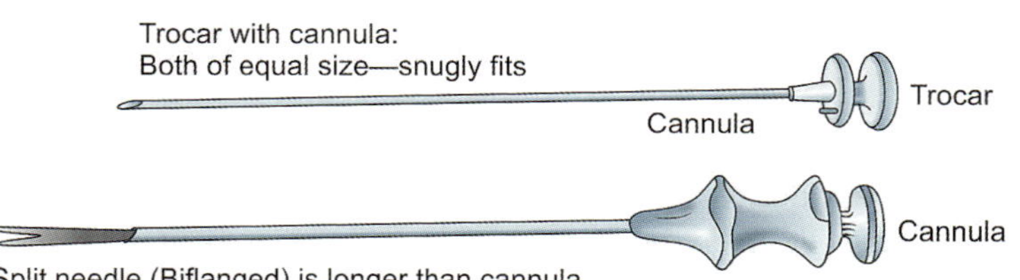

Fig. 7-53: Vim-Silverman needle.

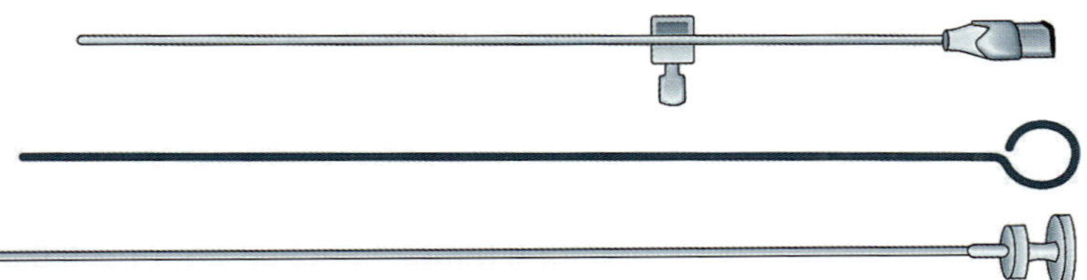

Fig. 7-54: Menghini needle.

The traditional Menghini needle is 6 cm long with an oblique tip slightly convex towards the outside. A retaining device is incorporated into its proximal end to prevent liver tissue from being aspirated into the syringe. The diameter of the needle usually does not exceed 1.4 mm. A penetration limiter is often utilised in children and thin adult patients to limit the depth to which the needle advances. The patient is asked to inhale slightly and exhale maximally and then hold his breath in a maximum exhaled position. At this point, steady suction is applied to the syringe, which is connected to the needle, and the needle is advanced into the liver and withdrawn.

Features of biopsied liver tissue are—floats in water in fatty liver; fragmented small pieces in cirrhosis; dull white coloured in malignancy; green coloured in biliary cirrhosis; chocolate coloured in Dubin-Johnson's syndrome.

Post-procedure Observation

Patient is monitored or hypotension, tachycardia, breathlessness. Patient is asked to lie down right lateral position for 2 hours. Usually procedure is done as OP procedure unless patient already is an inpatient.

Often complications develop within 24 hours. Rest, observation with monitoring of pulse, blood pressure and respiration is essential. Heavy work and exercise should be avoided for 7 days. Routine work after 24 hours is safer. Shoulder pain on right side may be warning sign and needs evaluation using chest X-ray and ultrasound.

Complications

Haemorrhage, bile leak and biliary peritonitis, infection, injury to gallbladder, colon, kidney. Hepatic coma/failure may be precipitated in cirrhotic patients.

Causes of Failure in Liver Biopsy

Cirrhosis, emphysema, uncooperative patient, improper technique.

KIDNEY BIOPSY

Kidney biopsy is done as diagnostic or prognostic indications.

Indications are—asymptomatic proteinuria, nephritic syndrome, glomerulonephritis. It is mainly used in medical causes.

Contraindications are—unilateral kidney, totally shrunken kidney, infections, cystic diseases, hypernephroma, bleeding diathesis. Prothrombin time and platelet count should be assessed. X-ray KUB (kidney, ureter and bladder), ultrasound is done to assess the size of the kidney.

Procedure is done *in prone position* under ultrasound guidance. Procedure is done on the diseased side; whereas in bilateral disease *left side* is preferred. Point of entry of needle is decided under US guidance. Xylocaine local anaesthesia is injected. Needle is passed across skin, subcutaneous tissue, and muscles. While patient is asked to hold the breath, needle is entered into the kidney. When patient breathes back needle moves with respiration. Tissue is aspirated with negative pressure. Needle is removed. In post-procedure period patient is observed for pain, haematoma and bleeding. Bed rest is needed for 24 hours.

Complications

Pain, haematuria, infection, abscess formation, perirenal haematoma, injury to colon, etc.

BONE MARROW ASPIRATION

It is done for diagnostic and prognostic purpose in various conditions like aplastic anaemia, aleukaemic leukaemia, lymphomas, myeloproliferative diseases, myelofibrosis, multiple myeloma, agranulocytosis. It can be done in refractory or iron deficiency anaemias, leukaemias, tropical diseases, storage diseases. Bone marrow transplantation is a therapeutic method. Blood dyscrasias are contraindications.

Usual *site* is sternum (mid manubrium). Other sites are—spinous process of lumbar vertebra, iliac crest. After injecting local anaesthesia, bone marrow aspiration needle with the guard at 1.5 cm from the tip of the needle is punctured through the skin at sternum perpendicularly. *Guard* prevents inadvertent deeper penetration of the needle. Needle is pushed in boring/screwing movements. Sudden giving way suggests the entry of the needle into the bone marrow. Stillete is removed. 0.5 mL of bone marrow fluid is aspirated using 1 mL syringe. Material is smeared in slides also. After removal of the needle, pressure is applied over the site to prevent bleeding and haematoma formation.

Complications

Bone pain, haematoma, infection, injury to great vessels. Normal compositions of bone marrow are—blood cells, blood vessels, reticulum and fatty tissue.

Causes for *dry tap*—technical; myelosclerosis, carcinoma, hyper or hypoplasias. *Analysis of bone marrow* is done for—erythropoiesis, leukopoiesis, megakaryocytes; cellularity, myeloid-erythroid ratio (3:1); presence of parasites and different bodies.

LUMBAR PUNCTURE

It is aspiration and collection of cerebrospinal fluid (CSF) from the spinal subarachnoid space by passing a needle into the space between lumbar 2nd and 3rd vertebra or 3rd and 4th vertebra.

Indications

Meningitis, subarachnoid haemorrhage, neurosyphilis, unexplained coma, Guillain-Barré syndrome, multiple sclerosis, during myelography, to introduce drugs into the CSF, for spinal anaesthesia, in hypertensive encephalopathy.

Contraindications

If lumbar puncture done in raised intracranial hypertension herniation of brain trough foramen magnum can develop leading to sudden death. Suspected cord compression is also a contraindication. Back pain, sciatica, syringomyelia, sepsis, allergy are other contraindications.

Procedure

Patient is positioned in lying down position turned to one side with knee fully flexed and head also flexed. Sitting and bending forward is another position often used. 3rd lumbar vertebra is at the level of highest point of iliac crest. Entire back is cleaned with savlon/povidone iodine and draped. Xylocaine injection is infiltrated (5 mL) subcutaneously and up to ligamentum flava. Lumbar puncture needle with stillete is introduced into the space. Cutting edge of the bevel of the tip of the needle should be parallel to fibres of ligamentum flava. It is directed upwards and forwards at 5° through resistance of supraspinous ligament. Needle is then passed through interspinous ligament, ligamentum flavum and dura mater of spinal cord. Giving way sensation of entering the subarachnoid space is typical. Stilette is withdrawn. *Spinal fluid* is collected for biochemical, cytological and serological studies. Fluid will be clear with continuous flow of drops (0.5 mL/second flow rate). A manometer is attached to lumbar puncture needle; pressure is applied over one jugular vein and then the other which causes raise in intracranial venous pressure and then intraspinal venous pressure which is reflected in manometer. There is raise in fluid level in manometer quickly for about 100 mm and falls down slowly. It is possible only if pathway between lumbar puncture site and cranium is patent. Delay in this means spinal block—*Queckenstedt's test* **(Figs. 7-55 and 7-56)**.

Normally CSF is formed at choroid plexus of lateral ventricle (95%), of 3rd and 4th ventricle, perivascular spaces of brain. It circulates from choroid plexus of lateral ventricle → foramen of Monro → lateral ventricle → Sylvian duct → 3rd ventricle → 4th ventricle → foramen of Luschka and Magendie → subarachnoid space → basal cisterns → circulates over brain and spinal cord. CSF is *absorbed* by arachnoid villi. *CSF* maintains intracranial pressure and temperature acting as shock absorber, and gives nutrition and help in dispose of metabolic waste. *Normal CSF* formation is—1500 mL/day; total volume of CSF is 150 mL; clear in colour; 60–150 mm is the pressure in lying down and 200 mm in sitting position; pH is 7.35; specific gravity is 1.007; proteins is 20–40 mg%; sugar is 40–60 mg%; chlorides is 720–750 mg%; cells are 0–5 epithelial lymphocytes like cells. In CSF sugar, proteins, cholesterol, urea, calcium and phosphorus are less than that of blood; chlorides and magnesium are more than that of blood. Antibodies and enzymes are not seen in CSF. Penicillins, streptomycin will not cross blood-brain barrier and so not found in CSF.

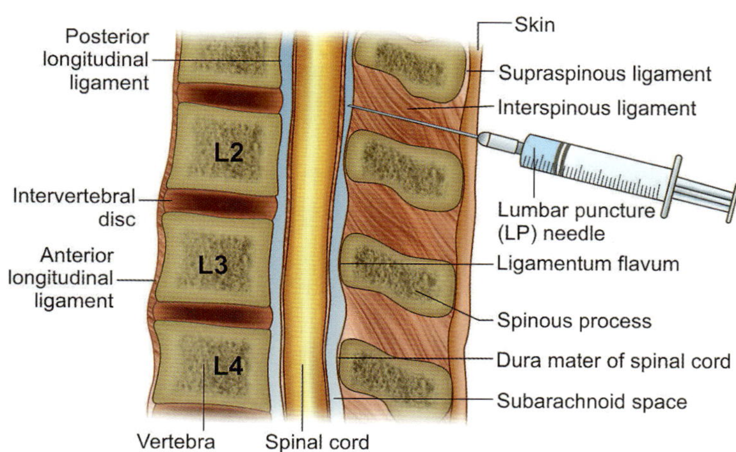

Fig. 7-55: Diagram showing lumbar puncture needle passing through different layers.

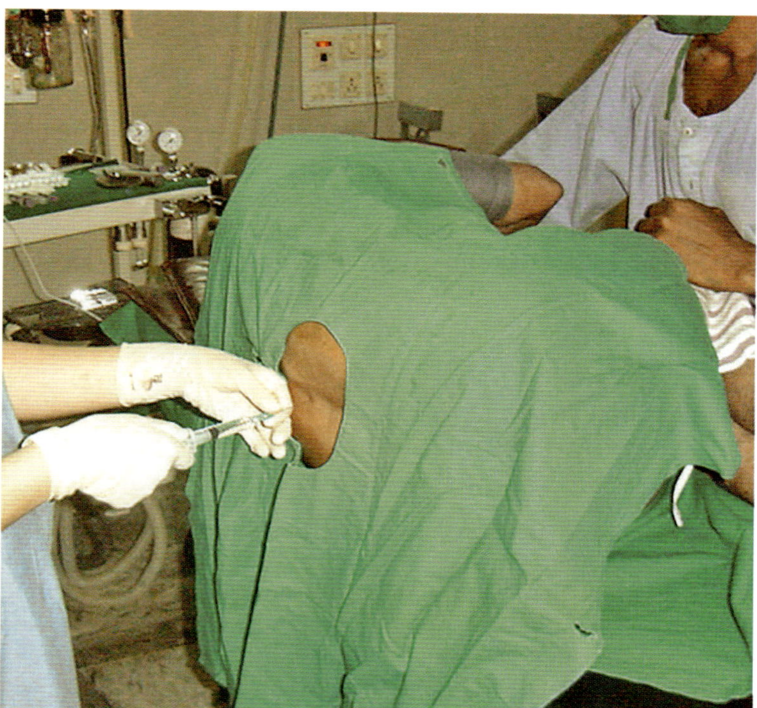

Fig. 7-56: Photograph showing position and aspirating the CSF through lumbar puncture.

Findings

CSF is turbid in pyogenic meningitis; cobweb appearance in tuberculous meningitis; bloody in subarachnoid haemorrhage/trauma/bleeding disorders. Yellow CSF *(xanthochromia)* is due to presence of bilirubin in CSF seen in haemorrhage into subarachnoid space; high protein content like Guillain-Barré syndrome, spinal block or neurofibroma; jaundice patients; spinal tumours. *Proteins* in CSF are raised in meningitis, Guillain-Barré syndrome, intracranial tumours, spinal cord compression, disseminated sclerosis. Sugar in CSF is increased in diabetes mellitus, encephalitis. It is decreased in meningitis. Chlorides in CSF are decreased in meningitis and metabolic conditions.

Cohen's law of meningitis: Substances which are more in CSF than blood will reduce in meningitis and substances which are low in CSF than blood will raise with exception of sugar (sugar is less in CSF than blood normally; it reduces further in meningitis).

While giving *spinal anaesthesia* (xylocaine 5% in 6% dextrose of 2 mL; or bupivacaine 0.5% in 5% dextrose of 3 mL), bevel should face upwards (360° rotation). Syringe is aspirated to get clear CSF into it and the anaesthetic drug is injected. Needle is removed, area is cleaned and sealed.

Complications

Headache is the commonest complication. Plenty of oral fluids, intravenous fluids, head down position, bed rest, and analgesics are used to control it. Back pain, infection, meningismus, coning, bleeding, rarely paraplegia, converted to total spinal in spinal anaesthesia are other complications.

PLEURAL TAP (THORACOCENTESIS)

Indications

In pleural effusion both diagnostic as well as therapeutic purpose. The fluid is sent for culture, cytology, microscopy, specific gravity, biochemical analysis like proteins for diagnosis of tuberculosis, malignancy. In empyema thoracis, for diagnostic purpose before placing an intercostal tube (ICT), intrapleural administration of drugs pleural tap is being done.

Position

In sitting position, leaning forward over a wooden support.

Site

Tip of scapula at 7th intercostal space (posteriorly—scapular line), in midaxillary line.

Procedure is done with patient in sitting position and leaning forward over a support. Tapping is done from behind. After giving local anaesthesia (xylocaine 2% into skin, subcutaneous tissue, up to parietal pleura) wide bore needle (Abraham needle) is used to tap the fluid. Needle is passed at right angles to the skin; in the intercostal space between two ribs; typical '*giving way*' feel of puncturing the parietal pleura is felt. Needle with stopcock (3-way) is used. 50 mL syringe is connected to the stopcock. Fluid is aspirated from the pleural cavity with stopcock in straight position. Then the knob is turned to right angle to empty the syringe to reservoir. Procedure is repeated to clear the fluid **(Fig. 7-57)**.

For diagnostic tap, 50 mL of fluid is aspirated and sent for biochemical/cytological analysis and culture.

For therapeutic aspiration—750-1000 mL per day is aspirated. Pulmonary oedema may develop if more quantity is aspirated rapidly, leading to often ARDS which may be life threatening.

Post-tapping, patient should be monitored for change in breathing, tachycardia **(Figs. 7-58A to F)**.

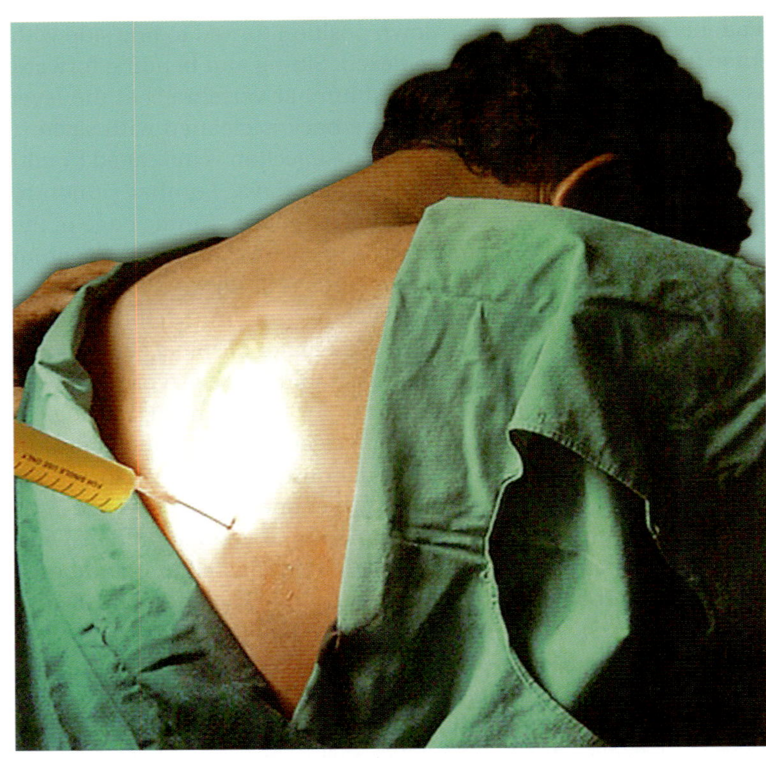

Fig. 7-57: Pleural tap. Note the position of the patient and placement of the needle.

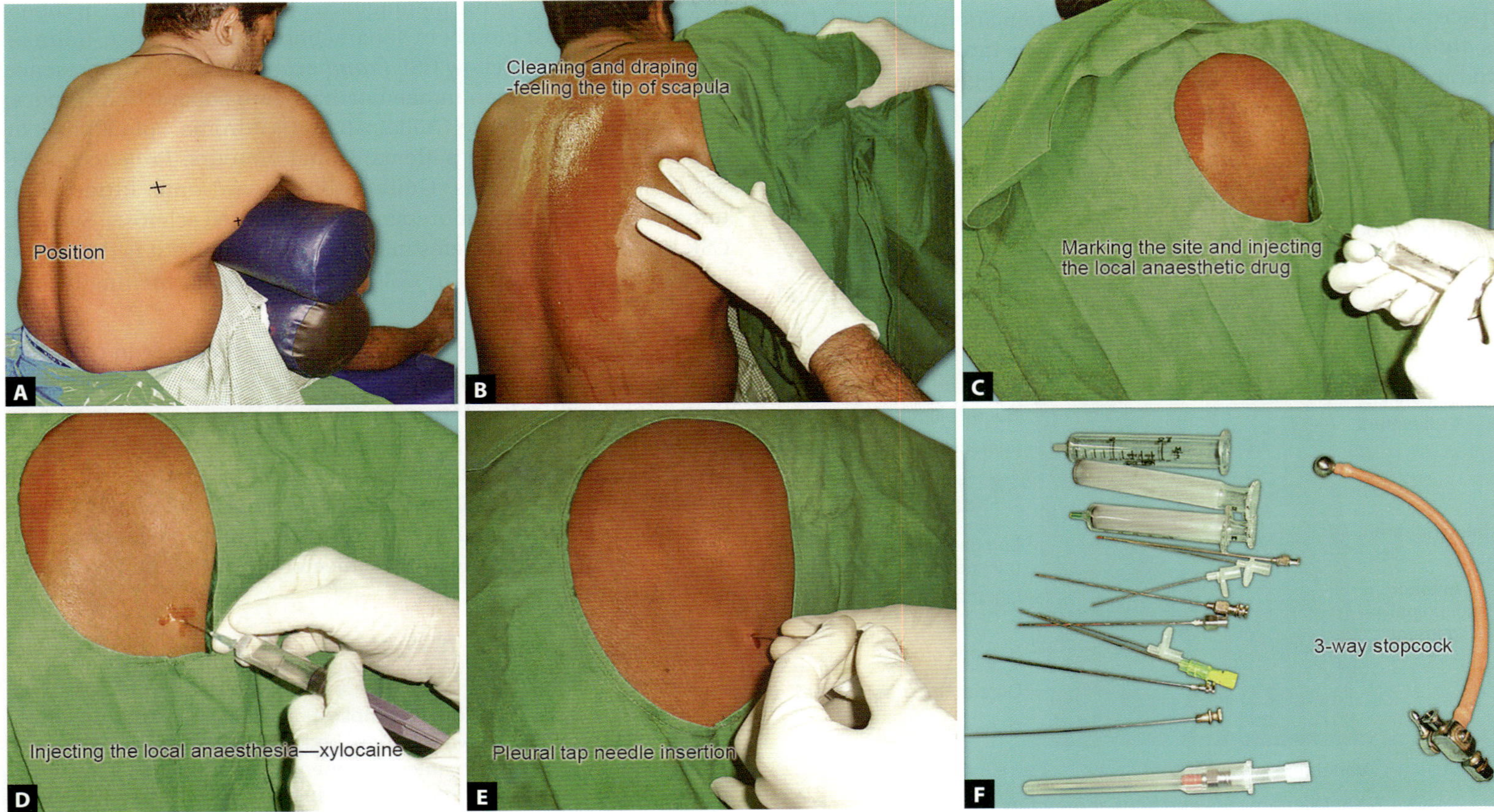

Figs. 7-58A to F: Steps in pleural tapping with instruments used—needle, syringes, 3-way stopcock.

Complications

Complications are infection, dry tap or bloody tap, bleeding, development of pneumothorax occasionally, sudden vagal shock, pain and respiratory distress.

PERICARDIAL TAP (PERICARDIOCENTESIS)

Indications

Pericardial effusion due to any cause—viral, tubercular, rheumatic (rapidly progressive or not regressing in 4 weeks); haemopericardium; purulent pericardium **(Fig. 7-59)**.

Procedure

Injection atropine 0.6 mg with injection pethidine 100 mg is given intramuscularly half an hour prior to tapping. In supine position after injecting xylocaine local anaesthesia 1–2% needle is passed. A 16 or 18-gauge needle is passed into the pericardium just below the xiphoid process directing upwards and backwards towards left side—in the direction of midclavicular line with an angle of 45° to the surface. Under ECG and US guidance needle position is confirmed. Negative deflection in the ECG means needle is touching the heart and so needle should be withdrawn a little. ECG should show normal tracing. Post-procedure monitoring is a must.

This site is used because it is—most dependent for aspiration; unlikely to traumatise heart; pleura is not punctured; coronary vessels are not injured. Occasionally other sites are used—anteriorly in the left 5th intercostal space just outside the apex beat but within the cardiac dullness; posteriorly near inferior angle of scapula; in the left 4th intercostal space lateral to the sternum.

Complications

Injury to heart causing bleeding/ventricular fibrillation; infection; injury to coronary vessels. Life-threatening haemopericardium may develop which may need immediate thoracotomy, pericardiotomy by cardiothoracic surgeons. Air embolism, pulmonary oedema, vagal shock, circulatory collapse, injury to intercostal vessels, pneumothorax are other complications.

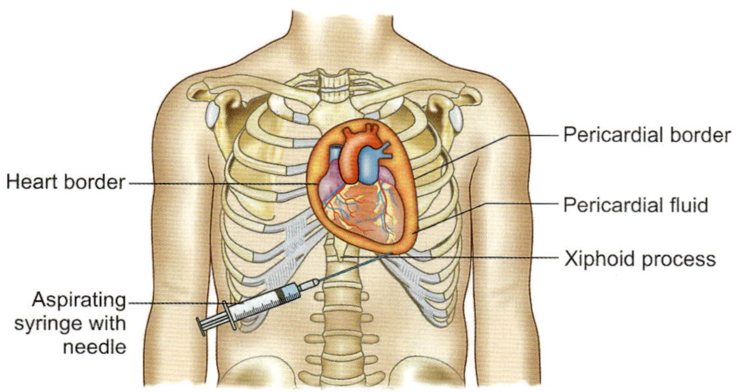

Fig. 7-59: Pericardial tap—diagrammatic look.

PERITONEAL TAP (ASCITIC TAP)

Indications

For diagnosis: Abdominal tuberculosis, peritoneal secondaries, ascitic fluid study.

For therapy: In massive ascites to relieve distress and cardiopulmonary discomfort by removing fluid—as seen in malignancy, portal hypertension. It is done in refractory ascites with failure of medical line of therapy.

Site

In the spinoumbilical line lateral to rectus abdominis muscle **(Fig. 7-60)**.

Procedure

Patient is asked to *empty the urinary bladder* or should be catheterised. Abdomen is percussed to confirm the dullness in the flank. Site of tapping is marked. Injection xylocaine 1% local anaesthetic is infiltrated. 20 gauge long needle is inserted into the peritoneal cavity. Ascitic fluid comes into the syringe. Syringe is connected to the 3-way stopcock to have controlled tapping.

For diagnostic purpose 50 mL of fluid is aspirated. Fluid is sent for culture/cytology/acid fast bacilli (AFB)/biochemical analysis.

To relieve distress 1,500 mL/day is aspirated. If more quantity is aspirated sudden hypotension and cardiac arrest can occur. It is always safer to do procedure with an intravenous line with fluid flowing.

Complications and Difficulties

Infection and peritonitis can occur. Bleeding from the puncture site into the peritoneal cavity causing haemoperitoneum. Puncture into the bowel causing bowel injury. Protein depletion occurs after tapping of large quantity of fluid. Tapping may precipitate hepatic failure and coma in patients with jaundice and severe liver cell dysfunction.

Negative tapping: In *loculated ascites* due to (commonly) abdominal tuberculosis, fluid may not get aspirated and so ultrasound guidance is needed to aspirate fluid. In females, tense ascites should be differentiated from *large ovarian cyst* before tapping.

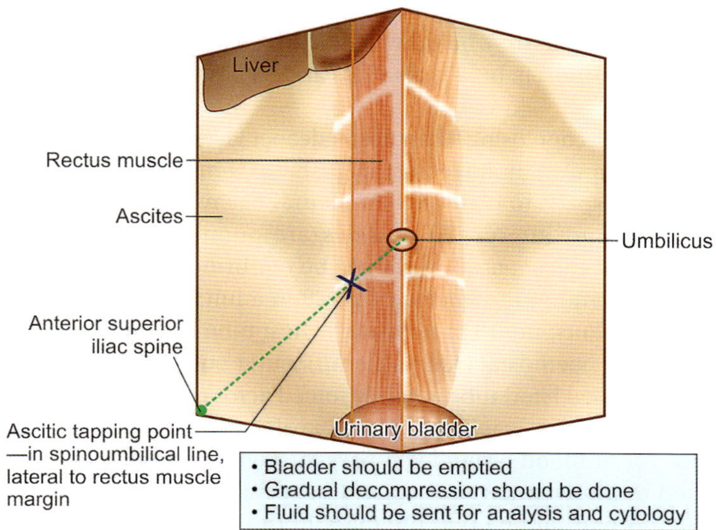

Fig. 7-60: Ascitic tap.

INTERCOSTAL TUBE DRAINAGE (ICT DRAINAGE)

It is the method of draining collections in the pleural cavity safely so as to make the lung to expand. Technique is also called as ***tube thoracostomy***; tube is called as chest or intercostal tube or drain (Bulau drain). Concept was first introduced by Hippocrates to drain empyema but popularised by Dr C Pope in 1922.

Chest tube is made up of clear plastics or polyvinyl chloride (PVC); it has got multiple fenestrations on the side which resides inside the thoracic cavity. Ranges from 6 French to 40 French sizes are available. Tube has got a radio-opaque strip. Silastic channel styled chest drains (Blake drains) are available which drain through capillary action and suction; it is less painful.

Indications

Haemothorax (trauma/malignancy), pneumothorax, haemopneumothorax, empyema thoracis, traumatic lung contusion, after thoracotomy to drain pleural cavity.

Contraindications

Refractory coagulopathy, traumatic diaphragmatic hernia, pleural adhesions, emphysematous bullae are contraindications for ICT drainage.

Procedure

Patient is in 30–45° partial lying position with backrest support. Under local anaesthesia (5 mL of 1% xylocaine injection), an ICT is placed in 5th or 6th intercostal space in case of haemothorax and in 2nd or 3rd space in pyothorax and in pneumothorax.

A small (3 cm) transverse incision is made just in front of the midaxillary line (as the muscle bulk is less here and so passage of ICT is easier) using no. 11 blade, parallel to intercostal space (above the rib, i.e. lower part of intercostal space to avoid injury to neurovascular bundle which are located in the groove in the lower part of rib). [***Site: Triangle of safety***—British Thoracic Society describes the *safe zone* as—bounded by the lateral border of pectoralis major, a horizontal line inferior to the axilla, the anterior border of latissimus dorsi and a horizontal line superior to the nipple; commonly the tube is inserted into the 5th intercostal space slightly anterior to the midaxillary line; but it may be in 6th space below in haemothorax or empyema or it may be upwards in 4th space in pneumothorax. At this point muscle bulk is also less and so easier to pass the intercostal tube].

Blunt dissection using a haemostat deeper layer is dissected; pleura is punctured. Air/blood/pus may gush out. Finger is inserted into the pleural space to confirm that pleural cavity has been reached. OR fascia and intercostal muscles are opened and separated; adequacy of the separation should be confirmed using finger tip; fenestrated end of the selected (no. 28 in adult; no. 18 in children; no. 12 in infants; no. 10 in neonates) chest tube is held firmly using long curved haemostat (Kelly's clamp); outer end is clamped which will be released later; tube is gently forced across the parietal pleurae which gives 'a give way' feel. Tube is easily pushed into the thoracic cavity. Air or blood or fluid will pass through the tube; tube is connected to under water seal apparatus which should be filled with sterile normal saline up to the mark in the canister (Tube is often clamped prior to insertion and released after that). ICT is sutured to the skin using non-absorbable polyethylene suture; often additional suture bites are taken around and kept untied which will be tied immediately firmly after removal of the ICT (central vertical mattress suture—*sealing suture*). Airtight plaster dressing is placed around to keep the ICT in position.

20 French size tube for air; 32 French size tube for blood is used. Tube with side openings is pushed into the pleural cavity. Other end is connected *to under water seal (200 mL of sterile normal saline/water). Air-water column moving* with respiration can be observed. Tube is fixed with skin sutures. *Heimlich valve* is a plastic container with collapsible rubber tube that acts as a one-way rubber tube is also can be used. Ultrasound or CT-guided placement of chest tube is done in posterior or inferior loculated pleural collection. Patient should be in sitting position in this posterior tube placement. *Three bottle chest drain system* is also often used **(Figs. 7-61 and 7-62)**. First one is fluid collection chamber; second one is under water seal to prevent air entering into the pleura; third one acts as manometer for adjusting the suction transmission to the patient. Moulding disposable plastic units are available.

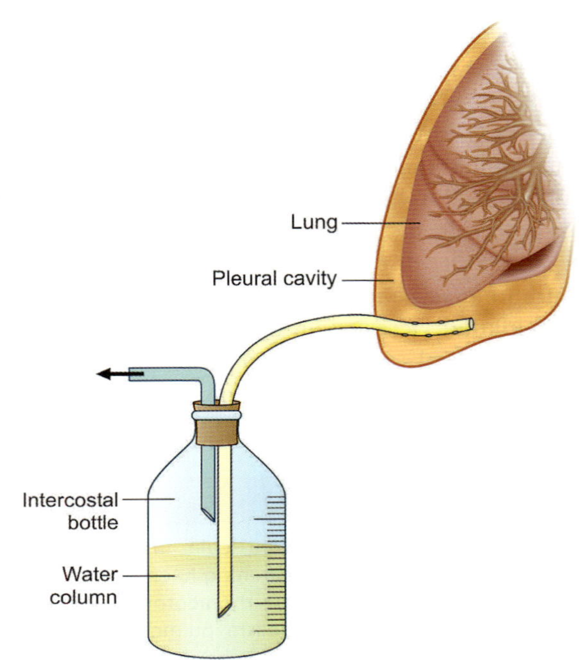

Fig. 7-61: Intercostal tube drainage.

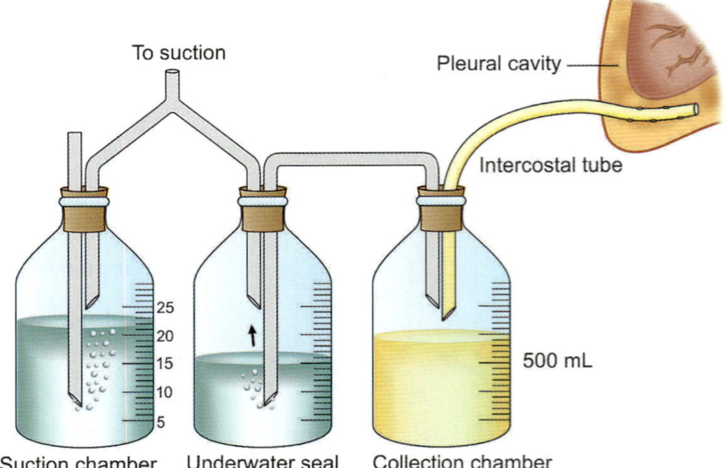

Fig. 7-62: Intercostal tube drainage using three bottle thoracic drainage.

Drainage canister is used to collect the blood, air, fluid and so on through a water seal apparatus. *Triple chamber canisters* are often used for better function; here first chamber collects the fluid content. Second chamber acts as water seal which allows the air escape acting as one way valve; it also indicates the air leak from pleura or lung. Third chamber is the suction control chamber; height of water column in this regulates the negative pressure so controls the suction system **(Fig. 7-63)**. Only water seal and water column regulator system is 'wet' type; water seal with mechanical regulator is 'wet-dry' type; system without water seal but uses mechanical check valve and mechanical regulator is called as 'dry' system.

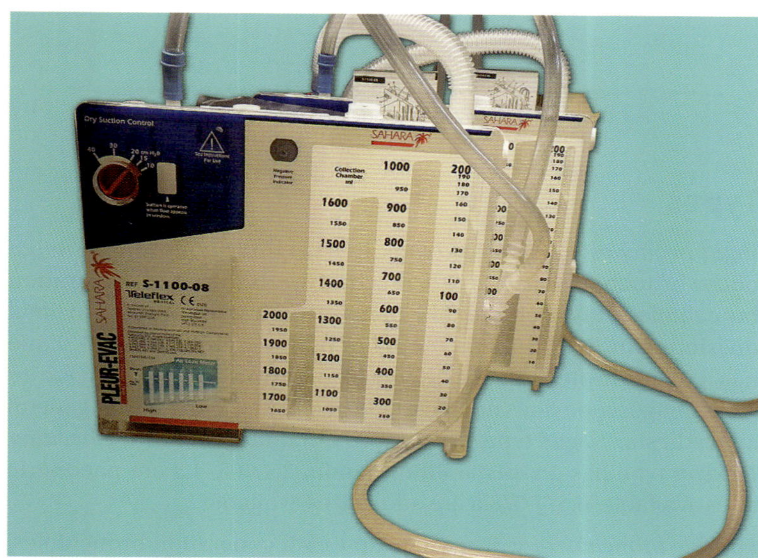

Fig. 7-63: ICT canister—three chambers.

Usually for pneumothorax ICT is kept for 2–3 days (until lung expands—confirmed by check chest X-ray and air leak is not observed). For haemothorax and pyothorax it is kept for 4–6 days or until it stops draining (less than 100 mL/24 hours) and lung expansion is confirmed by repeat chest X-ray. To have a proper expansion of lungs patient is asked to blow football bladder/spirometer (balloon) breathing exercise). If there is bronchopleural fistula, ICT should be placed for longer time until fistula heals **(Fig. 7-64)**.

Trocar ICT or guide wire directed ICT placement is also used in few centres but they are not popular.

Complications and Problems

Different complications are—infection, displacement and inadequate functioning, injury to intercostal vessels and bleeding, injury to intercostal nerves, lung and mediastinum and pain at the site of ICT placement **(Fig. 7-65)**.

Post-operative Care

ICT care is crucial. Movement of the column, quantity of fluid collected should be observed. *Mechanical manipulation* (tapping, milking) gently may be done to correct kinking, clot inside or to facilitate free flow of fluid but they are painful. *Movement of the air column* during respiration (and during the act of coughing) should be checked; quantity of fluid or blood collecting also should be observed. *Check chest X-ray* should be taken *immediately* to assess the position of the ICT. O_2 supplementation is needed often; patient should be monitored throughout. Canister or underwater seal bottle or bag should be kept *100 cm below* the patient level.

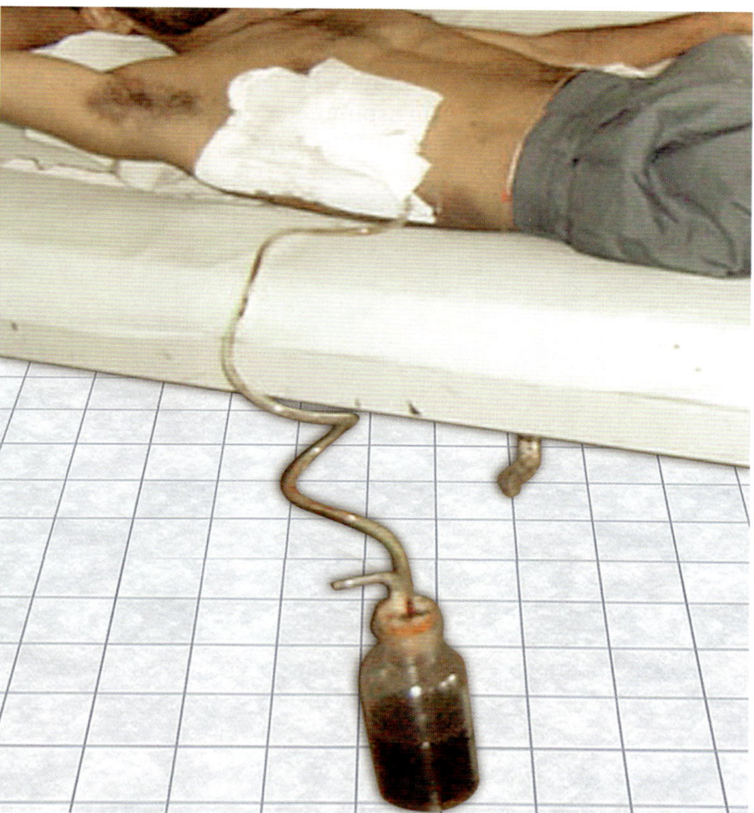

Fig. 7-64: Intercostal tube drainage in a patient with haemothorax.

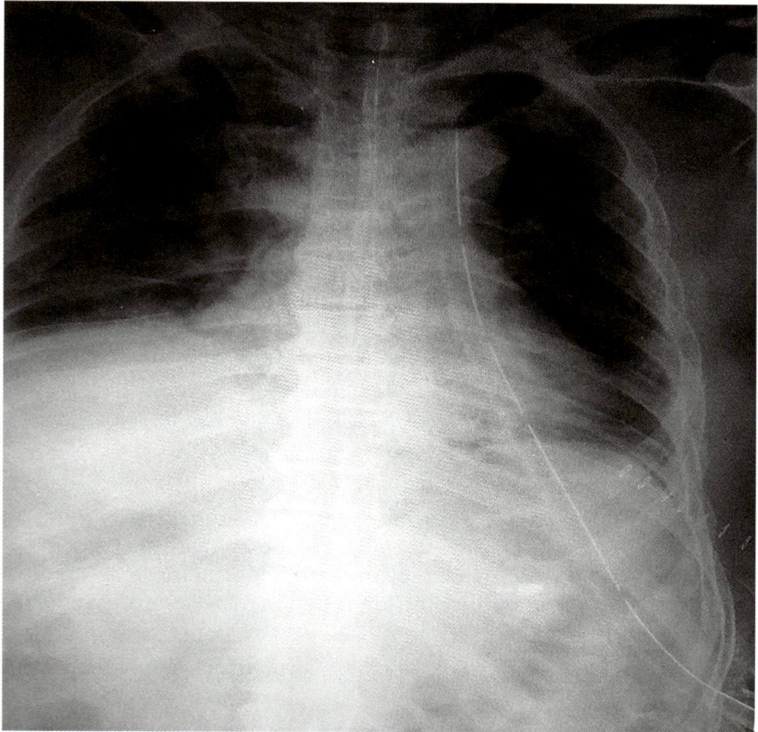

Fig. 7-65: Immediate check chest X-ray should be done to confirm the position of the ICT.

Closed chest tube clearing device using sterile magnetically wired loops can prevent clogging and blocking of the tube which prevents formation of retained blood syndrome (haemothorax, pleural effusion, tamponade, atrial fibrillation). Lung expansion should be checked at regular intervals. Usually ICT is placed for 3–5 days for pneumothorax until lung expands adequately which should be confirmed by chest X-ray; for haemothorax for 4–7 days. For bronchopleural fistula ICT should be kept for longer period. *Respiratory physiotherapy* using spirometer or football balloon and breathing exercise should be done **(Fig. 7-66)**.

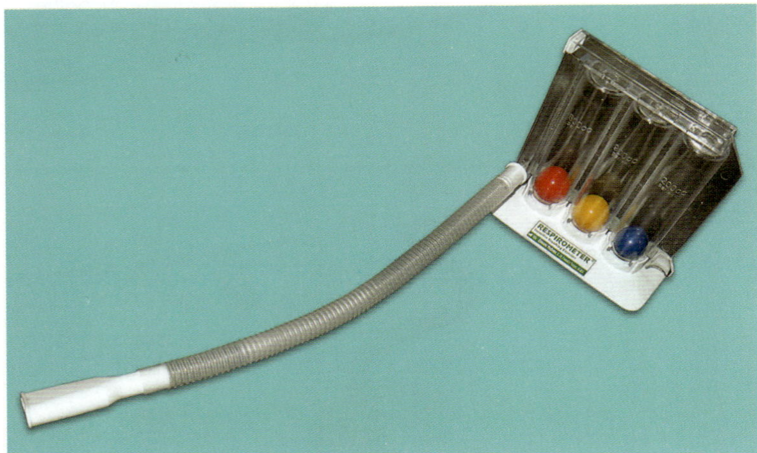

Fig. 7-66: Spirometer. Respiratory physiotherapy should be done using spirometer.

ICT Removal

It is done once chest X-ray confirms that lung has expanded properly, pleural fluid drain becomes serous and less than 25 mL/day for 3 consecutive days, water column movement becomes less than 1 cm. It is removed under all aseptic precaution; suture is removed; patient is asked to take deep inspiration; often outer end of the tube may be connected to low volume suction. At the summit of deep inspiration, tube is pulled out; wound is cleaned quickly and if sealing suture is present it should be tied firmly; sealed plaster dressing is placed to avoid air reentry into the plural cavity.

Complications

Clogging of the ICT (40%) is the main complication which is commonly unnoticed as part inside the thoracic cavity is getting clogged commonly. It can cause retained blood syndrome, tension pneumothorax, effusion, haemothorax.

Injury to intercostal nerve and vessels, diaphragm, liver, spleen, aorta and heart can occur.

Improper placement of the tube.

Reexpansion pulmonary oedema can occur if large quantity of fluid or pus drained in effusion or empyema; it may cause sudden onset cough, breathlessness and respiratory arrest (potentially fatal). In such situation gradual decompression is better. 500–800 mL at regular intervals.

Subcutaneous haematoma, seroma, subcutaneous emphysema can occur.

Displacement, pain, intercostal neuralgia, dyspnoea, cough, infection can occur.

BRONCHOSCOPY

Indications

Diagnostic: To take biopsy in carcinoma lung, lung abscess, pulmonary tuberculosis.

Therapeutic: To remove foreign body, to suck out the bronchial secretions, tracheobronchial stenting in fistulas like tracheo-oesophageal fistula, malignancy, etc. **(Fig. 7-67)**.

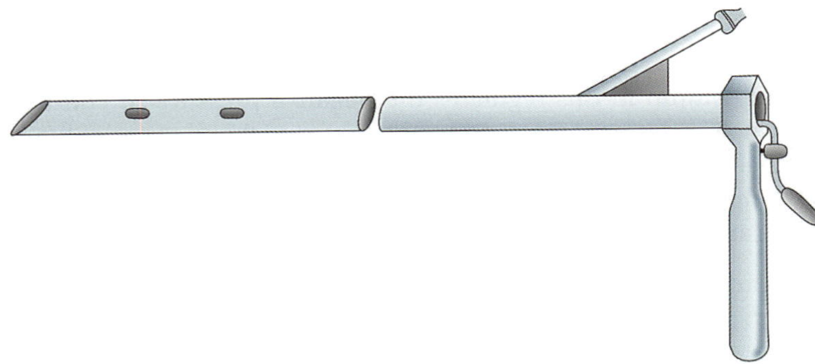

Fig. 7-67: Bronchoscope.

Types

Rigid bronchoscopy (Negus type): It is used for removal of foreign body, bronchial wash, etc. It reaches up to the third generation bronchioles. It is useful to take biopsy from carcinoma of proximal divisions but not from carcinoma of peripheral lung. Rigid scope has got multiple holes to allow ventilation during procedure (oesophagoscope does not have side holes). It is done under general anaesthesia. *Negus* type has got proximal illumination. *Chevalier Jackson* type has got distal illumination. 2.4/3.5/4.5 are paediatric sizes available. 6.5/7.5/8.5 are adult sizes available.

Flexible bronchoscopy: It reaches up to 5th generation bronchioles. It can be done under local anaesthesia. It is mainly used for diagnosis, biopsy and suctioning, removal of clot from the trachea, endotracheal tube clearing, clearing of tracheobronchial tree through tracheostomy. It is also used to facilitate difficult endotracheal intubation.

Complications

Bleeding, infection, perforation of trachea and bronchospasm.

VASECTOMY

Indications

Vasectomy is done commonly for family planning purpose. Consent of both partners is needed. One should look for any hernia/hydrocele—if present vasectomy should be done along with specific surgeries for these conditions. Previously while doing prostatectomy vasectomy was done as the procedure to prevent retrograde infection of testes. Occasionally, in specific diseases like tuberculosis of vas, vasectomy may be done for biopsy purpose.

There are no specific contraindications for vasectomy but if patient is having hernia or hydrocele, it is better to do vasectomy along with surgery for hernia or hydrocele.

Types

Classical method—Scalpel technique.
No scalpel technique (Shunqiang Li—China).

Classical method: After cleaning and draping the scrotum, 2–5 mL of xylocaine plain 1% is injected into root of the scrotum on lateral aspect. Skin, dartos are incised (1–2 cm vertical incision). Once spermatic fascia is incised cord structures are identified. Vas deferens is seen and felt as thickened whitish cord like structure. It is dissected using mosquito artery forceps. It is held using Babcock's forceps as loop outside the wound. Vas is clamped in two different places using two artery forceps with a gap in between. A piece of the vas (5–10 mm) is excised in between the clamps. Cut ends are ligated using non-absorbable sutures like silk. Skin is closed with sutures. Procedure is repeated on the other side. Dressing is placed. Sutures removed after 7 days **(Fig. 7-68)**.

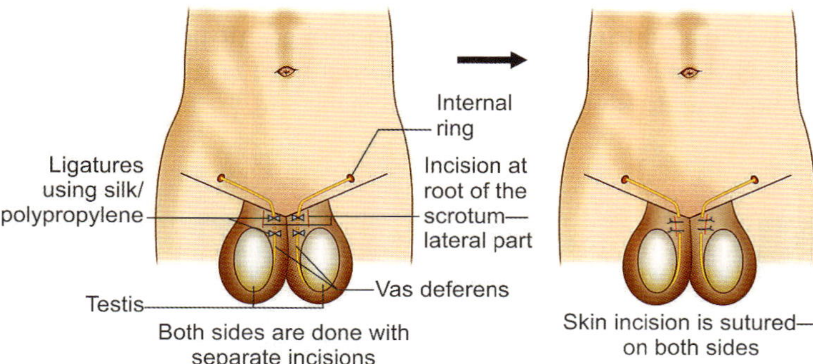

Fig. 7-68: Classical method of vasectomy.

No scalpel technique: Two special instruments are used here—an extracutaneous ring clamp and Chongquing's sharpened curved mosquito clamp. After cleaning and draping, 2–3 mL of xylocaine 2% is injected under the skin of midline raphe on proximal aspect. Vas deferens of one side is felt and pushed under the raphe. It is carefully held with extracutaneous ring clamp. Skin is incised using sharp tip of the curved mosquito clamp. Whitish cord-like vas which is held with ring clamp is dissected → clamped → a small piece of 5 mm is cut. Cut ends are ligated using silk. Opposite vas is also similarly brought out into the same wound by manipulation, clamped and ligated after cutting. Skin is not closed. It gets apposed automatically and heals on its own. Post-operatively antibiotics and analgesics are given **(Figs. 7-69A to K)**.

Excised small pieces of both sides vas should be sent for histology for confirmation.

Advice: Additional contraception should be used to have protected intercourse for a minimum period of 6 weeks/15 ejaculations.

Complications

Infection, pyocele, bleeding, haematoma, haematocele, sperm granuloma, recanalisation and failure.

VASOVASOSTOMY (RECANALISATION PROCEDURE)

Indications

Patient who has undergone vasectomy earlier if needs fertility (one more child) again.

Technique

Under general/spinal anaesthesia incision over the front of the scrotum is made. Cord is dissected. Cut ends of the vas are identified. Both ends are carefully mobilised. Cut ends are trimmed to see the clear lumen. Fine 3-zero polypropylene suture material is passed through the lumen to act as a stent. Cut ends are sutured using 4-zero polypropylene continuous sutures. Stent is brought out through vas and through scrotal skin away from main wound. Skin is closed with sutures. Procedure is commonly done on both sides. Stent is kept for 3 weeks and removed. Success rate of vasovasostomy is 30%.

Complications

Infection, haematoma and failure.

STAPLERS IN SURGERY

Staplers are used for apposition of tissues. It is used in skin, bowel, lungs, etc. It is useful in depth and quick surgery. It is equal to suturing as far as final outcome is considered (neither better nor worse).

Types

Cutaneous staplers give clean apposition. It is faster and technically easier. Problem is removal as it requires specific instrument and costlier than sutures **(Fig. 7-70)**.

Linear staplers are used to close the bowel either completely or partially.

Circular staplers also called as EEA Stapler—**E**nd to **E**nd **A**nastomosis. It is commonly used for colorectal anastomosis in anterior resection for carcinoma rectum, oesophagogastric (OG) anastomosis after oesophagogastric resection in case of carcinoma at OG junction.

Parts are *stapler gun,* and *cartridge* with two rows of stapler pins for apposition. Loaded cartridge is detachable. Cut ends of bowel are placed over *gun and cartridge.* Once gun is shot, cartridge moves to the gun and creates anastomosis **(Fig. 7-71)**.

GIA stapler (Gastrointestinal anastomosis stapler) for *side to side* anastomosis like small bowel or ileocolic anastomosis.

Stapler for lung apposition.

Endostaplers: Staplers used during laparoscopic surgeries. It is commonly used for bowel anastomosis. ***Endovascular staplers*** are used to ligate vascular pedicles like renal pedicles during laparoscopic nephrectomy.

Disposable staplers are available but are costly.

Advantages

It is technically easier and faster. Main advantage is speed. Stapler gastrointestinal anastomosis takes 2–5 minutes which saves lot of time especially in critically ill patients. It is useful in the depth.

Disadvantages

Cost factor, availability are the problems. It is not completely haemostatic and so bleeding can occur. Leak from anastomosis, improper apposition, intestinal obstruction are other problems. It is uncomfortable to use stapler in biliary anastomosis, pancreatic anastomosis. Staplers are not safer in too thick or too diseased bowel like in Crohn's disease. Suture anastomosis is more appropriate and accurate in such situations.

Principle

Staples enter the tissue straight and then made to bend to 'B'. Blood flow to tissues is maintained through the gap. Standard linear stapler is available in two standard staple sizes—3.5 mm and 4.8 mm size. Each is 4.0 mm in width and 3.5 mm and 4.8 mm leg length respectively. 4.0 mm × 3.5 mm closes to a size of 1.5 mm (used for small and large bowel); 4.0 mm × 4.8 mm closes to 2 mm size (used for stomach). These cartridges are coloured differently for identification purpose. Endoscopic linear stapler compresses tissues up to 1.75 mm thickness. Stapling can be done in inversion or in eversion. Circular and linear cutting stapler creates inverted staple line. Stapling in eversion is used in anastomosis **(Fig. 7-72)**.

Linear Devices

Linear stapling devices are of 55 mm or 90 mm or rarely 30 mm (smaller only for short sutures). Each applies two staggered row of staples of 55 mm/90 mm/30 mm length respectively. Staples could be 3.5 mm or 4.8 mm depending on need and thickness of the tissue. Aligning pin on the tip confirms the proper meeting of the anvil accurately on either sides of the tissue which device is holding. The device that just staples without cutting is called as a *linear stapling device without cutting*. It is used in closure of duodenal stump, during partial gastrectomy and gastrojejunostomy in creation of new lesser curve, closure of bowel in end to side or side to side anastomosis, during ileostomy, creation of gastric pouch in morbid obesity. Laparoscopic linear stapling device is used for stapled ligation and division of the vessels.

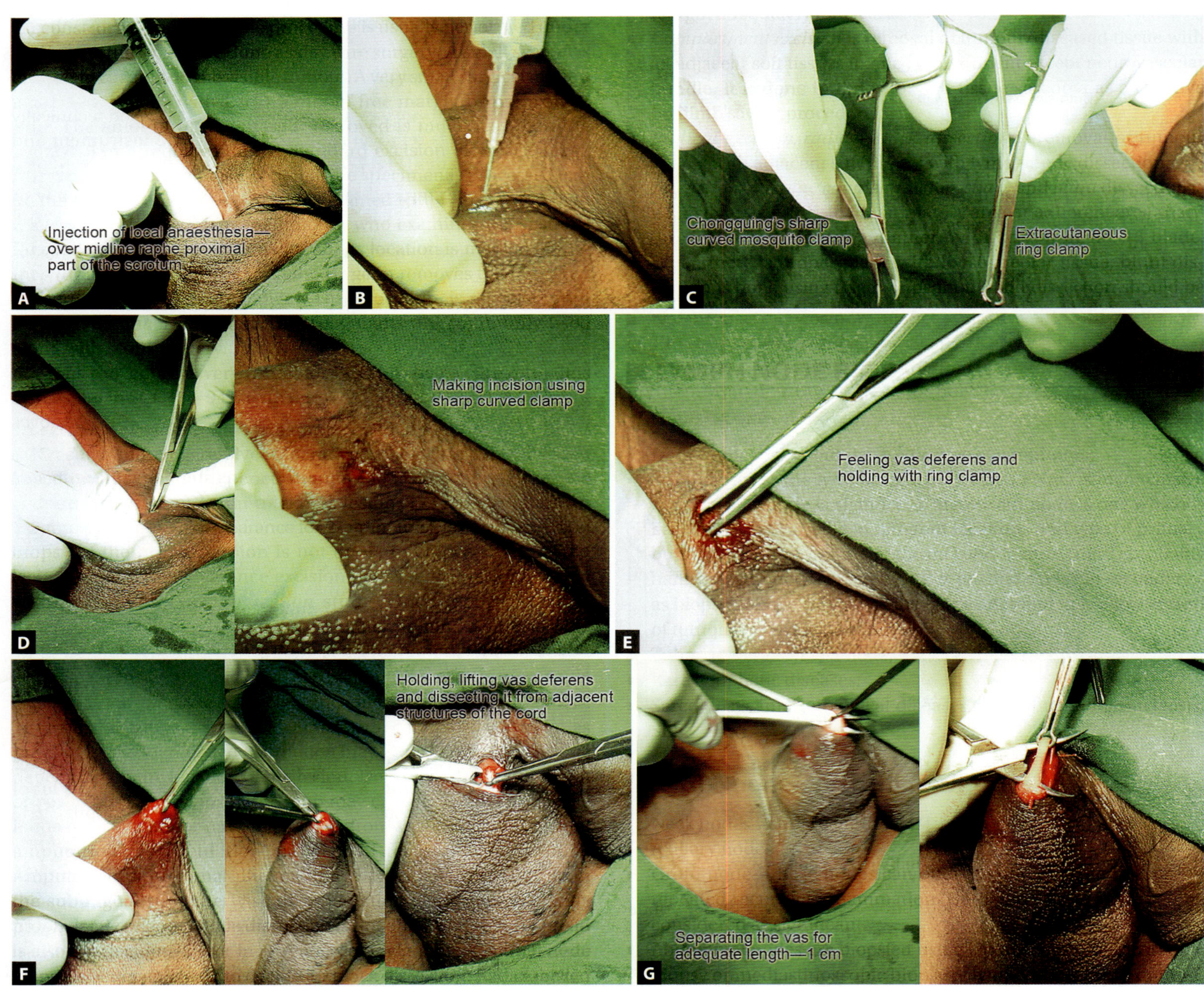

Figs. 7-69A to G

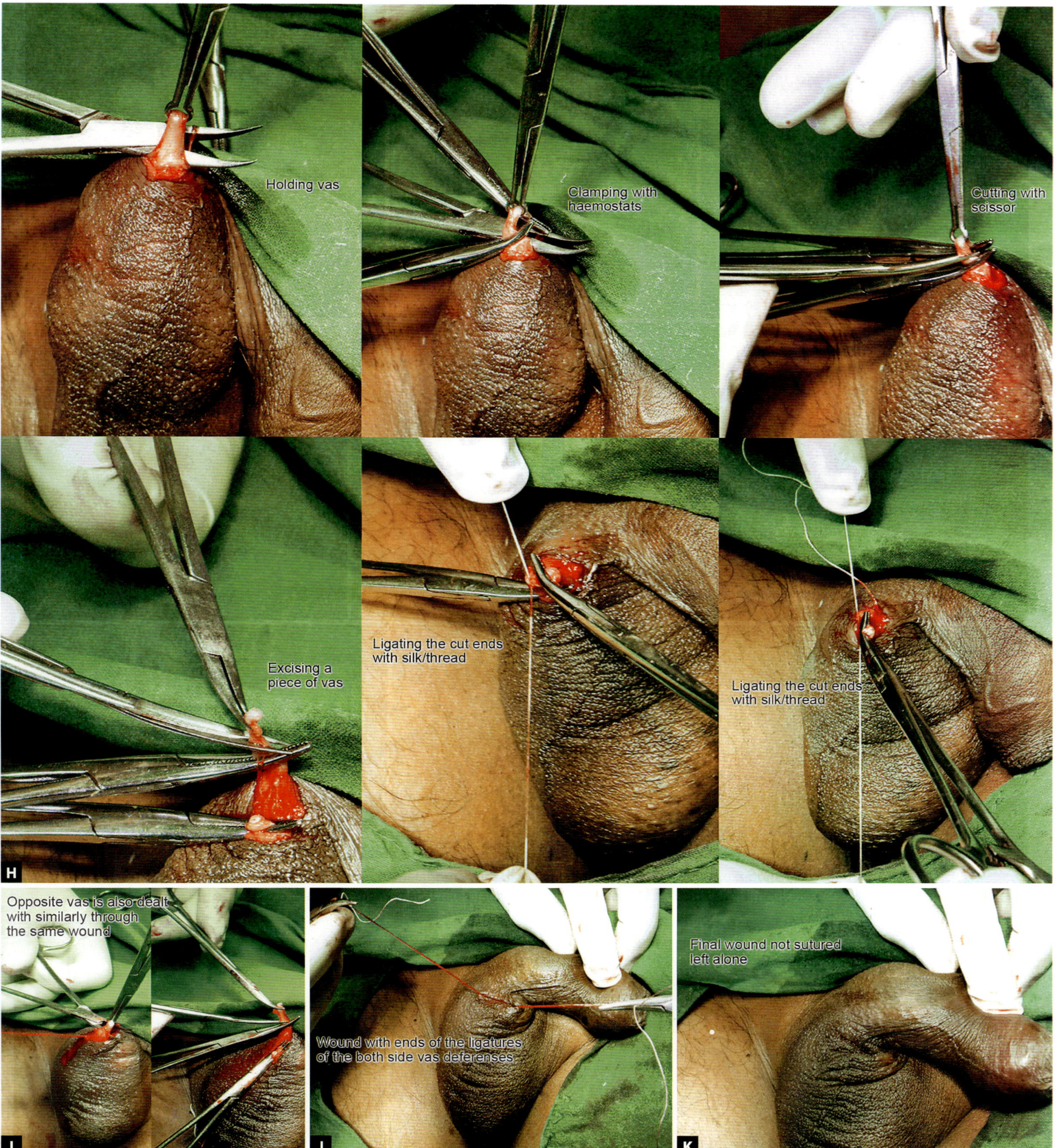

Figs. 7-69H to K

Figs. 7-69A to K: Technique of no scalpel vasectomy—it is done with single incision as sutureless procedure.

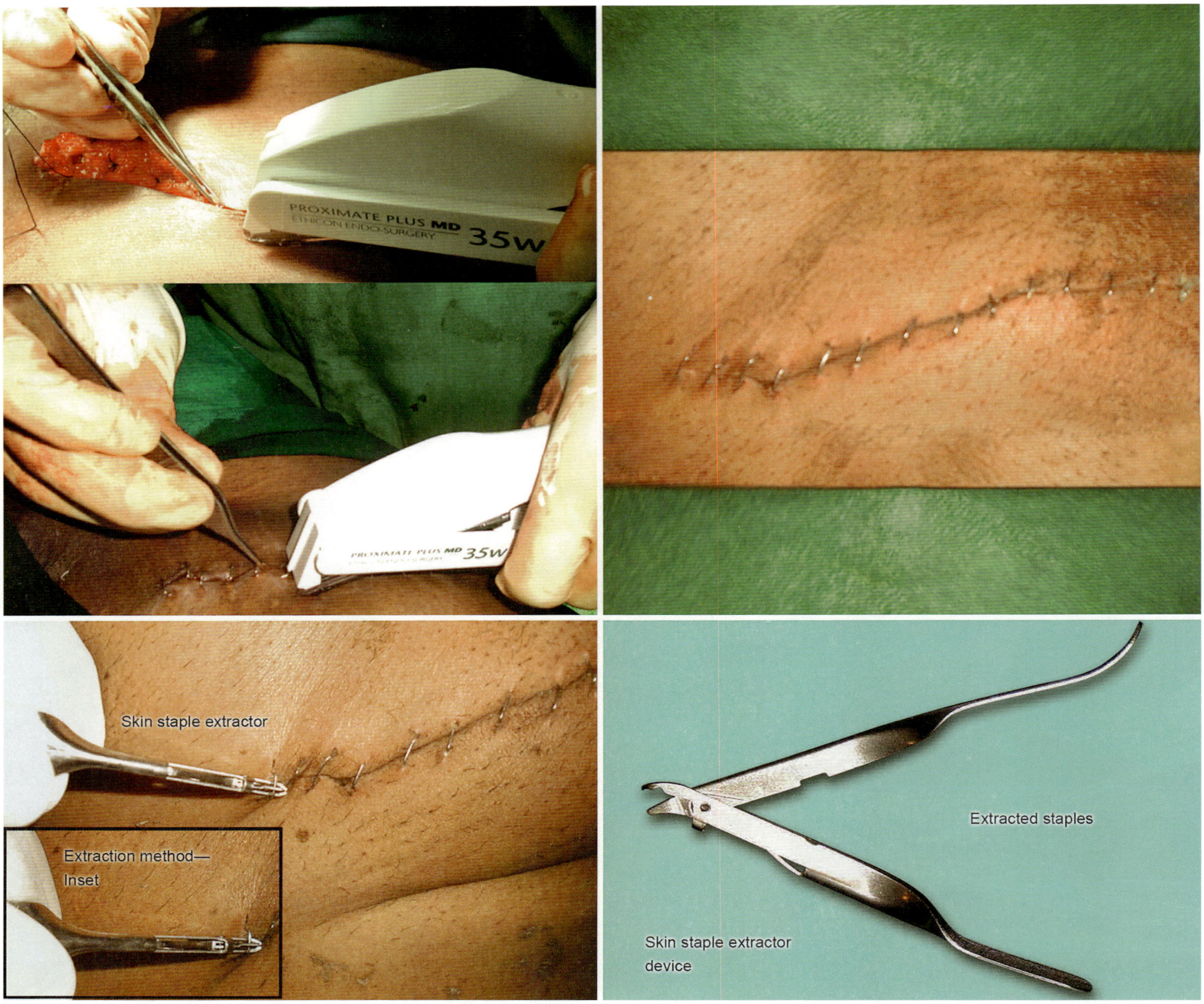

Fig. 7-70: Skin stapler, technique and stapler extraction instrument.

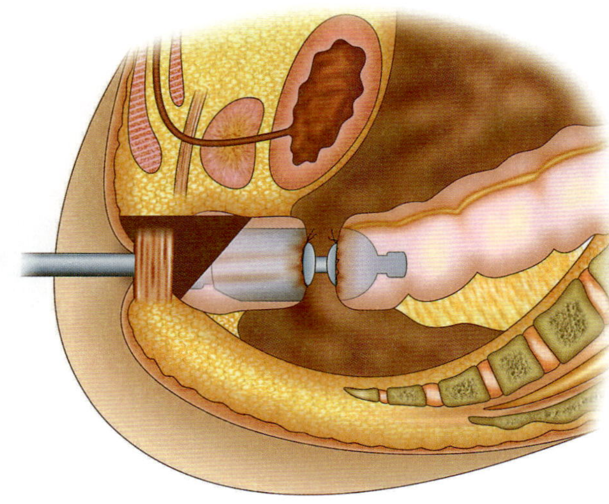

Fig. 7-71: Circular stapler is used for colorectal anastomosis.

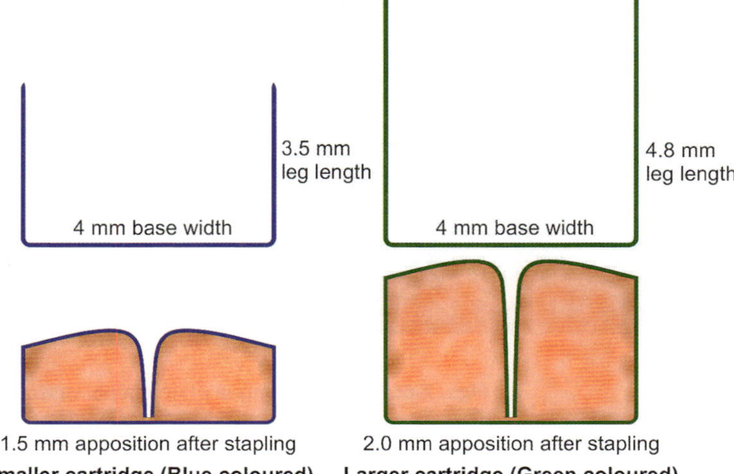

Fig. 7-72: Usually two sized stapler pins are available. 4 mm × 3.5 mm is smaller sized, blue coloured. 4 mm × 4.8 mm is larger sized, green coloured.

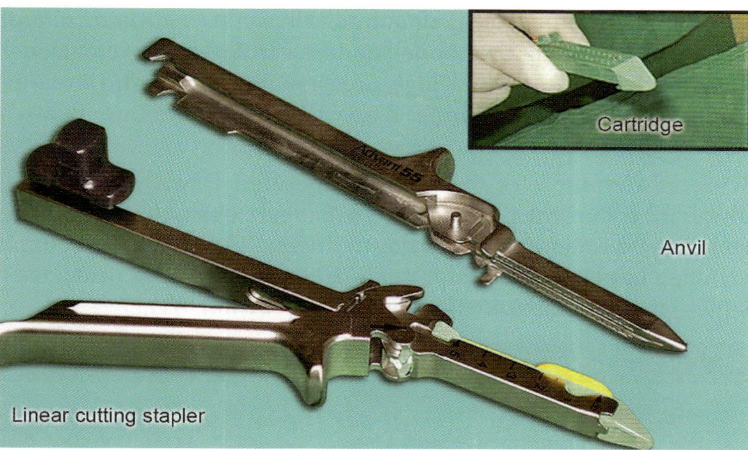

Fig. 7-73: Linear cutting stapler device.

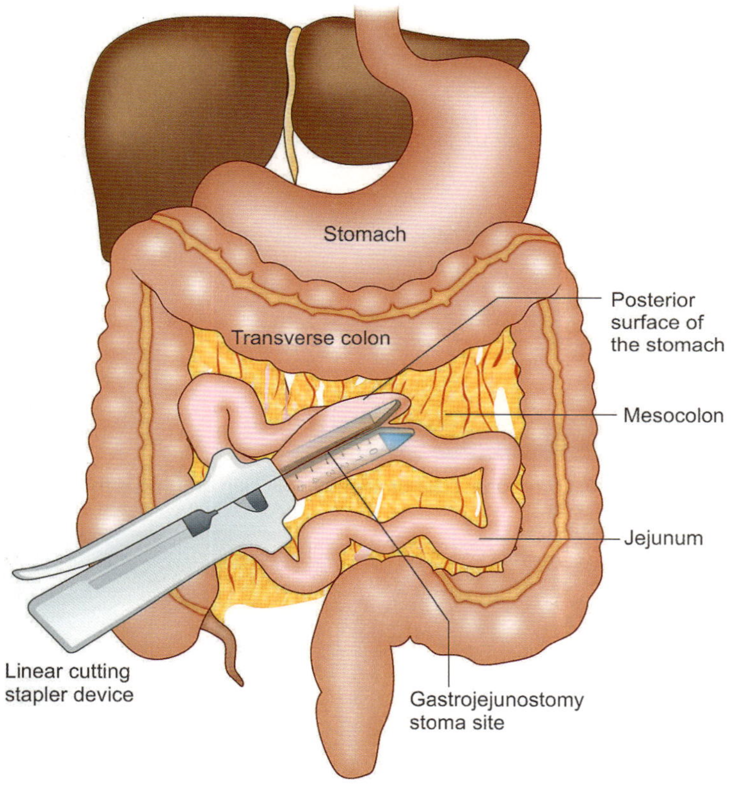

Fig. 7-74: Posterior gastrojejunostomy is being done using linear cutting stapler device.

Linear cutting stapler device is used for cutting and anastomosis simultaneously. Knife within it divides the tissue; cartridge places two rows of staples on either side of the cut tissue. This linear cutting device is used for side to side anastomosis. It is very useful for gastrojejunostomy, colonic anastomosis, pouch creation, etc. Incisions made to pass the blades into bowel parts need to be closed **(Figs. 7-73 and 7-74)**.

Circular Stapling Device

It is used for end to end anastomosis. It creates a two layered stapled anastomosis with inversion, with a circular knife inside the device cutting the tissue between, completing the anastomosis. It is very useful for low colorectal anastomosis after low anterior resection for carcinoma of rectum, sigmoid resection, oesophagogastric/

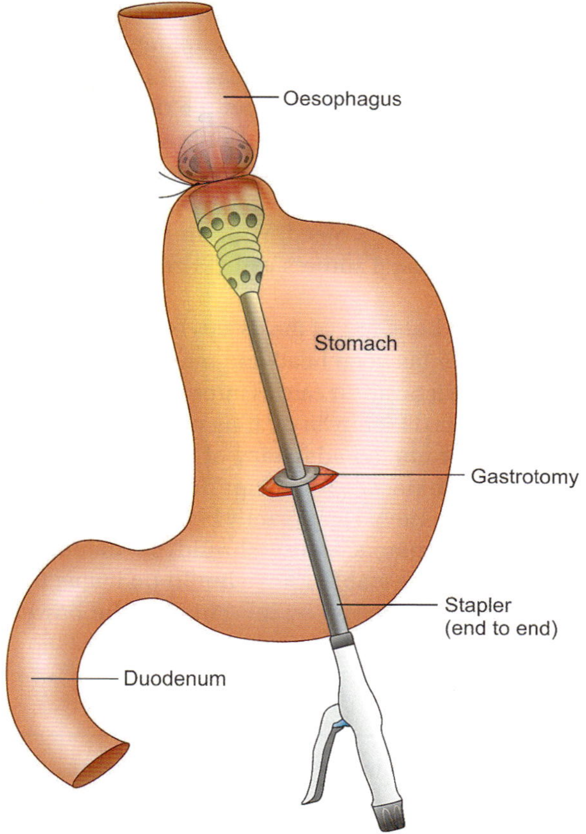

Fig. 7-75: Oesophagogastric anastomosis with resection using end to end circular stapler device.

oesophagojejunal anastomosis, gastroduodenal anastomosis (Billroth I). Device is available at varying sized ranges from 12 to 24 mm. Usually 20 mm is used. Thickness of apposition achieved is usually 2.0 mm. Thickness here can be adjusted in some devices. It has got two parts—head/anvil and cartridge which fires and cuts. Head is inserted into the cut end of the colon in colorectal anastomosis from above **(Fig. 7-75)**. Bowel is firmly fixed into the proximal part of head using purse string suture or using a device called *furnace* through which polypropylene suture is passed. Large main instrument is passed above through the anal canal towards the abdominal cavity. Distal rectal stump is fixed to this using spike in the instrument or by another purse string suture. Care should be taken not to leave excess tissue protruding to prevent incomplete stapling. Two spikes on either side are locked; two parts are apposed; device fired for completing the anastomosis. Device with head is removed through the anus. Doughnut should be carefully removed from the device for inspection for completed circular intact piece which suggests proper anastomosis.

Stapler haemorrhoidopexy (PPH) instrument is a circular stapling device.

Prerequisites for Stapling

- Adequate blood supply in the tissue is the essential part of stapling.
- Thickness of the tissue stapled is also an important factor. Thicker the tissue, more chance of tissue strangulation.
- Selection of the size of cartridge and size of the staple should be proper for ideal stapling result.
- Avoidance of linear tension, if needed few additional supportive seromuscular sutures over stapled line often makes a big difference.

- Technical problems in the instruments which may occur rarely may cause failure in spite of proper stapling. Improper firing of the staples may cause anastomotic leak.
- Often knife in cutting device may cut the tissue partially leading into narrow lumen and obstruction at the anastomotic site.
- Avoid incorporating mesentery or mesenteric fat in the anastomosis.
- After stapling, if there is bleeding point on the staple line one should place additional sutures using 3-zero polyglycolic suture or PDS.
- One should avoid bunching of the tissues between cartridge blades in linear device or between head and main instrument in case of circular device. If it occurs it causes improper stapling and leak.
- Stapled stoma has difficulty in dilating naturally while food/stool passes through it and so adequacy of stoma size is important. In sutured anastomosis, stoma can dilate, accommodate and allow passage of content significantly better.
- Doughnut in circular stapling should be inspected. Entire circumference of the stapled line should be inspected. Lumen patency should be checked by invaginating the bowel into the stoma using index finger.

GRAFT

It is transfer of tissue from one area to another without its blood supply or nerve supply. *Autograft* is tissue transferred from one location to another on the same patient. *Isograft* is tissue transfer between two genetically identical individuals, i.e. between two identical twins. *Allograft* is tissue transfer between two genetically different members, e.g. kidney transplantation. *Xenograft* is tissue transfer from a donor of one species to a recipient of another species. Composite graft is graft with skin, fat and other tissues like cartilage.

Skin Grafting

It is transfer of skin from one area (donor area) to the required defective area (recipient area). It is an autograft.

Ollier's—Thiersch split skin graft is originated in 1872–1886. Wolfe and Krause's full thickness graft started in 1875–1893. Reverdin pinch graft started in 1869.

Punch graft is used for hair transplantation (full thickness graft) and in depigmented skin lesions. Suction blister grafts are used to cover cavities like nostrils, orbits, etc.

Types

1. Partial thickness graft (Split thickness graft, SSG)

It is also called as **Thiersch graft**, which is removal of full epidermis + part of the dermis from the donor area. It may be *thin* SSG, *intermediate* SSG or *thick* SSG—all depends on the amount of thickness of dermis taken. Thick SSG withstands late trauma to recipient area better than thin SSG. It may be thin (0.008 to 0.0012 mm); medium/intermediate (0.0012 to 0.0018 mm); or thick (0.0018 to 0.03 mm) SSG—all depends on thickness of dermis taken. *Indications:* (1) Well-granulated ulcer. (2) Clean wound or defect which cannot be apposed. (3) After surgery to cover and close the defect created, e.g. after wide excision in malignancy, after mastectomy, after wide excision of squamous cell carcinoma, etc. Graft can survive over periosteum or paratenon or perichondrium. *Prerequisites:* (1) Healthy granulation area. (2) Streptococci load less than 10^5 per gram of tissue, otherwise graft failure will occur. *Contraindications:* SSG cannot be done over bone, tendon, cartilage, joint, etc. *Donor areas used are*—commonly *thigh,* occasionally arm, leg and forearm. Knife used is *Humby's Knife*. Blade is *Eschmann blade*, Down's blade **(Figs. 7-76 to 7-80)**.

Powered dermatomes like battery-operated Davol dermatome, alternating current (AC) operated Padgett dermatome and the compressed water pumped nitrogen driven Zimmer air dermatome are often used to harvest large grafts. Humby knife, Weck blade, Blair knife—are other instruments used **(Figs. 7-81 to 7-84)**.

Different instruments used to harvest the skin graft

- Humby knife.
- Watson modification of Humby knife.
- Power dermatome is also used (Brown).
- Sterilised razor blade can be used with a specialised device to harvest small grafts under local anaesthesia—Silver knife.

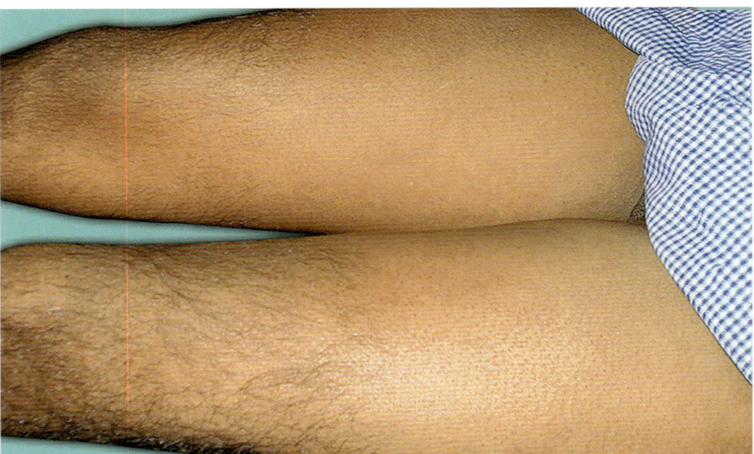

Fig. 7-76: Commonest donor area for spilt skin grafting is thigh.

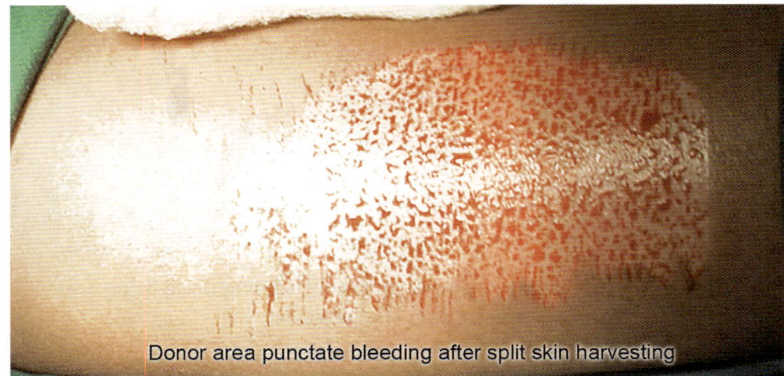

Fig. 7-77: Donor area of split skin graft immediately after harvesting graft showing punctate bleeding.

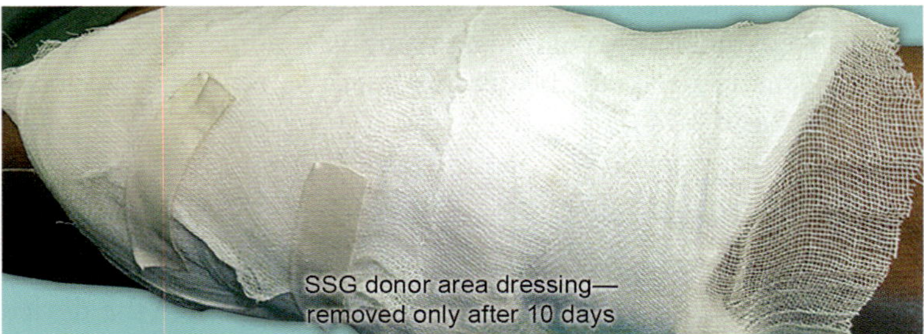

Fig. 7-78: Donor area dressing is not removed for 10 days. If soakage is observed an over dressing is done on earlier dressing without removing it.

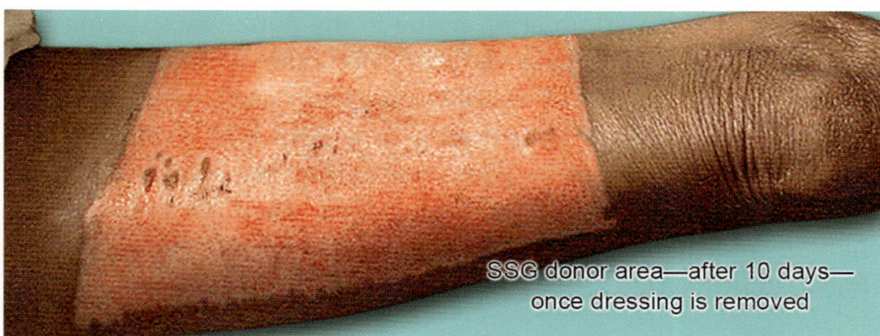

Fig. 7-79: Split skin graft donor area—10 days after removal of the dressing. Dressing from donor area is removed only after 10 days and left open after that.

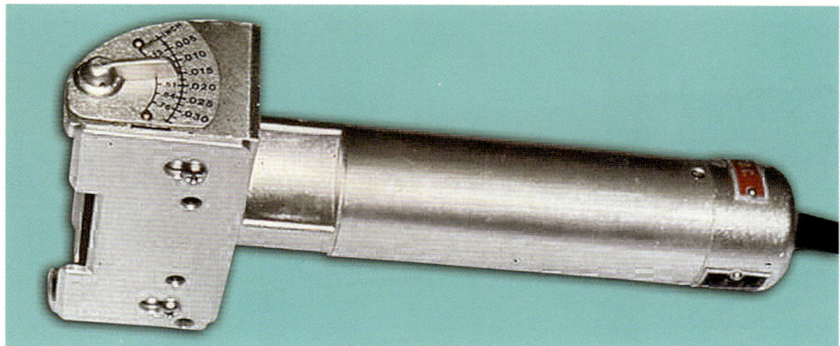

Fig. 7-82: Padgett dermatome.

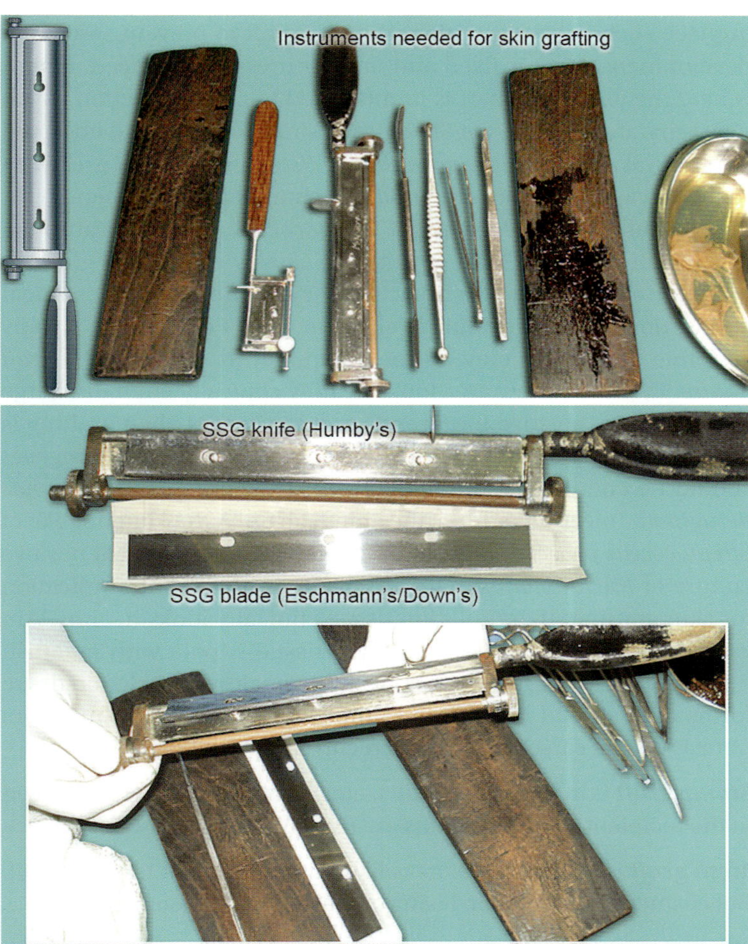

Fig. 7-80: Instruments needed for split (Thiersch) skin grafting. Humby's knife, Eschmann blade; skin spreader; wooden boards; scoop; kidney tray; saline to keep harvested split skin; forceps; scissors.

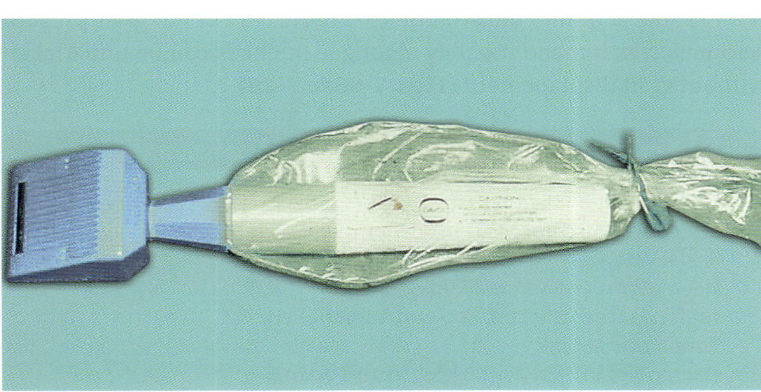

Fig. 7-81: Davol dermatome.

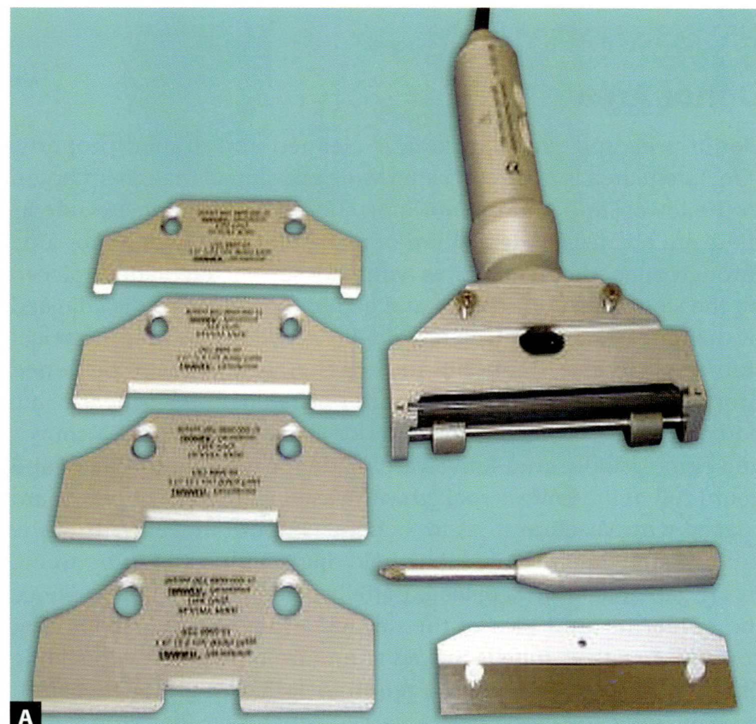

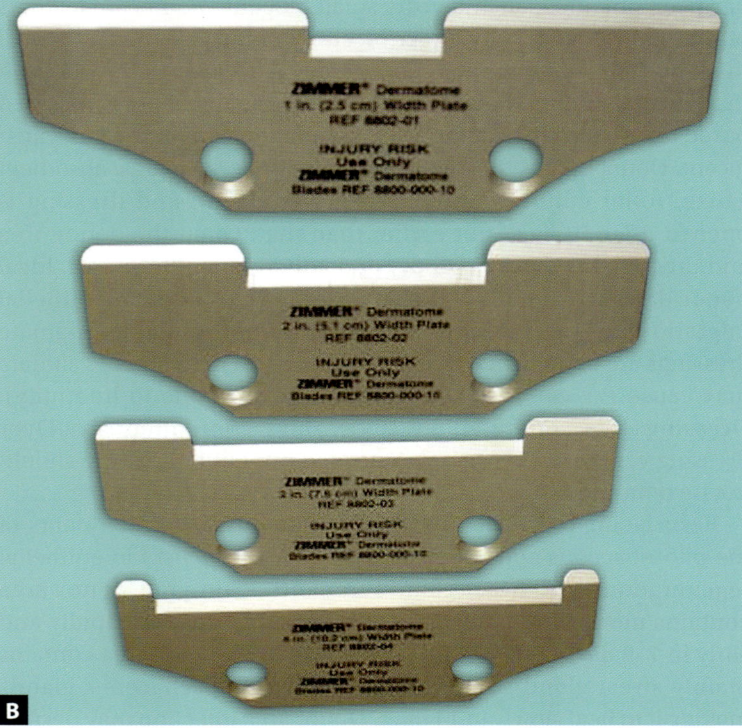

Figs. 7-83A and B: Zimmer's dermatome and guard.

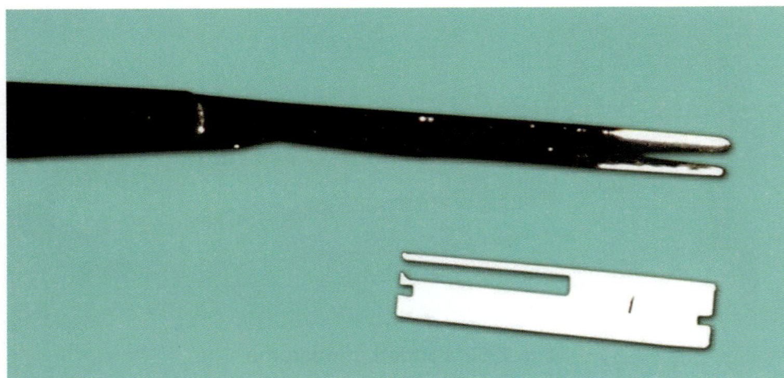

Fig. 7-84: Weck's skin grafting knife.

Donor Area

Donor area and recipient area is cleaned and draped properly. If recipient area is a raw area after wide excision of malignant lesion in the lower limb, then donor area should be on opposite side as there are chances of deposition of malignant cells over donor area through opened up cutaneous lymphatics. Selected blade is placed on the slot of the knife. Blade and gap in the sliding rod is adjusted by markings on the knob on the handle. Markings are made to select thin/intermediate/thick split thickness graft. Knobs are tightened properly. Assistant holds the thigh on its posterior aspect using both his hands firmly making anterior aspect or donor area convex and firm. Usually graft knives are made for right hand. Blade and guard rod of the knife is soaked with Vaseline. Using wooden board soaked with Vaseline so as to facilitate smooth movements of the boards, stretched donor skin is held apart with a gap in between. In the gap graft knife is placed. Initially blade is deepened to pierce the epidermis and part of the dermis and with continuous firm constant pressure knife is moved to and fro repeatedly with sliding progressively forward to get a required split skin graft. Once graft is taken, *punctate bleeding* is observed which says that proper graft has been obtained. High density small bleeding points are features of thin graft; low density larger bleeding points are the features of thick graft. In the thigh, lateral and distal area gives thicker graft than medial and proximal. Clinically on table thickness is assessed based on translucency of the graft. Thinner the graft more it is translucent. Donor area is dressed (using Sofra-Tulle/bactigras, absorbent gauze, roller cotton, crepe bandage/bandage), and dressing is opened *after 10 days*, not earlier than that. Often the donor area and dressing becomes hard, dry and adherent to donor area. Ideal donor dressing should be moist, absorbent to promote epithelial migration but such aseptic dressings are not available. Alginate dressings are better when available (Moist area in temperate climate may cause *Pseudomonas aeruginosa* infection due to humidity). Dressing gets separated in 10–12 days spontaneously. Over dressing can be done whenever needed but entire dressing should not be removed.

Resurfacing of the donor area occurs on its own. Remnants of the pilosebaceous apparatus are the *active component* in epithelial regeneration than sweat gland remnants. Thin graft donor area contains more pilosebaceous glands making it to heal rapidly and early in 7–9 days; whereas thick split skin graft donor area contains mainly sweat gland components with less pilosebaceous glands making it to heal slowly in 14 days. Donor area infection may destroy the pilosebaceous or sweat gland remnants causing inability to resurface leaving a granulation tissue in the floor. Once donor area dressing is removed healing raw area is left open with application of emollients/oil for 4 weeks. *Problems in donor area*—post-operative pain is more in donor area than in recipient bed. Pain subsides in 5–7 days. Deep raw area when not epithelialised leave an ulcer which may require regular dressing later. Pigmentation, colour changes and hypertrophic scar formation are the usual problems **(Figs. 7-85A to H)**.

Recipient Area

Recipient area is scraped well and graft is placed after making *window cuts* (fenestrations with multiple cuts; it is not mandatory to place such cuts; it is optional) in the graft to prevent seroma of development. Graft is fixed and *tie-over* dressing is placed. If graft is near the joint, then part is immobilised to prevent friction which may separate the graft. On *5th day* dressing is opened and observed for graft take up. *Healthy granulation tissue* in recipient area with red, flat, vascular look with good marginal healing is essential for proper graft take up. Presence of *Streptococcus pyogenes* is absolute contraindication for skin grafting. It causes gelatinous glaze in granulation tissue. Slough excision, systemic antibiotics, local application of chlorhexidine is effective way of eradicating it (only systemic antibiotics may not be adequate). It causes *100% graft failure*. Even when raw area looks healthy clinically but if discharge culture shows positive for *Streptococcus pyogenes*, then grafting is contraindicated as graft will not take up. *Streptococcus pyogenes* should be completely eliminated prior to grafting. *Pseudomonas aeruginosa* infection reduces the graft take up by *10%* but not like of *Streptococcus pyogenes* infection. One has to remember that positive culture of *Pseudomonas* in the discharge is not a contraindication for skin grafting. If granulation tissue clinically looks healthy skin grafting can be done. If granulation tissue is pale with greenish discharge then grafting is not done. Once healthy granulation tissue forms area should be grafted at the earliest otherwise infection, fibrosis of area can occur causing recurrent problems.

Stamp graft is in perineum, axilla, etc. It is small-sized grafts placed in the recipient bed. Such grafts are usually not fixed.

Mesh graft is used in wide areas like burn wounds. It takes up well. But cosmetically it is poor. Fixing of mesh is cumbersome.

Quilted grafting: It is commonly used in places where immobilisation is impossible like in oral cavity (cheek) and tongue after wide excision. Split skin graft is placed over the defect. Edge is sutured to the margin of the defect. Multiple additional sutures are placed through the graft to the muscle underneath to anchor both together. It looks like a 'quilt.' Fenestrations/window cuts in the graft prevent seroma formation and mobility of tongue or cheek can be undertaken without graft displacement **(Figs. 7-86 to 7-89)**.

Causes for poor graft take up/contraindications for skin grafting

- Unhealthy granulation tissue.
- Infection—*Streptococcus pyogenes* mainly, *Pseudomonas aeruginosa* less severely.
- Haematoma and seroma formation.
- Graft over the joint surface—not immobilised.
- Poor blood supply.
- Haemoglobin of patient if less than 10 gram%.
- Poor nutrition, hypoalbuminaemia (Albumin level less than 3 gram %).

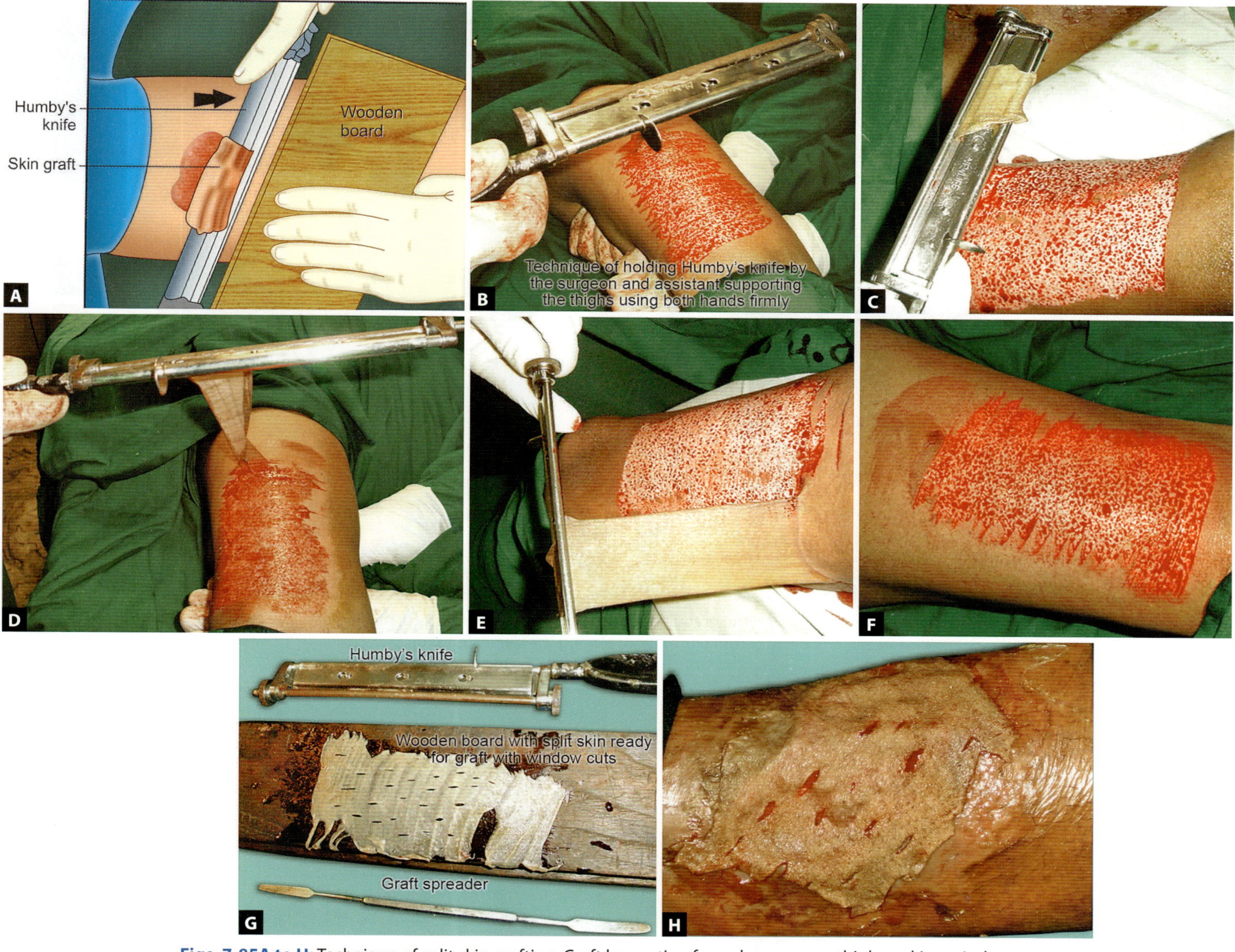

Figs. 7-85A to H: Technique of split skin grafting. Graft harvesting from donor area—thigh; making window cuts; placing graft over recipient area.

Graft Application and Stabilisation

Applied graft is stabilised into the recipient bed by various methods (or dressings). They are:

Bolus dressing/bolus grafting: If there is ooze and chances of haematoma or seroma formation, commonly observed over granulation tissue, then pressure dressing is used. It is done using 'tie over' dressing and crepe bandaging. Tie over dressing over a graft is called as *bolus grafting*. Crepe bandage over 'tie over' gives immobilisation and additional pressure. In full thickness grafting, graft edge is properly apposed exactly over the recipient area without any overlapping. Few sutures, all round are kept long to place tie over. In split thickness grafting graft is kept *overlapping over the defect* and tied over from the defect edge. Overlapped skin is trimmed during graft inspection on 5th post-operative day. After placing the tie over sutures all round the edge, tulle gras layer is applied. Later bolus material consisting of cotton soaked in saline dilute povidone iodine or cotton soaked in liquid paraffin or polyurethane or flavine wool material (flavine emulsion, Gamgee, cotton wool are used here. Cotton wool sheet is soaked with warmed flavine emulsion to impregnate over it and Gamgee is placed over it, dried and autoclaved) placed firmly. Long sutures tied over it at different places. Further cotton roll is placed over it. Roller bandaging and crepe bandaging is done over it to diffuse equal effective pressure and also immobilisation. Bolus grafting is used in limbs and face. It is often difficult to place in trunks and groin. *Tie over also can be* achieved in limbs by placing continuous circular ties circumferentially over the dressing pads kept on the graft. It is quicker and easier. It does not require placement of any sutures over the edge **(Fig. 7-90)**.

Exposed grafting: It is often used in trunk and groin. By exposed method shearing movements between recipient bed and graft are prevented. Here natural fibrin formation prevents to and fro movement between bed and graft. Exposed grafting is used mainly in raw area created after excision of a lesion wherein haemostasis is

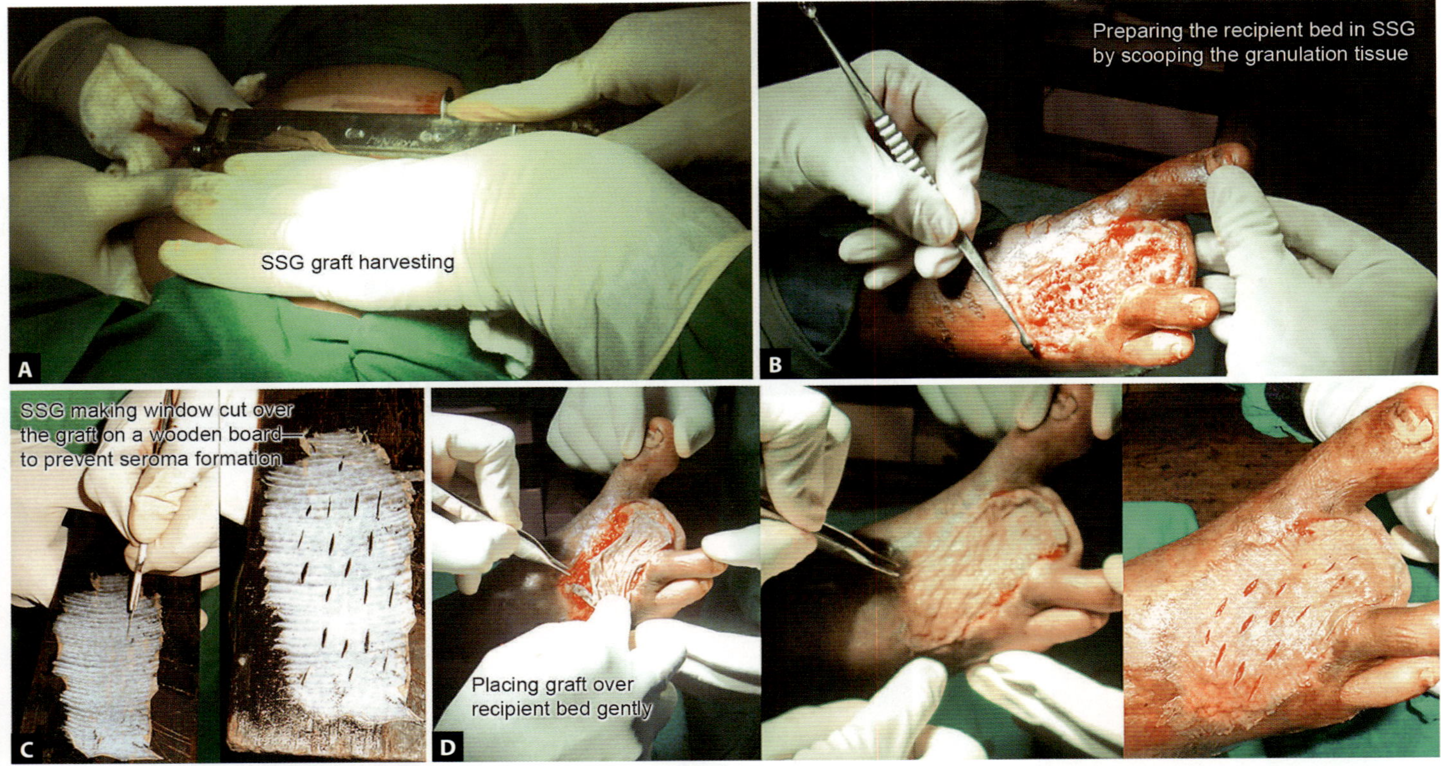

Figs. 7-86A to D: Harvesting skin graft; scooping the granulation tissue from the recipient bed; making window cuts over the graft to prevent seroma formation; placing the harvested skin.

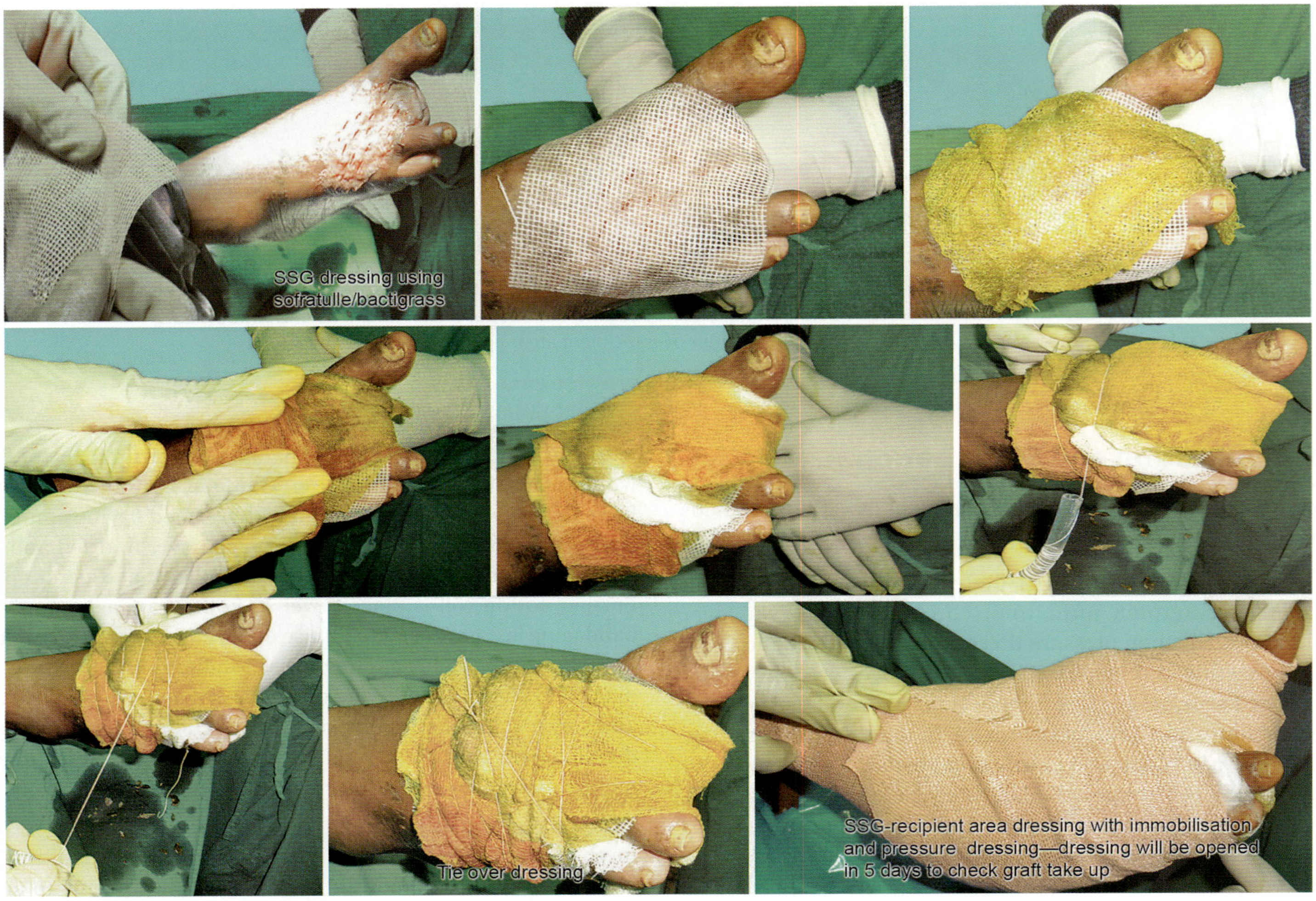

Fig. 7-87: Split skin grafting and covering the grafted area with sofratulle, povidone iodine soaked dressing pads, tie over dressing, bandaging, crepe bandage or immobilisation using plaster of Paris slab/cast.

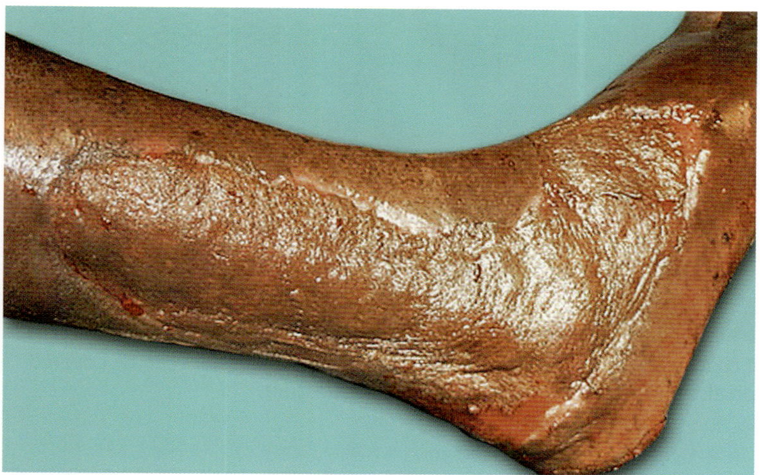

Fig. 7-88: Split skin graft in the leg—taken up well observed in 5 days.

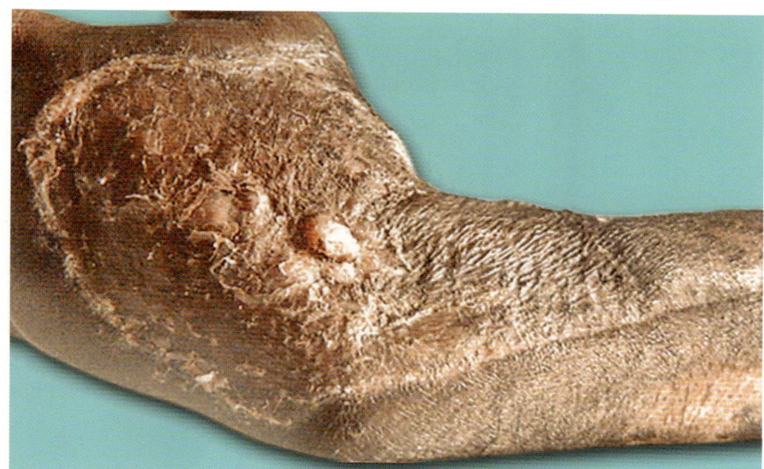

Fig. 7-89: Split skin grafting taken up which is observed after one month.

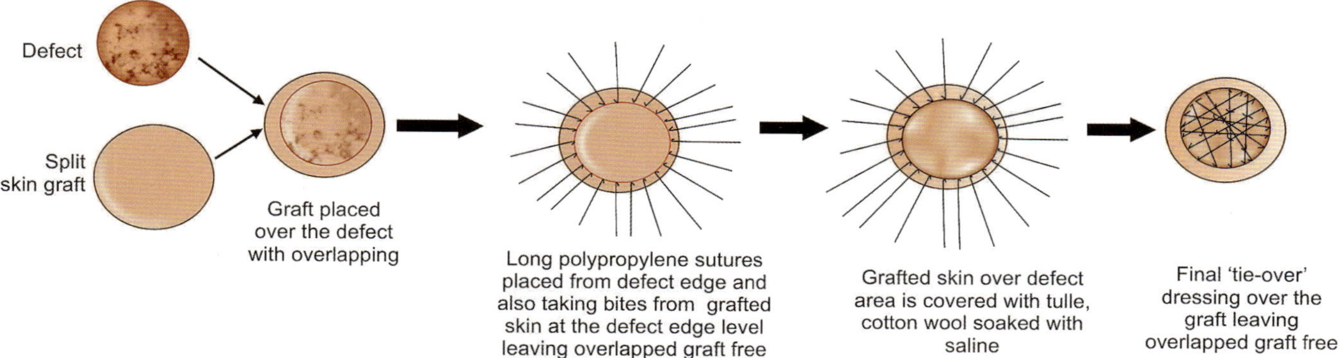

Fig. 7-90: 'Tie-over' dressing after split skin grafting.

achieved properly by cautery or ligation. Often after initial excision of the lesion, dressing is done for 48 hours and then graft is placed with *delayed exposed grafting.* As haematoma and seroma formation *cannot* be prevented in this method it is not usually used in ulcer bed. Patient cooperation is essential in this type of graft management. This method is useful for single safe surface. It is not useful in circumferential or wide raw areas.

Stages of Graft Intake

Stage of Plasmatic imbibition: Thin, uniform, layer of plasma and fibrin forms between recipient bed and graft.

Stage of inosculation: Linking of host and graft which is temporary.

Stage of neovascularisation: New capillaries proliferate into graft from the recipient bed which attains circulation later.

Disadvantages of SSG

(1) Contracture of the graft—it is of two types: (A) *Primary contracture* means SSG contracts significantly once graft is taken from donor area (20–30%). Thicker the graft more is the primary contracture. (B) *Secondary contracture* occurs after graft has taken up to recipient bed during healing period, due to fibrosis. Thinner the graft more is the secondary contracture. (2) Seroma and haematoma formation will prevent graft take up. (3) Infection. (4) Loss of hair growth, blunting of sensation. (5) Dry, scaling of skin due to non-functioning of sebaceous glands. So after healing oil (coconut oil) should be applied over the area. (6) Graft failure.

Advantages

(1) It is technically easier. (2) Wide area of recipient can be covered. To cover large area like burns wound, graft size is increased by passing the graft through a ***Mesher*** which gives multiple openings to the graft which can be stretched on the wider area like a net. It can cause expansion up to 6 times. (3) Graft take up is better. (4) Donor area heals on its own **(Figs. 7-91 and 7-92)**.

Note:
Graft can be stored in low temperature 4°C for up to 21 days. It is stored in normal saline. But usually it is not used beyond 10 days.

Full Thickness Graft (Wolfe Graft)

It includes both epidermis + entire dermis. It is used over the face, hands, fingers, over the joints or for small defects like ectropion, eyelid/nasal/cheek defects and deformities, injury and contractures of fingers, syndactyly. It is removed using scalpel blade. Underlying *fat should be cleared* off properly. No epidermal elements are found in left out donor area. So resurfacing of the donor area cannot take place on its own. Deeper raw area is closed by primary suturing. If larger area is taken then that donor area has to be covered

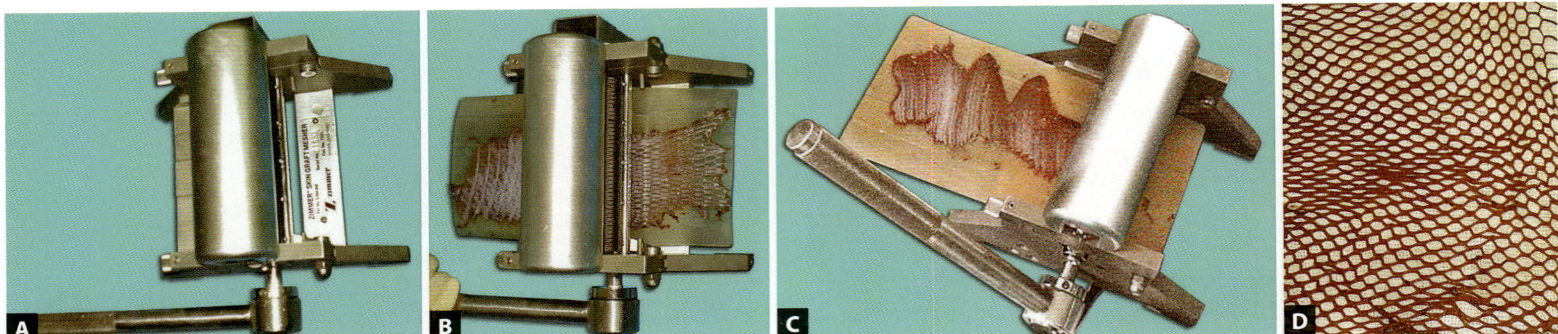

Figs. 7-91A to D: Mesher used in split skin grafting to increase its surface area of coverage for wider areas like burns wound. A large defect can be covered by this. It can cause expansion up to six times. Photograph also shows exact look of meshed split skin graft.

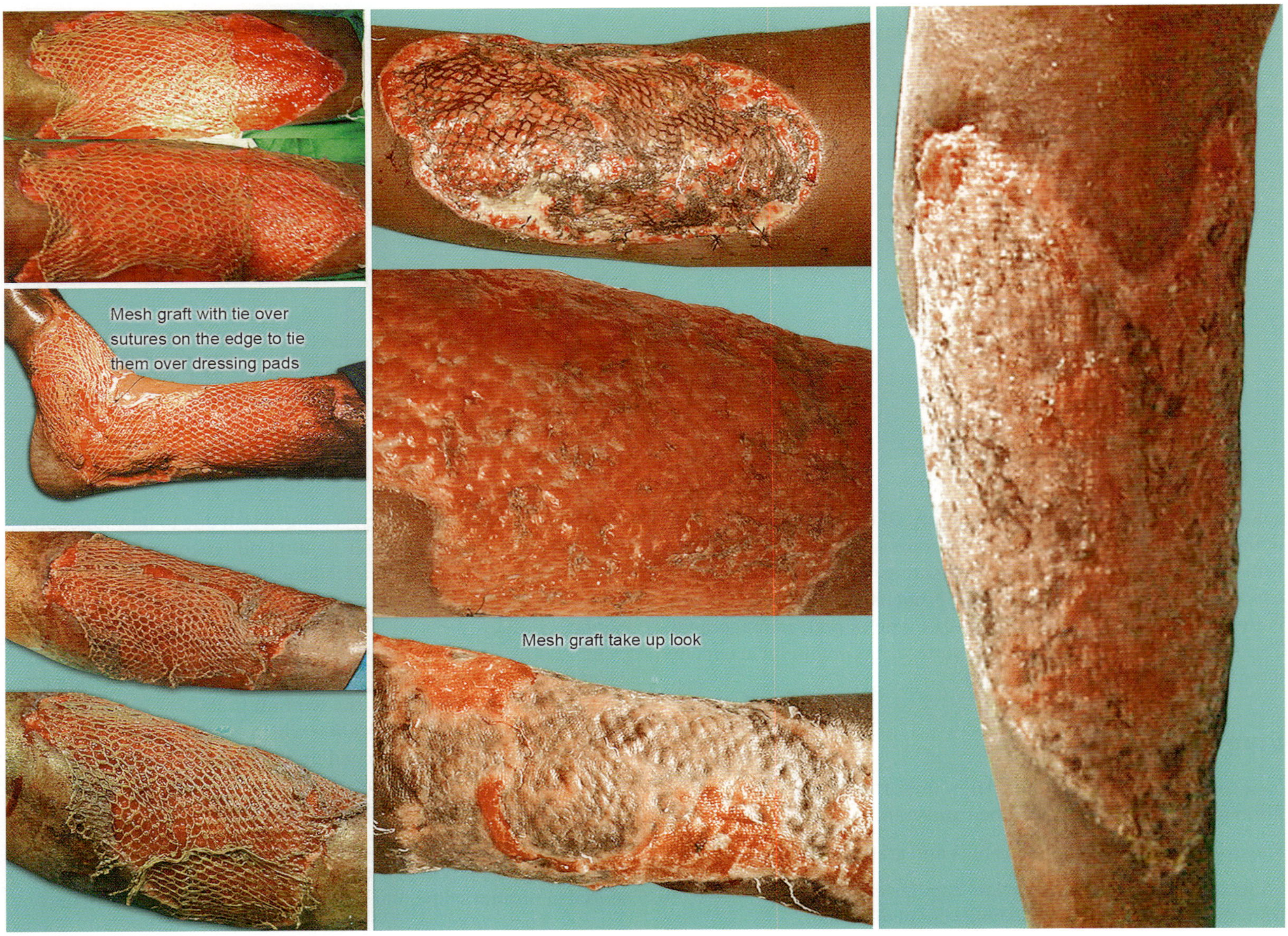

Fig. 7-92: Mesh grafts placed over donor areas and their take up look.

with SSG which is a disadvantage in full thickness graft. Defect and donor site of required size should be marked using Bonney's blue properly. Size matching is important. Area may be infiltrated with normal saline with or without 1 in 2,00,000 noradrenaline to balloon the skin which will facilitate the raising of the graft. While raising the graft using blade, with skin hooks, the edge of the graft should be held. Full thickness graft has got colour and look of cadaver skin. Graft edge is properly apposed exactly over the recipient area without any overlapping. Few of sutures all round are kept long to place tie over. Tie-over dressing is a must in full thickness graft. Common sites of donor area are—(1) Post-auricular area. (2) Supraclavicular area. (3) Other areas like—infraclavicular, lateral groin, upper eyelid part, antecubital fossa, inframammary area in females often also used **(Figs. 7-93 to 7-95)**.

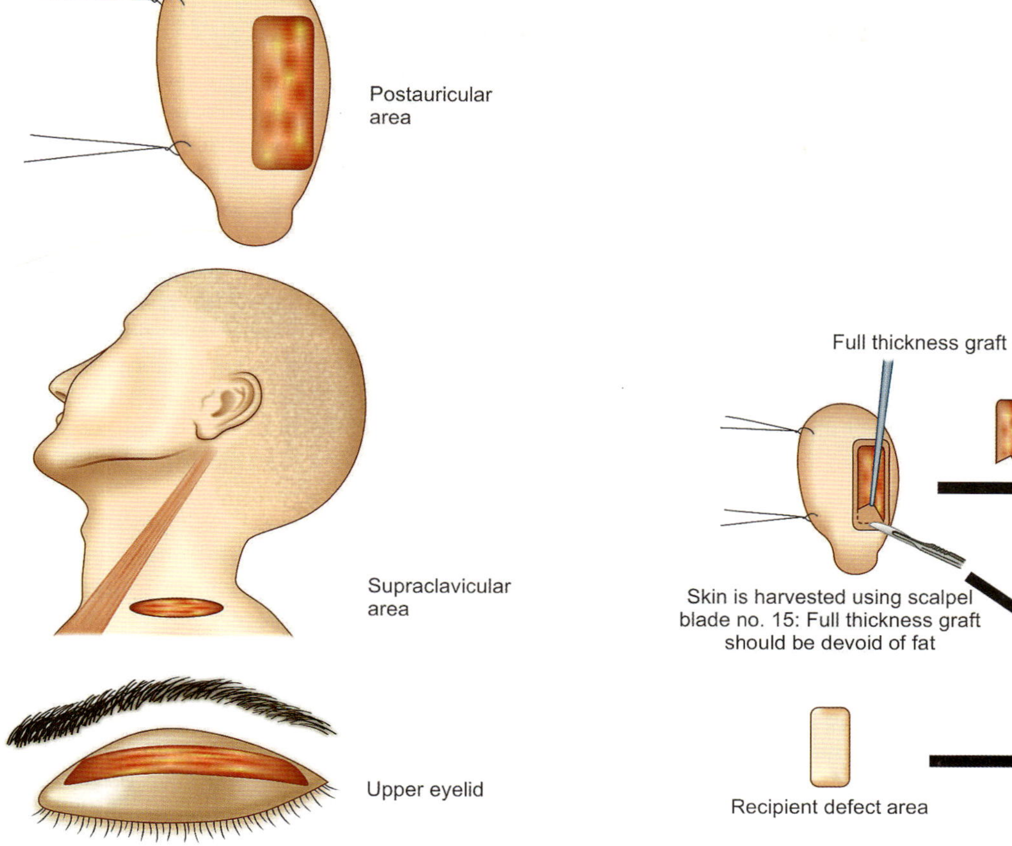

Fig. 7-93: Common donor areas for Wolfe graft.

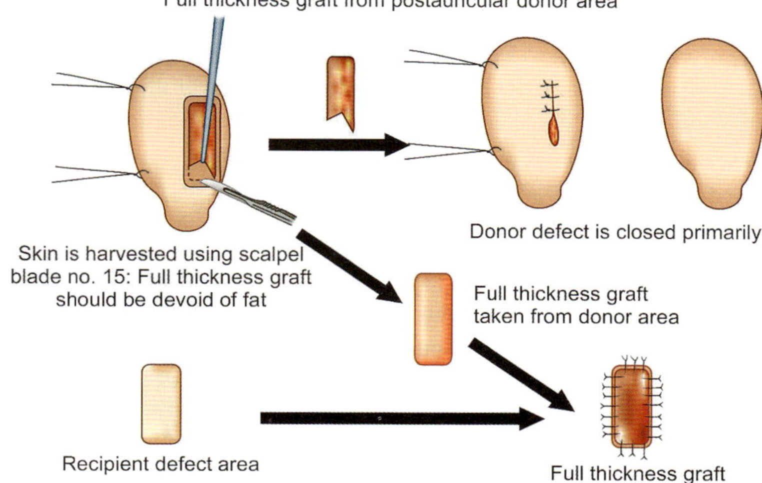

Fig. 7-94: Technique of Wolfe—full thickness graft.

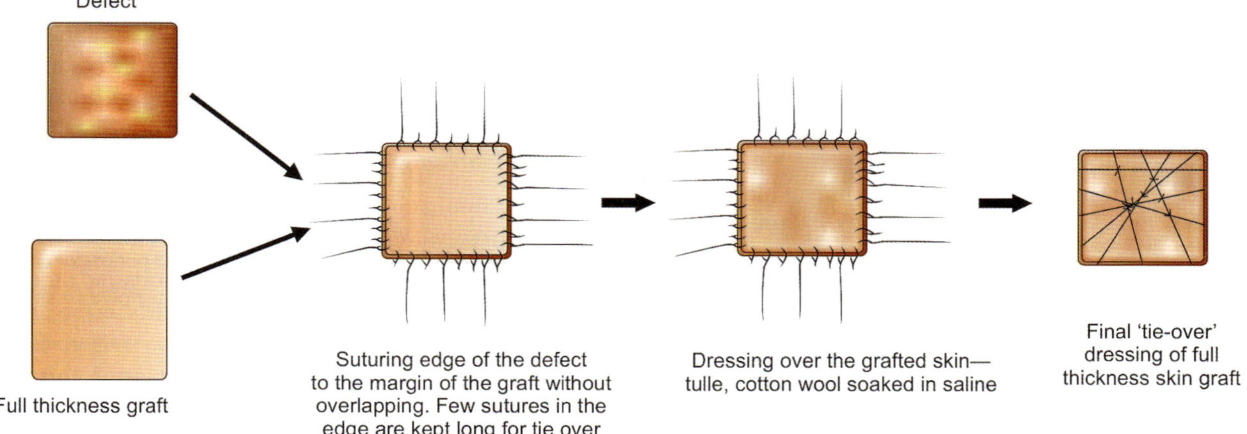

Fig. 7-95: 'Tie-over' dressing for Wolfe graft (full thickness graft).

Advantages

(1) Colour match is good especially for face. (2) No contracture (unlike in SSG) and so remains in its original size. (3) Sensation, functions of sebaceous glands, hair follicles are retained better compared to SSG. Texture, colour, durability is better.

Disadvantages

(1) Only for small area it can be used. (2) Wider donor area has to be covered with SSG to close the defect. (3) It cannot be used to cover ulcers.

FLAPS

Flaps are transfer of tissues from one area to another with their blood supply.

It is transfer of donor tissue with its blood supply to the recipient area.

Parts of flaps: Base, pedicle, tip of flap. Vasculature is usually through the pedicle in the centre of the flap. Tip is the place where often flap goes for necrosis **(Figs. 7-96A to C)**.

Congruity, configuration, components, circulation, conditioning are the *different aspects* of the flap.

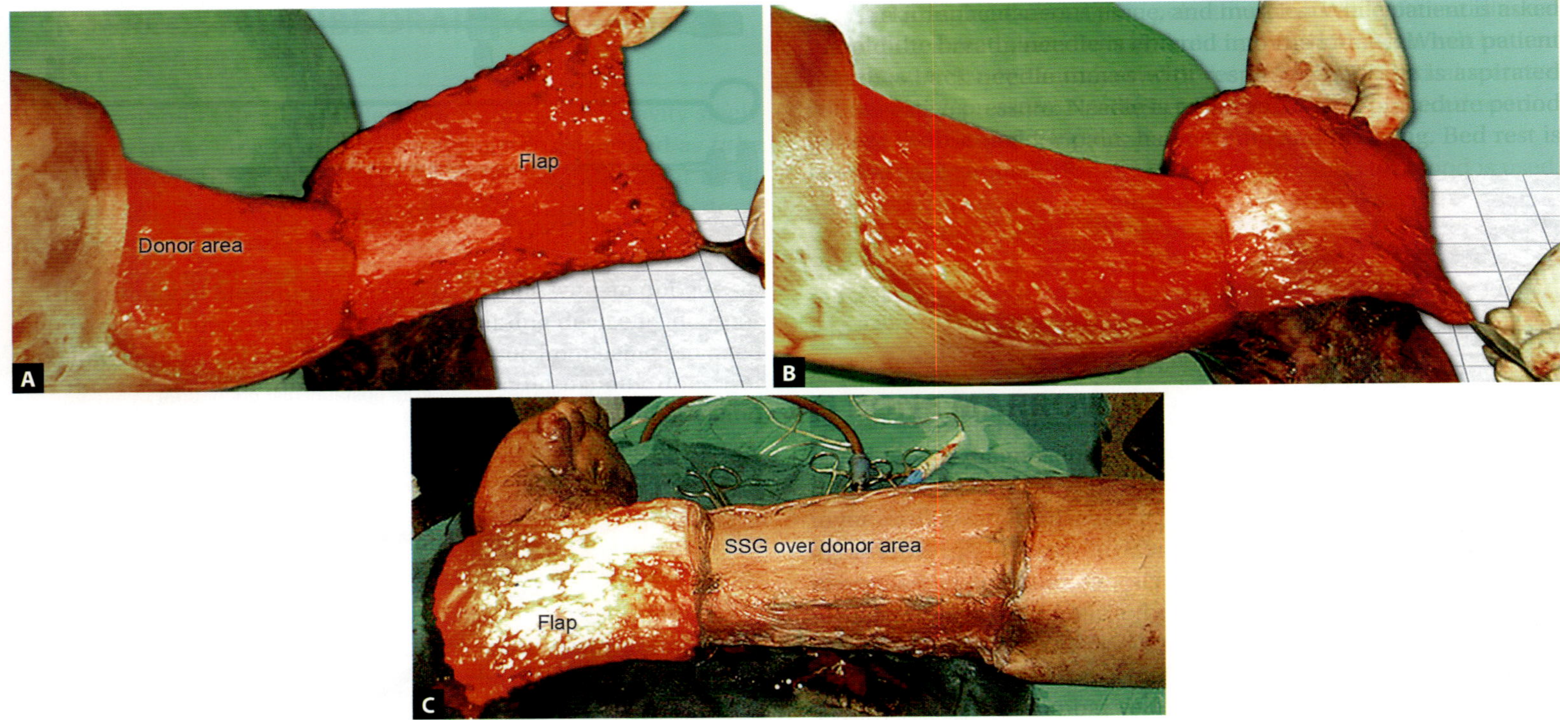

Figs. 7-96A to C: Typical flap, method of raising it; and donor area being wide is covered with split skin graft.

Indications

(1) To cover the wider, deeper defects. (2) To cover over bone, tendon, cartilage. (3) If skin graft repeatedly fails.

Types

(1) *Random pattern flaps:* Here vascular basis is subdermal plexus of blood vessels. Known blood supply is not present. It is usually a rectangular flap with length to width ratio is ***1:1*** or 1.5:1. This flap has got limitations in its dimensions. (2) *Axial pattern flaps:* Here superficial vascular pedicles pass along their long axes, e.g. forehead flap, deltopectoral flap, groin flap. A known anatomical blood vessel supplies the flap. It is *long lengthy* flap **(Figs. 7-97 to 7-100)**.

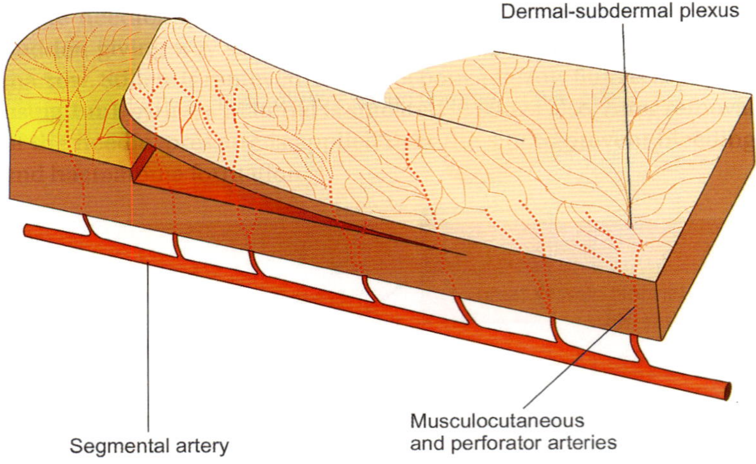

Fig. 7-97: Anatomy and blood supply of a skin flap.

Anatomical Types Depending on the Types of Tissue in the Flap

(1) Cutaneous flap: Forehead flap, deltopectoral flap. (2) Fasciocutaneous flap: Radial forearm flap, scapular flap, lateral arm flap. (3) Muscle flap: Gluteus maximus muscle flap, gracilis flap, tensor fascia lata muscle flap. (4) Myocutaneous flap: Pectoralis major myocutaneous flap, latissimus dorsi flap. (5) Osteomyocutaneous flaps: Radius with brachioradialis and skin; rib with intercostal muscles and skin. (6) Local rotation flaps. (7) 'Z' plasty. (8) Free flaps: Vascular pedicle of the flap both artery and vein are anastomosed to recipient vessels using operating binocular microscopes. (9) Omental flaps. (10) Island flap **(Figs. 7-101 and 7-102)**.

Areas where Commonly Flaps are Used

Oral cavity, neck, breast, limbs (leg), buttock, bedsores, etc.

Flaps mobilised from donor area with its pedicle is placed and sutured to recipient area. Once flap gets taken up usually in 3–6 weeks, base of the flap is cut and sutured to recipient area.

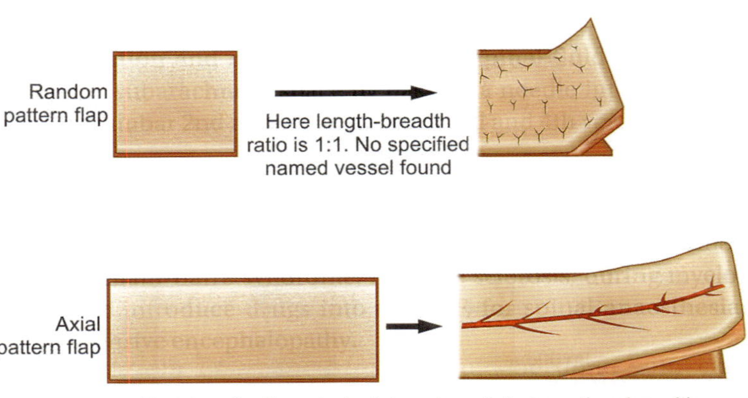

Fig. 7-98: Types flap based on vascular pattern—random pattern and axial pattern.

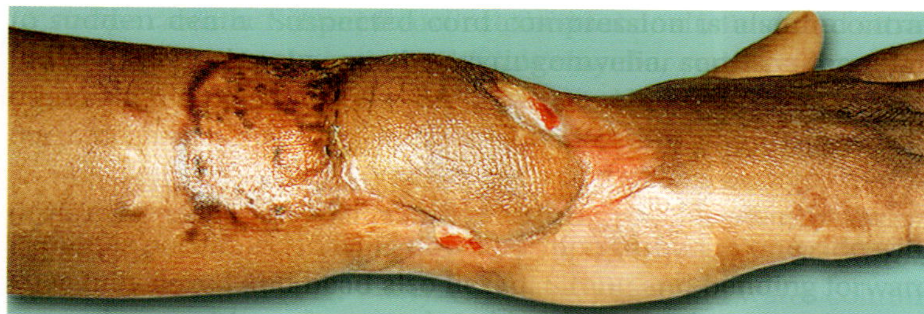

Fig. 7-99: Flap which has taken up well placed over the defect on the bone with osteomyelitis.

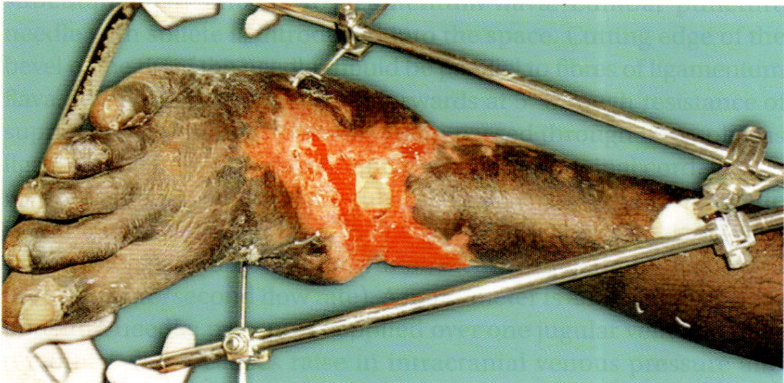

Fig. 7-100: Traumatic exposure of the bone. Flap is needed to cover this defect. It could be cross leg flap or rotation flap. Skin grafting is not possible in this situation.

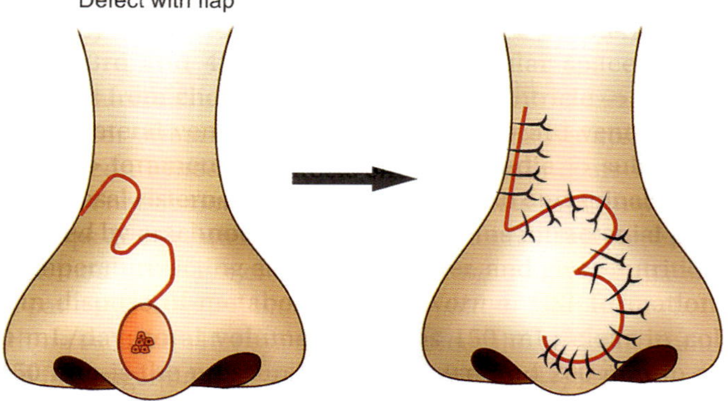

Fig. 7-101: Bilobed flap is used in lesions of the nose commonly.

Saltatory flap is mobilising the flaps in stages from distant donor area towards recipient area. It requires many staged surgeries and long-term hospitalisation. Intermediate tissue is used as '***carrier***' **(Figs. 7-103 and 7-104)**.

Advantages of Flaps

(1) Good blood supply, good take up. (2) It gives bulk, texture, and colour to the area. (3) Allowing the required movements in the recipient area, e.g. jaw movements after pectoralis major flap following wide excision with hemimandibulectomy for carcinoma cheek. (4) Cosmetically better.

Disadvantages of Flaps

(1) Long-term hospitalisation is needed. (2) Infection. (3) Kinking, rotation and flap necrosis. (4) Staged procedure.

Positioning of the patient for long time is important to have a good flap take up which is a real discomfort to the patient.

Waltzing is a technique wherein flap is moved from donor area and attached adjacent to the recipient defect area. Later in 2nd stage it is moved towards the defect formally. It reduces the tension on the flap and increases the success rate **(Fig. 7-105)**.

Delaying of the Flap/Conditioning the Flap

Flap is raised properly as required and re-sutured to same place so as to allow the formation of reorientation of vasculature near the tip of the flap. *This delayed flap* is raised again in 10–14 days to place in required area. It is used both in random pattern as well as axial pattern flap. In random pattern flap delay improves the length-breadth ratio. In axial pattern flap, delaying enhances the blood flow across the distal attachment of the flap. It is often used in deltopectoral flap **(Fig. 7-106)**.

Different Flaps

Flap lying immediately adjacent to the defect is called as *local flap*. Flap moved from adjacent anatomical area is called as *regional flap*. Flap when moved from distant anatomical site is called as *distant flap*.

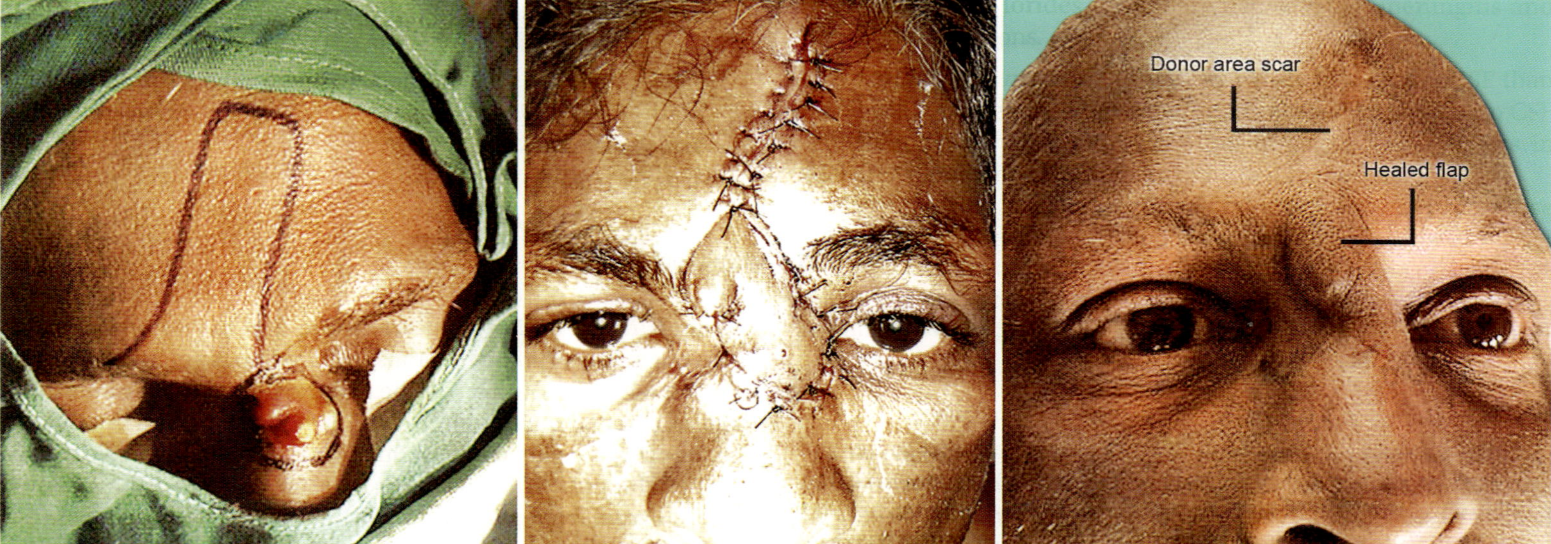

Fig. 7-102: On table marking of glabellar flap to place after excising a lesion in the root of the nose.

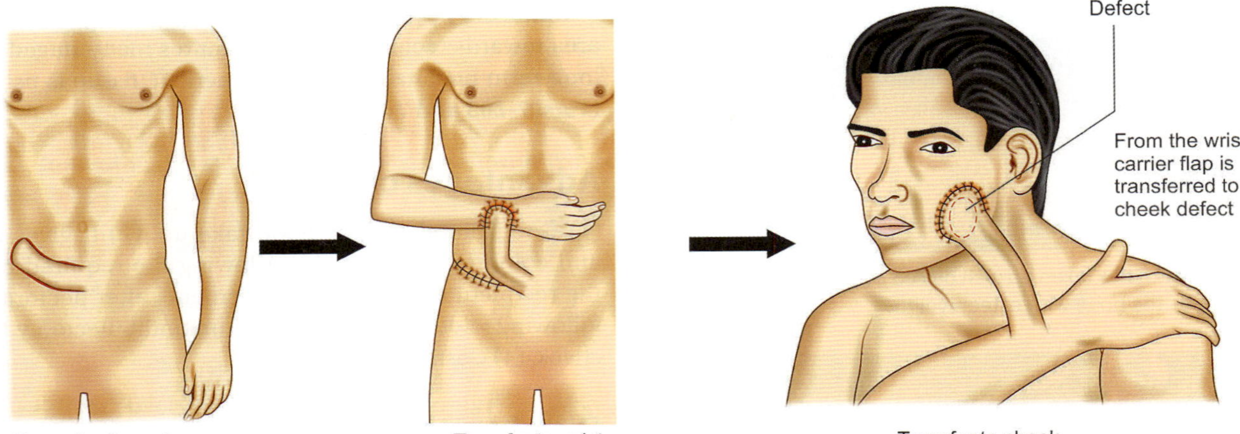

Fig. 7-103: Saltatory flap. Flap raised from the abdomen is reached to the cheek in stages—from abdomen to wrist; from wrist to cheek.

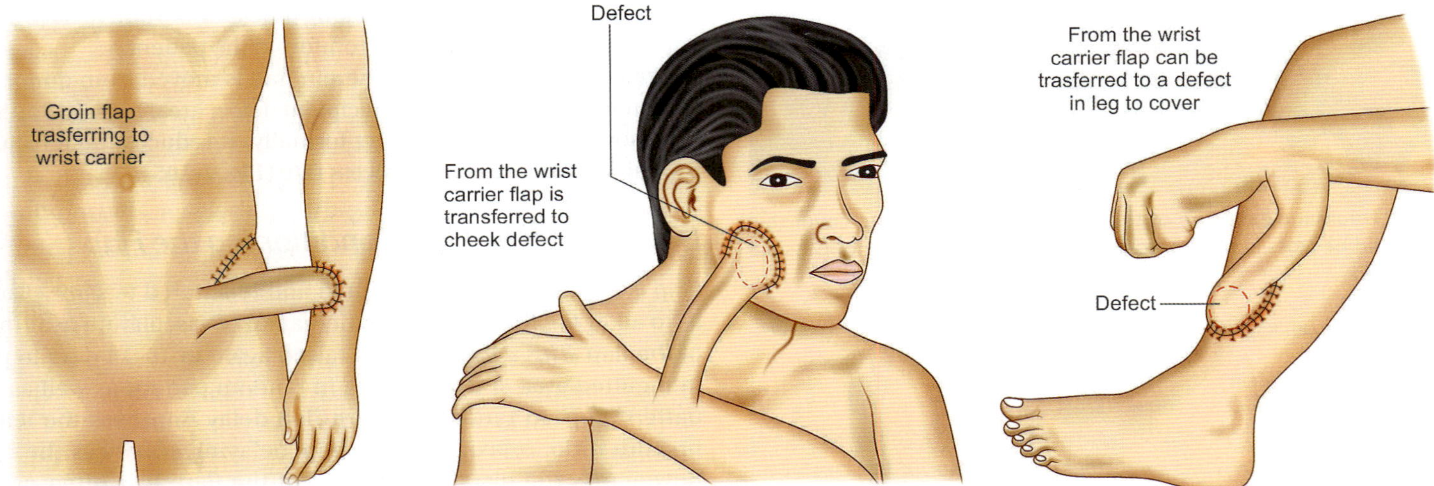

Fig. 7-104: Transferring the groin flap to the defect area either in cheek or in leg using wrist as carrier. It is the staged procedure. In each stage flap is divided in 3 weeks period.

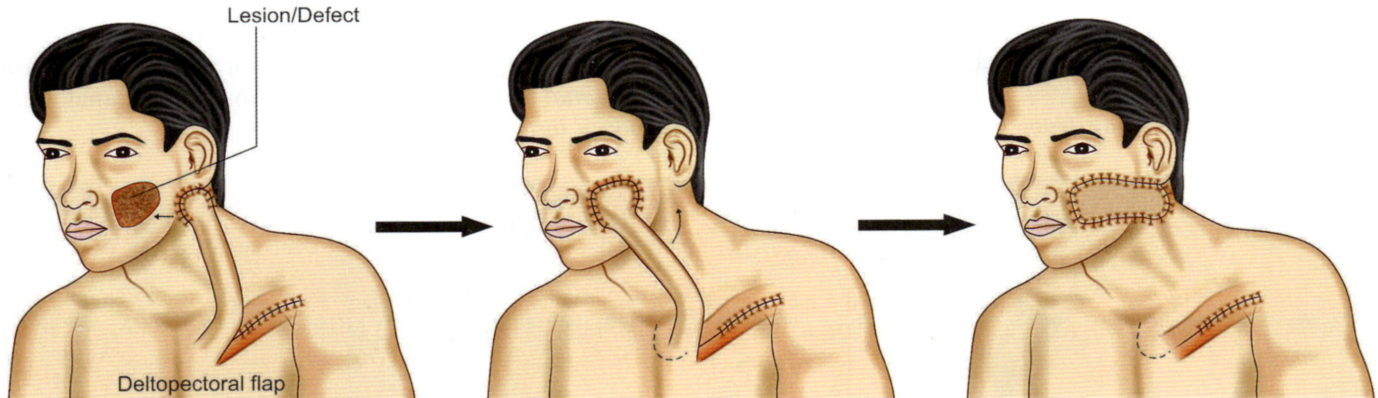

Fig. 7-105: Waltzing flap.

Pedicled flap is a flap which is moved with intact tissue bridge to support it. Deltopectoral flap is a pedicled flap.

Islanded flap is a flap which is moved to a site which is non-contiguous from the donor flap area but flap is moved under the skin bridge through a tunnel. Pectoralis major myocutaneous flap is an islanded flap. Localised flap is swung around a stalk from the donor area to the recipient area often with the pedicle buried underneath the skin bridge in between.

Transposition/rotation flap: When the flap moves laterally it is called as *transposition flap*. Transposition flap is squarely designed which moves laterally to close the defect creating a larger area on its original place which can be covered with split skin graft. Mobility of the transposition flap depends on the laxity, flexibility, mobilisation and blood supply. When the flap rotates laterally towards defect it is called as *rotation flap.* It is commonly used to cover bedsores over buttock, sacral region and also on scalp. Flap needed is much wider in relation to the size of the defect **(Figs. 7-107 to 7-110)**.

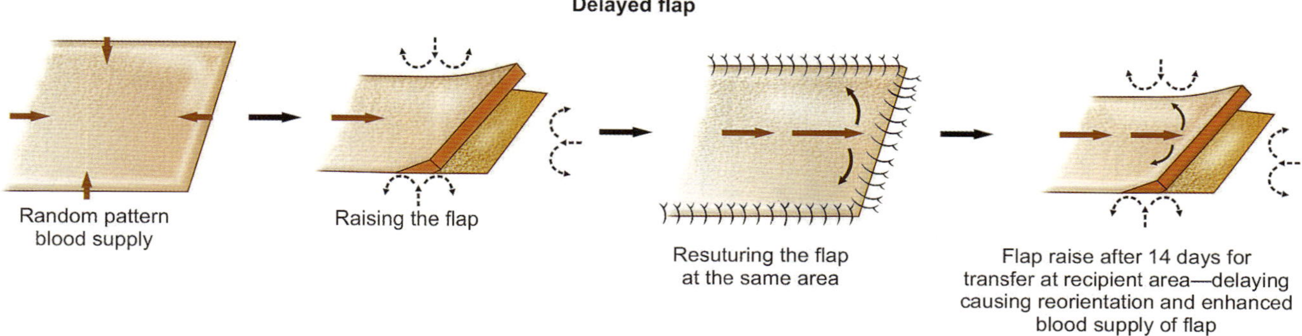

Fig. 7-106: Delaying the flap for 10–14 days to reorient the blood supply. It is done in random pattern flap to improve length to breadth ratio or in axial pattern flap to improve distal blood supply.

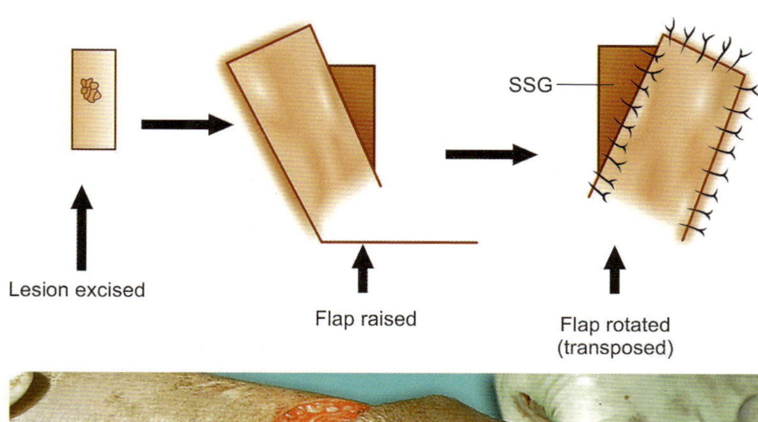

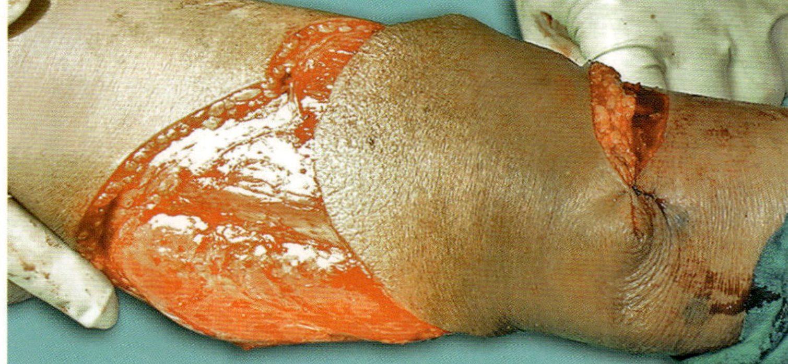

Fig. 7-107: Transposition flap.

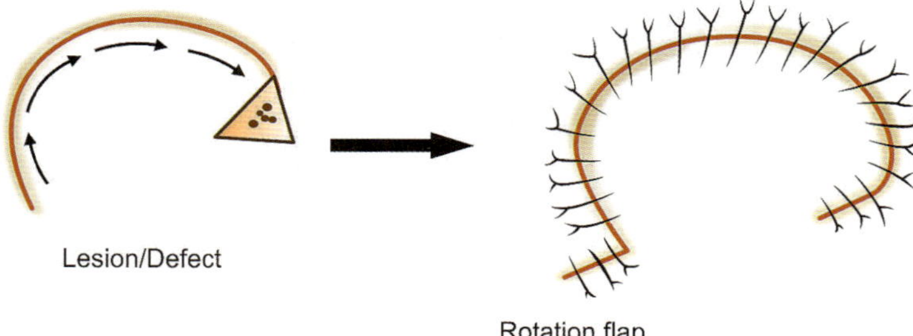

Fig. 7-108: Rotation flap. It is commonly used in gluteal region in managing bedsores.

Advancement flap: It is advancing the flap from one angle towards the defect in longitudinal direction. Here flap transferring area is less but useful. It is used commonly in fingers **(Figs. 7-111 and 7-112)**.

'Z' plasty: It is a procedure which involves transposition of two interdigitating triangular flaps. There is change in direction as well as gain in length of the common limb of Z. Angle size and length of the limb is the most important factors. With an angle of 60° there will be increase in length by 75%. It is used in managing contracted scars, facial scars, Dupuytren's contracture and cover the excised defects like pilonidal sinus (example). There should be transverse skin slack available equal to the length between the axes of Z. It can be single or multiple Z plasty. Multiple Z plasty shows overall 2 cm lengthening but shortening only of 0.5 cm in transverse axis whereas single Z plasty causes 2 cm lengthening and 2 cm shortening in parallel line. Lateral tension is diffused in multiple Z plasty but it is concentrated in single Z plasty. Complications are flap necrosis near the angle tip, infection, failure. Vascularity of the flaps is essential need. Side limbs of the flaps can be curved and broadened to improve the blood supply **(Figs. 7-113 and 7-114)**.

Deltopectoral flap (Bakamjian flap): It is a *fasciocutaneous flap* (axial pattern) based on first three perforating branches of the internal mammary artery (mainly 2nd perforator) **(Fig. 7-115)**. Flap runs horizontally across the chest wall anteriorly towards shoulder tip from its base over the sternal border. Its upper border is along the line of the clavicle; its lower border is along the anterior axillary fold line. Raw area often requires a spilt skin grafting. It is usually rotated upwards often with waltzing. It is tubed and attached above. Tube is drained to prevent any collection to occur. Rotation angle is important to prevent any kinking on the pedicle. It is usually used to cover the defects in cheek, chin, mastoid and parotid region. *Pivot point* of rotation is located in upper medial aspect. Often flap is delayed to get adequate length. Upper medial point is rotating pivot point. It moves a *quarter circle*. Flap can be reached as high as defect over the zygomatic region, as rotating lower border of the flap is slack and lax (as it is near anterior axillary fold which is lax). Occasionally it is also used to transfer below to the chest or abdomen.

Groin flap: It is a *cutaneous flap* (axial pattern) based medially on *superficial circumflex iliac artery* which is 2–3 cm below and parallel to the inguinal ligament. Artery originates from femoral artery over medial border of the sartorius and ends at anterior superior iliac spine. Deep branch is at the margin of the sartorius and superficial branch continues towards anterior superior iliac spine. 1:1 rectangular flap with deep fascia is used. Dissection of raising the flap is done up to the medial border of the sartorius. Secondary defect can usually be closed with sutures. It is used mainly for defects in wrist/forearm where positioning is easier. Often *tubed groin flap* can be transferred to cheek or leg using wrist as carrier **(Figs. 7-116 and 7-117)**.

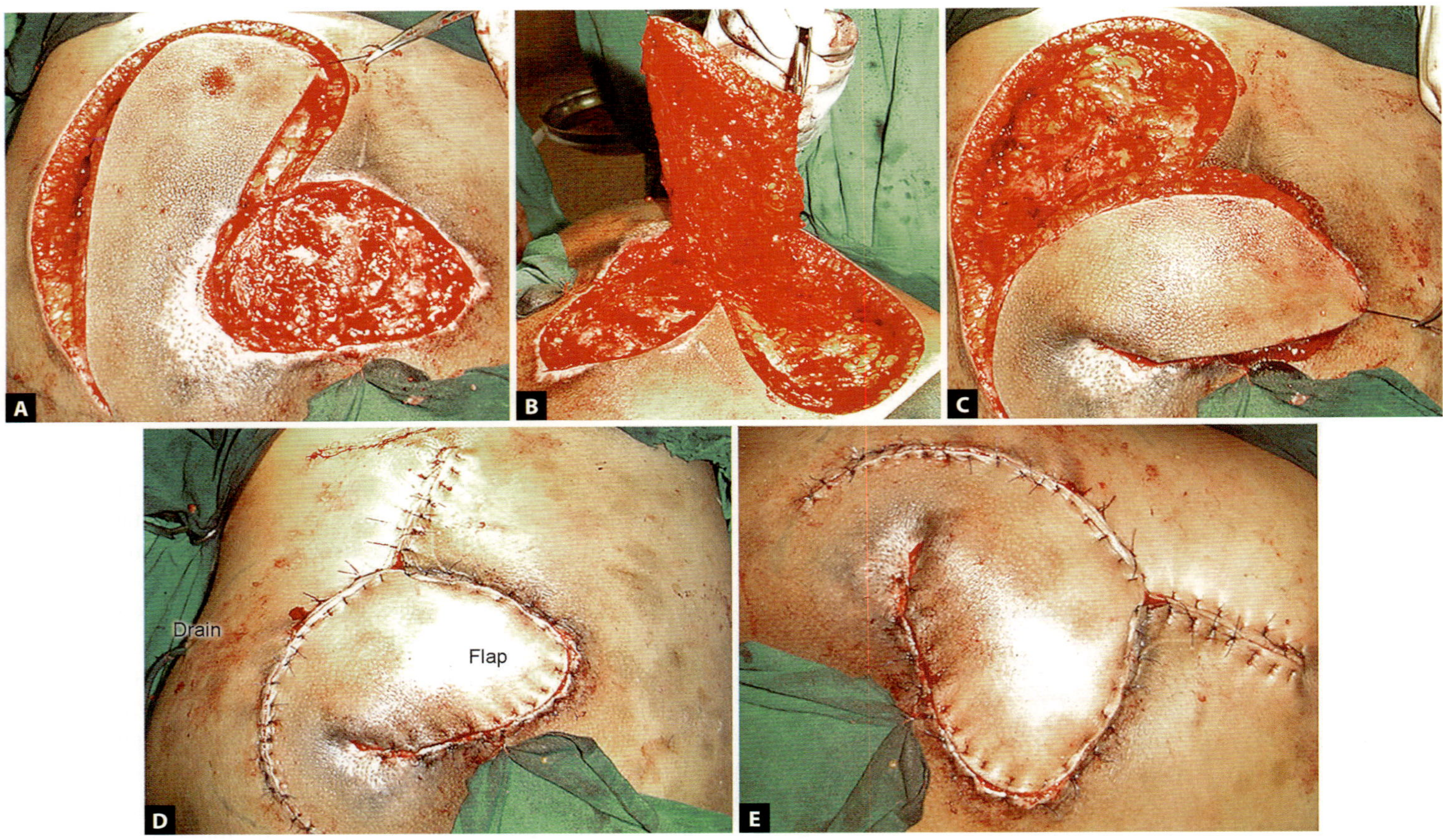

Figs. 7-109A to E: Rotation flap for gluteal defect/bedsore.

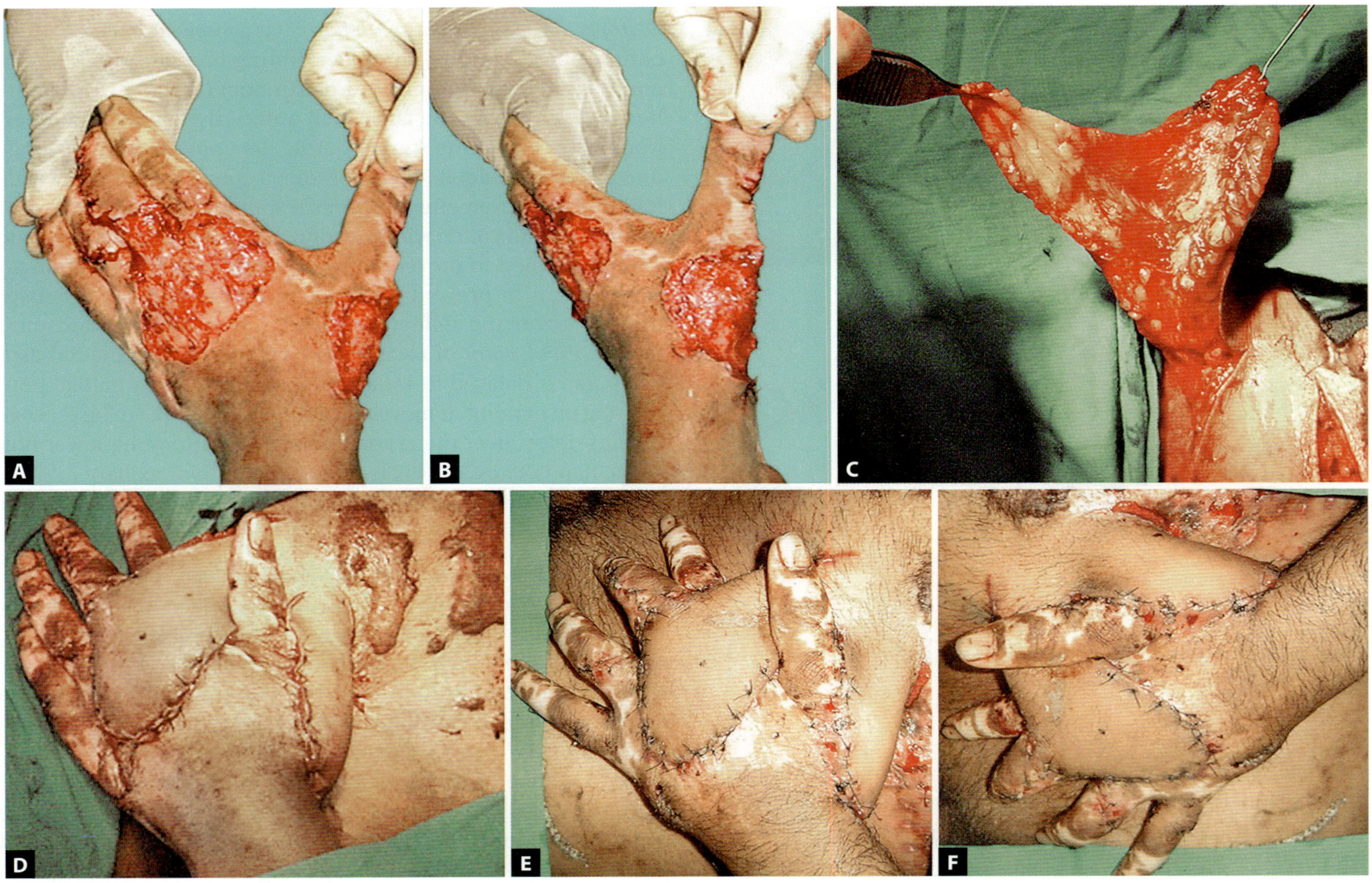

Figs. 7-110A to F

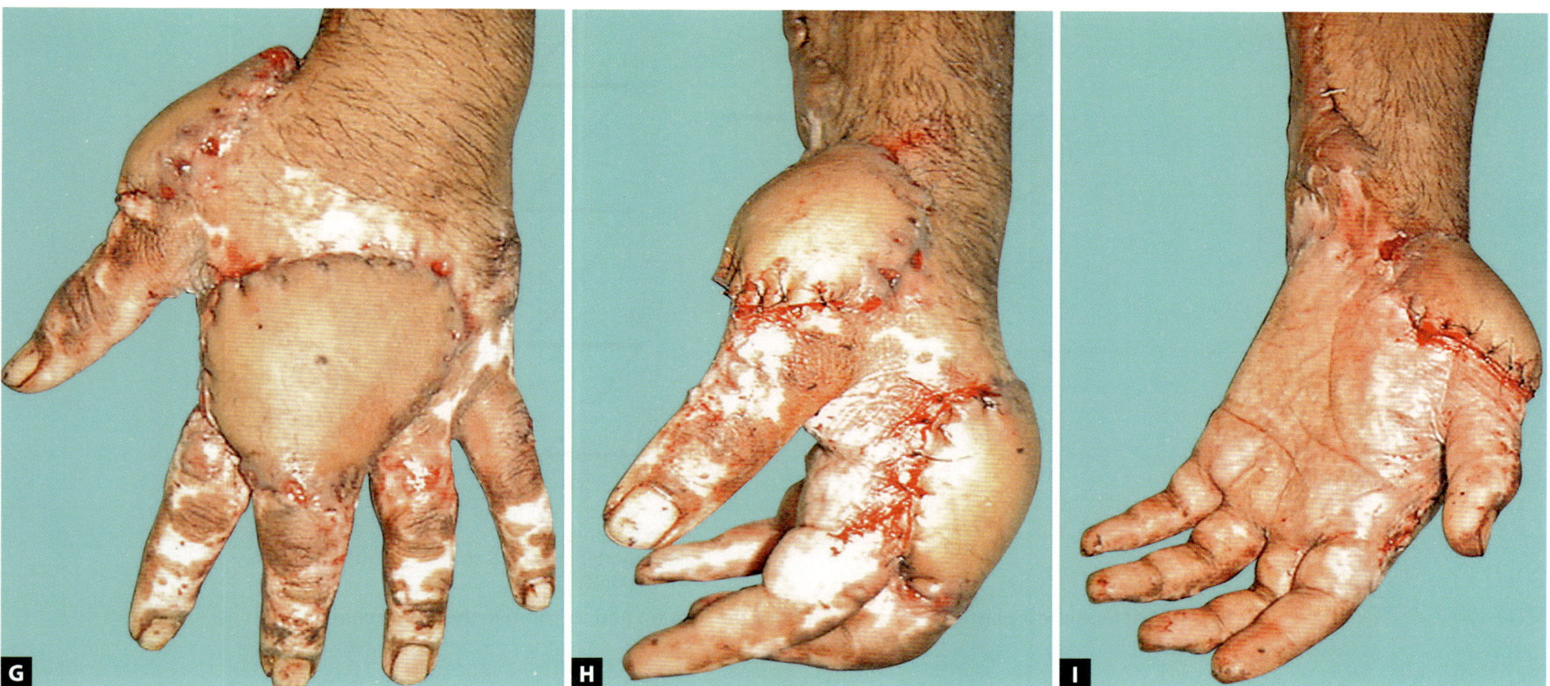

Figs. 7-110G to I

Figs. 7-110A to I: Bilobed flap taken from abdominal wall and placing to the hand and wrist area over two defects.

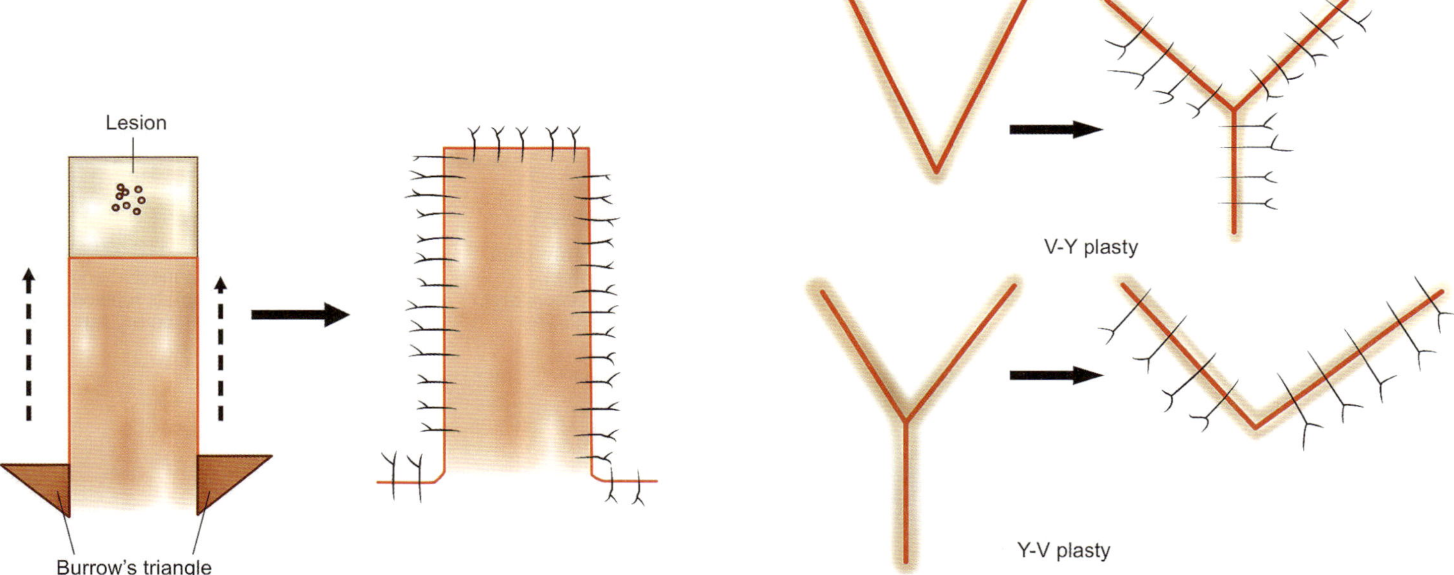

Fig. 7-111: Advancement flap is used in distal defects.

Fig. 7-112: Technique of V-Y plasty and Y-V plasty.

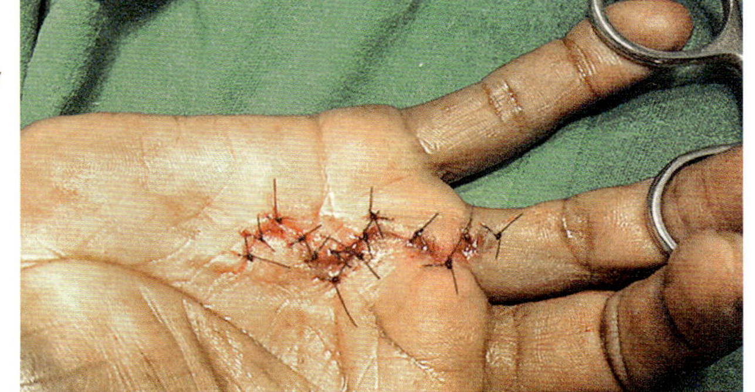

Fig. 7-113: Technique of 'Z' plasty. It is used in contracture release; Dupuytren's contracture and pilonidal sinus. Angle of rotation here is 60°. Note the Z plasty done for Dupuytren's contracture. Fingers can be retracted using finger bows of the haemostats.

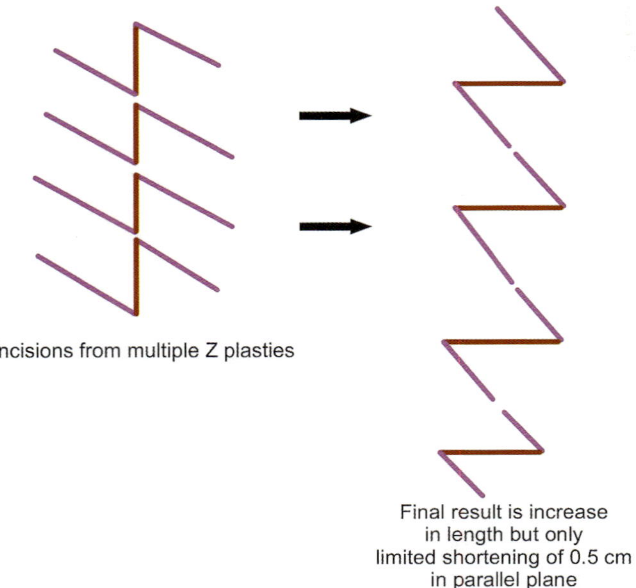

Fig. 7-114: Multiple Z plasties are done to diffuse the tension and to improve the lengthening.

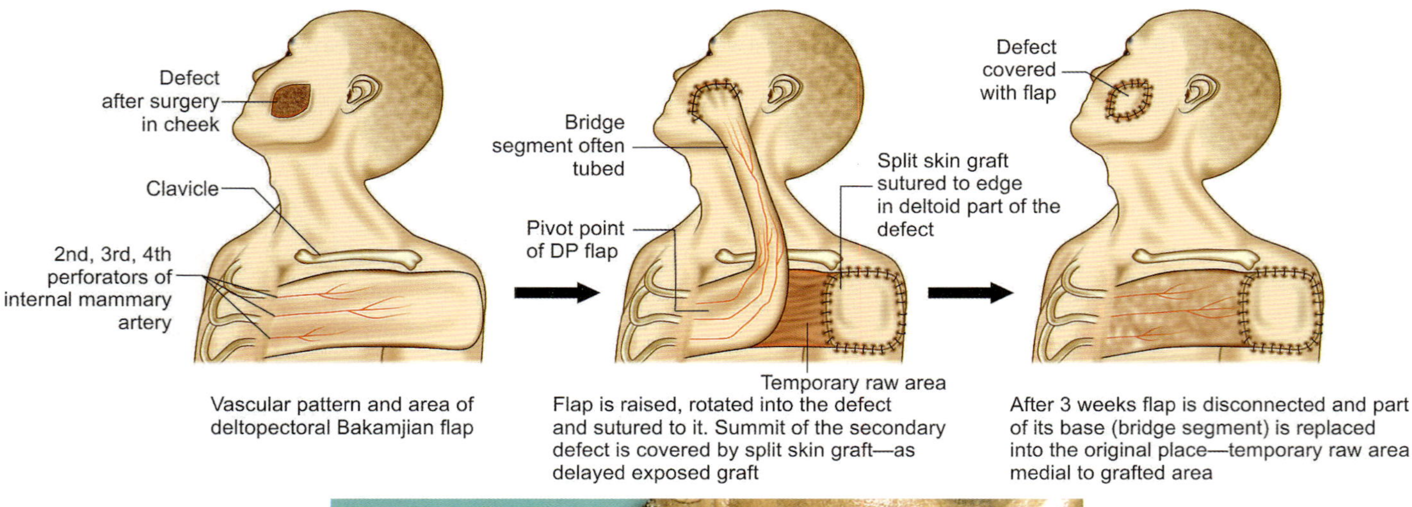

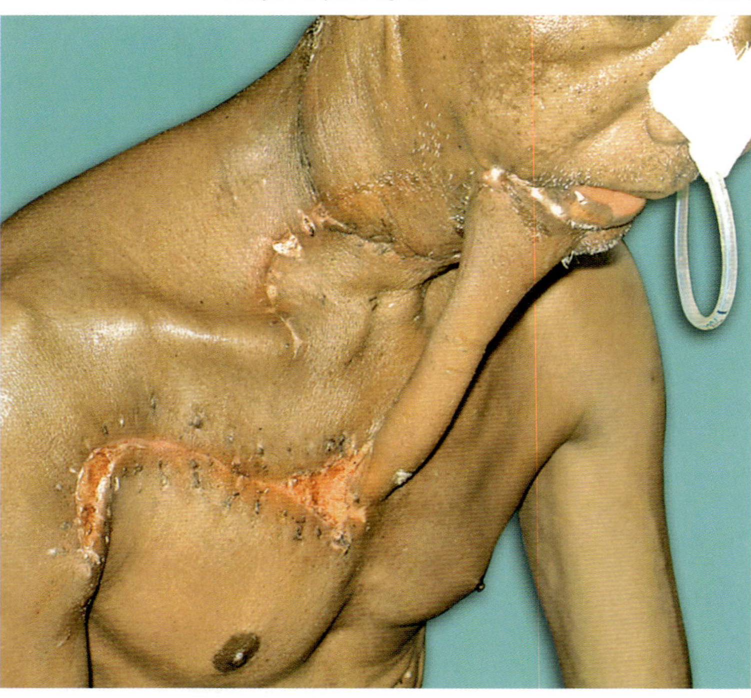

Fig. 7-115: Deltopectoral cutaneous flap (Bakamjian flap).

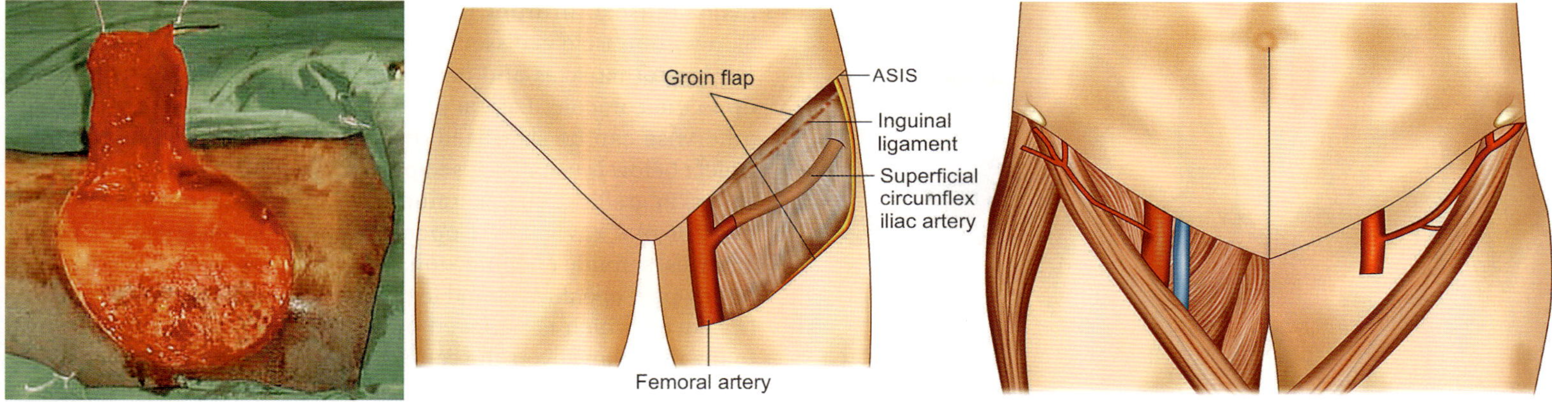

Fig. 7-116: Groin flap is based on superficial circumflex artery. It can be used for defects in hand and forearm. It is a cutaneous flap.

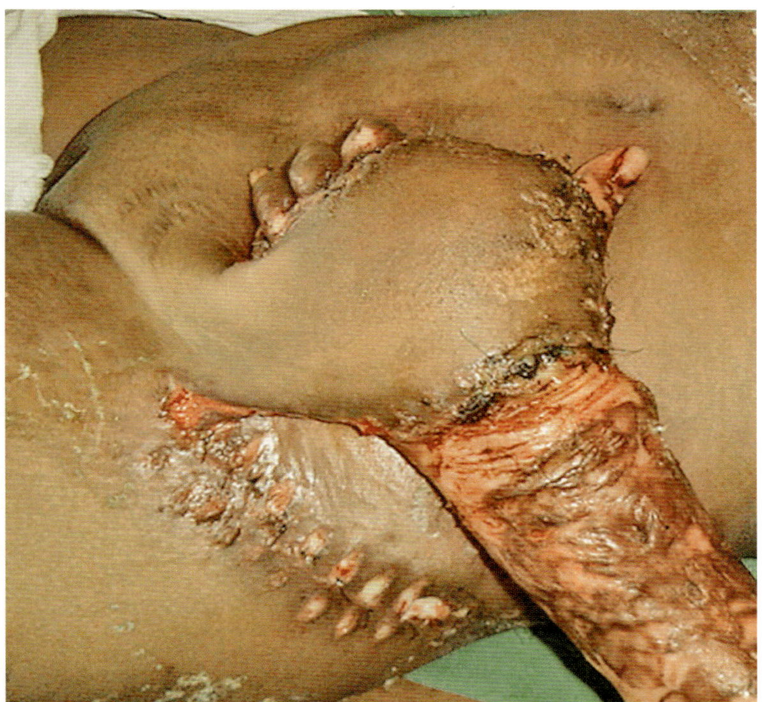

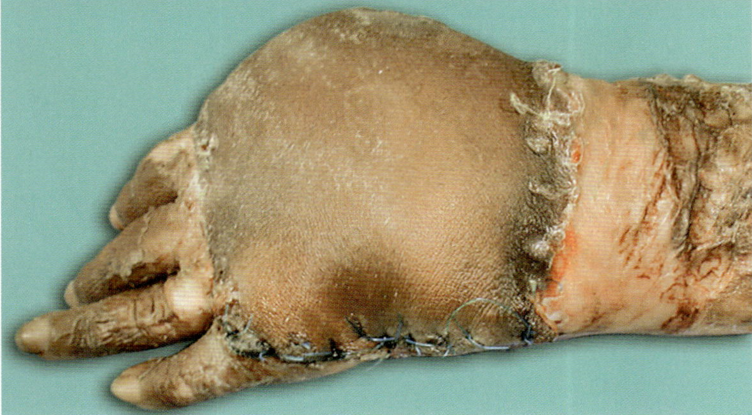

Fig. 7-117: Groin flap used for defect due to burns in the hand.

Hypogastric flap: It is a *cutaneous flap* (axial pattern) based on superficial epigastric vessel directing upwards from the inguinal ligament in the lower abdomen. It is used for wrist in similar way like groin flap **(Fig. 7-118)**.

Latissimus dorsi muscle/myocutaneous flap: It is based on thoracodorsal artery, a branch of subscapular artery. Skin over the upper

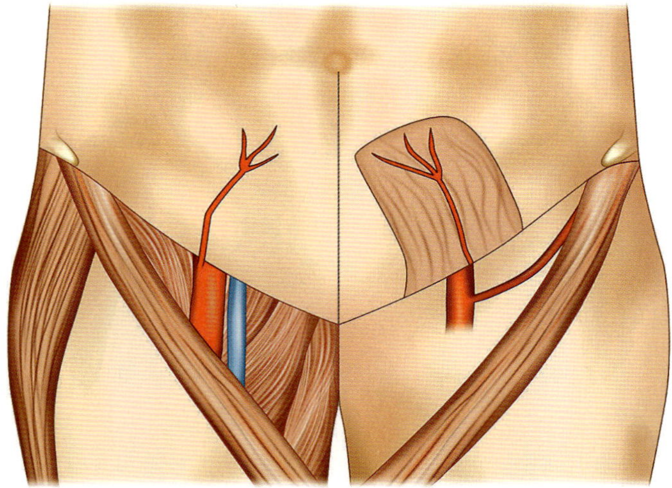

Fig. 7-118: Diagram showing hypogastric flap based on superficial epigastric artery.

and anterior border of the muscle is used for transfer **(Fig. 7-119)**. It is commonly used to cover the defect after mastectomy. But it does not give the bulk. It is technically easier. It can be used as muscle flap also. It helps as skin cover. Prosthesis (submuscular silicone) is needed to place underneath to provide the bulk in post-mastectomy defect. Muscle arises from iliac crest upwards to mid-thoracic spine. Muscle is like a fan below forming tendinous fibres above to insert into humeral shaft. Subscapular artery a largest branch derived from 3rd part of axillary artery runs along posterior wall of the axilla giving circumflex scapular vessels at 4 cm distance and later continuing as thoracodorsal artery for about 6 cm enters the muscle giving many branches. Flap is usually taken as myocutaneous flap with elliptical skin on the surface. Skin part is either horizontal ellipse when taken from upper margin of the muscle or vertical when taken from the anterior margin of the muscle. Point of origin of the subscapular artery is the pivot point of the flap. Artery accompanies the vein also. During raising the flap after islanding it with skin, only pedicle can be retained cutting muscle above to attain extra length (but commonly anterior attachment is retained) and flap is rotated to the needed area. Donor area can be sutured primarily or covered with a split skin graft. In LD flap nerve is not retained (as if retained it causes unpleasant muscle contractions) and so it will not maintain the bulk but gives well coverage of the defect. Flap harvesting is done in lateral position. Subscapular vessels maintain the adequate length and calibre and so it is often used as *free flap* based on subscapular vessels.

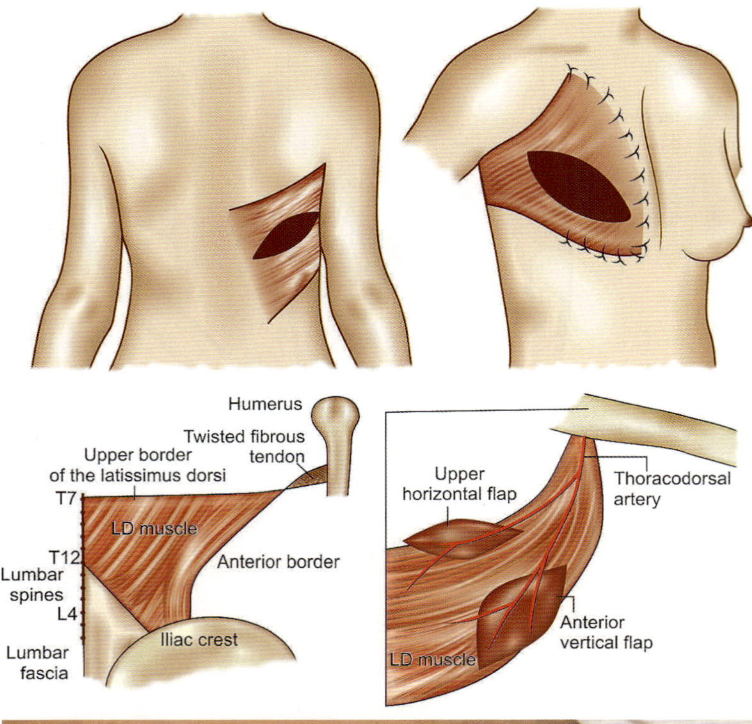

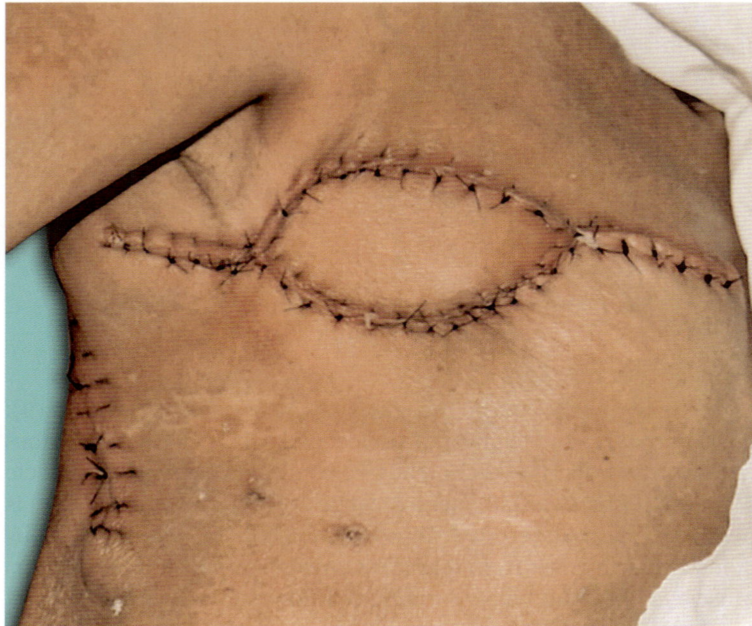

Fig. 7-119: Latissimus dorsi myocutaneous flap.

Pectoralis major myocutaneous flap (PMMF): It is based on the pectoral branches of *thoracoacromial artery*. Usually, skin below and medial to nipple over the muscle is used. Muscle pedicle is made as broad as skin. It is used to cover the defect over the cheek/neck/pharynx/intraoral lesions after wide excision with removal of skin over the tumour. Vessel marking is 2 cm medial to coracoid process, obliquely below the clavicle at the junction between middle third and outer third. Line runs towards the xiphoid process. Oblique downwards incision is placed encroaching the ellipse of the needed skin in the flap. Often skin incision begins below the line of 3rd rib to retain the deltopectoral flap area in case of need in future. Lower border of the muscle is raised by dissecting beneath the pectoral fascia. While raising the flap of the chest wall thoracoacromial vessels can be visualised. Enough care should be taken not to injure it. Flap is raised over the medial and lateral margins of the pectoralis major muscle. In front it is dissected off from the deep fascia. Skin with muscle is dissected from the deeper structures like ribs, intercostal muscles and pectoralis minor. Flap is raised upwards up to the coracoid. Lateral pectoral vessels if possible are retained otherwise can be sacrificed. Pectoral nerves should be retained. Defect below is usually closed primarily with sutures. Often it needs spilt skin grafting. Flap is tunneled in subcutaneous plane towards neck or oral cavity. Post-operatively flap is observed for colour changes, seroma, and infection. Neck is flexed towards the flap side during post-operative period to prevent tension. Suction drain should be placed which is removed once drainage stops or in 72 hours. In the neck flap covers the carotids protecting it. In oral cavity if flap is of large size, its skin can be split into half to cover both inner and outer aspect of the oral cavity. It gives bulk and adequate movements of the jaw. Pectoralis major flap can be used along with deltopectoral flap with proper planning **(Figs. 7-120 to 7-122)**.

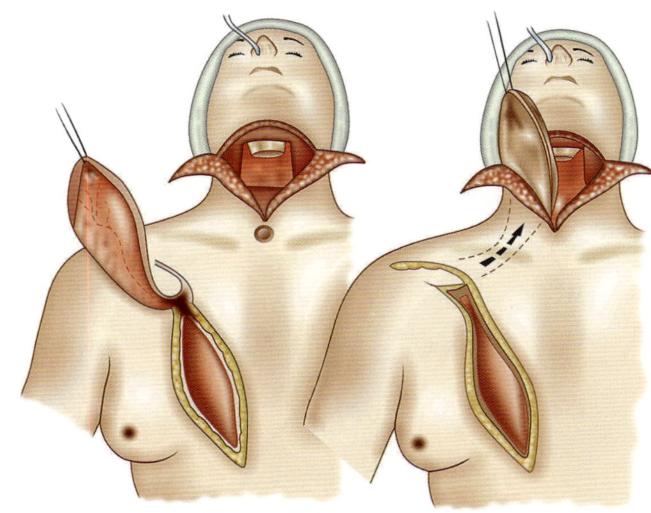

Fig. 7-120: Diagrammatic look of pectoralis major myocutaneous flap.

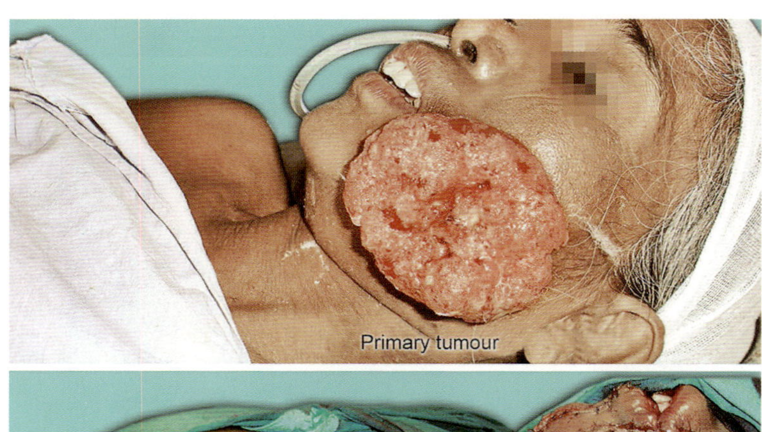

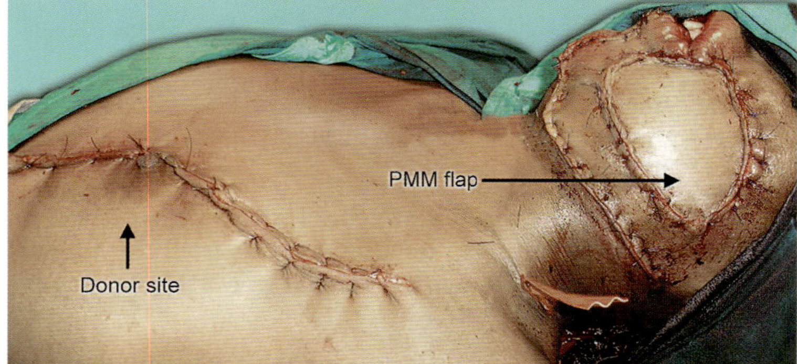

Fig. 7-121: Pectoralis major myocutaneous flap used for carcinoma cheek.

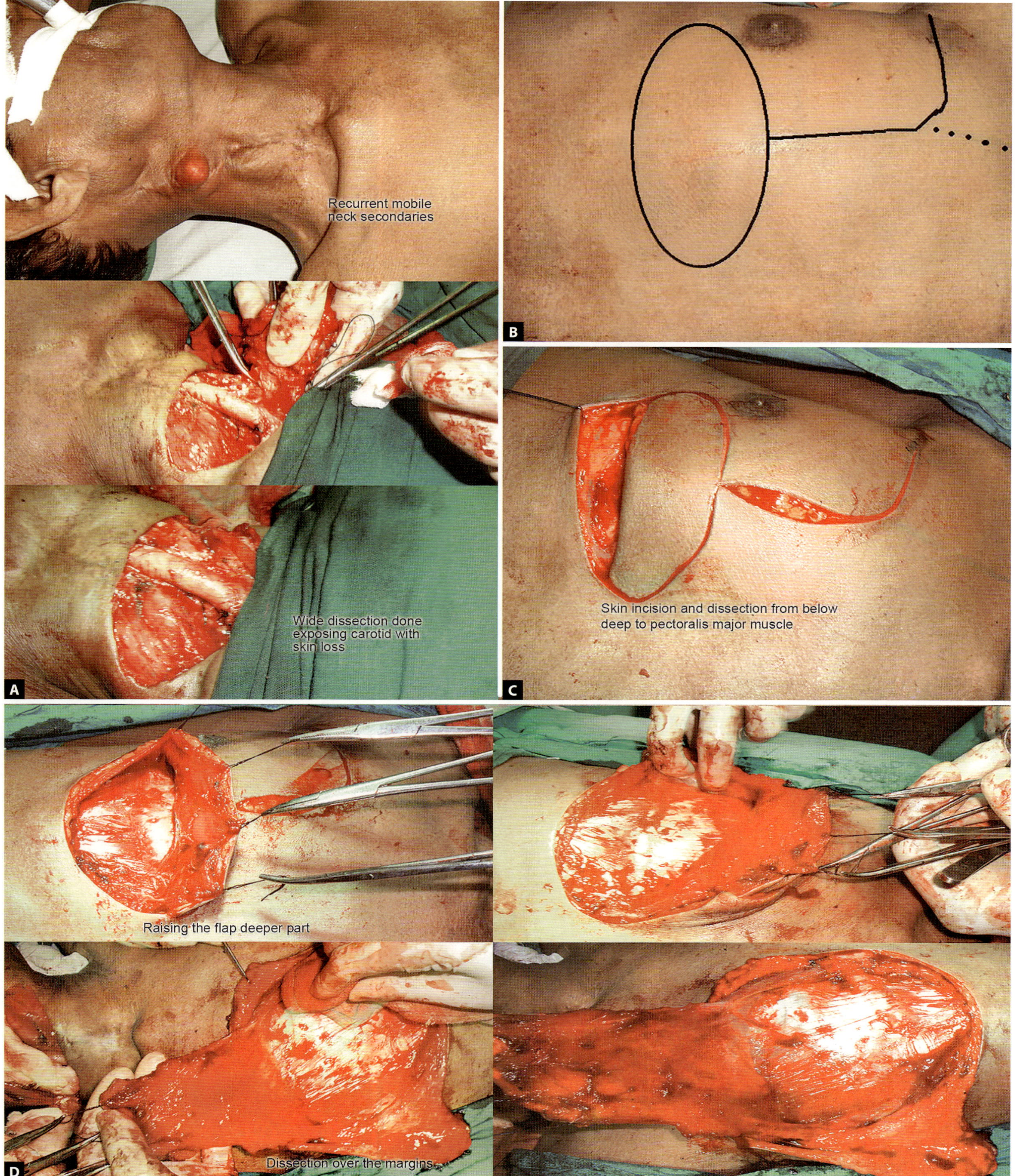

Figs. 7-122A to D

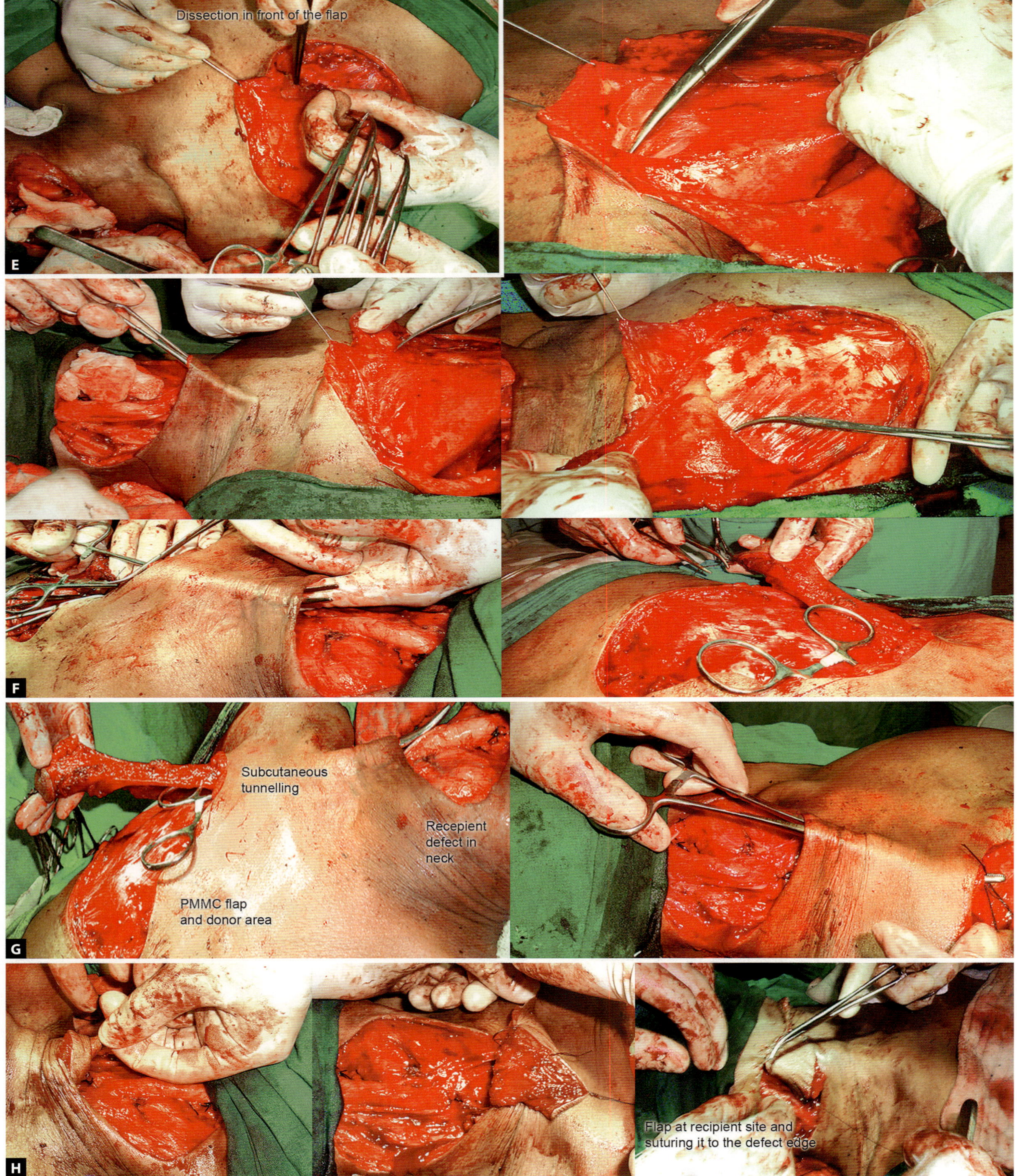

Figs. 7-122E to H

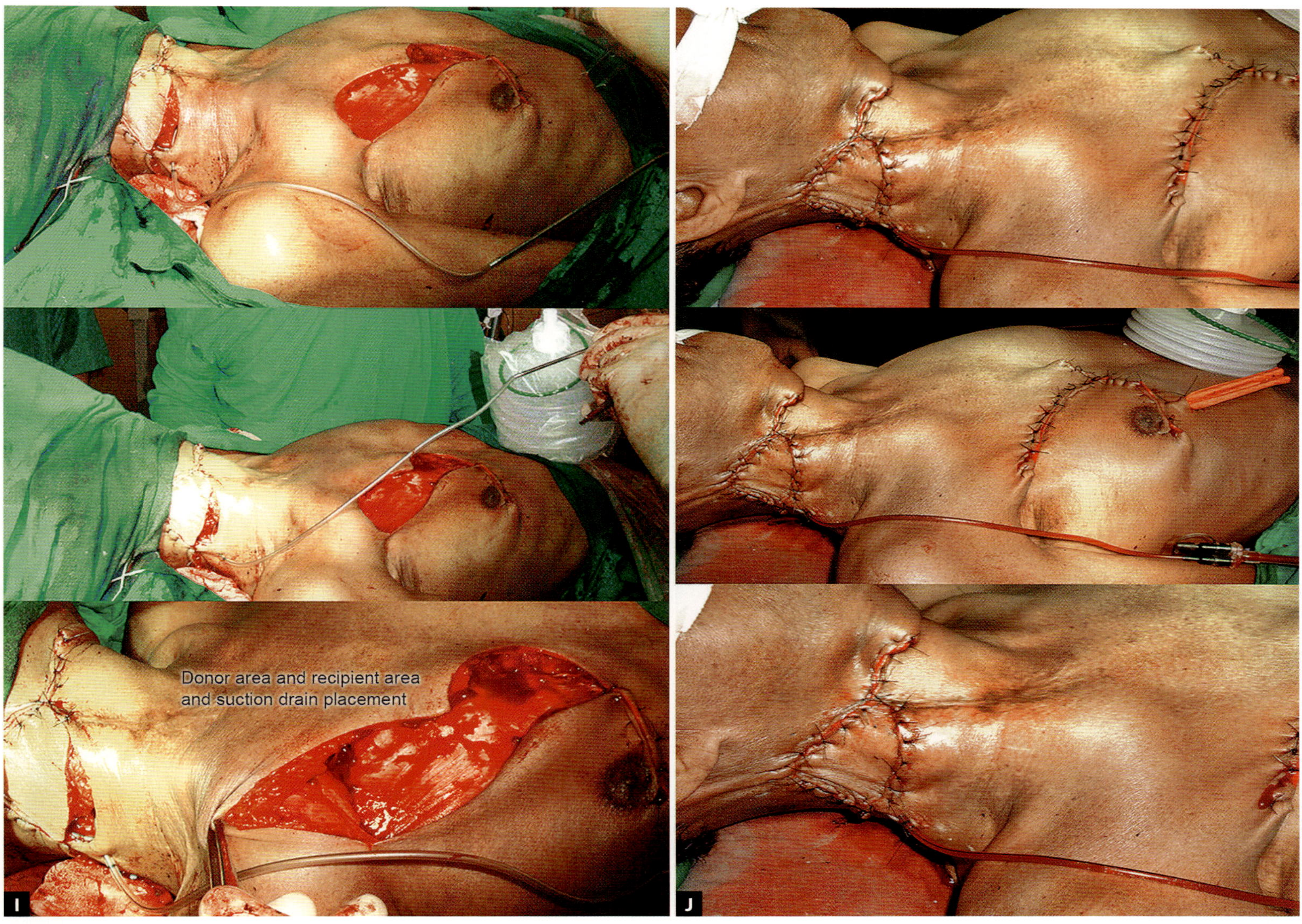

Figs. 7-122I and J

Figs. 7-122A to J: Incision marking, flap raise and steps in pectoralis major myocutaneous flap.

Gastrocnemius muscle flap: It is either medial or lateral and is commonly used to cover the upper part of the tibia and knee joint. It is technically easier and functional deficit occurring at donor area is insignificant. It is rarely used as myocutaneous flap.

Transverse rectus abdominis muscle flap (TRAM flap): It is either superior pedicle based on the superior epigastric vessels or inferior pedicle based on the inferior epigastric vessels. Superior pedicle based flap is used to cover post-mastectomy area or chest wall defect. To cover post-mastectomy area opposite sided superior pedicle is used to reduce the arc through which flap has to rotate (but rotating from opposite side is technically difficult). Inferior pedicle flap is used to cover the defects in groin and thigh. Proper marking of the flap is essential **(Fig. 7-123)**. Skin incision is made like an ellipse. Anterior rectus sheath is cut in the line of incision and is raised upwards carefully off the rectus muscle up to the xiphisternum. Muscle is gently separated off the posterior rectus sheath with care not to injure the epigastric vessels. Once dissection is complete lower part of the muscle is cut in superior pedicle to rotate upwards carefully. In the upper part again anterior rectus sheath is opened to pass the flap towards the defect in subcutaneous plane. TRAM flap gives bulk and contour to the defect. But it is technically difficult. Usually opposite side of the defect is taken as flap as it is easier to rotate from opposite side. Defect in the abdomen usually needs mesh to support and close. It is not possible to do this flap in obese and if patient has underwent laparotomy earlier (with a lengthy scar). Below the flap cut end of the inferior epigastric artery in superior pedicle flap can be anastomosed to a vessel in recipient bed to improve the perfusion *(supercharging)*. Inferior epigastric artery in inferior pedicle can be additionally perfused using opposite inferior epigastric artery *(recharging)*.

Radial forearm flap: It is perfused from the radial vessels and raised on the flexor aspect of the forearm. Perforating branches of these vessels supply deep fascia and skin over it. Flap can be fasciocutaneous or osteofasciocutaneous/osteomyofasciocutaneous if radial bone is also used as part of the flap. Radial forearm free flap is commonly used for mandible defects. It is technically easier and safer. Flap is raised along with skin, segment of the radius along its intermuscular septum through which vessels pass and brachioradialis as components. Care is taken in dissecting vessels of the bed and not to injure the radial nerve. In free flap artery is sutured to the recipient artery like facial artery using microscope. Other similar flaps are—ulnar forearm flap, scapular flaps, and vascularised fibular transfer.

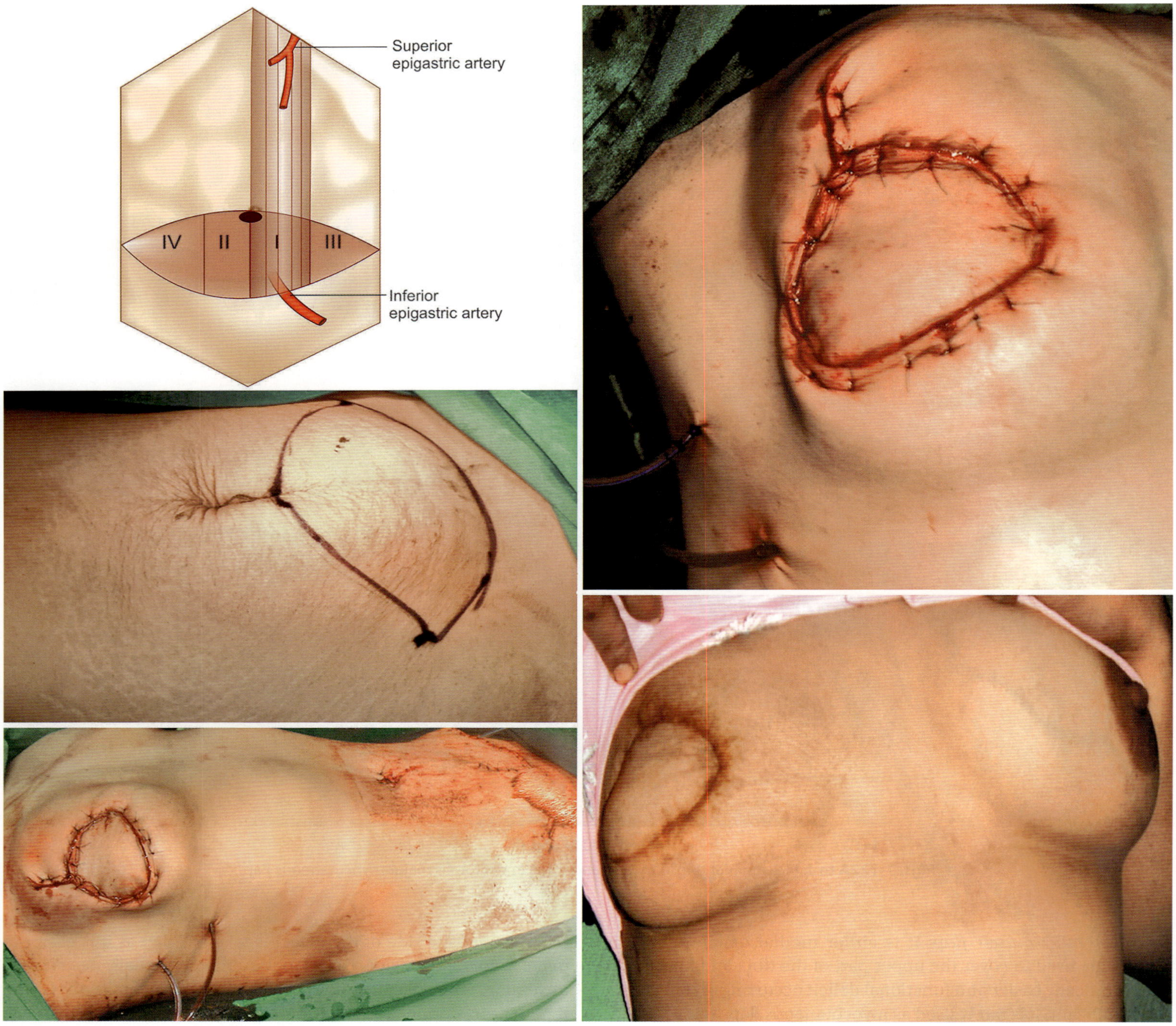

Fig. 7-123: Transverse abdominis myocutaneous flap to cover post-mastectomy area.

Limberg flap is a type of rhomboid flap used in—pilonidal sinus with base at gluteal skin; defects in face after surgical wide excision **(Fig. 7-124)**.

Cross leg flap: It is commonly used to cover the defect in the opposite foot/leg. It is random pattern flap. Limb should be immobilised for 3 weeks by plaster of Paris or external fixation. Raw donor flap area needs split skin graft cover. It is direct flap with 1:1 length breadth ratio **(Fig. 7-125)**. It is commonly used in post-trauma defects in younger individuals. Joint stiffness due to immobilisation may be a problem.

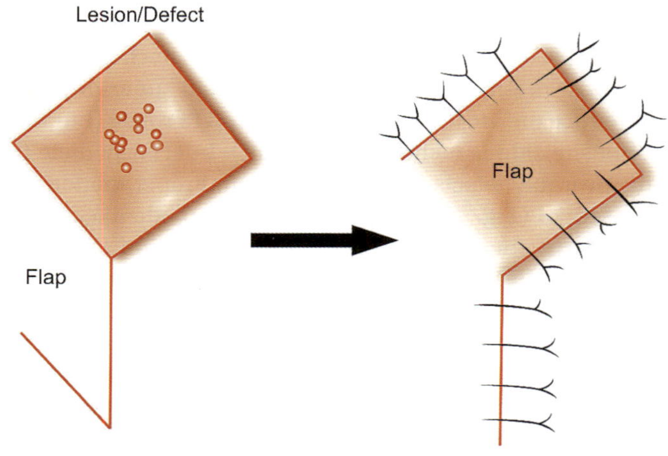

Fig. 7-124: Rhomboid flap.

Free Flaps

Flap with a single lengthy wide calibered arteriovenous system is transferred with its vascular pedicle. Here vascular pedicle is

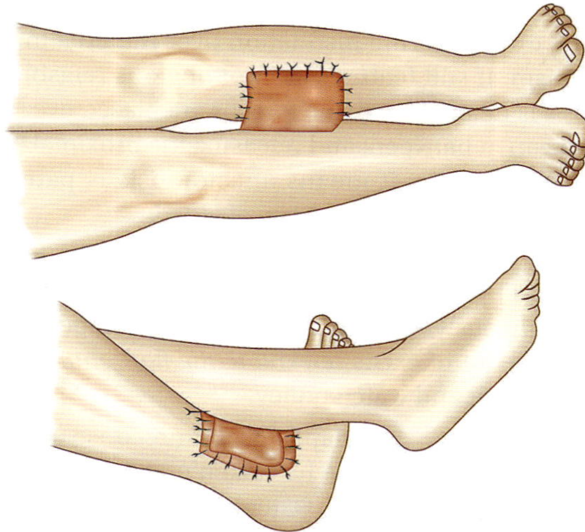

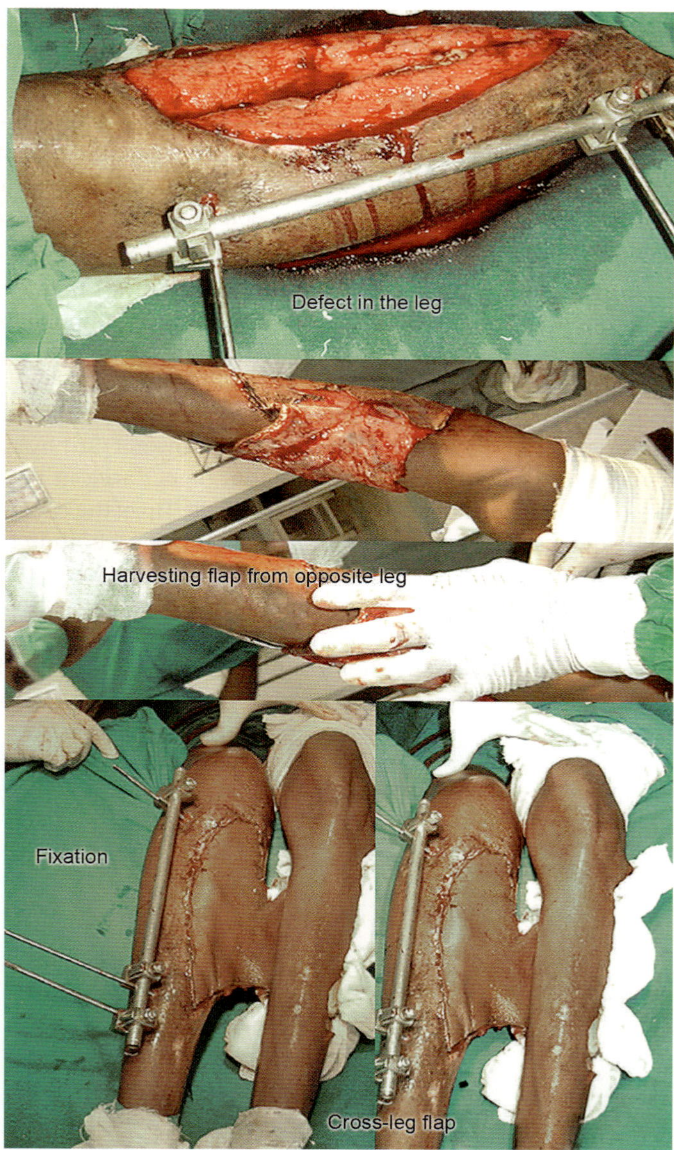

Fig. 7-125: Cross-leg flap.

transected with flap; both artery and vein of the flap is anastomosed to the specific artery and vein at recipient area to re-attain its perfusion through newer blood vessel. *Length and calibre of the vessels* are deciding factors here. Often associated nerves either motor or sensory are also anastomosed. *Healthy vessel wall and adequate pulse volume* are essential in recipient vessel. Presence of *infection* in recipient area is *absolute contraindication*. It can cause thrombosis of the vessel and flap necrosis. Vein ideally should be as large as artery. Often if possible a second vein is also anastomosed. Calibre of the vessels of both recipient and donor parts should be reasonably corresponding. Recipient bed and vessel preparation and raising of donor flap should all be done simultaneously. *The ischaemic time* (time between division of the donor vessel and restoration of perfusion at recipient) should be kept minimum as much as possible.

Factors deciding the adequacy of a flap

- Blood supply of the flap.
- Avoiding mechanical tension and kinking.
- Flap geometry with limited angulation at pivot point of the flap.
- Marking the flap and using gauze cut equal to the size of the flap mock transfer and placing of the flap.
- Post-surgery positioning, prevention of infection.
- Compression of flap should be avoided while passing through a tunnel-like pectoralis major myocutaneous flap.
- Avoiding injury to feeding vessel while raising the flap.
- Thinning of flap if needed should be done with utmost care.
- Prevention of haematoma formation.
- Proper placement of suction drain under the flap.
- Dressings should not be too tight to compromise the blood vessel.
- Delaying the flap especially in random pattern flap.
- Careful tubing of the flap, proper selection of carrier site when needed.
- Positioning of the part and immobilisation.

Anastomosis is done *end to end or side to end* to the flap vessel from recipient vessel (side of the recipient vessel to end of flap vessel). When diameters of the both vessels are equal end-to-end anastomosis is done. When diameter is unequal, then side to end anastomosis is done. End to end in such situation may cause turbulence in blood flow due to unequal diameter and leads to thrombosis of the vessel. Instruments used for anastomosis are—spring handled needle holder; spring handled scissors; fine dissecting and cutting scissors; blunt tipped forceps as vessel dilator; microclamps.

Vessel wall should be healthy, atheroma free, without any branches near to the suturing site, without any valves in veins near the site. Any factor which is likely to cause turbulence should be avoided. Vessel should be held using fine forceps on the periadventitia. *Only bipolar cautery* should be used. Main vessel should not be handled directly. Unnecessary handling of the vessel may cause *vasospasm* which should be avoided. During dissection of the vessel, vascular spasm prevented by irrigating the area local anaesthetic agents (lignocaine) or using papaverine. Tension, kinking, torsion of both recipient and flap vessels should be carefully avoided. Only when recipient vessel is ready, flap vessel is divided after applying a *microclamp*. Once vessels are ready then only microscopy should be used for anastomosis. Now periadventitia is removed for 3 mm from the cut margin in end-to-end anastomosis and 1 cm in end to side anastomosis. Entrapment of periadventitia into the suture line will induce thrombosis. Final trimming of the cut ends is done. *Flushing of the lumen* with heparinised Ringer lactate or Hartmann's solution is done to remove small thrombi and to maintain wet operating field. Vessel ends are *dilated using forceps* to prevent spasm.

Suturing is done using 8-zero/9-zero *monofilament polypropylene* suture material. *Interrupted sutures* are used. Distance of the needle bite from the cut margin should *be twice* the thickness of the vessel wall. Bite is taken from adventitia outside into the lumen on one side then from lumen towards outside through adventitia on opposite side. Knot should *be always outside*. Carrel's triangulation technique with placement of three key stitches at equidistance in the circumference of the cut edges of the vessels. First two key stitches are placed at 120° gap; additional sutures are placed in this gap; vessels are turned over to visualise the remaining gap; in the middle 3rd key stitch is placed; further stitches are placed in the gap. Vessels should be completely apposed to prevent blood leak. Knots should be *on one side* of the suture line in end to end anastomosis; and should be on the *flap vessel side in end to side* anastomosis. In end to side suturing first posterior row is sutured; then followed by anterior row. Deeper vessel in the area should be sutured first; then superficial one. Only after suturing of both artery and vein are completed, microclamps are then released. Always microclamp distal to the suture line should be released. Again venous clamps should be released first followed by arterial. Last clamp to be released is arterial microclamp proximal to anastomosis. After release small leak at suture site will subside **(Fig. 7-126)**. Significant blood leak when observed is controlled by few additional sutures. *Bounding arterial pulse, pink flap, filled vein* suggests good perfusion. Local anaesthetic or papaverine instillation over the area may relieve or prevent spasm. If still features are not obvious refashioning of the anastomosis is needed. Two fine forceps are placed over the emptied vein with a gap in between; and releasing the proximal one if causes filling of vein distally, it means anastomosis is patent. Kinking, compression over the site should be avoided.

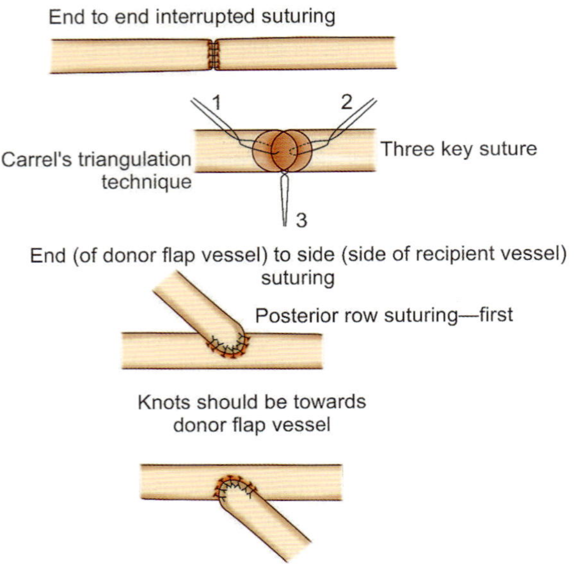

Fig. 7-126: Technique in end-to-end and end-to-side vascular anastomosis in free flap.

Complications are flap oedema, cyanosis, venous block, arterial spasm/block, flap failure. Flap temperature, oxygen tension assessment percutaneously, Doppler study are the methods used to assess the flap. When doubt exists *re-explore the flap immediately*; do not waste time by wait and watch policy.

Uses and advantages—free flap is used in reconstruction of cheek, mandible, neck, etc. Once flap has taken up it is cosmetically better. Perfusion is well maintained. Osteomyocutaneous flap like radial forearm flap, myocutaneous flap, fasciocutaneous flaps can be used as free flaps.

EARLOBE REPAIR

It is commonly used cosmetic simple surgical procedure. Ear stud pierced point gets widened and will not hold the earring any more and lobule sags downwards. Problem is common in those who use overweight earrings/studs; in old people.

Technique: Xylocaine 1% plain (without adrenaline) is injected into the root of lower part of the ear lobule (lobule is supplied great auricular nerve) and directly over the margin of the defect (upper 2/3rd of lateral surface of external ear is supplied by auriculotemporal nerve and lower 1/3rd by great auricular nerve; upper 2/3rd of medial surface is supplied by lesser occipital nerve; lower 1/3rd by great auricular nerve). Elliptical circumferential defect area in the ear lobule is excised using no. 11 sharp pointed blade. Tip of the ear lobule is held using a stay suture. Skin part of the cut wound both in front and behind are approximated using 4-zero polypropylene sutures (interrupted mattress). Bites should not be taken from the cartilage. Dressing is placed. Sutures are removed after 5–7 days. Re-piercing of the ear lobule is done only after 3 months **(Figs. 7-127 to 7-129)**.

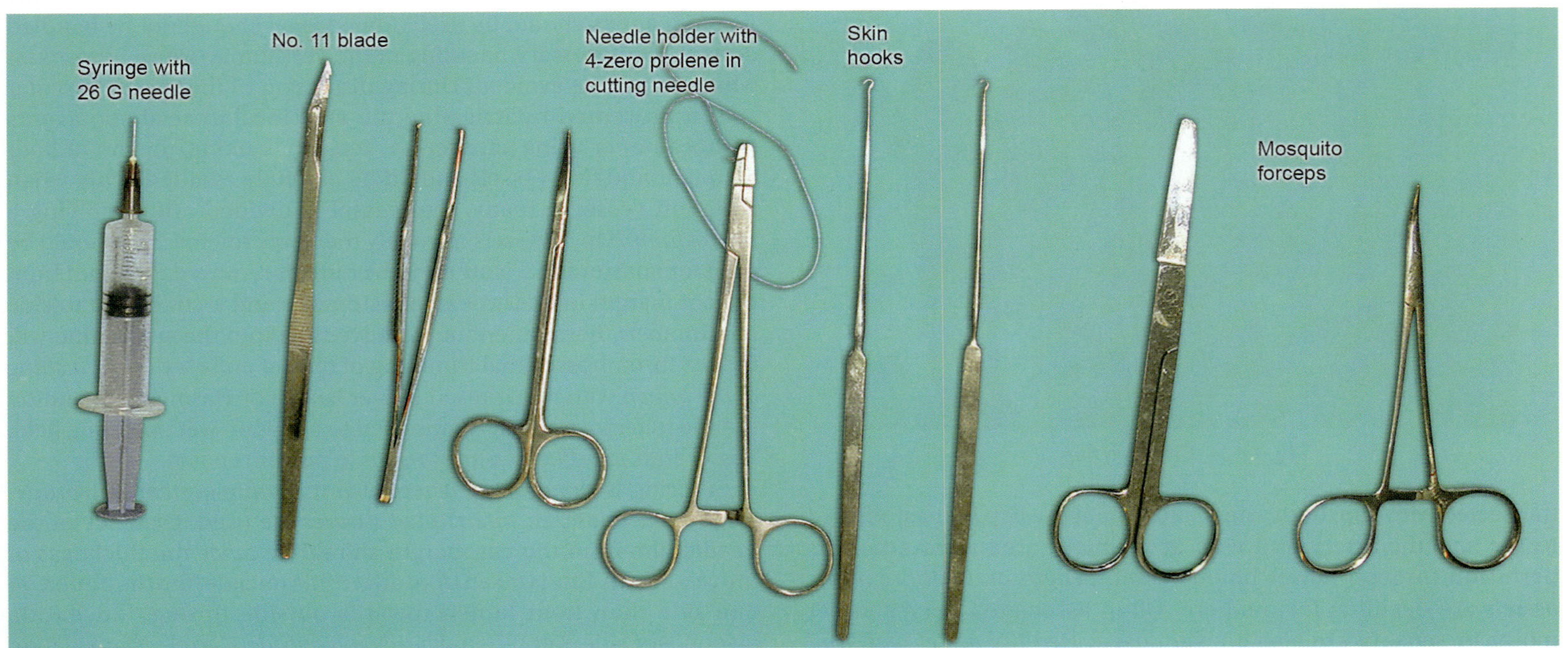

Fig. 7-127: Instruments used in earlobe repair.

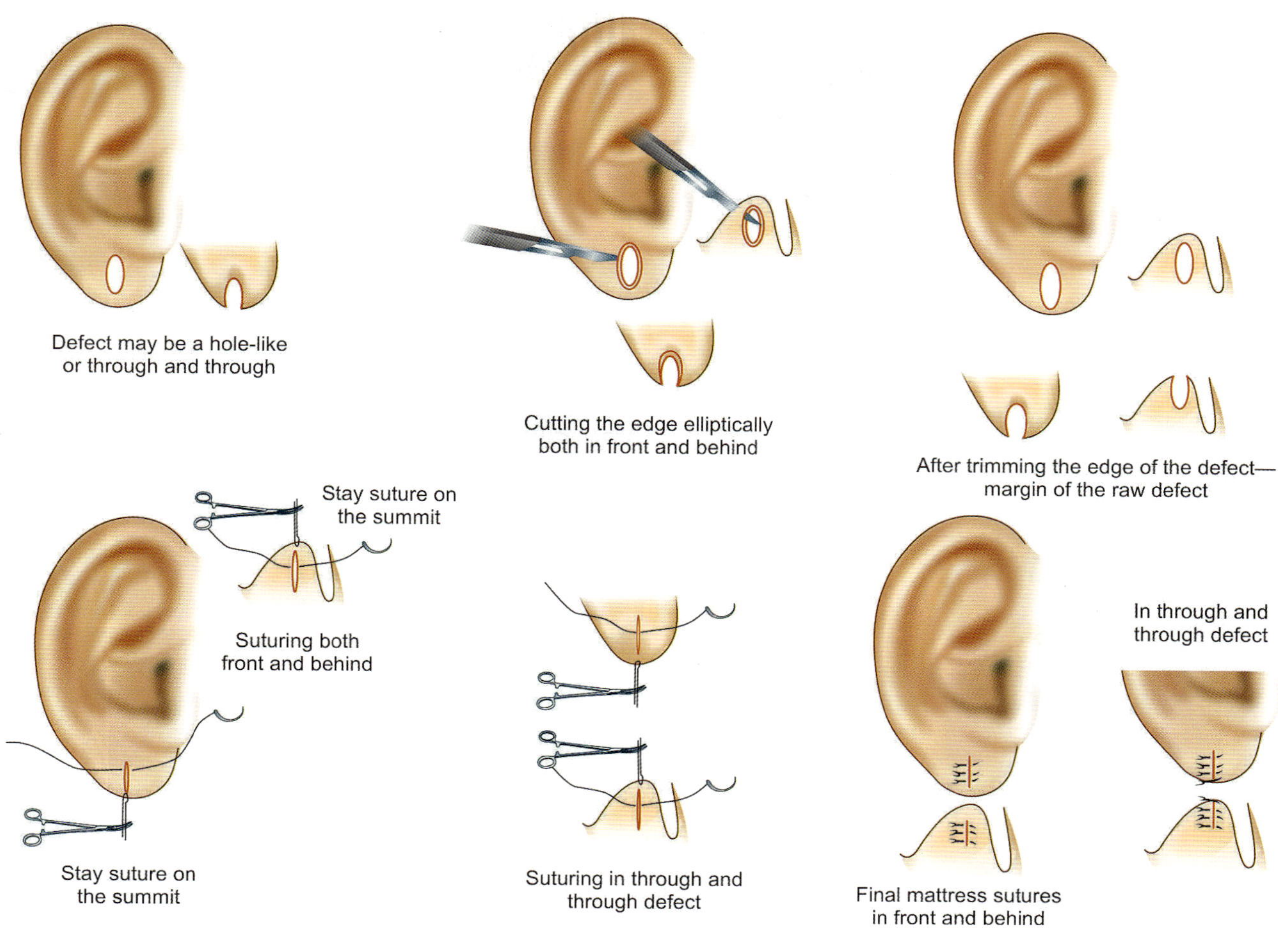

Fig. 7-128: Diagram showing steps in earlobe repair.

TOE NAIL EXCISION

Partial or complete matrixectomy: In recurrent disease or in stage 3 disease partial or complete matrixectomy is done. In partial matrixectomy, soft tissue resection is done; then ingrown toe nail with that part of the nail root (germinal matrix) is excised properly. In complete matrixectomy, entire nail with its root is removed. Incisions may be 45° angled with root flap (Zadik's/Fowler's) or with L shaped incision (Frost) or 'D' shaped excision of the nail root (Winograd) or 'H' shaped incision with removal of the entire nail, nail root, nail bed with diseased soft tissue resection (Kaplan). *Zadik-Fowler's radical nail excision* (1950) as partial or complete matrixectomy is commonly used with flap elevation at angles. Phenol matrixectomy, laser and radiosurgical matrixectomy are also currently in use.

Note:
Different names are used with slight technical modifications; it is the matrixectomy that is most important; rest (names) is only of academic interest. Staging of ingrowing toenail: (1) Embedded toenail edge with swelling and erythema; (2) Infection, painful discharge from nail edge; (3) Soft tissue hypertrophy, chronic infection, granulation tissue formation.

It is done for trauma, infection and in ingrowing toe nail. *Ingrowing toe nail* is a real problem as it is often recurring, distressing due to pain, infection and tenderness. Hypertrophy of soft tissue with formation of protruded unhealthy granulation tissue is common. Often foul-smelling pus exudes out. Medial or lateral or both margin/margins are ingrown on the edge causing soft tissue injury and irritation. It is common in great toe often bilateral.

Zadik's excision (Frank Raphael Zadik) of the toe-nail is done. Procedure is done using finger tourniquet under digital local anaesthesia block using injection xylocaine 2% plain without adrenaline. Nail from the margin is carefully lifted using haemostat or Allis forceps and is avulsed off the nail bed. Here after avulsion of the nail, germinal matrix is also removed. Germinal matrix is located on the proximal third of the nail bed. It extends proximally under the skin fold and extending much more over the proximal corners. Entire germinal matrix should be removed carefully. Incision should extend more proximally near the edge. Flap is raised from the skin fold. Glistening whitish germinal matrix is identified and it is excised. Flap is placed back. Suturing is not done. Careful phenolisation of the specified area without any spillage into the surrounding tissues prevents the recurrence. Phenol applied is allowed to settle for 5 minutes and is neutralised using alcohol. Application of phenol is useful in presence of infection. Often only medial or lateral margin of the nail is removed. Here nail is retained in the centre. But problem here, even though cosmetically better, recurrence of ingrowing toe nail **(Figs. 7-130 to 7-132)**.

DERMABRASION

Dermabrasion is a cosmetic medical procedure in which the surface of the epidermis of the skin (the stratum corneum) is removed by abrasion (sanding). The instrument used to perform the procedure is called a dermabrader. It is used to remove sun-damaged skin, to remove or lessen scars and dark spots on the skin. The procedure is very painful and usually requires a general anaesthesia or twilight anaesthesia, in which the patient is still partly conscious.

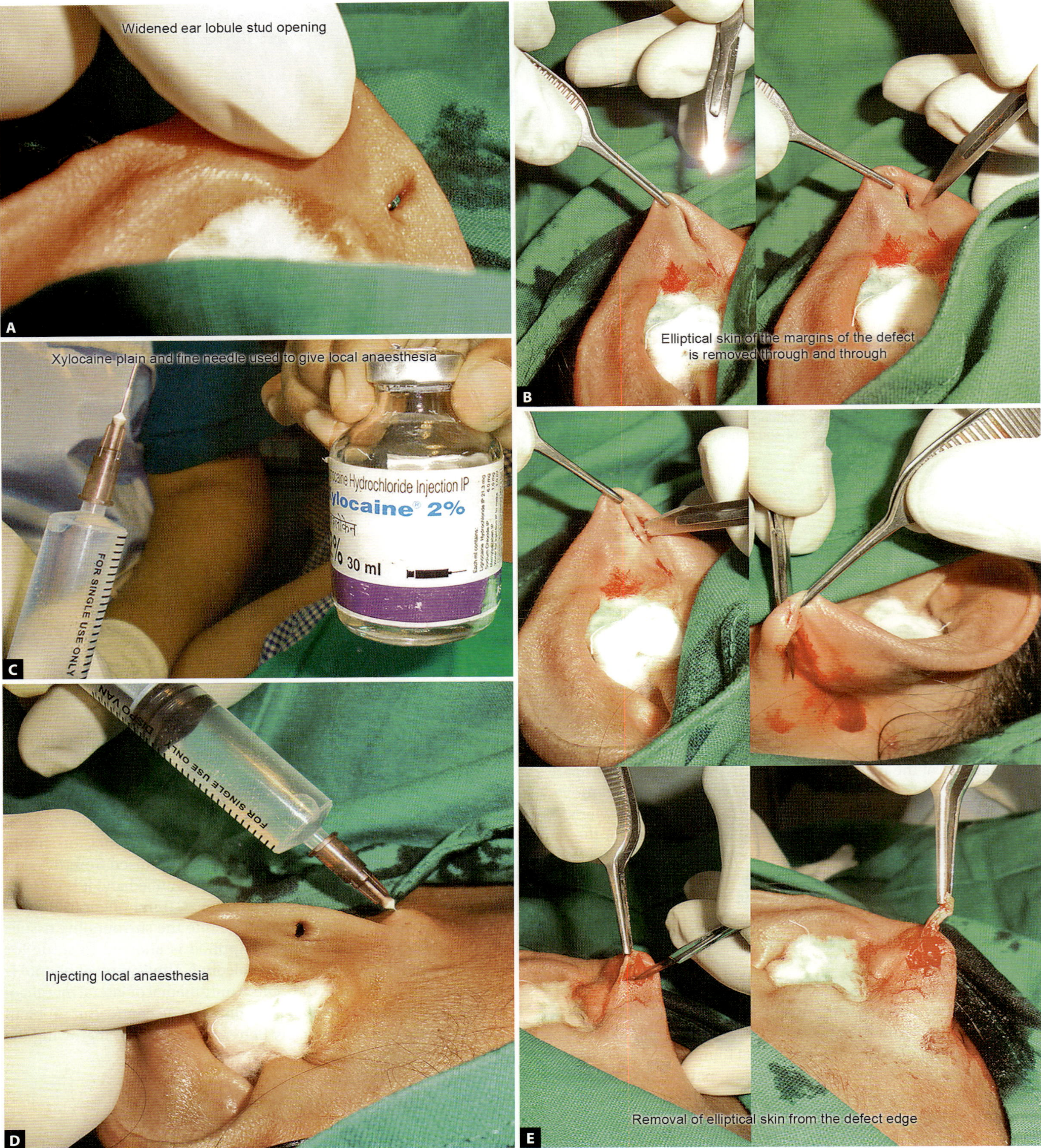

Figs. 7-129A to E

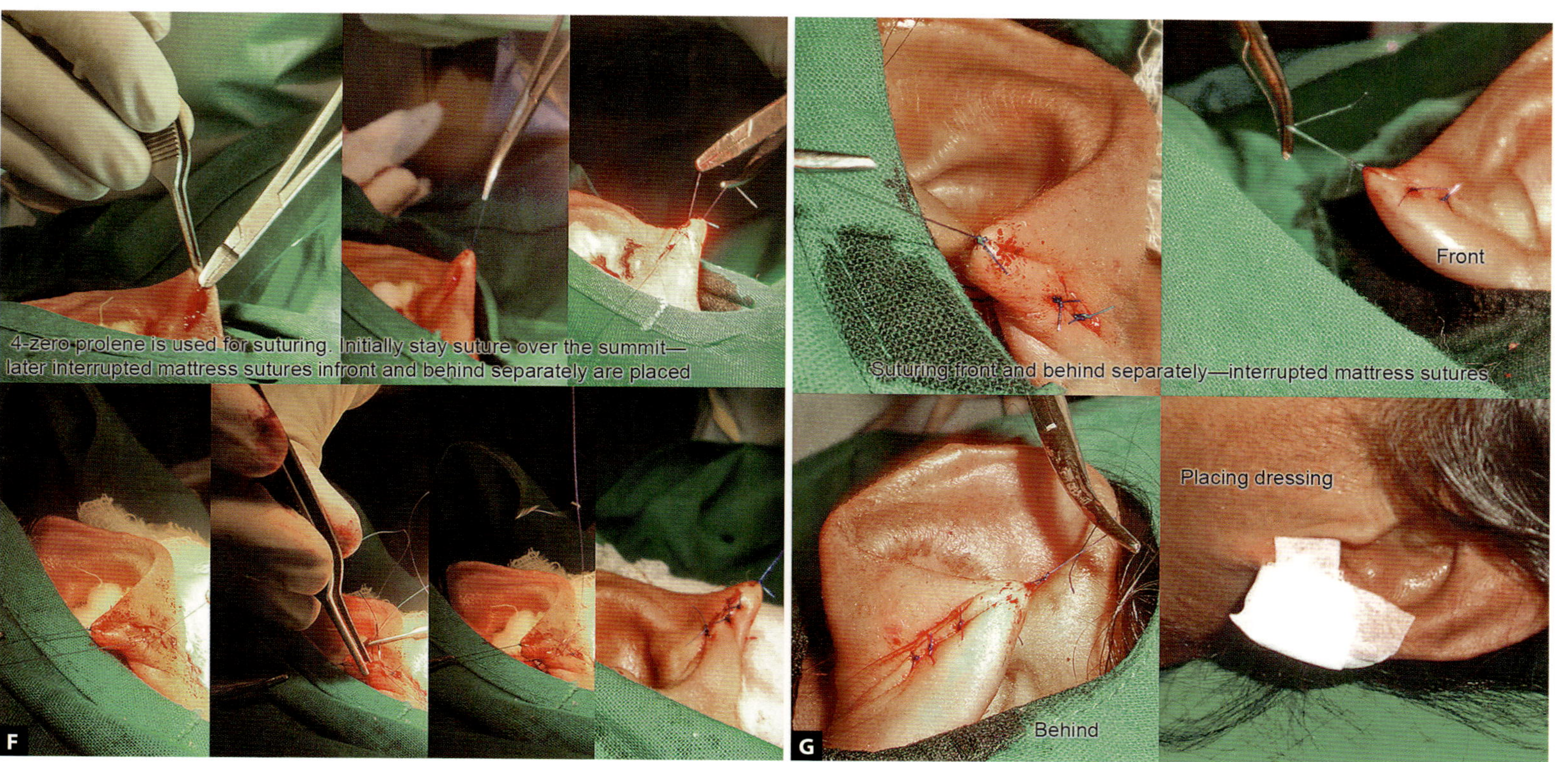

Figs. 7-129F and G

Figs. 7-129A to G: Operative steps in earlobe repair.

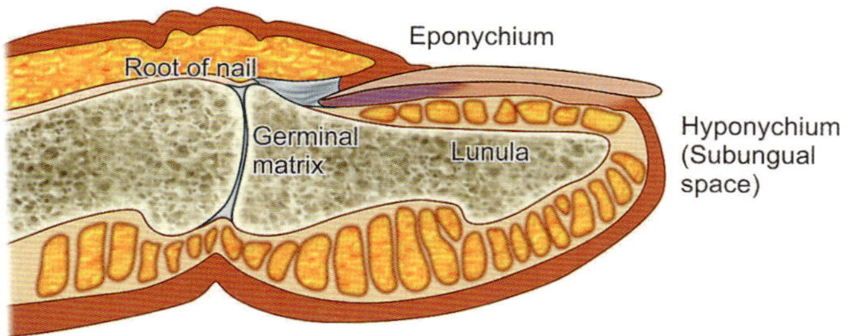

Fig. 7-130: Anatomy of the nail.

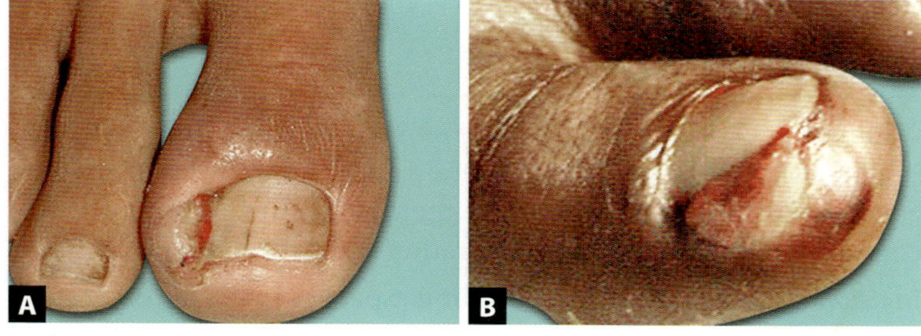

Figs. 7-131A and B: Ingrown toe nail with hypertrophied soft tissue.

After the procedure, the skin looks very red and raw, and takes several months for the skin to regrow and heal. Dermabrasion is useful for removal of scars especially when the scar is raised above the surrounding skin, but is less effective in sunken scars. In the past, dermabrasion was done using a small, sterilised, electric sander. In the past decade, it has become more common to use a CO_2 or Erbium:YAG laser. Laser dermabrasion is much easier to control, much easier to gauge, and is practically bloodless compared to classic dermabrasion. Microdermabrasion, crystal dermabrasion, diamond dermabrasion are different types. Even though healing is slow, eventual result is cosmetically better **(Figs. 7-133A and B)**.

VENEPUNCTURE

Forearm veins are commonly used. Venepuncture is needed for fluid therapy, parenteral drug therapy, transfusions, etc. Clothing of the arm and forearm is removed. Hairs are shaved from the site. Area is cleaned with spirit. Tourniquet is applied above in the arm. Patient is asked to fist the fingers. Needle is passed obliquely into the skin with its bevel facing front and to the prominent vein. Skin puncture is 5 mm distal to the site of entry of the vein. Blood will enter the syringe. Intravenous cannula when used needle is removed once it is inside the vein which is confirmed by the blood flow; cannula is pushed into the vein entirely; needle is removed; cannula is connected to IV set and fluid. Cannula is fixed using plasters. Small dose of heparin should be flushed into the cannula daily to prevent thrombophlebitis.

Problems with venepuncture: Veins may not be visible. Flow may not be sufficient. Circulatory overload, thrombophlebitis, local haematoma, infection are common problems. Infection may be often hospital acquired and severe enough to cause septicaemia. Abscess at local site, oedema are also common. There is a real danger of air embolism if IV set is not closed once drip fluid gets over.

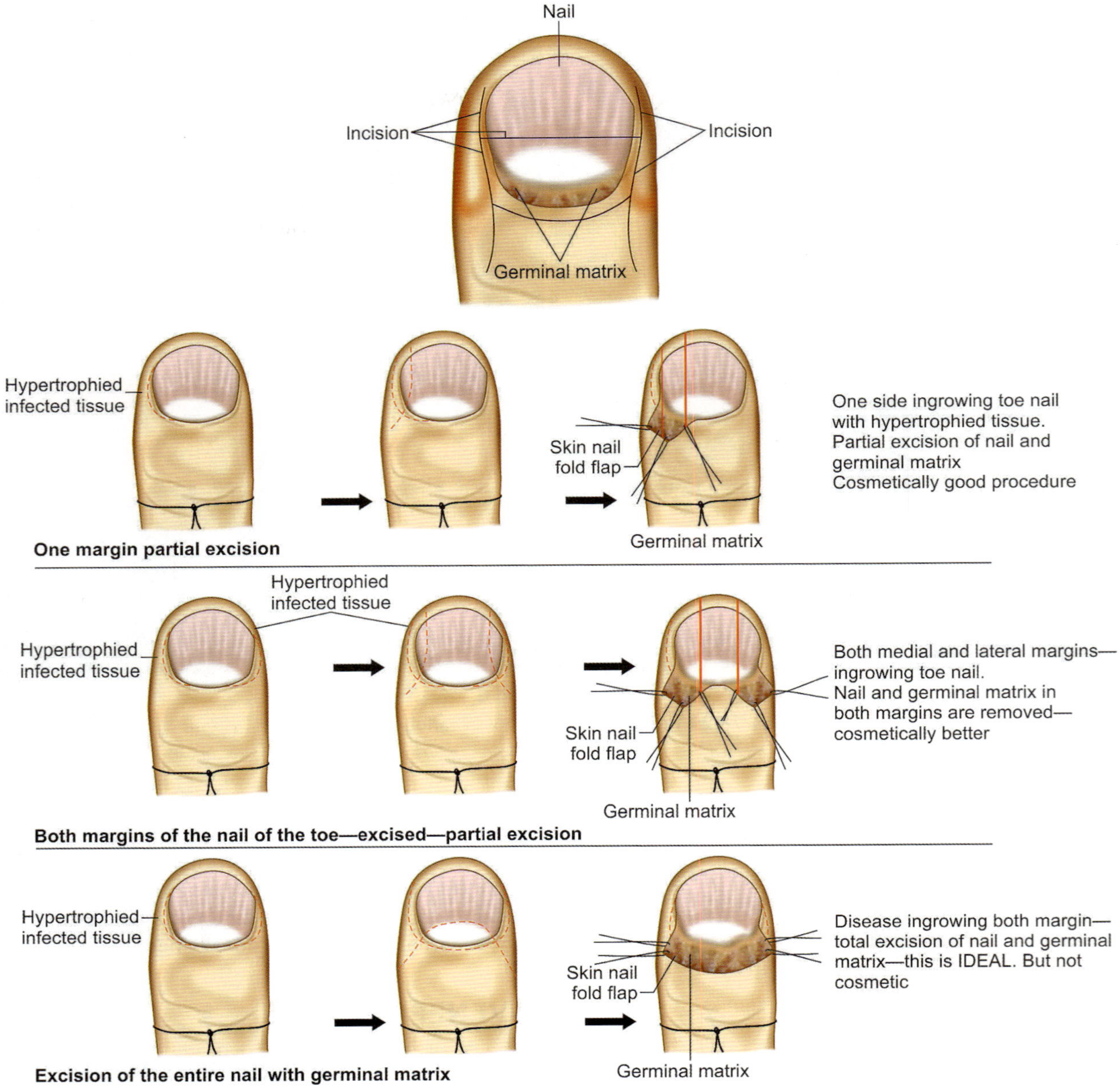

Nail

Incision

Incision

Germinal matrix

Hypertrophied infected tissue

Skin nail fold flap

Germinal matrix

One side ingrowing toe nail with hypertrophied tissue. Partial excision of nail and germinal matrix Cosmetically good procedure

One margin partial excision

Hypertrophied infected tissue

Hypertrophied infected tissue

Skin nail fold flap

Germinal matrix

Both medial and lateral margins—ingrowing toe nail. Nail and germinal matrix in both margins are removed—cosmetically better

Both margins of the nail of the toe—excised—partial excision

Hypertrophied infected tissue

Skin nail fold flap

Germinal matrix

Disease ingrowing both margin—total excision of nail and germinal matrix—this is IDEAL. But not cosmetic

Excision of the entire nail with germinal matrix

Fig. 7-132: Technique of excision of nail, partial and complete with removal of adjacent or entire germinal matrix. Note the incision used for removal of the germinal matrix.

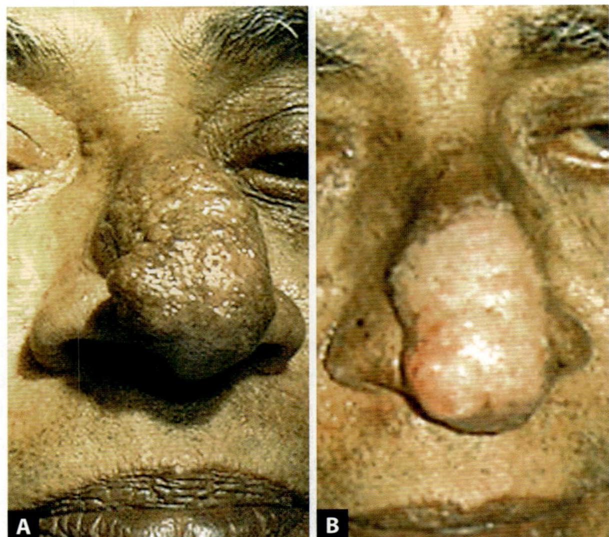

Figs. 7-133A and B: Rhinophyma—typical look. Also observe after scraping/dermabrasion.

VENESECTION

It means accessing the vein by *open surgical* approach. It is done in patient in shock where peripheral vein or central vein cannot be cannulated. It aids in rapid fluid therapy in shock, monitoring of central venous pressure, administration of different drugs.

Incision: Usually upper arm on lateral aspect or in the leg on medial, posterior lower aspect is used. In the upper arm cephalic vein is used (if CVP monitoring is needed cephalic vein is selected); in the leg long saphenous vein is used. Cephalic vein is used in upper/mid-arm aspect, laterally between triceps and biceps muscles. Long saphenous vein is cannulated 1–2 cm above and anterior to the medial malleoli. *Saphenous vein* is superficial in the subcutaneous plane. But *cephalic vein* is deep and needs deeper dissection. Inadvertent dissection may cause injury to brachial vessels and so one should be careful.

Procedure: Area is cleaned and draped with aseptic precautions. *Transverse incision* is made. Skin, subcutaneous tissue is incised. Vein is identified by its bluish nature. It is dissected using mosquito forceps and freed from adjacent tissues for 2 cm. Two thread or silk sutures are passed under the vein, each with 1 cm gap. Distal thread is ligated. Aneurysm needle may be helpful for proper dissection and passing ligatures around the vein. Front aspect of the vein is opened using a scalpel blade no 11. Venous cannula or venous catheter or polythene tube or infant feeding tube with cut tip is passed adequately. Its tip is empirically adjusted to place at subclavian vein or at superior vena cava. C-arm monitoring may confirm it if needed (usually not used). Patency of the vein is confirmed by pushing the saline and rapid flow of fluid through the drip. Proximal thread is tied around the cannula. Skin is closed and cannula is secured firmly **(Figs. 7-134 and 7-135)**.

Complications (Problems): Often difficult to get vein as vein may be collapsed due to shock or vein may be thrombosed due to repeated earlier venepuncture. Thrombosis of vein, blockage, bleeding, sepsis, failure, displacement of cannula are other complications.

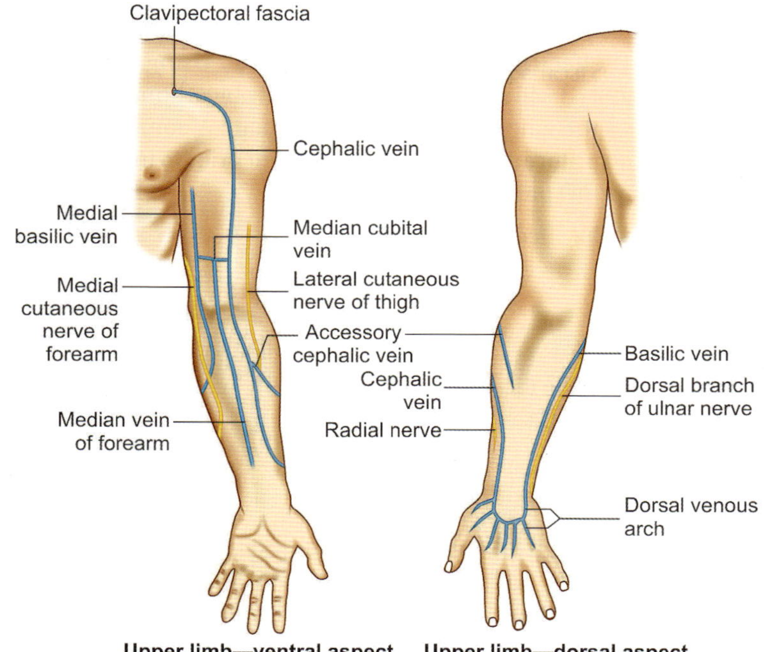

Fig. 7-134: Venous anatomy of the upper limb. *Cephalic vein* (pre-axial vein of upper limb) is formed at lateral part of the dorsal venous arch runs upwards along the anatomical snuff box, lateral part of the forearm, lateral margin of the biceps brachii, lateral aspect of the arm. At lower margin of the pectoralis major, after piercing the deep fascia, it passes through deltopectoral groove, clavipectoral fascia to enter the cephalic vein. *Median cubital vein* is a large communicating vein begins from cephalic vein 2.5 cm below the elbow crossing obliquely from lateral to medial side to reach the basilic vein 2.5 cm above medial epicondyle. Median cubital vein is located in front of the bicipital aponeurosis, through which a constant perforator vein from deep veins pierces. This perforator vein fixes the median cubital vein making this vein ideal for intravenous injections, drawing blood. Median cubital vein is absent in 30% of individuals; in such occasions basilic vein is used for drawing blood than cephalic vein as it is more efficient. Cephalic vein is mainly used for venesection. *Basilic vein* is post-axial upper limb vein; begins at lateral aspect of the dorsal venous arch; runs medially along forearm, elbow, medial border of the biceps brachii, medial part of the arm. In middle of the arm it pierces the deep fascia running along the medial aspect of the brachial artery; continues as axillary vein at the lower margin of the teres major.

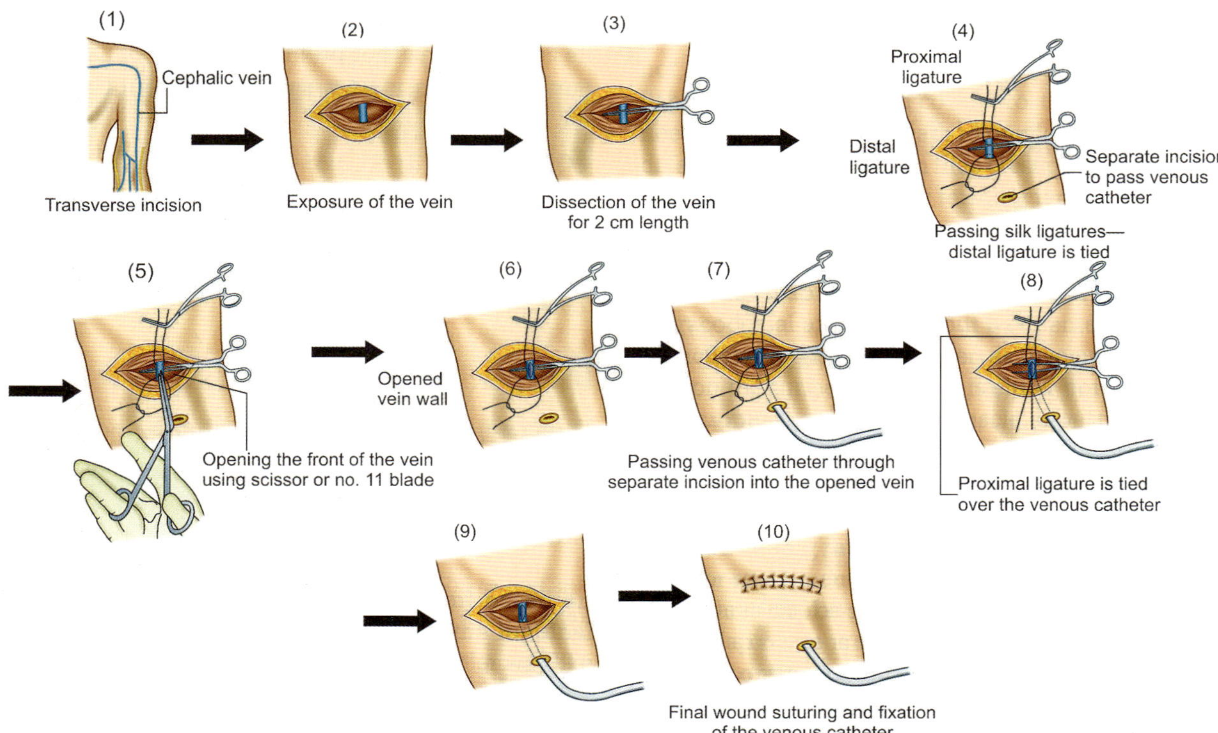

Fig. 7-135: Venesection—steps (Venous cutdown)—shown here is in cephalic vein.

INTRAOSSEOUS FLUID THERAPY

Intraosseous fluid therapy is useful in children whenever intravenous access has failed completely. Through vascular bone marrow fluid is infused which reaches main circulation in 10 seconds. Specific needles *(Sussmane-Raszynski needle)* are available for this purpose. 18 G spinal or bone marrow aspiration needle also can be used. Local anaesthesia is injected under the skin. Tibia is ideal site. In children *below* 5 years, *upper end of tibia* is used—anteromedial aspect just below the tibial tuberosity with direction of the needle being *caudal*. In *children above 5 years* and in adults, *lower end of tibia* 5 cm above the medial malleolus is used. Here direction of needle will be *cephalad*. This part of the bone is thin and flat and so it is easier to puncture. Lower end is not used in children below 5 years. Intraosseous fluid flow is usually at the rate of 10–15 mL/minute **(Fig. 7-136)**.

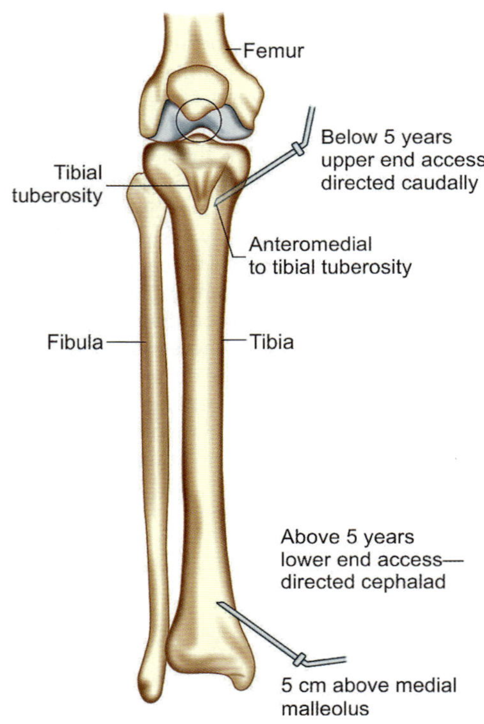

Fig. 7-136: Intraosseous fluid therapy sites.

SUBCUTANEOUS INFUSIONS AS FLUID THERAPY

It is rarely used but in dire time can be used only for fluid therapy. Sites used are—outer aspect of the thigh, abdominal wall, and lateral chest wall. After cleaning the wide skin area, needle is inserted (20 G needle) into the subcutaneous tissue and is connected to drip. Usual infusion rate possible is 80 mL/minute. *Problems are*—pain, swelling, infection and slow absorption of the fluid.

LOCAL/REGIONAL ANAESTHESIA

Carl Koller, an *ophthalmologist* introduced cocaine as local anaesthetic in ophthalmic practice. Mode of action: It causes temporary conduction block of the nerve, thus preventing the propagation of nerve impulse. *Advantages* of local anaesthetic agents are—it is technically simpler; general anaesthesia is avoided; patient's consciousness is retained; patient can have food soon after surgery.

Drugs used:

Cocaine, procaine, cinchocaine—amino esters.

Lignocaine, prilocaine, bupivacaine, ropivacaine—amino amides.

Lignocaine/lidocaine/xylocaine: It is the commonest local anaesthetic agent used. It is available as 0.25–5% concentrations. It is metabolised in the liver and excreted in the kidney as xylidines. It is also an anti-arrhythmic drug and so commonly used in cardiology and cardiac surgery.

Side effects: Giddiness, headache, postural hypotension, tinnitus, circumoral anaesthesia, rarely anaphylaxis, convulsions and cardiac arrest if it becomes inadvertently intravenous.

Local anaesthesia infiltration is painful; intradermal injection of the drug is effective but much more painful. Using fine gauge needle (24 G/26 G) will reduce the pain. Adding bicarbonate into the drug increases the efficacy and reduces the pain. A combination of lignocaine and prilocaine (EMLA) topical agent prior to injecting the drug (1 hour prior) prevents such pain.

Dose: 4 mg/kg. Its effect lasts for 90 minutes.

Uses

- Topical: 4%.
- Infiltration block: 0.5–2%.
- Field block: 0.5–2%.
- Nerve block: 1.0%.
- Epidural: 1.5, 2.0%.
- Spinal: 5%.

It can be used with or without adrenaline. Xylocaine with adrenaline (1 in 2,00,000) has got longer duration of action. It creates relatively bloodless field. Higher dose can be injected as absorption is slow (7 mg/kg). But it should not be used in places where end arteries are present like glans penis, ear lobule, tip of the nose, lip, fingers and toes.

Bupivacaine (Marcaine): It has got prolonged action. It is a vasodilator also. It is used as 0.25–0.5%. It takes more time to begin its action but has got prolonged action of 8 hours. Dose: 3 mg/kg. For epidural block: 0.5%; spinal 0.5% of 3 mL solution.

Topical Anaesthesia

It is used for minor surgeries of eye, laryngoscopy, bronchoscopy, cystoscopy, gastroscopy, submucus injection. It is available as instillation, spray, viscous, ointment, gel, *EMLA* (Eutectic mixture of local anaesthetic).

Infiltration Block

Direct injection of local anaesthetic under the skin for small procedures.

Field Block

It is achieved by blocking the entire field of excision where lesion is located.

Nerve Block

- Block of inferior dental nerve and lingual nerves in the region of the mental foramen for extraction of teeth.

- Finger block of digital nerves. Here plain xylocaine is used (without adrenaline)—*digital nerve block*. It is injected just distal to web space near base of the finger on either side into palmar and dorsal digital nerves.
- Intercostal block.
- Ankle block.
- Median and ulnar nerve block.
- Brachial plexus block (Winnie's block): It can be given through interscalene, axillary, supraclavicular approaches. Supraclavicular approach is commonly used. 1 cm above the midpoint of the clavicle, needle is passed downwards, backwards and medially towards first rib. Once needle hits the first rib, 15–20 mL of 1.5% xylocaine is injected (with walking or stepping over the first rib). Complications are pneumothorax and injury to the great vessels.

Other Blocks

Cervical plexus block; sciatic nerve block; femoral nerve block.

Intravenous Regional Anaesthesia (Bier's Block)

Limb is exsanguinated and occluded with tourniquet. Pressure in the tourniquet must be 30 mm Hg more than the systolic pressure of the patient. Needle is placed in the selected vein. 40 mL of 0.5% xylocaine for upper limb and 80 mL of 0.25% of xylocaine for lower limb is injected into the vein. *Xylocaine with adrenaline should not be used.* It gives very good analgesia for 2 hours. Side effects: Sudden release of drug into the circulation can cause hypotension, convulsions and often death. Bupivacaine should not be used.

Indications: For upper and lower limb surgeries it can be used without general or spinal anaesthesia.

Spinal Anaesthesia

Xylocaine or bupivacaine is injected into subarachnoid space using long (disposable needles are available now) needle (***Quincke spinal needle***). It is 10 cm long with stillete inside it. Transparent hub needle is available now. 25 G/27 G needles are finer and better with lesser complications especially headache and backache. *Refer lumbar puncture* for details.

Saddle block: It is used for surgeries in perineal and anorectal region. It is spinal anaesthesia using xylocaine or bupivacaine given in sitting position. It is low spinal block.

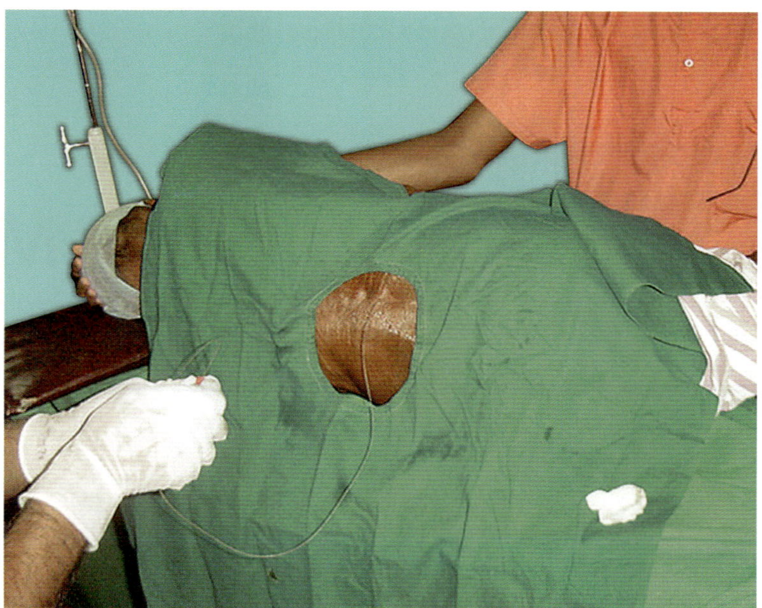

Fig. 7-137: Epidural anaesthesia is being given.

Epidural Anaesthesia

It is a potential space between dura anteriorly and ligamentum flavum posteriorly which has got negative pressure inside. It extends from foramen magnum to sacral haitus. ***Touhy needle*** is used for epidural anaesthesia. Once the needle is in the space there will be sudden indrawing of air or saline drop. An epidural catheter is placed in the space and fixed. 2% xylocaine with adrenaline or 0.5% bupivacaine is injected into the space to achieve anaesthesia up to the desired level **(Fig. 7-137)**.

Advantages: It can be used for continuous repeated prolonged anaesthesia. It can be used for post-operative analgesia. It can be kept for several days.

Caudal Anaesthesia

Caudal space is the sacral component of *epidural space* and access is through the sacral hiatus. *Indications:* Haemorrhoidal surgery; circumcision; small procedures in the perineum like cystoscopy. *Procedure:* It is given in lateral position. Needle is inserted through the sacral hiatus to enter the caudal epidural space. Drug is then injected into the space. It takes 20 minutes to act and so surgeon has to wait for this to act. *Complications:* Trauma to anal canal, intravascular injection, failure of caudal block is common.

8

CHAPTER

Principles of Surgical Management in Trauma

Trauma is the major cause of death worldwide. It can be road traffic accidents, stab injuries, thermal injuries, and gunshot-related injuries.

Inexperienced motor skills, alcohol consumption; aggressive driving, influence of drugs are the common factors for RTA. Gun shot injuries is becoming more common nowadays due to usage of guns for fights. Gun shot can cause local injury, compression injury, cavitational injury (10 times the diameter of the bullet), burn injury. Fall from height is also a major cause as it leads into spinal injury, internal organ injury. Fall from 10 meters height has got impact velocity of 50 kph. Fall from more than 15 meters height carries more than 50% mortality. Nature of landing surface, part of the body coming into contact with the surface first, deceleration force, body's position during landing.

Trauma is categorised as group trauma like in earthquake, train accidents, fire injury, etc. or individual trauma **(Fig. 8-1)**.

War injuries are of special type could be missile wounds, low velocity missile wounds or high velocity missile wounds or blast injuries.

Dictum in trauma is '*first save life; then think of limbs; later worry about sufferings*'.

ASSESSMENT OF SEVERITY OF THE INJURY

AIS (Abbreviated Injury Scale) scoring system is used once all injuries of the patient is identified. Each injury is scored from 1 to 6. An AIS score of 6 anywhere in the body is not compatible with life. So maximum score assessed in a live patient is 5. Square of three highest AIS scores within six areas in the body—head and neck; abdomen and pelvic contents; bony pelvis and limbs; face; chest and body surface is called as *Injury Severity Score* (ISS). Maximum ISS score is 5 × 5 + 5 × 5 + 5 × 5 = 75. Glasgow coma scale and revised trauma scale [RTS = respiratory weight × 0.2908 + systolic blood pressure weight × 0.7326 + GCS (Glasgow Coma Scale) **(Table 8-1)** weight × 0.9368] are commonly used in head injury patients.

Trauma and Injury Severity Score (TRISS) system is used by combining anatomical and physiological injuries **(Figs. 8-2 and 8-3)**.

Severe trauma may be entrapment, high speed impact, collision, fall from height of more than 3 meters, ejection from a moving vehicle and penetrating injuries.

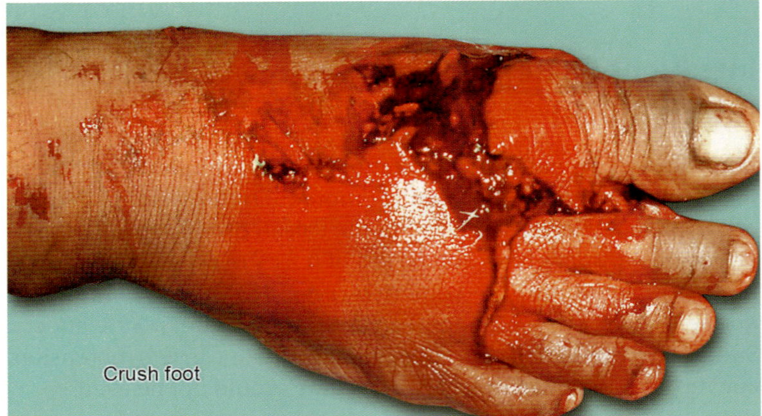

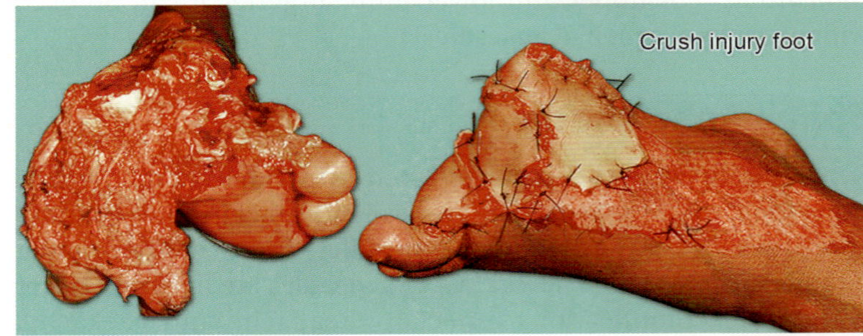

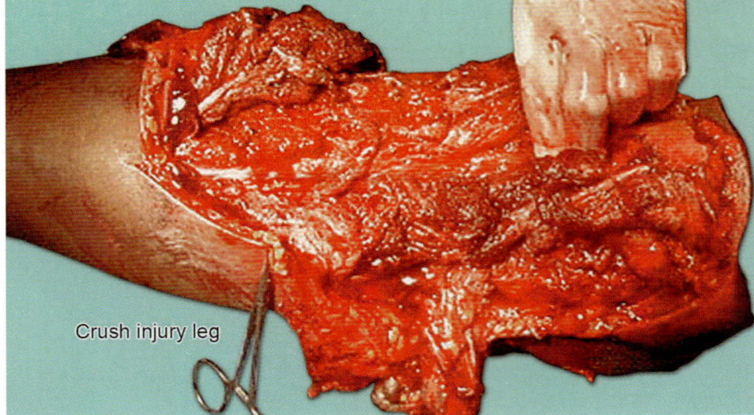

Fig. 8-1: Thorough warm saline wash is a must to all open wound. Wound excision is done by removing all devitalised tissue. Viable skin part should be retained for future reconstruction. Often such flap can be rotated as quilting into the defect area.

TABLE 8-1: Glasgow coma scale (GCS).

Eye opening		*Verbal response*		*Motor response*	
Spontaneous	4	Oriented	5	Obeys commands	6
To Speech	3	Confused	4	Localises pain	5
To Pain	2	Inappropriate words	3	Flexion to pain	4
None	1	Incomprehensible words	2	Abnormal flexion	3
		None	1	Extension to pain	2
				None	1
Total score: 15. Mild head injury: 13–15. Moderate head injury: 9–12. Severe head injury: Less than 8 [3–8].					
Score 1—dead or dying. Score 2—vegetative state. Score 3—severe disability. Score 4—moderate disability. Score 5—good recovery.					

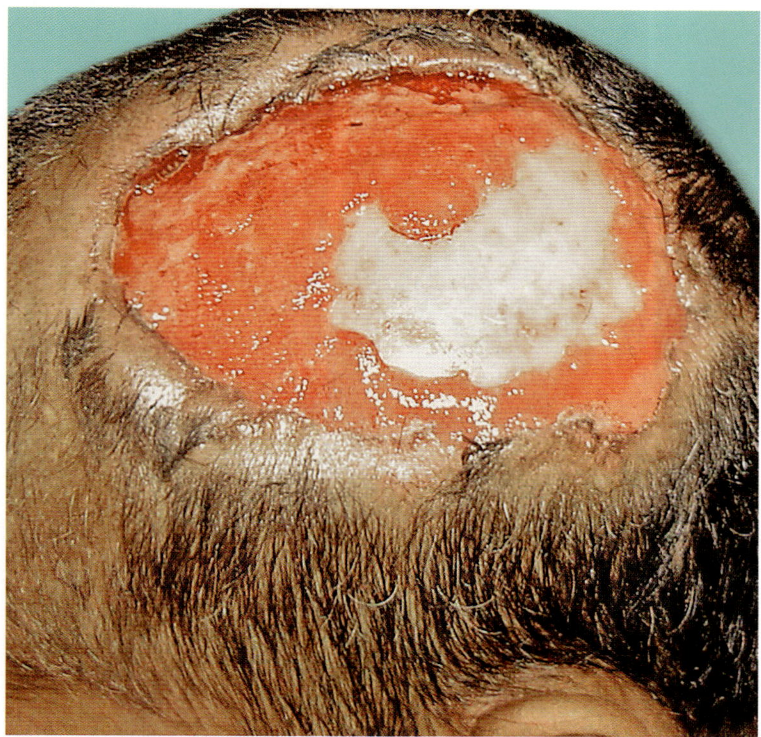

Fig. 8-2: Scalp trauma exposing outer table partly.

Baton round injury occurs during police firing in mob dispersion. It is rubber bullet/plastic compound injury occurring during police firing. It can cause bruising, lacerations or life-threatening blunt injuries/penetrating injuries also. So *baton round injury* cannot be ignored.

PREHOSPITAL TRAUMA CARE

It is the initial safe resuscitation and proper arrangement and planning for transport as early as possible. It is done by police and fire service people. They should be trained for initial resuscitation. Transportation and ambulance service is essential. Well-equipped ambulance should be available. Transport is done by vehicles, ambulances and helicopters. Careful transport is essential depending on the type of trauma. It is essential in spine injury, chest/abdominal/head injuries. A dedicated resuscitation team is ideal. 3 doctors, 2 nurses, 2 technicians are essential in the team with all essential facilities like central line, fluid therapy, emergency drugs, etc.

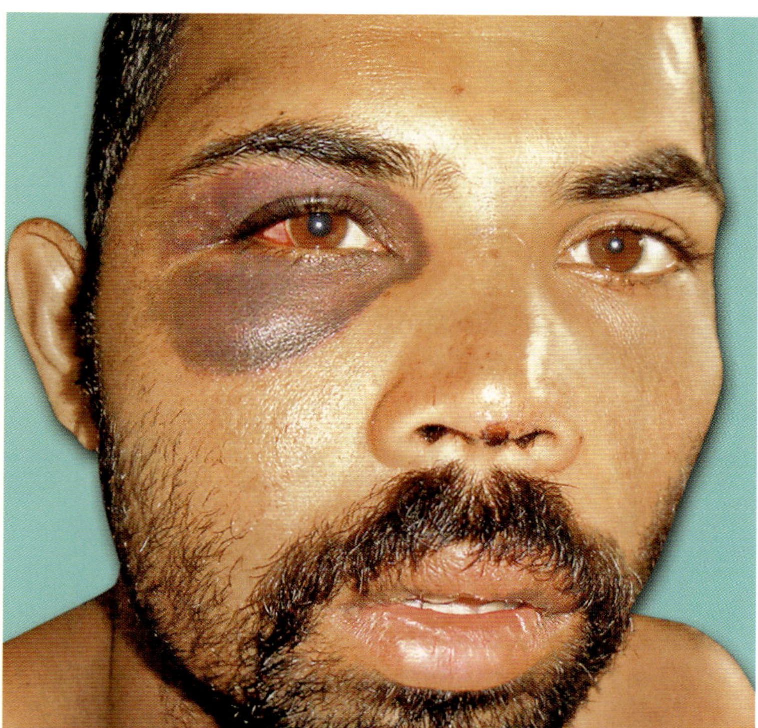

Fig. 8-3: Black eye. It may be a sign of intracranial bleed.

TERTIARY HOSPITAL CARE

Airway: Suctioning, clearing throat, clearing foreign bodies/dentures, oxygen, endotracheal intubation, percutaneous cricothyrotomy, tracheostomy are done, depending on need.

Breathing: Breathing is assessed and if needed intercostal tube drainage in case of pneumothorax or haemothorax should be inserted.

Circulation: It is assessed by pulse, blood pressure, capillary filing and monitoring. Proper perfusion and blood transfusion is needed. Two 12 or 14 G cannulas should be passed to have proper intravenous access. In difficult situations when patient is in shock with collapsed peripheral veins, long saphenous vein, cephalic vein, basilic vein, external jugular vein or femoral vein cannulation should be tried. Definitive venous cut down of long saphenous vein or cephalic vein should be done. Percutaneous puncture of internal jugular vein is also possible. Blood samples should be collected for electrolyte estimation, haematocrit, blood urea and creatinine, blood group and cross matching. Central venous catheter should be passed after that in all patients. It is passed through subclavian vein or through internal jugular vein. In children *intraosseous* route is possible to perfuse in emergency **(Fig. 8-4)**.

Initially isotonic crystalloid such as normal saline/Ringer's lactate is used. Once around 1,500 mL of crystalloids are infused to bring up the volume, then colloids and blood are given. Dextrans, other volume expanders are also used in emergency but

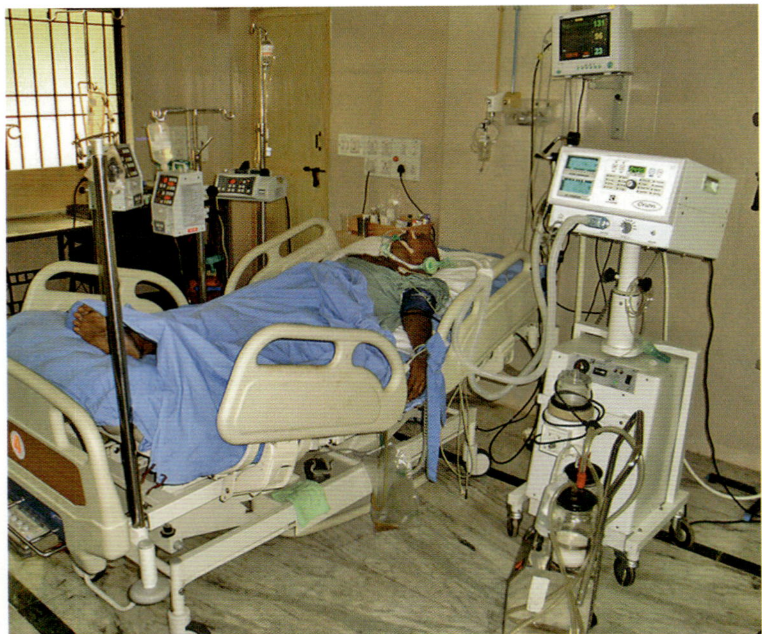

Fig. 8-4: Intensive care is needed in critical trauma patient.

not more than 1,500 mL. It is better to give warmed fluid of any of these forms to prevent hypothermia. Intravenous warmer devices are available. If patient is responding for initial 2 L of fluid therapy means blood loss is more than 40% suggesting severe circulatory failure. *Blood transfusions* are given to maintain haematocrit at 30%.

Nasogastric tube and urinary catheter placement is a must.

Monitoring is done by pulse, oxygen saturation, urine output with a indwelling catheter in situ (should be >1 mL/kg/hour), platelet count, coagulation factors, serum electrolytes estimation, ECG monitoring, CVP and PCWP assessment, arterial blood gas analysis.

Further assessment is done by assessing neurological status, specific injuries in head, skull base, thorax, abdomen, pelvis and fractures. CT of part is ideal investigation. Usually plain CT without contrast is done. Hypoxia, hypercapnia, hypotension are the important critical factors. Spine injury may be missed very often in initial assessment. It should be carefully assessed and if needed/suspected should be evaluated by CT imaging. MRI is not possible in initial phase of resuscitation which should be done at later period.

Often endotracheal intubation, ventilator or tracheostomy may be needed and should be utilised without any hesitation to save the life.

Adequate analgesia is important. Morphine/dimorphine/non-steroidal anti-inflammatory drugs (NSAIDs) intramuscularly can be given. *Temporary immobilisation* using proper splintage for long bone fractures reduces the pain severity. Fixation in pelvic fractures with external fixator reduces the pain. Medical anti-shock trouser (MAST) is used for shock.

Three primary X-rays are done even though they have got limitations. Chest X-ray to see pneumothorax/haemothorax/fracture ribs. But 30–40% of fracture ribs will be missed in X-ray. Cervical spine lateral X-ray and pelvis anteroposterior X-rays are taken.

Ultrasound abdomen, CT of chest, pelvis and abdomen is ideal. Diagnostic peritoneal lavage (DPL) is useful in blunt injury abdomen.

ASSESSMENT OF THE WOUND

Size of the injury; extent of the damage—nerve, vessels, viscera, peripheral ischaemia especially in the limbs, presence of haematoma, extent of deeper injury including bones, entry wound and exit wound in missile injury are carefully assessed **(Fig. 8-5)**.

First Aid Management of the Wound

Large occlusive firm pressure dressing of the wound, compression bandage, control of haemorrhage, occasionally tourniquet application, positioning of the patient are the first aid measures often required.

Wound will be minimally contaminated in 0-6 hours; significantly contaminated in 6–12 hours; grossly contaminated in more than 12 hours **(Fig. 8-6)**.

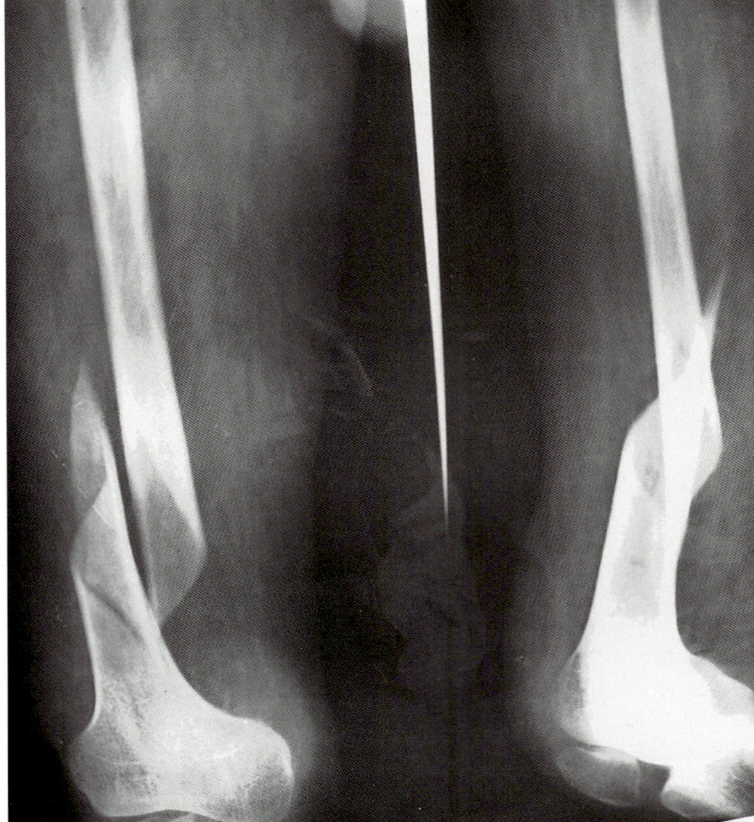

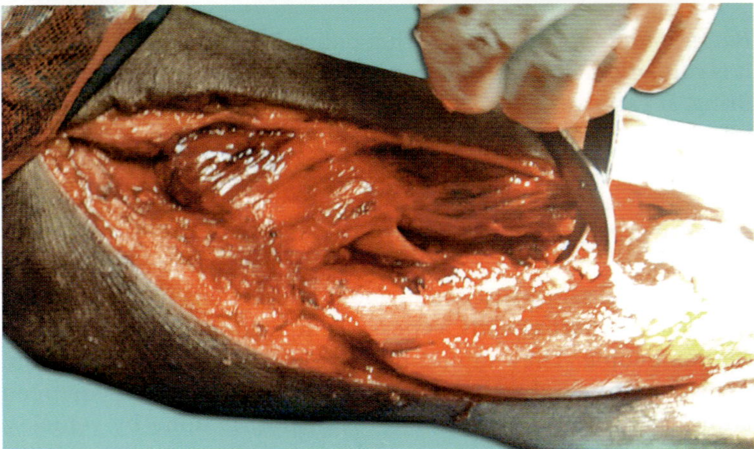

Fig. 8-5: X-ray should be taken to see the fracture. Soft tissue injury should be assessed properly.

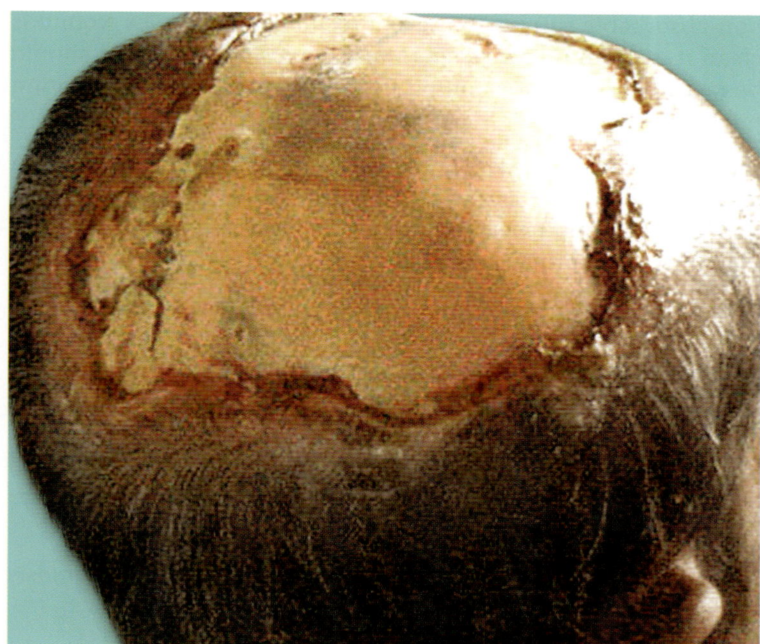

Fig. 8-6: Skull bone is exposed without any retained periosteum. Such bone will not show any granulation tissue. Burr holes in many places on the outer table allow marrow to proliferate as granulation tissue; later area is covered with flap. Care should be taken while doing burr drills to avoid injury to the venous sinuses.

WOUND EXCISION AND MANAGEMENT

Wound excision should be done under *general* anaesthesia. Local anaesthesia should be avoided. Here dead/damaged or contaminated tissues are excised. All foreign bodies should be removed. Exception for this is probably bullet injuries/pellet injuries. It is often difficult to remove a bullet or multiple pellets. They may lie in close proximity to any major vessel or often difficult to identify and remove. During entry they are in high temperature and so are absolutely sterile; will not precipitate any contamination. Control of bleeding is also an essential part in wound excision.

Tourniquet during surgery (wound radical excision) is used only if it is inevitable; otherwise should be avoided as it is difficult to differentiate dead and living tissue under tourniquet. Hairs should be removed 1 cm beyond the margin of the wound. Skin and wound should be thoroughly scrubbed with soap, water and saline for 5–10 minutes until it appears clean and then area is widely cleaned with povidone iodine before draping. Proper initial irrigation of the contaminated wound often using pressure device is important to remove dirty particles from the surface. Incision placed in the wound should be enlarged/extended liberally without any hesitation especially in penetrating wounds, war wounds, bullet wounds, crush wounds, entry wound of bullet, multiple deep wounds. Exploring the entire wound is very important. Excision is done until healthy bleeding live tissue is reached. Excision should be done by sharp dissection using knife or scissor. Underlying nerves and major feeding vessels should be protected. Skin is excised for 2 mm from the contaminated edge. There is no use in retaining the dead tissue and no point in cutting healthy skin which is again essential for future closure or reconstruction. Wound can be re-inspected for further wound excision if needed especially skin after 48 hours.

Often *flap-like injury* when found with a wide base can be retained provided it is relatively healthy. Crushed skin may not be vital for placing. Flap should be washed, irrigated and placed over the raw area. When such flap sustenance is not sure, the flap can be cut completely, fat underneath should be cleared and sutured like a free full thickness graft. If possible split thickness graft is taken from the surface of such flap using a Humby's knife, and is very well placed on the defect area which often takes properly. Fat in the entire area should be excised otherwise it is a sure way of causing necrosis and contamination of the area in later period. Fascial layers should be split. Ragged devitalised part should be excised. Oedema underneath the fascial layer causes initial impairment of venous and lymphatic drainage later blocking arterial function leading into distal ischaemia, necrosis and gangrene. Lengthy liberal fasciotomy is a must in these patients. All *devitalised, dying and dead muscles* should be excised without fail. There is no reason to retain the dead muscle at all. Dead muscle is a sure way for infection like *Clostridium* bacteria. All haematomas should be evacuated liberally. After radical wound excision if there spurting bleeders, it should be ligated securely using fine absorbable sutures **(Figs. 8-7 to 8-10)**.

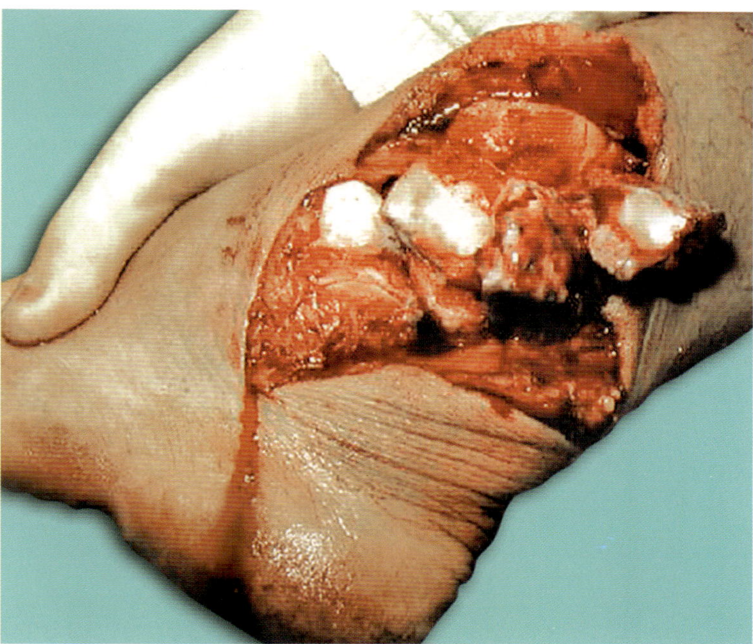

Fig. 8-7: Crush injury of ankle.

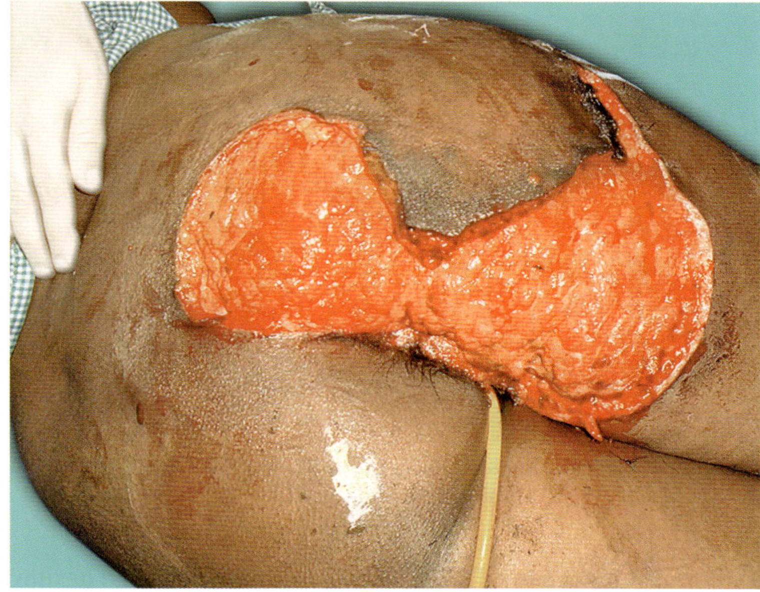

Fig. 8-8: Degloving injury of buttock region. It is eventually covered using a flap.

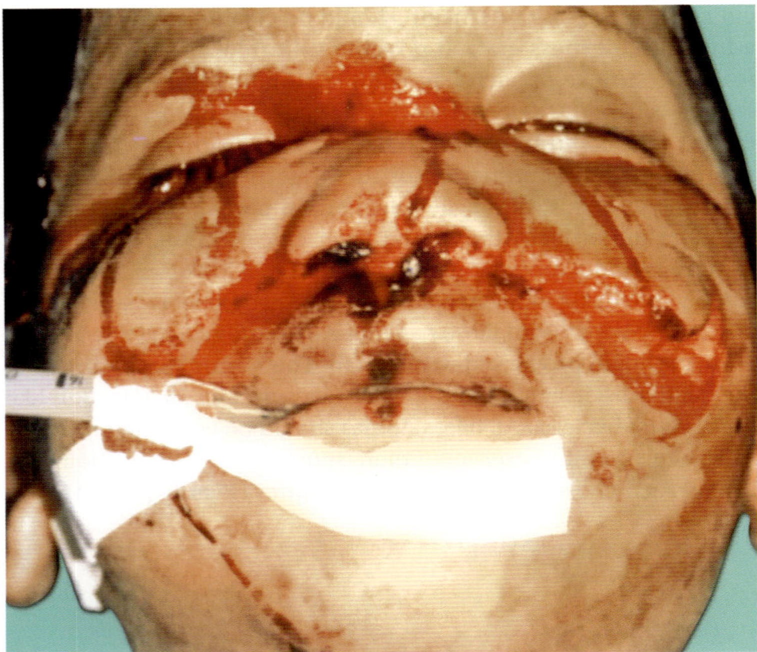

Fig. 8-9: Extensive injury in a child due to dog bite. Wound debridement should be done under general anaesthesia.

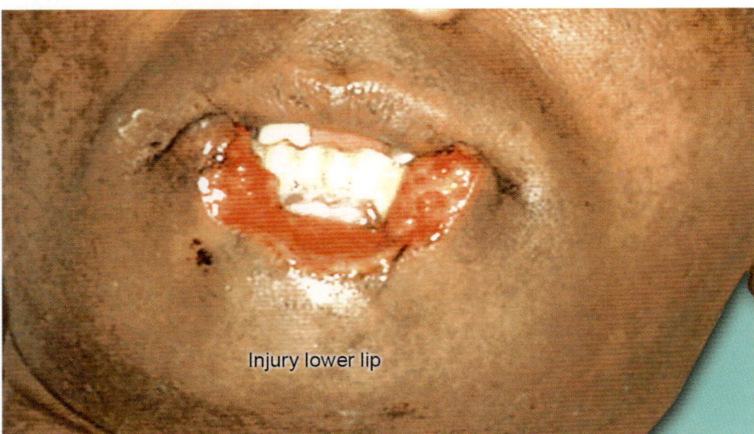

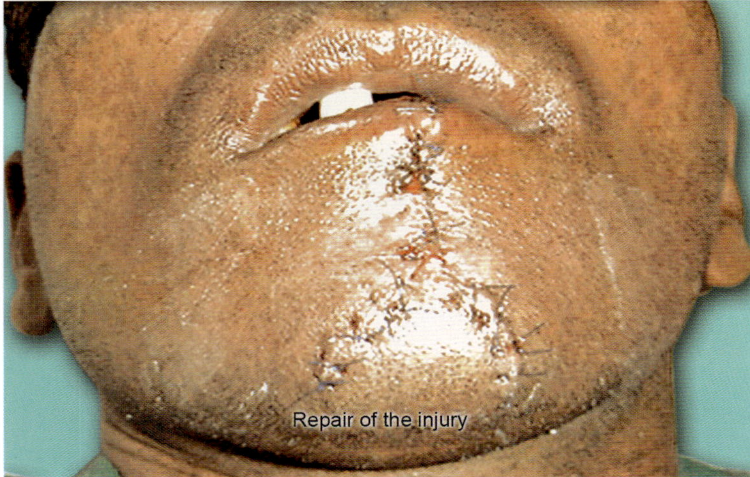

Fig. 8-10: Injury to the lower lip causing defect in its central part which is primarily repaired.

Nerve injury is dealt in different ways. If wound is clean and healthy it is sutured primarily with non-absorbable sutures; otherwise it is trimmed and tethered to the adjacent soft tissues loosely using non-absorbable sutures to prevent recoiling. Later once wound is clean it is taken up for repair. Many nerves when injured should be tagged in different coloured sutures for eventual identification purpose.

Exposed tendons can be left alone; but if paratenon is denuded it should be excised as tendon will necrose. Repair of tendon may be done at later period in such occasion. If it is a clean incised tendon injury then only primary repair of tendon is done.

Bone even though injured until periosteum is intact, it heals well. Skin can be covered over periosteum. If periosteum is denuded then flap is needed to cover it. Bone fixation, prevention of sepsis and flap cover is the needed plan in these patients.

Joint injury needs early immediate cover to prevent from anticipated infection. Synovium should be sutured with interrupted sutures. Proper wound cleaning with adequate ideal antibiotics are mandatory.

Major vessel injury should be sutured as per vascular anastomosis rule.

Body cavities when opened by trauma should be closed. Dura should be closed by temporalis fascia graft.

Primary closure means closure done immediately after wound excision. Delayed primary closure is done in 5 days after wound excision. Secondary late closure is closure done after 5 days. When in doubt do not close the wound immediately—is the principle.

PRINCIPLES IN USAGE OF ANTIBIOTICS

It is a debate whether to use it or not. In minor wounds it is not necessary to take antibiotics or a single intravenous dose is sufficient. In major wounds it is essential to give antibiotics intravenously; an oral antibiotic in initial phase of therapy is less preferred one than intravenous one. Intravenous penicillin or cephalosporins are given conventionally. Higher generation antibiotics are used depending on the need and contamination.

One should remember that antibiotics are not a substitute for adequate wound care. There is no short coming in proper wound care to have a good final outcome.

Gas gangrene is more common in deep ragged wounds, crush injuries, war wounds, blast injuries. Radical wound excision and closure of wound only at later period are the important preventive measures. In suspected cases anti-gas gangrene serum should be injected.

Immobilisation is often very important in major wounds even if there is no bone injury. Immobilisation improves healing; reduces the pain; possibly decreases the infection rate.

MANAGEMENT OF FOREIGN BODY

Unlike many think it is usually not an emergency procedure unless it is causing life-threatening problems. Image intensifier (C-arm) should be used to remove foreign body. It should be done under general anaesthesia. Tourniquet is used when it is in the limbs. Adequate incision with wide exposure is a must. Gentle finger exploration is better than by instruments as feel of the foreign body by fingers is more appreciable than through the instrument. Every foreign body need not be removed (like bullets/pellets). Foreign body if not retrieved in 45 minutes of exploration, procedure should be abandoned.

TRIAGE

Triage: Triage means *'To sort' in 'French'*.
Triage was formulated by a committee of Trauma of the American College of Surgeons.

Advanced Trauma Life Support (ATLS) *is essential for first hour care of an injured patient.*

Pre-hospital Trauma Life Support (PHTLS) *is to prevent deaths while injured patients are transported to the hospital.*

Types of Triage System

Multiple casualties: Staff and facilities are sufficient, net priority is given to life-threatening injuries.

Mass casualties: Staff and facilities are not sufficient to manage. Here those who are likely to have highest chance of survival are given priority.

CONCEPTS IN TRAUMA MANAGEMENT

Concept of 'golden hour' to treat the trauma patient is important. Multidisciplinary approach; planning, setting up, organising, team work; assessing respiratory system; circulation; bleeding areas—as priority; assessing also whether patient is haemodynamically stable or unstable; arranging fluids, blood, catheters, ventilator, etc. Further definitive therapy is undertaken depending on severity and site of injury.

DAMAGE CONTROL SURGERY

It includes—resuscitation and early therapy in operation theatre itself; minimum but essential surgery to control bleeding and prevent contamination; secondary definitive surgery at a later period to have final control.

Assessing four components

i. Physiologic response.
ii. Anatomical injury.
iii. Biomechanical injury.
iv. Comorbid factors.

Triage algorithm

STEP ONE (Assess physiological impact)
- Measure vital signs and level of consciousness.
  - By Glasgow coma scale.
  - Systolic blood pressure.
  - Respiratory rate.
  - Revised trauma score. It is based on airway, laryngeal injury, spine injury, maxillofacial injury.

STEP TWO (Assess anatomical impact)
- All penetrating injuries to head, neck, thorax, major burns, fracture bones, pelvic fractures, paralysis.

STEP THREE (Assess mechanism)
- Automobile accidents, crash or blast injuries, high energy injuries, fall from more than 20 feet.
- Bullet injury.

STEP FOUR (Assess history)
- Patient's age below 5 years or age more than 55 years.
- Cardiac diseases, respiratory and metabolic diseases.

Contd...

Contd...

- Pregnancy.
- Patients with bleeding disorders.
- Immunosuppressed individuals.

BASED ON THE STEP CONSIDER TO SHIFT THE PATIENT TO TRAUMA CENTRE & TRAUMA TEAM SHOULD BE KEPT ALERT.

It is important in multiple and mass casualties (fire, blasts, automobile accidents, train accidents).

Management includes: Goals; primary management; investigations; secondary survey; definitive care.

Tag the patient accordingly

Red colour: Immediate treatment is required.
Yellow colour: Urgent treatment is required.
Green colour: Delayed treatment is required.
Blue colour: Expectant treatment is required.
Black colour: Deceased.

Primary management—ABCDEF

AIRWAY
- Chin lift.
- Jaw thrust.
- Nasal airway.
- Oral airway.
- Endotracheal intubation.
- Tracheostomy.
  [Assess airway patency].

BREATHING
- 100% oxygen.
- Assess bilateral chest raise.
- Assess breath sounds.
- Use pulse oximetry.
- Treat flail chest, pneumothorax.
- Intercostal tube drainage.

CIRCULATION
- Monitor vitals.
- Heart sounds.
- Electrocardiogram
- IV fluids blood transfusion.
- Treatment of shock.
- Control of external bleed.
- Use two IV lines—14G/16G.

DISABILITY EVALUATION
- Neurological examination.
- Glasgow coma scale.
- Pupillary reaction.

EXPOSE THE PATIENT FULLY
- Undress the patient.
- Hypothermia assessment.
- Assess injuries.
- Examine joints, bones, abdomen, other systems.
- Look for identification marks.

FINGERS and TUBES
- Examine all orifices like P/R,P/V, etc.
- Use required tubes like catheter, Ryle's tube.

Goals	*Investigations*
Identify life-threatening conditions.	X-ray spine, chest, pelvis, extremities.
Decide and implement appropriate treatment to the area of trauma.	CT scan.
First think of salvage of life, then think of salvage of limb.	Blood group and cross matching.
Rapid assessment, rapid resuscitation, rapid stabilisation.	Arterial blood gas analysis.
Optimum, complete care.	Serum electrolytes.
Transport efficiently to higher trauma centre.	Ultrasound abdomen.

Categorise the patient.

i. Deceased.
ii. Walking wounded.

Contd...

Contd...

iii. Immobile wounded.	
iv. Trapped wounded.	
Secondary survey	*Definitive care*
Re-evaluate the patient completely again.	

NECK INJURIES

Neck is divided into zones for managing neck injuries. *Zone I* is from clavicle to cricoid cartilage. Injury here may extend into the mediastinum/thorax. *Zone II* is from cricoid cartilage to angle of the mandible. *Zone III* is above the angle of the mandible. Injury here may extend into cranial cavity or skull base; extended vascular injuries here are quite difficult to manage **(Fig. 8-11)**.

Indications for neck exploration in injuries are: Expanding haematoma; uncontrolled external haemorrhage; decreased carotid pulse; stridor, hoarseness, dysphonia, haemoptysis; severe dysphagia, odynophagia; blood in oropharynx. Vital structures in compact area make neck injury an area of priority. Penetrating injuries of major vessels (20%), trachea, oesophagus, thyroid, and nerve plexus can cause severe problems. Exact anatomical extent of the injury should be assessed. Extension into pharynx, larynx, chest or mediastinum should be thought of. Anterior triangle injuries pose a high threat than posterior triangle injury. CT neck is the ideal investigation for neck injuries. One must also think of possible injuries like Le Fort facial injuries; cervical spine injuries; skull base injuries which should be assessed clinically and radiologically properly before jumping into hurried intervention.

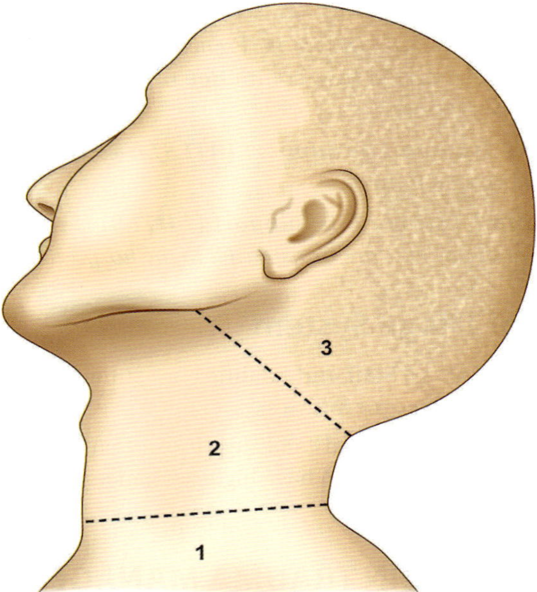

Fig. 8-11: Neck zones used in neck trauma.

Treatment

Patient with aerodigestive and vascular injury needs neck exploration. It is the exploration of the neck rather the wound as such is important. Oblique incision along the anterior border of the sternomastoid is done in unilateral injury. Bilateral connecting collar incision along the anterior borders of the both sternomastoid muscles is used for bilateral injuries of the neck **(Fig. 8-12)**.

Intraoperative endoscopy to identify injuries of trachea and oesophagus is beneficial. Methylene blue instillation into the oesophagus will identify the oesophageal tear. Neck is explored with adequate incision under general anaesthesia. Suturing of the injured structure like carotid, oesophagus, trachea, muscles, etc. is done. External carotid artery can be safely ligated. Internal carotid or common carotid requires repair often using vein or polytetrafluoroethylene (PTFE) graft. Tracheal injury up to two rings can be repaired primarily using interrupted non-absorbable sutures like polypropylene. Loss of more than two rings needs tracheostomy. In laryngeal injuries cartilage fractures should be reduced; mucosal lacerations should be sutured. Oesophageal injury if identified within 12 hours sutures of injury is repaired primarily in two layers of interrupted PDS/vicryl sutures with nasogastric tube in situ. Drain to the wound is a must. Injury identified after 12 hours of trauma or extensive injury of cervical oesophagus needs initial cervical oesophagostomy and later reconstruction. Often total oesophagectomy with gastric/jejunal colonic interposition may be needed. Antibiotics, blood transfusion, nasogastric tube passing—as required.

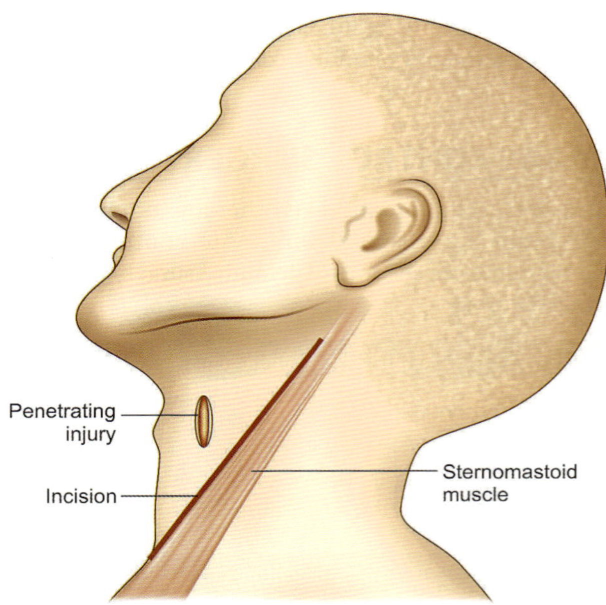

Fig. 8-12: Incision in neck trauma is oblique one along the anterior border of sternomastoid muscle.

THORACIC TRAUMA

Thoracic trauma is the cause of 25% of all trauma deaths. Cardiac injury is the cause for early deaths. Airway obstruction, tension pneumothorax, massive haemothorax, cardiac tamponade are other causes of death which are actually preventable in *golden hours*. Chest trauma causes *hypoxia, hypercapnia and acidosis*. Chest X-ray, CT chest and ultrasound chest are diagnostic methods in chest trauma. But in severe critical cases one should not wait for these investigations. Instead it is better to take up straight a way the therapeutic measures like *intercostal tube drainage* (tube thoracostomy), aspiration of tension pneumothorax and cardiac tamponade.

The thoracostomy (ICT drainage) is done in midaxillary line in 6th intercostal space. In slight head up position, after injecting xylocaine 1% local anaesthesia, 1 cm incision is made in the space in lower part of the space to avoid injury to the intercostal vessels. External and internal intercostal muscles are split; pleura is opened; finger is inserted and blunt finger dissection is done; mattress stay suture is loosely placed using polyethylene suture; 40 French intercostal tube with end and side holes is introduced. Tube is directed above and posteriorly. Tube is secured to the skin by tying the tube. Tube is connected to under water seal apparatus. If pre-insertion suture is not placed, suture is placed later after inserting the tube. Post-operative air column movement is observed. *Absence of air leak; fluid drain less than 100 mL/day; chest X-ray* if shows adequate expansion then tube can be removed safely.

Twenty percent of patients with chest trauma *need thoracotomy* and definitive repair of injured intrathoracic structures. *Indications are*—massive haemothorax with more than 1,500 mL of blood in ICT when passed or hourly drainage if more than 300 mL/hour; pericardial/cardiac injuries; thoracic cage open wounds; thoracic vascular injury; tracheobronchial tree injury; oesophageal injuries. All these indications are critical and life-threatening situations. But still if proper cardiothoracic set up is available and timely intervention is done, life can be saved **(Fig. 8-13)**.

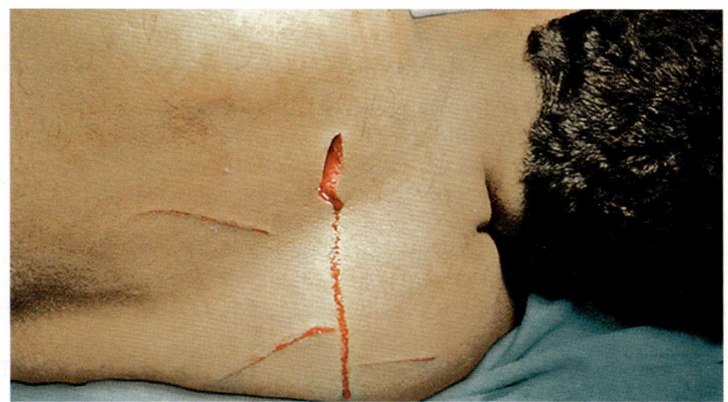

Fig. 8-13: Open communicating wound in thorax/chest wall.

Rib fractures are the commonest type of chest trauma. But commonly it does not cause problem unless there is haemothorax or pneumothorax. 4th to 10th ribs are commonly fractured. Rib fracture causes severe *pain, reduces the ability to cough, and reduces vital capacity causing atelectasis and pneumonia*. Pain on *inspiration* is the main feature in rib fracture along with *crepitus*. Proper pain control is essential using intravenous analgesics, epidural analgesia. *Flail chest* (15%) with fractures in two or more ribs, with each rib having two or more fracture sites causes chest wall instability → paradoxical movement of the chest wall (during inspiration flail segment is drawn in) → pendular movement of the air → mediastinal flutter → sudden kinking of great vessel → respiratory failure and cardiac arrest. It can be anterior, lateral or posterior. Pain and pulmonary contusion is common. Endotracheal intubation, ICT placement, tracheostomy, prevention of movements of flail segment is needed.

Pulmonary contusion is a different typical recognised entity. It can be commonly due to blunt trauma or often due to penetrating injury. It commonly causes respiratory failure. So along with management of mechanical problem, respiratory problems also should be dealt with carefully. Arterial blood gas analysis is a must. *Measures are*—crystalloid infusion, oxygen support, avoiding fluid overload, maintaining the tissue perfusion, blood transfusion, ventilator support, transfusion of packed cells and blood products.

Pneumothorax: It can be *small* pneumothorax with volume loss is 1/3rd of normal lung volume; *large* pneumothorax with complete collapse of the lung on one side but without any tracheal/mediastinal shift; *tension* pneumothorax which is a critical emergency situation with tracheal and mediastinal shift towards opposite side causing *hypotension* decreased cardiac venous return, cardiac arrest and acute respiratory distress or *open pneumothorax* with a large chest wall *sucking open wound*. Pneumothorax needs ICT placement in 4th space in midaxillary line. Tension pneumothorax needs emergency placement of *wide bore needle in midclavicular line in 2nd intercostal space* with a glove finger placed over the hub of the needle to prevent air getting sucked inside during expiration; later ICT should be placed. Open pneumothorax needs open *surgical closure* of the chest wall defect with an ICT in place **(Fig. 8-14)**.

Haemothorax: 80% of haemothorax is treated by ICT placement. Remaining 20% needs thoracotomy and control of bleeding like resection of lung.

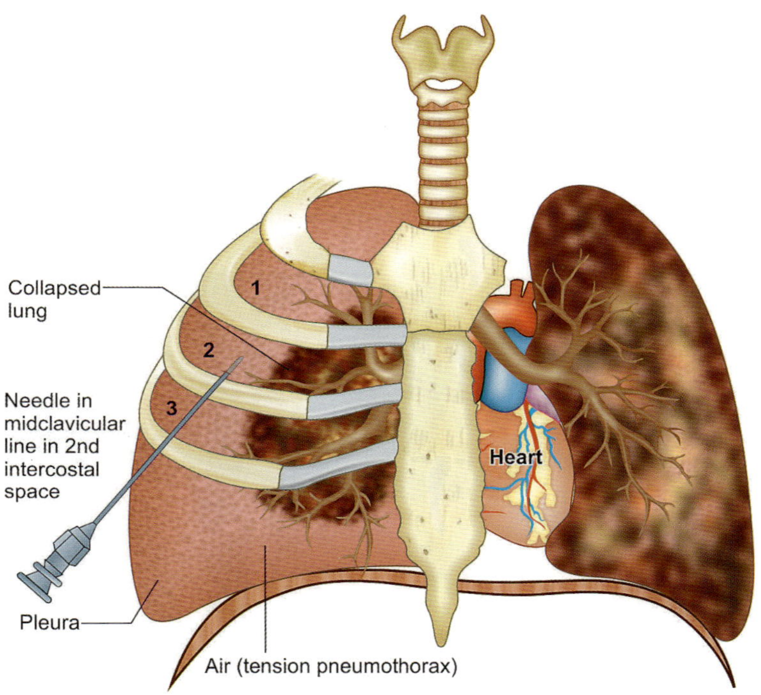

Fig. 8-14: Emergency aspiration through 2nd intercostal space in midclavicular line is life saving measure in tension pneumothorax.

Intercostal Tube Drainage (For Details—Refer Chapter 7)

It is done head up lying down position or supine position. Chest should be done and if possible ultrasound thorax. Cleaning and draping is done. After injecting the local anaesthesia in safety zone, skin is incised transversely for 3–4 cm in 5th space in its lower part (to avoid neurovascular injury); fascia is incised, external and internal intercostal muscles are incised and split using Kelly's haemostat; gentle push across the pleura feels 'the giving way' of entering the pleura. Pathological fluid (blood/air/fluid) will gush out. Required sized ICT tube with multiple fenestra (8 or 32) is passed across the wound into the pleural cavity. Tube is sutured to skin using monofilament non-absorbable suture; it is often better to place and keep ready the suture in place prior to insertion of the tube. Other end is connected to the ICT bag/bottle or canister. ICT bag should be filled with normal saline as specified up to the mark. Column movement and bubbling and quantity collected immediately should be noted. Check chest X-ray should be done **(Figs. 8-15 and 8-16)**.

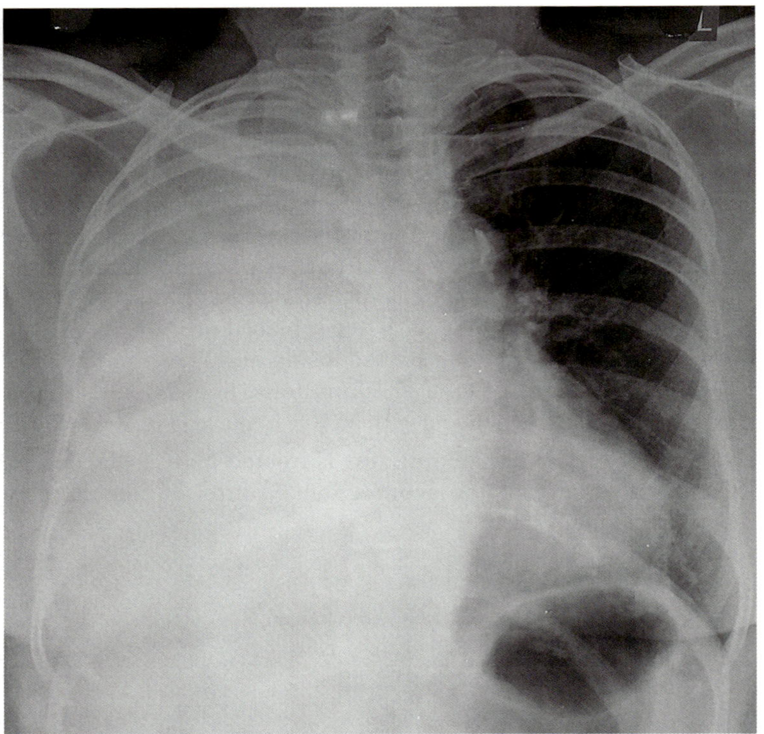

Fig. 8-15: Chest X-ray showing right-sided haemothorax.

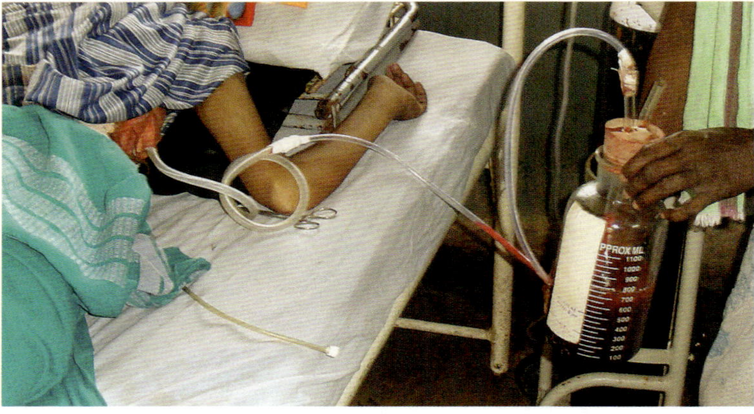

Fig. 8-16: ICT placed for haemothorax after chest trauma.

'C S" Perspectives on ICDs

The Intercostal Drain (ICD) is a CRUCIAL SAVIOUR for All Thoracic Surgical Pathology (By Professor CS Rajan, Bengaluru)

ICDs Need—14 *CORRECT STEPS* (7 + 7)

- **Cautious Siting (Insertion)**
  1. **C**orroborate the **S**ide (clinical and check chest X-ray).
  2. **C**hoose **S**ite (triangle of safety).
  3. **C**opious **S**oother (use large amounts of local anaesthesia/LA).
  4. **C**reate **S**haft (blunt track dissection, use finger to confirm).
  5. **C**apable **S**utures (to anchor tube to chest wall).
  6. **C**ontrolled, **S**oft Entry (*no force to be used*).
  7. **C**heck **S**napshot (check X-ray, to confirm entry into chest).
- **Caboxreful Scrutiny (Management)**
  1. **C**ontinuous **S**wing (respiration related oscillations in tube below water level).
  2. **C**onnections **S**ecure (between emerging drain from chest, tubings and bottle).
  3. **C**onstant (Under Water) **S**eal (the non-reflux valve, kept 1 metre below).

Contd...

Contd...

  4. **C**onsider **S**uction (if needed).
  5. **C**ommend **S**pirometry (chest physiotherapy is a must).
  6. **C**ondition and **S**hadow (check X-ray) Improvement.
  7. **C**o-ordinated **S**eparation (timing and method of removal of the ICD).

Complications and Solutions for ICDs

1. **C**rooked **S**tationing [wrong position of tube (subcutaneous or abdominal)]—will need full re-insertion of tube under aseptic precaution.
2. **C**entral **S**tructure and Visceral Injury (during insertion) a true catastrophy, call for cardiothoracic help and react fast to treat the shock.
3. **C**onduit **S**huts down (tube gets blocked), needs proper/frequent 'milking' and clearing of blood clots/fibrin plugs in the tube.
4. **C**hest (tube) **S**lippage (drain/drain holes come out of chest cage), reposition the chest tube into the chest under aseptic precaution.
5. **C**repitus **S**ubcutaneous (surgical emphysema), usually settles with time, but if air leak around chest drain site, may need a deep skin suture to make site air tight.
6. **C**onfused **S**hift (paradoxical/re-expansion pulmonary oedema), especially in long standing effusions/empyema, avoided if drainage is controlled to empty out of the chest gradually, and not all at one time.
7. **C**hannel (wall) **S**uppuration (chest wound/chest cavity infection), both insertion and subsequent daily management need full aseptic technique at all times.

'C S' Perspectives about Thoracic Empyema (and Pneumothorax too)….!

The 'Comprehensive Suggestions'

1. **Complete Story** to be elicited. All details of the history of the illness, especially duration of the chest symptoms.
2. **Clinical State** to be assessed. It involves complete general examination and a full assessment of the chest following the set pattern of inspection, palpation, percussion and auscultation.
3. **Chest Skiagram,** or the radiography of the chest is the first imaging modality to be asked for and read carefully.
4. **Confirm Status,** by the diagnostic aspiration, better under image control localisation, with fluid analysis to give stage of disease.
5. **Culture and Sensitivity,** of aspirated fluid including a smear for AFB
6. **Check Sputum** for infection and also for AFB by the ZN stain.
7. **Computerised Scan,** to get cross sectional with sagittal and coronal reconstructions to get the 3D evaluation of the disease process in the chest. It is important to look at both, the 'lung' and the 'mediastinal' windows. The HRCT of the chest is NOT ideal for assessing empyemas.
8. **Confirmatory Scopy** (fibreoptic bronchoscopy) is needed to rule out endobronchial lesion and obstruction. Laboratory analysis and stains of bronchoalveolar lavage give a better yield for Koch's.
9. **Choose Strategy.** This is crucial, and determines outcome. It is a planned intervention in discussion with the medical and radiological teams. *Within the first 2 weeks, minimal access by VATS is now the standard of care.* When the clinical duration is over 2 weeks and scans suggest development of a cortex, then a formal thoracotomy is indicated to achieve complete decortication.
10. **Closed Solution** of either just an ICD or the VATS procedure is chosen when the disease is in early presentation and there is no cortex seen on imaging.
11. **Cut** (with) **Scalpel,** or the open procedures is offered to those with complex collections/loculations, especially in inaccessible parts of the chest (Mediastinal/Hilar). A rib resection over the collection, a mini-thoracotomy and clean up or the formal thoracotomy with decortications is the open procedures.
12. **Clean and Scavenge.** The opportunity to enter the chest must ensure complete removal of all toxic material, pus, flakes, cortex from ALL aspects of the lung, costal, apex, diaphragmatic, mediastinal and interlobar fissures. Closure is ALWAYS with a wide bore intercostal chest drain (the ICD) with the underwater seal.

Contd...

Contd...

13. **Combined Support,** of the anaesthetists for pain relief, physiotherapist for breathing exercises to inflate the collapsed lungs, and nursing to ensure proper care of the ICD, the other vitals and the nutrition.
14. **Conduit Supervision.** It is mandatory the surgeon has a personal review of the ICD during the entire length of its stay in situ. The look for the air leak, the quality and quantity of drainage, and the ensuring of patency are vital to the outcome. Removal may often be delayed, and patients are sent home to allow time for recovery.
15. **Continued Surveillance.** This often goes well beyond the hospital stay of the patient, and involves loads of encouragement and solace giving to the patient.

By the use of the above 15 'C S', the benefits are....more 'C S'...!

1. **Control** (of) **Sepsis.**
2. **Clean Shadows**, meaning radiological improvement.
3. **Clear Sounds** on auscultation showing equal and clear air entry in both lung fields.
4. **Customer Satisfaction,** with the patient being able to return to full activity soon.
5. **Comforting Sleep** for all..!

With permission from Professor, Dr CS Rajan MS, FRCS, Consultant Surgeon, Mallya Hospital and Annaswamy Mudaliar General Hospital, Bengaluru; Ex-HOD of Surgery, St. Martha's Hospital, Bengaluru (2003-2013), authentic teacher, guide, mentor to many more students and postgraduates, examiner for MS, DNB and other examinations, an excellent sports person and orator; but a simple, humble person with humility.

Pulmonary injury: Small lacerations of the lung are common but are treated with ICT. 10% of patients will have large significant lacerations with massive air leak through ICT. It needs thoracotomy, lung sparing resections like non-anatomic resection or tractomy using stapling device. Extensive lung injury occasionally needs lobectomy or pneumonectomy as life-saving measure. Persistent air leak in ICT may be due to bronchopleural fistula.

Tracheobronchial tree injury is difficult to manage. It needs initial bronchoscopy to identify the site and extent. Later thoracotomy is done to explore entire tracheobronchial tree, depends on the side of injury. Small injury heals spontaneously. Injury more than 1/3rd of the circumference of the tracheobronchial tree needs primary repair using polypropylene interrupted sutures with selective intubation of the opposite bronchus. Collapse of lung, stricture of tracheobronchial tree, pneumonia and septicaemia are distressing complications.

Cardiac injury: Blunt injury to anterior chest wall causes cardiac trauma. It may be minor contusion of the wall, major contusion, cardiac chamber rupture, haemopericardium and death. Right ventricle is commonly affected as it lies near to the anterior chest wall. If patient reaches the hospital it is diagnosed by US chest, echocardiography, CT chest and ECG. ECG and raised serum troponin I level suggests early or late myocardial damage. *Treatment* in small contusions is continuous ECG monitoring and observation. Major injuries need *urgent thoracotomy* and surgical repair by cardiac surgeons. *Pericardial tap* may be helpful in haemopericardium. Mortality rate is more than 80% in major cardiac injuries. During admission if pulse is felt survival rate increases to 70% with proper intervention and care. Even cardiac tamponade due to haemopericardium needs early open surgical intervention as tamponade itself is a temporary natural haemodynamic compensatory mechanism.

Oesophageal injuries: Thoracic oesophageal injuries are rare as it is located in posterior mediastinum. It occurs due to deep penetrating injuries. It is often difficult to diagnose. It is always associated with other thoracic injuries. Oesophagoscopy and oesophagography, increased oesophageal pressure, CT chest may reveal oesophageal injury. Problems with oesophageal injury are—empyema, mediastinitis and septicaemia. If identified within 24 hours of trauma, early debridement, primary repair, and drainage with nasogastric placement is the treatment. If identified after 24 hours, mediastinal sepsis is likely and so needs diversion with cervical oesophagostomy, feeding jejunostomy, oesophageal resection, later colonic/gastric transposition.

Diaphragmatic injury: It can occur in thoracic or abdominal injuries. It can be diagnosed by CT scan. But more often it is identified during laparotomy or thoracotomy. It is sutured using interrupted horizontal mattress sutures with polypropylene sutures.

ABDOMINAL TRAUMA

Abdominal trauma is a major emergency surgical problem which surgeons face. It is often associated with head, chest, pelvic and bone injuries. Often patient may be unconscious causing difficulty in diagnosing the condition. Often while giving more importance to other systems like head, thorax and bones and abdominal injury is not addressed properly causing life-threatening consequences. When patient is conscious, history related to abdominal trauma is useful. Abrasion over the abdominal skin suggests possibility of internal injury (*London's sign*). Distension, tenderness, rebound tenderness, fullness and dullness in the flank, when present one should presume internal injury. Tachycardia, hypotension, shock may be evident when there is significant haemoperitoneum. Injuries may be organ injuries like of liver, spleen, kidney, pancreas. etc; or bowel injury or retroperitoneal injury which is often underdiagnosed or missed. Major vessel injury like inferior vena cava, mesenteric vessels can cause real threat to life unless it is identified and managed early. 25% of entire trauma patients need surgical exploration of the abdomen.

Abdominal trauma can be *blunt or stab/penetrating or abdominal wall injuries.* Spleen is the commonest organ involved in *blunt trauma.* Often in blunt trauma first part of the jejunum or ileocaecal junction gives way (blow-out effect) due to traction causing often complete transection of bowel horizontally close to the junction. It is due to force of the mobile part of the bowel over fixed part of the bowel. Liver is the commonest organ involved in *penetrating injuries* **(Fig. 8-17)**.

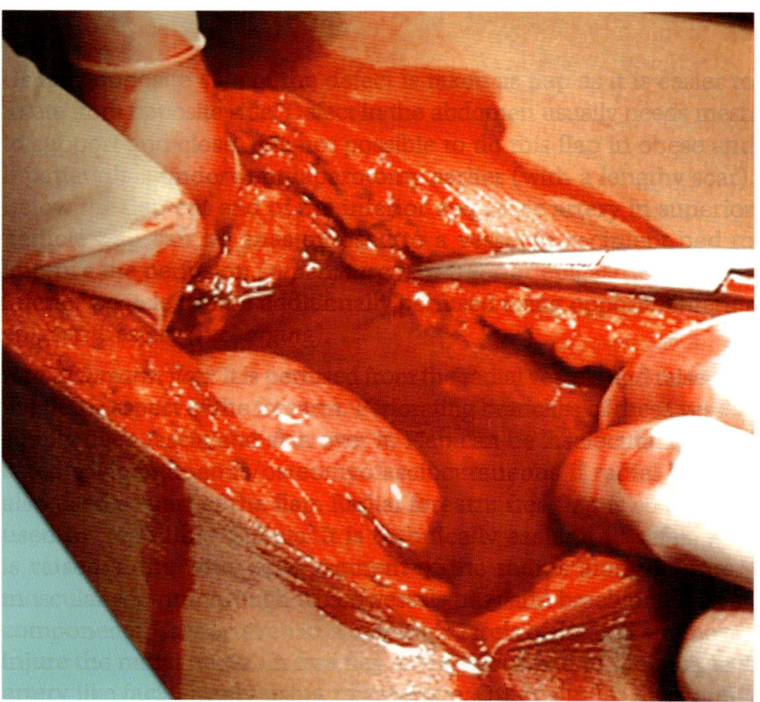

Fig. 8-17: Haemoperitoneum on table.

Injuries of the abdomen may be *closed injuries, compression injuries and penetrating injuries*. Penetrating injury may be low velocity injury like stab or high velocity injury like gunshot injury. Blunt weapon penetration causes lesser deep trauma than sharp weapon trauma (sickle, knife). In sickle injury tip and sharp edge moves in curved pattern and so it is often difficult to predict the depth, track and organs injured **(Figs. 8-18 and 8-19)**.

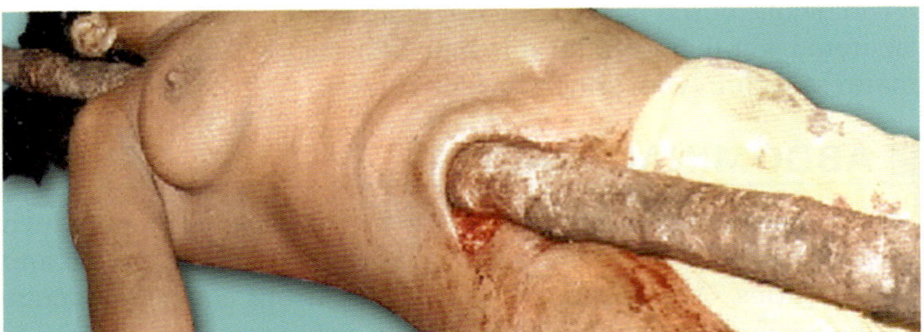

Fig. 8-18: Penetrating injury of the abdomen and chest right sided. Patient fell over a tree which had its top end cut. Tree has penetrated into her abdomen and chest wall. Patient was brought after cutting the tree from its root. Patient survived after surgery.

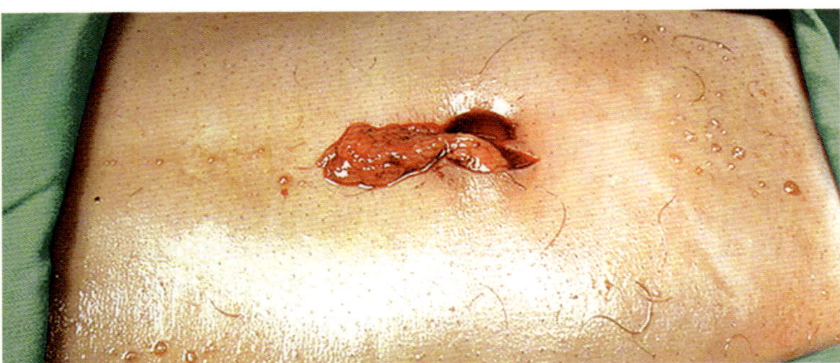

Fig. 8-19: Stab wound in the abdomen with omentum protruding through the wound.

Blunt trauma is common in accidents. It is often missed or lately diagnosed. Ultrasound/CT abdomen or diagnostic peritoneal lavage (DPL) is useful. In many cases on clinical grounds direct exploratory laparotomy is done. Plain X-ray abdomen may show gas under diaphragm.

Difficulty arises in *deciding about the need for laparotomy* in abdominal trauma in *unconscious* patients. If external injury is not severe in proportionate to the existing severe shock then exploratory laparotomy is indicated in an unconscious patient. It is also often difficult to diagnose bowel injury in such patients. If it is suspected laparotomy should be undertaken in such patients.

Routinely followed indications in abdominal trauma are—hypotension without any other cause; bleeding through wound; continuous bleeding from nasogastric tube; evisceration of abdominal content through the open wound except in case of protruded omentum without any hypotension and features of peritoneal irritation; air under diaphragm in blunt abdominal injury (not in penetrating injury as external air gets sucked into the peritoneal cavity through the wound).

Ultrasound abdomen is very useful, simpler, non-invasive method of evaluating the abdomen. Negative ultrasound means no immediate further work is needed and also can be treated conservatively. *Advantages of ultrasound are*—there is no danger of radiation; it can be done at bedside; it can be repeated many times; it is cost effective. It is less useful in obesity, with gas interposition, intraperitoneal fluid less than 500 mL; retroperitoneal injuries and bowel injuries. Its sensitivity is 90%; specificity is 98%. Focused Abdominal Sonar (ultrasound) for Trauma *(FAST)* is very useful method. FAST is rapid, non-invasive, portable bedside method of investigation focusing on pericardium, splenic, hepatic and pelvic areas. Blood more than 100 mL in cavities can be identified. It is not reliable for bowel or penetrating injuries. It often needs to be repeated.

Diagnostic peritoneal lavage (DPL) (by Perry) is useful in *blunt injury* abdomen. It is not very useful in penetrating injury, bowel injury, retroperitoneal and pelvic injuries. It is the *procedure of choice in physiologically unstable patient* with blunt abdominal injury (like with spinal injury, unconscious patient, in situations where clinical signs cannot be interpreted, where injuries of more priority are in other areas like head or chest). 10 French polyvinyl catheter is used. Urinary bladder is emptied by passing a catheter. After injecting xylocaine local anaesthesia in subumbilical region, 2–3 cm vertical subumbilical midline incision is made. Skin, linea alba is incised. Local anaesthesia is infiltrated into the peritoneum again. Peritoneum is held with two haemostats and a purse string suture is placed using polylactic acid absorbable suture material. Peritoneum is incised for 3 mm length. Catheter (standard peritoneal dialysis catheter) is introduced into the peritoneal cavity. If blood enters the catheter immediately, it means early laparotomy is needed and carried out without continuing the peritoneal lavage. If otherwise, one liter of normal saline is infused into the peritoneal cavity rapidly in few minutes through the catheter using a drip set with elevation of the fluid bottle/bag. Patient is moved well to mix the fluid in all four quadrants. Now bag is lowered below so that fluid from the peritoneal cavity reenters/siphoned into the bag. Collected fluid is analysed for red cells, leukocytes, etc. (see box). DPL may not be

Diagnostic peritoneal lavage (DPL)

Significant positive lavage:
- 10 mL of gross blood.
- Red cells more than 1, 00,000/cu mm.
- WBC count more than 500/cu mm.
- Amylase more than 175 mL/dL.
- Presence of bacteria, bile, food particles, foreign body.

Indeterminate lavage:
- Red cells between 50,000 to 1, 00,000/cu mm.
- WBC between 100 and 500/cu mm.

Lavage not significant:
- Red cells less than 50,000/cu mm.
- WBC less than 100/cu mm.

Strongly positive means:
- Red return solution in the bag.
- Always needs laparotomy.
- Features mentioned above.

Weakly positive means:
- Pink or just red tinged fluid.
- Laparotomy chances are 10%.
- Observation/repeat investigations/repeat DPL later.
- Retroperitoneal haematoma may be present.

Lavage negative:
- Return fluid is crystal clear.
- No need of laparotomy here. Patient is observed.

False positive:
- Occurs when bleeding from retroperitoneum into peritoneal cavity occurs.
- It may lead into negative laparotomy.
- Abdominal wall bleeding into the peritoneal cavity can cause false positive result.

Contraindications for DPL:
- When laparotomy is indicated definitely.
- Previous laparotomy history.
- Pregnancy and obesity.

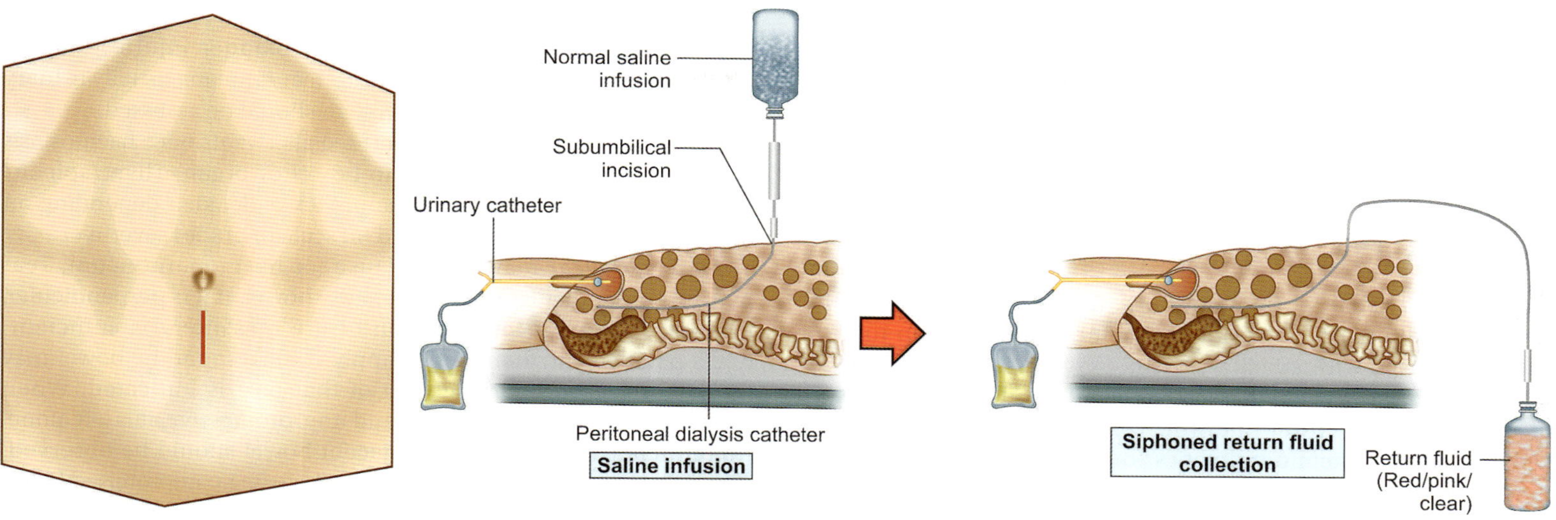

Fig. 8-20: Diagnostic peritoneal lavage—incision and technique.

useful in bowel injury, retroperitoneal injury, diaphragmatic injury, organ haematoma (subcapsular splenic haematoma). If patient is decided for observation catheter can be left in situ for repeat DPL after 6 hours. One has to remember that DPL is not a substitute for clinical assessment and monitoring. In *Lazarus-Nelson approach* Teflon catheter with a guidewire is used **(Fig. 8-20)**.

CT scan of abdomen is most commonly used and better investigation for abdominal trauma. It is useful in blunt/penetrating trauma, suspected pancreas, spleen, liver, duodenal, retroperitoneal injuries. Smaller injuries, early haemoperitoneum are better detected. It is non-invasive, highly specific, highly accurate (96%), with low false positive/low false negative, non-invasive. It is very essential investigation when solid organ injuries are treated non-operatively. Three dimensional helical CT is needed to identify mesenteric or bowel injury and to find out site of injury. It is obviously not necessary to do CT when there is clear indication for immediate laparotomy. In such occasions ultrasound is more than sufficient.

Other investigations are—(1) *Abdominal diagnostic paracentesis* (Drapanas and McDonald): Here 18 G short bevel spinal needle is inserted into the peritoneal cavity after injecting local anaesthetic agent into the abdominal wall. With continuous suctioning through syringe needle is passed at various sites. Positive tap means return of minimum of 0.1 mL of non-clotted blood. False-positive result occasionally can occur due to needle puncture of abdominal wall vessels. Needle should not be inserted close to previous abdominal scar as bowel may be adherent underneath the scar. Change of direction of needle is done by withdrawing the needle tip outer to peritoneum and again puncturing the peritoneum. Puncture of non-distended bowel will seal without any leakage in 18 G needle. If there is distended bowel peritoneal tap should be avoided **(Fig. 8-21)**. *Bilateral flank tap/four quadrant tap* is also done with similar result. Rectus sheath haematoma and false-negative results are problems **(Fig. 8-22)**. (2) *Diagnostic laparoscopy* is very useful. It can be done under local anaesthesia. Haemoperitoneum and solid organ and diaphragmatic injuries are well assessed. But bowel and retroperitoneal injuries are more likely to be missed. (3) *Arteriography* through Seldinger technique is useful in suspected cases of renal arterial injury (thrombosis/spasm); intimal tears, traumatic aneurysm and aortic occlusion (after seat belt injury) are well diagnosed with arteriography. Often it can be therapeutic also. Pelvic bleed extending into retroperitoneum is not uncommon which can be assessed by arteriography to

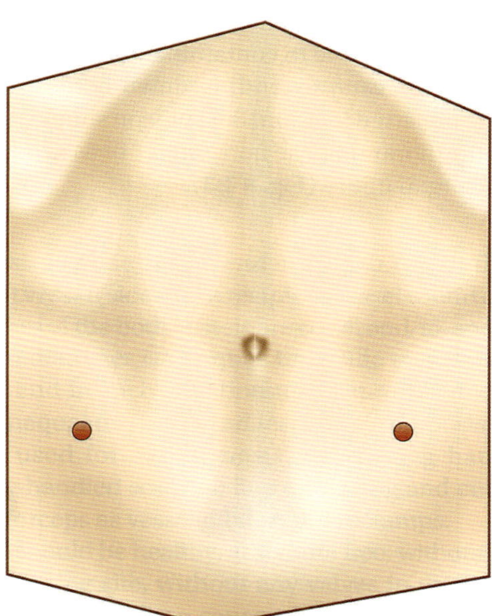

Fig. 8-21: Abdominal paracentesis.

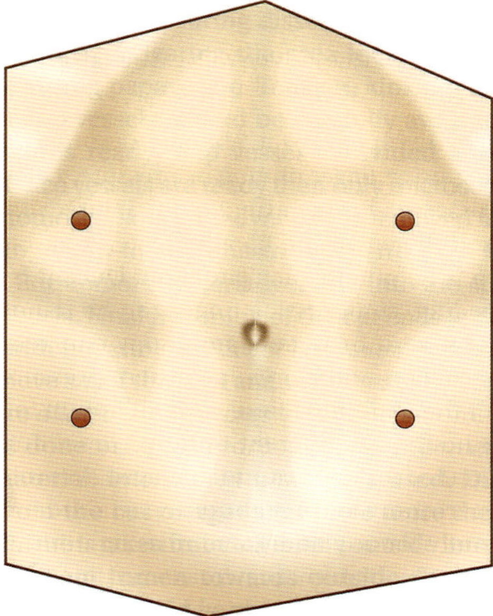

Fig. 8-22: Four quadrant aspiration of the abdomen.

identify the bleeding vessel. But venous bleed cannot be assessed by this. (4) *Doppler assessment of major vessels* may be beneficial especially for inferior vena cava (IVC), aorta, iliac vessels, portal system; but with haemoperitoneum visualisation window may be poor and vessels can be better identified by contrast CT scan.

Management Concepts in Abdominal Trauma

Evaluation of extent of the injury; number of organs injured and severity; haematocrit assessment (haemoglobin drop up to 6 g% is tolerated well with adequate tissue oxygenation. Rapid drop of haemoglobin needs adequate number of blood to be kept ready like 5/10/more); central line with volume replacement; urinary catheterisation; systemic antibiotics administration.

Autotransfusion of blood is very useful in such situation as a life-saving procedure. Blood from the cavity is sucked out into a sterile bottle which contains 150 mL of 3.8% sodium citrate dextrose solution. This blood is strained/filtered through gauze and retransfused. If there is colonic and small bowel injuries autotransfusion is not possible in fear of sepsis due to contamination.

Upper midline incision extending down across the left of the umbilicus is the preferred incision. But surgeon should not be hesitant to extend into the thorax or make horizontal T or as needed depending on the internal organ injury **(Fig. 8-23)**.

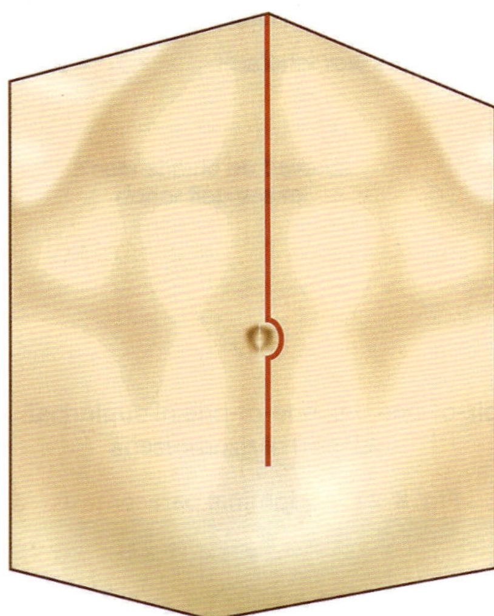

Fig. 8-23: Lengthy midline incision with extension on the left side of the umbilicus is used.

First priority after opening the abdomen *is immediate control of profuse bleeding using finger or mop* or pressure. Later once field is clean; area is assessed for the extent of the injury without releasing the compressed finger on the bleeding site. A vascular clamp or bulldog clamp is helpful in such situation. Once it is applied over the site of bleeding, compressing finger can be removed. Vascular suturing using 4-zero or 6-zero polypropylene/resection of the tissue; reconstruction of the area; persistent pressure mop in situ with closure of the abdominal wall with an option for second look surgery in 48 hours are different options. Individual organs are assessed and graded for injuries and managed accordingly.

During laparotomy entire abdomen should be inspected/ palpated carefully for any additional missing injuries. Lesser sac, retroperitoneum, duodenum, pancreas and diaphragm should be checked for. Often peritoneum on the margin of the duodenum and right side colon is incised and duodenum and colon are reflected medially to visualise the retroperitoneum. Pelvic structures need special attention. Rectum and urinary bladder injuries may be missed. If on catheterisation, urine is clear it means usually urinary system is normal. Portal venous system should be assessed.

Resection or repair should be decided afterwards once haemostasis is maintained. Whether injury to bowel or organs (liver/spleen/ kidney, etc.) resection or repair approach is decided depending on the individual organ injury (based on scale or grade) severity.

Mesenteric tear may be the cause for haemoperitoneum. Tear may be perpendicular or parallel to the bowel. If it is perpendicular, haemostasis and approximation of the mesentery is sufficient; if it is parallel tear, then blood supply to corresponding bowel may be compromised and resection of that part is indicated. When mesenteric haematoma is small and non-progressive, it is left alone. Colour changes if any in the adjacent bowel should be observed. If haematoma is large and is progressive causing compromised blood supply of the adjacent bowel, then it should be gently evacuated. Mesenteric leaf is opened using curved scissor; using gentle finger dissection clot is evacuated; bleeder is identified and ligated. If there is compromised bowel function, it should be resected. Bleeding from the major vein like superior mesenteric vein is disastrous as tear may not be localised but may be extensive and even gentle dissection may cause more tear. It is carefully mobilised; vascular clamps are applied and repaired using 5-zero polypropylene sutures **(Figs. 8-24 to 8-26)**.

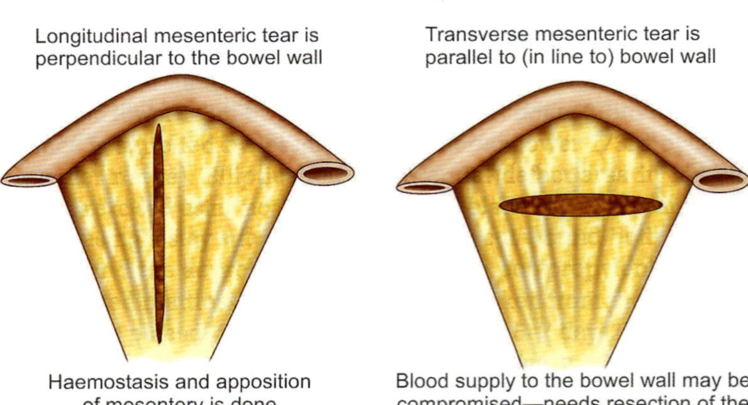

Fig. 8-24: Transverse mesenteric tear is risky as it may compromise the blood supply of adjacent bowel. In such tear adjacent bowel should be resected.

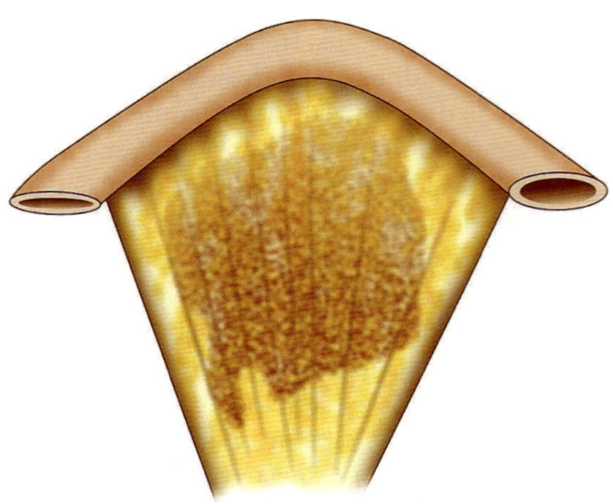

Fig. 8-25: Large mesenteric haematoma which is progressive needs to be intervened. Gentle evacuation by finger dissection and ligation of bleeding vessel is the option.

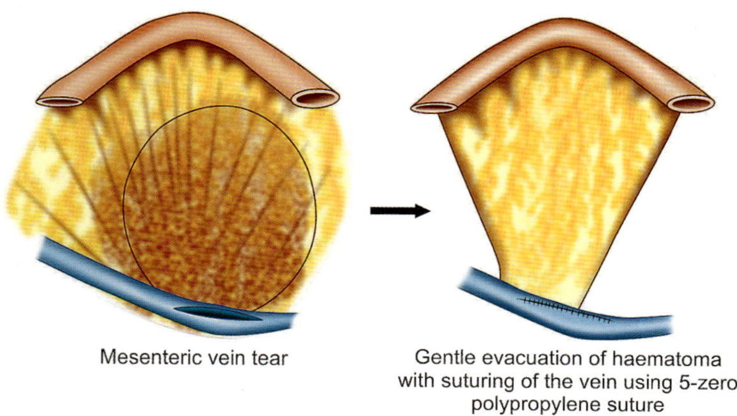

Fig. 8-26: Major mesenteric vein tear should be sutured using 5-zero polypropylene. Vascular clamps should be used to control bleeding. Gentle approach is needed as tear may extend and get worsened.

Aortic Clamping

Catastrophic bleeding found after opening the abdomen which cannot be controlled and bleeding with profound hypotension are the indications for aortic clamping. Profuse intraperitoneal bleed comes under control temporarily by tamponade effect of tense abdominal wall and it itself temporarily helps the patient. The moment abdomen is opened tamponade is released causing further rapid bleed leading into critical catastrophe. If such event is expected prior to opening the abdomen a very quick rapid thoracotomy (*prelaparotomy thoracotomy*) through left 5th intercostal space is done; left lung is deflated and displaced; pleura over the thoracic aorta is incised; aorta is dissected using finger; vascular clamp or soft intestinal occlusion clamp is applied to occlude the thoracic aorta. Later laparotomy is performed to go ahead with management of the bleeding. If profound bleeding is observed after laparotomy necessitating the aortic clamping, it is done by applying the clamp in infradiaphragmatic part of the aorta. Peritoneum is incised on the right of the abdominal oesophagus in infradiaphragmatic area; aorta is dissected using finger high up close to diaphragm to avoid injury to celiac plexus; clamp is applied across (infradiaphragmatic aortic occlusion) **(Figs. 8-27A and B)**.

Usually drainage using tube drains on either side of the abdomen is used even though it is controversial. ICT should be placed if thoracotomy is also undertaken.

Jejunostomy for enteral nutrition is ideal in all major abdominal injuries. Often gastrostomy is also done along with jejunostomy in case of duodenal and pancreatic injuries.

LIVER INJURY

Liver is the commonest organ injured in penetrating abdominal trauma. Mortality is 10%. It is less in isolated liver injury but increases up to 25% when it is associated with other injuries.

Grade and type	*Injury*
I – Haematoma – Laceration	Subcapsular haematoma less than 10% surface area. Capsular laceration less than 1 cm in depth.
II – Haematoma – Laceration	Subcapsular haematoma 10–50%; intraparenchymal less than 10 cm diameter. Capsular laceration 1–3 cm in depth; less than 10 cm length.
III – Haematoma – Laceration	Subcapsular haematoma more than 50%; intraparenchymal more than 10 cm diameter—expanding. Capsular laceration 3 cm in depth.
IV – Laceration	Parenchymal disruption 25–75% hepatic lobe; 1–3 Couinaud segments.
V – Laceration – Vascular	Parenchymal disruption more than 75% or more than 3 Couinaud segments. Major hepatic veins or retrohepatic vena caval injuries.
VI – Vascular	Hepatic avulsion.

Management

Initial Conservative Non-operative Management

It is done in non-progressive liver injuries who are haemodynamically stable, low grade liver injury, need for transfusion less than 2 units. However, CT abdomen (absence of contrast extravasation during arterial phase can be treated non-operatively) and repeat CT or regular ultrasound follow up is a must. Replacement of lost blood; prevention of sepsis; regular monitoring by haematocrit, liver function tests,

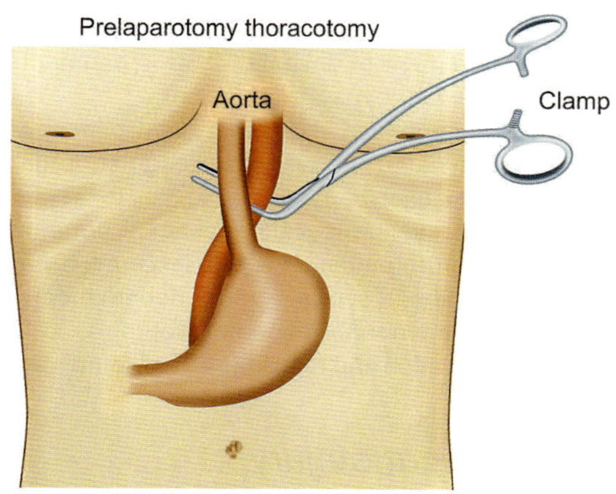

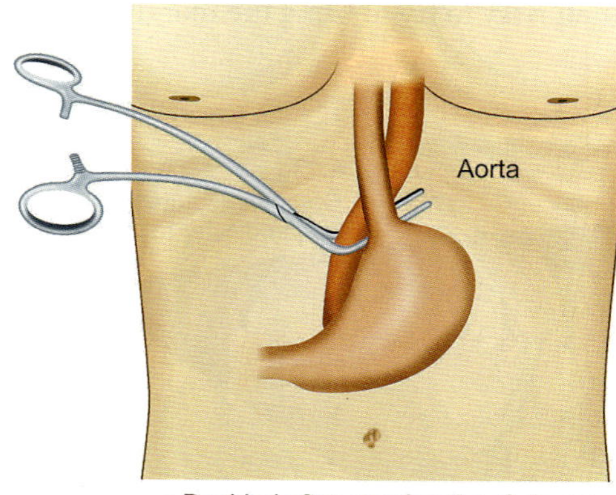

Figs. 8-27A and B: Aortic clamping is done when there is dangerous bleeding. Prelaparotomy thoracotomy is done just before laparotomy in anticipation through left sided 5th intercostal space. Aorta is clamped in the thorax. Abdomen is opened later. Infradiaphragmatic aortic clamping is done just above the celiac plexus level; it is decided after laparotomy because of the torrential uncontrollable bleeding. Vascular clamp is placed behind the abdominal oesophagus from right side.

prothrombin time are needed. *Angiographic embolisation* increases the success rate of non-operative therapy. Initial critical care (ICU) management for 2–5 days; repeat CT scan after 5 days; bed rest to be continued; patient can have normal activity only after 3 months. When any time patient's condition worsens, he should be taken up for laparotomy.

Surgical Management

If bleeding continues, if patient deteriorates, if major hepatic injury with vascular lacerations, has occurred surgical intervention is done. Lengthy midline incision is better if other parts of the abdomen like bowel also need intervention. Bilateral subcostal/bucket handle or often thoracoabdominal incision is also needed **(Fig. 8-28)**.

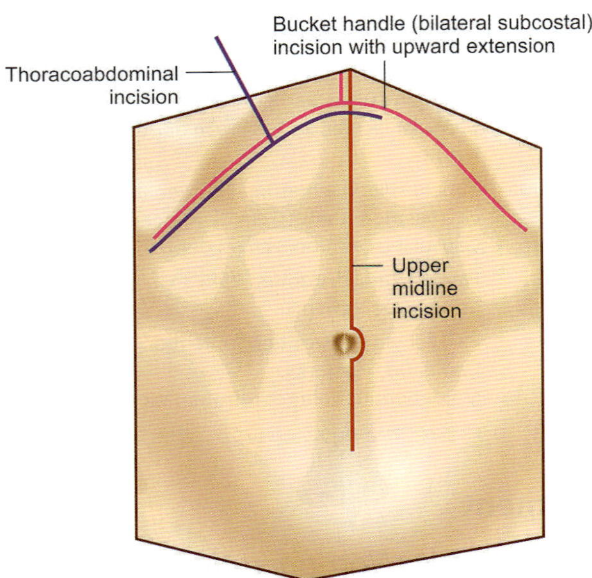

Fig. 8-28: Incisions used for different liver injuries. Wide exposure is the basic need in these patients.

Small lacerations are apposed using simple sutures with haemostatic agents. Polyglactic or PDS is used with a gel foam or surgicel support. *Kous Netzof aluminium needle* is used for these *co-opting sutures*. Initially mattress sutures parallel to the tear is placed. Row of sutures perpendicular to the tear to co-opt these mattress sutures are placed. Large lacerations need deep suturing. It is not necessary or often risky to try to bring the margins together **(Fig. 8-29)**.

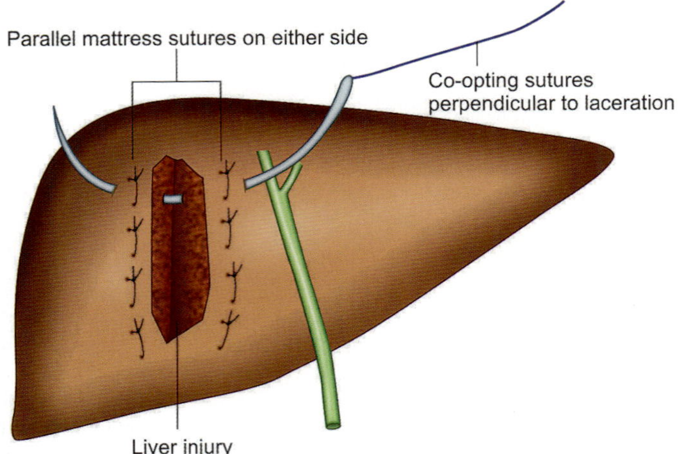

Fig. 8-29: Co-opting sutures are placed perpendicular to already placed parallel mattress sutures.

Packing is a good old method of controlling bleeding in critical patients. It can be done quickly, controls bleeding well by *tamponade*. Reexploration is done in 48-72 hours. Pack is removed. Necrotic tissues are removed. Proper saline irrigation is done. Haemostasis is achieved using bipolar cautery, argon beam ligaseal, harmonic, etc. Risk of abscess formation in packing is 15%.

In *deeper lacerations*, ligation of bleeding vessel individually on the cut surface is needed and is called as *tractotomy*. Biliary ductules are also ligated. As vessels are supported by *fibrous adventitia* suture ligation holds well in these vessels even though liver parenchyma is soft and friable.

Pringle manoeuvre is occluding the porta at foramen Winslow to control bleeding temporarily. It is done using fingers and thumb or vascular clamps or vascular loops. During Pringle manoeuvre, if bleeding gets controlled it means bleeding is from portal vein or hepatic artery branches, and if bleeding continues it is due to hepatic vein or retrohepatic IVC injury. It needs bypass (venovenous bypass between femoral vein and superior vena cava) and vascular repair. As access is technically difficult in these patients with retrohepatic caval injury, a wide tube placed across from atrial appendages to IVC just above the renal vein level may be appropriate (*intracaval catheter placement*). Pringle manoeuvre can be used continuously maximum for only one hour beyond that hepatic ischaemia may occur. But usually it is wiser to release the occlusion once in 10 minutes to reperfuse the liver and clamp the porta again. Pringle manoeuvre also helps to control bleeding while suturing the liver surface. In surface injury, liver can be wrapped with absorbable mesh (*mesh hepatorrhaphy*) to achieve haemostasis. Segmental resection is done often when needed. Hepatectomy and hepatic artery ligation is *rarely used* nowadays. Such an extensive injury can be treated initially by packing and further therapy is planned at later dates. *Push* (direct compression), *plug* (plugging the deep track injuries using silicone tube or SB tube), *Pringles*' manoeuvre, *pack* (liver wound is directly packed with mop) are basic principles in initial management **(Figs. 8-30 to 8-32)**.

Management of liver trauma

- Control of haemorrhage—packing; tractotomy; mesh hepatorrhaphy; debridement of devitalised tissue; segmentectomy, vein repair with venovenous bypass; transfusions.
- Management of metabolic disturbances—prevention of acidosis, disseminated intravascular coagulation (DIC), fresh frozen plasma (FFP); platelets.
- Monitoring—repeat US; repeat CT; urine output; liver function test (LFT); prothrombin time; platelet count; haematocrit.
- Prevention of sepsis—proper debridement; irrigation of liver wound with warm normal saline; antibiotics.
- Identification and management of complications of liver injury.

Porta Hepatic Injury

It is life threatening even though rare. Penetrating injuries commonly cause this injury. It is commonly associated with organ injuries. Isolated porta injury is rare. It is difficult to manage with mortality 50–80%. Portal vein is sutured after venovenous bypass. Common bile duct injury involving less than half the circumference can be sutured over a T tube. Injury more than 50% or transection needs choledochojejunostomy.

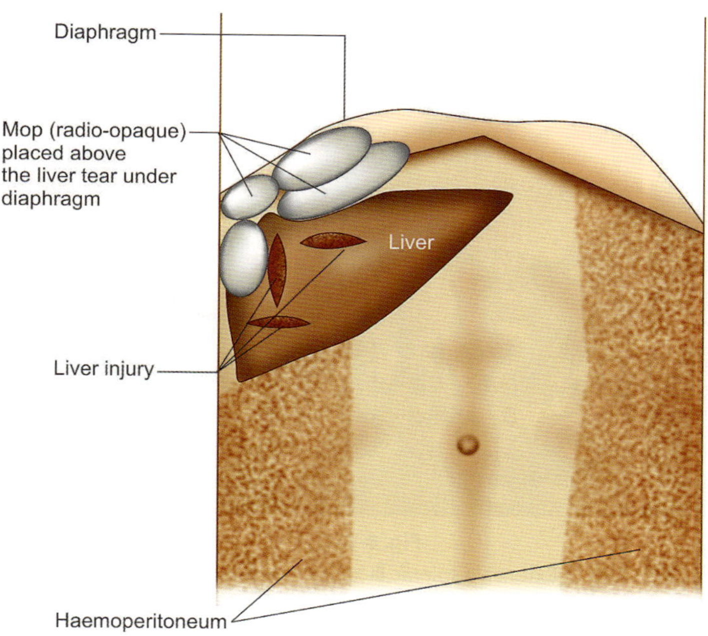

Fig. 8-30: By placing 3–5 mops between injured liver and diaphragm tamponade effect can be achieved to control bleeding from the liver. After 48–72 hours electively abdomen is reexplored for further intervention. Often bleeding will be controlled by then and further management becomes easier. Sepsis should be taken care of by higher generation antibiotics.

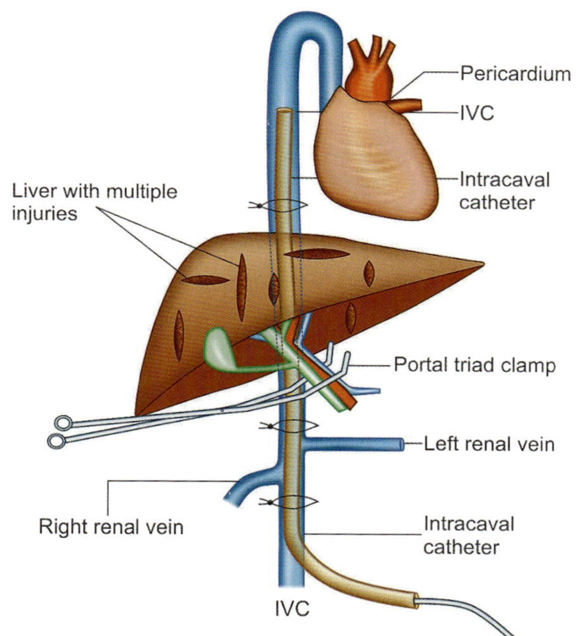

Fig. 8-31: Intracaval catheter placement is the only life-saving option in case of hepatic vein or retrohepatic inferior vena cava (IVC) injuries.

Complications of Liver Injury

Shock, blood loss, DIC, sepsis, intraabdominal abscess or liver abscess formation, bile leak, biliary peritonitis, biliary fistula, hepatic artery aneurysm, haemobilia, hypoalbuminaemia, electrolyte imbalance, respiratory problems, liver failure, stricture of common bile duct are common complications.

SPLENIC INJURY

It is the most commonly affected intra-abdominal organ in blunt injury. Any injury towards left side of the chest or abdomen should

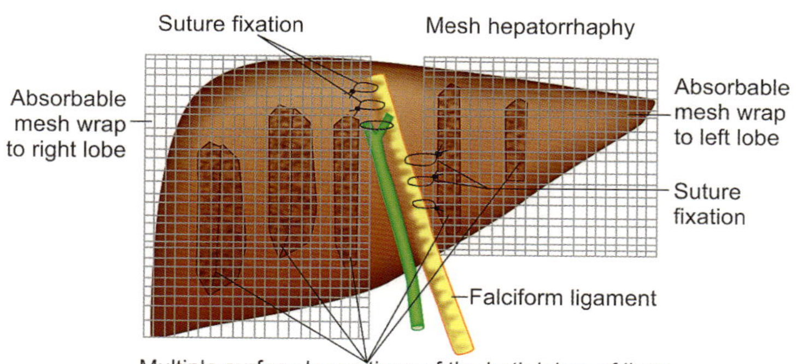

Fig. 8-32: Mesh hepatorrhaphy using absorbable mesh wrap around the liver surface. Right and left lobes are separately wrapped with mesh and fixed to falciform ligament.

suspect splenic trauma. Stab injuries also can cause splenic injury. Splenic injury is often associated with fracture lower ribs (30%), haemothorax, liver injury (left lobe), jejunal, pancreatic and left kidney injuries. Left side diaphragmatic injury is also known to occur. Injury is more common and severe in already enlarged spleen like of malaria, tropical splenomegaly, etc. Spontaneous rupture of spleen can occur in malaria. *Larang* was used for killing by the murderers in Far East where malaria is endemic leading to splenomegaly, ruptured spleen more easily **(Fig. 8-33)**.

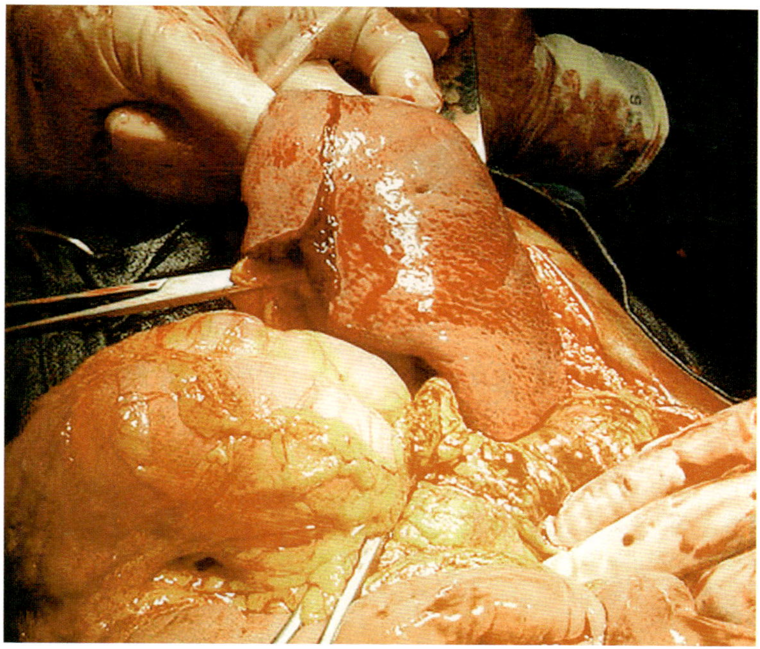

Fig. 8-33: Splenic laceration on one side. Splenorrhaphy/partial splenectomy is possible here.

Types of Splenic Injury

Splenic subcapsular haematoma: After initial injury patient remains asymptomatic for a short period. But this haematoma may rupture often later after few days—causing torrential haemorrhage. *Clean incised wound on the splenic surface* may be treated by non-operative methods or by splenorrhaphy. *Splenic lacerations* when occur its extent of involvement and depth is important. If it is less than 50% part of the spleen can be salvaged by partial splenectomy. *Splenic hilar injury* often needs emergency splenectomy **(Figs. 8-34 and 8-35)**.

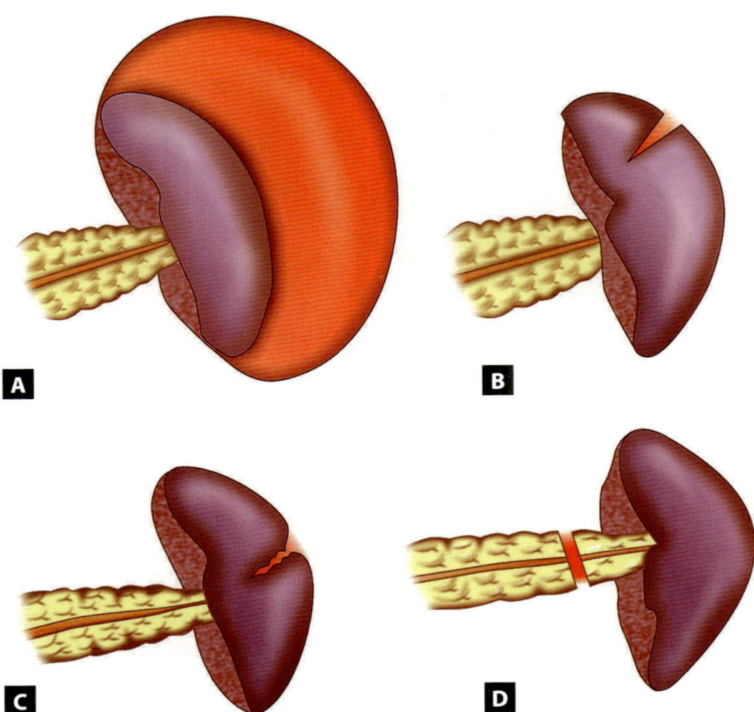

Figs. 8-34A to D: Types of splenic injury: (A) Subcapsular haematoma; (B) Incised tear/wound on the surface; (C) Lacerated wound; (D) Hilar injury.

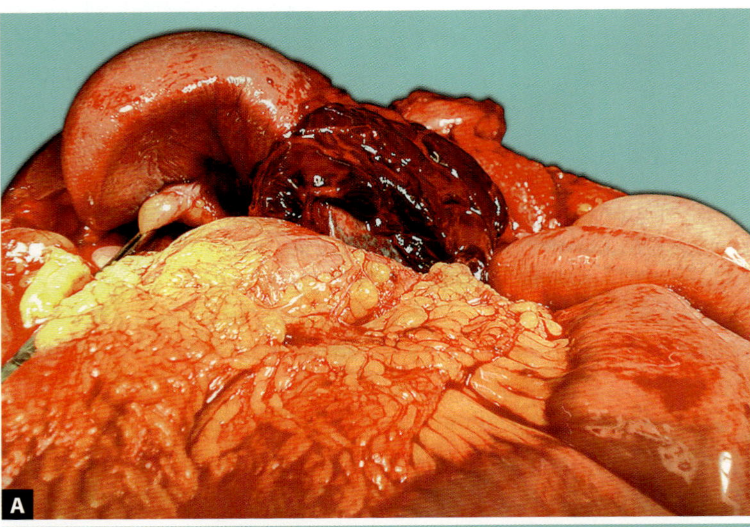

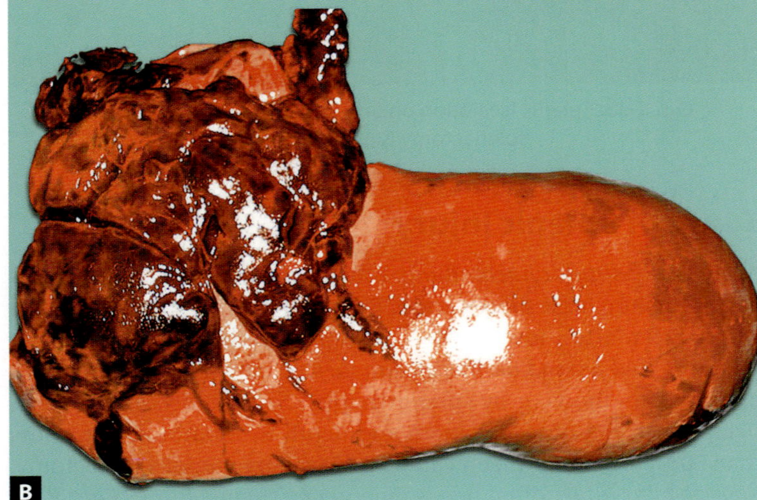

Figs. 8-35A and B

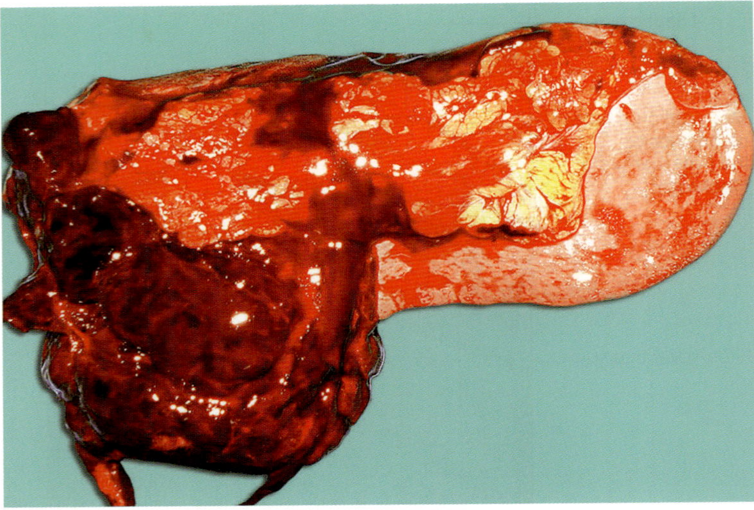

Fig. 8-35C

Figs. 8-35A to C: Extensive splenic laceration which needed splenectomy.

Presentations

Common presentations in severe splenic injury are features of shock; left upper abdominal pain and tenderness; referred pain over left shoulder due to irritation of left side diaphragm and left phrenic nerve (Kehr's sign); dullnes over left side abdomen which is not shifting due to presence of clot formation (Ballance's sign); tenderness between left sternomastoid and scalenus medius (Saegesser's tender point); formed haematoma in perisplenic area is initially localised by omentum and bowel and so patient shows delayed presentation of severe haemorrhage once clot dislodges off the omentum (latent period of Bandet).

Splenic organ injury scale		
Grade I	Haematoma	Non-expanding subcapsular haematoma <10% surface area.
	Laceration	Non-bleeding capsular laceration with <1 cm depth.
Grade II	Haematoma	Non-expanding subcapsular haematoma 10–50% surface area. Non-expanding intraparenchymal haematoma <5 cm.
	Laceration	Capsular tear; 1–3 cm depth parenchymal injury not involving trabecular vessel.
Grade III	Haematoma	Expanding subcapsular or intraparenchymal haematoma. Bleeding subcapsular haematoma or subcapsular haematoma >50% area or intraparenchymal haematoma >5 cm.
	Laceration	Parenchymal laceration >3 cm depth.
Grade IV	Laceration	Ruptured intraparenchymal haematoma with active bleed; laceration involving segmental or hilar vessels with >25% devascularisation.
Grade V		Shattered or avulsed spleen; hilar devascularisation with separation of entire spleen.

Complications

Complications of splenic injury are—haemorrhage and its consequences; disseminated intravascular coagulation; sepsis like subphrenic abscess, pancreatitis; splenic artery pseudoaneurysm; splenic arteriovenous fistula.

Investigations

Ultrasound is the basic investigation initially to identify splenic trauma.

CT scan should be done in all patients to confirm the type of injury. CT with contrast to see blush in arterial phase of the contrast is very significant.

Haematocrit, blood grouping and cross-matching samples often to keep needed quantity of blood ready are basic requisites. Angiogram with possible need for angiographic embolisation is commonly used in some centres as diagnostic as well as a non-operative method of treatment. Diagnostic peritoneal lavage as discussed earlier is also helpful.

Chest X-ray with plain X-ray abdomen is older method of evaluation with higher chances of missing the splenic injury. However, features to be looked for in X-ray are—obliteration of splenic outline and left sided psoas shadow; indentation of fundic gas shadow; fracture ribs; elevation of left sided diaphragm; dilated intestinal coils on the left side.

Treatment

Initial Management

Central venous line for perfusion and monitoring; transfusion of blood as needed; antibiotics coverage; urinary catheterisation; nasogastric tube aspiration.

Non-operative Management

When facilities are available, splenic injury can be managed conservatively by non-operative method. Clinically close observation, serial haematocrit evaluation, serial CT abdomen/US abdomen at regular intervals to assess the progress or regress of the bleeding spleen has to be done. Initial abdominal CT with intravenous contrast is essential to see contrast extravasation and contrast blush in arterial phase. If in later period bleeding persists it is again repeated. Presence of blush is whether an indication for surgical intervention or not is a controversy. In a set up where all facilities are available for intervention, patient can be managed with non-operative method. Absolute bed rest, sedation, antibiotic coverage and proper monitoring are needed. It is often supported by angiographic embolisation to improve the splenic salvage rate. But it may cause pain, splenic abscess or infarction. Routine angiographic embolisation is also advocated but whether it is needed is a doubtful entity. 70% of stable splenic injury patients can be treated by non-operative method. Decreasing haematocrit, hypotension, and persistent paralytic ileus may be an indication for surgical intervention. *Indications for non-operative treatment:* Only splenic injury—no other associated injuries; Grade I, II and selected grade III injuries. Absolute bed rest for 10 days and avoiding excess physical activity for 3 months is mandatory.

Surgical Management

Splenorrhaphy

Especially in a clean incised wound spleen can be salvaged by suturing the wound carefully with placement of gel foam, topical thrombin, absorbable mesh wrap over the wound. PDS or vicryl is used as interrupted horizontal mattress sutures. Fibrin glue and use of argon beam coagulator on the surface is also beneficial. But in class/grade III, IV or V injuries splenorrhaphy is not possible **(Fig. 8-36)**.

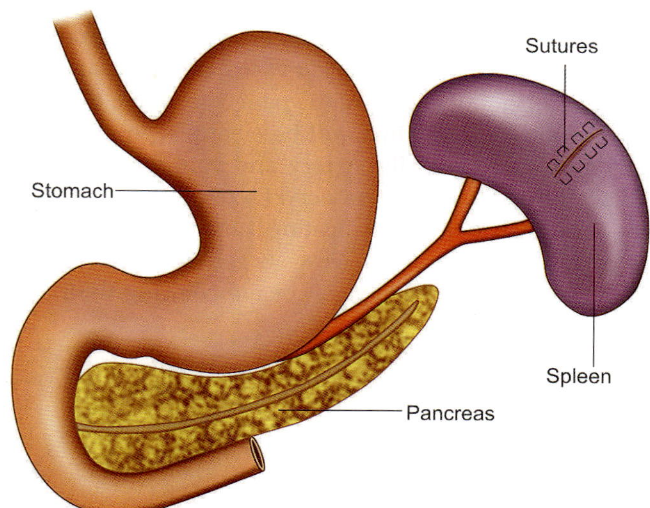

Fig. 8-36: Splenorrhaphy is ideal in surface injury and simple injuries.

Advantages of splenorrhaphy

- It avoids OPSI.
- It avoids dead space and so prevents potential space for subphrenic abscess.
- Cellular components of blood are better maintained.

Partial splenectomy (upper/lower)

It can be done by retaining either of the upper or lower polar branches of the splenic artery depending on the location of the injury whether in lower or upper part of the spleen. Hilum is carefully dissected to identify the division of the splenic artery into polar vessels. Isolated artery is individually ligated. Accompanying veins are also ligated. Injury extending across both poles is difficult to manage by partial splenectomy. Surface of the spleen is sutured with PDS or vicryl and cut surface is cauterised or small bleeders are controlled using Ligaseal. Gelfoam/spongistan are placed over the raw area **(Fig. 8-37)**.

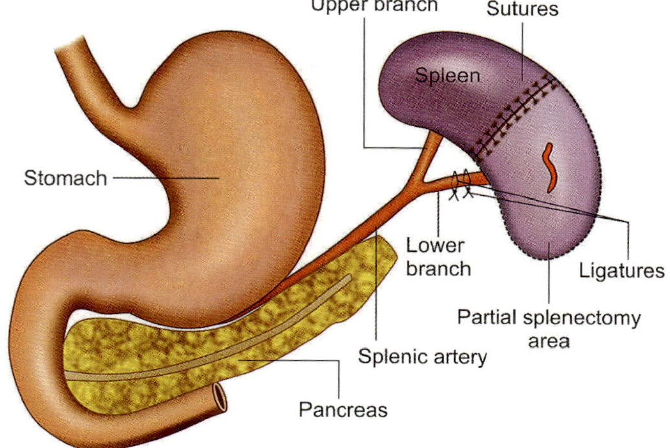

Fig. 8-37: Partial splenectomy can be done if injury is on one pole of the spleen.

Emergency splenectomy

It is done through midline/left subcostal incision. Thoracoabdominal extension of incision may be needed for rapid control of bleeding for injury to a large tropical spleen with severe bleeding. Other associated injuries should be looked for and dealt with (injury to left lobe liver/pancreas/intestine/colon). Abdomen is opened rapidly; splenic hilum is held between thumb and fingers to control bleeding immediately; blood/clots in the peritoneal cavity is sucked out and washed to clear the field; often a soft vascular clamp can be placed across hilum including the tail of the pancreas to free the surgeon's hand. With this splenic hilum will be clearly seen and bloodless hilum is dissected carefully. Artery and vein and branches are individually ligated using silk or vicryl (2-zero). Spleen is dissected from the short gastric vessels by ligating it and also from splenorenal and phrenicocolic ligaments. Few surgeons also prefer to use polypropylene but knot holding may be difficult **(Fig. 8-38)**.

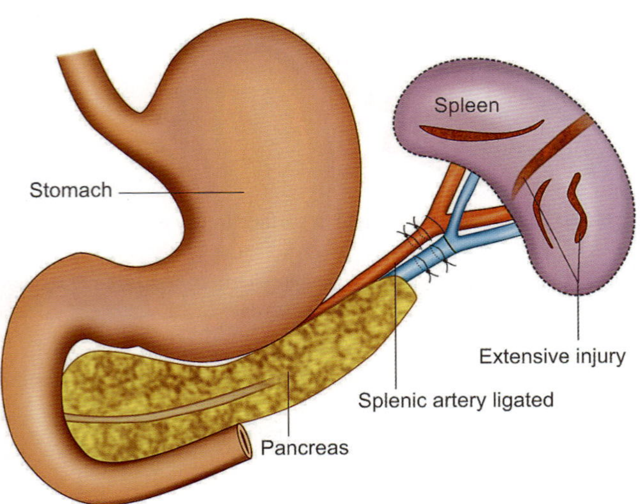

Fig. 8-38: Technique of splenectomy.

Mass ligature of the entire splenic hilum, even though is commonly used by many surgeons, is a controversial and not universally accepted; however, if patient is haemodynamically *unstable* due to exsanguination and adequate quantity of blood is not available, quick mass ligature can be done using silk. In such situation abdomen is also closed as single mass closure instead of layer by layer **(Fig. 8-39)**.

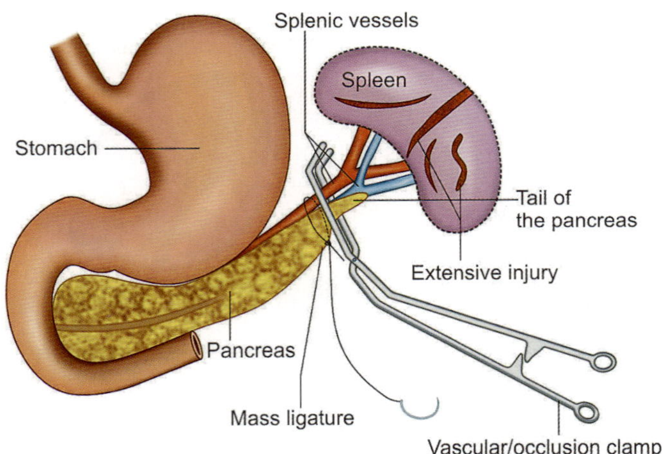

Fig. 8-39: Mass ligature of the splenic pedicle is often used in emergency splenectomy in splenic trauma.

Salutary effect

In traumatic rupture of spleen, spleen is cut into pieces of 0.5 cm and placed in omental pockets. This autotransplantation is still experimental and controversial.

Complications of Splenic Injury

Metabolic imbalance, acidosis, shock, renal failure, sepsis, DIC, splenic artery pseudoaneurysm, splenic arteriovenous fistula.

Splenectomy can cause DVT, OPSI, haematemesis, left sided pleural effusion, pancreatitis, pancreatic fistula, subphrenic abscess left sided, left lung atelectasis (commonest), left colonic and rarely gastric injury, severe sepsis.

PANCREATIC INJURY

It is rare entity as pancreas is retroperitoneal and well protected. However, penetrating injury and blunt seat belt injury (due to close proximity to vertebral column) can cause pancreatic trauma. It is commonly associated with other abdominal injuries and so commonly missed. It is often difficult to diagnose the pancreatic trauma clinically, sonologically or by CT scan. DPL is also not much beneficial. High degree of suspicion is needed. Isolated pancreatic injuries are rare. It is usually associated with duodenal injury. Superior mesenteric vessel injury is common association. Repeat CT, persistent elevation of serum amylase (repetitive assessment of serum amylase) is helpful in diagnosis. MRI/MRCP may be beneficial. *Pancreatic duct injury* is the main deciding factor in managing and predicting the outcome. If injury is right of the superior mesenteric vein, it is called as *proximal pancreatic injury*. If it is towards left it is called as *distal pancreatic injury*.

Proximal injury is treated by surgical debridement; suture ligation of bleeding area; drainage of the pancreatic bed. If there is associated duodenal injury, then pancreaticoduodenectomy is also done. Debridement, closure of duodenal wound and pylorus exclusion is also done. Pancreatic fistula (40%), pancreatic abscess, pancreatitis (15%) septicaemia, pancreatic ascites, pancreatic pleural effusion are common complications which can occur in survived patient.

Distal injury is managed by distal pancreatectomy. Role of pancreaticojejunostomy, ERCP stenting is controversial.

Pancreatic injury		
Grade I	Haematoma Laceration	Minor contusion without duct injury. Superficial laceration without duct injury.
Grade II	Haematoma Laceration	Major contusion without duct injury or tissue loss.
Grade III	Laceration	Distal transection or parenchymal injury with duct injury.
Grade IV	Laceration	Proximal transection or parenchymal injury involving the ampulla.
Grade V	Laceration	Massive disruption of the parenchymal head.

DUODENAL INJURIES

Duodenal injuries are 5% common; commonly penetrating; commonly associated with other abdominal injuries like liver, pancreas, major vessels, etc. Isolated injury of the duodenum even though is rare, causes difficulty in diagnosing as it does not cause early peritonitis or haemodynamic instability. But late life-threatening complications like intra-abdominal abscess or peritonitis develops. Raised serum amylase; plain X-ray abdomen showing mild scoliosis, obliteration of psoas shadow, *presence of air in retroperitoneum around kidney*, absence of air in duodenal bulb; gastrograffin study; CT abdomen with oral intravenous contrast; or dilute barium (microbar solution) study are the investigations needed. CT may show extravasation which is an absolute indication for laparotomy. *Extraluminal air in the CT is diagnostic* **(Fig. 8-40)**.

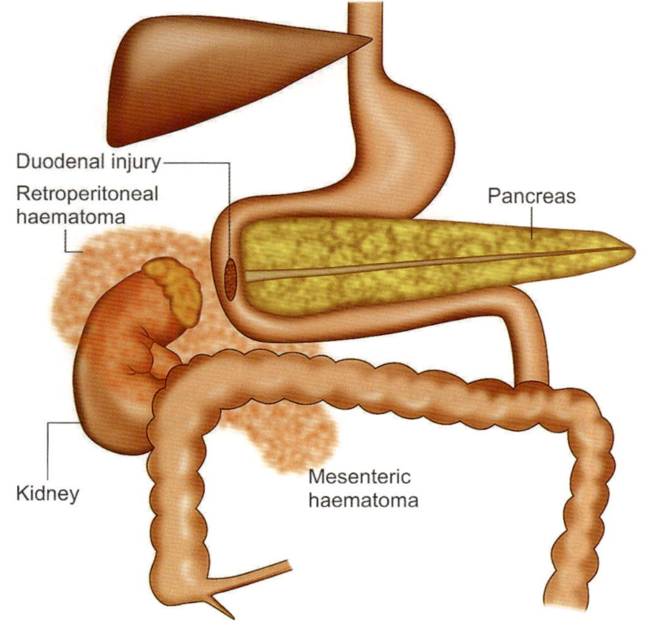

Fig. 8-40: Duodenal injury often associated with pancreatic injury; haematoma in duodenum, and retroperitoneum, around right kidney, mesentery.

Duodenal haematoma causes radiologically coiled spring or stacked coin sign; but is not a sign to do surgery; only haematoma causing obstruction is operated. It occurs on the convex surface of the duodenum extending into the retroperitoneum. If it is causing obstruction, it can be carefully evacuated without opening the mucosa; gastrostomy and jejunostomy is a must **(Fig. 8-41)**.

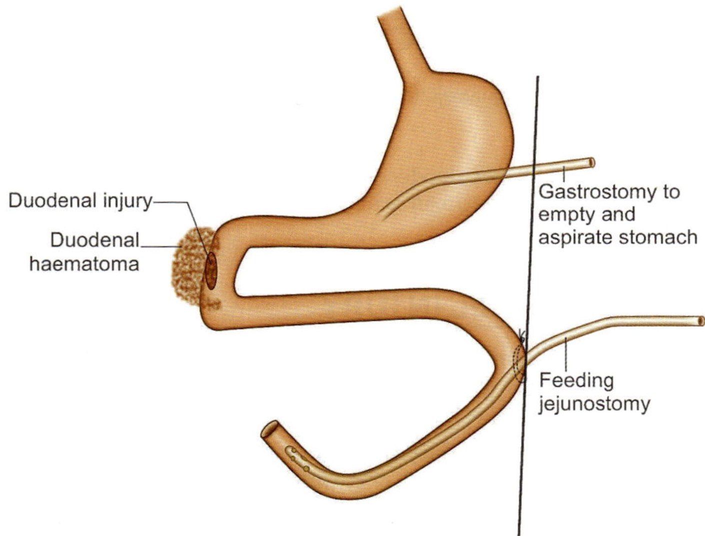

Fig. 8-41: Duodenal haematoma. It is treated by gastrostomy; feeding jejunostomy. It is intervened when it causes duodenal obstruction.

Duodenal injury grading		
Grade I	Haematoma Laceration	Involving single portion of the duodenum. Partial thickness injury without perforation.
Grade II	Haematoma Laceration	Involving more than one portion. Disruption less than 50% circumference.
Grade III	Laceration	Disruption 50–75% of the circumference of 2nd part of the duodenum; disruption 50–100% of the 1st, 3rd or 4th part of the duodenum.
Grade IV	Laceration	Disruption more than 75% of 2nd part of the duodenum and involving the ampulla or distal common bile duct.
Grade V	Laceration Vascular	Severe disruption of duodenopancreatic complex. Duodenal devascularisation.

Procedure

When decided for surgery; after laparotomy with a lengthy midline incision, extended Kocherisation is done (peritoneum on the right of the 2nd part is cut and duodenum is mobilised in front and medially in front of the IVC and up to left margin of the aorta completely); hepatic flexure and right part of the transverse colon is mobilised fully; 3rd and 4th parts of the duodenum are visualised properly. Any haematoma or injury or presence of associated pancreatic injuries is looked for. Duodenojejunal junction is mobilised more proximally by dissecting the peritoneal fold to get the proximal length.

Eighty percent of duodenal injuries are *sutured primarily* using polyglactic acid or PDS interrupted sutures horizontally **(Fig. 8-42)**.

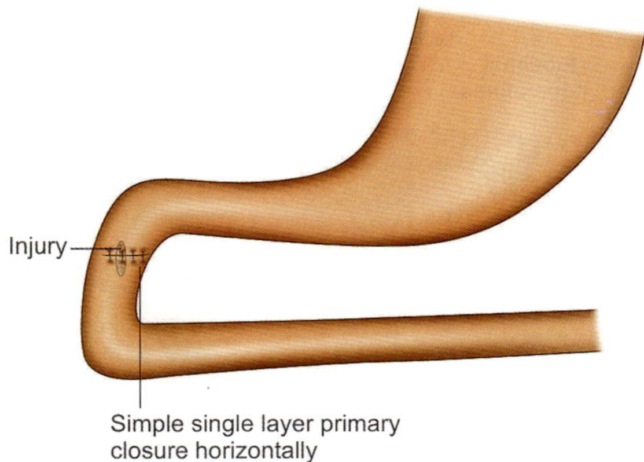

Fig. 8-42: Simple duodenal injury is closed using interrupted single/double layer sutures horizontally. Jejunostomy is usually needed.

Single layer suturing is proved to be sufficient. But many advocates two layer suturing. Often many use silk; silk holds the bowel wall well with low rate of leak; but being a non-absorbable multifilament braided suture it has got tendency to form small granulomas in the anastomotic line even though said to be safer.

Injury on the medial/inner aspect of the duodenum especially in 3rd and 4th parts is sutured transduodenally using continuous single layer PDS sutures. Incision made in the anterior wall is closed horizontally **(Fig. 8-43)**.

In grade I and II injuries: Just suturing is sufficient if opened within 6 hours but if opened after 6 hours suturing along with jejunostomy is required. Often tube duodenostomy is preferred by many **(Fig. 8-44)**.

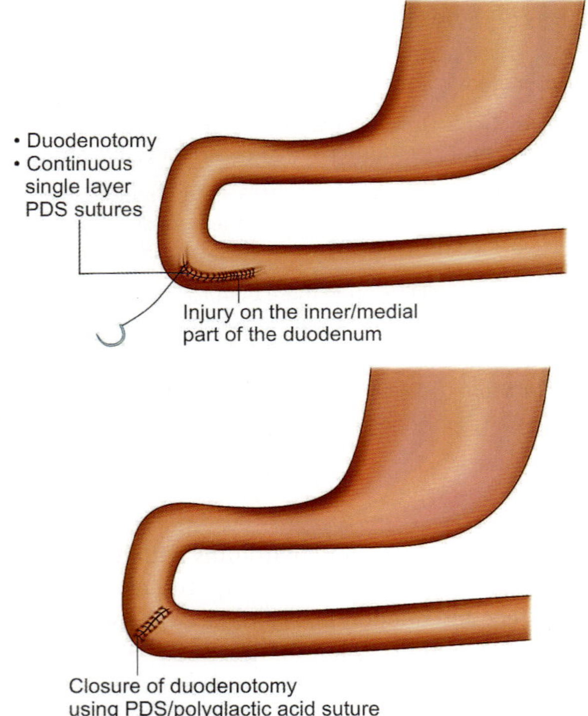

Fig. 8-43: Injury on the medial wall of the duodenum is closed with continuous PDS sutures after doing duodenotomy. Duodenotomy is closed with interrupted vicryl sutures.

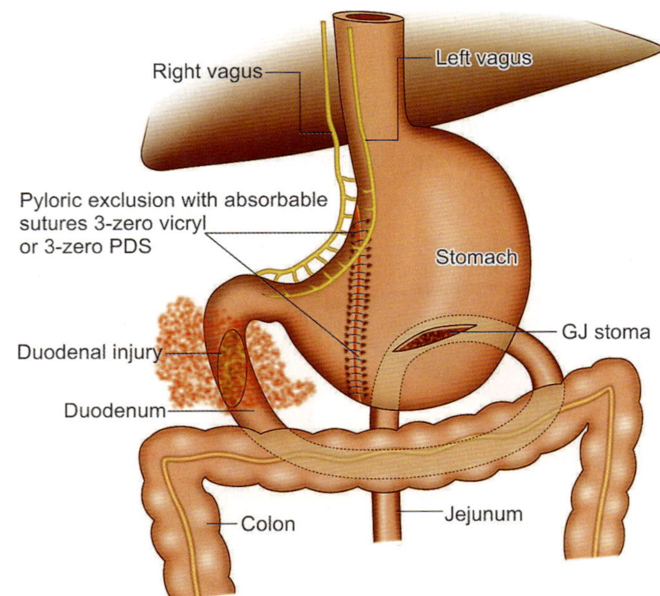

Fig. 8-45: Pyloric exclusion with gastrojejunostomy (GJ) with feeding jejunostomy is one of the options can be used in duodenal injury. Just doing gastrojejunostomy is not advised.

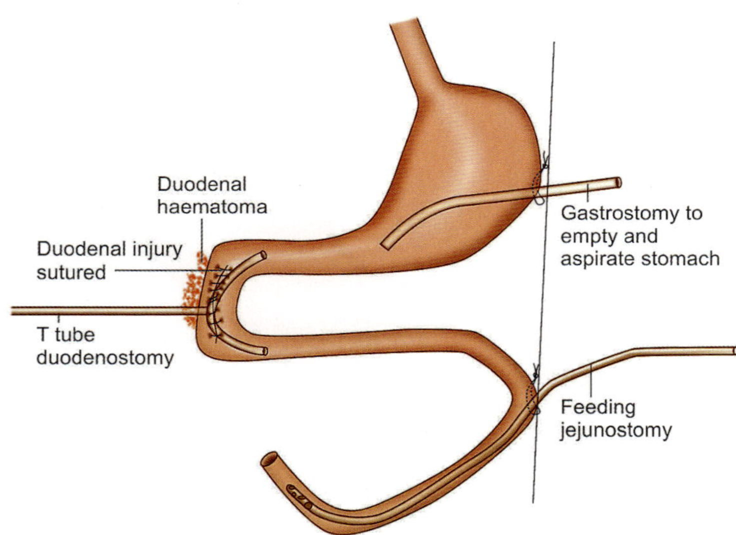

Fig. 8-44: Duodenal injury with T tube duodenostomy; closure of the injury; gastrostomy and feeding jejunostomy.

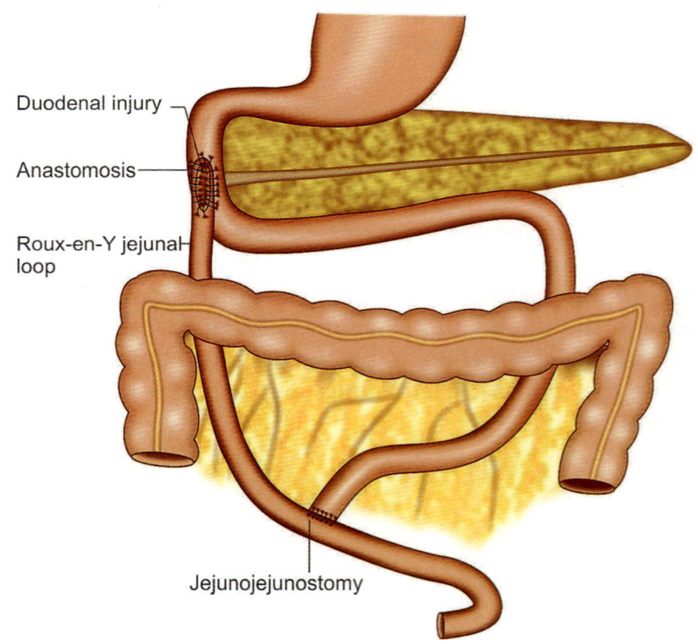

Fig. 8-46: Roux-en-Y loop duodenojejunostomy on to the site of the injury with a feeding jejunostomy is another alternative.

In grade III injury: Duodenojejunostomy or pyloric exclusion with gastrojejunostomy drainage procedure is done. Serosal patch of the jejunum is useful. Roux-en-Y duodenojejunostomy with feeding jejunostomy is also beneficial **(Figs. 8-45 to 8-47)**.

In grade IV injuries: Duodenal repair; repair of CBD with T tube having lower part of the horizontal limb of T tube into the duodenum across the injury is done. Other option is duodenal repair with or without pyloric exclusion with ligation of the CBD; later during second stage dilated proximal CBD is used for choledochoenteric anastomosis.

Grade V injury needs pancreaticoduodenectomy. It carries high mortality. But one has to remember that if overall duodenal injuries are considered, pancreaticoduodenectomy is rarely needed **(Fig. 8-48)**.

SMALL BOWEL INJURY

Blunt injury abdomen causing small bowel trauma is often difficult to identify at initial phases when patient arrives to the hospital. London's sign (abrasion over the abdominal wall), Monk's localising zones in the abdomen may be useful features but not clear cut evidence of small bowel injury. Once peritonitis develops patient presents with typical features. Junction of fixed proximal jejunum or terminal ileum is commonly injured due to shearing force. Often it is like a blow-out injury causing complete transection of the bowel at the junction **(Fig. 8-49)**.

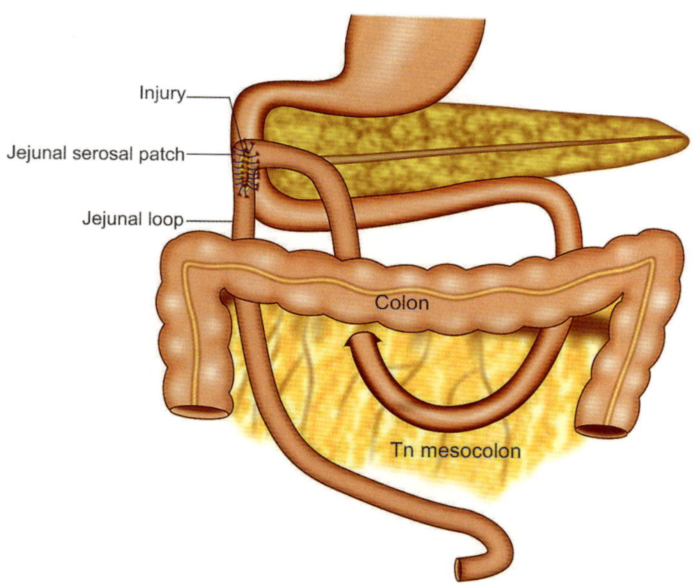

Fig. 8-47: Jejunal serosal patch over the injury site reduces the risk of duodenal leak. Feeding jejunostomy is also added.

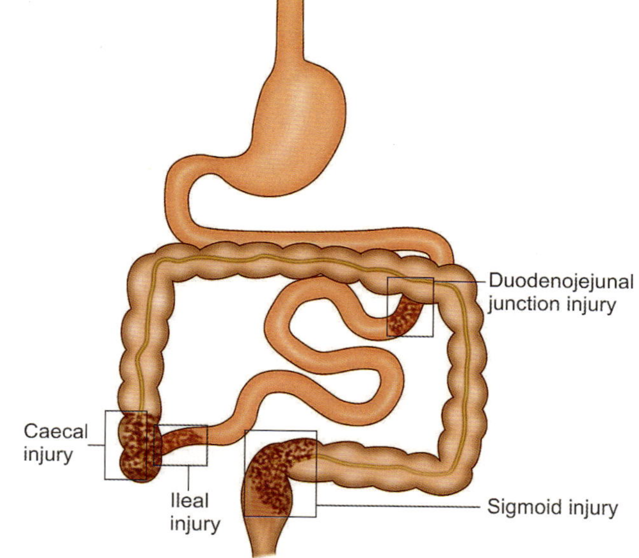

Fig. 8-49: Sites of bowel injury in blunt trauma abdomen. Proximal jejunum, terminal ileum, caecum, sigmoid are the common sites.

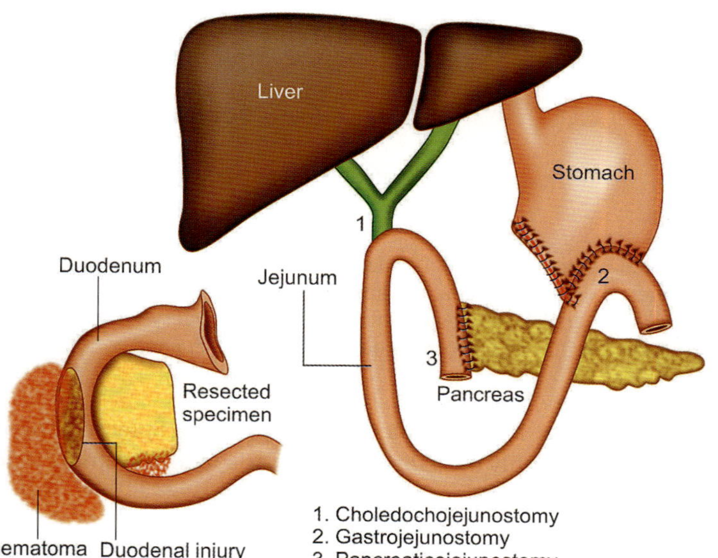

Fig. 8-48: In extensive injury only pancreaticoduodenectomy is done.

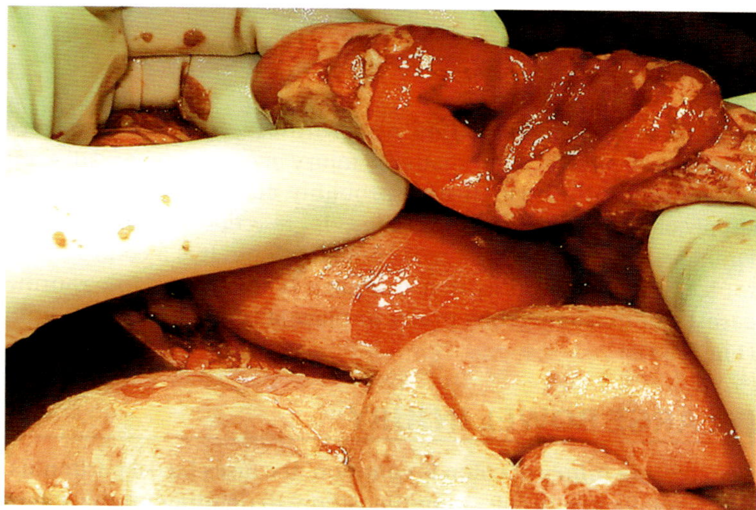

Fig. 8-50: Transection of the jejunum in blunt injury abdomen due to shearing force/blow out effect.

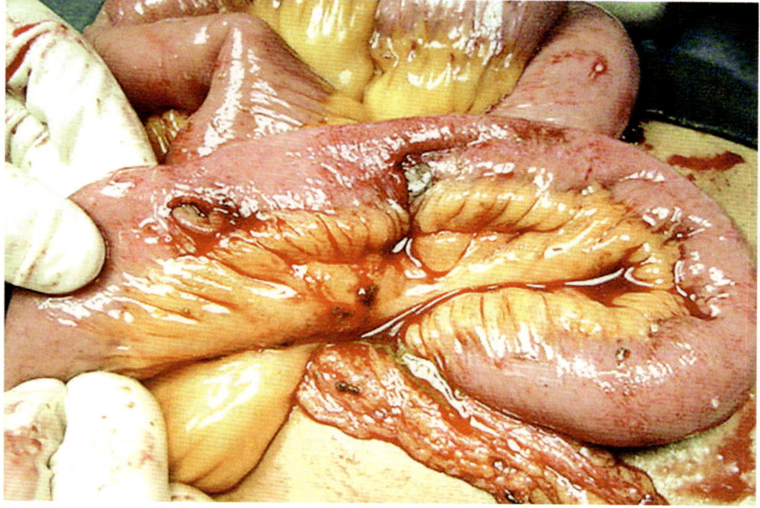

Fig. 8-51: Small bowel injury causing multiple perforations due to penetrating trauma.

Penetrating injury can often cause not just single perforation **(Fig. 8-50)** but multiple perforations with mesenteric injury **(Fig. 8-51)**.

Plain X-ray abdomen shows gas under diaphragm in blunt injury abdomen. DPL may not be diagnostic. CT may be useful. Best way is to explore if there are features of peritonitis.

Formal laparotomy is done using midline incision. Entire small and large bowel mesentery and other organs are examined for any injury.

Small single tear in the small bowel is sutured horizontally using polyglactic acid (vicryl) interrupted *single layer* sutures (preferred). In *two layer method*—inner continuous absorbable sutures with outer interrupted seromuscular mattress sutures can be placed. One should not miss additional tears in other part of the bowel **(Fig. 8-52)**.

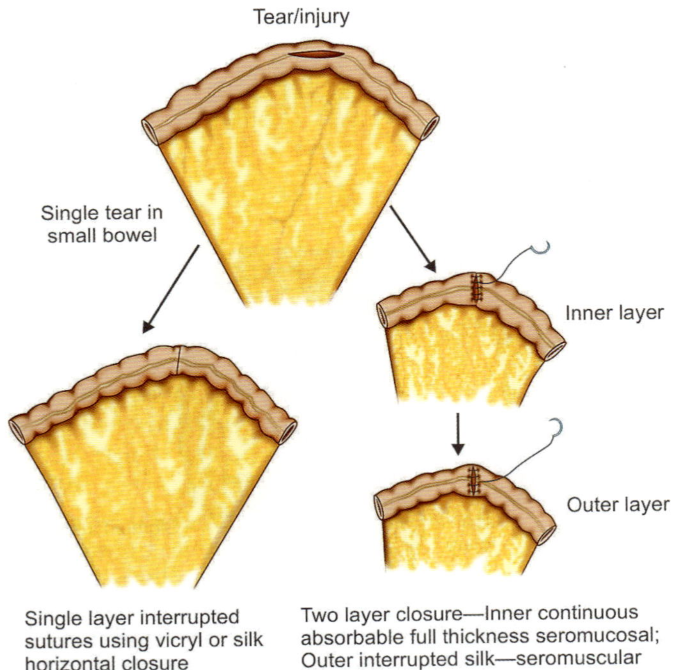

Fig. 8-52: Single small tear in the small intestine is closed horizontally using silk/vicryl either as single layer interrupted sutures or two-layer closure with inner continuous suture and outer interrupted sutures.

When there are *multiple perforations (10%)* located very closely in the bowel loop; shattered injury in one segment; adjacent mesenteric injury which may probably compromise the blood supply of the bowel are the indications for *resection* and anastomosis. Drainage is used only if there is contamination. It is a controversial topic. Literature opines that drainage is not needed in routine cases; but most surgeons prefer to place a tube/corrugated drain **(Fig. 8-53)**.

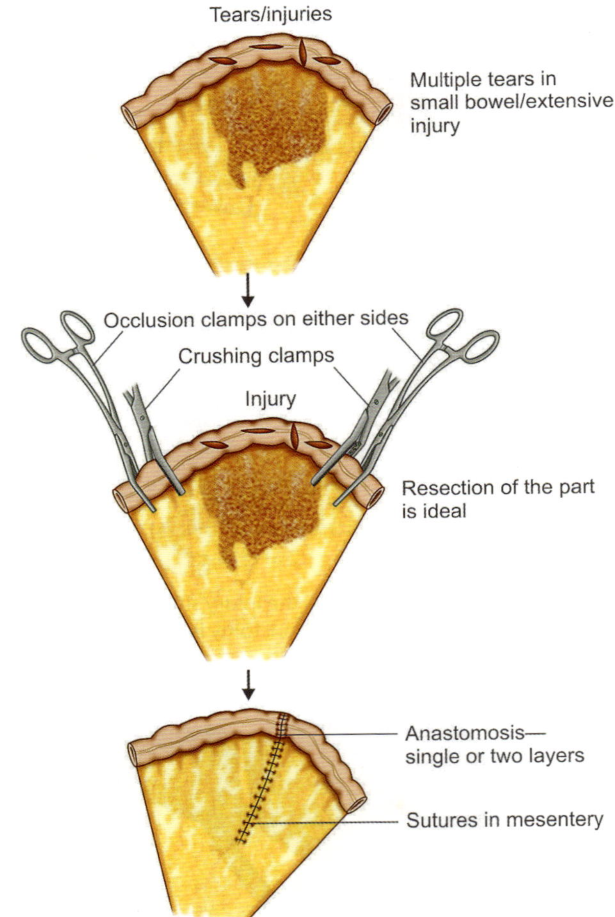

Fig. 8-53: When extensive/multiple tears at close proximity, resection of the involved bowel segment and anastomosis is done. But one should remember that massive small bowel resection may cause short gut syndrome due to less than required (120 cm) length of the small bowel is retained.

LARGE BOWEL INJURY

Penetrating injury of colon is common. It causes faecal peritonitis. It essentially needs colostomy/ileostomy depending on the site of injury. Small tear can be closed primarily using silk/vicryl horizontal interrupted mattress sutures. Primary repair is done only if early diagnosis is done in 6 hours of injury; without any hypotension; without gross contamination of the peritoneal cavity; without colonic vascular injury.

Low risk colonic injuries are one without much contamination of peritoneal cavity and without vascular injury. It is treated by primary closure or resection and primary anastomosis. Stapled or hand anastomosis has equal results in colonic trauma.

Plain X-ray abdomen, presence of blood during digital examination is typical and one can suspect colonic injury.

Blunt trauma of colon is rare. Caecum and sigmoid colon are commonly affected. Pericaecal haematoma can cause late bowel wall ischaemia → necrosis → perforation → peritonitis. In critically ill patient due to trauma, initially there is only serosal injury without mucosa, but due to persistent hypotension and hypoperfusion late ischaemic necrosis and perforation can occur. It is common in sigmoid colon.

Exteriorisation either ileostomy or colostomy should be always kept in mind by the surgeon whenever needed. If extensive injury is found right or left hemicolectomy is the need. Splenic or hepatic flexure is commonly used for colostomy as a loop. Ileostomy is done usually as end type **(Figs. 8-54 to 8-56)**.

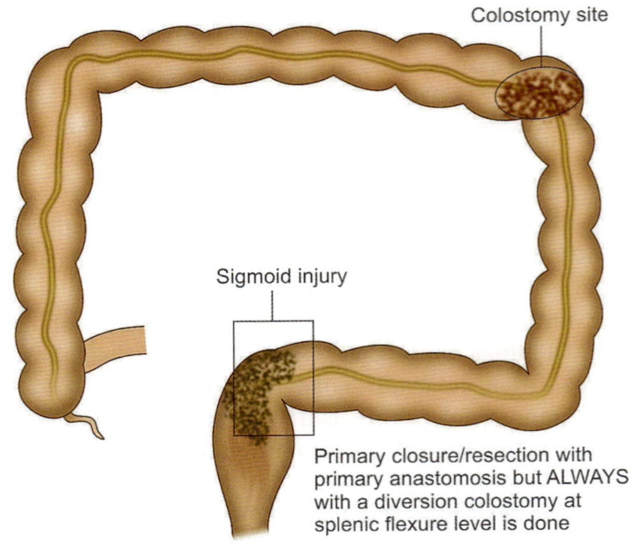

Fig. 8-54: Injury to sigmoid colon needs diversion colostomy at splenic flexure or proximal level. Tear in the sigmoid colon is sutured using interrupted silk/vicryl. Often sigmoid resection and anastomosis is done if injury is extensive.

Maintenance of nutrition, total parenteral nutrition (TPN), antibiotics, fluid and electrolyte management are the other main required management for good outcome. Transfusion of blood may be required.

Rectal injury when it is high needs colostomy for 6 weeks. If it is low rectal injury, primary repair can be done perineally after thorough wound debridement and wash using warm normal saline.

Closure of the exteriorisation is done once sepsis is under control; patient recovers well.

Complications after surgery are—anastomotic leak; pelvic/intraperitoneal abscess, sepsis, wound dehiscence, mortality.

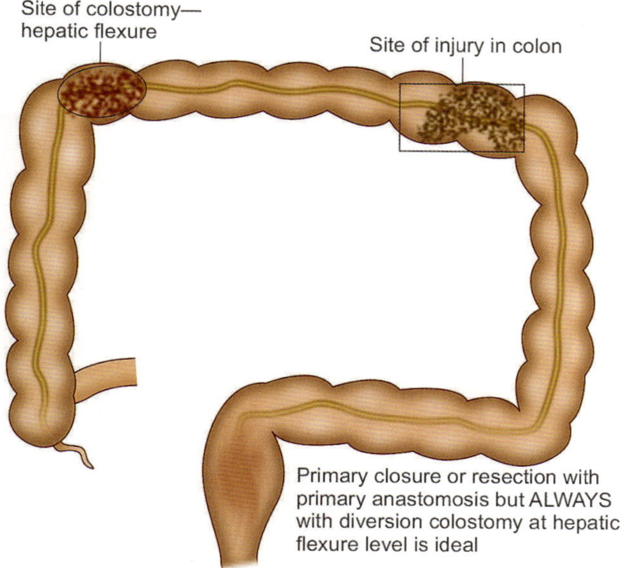

Fig. 8-55: If injury is in the splenic flexure level then colostomy is done at hepatic flexure level.

RECTAL INJURIES

Rectal injuries are commonly penetrating type. It is often associated with pelvic injuries, urinary system injuries. It is difficult to manage. Blood on rectal examination is diagnostic. Injury should be assessed under general anaesthesia. Prior to that associated injuries and ultrasound abdomen for haemoperitoneum should be checked. Haematuria when present suspects associated bladder injury. Proctosigmoidoscopy should be done for proper assessment of rectal injuries.

Rectal injury can be *extraperitoneal or intraperitoneal.*

Treatment

Treatment is diversion colostomy, proper saline wash (very important), primary closure of the accessible rectal injury either perineally or through laparotomy. Unless rectal injury is small and low, diversion colostomy is a must. Presacral drainage after thorough wash of this space is a must. Otherwise retrorectal abscess may develop which is rather difficult to manage. Colostomy closure is done only after sepsis settles down and one must confirm that rectal or urinary fistulas will not develop **(Fig. 8-57)**.

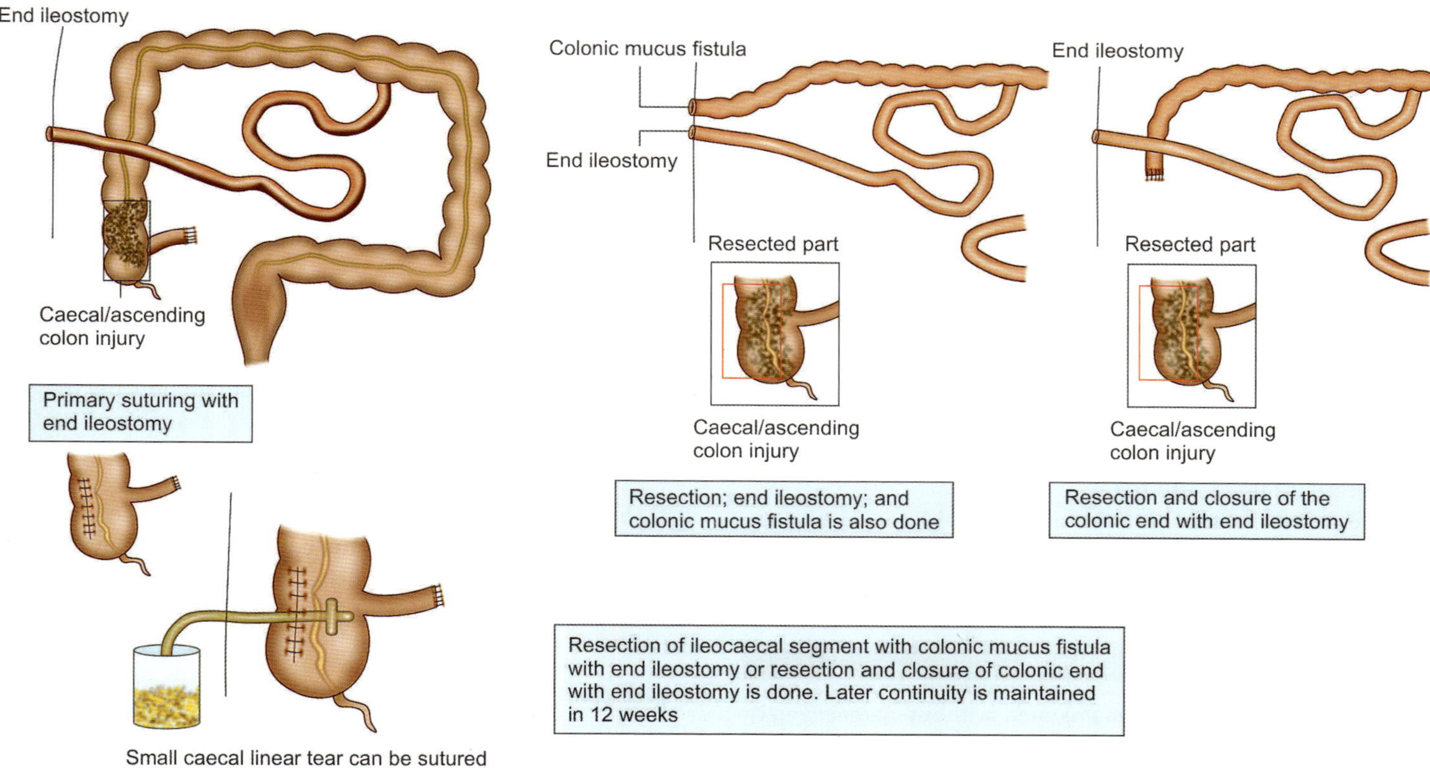

Fig. 8-56: Injury at caecal level needs ileostomy. Ileocaecal resection with end ileostomy with colonic mucus fistula or after resection colonic end is closed with end ileostomy. Ileostomy is closed in 3 months. If injury is not extensive tear can be sutured primarily with an end ileostomy. If linear small tear is present in the caecum without peritoneal contamination then closure of the caecal tear around a tube caecostomy can be done. All decisions are taken on table during surgery on individual case basis.

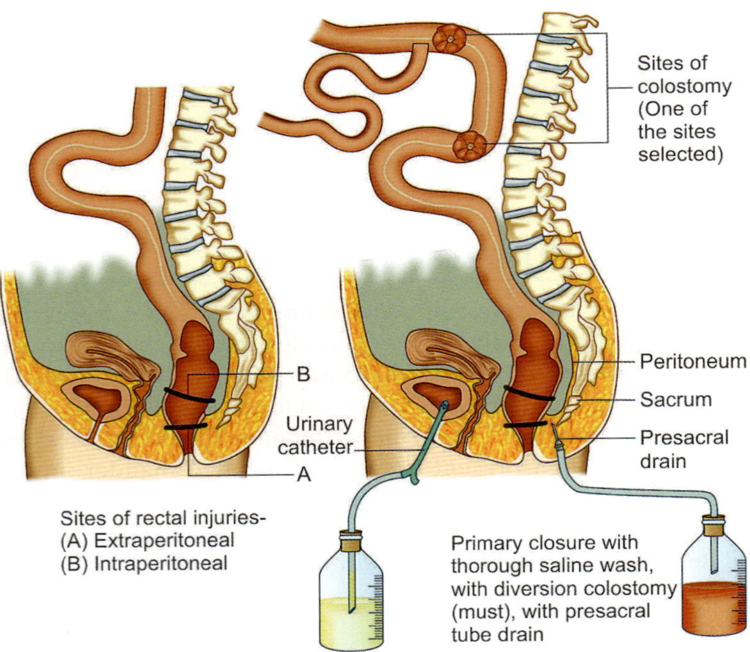

Fig. 8-57: Rectal injury can be intraperitoneal or extraperitoneal. Diversion colostomy; thorough saline wash; presacral drainage are the essential steps.

Associated urinary injury should be dealt with the help of urologists. Rectourinary fistula as a late complication is not uncommon.

Complications

Complications are abscess, sepsis, fistula, rectal incontinence, rectal stricture, sexual dysfunction, associated urinary incontinence due to damage to nerves and puborectalis.

RENAL INJURIES

Commonly it is due to a blunt injury. Often it is associated with other abdominal injuries—of liver, spleen, bowel, mesentery, etc. *Per se renal injury is extraperitoneal.*

Types

Small subcapsular; large subcapsular; cortical laceration; laceration with perinephric haematoma; medullary laceration with bleeding into the renal pelvis; corticomedullary complete rupture; hilar injury (most dangerous) **(Figs. 8-58A to G)**.

Eighty five percent of renal injuries are minor. Minor injuries are treated non-operatively. Major injuries means—deep corticomedullary injury with extravasation and renal pedicle injuries.

Grading of renal injury

1. Subcapsular non-expanding haematoma without parenchymal laceration.
2. Cortical laceration <1 cm of parenchymal depth, no extravasation; perirenal haematoma.
3. Cortical laceration >1 cm depth; no urine extravasation.
4. Parenchymal laceration extending through cortex and medulla with collecting system; with extravasation of urine.
5. Renal pedicle avulsion; shattered kidney.

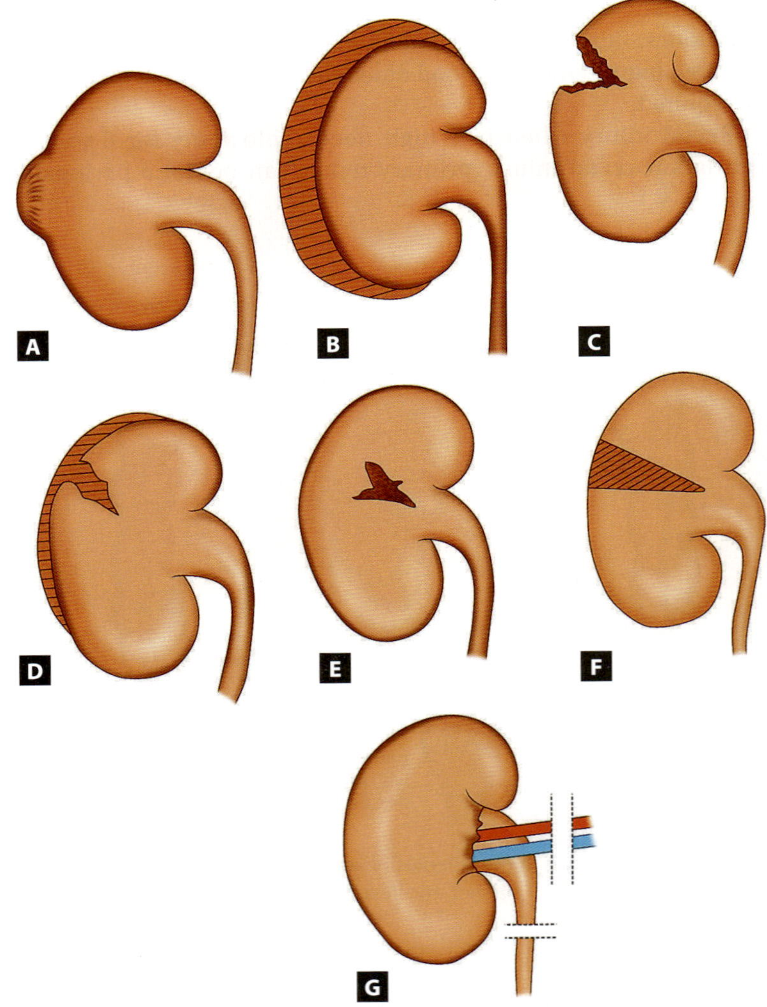

Figs. 8-58A to 'G: Renal injuries: (A) Small subcapsular; (B) Large subcapsular; (C) Cortical laceration; (D) Laceration with perinephric haematoma; (E) Medullary laceration with bleeding into the renal pelvis; (F) Corticomedullary complete rupture; (G) Hilar injury—most dangerous.

Clinical Features

Features of shock; haematuria—may be mild to profuse depending on the type of injury; clot colic; bruising, swelling and tenderness in the loin; paralytic ileus with abdominal distension occurs due to retroperitoneal haematoma implicating splanchnic nerves.

Investigations

IVU (high dose): It is the investigation of choice. Function of not only the injured kidney but also of the contralateral kidney can be seen. Often it is observed that opposite renal artery undergoes a reflex spasm, temporarily ceasing of function of the contralateral kidney occurs.

US abdomen: It is done to see the type of injury, amount of haematoma and other associated injuries in the abdomen. US should be repeated at regular intervals to see the progress (at 12–24 hourly). Blood urea and serum creatinine should be repeated again at regular intervals. Acute renal failure is known to occur even in one sided renal injury; it responds well for temporary few haemodialysis until same side or/and opposite side kidney start functioning. Blood grouping and cross matching is needed for blood transfusion.

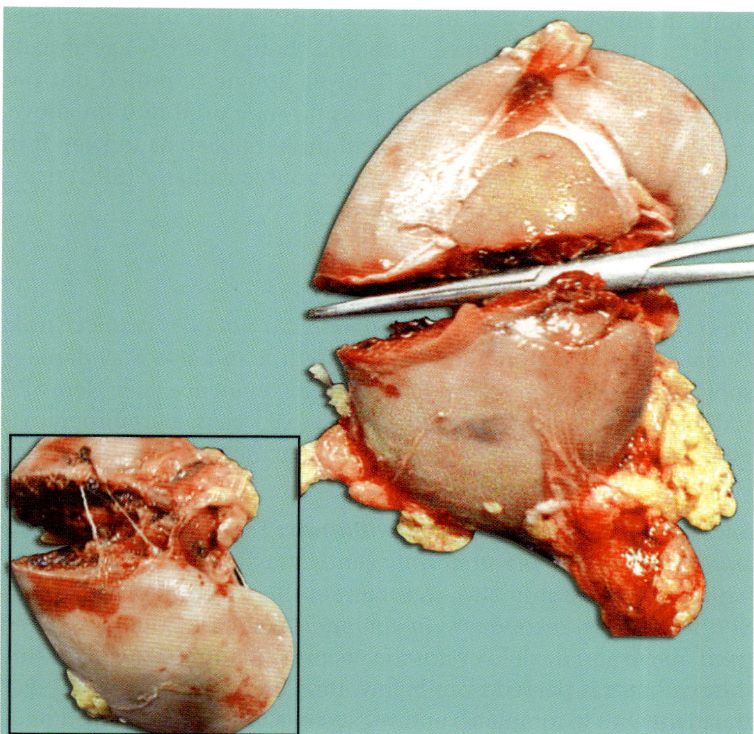

Fig. 8-59: Injury to the kidney causing near transection requiring emergency nephrectomy.

Treatment

I. Initially always conservative—patient is catheterised and urine colour and output is observed; blood transfusion; strict observation with regular monitoring of the pulse, blood pressure, temperature; sedation, analgesic and antibiotics. 75% of patients respond to conservative management. While treating conservatively, regular monitoring of blood urea and serum creatinine is a must. If the patient goes in for renal failure, haemodialysis should be done for 6–8 weeks. Meanwhile, the other kidney will start functioning again and patient will recover without any further problem.

II. *Indications for surgical intervention* **(Fig. 8-59)**:
  1. When there are signs of progressive blood loss with the condition of the patient deteriorating.
  2. Formation of progressive perinephric haematoma.
  3. When there are associated other injuries.
  4. Hilar injury.

Surgery

Options:

a. Gentle suturing of the laceration. Often as kidney is friable, this is not easier technically. Here initially before opening Gerota's fascia and evacuating the haematoma, *renal vessels should be isolated* and either bulldog clamp or umbilical tape should be placed around. Suturing, wrapping, gelfoam, spongiston are other materials tried **(Fig. 8-60)**.
b. Then nephrostomy (Cabot's) is done.
c. When the injury is in the poles—partial nephrectomy.
d. In hilar injury and severe laceration nephrectomy is the only choice **(Fig. 8-61)**.

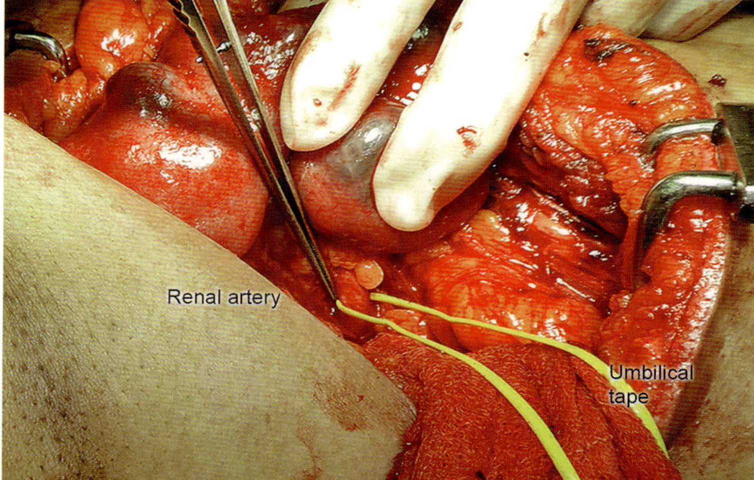

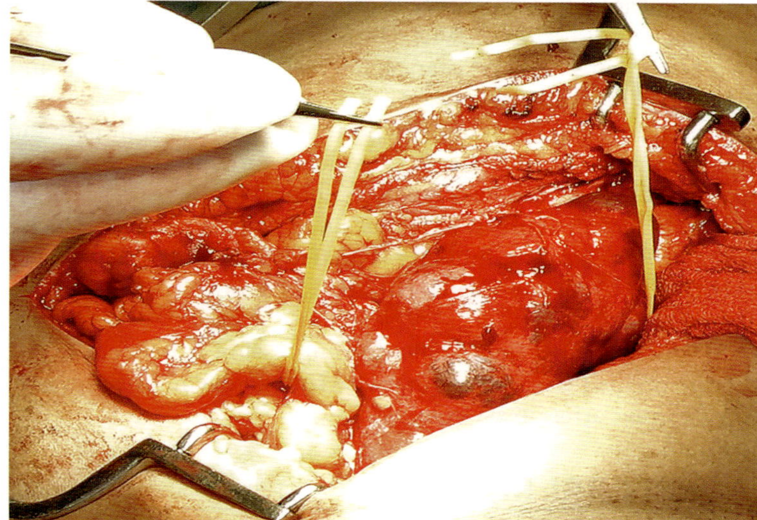

Fig. 8-60: Renal pedicle should be isolated and either using bulldog clamp or vascular clamp or umbilical tape renal artery and vein should be individually clamped. Renal artery clamp is most important.

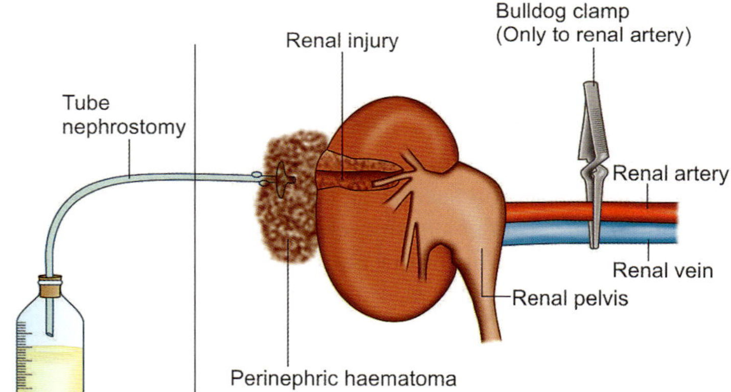

Fig. 8-61: Tube nephrostomy is better when there is significant renal and perinephric haematoma.

Type	*Treatment*
1. Only bruise/contusion	Conservative
2. Breach in calyceal system/rupture of one of the small branches of renal artery.	Conservative/nephrectomy
3. Rupture of pelvicalyceal system/renal substance.	Nephrectomy

Complications of renal injury

1. Clot retention in the bladder and may go for renal failure.
2. Pararenal pseudohydronephrosis.
3. Infection.
4. Perinephric abscess.
5. Aneurysm of the renal artery.
6. Renal failure.
7. Post-injury renal hypertension.

ABDOMINAL COMPARTMENT SYNDROME

It is increased intra-abdominal pressure more than 12 mmHg. It is common in multiple traumas. Ileus and bowel oedema are the factors causing it. It is also seen in retroperitoneal haemorrhage, pancreatitis, long-standing hernia after reduction into the peritoneal cavity. Upward displacement of the diaphragm, hypoxia, hypercapnia, acidosis, compression of IVC, decreased venous return to heart, increase in peripheral resistance, decrease in cardiac output and right atrial pressure, decreased renal blood flow and glomerular filtration, mesenteric venous hypertension, bowel wall oedema and ischaemia—are the effects. Oliguria, respiratory failure, cardiac arrest ensures if abdomen is not decompressed.

Intra-abdominal pressure is measured using a *urinary catheter in the urinary bladder*. Pressure is graded *(Busch)* as (I) 10–15 cm of H_2O; (II) 16-25 cm of H_2O; (III) 26–35 cm H_2O; (IV) more than 36 cm H_2O.

Beyond grade III immediate decompression is needed. Initial volume preload is essential otherwise sudden decompression may cause cardiac arrest in asystole.

URETHRAL INJURY

It can be in membranous or bulbar urethra. It can be complete/incomplete; total/partial.

Rupture of Membranous Urethra (Posterior Urethra)

It is usually associated with pelvic fractures. Instrumentation, catheterisation, stone, obstetric causes are other etiologies. In complete rupture urethra puboprostatic ligament may be disrupted causing *floating prostate—Vermooten's sign. Maccullum-Colapinto classification* is based on ascending urethrogram findings—Type I: Elongation but intact of posterior urethra; Type II: Floating prostate; Type III: Total disruption of the urethra with extravasation urine above and below the sphincter.

Features

Difficulty and failure in passing urine; blood in external meatus; urinary extravasation into perineum/scrotum/abdominal wall are typical features. Digital examination of rectum reveals impalpable prostate—floating. X-ray pelvis shows fracture. Urethrogram is diagnostic.

In Floating Prostate

As rupture is complete, bladder is opened from above. A metal bougie is passed from above through the bladder and one more metal bougie is passed from below through urethra and both are manipulated so as to meet each other. Lower bougie is negotiated along the upper one and so into the bladder. Red rubber catheter is tied to the tip of the lower (urethral) bougie which has already entered into the bladder. When lower bougie is pulled out per urethrally, catheter tied to it will pass through urethra from above, to which Foley's catheter is tied and pulled up, so as to keep it in position. Bladder is closed with a suprapubic catheter (SPC) using Malecot's catheter—***Railroad technique***.

In Incomplete Rupture

Two approaches:

First approach proposed by Mitchell: *Do not pass catheter from below* as it may further damage the urethra and also may damage sphincter mechanism and so may cause incontinence later. Here SPC is done using Malecot's catheter. After 3 to 6 weeks, a urethrogram is done. Using endoscopy or along with open method Foley's catheter is passed, often after dilatation.

Second approach advocated by Blandy: *Single attempt to pass a small soft catheter per urethrally* gently may lead into the bladder, which will be kept in situ, to maintain the continuity. If this fails SPC is done. On second day, in operation theatre, bladder is opened from above and flexible cystoscope is passed from below and using this, catheter is passed from below. Bladder is closed with an SPC. If patient with incomplete rupture presents later, it is managed once a stricture forms, accordingly as for stricture urethra, after 3 months. Until then patient may require SPC. Other measures: Antibiotics, blood, fluid replacement, treat other injuries.

Complications

Urinary incontinence; impotence; stricture urethra; infection.

Rupture of Bulbous Urethra (Anterior Urethra)

Usually due to a fall astride a projecting object, like in sailing ships, cycling, over loose manhole cover, gymnasium.

Clinical Features: Triad

(1) Blood in external meatus (urethral haemorrhage). (2) Perineal haematoma. (3) Retention of urine. X-ray pelvis and US abdomen are investigations. Condition is diagnosed clinically **(Figs. 8-62 and 8-63)**.

Treatment

Patient should be told not to try to pass urine, if passed, then extravasation of urine occurs. In operation theatre, *one attempt of urethral catheterisation is tried gently*. If able to pass a catheter, then it is left in place. Often perineal haematoma which occurs has to be drained. Antibiotics should be given to prevent sepsis. *If catheter fails to pass*, then under general anaesthesia, in lithotomy position, SPC is done. Bulbous urethra is exposed through perineal midline incision and tear is sutured with an indwelling Foley's catheter. Drain is then placed into the perineum. If suturing is not possible (sometimes), then *perineal urethrostomy* is done and at later stages continuity is maintained (usually after 3 months).

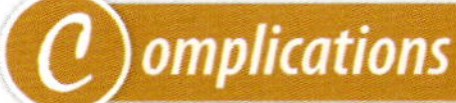

Infection, extravasation of urine, stricture urethra.

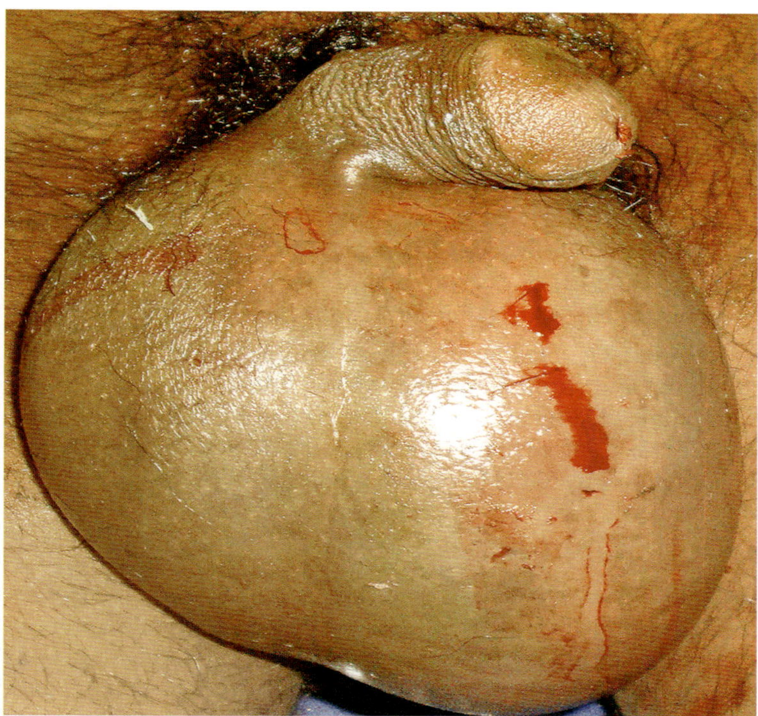

Fig. 8-62: Urethral injury showing blood in the external meatus with extravasation.

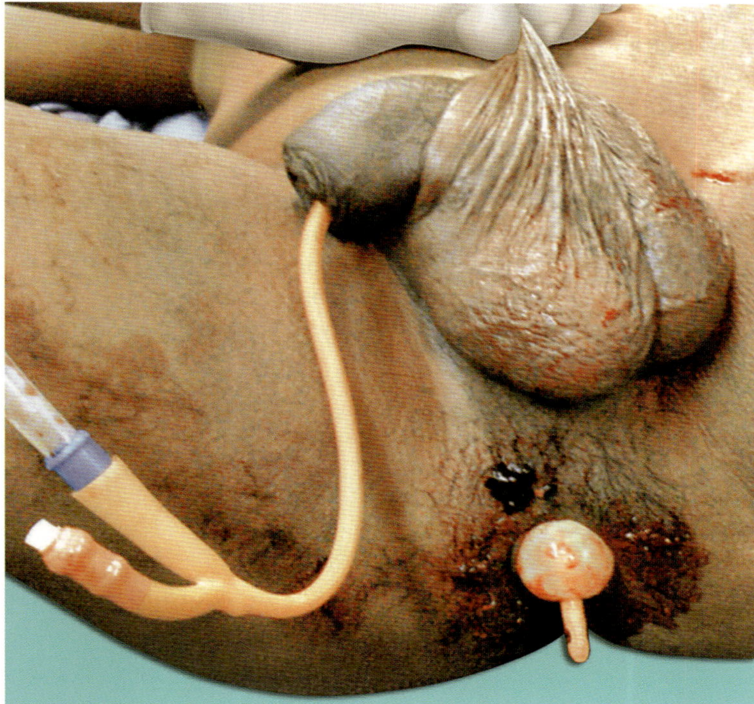

Fig. 8-63: Penetrating injury in the perineum causing rectal and urethral injury which is communicating. Note the catheter passed per urethral has gone into the rectum and come out into the anal canal. It needed colostomy and suprapubic cystostomy diversions.
Courtesy: Dr Ashfaque Mohammad, DNB, KMC, Mangaluru.

RUPTURE BLADDER

Causes

Blow, kick or fall; road traffic accidents; stabs, gunshot injuries; endoscopic trauma; instrumentations. **Bladder injury can also occur** during hysterectomy both abdominal and vaginal, surgery of colon or rectum, repair of direct inguinal or femoral hernias.

Types

I. *Intraperitoneal rupture*—20% common. It occurs in fully distended bladder due to blow, kick, or fall.
II. *Extraperitoneal rupture*—80% common. It is due to road traffic accidents, golf playing, fall over the manhole. Its features and management are same as rupture of posterior (membranous) urethra **(Figs. 8-64 and 8-65)**.

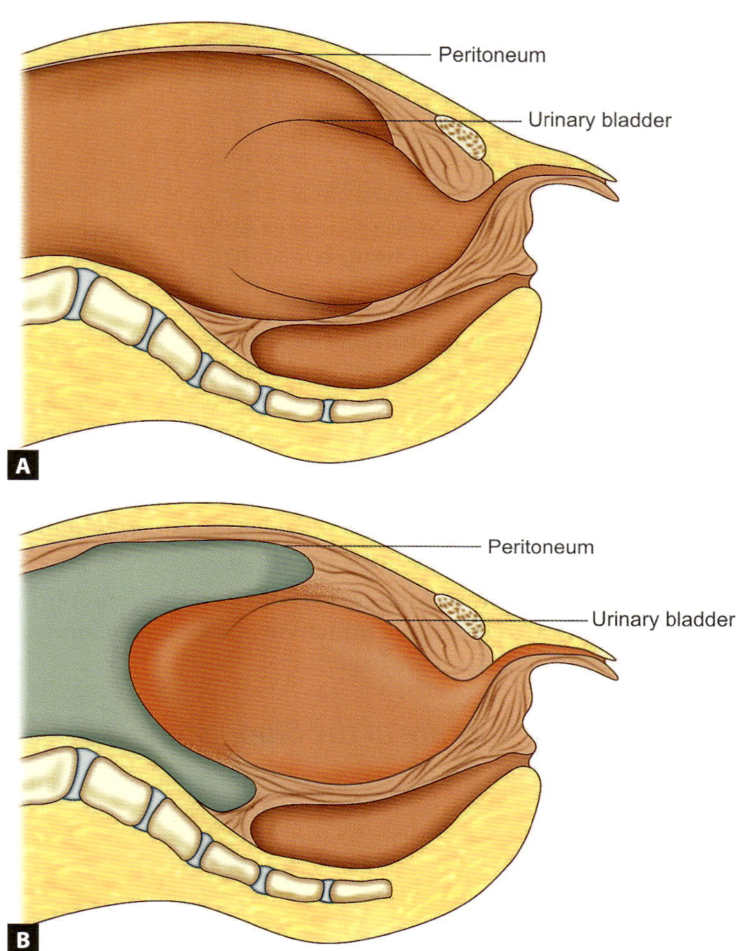

Figs. 8-64A and B: Bladder rupture: (A) Intraperitoneal rupture; (B) Extraperitoneal rupture.

Intraperitoneal Rupture

It is 20% common. *It occurs in full bladder.*

Features: Sudden pain in suprapubic region; shock and syncope; diffuse abdominal pain; urine leaks into the abdominal cavity causing distension of abdomen; later it causes features of peritonitis, with guarding, rigidity, tenderness and rebound tenderness, dull flank. *Patient does not have the desire to micturate.*

Investigations: (1) Plain X-ray shows ground glass appearance. (2) Peritoneal tap to collect urine. (3) After passing a small catheter gently per urethra, water soluble iodine dye is passed to visualise the tear in the bladder and entry of the dye into the free peritoneal cavity. This can be done now through C-arm image intensifier easily. (4) US abdomen to look for other injuries in the abdomen.

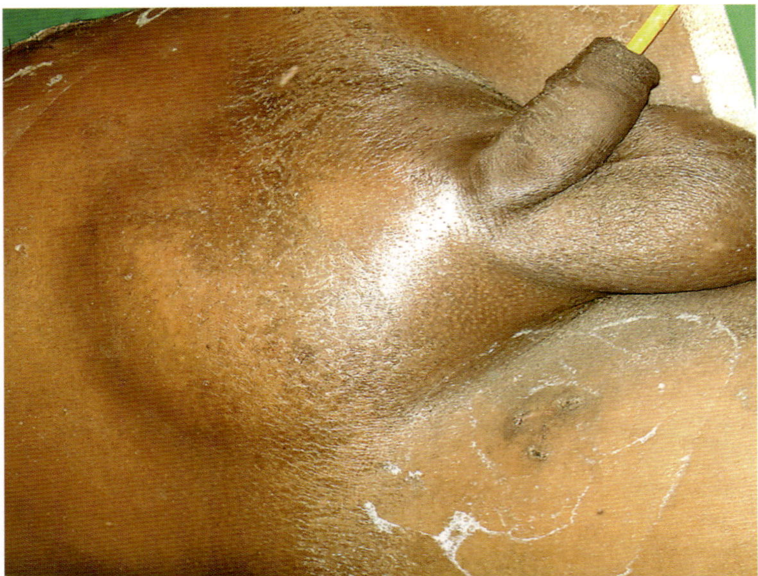

Fig. 8-65: Extraperitoneal bladder rupture with extravasation of the urine.

Treatment: Emergency laparotomy is required. Bladder tear is sutured using polyglactic acid (vicryl) in two layers. Peritoneal wash is given. Malecot's catheter is placed from above as SPC. Prevesical space and peritoneal cavity are drained separately. Foley's catheter from below is also passed. Adequate specific antibiotics are given to prevent sepsis.

Surgery is the only treatment for intraperitoneal rupture of the bladder. Without surgery mortality is 100%.

Complications of rupture bladder: Cystitis/and pyelonephritis; peritonitis; pelvic abscess; fistula formation (vesicovaginal or recto-vesical); paralytic ileus; haemorrhage.

Extraperitoneal Rupture of the Bladder

It is 80% common. It occurs in road traffic accidents, in a non-distended bladder.

Features: There is collection of urine and blood in the extraperitoneal space in front, with fullness, diffuse pain and tenderness in lower abdomen; swelling in the scrotum or labia and abdominal wall; strangury and inability to pass urine; often blood in the external meatus is noted. Features of shock and of other associated injuries may be noted.

Investigations: Plain X-ray pelvis shows fracture pelvis. Cystogram shows leak from the bladder. **During cystoscopy:** (1) Bladder cannot be distended; (2) Endoscopy light may be shining through the abdominal wall; (3) Irrigating fluid cannot be retrieved back.

Treatment: The bladder is exposed extraperitoneally, the tear is identified and sutured and the extraperitoneal space is irrigated with saline. Bladder is closed with an SPC using Malecot's catheter and a drain is placed in prevesical space (cave of Retzius). If there is urethral injury it should be treated accordingly.

Seat Belt Injuries

In an individual with tied seat belt, during impact *violent deceleration* of human body occurs. Seat belt impinges heavily on its point of contact with trunk and viscera continue to move forward. It leads into severe contusion of abdominal contents; *detachment of bowel from its mesentery* due to free forward rapid mobility of the bowel over a relatively fixed mesentery. Solid organ injury occurs only occasionally.

Two point anchorages causes solid organ injuries like of liver/spleen. *Lap belt* causes contusion and bowel injury commonly.

It is often difficult to identify the injuries due to presence of more obvious other injuries. CT chest and abdomen diagnostic peritoneal lavage (DPL) are very useful.

Petechiae around iliac crest or costal margin are signs wherein one can suspect seat belt injuries.

Distraction fracture of lumbar spine (*chance fracture*) with hyperesthesia of T12 and L1 level is often associated. 10% of such fractures are associated with intra-abdominal injuries.

Treatment is immediate laparotomy and proceed—bowel suturing/resection/suturing of the organ injuries/splenorrhaphy/splenectomy.

9

CHAPTER

Principles of Surgical Treatment in Infections

Infections in different parts of the body are dealt in different ways. Infections may be in limbs, in body cavities or extending from outside to inside or multiple site infections.

It can be surface infections in skin and subcutaneous tissue. It can be deeper infection in the muscle, bone, joint and fascial planes. It can be infection in cavities like in peritoneum, pleura and cranial cavities.

PRINCIPLES

Once there is abscess, it should be drained. Abscess should be formed before drainage in most of the places except in breast, parotid, ischiorectal fossa, hand, and thigh. Pointing pus, excruciating pain, fluctuation, induration are the features of formed abscess. Pus is drained under general or regional anaesthesia. Digital block, brachial plexus block, Bier's block, wrist block, ankle block, sciatic block can be used for anaesthesia. Local infiltration at the site even though is commonly practiced is unsatisfactory as it may not act due to acidic pus media and also due to oedema at the site. Hilton's method of drainage is used to drain an abscess **(Figs. 9-1 and 9-2)**.

Digital block is given using xylocaine 1–2% *without adrenaline* (plain) 1–2 mL on each prick site. By diluting with equal quantity of normal saline 0.5% strength can be made. 3 mg/kg is the dose.

Tourniquet should be used in limbs while draining or doing fasciotomy. Pneumatic tourniquet is used. Limb is elevated for 2 minutes for venous emptying prior to applying the tourniquet. Tourniquet is inflated to a pressure 30 mm Hg more than systolic pressure of the patient. Tourniquet time for upper limb is 60 minutes; for lower limb it is 90–120 minutes.

Principles

- Always pus should be aspirated for confirmation.
- Adequate incision is the priority. One should not compromise the incision.
- Expose all layers in deeper abscess like psoas abscess, groin abscess, loin abscess.
- Drain should be placed—wick/tube/corrugated depending on need.
- All loculi should be broken. All communications should be drained.
- Proper saline (warm) irrigation to the cavity is essential.
- Pus should be sent for culture.
- In superficial/surface abscess wound is left open. In deep abscess like psoas abscess wound is closed in layers or single layer with a drain.
- Antibiotics should be started prior to drainage.
- General/regional anaesthesia is used.
- Deeper abscess can be confirmed by CT scan or ultrasound. Repeat ultrasound/CT scan for completion of drainage may be needed.

Hand Infection

Hand should be properly examined clinically for tendon functions; neurological problems—sensations (sweat test, two point discrimination test); for circulation (Allen's test); joint movements; examination of entire upper limb; opposite hand; axillary lymph nodes and relevant systemic examinations.

The principles of treatment are elevation of hand to reduce oedema; splintage to prevent contracture; rest during initial stage of diffuse infection; early movements once inflammation subsides; early exploration of wound or surgical drainage of infective area; regional anaesthesia; usage of tourniquet; incisions when cross the flexor creases, it should be at 45° angle.

Rest is achieved by *plaster of Paris* applied on the ventral aspect of the hand. Elevation is achieved by suspending the arm from an overhead support. Flucloxacillin 500 mg 6th hourly, metronidazole 400 mg 8th hourly orally is given initially until pus culture sensitivity report is available.

During surgical drainage *site of incision should be marked* properly prior to anaesthesia. Length of the incision should be adequate. Superficial part of the deep abscess should be drained initially (collar stud part); and then deeper part is reached and drained properly. Pus should be collected for culture and sensitivity. Skin edge is trimmed using a fine scissor to create a *diamond-shaped opening*. Thorough saline irrigation is done. Dressing is placed. Tourniquet is released. Arm is elevated. Dressing is opened and wound is inspected after 24 hours. Further dressings are done once in 1–2 days, depending on need. Continuation of antibiotics for longer period is done only if abscess is large; signs of bone infection or spreading infection **(Figs. 9-3 to 9-6)**.

Apical Subungual Infection

It is infection of the space between subungual epithelium and the periosteum. It occurs after minor trauma or rarely after formation of subungual haematoma. Beneath the free edge of the nail, pus comes to the surface. Excruciating tenderness with small visible pus under the tip (summit) of the nail is the feature. Drainage with transverse incision at the tip of finger with removal of V shaped of wedge of nail over the summit is the treatment along with antibiotics. Osteomyelitis is *not common* here **(Fig. 9-7)**.

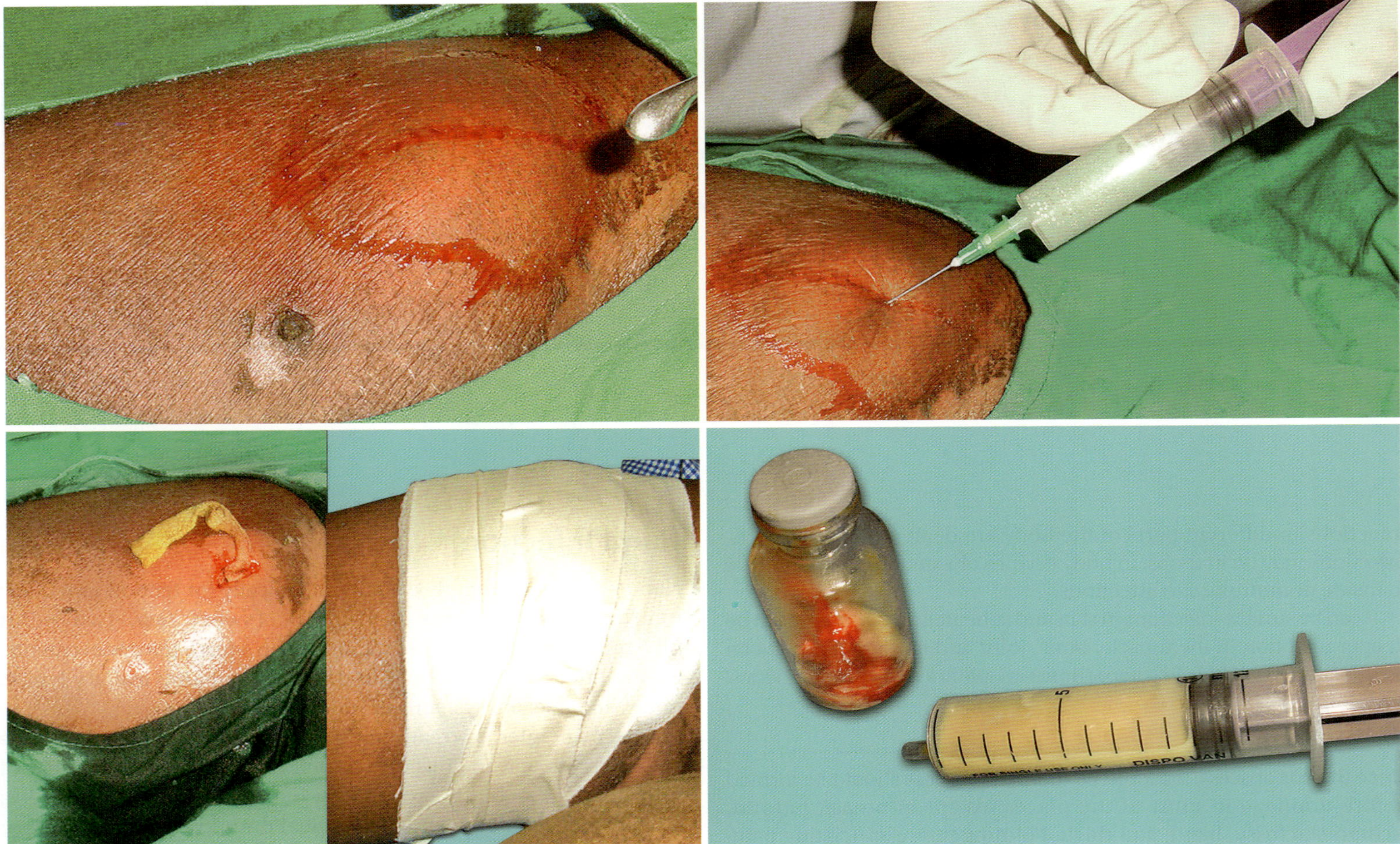

Fig. 9-1: Abscess is drained by Hilton's method of drainage. Abscess should be aspirated prior to making incision. Longitudinal adequate length incision is made over the skin. Pyogenic membrane is opened using sinus forceps. All loculi are broken using little finger or sinus forceps. Warm saline wash is given. Cavity is packed with gauze or drain. Pus should be sent for culture and sensitivity.

Paronychia

It is infection of nail fold. It can be acute or chronic. Acute is usually bacterial. Chronic is commonly fungal. Acute is usually due to *Staphylococcus* or *Streptococcus*. It occurs under the eponychium. Pus spreads under the nail causing hang nail or floating nail. Condition is precipitated by minor trauma. Excruciating throbbing pain and tenderness under nail root are the features. Digital block anaesthesia is used. Using fine scissors lateral nail fold is elevated; loose skin portion is removed; pus extrudes out; portion of this base of nail should be removed in floating nail as it is usually dead. Keeping drain or gauze wick is not needed. Pus is sent for culture. Dressing is done. In chronic paronychia entire nail may required to be removed **(Figs. 9-8A to E)**.

Pulp Space Infection (Felon)

Terminal pulp space infection is common. Throbbing pain is common; but pointing pus may not be clear initially. It is initially treated by rest, elevation and antibiotics. Once pus points or maximum tender point is determined, drainage is done. But undue delay in draining should be avoided as osteomyelitis of terminal phalanx can occur due to blockage of the end artery of the terminal phalanx by infective thrombosis. Oblique deep incision directly over the pulp is needed. Superficial collar stud part is opened; then deeper part is opened adequately **(Fig. 9-9)**.

Web Space Infection

It is initially treated with splinting, elevation and antibiotics. It is drained under general or regional anaesthesia. A transverse incision is placed on the palmar aspect opposite the interdigital space and 1 cm proximal to the free edge of the web. Only skin is incised using no. 11 blade. Deepening of the wound is done using sinus forceps by blunt dissection. It is important to go deeper to palmar aponeurosis otherwise drainage is incomplete. Dorsal counter incision is not needed. Vertical incision in the web should not be placed as it will cause bad contracture **(Figs. 9-10 and 9-11)**.

Deep Palmar Space Infection

Midpalmar Space Infection

Midpalmar space (triangular shape) is bound by palmar aponeurosis in front; medial three metacarpals behind; a vertical line from lateral margin of middle finger (intermediate palmar septum) laterally; medial palmar septum medially **(Figs. 9-12 to 9-14)**.

Proximally it begins from flexor retinaculum; distally it extends into distal palmar crease along 3rd and 4th lumbrical canals. It is on the inner half of the hollow of palm. It contains flexor tendons, lumbricals and neurovascular bundles. Posteriorly it is bounded by 3rd, 4th, 5th metacarpals and fascia covering interossei muscles of 3rd and 4th intermetacarpal spaces. Pain and tenderness in the palm;

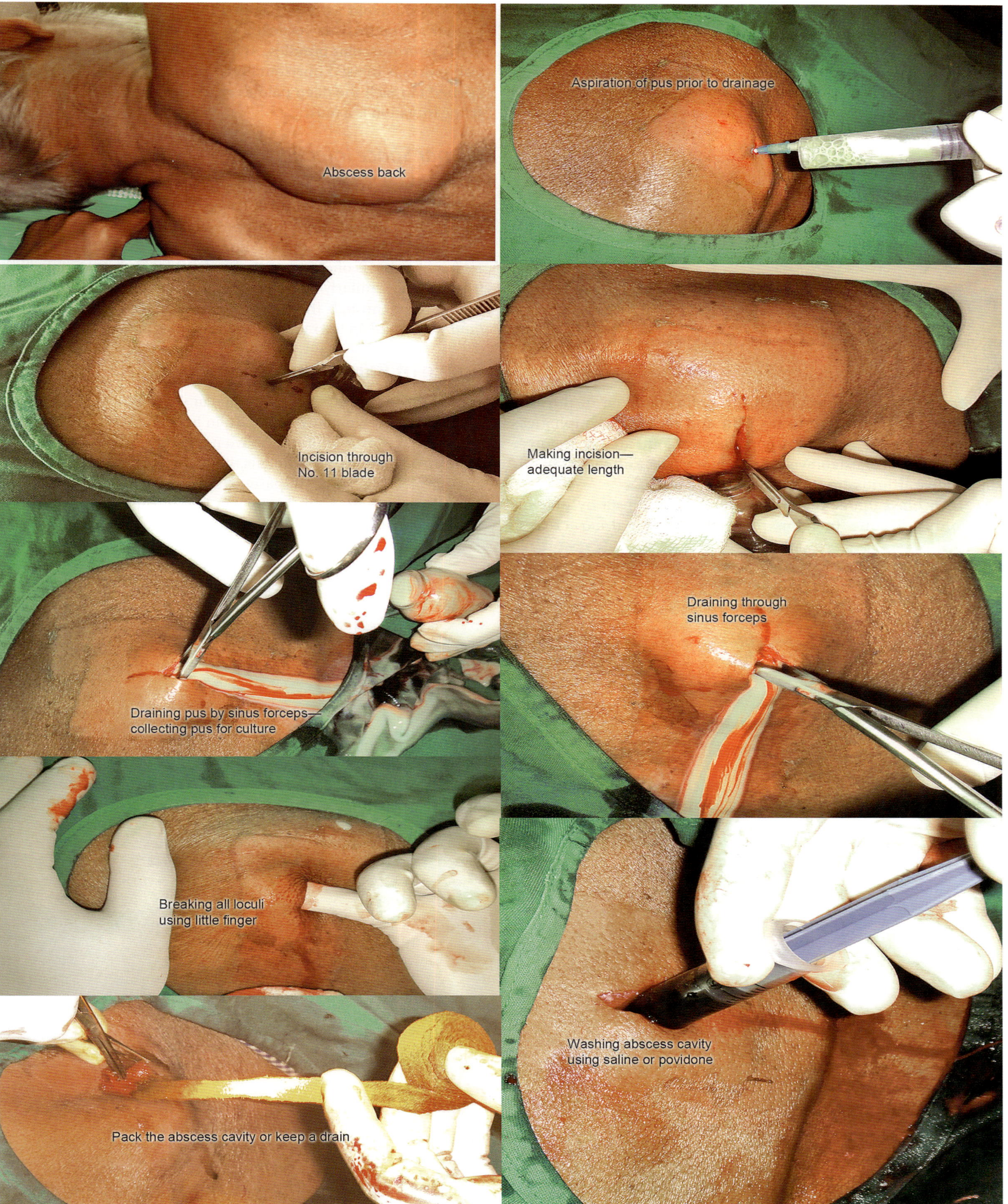

Fig. 9-2: Drainage of an abscess in the back.

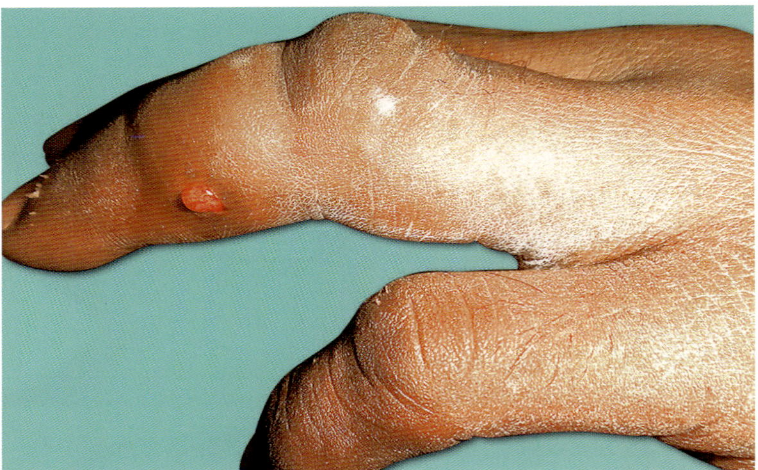

Fig. 9-3: Finger infection causing oedema, discharge. It can lead into stiffness, osteomyelitis, and gangrene of the digit due to infective thrombosis of the digital artery.

obliteration of the concavity of the palm; oedema of dorsum of hand (frog hand) due to lax skin and plenty of lymphatics; painful movements of metacarpophalangeal joint are the features. *Complications* like osteomyelitis of metacarpals, stiffness of hand, suppurative arthritis are common.

It is *drained* under regional/general anaesthesia by placing horizontal/oblique incision parallel to the palmar crease. One should avoid as much as possible to cross the crease line. Palmar aponeurosis is vertically incised carefully to avoid injury of the neurovascular bundles. Alternatively, one of the *interdigital web spaces* is incised horizontally; *lumbrical canal* (3rd or 4th) is opened to reach the deep palmar space. Pus is drained. Thorough saline irrigation is a must.

Thenar Space Infection

Thenar space (triangular shape) is located anterior to the lateral two metacarpals. It is on the outer half of the hollow of the palm. Proximally it extends from flexor retinaculum; distally it extends to transverse palmar crease. It communicates to fascial sheath of 1st lumbrical. It is often associated with midpalmar space infection. It is drained similarly by placing incision on the lateral aspect of the palm or through the first web space incision along the *first lumbrical canal* on the radial side of the index finger **(Fig. 9-15)**.

Space of Parona Infection

Forearm space of Parona is a rectangular space situated in the lower part of the forearm above the wrist, in front of pronator quadratus, deep to long flexor tendons. Above it extends up to oblique origin of flexor digitorum superficialis, below up to flexor retinaculum communicating with midpalmar space. Flexor tendon sheath extends proximally into this space. Pus in this space is drained through lateral incisions in the lower part of the forearm.

A

B

C

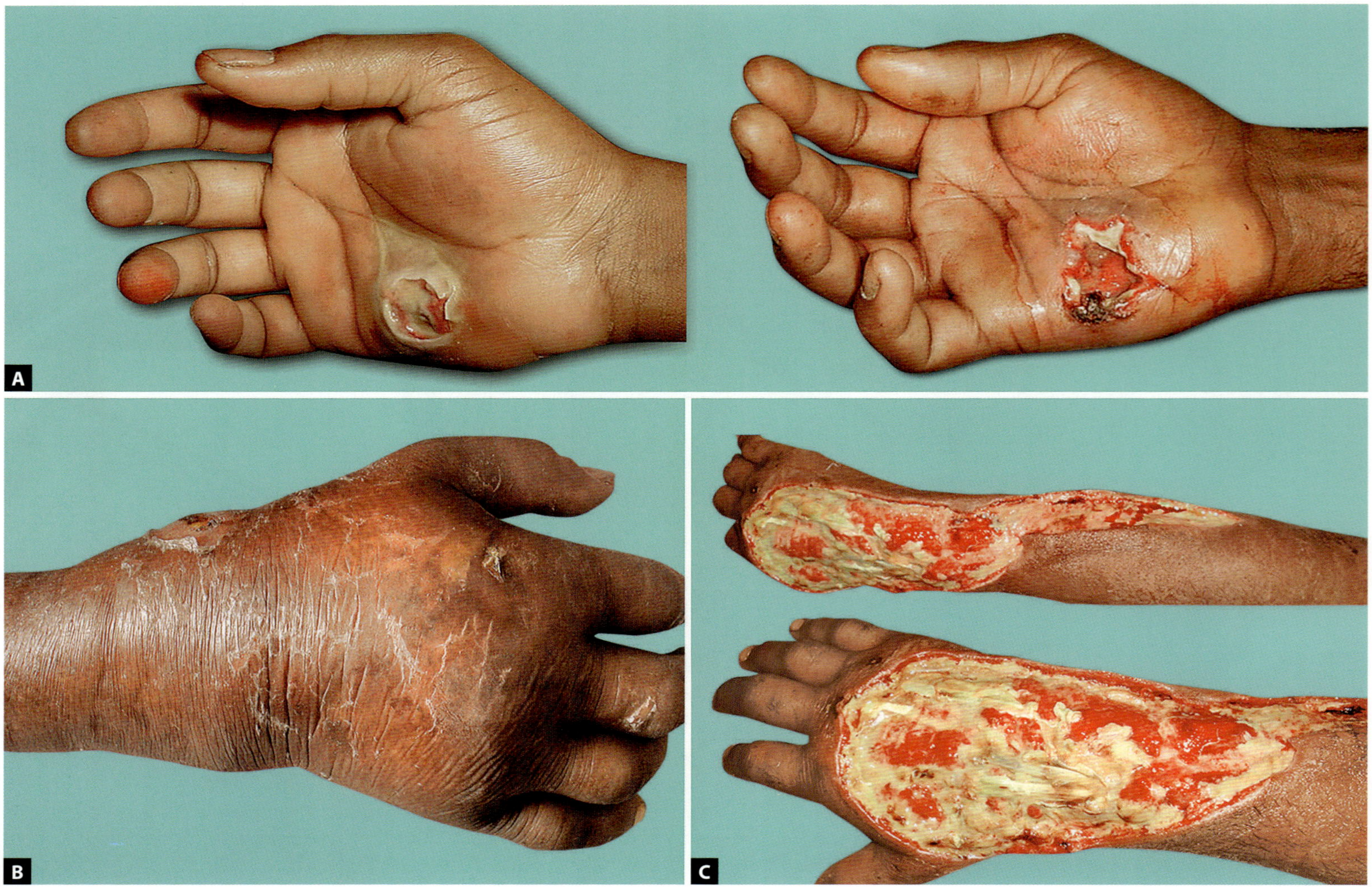

Figs. 9-4A to C: Different types of hand infections—ulcer, abscess, ulcers.

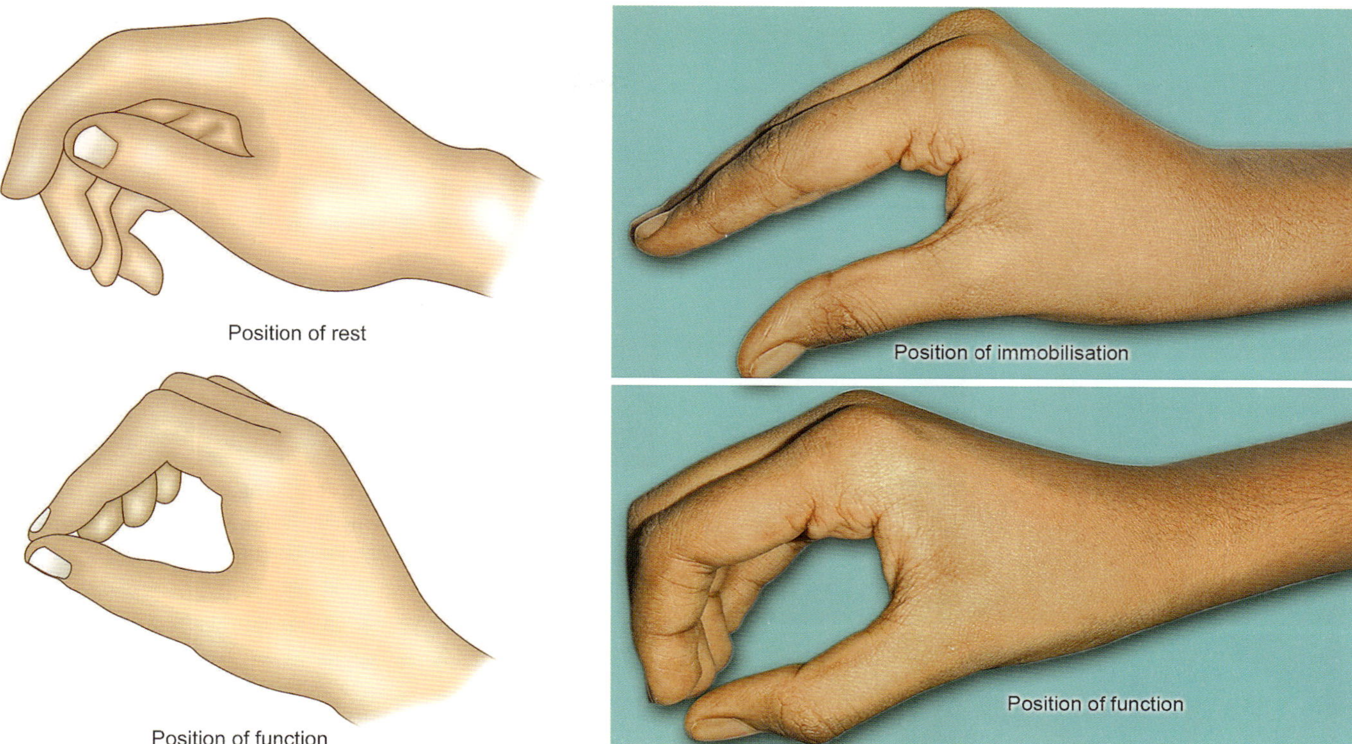

Fig. 9-5: Position of rest, function and immobilisation. Position of rest and immobilisation are same.

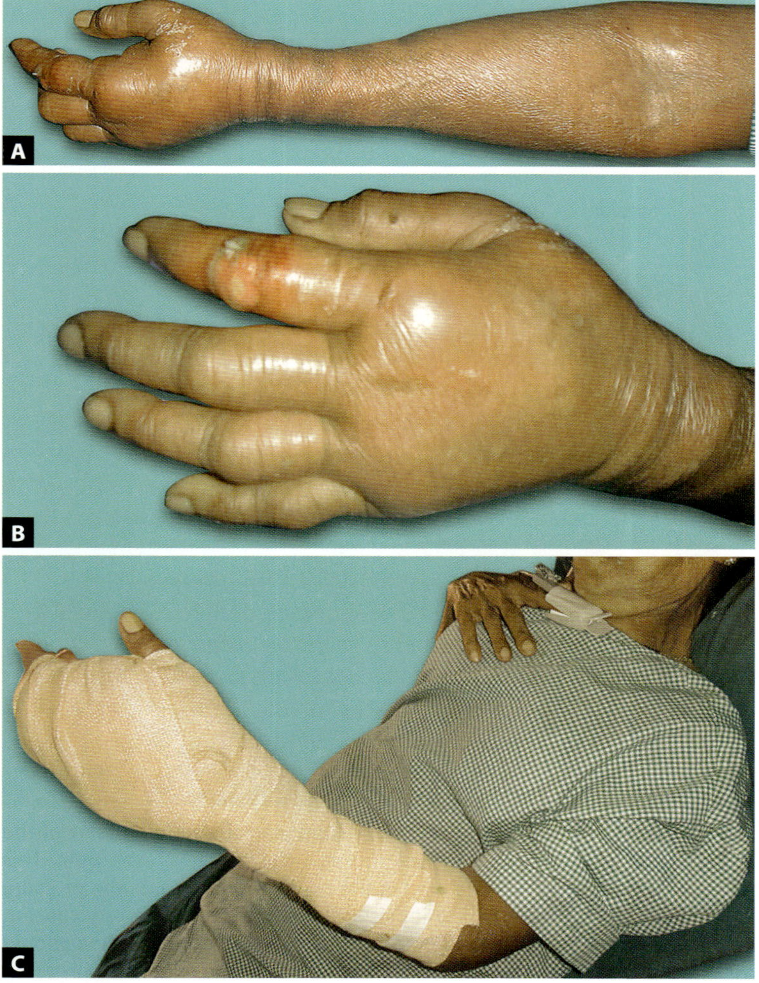

Figs. 9-6A to C: Hand infection showing oedema, swelling and elevation after drainage.

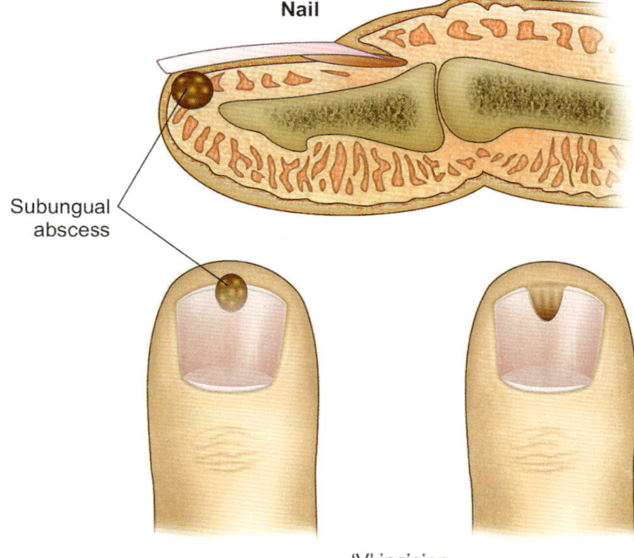

Fig. 9-7: Apical subungual infection and pus formation. Note the 'V' shaped incision to drain the same.

Acute Suppurative Tenosynovitis (Tendon Sheath Infections)

Radial bursa is synovial sheath of flexor tendon of thumb which extends into the *digit*. Ulnar bursa is synovial sheaths of the medial four flexor tendons of hand which extends into the digit of the *little finger*. Radial and ulnar bursae communicate with each other in 80% of cases. Extensor tendons are *devoid* of sheaths. It presents with symmetrical swelling of entire finger. *Hook sign* with flexion of finger is typical. Oedema of the dorsum of the hand,

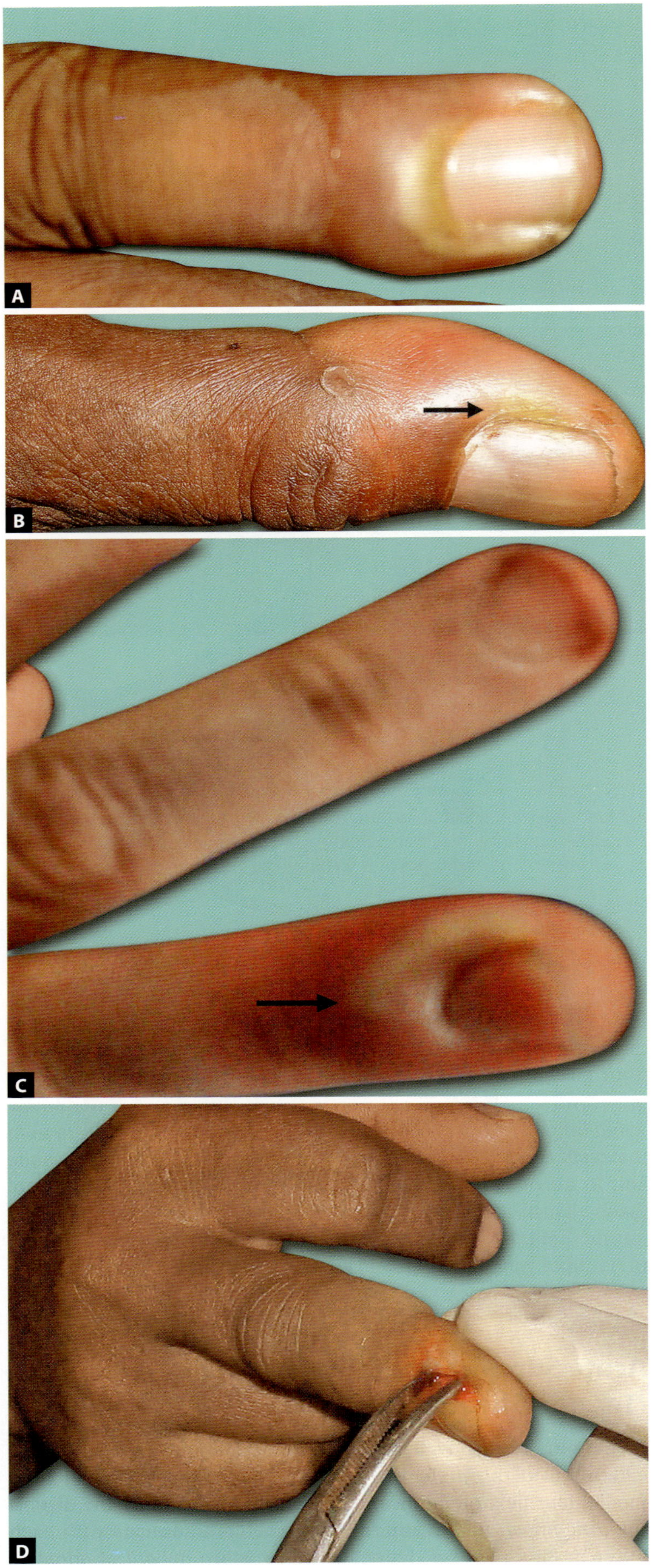

A

B

C

D

Figs. 9-8A to D

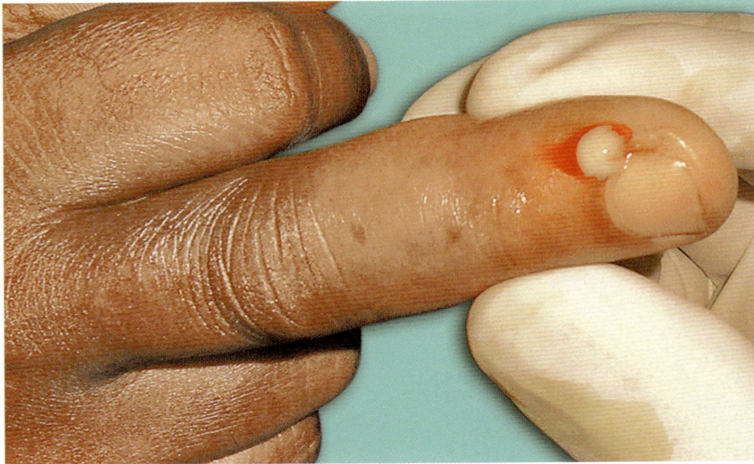

Fig. 9-8E

Figs. 9-8A to E: Acute paronychia. Pus even though is in small quantity, it should be drained.

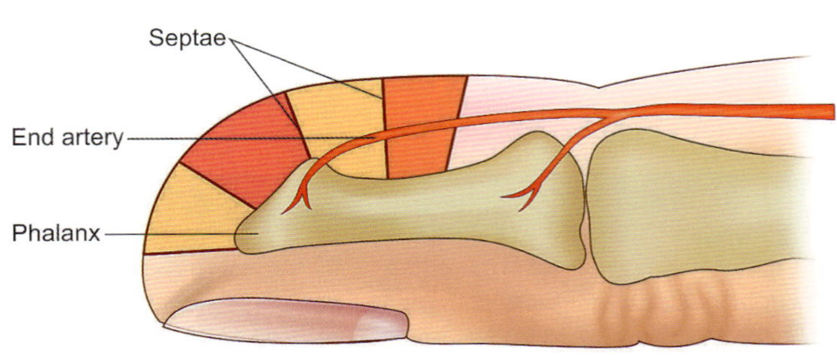

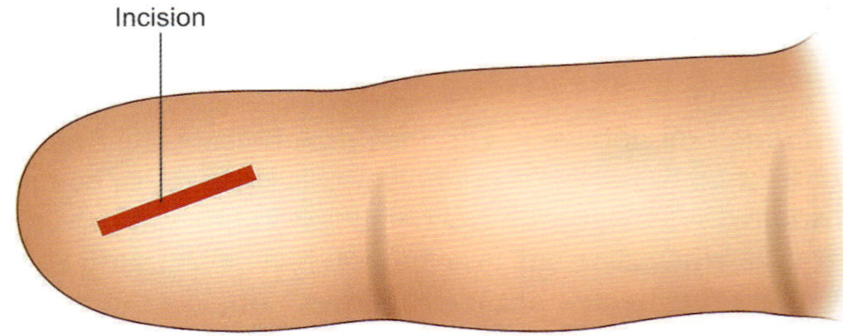

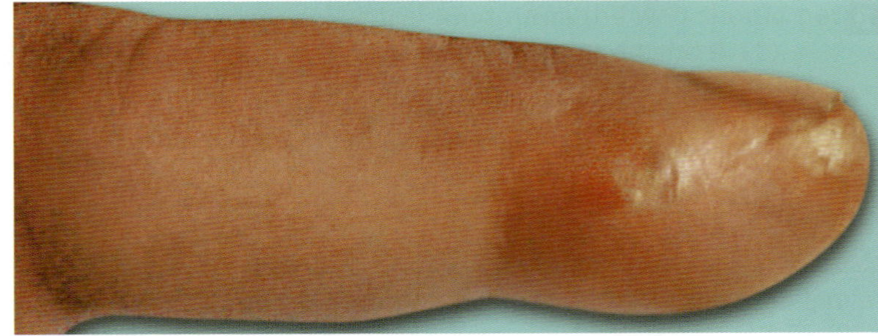

Fig. 9-9: Anatomy of pulp space. Artery supplying the terminal part of the distal phalanx of the finger passes through the septae on the pulp. This artery is an end artery. So, infection in the pulp space increases the pressure inside leading to infective thrombosis and blockage of end artery causing osteomyelitis of the terminal phalanx. Terminal pulp space infection should be drained through an oblique pulp incision. Decompression with breaking of septae is important.

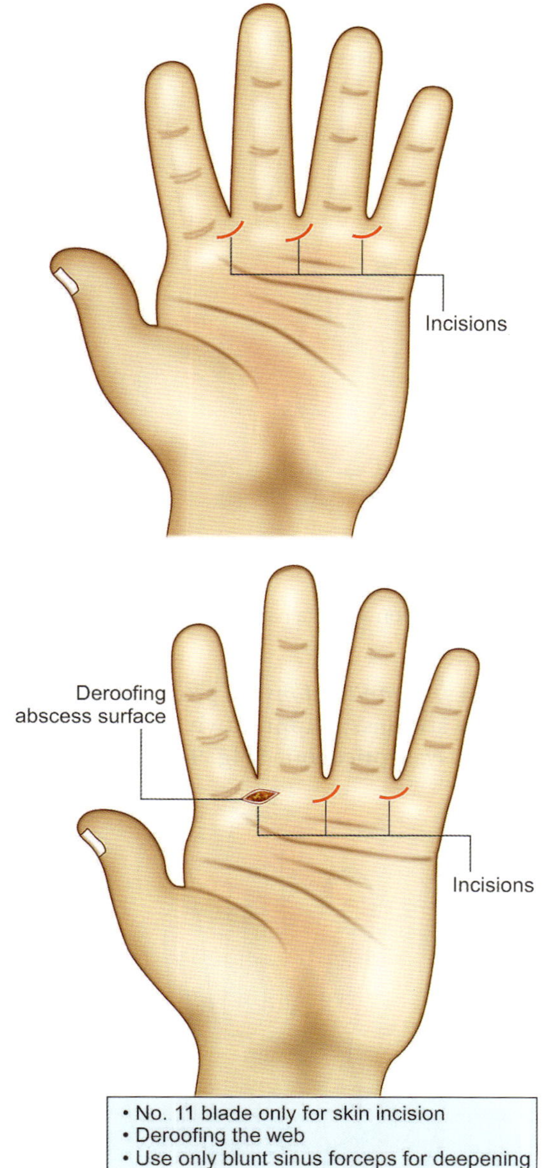

Fig. 9-10: Transverse incision is used to drain web space infection. Deroofing of the incision and web space is done.

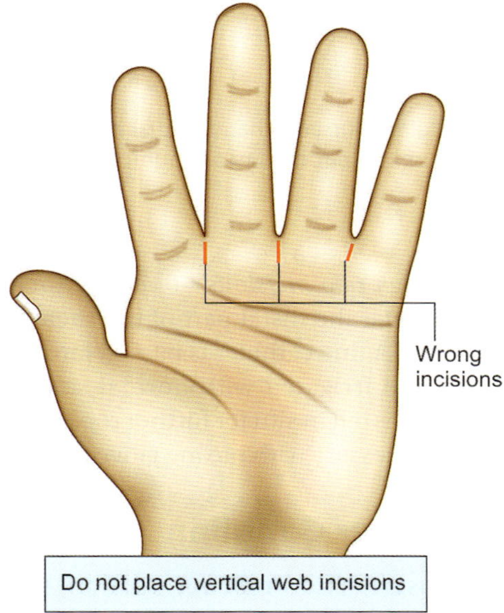

Fig. 9-11: Vertical incision to drain web space infection is avoided.

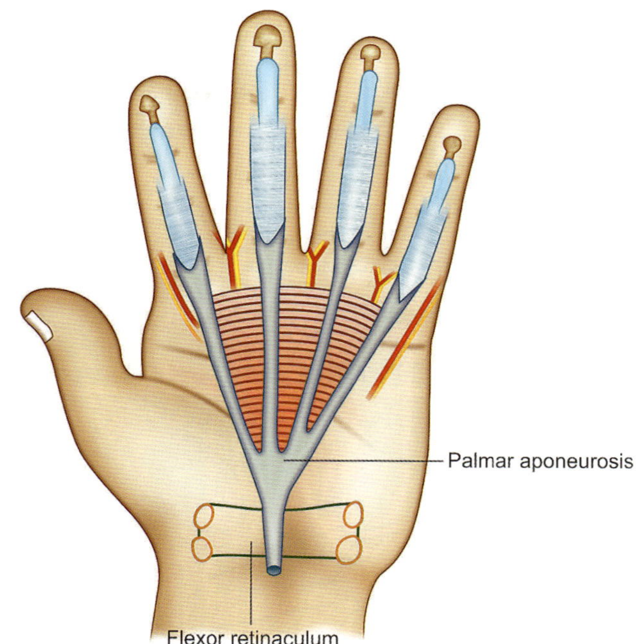

Fig. 9-12: Flexor retinaculum—anatomy.

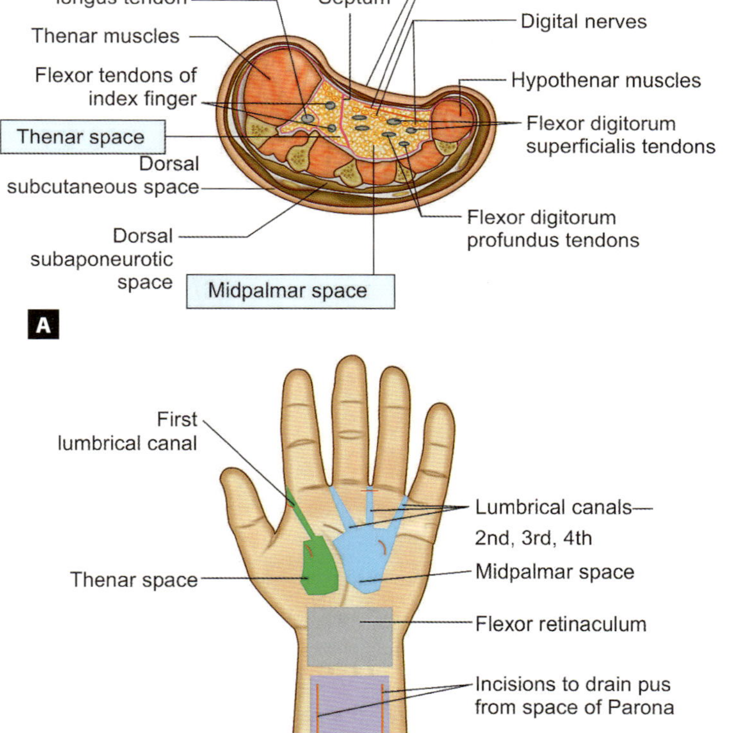

Figs. 9-13A and B

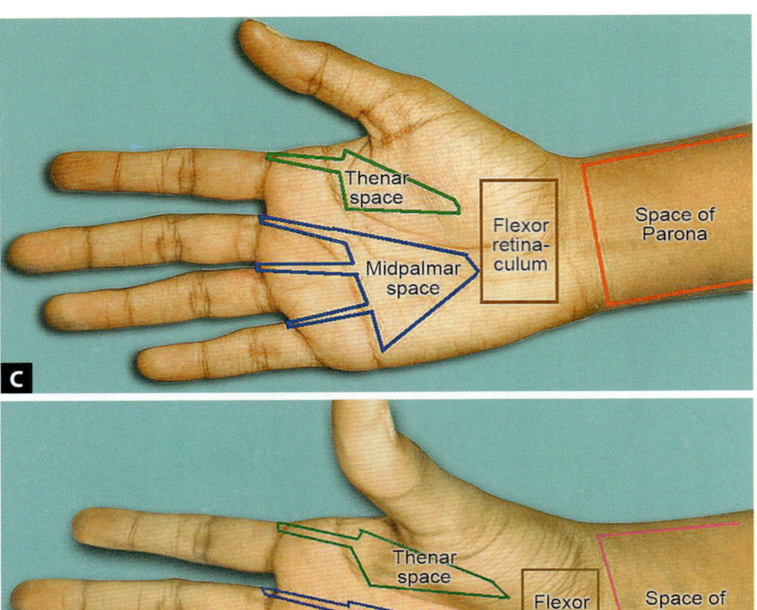

Figs. 9-13C and D

Figs. 9-13A to D: Anatomy of palmar spaces of the hand and forearm. Midpalmar space is on the medial aspect; thenar space is on the lateral aspect. Space of Parona is on the lower forearm.

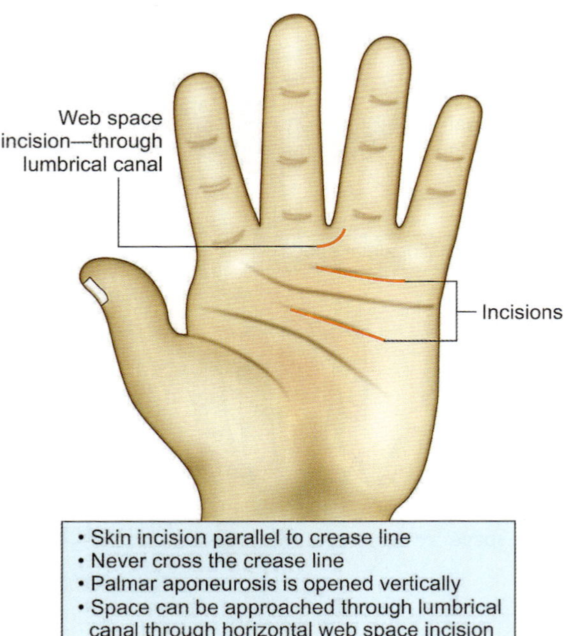

Fig. 9-14: Incisions to drain midpalmar space infection.

tenderness extending into the little finger in infection of ulnar bursa; extending into the thumb in infection of radial bursa; swelling extending proximal to flexor retinaculum; positive Kanavel signs are obvious. *Kanavel signs*—swollen finger held in flexion; exquisite pain on passive extension; tenderness over tendon sheath; greatest point of tenderness is between two

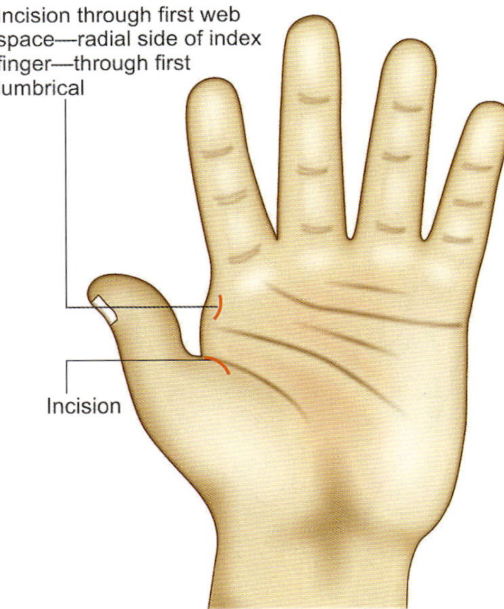

Fig. 9-15: Incision and drainage of thenar space abscess.

transverse creases. *Complications* are proximal spread to forearm; hand and finger stiffness; suppurative arthritis; osteomyelitis; median nerve palsy; septicaemia **(Fig. 9-16)**.

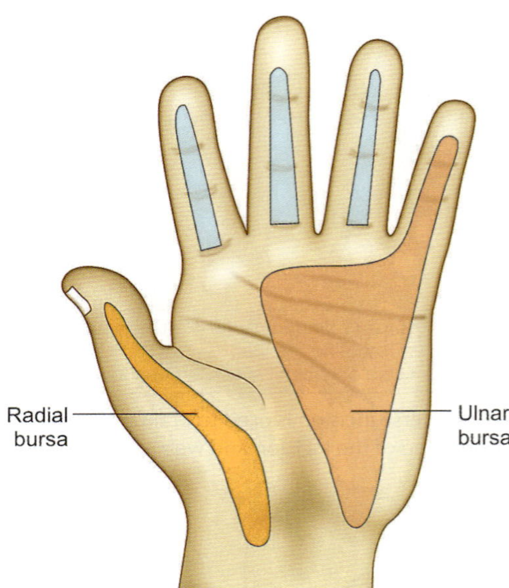

Fig. 9-16: Radial and ulnar bursae in hand. Radial bursa communicates with the sheath of the thumb; ulnar bursa communicates with sheath of little finger.

It is *drained through two incisions*—one over the proximal part of the sheath; other over the distal part of the sheath in the digit—along the crease lines. A fine catheter is passed into the sheath from proximal incision and irrigated with normal saline through this catheter. This catheter is left in situ for further regular irrigations, and splinting of hand is necessary with boxing glove dressing **(Fig. 9-17)**.

Compound Palmar Ganglion

It is chronic tenosynovitis of flexor tendon sheaths due to tuberculosis or rheumatoid arthritis. Smooth, soft, non-tender cross fluctuant swelling in the hollow of palm is typical. *Melon seed bodies*

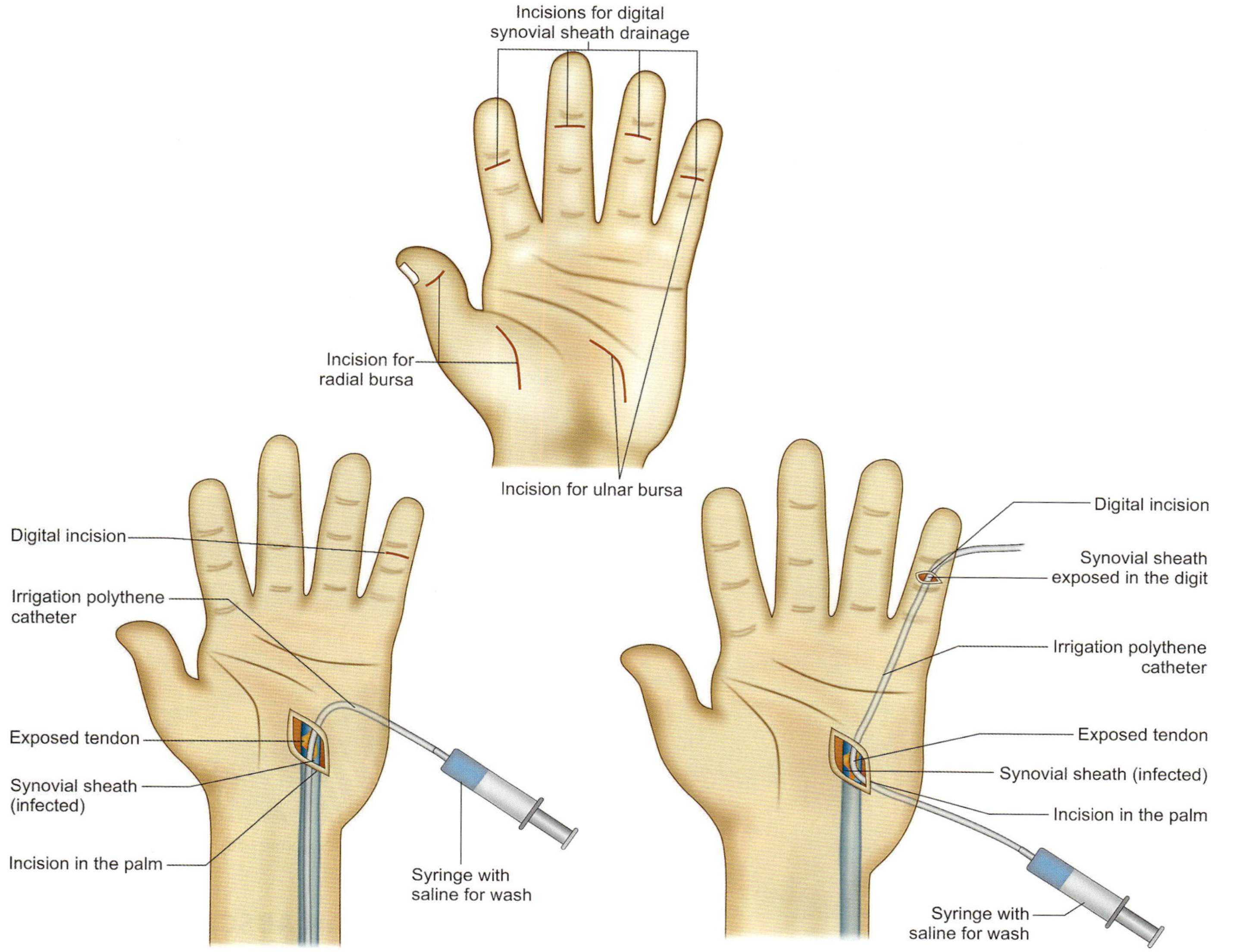

Incisions for digital synovial sheath drainage

Incision for radial bursa

Incision for ulnar bursa

Digital incision

Irrigation polythene catheter

Exposed tendon

Synovial sheath (infected)

Incision in the palm

Syringe with saline for wash

Digital incision

Synovial sheath exposed in the digit

Irrigation polythene catheter

Exposed tendon

Synovial sheath (infected)

Incision in the palm

Syringe with saline for wash

Fig. 9-17: Suppurative tenosynovitis is drained through incision at proximal part and another at digital sheath. Often by placing fine polythene catheter into the sheath saline wash is given into the area.

are characteristic. It is treated surgically after starting the antituberculous drugs. But surgical treatment is not easy. With tourniquet in place, under general anaesthesia, tendon sheath is exposed widely by a vertical incision. Diseased tendon sheath shows adhesions and ramifications on the median and ulnar nerves. With meticulous careful dissections, tendon sheath is excised. All diseased tissues and melon seed bodies are removed. Thorough irrigation is given. Often fine polythene catheter is placed over the sheath for further irrigations post-operatively. Streptomycin irrigation is often used in case of tuberculosis.

Fasciotomy for Compartment Syndrome

Compartment syndrome is a special entity; common in leg, forearm, thigh and arm; is due to increased intracompartmental pressure within a limited space area. *Causes* are—narrowed space due to tight dressings/plaster cast, lying on one limb in comatous patient; increased content of the compartment due to trauma/fractures, oedema, ischaemic injury, haematoma, positioning after trauma, burn injury, etc; high pressure injection injuries like gun injury, oil-based material injury as in extravasation of chemotherapeutic drugs; snake bite. It compromises circulation mainly of muscle and nerves. It often maintains the normal colour and temperature of the fingers and distal pulses may not be obliterated in spite of severe muscle ischaemia. Muscle ischaemia for more than 4 hours causes muscle death and myoglobinuria. Irreversible nerve damage develops if ischaemia persists for 8 hours. Progressive, persistent severe pain which is aggravated by passive muscle stretching is the diagnostic sign. Tense tender regional lymph node is typical. Pulse is usually normally felt in compartment syndrome; but may become absent if there is associated arterial injury. Compartment pressure more than 30 mmHg is an indication for fasciotomy **(Fig. 9-18)**.

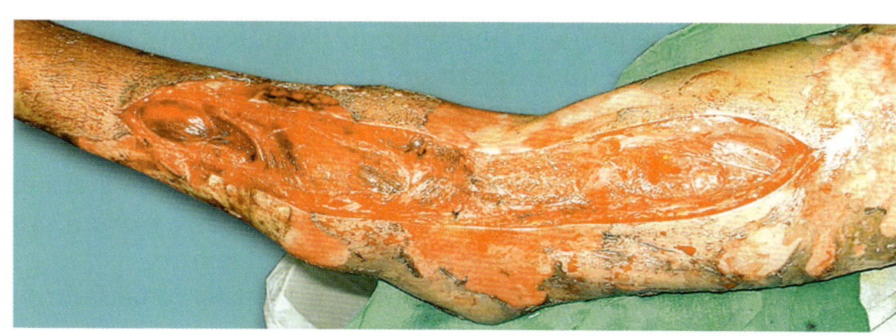

Fig. 9-18: Fasciotomy is done in compartment syndrome. Often incision has to be extended into the arm also.

Fasciotomy of anterior compartment of forearm is specific method. Carpal tunnel *should be released* by *cutting flexor retinaculum*. Incision begins at the junction of the thenar and hypothenar area; extends proximally initially transverse across flexion crease of the wrist at the ulnar border; then across forearm towards radial side of forearm; then in proximal forearm towards medial side creating convex flap towards lateral side. In the elbow it crosses along the medial border to reach the arm where it runs along the medial side of the anterior arm. Injury to major nerves, palmar cutaneous branch of median nerve should be avoided while placing the incision. Incision should be deepened by cutting the deep fascia along the entire length of the incision **(Fig. 9-19)**.

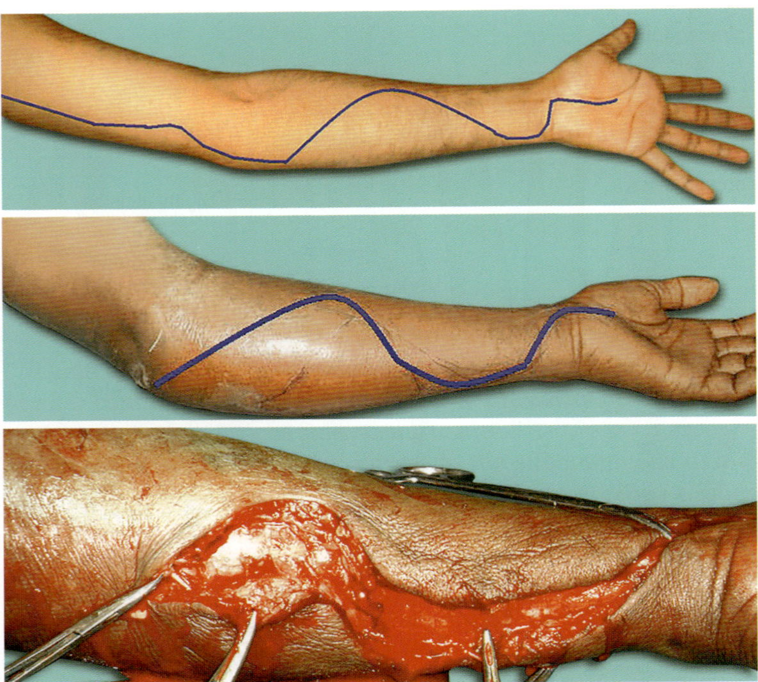

Fig. 9-19: Incision for fasciotomy in upper limb begins at flexor retinaculum extending into the forearm with a convex flap towards radial side eventually leading towards medial epicondyle of the elbow joint.

Dorsal fasciotomy should be added by placing longitudinal lengthy incision in the midline. Two longitudinal incisions on the dorsum of the hand also should be made **(Fig. 9-20)**.

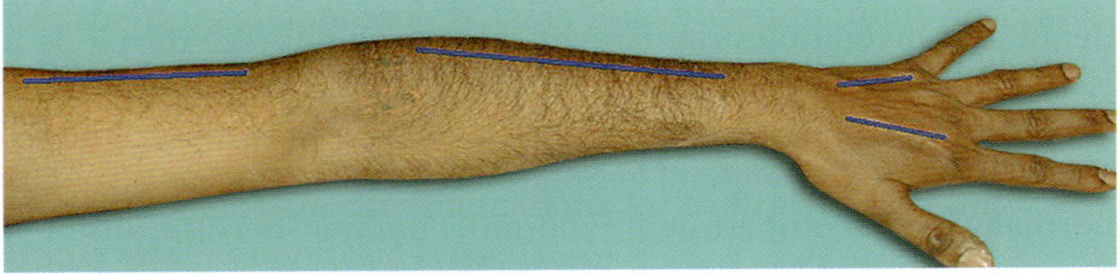

Fig. 9-20: Fasciotomy on the dorsum of forearm.

In lower limb also lengthy fasciotomy is done. Often multiple fasciotomies are required. Longitudinal, deep, lengthy incisions to expose the muscle underneath are required. Fasciotomies are done in different compartments—anterior, posterior and lateral **(Fig. 9-21)**.

Delayed secondary suturing in 5–10 days with split skin grafting is needed. Blood transfusions, antibiotics, hyperbaric oxygen are needed. Mannitol may be needed to prevent renal failure.

Chronic ischaemic contracture, gangrene, sepsis, renal failure, disability are the complications.

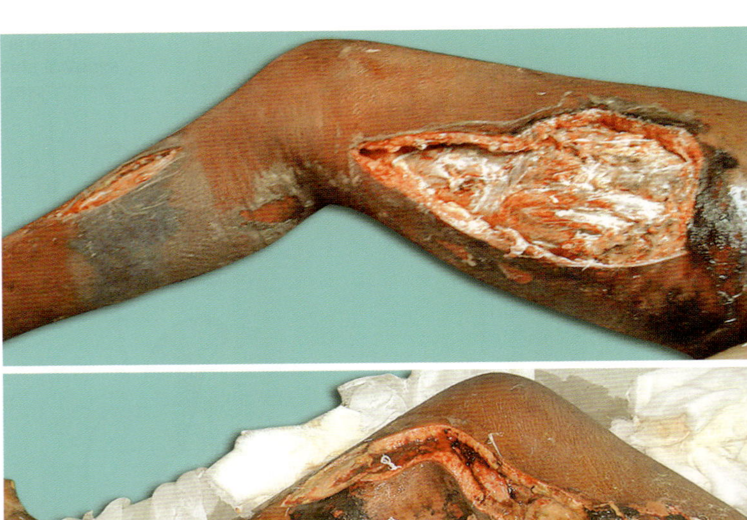

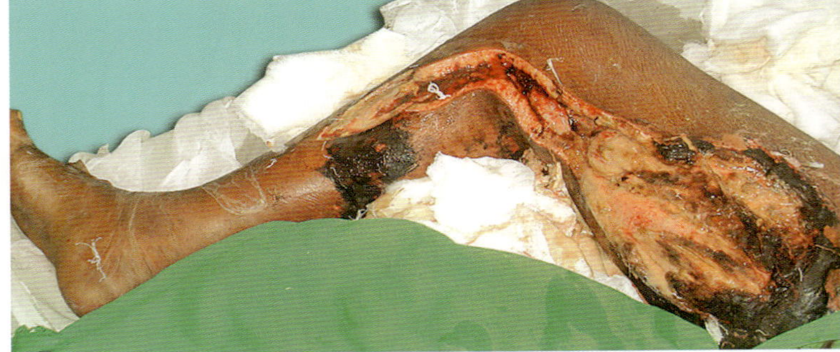

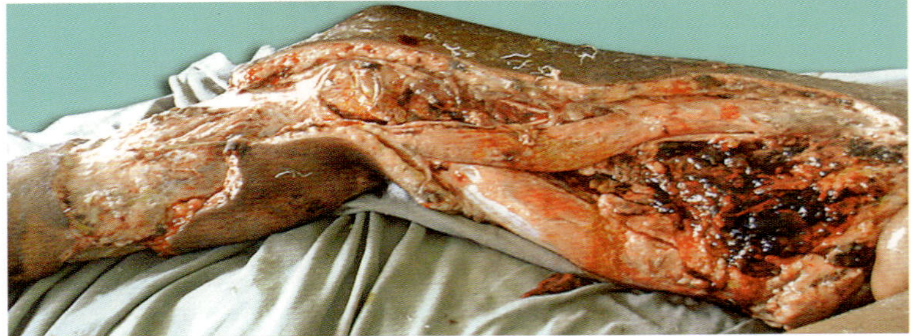

Fig. 9-21: Fasciotomies done for lower limb.

DRAINAGE OF AN ABSCESS

Drainage of an abscess depends on location of the abscess; whether abscess is formed or not. Superficial/surface abscess is drained by *Hilton's method* of drainage.

Deeper abscess: It is drained after confirmation by CT scan/MRI, etc. It is approached by layer-by-layer incision and drainage. Thorough warm saline irrigation is given. Drain is placed and closed in layers. Pus should be sent for culture.

Pus in the joint: It is confirmed by X-ray/total count, MRI features like pain, warmness, swelling, tenderness, oedema, restriction and pain in all movements of joint. It is usually aspirated under guidance. **Arthroscopy** and wash can be given. Often open drainage is done.

Intra-abdominal Abscess

It can be drained percutaneously by placing percutaneous catheter under guidance. Open drainage when needed should be undertaken if aspiration or percutaneous drainage fails.

Laparotomy is done to drain intra-abdominal abscesses. Abscess may be located in bilateral subphrenic space, lesser sac, prepancreatic space, interloop, anastomotic site, mesenteric or pelvic region. Except pelvic abscess all are drained transperitoneally, and is through upper midline incision **(Figs. 9-22 to 9-24)**.

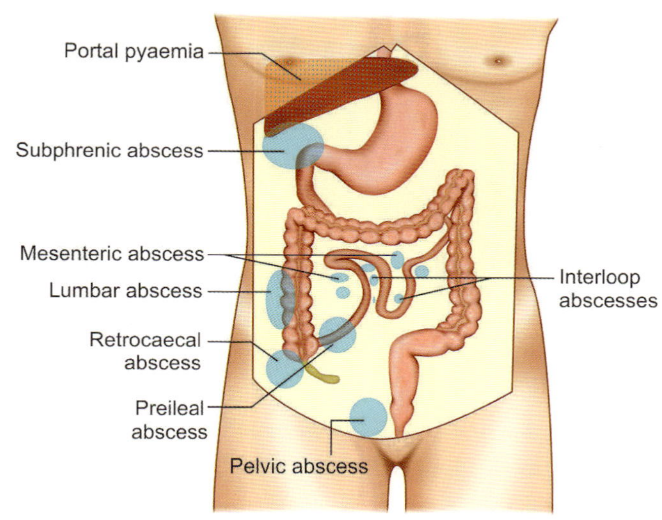

Fig. 9-22: Different intra-abdominal abscesses.

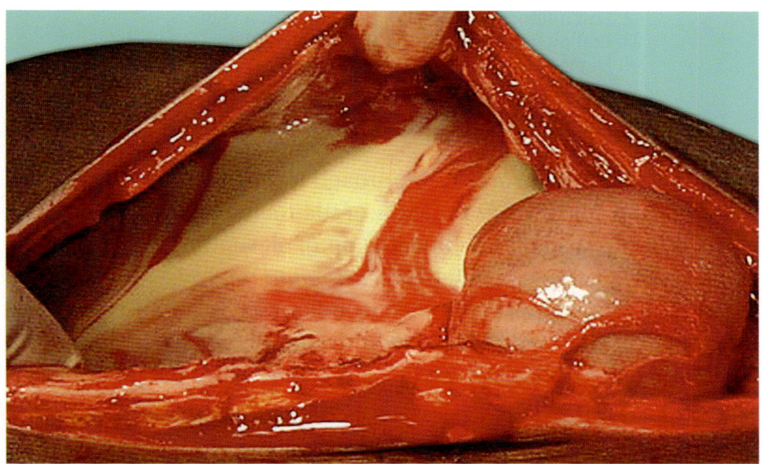

Fig. 9-23: Pus in the peritoneal cavity is drained through laparotomy incision.

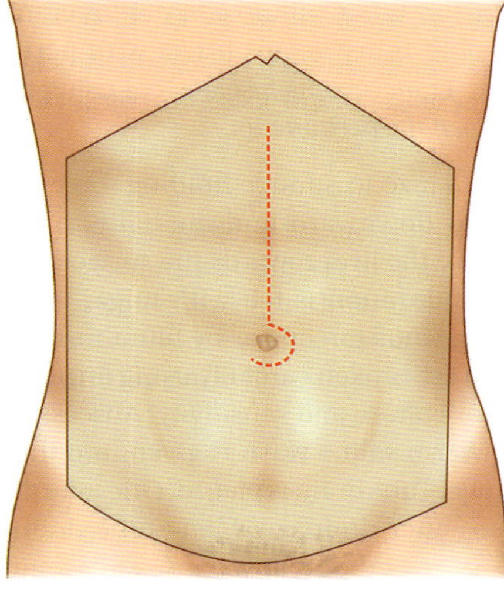

Fig. 9-24: Upper midline laparotomy incision is used for transperitoneal drainage of intra-abdominal abscesses. It is also used for open drainage of liver abscess, transperitoneal drainage of subphrenic abscess when needed.

Technique

Urinary catheter and nasogastric tube should be passed. Anaesthetist often prefers a central line. General anaesthesia with epidural support is used. Lengthy midline incision is used. If patient has undergone recent laparotomy, same incision with extension above and below is used. Peritoneum is opened over new extended part of the incision as it is virgin and chances of bowel adhesions underneath is less likely. Falciform ligament is identified and used as a guide for further dissection. By lifting the ligament dissection is carried out gently using pulp of the finger and gauze. Care should be taken as much as possible to avoid opening of bowel lumen during separation. Right and left suprahepatic and infrahepatic spaces are reached to clear the pus. Lesser sac is approached through gastrohepatic ligament along the lesser curvature of the stomach or through the omentum along the greater curvature of the stomach. Both right and left paracolic gutters are exposed to clear the pus. Often entire small bowel should be freed to clear the pus from interloop areas. Pelvis is reached by pulling the entangled bowel upwards from the pelvis. Pus should be sent for culture and sensitivity. Thorough warm saline wash (10 litres) is given. *Feeding jejunostomy is always* better to be done. Two tube drains/sump drains are placed on either side. Abdomen is closed by *Smead-Jones closure* method.

Subphrenic Abscess

Early diagnosis; considering that subphrenic abscess is thoracoabdominal in extension; drugs and early drainage; initial percutaneous ultrasound/CT-guided catheter placement; when needed open surgical drainage are essential parts always to be remembered in dealing with subphrenic abscesses **(Figs. 9-25 to 9-27)**.

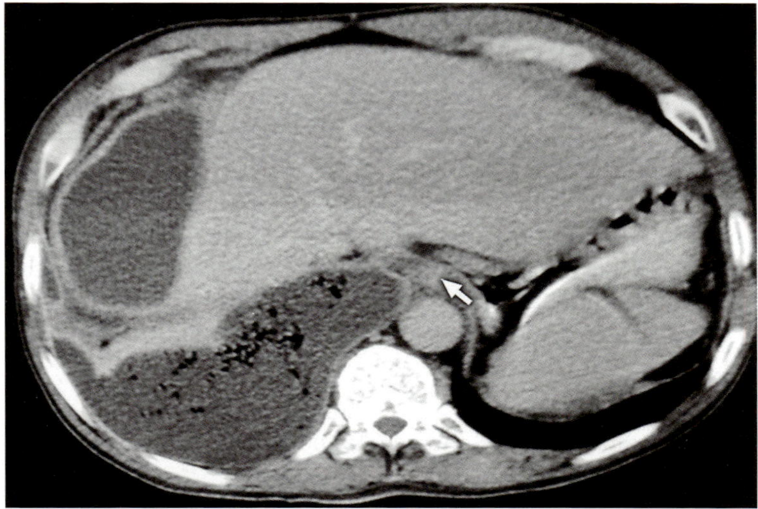

Fig. 9-25: CT scan showing subphrenic abscess.

Percutaneous Catheter Drainage

It is the standard initial treatment for subphrenic abscess. US or CT guided placement of catheter is done. One has to remember that *aspiration alone is not done* in subphrenic abscess.

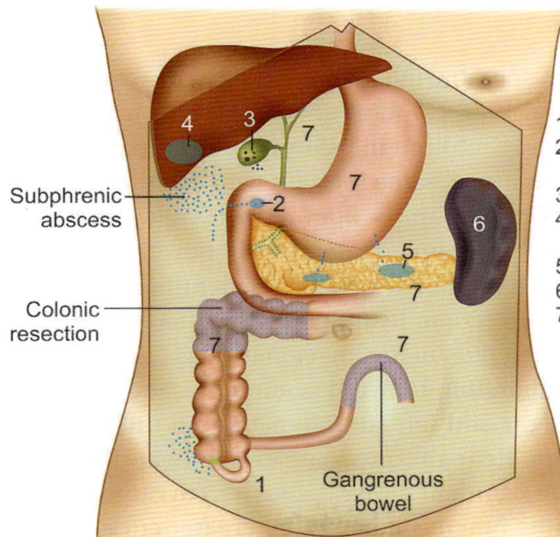

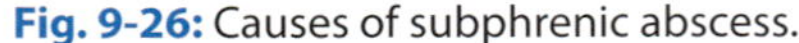
Fig. 9-26: Causes of subphrenic abscess.

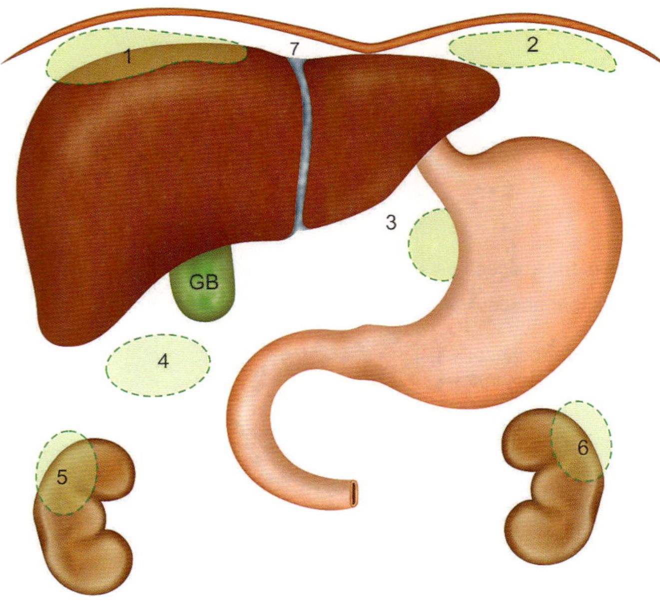

Fig. 9-28: Subphrenic spaces anatomy.

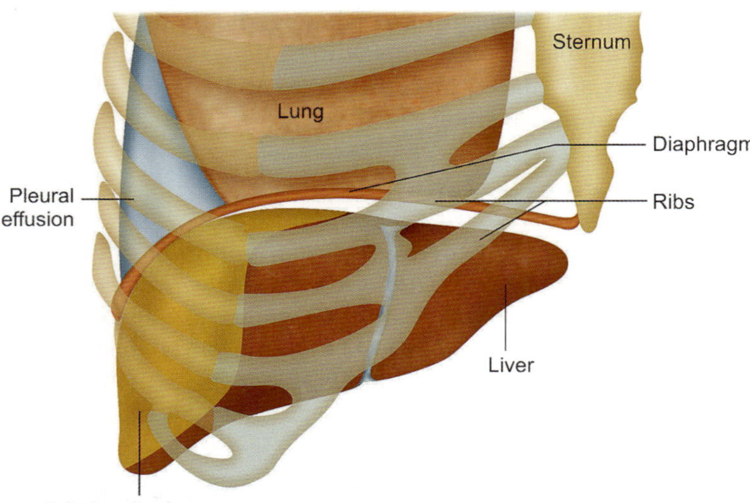

Fig. 9-27: Subphrenic abscess—common site.

Open Drainage

It is drained by extraperitoneal and extrapleural (*extraserosal*) approach. Aspiration/placing percutaneous catheters under guidance (CT/US) are also used. *Pre-operative preparation*—CT scan is very essential diagnostic. Antibiotics should be given—aminoglycosides, amoxicillin, metronidazole. Nasogastric tube should be placed.

Anaesthesia: Procedure is done under general anaesthesia with epidural support for post-operative pain relief.

Technique: Subphrenic abscess is second common intra-abdominal abscess. 30% of patients with subphrenic abscess can be asymptomatic. *Boyd* classified subphrenic spaces into right suprahepatic and infrahepatic; left suprahepatic and infrahepatic **(Fig. 9-28)**.

Position: Lateral position with body kept obliquely on the table. Patient should be supported properly before cleaning and draping.

Incision: Anterior extraserous approach is like a subcostal incision (10–12 cm) from the outer margin of the rectus muscle laterally up to the anterior axillary line towards tip of eleventh rib. *Left anterior extraserous* approach is called as *Clarimount approach.*

Posterior extraserous approach is oblique incision 2 cm from the midline over the bed of 11th rib with opening of periosteum and resection of the rib. Care must be taken not to enter the pleura.

Layers: Skin, subcutaneous tissue, superficial fascia, external oblique muscle, internal oblique muscle are cut. Skin is incised using no. 22 blade. Remaining layers are cut using cutting and coagulation monopolar cautery. 9th intercostal nerve is visualised and often need to be cut. Transverse abdominis muscle is usually split but can be cut if needed. Splitting is started from behind from posterior aspect as here muscle is not adherent to peritoneum unlike in front. Once muscle is split transversalis fascia with peritoneum can be visualised clearly. Transversalis fascia is cut using blade. One must take care *not to open the peritoneum.*

Technique: Using gauze in sponge holding forceps or finger peritoneum is pushed downward and medially to reach under the costal margin above the liver towards the surface of the subphrenic abscess. Area of induration is felt with finger. Abscess surface is opened using long sinus forceps or by blunt finger dissection. Pus gushes out. Loculi are broken carefully using finger or sinus forceps. Pus is collected for culture and sensitivity. Abscess cavity should be opened widely. Warm saline wash is given into the abscess cavity using 50 mL syringe. Tube drain is placed. One tube drain is sufficient if cavity collapses after drainage. Many tube drains are placed if abscess cavity is large and do not collapse after drainage. Wound is closed in layers using polyglactic acid zero or no. 1 suture. Layer by layer closure is done. Many advocate a mass single layer continuous suture which is also accepted. Skin is closed with interrupted sutures or using skin staplers **(Figs. 9-29 and 9-30)**.

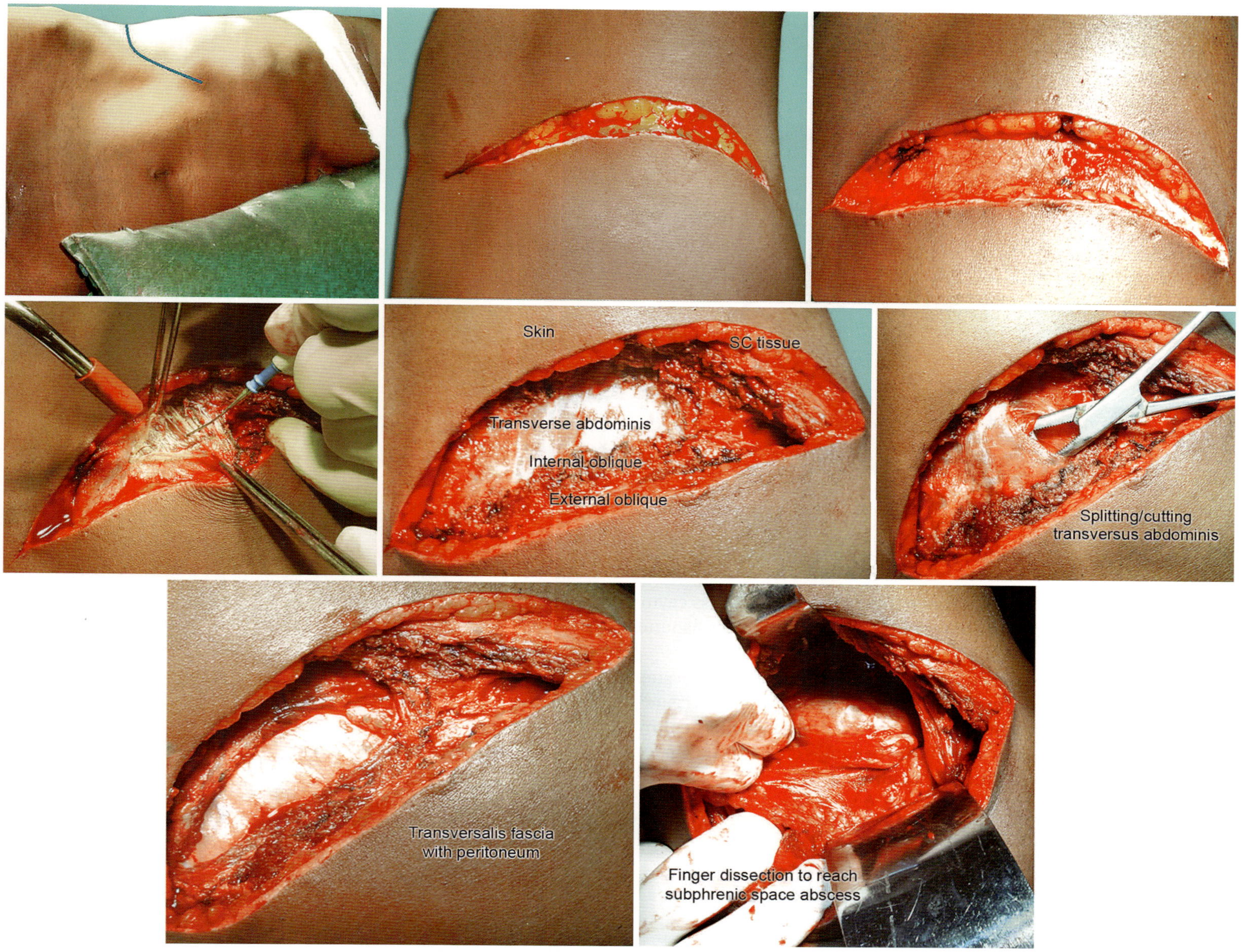

Fig. 9-29: Subphrenic abscess—open drainage steps—extraserosal approach.

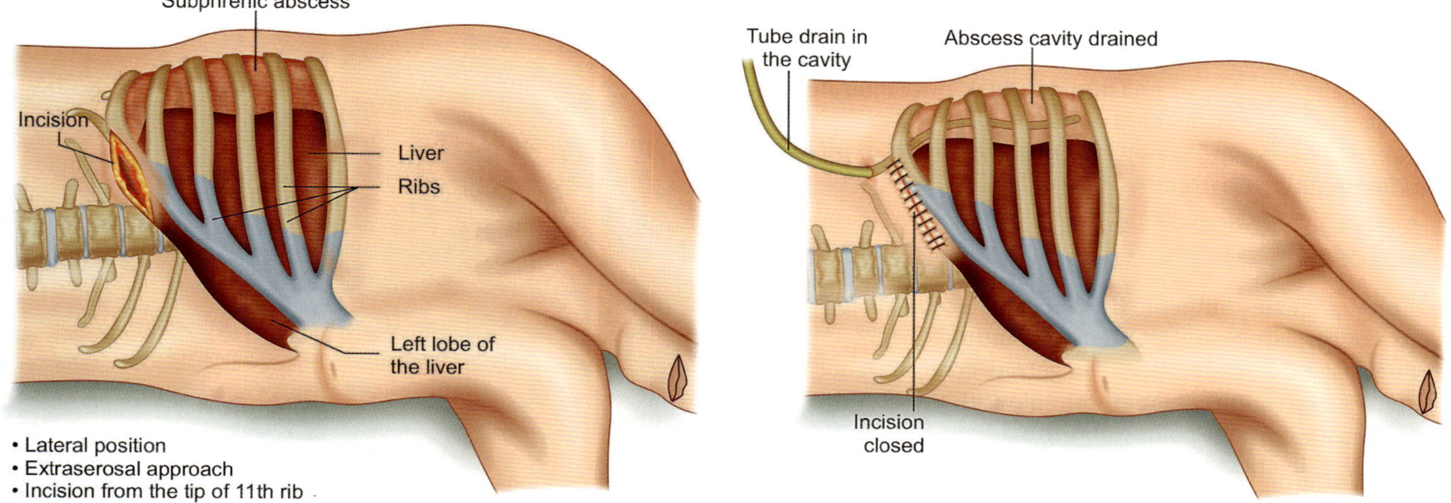

Fig. 9-30: Subphrenic abscess—incision, approach and closure.

If the abscess cavity has large thick rigid wall, it takes long time to collapse and often needs regular irrigation of the cavity using one of tube drains **(Fig. 9-31)**.

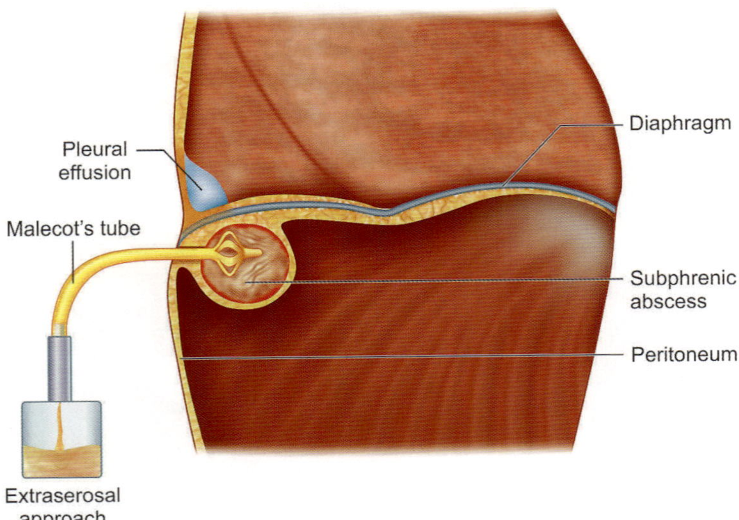

Fig. 9-31: Subphrenic abscess—open drainage by placing a tube.

Drain is *removed* in 10–14 days or after collapse of abscess cavity or after confirmation of the obliteration of the cavity by ultrasound or CT scan or contrast dye study using C-arm.

Often it is advised to keep a drain in the subcutaneous tissue. If there is more contamination, skin and subcutaneous tissues are left without suturing but covered with a dressing until healthy granulation tissue develops and wound becomes clean to take up for secondary suturing. Antibiotics are continued.

Complications

Injury to pleura, colon, liver, spleen; bleeding; sinus/fistula formation; incomplete drainage. Other intraperitoneal abscesses may be missed through extraserosal approach.

Transperitoneal Approach

Often transperitoneal approach is needed. Now it is proved that transperitoneal approach is safer. Bilateral subphrenic abscesses, multiple abscesses/more than one cavity or more loculations or subphrenic abscess due to anastomotic leak post-operatively (wherein leak site can be inspected and necessary repair can also be undertaken) are sure indications for *transperitoneal approach*. Upper *midline* approach is used.

Liver Abscess

In developing countries amoebic liver abscess accounts for 80%. In western countries pyogenic abscess accounts for 80%. Fever, chills, abdominal pain, tender hepatomegaly, decreased right sided diaphragmatic movement, sympathetic pleural effusion are the presentations. Raised total count; abnormal liver function tests; anaemia; effusion in chest X-ray are common. US (90% sensitivity) and CT (95% sensitivity) are useful methods. MRI is useful when associated biliary pathology is suspected and when multiple follow-ups are needed **(Figs. 9-32 to 9-35)**.

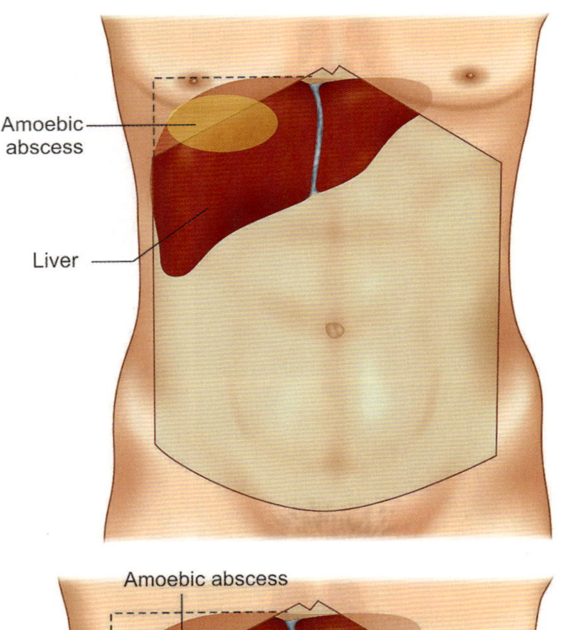

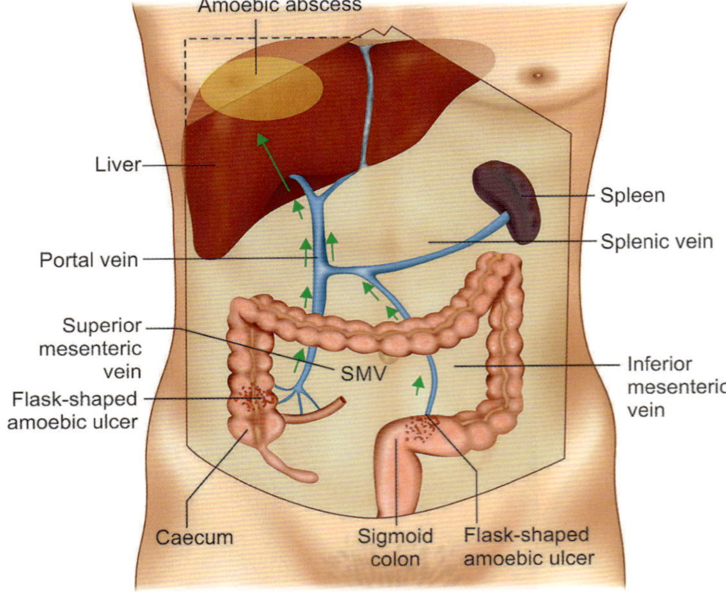

Fig. 9-32: Amoebic liver abscess is common in right lobe of the liver. Trophozoites reach liver from the colon.

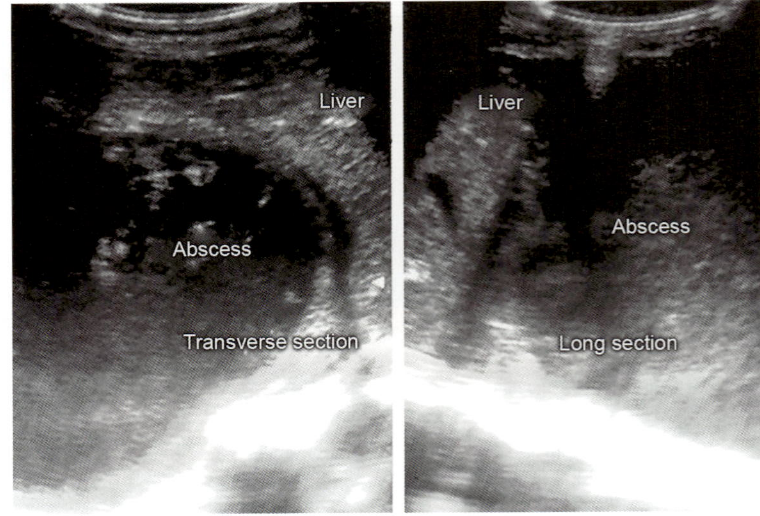

Fig. 9-33: Amoebic liver abscess ultrasound picture.

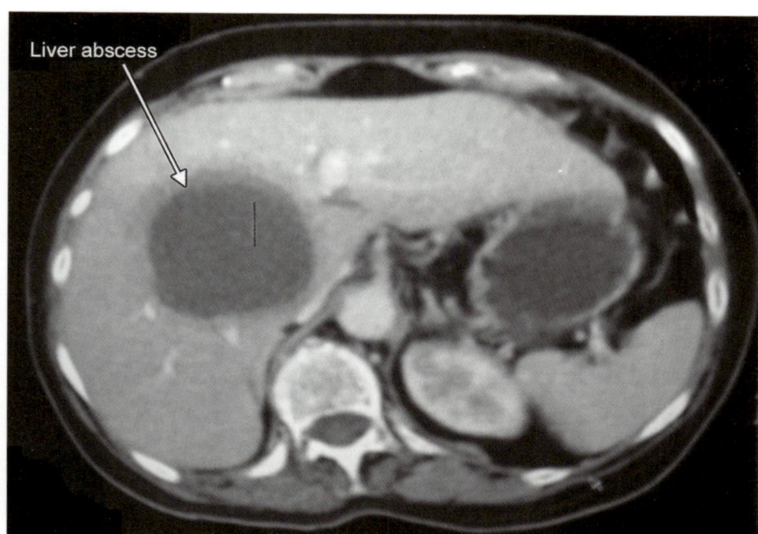

Fig. 9-34: Amoebic liver abscess—CT showing single abscess in right lobe of the liver.

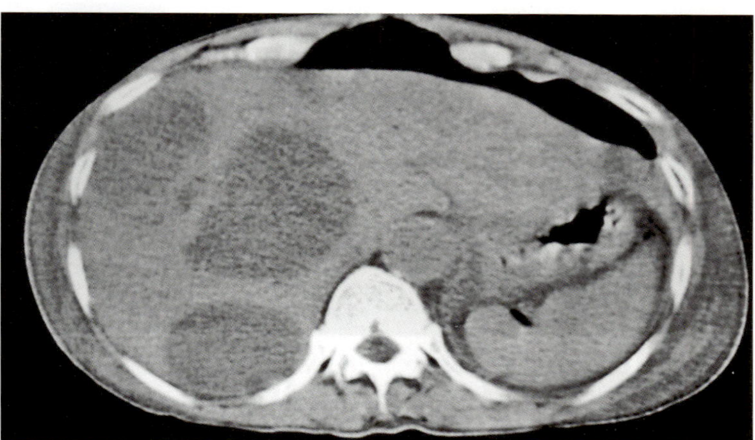

Fig. 9-35: CT scan showing multiple liver abscesses.

Aspiration

It is aspirated under US/CT guidance. Wide bore needle is used. Prothrombin time should be corrected if elevated using transfusion of FFP or by injection vitamin K. Needle is placed directly over the abscess or in right intercostal space in midaxillary line **(Fig. 9-36)**.

Percutaneous Drainage

Under US guidance pigtail catheter is placed into the abscess cavity percutaneously to drain the pus. Catheter tube and abscess cavity has to be washed and irrigated at regular intervals with normal saline. It may fail if there is thick pus, multiloculated abscess, and multiple abscesses. Procedure may cause bleeding and infection **(Fig. 9-37)**.

Surgery

Open drainage is done only when indicated. Indications are—filling of cavity after repeated aspirations; thick pus; multiloculated pus; left lobe abscess; ruptured abscess; caudate lobe abscess; multiple abscesses. It is done usually transperitoneally.

Procedure: Through transperitoneal approach, abscess area is opened, pus is evacuated. Malecot's catheter/suction tube drain/sump drain is placed and brought out through a separate wound. The catheter/tube is kept in situ until it completely stops draining. Complete drainage of

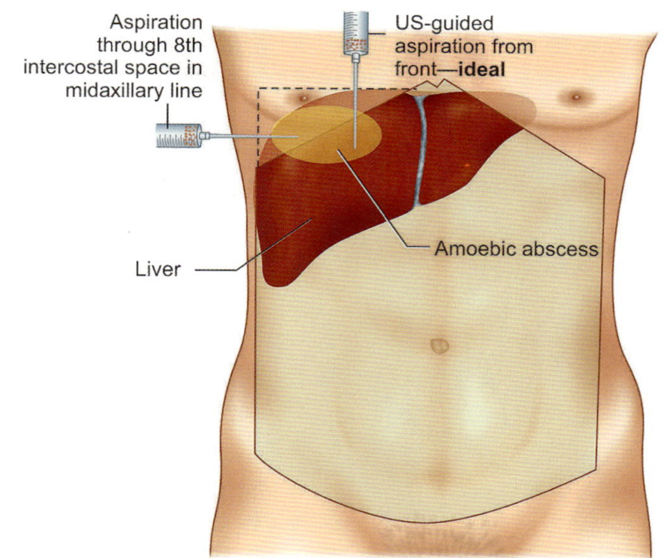

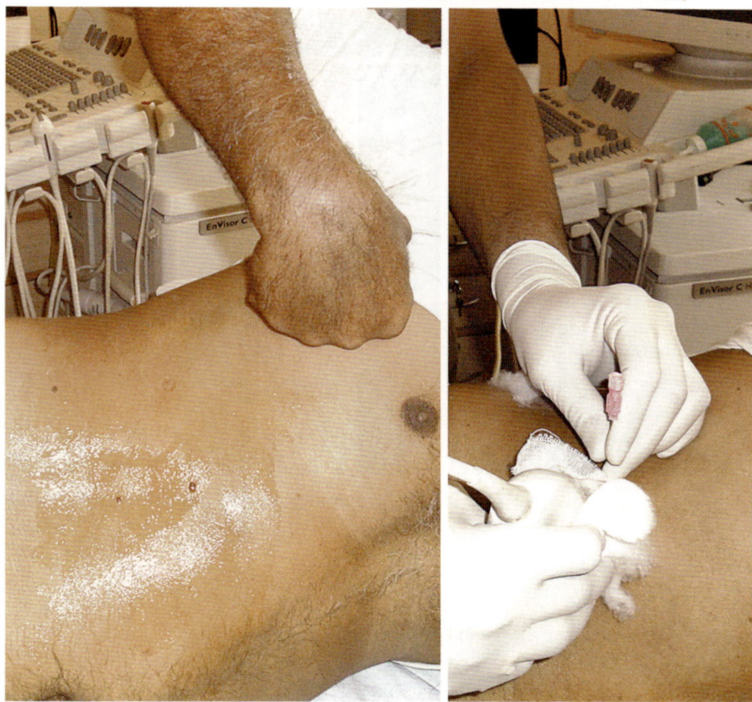

Fig. 9-36: Amoebic liver abscess aspiration is commonly done under ultrasound guidance. Prothrombin time should be normal prior to aspiration; if it is widened injection vitamin K 10 mg IM once a day for 5 days or 3 units of FFP should be given to make prothrombin time normal. While passing the needle into the abscess cavity, patient should hold the breath. After aspiration patient is monitored for 6–8 hours. Repeat US is needed after 7 days and 14 days to confirm that abscess has not reformed again.

pus will be confirmed by repeat US. During discharge, advice is given to avoid alcohol. Chloroquine 250 mg bd for 10 days and Diloxanide furoate 500 mg tid is given for 10–14 days **(Figs. 9-38 and 9-39)**.

Complications

Anaesthetic problems; bleeding; liver failure (in cirrhotic patients); intra-peritoneal abscess formation; bile leak—biliary peritonitis and fistula.

Follow-up: At regular intervals is important. Avoiding alcohol; repeat LFT; repeat ultrasound to confirm the complete resolution of the abscess cavity.

Laparoscopic drainage of liver abscess is becoming popular.

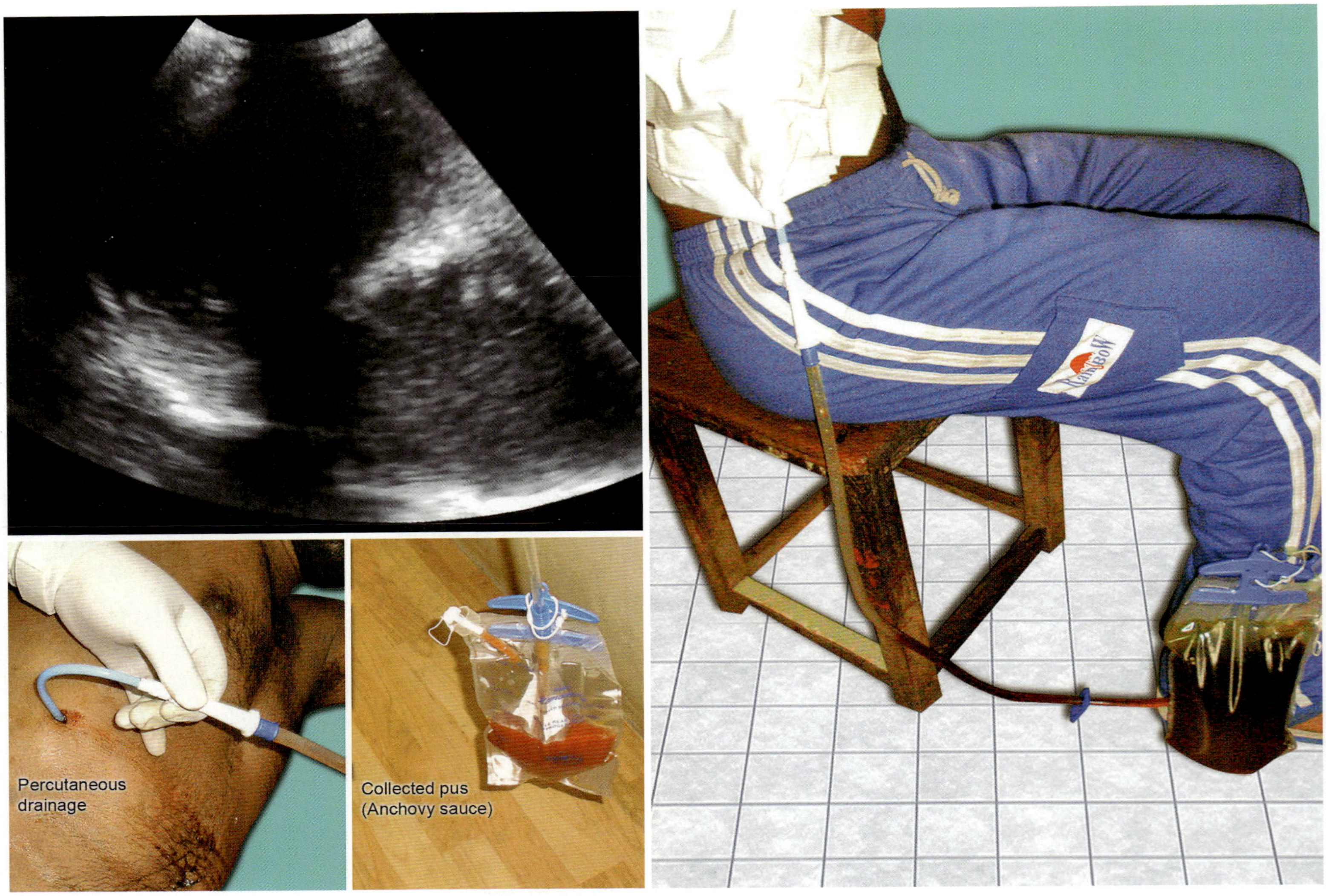

Fig. 9-37: Ultrasound-guided percutaneous drainage is commonly used in amoebic/pyogenic liver abscess.

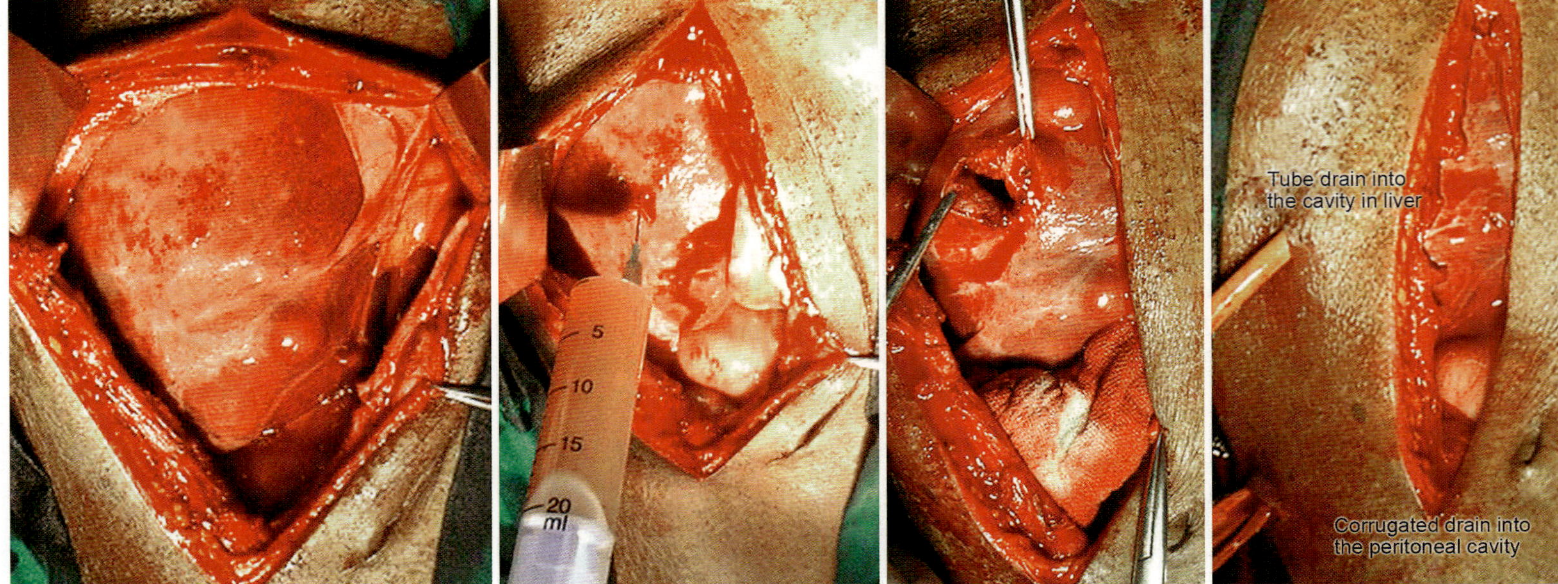

Fig. 9-38: Amoebic liver abscess on table look. Upper midline transperitoneal approach is used. Abscess is identified. Often on table ultrasound may be useful. Initially abscess cavity is aspirated and confirmed. Liver tissue on the surface is incised using cautery. Anchovy sauce pus is drained; collected for culture; last part of the pus should be collected for trophozoites. saline/metronidazole wash is given to the cavity by separate tube. Malecot's catheter drain is placed into the abscess cavity. Peritoneum is drained separately using a tube. Abdomen is closed in layers.

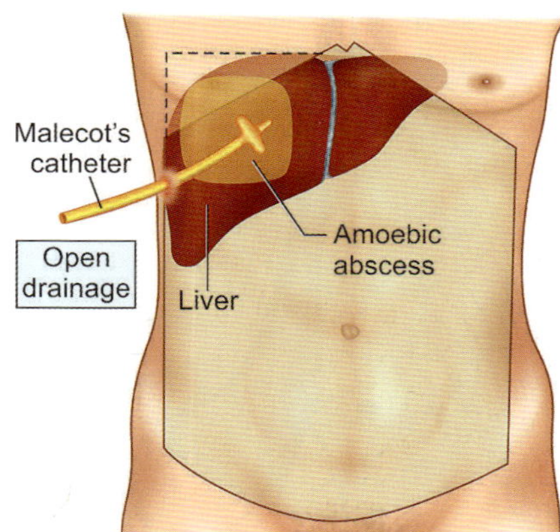

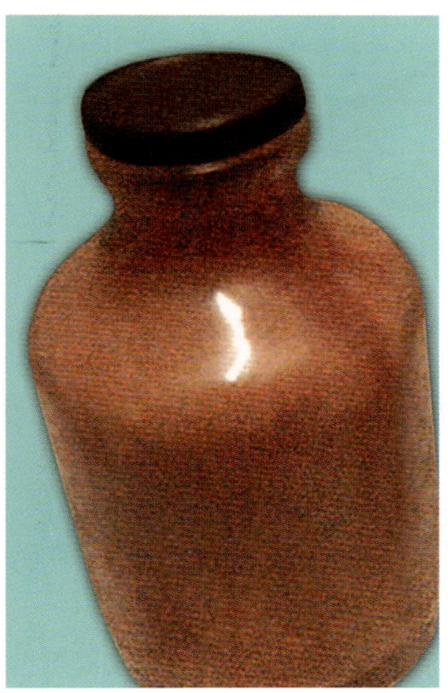

Fig. 9-39: Open drainage of amoebic liver abscess. Typical Anchovy sauce pus of amoebic liver abscess contains dead liver cells, RBCs, necrotic material.

Pelvic Abscess

It is commonest intra-abdominal abscess. Post-operative being the commonest cause, pelvic diseases, pelvic surgeries, gastrointestinal causes, perforation and peritonitis are other different causes. Tenesmus, diarrhoea, lower abdominal pain, tenderness, guarding and rigidity, fever and tachycardia are the features. US/CT is diagnostic. It is initially treated with antibiotics. When it is progressive or symptoms persist it should be drained.

It is drained pervaginally through posterior colpotomy in females or per rectally in males. Urinary catheter should be passed prior to surgery. Under general or spinal anaesthesia cleaning and draping is done in lithotomy position. Gloved finger is passed into the rectum to feel the soft boggy swelling in front above the prostate level. Incision is made over the swelling in the rectal mucosa to reach the abscess cavity. Pus is drained; collected for culture. Thorough saline irrigation is given. Often tube drain is placed in the cavity across rectum, which is removed in 24 hours. Follow-up ultrasound in 4–5 days is needed to confirm the resolution of the abscess cavity. In females it is drained in lithotomy position. Incision is made over the posterior fornix pervaginally; pus is drained **(Figs. 9-40A to C)**.

Drainage through laparotomy is usually not necessary.

Perinephric Abscess

It is pus in the perinephric region. Trauma, haematoma, tuberculosis of kidney, blood spread, extension from other area and lymphatic spread are the causes. Fever, loin fullness, tenderness and rigidity, scoliosis towards same side are the features. Loss of downward displacement of kidney is observed in intravenous urogram (*Mathe's sign*). CT is useful to confirm. It is drained percutaneously by placing catheters or by open drainage. Lateral position is used for open drainage. Lumbotomy incision is placed behind over the loin (lumbar incision) to reach the perinephric area. Drain (tube drain/ *Malecot catheter*) should be placed **(Fig. 9-41)**.

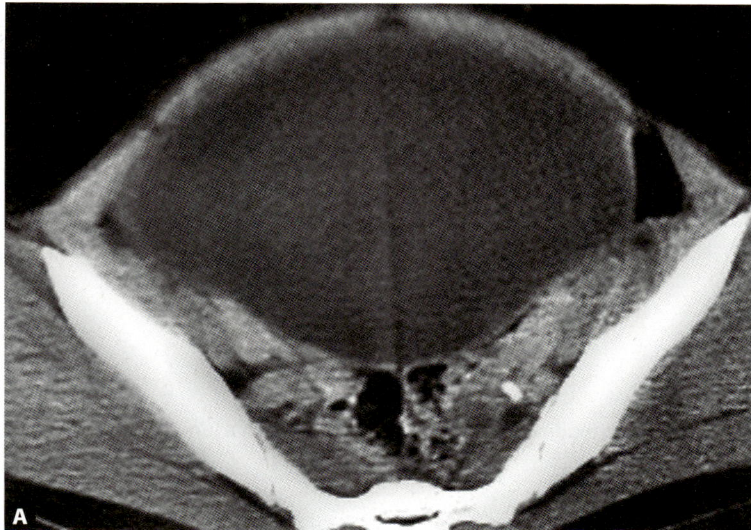

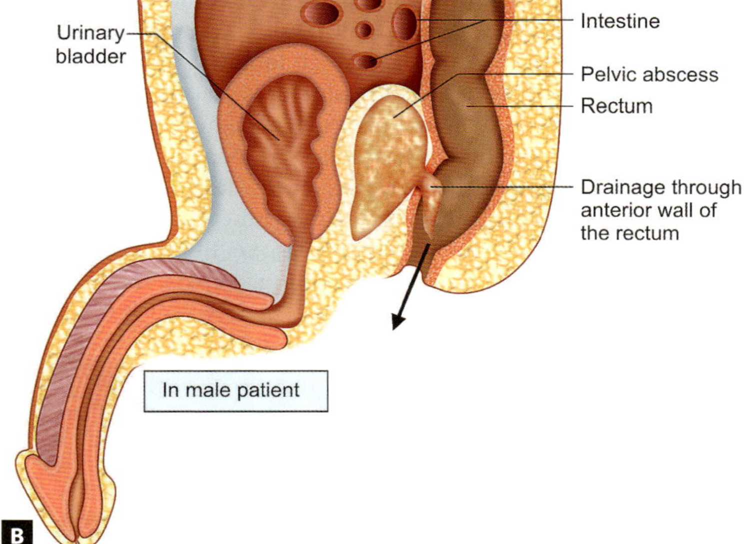

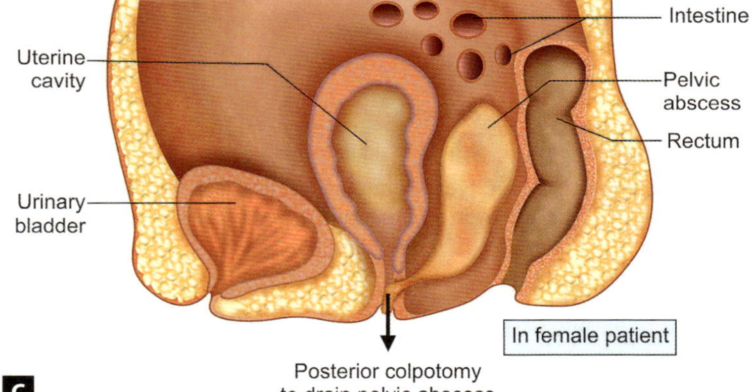

Figs. 9-40A to C: CT scan of pelvic abscess. Pelvic abscess is drained through rectum in males and through posterior fornix of the vagina in females.

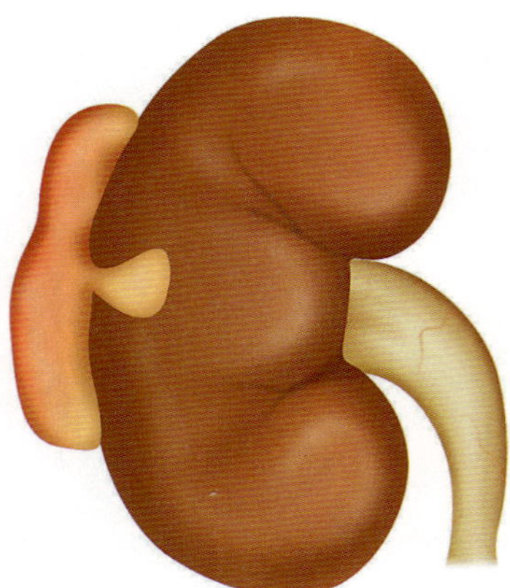

Fig. 9-41: Perinephric abscess. It is drained through a lumbotomy incision.

Pyonephrosis

It is drained by nephrostomy—***Percutaneous/Cabot's open method/Tresidder's method***. Percutaneous method is done under ultrasound guidance. Cabot's nephrostomy is open method; is done under general anaesthesia through loin incision with patient in lateral position. Tube/Malecot's catheter is placed into the renal pelvis across posterior convex surface of the kidney parenchyma. In Tresidder's method, tube is passed across renal parenchyma and pelvis and it comes out through two places. Its advantages are—it drains from two places through a single tube; it can be replaced with a similar new tube by railroad technique. But it is technically more difficult. *Complications*—bleeding, sepsis, blockage of nephrostomy tube **(Figs. 9-42A to C)**.

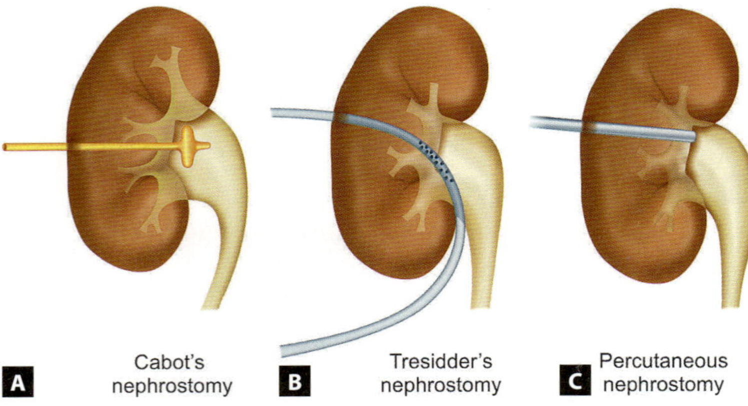

Figs. 9-42A to C: Different types of nephrostomies used to drain pelvis of the kidney in obstruction/pyonephrosis.

Psoas Abscess

It can be pyogenic or tuberculous origin. *Psoas spasm*, with typical flexion position, tender swelling in the iliac fossa are *typical* features. It should be differentiated from iliac artery aneurysm, ovarian cyst, and soft tissue tumour. It is drained extraperitoneally through an incision in lumbar region **(Fig. 9-43)**.

CT confirms the diagnosis **(Figs. 9-44 and 9-45)**.

It is drained under general anaesthesia or spinal anaesthesia.

Position of the patient is slight lateral tilt. *Urinary catheter* should be passed. Antibiotics should be started.

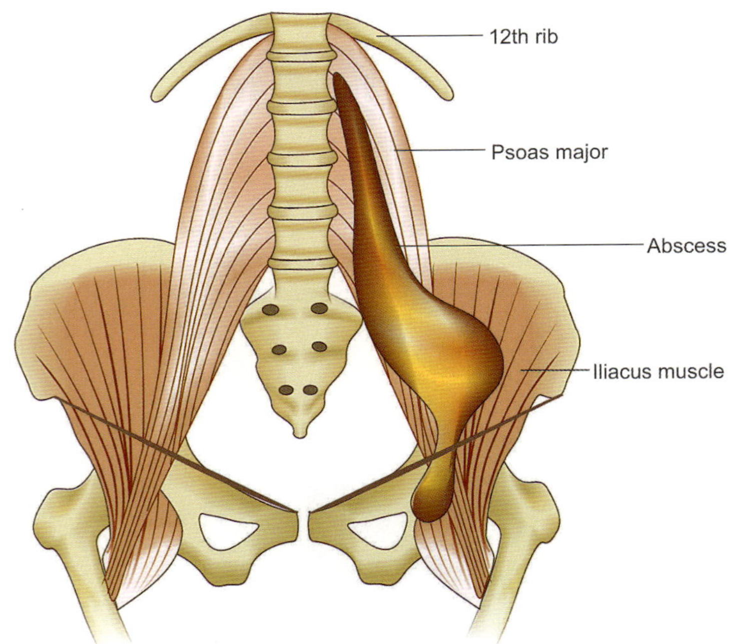

Fig. 9-43: Anatomical location of psoas abscess.

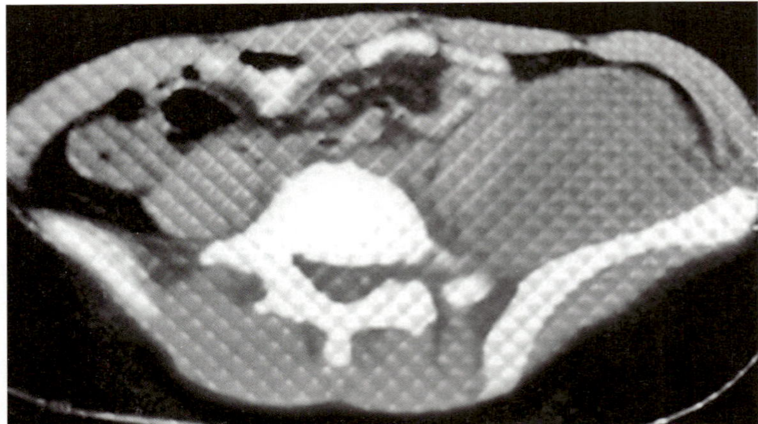

Fig. 9-44: CT scan showing left-sided psoas abscess—unilateral.

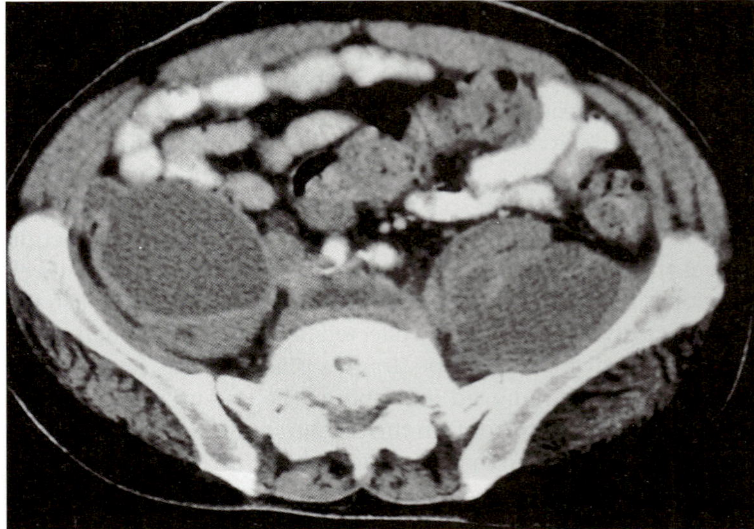

Fig. 9-45: CT scan showing bilateral psoas abscess.

Technique: Oblique incision at the level of the umbilicus extending medially and downwards up to the rectus muscle. Skin, subcutaneous tissue, superficial fascia, external oblique, internal oblique is incised in the line of incision using cautery. Transverse abdominis is split or cut. Often abscess wall is adherent to transverse abdominis and opens while incising the transversus abdominis. Peritoneum is pushed medially without opening it—*extraperitoneal approach*. Abscess cavity is opened. Pus drained and collected for culture and AFB. Often biopsy from the abscess wall is taken. Occasionally psoas abscess will be located within the psoas muscle sheath or in the muscle. In such occasions sheath is opened longitudinally or muscle fibres are split to reach the abscess cavity. After draining pus properly, thorough warm saline wash is given. In tuberculosis of spine anterolateral decompression of the vertebra followed by vertebral fixation is done. Antituberculous drugs should be started. Tube drain is placed; wound is closed in layers **(Fig. 9-46)**.

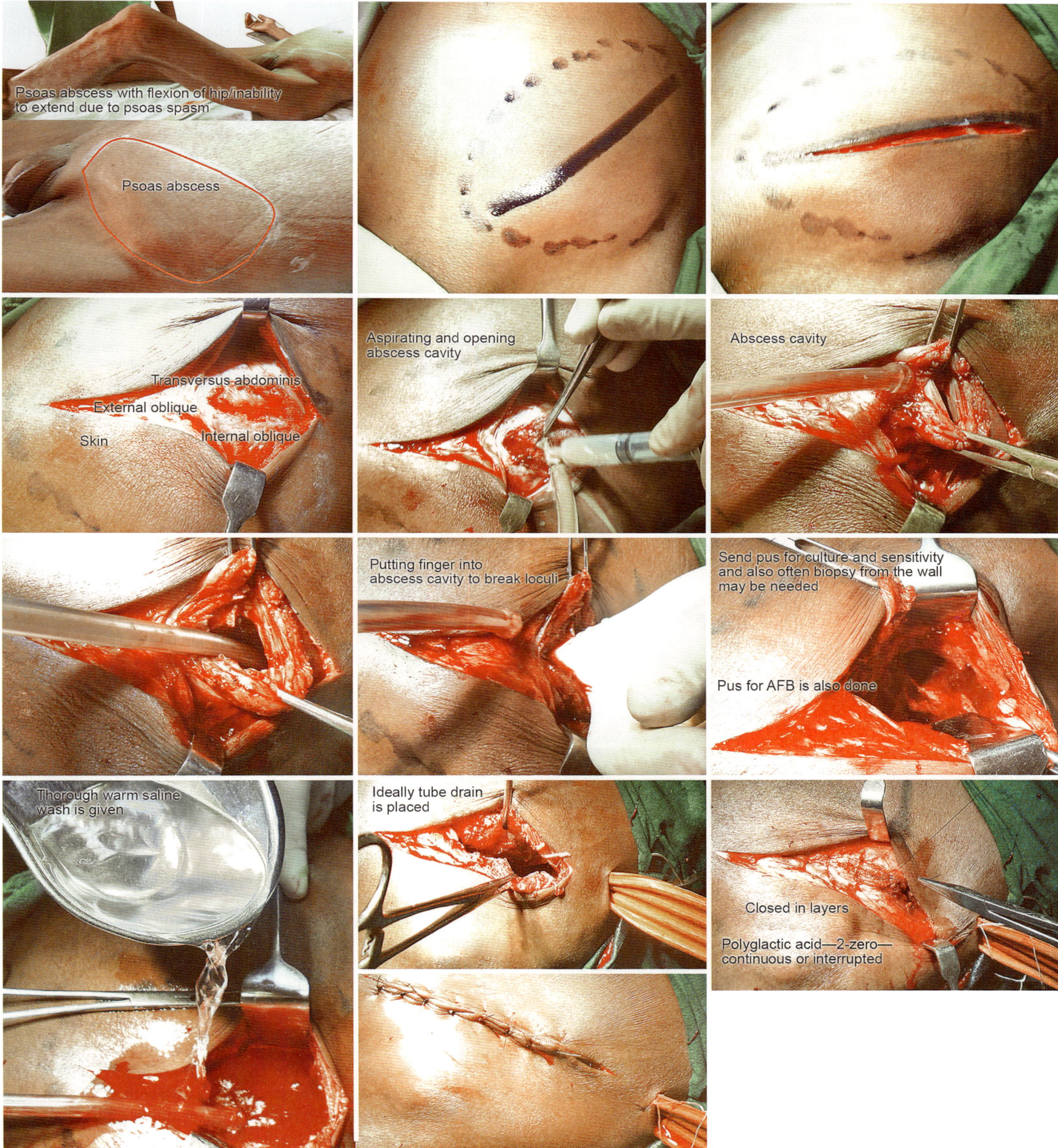

Fig. 9-46: Drainage of psoas abscess is done extraperitoneally through oblique incision at the level of the umbilicus.

Drain is removed in 10–14 days after confirming of obliteration of the cavity **(Fig. 9-47)**.

Complications

Peritoneal opening may cause peritoneal contamination. Injury to iliac vessels often can occur. Often iliac vein wall undergoes pressure necrosis and causes life-threatening haemorrhage. In such occasions it is difficult to repair the vein with sepsis underneath. Best way is to put a pack or ligated the vein.

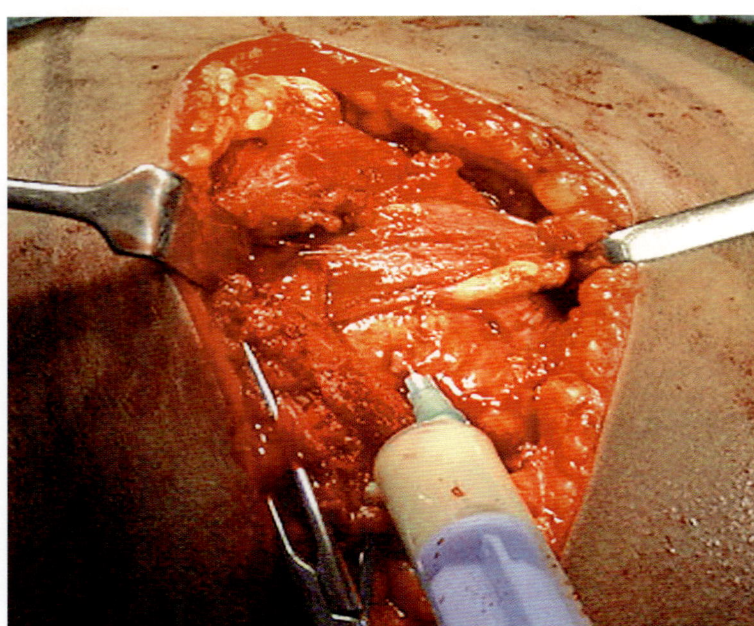

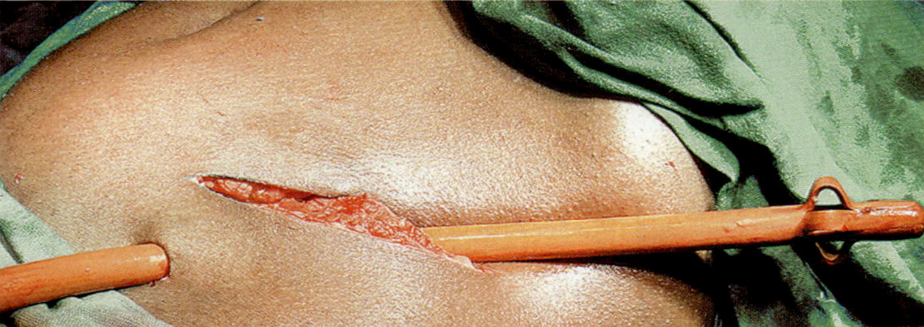

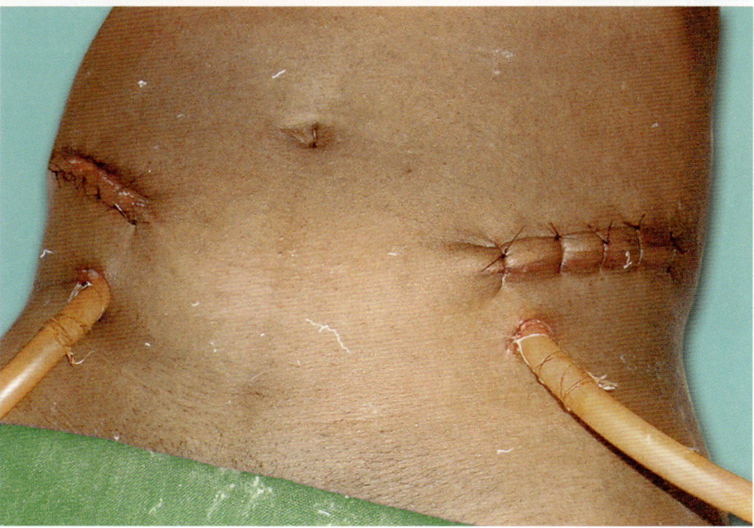

Fig. 9-47: Confirmation of pus in psoas abscess by needle aspiration. Drainage of psoas abscess by placing Malecot's catheter.

Other Abscesses

Pancreatic abscess is aspirated under CT guidance or drained by transperitoneal open drainage method or laparoscopic method.

Mesenteric abscess/bowel interloop abscess are drained through laparotomy—midline incision.

Abscess neck is drained under general anaesthesia. Usually horizontal incision is placed.

Abscess in the axilla is drained under general anaesthesia through crease incision placed in the lower part of the axilla.

Intracranial abscess is drained through craniotomy/burr holes using Dandy's brain cannula. It may be due to trauma, infective endocarditis, spread from infected sinus, untreated suppurative otitis media. CT brain localises the site of abscess. Headache, fever, localising symptoms, convulsion, systolic hypertension, vomiting and drowsiness are the typical clinical features. Antibiotics, anticonvulsants, supportive treatment are essential **(Fig. 9-48)**.

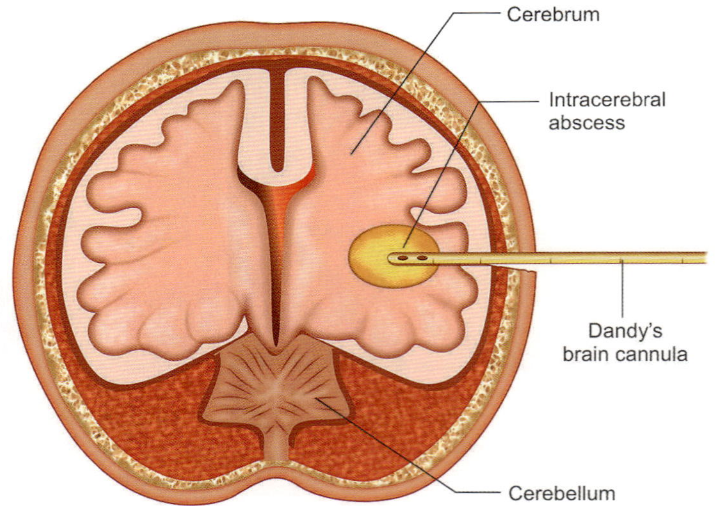

Fig. 9-48: Intracerebral abscess is drained by burr hole and passing Dandy's brain cannula into the abscess cavity.

Lung abscess is difficult to drain. It needs thoracotomy; exploration; often lobectomy. Empyema is drained using intercostal tube drainage.

Brodie's abscess is abscess in the bone (metaphysis). It is drained by open methods—saucerisation and sequestrectomy.

Bartholin cyst is retention cyst due to blockage of duct of the gland. Bartholin glands are greater vestibular glands (similar to Cowper's glands in males) lying in superficial perineal space, overlapped by the posterior ends of the bulbs of the vestibule. Each gland on either side has a 2 cm long duct which opens on either side on the margin of the labia minora posteriorly. Once it gets infected abscess forms. Drainage with marsupialisation is the treatment. 2 cm elliptical incision is made on the skin over the inner side of the cyst. Skin is excised; corresponding elliptical incision is also made over the cyst wall. It is often difficult to incise skin and cyst separately even though it is ideal; in such situation both skin and cyst wall are incised together. Cyst content with pus is drained. Edge of the incised cyst wall is sutured to the corresponding part of the incised edge of the skin using fine—4-zero absorbable polyglactic acid to create a stoma. *Marsupialisation*—stoma drains, granulates and heals with less chances of recurrence **(Fig. 9-49)**.

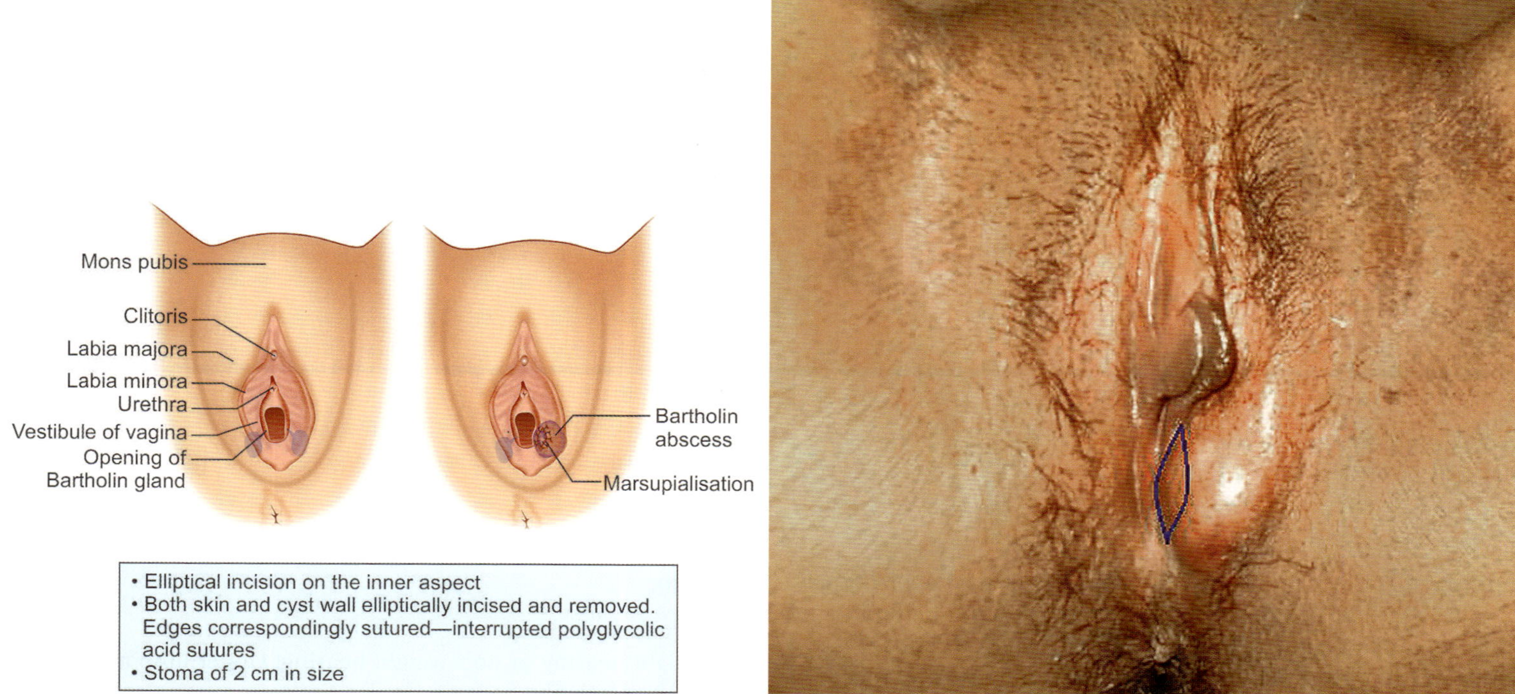

Fig. 9-49: Bartholin abscess occurs on the posterior aspect of the vestibule over labia minora. It is drained by marsupialisation.

10

CHAPTER

Amputations

Amputation is done as life-saving procedure especially in sepsis, diabetic gangrene, gas gangrene, etc. It is also often a therapeutic approach for malignancies in distal limb wherein conservative approach is not possible. Olden days amputation was a procedure done for leprosy and ergotism. Amputation needs proper planning of the flaps, prosthesis, initial mobilisation later rehabilitation and psychological support. It is one of the ancient surgical procedures. Sir William Fergusson in 1867 said, "Amputation is one of the meanest, yet one of the greatest operations in surgery; mean, when resorted to where better may be done great, as the only step to give comfort and prolong life". Ambroise Pare in 16th century did functional stumps and used the ligatures for major vessels. In World War I and II amputations were commonly done procedures along with invention of prosthesis.

Amputation is a procedure that removes a part through one or more bones, with exception of penectomy for carcinoma of penis which is called as amputation of penis.

Disarticulation is removal of part through the joint.

INDICATIONS

(Dead, dying, devitalised or dead, deadly/dead loss)

Gangrene due to atherosclerosis, embolism, thromboangiitis obliterans, diabetes, ergots, frostbite, trauma (complete devitalised distal tissues); to save life in crush injuries; severe electric burns; neoplasms; osteosarcomas; Marjolin's ulcer; melanomas; gas gangrene; severe sepsis; after nerve injury if part of the limb is completely paralysed with disabling trophic ulcers occasionally severe elephantiasis, madura foot, osteomyelitis, septic arthritis when all other methods were not of help. Disabling congenital deformities like complete fibular hemimelia, tibial hemimelia, femoral deficiencies and severe acquired deformities are also rare indications for amputations.

To salvage limb different scores are used: Predictive salvage index, limb injury score, mangled extremity syndrome index and mangled extremity severity score. If severely injured limb is attempted to salvage, then metabolic complications with secondary organ failure is likely. Limb injury score more than 50% or mangled extremity severity score more than 7 suggests need for amputation.

Reasons for amputation are: To preserve life (life saving), to improve general health, to relieve pain, to restore the function of the limb if needed by appropriate prosthesis.

Types

Amputation can be:

- Weight bearing or non-weight bearing: Upper limb amputations are non-weight bearing; lower limb amputations are weight bearing except forefoot amputation.
- Side bearing (non-end bearing): Here weight is taken up by the joint; end bearing (cone bearing): Here weight is taken up by the body of the patient (below knee amputation). Syme's amputation is cone bearing. End bearing is better for weight bearing like in lower limb.

Types of Flaps

Long posterior flap like in below knee amputation **(Fig. 10-1)**.
Equal flaps like in above knee amputation.

Elective amputation is planned one with flap. Infection should be absent. Viability of muscles and healthy skin are basic requisites for elective amputation. Level of amputation should be decided properly. Major blood vessels are ligated individually at same level. Nerve is pulled down adequately and cut without ligation. Cut bone

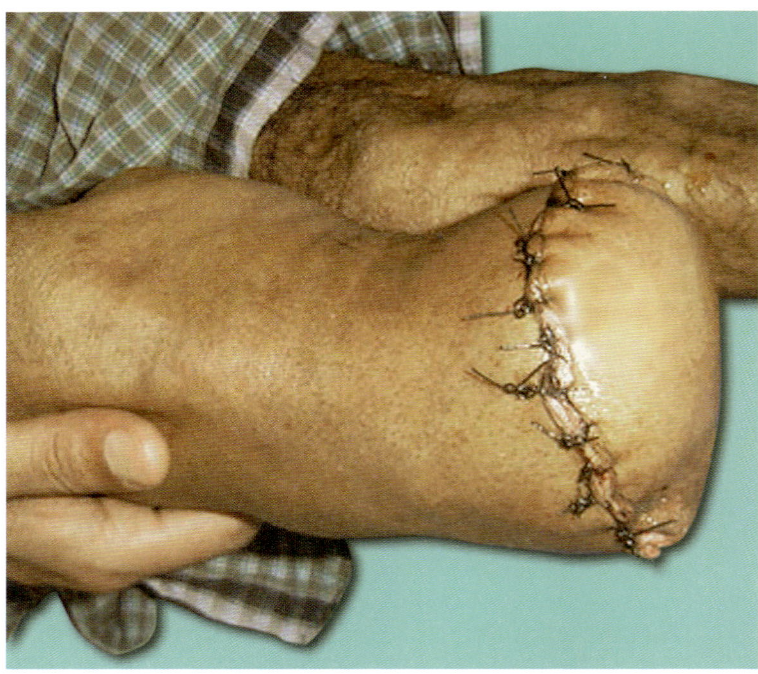

Fig. 10-1: Below knee amputation stump with long posterior flap.

margin should be made smooth using a rasp. Muscles should be closed over the bone. Suction drain ideally or corrugated drain is inserted on the lateral margin of the same wound which is removed in 48 hours. After removal of drain, firm pressure dressing is applied to control oedema and to prevent haematoma formation and which is left in situ undisturbed for 5 days. Early temporary prosthetic device may be used. Later permanent prosthesis is used after 3 months once stump forms a smooth round surface.

Emergency amputation is done in trauma, gangrene leg or severe sepsis. Here skin, muscles and bone are cut at the same level without suturing as in *guillotine amputation*. Later once sepsis subsides and patient recovers stump is revised for a proper flap.

In vascular diseases tourniquet should not be used during amputation.

Present Classification of Amputation

Present classification of amputation is as:

Open or closed amputation:

Amputation may be open, closed, revised, and planned. It may be guillotine (circular/linear/flapless) or modified guillotine or flap type. In acute conditions guillotine amputation is done [Guillotine is a device used to behead a person during execution by French in 1791; (French humanitarian physician Joseph Ignace Guillotin in 1789 recommended/urged to use it; surgeon Antoine Louis in 1792 first designed to get first guillotine execution)]. Open amputation is done in emergency situation like life-threatening sepsis, spreading fasciitis, critically ill patient, crush injuries of the limb. Such open guillotine method may be circular wherein limb is transected at the desired level with skin to bone all tissues are cut and left open; later skin grafting, secondary suturing or revision amputation is done. In modified guillotine amputation open amputation is done with inverted skin flap. In closed method, tourniquet is used except in diabetes and ischaemic limbs. Skin flap should be properly designed. Muscle coverage should be checked. Usually muscle is cut 5 cm distal to the level of the bone stump. Muscle is either sutured to the bone using drills (myodesis) or muscle sutured to the opposite group of muscles or fascia (myoplasty). Nerves are retracted and cut proximally; muscles are cut distally unless it is ischaemic. Bones are beveled using bone file.

The energy required for walking is inversely proportionate to the level of the amputation; higher the level of amputation greater the energy required.

Open Amputations

- Open amputation with inverted skin flaps.
- Circular open amputation.
- Guillotine amputation.

Open amputation with inverted skin flaps: Skin flaps are elevated longer than normal. Muscles are divided distal to the intended level of bone transection. After amputation, edge of skin flap is sutured at the corresponding level along with subcutaneous tissue and fascia using interrupted absorbable sutures creating rolled flaps. Once good granulation tissue appears, infection subsides, flaps are closed after 14 days.

Circular open amputation: Skin and muscles are divided circularly at a lower level than bone and left alone. Flap is closed at a later date once sepsis comes under control.

Guillotine amputation: Here all tissues of the limb are divided at the same level and left exposed. It is used in machinery trapping or severe sepsis. It is primitive type of amputation. Revision amputation is needed at a later period. *Definitive closure* is done using reamputation at proximal level; revision amputation; repair of the stumps.

Closed Amputations

It is widely used definitive amputation wherein stump is covered with flaps which should be ideal, highly functional and suitable for proper prosthesis. *Tourniquet* is used except in vascular cases. General/spinal/epidural anaesthesia is used.

Level of amputation is decided based on the identification of the level of adequate perfusion. It is assessed by skin temperature; systolic pressure (ankle systolic pressure should be more than 40 mmHg); Doppler; transcutaneous oxymetry (PO_2 more than 40 mmHg); arteriography; digital plethysmography; thermography; isotope clearance and dye attenuation studies.

IDEAL STUMP

- It should have adequate blood supply. It should heal adequately by first intention.
- It should have rounded gentle contour; with adequate muscle padding, conical shape with distal tapering is better. Stump should be free from tenderness and conical.
- Opposing groups of muscles should be fixed together over the end of the bone to attain optimum power and control of the muscles at the stump. Smooth, pain free/tenderness free stump should be obtained.
- Joint proximal to the amputation stump should show full range of movements without any contractures. Skin should have a clean incision which should be sutured tension free. Freely mobile skin over the bone and soft tissues should be achieved to get free movement of the prosthesis to be placed later. Socket of prosthesis with mobile skin creates a piston to bone to move like a joint. Transverse posterior scar is better which will not expose to pressure.
- It should have sufficient (optimum) length to bear prosthesis. For below knee amputation (B-K) 7.5 (minimum) to 12.5 cm from ischial tuberosity; for above knee amputation (A-K) 23 cm from greater trochanter. For above and below elbow 20 cm stump is used.
- It should have thin scar which does not interfere with prosthesis function. Scar should be in a place where it is not exposed to pressure. Skin should not be folded. Redundant soft tissue should not be present.
- It should have adequate adjacent joint movement.

Conical bearing

- Here healing is by primary intention.
- Bone should not be projecting.
- Myoplastic.
- Neuroma formation is not there.
- Scar should not be tender.
- Proximal joint should be supple.

Postoperative Period

Physiotherapy is advised. Regular dressings are done. Crutch is used initially, after 3 months prosthesis is placed. Rehabilitation is important.

COMPLICATIONS OF AMPUTATIONS

- **Early**
  Haemorrhage, haematoma, infection.
- **Late**
  Pain, ulceration of stump, ring sequestrum formation, flap necrosis, painful scar. ***Phantom Limb***—feeling of amputated part in toto or partially with pain over it.

Haematoma is identified by pain, swelling over the stump underneath the flap. It is aspirated using a wide bore needle. Haematoma may delay healing; may precipitate infection or flap necrosis due to pressure. After aspiration, pressure dressing is needed. If haematoma reforms after 2-3 aspirations, it should be drained by opening the wound on one corner and inserting haemostat into the wound.

Infection of the stump may cause abscess formation, delay in healing of wound, flap necrosis, giving way of the wound. Removing few or all sutures to relieve pressure and draining the pus underneath is needed. Infection may also lead into poor scar, adherent scar which causes difficulty in placing the prosthesis **(Fig. 10-2)**.

Flap necrosis is *common* complication. Main causes for flap necrosis are poor blood supply, infection, haematoma underneath, inadequate length of the flap causing stretching of flap. Small area of necrosis can be excised. Wider area needs laying open of the wound or revision of the stump or higher level amputation. Anaemia, poor nutrition, deficiencies, diabetes mellitus, immunosuppression, smoking and old age are other factors causing flap necrosis.

Stump neuroma can occur due to proliferation of the nerve fibrils beyond the point of nerve division and is usually due to failure of cutting of the nerve more proximal to the level of division of the bone. It causes pain and tenderness over the stump. It is usually relieved by analgesics, reassurance and prosthesis. Occasionally it may require reexploration of the wound, excision of end neuroma and also cutting of nerve more proximally.

Stump pain after amputation is *a common problem*. Causes are - infection, poor blood supply, causalgia, stump neuroma, phantom pain/limb, deep vein thrombosis, adherent scar, formation of spurs and osteophytes at amputated bone end. Scar adhesion to bone is prevented by keeping adequate length of deep fascia underneath intact. Spurs and osteophytes are confirmed by X-ray and needs removal using bone nibbler after appropriate skin incision.

Phantom limb is *typical* awareness of sensation that as if amputated part is still present; often such part may be painful or disturbing or hyperaesthetic. Exact cause is not known; but it is probably due to presence of severe pain at the amputated part just prior to amputation making brain area representing the part in alert situation causing phantom limb. Reassurance, prosthesis, analgesics control the condition. It is said that it can be prevented by proper pain control for 24 hours prior to amputation; but it is often difficult.

Ulceration over the stump is *not uncommon*. It is due to necrosis, infection, lengthy bone stump pressing on the summit of the flap, prosthesis, deficiencies, diabetes mellitus, ischaemia. Ulcer may be small/large; superficial/deep. Callous chronic ulcer at the end of the stump is called as *Douglas ulcer*. Small ulcer is treated by regular dressings and suturing later. Large ulcer needs flap to cover the defect. *Osteomyelitis of the stump* should be ruled out in chronic stump ulcer. *Ring sequestrum* may be typical in such situation. Revision amputation is needed for stump amputation **(Fig. 10-3)**.

Contracture of the joint proximal to the amputated stump is *common*. It is mainly due to improper positioning after amputation; due to pain, poor exercise and occasionally due to inflammation of surrounding soft tissues. Contracture interferes with proper fitting and functioning of the prosthesis and delays rehabilitation. Proper positioning, passive stretching and strengthening exercises correct it. Rarely needs surgical release of the contracture.

Other complications like scar hypertrophy, skin thickening, hyperkeratosis, papilloma, eczema, lymphoedema, boils, bursae over bony point, new bone formation at the stump, flexion deformity, hyperaesthesia, stump oedema, causalgia, painful adhesive scar formation can occur, which are treated accordingly.

Evaluation of the patients who need amputation

- Haematocrit, control of anaemia by transfusing blood/packed cells.
- Control of infection using antibiotics.
- Decision of level of amputation by skin temperature, arteriography, arterial Doppler, transcutaneous PO_2, laser evaluation.
- Informed consent.
- Plan for prosthesis and rehabilitation by physiotherapist and rehabilitation team.

Different incisions for amputations

- *Circular incision amputation*—skin and muscles are divided circularly at a lower level than that of bone.
- *Elliptical/oval incision* amputation.
- *Racquet incision amputation*—for digital disarticulation.
- *Amputation using flaps*—it may be of equal flap (above knee amputation) or with long posterior single flap (below knee amputation). Total length of single flap or combined length of two flaps should be equal to 1½ times the diameter of the limb at the line of amputation. Flap should be semicircular to get a conical stump, not rectangular.

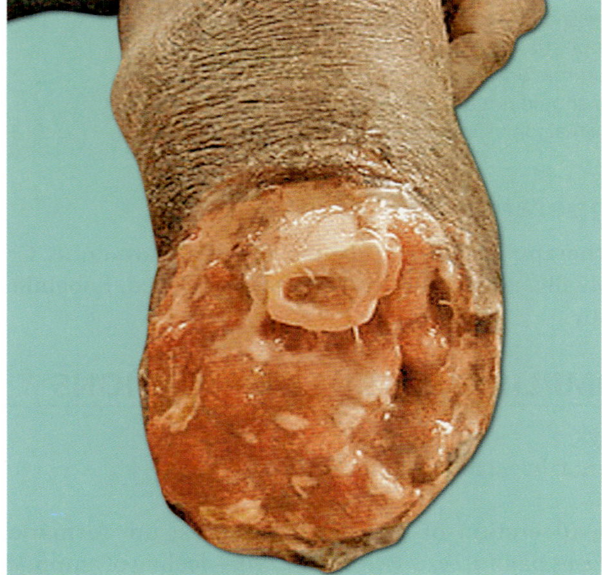

Fig. 10-2: Infection of the below knee stump exposing the cut end of tibia.

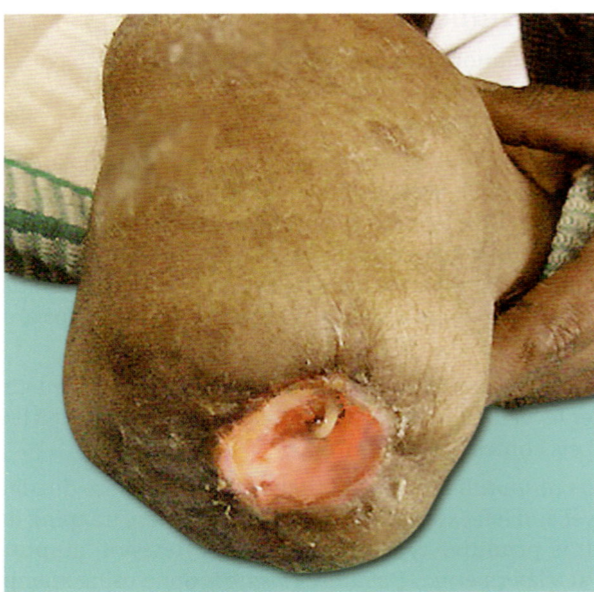

Fig. 10-3: Ulcer in amputated stump.

PRINCIPLES IN AMPUTATION

- Adequate blood supply of the flap should be maintained.
- Proper marking of the skin incision is essential. Skin should not be crushed or traumatised. Clean cut on the flap is essential. Opposing two equal flaps or long single flap is used. Total length of single flap or combined length of two equal flaps should be 1½ times the circumference of the limb at the level of bone section. Equal anterior and posterior flaps (above knee amputation) or long posterior flap (below knee amputation) is commonly used. Tension free flap suturing should be achieved.
- When unequal flaps are used, shorter flap should be broader than longer flap so that skin edges sutured as equal length. Adequate blood supply of the flap should be ensured.
- Tourniquet *should not be used* if amputation is done for vascular diseases. In other conditions like in trauma and tumour it can be used. When it is used, it should be released before skin closure to achieve proper haemostasis.
- Proximal part of the flap contains muscle component but distal part should contain only skin and deep fascia. Deep fascia is cut along with the skin and reflected along with skin. Earlier in conventional amputations, muscles are cut at the level of transection of bone. But now myodesis or myoplasties are routinely done. In *myodesis,* opposing muscle groups are sutured/anchored to bone end using drill holes. Myodesis is contraindicated in peripheral vascular disease. In *myoplasty*, opposing muscles which are divided 5 cm distal to bone transection are sutured to one another adjacent to bone end. It is preferred in peripheral vascular disease.
- Flap length should be adequate; not short. It should be ideally *semicircular* not rectangular to get a conical stump.
- Nerve should be pulled down and cut using a sharp knife and allowed to retract into the soft tissue otherwise neuromas may develop.
- Major vessels should be individually isolated and ligated. Mass ligature should be avoided.
- In crush injury/entrapment injury/sepsis—*guillotine amputation* is done. Later skin is pulled down by using skin traction, eventually to have better skin coverage.
- Bone should be cut with beveling and all sharp margins should be rounded using rasp. *Osteoplasty* can be done by raising a sleeve of periosteum over the bone; after cutting the bone, periosteum is closed over the bone end.
- Usually drain is placed (tube drain) through the wound which is removed in 48–72 hours. *Conventional soft dressing* using gauze, wool and crepe bandage is used. Amputation in weight-bearing area like lower limb, *rigid dressing* using plaster of Paris cast is used to reduce oedema, stump pain, early stump maturation and proper healing. Rigid dressing may cause pressure necrosis, ischaemia and infection. *Intermittent pressure* as a controlled environment chamber in a plastic sleeve is also used. A *true prosthetic cast* may be used if weight-bearing ambulation is anticipated in immediate postoperative period **(Fig. 10-4)**.
- Postoperatively patient is mobilised using axillary crutches. After 3 months, once scar has matured and stump has become supple, proper prosthesis is fit. *Berlamont* first started immediate postoperative fitting of prosthesis to leg for early mobilisation. *Plaster pylon* is applied to the stump and a prosthetic extension is fit to facilitate partial weight bearing immediately after surgery. It has got more stump complications and so has not become popular **(Fig. 10-5)**.
- Position of the stump in postoperative period is important. Stump should be elevated by raising the foot end of the bed. In above knee amputation avoid placing pillow below or on inner aspect of the stump so as to prevent fixed flexion or abduction contracture.

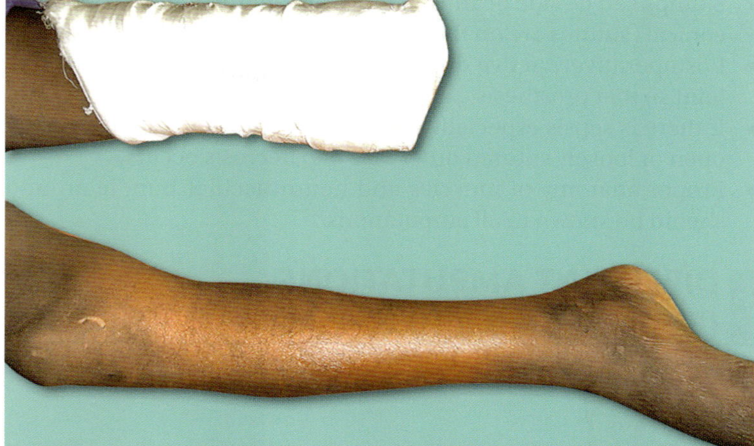
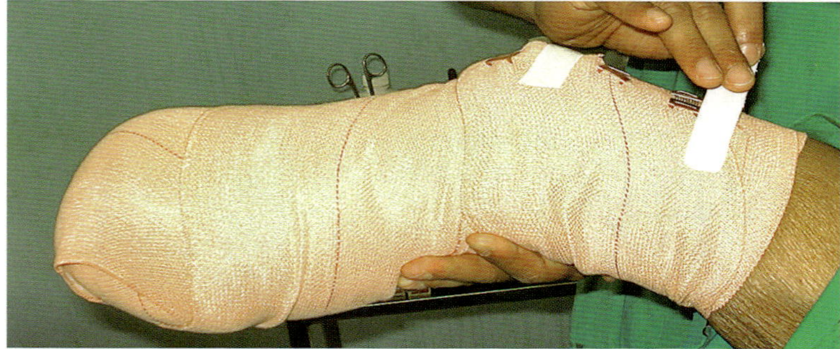
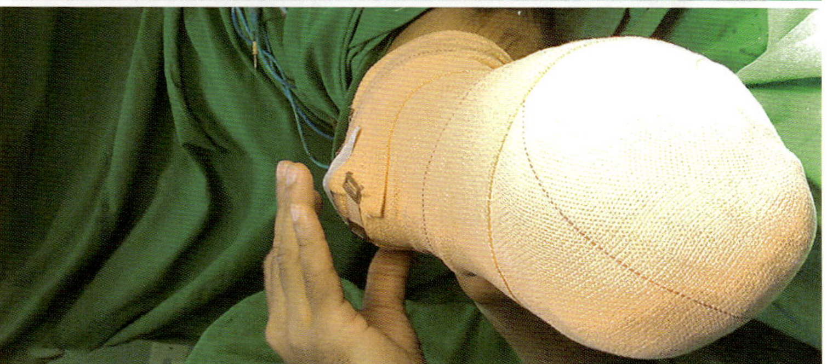

Fig. 10-4: Rigid and soft dressings used for amputation stump.

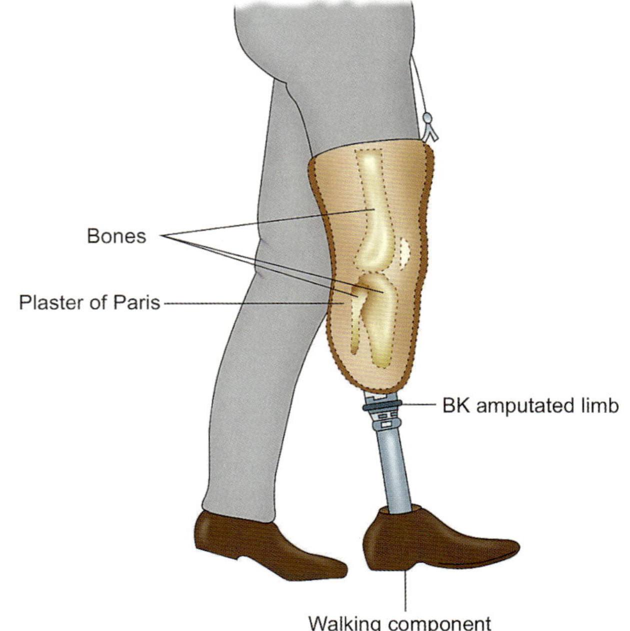

Fig. 10-5: Pylon is plaster cast with walking component used for immediate mobilisation after below knee amputation.

- Stumps can be side bearing (sutures are on the side); end bearing/ conical (sutures are on the end) or cylindrical.
- Postoperatively active exercise should be given to the proximal joint so that prosthesis can be fit to it properly.
- If there is sepsis especially in gangrene limb, flaps should be left open or loosely sutured otherwise flap necrosis occurs.
- Proper anatomy of muscles and neurovascular bundle around should be known in all amputations.

DIFFERENT AMPUTATIONS (FIGS. 10-6 AND 10-7)

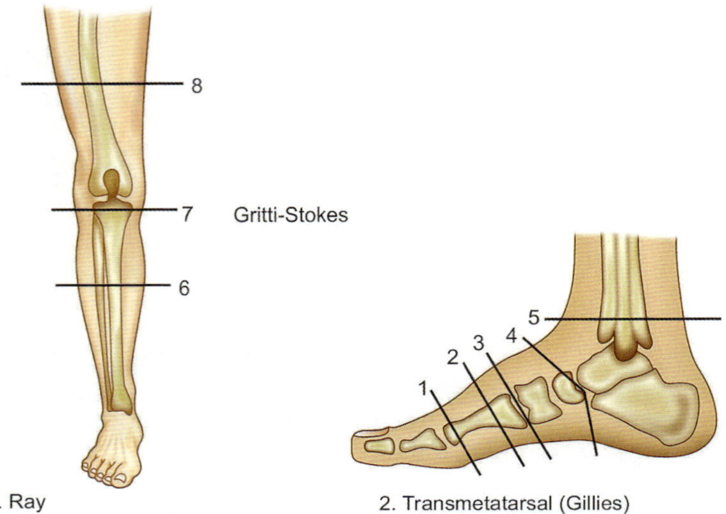

Fig. 10-6: Different levels of amputation in lower limb.

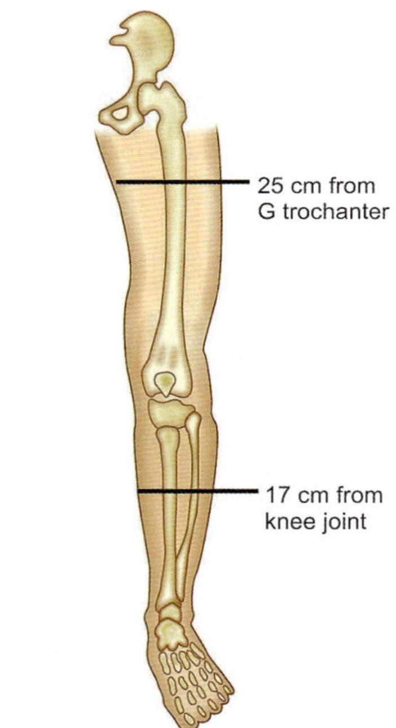

Fig. 10-7: Levels of bone transactions in above knee and below knee amputations.

Toe Amputation

In conditions like trauma, other than vascular or septic causes toe can be amputated at the base of first phalanx so the joint capsule of metatarsophalangeal joint is kept intact. One or two toes can be amputated with retaining of remaining toes. If three or more toes need amputation then all toes should be amputated. When only 2nd toe is amputated it is done at or close to the first interphalangeal joint, otherwise if amputated more proximally it will cause valgus deformity of great toe which can be distressing **(Figs. 10-8 to 10-10)**.

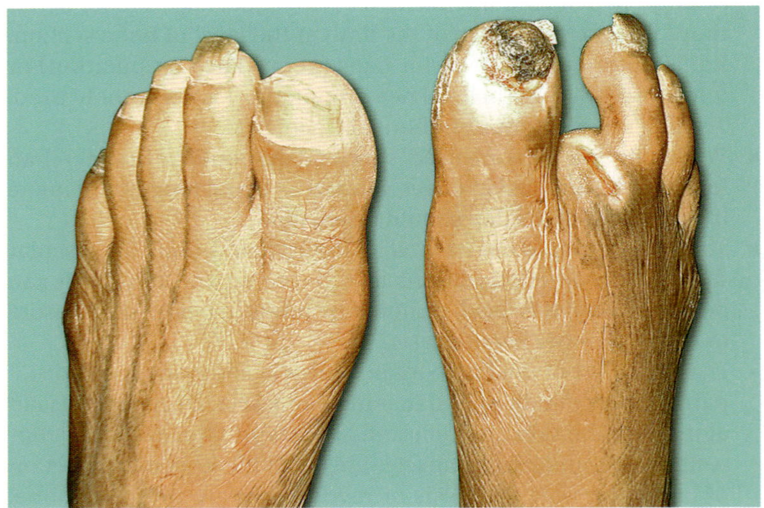

Fig. 10-8: Second toe amputation.

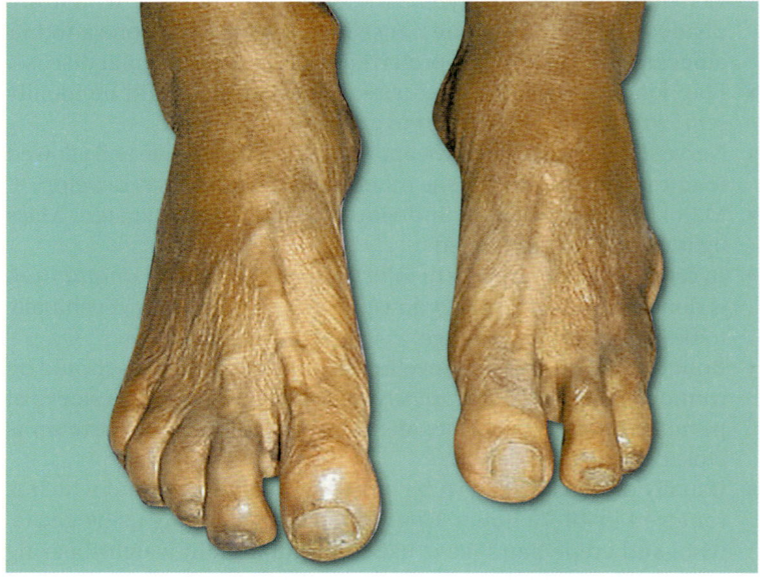

Fig. 10-9: Lateral two toes (4th and 5th) amputation.

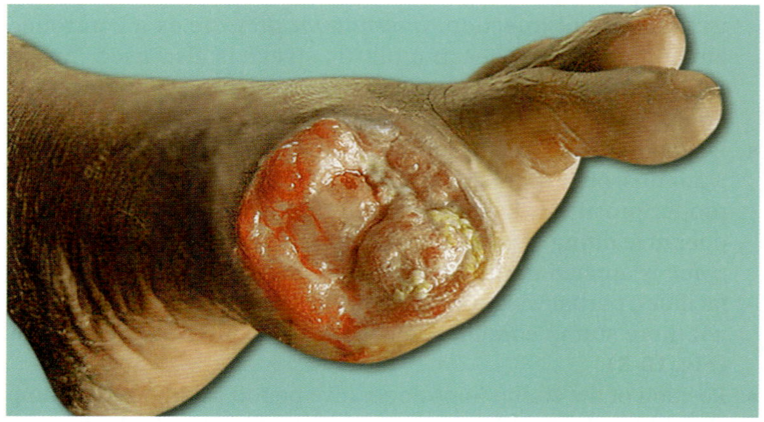

Fig. 10-10: Great toe amputation in vascular disease. Here flap is kept open; not sutured.

Ray Amputation

Amputation of toe is done with removal of corresponding head of metatarsal or metacarpals. Amputation of one or more toes causes loss of push off power during walking. Racquet incision is placed at metatarsophalangeal joint. Incision is deepened directly to the bone; then proximally flap is raised close to the bone. It is important to keep the scissor/knife blade close to the bone to maintain the blood supply of flap. Digital vessels of the toe are ligated near distal end of the wound. Head of the respective metatarsal should be removed as granulation tissue may not form over it when wound is left open like in vascular cases; or necrosis of metatarsal head can occur; or extra callus may be formed once walking is started. Metatarsal head can be cut using bone cutter. Alternatively toe is amputated with same racquet incision initially at the metatarsophalangeal joint level; then head of the metatarsal is removed by piecemeal using bone nibbler. In vascular cases it is better not to suture the flap rather than closing it. Suturing when done, only skin flap is closed using 3-zero polypropylene or polyethylene sutures. Dressing placed. Sutures removed in 7–10 days **(Fig. 10-11)**

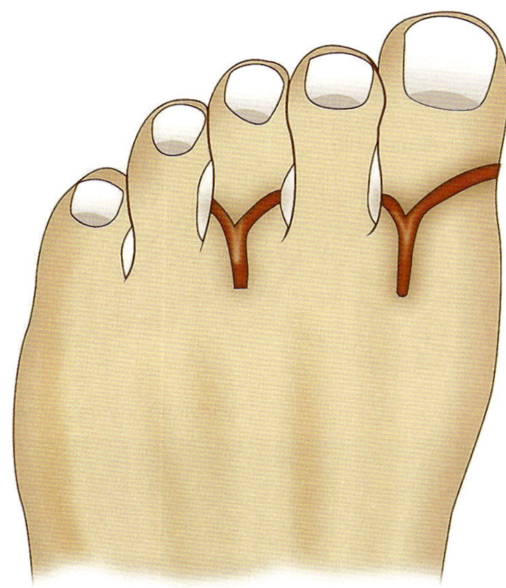

Fig. 10-11: Ray amputation for toes—racquet incision.

Transmetatarsal Amputation (Gillies')

Here amputation is done proximal to the neck of the metatarsals, distal to the base. It is done if skin over the distal part of the dorsum of foot between toes is necrosed and non-viable. Patient can wear a normal shoe with this amputation. But volar and proximal parts of the foot should be viable for this amputation. Plantar part of the incision is close to digits. Dorsal part of the incision is much more proximal than plantar one—3 cm distal to the base of toes. First plantar incision is placed which is deepened up to the metatarsals and flexor tendons. Flexor tendons are individually divided. Volar flap is raised close to the metatarsals. All metatarsals are transected 2 cm from the base. Dorsal incision which is much proximal is deepened to cut soft tissues to remove the distal part of the foot to retain the stump. Deep fascia is sutured. Skin is sutured with suture line on the dorsal aspect. Drain is placed underneath **(Fig. 10-12)**.

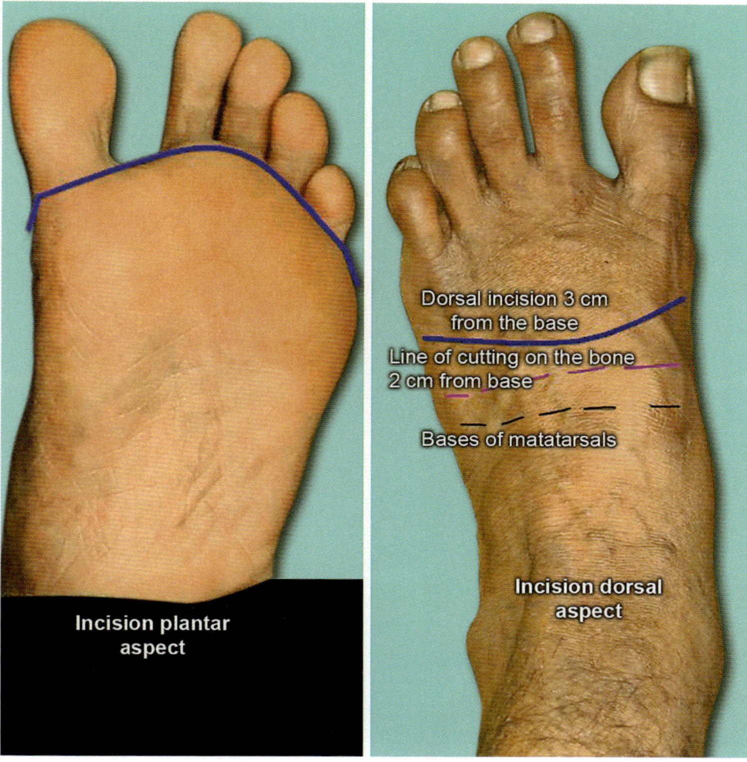

Fig. 10-12: Transmetatarsal amputation.

Lisfranc's Amputation

Tarsometatarsal amputation: Here tarsometatarsal joint is disarticulated with a long volar flap (between tarsals and metatarsals). Long plantar sole flap is used. Tarsometatarsal joint is disarticulated. Flexors and extensors are sutured to soft tissues. It needs a surgical boot. But there is inevitable development of equinovarus deformity. So stabilisation of midtarsal and ankle joints is needed. In *Hey's modification*, 2nd metatarsal is cut at base instead of disarticulation.

Chopart's Amputation (Midtarsal Amputation)

Here talonavicular joint and calcaneocuboid joints are disarticulated (only talus and calcaneum are preserved). Tibialis anterior muscle is sutured to drilled neck of the talus bone. A long volar flap is used and limb is immobilised for 6 weeks after surgery with ankle in neutral position. *Equinovarus deformity* is the problem **(Figs. 10-13A to C)**.

Syme's Amputation

It is removal of the foot with calcaneum and cutting of tibia and fibula just above the ankle joint with retaining heel flap (dividing both malleoli). Heel flap is supplied by medial and lateral calcaneal vessels (branches of posterior tibial artery). *Elephant boot* is used for the limb after Syme's which is inexpensive. Many patients walk well with Syme's stump without difficulty. It is presently mainly used in trauma (crush injury), congenital deformities of foot wherein amputation is inevitable, non-ischaemic damage of foot and malignancies in distal part of the foot. In vascular diseases, calcaneal vessels may not be adequate to maintain the viability of the flap. Ulcer in the heel, cosmetic view if considered, Syme's amputation cannot be done.

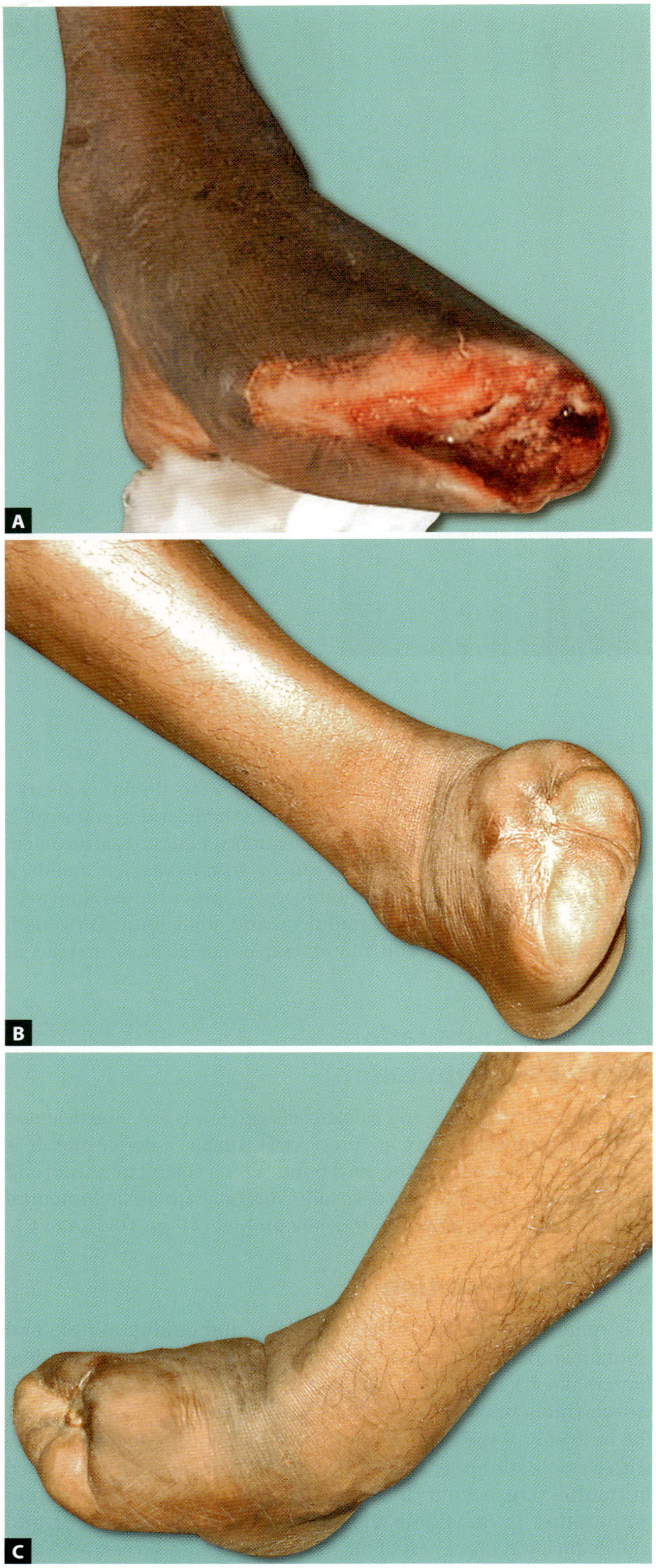

Figs. 10-13A to C: Forefoot amputation.

Incision is from the tip of lateral malleolus to a point 2 cm below the medial malleolus. While raising the flap knife should be very close to the calcaneum so as to avoid injury to calcaneal vessels and to maintain the flap vessels viable—subperiosteal dissection of the calcaneum along posterior flap. Anteriorly retinaculum and tendons are divided. Anterior joint capsule of the ankle is incised; medial and lateral ligaments are divided. Tibia and fibula are cut just 0.6–1.0 cm above the ankle. Plantar fascia is sutured to soft tissues in front of tibia. In *Wagner's method* deep fascia of heel is sutured to drill holes made on the anterior edge of tibia and fibula. *Above knee cast* is essential. Drain placed is removed after 48 hours. Plaster cast to heel pad in 7th day; weight bearing rocker is added in 3rd week; definitive prosthesis is used after 8 weeks.

Advantages are: It is an end bearing stump having good proprioception. Patient can walk without prosthesis. Low energy consumption ambulation is possible.

Disadvantages: Posterior displacement of heel pad; poor cosmesis **(Figs. 10-14 to 10-16)**.

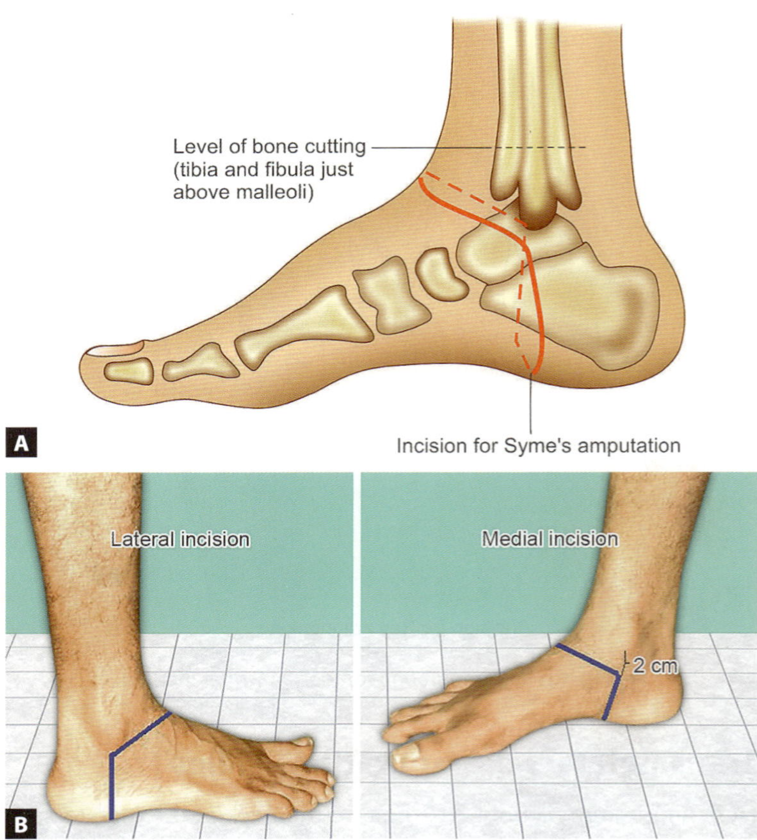

Figs. 10-14A and B: Incision for Syme's amputation and level of amputation.

Two stage Syme's amputation is done when there is gross forefoot infection. First stage—with an incision 1 cm distal and anterior to malleoli, ankle joint is disarticulated with closure of flaps with suction irrigation. Second stage—formal elliptical incision and removal of malleoli.

Boyd's amputation: Anterior part of the calcaneum is excised (osteotomy) just distal to the peroneal tuberosity and calcaneotibial arthrodesis is created. It is done to prevent posterior migration of heel pad.

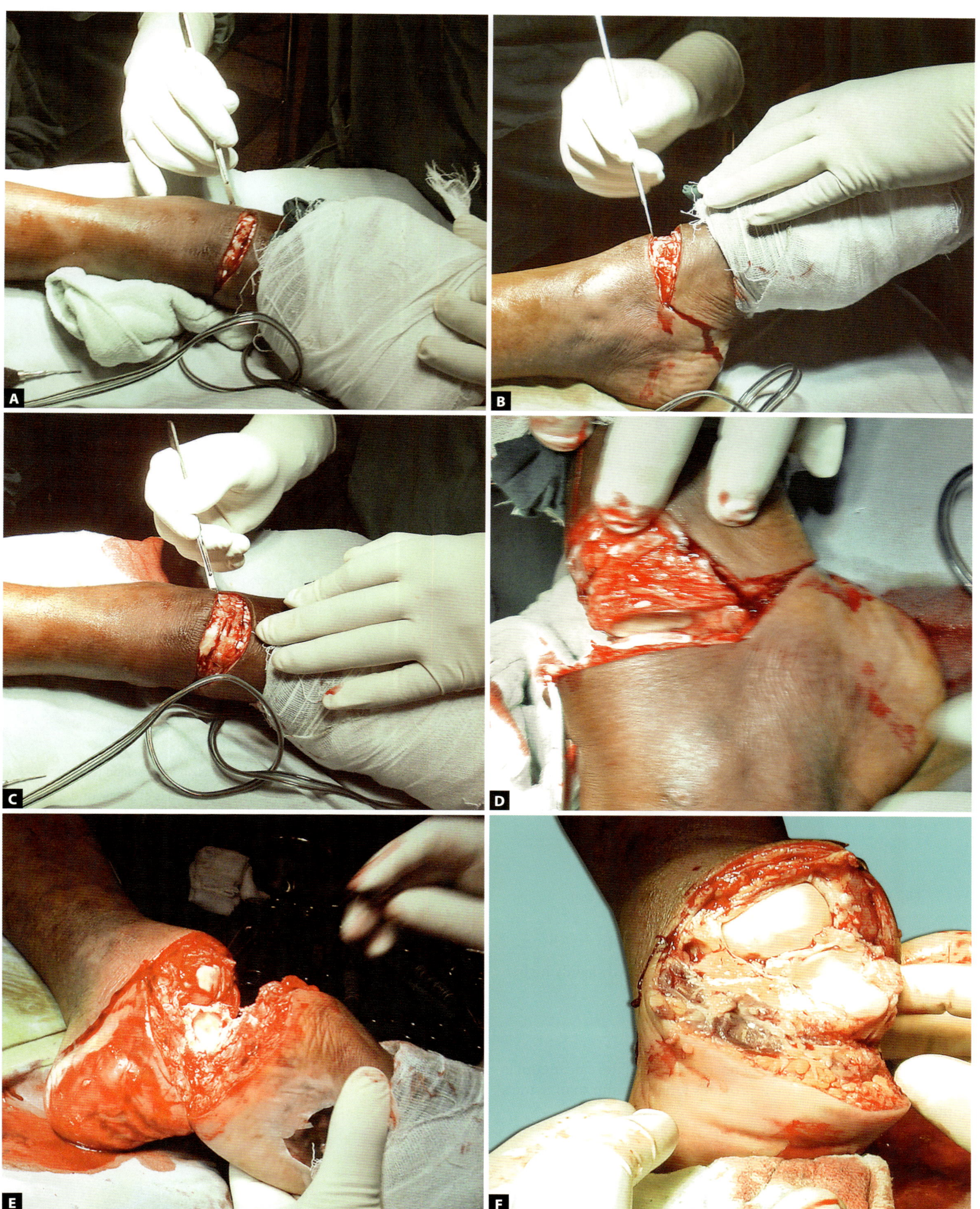

Figs. 10-15A to F

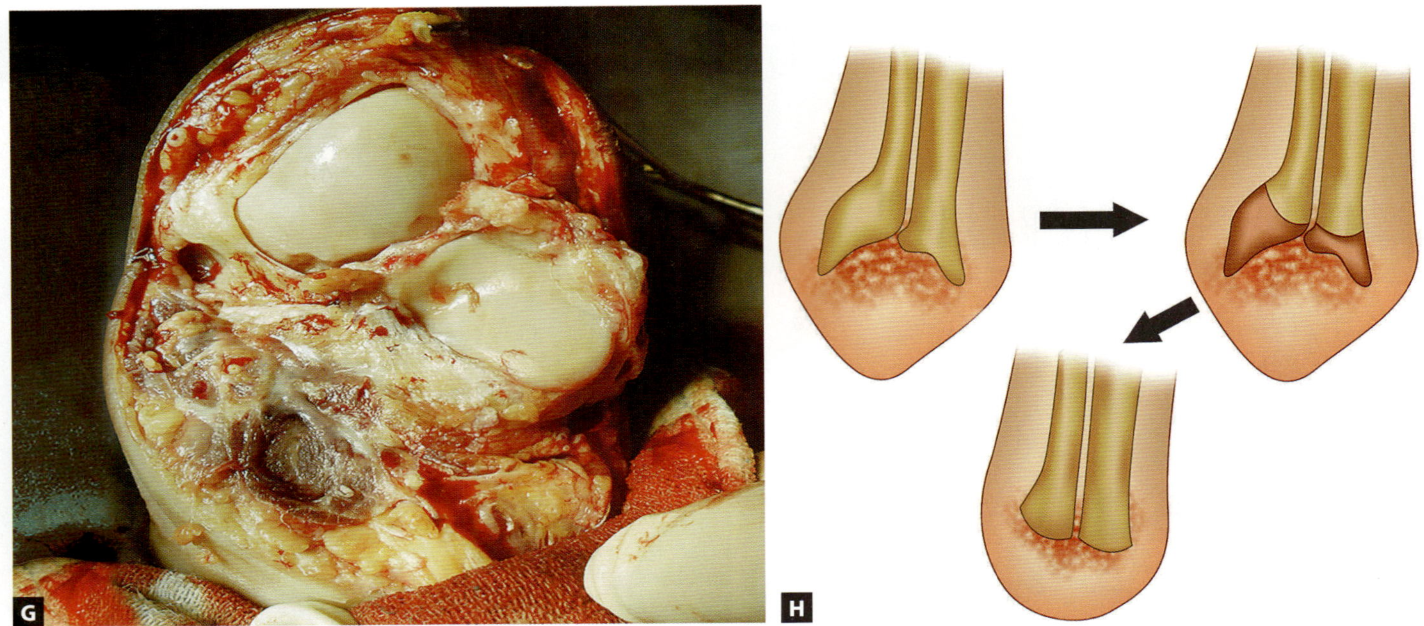

Figs. 10-15G and H

Figs. 10-15A to H: Syme's amputation technique.

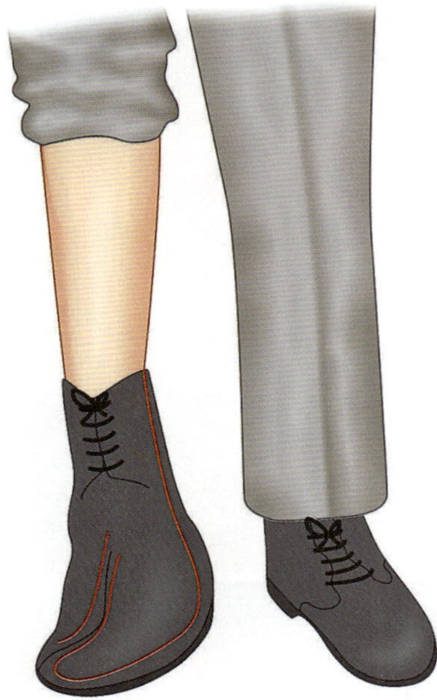

Fig. 10-16: Elephant boot used after Syme's amputation.

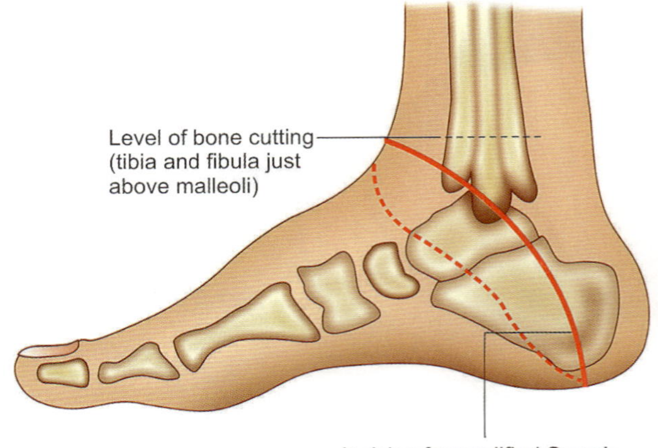

Fig. 10-17: Modified Syme's incision is elliptical one.

Modified Syme's Amputation

Here heel flap is elliptical. Tibia and fibula are divided slightly higher. But variation here is the elliptical flap **(Fig. 10-17)**.

Pirogoff's Amputation

It is like Syme's amputation except posterior part of the calcaneum is retained along with heel flap. It provides longer stump than Syme's amputation **(Fig. 10-18)**.

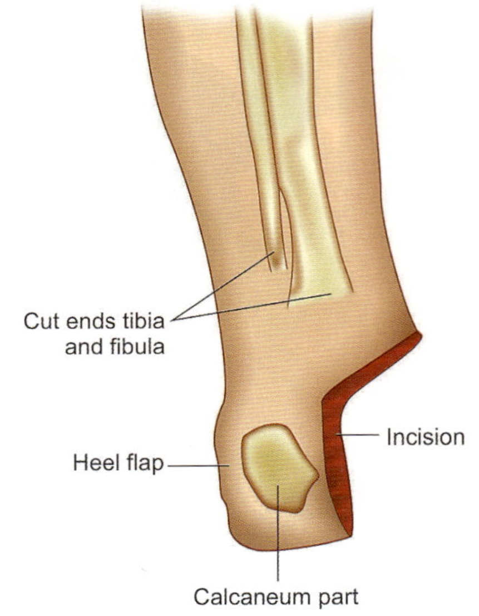

Fig. 10-18: Pirogoff's amputation.

Below Knee Amputation

It is done in peripheral vascular disease, trauma, infections and tumors. In peripheral vascular disease, posterior flap is used. In trauma equal flap may be a choice. It is contraindicated in stump if becomes less than 7.5 cm, flexion deformity of 30° or more, restricted knee joint movement, motor neurological diseases which prevents prosthesis function.

Here long posterior flap with scar placement over anterior aspect is used. Prosthesis placement is better here with greater range of movements without limp and without support. It is also called as *Burgess amputation*. Fibula should be divided first; higher (1 cm) than the proposed site of cut of tibia otherwise its sharp end will press on the skin flap. Tibial stump should be beveled anteriorly. Its edge is smoothened using rasp. Vessels are isolated and individually ligated using silk at the level of the stump. Nerve is pulled down sufficiently and cut at more proximal level without any ligature. Muscle is cut tapering towards the distal end of the flap. Soleus muscle is cut, gastrocnemius is trimmed on the edge to reduce the bulk. Posterior muscles are sutured across the bone end, to the periosteum in front. In more proximal type of below knee amputation, fibula often is removed to allow the proper use of flap. Length of the flap should be 1½ times the circumference of the site (around 12 cm). Stump length is 14–17 cm from knee joint. Minimum length required for prosthesis is 8 cm. For anything proximal, it is better to do above knee amputation. Suction drain ideally or corrugated drain on the edge of the same wound is placed and kept for 72 hours. Adequate dressing pads should be placed over the stump and pressure bandage using crepe is placed. Often posterior slab/cast are used up to mid-thigh to prevent patient from keeping the knee in flexed position. Stump maturation occurs in 8 weeks. Modern artificial limbs like *suction socket prosthesis* are used now **(Figs. 10-19 to 10-21)**.

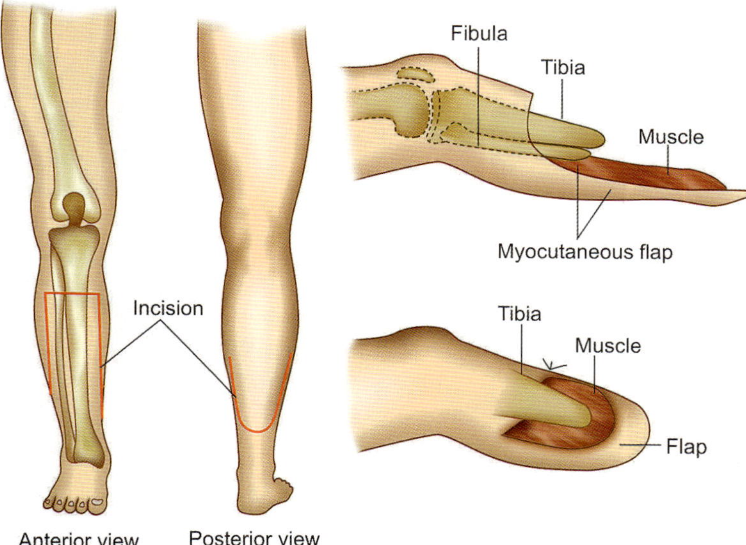

Fig. 10-19: Below knee amputation technique—incision, flap and levels of cutting bones.

Skew flap with skin flaps are equal on medial and lateral aspects but single posterior muscle flap is sutured anteriorly to the tibia. Flap is along long saphenous vein and saphenous nerve medially; and along small saphenous vein and sural nerve laterally **(Fig. 10-22)**.

Periosteum from tibia can be raised from distal to the level of transection of the tibia which is swung over the cut end of fibula to create a synostosis bridge of periosteum between tibia and fibula. This is used when amputation is done in young individual.

Prosthesis fit to below knee stump makes patient to walk normally **(Figs. 10-23 to 10-26)**.

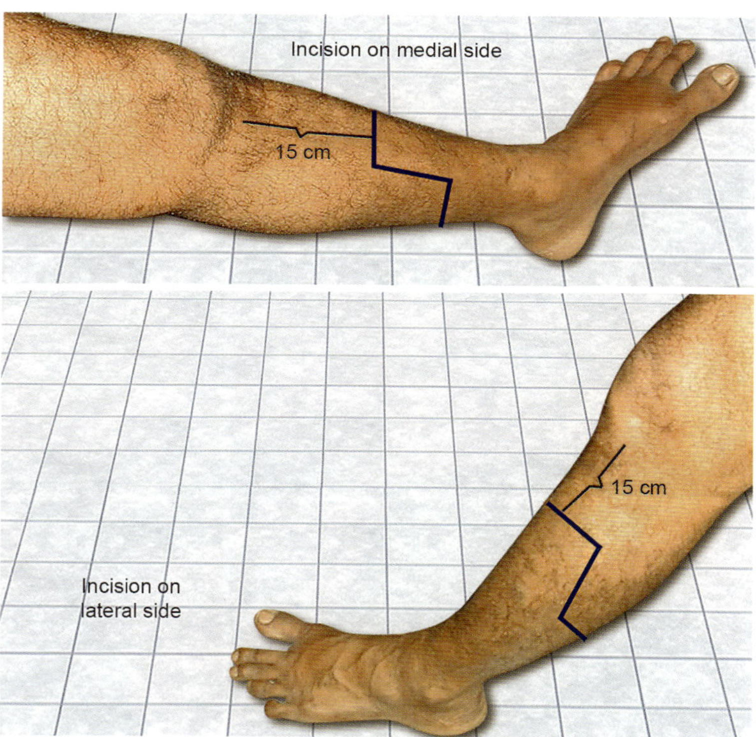

Fig. 10-20: Incision for below knee amputation.

'Peg-Leg' Amputation

It is amputation 5 cm below the knee level—most proximal below knee amputation. It is *not practiced* nowadays. Here anterior flap is rotated posteriorly like a hood and patient kneels and bears weight which is well accustomed to pressure. It is done whenever prosthesis cannot be used probably due to economic causes (in developing countries) **(Fig. 10-27)**.

Knee Joint Disarticulation

It is done in non-functional damaged knee joint wherein below knee amputation is not possible; amputation in non-ambulating bedridden patient; very ill patients; patients who need locked knee prosthesis or *end-bearing stump*. It is *preferred in children*, than doing above knee amputation. Its bulbous end allows suspension of prosthesis without thigh corset.

It is contraindicated in ischaemic conditions. It is cosmetically inferior; less vascular; poor healing; prosthesis controlled gait is difficult to achieve **(Fig. 10-28)**.

It is done in *prone position* through an anterior incision from a point mid-way between lower pole of patella and tibial tubercle to a point 5 cm laterally below the joint line. Incision posteriorly curves towards midline in popliteal fossa 2.5 cm above joint line. Flaps are *medial and lateral*; medial is larger. Incision is deepened in posterior aspect first; vessels and nerves are divided; posterior muscles and joint capsule is cut; joint is opened; cruciate, medial and lateral ligaments are cut; patellar tendon is cut; patella is retained. Once joint is disarticulated patellar tendon is sutured to cruciate ligaments and retinaculum is sutured to hamstrings. Anteroposterior longitudinal scar is formed. Drain should be placed.

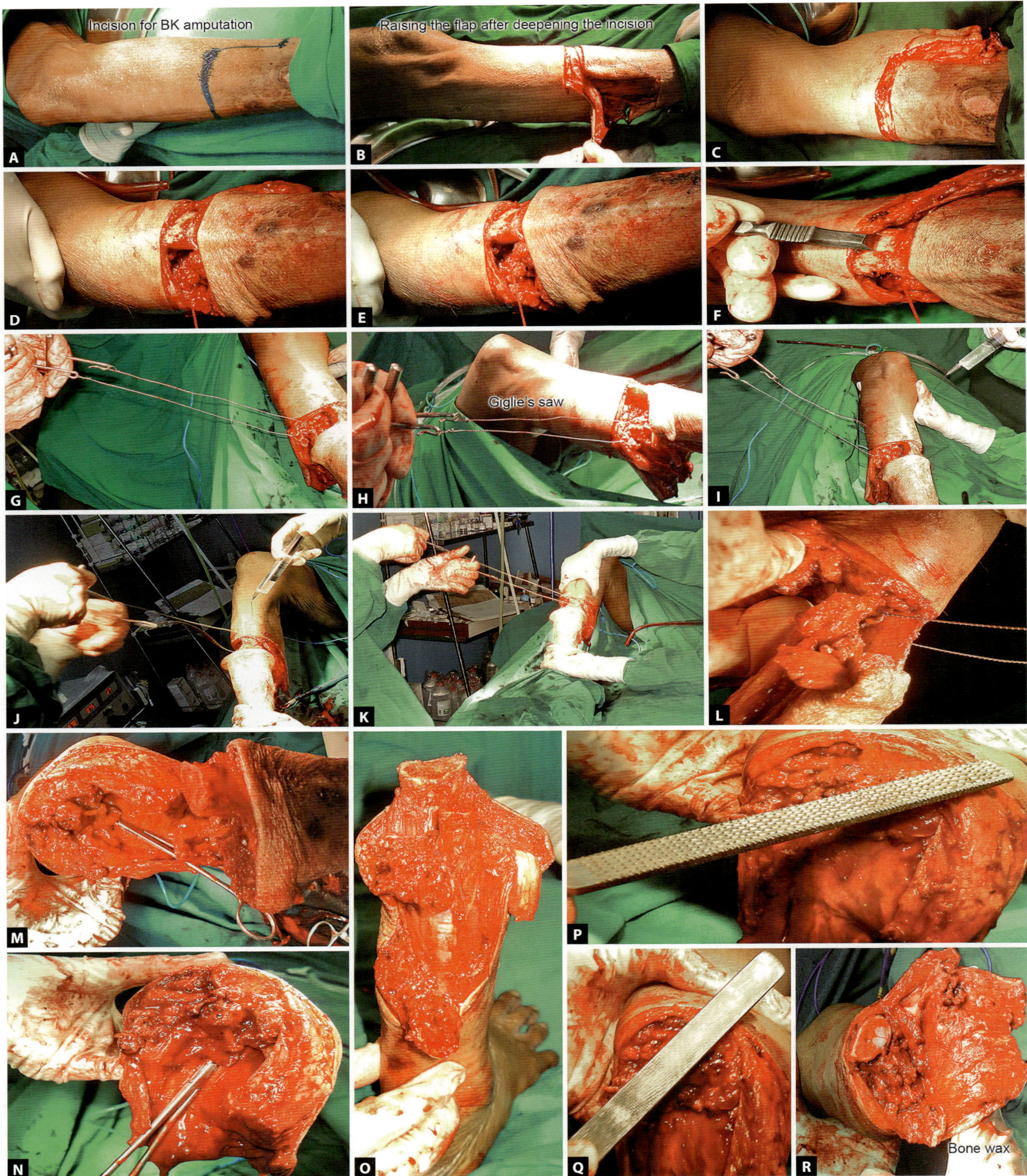

Figs. 10-21A to R

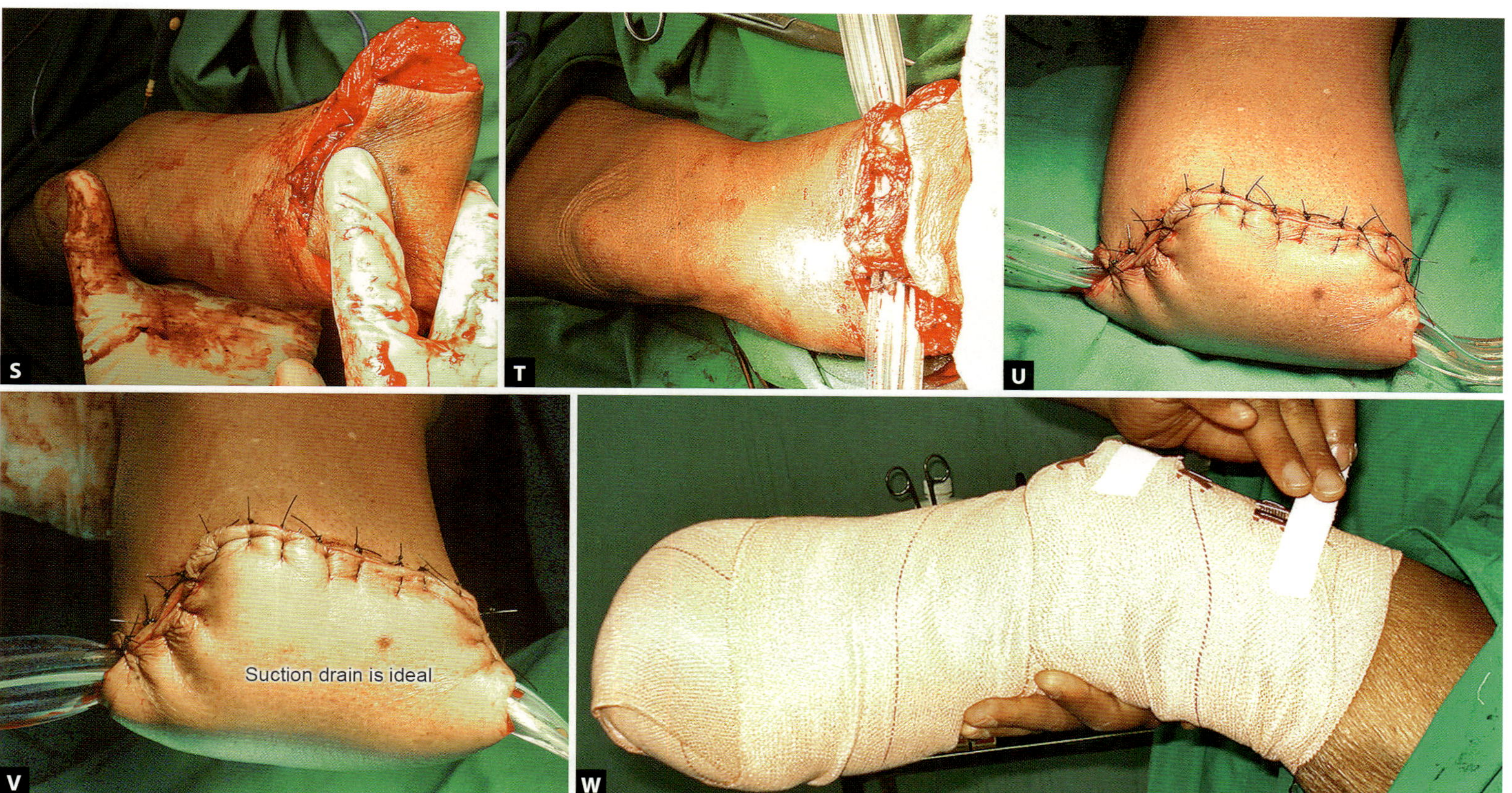

Figs. 10-21S to W

Figs. 10-21A to W: Technique of below knee amputation.

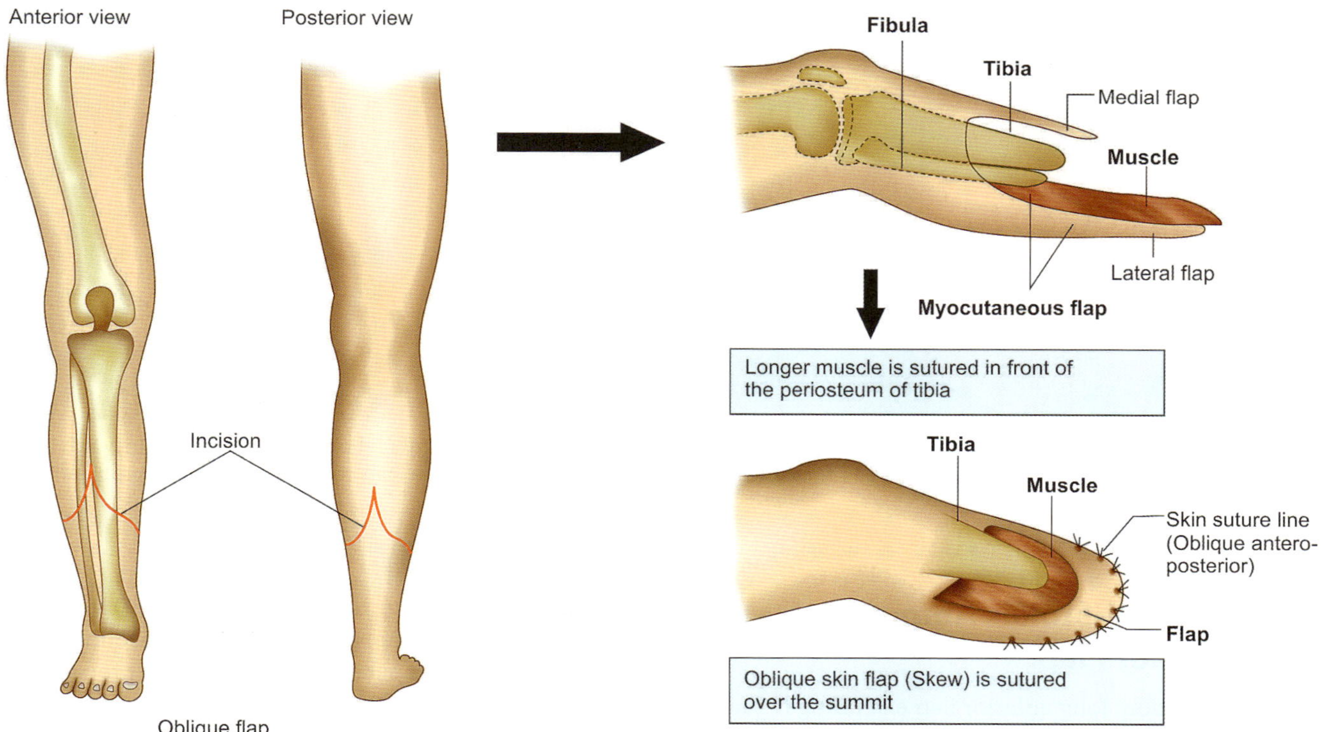

Fig. 10-22: Skew flap for below knee amputation.

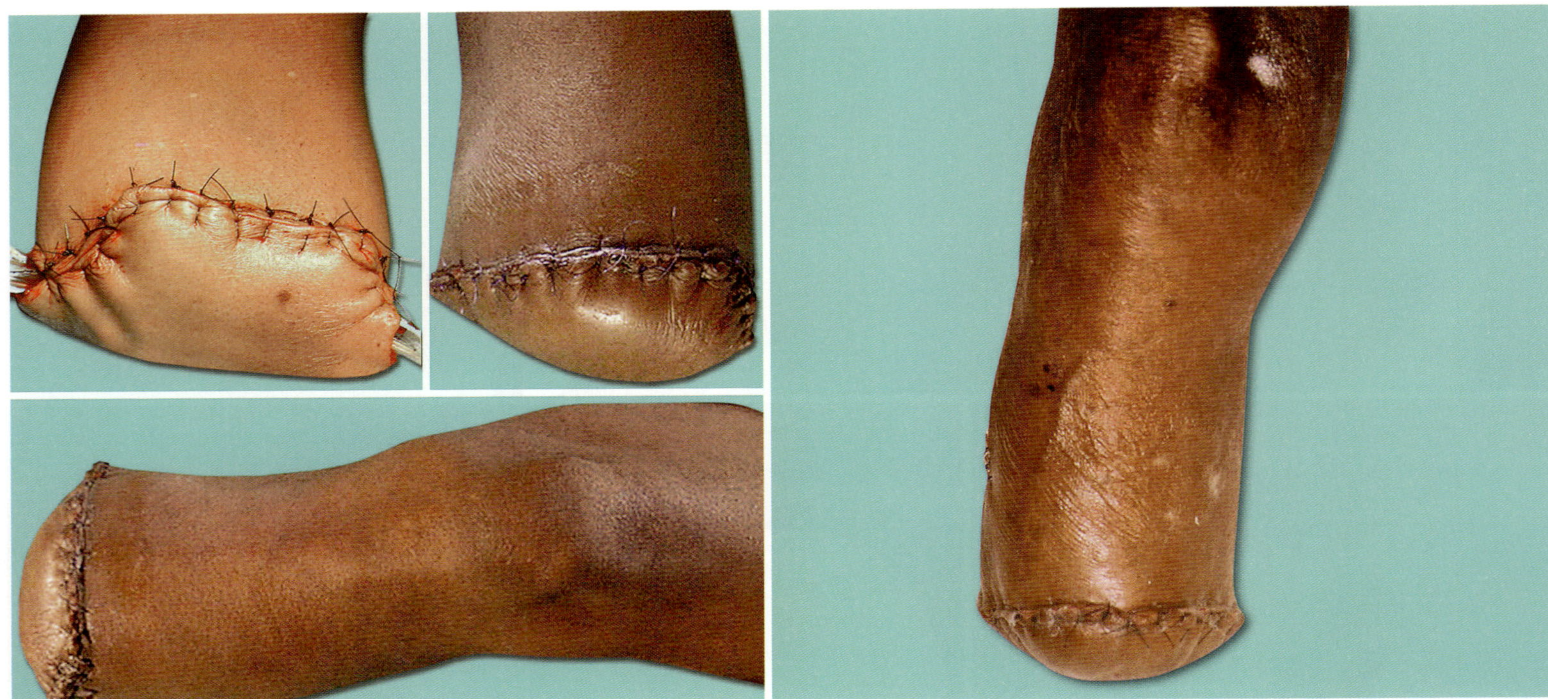

Fig. 10-23: Below knee amputation—long posterior flap. Note the placing of the drain.

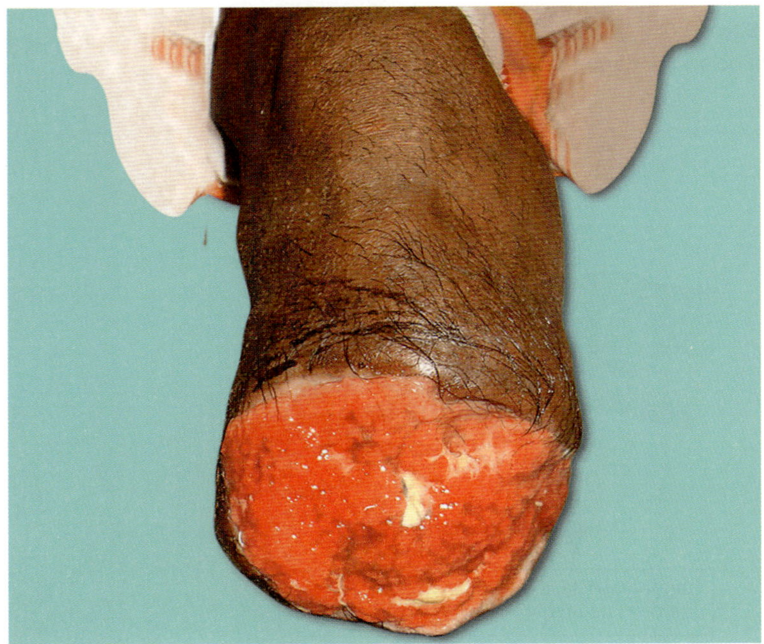

Fig. 10-24: Below knee amputation flap necrosis has occurred which eventually granulated with regular dressings. Area is ready for skin grafting.

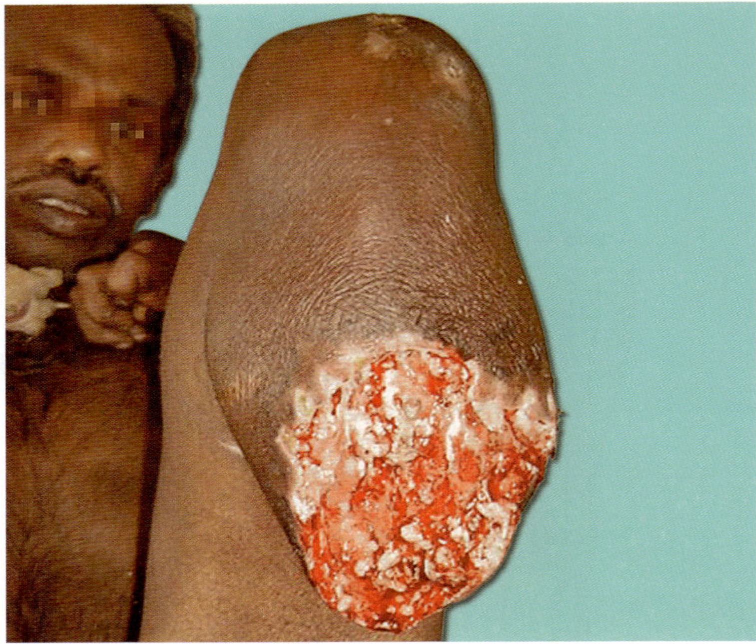

Fig. 10-25: Below amputation with flap necrosis in which later wound got granulated well. Knee joint contracture is a great problem in rehabilitation.

Transcondylar/Gritti-Stokes Amputation with Long Posterior Flap

It is done in supine position; long anterior flap extending below the patella is used (flap is not raised posteriorly). Patellar tendon is cut; joint is entered from front; posterior soft tissues and muscles are divided. Femur is divided just above the articular surface; articular surface of the patella is shaved off; patella is anchored to the divided femur through drill holes with wires passed through drill holes; patellar tendon is sutured to hamstrings. Femur may be divided 30° obliquely anteroposteriorly as a modification. There is risk of non-union between patella and femur. This procedure is *no longer performed* **(Figs. 10-29 and 10-30)**.

Above Knee Amputation

It is done in ischaemia, trauma, sepsis and gangrene which is spreading above. Often patient might have undergone below knee

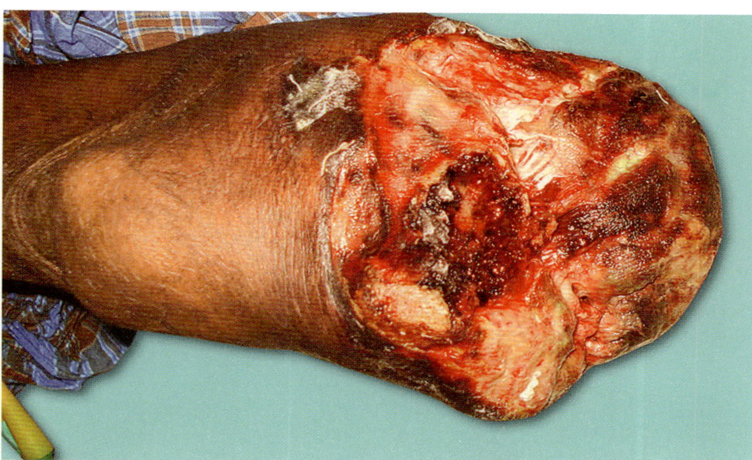

Fig. 10-26: Below knee amputation stump which is badly infected, this may need above knee amputation.

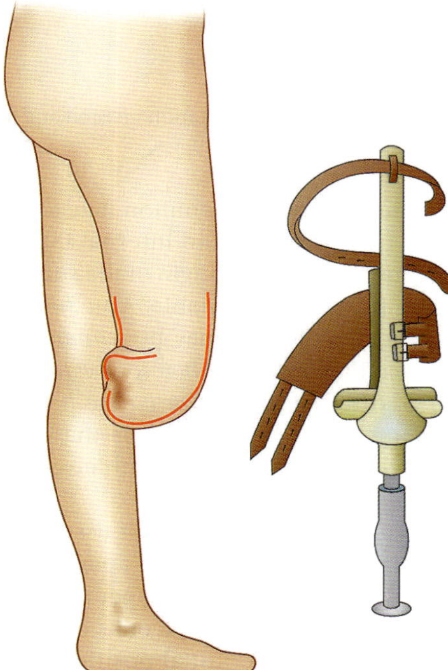

Fig. 10-27: 'Peg leg' amputation is below knee amputation done close to the knee joint (5 cm stump) with folding flap and metallic support down. It is not used now.

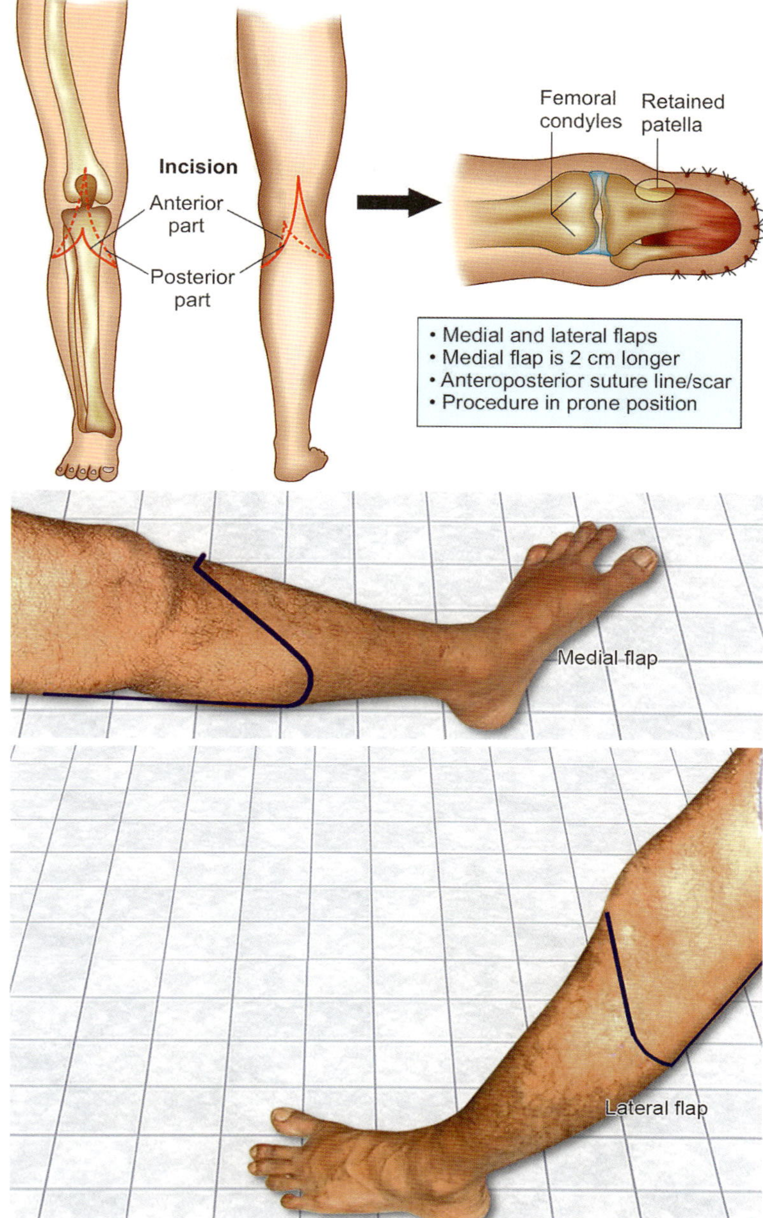

Fig. 10-28: Technique of knee disarticulation.

amputation earlier but now as indicated for above knee amputation as either BK flaps are not good or sepsis is extending above. It is usually contraindicated in children (done only in undue definitive indication) or if stump is less than 7.5 cm.

Advantages are technically easy, healing chances are better and faster. Disadvantages are cosmetically poor, rehabilitation is difficult, and prosthesis fitting is not proper, patient needs a third support for walk with often a limp.

Usually equal anterior and posterior flaps are used. Alternatively long anterior flap may be used.

Lower third and middle third level amputations are done. Ideally the required length of the femur as stump is 25 cm from the tip of the greater trochanter. Length lesser than 10 cm is not possible and one needs to do hip disarticulation. In children as growing epiphysis of femur is at the lower end, as much length of femur as possible should be preserved.

Femoral vessels are individually ligated two times. Femur is cut with anterolateral bevel. Sciatic nerve is pulled and cut; accompanying artery, arteria nervi ischiadii when needed should be ligated separately not along with sciatic nerve. Quadriceps is sutured to hamstrings or the drill holes made in cut distal end of the femur. This myodesis prevents muscle imbalance. Suction drain and soft crepe bandage dressing is placed. Patient is advised to lie prone for 15–30 minutes a day to prevent flexion contracture of hip joint **(Figs. 10-31 to 10-34)**.

Hip Disarticulation

It is done whenever it is not possible to save the minimum 10 cm length of the femur. Incision used is either single posterior flap—Solcum's approach (better) or anterior racquet incision—Boyd's approach. Posterior flap stump is better to fit prosthesis. Anterior racquet incision begins as a vertical incision along the femoral vessels with medial and lateral flaps curving posteriorly; medial flap is longer. Scar here will be away from perineum. In the posterior

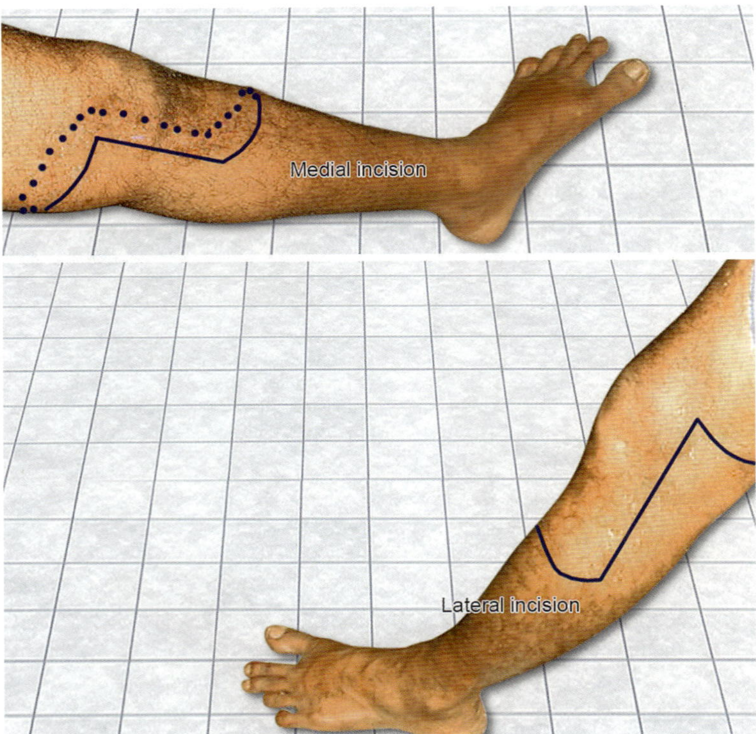

Fig. 10-29: Incision for Gritti-stokes amputation.

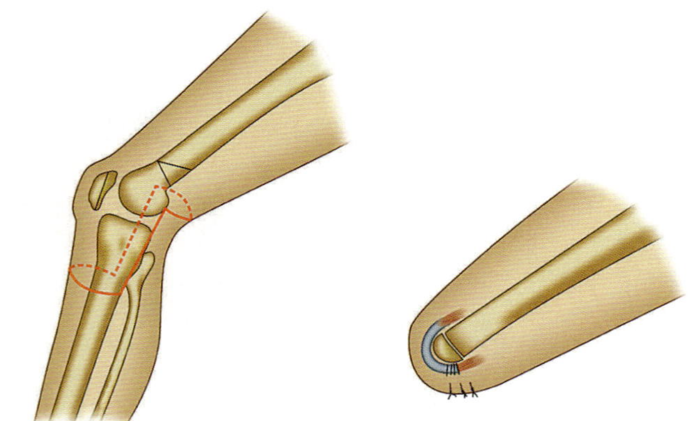

- Long anterior flap
- Femur is cut just above the condyles straight or obliquely
- Patellar articular surface is shaved and apposed to cut surface of femur
- Quadriceps/patellar tendon is sutured to hamstrings
- Procedure is done in supine position

Fig. 10-30: Gritti-stokes amputation.

flap the length of the flap should be 1½ times the anteroposterior diameter of the limb at hip joint level. The anterior part of the incision is 2.5 cm below and parallel to inguinal ligament. Anterior part of the incision is deepened; muscles are divided in the line of incision; joint is opened from front; adductors, hamstrings and gluteus maximus are divided with retaining part of it in posterior flap. Joint capsule and short muscles are cut to complete the disarticulation. Muscles and flaps are sutured to create a stump **(Fig. 10-35)**.

Hind Quarter Amputation

Interinnominoabdominal amputation (Sir Gordon Taylor amputation): Removal of one side pelvis with innominate bone, pubis, muscles

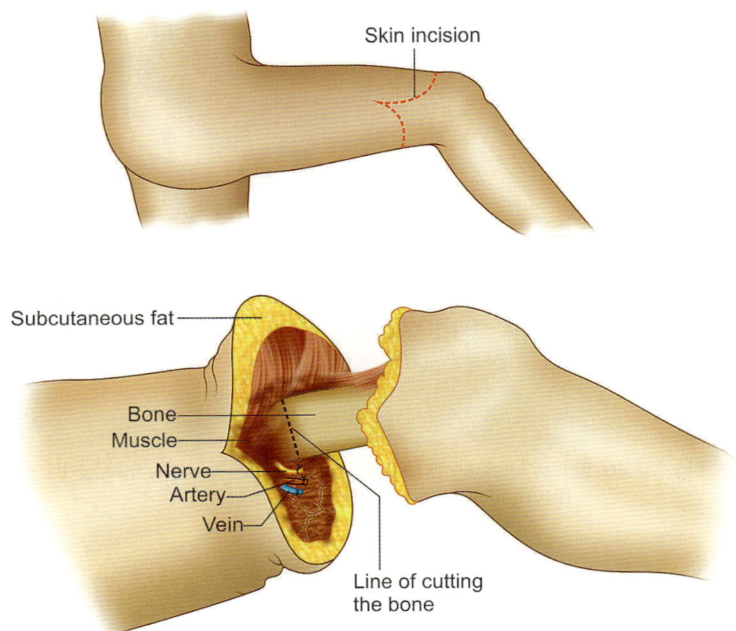

Fig. 10-31: Above knee amputation incision and approach.

and vessels. Original ligation of common iliac artery is modified to individual ligations of external and internal iliac vessels. Internal iliac artery is ligated beyond the origin of the superior gluteal artery to keep the large posterior flap viable. *Now hind quarter name is replaced by hemipelvectomy*. It may be *standard hemipelvectomy* with classic gluteal flap; *extended hemipelvectomy* with removal of posterior part of the sacrum; *conservative hemipelvectomy* with retaining part of the pubis, ilium bones on that side. *Internal hemipelvectomy* is new method wherein hemipelvectomy is done with preserving the limb.

It is done in malignant diseases of soft tissues of pelvis or thigh; severe congenital malformations; failed above knee amputation or hip disarticulation. Procedure needs proper prior preparation of the perineum and limb to prevent sepsis. 6 units of blood should be kept ready as bleeding is common. Initial position is supine with long narrow sand bags placed under shoulder and buttock of same side. Later patient is rolled to lateral position for posterior flap dissection.

Standard hindquarter amputation is done with an elliptical incision with anterior abdominal muscles being divided in the line of incision. Inferior epigastric vessels are ligated. Pubic symphysis is divided. Peritoneum and ureter are pushed medially with blunt dissection. Internal iliac artery is ligated distal to the origin of the superior gluteal artery. External iliac vessels are divided. Ilium is divided across greater sciatic notch. Main part of the gluteus maximus is retained in the flap supplied by superior gluteal artery. Remaining soft tissues and nerves are cut. Obturator, pudendal, other gluteal vessels are ligated. Flap is sutured after proper haemostasis **(Fig. 10-36)**.

UPPER LIMB AMPUTATIONS

Upper limb amputations are less commonly done (3–15%) as compared to lower limb amputations. Trauma, malignant tumour, gangrene are the indications. All possible length should be preserved to improve the efficacy of the prosthesis. In distal amputations, prosthesis function will be better **(Fig. 10-37)**.

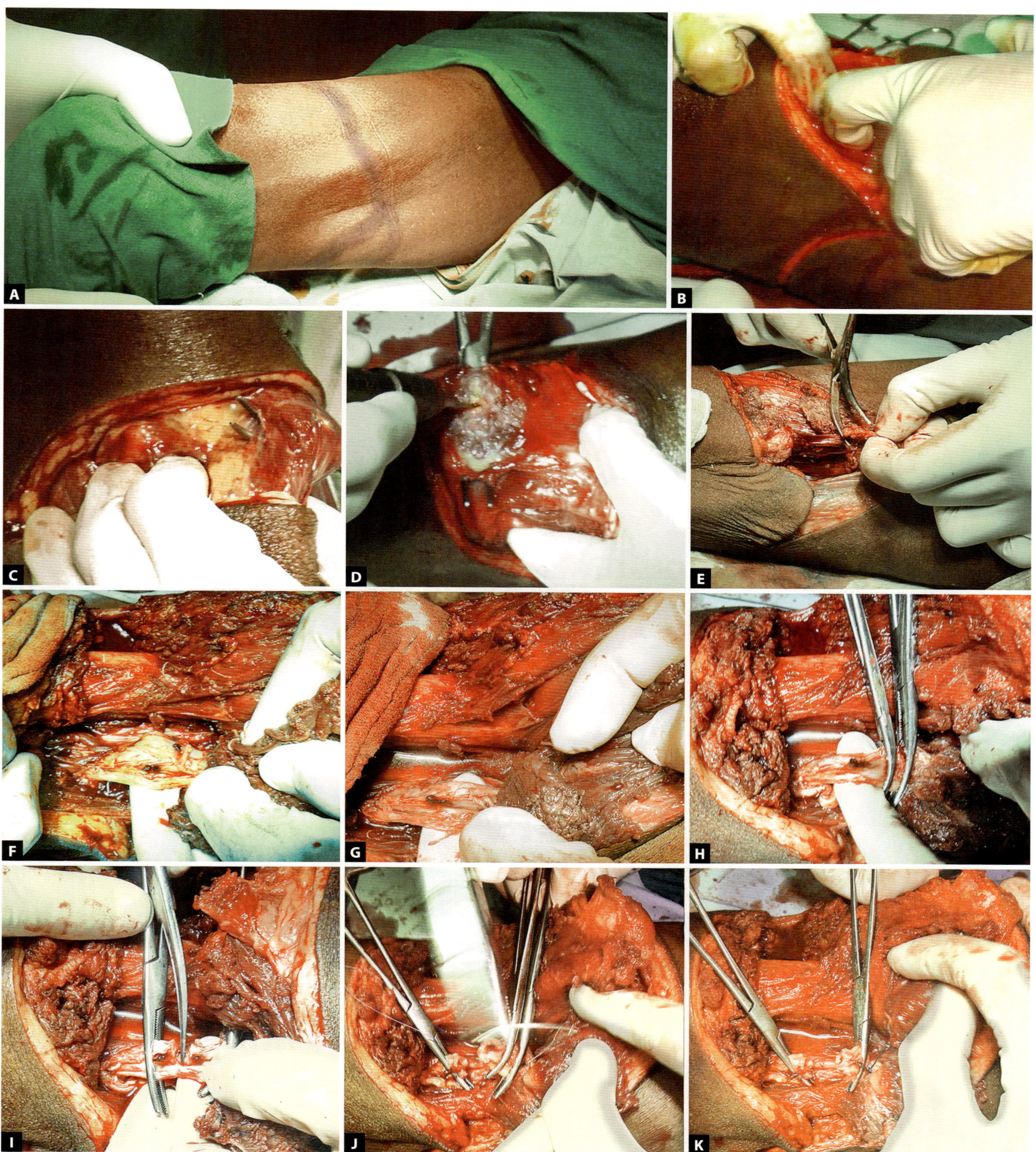

Figs. 10-32A to K

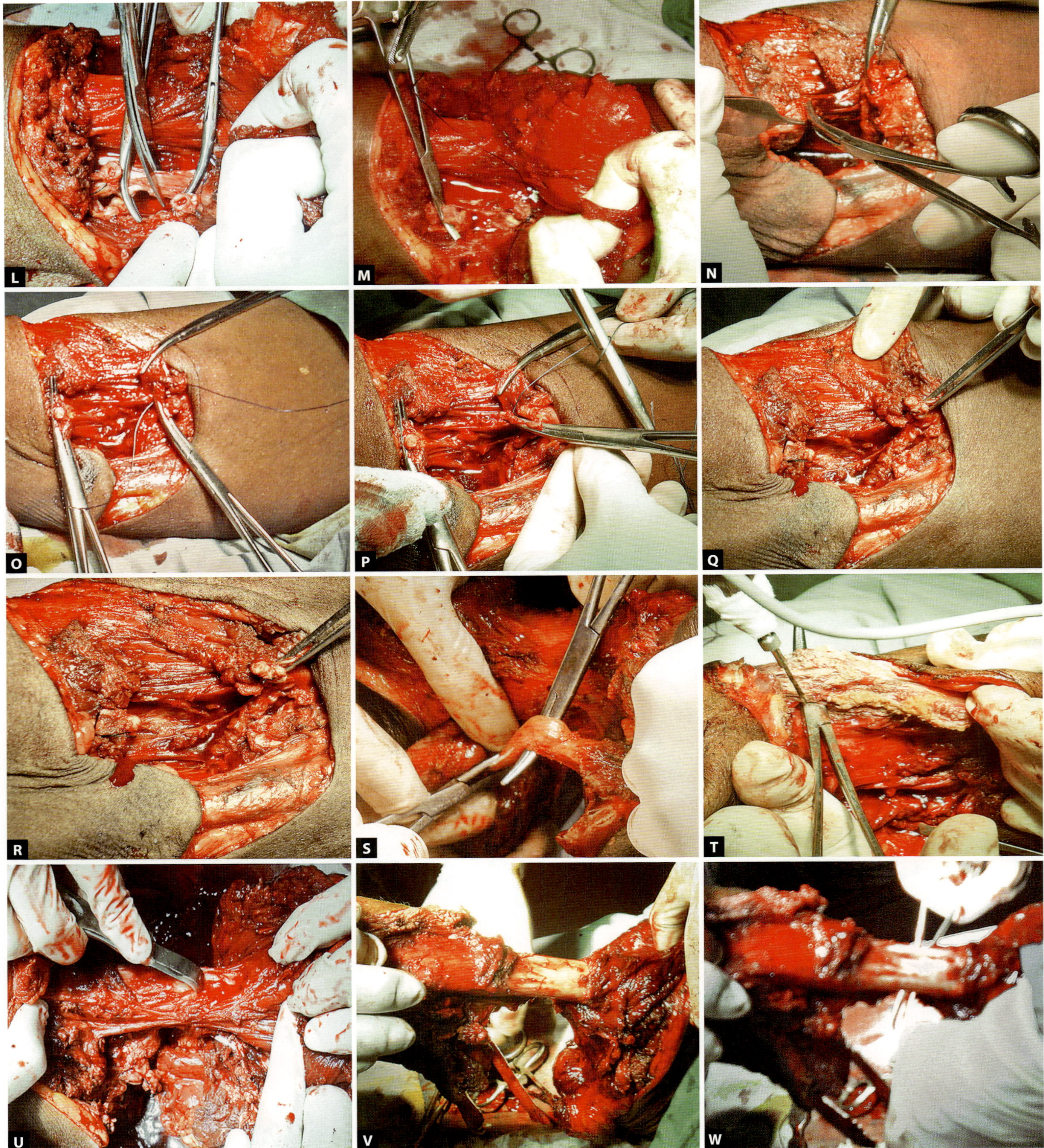

Figs. 10-32L to W

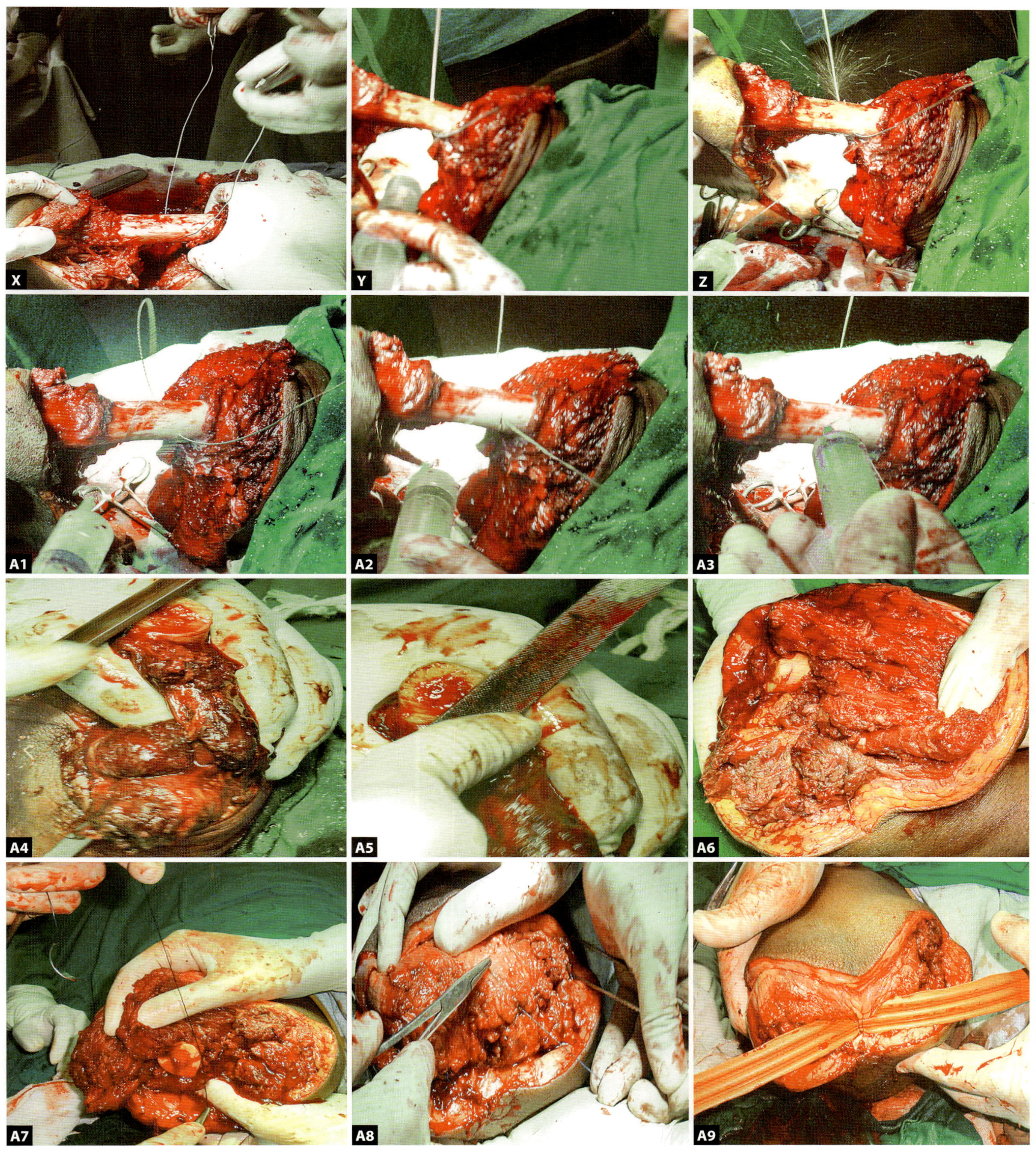

Figs. 10-32X to A9

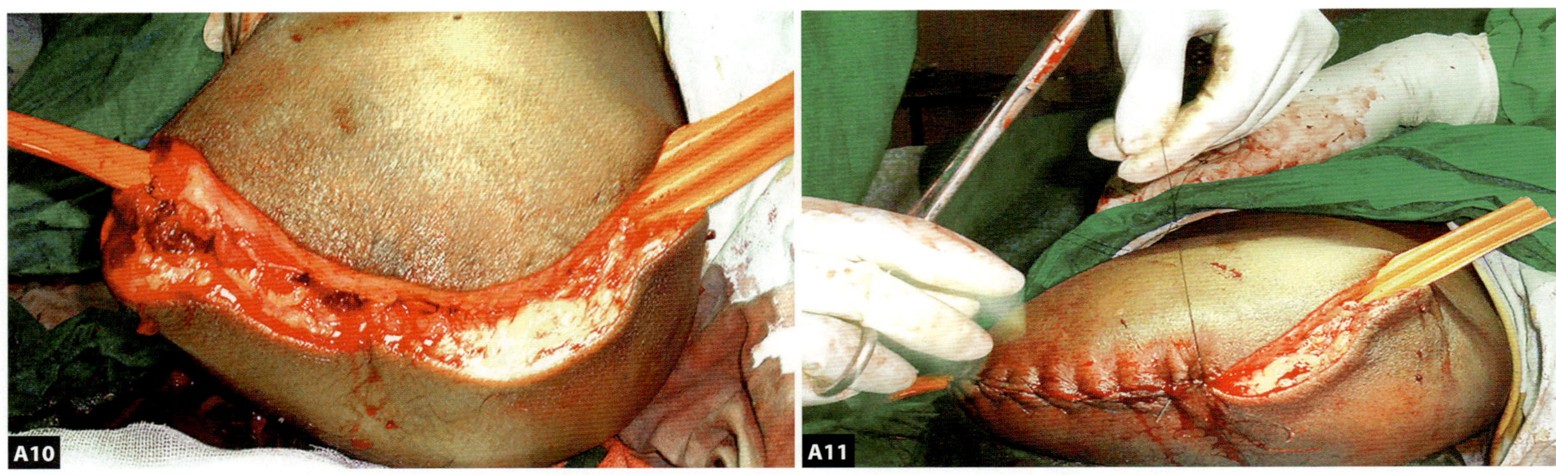

Figs. 10-32A10 and A11

Figs. 10-32A to A11: Steps in above knee amputation.

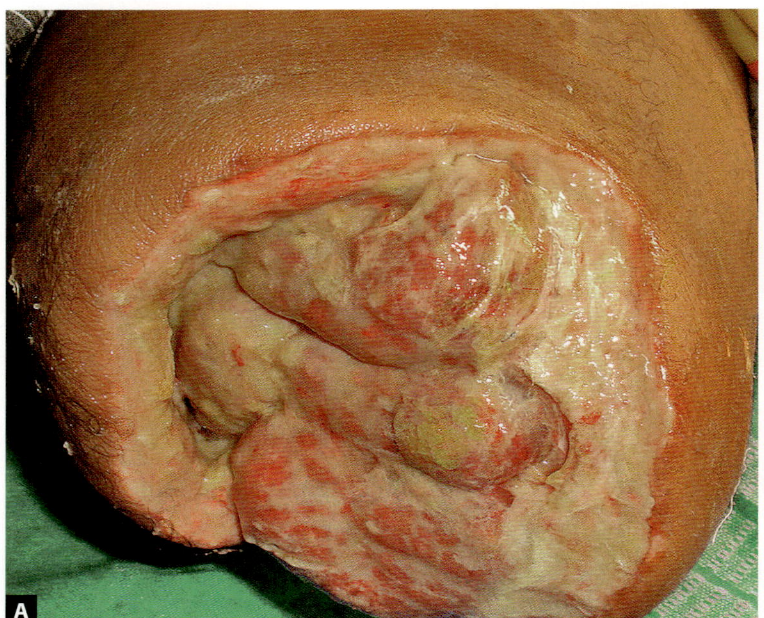

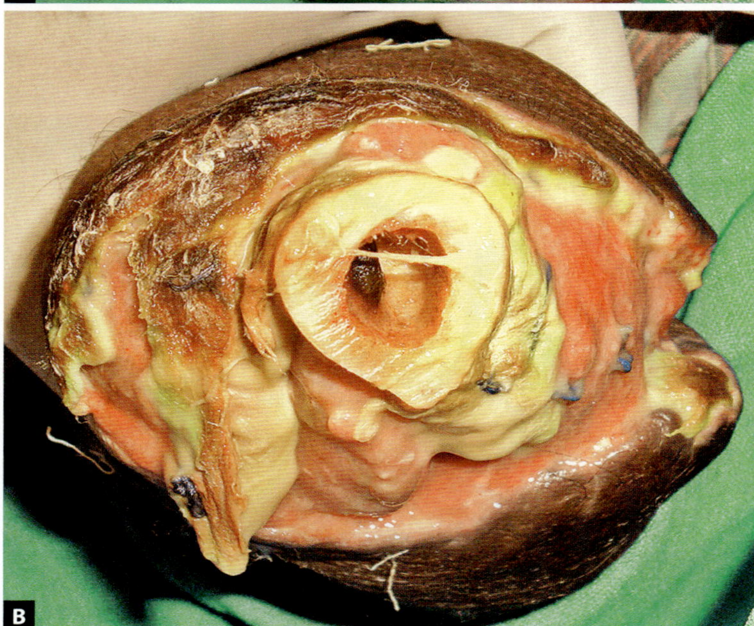

Figs. 10-33A and B: Above knee amputation wound which is infected in a diabetic patient with exposed cut end of femur. after above knee amputation is seen in another photograph.

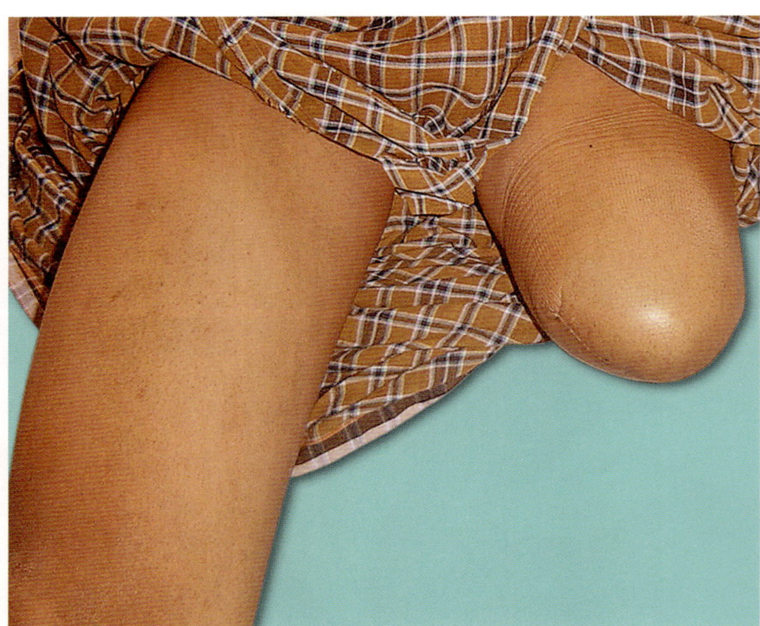

Fig. 10-34: Above knee amputation for osteosarcoma of upper end of tibia.

HAND AMPUTATIONS

Loss of blood supply is the only absolute indication. Five tissue areas are observed—skin, tendon, nerve, bone and joint. If three or more tissues are damaged then amputation may be needed. In traumatised finger if skin is retained but not bone and tendons, then this skin with its blood supply can be used to cover defect locally. Any retained tissue may be used for reconstruction in the hand elsewhere like bone, tendons.

Flaps used for amputations in hand are usually long volar with scar on the dorsal aspect. Digital nerves should be cut 6 mm proximally. Digital arteries are ligated using 3-zero polyglactic acid or cauterised using bipolar cautery. Tendons are drawn distally to divide and later to retract proximally. Condyles should be trimmed when amputation is done through joints. In amputation of distal phalanx distal interphalangeal joint is preserved so that tendon functions are retained; in middle phalanx proximal interphalangeal joint is preserved. In middle and ring fingers amputations of proximal

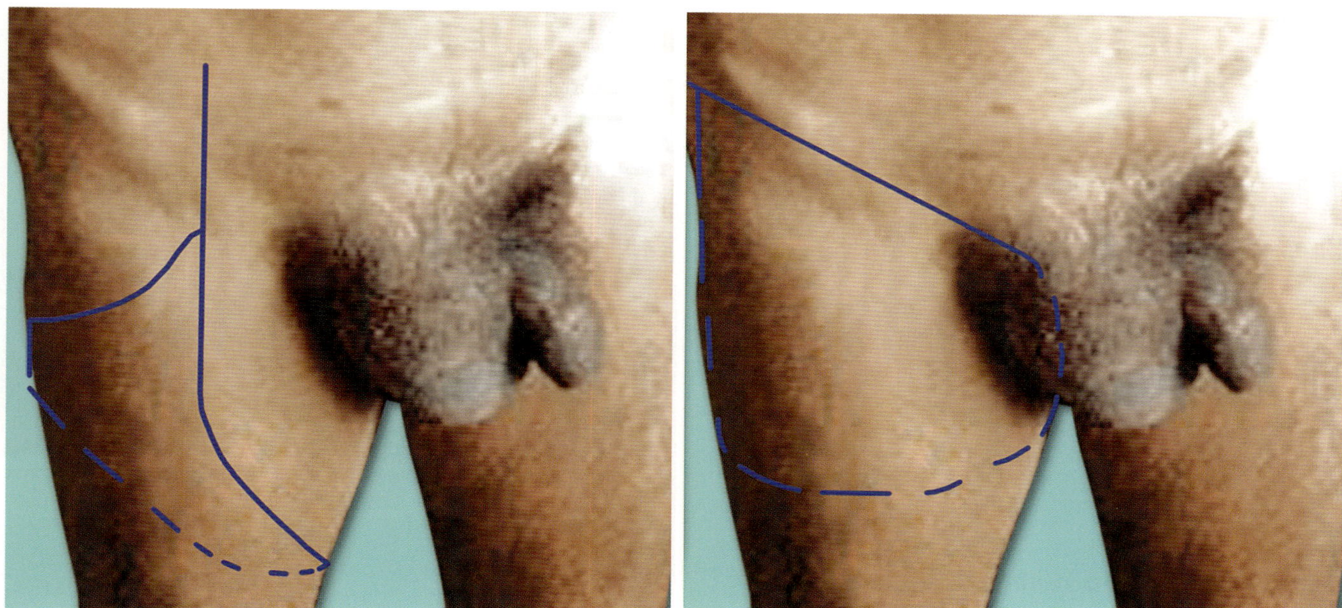

Fig. 10-35: Anterior and posterior incision in hip disarticulation procedure.

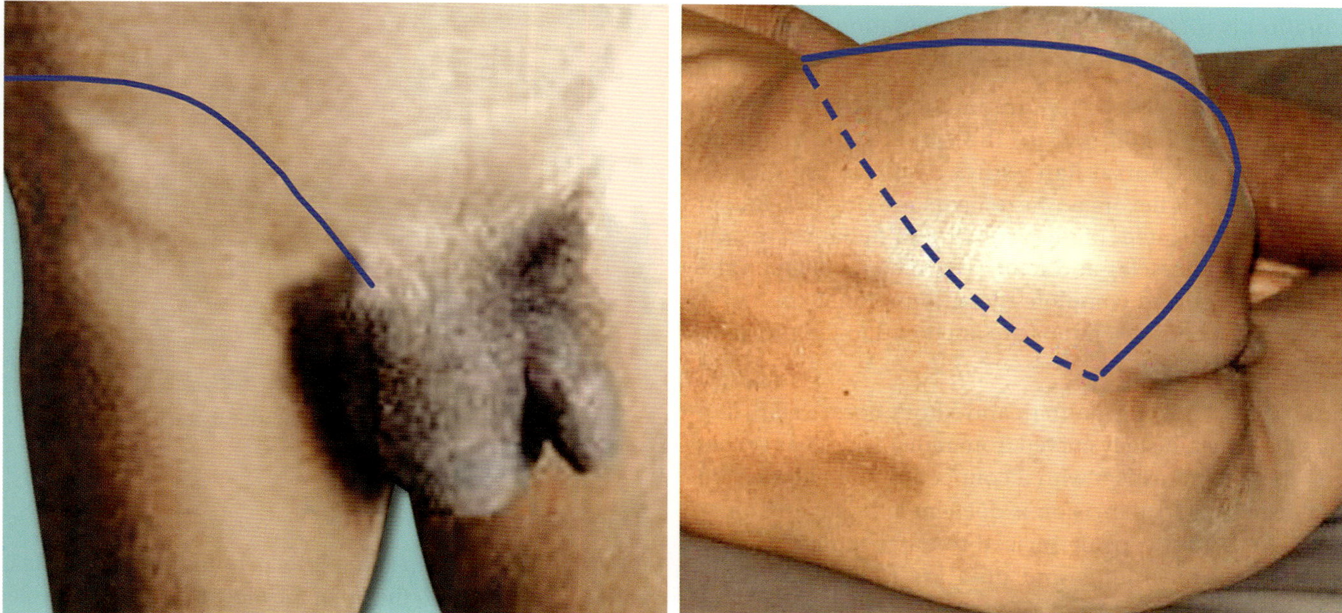

Fig. 10-36: Incision for hindquarter amputation.

phalanx are done so that stump retained in proximal phalanx can be used for power grip of hand using active flexion by intrinsic muscles. In index and little fingers proximal phalanx amputation is a waste and such stump prevents the proper pinch by thumb and fingers. So amputation through respective metacarpals is done **(Fig. 10-38)**.

Amputation of Index Finger

Here proximal phalanx is never retained. Second metacarpal is divided at its distal part proximal to metacarpophalangeal joint. Volar flap incision is placed. Dissection is started from dorsal aspect. Dorsal digital nerve and digital vessels are divided. Extensor digitorum and extensor indices tendons of index finger are divided. Dorsal and palmar interossei of 2nd metacarpal is divided; distal transverse metacarpal ligament is cut; 2nd metacarpal bone is divided obliquely 2 cm from the end (one should not disarticulate the metacarpophalangeal joint). Flexor tendons, palmar digital nerve and vessels are divided. Dorsal interossei tendon is anchored to base of 3rd proximal phalanx (of middle finger). It should not be attached to severe extensor tendon. Other muscles are sutured each other and skin is closed.

Middle and Ring Finger Amputations

Here proximal phalanges should be preserved to maintain the grip of fingers and hand. 3rd and 4th metacarpals heads are important as they provide attachment to metacarpal arch. Here transverse volar flap is used. Digital neurovascular bundles are cut. Extensor tendon/hood, flexor tendons are divided. Bone is cut near the base. Muscles/tendons are sutured. Flap should not have any tension as if tension develops it interferes with functioning of adjacent fingers also.

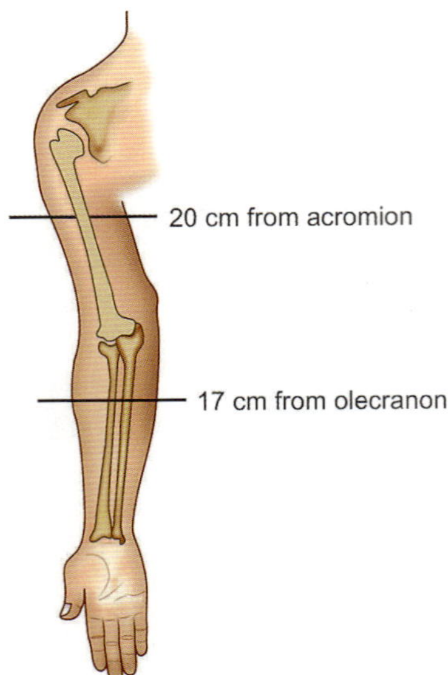

Fig. 10-37: Level of bone transaction in upper limb amputations.

Wrist Amputations

Wrist amputation is preferred to forearm amputation as retained distal radioulnar joint facilitates pronation and supination.

Transcarpal amputation: It is the amputation—disarticulation between proximal and distal rows of the carpal bone complex. Long palmar and short dorsal flap with 2:1 ratio is used. Once incision is deepened all flexors and extensors are divided. Radial and ulnar arteries are ligated. Median, ulnar and radial nerves are cut. Remaining small muscles and tendons are divided. Open the transcarpal joint space and complete the amputation. Skin flap is sutured. Flexor and extensor tendons are anchored to the proximal carpal bones.

Wrist disarticulation: Long palmar and short dorsal skin flap incision which is 1.3 cm distally curved from radial and ulnar styloid processes on the palmar aspect with a connecting straight incision on the dorsal aspect. Dorsal incision is deepened; radial and ulnar arteries are ligated; joint capsule incised to enter the wrist joint; styloid processes of the radius and ulna are resected without opening the radioulnar joint. Median, radial, ulnar nerves are cut after pulling it distally. All tendons are divided at wrist joint level circumferentially. Long palmar flap is sutured back on the posterior aspect after placing a suction drain.

Forearm Amputations

In forearm amputation length as much as possible should be preserved. Distal amputation is done at the junction of distal ⅓ and proximal ⅔ of the forearm. In proximal amputations as proximal as 3.8 cm stump is retained. Both distal and proximal amputations are done with equal flaps **(Figs. 10-39A to C)**.

Krukenberg Amputation

It is done in upper limb following any trauma. Here forearm amputation is done in such a way that it creates a gap between radius and ulna like a claw to have a hold or grip. Krukenberg amputation does not require any prosthesis. But it is cosmetically poor.

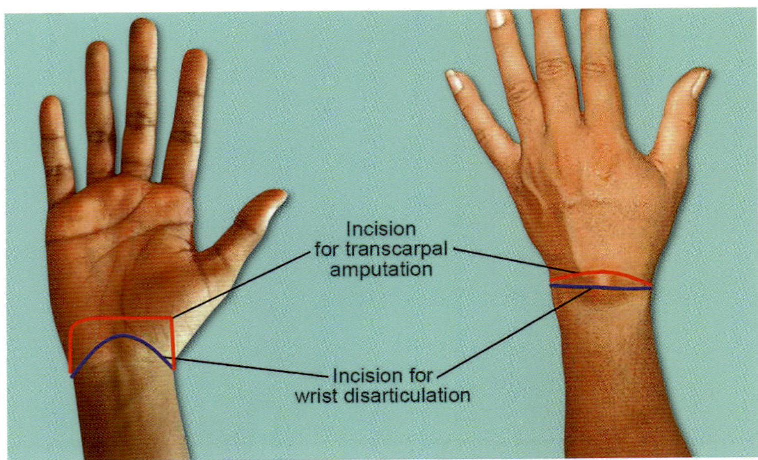

Wrist amputation are preferred than forearm amputation as pronation and supination are preserved

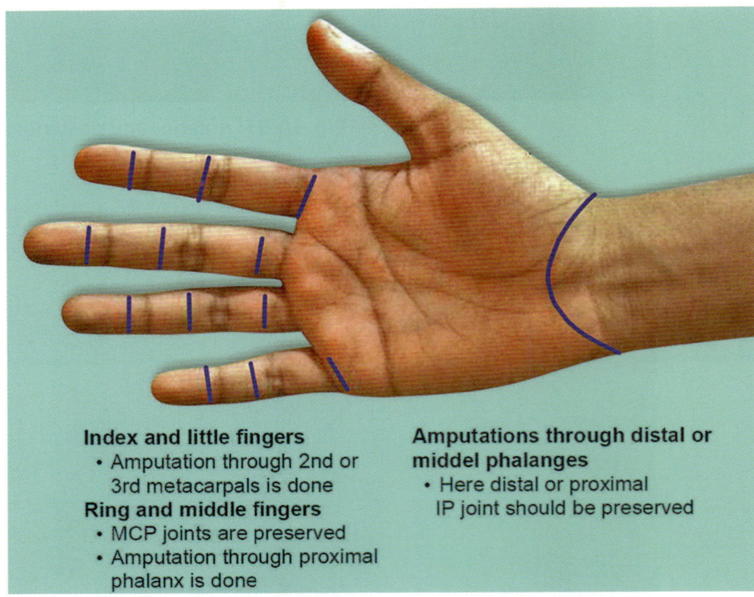

Fig. 10-38: Different amputations in the hand.

Elbow Disarticulation

It is done as equal flap at the level of humeral epicondyles. Posterior flap is 2.5 cm distal to the tip of the olecranon process. Anterior flap is just distal to the attachment of bicipital aponeurosis. Brachial artery is ligated medial to the biceps tendon. Triceps is divided near the tip of olecranon. Triceps is sutured to tendon of brachialis and biceps after disarticulation. Common extensor origin with remnants on the lateral epicondyle which is kept about 6 cm length is sutured to retained remnant of common flexor origin on the medial epicondyle.

ARM AND SHOULDER AMPUTATIONS

Amputation in the arm can be done at any level from supracondylar region to axillary fold proximally. Usual/ideal level is 20 cm from acromion. Distal amputation close to condyles function like elbow disarticulation. Amputation proximal to axillary fold functions like shoulder disarticulation. Prosthesis placement for arm amputation should contain elbow lock mechanism to stabilise the joint in extension/flexion/varying positions; hernatable mechanism as a substitute for humeral rotation. Usually amputation is done as equal flap with length of the flap 1½ times the circumference of the arm.

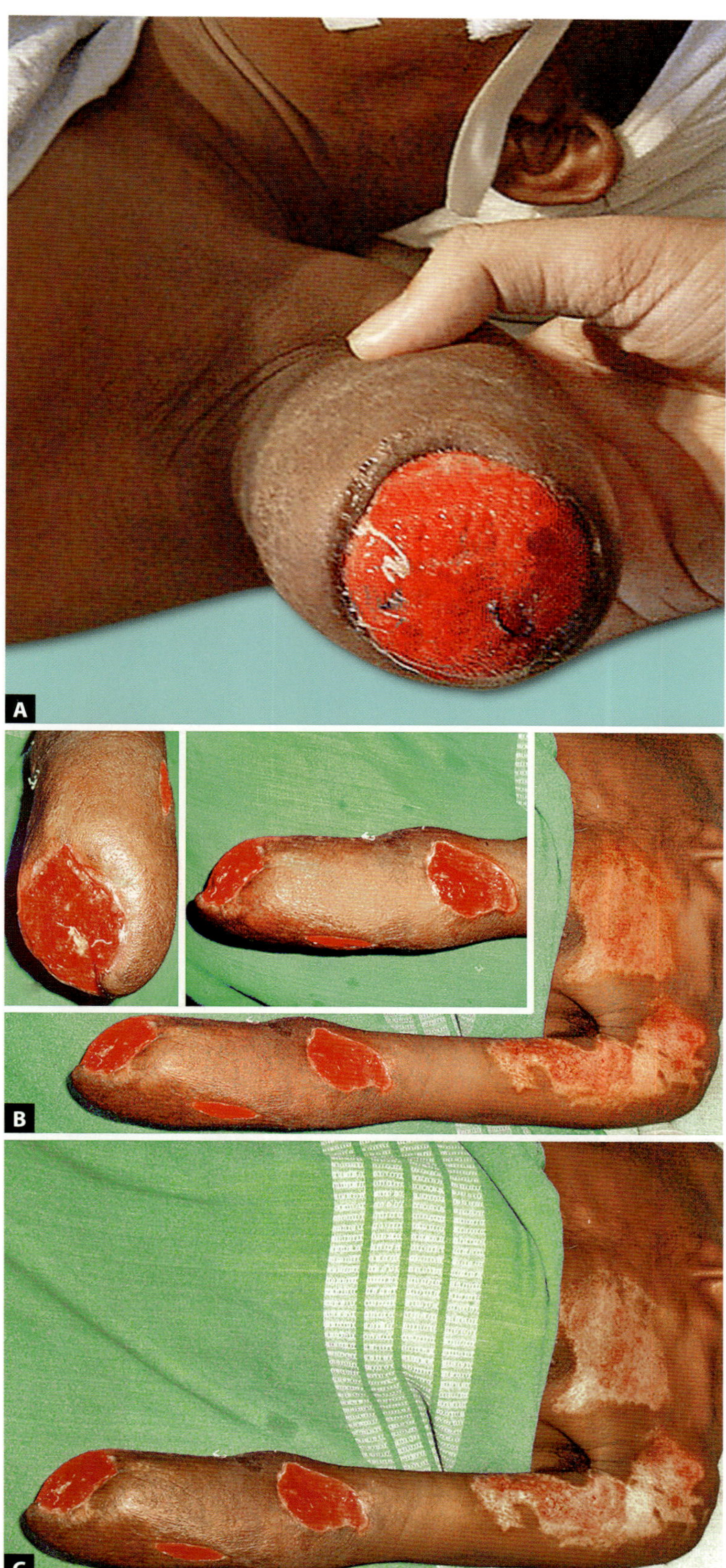

Figs. 10-39A to C: Various upper limb amputations.

Elbow lock mechanism of prosthesis if needed then amputation level should be 3.8 cm proximal to the elbow joint. Brachial artery, nerves and muscles are cut. Bone is divided using Giglie's saw. Triceps muscle is kept long to rotate across cut bone end to suture to anterior fascia or muscles **(Fig. 10-40)**.

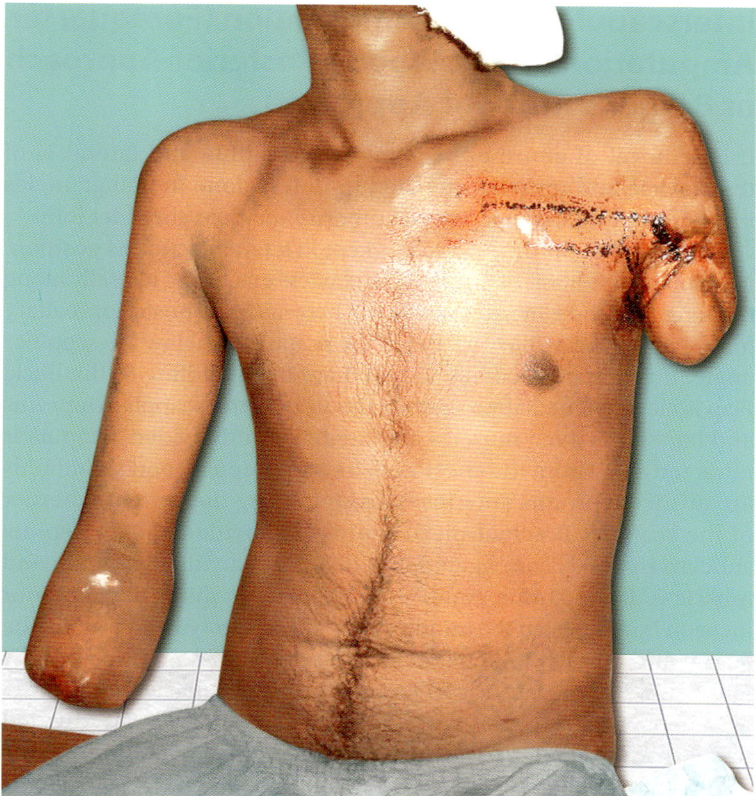
Fig. 10-40: Upper limb amputations of both sides in a patient due to trauma. Right side he underwent forearm amputation; left side amputation at arm level.

Shoulder Amputation

It is amputation at the level of surgical neck of humerus. Incision is made anteriorly from coracoid process along the anterior border of the deltoid muscle to its insertion; then superiorly along the posterior border of the deltoid muscle to reach posterior axillary fold; two anterior and posterior incisions are joined by one more incision passing through axilla. Cephalic vein in deltopectoral groove is ligated. Deltoid and pectoralis major muscle is separated. Deltoid is retracted laterally. Pectoralis major muscle is divided at its insertion to lateral lip of bicipital groove of the humerus. Axillary vessels located between coracobrachialis and pectoralis minor are ligated individually (double ligation with transfixation) distal to the level of pectoral nerves. Deltoid muscle is divided at its insertion. Teres major and latissimus dorsi muscles are divided at their insertion to bicipital groove. Biceps, triceps and coracobrachialis are cut 2 cm distal to the line of bone division. Humerus is cut at its surgical neck. Biceps, triceps and coracobrachialis are sutured over the end of the cut humerus. Pectoralis major is swung laterally to suture to bone. Skin flaps are closed.

Shoulder Disarticulation

It is similar like shoulder amputation but at later period by keeping arm in internal rotation external, rotator muscles and posterior joint capsule is divided. Anterior aspect of the joint capsule and subscapularis and triceps are cut. At the end inferior part of the joint capsule is cut. Unduly prominent acromion process may be trimmed to achieve smooth rounded contour. Muscles are sutured into the glenoid cavity.

Interscapulothoracic Amputation (Forequarter Amputation) (Little Wood's Posterior Approach or Berger's Anterior Approach)

It is removal of entire upper limb with scapula and lateral ⅔ of the clavicle and muscles attached to it. It is done in malignancies involving scapula, upper part of humerus and near shoulder joint.

In posterior approach patient is kept in lateral decubitus position. Incision begins at medial end of the clavicle extending laterally along the length of the clavicle → over the acromion → posterior axillary fold → along the axillary border of the scapula → below the scapular angle. It is curved medially to end 5 cm from midline of the back. Flap is elevated medially to vertebral border of the scapula. Trapezius and latissimus dorsi muscles are identified and divided. Scapula is retracted away from the chest wall, levator scapulae and rhomboids are divided. Serratus anterior is divided along the vertebral border of the scapula. Brachial plexus cords are divided close to spine; subclavian vessels are ligated and divided individually; omohyoid muscle is divided. After completion of posterior dissection, anterior incision is made from the middle of the clavicle downwards along the lateral and parallel to deltopectoral groove across anterior axillary fold below and posteriorly to join the posterior incision at lower ⅓ of axillary border of the scapula. Pectoralis muscles are divided to complete the forequarter amputation. Flaps are sutured with a suction drain **(Figs. 10-41A and B)**.

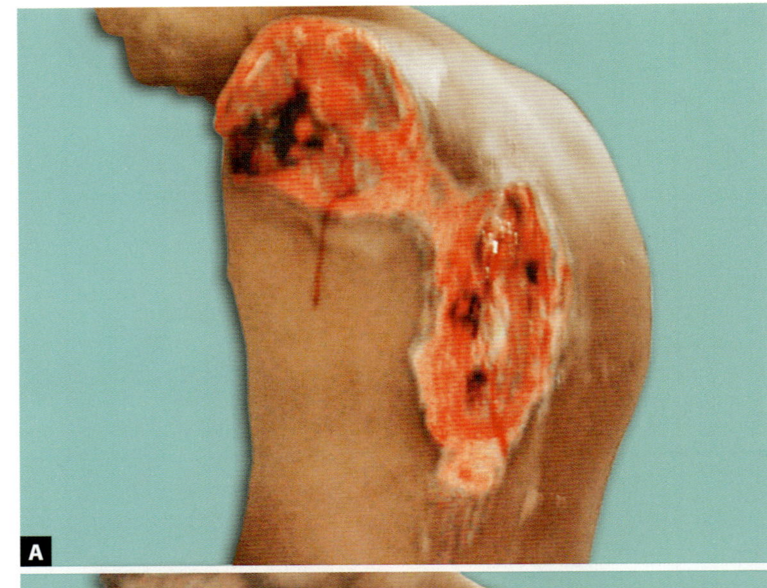

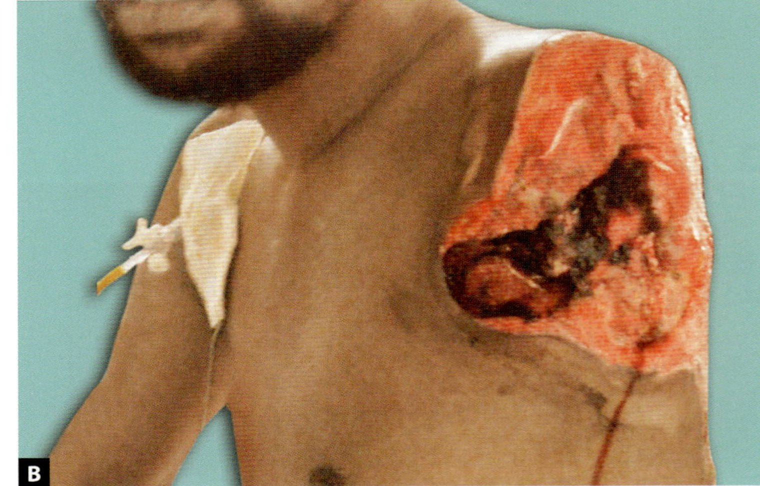

Figs. 10-41A and B: Forequarter amputation.

Some Special Type of Amputations

Dupuytren's amputation—amputation of the arm at the shoulder joint. *Hey's amputation*—amputation of the foot between the tarsus and metatarsus. *Larrey's amputation*—amputation at the shoulder joint. *Spontaneous amputation*—loss of a part without surgical intervention, as in diabetes mellitus, leprosy, aihnum. *Sarmiento's amputation*—level is 1.3 cm proximal to ankle joint line. *Teale's amputation*—amputation with short and long rectangular flaps; Tripier's amputation—amputation of the foot through calcaneum.

REHABILITATION

Rehabilitation after amputation needs a team approach—surgeon, physiotherapist, occupation therapist, psychologist, social worker, etc.

Exercises should be started by physiotherapist from the 2nd or 3rd day after surgery. It is for both muscle setting and joint mobilisation.

Construction of a new organ of locomotion is essential and should be a planned one. Preservation of joint is more important then only of length. Level of amputation should eliminate pathology for which amputation was done.

Split skin grafting over the raw stump area is often done only as a temporary measure. Otherwise it should be avoided as it may repeatedly breakdown by prosthesis.

Joint movement especially adequate extension is a pre-requisite for good prosthesis. More than 30° fixed flexion at knee is contraindication for below knee amputation. Flexion contracture development after amputation is common and it should be avoided by proper rigid dressing (cast/posterior slab using plaster of Paris) and exercise (quadriceps exercises).

Proper tension free skin flap over the stump and thin linear scar are important for proper prosthesis placement **(Figs. 10-42 and 10-43)**.

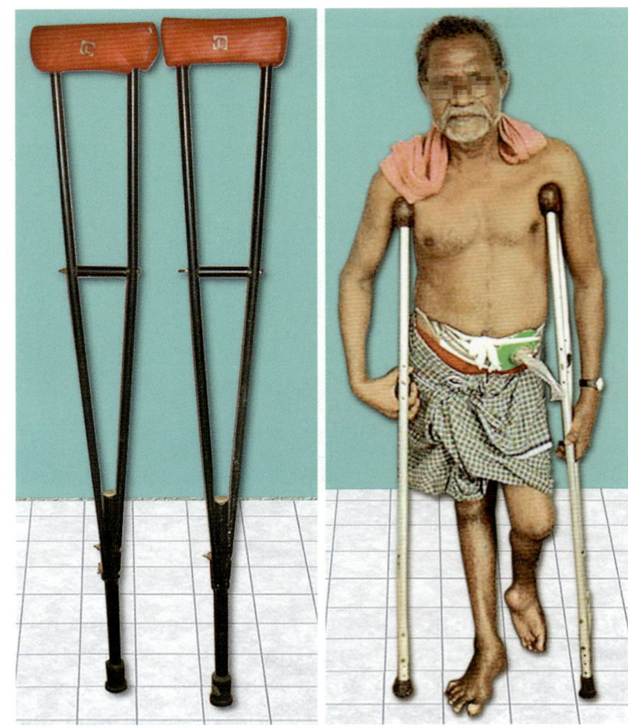

Fig. 10-42: Crutches used for lower limb amputation.

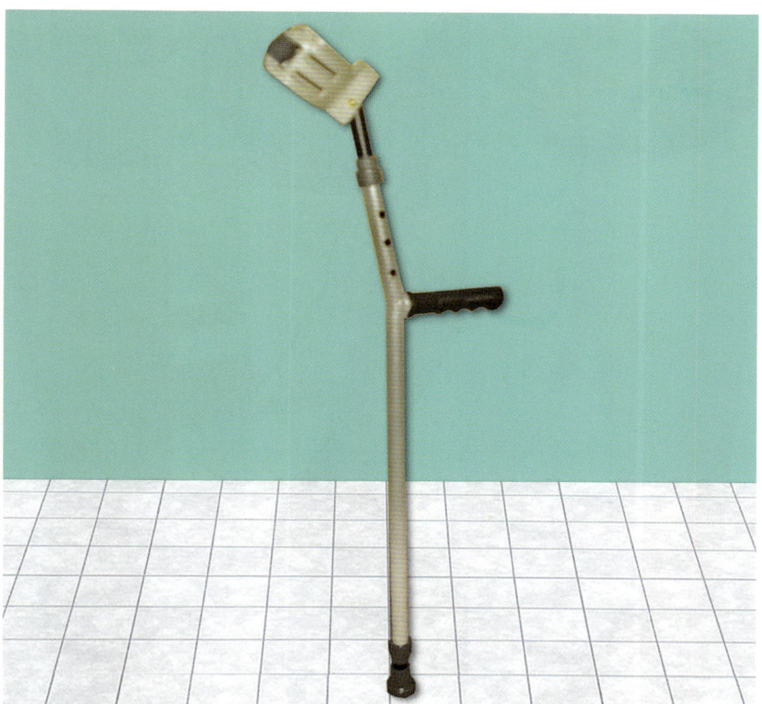

Fig. 10-43: Elbow crutches are used as support after lower limb joint/bone surgeries during rehabilitation.

Prosthesis

Prosthesis is *the substitution* to a part of the body to achieve its optimum function (Orthroses are *supplement* for limb function). It can be *end bearing* or *side bearing*. Prosthesis can be suction type or non-suction type. *Suction type* is placed above the stump. It is better and well tolerated. *Non-suction type* prosthesis is placed at the ends. It requires additional support. Prosthesis can be *external* where prosthesis is placed outside; or *internal* where prosthesis is placed inside into the joint or structure related by open surgery method **(Figs. 10-44 and 10-45)**.

Its functions are—cosmesis, relative achievement of the function of the part, ambulation in lower limb prosthesis. Infection, pressure ulcers, joint instability are the disadvantages.

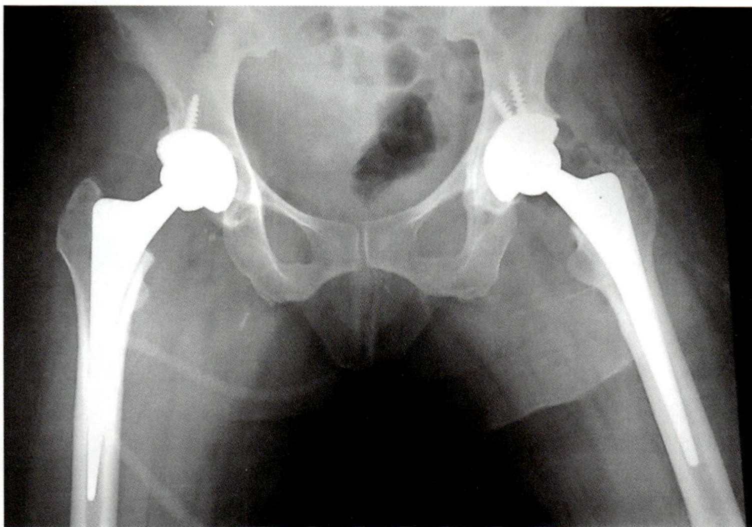

Fig. 10-44: X-ray showing bilateral hip prosthesis.

- *Syme's amputation:* Elephant boot.
- *Below-knee amputation:* Patellar tendon bearing (PTB) prosthesis.
- *Above-knee amputation:* Suction type prosthesis. It is placed above the stump. It is better and well tolerated.
- *Hind-quarter amputation:* Tilting table prosthesis (TTP) is used here or Canadian prosthesis

Prosthesis gives structural strength to the limb. Three groups of prostheses are available: (1) *Endoskeletal/modular limb:* It has got central structural tube to which socket and joints are attached and covered with shaped form to match the contour of the contralateral limb as closely as possible. The foam is covered by skin of silicone, PVC woven material. Load bearing tube is made up of carbon graphite fibre or aluminium in conjunction with titanium for highly stressed components. (2) *Exoskeleton/conventional limb:* The outer visible skin is main structural element and such limbs are hollow. Materials used are willow, plastic laminates. Upper limb prostheses are commonly exoskeletal type. (3) *Temporary pylon type:* It is used for lower limb with two self-locking jointed side struts, resembling a traditional above knee calipers.

Socket of the prosthesis transmits all loads in both swing and stance phases of walk between prosthesis and stump. Socket is the most important part of the prosthesis. Women take time to adjust to prosthesis as they are having less muscle bulk and more subcutaneous fat and stump volume may fluctuate due to hormonal changes during menstrual cycle and pregnancy. Sockets have got tolerant areas for increased loading pressure like ischial tuberosity or patellar tendon and intolerant areas for reduced pressure like head of fibula or adductor tendon. Polypropylene, fibre glass, aluminium alloy, plastic are different materials used for sockets. Socket is worn over a stump sock of cotton or wool. Thickness of sock for proper fitting of the socket is important. Sock is not used in suction or myoelectric sockets. Polyurethane gel layer incorporated or silicone impregnated socks are also used to reduce the skin shearing and stump sweating.

Prosthesis requires *suspension* to hold it place with a belt, cuff or sleeve. Self suspending or suction sockets are also available. Rotational alignment around the central axis of the limb, angular alignment in coronal and sagittal planes and mediolateral and anteroposterior shift must be optimised.

Prosthesis for Below Knee Amputation

Ideal below knee stump is 15–18 cm. Longer stump causes alignment problem. Minimum length is 9 cm. If after flexing the knee joint to right angle, residual tibial length more than three fingerbreadth beyond the hamstring insertion, it means stump is adequate for use. Robinson skew flap is better for fitting early definitive prosthesis. Bone bridge between tibial and fibular cut ends is better for prosthesis. Excess bulbous soft tissue on the end of the stump is not good for prosthesis. Stable mobile knee joint is essential for proper prosthesis.

Patellar tendon bearing prosthesis (PTB prosthesis): Here all the weight bearing is done below knee; movement is controlled by his own knee joint. Patellar tendon is the main key weight-bearing area within the socket; stump posteriorly up to the popliteal fossa is also important to provide counter pressure so that patellar tendon is kept in place. Medial and lateral paratibial areas and medial condylar flare also bear significant weight. Head of the fibula, tibial tubercle, cut ends of tibia and fibula are pressure intolerant areas. Socket should have proper relief areas to these intolerant parts.

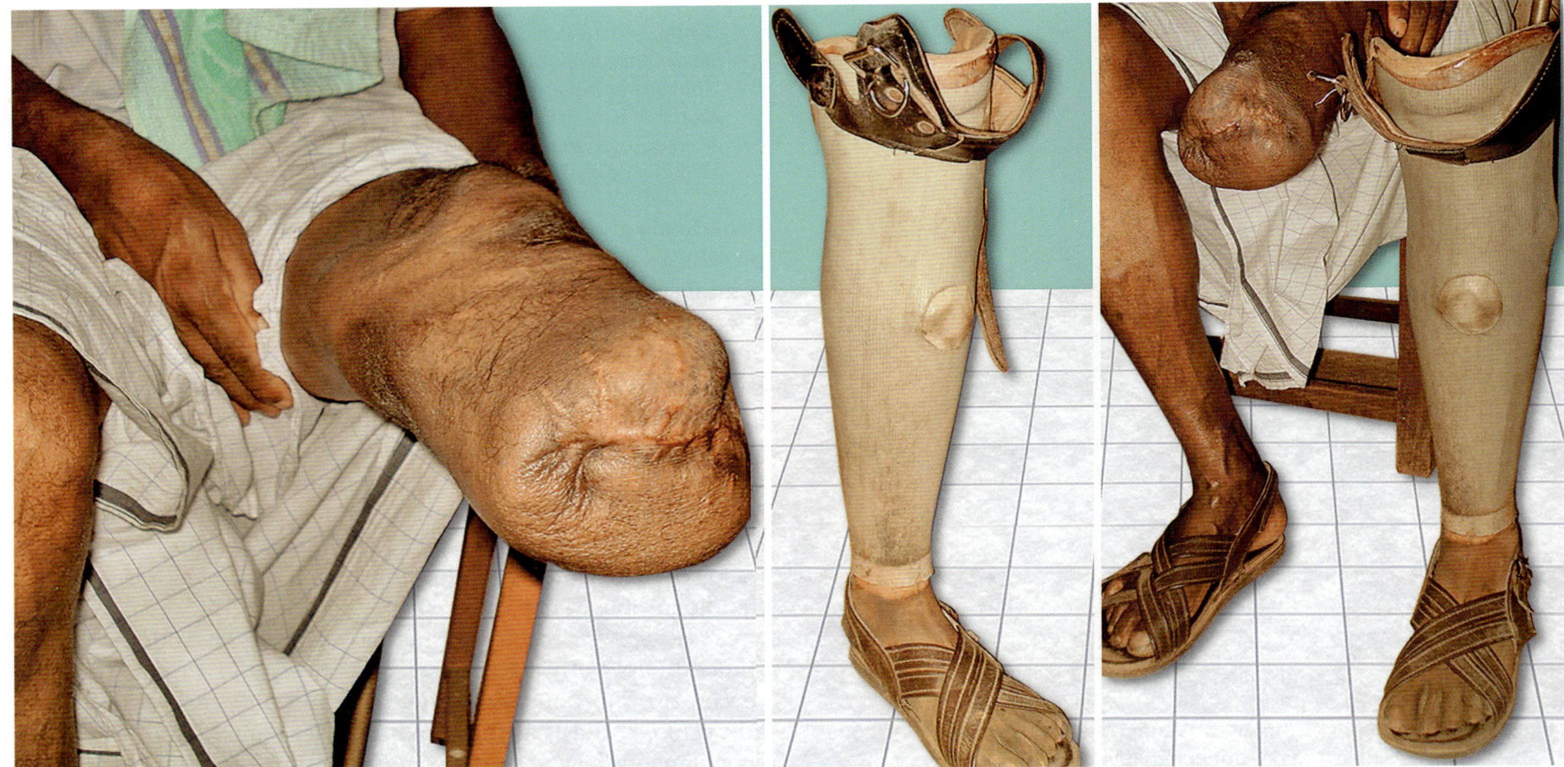

Fig. 10-45: Below knee amputee with prosthesis. It gives good range of movements, normal walk and comfort.

Computer-assisted designing and computer-assisted manufacturing (CAD-CAM) socket is an automated processing method which fulfills all above criteria accurately with modifications. It is more comfortable and is made up of thermoplastic or laminated plastic with closed cell polyethylene foam.

Suspension for below knee amputation prosthesis is leather cuff strap above femoral condyles. Exoskeleton or endoskeleton is used. For athletics endoskeleton is preferable.

SACH (Solid Ankle Cushion Heel) foot: It is multiaxial, optimises gait, and facilitates walking on rough ground. It needs minimal maintenance. It is preferred in old people. Energy storing foot is often used wherein ankle joint is replaced by a plastic spring **(Fig. 10-46)**.

Below knee prosthesis with a thigh corset is used in patients who cannot bear full weight below knee may be due to extensive scarring, presence of skin graft, loss of sensation, damaged knee. Leather thigh corset is joined to lower part of the prosthesis by side steel incorporating joints at knee level to transmit body weight above knee; but retaining entire knee movement and control. Ischial tuberosity is also used often additionally to high corset to minimise below knee weight bearing **(Fig. 10-47)**.

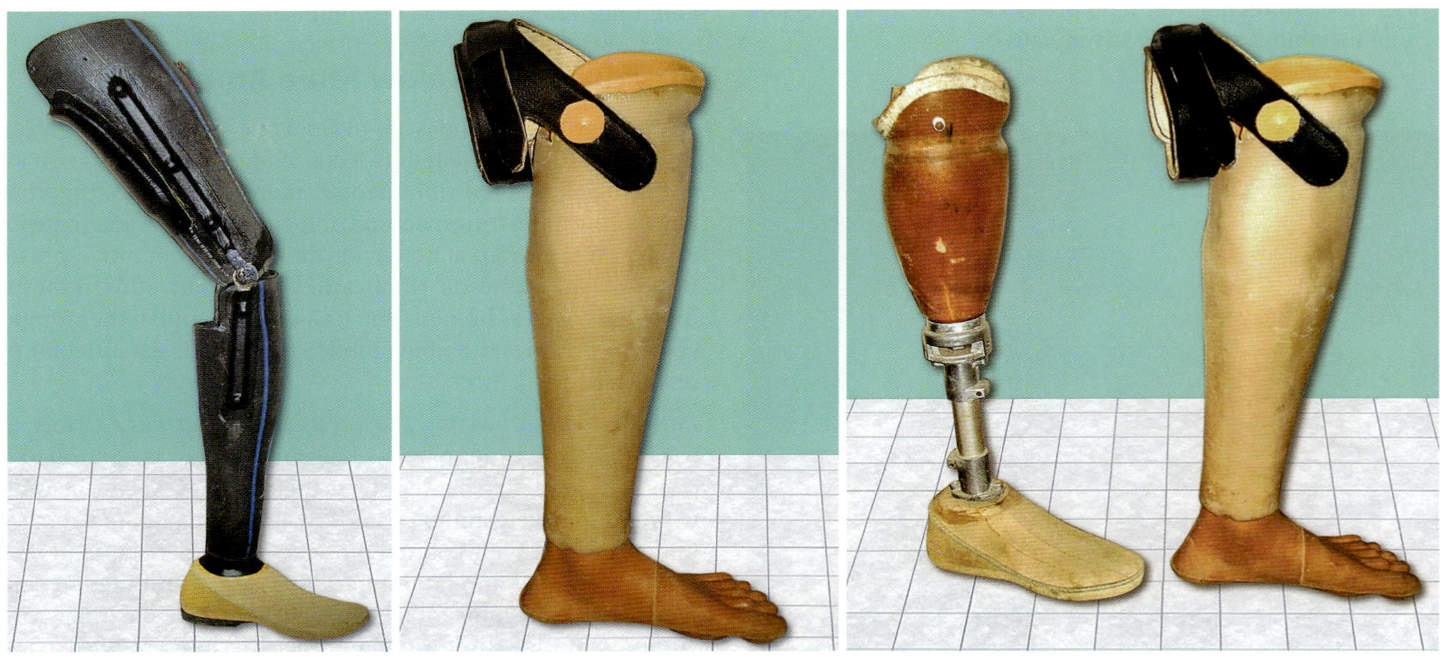

Fig. 10-46: Prosthesis used for lower limb amputation.

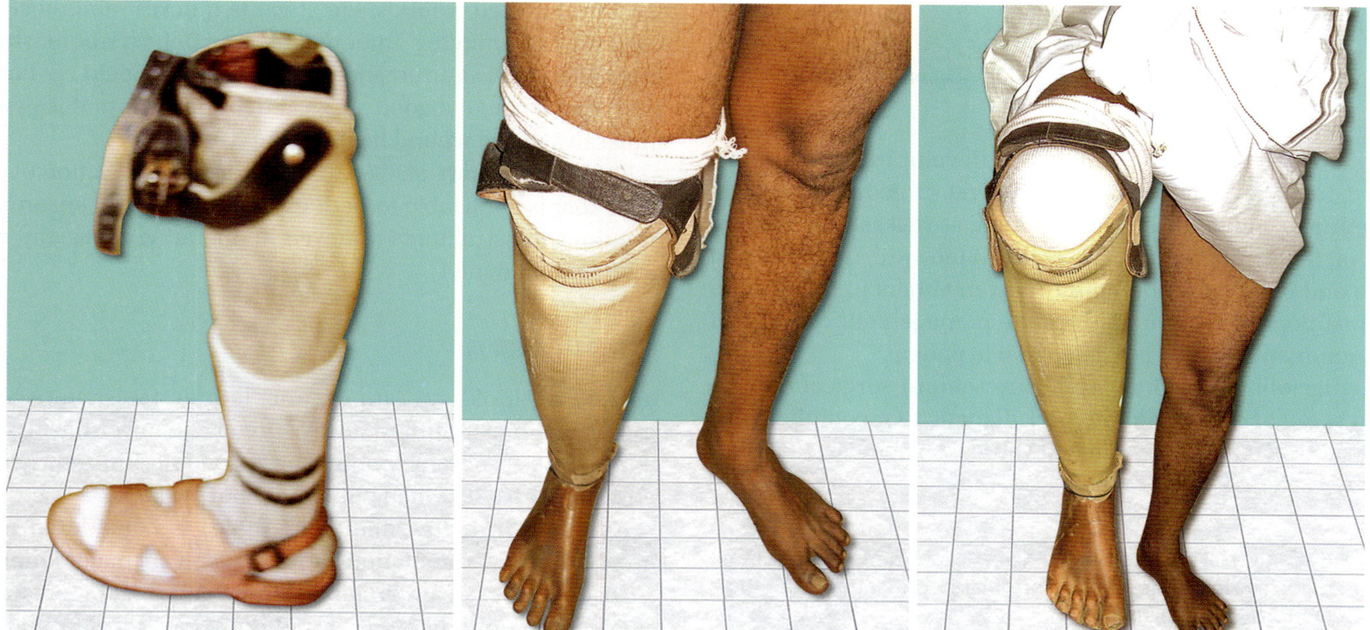

Fig. 10-47: Below knee amputation—prosthesis.

Prosthesis for Above Knee Amputation

Above knee prosthesis is heavier and bulkier and needs more energy for walk (50% more than normal). Minimum length of the above knee stump needed for placing prosthesis is 8 cm measured from the origin of the adductor longus on pubis to the cut end of the femur. *Ischial tuberosity* is the key weight-bearing part for above knee amputation prosthesis. Anterior wall of the socket must extend more proximal than ischial tuberosity to prevent slipping. Rigid plastic or Ireland Sweden Newyork (ISNY) socket is used. ISNY socket contains a flexible plastic liner in a rigid carbon fibre reinforced frame. It controls the shape of the socket brim extending down the medial side of the socket as narrow strut to provide strength and attachment to knee mechanism. Contoured adducted trochanteric controlled alignment method socket (CAT-CAM) has main weight bearing in ischial tuberosity but the stability of the stump is in coronal plane with a bone lock between medial aspect of the ischial tuberosity and greater trochanter.

Knee joint mechanism system is added to all above knee prosthesis. Locked prosthesis knee which flexes on sitting is used in elderly. Simple friction system with a spring or pneumatic unit to assist extension may be used. Self-retaining suction socket or soft neoprene leather belt or rigid pelvic band or shoulder brace is used for suspension system for above knee amputation prosthesis.

Prosthesis for other Lower Limb Amputations

Lisfranc's and Chopart's amputations have tendency to develop equinovarus deformity. So they need ankle joint fixation/obliteration.

In Syme's amputation, person can walk for short distances without prosthesis. Preservation of heel pad fat is very important. Projections of malleoli should be preserved to act as suspension. Compliant linear closely fitting polyethylene foam prosthesis is used. Sockets are end weight bearing but extends proximally to patellar tendon level. SACH foot variant is used.

Through knee disarticulation is cosmetically poor. Endoskeletal prosthesis is longer than the natural side and causes limp. Exoskeletal prosthesis with hinge knee joint shows poorer knee control. Rigid plastic socket with compliant linear inside which suspends condyles is used.

In Grittistokes amputation lateral/side weight-bearing prosthesis over ischial tuberosity is used.

In through hip amputation endoskeletal prosthesis is used with ischial tuberosity as weight bearing. Socket wrap around both iliac crests in through hips and self suspending is used.

In hind quarter amputation endoskeleton prosthesis with contralateral ischial tuberosity as weight bearing point is used. Socket wrap around with shoulder brace is needed.

Prosthesis for Upper Limb Amputations

Upper limb prosthesis provides grip. But sensation and movements are limited. It is very difficult to achieve complex movements of the natural hand. Every part of the upper limb should be tried to be preserved. More the preservation betters the rehabilitation outcome. Pinch grip is totally lost if there is loss of thumb. Opposition prosthesis is helpful. Even when all digits are lost wrist should be preserved for prosthesis plate suitable for pinch and oppose.

In forearm/below elbow amputation ulna length should be at least 8 cm from tip of the olecranon. This gives 4 cm flexor stump beyond the insertion of the biceps tendon. There is not much problem if radius is not preserved. Junction of middle and distal third level is the ideal level of amputation in the forearm to achieve proper function. Laminated prosthesis and socket with cotton sock is used. Prosthesis may be—body powered split look operated; or mechanical hand with active three point grip between thumb, middle and index finger; or myoelectric hand wherein electrical signals are picked up by skin electrodes placed over common flexor or extensor origin; powered wrist rotation.

Above elbow amputation should have stump length of 3 finger width below the anterior axillary fold measured with arm by side. Clearance from stump end to the tip of olecranon should not be less than 9 cm. Prosthesis for above elbow is heavier and bulkier with poor and variable functional outcome. Plastic exoskeleton functional prosthesis with plastic/leather socket over the top of the shoulder is used.

DIABETIC FOOT AND DIABETIC FOOT SURGERY

Amit Jain

Diabetic foot is extremely common in developing and underdeveloped countries like India and as general surgeons, this is one of the common conditions seen in outpatient as well as emergencies. In spite of being common, it is underrated and undervalued condition and often left upon junior most members in the team to handle unsupervised and inappropriate management could lead to major amputation which is detrimental to patient.

Distinct lesions **(Flowchart 10-1)** are seen in surgical department and some of the common type 1 diabetic foot complications requiring surgical management include abscess, necrotising fasciitis, wet gangrene, etc.

Flowchart 10-1: Universal classification for diabetic foot complications (Amit Jain's) as whole. This simple descriptive original classification from India includes most lesions seen in diabetic foot.

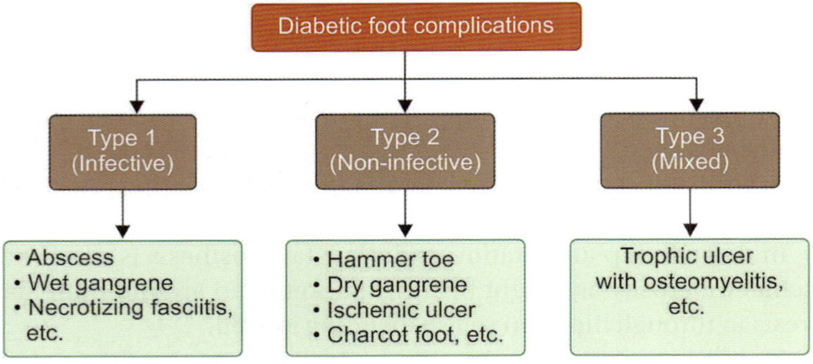

Among various surgical procedures performed on diabetic foot **(Flowchart 10-2)**, Category 1 surgical procedures like debridement, amputation, skin grafting, etc. are most frequently performed procedures by every surgeon on foot.

Flowchart 10-2: Amit Jain's classification for diabetic foot surgeries (SCC classification).

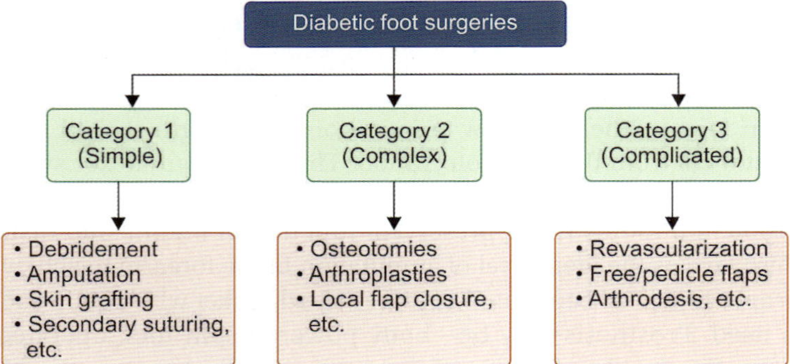

Debridement

Debridement is removal of dead, non-viable or contaminated tissue from the wound in order to control infection and help in wound healing. Debridement can be mechanical like surgical debridement or non-mechanical debridement like enzymatic or autolytic.

Surgical debridement is a commonly performed procedure by general surgeon and often done in case of abscess, necrotising fasciitis, infected wounds, etc. It is the quickest and most efficient method of removing infected tissue. Debridement should be considered both as an art and science and one should not undervalue the importance of a good surgical debridement that is essential in limb salvage and wound healing **(Fig. 10-48)**.

Table 10-1 shows an easy and practical classification of debridement that is applicable to both extremities. Always ensure that one mentions the structures removed in operating notes and extent of debridement done.

Amputation

When one looks at Amputation ladder (Destructive ladder) applicable to extremities, always prefer the lowermost rung as far as possible to obtain biomechanical viable limb and climb the ladder **(Fig. 10-49)** when options are not available.

Amputation below malleoli (Ankle) is considered as minor amputation and amputation above malleoli are major amputation.

Distinct types of amputation **(Fig. 10-50)** exist in foot and type 1 foot amputations like toe amputation, ray amputation, etc. are commonly performed foot amputations.

Even in upper limb amputation, one can use the ladder approach **(Fig. 10-51)**.

SURGICAL OFFLOADING

Diabetic foot ulcers are extremely common in clinical practice. Often, non-infected ulcers are treated by conservative management that includes cleaning and dressing. Plantar ulcers also require some form of offloading and some of them includes total contact cast, removable cast walkers, footwear, etc. There are times when some of the complex ulcers **(Flowchart 10-3)** do not heal due to intrinsic causes which could be either due to ischemia or due to bony issues and many of them frequently recur. Ulcers that are not healing due to ischemia requires revascularisation.

In ulcers caused due to underlying deformities, one may have to resort for correction of underlying biomechanical deformities that is through surgical offloading. Amit Jain's classification for surgical offloading is a new, easy to remember practical descriptive classification for surgical offloading **(Table 10-2)**.

However, one needs to be cautious while considering some of the surgical offloading procedures in view of high post-operative complications like infection, wound dehiscence, recurrence, transfer ulcer, deformities, etc. Guidelines recommend surgical offloading to be the last resort when other conservative methods of offloading do not heal ulcers. Further, long-term studies are lacking on it.

Some of the commonly done procedures are as follows:

Tenotomies

This is performed in cases of non-healing ulcers over the distal part of the toes due to hammer or claw toe. The flexor tenotomy **(Fig. 10-52)** is an easy and minimally invasive technique and can be done by open or percutaneous method wherein no. 18 gauge needle or blade is used to transect the flexor tendon. Complication of this procedure includes wound infection, vessel injury, re-ulceration, and transfer ulcer.

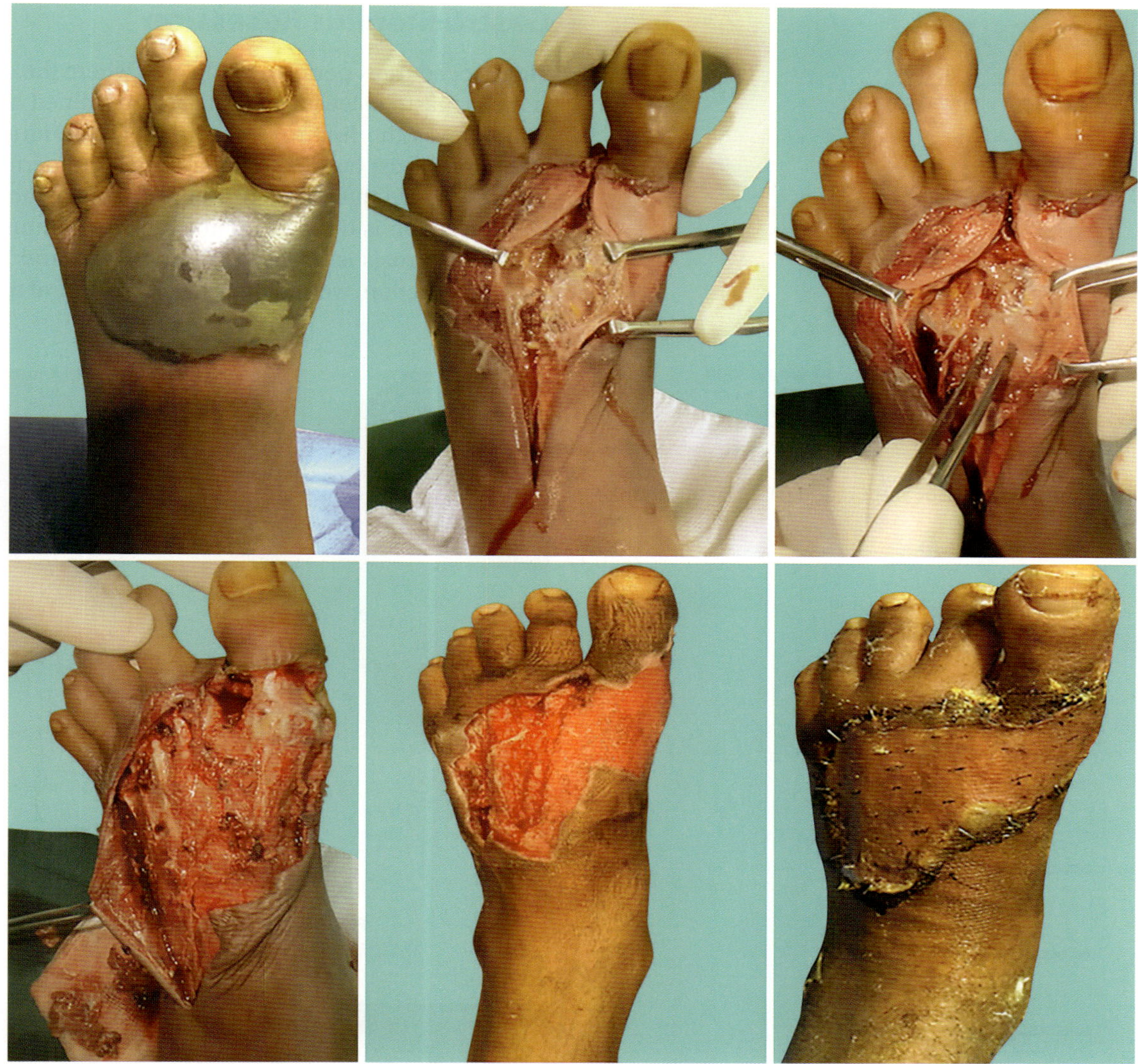

Fig. 10-48: Debridement in diabetic foot. Patient underwent AJ G3E1R0 debridement and once a good granulation tissue was obtained, he underwent split skin graft (SSG).
Courtesy: Dr (Prof) Amit Jain, Founder of Modern Diabetic Foot Surgery, Bengaluru.

TABLE 10-1: Amit Jain's grading of debridement.

Parameters	*Coding*	*Description*
Grade of debridement	G1	Removal of sloughs from the ulcer, callus removal, deroofing the large blisters/blebs, removal of desiccated tendons, etc.
	G2	Removal of necrotic/unhealthy skin and subcutaneous tissue
	G3	Removal of infected/necrotic skin, subcutaneous tissue along with either tendons/retinaculum/deep fascia
	G4	Removal of infected/necrotic skin, subcutaneous tissue, tendon/retinaculum/deep fascia along with necrotic/infected muscle
Extent	E1	Only one site (foot/leg/thigh)
	E2	Two sites (foot + leg, leg + thigh)
	E3	Three sites (foot + leg + thigh)
Repetition	R0	Debridement not repeated
	R1	Debridement repeated once
	R2	Debridement repeated twice
	R3, etc.	Debridement repeated thrice, etc.

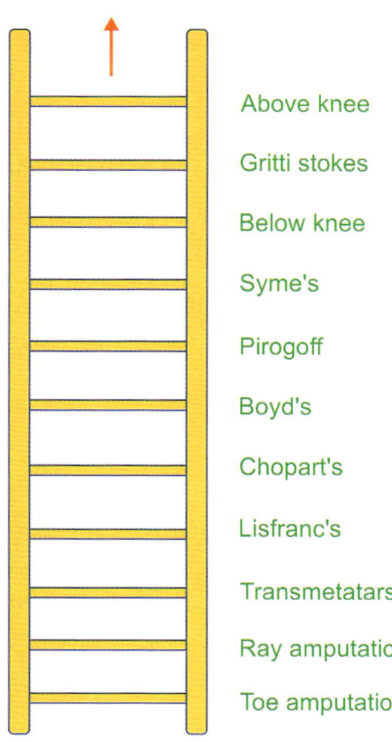

Fig. 10-49: Destructive ladder (Amit Jain's) akin to reconstructive ladder. One can even utilise the Elevator approach in amputation.

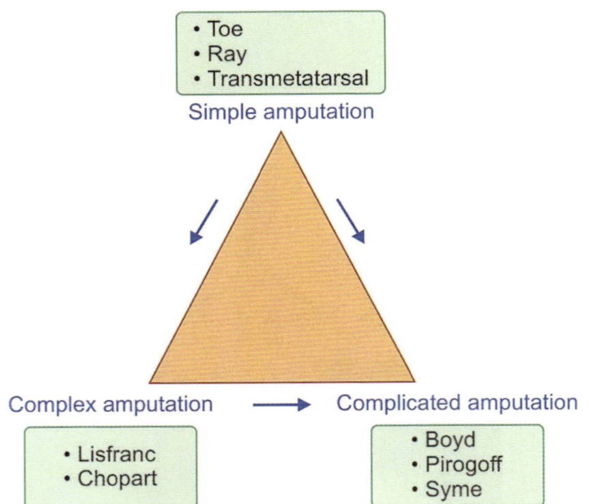

Fig. 10-50: Amit Jain's classification of foot amputation (SCC classification).

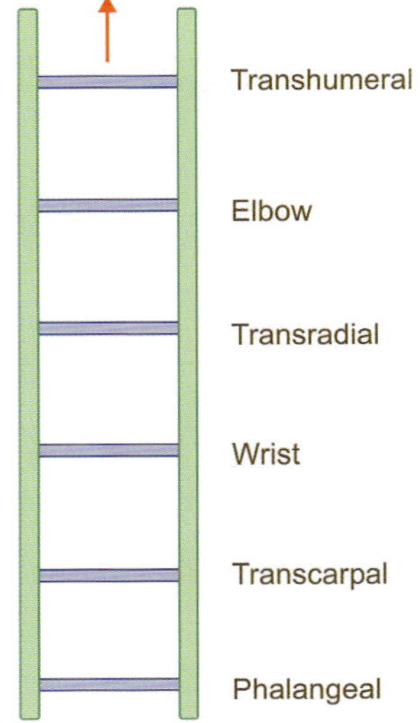

Fig. 10-51: The amputation ladder approach in upper extremities.

Flowchart 10-3: Amit Jain's diabetic foot ulcer classification (SCC classification).

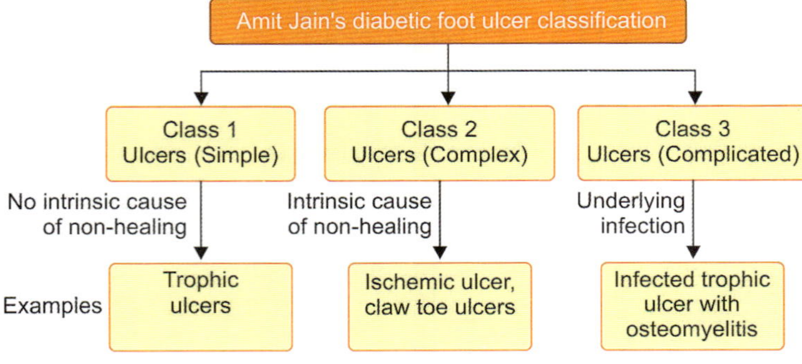

TABLE 10-2: Amit Jain's classification for surgical offloading (SCC classification).

Amit Jain's type of surgical offloading	*Description*	*Examples*
Type 1 surgical offloading	Simple	Tenotomies, Tendo-Achilles Lengthening, gastrocnemius recession, etc.
Type 2 surgical offloading	Complex	Osteotomies, arthroplasties, tendon transfers, etc.
Type 3 surgical offloading	Complicated	Arthrodesis, joint stabilisation procedures, etc.

Gastrocnemius Recession

This procedure is performed in cases where the equinus of the foot is due to gastrosoleus tightening as determined by Silfverskiold test. Vulpius was the first to describe this technique and many other techniques exist but common and easier to perform is Strayer type of recession. In this technique, posteromedial incision is used in the leg, dissection is done to identify gastrocnemius aponeurosis and this aponeurosis is released **(Figs. 10-53A and B)**. Complications include infection, wound dehiscence, and sural nerve injury.

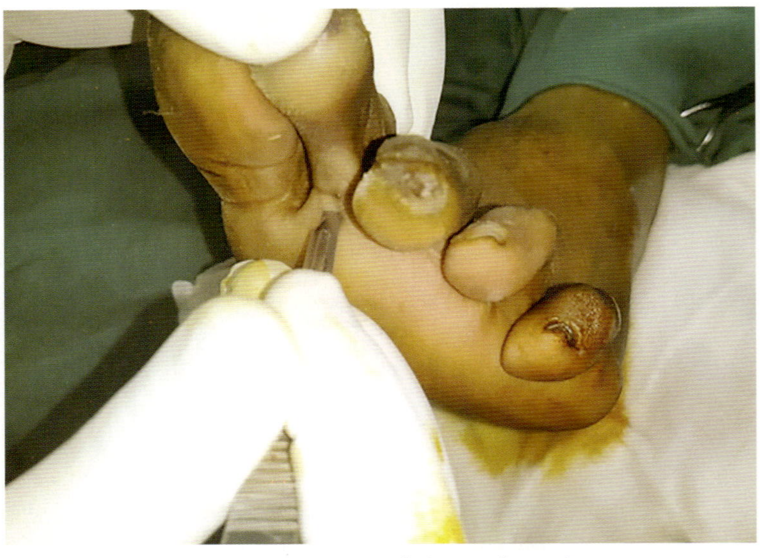

Fig. 10-52: Tenotomy being performed.

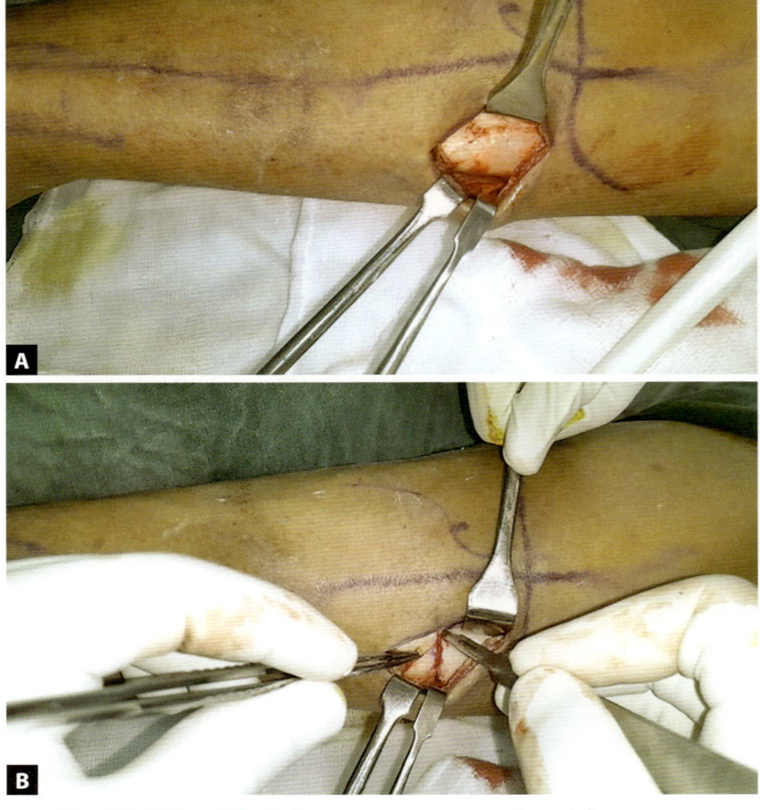

Figs. 10-53A and B: Gastrocnemius aponeurosis and the recession being performed.

Tendo-Achilles Lenthening (TAL)

This procedure is performed in cases where the equinus of the foot is due to Achilles tendon tightening as determined by Silfverskiold test. Percutaneous technique (Triple hemisection) with help of surgical blade 15 remains an effective surgical option **(Fig. 10-54)** though this method is associated with many complications especially tendon rupture, calcaneal gait and ulcer that can be difficult to treat later. One should be adequately trained before performing this procedure.

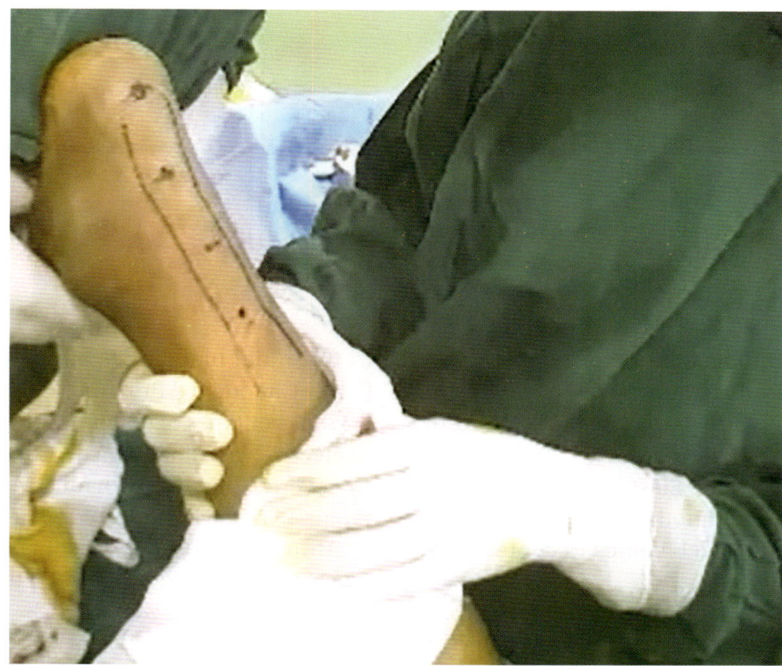

Fig. 10-54: The marking and percutaneous triple hemi-section of tendo-Achilles.
Courtesy: Dr (Prof) Amit Jain, Founder of Modern Diabetic Foot Surgery, Bengaluru.

11

CHAPTER

Surgeries in Arterial Diseases

Surgery for arterial diseases is a complicated one. Artery is always surgically mobilised deep to the adventitia. Tunica adventitia contains fibrous and elastic tissue with periarterial sympathetic nerves. It is attached loosely to the tunica media. Tunica media contains smooth muscle and elastic tissue. Elastic tissue is more in large vessels. Tunica intima is inner thin endothelial layer that lies on an elastic tissue basement membrane which comes in contact with tunica media.

Alexis Carrel in 1912 got Nobel Prize for establishing principles of vascular suturing. Arterial repair is needed in trauma, aneurysm, and block surgery for malignancy in many anatomical places like neck, axilla, abdomen; limbs may need vascular reconstruction while doing radical surgery. All general surgeons should know the technique of vascular suturing which will be handy while operating.

PRINCIPLES IN VASCULAR SURGERY

Gentle handling of all vessels using non-toothed fine forceps is essential. Intima can get damaged without adventitial injury which may lead to thrombosis.

Artery should be mobilised adequately including proximal branches to have adequate control.

In emergency situation like bleeding speed of surgery is very important especially in major arterial injury. Rapid access, quick proximal control is essential to save the life.

Blind clamping of bleeding area in a hurry due to stress should be avoided. It may damage more or injure adjacent structures.

Resuscitation should be undertaken simultaneously by a critical care team with adequate venous accesses including a central line in major vascular bleeding.

Precision and gentle handling is essential in vascular surgery.

Vascular clamps or tapes are used at the site of an arteriotomy. While applying clamps, adjacent vein should be taken care off as thin-walled vein may get injured. Vascular clamps available occlude lumen to control bleeding without injuring the vessel wall; but diseased atheromatous vessel may develop breakage of the plaque often causing embolus. Injury to the plaque itself may precipitate the thrombosis of the vessel. Clamp should be held properly or should be fixed to the drape as twisting or traction of the instrument may injure the vessel. Side clamp is also used often in major vessels like in aorta, and inferior vena cava. Prelaparotomy thoracotomy for aortic clamping or intra-abdominal per laparotomy aortic clamping in torrential bleeding is often advocated as life-saving procedure (Refer Chapter 8—Principles of Surgical Management in Trauma).

Slings or tapes of different colours are used to control haemorrhage in elective vascular surgical procedure **(Figs. 11-1 and 11-2)**.

Severe ischaemia with muscle death is contraindication of arterial repair. It is also better avoided in presence of sepsis.

Atraumatic but firm vascular clamps should be used. Size and type of clamps should be selected depending on need, site, size of the vessels **(Figs. 11-3 to 11-5)**.

Needle holder for arterial suturing should be of high quality material like tungsten with fine points. Monofilament non-absorbable synthetic suture material is used. 3-zero to as fine as 7-zero suture materials are used. For aorta 3-zero or 4-zero is used; for iliac arteries 4-zero; for femoral artery 5-zero; for popliteal and brachial arteries 6-zero; for distal vessels 7-zero is used. Always atraumatic needle is used. Polypropylene suture material is ideally used. It is very smooth, slips through tissues easily. Brittleness, memory, knot slipping should be taken care of. Minimum 5 knots should be placed. Polytetrafluoroethylene (PTFE) sutures are very strong but knot slips easily.

Usually continuous sutures are placed as it is haemostatic. But often interrupted sutures are also placed safely especially in medium sized and small sized arteries. Single needled suture material is used for closure of longitudinal arteriotomy; double needled suture material (double armed suture with needle at both ends) is used for end-to-end closure or patch closure.

Use of magnifying loops may be necessary for fine suturing. But once habituated it is difficult to do suturing in the absence of loops.

In suturing of diseased vessels thicker suture material is used (3-zero/4-zero). Needle should be passed from within outside of the artery.

During arterial suturing, interposition of the adventitia should be avoided as it may initiate thrombosis.

End of the suture material should not be held directly by fine haemostat but with jaws protected by fine rubber or plastic tubes. Unprotected metal instruments should never be used to hold the end of fine suture.

Before application of clamps 5,000 IU of heparin is given intravenously. Often half the dose is reversed using protamine sulphate but not necessarily always. Heparinised saline solution should be used for irrigation of opened vessels. 5,000 IU of heparin is mixed with 500 mL of normal saline to prepare such solution.

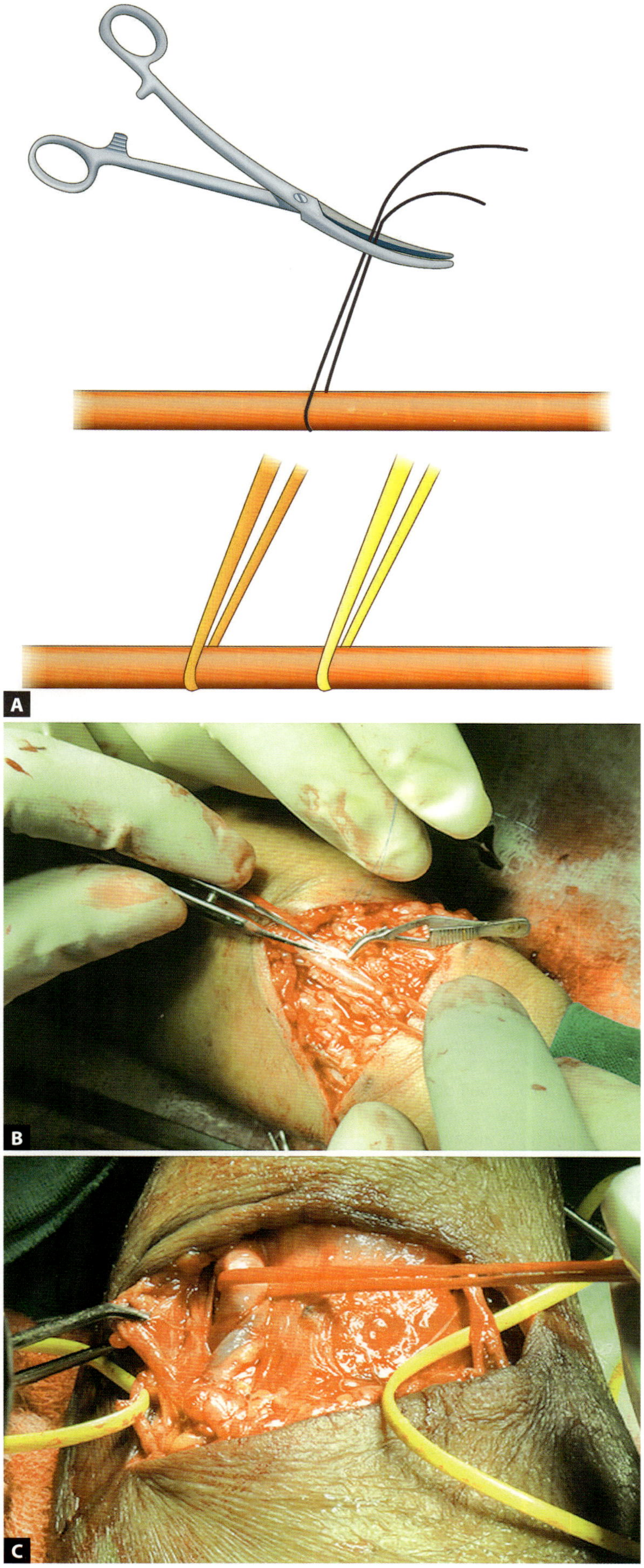

Figs. 11-1A to C: Silk slings or fine coloured rubber or synthetic slings/loops can be used to control haemorrhage.

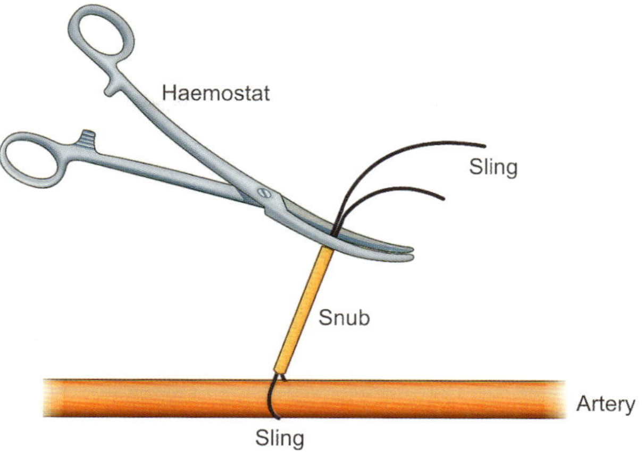

Fig. 11-2: Sling with snub also can be used to control the haemorrhage.

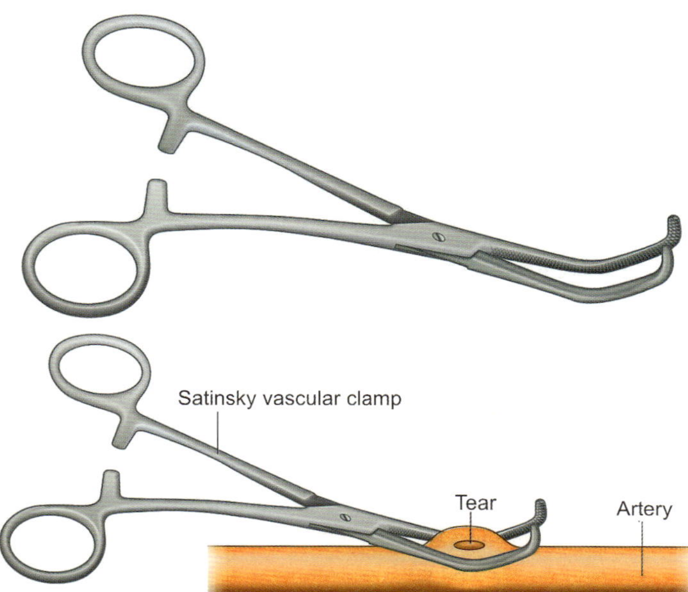

Fig. 11-3: Satinsky vascular clamp and its use in vessel tear.

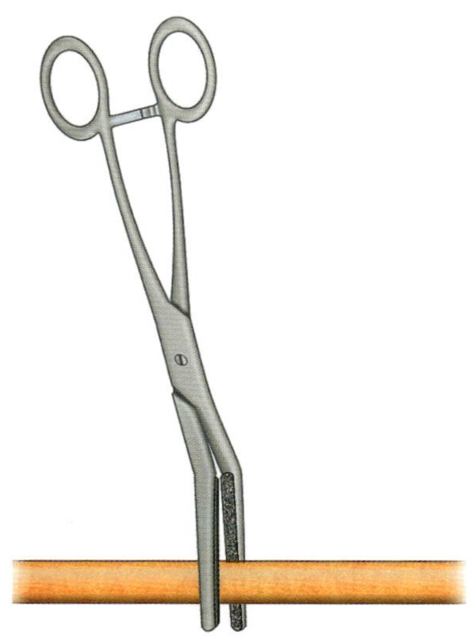

Fig. 11-4A

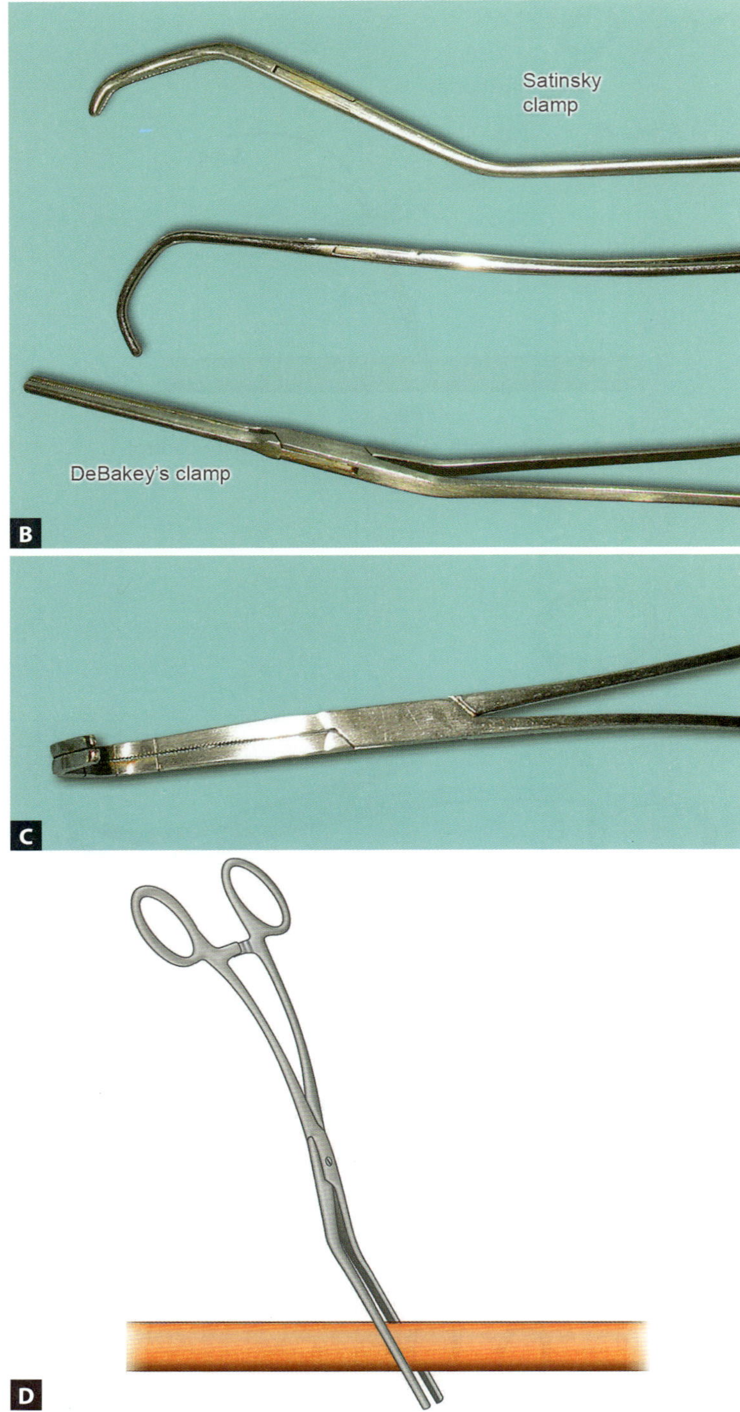

Figs. 11-4B to D

Figs. 11-4A to D: Different vascular clamps—soft jaw Fogarty clamp; Satinsky vascular clamp.

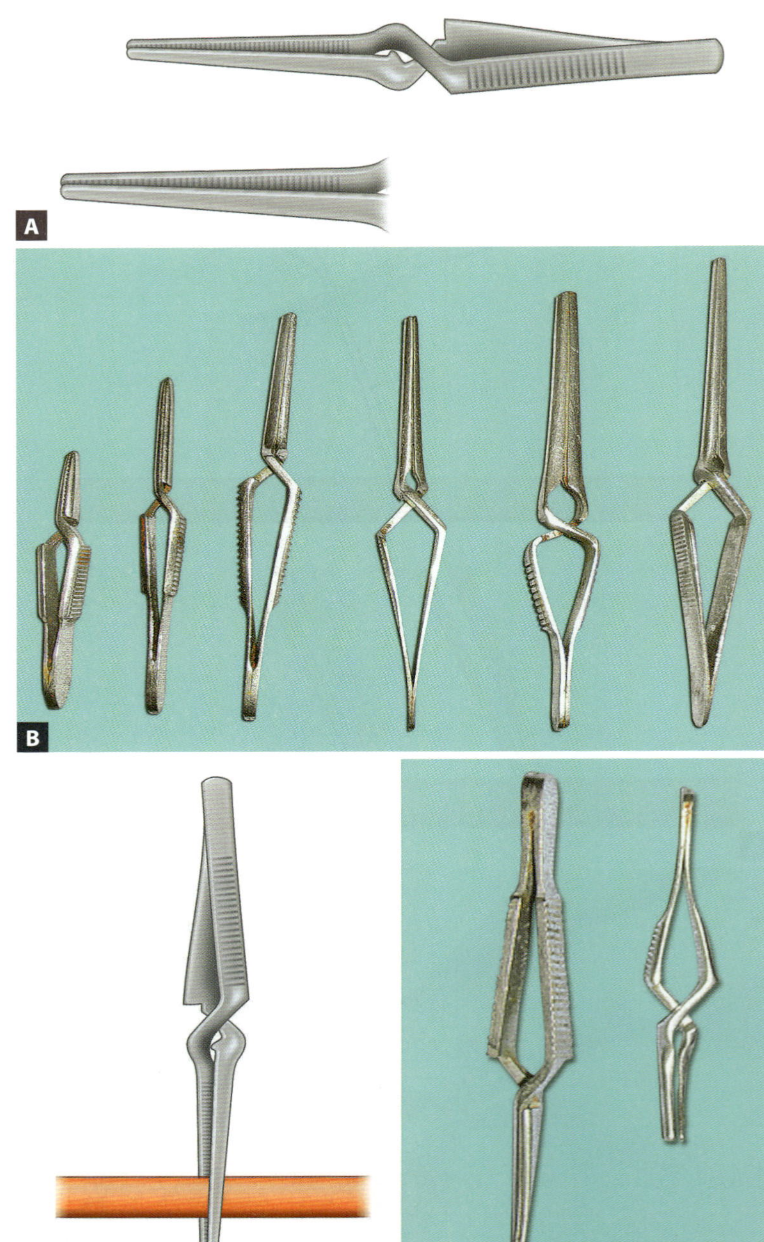

Figs. 11-5A to C: Bull dog clamp and its application. It temporarily occludes vessel firmly and completely. Different sized and type of clamps—straight and curved types are available.

Arteriotomy

Artery is opened (*arteriotomy*) longitudinally. *Longitudinal arteriotomy* is easier to close. Thrombus formed in suture line will be thin and longitudinal and so will not block the lumen. Longitudinal arteriotomy is easy to extend as needed. It is commonly used in thrombectomy and endarterectomy. *Transverse arteriotomy* is difficult to appose. Circular suture line thrombus formed at one place may block the lumen. Intima retracts much more than deeper layers so that often it is difficult to take suture bite. Intima may get dissected in transverse arteriotomy. But in many situations like in trauma, in surgeries of malignancies end-to-end anastomosis is needed. Often it is done using interrupted sutures especially in medium-sized vessel of less than 4 mm size **(Figs. 11-6A and B)**.

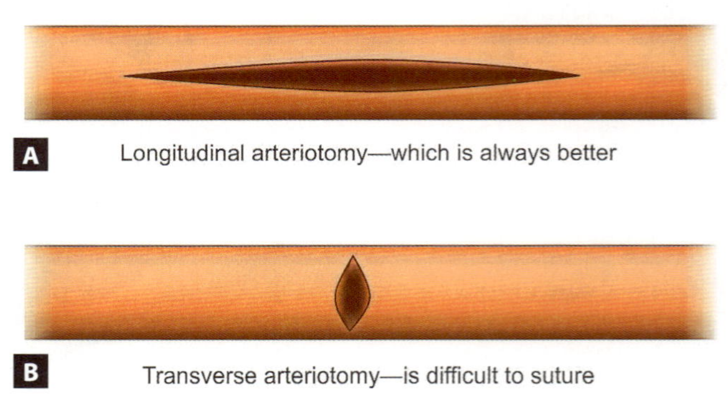

Figs. 11-6A and B: Arteriotomy is opening of artery surgically. Longitudinal arteriotomy is better than transverse one.

Sterile field, good retraction, light and access, control of bleeding are essential parts of vascular surgery. Non-absorbable monofilament polypropylene is used as a suture material. Round body needle is used for arterial anastomosis. Tapercut needle can be used if suturing is done through a thick graft.

Intima should be included in all bites during sutures except in endarterectomy. Needle should be passed from within out across the vessel to prevent intimal flap formation and dissection. When bite is taken from without in towards intima, intima should be supported firmly using fine instrument to prevent intimal separation.

Arterial ligation is done in different methods: (1) Direct ligature of the vessel using non-absorbable or delayed absorbable sutures. Silk/polyglactic acid/thread may be used. (2) Transfixation sutures across the vessel using polypropylene or polyglactic acid sutures. (3) Over sew technique is continuous running sutures over a large vessel to have a firm safe/secure closure of the vessel **(Fig. 11-7)**.

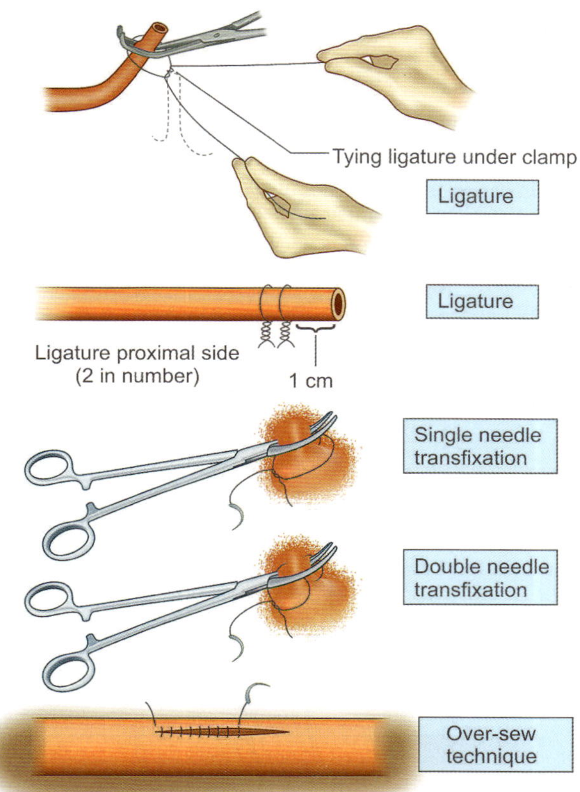

Fig. 11-7: Different methods of arterial ligation. Secure ligation is important. Type of ligation is used individually in each surgery. For definitive arteries like uterine or cystic or gastric, proper 2 or 3 ligatures should be placed. Transfixation suture also can be placed. In bulky tissues bleeding is controlled by double transfixation or over sewing method.

DIFFERENT METHODS OF ARTERIAL SUTURING

All layer simple lateral sutures are used for closure of longitudinal arteriotomy. Turning intima outwards, firm uniform tension on suture line, proper spacing of the bite and optimum width of the bite are essential.

Closure using a venous (autologous) or prosthetic (Dacron or PTFE) patch is used in smaller arteries like brachial artery or deep femoral artery (profundaplasty). Oval or rectangular patch should be used; not elliptical one with sharp point which may narrow the artery at the corners **(Figs. 11-8A and B)**.

End-to-end suturing of the cut ends of artery is done by Carrel's triangulation technique. Three sutures are placed; one on the posterior deeper part; one on each at equidistant on the corners. Continuous sutures are placed keeping these three stay sutures as guiding points. Everting mattress sutures also can be placed. Deepest parts of the triangulation should be sutured first. Larger arteries are sutured with continuous sutures; medium and small arteries are sutured with interrupted sutures. Whether continuous or interrupted sutures are used, triangulation should be done at the beginning **(Figs. 11-9 and 11-10)**.

Single stitch, end-to-end suturing of large artery can be done by placing continuous sutures beginning from the nearest cut end progressing posteriorly towards other cut end and commencing later on anterior aspect to complete the end-to-end suturing. Double needle suture may be used which is started at midpoint posteriorly proceeding on either sides towards in front to complete the end-to-end suturing.

Inlay method of suturing is usually practiced in reconstruction of abdominal aorta using graft wherein horizontal mattress sutures are placed with needle passing from graft to aorta. Parachute technique is a method where double end sutures are placed without initial tying of the knot.

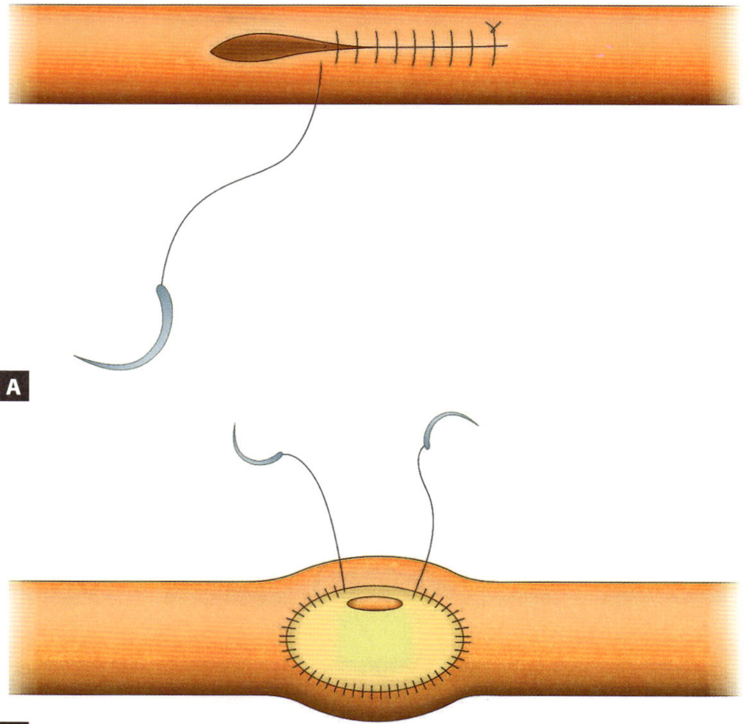

Figs. 11-8A and B: Simple suturing of the vessel; often venous or prosthetic patch may be required in smaller arteries.

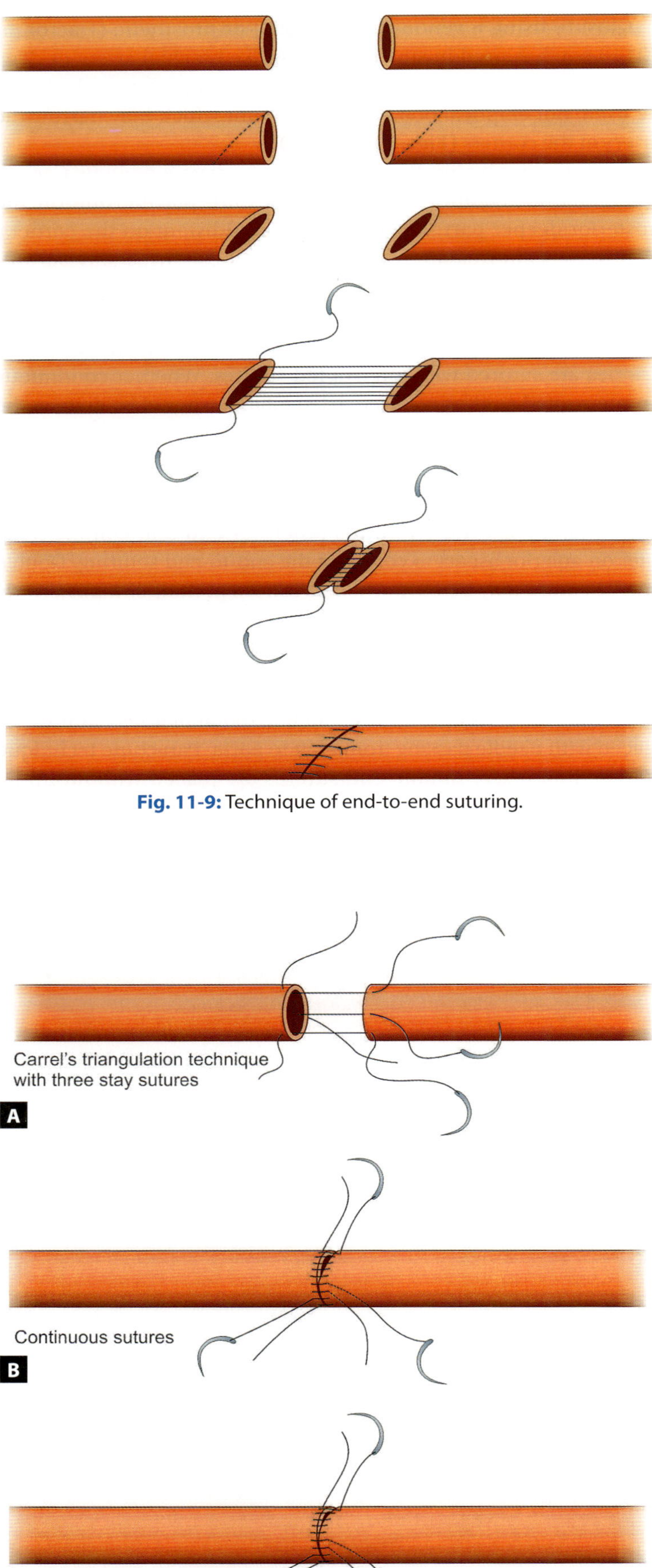

Fig. 11-9: Technique of end-to-end suturing.

Figs. 11-10A to C: Carrel's triangulation technique in arterial suturing.

End-to-side suturing of the arteries is done in arterial bypass procedures with oblique stoma which is twice the diameter of the artery/graft to have a spatula end with cobra head look.

Four quadrant technique with double ended suture at the heel of the anastomosis; the end with acute angle of the anastomosis is called as *heel* and the end with obtuse angle is called *as toe* of the anastomosis.

Parachute end-to-side suturing is also done whenever there is poor access or poor visualisation; is done using double-ended vascular running stitches continuously which later is pulled tight for approximation of the vessel/graft parts **(Figs. 11-11A and B)**.

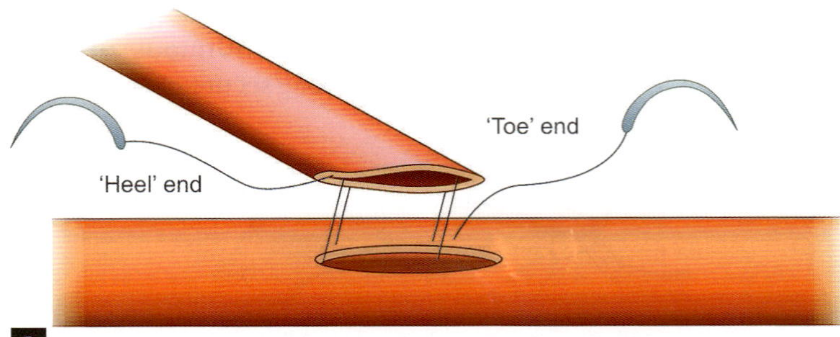

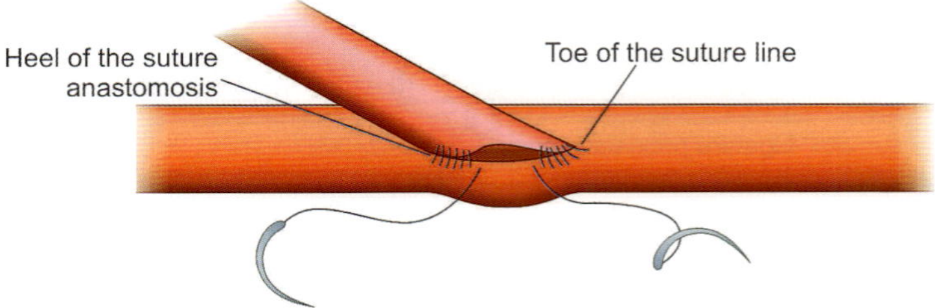

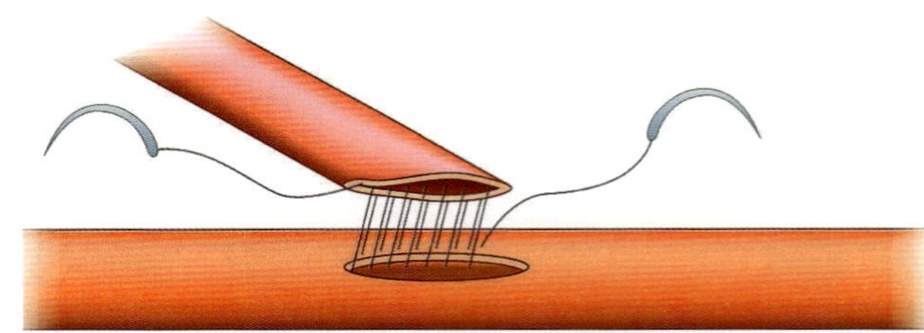

Figs. 11-11A and B: Different end-to-side suturing technique. Note the *heel and toe end* of the arterial suturing.

In an endarterectomy special ***Kunlin suture*** is inserted to prevent intimal dissection. Suture initially passed from outside to inside through endarterectomised part then from inside out through atheromatous part to tie outside. It fixes the intima properly **(Fig. 11-12)**.

In calcified artery often additional fine adventitious sutures may be required. In a friable artery suture holding may be inadequate; so to hold sutures and to prevent haemorrhage, additional *buttressing under the sutures* is done using Dacron in larger artery or muscle piece in small artery **(Fig. 11-13)**.

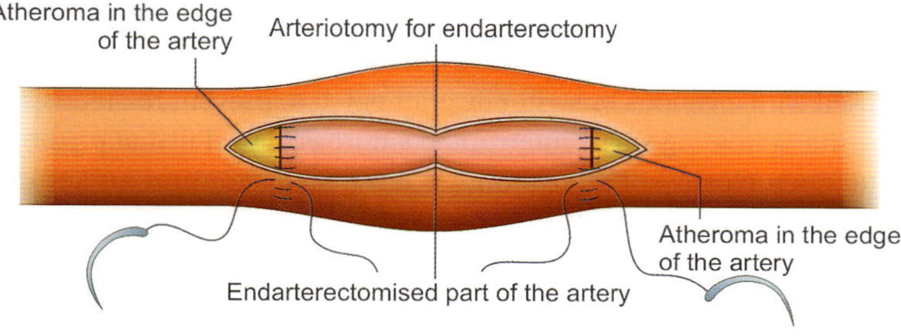

Fig. 11-12: Kunlin suture.

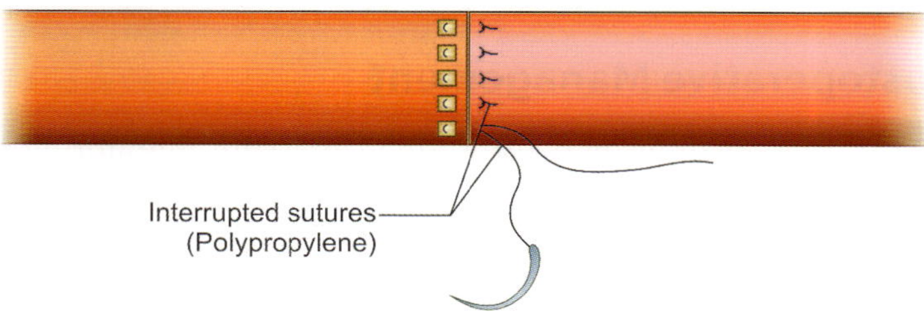

Fig. 11-13: Buttressing under suture is done using Dacron or muscle piece.

Non-sutured anastomosis is a new method used in aorta during surgical treatment of aneurysm to keep in place of a synthetic graft. A rigid Dacron covered polypropylene ring is passed using an applicator within the lumen. Tapes are ligated outside the aorta also.

Peripheral aneurysms are approached by different methods—Matas aneurysmorrhaphy; excision of aneurysm and Dacron graft; ligation and exclusion using vein; excision of aneurysm and bypass using autologous vein **(Figs. 11-14 and 11-15)**.

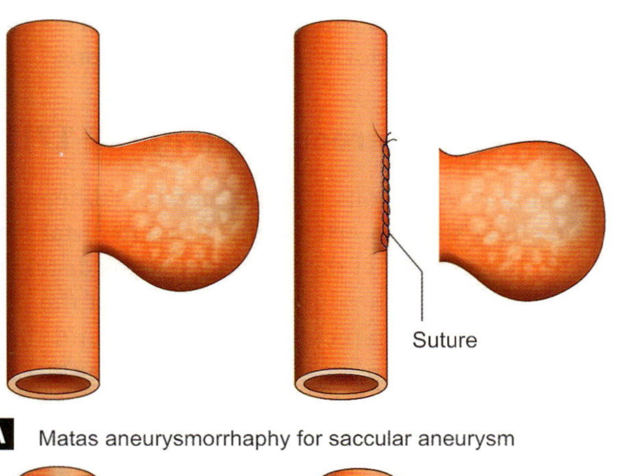

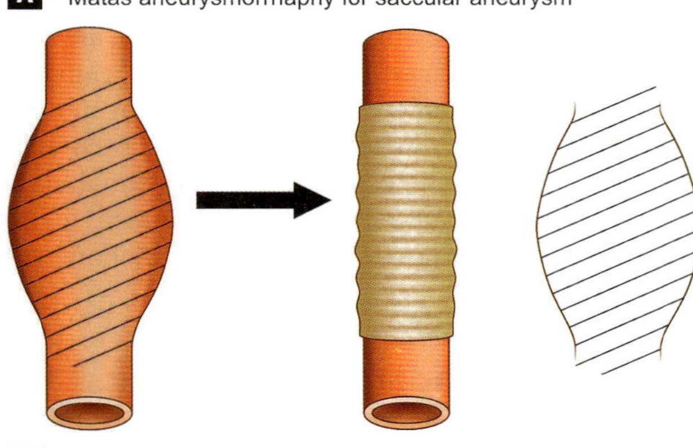

Figs. 11-14A and B

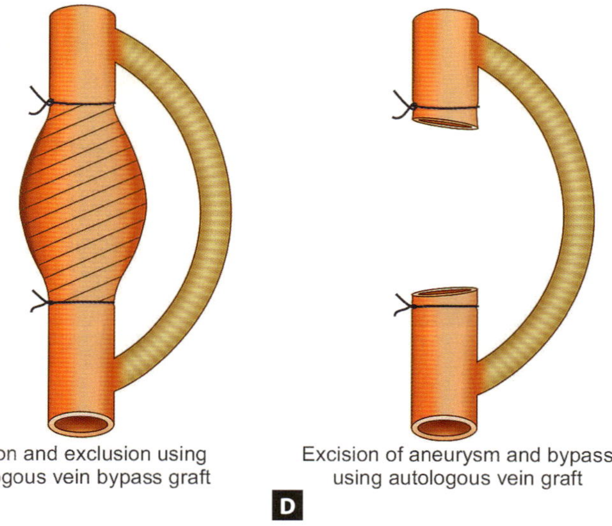

Figs. 11-14C and D

Figs. 11-14A to D: Different surgical approaches for managing peripheral aneurysm. Basic principles are similar—meticulous dissection proximally and distally; heparinisation on table; proper clamping of artery on either ends; right selection of the technique; avoidance of sepsis; synthetic (Dacron or PTFE) or venous graft placement; proper postoperative positioning; prevention of postoperative sepsis and thrombosis.

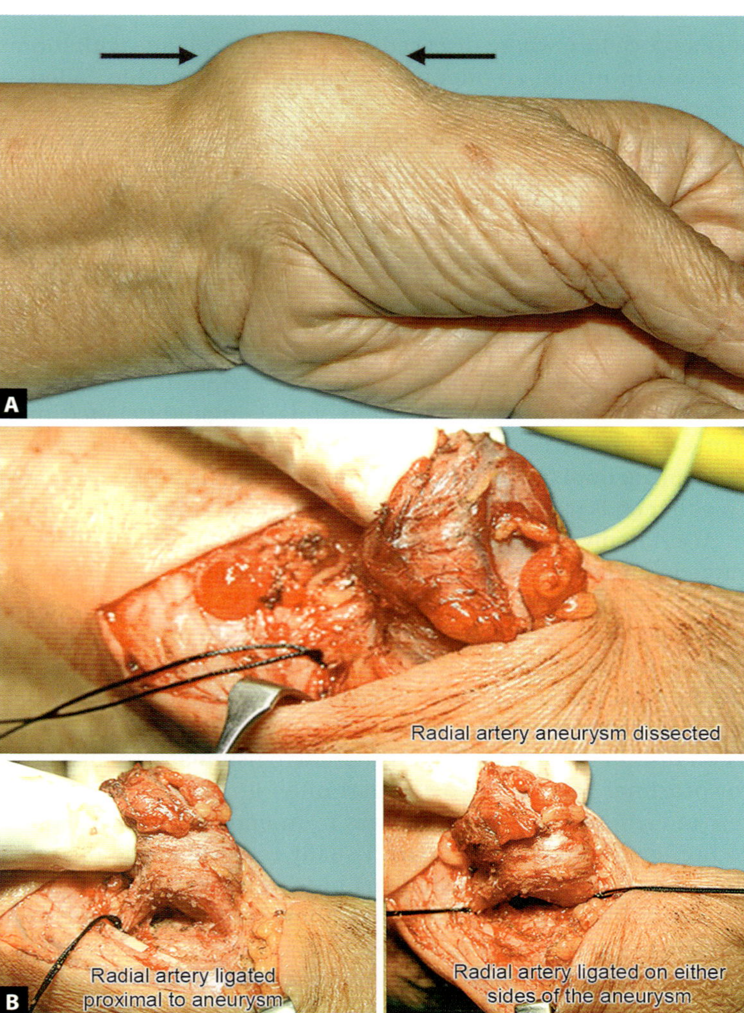

Figs. 11-15A and B

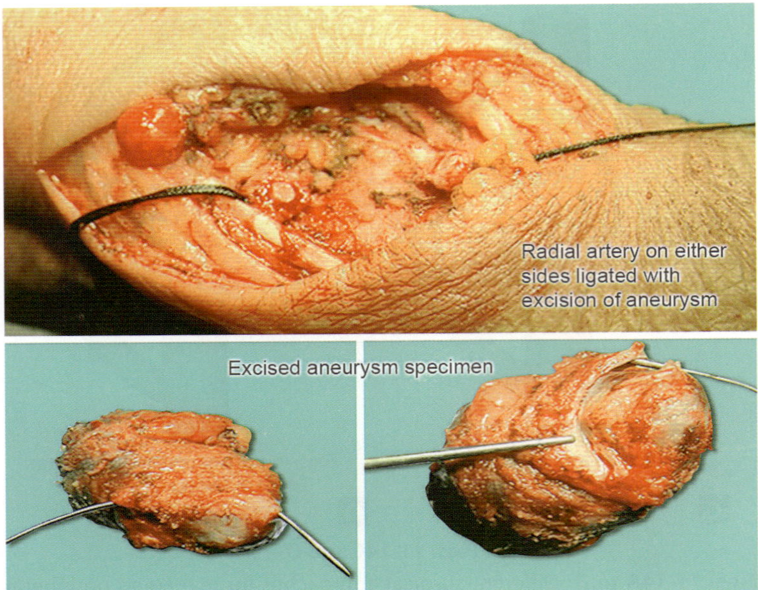

Fig. 11-15C

Figs. 11-15A to C: Radial artery aneurysm. It is excised with ligation of the artery proximally and distally. Usually there is no need to repair as collateral circulation through ulnar artery and palmar arch will maintain the distal circulation.

ENDARTERECTOMY

It is a procedure where diseased atheromatous plaque with intima is excised through an adequate arteriotomy. It is often called as *reboring/disobliteration*.

It is done in short stenotic lesion commonly; often it is done in long arterial blocks where graft is contraindicated. It is done commonly in *carotid artery*.

Preoperative *angiogram* is a must to evaluate exact site, extent and nature of the arterial stenosis.

Procedure

Artery is exposed with proper incision. Patient is heparinised. Arterial clamps are applied on both ends. Longitudinal incision is made over the artery using No. 15 blade. Incision deepened with same blade until fresh blood oozes out. Incision is further extended on either ends using *Pott's* scissor.

Arteriotomy edges are held and lifted using fine instruments by surgeon and assistant. A plane between arterial wall and diseased intima with plaque is created.

Dissector is passed at distal end around the plaque which is then continued proximally. Proximal end of the plaque is cut circumferentially. Proximal to this point of cut, intima should never be lifted off and if done it will cause flap dissection as complication. Then distal end of the plaque is cut taking similar care like done for proximal part. In the distal part often it is necessary to place few interrupted anchoring sutures from endarterectomised part to non-endarterectomised part. Usually removal of the plaque is done from proximal to distal part of the artery. Only in difficult situations like in carotid endarterectomy (often), it is done from distal to proximal part **(Fig. 11-16)**.

Each clamp is released once and reapplied to check the forward flow and backflow.

Arteriotomy is closed using 3-zero polypropylene in large artery, 5-zero polypropylene in small arteries. Artery lesser than 5 mm is closed with a venous or synthetic graft patch to prevent re-stenosis at the site. A holding single interrupted suture is placed first at proximal site. Then closure of arteriotomy is done using continuous sutures from *distal to proximally*.

Always proximal vascular clamp is first released to empty the air from the arteriotomy segment. Then distal clamp is released. Artery distal to the arteriotomy is palpated for adequate pulsation. Distal part of the arterial wall is inspected for few minutes for possible formation of bluish discoloration as an evident of intimal flap lift distally. Here distal pulse is absent but pulsation may be well felt over dissected intimal flap part.

Postoperative Management

Closed suction drain is placed. Blood pressure monitoring to prevent/control hypertension is needed so that to reduce hyperperfusion syndrome. Heparin should be given for 5–10 days. Later warfarin may be needed. Infection should be prevented. If infection develops proper antibiotics should be given. One should watch the area for haematoma. Distal pulse, limb warmness, should be checked at regular intervals. Postoperative Doppler should be done for assessment. Immobilisation of the part and positioning is required for 2 weeks.

Problems and Complications

Intimal flap dissection is an on table problem. Procedure may be insufficient and on table decision may be taken to change over to graft interposition.

Haematoma, torrential bleeding, infection, reblock, thrombosis formation and suture breakdown are the complications.

Semiclosed Endarterectomy (Fig. 11-17)

It is used in lengthy occlusions of the artery. Initial heparinisation → clamps on either sides → arteriotomy distal to distal part of the occluded part → extension of the incision towards distal occluded part → dissection and cutting of the distal part of the plaque → passing of the loop endarterectomy stripper around the plaque towards proximal part (often arc stripper is also used) → plaque is broken gently using artery forceps or using thumb and fingers → care must be taken that outer wall of artery is not damaged → plaque is gently removed using loop. If fragments of plaque are left in the wall, which can be confirmed by feeling, can be removed using Martin's thrombectomy forceps. Undue traction or more should not be executed as it may injure the vessel wall. In such difficulties another arteriotomy may be made over the proximal end of the occluded artery. Arteriotomy is closed from distal end to proximal end. When two arteriotomies are present, proximal one is closed first, then the distal one.

Wiley's Eversion Endarterectomy (Fig. 11-18)

Here artery is transected completely (transversely) so that right plane between diseased intimal plaque and media is created

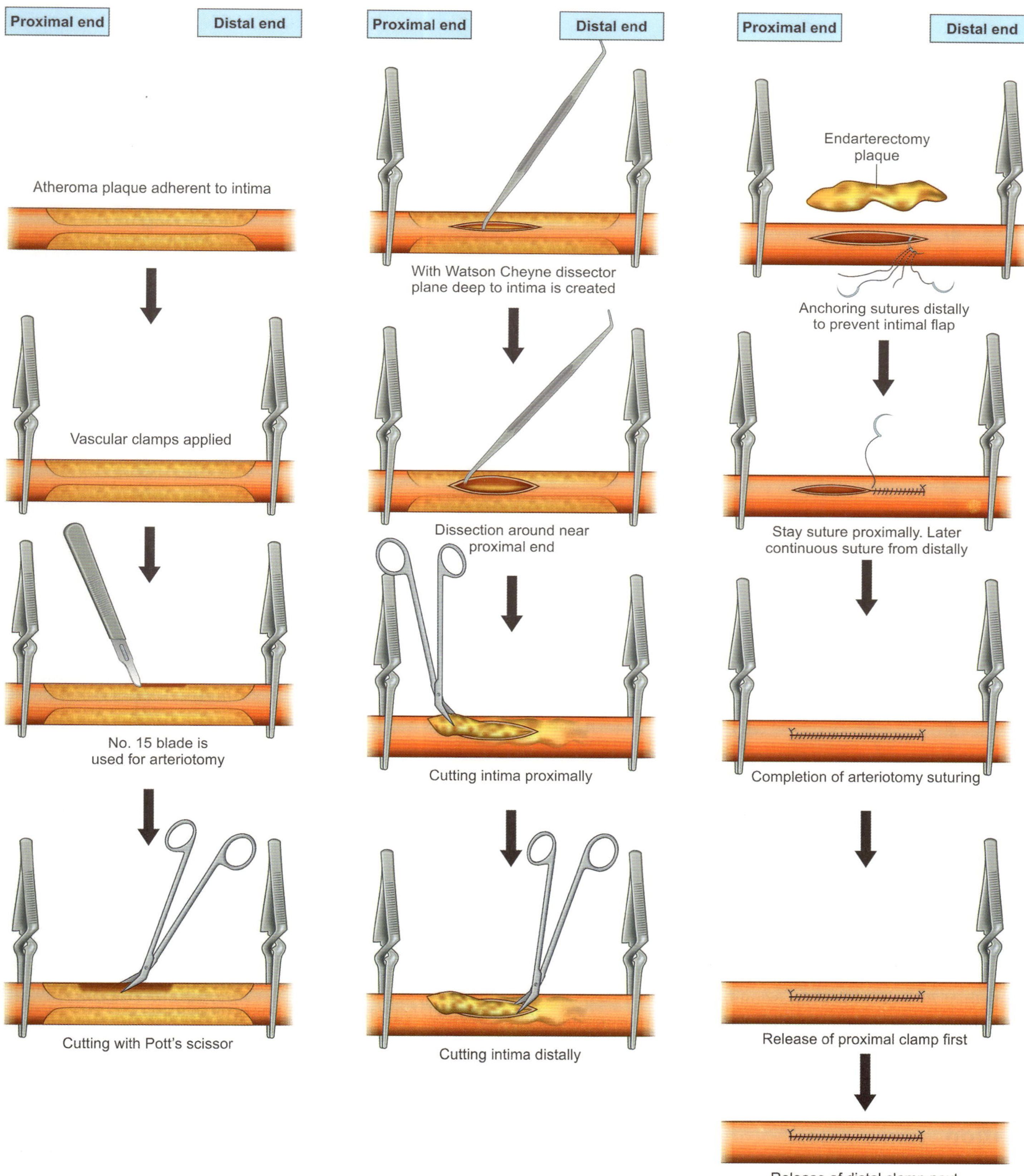

Fig. 11-16: Open endarterectomy technique.

circumferentially. Once plane is created all around arterial wall is everted to exteriorise the plaque completely. Everted artery is reduced later. Cut ends of the artery is sutured using polypropylene interrupted sutures with bite taking from outside-in of the endarterectomised segment to inside out of the unendarterectomised segment.

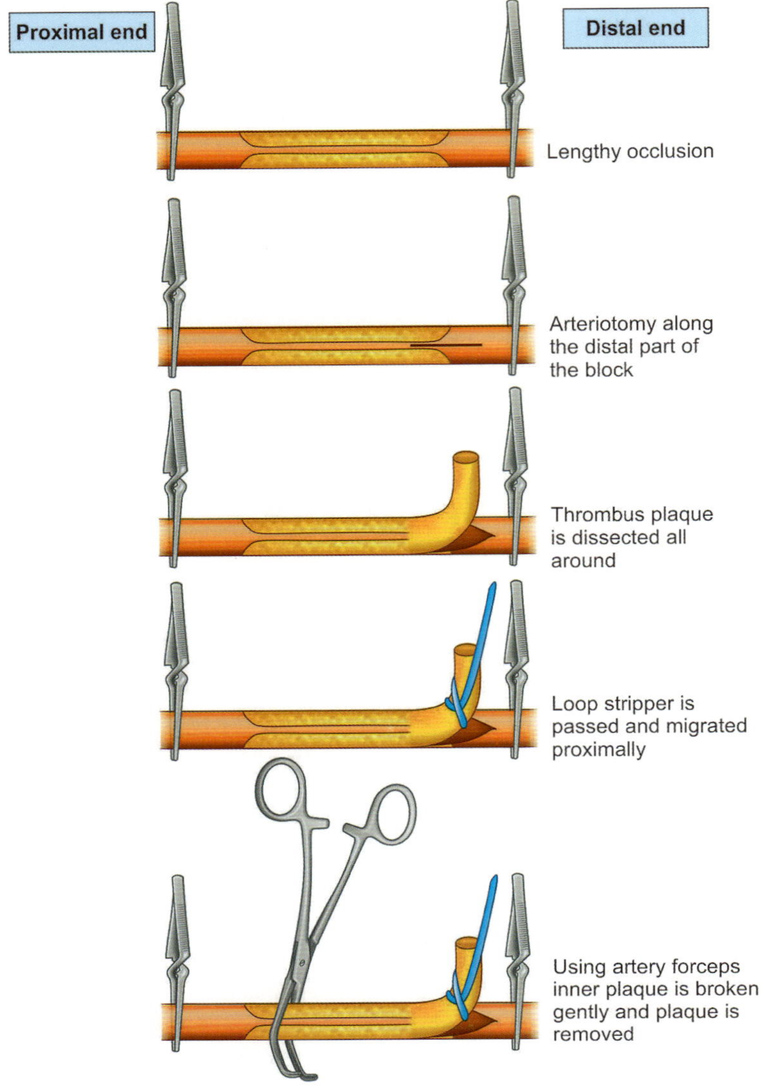

Fig. 11-17: Semiclosed/semiopen endarterectomy.

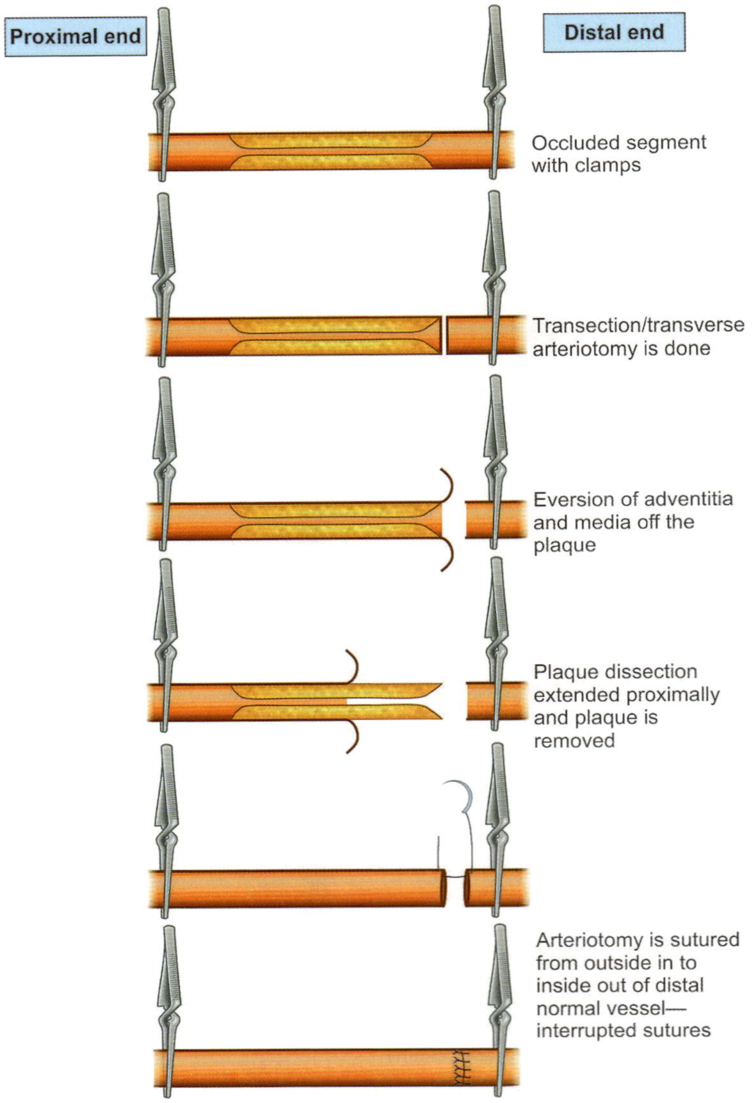

Proximal end
Distal end
Occluded segment with clamps
Transection/transverse arteriotomy is done
Eversion of adventitia and media off the plaque
Plaque dissection extended proximally and plaque is removed
Arteriotomy is sutured from outside in to inside out of distal normal vessel—interrupted sutures

Fig. 11-18: Eversion endarterectomy technique.

CAROTID ENDARTERECTOMY

Indications

- Asymptomatic carotid stenosis more than 60% by angiography or more than 70% on Duplex ultrasound.
- Symptomatic carotid stenosis with cerebrovascular accident/transient ischaemic attacks/amaurosis fugax with >50% block.

Carotid endarterectomy *prevents development of stroke* for significantly long period.

Evaluation

Blood parameters, lipid profile, duplex ultrasound are the usual needed investigations. Duplex ultrasound is sensitive method of assessing the carotid artery. Angiogram is done only in selected patients with re-stenosis, neck irradiation, earlier neck lymph node block dissection, and atypical cases.

Procedure

Patient is placed in semi-sitting position with round pillow under shoulder to extend the neck. Head is rotated towards opposite side. Arm on the same side is tucked over the chest or side of the table. Earlobe, mastoid, mandible, sternal notch and clavicle area should be prepared and exposed as landmarks.

Procedure is done under general anaesthesia with routine or selective shunting as needed. Intraoperative EEG monitoring is essential. Regional anaesthesia is often used.

Incision is oblique one along the anterior margin of the sternocleidomastoid muscle. Transverse incision is also often used. But it is not useful in higher lesions. Platysma once divided; medial margin of the sternomastoid muscle is dissected from its upper tendon part to the level of the omohyoid. Internal jugular vein is dissected by sharp dissection along its medial edge. Common facial vein, middle thyroid vein and hypoglossal veins are ligated carefully. Sternomastoid and IJV are retracted laterally. Ansa cervicalis is cut near its origin. Superior thyroid artery is dissected near its origin. Common, external and internal carotid arteries are dissected all round circumferentially at the confluence. Each artery is held with vascular tape (sling with snub). Superior thyroid artery is held with a loop of silk suture. Hypoglossal nerve is identified by tracing the ansa hypoglossal part above. It is further mobilised after ligating the occipital and sternomastoid arteries. Digastric muscle is divided only when there is a need to expose distal part of the internal carotid artery. Internal carotid artery *should be exposed adequately when needed prior to arteriotomy.* It is difficult to expose internal carotid artery distally once arteriotomy is already done.

Internal carotid artery distally is occluded with a vascular clamp/clip. Routine or selective shunting of the carotid (internal) artery is done. Longitudinal arteriotomy is done → plaque is dissected off the media → proximal portion is first dissected circumferentially → extended towards distal part of the internal carotid artery → eversion endarterectomy is done in external carotid artery plaque → heparinised saline irrigation of the bed of the opened artery is done → with fine forceps small pieces of plaques are removed → Dacron or bovine pericardium patch graft is placed over the defect → sutured to vessel using polypropylene suture material 4-zero or 5-zero. Prior to completion of suturing near the end shunt is removed and back bleed is allowed. First blood flow is allowed to external carotid artery then only internal carotid artery.

Nasotracheal intubation and mandibular subluxation may be needed in difficult cases.

Risk and Problems

It is not possible to do endarterectomy for most distal part of the internal carotid artery in the neck.

Perioperative stroke risk is 1.5%.

Hypoglossal nerve injury, non-recurrent laryngeal nerve (anomaly) injury (it is mistaken for ansa cervicalis and is cut), superior laryngeal nerve injury, marginal mandibular branch (facial nerve) injury, glossopharyngeal nerve injury and spinal accessory nerve injury are neurological complications in relation to cranial nerves.

Distal end of the stenosis should be assessed properly as distal exposure is often difficult. It is quite difficult to expose unusual high bifurcation of the carotid.

Postoperative bleeding, myocardial infarction and carotid re-stenosis are other complications.

Eversion Carotid Endarterectomy

It is done in well-localised severe lesions. Type I transection is done as oblique near vertical cut when main block is in the internal carotid artery. Type II transection is done as oblique near transverse cut when main block is in common carotid artery. Shunt is needed during the procedure. After endarterectomy end-to-end anastomosis is done often with a synthetic patch.

AORTOILIAC THROMBOENDARTERECTOMY

Open (Dos Santos), semi-closed, eversion methods are used. Often aortofemoral bypass has replaced this procedure. Even though commonly performed procedure is bypass graft in cases with localised disease at distal aorta and iliac arteries, thromboendarterectomy is also done. In a *contaminated field* endarterectomy is *better* than graft.

Evaluation is done with duplex ultrasound, angiography of entire abdominal aorta, visceral and renal branches. Both anteroposterior and lateral views are essential as origin of the celiac and superior mesenteric arteries and posterior aortic plaques are well identified by lateral views. To assess the extent of the disease oblique films are taken. Distal tibial films are taken to check distal run off. Pull back pressure gradient more than 10 mmHg after injection of vasodilator like papaverine suggests significant block. Transfemoral Seldinger method is used for both angiogram and pressure gradient assessment. If there is complete block, transbrachial or lumbar transaortic approach may be used. Arterial digital subtraction angiography can be used. Venous DSA is less informative. Systemic assessment like of renal, cardiac and respiratory should be done.

Prophylactic antibiotic is given intravenously one hour before surgery.

General anaesthesia with epidural supplements is used.

Approach: Retroperitoneal standard or transabdominal approach is used.

Procedure

Left side 45° elevated position is used. Break table (reverse flexion/jack knife) position will give additional access.

↓

Incision is from a point just medial to the lateral margin of the left rectus muscle just below the umbilicus level extending laterally to the tip of the 12th rib. Incision is deepened to superficial fascia and fat.

↓

Anterior rectus sheath is incised to expose rectus muscle. Rectus muscle is either transected or retracted medially. Care should be taken not to open the peritoneum.

↓

External oblique, internal oblique and transverse abdominis muscles are cut in the line of incision. Glistening peritoneum is visualised. It is swept/pushed using gauze or finger and retracted medially. Psoas major muscle and genitofemoral nerve is identified **(Fig. 11-19)**.

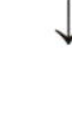

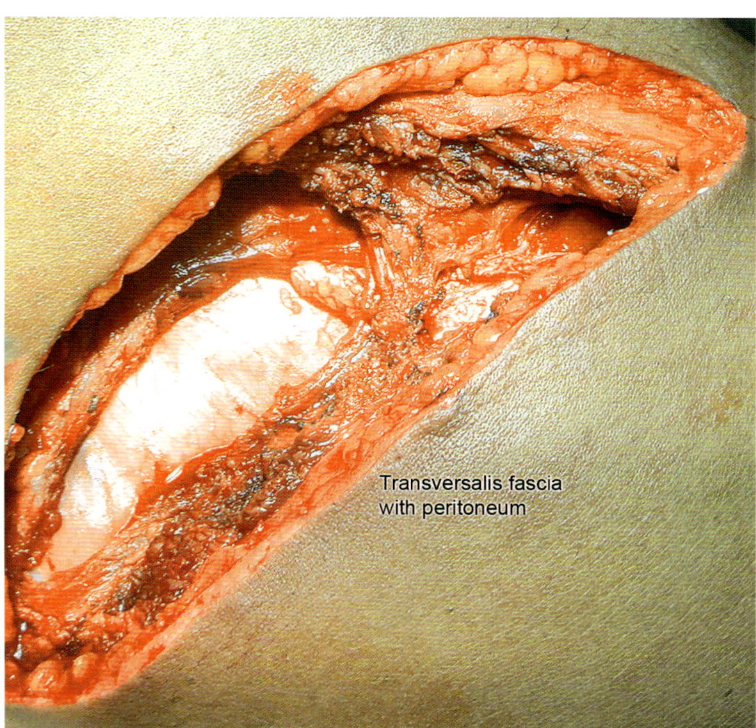

Fig. 11-19: Extraperitoneal approach for aortoiliac segment.

Inferior mesenteric artery is identified, ligated and divided. Aorta and iliac arteries are mobilised properly along full/adequate length. 3 cm proximal and 3 cm distal to the level of occlusion should be isolated.

↓

Common, external and internal iliac arteries are dissected; middle sacral and lumbar arteries are identified.

↓

Vascular clamps are placed at all ends.

↓

Arteriotomy incisions are made in the aorta and iliac arteries in different methods. (A) Here two incisions are used—(1) From right of the inferior mesenteric artery extending down along the origin of right common iliac artery. (2) Second incision is separately along the left common iliac artery. This is done to avoid injury to preaortic autonomic plexus which is located to the left side of aortic bifurcation. (B) In this type three separate arteriotomies are made in the aorta and both common iliac arteries. Arteriotomy incisions in iliac arteries should extend beyond their bifurcations.

↓

Endarterectomy is begun at proximal part using a spatula circumferentially; then extending distally along the diseased segment of the artery.

↓

Initially it is cut transversely at proximal point; later at distal point using Pott's scissor.

↓

Endarterectomised part of the vessel is inspected, loose debris and thrombus are removed, and part is irrigated with heparinised saline solution.

↓

Often intima at distal cut margin should be anchored to the artery using non-absorbable polypropylene interrupted mattress sutures which are tied outside. It is done to prevent *intimal flap* dissection.

↓

Repeated irrigation using heparinised solution is needed.

↓

Arteriotomies are closed using continuous 4-zero polypropylene sutures from proximal to distal. Vascular clamps are released just prior to last suture bite; first distal clamp is released then proximal clamp is released.

↓

Arteriotomy often is closed using Dacron or PTFE (Polytetrafluoroethylene) graft as a patch.

↓

Once after release of vascular clamps if bleeding points are found over the sutured arteriotomy, then it is controlled by interrupted 6-zero sutures/liquid thrombin/collagen/light pack and pressure **(Figs. 11-20A to I)**.

Anticoagulant effect is reversed using protamine sulfate.

Postoperative Care

ICU monitoring for 2 days. CVP line, pulmonary artery catheter line, radial artery line, urinary catheter is a must.

Complications

- It is technically more demanding. It is done in only selected localised disease.
- Bleeding can occur which occasionally requires re-exploration. Hypovolemia is common.

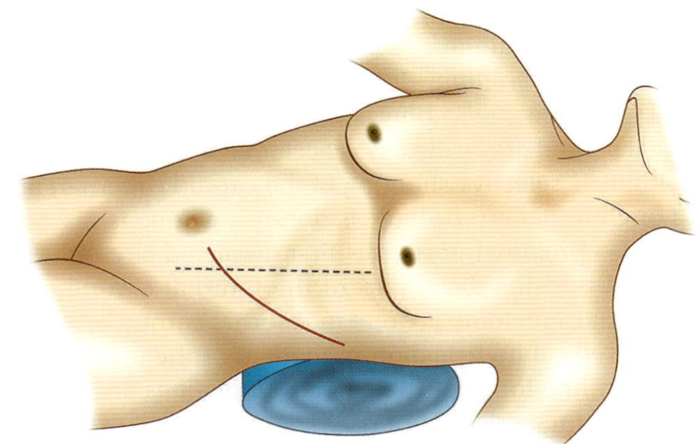

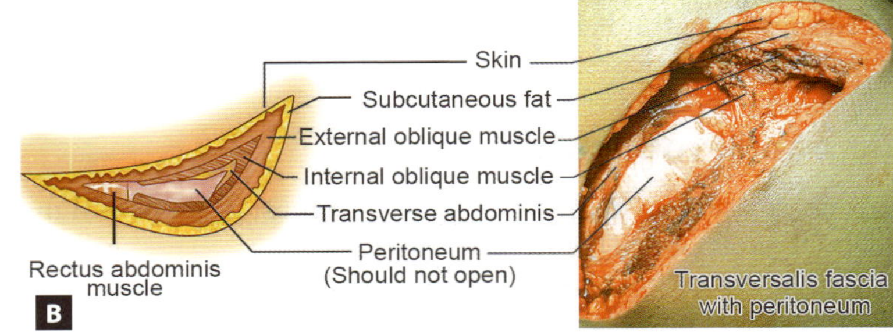

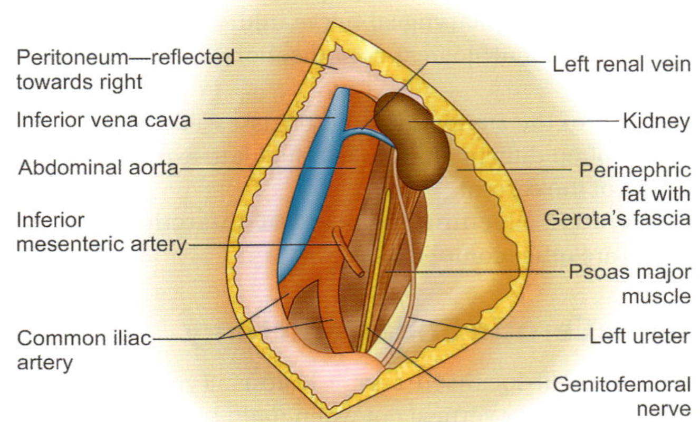

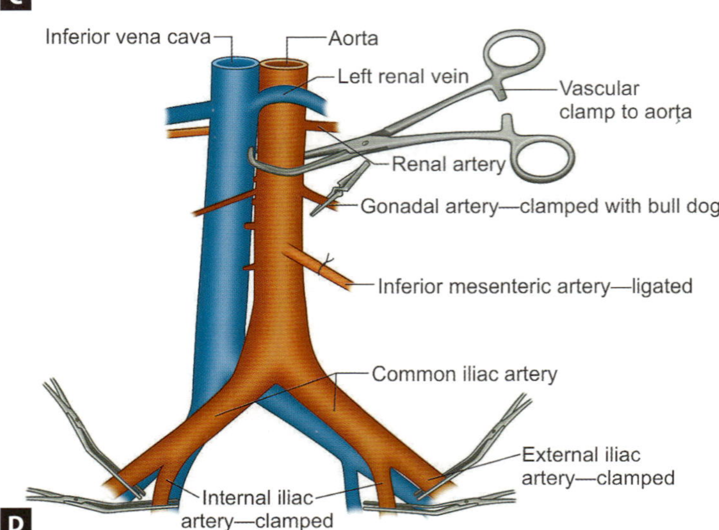

Figs. 11-20A to D

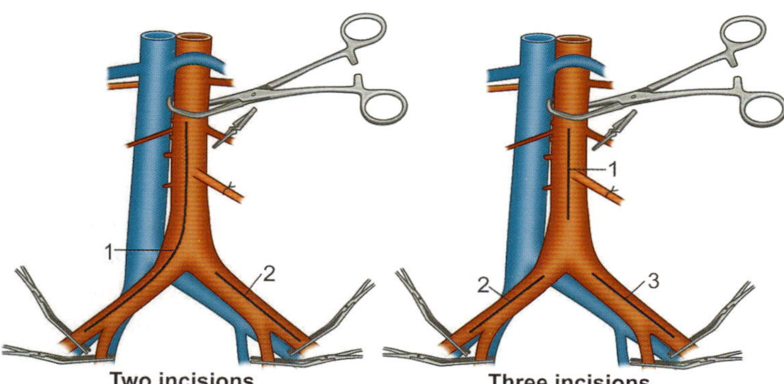

Two incisions

1. First incision is on the aorta along the right of origin of the inferior mesenteric artery extending along the right common iliac up to external iliac artery
2. Second arteriotomy incision along left common iliac artery

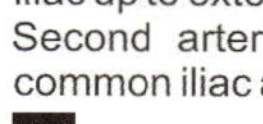

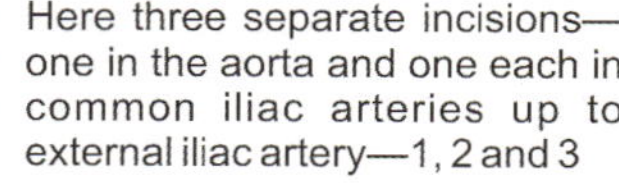

Three incisions

Here three separate incisions—one in the aorta and one each in common iliac arteries up to external iliac artery—1, 2 and 3

E

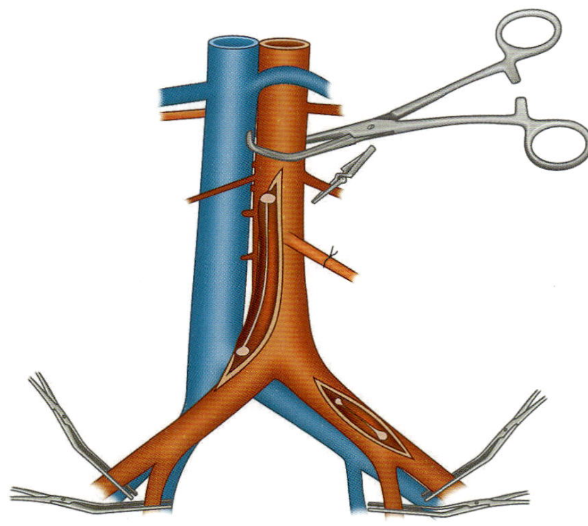

Intima with thrombus (endarterectomy) is separated from media throughout the length of the arteriotomy incisions both proximally and distally and cut across on both ends

F

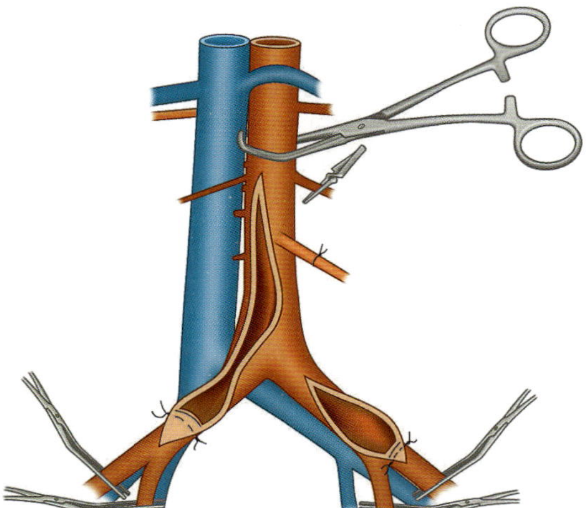

After extraction of endarterectomy specimen, mattress anchoring sutures at the distal end intima with knots outside—are placed to prevent intimal flap

G

Figs. 11-20E to G

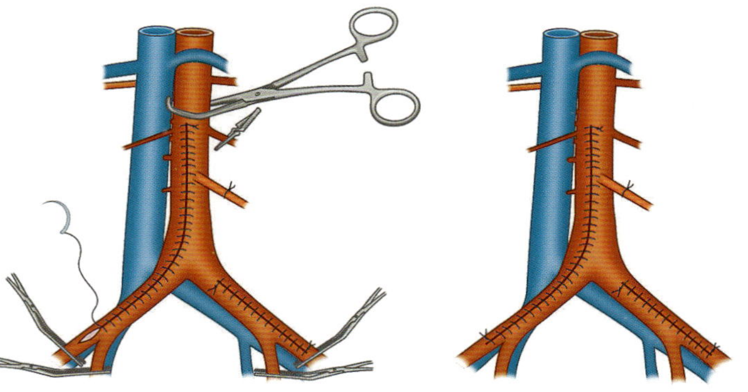

Closing the arteriotomy using continuous polypropylene 4-zero sutures

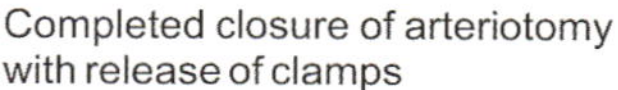

Completed closure of arteriotomy with release of clamps

H

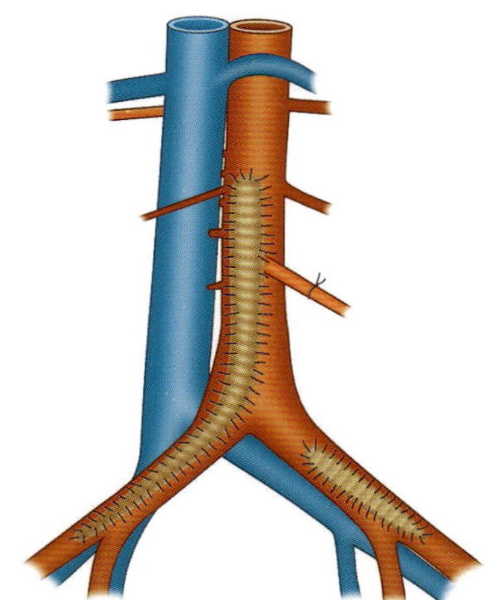

When the lumen is narrow arteriotomy can be closed with PTFE/Dacron vascular graft patch to widen the lumen

I

Figs. 11-20H and I

Figs. 11-20A to I: Technique of aortoiliac endarterectomy.

- Rethrombosis and failure is also a known complication.
- Distal ischaemia and gangrene can occur. Doppler study of limbs is done to assess the distal perfusion.
- Embolism due to atheroma dislodged when it occurs with intact pulse needs embolectomy.
- Injury to aortic nerve plexus may cause impotence but it is less common.
- Wound infection, haematoma and abscess formation are other complications. Progressive haematoma needs re-exploration.
- *Colonic ischaemia* mainly left sided (sigmoid) can occur. Only mucosal ischaemia is treated by nasogastric aspiration; deeper level ischaemia needs laparotomy and resection.

ARTERIAL SUBSTITUTES

Ideal arterial substitute is not yet developed. Ideal arterial substitute should be strong, durable for patient's life, biocompatible, non-thrombogenic, should be resistant for infection, easily available, should have a long-term patency rate and elastic property of normal artery.

Features of ideal graft

- Strong
- Durable for patient's life
- Non-thrombogenic
- Biocompatible
- Resistant to infection
- Flexible
- Should maintain long-term patency
- Should have elastic property of normal artery
- Should be leakproof on restoration of blood flow
- Should not chemically or physically degenerate
- Should not cause any abnormal reaction to surrounding tissues
- Should not occlude when flexed
- Should not damage blood contents

Carrel and Guthrie first did venous autograft into arteries of dogs. They did extensive histological study of viable and non-viable grafts. Lexer in 1907 used saphenous vein for axillary artery repair. Murray started to use intraoperative heparin. Enaz Moniz and dos Santos originated technique of arteriography. Gross and his colleagues in 1948 started to use viable arterial allografts. Later it was found that as far as graft is considered tissue viability is not essential for success of graft take up.

Classification of Arterial Substitutes

1. Arterial allograft: Not used.
2. Arterial autograft: Internal mammary artery (common), internal iliac artery.
3. Arterial xenograft: Bovine carotid artery graft - not used.
4. Venous autograft: Long saphenous vein (common), small saphenous vein, basilic vein, cephalic vein.
5. Venous allograft: Umbilical vein graft.
6. Prosthetic grafts:
   a. Textile grafts
      - Dacron graft: Knitted or woven or crimping or velour types.
      - Teflon graft: Knitted or woven or crimping or velour types.
   b. Non-textile semi-inert polymer graft
      - ePTFE graft: Expanded polytetrafluoroethylene graft.

Arterial Allograft

As aorta contains more collagen and elastin long-term graft function is more than in femoral artery which contains more smooth muscle. Arterial allograft loose endothelium rapidly with formation of platelet fibrin coagulum. Over the years graft becomes less cellular with thinning of the wall. Late thrombosis, calcification, aneurysm formation and rupture can occur. Arterial allografts are not used now.

Arterial Autografts

Arterial autografts has the *advantages of* intact blood supply, resistance for infection, maintenance of flexibility, absence of degeneration, growth potential when used in paediatric age group. Wylie in 1965 first used arterial autograft. There is very less incidence of intimal thrombosis in autograft. Small initial thrombus formed around suture line will get absorbed in 20 days.

Inner most 500 μ thickness of arterial wall gets its nutrition directly from luminal blood through diffusion. Thickness outer to this level gets its blood supply through vasa vasora, a complex system derived from arterial side branches. So in arterial autograft few side branches should be retained.

Arterial autografts are used in *coronary artery bypass*, renal artery bypass (in paediatric age group), in places where graft is needed in infected field.

Internal mammary artery is the commonest and *preferred autograft* used. Internal iliac artery can be used in paediatric age group and in adults if it is not atherosclerosed.

Internal mammary artery is commonly used for CABG (coronary artery bypass graft). It shows superior long-term patency (95%) and is very suitable in emergency situation. Both internal mammary arteries are used commonly. They are dissected from chest wall retaining wide pedicle. *Distal internal mammary artery anastomosis* is done as end-to-side into the coronary artery using 8-zero polypropylene interrupted sutures. *Sequential internal mammary artery grafting* is also done when more than two anastomoses are needed. Free internal mammary arterial graft also can be used wherein internal mammary artery is cut at its origin and is sutured to proximal part of the aorta if extra length is needed. A combination of bilateral internal mammary artery graft with sequential and free mammary graft is called as *complex mammary grafting.*

Internal mammary artery (internal intercostal) arises from inferior aspect of the first part of the subclavian artery 2 cm above the sternal end of clavicle. It runs downwards, forward and medially behind sternal end of clavicle, internal jugular vein, brachiocephalic vein, first costal cartilage and phrenic nerve. Below and behind the first costal cartilage artery runs vertically downwards up to 6th intercostal space. Here it is related in front to pectoralis major, upper six costal cartilages, external intercostal membrane, internal intercostal muscles and upper six intercostal nerves. Behind it is related to endothoracic fascia and pleura up to 3rd costal cartilage; further it is separated from pleura by sternocostalis muscle. At 6th intercostal space it divides into two terminal branches as superior epigastric artery and musculophrenic artery. Below 3rd intercostal space artery is accompanied by two venae commitantes which join together to form internal mammary vein which runs on the medial side of the artery to join brachiocephalic vein. Internal mammary lymph nodes are located along the artery. Its branches are—pericardiophrenic artery, mediastinal arteries, and two anterior intercostal arteries (upper and lower) for each upper six spaces, perforating branches and terminal branches **(Figs. 11-21 and 11-22)**.

Arterial Xenograft

Xenograft from other species causes immense immunologic reactions leading to graft rejection. A modified xenograft (*Rosenberg*) is derived from *bovine carotid artery* which is treated by proteolytic enzyme ficin. Ficin removes smooth muscle and elastic tissue retaining collagen tube which has got equal tensile strength and is non-antigenic. This collagen tube is tanned with dialdehyde starch. But this graft has got high rate of aneurysm formation (6%) and high infection rate (6%) and patency rate is 40% after 6 years. So this type is also inferior to autograft and synthetic grafts.

Venous Autograft

Saphenous vein autograft is commonly used autograft as arterial substitute successfully. Normal ***long saphenous vein*** in adult is 60 cm in length and thigh part is a single trunk. 8–12 valves of LSV is mainly located at below knee level. Its average diameter is 5.5 mm after gentle distension in thigh. Minimum diameter required for grafting is 4 mm. In 10% of individuals LSV is too small for grafting; in another 20% patients it cannot be used due to phlebitis, varicosity, and prior surgery. So only in 70% of people it is available for grafting. In 30% of non-available LSV category, small saphenous vein, basilic vein or cephalic vein can be used as a graft. But these alternate veins

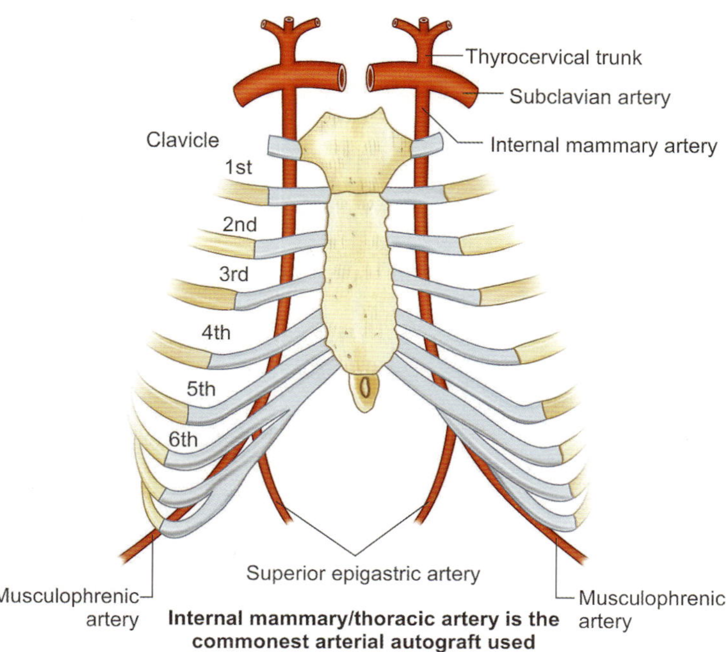

Fig. 11-21: Arterial autograft. Internal mammary artery is commonly used.

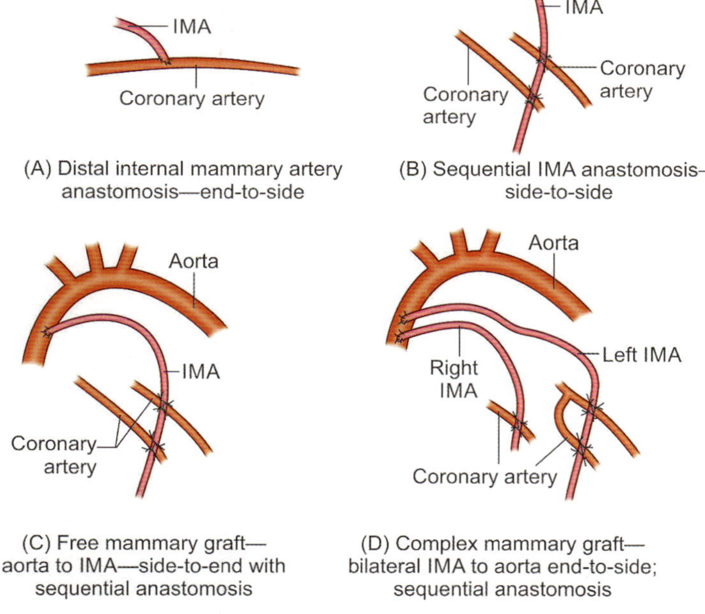

Fig. 11-22: Technique of internal mammary artery (IMA) graft to coronary artery.

are not as good as LSV. Saphenous vein graft is used for small and medium-sized arterial replacement—mainly in coronary artery bypass and lower limb bypass surgeries (superficial femoral and popliteal). *Standard reversed saphenous vein graft or modified in situ saphenous* vein grafts may be used. It is excellent for coronary and femoropopliteal artery bypass. Carrel observed that after vein graft there will be marked subintimal and medial hyperplasia of the venous graft called as 'arterialisation' of vein graft.

Venous Allograft

Saphenous vein allograft was not successful. ***Umbilical vein allograft*** is successful after glutaraldehyde tanning of the graft which increases collagen wall strength and also makes graft non-antigenic. Complications are aneurysm formation, separation and infolding of inner lining causing luminal narrowing. Its only advantage over prosthetic graft is availability and cost.

Prosthetic Grafts

Voorhees in 1952 developed nylon related porous textile graft Vinyon N and used as arterial replacement in animals.

Later Dacron and Teflon synthetic grafts were evoluted. Dacron looses up to 10% of its tensile strength. Teflon does not lose its tensile strength **(Figs. 11-23 and 11-24)**.

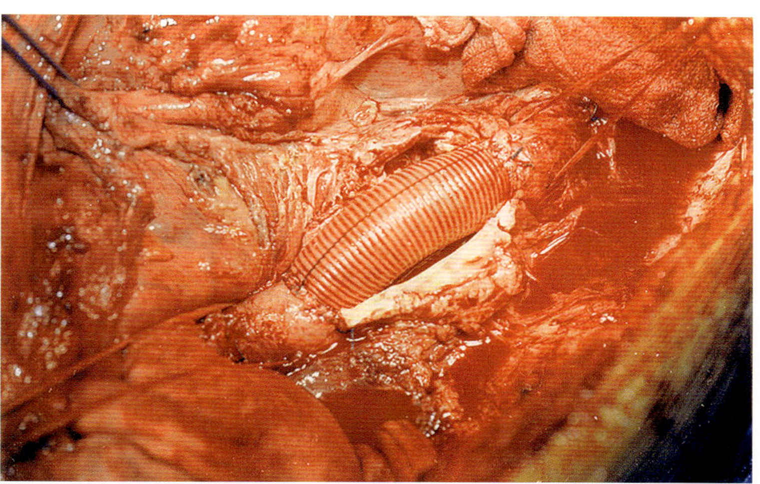

Fig. 11-23: Arterial prosthetic Dacron graft placed to aorta.

Prosthetic grafts are manufactured by weaving or knitting multifilament yarns of Dacron or Teflon.

Woven type is compact one with small interstices and low porosity. Woven graft has difficult in handling **(Fig. 11-25)**.

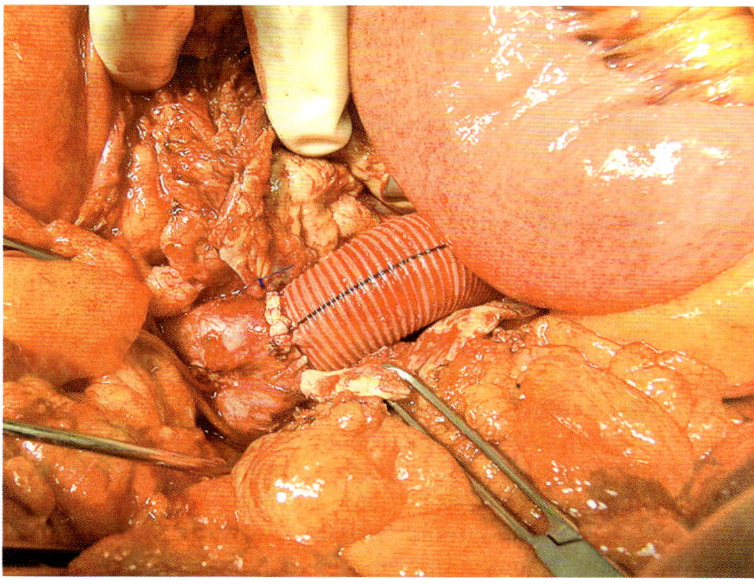

Fig. 11-24A

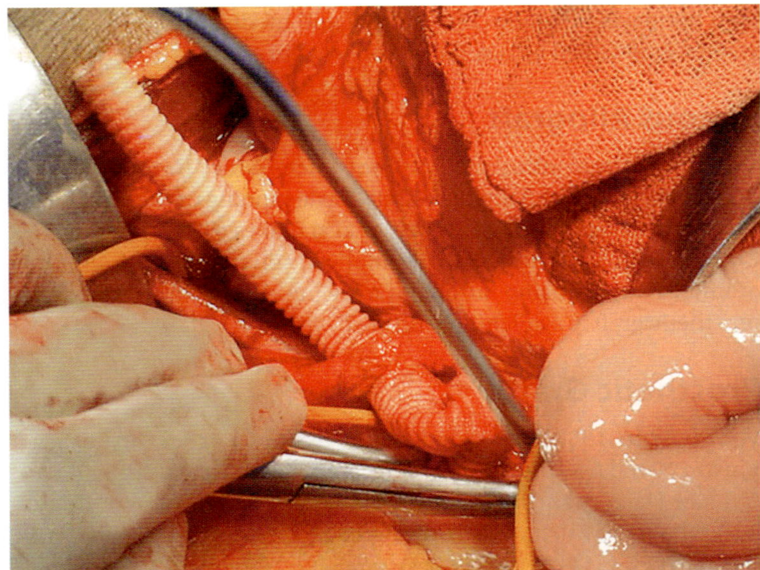

Fig. 11-24B

Figs. 11-24A and B: Dacron arterial graft placement.

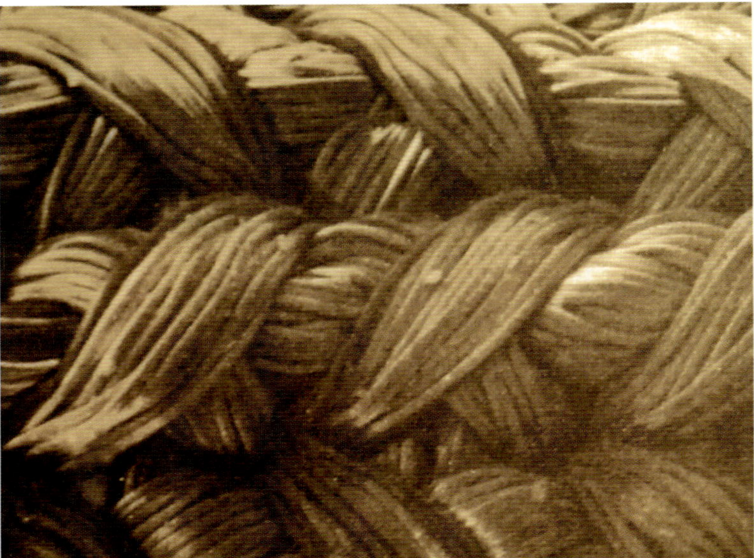

Fig. 11-26: Knitted Dacron graft.

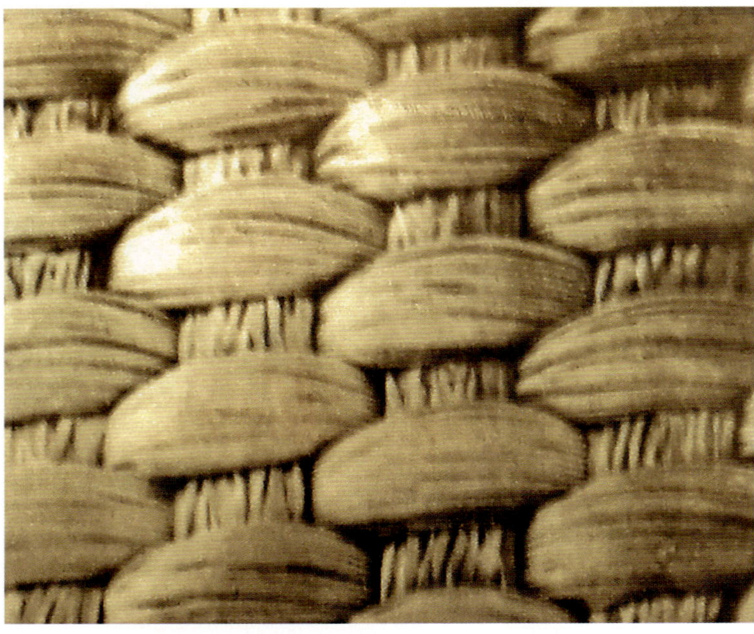

Fig. 11-25: Woven Dacron graft.

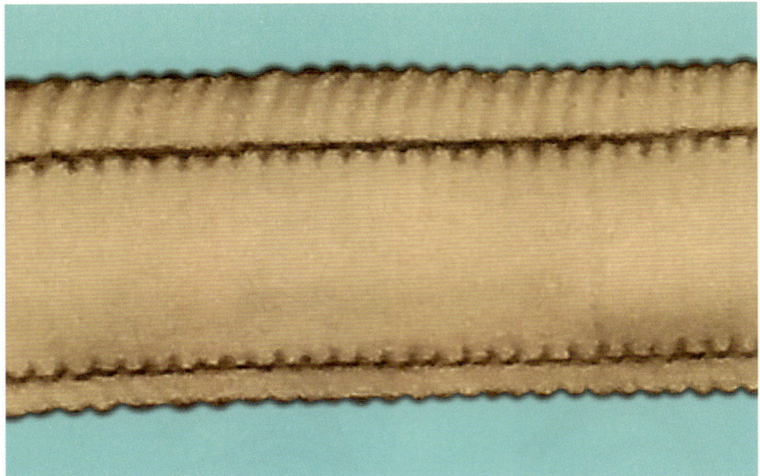

Fig. 11-27: Dacron crimping graft.

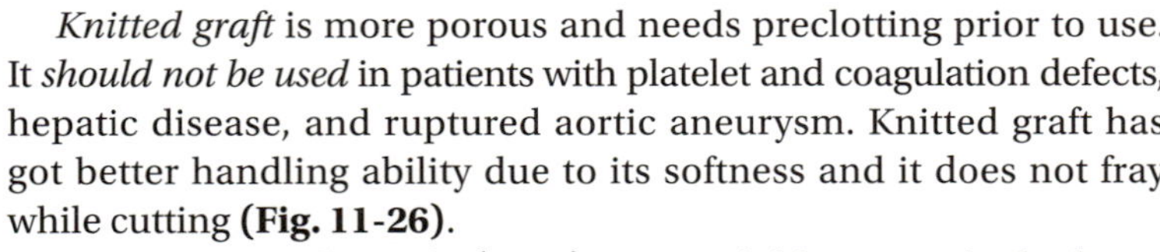

Knitted graft is more porous and needs preclotting prior to use. It *should not be used* in patients with platelet and coagulation defects, hepatic disease, and ruptured aortic aneurysm. Knitted graft has got better handling ability due to its softness and it does not fray while cutting **(Fig. 11-26)**.

Crimping textile grafts (1955) are available now which shows greater flexibility without kinking. But it may reduce the graft diameter and may be thrombogenic **(Fig. 11-27)**.

Velour surface graft (1960) was evoluted later with loops of yarn extending perpendicular to graft surface. It provides a better preclotting and gives scaffold for fibroblast proliferation and so makes graft firmly adherent to surrounding tissues **(Fig. 11-28)**.

Both knitted and woven grafts are commonly used. Surgeons prefer to preclot both grafts.

Preclotting the ***non-coated knitted*** or woven Dacron graft is done to seal the graft and to prevent leak and to create a smooth lining at graft-blood interface. This step is not necessary for PTFE

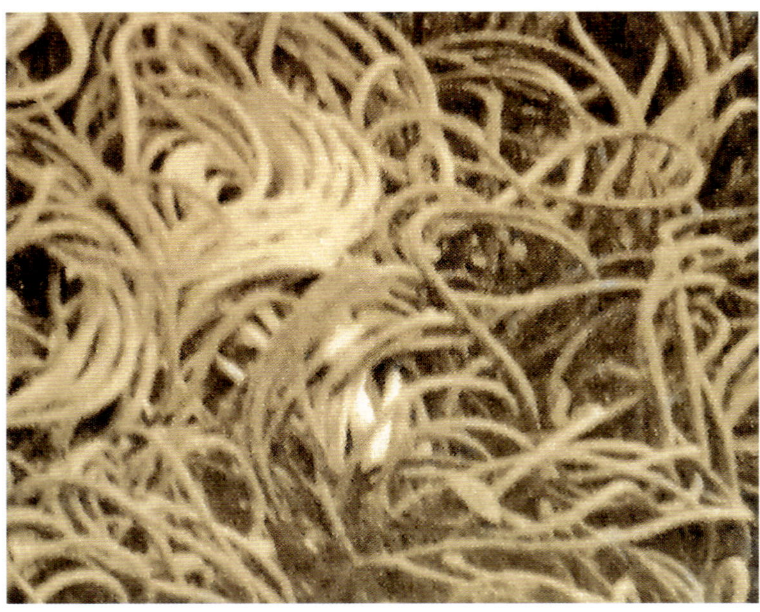

Fig. 11-28: Velour graft.

or newer grafts. Preclotting is done by collecting 100 mL of patients' blood prior to heparinisation from aorta or IVC using a syringe which is collected in a bowl. Selected graft is clamped at one end; from other end fresh blood collected in the bowl is forced into the graft using a fine catheter or syringe until leakage from the pores stops. Later graft is flushed using heparinised saline. Deposited platelet fibrin layer in the interstices on inner part of the graft after implantation is slowly replaced by fibrous in growth. Cooley described a *modified version of pre-clotting* of the prosthetic graft. Knitted Dacron graft is soaked with patient's own platelet-rich plasma and which is steam autoclaved for 5 minutes to produce a blood impervious graft in which denatured protein is slowly resorbed.

Expanded Polytetrafluoroethylene Graft (ePTFE)

Soyer (1972) first used ePTFE as arterial graft. PTFE is a fluorocarbon polymer manufactured by paste extrusion method containing solid nodules with interconnecting small fibrils. Standard pore size presently in use is 17 μ. Fluorine gives high electronegative surface charge to the polymer to prevent thrombosis. It is mainly used in lower limb arterial disease **(Fig. 11-29)**.

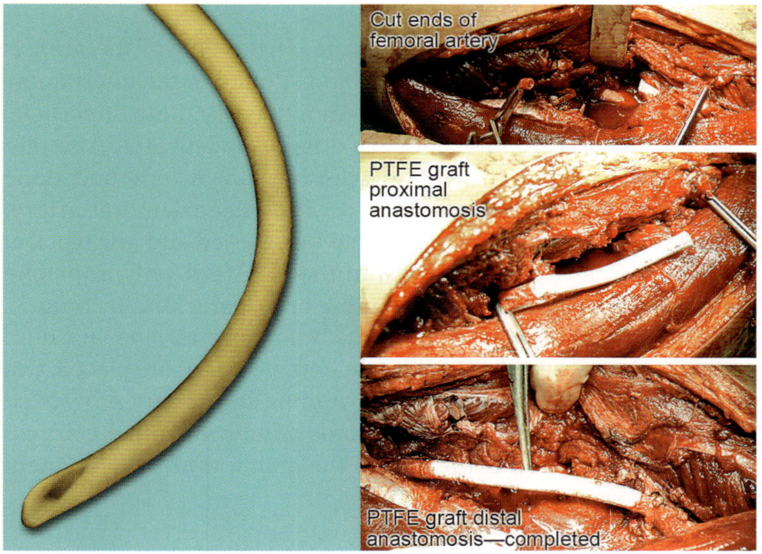

Fig. 11-29: PTFE graft. PTFE graft used in the lower limb in a patient.

Complications of Graft

Neointimal fibrous hyperplasia at suture lines of the graft is due to surgical trauma, PDFG, arterial smooth muscle proliferation.

Graft infection incidence is 2%. It is more in lower limb graft than abdominal graft. Peroperative cephalosporin administration reduces the rate of graft infection. If infection occurs graft should be removed and revascularisation is achieved using a saphenous vein graft.

Graft failure is rare but can occur. It is due to fibre degeneration, manufacturing defect, diffuse dilatation of graft (is due to expansion of the knit in knitted Dacron).

Anastomotic false aneurysm (3%) occurs just adjacent to suture line towards host artery. It is tearing of the artery adjacent to suture line due to mismatched graft artery compliance, improper suture placement, and arterial degeneration. There will be partial or total separation of the graft from the host with blood collection in a covering of the fibrous capsule. It eventually will rupture/may cause thrombosis and embolism. Treatment is graft–artery re-anastomosis with insertion of additional piece of graft **(Fig. 11-30)**.

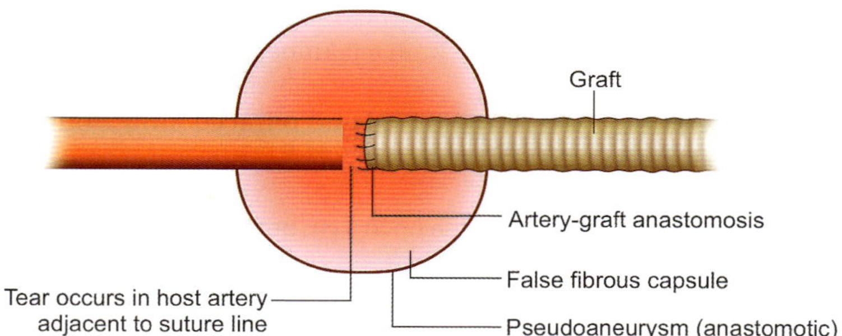

Fig. 11-30: Anastomotic pseudoaneurysm can occur at disrupted suture line.

Basic Principles in Arterial Graft Surgery

Type of surgery should be selected properly based on site, extent and severity of block.

Site for inflow anastomosis should be having adequate inflow of blood. Site of outflow anastomosis is also important to accommodate the graft blood flow. If it is too diseased graft failure can occur.

Type of graft selected is also important. Size, quality, length, preclotting should be proper.

Adequate imaging in the form of Duplex scan, angiogram, CT angiogram and MR angiogram (contrast or non-contrast) are needed. In critical limb with extensive arterial involvement contrast may precipitate total block and gangrene and in such situation non-contrast MR angiogram is ideal to delineate the site. However, much hope cannot be given to the patient as far as limb salvage is considered.

AORTOFEMORAL BYPASS GRAFT

It is commonly used technique at present. Aortofemoral bypass is preferred as often block extends to distal iliac arteries. Dacron or PTFE is commonly used. Knitted/woven Dacron when used needs preclotting before use. Collagen impregnated Dacron/PTFE does not require preclotting.

Transperitoneal approach: Transabdominal/transperitoneal approach is ideal for graft placement. Lengthy midline incision from xiphisternum to pubic symphysis is needed. Femoral arteries are exposed from above the level of the inguinal ligament down, below and beyond the level of the common femoral bifurcation. When there is a need to expose the external iliac artery additionally, it is achieved by extending the femoral incision above, laterally curving parallel to inguinal ligament with or without cutting the inguinal ligament.

↓

Omentum and transverse colon are pushed upwards; small intestine is shifted towards right; duodenojejunal junction is exposed properly. Retroperitoneum is incised adjacent to duodenum lateral to fourth part of the duodenum. Duodenum is mobilised to expose the aorta. Lymphatic vessels are ligated. Proximal aortic clamp is placed here *from left side* after heparinisation and after clamping distally at femoral vessels.

↓

Proximal dissection is done up to the level of renal vein. It is identified by left renal vein crossing the aorta *in front* to reach IVC. Occasionally as a variation left renal vein may be retroaortic. Left renal vein should be mobilised adequately without division by ligating left gonadal and left adrenal veins. Rarely in high lesions left renal vein may need to be divided at its entry into the IVC. In such occasion ligation of left gonadal and left adrenal veins should be avoided as these two veins are essential to drain left kidney.

↓

Inferior mesenteric vein is mobilised and retraced away from the field.

↓

Infrarenal aortic dissection is done up to 3 cm beyond the block or level of graft anastomosis. During dissection care should be taken not to injure IVC and lumbar veins. Lumbar arteries can be ligated if needed.

↓

Preclotting the non-coated knitted or woven Dacron graft is done to seal the graft and to prevent leak and to create a smooth lining at graft-blood interface. This step is not necessary for PTFE or newer grafts. Preclotting is done by collecting 100 mL of patient's blood prior to heparinisation from aorta or IVC using a syringe which is collected in a bowl. Selected graft is clamped at one end; from other end fresh blood collected in the bowl is forced into the graft using a fine catheter or syringe until leakage from the pores stops. Later graft is flushed using heparinised saline.

↓

Retroperitoneal *tunnel* is made by blunt finger dissection extending down into the femoral incision. This tunneling should pass *behind ureter* and *in front* of iliac artery. Umbilical tape on each side is placed along the length of the tunnel.

↓

Intravenous heparin is injected 150 units/kg body weight to anticoagulate the patient. First distal part of the artery is clamped to prevent embolism; then proximal part.

↓

Proximal anastomosis: End-to-end or end-to-side anastomosis can be done. *End to end is preferred* as it causes uniform blood flow with less turbulence and stable accurate suturing is possible. It also allows proper inspection of the proximal part with limited endarterectomy at proximal site which gives more stable suture line. Aorta is transected between two vascular clamps at the site of anastomosis; distal cut end of the aorta is sutured with double layer 4-zero polypropylene continuous sutures—first like a sewing machine method; second as a oversewing/over and over sutures at cut edge (like closure of duodenal stump in gastrectomy).

↓

Graft should be of *same size or smaller than the size* of the aorta. Ideally it should not be larger. 4-zero polypropylene continuous sutures are placed posteriorly and anteriorly. Needle bites should be smooth, single stroke, precise with needle piercing the aorta *from intimal side towards adventitia*; in the graft *from outside towards inside.* Interrupted mattress sutures are often used but it is not popular.

↓

Once proximal anastomosis is completed, graft is filled with blood by releasing the proximal clamp and later clamp is reapplied to the aorta proximal to suture line. Another vascular clamp is applied on the graft distal to suture line and proximal clamp over aorta is again released for short period to check the bleeding at the site suture line. Small bleeders can be controlled by pressure; persistent or large leaks are controlled by additional interrupted sutures. Proximal aortic clamp is reapplied and clamp over the graft just distal to proximal suture line is also released. Repeated clamping of the graft is not advisable. Often a cuff of graft additionally placed over the graft to prevent aortoenteric fistula as complication.

↓

Distal anastomosis: It is done over *common femoral artery commonly;* near the origin of the deep femoral artery to improve the long-term patency rate. Allowing an area of flexion along the length of the graft at groin is small but less significant drawback (In aortoiliac graft such flexion problem is not present).

↓

Tunneling is completed by passing long vascular clamp from thigh wound below towards abdominal wound above. It is done on both sides. An index finger is passed gently in front of common femoral artery; gentle finger dissection upwards is done to create a tunnel. Deep circumflex iliac vein runs over external iliac artery which should be taken care of as injury to it can cause torrential bleeding. Tunnel usually of two fingerbreadth size is created deep to inguinal ligament. Peritoneum is pushed upwards from upper wound; ureter is also pushed aside. A long Robert clamp is passed from thigh wound across groin to abdominal wound. Often umbilical tape is kept in place on the tunnel till graft is passed down.

↓

Through the vascular clamp each side limb of the aortofemoral graft is pulled gently downwards towards thigh (femoral) wound on respective sides avoiding any twist or undue pull **(Figs. 11-31A to L)**.

↓

Distal anastomosis is *end-to-side* one. Distal end of the graft is bevelled like 'S' using heavy scissor and sutured to the arteriotomy made at the junction of common femoral artery. Both superficial and deep femoral arteries should be dissected adequately. Vascular clamps are placed on the two branches distally. Arteriotomy done at the junction can be extended towards deep femoral artery, if needed. Orifices of branches should be exposed and any block at the orifices can be cleared. Continuous 6-zero polypropylene sutures are placed either tied running or as parachute technique. Suturing should be done from inside out at arterial side and from out to inside at graft side. Usually four corner sutures are placed; two in middle and two at angles. Then running sutures are proceeded towards angle posteriorly then towards anteriorly. Initial mattress suture may be placed at the heel of the graft for proper alignment of the graft over the artery.

↓

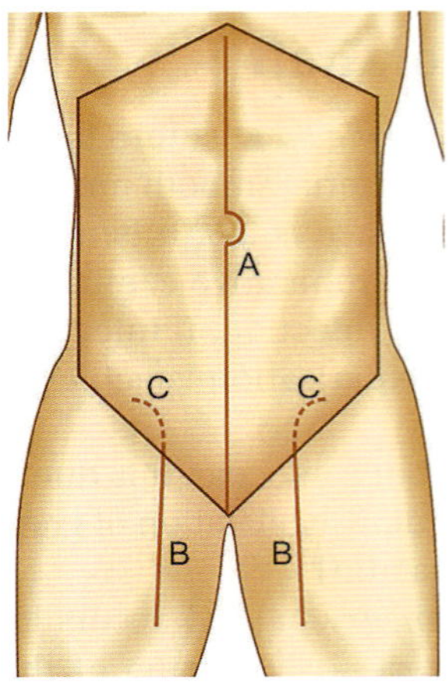

Incision:
(A) Lengthy midline incision from xiphisternum to pubic symphysis
(B) Femoral exposure is vertical incisions on both sides from inguinal ligament along mid-inguinal point in on thigh
(C) If external iliac artery need to be exposed then lateral upward extension is needed

Fig. 11-31A

1. Inferior phrenic artery
2. Middle suprarenal artery
3. Coeliac trunk:
   3a. Hepatic artery
   3b. Splenic artery
   3c. Left gastric artery
4. Superior mesenteric artery
5. Renal artery
6. Gonadal artery
7. Lumbar artery
8. Inferior mesenteric artery
9. Median sacral artery
10. Common iliac artery

11. Inferior vena cava (IVC)
12. Left renal vein
13. Left adrenal vein
14. Left gonadal vein
15. Common iliac vein
16. Liver
17. Diaphragm
18. Oesophagus
19. Right kidney
20. Duodenum: 20a—1st part; 20b—2nd part; 20c—3rd part; 20d—4th part

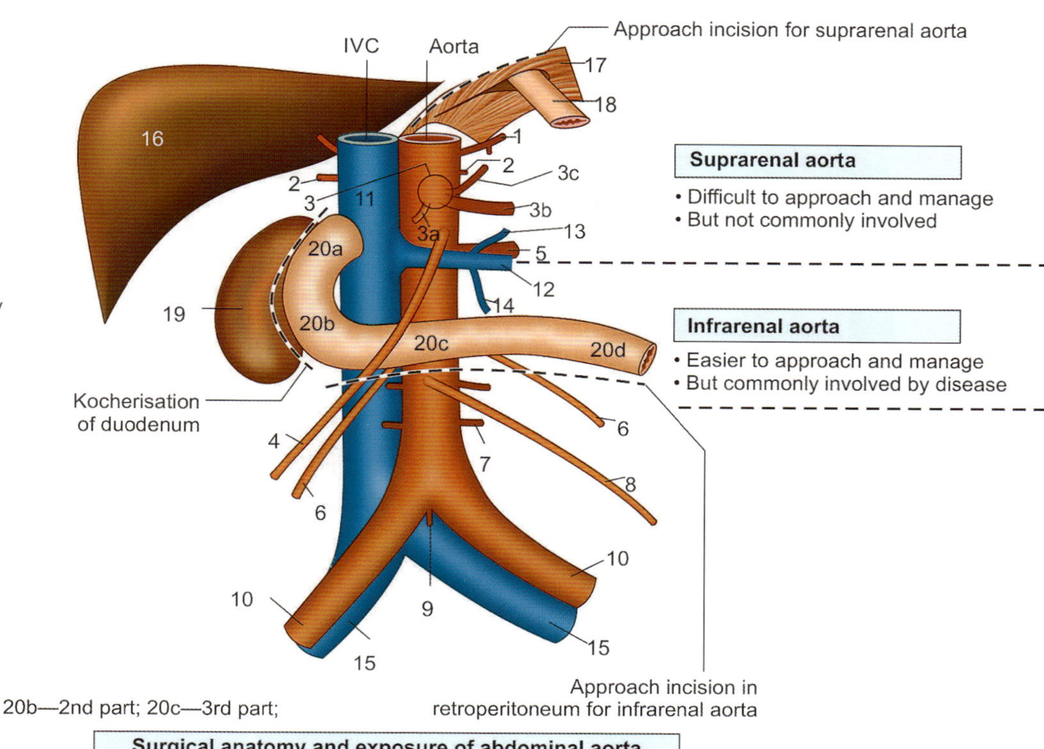

Surgical anatomy and exposure of abdominal aorta

Fig. 11-31B

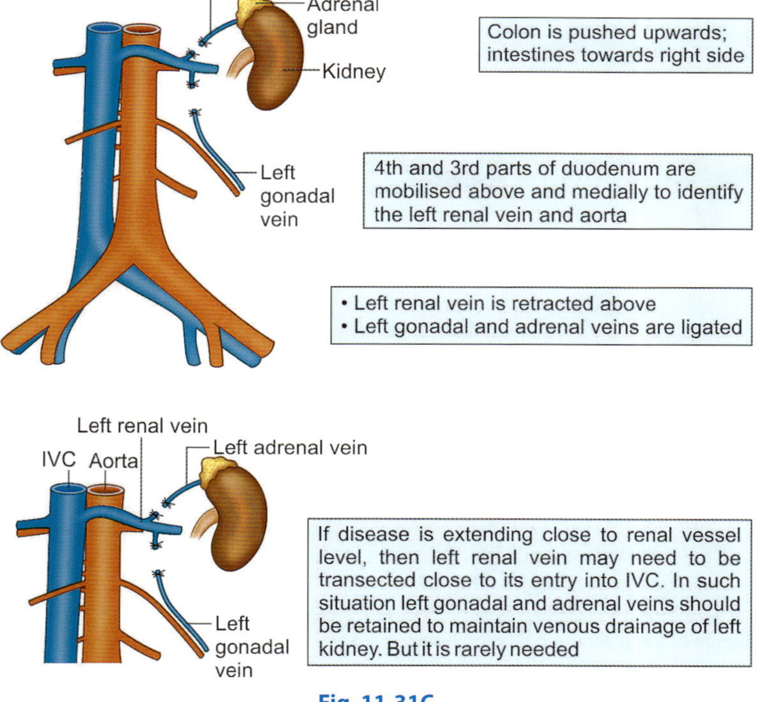

Fig. 11-31C

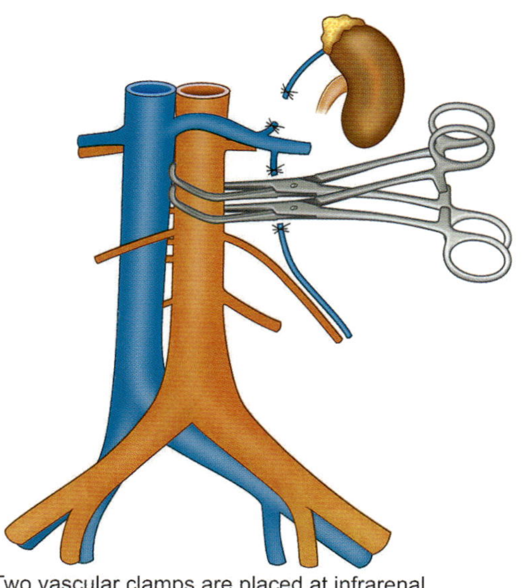

Two vascular clamps are placed at infrarenal portion of the aorta from left side

Fig. 11-31D

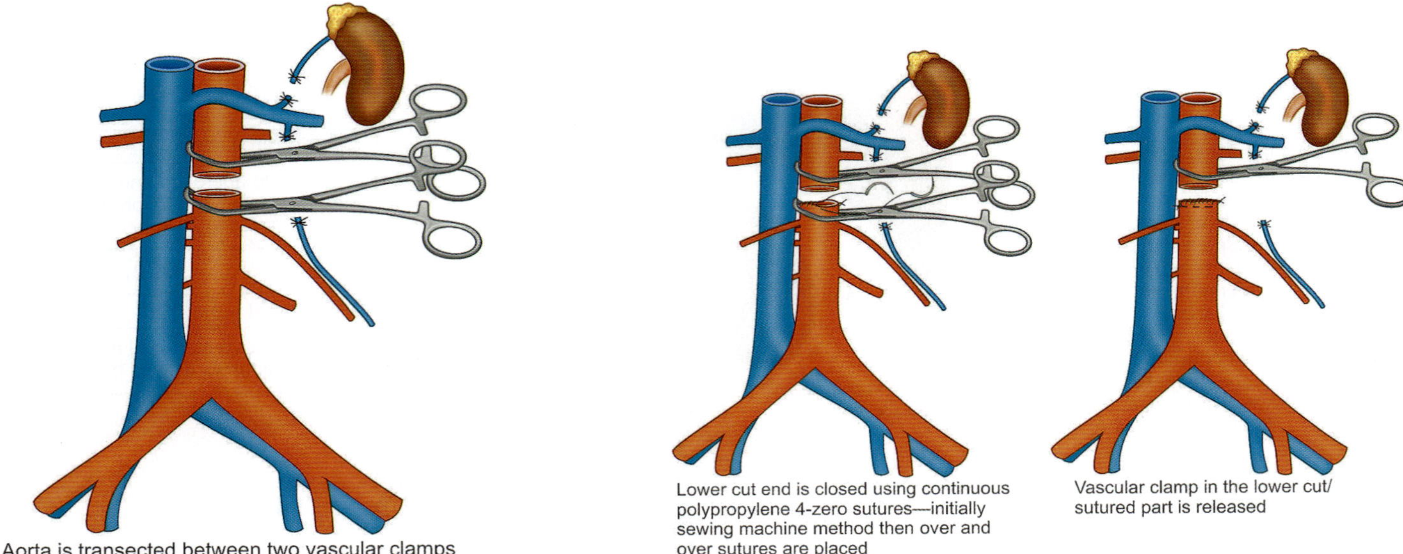

Fig. 11-31E

Fig. 11-31F

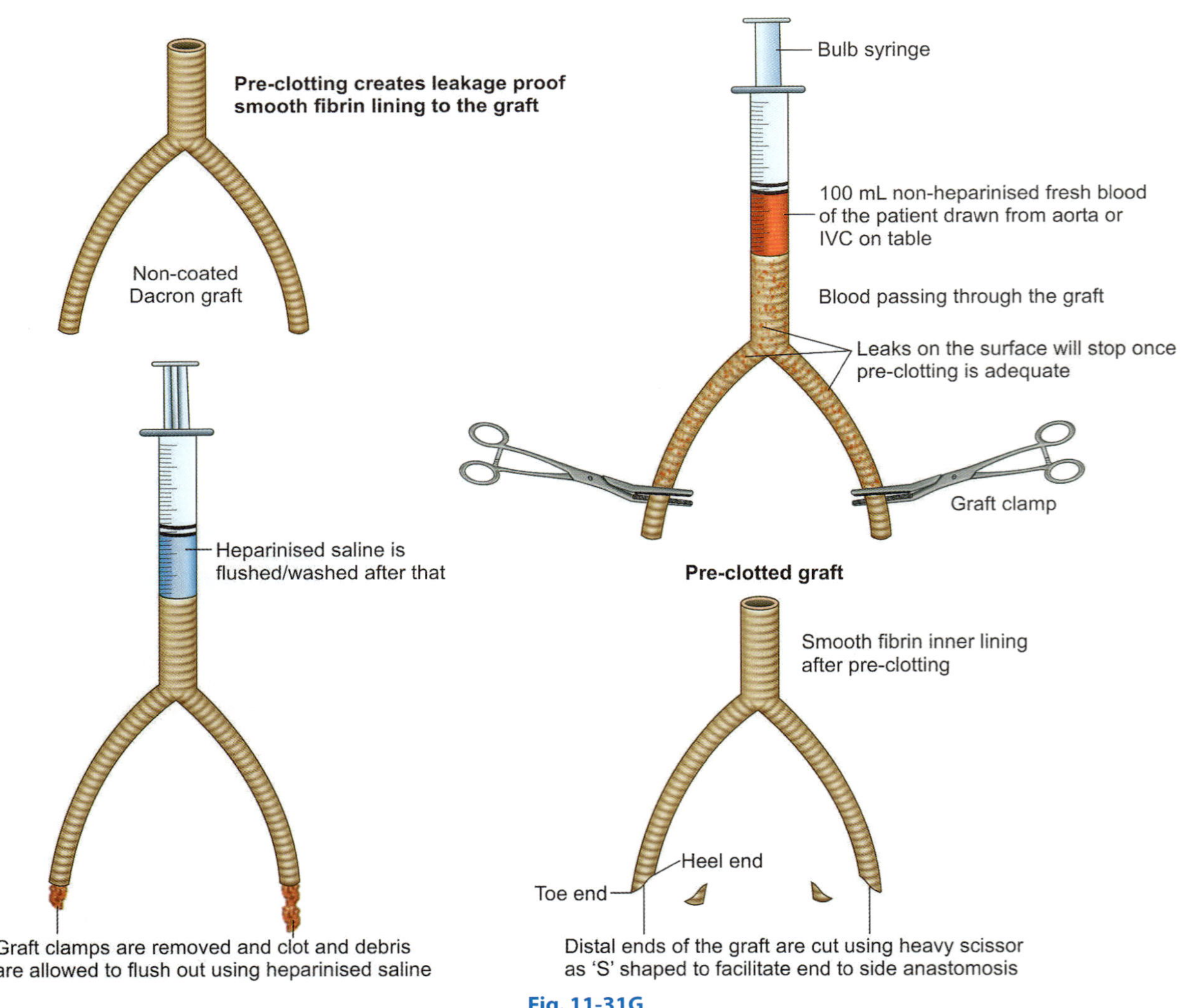

Fig. 11-31G

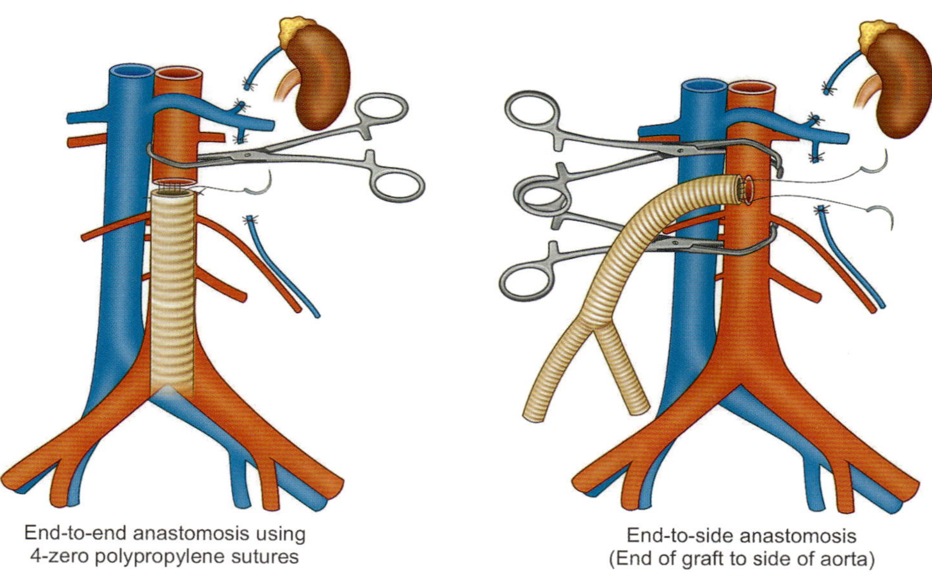

End-to-end anastomosis using 4-zero polypropylene sutures

End-to-side anastomosis (End of graft to side of aorta)

Fig. 11-31H

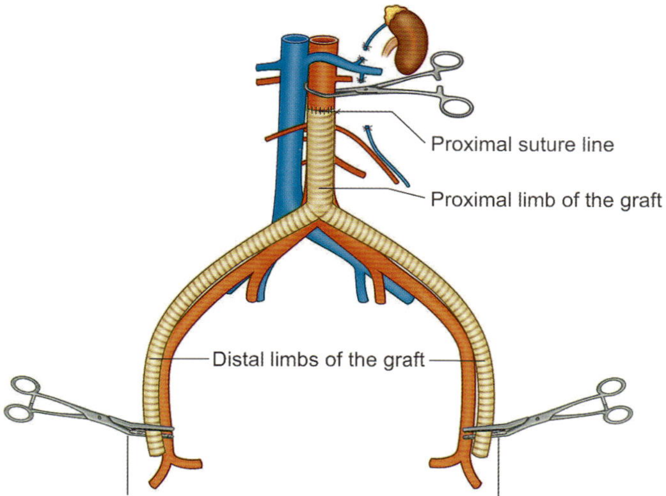

Proximal suture line

Proximal limb of the graft

Distal limbs of the graft

Peripheral/distal limbs of the graft are clamped

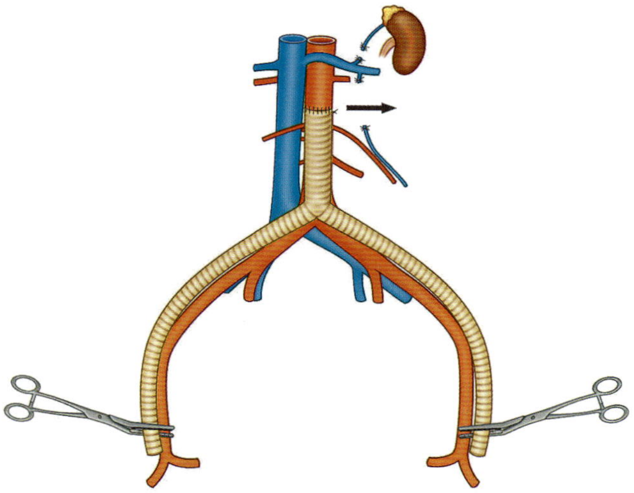

Proximal aortic clamp is released for short period to fill the graft with blood

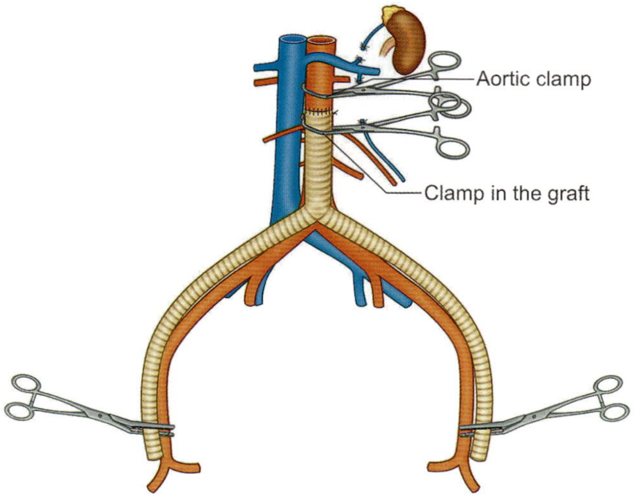

Aortic clamp

Clamp in the graft

Aorta is reclamped and graft just distal to the graft—aorta suture line is also clamped gently

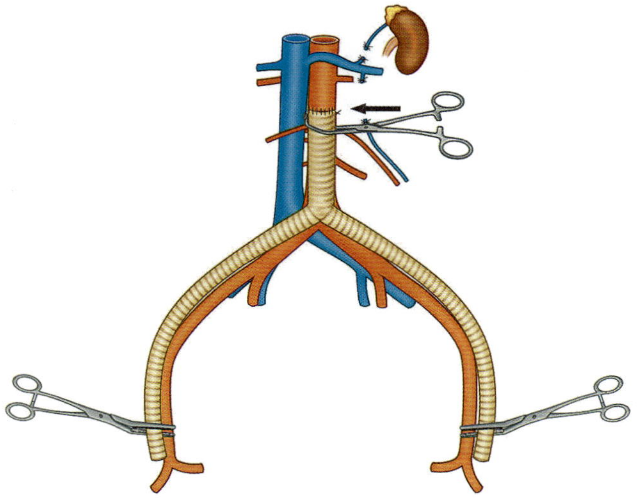

Aortic clamp is released to check the graft suture line security. If needed additional sutures may be added

Fig. 11-31I

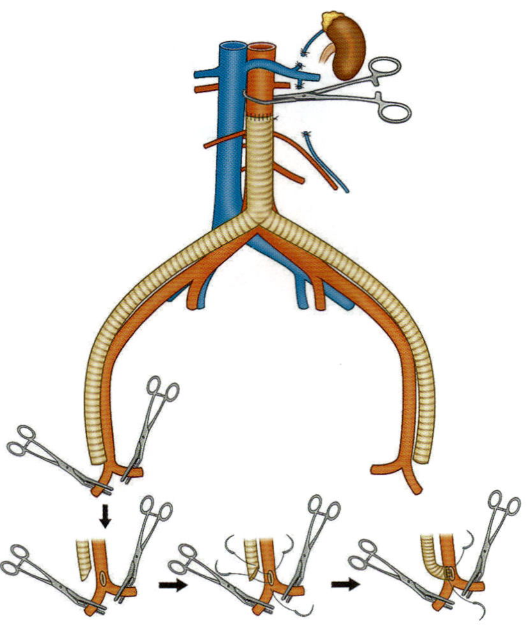

Vascular clamps are applied to both branches of femoral artery of one side. Aortic clamp is kept in place. End-to-side anastomosis is done

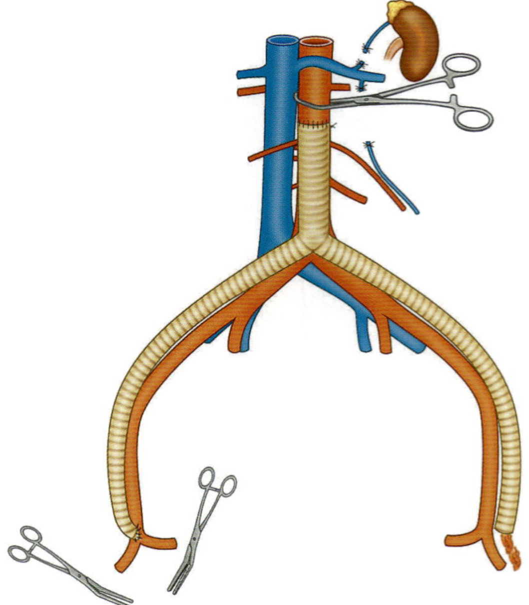

Clamps over the femoral branches are released to allow retrograde flow of blood to opposite limb of the graft to remove clots and debris. Aortic clamp should be in situ

Fig. 11-31J

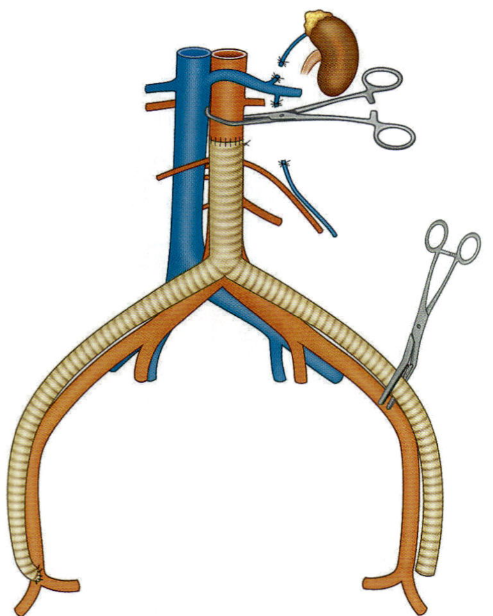

Clamp applied over to the opposite limb of the graft

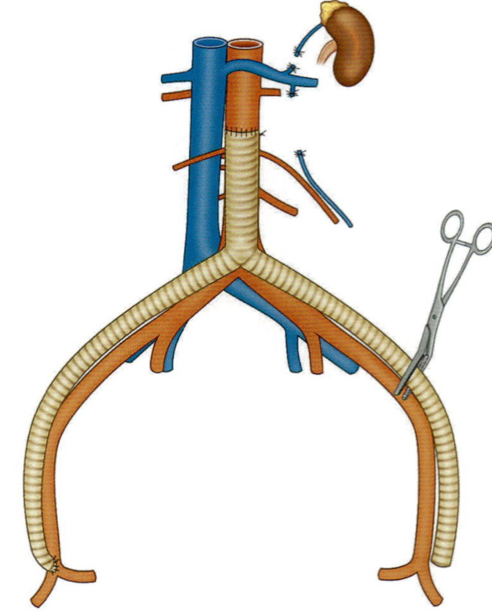

Aortic clamp is released to allow blood flow to sutured limb

Fig. 11-31K

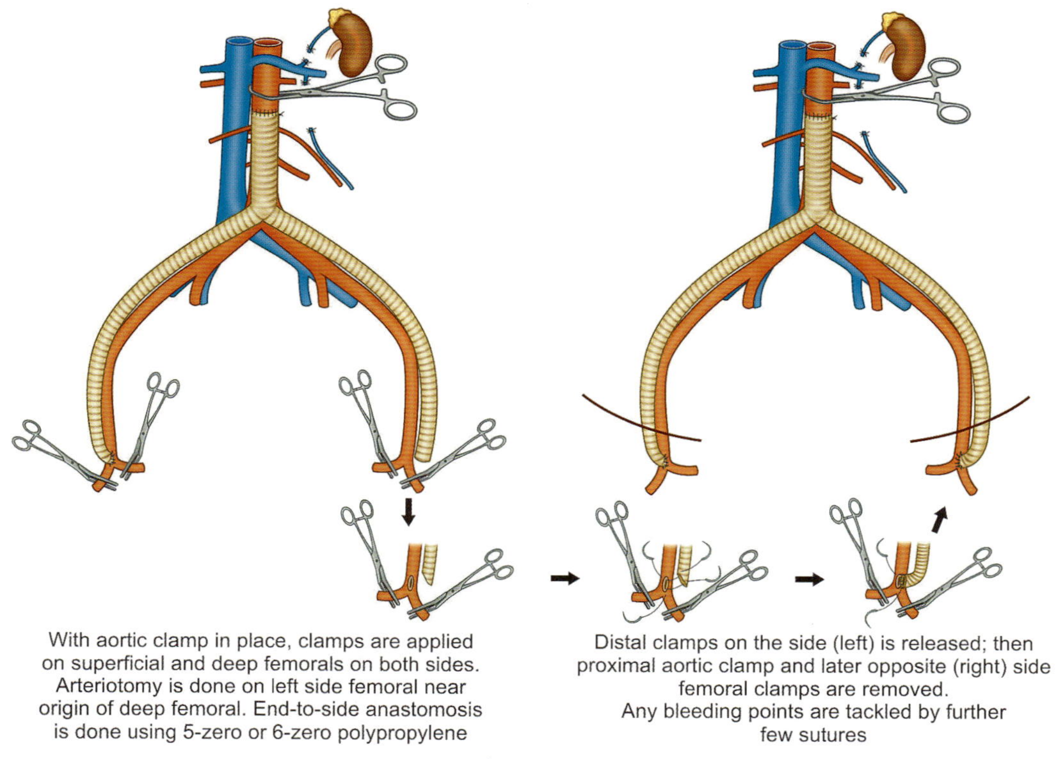

Fig. 11-31L

Figs. 11-31A to L: Aortofemoral bypass graft.

Distal clamps of the superficial and deep femoral arteries are released to allow retrograde flow of blood along the limb of the same side of the graft; towards the limb on the opposite side of the graft to clear clots and debris.

↓

Now opposite limb of the graft is clamped near its bifurcation/origin of the branching. Proximal aortic clamp is slowly released so as to avoid sudden fall in blood pressure beyond 20 mmHg.

↓

Opposite side superficial and deep femorals are clamped; arteriotomy is done near its origin; opposite graft limb is trimmed as 'S'. Anastomosis is done similarly. Femoral clamps are released just before last sutures. Proximal clamp at the graft limb is slowly released to perfuse across the graft. Any leak is dealt with similarly.

↓

Inferior mesenteric artery, if needed, should be reimplanted into the proximal limb of the graft. Large artery, artery with less back bleeding after transection, and when there are poor collaterals need reimplantation of inferior mesenteric artery. Colour of the bowel wall and Doppler study by placing the probe on the antimesenteric part of the bowel after clamping the artery will decide the need for reimplantation.

↓

Retroperitoneum is *closed over the graft*. It prevents the contact of the graft into intestines or duodenum to prevent aortoduodenal or aorto- intestinal fistula. Omental pedicle may be placed between aorta and intestines. Meticulous haemostasis in all layers is important **(Fig. 11-32)**.

Complications

Bleeding can occur which occasionally requires re-exploration. Hypovolaemia is common.

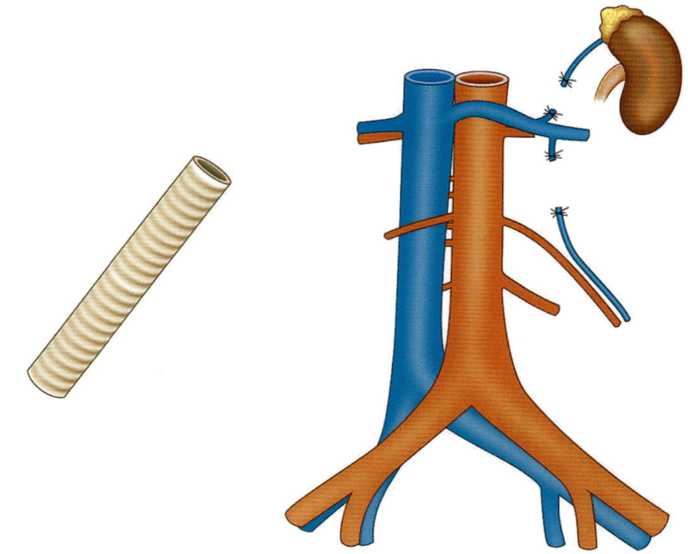

Fig. 11-32: End-to-side aortic graft. It is not commonly used; but it maintains the spinal cord blood supply to reduce the chance of spinal cord ischaemia.

Re-thrombosis and graft failure are also known complications.

Distal ischaemia and gangrene can occur. Doppler study of limbs is done to assess the distal perfusion.

Embolism due to dislodged atheroma when occurs, with intact pulse needs embolectomy.

Injury to aortic nerve plexus may cause impotence but it is less common.

Wound infection, haematoma and abscess formation are other complications. Progressive haematoma needs re-exploration.

Colonic ischaemia mainly left sided (sigmoid) can occur. Only mucosal ischaemia is treated by nasogastric aspiration; deeper level ischaemia needs laparotomy and resection. If preoperatively suspected by wider diameter of inferior mesenteric artery or artery with poor back bleeding then *reimplantation of inferior mesenteric artery is done.* Inferior mesenteric artery at its origin is cut with cuff/button of adjacent aorta. Corresponding graft at the site is opened like a buttonhole to which origin cuff of inferior mesenteric artery is sutured using polypropylene to achieve reimplantation **(Fig. 11-33)**.

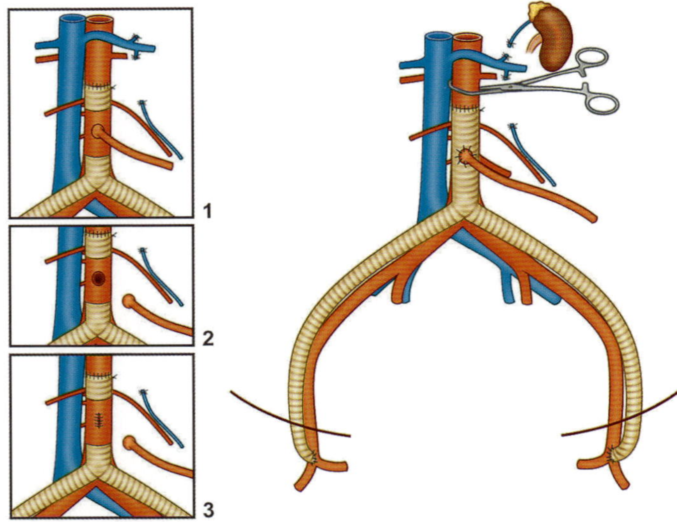

Fig. 11-33: Inferior mesenteric artery origin can be reimplanted into the aortic graft in case if possibility of colonic ischaemia is suspected.

Graft failure and leak when occurs, needs re-exploration and regrafting. Sepsis is the major cause for graft failure.

Disruption of the parasympathetic nerves near aortic bifurcation leads into impotence or retrograde ejaculation. Care is taken during the dissection around bifurcation so as not to injure the nerve plexus **(Fig. 11-34)**.

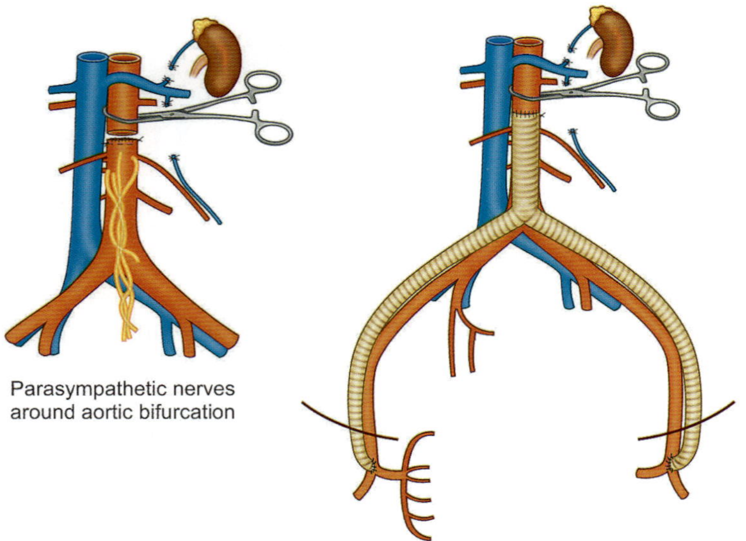

Fig. 11-34: Impotence can occur after aortofemoral grafting due to parasympathetic disruption.

Spinal cord ischaemia can occur due to severe arterial insufficiency. It leads into paraplegia. It is more common in end-to-end anastomosis of the proximal part of the graft into aorta. In *proximal end-to-end anastomosis,* distal to distal cut end of the aorta gets its perfusion through retrograde blood flow along hypogastric arteries. But in severe bilateral iliac disease, such retrograde perfusion is not adequate as it leads to poor perfusion of the lower spinal arteries causing spinal cord ischaemia. It can be identified prior to surgery by preoperative angiogram; if detected it is better to add on revascularisation procedure of the hypogastric artery. In *end-to-side proximal graft—aorta anastomosis* incidence of spinal cord ischaemia is less **(Fig. 11-35)**.

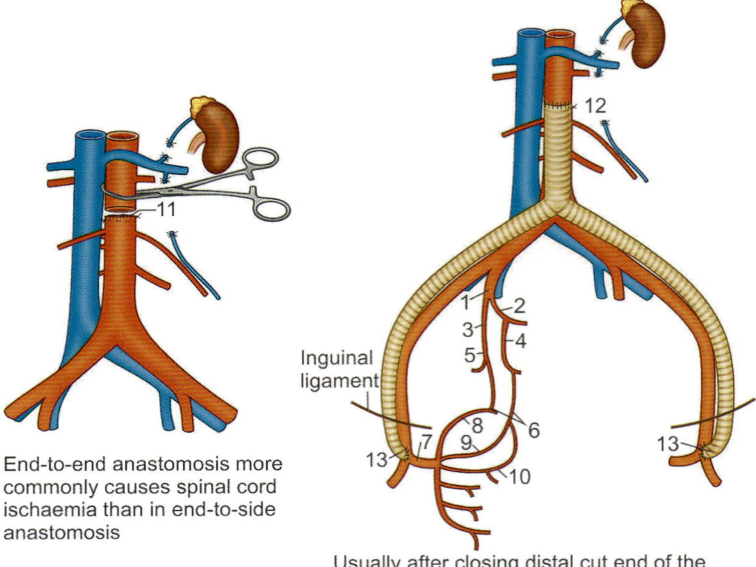

Fig. 11-35: Diagrammatic representation of collaterals and possibility of developing spinal cord ischaemia.

Aortoduodenal/aortointestinal/aortovenacaval fistula can occur which is often life threatening. It is treated by immediate surgery, redoing of graft, resection, etc., but it is technically demanding with high mortality.

OTHER GRAFT PROCEDURES

Other grafts in the lower limb/aortoiliac femoral segments can be done using same principles. Bypass grafts are classified as anatomical bypass graft and extra-anatomical bypass graft.

Anatomical bypass graft is the one which is along the normal course of the artery. Examples are aortobifemoral, aortoiliac, iliofemoral, femoropopliteal grafts.

Extra-anatomical bypass graft is the one which traverses through different than normal arterial pathways. Examples are cross over femoral graft, axillofemoral bypass graft.

Duplex ultrasound scanning, segmental limb pressures and segmental limb plethysmography are needed investigations to assess accurate physiological status of the vessel. Cardiac assessment is essential in all these patients.

Prophylactic antibiotics are started 24 hours prior to surgery; entire abdomen both lower limbs and chest below nipples should be prepared.

AORTOILIAC BYPASS GRAFT

Aortoiliac bypass graft can be done if there is unilateral common iliac artery block. Often unilateral aortofemoral graft is preferred although graft has to pass across groin crease.

Aorta and iliac artery is exposed *through retroperitoneal* (occasionally transperitoneal) approach using oblique groin muscle cutting incision (peritoneum is not opened, instead is pushed above towards left). Lower end of aorta with bifurcation and common, external and internal iliac arteries on that side are exposed and dissected. Vascular clamps are applied over aorta above the level of aortic anastomosis, on to opposite common iliac artery to prevent retrograde flow, and distal part of the external iliac artery distal to the line of anastomosis **(Figs. 11-36A and B)**.

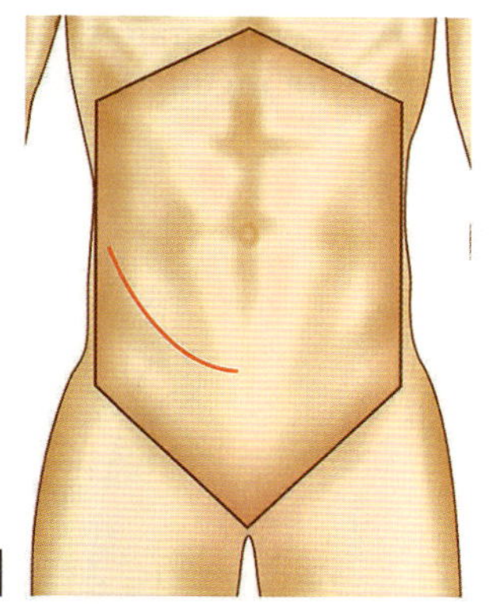

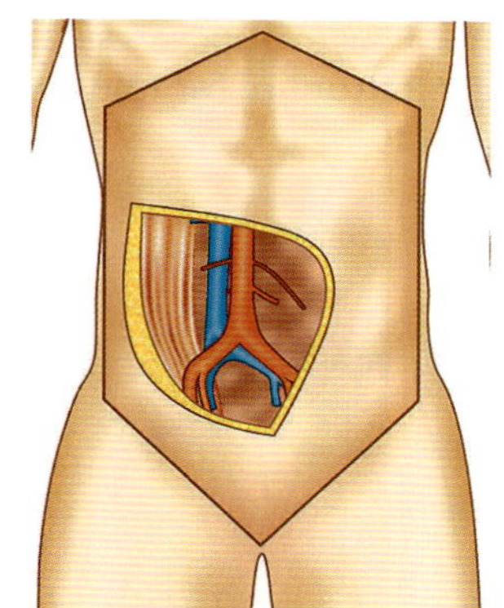

A

An oblique lower abdomen incision is made. Muscles (all three and rectus) are cut. Peritoneum is pushed upwards and towards left to expose the aorta and iliac vessels. Opposite iliac artery is also exposed to place vascular clamp if needed. Aortoiliac graft is done as side-to-side anastomosis

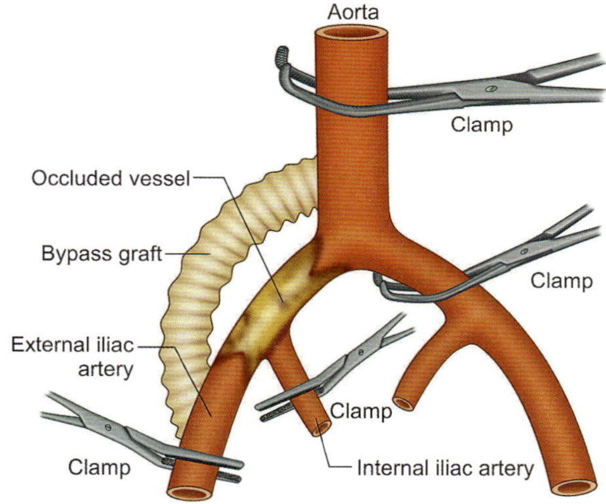

B

Figs. 11-36A and B: Aortoiliac graft.

Pre-clotting of the selected graft is done. Aorta is opened longitudinally and side-to-side graft to aorta anastomosis is done. Its integrity is confirmed by once releasing aortic clamp for a short period and later reapplied. External iliac artery just proximal to distal clamp is opened and side-to-side anastomosis is done between lower end of graft and external iliac artery. Just prior to completion of last suture distal clamp is released to remove clot and debris. Proximal clamp and clamp on the opposite common iliac artery is released. Suction drain is placed and kept for 72 hours. Complications are similar to other graft procedure.

ILIOFEMORAL GRAFT

It is done when disease is limited to one common iliac artery. Common iliac artery near its origin should be patent and free of disease to do iliofemoral graft. Aortic bifurcation also should be normal. It is often preferred method than cross femoral graft as opposite limb dissection is avoided here.

Incisions may be suprainguinal (*retroperitoneal commonly,* transperitoneal occasionally) to expose the aorta and common, external and internal iliac arteries; or vertical thigh incision along midinguinal point across inguinal ligament. External and internal oblique and transversus abdominis muscles are split to reach retroperitoneal area; by blunt finger dissection, vessel is dissected adequately; common iliac or external iliac artery is used for proximal graft placement **(Figs. 11-37 to 11-39)**.

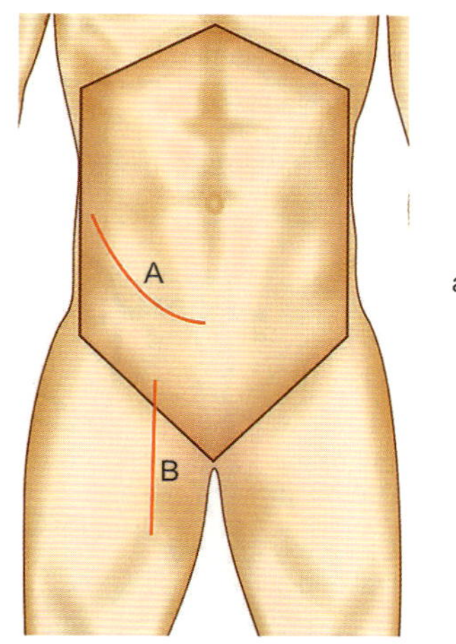

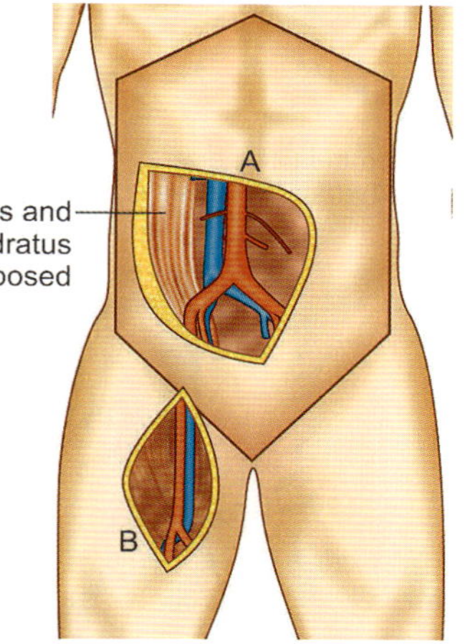

Incision:
(A) In the abdomen obliquely from lateral above downwards towards midline just above the pubic symphysis. Usually retroperitoneal approach is used. After cutting all three layers of muscles and rectus abdominis, peritoneum is pushed above and towards left to expose the aorta and iliac vessels fully. In difficult situation trasabdominal approach is used by opening the peritoneum
(B) Vertical thigh incision at midinguinal point across inguinal ligament

Exposure of the both wounds to delineate the aorta, IVC, iliac vessels and femoral vessels

Fig. 11-37: Incision and exposure for iliofemoral graft.

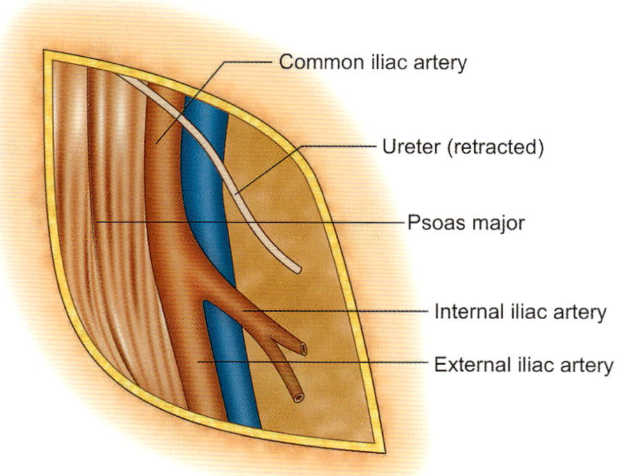

Fig. 11-38: Iliac artery exposure.

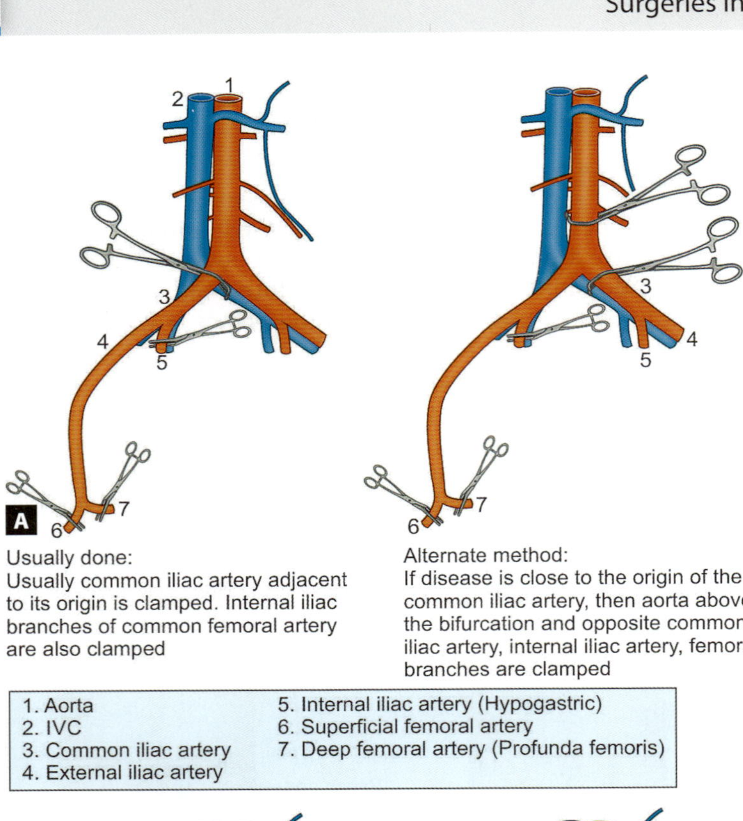

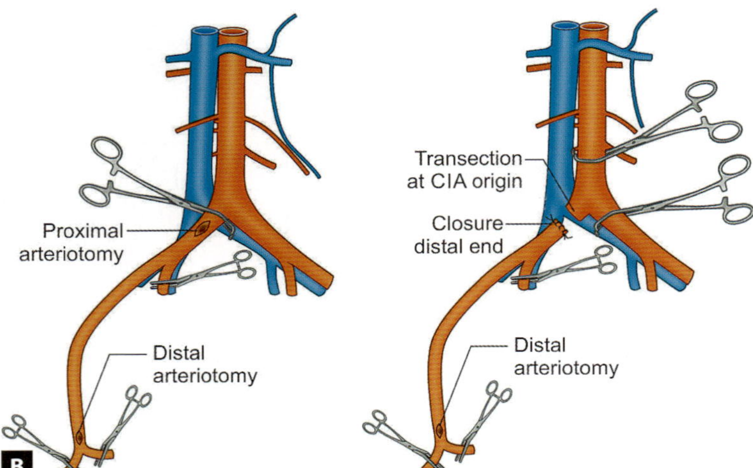

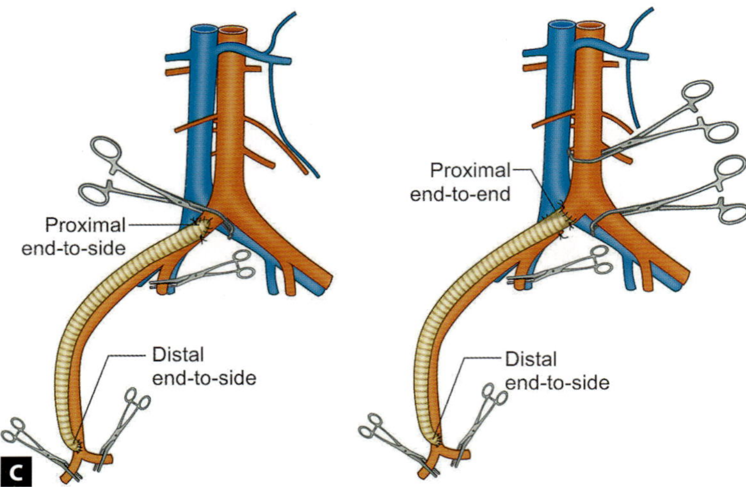

Figs. 11-39A to C: Iliofemoral graft—technique.

Initial heparinisation is done. Vascular clamps are applied on the origin of the common iliac artery, internal iliac artery and femoral branches. If the origin of iliac artery is diseased then clamps are placed on aorta above the bifurcation and on opposite common iliac artery to prevent retrograde blood flow from opposite common iliac artery. Cut end of its origin is sutured using 4-zero polypropylene sutures (if end-to-side anastomosis is proposed method, transection of artery is not done). Usually 10 mm graft is used. Internal iliac, superficial and deep femoral arteries are also clamped beyond their origin.

Proximal anastomosis can be done as end-to-side or end-to-end if common iliac artery is transected. Continuous 4-zero polypropylene sutures are placed. Distal part of the graft is tunneled deep to inguinal ligament across femoral triangle into common femoral artery near its division towards deep femoral artery. Distal anastomosis is done as end-to-side using 4-zero polypropylene continuous sutures.

Wounds are closed with a suction drain. *Complications* are bleeding, graft leak, haematoma, thrombosis of graft, intimal dissection, infection and impotence.

Iliofemoral cross-over graft is used from one side common or external iliac to opposite side femoral artery wherein graft is passed usually in front of (or underneath) the opposite inguinal ligament **(Fig. 11-40)**.

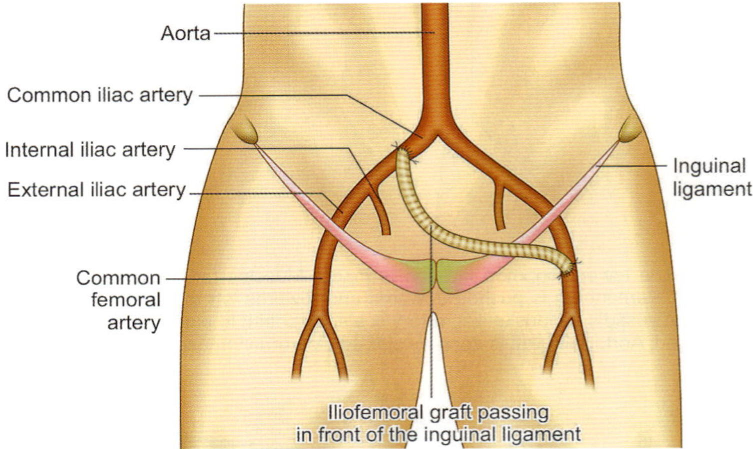

Fig. 11-40: Iliofemoral cross-over graft.

FEMOROPOPLITEAL BYPASS GRAFT

It is done in lower limb ischaemia as a limb saving procedure if disease segment is in superficial femoral artery from its origin to below knee popliteal segment. There should be adequate good blood flow in iliac arteries to do femoropopliteal bypass. *Adequate distal run off* is also needed. If there is associated localised profunda femoris (deep femoral) artery block, then profundaplasty with a vein or graft patch should also be added to improve collateral circulation. Vein graft is always better than prosthetic graft in below knee segment revascularisation. Main artery is left in situ to retain whatever existing functions as it is. Side-to-end femoro graft anastomosis proximally and end-to-side graft to popliteal anastomosis is done **(Fig. 11-41)**.

Procedure

Under regional/general anaesthesia preparation of entire limb from umbilicus up to ankle is done.

First *recipient popliteal segment* is dissected. *Medial approach* is commonly used. Initially *proximal segment of artery* is exposed.

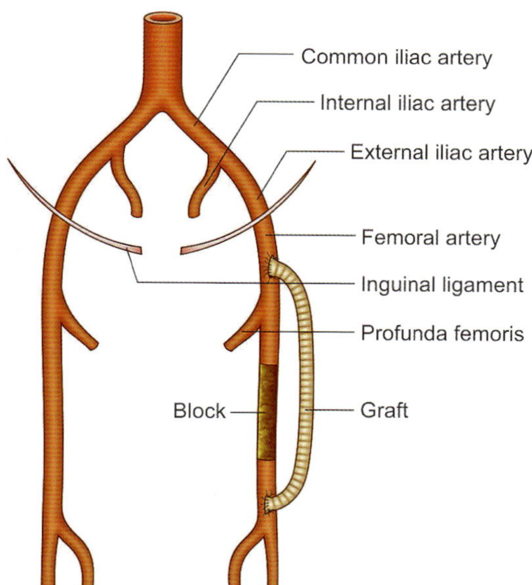

Fig. 11-41: Femoropopliteal bypass graft.

Incision is on the medial aspect from upper part of femoral condyle proximally for 10 cm. Dissection is deepened between vastus medialis and hamstring muscles (semitendinosus, semimembranosus). Sartorius, gracilis, vastus medialis are retracted in front. Artery passing through the adductor hiatus under femur is found. In popliteal fossa artery is found in a fatty area. It is separated from popliteal vein. Genicular branches are identified and safeguarded **(Figs. 11-42A to C)**.

Distal segment of artery is dissected next by medial approach through an incision which is vertical and 1 cm posterior to medial subcutaneous border of the tibia. Often flexion and abduction of hip joint and flexion of knee joint at 90° is needed. As long saphenous vein is very close to this incision it should not be injured as it is needed to use as a graft for bypass. After skin incision, long saphenous vein is fully mobilised. Medial head of the gastrocnemius is retracted posteriorly. Dense fascia connecting it to tibia is divided to expose the lower part of the popliteal fossa **(Fig. 11-43)**.

Division of guy ropes (semitendinosus, semimembranosus and gracilis) is only occasionally needed; retraction only suffices. Anterior tibial vein is ligated; artery is dissected carefully including its divisions—anterior tibial artery and tibioperoneal trunk. Popliteal artery is medial to posterior tibial nerve and popliteal vein. Small tributaries are ligated using double loop silk sutures *(Pott's sutures/ties)*. Both branches are isolated and occlusion slings are placed. Fascia anterior to sartorius is incised and using blunt finger dissection tunnel is created to pass the graft **(Figs. 11-44A to D)**.

Adductor canal is an intermuscular space (*Hunter's canal*, John Hunter—1793) situated on the medial side of middle ⅓ of the thigh extending from apex of femoral triangle to tendinous opening (adductor magnus hiatus) in the adductor magnus below. It is formed anteriorly by vastus medialis; posteriorly (floor) by adductor longus above and adductor magnus below; medially (roof) is formed by strong fibrous membrane joining anterior and posterior walls, which is covered by sartorius. Canal contains femoral artery and vein, saphenous nerve, nerve to vastus medialis, two divisions of obturator nerve. Descending genicular artery originates in the canal from femoral artery which divides into saphenous artery which accompanies the saphenous nerve and muscular branch to vastus medialis **(Fig. 11-45)**.

Proximal dissection at femoral artery level is done through a vertical incision with convexity laterally at midinguinal point. Convexity towards lateral side prevents damage to lymphatic vessels. Lymphatic vessel disruption can cause lymphorrhoea, lymphocele, lymph fistula and wound infection. If lymph vessels are injured, it should be ligated with fine silk suture. Long saphenous vein (LSV) can be dissected through same incision on its medial margin. Long saphenous vein may be dissected through a separate vertical incision 1 cm below and lateral to the pubic tubercle directly on LSV. Skin flaps should not be raised as much as possible to prevent development of skin necrosis.

Usually vein graft is used. Long saphenous vein is commonly used. If it is not available by disease or previous surgery, then small saphenous vein or cephalic vein is used. Vein graft is better than prosthetic graft in relation to graft take up and long-term efficacy in femoropopliteal bypass. However, technical precision and availability of good graft makes prosthetic graft also equally effective **(Figs. 11-46A to F)**.

SAPHENOUS VEIN GRAFT

Both in situ and reversed vein graft is used. LSV is divided in the wall of the common femoral vein to achieve maximum width at the LSV opening. Junction is clamped using Satinsky vascular clamp. All tributaries are ligated at 1 mm distance. It should not be less nor more than 1 mm; if less, it may narrow the graft or block; if more, it may precipitate the thrombus at the stump of the tributary. Care should be taken not to injure the adventitia of the vein **(Figs. 11-47 to 11-51)**.

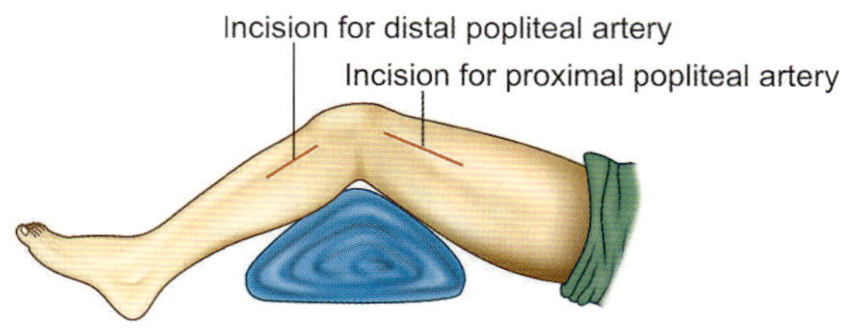

A Medial incision in supine knee flexed position

Distal incision/incisions for recipient artery site—Popliteal artery is made first. Supine semiflexed knee with medial incision is preferred. Incision for proximal popliteal artery is vertical just above the femoral epicondyle two fingerbreadths behind the femur along the anterior margin of sartorius. Incision for distal popliteal artery is vertical, medial and just behind the tibial margin of 15 cm length

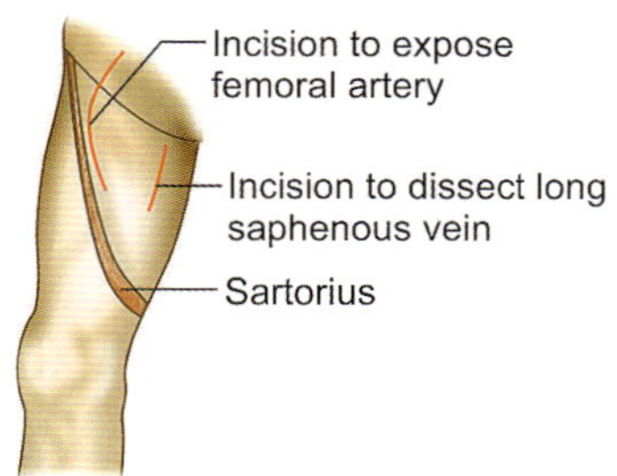

B Proximal incision to expose femoral artery—It is vertical incision in the thigh at midinguinal point with lateral convexity to avoid disruption of lymphatics. LSV can be dissected through same incision on medial flap or through separate vertical incision below and lateral to pubic tubercle

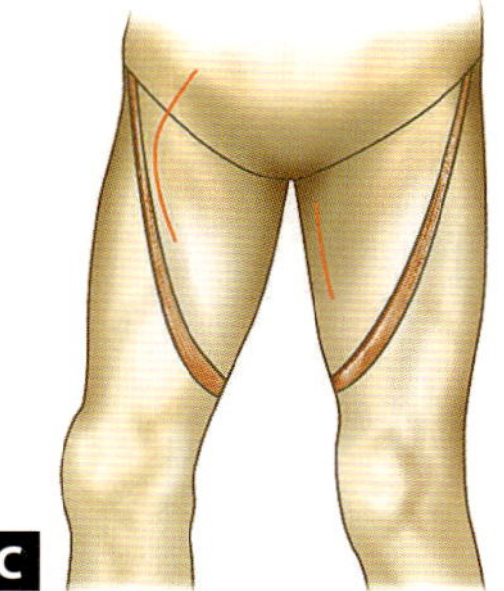

C Donor LSV may be taken from opposite side if same side LSV is not amenable for graft

Figs. 11-42A to C: Incisions and approaches for femoropopliteal bypass graft.

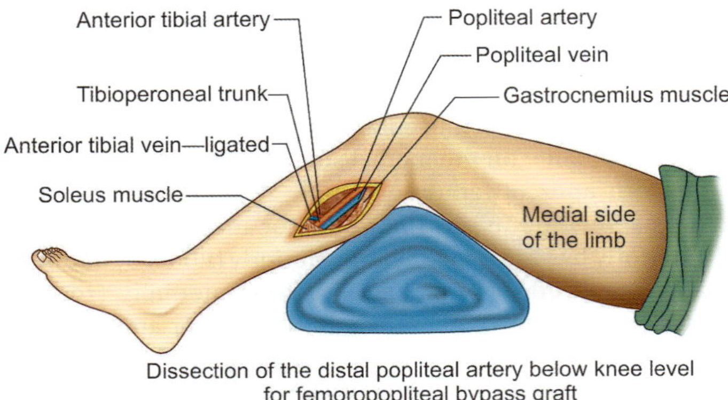

Fig. 11-43: Dissection of the distal artery for femoropopliteal artery bypass.

In Situ Saphenous Vein Graft

Here proximal part of the graft is anastomosed to the femoral artery above the level of the block without disturbing the LSV graft anatomical location. But as LSV junction is often at lower level than site of anastomosis to artery, proximal part of the LSV often needs to be mobilised.

Since valves are present in the LSV graft, they need to be destroyed using valvulotome. First valve is usually at 1 cm from saphenofemoral junction (SFJ). Its translucent central part is excised under direct vision using Pott's scissor. Second valve is 3-5 cm from SFJ. If saphenous vein is 3 mm or more in diameter *valve cutter method* can be used to destroy the valves. A guide catheter is passed from ankle level of the saphenous vein upwards towards proximal cut end of the LSV. Proximal pulled out catheter is connected to a heparinised saline delivery system which inflates up to the next proximal valve and valve cutter should float in the lumen freely. Vascular loop kept around proximal part of the saphenous vein is snugged. Valve cutter is rotated 90° to cut the valve leaflets using cutting edge. Once valve is cut, distal next level valve will become prominent due to saline distension and cutter is gently pulled down distally to feel the resistance by the valve. Valves are cut to feel a popping sensation with vein getting distended below up to the next valve level **(Figs. 11-52A and B)**.

During valvulotomy, intima of the vessel may be damaged. Retained tributary of in situ saphenous graft is a potential anatomical area of *arteriovenous fistula* formation.

Vascular clamps are applied on proximal part of the femoral artery and proximal cut end of saphenous vein. Distal part of the popliteal artery is also clamped. *Side-to-end proximal anastomosis* is done between side of the femoral artery and proximal cut end of saphenous vein (cobra head) using 6-zero polypropylene sutures first 'heel' of the graft is sutured; then sides and at the end 'toe' of the graft. Often parachute technique is used. Arterial vessel loops/ slings/clamps are released to allow blood flow through saphenous vein up to proximal valve. It is confirmed by pulsation which stops at first valve level. Venotomy is done at the side branch of distal end of the vein. *Valvulotomy* instrument (*Le Maitre's valvulotome*—blunt tipped) is passed carefully through it with 90° rotations without traumatising the intima. Proximal graft anastomosis is pinched by assistant's finger to prevent valvulotome entering into the anastomotic site. If it enters anastomotic site, it will snag the sutures and cut. Valve with distended proximal vein segment is identified; valve is cut carefully by rotating the valvulotome 90°. Blood now flows towards next level of valve which is cut again and is repeated until all valves are cut. *All tributaries should be identified carefully and ligated.* Full length of the vein is exposed and tributaries are ligated. Tributaries in the deeper aspect of the vein should be

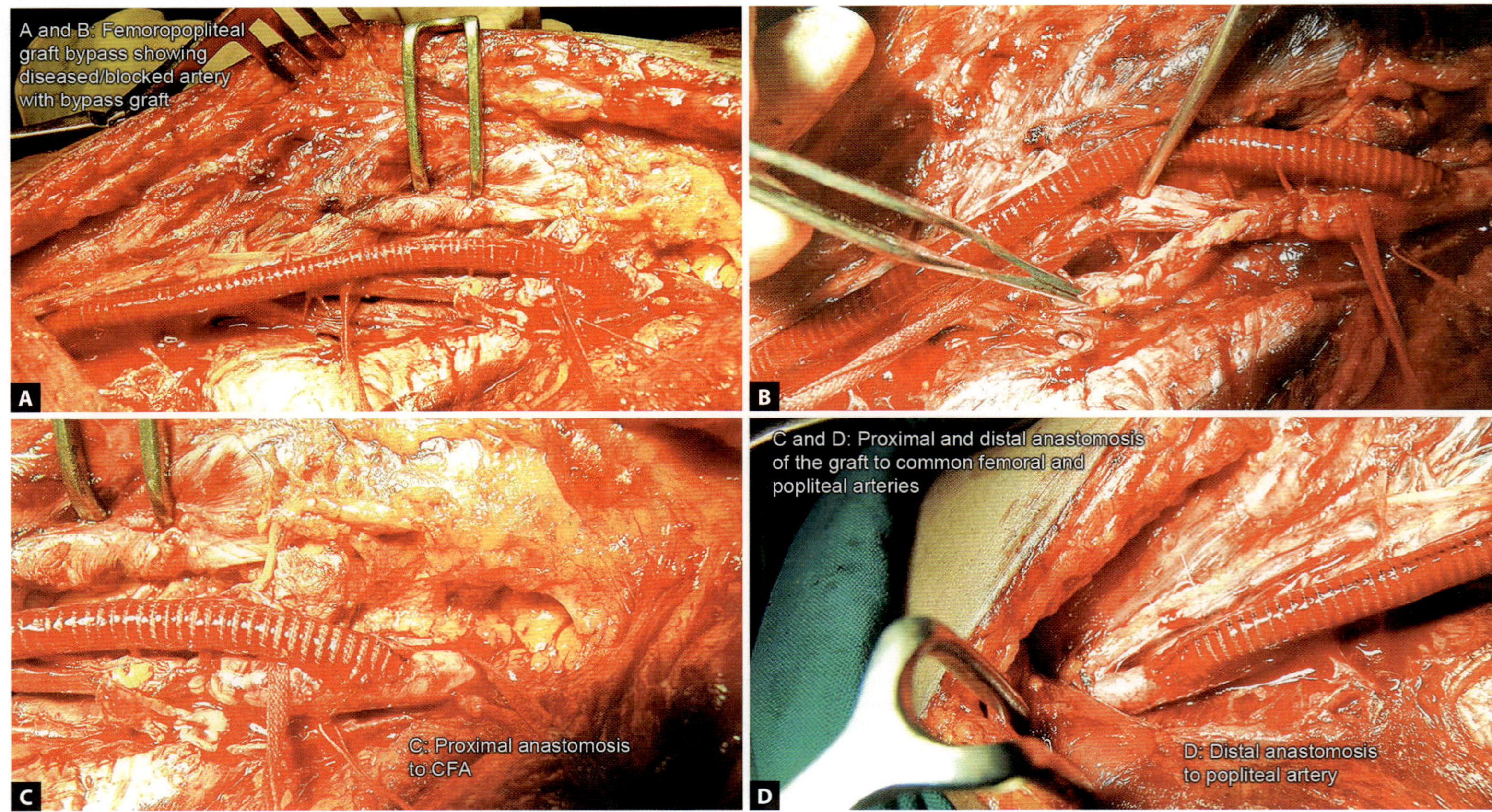

Figs. 11-44A to D: Femoropopliteal bypass graft.

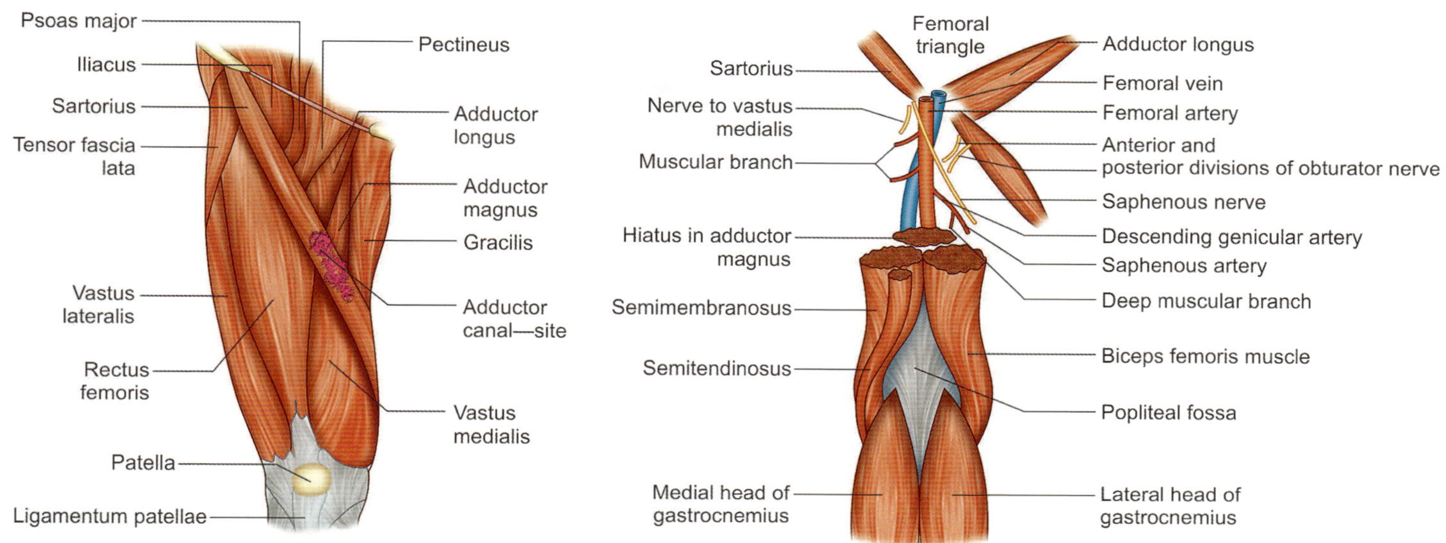

Fig. 11-45: Anatomy of femoral triangle and adductor canal in relation to femoropopliteal bypass graft.

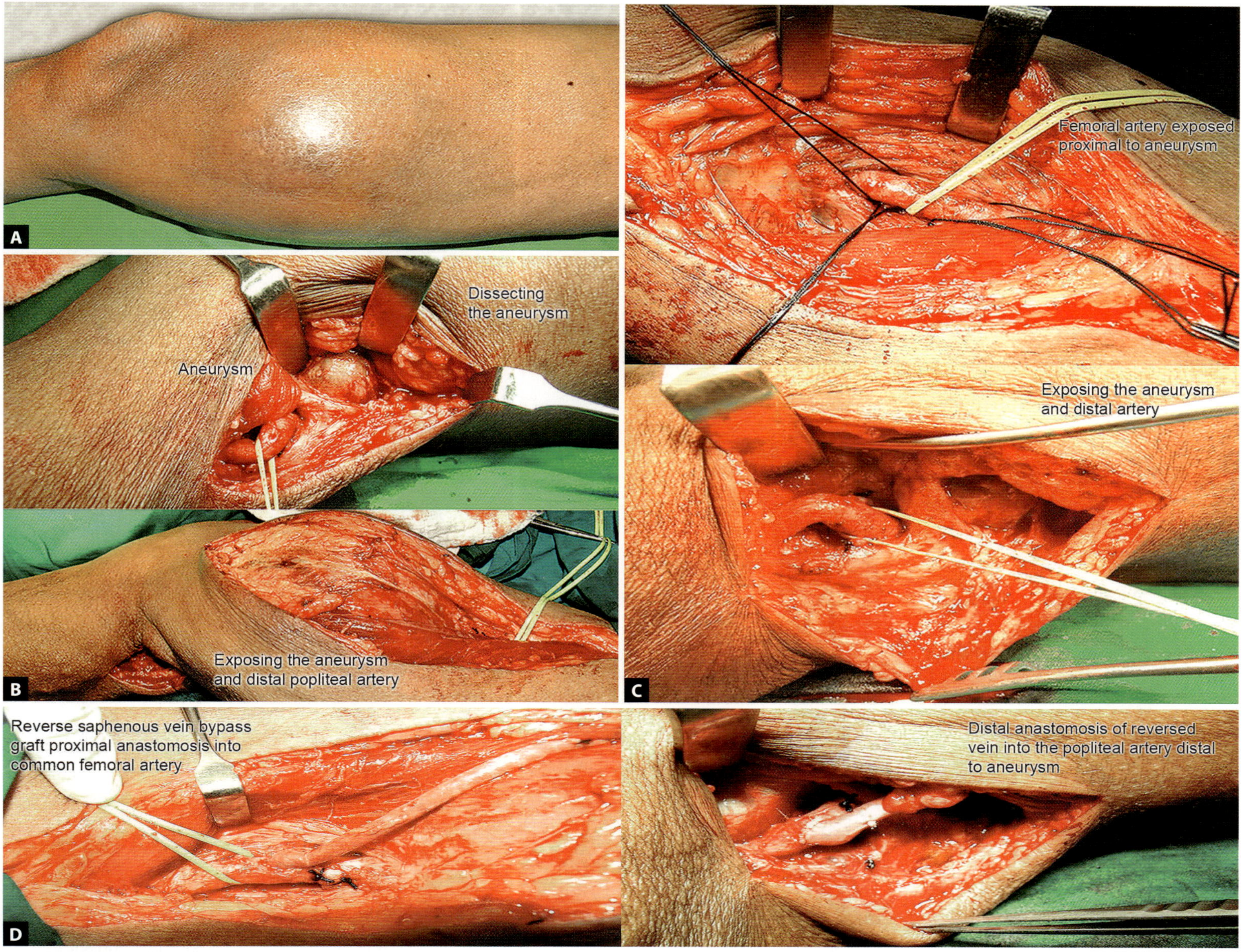

Figs. 11-46A to D

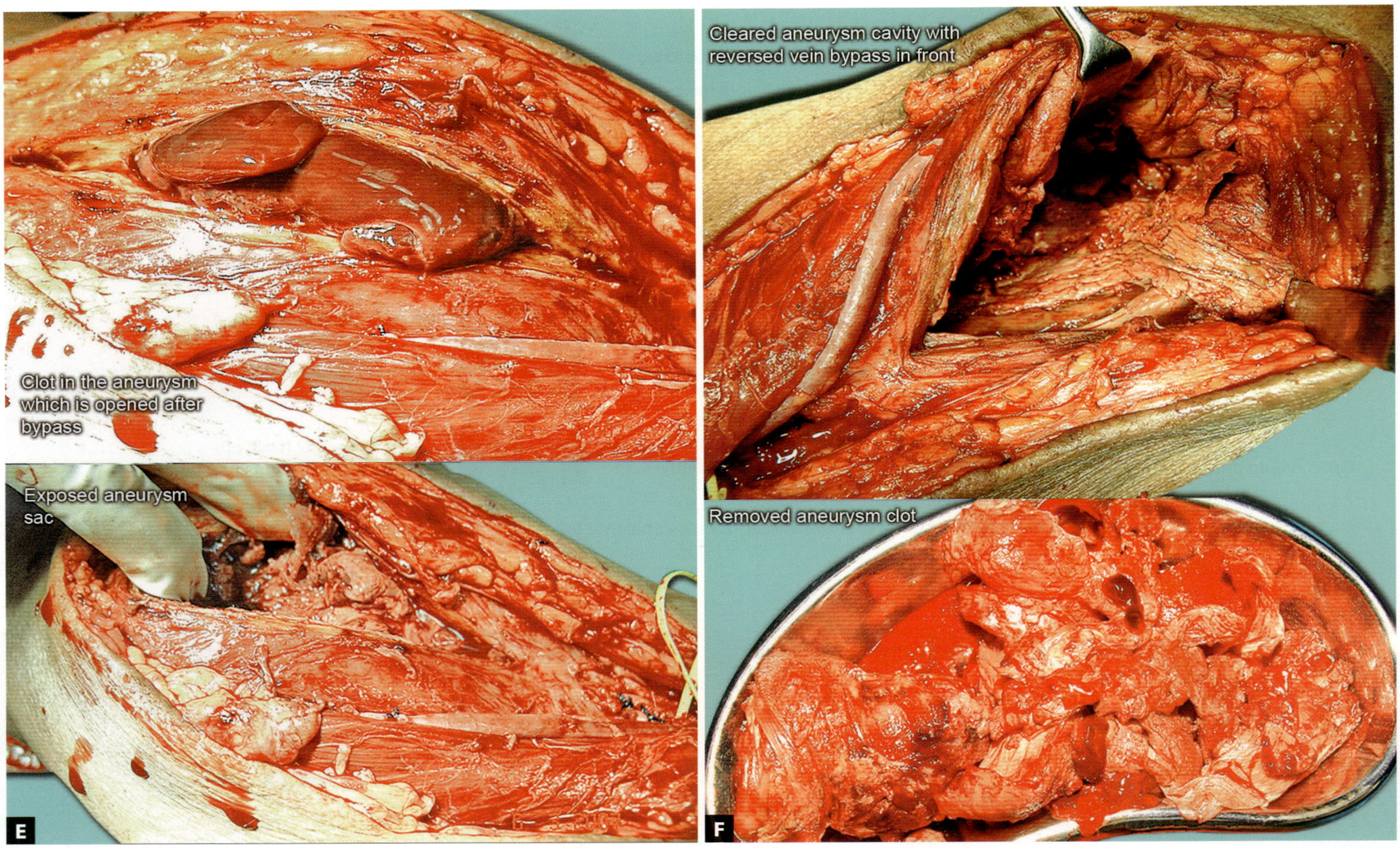

Clot in the aneurysm which is opened after bypass

Cleared aneurysm cavity with reversed vein bypass in front

Exposed aneurysm sac

E

Removed aneurysm clot

F

Figs. 11-46E and F

Figs. 11-46A to F: Femoropopliteal aneurysm—clot evacuation after placing reverse saphenous vein femoropopliteal venous bypass graft.

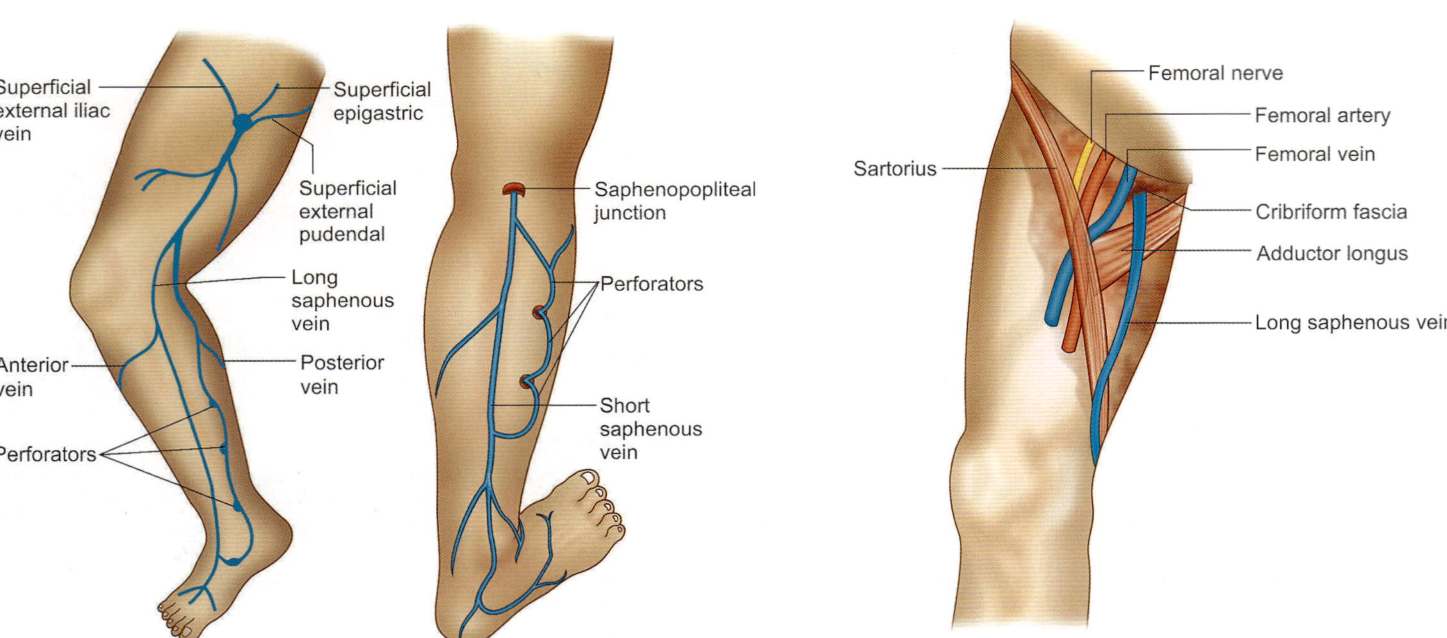

Fig. 11-47: Anatomy of long and short saphenous vein.

Fig. 11-48: Surgical anatomy of saphenofemoral junction and femoral triangle.

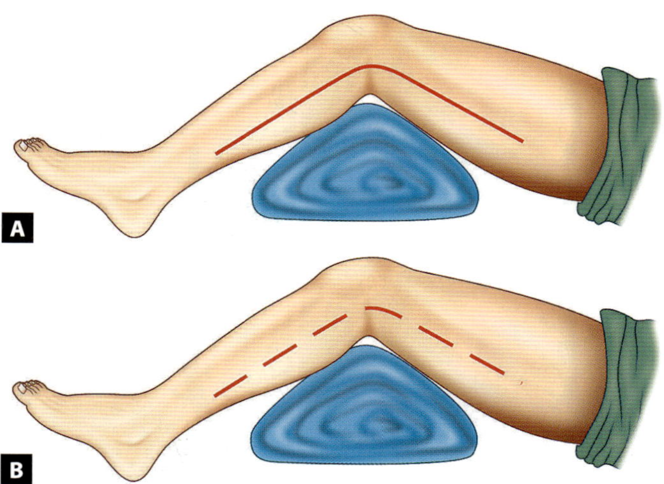

Incisions for long saphenous vein harvesting for saphenous vein femoropopliteal graft. LSV may be exposed by (A) longitudinal incision along the LSV or (B) by multiple small longitudinal incisions. It is technically easier with single lengthy incision. In situ saphenous vein graft cab be done with multiple incisions. All tributaries should be ligated at 1 mm distant from the surface of the LSV using 4-zero polypropylene sutures

Figs. 11-49A and B: Incision for exposing the long saphenous vein.

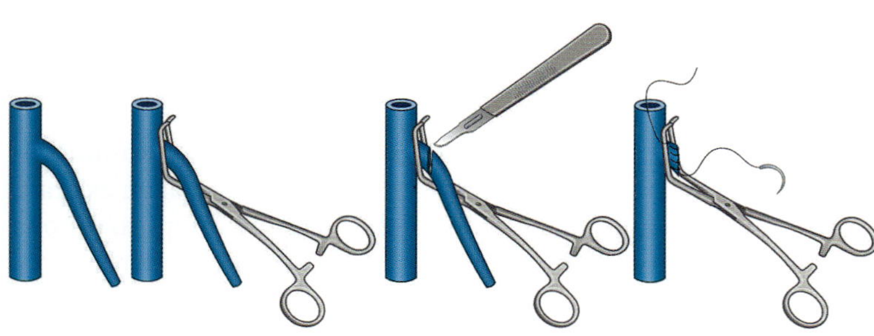

Harvesting of LSV is done by ligating the saphenofemoral junction very close to the femoral vein so that to achieve wide LSV opening for proximal (in 'in situ' graft) or distal (in reverse graft) anastomosis to artery. Satinsky clamp is applied at SFJ; LSV is cut using No. 15 blade; continuous underrunning over and over sutures on the Satinsky clamp is done using 4-zero polypropylene suture to close the SFJ

Fig. 11-50: Saphenofemoral ligation for harvesting the LSV graft.

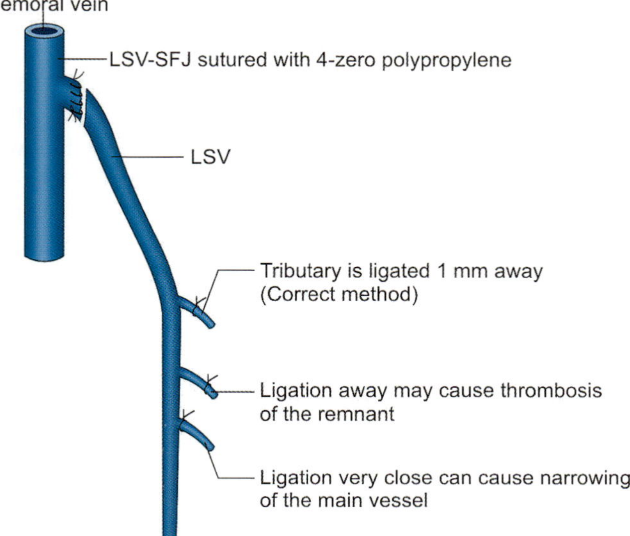

Fig. 11-51: Proper ligation of tributaries is essential in harvesting the saphenous vein.

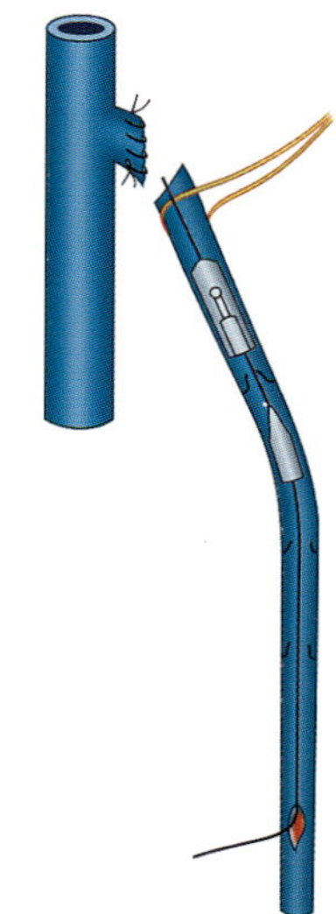

SFJ is ligated close to the femoral vein; proximal saphenous vein is looped; through distal venotomy valvulotome is passed; next to proximal valve is cut gently

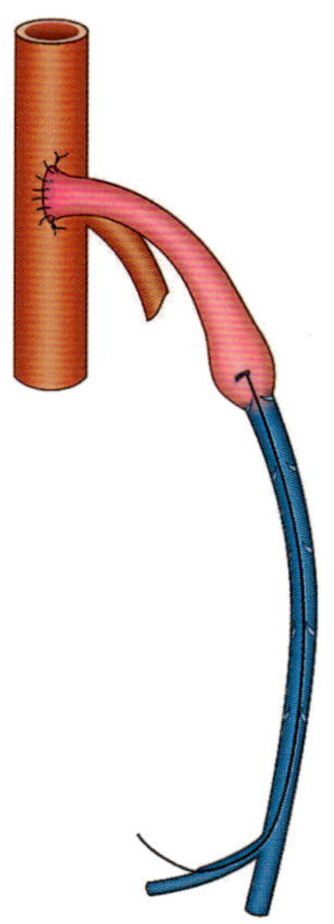

Proximal anastomosis is done into the common femoral artery; valvulotome is further pulled down along each valve to cut it; till lower end valves are cut

Figs. 11-52A and B: In situ saphenous vein graft for femoropopliteal bypass.

identified and ligated. Angiogram is done to identify and ligate the site of tributaries. Tributaries are identified using a Doppler probe; pinching the graft distal to probe, flow to the tributary proximally can be recognised **(Figs. 11-53A to D)**.

Distal anastomosis between end of the saphenous vein and side of the artery (end to side) is decided. It may be either lower popliteal, anterior tibial, tibioperoneal or posterior tibial depending on the site and extent of the block. Vein end is tailored like a cobra head. Magnifying loop or glass may be used for distal anastomosis. Small bulldog clamps or vascular loops are used to occlude the vessel all around prior to anastomosis. 6-zero or 7-zero polypropylene sutures are used for distal anastomosis. Any arteriovenous fistula in 'in situ saphenous graft' is carefully felt (by thrill); if present identified and ligated securely. It can also be identified by doing on table angiogram or on table Doppler study.

In 'in situ saphenous vein graft' usually *proximal anastomosis is done first*; later distal anastomosis.

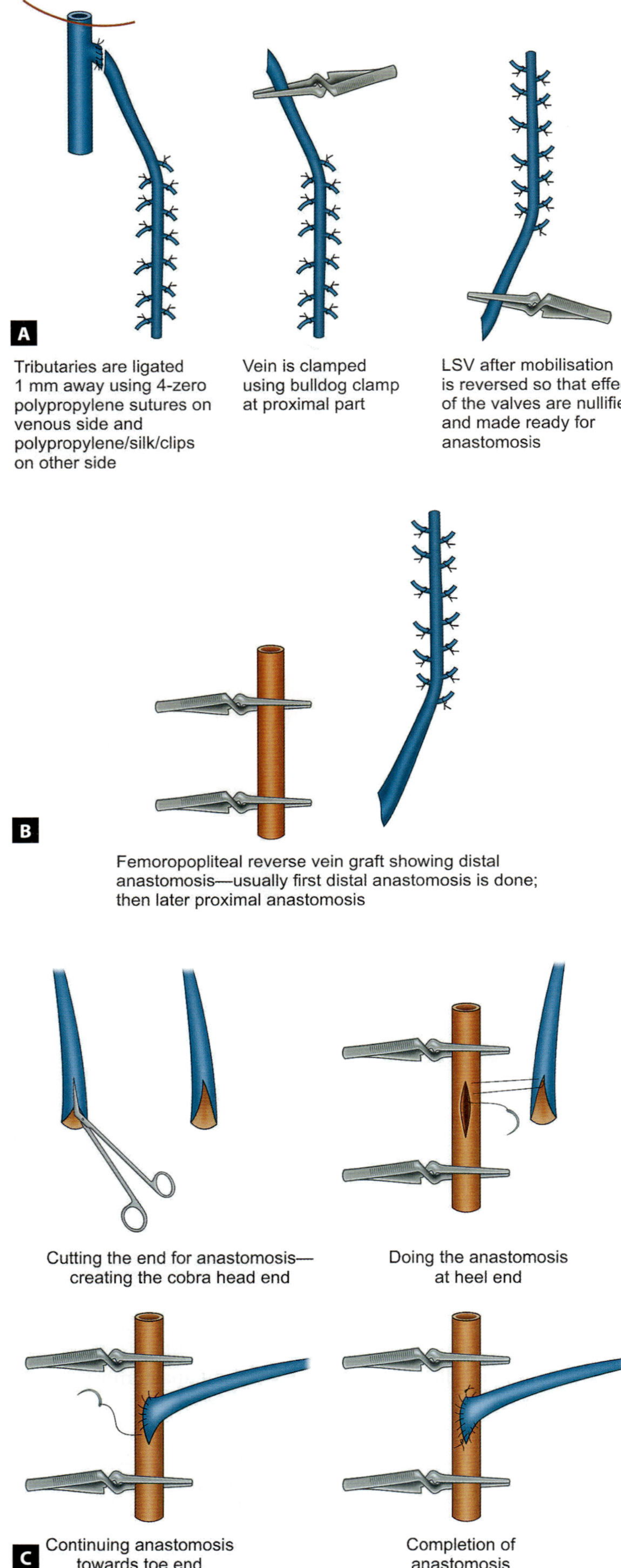

Figs. 11-53A to C

A B

(A) Reversed vein is filled and passed with cold heparinised patient's blood using syringe with ball tipped needle. Any bleeding point is sutured using fine 6-zero polypropylene suture to make vein ready (B) for graft

Fig. 11-53D

Figs. 11-53A to D: In situ saphenous vein graft for femoropopliteal bypass graft.

Free Reversed Saphenous Vein Graft

Long saphenous vein (LSV) is used commonly. LSV should be available as a normal vein. Opposite LSV can also be taken as graft. Diseased vessel cannot be harvested. Preoperative Duplex/venous Doppler scan should be done. Procedure is done under spinal/epidural anaesthesia. It may be a single long incision along the course of the vein or skip incisions or interrupted incisions. Saphenous vein is divided at saphenofemoral junction; cut vein end on femoral vein side is closed using 4-zero polypropylene suture.

Vein is dissected; all large and small tributaries are ligated at 1 mm distance. Creating flaps under the skin or undermining the skin should be avoided as necrosis of skin flap can occur. Vein should be irrigated continuously using saline to prevent desiccation. Vein should be held very carefully without causing any adventitial injury. Vein is completely dissected off the surrounding tissue and rotated 180° to reverse it. Fine needle (*ball tipped* needle) with syringe containing *cold heparinised patient's blood* is passed through the distal aspect of the vein (reversed vein proximal part). Plain saline solution should not be used. Solution containing saline, albumin, heparin and papaverine can be used. Vein is gently flushed with the heparinised blood causing distension of the vein. Care should be taken not to force blood/fluid rapidly to create over distension which may lead into intimal damage. A pressure over 200 mmHg is not advisable (rapid force in usual syringe creates pressure more than 200 mmHg). Any leaking points are identified and securely ligated using 8-zero polypropylene suture without narrowing the lumen. *Magnifying lens* may be used for suture ligation.

Short/small saphenous vein when needed is harvested in prone position. Flexion and inward rotation of the hip is also used which avoids change of position for graft suturing. Small saphenous vein which is located behind the lateral malleolus is identified. Longitudinal skin incision (from lateral malleolus up to mid calf level) is made; skin should not be undermined; identified vein is dissected off the adjacent tissues with ligation of tributaries.

In proximal ⅓ of leg vein penetrates the deep fascia. Continuous papaverine irrigation into the vein is needed to prevent spasm.

If both LSV and SSV are not good for graft then *cephalic vein* is used as autologous vein graft. Cephalic vein is harvested from lateral side of wrist to deltopectoral triangle. Anatomical variations are common in upper limb veins. Upper limb veins are more adherent to skin compared to lower limb veins and so it is more difficult to harvest them without traumatising. Both cephalic and basilic veins can be used as one conduit. Lateral lengthy single incision or multiple incisions may be used.

Tunneling to pass the graft is done either in deeper plane or superficial subcutaneous plane. Graft placed in deeper plane avoids kinking and block; but access for possible eventual stenosed area becomes difficult. Above knee popliteal graft is placed in superficial plane where vein is harvested upon. Below knee popliteal graft is passed through deeper plane to avoid kinking by hamstrings. *Twist in the vein should be avoided.* After proximal anastomosis clamp is released; twist can be made out during blood flow. Often *ink marking* is done on the surface of the vein to identify the twist if it develops. *Completion angiogram* also shows twist along with leak.

Common, superficial and deep femoral arteries are exposed properly through thigh incision. These arteries are occluded using vascular clamps. Arteriotomy is done (No. 11 blade) on the common femoral artery with lower end of incision *directed towards* deep femoral artery. Incision can be easily extended into deep femoral artery if there is localised stenosis of the orifice of the deep femoral artery.

Anastomosis is done either as distal anastomosis first and later proximal anastomosis or as proximal anastomosis first. Many surgeons prefer to do distal anastomosis first. Either way is acceptable.

Proximal side-to-end anastomosis is done. Proximal cut end of the vein is made oblique by cutting on one edge. It reduces the tension on the anastomotic line and also makes the stoma wider. Sutures are placed from inside of the artery towards outside to avoid intimal flap formation. 'Heel' *should be distal* part of the anastomotic stoma and *'toe' should be proximal* part. Before last suture, clamp is released to confirm the back flow and down flow. Anastomosis is irrigated with heparinised saline. Clamp is reapplied and anastomosis is completed. Clamp on the venous side distal to the anastomosis is applied.

Distal anastomosis is done as end-to-side. End of the vein is cut and spatulated like a *'cobra head'* to widen the stoma at end-to-side anastomosis into the arteriotomy of distal popliteal artery. Here *'heel' end* of anastomosis is proximal; *'toe' end* is on distal side. Arteriotomy is done in the popliteal artery either above knee or below knee. As anastomotic site is smaller than proximal part, three initial stay sutures are placed near 'toe end' to achieve perfect anastomosis. Parachute or sliding technique may be also used beginning at the 'heel' end of the anastomosis in difficult situation. Back flow is checked during completion of anastomosis and heparinised saline irrigation is done **(Figs. 11-54A to C)**.

Completion angiogram is a must to check for leak, adequate filling, and twist. 20 mL of water-soluble iodine dye is injected. C-arm imaging is used. Suction drain is placed and kept for 72 hours. Wound is closed.

Intraoperative heparin or dextran is given to prevent formation of clot. Heparin is given 100 units/kg body weight at cross clamping. It is continued daily for 4 days **(Fig. 11-55)**.

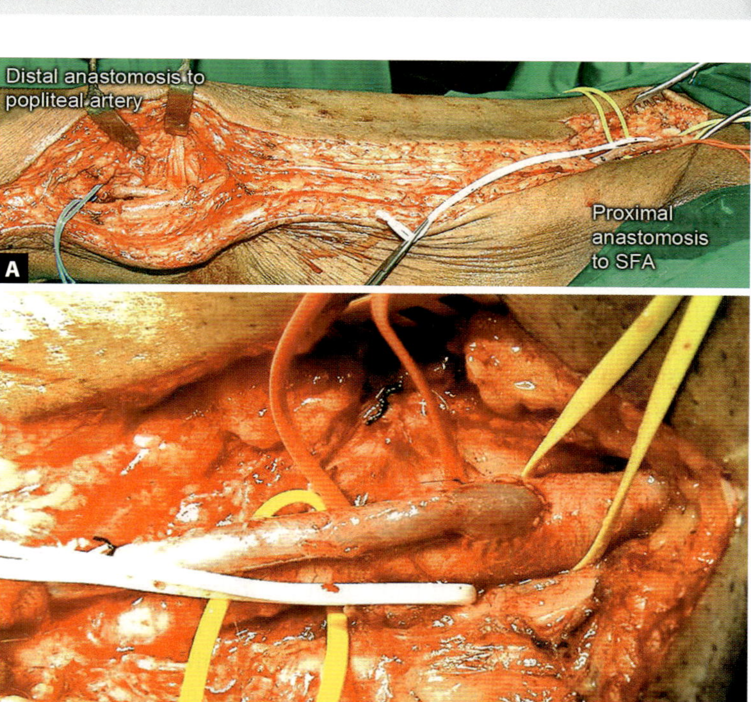

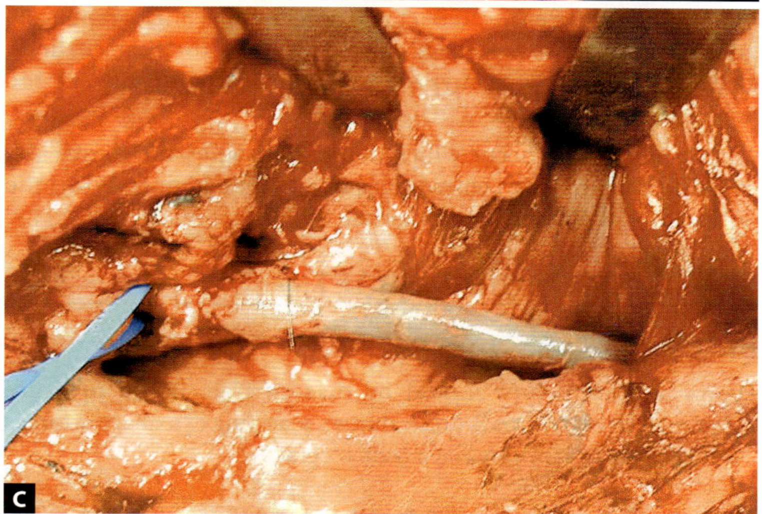

Figs. 11-54A to C: Femoropopliteal bypass reverse vein graft.

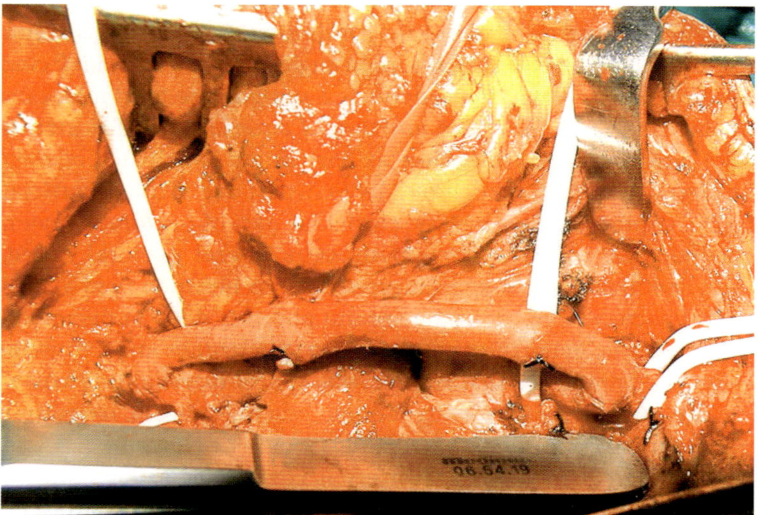

Fig. 11-55: Femoral artery to popliteal artery saphenous vein bypass graft.

Postoperative Care and Follow-up

It is common use to take oral anticoagulants and antiplatelet drugs even though graft survival by these drugs alone is not entirely proved.

ICU care, postoperative low molecular dextran are needed for 48–72 hours.

Smoking should be stopped to improve the graft survival.

Circulation should be checked by regular checking of pulse or using Doppler. Duplex scan is very useful to identify the stenosed areas. Stenosis is commonly observed at anastomotic site, at the level of valves. Duplex scan is done 3 weeks after surgery; then afterwards once in 3 months for 1 year. Late occlusions are less in 'in situ graft' than in reversed saphenous vein graft or synthetic graft.

Complications

Bleeding, thrombosis, graft leak, graft thrombosis, infection and failure are known complications.

Early occlusion of the graft: If occlusion occurs within 30 days of graft it is called as early occlusion. It is commonly due to technical cause, poor selection of patient, inadequate 'run-in' and/or inadequate 'run-off'. A revision procedure may be tried; but amputation is commonly needed in such patients as revascularisation is impossible. Catheter thrombectomy, angioscopy, angiographically guided thrombolysis are tried to revascularise the limb. Balloon angioplasty, short jump bypass graft are all tried to salvage the limb.

Late occlusion can occur which is due to progression of disease, smoking, persisting precipitating factors. Angiogram confirms the occlusion. It is difficult to manage late occlusion.

AXILLOFEMORAL GRAFT

Prerequisites

Donor axillary artery should be disease free. Blood pressure measuring in both arms is done; duplex scanning of axillary artery is essential. It is *extra anatomical indirect graft.*

Surgical Anatomy of Axillary Artery

It is the continuation of subclavian artery from outer border of first rib to lower margin of teres major muscle with its 1st part occupying superior, 2nd part behind and 3rd part is inferior to pectoralis minor muscle. When the arm is held at right angle to body with palm facing upwards, surface marking is done as a straight line from midpoint of clavicle to a point at the junction of anterior ⅓ and posterior ⅔ of lateral wall of axilla. Here axillary artery is palpated against humerus. Superficial relations in first part are skin, superficial fascia, supraclavicular nerves, clavicular part of pectoralis major, clavipectoral fascia with cephalic vein, lateral pectoral nerve, thoracodorsal vessels, communicating loop between medial and lateral pectoral nerves; in the second part it is deep to pectoralis minor muscle; in the third part it is deep to pectoralis major muscle. Deeper relations are first intercostals space, external intercostal muscle, serratus anterior digitations, brachial plexus, latissimus dorsi and teres major below. Axillary vein is below, medial and superficial to artery. Axillary artery is covered by axillary sheath which is derived from prevertebral layer of deep cervical fascia. Axillary vein is not covered by axillary sheath.

Of 6 *branches of axillary artery* one (superior thoracic) branch arises from first part; two (acromiothoracic/thoracodorsal and lateral thoracic) from 2nd part and three branches (subscapular {*largest branch*}, anterior circumflex humeral, posterior circumflex humeral) arise from 3rd part of axillary artery.

Incision: A small transverse incision below the middle of the clavicle extending laterally to a point below the medial part of the deltopectoral groove.

Procedure: Skin and pectoral fascia are incised; pectoralis muscle is split along the line of fibres and retracted. Clavipectoral fascia is identified and split to reach pectoralis minor muscle. Pectoralis muscle is cut or retracted to feel the axillary artery pulsation. Axillary vein is below and superficial to artery with close relation. Posterior minor branches of the artery should be ligated; fine sling is passed around the artery to have gentle traction over the artery **(Fig. 11-56)**.

Axillofemoral tunnel is created to place the prepared selected graft in the tunnel. Tunnel is created using finger under the pectoralis major in front of chest wall along the midaxillary line and later medial to anterior superior iliac spine to reach the groin below the inguinal ligament into common femoral artery. If both common femoral arteries are needed to perfuse then bifurcation axillofemoral graft can be used; or use a cross over graft from axillofemoral graft of one side to opposite common femoral artery. In between additional horizontal small incisions may be made as needed to facilitate the proper graft placement in the tunnel without kinking. Length of the graft should be adequate enough to prevent shortening and to allow adequate range of movements of shoulder and hip joints. Prior heparinisation is done; vascular clamps are placed to vessels; arteriotomy is done to both axillary and femoral arteries. Anastomosis is done first at proximal and then distally using polypropylene sutures.

Indications and Advantages

- It is done in conditions where already placed aortic graft is infected or as an alternate to aortofemoral graft.
- Advantages are major muscles are not incised; abdomen is not opened; aorta is not dissected and clamped.
- If it is done in case of infected aortofemoral graft original graft should be removed with ligation of aorta and proximal femoral arteries. Tunneling should avoid infected field.

FEMOROFEMORAL CROSSOVER GRAFT

It is done when one side vessel is diseased but other side is relatively normal with adequate perfusion. Initial angiogram and Duplex scanning are done to assess the flow and success of the procedure.

It is done in spinal or epidural anaesthesia as an *extra anatomical graft* technique.

Both sides' common femoral arteries are exposed through vertical groin incision. Arteriotomies are done in common femoral arteries. *Oblique* arteriotomies are preferred so as to place anastomosis obliquely to maintain the curve of the placed graft. Donor arteriotomy is slightly at higher level than recipient arteriotomy. Both arteries are clamped; tunnel is created in the suprapubic region with a curve; graft is placed in the tunnel. Care must be taken not to injure the urinary bladder (catheterisation is a must). Graft is anastomosed to donor artery and then at recipient artery in similar fashion as side-to-end. Clamps are released. Drains are placed on both wounds **(Fig. 11-57)**.

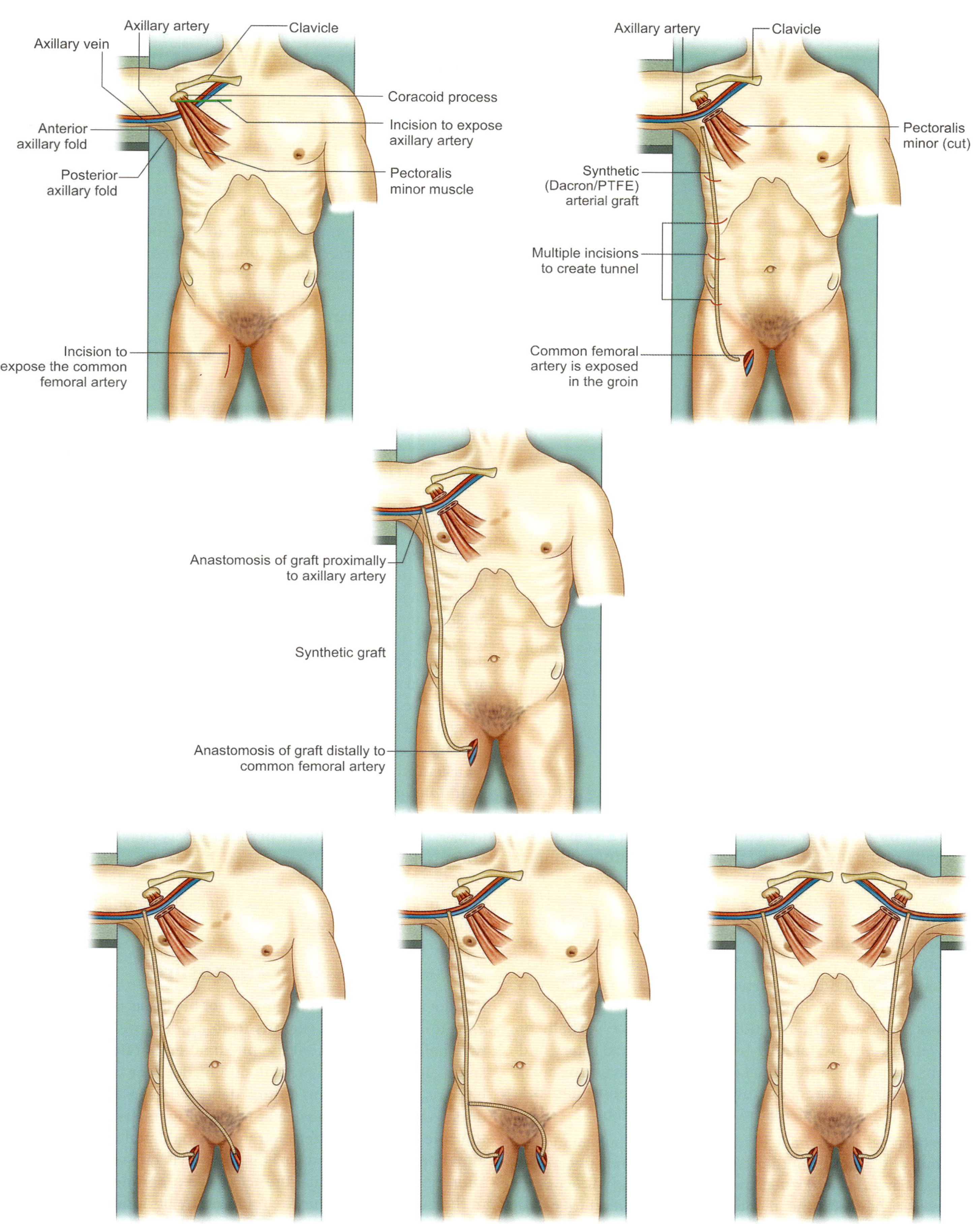

Fig. 11-56: Axillofemoral bypass graft. It is an extra anatomical graft.

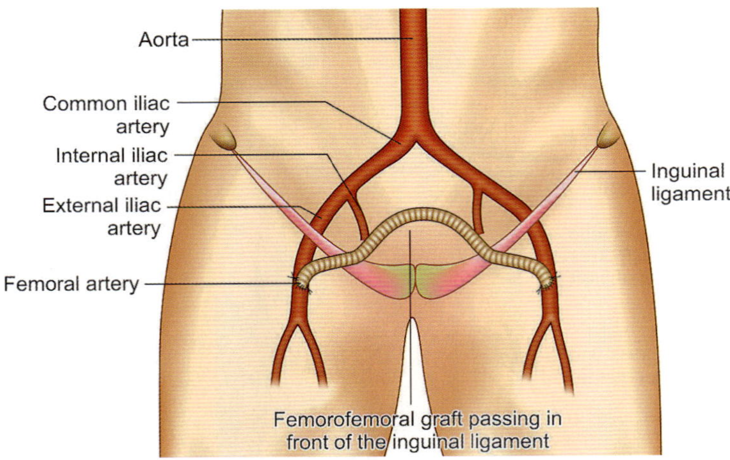

Fig. 11-57: Femorofemoral crossover graft.

Advantages

It is an extra-anatomical graft; easier to place; simple and effective.

Disadvantages

One side artery should be relatively adequate and normal to perfuse both limbs.

Injuries to urinary bladder, graft failure/blockage are the problems.

DISTAL ARTERIAL BYPASS

Block distal to popliteal artery is difficult to manage. Reconstruction is difficult and is possible only if artery distally is patent. Commonly it is done to anterior tibial, posterior tibial, peroneal arteries and rarely to dorsalis pedis artery.

Anterior Tibial Artery Exposure

It is small terminal branch of popliteal artery beginning at lower part of the popliteus opposite tibial tuberosity; enters the anterior compartment of the leg by passing close to the fibula (2.5 cm below the medial side of the fibular head) through an opening in upper part of the interosseous membrane. At midway between two malleoli it continuous as dorsalis pedis artery (at distal margin of superior extensor retinaculum). It lies between tibialis anterior and extensor digitorum longus; middle third between the tibialis anterior and extensor hallucis longus; lower third between extensor hallucis longus and extensor digitorum. Artery is crossed from lateral to medial side by extensor hallucis longus tendon. Deep peroneal nerve is lateral to artery. Anterior tibial artery may be partially or completely replaced by perforating branch of peroneal artery and perforating branch of posterior tibial artery. Artery gives muscular branches, anastomotic branches; medial and malleolar network branches. Artery is accompanied by two venae comitantes.

Incision: Vertical incision is made between the lateral subcutaneous margin of tibia and anterior border of fibula. Incision is deepened between tibialis anterior and extensor digitorum. Artery is exposed at various levels as needed either at middle third or lower third of the leg. Graft is passed from common femoral artery in thigh crossing from medial to lateral to pass onto lateral aspect of the knee joint to reach the leg. Alternatively graft can be crossed in the upper part or in the lower part of the leg.

Posterior Tibial Artery Exposure

It is larger terminal branch of the popliteal artery beginning at lower border of popliteus (in the midline on the back of calf at the level tibial tuberosity) between tibia and fibula deep to gastrocnemius; runs between medial malleolus and medial calcaneal tubercle deep to flexor retinaculum to divide as medial and lateral plantar arteries. It is related superficially to gastrocnemius, soleus and superficial transverse septum in the upper ⅔ of leg; it is in front and on medial border of tendo-Achilles in lower ⅓ of the leg. In the ankle it lies on capsule of ankle joint; between flexor digitorum longus and flexor hallucis longus. Artery is accompanied by two venae comitantes. Artery is accompanied and crossed by tibial nerve from medial to lateral side. It gives several branches—largest being peroneal artery; others are muscular artery, nutrient artery, anastomotic arteries, circumflex fibular artery, communicating branches, malleolar and calcaneal branches and terminal medial and lateral plantar arteries.

Incision: Vertical incision 1 cm posterior to medial subcutaneous border of the tibia extending like a 'hockey stick' under the medial malleolus. Lower down it is located between flexor digitorum longus and flexor hallucis longus. It is commonly used for 'in situ saphenous vein graft' **(Fig. 11-58)**.

Peroneal Artery Exposure

It is the largest branch of posterior tibial artery. It begins 2.5 cm below the lower margin of the popliteus; runs towards fibula → along the medial crest of the fibula → behind inferior tibiofibular joint and ankle joint → medial to peroneal tendons → ends as lateral calcaneal branches. Variations are common. It may replace posterior tibial/dorsalis pedis artery. It gives muscular branches, fibular nutrient artery, and anastomotic branches. Peroneal artery runs lateral to the tibial nerve in the groove between the fibular origin of flexor hallucis longus and tibialis posterior.

Both medial and lateral approaches are used. Graft placement is easier through medial approach.

In *lateral approach* incision is placed over lower part of lateral aspect of the leg; often segment of the fibula may need to be excised to pass the graft towards the peroneal artery. Once fibula is removed artery is directly seen.

In *medial approach*, as peroneal artery runs lateral to the tibial nerve in the groove between the tibialis posterior and fibular origin of flexor hallucis longus.

Dorsalis Pedis Artery Exposure

It is the main artery of dorsum of foot begins as continuation of the anterior tibial artery; extends from a point midway between the two malleoli to a point at the proximal end of first intermetatarsal space. It runs on the medial side of the foot lateral to extensor hallucis longus tendon to dip deep between two heads of first dorsal interosseous muscle at first intermetatarsal space to end in the sole as plantar arterial arch. It is palpated over intermediate cuneiform bone. Extensor hallucis brevis crosses the artery from lateral to medial. Medial branch of deep peroneal nerve is lateral to the artery. Artery may be replaced by perforating branch of the peroneal artery in 14% of individuals. It runs over talus, navicular and intermediate cuneiform bones. Branches are medial and lateral (larger) tarsal arteries; arcuate artery which gives 2nd, 3rd, and 4th dorsal metatarsal arteries and first dorsal metatarsal artery.

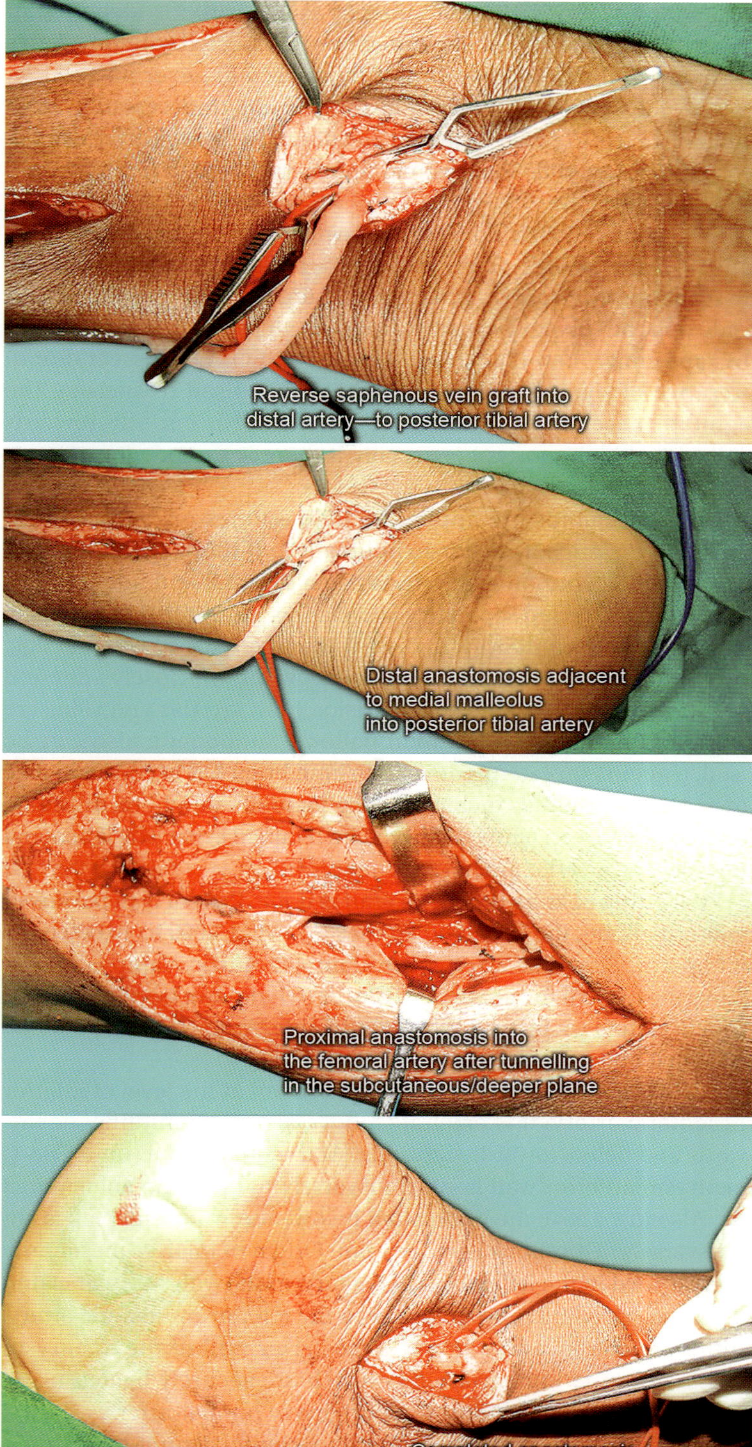

Fig. 11-58: Saphenous vein graft (reverse) into the posterior tibial artery through femoral artery.

Dorsalis pedis artery is exposed by vertical incision on the medial dorsal aspect of the foot for needed type of reconstruction.

ABDOMINAL AORTIC ANEURYSM

Indications for Surgery

Transverse diameter size more than 5.5 cm is an indication. Risk of rupture is 1% if size is less than 5.5 cm; raises to 20% if size is 7 cm. Mortality is 90% in rupture at community level; 50% if they reach hospital and undergoes surgery immediately.

Symptomatic aneurysm like pain/tenderness—whatever the size of aneurysm is.

Ruptured aortic aneurysm is *an emergency situation* with high mortality. It needs immediate surgery and aneurysm repair. Rupture may be anterior (20%) into the peritoneal cavity or posterior (80%) with formation of retroperitoneal haematoma.

Preoperative Preparation

It is essential in relation to cardiac, renal and pulmonary functions. Mass in the abdomen may be palpable clinically with a bruit over it. Lower limb ischaemia often may be evident on both sides. Thrombus from the aneurysm may cause emboli. CT abdomen or CT angiogram is a must. Size, thickness of the wall, course of ureter, site of left renal vein and status of visceral arteries are important findings to be assessed.

Preoperative bowel (colonic) preparation is essential **(Fig. 11-59)**.

Prophylactic antibiotics are given just during incision time.

Central line, an arterial line, nasogastric tube, warming blanket to upper body, urinary catheter—are needed **(Figs. 11-60 and 11-61)**.

Epidural catheter with general anaesthesia is used. Both hands are tied over chest wall.

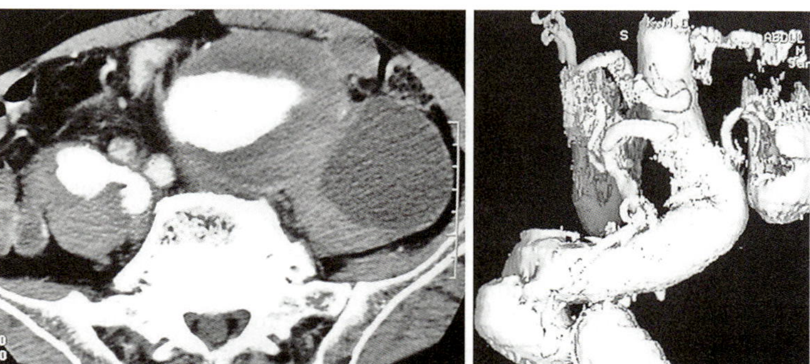

Fig. 11-59: CT scan showing abdominal aortic aneurysm.

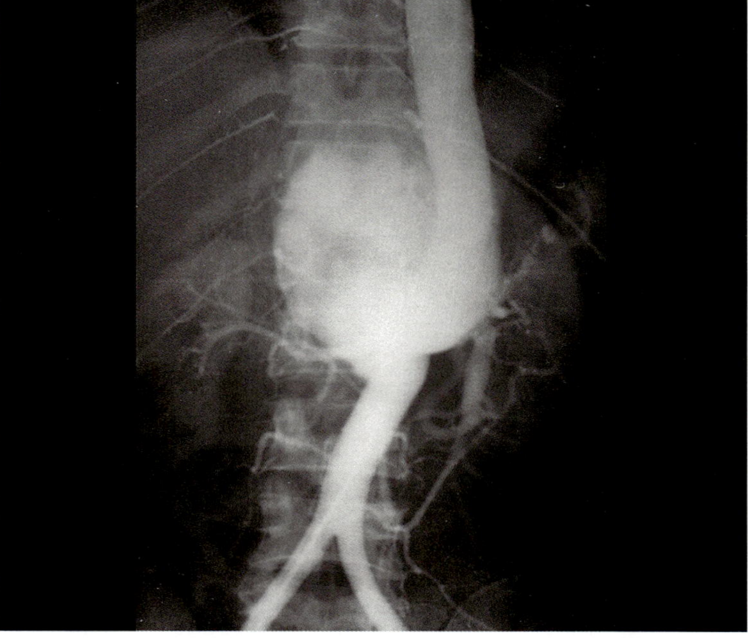

Fig. 11-60: Aortogram showing aortic aneurysm.

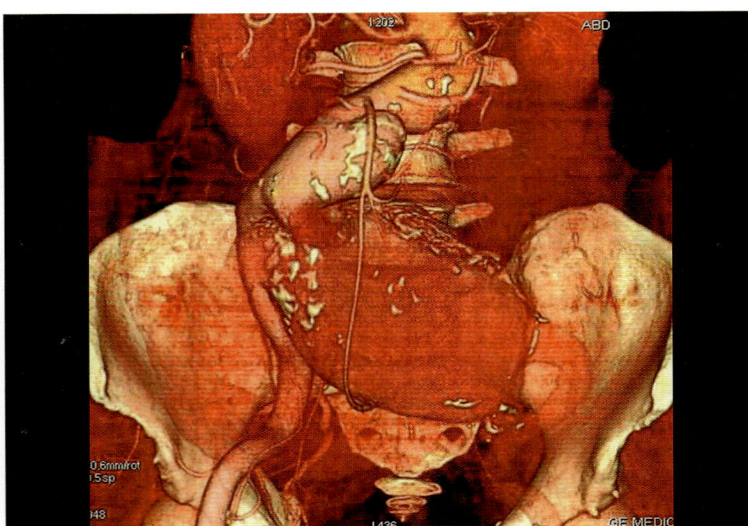

Fig. 11-61: Reconstructed CT angiogram showing abdominal aortic aneurysm.

Surgical Procedure

Midline incision from xiphisternum to pubic symphysis. Occasionally horizontal incision or midline incision extending across the costal margin is done. Abdomen is explored for additional pathologies, if any to confirm. Manipulation of the aneurysm should be avoided. Surgeon usually stands on left side of the patient but can stand on right side if he feels comfortable. Entire small bowel is mobilised towards the right side of the abdomen to visualise the base of mesentery; gut is wrapped with sterile towel and placed in a gut bag. Transverse colon is lifted above packed superiorly. Posterior peritoneum is divided at the junction of small bowel mesentery on right and large bowel mesentery on left. Division is continued up towards duodenojejunal junction which is identified by inferior mesenteric vein. Duodenum should not be injured. Left renal vein should be identified above, which runs usually in front of the aorta from left side. Rare anatomical variation of retroaortic left renal vein should be remembered. Inferior mesenteric vein is displaced above or ligated at its orifice. Left renal vein is usually above the level of the neck of the aneurysm. Left gonadal and left adrenal veins are not ligated but occasionally there will be a need to ligate left renal vein if neck of the aneurysm extends above this level. In such situation left gonadal and adrenal veins should be intact to drain left kidney **(Fig. 11-62)**.

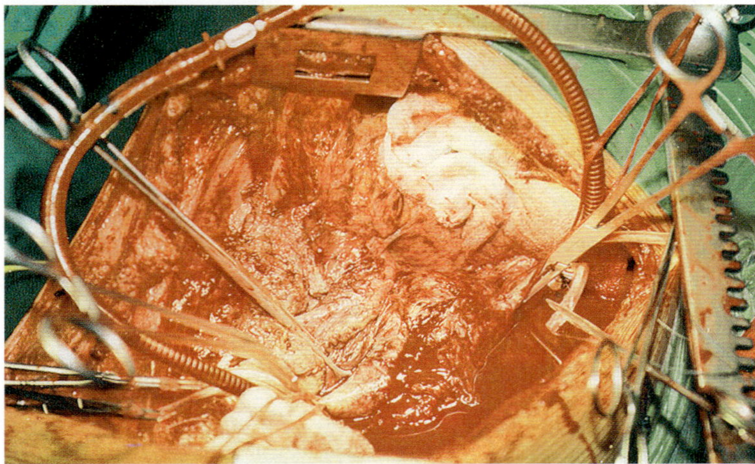

Fig. 11-62: Aneurysm if extensive blood flow can be diverted temporarily by placing arterial catheter from proximal to distal part.

Junction of aorta where it enlarges as aneurysm is identified in upper part. 1 cm of normal aorta above is dissected carefully. Sides of the normal proximal aorta is only dissected; never posteriorly. Posterior dissection by finger or instrument will unnecessarily injure lumbar vessels to cause torrential bleeding. Often renal arteries arise from the neck of the aneurysm at upper end. Renal arteries should be preserved.

Dissection below is done by exposing both iliac arteries. Ureters run in front of iliac arteries. Ureters should not be disturbed; dissection is done on either side of the ureter. Stretched ureter falls aside once aneurysm is dealt with. Blood supply of the ureter should be kept intact. Left iliac artery is often difficult to dissect due to presence of sigmoid colon. Sigmoid is mobilised by incising the sigmoid mesentery laterally and mobilising it entirely towards right side. It is important especially if there is extended aneurysm towards left iliac artery.

Vascular clamps are applied to iliac arteries on both sides at sufficient distance from aortic bifurcation. If there are aneurysms extending to common iliac arteries then external and internal iliac arteries are dissected separately and clamps are applied individually to them. It is often difficult to dissect the internal and external iliac arteries off their accompanying veins as veins are closely adherent to arteries at this level. In such occasion both arteries and veins are clamped together. Intraluminal balloon tamponade also can be used. If aneurysm extends down into both branches of common iliac arteries then femorals including deep femorals should be dissected for clamping. Deep femorals should be retained especially if bilateral internal iliac arteries are having aneurysm.

Preclotting of knitted Dacron graft is done. Patient is heparinised before clamping the aorta and arteries by giving 5,000 to 10,000 units of heparin. First iliac arteries are clamped. Aortic clamp is placed above the neck of the aneurysm. Glover's clamp can be placed easily from front to back instead from side-to-side. Aortic clamp should be tightened only to stop the distal pulsation.

Aorta is opened towards right side in front at the level of inferior mesenteric artery; it is extended above along the midline; downwards and below towards right side. At the neck of the (upper part) aneurysm anterior wall is cut transversely to open the aneurysmal sac. Also just above the bifurcation below, aortic anterior wall is cut transversely. Thrombus is scoped out. Origin of inferior mesenteric artery is held in the left flap of the aneurysm sac with vascular clamp to prevent bleeding (retrograde) from the inferior mesenteric artery. Initial profuse bleeding from the posterior wall of the aneurysm wall is from the lumbar arteries which are securely ligated using 4-zero polypropylene sutures. All origins of lumbar arteries should be ligated as once graft is placed its continuity cannot be restored **(Fig. 11-63)**.

Proximal part of the graft is sutured to the neck of the aneurysm using 3-zero polypropylene continuous sutures. Bites should be at 1 mm gap. Bite is taken from inside aorta to outside and from outside graft towards inside graft. Edge bite should be 2 mm from cut margin of aorta and also of graft. Knot should be towards left side to avoid closeness towards duodenum to prevent the possible aortoduodenal fistula.

Graft is clamped just distal to anastomosis and aortic clamp is released to check any leaks. Distal end of the graft is measured and cut adequately. It should not protrude beyond the bifurcation. Posterior bites of the suture material should be taken carefully as left common iliac vein lies close to its posterior wall. Continuous 4-zero or 3-zero polypropylene sutures are used often by parachute technique.

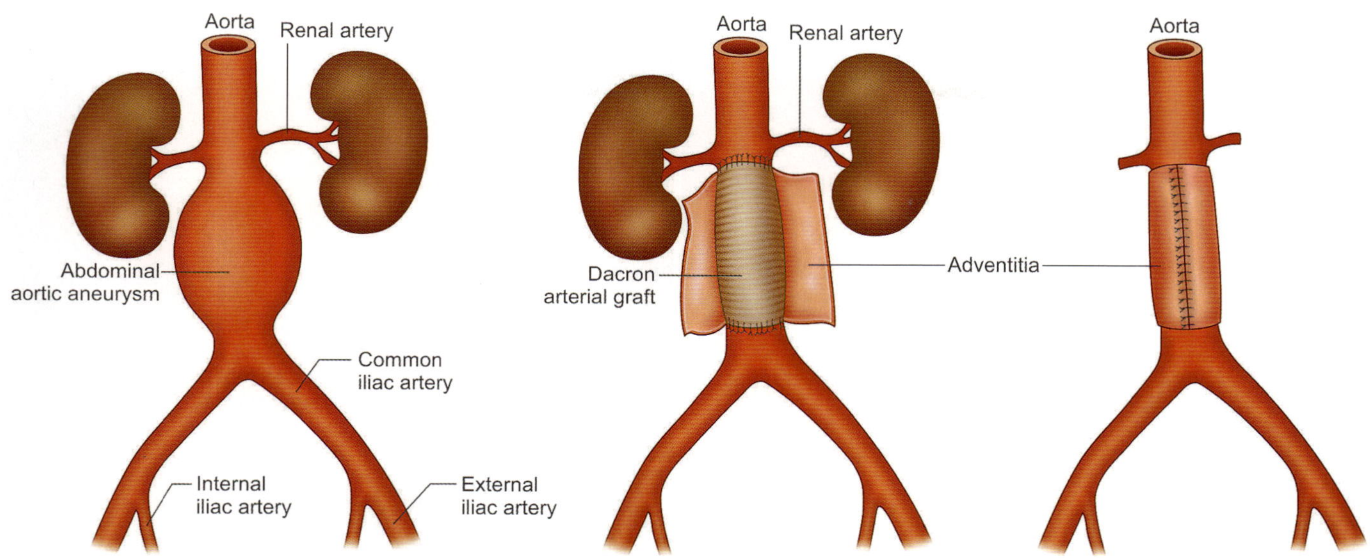

Fig. 11-63: Infrarenal aortic aneurysm repair.

Just prior to finishing the distal anastomosis, all clamps are released to clear clots and debris. First iliac artery clamp is released; and after few minutes clamp on other iliac artery is released. This is to avoid rapid fall in blood pressure after releasing the clamp which is due to return of cold deoxygenated blood, activated white cells, CO_2 and lactic acid causing cardiac depression and pulmonary vasoconstriction. A drop of 20 mmHg blood pressure is accepted. Back bleeding from inferior mesenteric artery is checked before ligating it. If it is not adequate then it needs to re-implant into the graft at proper place to maintain the adequate colonic perfusion. Sac is closed around the graft to prevent direct contact of the graft and gut **(Figs. 11-64A to M)**.

If aneurysm is extending into both common iliac arteries then bifurcation graft is placed; both distal ends are sutured at the junction of origins of external and internal iliac arteries. Graft should be placed within the aneurysmal sac. If there is aneurysm at iliac bifurcation but not involving internal iliac artery then external iliac artery distal to the aneurysm level is transected; its distal cut end is anastomosed to the similarly cut end of the internal iliac artery; graft is sutured to side of external iliac artery as 'end-to-side'. If internal iliac artery is also aneurysmal then it is ligated; graft is sutured to distal cut end as 'end-to-end' anastomosis **(Figs. 11-65A to J)**.

Postoperative Care

Intensive care unit (ICU) monitoring, measurement of output, assessment of clotting factors, pain management, antibiotic coverage are usual requirements in postoperative period. Heparin is used to prevent deep vein thrombosis (DVT). Fresh frozen plasma (FFP), platelet and blood are often needed. Patient is observed for bleeding and when suspected evaluation by haematocrit, US or CT abdomen is done. Any leak/disruption needs re-exploration.

Complications

Immediate Complications

Haemorrhage can occur from leak or bleeding from the branch vessels like lumbar arteries. Occasionally it may be due to injury to adjacent veins. It needs re-exploration and control of bleeding appropriately.

Later Complications

Colonic ischaemia (10%) develops if there is poor back bleeding in the cut inferior mesenteric artery origin. In such occasion, it is better to do re-implantation of the inferior mesenteric artery origin to the graft in front. Once ischaemia develops patient needs laparotomy and resection which carries high mortality due to sepsis.

Myocardial infarction is the commonest complication in first 2 days of surgery. Strict cardiac monitoring and management is required.

Renal failure is not uncommon especially if aneurysm extends up near the origins of the renal arteries. Patient may often require dialysis. It is the commonest non-cardiac complication.

Massive transfusion may cause complications like hyperkalaemia, electrolyte imbalance.

Tracheostomy may be needed for prolonged ventilation.

Sexual dysfunction may develop when internal iliac arteries are involved.

Aortoduodenal fistula/aortoenteric fistula at anastomotic site can occur. It is prevented by proper closing the sac over graft and placing knot of the suture away from the bowel site towards left side. It presents with haematemesis, melaena or hamatochezia which is often massive. It needs blood transfusion, exploration and correction of the fistula. It carries high mortality.

Infection is major problem which needs graft removal. It is often a challenging situation to manage.

Microemboli from aneurysm site are called as *'thrash' emboli.* Early clamping of the distal parts of the aneurysm area, flushing out of debris prior to placing last suture bite may prevent this. If it occurs then embolectomy or prostacyclin infusion may be required.

Graft leak, graft thrombosis and graft failure may require regrafting.

Spinal cord ischaemia can develop leading to paraplegia. It is due to block in the perfusion of spinal cord at its localised segment.

Prosthetic infection or migration may occur which needs graft removal.

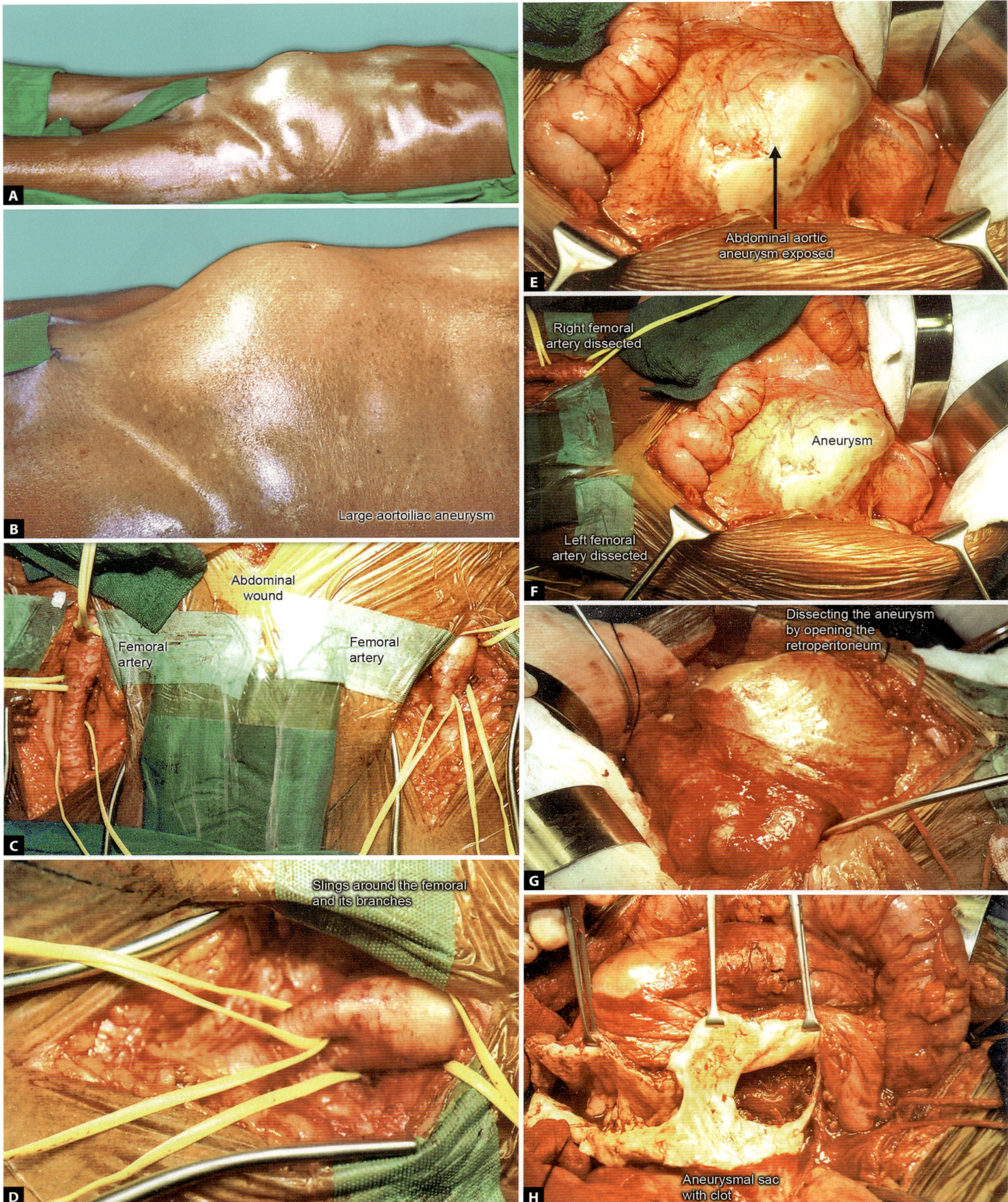

Figs. 11-64A to H

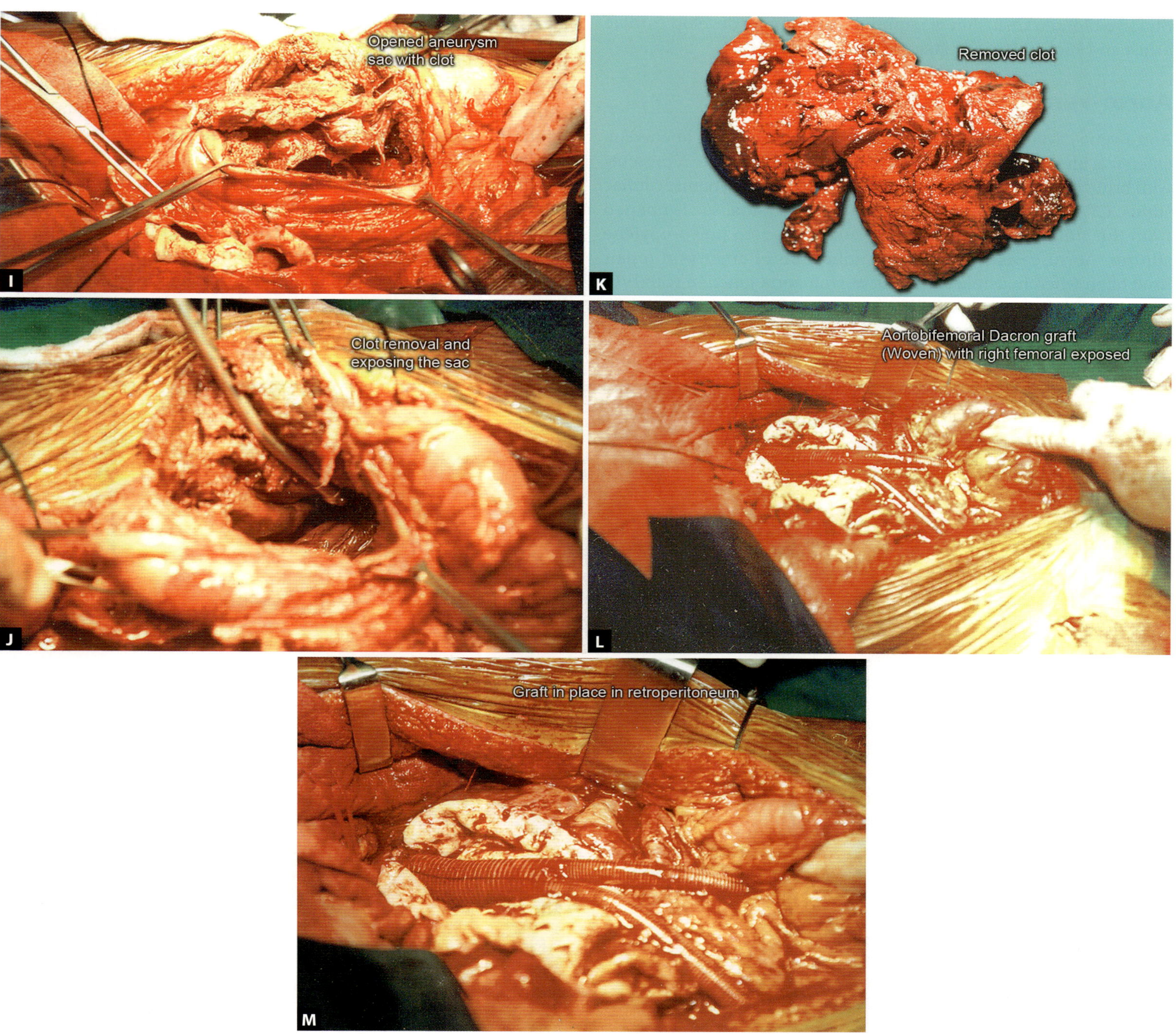

Figs. 11-64I to M

Figs. 11-64A to M: Abdominal aortic aneurysm. Operative steps.

Ruptured Aortic Aneurysm

Ruptured aortic aneurysm is a surgical emergency. Intraperitoneal rupture though less common (20%) has got very high mortality. In *retroperitoneal rupture* which is *more common,* after initial temporary bleeding, it stops due to tamponade effect of peritoneum and so patient can reach the hospital for definitive procedure on emergency basis. Central line, arterial line, urinary catheter and blood (10–20 bottles) for transfusion should be kept ready as preoperative measures. Emergency CT scan can be done if patient is stabilised.

Management of retroperitoneally ruptured aortic aneurysm is same as elective approach. But heparin is not given during procedure. It is administered only after clamping the aorta. Heparin solution can be flushed down the iliac vessels to prevent thrombosis of these vessels. Intraoperative complications like persistent ooze, disseminated intravascular thrombosis, myocardial infarction and cardiac arrest are dreaded complications which are not possible to reverse.

In intraperitoneal rupture which is much more critical as there is no temporary tamponade effect by peritoneum, emergency laparotomy is done. Direct pressure is applied over the neck of the aneurysm. A Foley's catheter may be passed into the aorta and inflated at the neck to control bleeding until patient is reasonably resuscitated. Alternatively vascular clamp may be applied directly over the aorta under the diaphragm at the level of crus to have an effective control. Once everything is under control, if patient is stable or reviving, then only repair of aneurysm may be undertaken.

Massive blood transfusion is required. Patient may develop cardiac arrest and succumb at any stage of the procedure.

Aorto-vena Caval Fistula

Aorto-vena caval fistula is a late dreaded complication of aneurysm. Often it is identified during ruptured aortic aneurysm also. It presents with bruit, poor perfusion of both lower limbs, hyperdynamic cardiac status. CT/MR angiogram is diagnostic. Aneurysmal sac is opened from the graft and is sutured using running 3-zero polypropylene sutures. Aorto-caval fistula is a complication of aneurysm repair itself often wherein fistula can occur at graft aorta junction with IVC. On table bleeding is controlled by vena caval finger occlusion or by passing a balloon over the fistula across saphenous vein.

ENDOVASCULAR ANEURYSM REPAIR (EVAR)

In 1991 Juan *Parodi* and Julio Palmaz first did endovascular aneurysm repair. It is less invasive, less morbid with less mortality rate and shorter hospital stay. It is basically aneurysm exclusion method. It is useful in old age and patients who are not fit for surgery. EVAR is basically a prophylactic procedure.

Femoral artery is cannulated; retrograde angiogram is done to evaluate the entire abdominal aorta including renal arteries. Cannulation → guidewire → stent device/graft placement are the steps. Special endovascular prosthesis/device is used and placed in place under guidance. First proximal part at infrarenal level is secured; then distal part of the prosthesis is secured on the femoral artery. Contralateral femoral artery is cannulated and

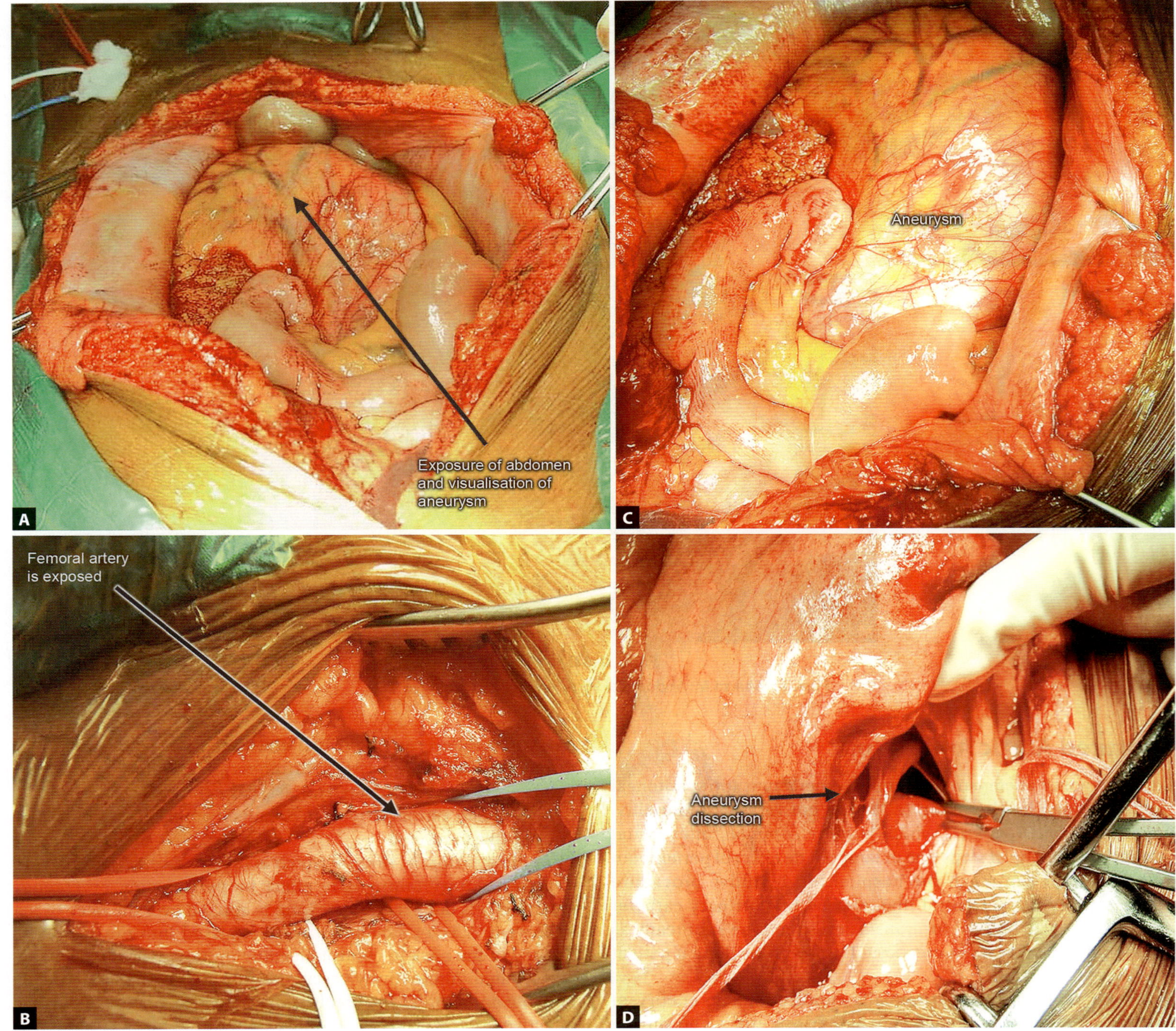

Figs. 11-65A to D

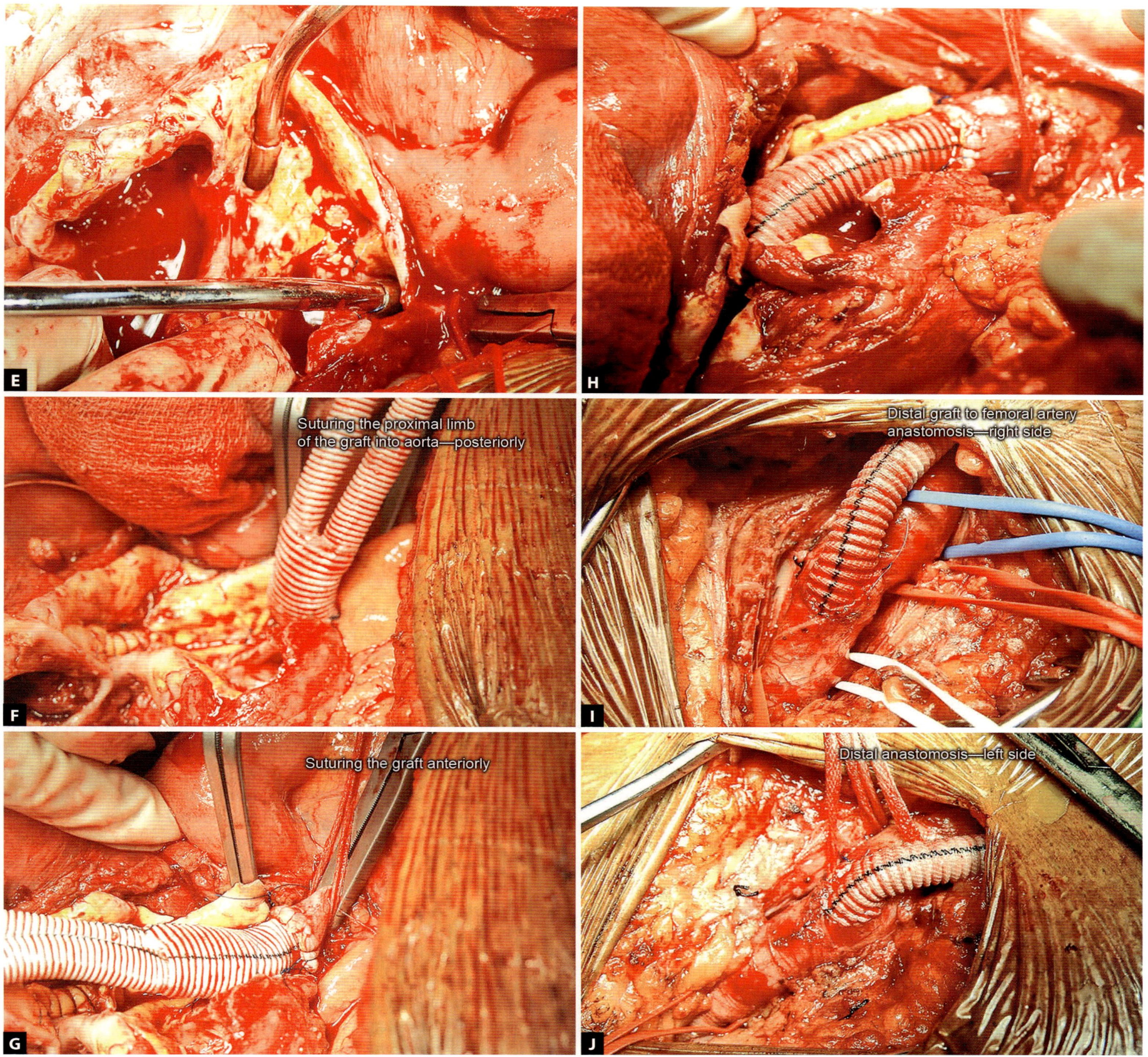

Figs. 11-65E to J

Figs. 11-65A to J: Aortic aneurysm exposure and placing aortofemoral graft.

prosthesis limb to opposite common iliac artery and femoral artery is placed. Suprarenal endovascular prosthesis needs fenestration for placement to maintain renal perfusion.

Percutaneous femoral artery puncture for device placement is also done. But open method is commonly advocated and safer.

Iliac vessels are also often used as access vessel.

EVAR is indicated if aneurysm is less than 5.5 cm in men and less than 5.0 cm in women. It is usually done in patients after 65 years.

Dacron or ePTFE is the material used as stent. Stent graft type, delivery system and skill for technique are essential. Many anatomical requirements are designed for successful EVAR.

Infrarenal neck is part of aorta between lowest renal artery and beginning of the aneurysmal sac. Anatomical requirements for effective EVAR are—proximal neck length should be more than 15 mm; diameter should be 18–32 mm; suprarenal angulation should be less than 60 degrees; infrarenal angulation should be less than 70 degrees; distal neck diameter should be more than 20 mm; common iliac vessel should be more than 15 mm in length; diameter is 8–25 mm.

Proper preoperative assessment is essential about site, extent and morphology of the aneurysm. Entire technique is done under radiological guidance and so C-arm and radiologist's help is essential.

Technique

General or spinal or epidural or local anaesthesia is needed. Abdomen and both groins are prepared. After exposing both common femoral arteries with a small vertical groin incision, using loops proximal and distal control is achieved. Heparin infused as 100 units/kg dose. Both side femoral arteries are cannulated using 18 gauge needle and flexible J guidewire is passed under C-arm guidance into thoracic aorta. Needle is removed; 7-9 French sheath is passed across guidewire; guidewire is removed; superstiff specialised guidewire (Meier wire) is inserted into the catheter and kept just below the left subclavian artery. Intra-operative intravascular ultrasound (IVUS) is very sensitive method of evaluating the aortic wall. Angioscaled pigtail catheter is passed through opposite common femoral artery into the abdominal aorta up to L_1, i.e. level of the renal arteries and aortogram is done to confirm the position of the renal arteries. Selected aortic endovascular graft is marked properly to identify upper part, right (same) side/limb and left limb. Graft is passed through *same side first* common femoral artery along superstiff guidewire; upper most part of the graft is positioned just below the level of renal arteries. Main body of the graft and same side limb of the graft are released and position is confirmed by C-arm image. Superstiff guidewire is removed from same side common femoral artery. Position of opposite limb gate of the graft is confirmed by passing an angled guidewire and guide catheter through opposite limb into main body of the graft followed by injecting contrast agent. A balloon catheter passed through opposite limb of the graft and once balloon is in the body of the graft its position can be confirmed if inflated. IVUS is also very useful to confirm the position across opposite limb gate. Superstiff guidewire is passed through opposite common femoral artery across graft and aorta unto left subclavian artery level. *Opposite limb of graft* is inserted and deployed. Using a compliant balloon inflation upper end and lower ends of the graft is made to seat and seal properly into the aortic wall. A final check angiogram is done to find out endoleaks and confirm position. Sheaths and wires are pulled out. Arterial puncture site may often need polypropylene suture closure. Wound is closed. Distal pulses are checked.

Patient is discharged in 2 days. In postoperative period patient is monitored for leak, thrombosis, embolism and infection.

In suprarenal aneurysms branched or fenestrated aortic grafts are placed. But it is technically demanding.

EVAR is under trial in ruptured aortic aneurysm **(Figs. 11-66A to D)**.

Problems and Complications

Problems are cost, displacement/malposition of graft, dissection, thrombosis, infection, iliac artery avulsion, need for replacement later often and endoleak. *Other complications* are—myocardial infarction; infection either local or wound or urinary or respiratory; ischaemia of sigmoid colon; distal embolisation; clamp injuries; renal failure; stent migration, stent fracture and kinking are other complications.

Endoleak is blood leak across the placed endovascular prosthesis material. Four types of leak can occur in abdominal aortic endovascular prosthesis leak. Type I—Leak from proximal or distal ends from sides of the graft into aneurysm (Ia—proximal; Ib—distal; Ic—iliac plug site). Type II—Back bleeding from lumbar or inferior mesenteric artery into the aneurysmal sac which is the most common leak (IIa—single vessel bleed; IIb—multiple vessel inflow and outflow bleed). Type III—Leak from inadequate graft to graft overlap at junctions (IIIa—modular junction leak or disconnection; IIIb—graft fabric tear). Type IV—Leak from graft itself due to porosity of graft. All type I and II leaks need intervention; type III is mostly treated conservatively.

COMPLICATIONS OF REVASCULARISATION IN ACUTELY ISCHAEMIC LIMB

- *Reperfusion* injury
- 'No reflow' phenomenon: It is due to severe capillary oedema causing poor peripheral tissue hypoperfusion in spite of major vessel revascularisation.
- Acute compartment syndrome can occur due to massive ischaemic oedema especially of skeletal muscles deep-to-deep fascia which compress on venules exceeding tissue interstitial pressure causing further compromise in tissue perfusion. Compartment pressure when measured using transducer needles will be more than 40 mmHg or >30 mmHg for 3 hours or above the mean arterial pressure. Muscle weakness, sensory changes, leg pain which is aggravated by dorsiflexion of toes.
- Other complications are—sepsis, reblock, bleeding and catheter related complications.

Reperfusion Injury

- It occurs after reestablishment of arterial flow to an ischaemic tissue bed which further leads to tissue death causing specifically *peripheral muscle infarction*. It is due to sudden release of oxygen free radicals which block the microcirculation, with release of high levels of potassium (hyperkalaemia) and myoglobin (myoglobinaemia and myoglobinuria). Haemodynamically patient becomes unstable with lactic acidosis, intracellular changes, interstitial oedema and cardiac dysfunction. It is often life threatening.
- *Haimovici triad* of revascularisation injury (1960): (1) Muscle infarction; (2) Myoglobinuria; (3) Acute renal failure.
- Severe ischaemia causes oedema in the muscular compartment with raise in compartment pressure more than the essential capillary perfusion pressure causing *acute compartment syndrome*. It is common in the anterior compartment of the leg. It is basically in the skeletal muscles deep-to-deep fascia. Compartment pressure when measured using transducer needles will be more than 40 mmHg or >30 mmHg for 3 hours or above the mean arterial pressure. Muscle weakness, sensory changes, leg pain which is aggravated by dorsiflexion of toes.
- *No re-flow phenomenon* due to tissue oedema causing capillary perfusion block. Even though compartment syndrome and 'no reflow' phenomenon are separate entities they are always seen together along with reperfusion injury.
- Metabolic acidosis, acute tubular necrosis causing acute renal failure and cardiac arrhythmias may set in and become life threatening.
- **Features are**—toxaemia; oliguria; persistent pain and oedema in the leg with muscular tenderness; raised blood urea and serum creatinine with features of acute ischaemia in the limb.
- **Treatment:**
  - Mannitol to prevent renal failure; fluid therapy.
  - Fasciotomy to reduce raised compartment pressure. All four compartments of lower limb should be decompressed surgically. Long vertical lateral deep fasciotomy incision in the calf behind the fibula along the deep fascia and its fibular

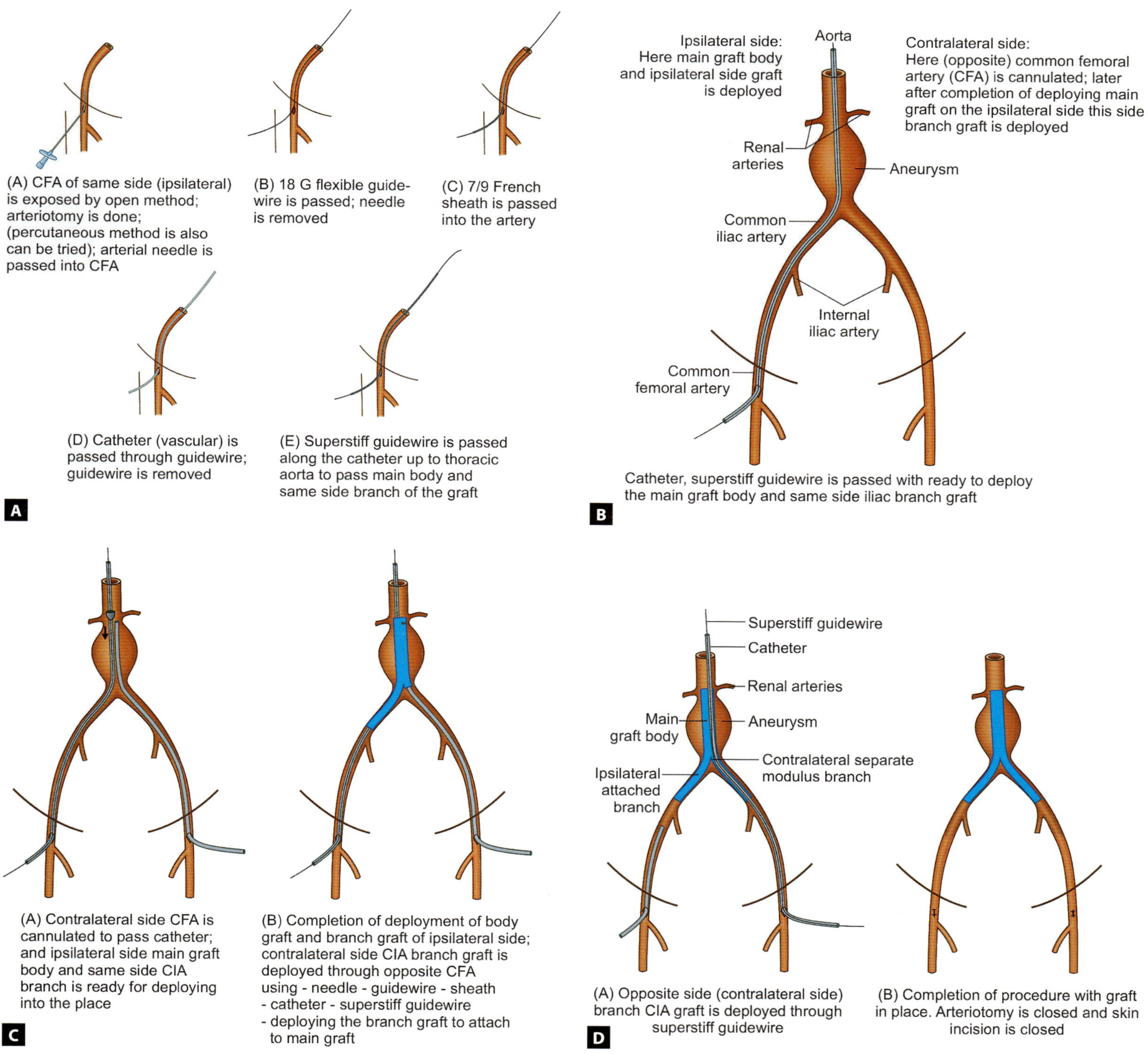

Figs. 11-66A to D: Technique of endovascular aneurysm repair (EVAR).

attachments is a must. Bleeding as patient is heparinised is common after fasciotomy. Infection of the wound can occur. Later once patient is stabilised and oedema subsides with healthy wound, secondary suturing or skin grafting is done. If fasciotomy is not done and if patient survives, eventual Volkmann's ischaemic contracture may develop.

– Antibiotics and supportive therapy.

ACUTE ISCHAEMIA

Acute ischaemia is a surgical emergency. It is common in lower limb but can occur in upper limb, mesenteric vessels, kidney, brain, etc.

Acute Limb Ischaemia

Acute limb ischaemia is either due to embolus or thrombosis. In embolic block critical period is 6 hours after which ischaemic damage is likely to occur. So early intervention to remove the block and to achieve revascularisation is needed. Once limb is non-viable and gangrenous attempt to revascularisation should be avoided as it will lead into multiorgan failure and death. Thrombolysis is not a suitable option in acute limb ischaemia as it takes time to act; before that limb becomes non-viable. Emergency Doppler is sufficient. If facilities are available angiogram can be done; but for the sake treatment cannot be delayed. On table angiography is very useful.

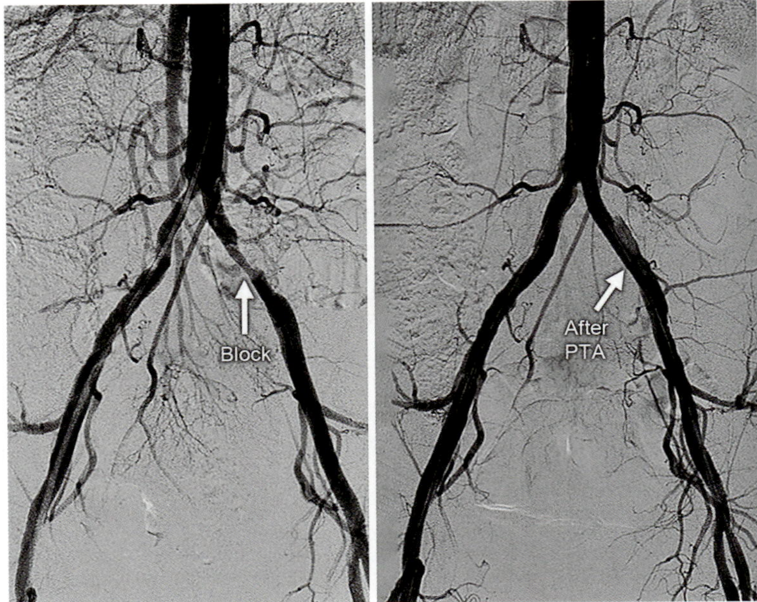

Fig. 11-67: Digital subtraction angiogram showing block in left aortoiliac segment. It is corrected by PTA (percutaneous transluminal angioplasty).

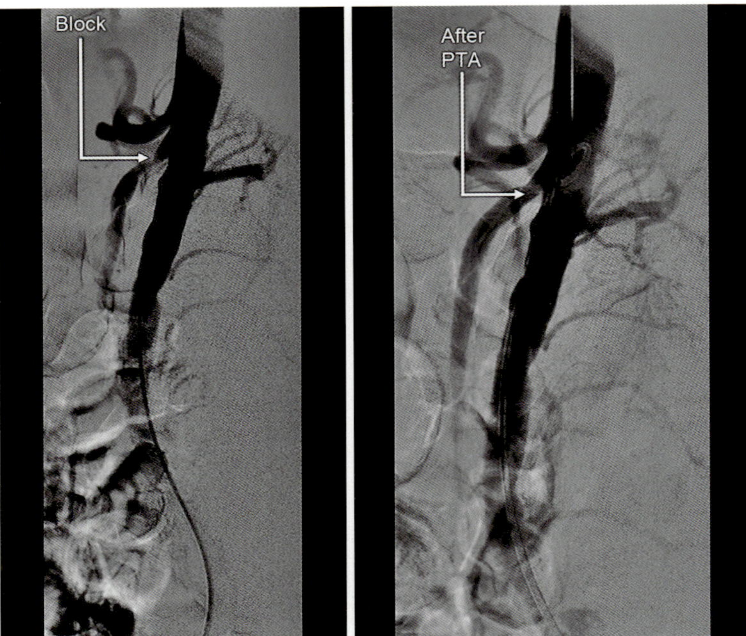

Fig. 11-68: Digital subtraction angiogram showing superior mesenteric artery block/stenosis which is corrected by PTA.

Immediate anticoagulation is done with 10,000 units of heparin. *Common sites of embolus block* in limbs are—common femoral artery in the groin and brachial artery in elbow. Embolus block precipitates thrombus formation proximally and distally which propagates on both directions **(Figs. 11-67 to 11-69)**.

Femoral Embolectomy

It is done under local anaesthesia. *C-arm imaging facility* should be there ideally in theatre while doing embolectomy. If additional procedure like bypass graft is required then spinal or general anaesthesia is needed. Entire limb should be prepared for the procedure to observe distal perfusion. Oblique or vertical incision is made in the thigh along the line of femoral artery; skin, subcutaneous tissue, Scarpa's fascia is incised. Common femoral, superficial femoral and profunda femoris arteries are identified; dissected and slings are placed around each. Longitudinal or oblique arteriotomy is done in the common femoral artery often extending into the profunda femoris artery in case if profundaplasty with venous patch is needed. Size 4 Fogarty catheter is passed along the iliac artery proximally to clear the thrombus to achieve good inflow; immediately iliac artery is flushed with heparinised saline (2,000 units in 500 mL of saline). Size 3 Fogarty catheter is passed distally along the superficial femoral artery; small fragments or ribbon arterial cast with propagated thrombus is extracted from distal part. It is repeatedly passed until all fragments are cleared with adequate back bleeding. Usually catheter is passed around 40 cm distally to achieve good embolectomy **(Fig. 11-70)**.

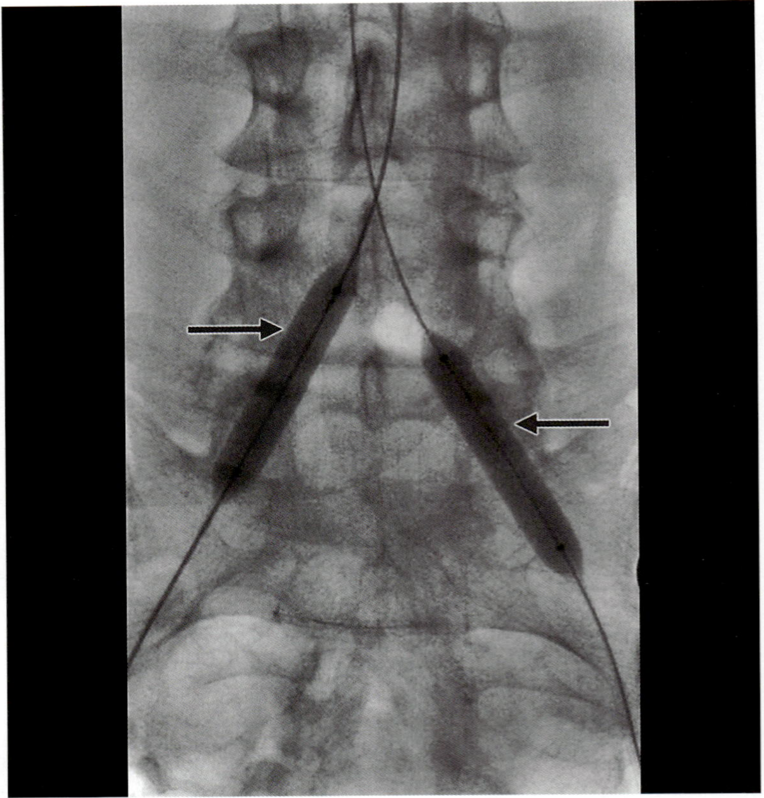

Fig. 11-69: Percutaneous transluminal angioplasty (PTA) balloon catheter in place.

A completion angiogram is done to confirm the adequacy of the flow, if reperfusion is poor, if Fogarty cannot be passed beyond adductor hiatus. Adherent clot can be lysed by direct injection of the tissue plasminogen activator (TPA) 10 mg in 20 mL saline, into the clot for 30 minutes. Profundaplasty may be added to prevent narrowing and rethrombosis.

Brachial Endarterectomy

Usual site of embolic block is at its bifurcation in antecubital fossa. Procedure is done usually under local anaesthesia. Entire limb should be cleaned from shoulder and axilla to hand. A lazy S incision is made from medial part of lower arm across biceps tendon down into the forearm. Brachial artery is deep to bicipital aponeurosis which can be divided. Median nerve should be taken care of and retracted. Brachial artery with its bifurcation branches is dissected

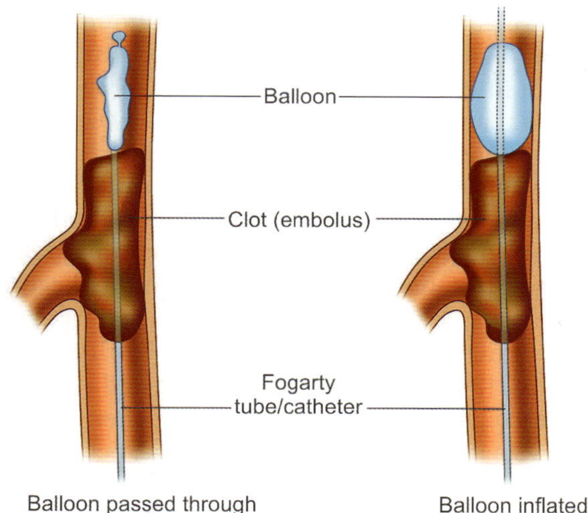

Fig. 11-70: Technique of arterial embolectomy.

and isolated with slings/loops. Bulldog clamps are applied to arteries. A transverse arteriotomy is made 1 cm proximal to bifurcation over brachial artery. Fogarty catheter is passed proximally and block is removed to clear inflow which is infused with heparinised saline. Distal arteries are also cleared by passing Fogarty catheter into ulnar and radial arteries. Clamps are released—first the proximal clamp and then distal clamps. Good back feeding should be achieved. Completion angiogram is done. Arteriotomy is closed using 6-zero polypropylene sutures.

Complications are—bleeding, thrombosis, infection and failure.

Saddle Embolus

It is the large embolus blocking at bifurcation of aorta presenting with acute ischaemic features in both limbs. Doppler and angiogram is diagnostic. It is usually due to large mural thrombus blocking at the bifurcation. Cardiology opinion and echocardiography is a must **(Fig. 11-71)**.

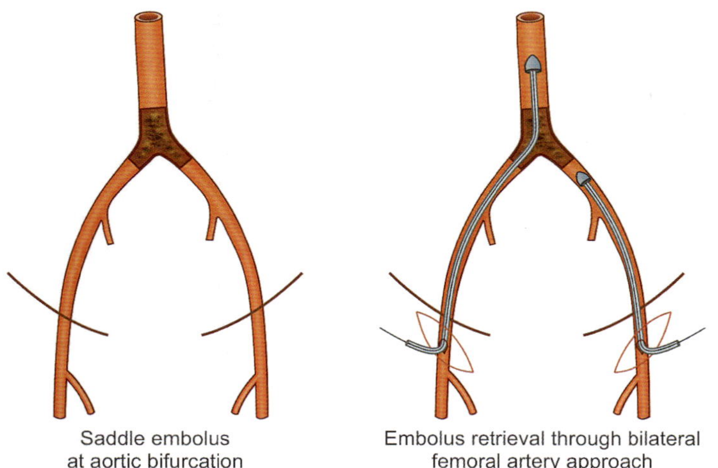

Fig. 11-71: Saddle embolus at the aortic bifurcation. It is retrieved by embolectomy from bilateral femoral artery approach.

Embolectomy is done by passing the balloon of Fogarty catheter through both femoral arteries. Patient should be heparinised. On table angiogram is a must.

THORACOABDOMINAL ANEURYSM

Type I: It involves descending thoracic aorta and abdominal aorta up to the origin of visceral vessels.

Type II: Aneurysm involving entire descending thoracic and entire abdominal aorta.

Type III: It involves lower part of descending thoracic aorta and entire abdominal aorta.

Type IV: Entire abdominal aorta including suprarenal portion (but aorta above the diaphragm is normal) **(Fig. 11-72)**.

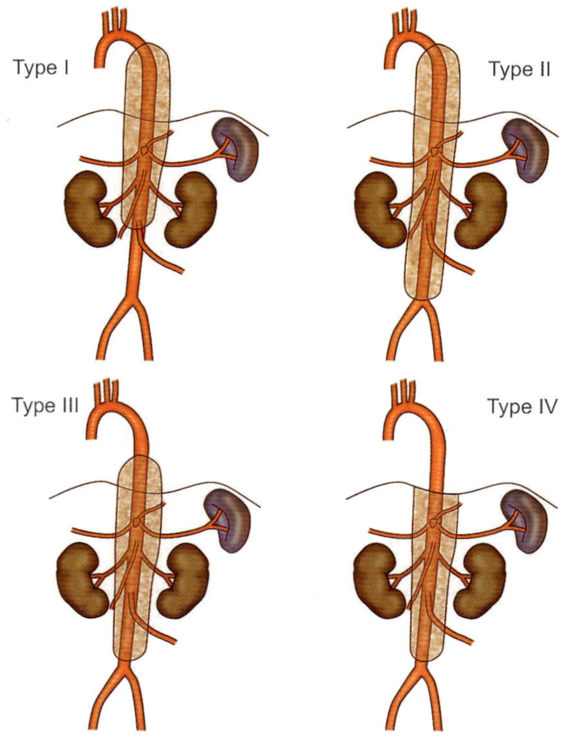

Fig. 11-72: Classification of thoracoabdominal aneurysm.

Exposure: Patient is placed such that left side thorax and abdomen are upwards for thoracoabdominal approach. Spleen with left kidney is rotated medially to access the upper part of abdominal aorta. Left lung is collapsed to visualise the thoracic aorta. Inflow may be maintained by temporary shunting or left heart bypass to femoral artery which will maintain visceral perfusion. Cooling of the kidneys and diuretics is needed as an additional protection. Aneurysm is opened. Pair of intercostal vessels is reimplanted into the graft first to maintain the blood flow of spinal cord. Graft is sutured proximally into the thoracic aorta after proximal clamping distal to bypass. Visceral arteries (coeliac trunk, SMA, IMA, right renal artery) are anastomosed with a part of native aorta at their origin into the hole made in the graft. Origin of left renal artery is separately implanted into the graft with a similar patch of native aorta. Distal end of the graft is anastomosed to distal end of the aorta distal to aneurysm level. Procedure is done usually by a cardiothoracic or vascular surgeon.

Problems are—spinal cord ischaemia with paraplegia; myocardial ischaemia; reperfusion injury.

RENAL REVASCULARISATION

Renal artery stenosis more than 70% will deteriorate the kidney function. Angioplasty is ideal in stenosis due to fibromuscular dysplasia.

Renal endarterectomy can be done with a venous patch over the stenosed area.

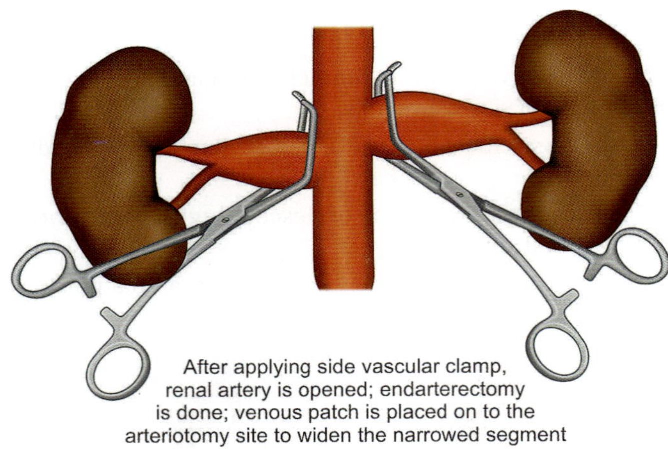

Fig. 11-73: Renal endarterectomy with venous patch over the stenosed area.

A graft can be used between terminal renal artery and infrarenal part of the aorta. Renal artery is ligated at its origin. Distal end of renal artery is anastomosed into the end of the arterial graft, the other end of it to side of the infrarenal portion of the aorta. If aorta is very much diseased, then right renal artery is anastomosed to hepatic artery and left renal artery is anastomosed to splenic artery after splenectomy **(Fig. 11-73)**.

EXPOSURE OF CAROTID ARTERY

It is indicated in endarterectomy to prevent stroke; excision of carotid body tumour; carotid artery aneurysm repair; in trauma of carotid artery.

Anaesthesia—general or local (in case of emergency).

Position—supine with head extended and turned away from the side of the surgery with sandbag under the shoulder.

Incision—from upper margin of the medial end of the clavicle along the anterior margin of the sternocleidomastoid muscle to the angle of the jaw extending above further backwards. Transverse skin crease/S-shaped incision are also helpful for a better cosmetic look.

Anatomy

Right CCA (common carotid artery) begins as a branch of brachiocephalic artery behind the right sternoclavicular joint. *Left CCA* arises from arch of aorta in the thorax in front of trachea and behind left of the manubrium to continue in the neck under left sternoclavicular joint. In the neck it runs upwards along and deep to inner border of sternocleidomastoid muscle; in front of transverse processes of lower four cervical vertebrae. At the level of thyroid cartilage it divides into external and internal carotid arteries. In front it is related to superior belly of omohyoid (crosses artery), descending hypoglossi nerve, superior thyroid vein, sternothyroid, ansa cervicalis, sternohyoid, anterior jugular vein, middle thyroid vein and sternomastoid. Behind the CCA sympathetic chain descends and ascending cervical artery ascends behind the CCA; inferior thyroid artery crosses medially behind the CCA; left side thoracic duct crosses CCA laterally behind. *Carotid sheath* encloses CCA, IJV (lateral to artery) and vagus nerve (behind). *Carotid sinus* is dilated terminal CCA and beginning of ICA which has got thin media and thick adventitia with rich glossopharyngeal and sympathetic innervations which act as baroreceptor. Carotid body is a small, oval reddish brown body located behind bifurcation of CCA with glossopharyngeal innervation; acts as chemoreceptor.

External carotid artery (ECA) begins as one of the terminal branches of CCA and runs anteromedial to internal carotid artery (ICA) in lower part and anterolateral to ICA in upper part. ECA is convex towards front in lower part; concave towards front in upper part. In the carotid triangle, ECA is crossed in front by cervical branch of facial nerve, hypoglossal nerve, facial, lingual and superior thyroid veins; deeply it is related to pharynx, superior laryngeal nerve with its external and internal branches. Above the carotid triangle ECA enters the parotid gland; here it is related in front to retromandibular vein and facial nerve; behind to (1) Internal carotid artery; (2) Styloglossus, stylopharyngeus, glossopharyngeal nerve, pharyngeal branch vagus, styloid process (which passes between ECA and ICA); (3) Superior laryngeal nerve and superior cervical sympathetic ganglion (are deep to ICA). Branches of ECA (8) are—in front are superior thyroid, lingual and facial; behind are occipital and posterior auricular; medial is ascending pharyngeal and terminal are larger maxillary and smaller superficial temporal.

ICA is one of the terminal branches of CCA beginning at upper level of thyroid cartilage opposite C3 and C4 vertebral disc entering into carotid canal to reach the cranial cavity. It has got 4 parts—cervical; petrous; cavernous; and cerebral. At the beginning there is dilatation called as carotid sinus. In the carotid triangle below it is related in front to sternomastoid muscle, hypoglossal nerve, descending hypoglossi, occipital artery, common facial and lingual veins, and ECA (anteromedial). In the digastric triangle above it is related in front to posterior belly of digastric, stylohyoid, posterior auricular artery, stylopharyngeus, styloid process, parotid, glossopharyngeal nerve, pharyngeal branch of vagus, cartilaginous part of auditory tube, tensor veli palatine. Posteriorly it is related to longus capitis, superior cervical ganglion, superior laryngeal nerve, carotid sheath, pharyngeal veins, vagus (posterolateral), glossopharyngeal, hypoglossal and accessory nerves. There are no branches to ICA in neck.

Exposure (Fig. 11-74)

Cervical branch of facial nerve should not be injured in upper most part of the incision especially in transverse incision (upper posterior part of the incision should be 1.5 cm below the angle of the mandible in transverse). Platysma and deep fascia are incised in the line of incision → external jugular vein is divided between ligatures → flaps are raised → anterior margin of sternomastoid is dissected and retracted behind → common facial vein which crosses CCA just below the bifurcation in front is identified and divided (supraorbital and supratrochlear veins join to form angular vein which continues as facial vein down and is joined by deep facial vein which is an extension vein from pterygoid plexus; this facial vein is joined by anterior division of retromandibular vein to form common facial vein which joins internal jugular vein (IJV). Posterior auricular vein joins posterior division of retromandibular vein to form external jugular vein which joins subclavian vein below) → IJV is identified as bluish tubular structure with thin wall and is retracted backwards → carotid is identified → descending branch of hypoglossal nerve (can be cut if needed) and main hypoglossal nerves (just above CCA bifurcation) are identified and retained. Thyroid and strap muscles are retracted anteromedially to expose superior thyroid artery and superior laryngeal nerve (deeper); posterior belly of digastric and parotid and greater auricular nerve are identified above. ICA above in the neck is dissected properly (if needed) by dividing digastric tendon, stylohyoid muscle; or often with subluxation of jaw in forward direction **(Figs. 11-75 and 11-76)**.

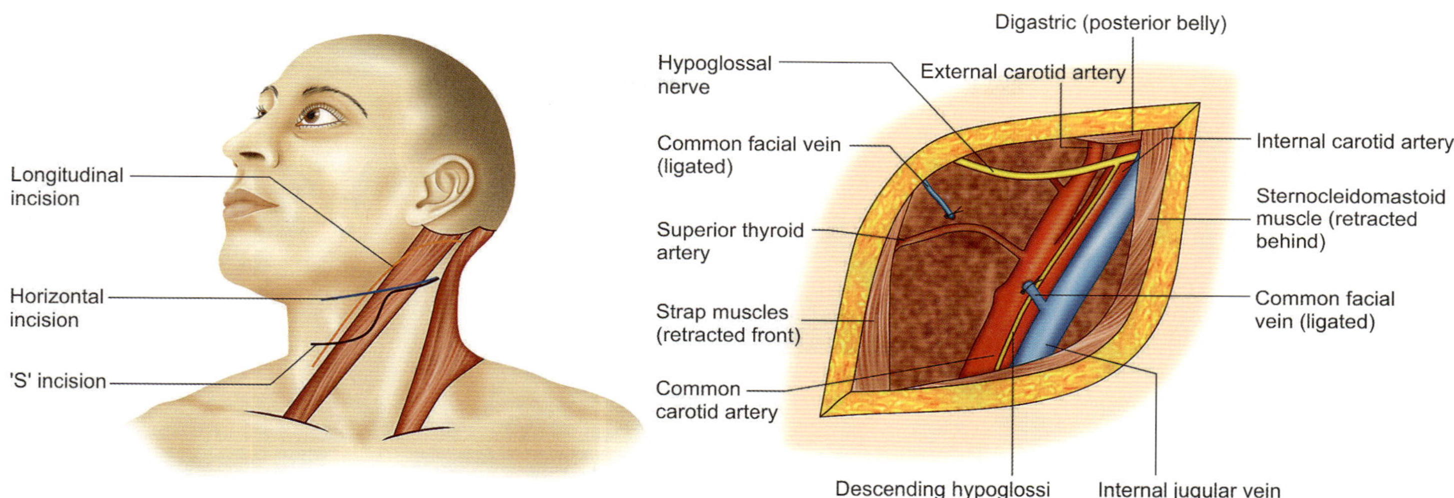

Fig. 11-74: Incision and exposure of carotid artery.

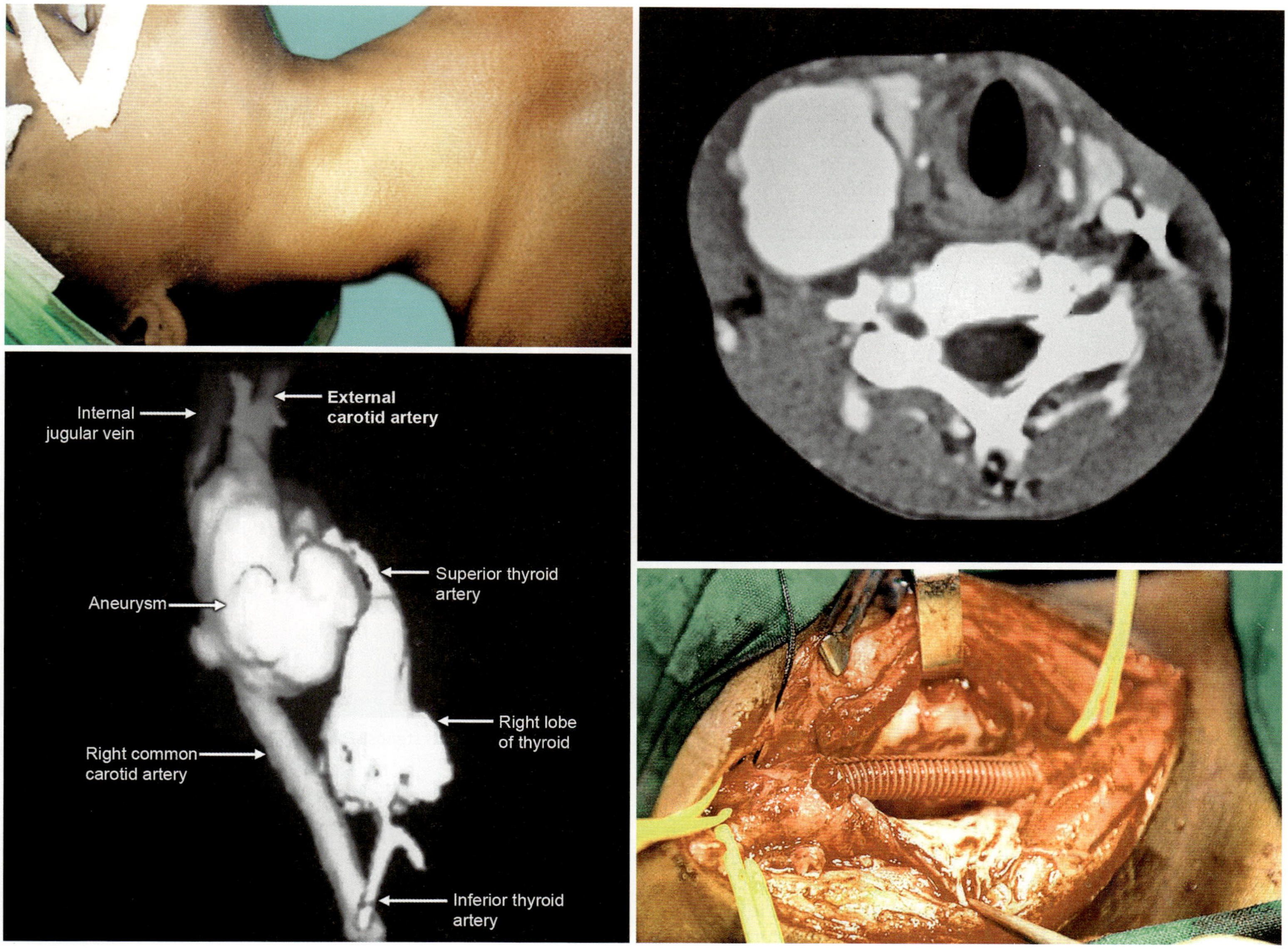

Internal jugular vein
External carotid artery
Superior thyroid artery
Aneurysm
Right lobe of thyroid
Right common carotid artery
Inferior thyroid artery

Fig. 11-75: Carotid artery aneurysm and its repair using graft.

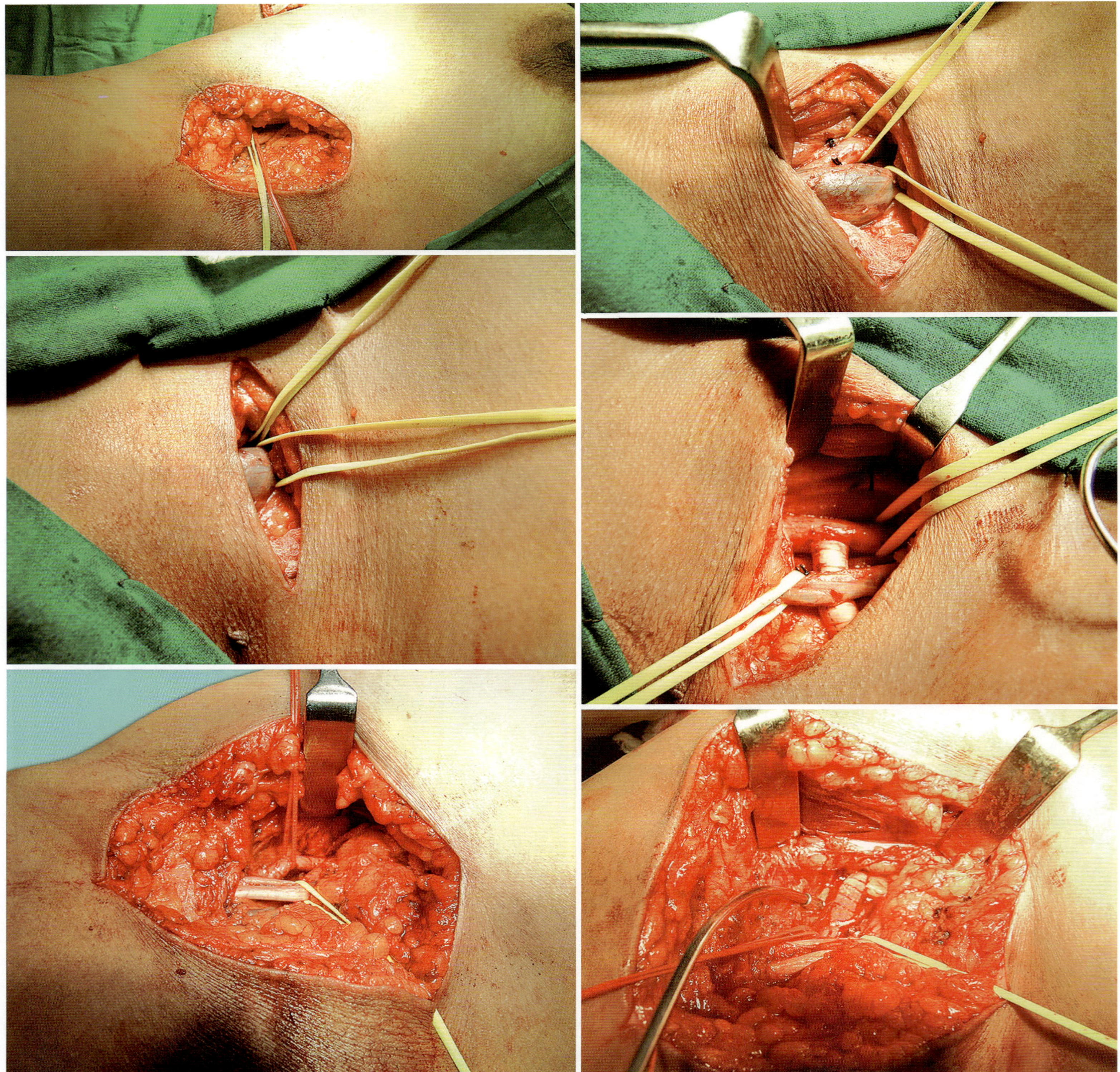

Fig. 11-76: Carotid axillary bypass. It bypasses the subclavian artery in its stenosis/blockage.

Different procedures of carotids can be undertaken like repair of carotid using venous patch, endarterectomy, carotid artery aneurysm repair using graft, graft reconstruction, ligation of ECA. *ECA ligation* is done just above the level of the superior thyroid artery to avoid turbulence effect on the carotid and so formation of thrombus proximally. ECA is ligated in torrential bleeding in face, antrum, larynx, traumatic damage of the ECA. CCA and ICA should not be ligated but should be reconstructed as chance of the person developing hemiplegia is 40%.

EXPOSURE OF VERTEBRAL ARTERY

Anatomy

It originates from first part of subclavian artery ends by joining the opposite vertebral artery to form basilar artery. It has got four parts. First part extends from its origin to transverse process of 6th cervical vertebra. First part is located in vertebral triangle bound by scalenus anterior and longus colli muscles; runs upwards and backwards;

related (anteriorly) to carotid sheath, vertebral vein, inferior thyroid artery and thoracic duct on left side; posteriorly to transverse process of C7 vertebra, inferior cervical ganglion and ventral rami nerves of C7,C8. Second part runs through foraminae of transverse processes of upper six vertebrae. It is accompanied by venous plexus and large branch of stellate ganglion. Third part lies in suboccipital triangle lying on the posterior arch of the atlas bone extending from transverse foramina of atlas to vertebral canal across lower arched margin of posterior atlanto-occipital membrane. It is related to atlas, vertebral muscles, and first cervical nerve. Fourth part extends from atlanto-occipital membrane to lower part of pons to join opposite vertebral artery to form basilar artery. It pierces the dura, arachnoid in front of roots of hypoglossal nerve, medulla to reach lower margin of pons. Branches are—spinal, muscular, anterior spinal, posterior inferior cerebellar (largest), often posterior spinal and medullary.

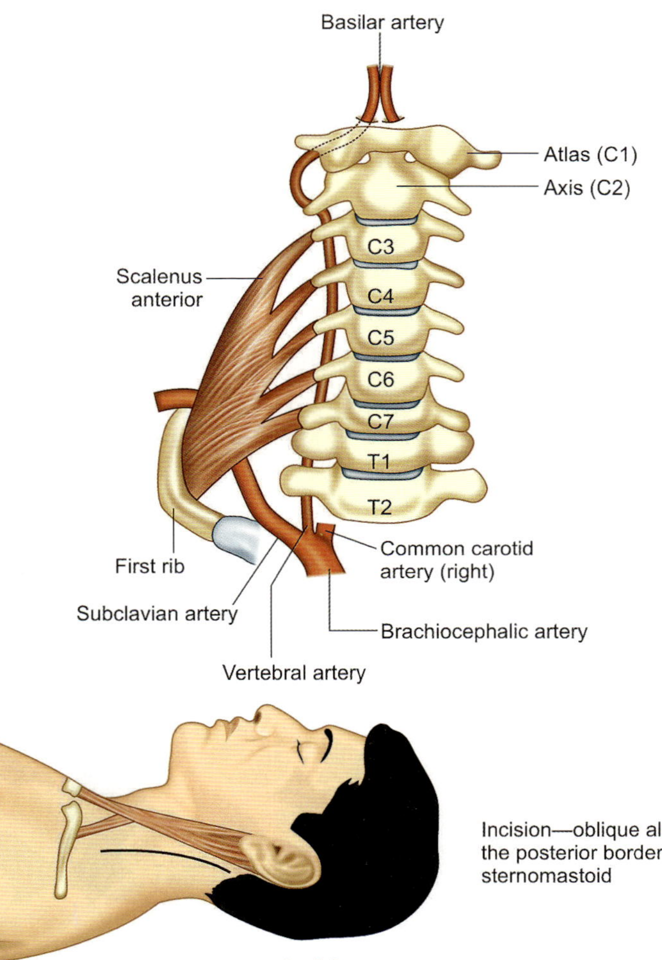

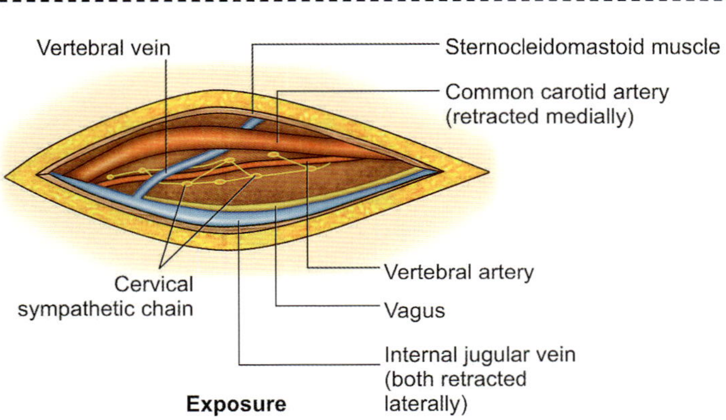

Fig. 11-77: Anatomy and exposure of vertebral artery.

Exposure

Oblique incision lateral to the sternocleidomastoid muscle → lateral part of the muscle is cut → IJV is exposed → vagus is identified → both IJV and vagus are retracted laterally → carotid artery is identified and dissected meticulously to retract medially → dissection is done between carotid and IJV → vertebral vein runs crossing the artery in front from medial to lateral → vertebral artery is identified behind the vein with crisscrossed cervical sympathetic chain. Vertebral vein can be divided to expose the artery properly. Sympathetic fibers crossing the artery can be divided **(Fig. 11-77)**.

Distal part of the artery is also exposed by extending the same incision above; levator muscle is identified and is divided after protecting the accessory nerve which crosses the muscle. Anterior ramus of C2 nerve is seen crossing the artery which can be divided.

EXPOSURE OF SUBCLAVIAN ARTERY

Anatomy

Subclavian artery arises on the right side from brachiocephalic artery and left side from arch of aorta. It begins behind the sternoclavicular joint curving with convexity upwards reaching outer part of the first rib to continue as axillary artery. Left artery has got thoracic part behind the left side of manubrium and left of left common carotid artery. Artery is divided into three parts by scalenus anterior muscle. First part is medial; second part is behind; third part is lateral to scalenus anterior.

Artery is related *in front* from medial to lateral to—CCA, ansa cervicalis, cardiac branches of vagus, sympathetic trunk, vagus, vertebral vein, IJV, phrenic nerve (left side it is in front of first part; right side it is in front of second part) and thoracic duct (left side), scalenus anterior, transverse cervical artery, suprascapular artery, subclavian vein, anterior jugular vein, suprascapular vessels, external jugular vein, transverse cervical vein, subclavius muscle, middle ⅓ of clavicle, sternocleidomastoid muscle.

Behind it is related to suprapleural membrane, cervical pleura, apex of lung, ansa subclavian, right recurrent laryngeal nerve (right side), scalenus medius, lower trunk of brachial plexus. *Above* it is related to inferior belly of omohyoid, upper and middle trunks of brachial plexus. *Below* it is related to first rib.

Branches are usually four—vertebral (largest), internal thoracic and thyrocervical arteries arise from first part of the subclavian artery. Thyrocervical artery gives inferior thyroid, suprascapular and transverse cervical branches. Costocervical artery arises from second part of the subclavian artery on right side (from first part on left side) which gives superior intercostal and deep cervical arteries. Occasionally dorsal scapular artery as a 5th branch may arise from third part of the subclavian artery.

Right subclavian artery may originate from descending thoracic aorta passing behind the oesophagus causing dysphagia called as *dysphagia lusoria*.

Exposure

Arm is placed to the side of the patient and drawn downwards to depress the shoulder with head turning to opposite side. Incision is made just above (1 cm) and parallel to clavicle from sternal head of sternocleidomastoid to anterior margin of trapezius. Superficial fascia, platysma and deep fascia are divided in the line of incision. External jugular vein is ligated. Supraclavicular nerve is identified and cut or retracted. Omohyoid is retracted above. Suprascapular artery, vein and nerve are identified crossing the third part of the subclavian artery superolaterally. Subclavian artery is identified along with upper and middle trunks of brachial plexus. To expose the 2nd and 3rd parts clavicular head of sternomastoid and scalenus anterior are cut. Care should be taken not to injure phrenic nerve which crosses the scalenus anterior in front from lateral to medial. Nerve is gently slinged and retracted. IJV is retracted medially to expose the subclavian artery. Division of sternal head of sternocleidomastoid and median sternotomy is needed to approach the origin of subclavian artery and brachiocephalic artery **(Figs. 11-78 and 11-79)**.

Distal 3rd part of subclavian and proximal 1st part of the axillary artery is exposed by infraclavicular incision or supraclavicular incision extending laterally and across the clavicle. Division of clavicle in this exposes the entire subclavian artery. In inevitable situation 3rd part of subclavian artery can be ligated.

EXPOSURE OF AXILLARY ARTERY

Axillary artery as a continuation of subclavian artery extends from outer border of first rib to lower border of teres major muscle.

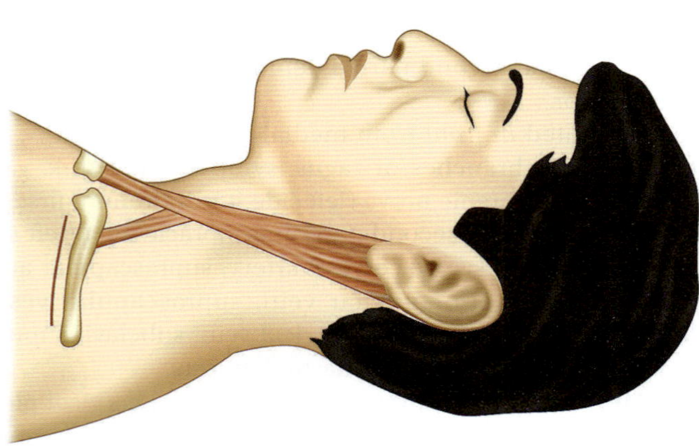

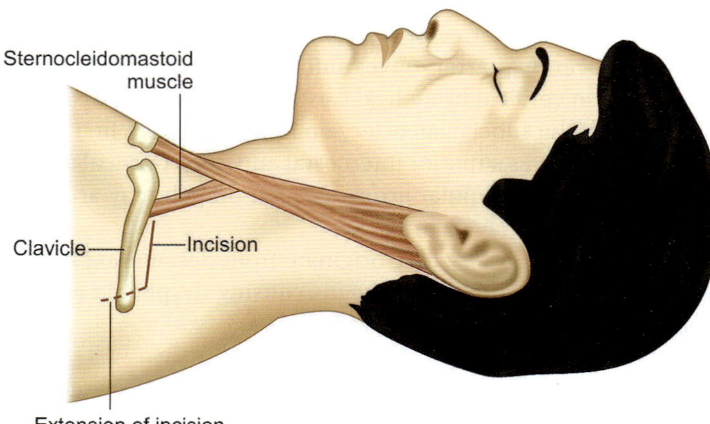

Fig. 11-78: Incision for subclavian and axillary artery exposure. If needed clavicle is cut.

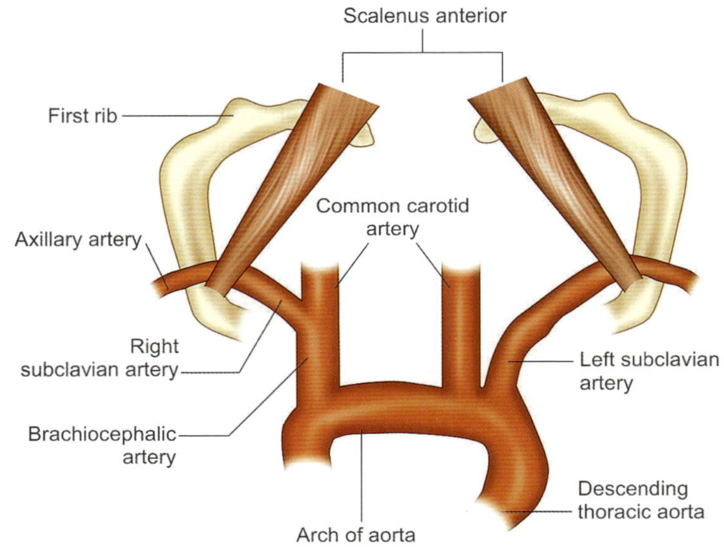

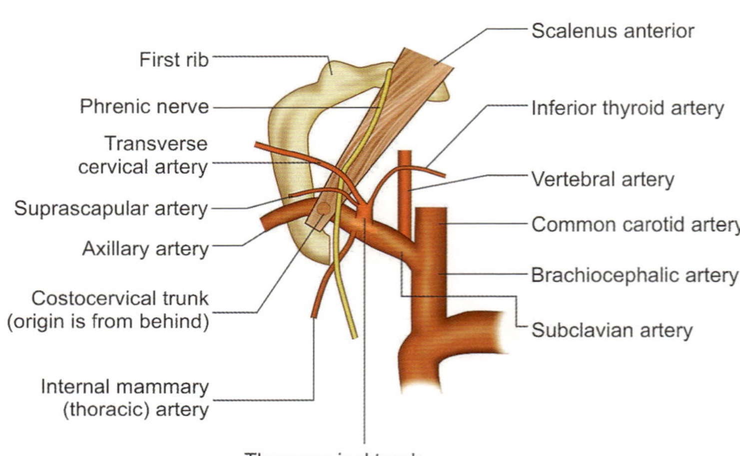

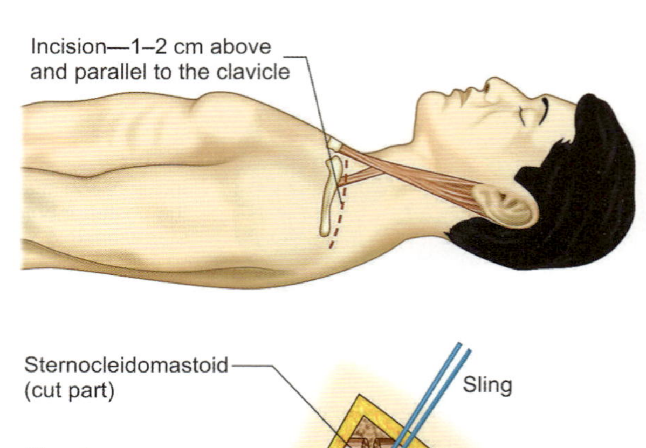

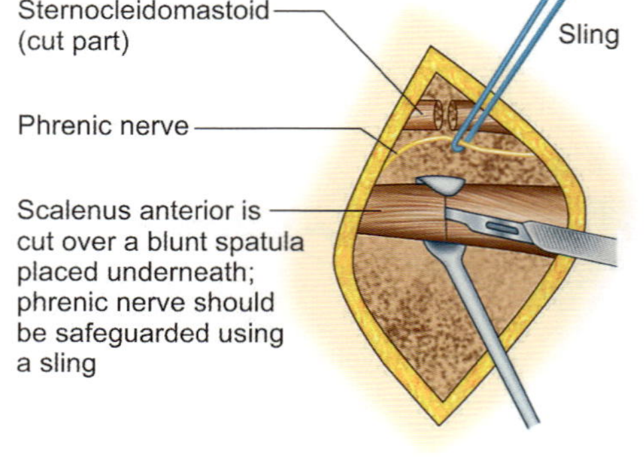

Figs. 11-79A to C

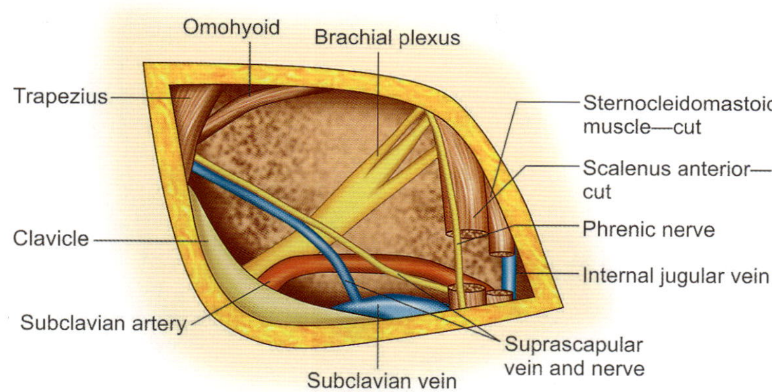

Fig. 11-79D

Figs. 11-79A to D: Anatomy and exposure of subclavian artery.

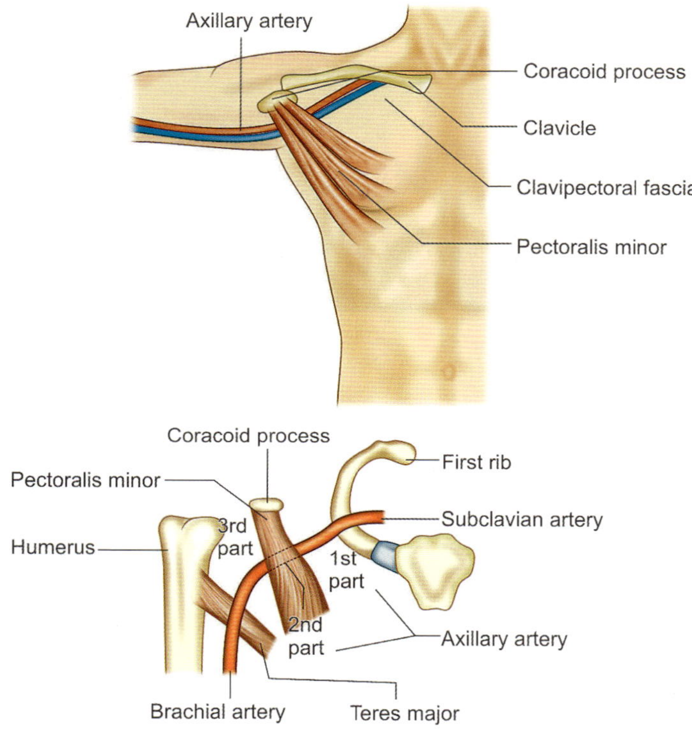

Fig. 11-80: Anatomy of the axillary artery.

It is divided into three parts by pectoralis minor as above (first part), behind (second part) and below (third part). It is related in front to skin, superficial fascia, platysma, supraclavicular nerves, deep fascia, pectoralis major, and clavipectoral fascia with cephalic vein, lateral pectoral vein and thoracoacromial vessels and pectoralis minor. Behind it is related to parts of brachial plexus, serratus anterior digitations, coracobrachialis, tendons of latissimus dorsi and teres major. Medially it is related to axillary vein. Axillary sheath encloses the axillary artery and brachial plexus which is derived from prevertebral layer of deep fascia. Axillary sheath *does not enclose* the axillary vein.

Branches of axillary artery are—superior thoracic artery (first part), thoracoacromial artery (second part), lateral thoracic artery (second part), subscapular artery (largest branch, third part), and anterior circumflex and posterior circumflex arteries (third part) **(Fig. 11-80)**.

Surface Marking of Axillary Artery

Arm is held at right angles to the trunk with palm facing forward; it extends from midpoint of the clavicle to a point at the junction of anterior 1/3rd to posterior 2/3rd of the lateral wall of axilla at its lower limit.

Exposure

Two incisions can be used. One is lengthy incision along the deltopectoral groove from lower border of clavicle to lower border of anterior axillary fold. Another is small incision in infraclavicular area horizontally placed along the clavipectoral fascia. This incision is also used to expose the third part of the subclavian artery. Often in trauma more extensive exposure of axillary and subclavian arteries together is needed and in such situation lengthy deltopectoral groove incision extending upwards into the neck across clavicle with resection of the middle third of the clavicle is done **(Fig. 11-81)**.

EXPOSURE OF BRACHIAL ARTERY

Anatomy

Brachial artery is the continuation of the axillary artery extending from lower border of teres major to a point in front of the elbow at the level of neck of radius just medial to the biceps brachii. It runs downwards and laterally to end in front of elbow bifurcating into radial and ulnar arteries. It is superficial throughout its extent and is accompanied by two venae comitantes. In the upper part it is related to medial cutaneous nerve of the forearm; in the middle part it is crossed by median nerve from lateral to medial side; in front of the elbow it is crossed/covered by bicipital aponeurosis (crosses artery from lateral to medial side). Posteriorly it is related to triceps, radial nerve, profunda brachii artery, coracobrachialis, brachialis. Medially in the upper part it is related to ulnar nerve, in the lower part to median nerve (crosses the artery from lateral to medial in front). Laterally it is related to coracobrachialis, biceps, median nerve in the upper part; tendon of biceps in the lower part. In the elbow, structures from lateral to medial are—radial nerve, biceps tendon, brachial artery and median nerve. It divides as terminal branches in *cubital fossa* in the elbow. It is a triangular hollow situated in front of the elbow; its lateral border is formed by medial margin brachioradialis; medial border is by lateral margin of pronator teres; base is directed upwards is formed by line joining the two epicondyles of humerus with apex pointing downwards **(Fig. 11-82)**.

It gives muscular branches, profunda brachii artery, superior ulnar collateral branch, nutrient artery, inferior ulnar collateral branch, radial and ulnar arteries. Brachial artery may divide into radial, ulnar, common interosseous branches at higher level than usual; or as radial and common trunk of ulnar and common interosseous branches.

Exposure (Fig. 11-83)

Incision is made in the upper arm along its medial border just behind the biceps muscle. Once skin and deep fascia is incised, identified biceps muscle is retracted in front; triceps posteriorly; artery is identified with median nerve lying superiorly and laterally which later crosses the artery in front towards medial side. Basilic vein will be lying medial to the artery in the upper part; two venae comitantes accompany the artery in the lower part. Basilic vein is retracted posteriorly to identify the ulnar nerve.

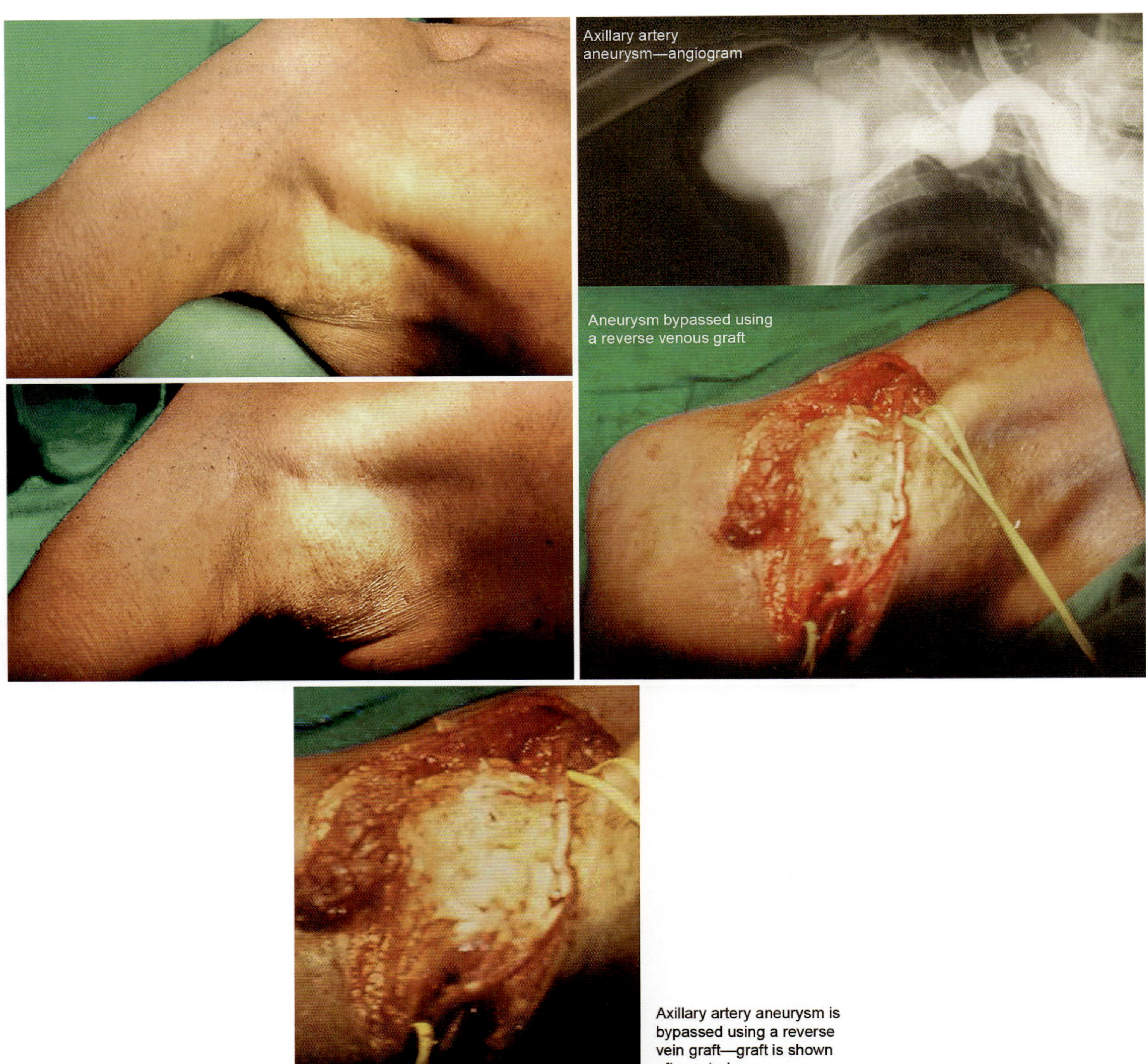

Fig. 11-81: Exposure of axillary artery aneurysm and repair and reconstruction using graft.

Bifurcation is exposed at cubital fossa using an S-shaped incision; not with vertical incision. A transverse incision can also be used. Bicipital aponeurosis which runs in front from lateral to medial side is divided. Median nerve will be posteromedial to the artery.

EXPOSURE OF RADIAL AND ULNAR ARTERIES

Anatomy

Radial artery is a smaller terminal branch (and more superficial compared to ulnar) of brachial artery extending from a point in front of the elbow at the level of neck of the radius medial to the tendon of the biceps brachii to a point at the wrist between anterior border of the radius laterally and the tendon of the flexor carpi radialis medially. It runs downwards to the wrist and enters the anatomical snuff box turning posteriorly. It is overlapped by brachioradialis above and skin, superficial and deep fascia below. Posteriorly it is related to biceps tendon, supinator, pronator teres tendon, radial origin of flexor digitorum superficialis (FDS) and flexor pollicis longus (FPL), pronator quadratus, lower end of radius. Medially it is related to pronator teres above and flexor carpi radialis in the lower 2/3rd; laterally to brachioradialis entirely and radial nerve in the middle third. Artery is accompanied by a pair of venae comitantes.

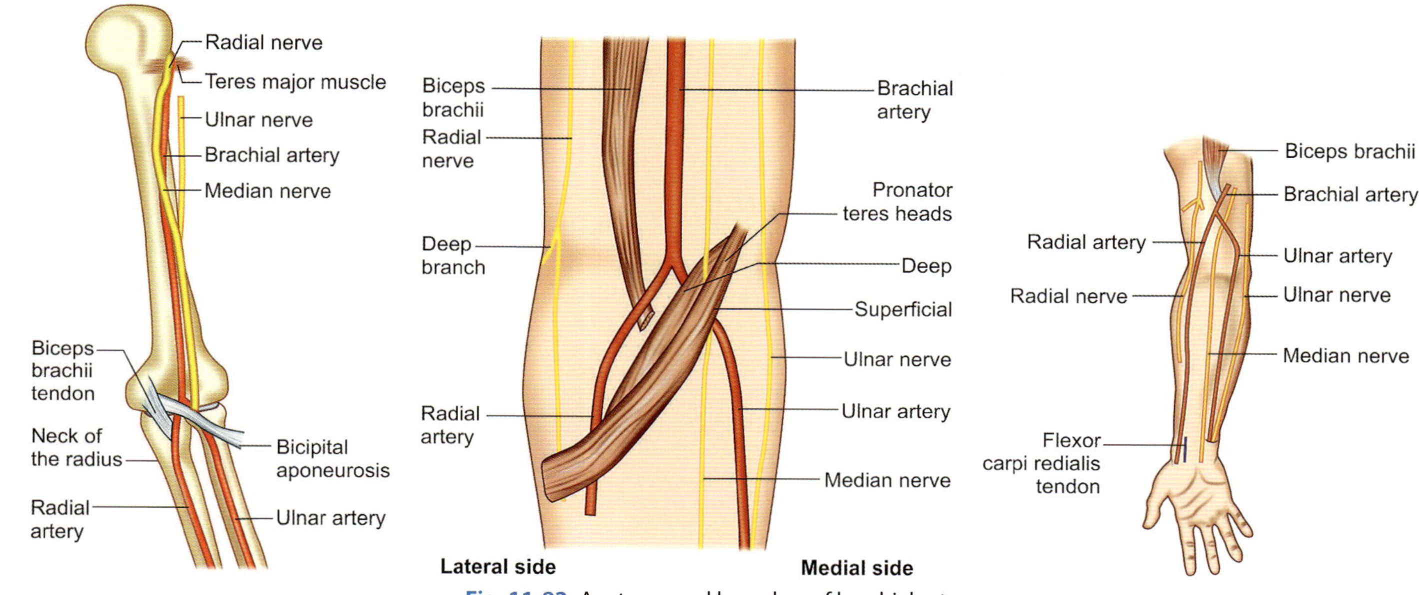

Fig. 11-82: Anatomy and branches of brachial artery.

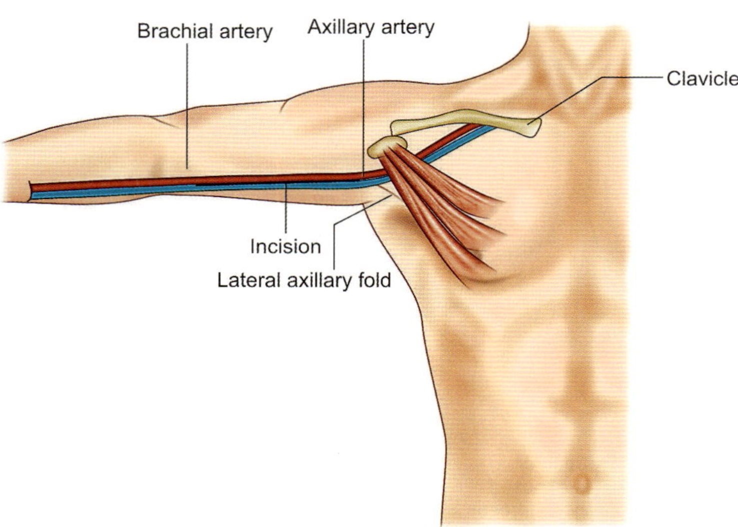

Fig. 11-83: Incision for exposure of brachial artery.

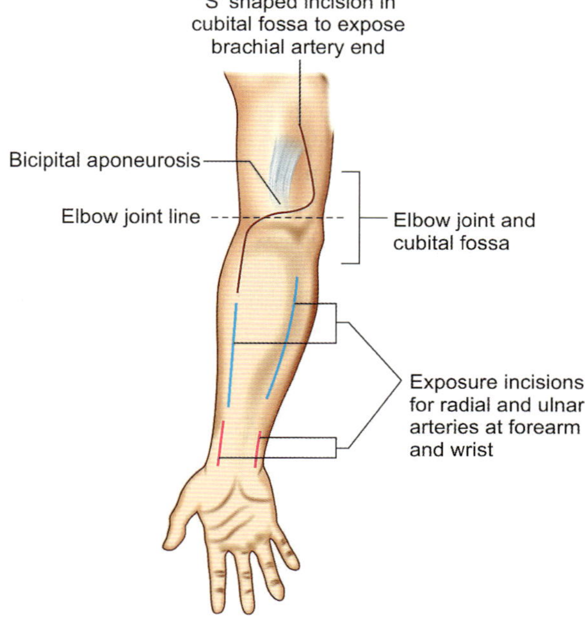

Fig. 11-84: Exposure of brachial bifurcation and branches (radial and ulnar arteries).

Branches are—radial recurrent, muscular, palmar carpal, superficial palmar.

Ulnar artery is the larger terminal branch of brachial artery beginning at cubital fossa running obliquely downwards and medially in upper 1/3rd of forearm; vertically in lower 2/3rd of forearm enters the palm by passing superficial to flexor retinaculum. At lateral part of the pisiform bone it enters the palm. Artery in its upper half is covered by pronator teres with median nerve, flexor carpi radialis, palmaris longus, flexor digitorum superficialis, flexor carpi ulnaris; lower half is covered by skin, superficial and deep fascia and palmar cutaneous branch of ulnar nerve; posteriorly above brachialis and below flexor digitorum profundus; medially to ulnar nerve and flexor carpi ulnaris; laterally flexor digitorum superficialis. *Branches are*—anterior and posterior ulnar recurrent arteries, common interosseous artery, anterior interosseous artery, muscular branches, palmar and dorsal carpal branches **(Fig. 11-84)**.

Both arteries are *exposed* through different vertical incisions on either side of the forearm. Radial artery is exposed by retracting the brachioradialis medially and flexor carpi radialis laterally. Ulnar artery is exposed by dissecting pronator teres and brachioradialis laterally and flexor digitorum medially.

EXPOSURE OF ASCENDING AORTA AND ARCH OF THE AORTA

Anatomy

About 5 cm long ascending aorta originates from upper end of left ventricle enclosed with pericardium; it begins at the level of lower border of 3rd costal cartilage behind the left half of the sternum, runs upwards, forwards and right continuing as arch of aorta at the upper border of the 2nd costal cartilage. At the root of the aorta there are 3 sinuses (dilatations)—right and left posterior and anterior.

Right coronary artery arises from anterior sinus; left coronary arises from left posterior aortic sinus.

Arch of aorta is situated in superior mediastinum behind the lower half of the manubrium sterni. From the upper end of ascending aorta it runs upwards, backwards and to left of trachea near carina, then passing behind the left bronchus arching over the root of left lung to continue as descending aorta at the level of left side of lower border of the body of 4th thoracic vertebra. It begins anteriorly and ends posteriorly. Anteriorly it is related to left phrenic nerve, lower cervical branch of left vagus, upper cervical cardiac branch of left sympathetic chain, left vagus; left superior intercostal vein between phrenic and vagus nerves; left pleura and lung, thymic remnants. Posteriorly it is related to trachea, deep cardiac plexus, tracheobronchial lymph nodes, oesophagus, left recurrent laryngeal nerve, thoracic duct and vertebra. Below to pulmonary trunk bifurcation, left bronchus, ligamentum arteriosus and left recurrent laryngeal nerve. Branches are—brachiocephalic artery, left common carotid and left subclavian arteries; often thyroidea ima artery and occasionally vertebral artery.

Exposure (Fig. 11-85)

Vertical sternotomy incision is used. After skin incision, a Robert's or Kocher's clamp is passed underneath the sternum along the free space underneath to pass a Gigli saw by which sternum is divided. Electric saw also can be used. Sternum is retracted using self-retaining retractor; brachiocephalic vein is retracted downwards. Aortic arch, roots of brachiocephalic, left carotid and subclavian arteries are exposed.

Aortic arch branches are exposed through an additional transverse neck incision on the upper part of the sternotomy. Through this transverse incision if sternocleidomastoid and scalenus anterior is divided, subclavian artery can be exposed at neck in its entire length.

EXPOSURE OF DESCENDING THORACIC AORTA

Anatomy

It is continuation of the arch of aorta at the level of 4th thoracic vertebral body, descending downwards with right side inclination in posterior mediastinum at the lower border of the 12th thoracic vertebra. It is related anteriorly to root of left lung, pericardium, heart, oesophagus in the lower part and diaphragm; posteriorly to hemiazygos vein and vertebrae; to the right side oesophagus in upper part, azygos vein, thoracic duct, right lung and pleura; to the left side left lung and pleura. Branches are—3rd to 11th intercostal arteries (total 9 × 2 = 18); two subcostal arteries one on each side; two left bronchial arteries (*Note:* Right bronchial artery is arising from right 3rd posterior intercostal artery usually, occasionally from upper left bronchial artery); oesophageal branches; pericardial branches; superior phrenic arteries.

Exposure

Descending thoracic aorta is exposed through left posterolateral thoracotomy through 5th or 8th intercostal space. Usually rib is removed and thoracic cavity is entered; lung is displaced forward; descending aorta will be seen posteriorly running vertically **(Fig. 11-86)**.

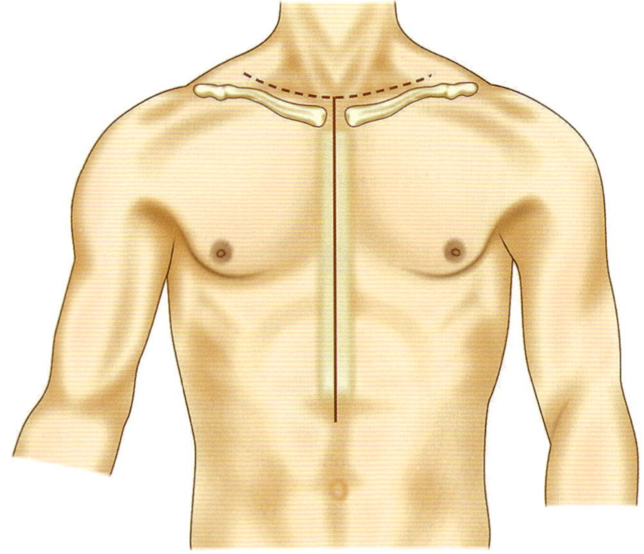

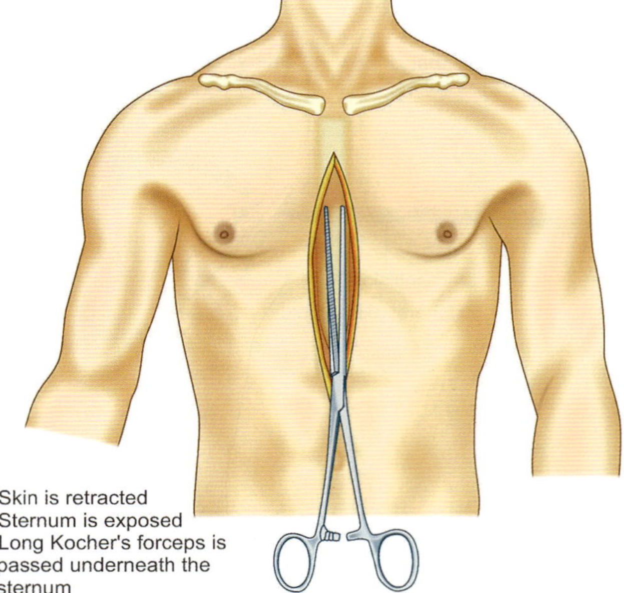

Fig. 11-85: Exposure of ascending aorta technique.

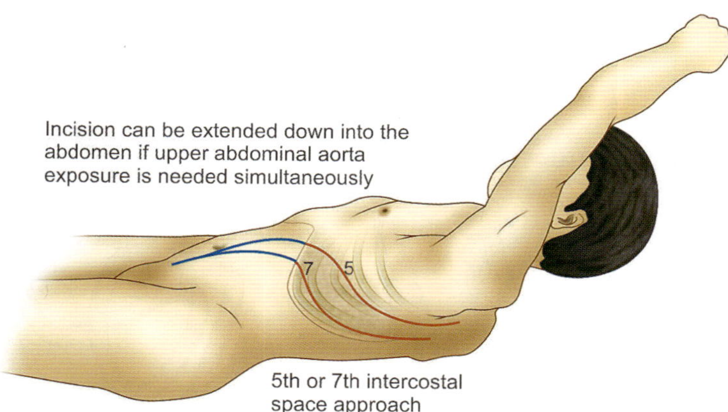

Fig. 11-86: Exposure of descending thoracic aorta either through 5th or 7th intercostal space which can be extended down into abdomen if needed to expose the proximal abdominal aorta also.

Same incision can be extended down in middle over the abdomen to expose the *upper abdominal aorta along with thoracic aorta.* Diaphragm is divided transversely close to the costal margin to avoid damage to phrenic nerve. Vertical incision in the costal margin will expose better but often damages the phrenic nerve. Through the wound liver, spleen, abdominal contents are visualised; peritoneum lateral to the spleen is incised to mobilise the spleen, colon, pancreas towards the right. It exposes the upper abdominal aorta with its branches in the upper part namely coeliac artery, superior mesenteric artery and renal vessels with left renal vein crossing the aorta in front towards IVC.

EXPOSURE OF ABDOMINAL AORTA AND BRANCHES

Anatomy

Abdominal aorta begins from aortic opening of diaphragm at the level of lower border of T12 vertebra, running downwards and slightly left in front of lumbar vertebra ending at the lower border of L4 vertebra about 1 cm left of midline by dividing into two common iliac arteries.

Its surface marking is—from a point 2.5 cm above the transpyloric plane in midline to a point 1.25 cm below and left of the umbilicus.

Anteriorly abdominal aorta is related to celiac plexus, aortic plexus, body of pancreas, splenic vein, left renal vein, 3rd part of the duodenum, retroperitoneum and intestine in abdominal cavity. Posteriorly it is related to bodies of upper four lumbar vertebrae, anterior longitudinal ligament, left lumbar veins, origin of lumbar arteries; towards the right related to IVC with sympathetic chain behind, right crus of diaphragm, cisterna chyli, azygos vein, lumbar lymph node; towards left it is related to left crus of diaphragm, pancreas, 4th part of the duodenum, left sympathetic chain, lumbar lymph nodes.

Branches of abdominal aorta—*Ventral (supply gut):* Coeliac trunk, superior mesenteric artery (SMA), inferior mesenteric artery (IMA); *Lateral (supply structures from intermediate mesoderm)*: Inferior phrenic arteries, middle suprarenal arteries, renal arteries, gonadal arteries; *Dorsal (somatic)*: 4 pairs of lumbar arteries, median sacral artery.

Infrarenal aorta is more mobile and accessible than suprarenal. IMA and gonadal arteries can be sacrificed. Origins of major arteries prevent mobilisation of upper abdominal aorta. Celiac trunk, pancreas, splenic vein, left renal vein, duodenum all obscure proper mobilisation.

Exposure

Lengthy midline (common) or transverse or oblique incision is used. Once peritoneum is opened, omentum and transverse colon is pushed upwards; small bowel is displaced to the patient's right; duodenojejunal flexure is identified and an incision is made lateral to the 4th part of duodenum; retroperitoneum is opened; entire small bowel with duodenojejunal flexure is mobilised medially towards right (medial mobilisation of the viscera). Aorta is identified and mobilised; infrarenal aorta is occluded with vascular clamp with finger guidance with care about IVC and left renal vein.

Coeliac axis is exposed through lesser omentum. Crura are dissected and divided. With careful blunt and sharp dissections coeliac trunk is identified **(Figs. 11-87 and 11-88)**.

It is artery of foregut supplying lower oesophagus, stomach, duodenum up to sphincter of Oddi, liver, pancreas and spleen. It originates just 1 cm below the aortic opening (T12 vertebra) at intervertebral disc level between T12 and L1. Trunk is *very short* in length (1.25 cm). It divides into three terminal branches—left gastric, common hepatic and splenic arteries. *Smallest left gastric artery*

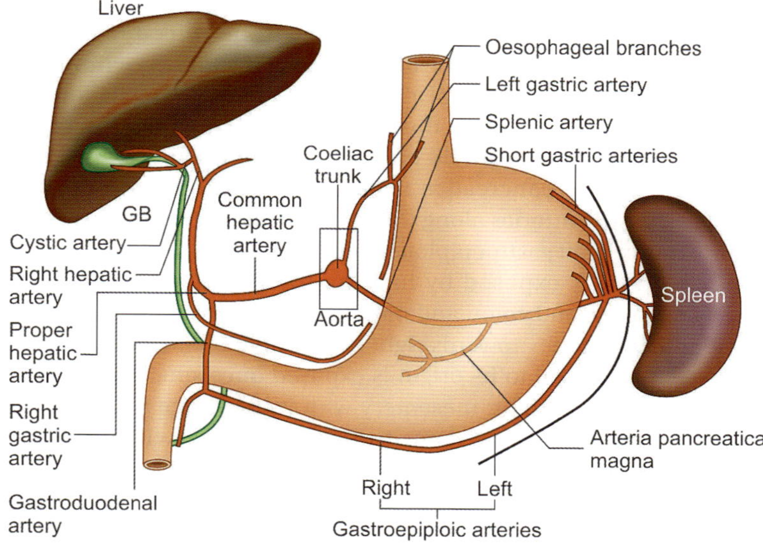

Fig. 11-87: Anatomy of coeliac trunk and branches.

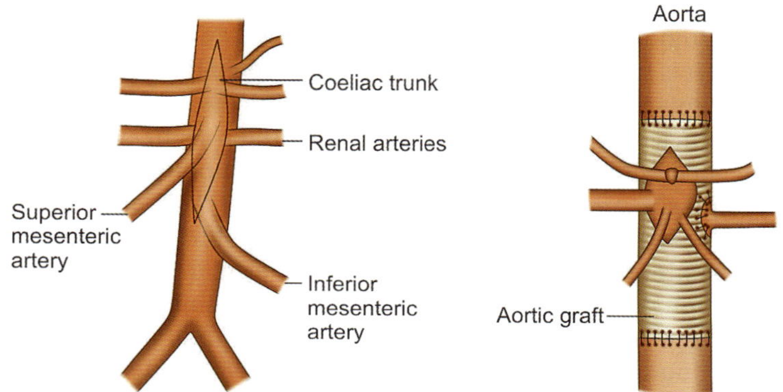

Fig. 11-88: Origin of visceral branches of aorta with a cuff of native aorta can be removed and reimplanted into the aortic graft.

runs upwards to the left behind the lesser sac to reach OG junction where it turns forwards into the lesser omentum along the lesser curve towards right to anastomose with the right gastric artery. It gives oesophageal branches and gastric branches. Once branch enters the lesser omentum, it is often called as descending branch of left gastric artery. *Common hepatic artery (CHA)* runs forward, downward and towards right behind the lesser sac and at upper border of the duodenum it enters the lesser omentum in front of the portal vein and left of CBD to end as right and left hepatic arteries. Gastroduodenal artery is the first main branch of the CHA which arises at upper part of the first part of the duodenum as a large branch, runs downwards behind the 1st part of the duodenum dividing at its lower border as right gastroepiploic artery (runs along the greater curvature in the greater omentum to anastomose with left gastroepiploic artery) and superior pancreaticoduodenal artery (often 2 in number as anterior and posterior; runs in the pancreaticoduodenal groove ending by anastomosing with inferior pancreaticoduodenal artery, a branch of SMA). CHA distal to gastroduodenal artery is called as proper hepatic artery (PHA) which gives right gastric artery just distal to the origin of gastroduodenal artery runs towards left along the lesser curvature to anastomose with left gastric artery. *Small supraduodenal artery* often may be present to supply proximal duodenum. Cystic artery arises from right hepatic artery, runs behind the CHD and cystic duct to reach neck of the gallbladder and dividing into superficial and deep branches. *Splenic artery is the largest branch* of the coeliac trunk runs transversely towards left along the upper border of the pancreas behind the lesser sac crossing left adrenal gland and kidney entering lienorenal ligament and splenic hilum dividing into many branches to enter into the spleen. Splenic artery branches are—numerous pancreatic branches; arteria pancreatica magna; arteria caudae pancreatis; 5–7 short gastric arteries along the gastrosplenic ligament to supply gastric fundus; left gastroepiploic artery **(Fig. 11-89)**.

SMA origin is exposed by incising the peritoneum vertically lateral to spleen and colon and mobilising the spleen and pancreas in front of left kidney towards right side. Origin of SMA will be well exposed. SMA distal to its origin is exposed once small intestine is mobilised towards right; mesentery with its free edge is identified; mesenteric leaf is incised to expose the artery with superior mesenteric vein. SMV is towards the right of the SMA. SMA is the artery of midgut. It originates from the front of the aorta at the level of L1 behind the body of pancreas usually 1.0 cm below the origin of coeliac trunk. It descends down behind the pancreas body, in front of the uncinate process crossing the duodenum to enter the root of mesentery directed towards right with a convexity towards left, ends by anastomosing with ileocolic artery at right iliac fossa. Above and in front it is related to the body of pancreas, splenic vein; above and behind to aorta, left renal vein, uncinate process and duodenum. In the mesentery it crosses IVC, right ureter, right psoas; it is associated with SMV which is towards right. Superior mesenteric nerve plexus surrounds the artery. *Branches of SMA are*—middle colic artery originates from the right side of SMA just below the pancreas level, runs downwards and forwards in the transverse mesocolon dividing into right and left branches. Inferior pancreaticoduodenal artery arises from SMA at the upper margin of 3rd part of the duodenum running in the pancreaticoduodenal groove divides into anterior and posterior branches; later anastomose with its superior counterpart. Right colic artery arises from SMA occasionally from a common trunk with middle colic artery directs towards the ascending colon divides into ascending and descending branches. Ileocolic artery arises from SMA close to caecum divides

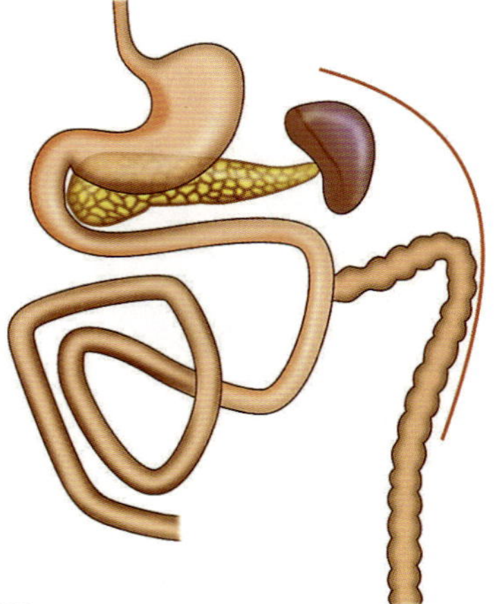

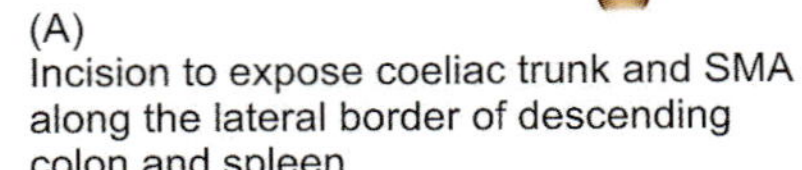

(A)
Incision to expose coeliac trunk and SMA along the lateral border of descending colon and spleen

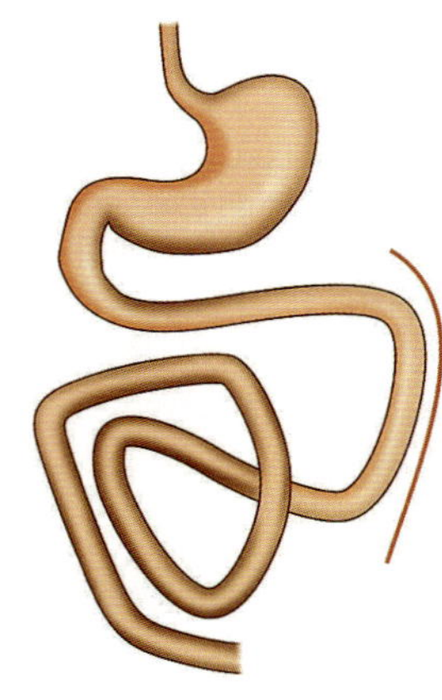

(B)
Incision to expose SMA along the margin of duodenojejunal flexure

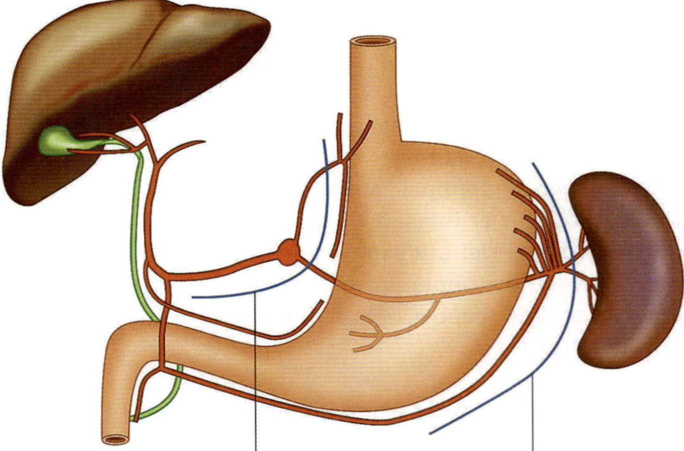

Fig. 11-89: Exposure of coeliac axis and its branches.

into superior and inferior branches; inferior branch apart from anastomosis into the terminal branch of SMA also gives ascending colic, anterior caecal, posterior caecal and an appendicular and ileal branches. SMA from its left side gives around 15 jejunal and ileal branches.

EXPOSURE OF ILIAC ARTERIES

Anatomy

Common iliac arteries are terminal branches of abdominal aorta; right is longer than left. It begins at the level of L4 vertebra 1.25 cm to left of the midline passing downwards and laterally ending at the level of lumbosacral intervertebral disc over the sacroiliac joint by dividing into external and internal iliac arteries. Right CIA passes in front of lower end of IVC, right common iliac vein which is medial to artery below. Left CIA is crossed by inferior mesenteric vessels at its middle.

Internal iliac artery (IIA) is smaller, 4 cm long supplying mainly pelvic organs (other than ovaries and superior rectal artery), perineum, gluteal region, iliac fossa. It begins in front of the sacroiliac joint at the level of L5 – S1 disc, medial to psoas major muscle running downwards and backwards ends at upper margin of greater sciatic notch by dividing into anterior and posterior divisions.

It is related in front to ureter and ovaries and Fallopian tube (in females); behind to internal iliac vein, lumbosacral trunk and sacroiliac joint; laterally to external iliac vein and obturator nerve; medially to peritoneum. Branches of anterior division are—superior vesical; obturator; middle rectal; inferior vesical; inferior gluteal (largest branch of anterior division) and internal pudendal (In females inferior vesical artery is replaced by vaginal artery; also uterine artery as an additional branch). Posterior division branches are—iliolumbar, two lateral sacral, superior gluteal arteries.

External iliac artery continues downwards and laterally on the psoas major muscle; under the inguinal ligament continues as femoral arteries. Branches are—inferior epigastric artery and deep circumflex iliac artery. External iliac vein is medial to the artery.

Exposure

Transabdominal approach is used for emergency situation like aorto-iliac surgery, trauma and ruptured aneurysm. Abdomen is opened through midline or oblique incision depending on whether only one side or both sides' iliac arteries need to be exposed. Peritoneum over the vessels is incised and dissected to expose the vessels. Ureter overlies the vessel. On left side sigmoid should be mobilised medially by dividing the pelvic mesocolon laterally to expose the vessel.

Extraperitoneal approach is used for isolated exposure of the iliac vessel in iliofemoral bypass or reconstruction. Oblique incision is placed in the skin above the inguinal ligament below the umbilicus with patient tilted 45° towards opposite side after placing sandbags behind. Skin, two layers of superficial fascia, external oblique and internal oblique are incised; transverse abdominis is split to visualise the peritoneum; it is swept above and medially using blunt finger or gauze dissection to expose the retroperitoneum. Ureter is safeguarded. Artery is exposed adequately as needed. Care should be taken while dissecting close to iliac veins.

EXPOSURE OF FEMORAL ARTERY AND BRANCHES

Anatomy

It is the continuation of external iliac artery behind the inguinal ligament at mid-inguinal point, coursing downwards and medially in the femoral triangle and adductor canal; at lower end of adductor canal at the junction of middle and lower third of thigh it passes through the opening in the adductor magnus to continue as popliteal artery. In front it is related to skin, superficial and deep fascia and femoral sheath; behind it rests on psoas major, pectineus and adductor longus. Femoral artery proximal to origin of profunda femoris artery is called as *common femoral* and distal to that is called as *superficial femoral artery*. Femoral vein is medial to artery to begin with, but at the apex of the femoral triangle it lies posterior to artery and later lies lateral. Femoral nerve is lateral to artery. Femoral branch of genitofemoral nerve is lateral to the femoral artery. *Branches*—Superficial: superficial external pudendal, superficial epigastric, superficial circumflex iliac; Deep: profunda femoris, deep external pudendal and muscular.

Profunda femoris is the largest branch of femoral artery, arising from the lateral part of the femoral artery 4 cm below the inguinal ligament in front of the iliacus muscle; it passes behind the femoral vessels leaving the femoral triangle deep to adductor longus, then between adductor longus and brevis, then between adductor longus and magnus with terminal part piercing the adductor magnus to anastomose muscular branches of popliteal artery. *Branches are*—medial and lateral circumflex femoral arteries and four perforating branches **(Figs. 11-90 to 11-92)**.

Popliteal artery begins at the junction of the lower third and middle third of the thigh from the opening/hiatus of the adductor magnus, running downwards and laterally to reach lower border of the popliteus muscle ending as anterior and tibioperoneal trunk which gives perineal artery and posterior tibial arteries. Superficially it is related to the tibial nerve which crosses the artery from lateral

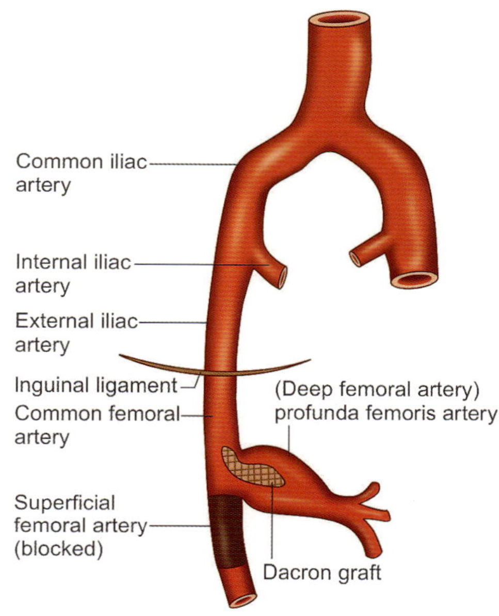

Fig. 11-90: Profundaplasty. It is done when there is localised stenosis at the origin of deep femoral/profunda femoris artery. It is done after proper exposure of the common femoral bifurcation through a vertical thigh incision. Proximal and distal parts of superficial and deep femoral arteries should be exposed to apply vascular clamps. Heparinisation is done. Arteriotomy is done at profunda femoris origin. Endarterectomy is done at the orifice adequately. A venous or prosthetic graft is sutured continuously into the arteriotomy wound to widen the origin of profunda femoris. Clamps are released. Check angiogram may be ideally done afterwards.

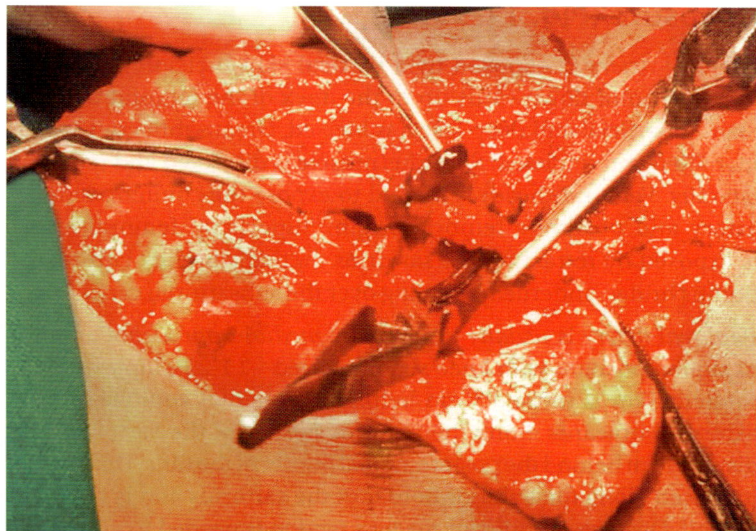

Fig. 11-91: Thrombectomy of femoral artery. It is not a common technique. Thromboendarterectomy is commonly done procedure.

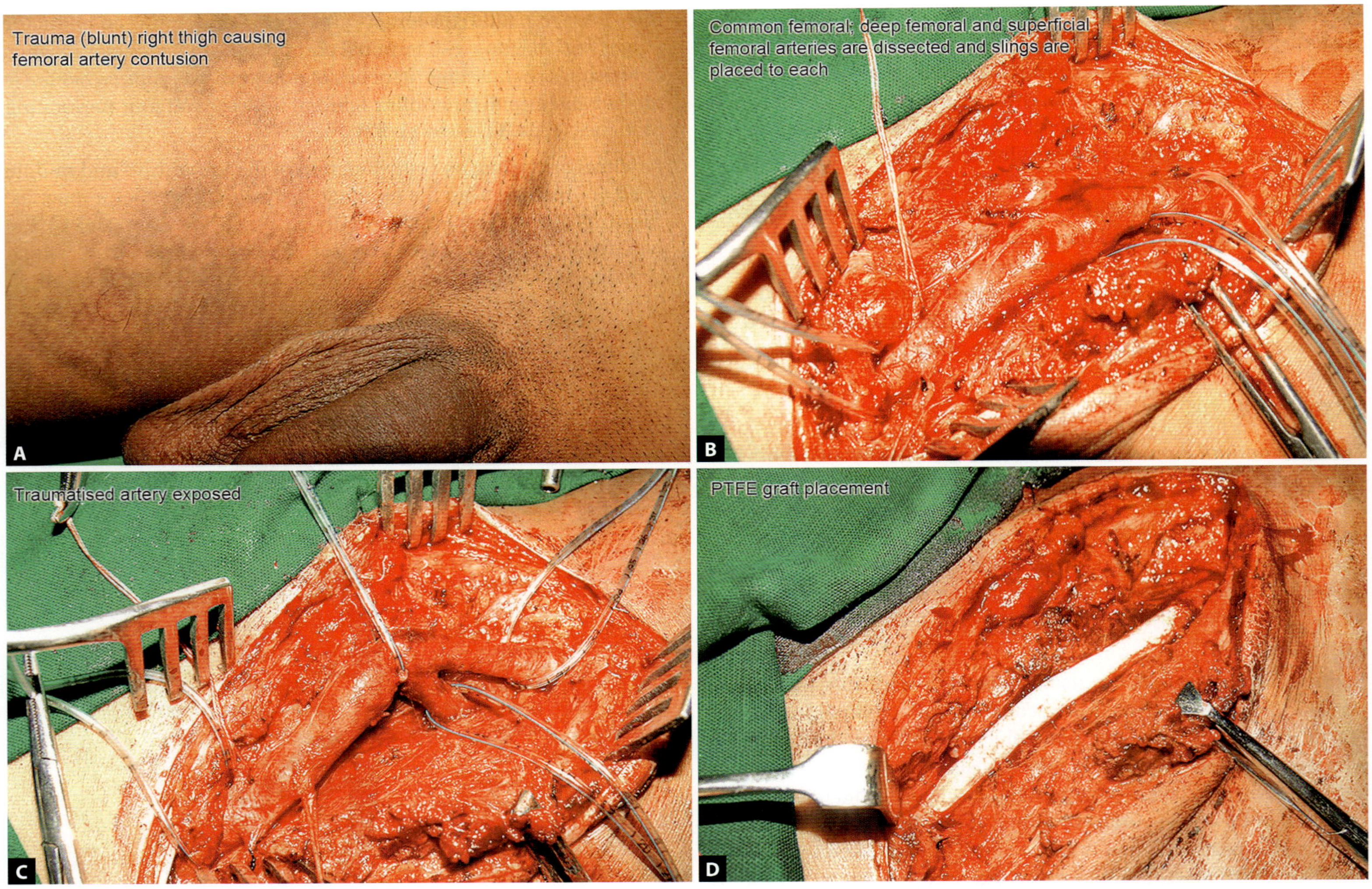

Figs. 11-92A to D: Femoral artery trauma causing arterial contusion which is corrected by polytetrafluoroethylene (PTFE) graft.

to medial side; popliteal vein which also crosses the artery from lateral to medial. Popliteal artery is overlapped by semimembranosus in the upper part and medial head of the gastrocnemius in the lower part. It lies on the knee joint and popliteus muscle in the deeper plane.

Exposure (Fig. 11-93)

Femoral artery is exposed by a vertical skin incision from mid-inguinal point downwards up to the apex of the femoral triangle. Skin, superficial and deep fascia is incised. Great saphenous vein is identified and retracted. Sartorius muscle is dissected and retracted laterally. Femoral sheath is incised to expose the common femoral artery and profunda femoris origin. Superficial femoral artery is exposed by retracting the sartorius medially and by cutting the fibrous bridge underneath roofing over the subsartorial canal.

Popliteal artery is *usually* exposed by *medial approach*. Patient is in supine position with knee slightly flexed—15–25°, hip externally rotated. Skin is incised 1 cm behind the medial condyle of tibia extended upwards along the anterior border of the sartorius and distally 1 cm behind the posteromedial border of the tibia. Deep fascia is incised along the anterior border of the sartorius and is retracted behind. Division of adductor magnus tendon is needed to expose the femoropopliteal junction. Below deep fascia along the tendinous part of three muscles sartorius, gracilis and semitendinosus is incised;

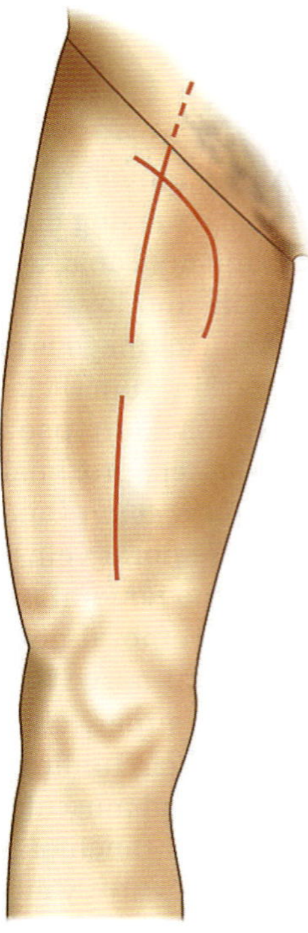

Fig. 11-93: Incision for exposure of femoral artery.

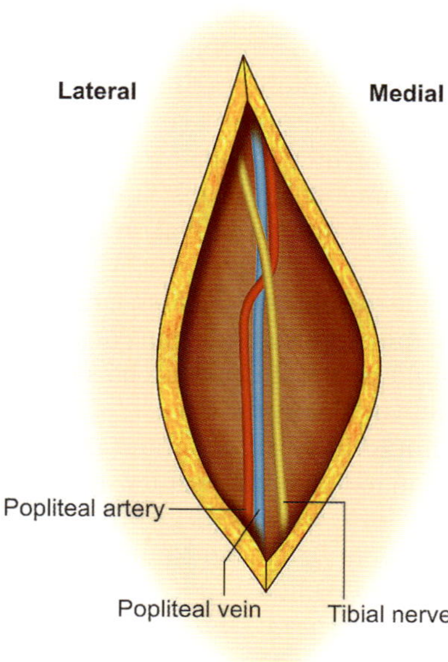

Fig. 11-94: Popliteal fossa anatomy.

tendinous insertion is retracted in front. Medial head of the gastrocnemius is retracted posteriorly **(Figs. 11-94 and 11-95)**.

Extensive exposure of popliteal artery needs division of tendinous insertion and medial head of gastrocnemius. After separation of popliteal fat, popliteal fascia is incised longitudinally to expose the popliteal vein which should be dissected very carefully and gently as its tear leads into torrential bleeding. Tibial nerve is dissected and retracted with a sling. Bifurcation or trifurcation of the popliteal artery can be exposed by dividing soleus muscle and tibial vein. Anomalies of popliteal vein should be remembered. *Posterior approach* is limited and is used in treating popliteal entrapment. A transverse skin crease incision with medial upward and lateral downward extensions is used. Deep fascia is incised vertically to reach the popliteal fossa.

ARTERIOVENOUS FISTULA FOR HAEMODIALYSIS (HAEMODIALYSIS ACCESS)

End stage renal failure needs haemodialysis. For regular haemodialysis well-perfused venous access is essential. Arteriovenous (AV) fistula is created at different levels to achieve this hyperdynamic circulation so that regular venous access will not be a problem.

Scribner shunt (1921) is the shunt created by Dr Belding H Scribner and Dr Wayne Quinton (Quinton-Scribner shunt) using *Teflon tubes* as circulatory access placed into the adjacent artery and vein. Access is kept patent by connecting two tubes outside the body with a *U-shaped Teflon tube*. It will shunt the blood from arterial side to the venous side. Infection and subcutaneous erosion of the tube are the complications. In 1962 Scribner started his first dialysis centre (*Seattle Artificial Kidney Center*).

Dr Willem Kolff did first successful dialysis in 1943 to a 67-year-old woman with uremic coma for 11 hours. Dr Nils Alwall also did extensive work on dialysis in University of Lund from 1946 to 1960.

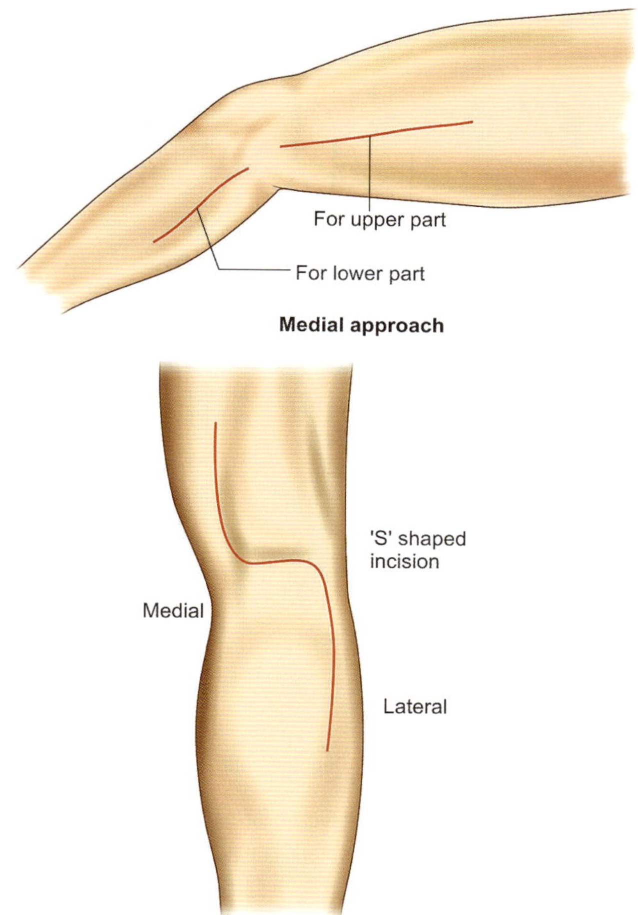

Fig. 11-95: Incision and exposure of popliteal artery.

Anatomy

Dorsal venous arch is formed from dorsal digital veins and dorsal metacarpal veins. Its efferent veins are cephalic (laterally; preaxial vein like GSV of lower limb) and basilic vein (medially; post-axial like SSV of lower limb) **(Fig. 11-96)**.

Cephalic vein begins at the lateral border of dorsal venous arch running upwards along the roof of the anatomical snuff box, lateral border of distal part of forearm, in front of the elbow, along the lateral border of the biceps brachii, piercing the deep fascia at lower margin of the pectoralis major muscle. Then it runs in the deltopectoral groove up to the infraclavicular fossa, piercing the clavipectoral fascia to join the axillary vein. Cephalic vein is accompanied by lateral cutaneous nerve of forearm and terminal branches of radial nerve. It communicates into basilic vein through median cubital vein. *A communicating vein* between cephalic vein and external jugular vein (neck) is present which runs across the clavicle. It is important for draining the upper limb in axillary vein removal (in carcinoma breast segment may be removed)/blockage.

Basilic vein begins at the medial side of the dorsal venous arch running upwards along the medial border of the forearm, near the elbow winds round towards the ventral aspect, continues upwards along the lateral border of the biceps brachii, in the middle of the arm it pierces the deep fascia, running along the medial side of the brachial artery becoming axillary vein at the lower border of the teres major. It is accompanied by posterior branch of the medial cutaneous nerve of the forearm and terminal part of the dorsal

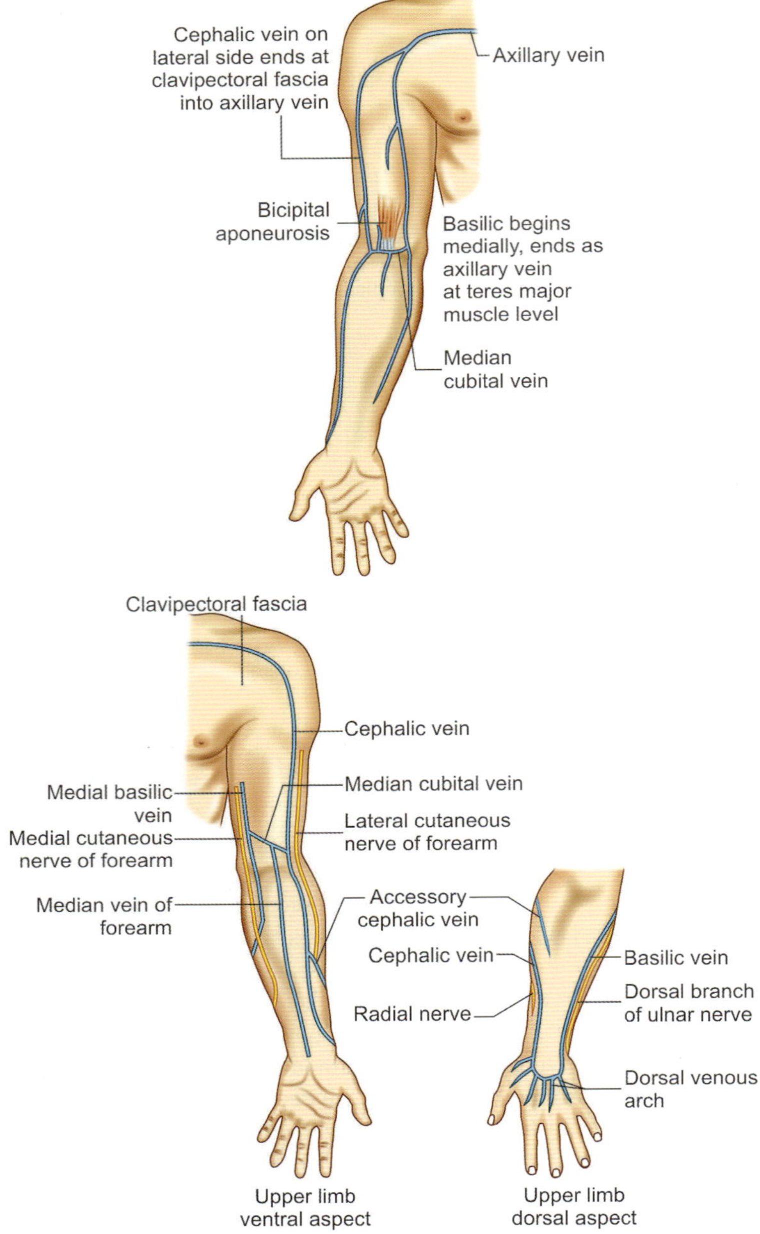

Fig. 11-96: Venous anatomy of upper limb to have vascular access for haemodialysis. Proper venous mapping is essential to create AV fistula.

branch of the ulnar nerve. Basilic vein is the more efficient venous channel than cephalic vein.

Median cubital vein begins 2.5 cm below the lateral part of the elbow as a large communicating vein from the cephalic vein running obliquely upwards and medially in front of the bicipital aponeurosis (deep to this brachial artery is present) ending at basilic vein 2.5 cm above the elbow (medial epicondyle) at medial aspect of the arm. Perforator veins from deep veins pierce the bicipital aponeurosis to enter the median cubital vein which fixes the vein firmly to make the IV cannulation easier and stable. Median cubital vein is absent in 30% of individuals.

Median vein of forearm begins at palmar network ending at cephalic or basilic vein.

Variations: Entire cephalic vein may drain into basilic vein (20%); separate cephalic and basilic veins without communications (10%).

Principle

Usually upper limb is used for creating of AV fistula (*Cimino-Brescia fistula*). Radiocephalic; brachiocephalic; brachiobasilic; PTFE forearm graft prosthesis and upper arm prosthetic graft fistula are different sites for creation of AV fistula.

Fistula should be done initially as distal as possible (radial artery). Even first fistula may be at anatomical snuff box level (snuff box fistula).

Non-dominant side should be used first. One should avoid placing any venous lines in the proposed side/part of the fistula.

Graft fistula should be avoided as much as possible; it should be kept as reserve in inevitable need.

Donor artery should have an adequate pulsation, volume and devoid of calcification to make successful fistula.

Intravenous 3,000 units heparin is given in all these patients on table. *Heparinised saline irrigation* to target artery and vein and wound is used during procedure.

Venous mapping and arterial Doppler is necessary in all patients **(Figs. 11-97 to 11-99)**.

Radiocephalic AV Fistula (Cimino–Brescia)

Doppler is done to evaluate cephalic vein and radial artery. Preoperative vein mapping is a must. Ideally *target vein* should be 3 mm or more in diameter. But adequate good flow with proper patency

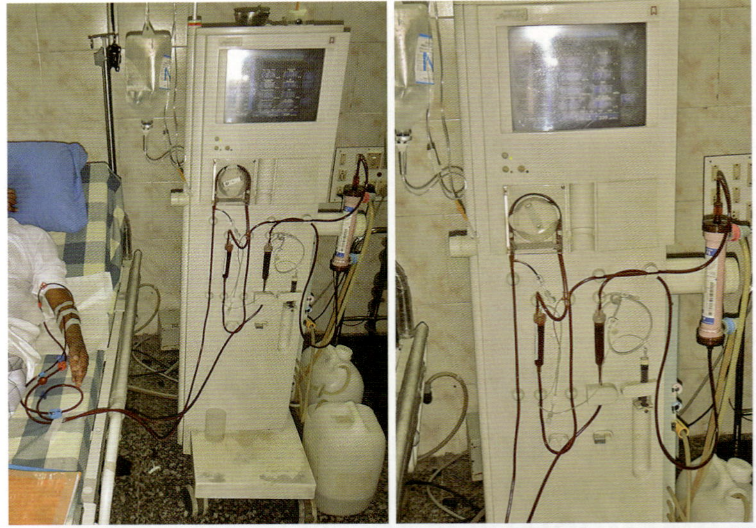

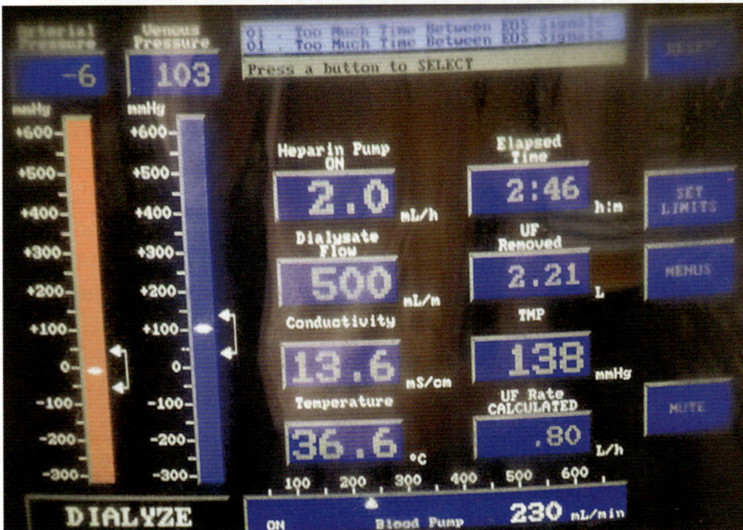

Fig. 11-97: Dialysis machine used for haemodialysis.

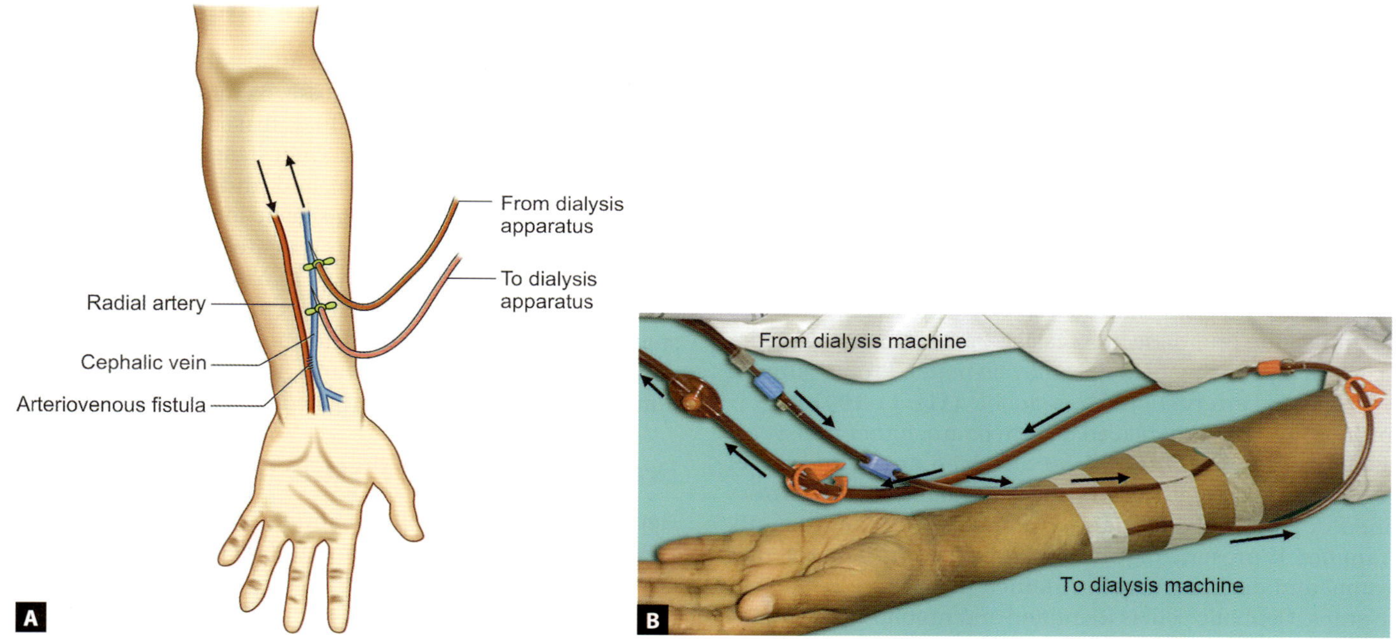

Figs. 11-98A and B: AV fistula access during haemodialysis.

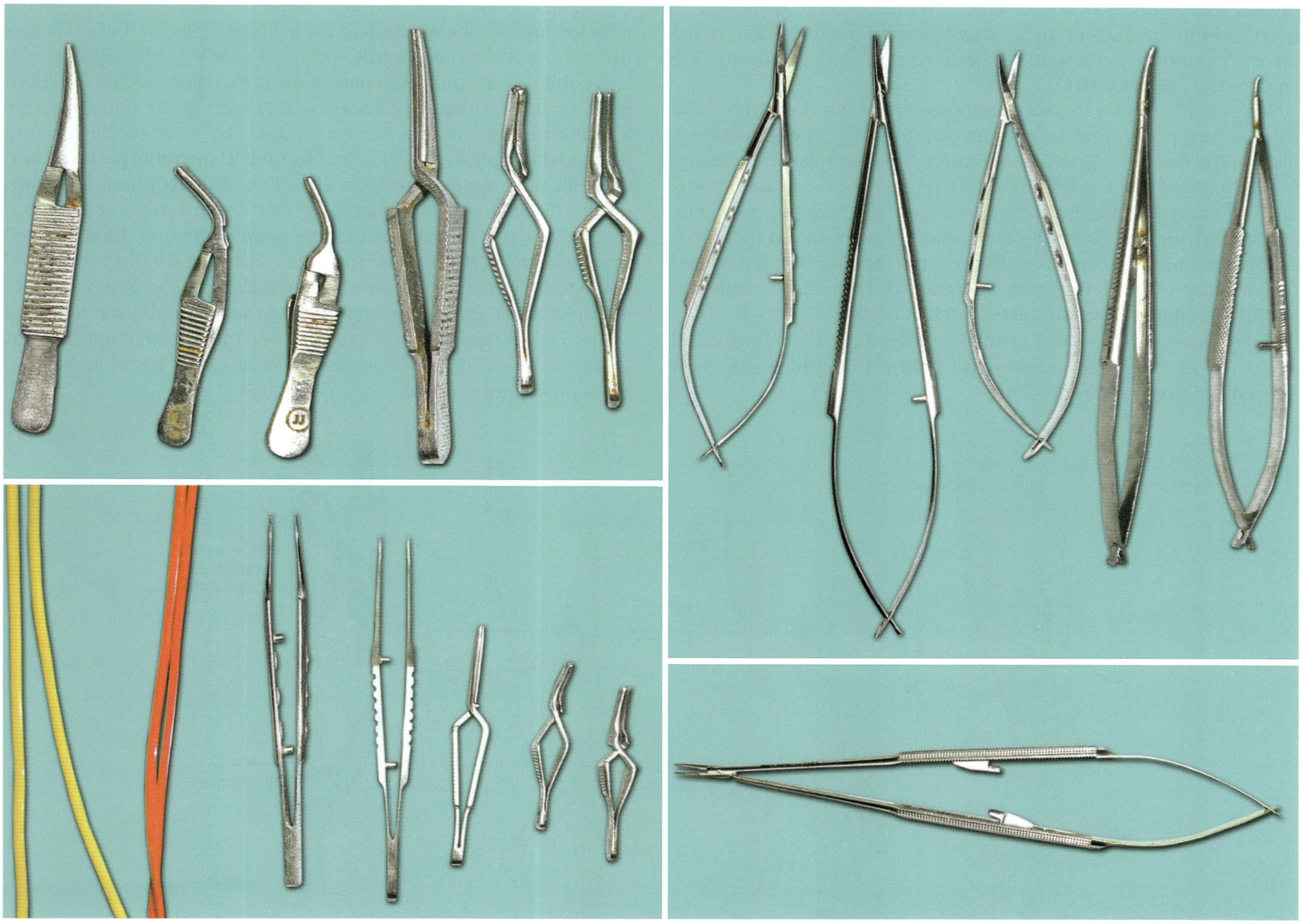

Fig. 11-99: Instruments used for AV fistula creation.

may be sufficient. Allen test is done to confirm adequacy of ulnar artery blood flow to the hand. It is better to avoid any cannulation or needle prick for IV injections in the planned limb for several weeks. Access fistula is created first in non-dominant upper limb; should begin always from distal to proximally. Vein transposition, PTFE graft fistula are the other alternatives should be kept in mind.

Procedure

It is done usually under local anaesthesia; brachial block can be given if needed. Regional anaesthesia causes venous dilatation to make venous identification and dissection easier. Preoperative antibiotics are given. Good light, using of loupes may be better. Proper surgical anatomy of vein and artery should be valuable **(Fig. 11-100)**.

Patient is supine with arm placed on arm board. Either transverse skin incision or ***longitudinal incision*** between artery and target vein area is used. Skin flaps are raised adequately. Radial artery is identified deep to deep fascia and mobilised for 2 cm length. Small branches if present requires secure ligation using 4-zero silk. Proximal and distal control is obtained using silastic loops or bulldog clamps. Cephalic vein is identified and mobilised as distally as possible. Small tributaries are ligated using 4-zero vicryl or silk. Vein is also secured with silastic loops if needed. It is flushed with heparinised saline. Intraoperative US may be useful to identify and assess the patency of the vein. Cephalic vein may be divided as distally as possible if needed. Vein is brought close to the artery to keep without any tension or kinking. Arteriotomy is done in radial artery. Venotomy is done in cephalic vein in case of side-to-side anastomosis **(Fig. 11-101)**.

End-to-side or side-to-side anastomosis (*Cimino-Brescia*) is done using 6-zero polypropylene sutures continuously. In end-to-side—distal end of the vein is ligated; proximal cut end is spatulated and its end is anastomosed to the side of radial artery. In side-to-side arteriotomy and venotomy wounds are approximated using 6-zero polypropylene continuous sutures. Once clamps (bulldog) are removed (proximal clamp is removed first and then distal clamp) cephalic vein is palpated for presence of thrill. On table venogram or Doppler is needed to confirm adequate flow. Wound is closed in layers.

Complications are—steal syndrome; bleeding; thrombosis and occlusion of the fistula; sepsis and failure to achieve sufficient arterialisation of venous network.

Brachiocephalic AV Fistula (Fig. 11-102)

After cleaning and draping, local anaesthesia xylocaine 0.5% plain is injected into the antecubital fossa. 6 cm transverse skin incision is made. Cephalic vein is identified; dissected for 5 cm length and stabilised with silastic loops. Deep fascia is opened; tendinous bicipital aponeurosis is identified and incised. Brachial artery is dissected and isolated using silastic loops. 3,000 IU of heparin is injected intravenously. Area is irrigated with heparinised saline. Cephalic vein is ligated distally. 6 mm arteriotomy over the isolated brachial artery is done. Proximal cut end of the cephalic vein is spatulated and anastomosed to the brachial artery using 6-zero polypropylene continuous sutures. Forward flush and back bleed is done. Fistula and wound is irrigated with heparin saline.

Brachiobasilic AV Fistula (Fig. 11-103)

Here basilic vein is mobilised and tunneled in subcutaneous plane and then fistula is created through brachial artery. Initial Doppler venous mapping is done. Basilic vein is not superficial; it is deep in the basilic tunnel in the medial aspect of the arm. So it should be kept in the tunnel in subcutaneous plane to have access.

It is done in brachial block or general anaesthesia. With supine 90° outstretched arm position, after cleaning and draping, longitudinal incision is made in arm medially from antecubital fossa to axilla. Basilic vein in the lower part of its tunnel is identified and dissected with freeing all tributaries up to the axilla. It is also mobilised across the cubital fossa downwards. Brachial artery is identified in the antecubital fossa and distal part of the arm; it is dissected for about 3 cm circumferentially. IV heparin 3,000 units given; heparin saline irrigation into the vessels and wound is also needed. Basilic vein distal to the cubital fossa is cut and ligated. Its proximal part is passed through the created tunnel in the subcutaneous plane (at 4 mm depth) in the anterior aspect of the arm downwards to the cubital fossa where it is passed through the deep fascia into the mobilised brachial artery. It is dilated manually. Kinking should be avoided while tunneling it. 6 mm arteriotomy is done in the brachial artery after placing silastic loops; spatulated proximal mobilised tunneled cut end of the basilic vein is anastomosed into the brachial artery as end-to-side. Thrill is checked in the venous side. Distal, radial and ulnar pulses are checked.

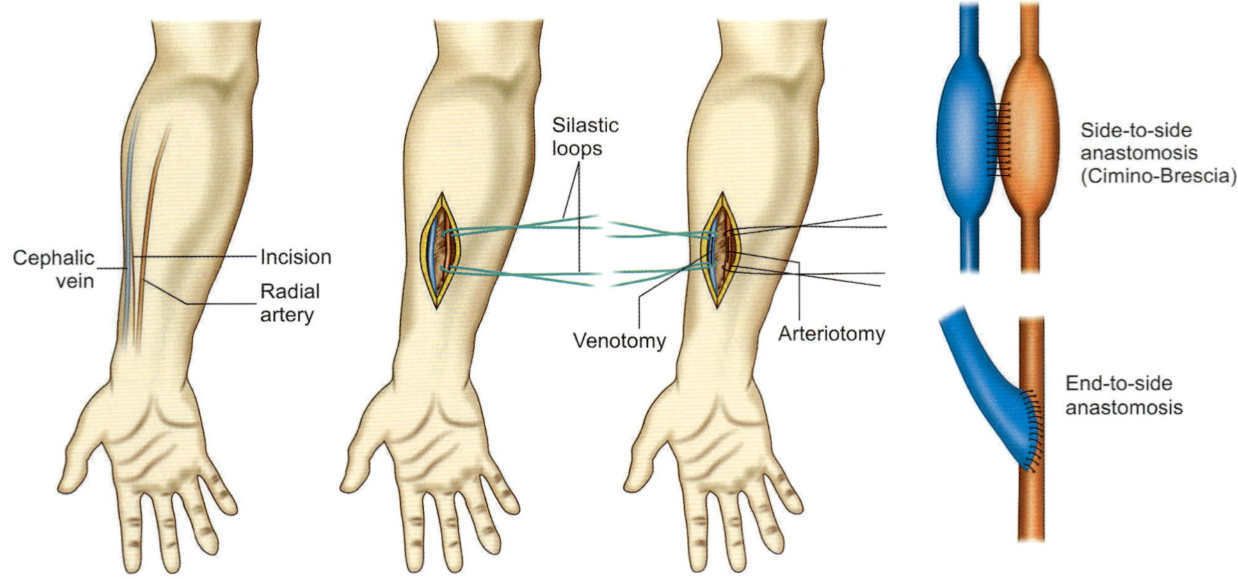

Fig. 11-100: Radiocephalic AV fistula creation.

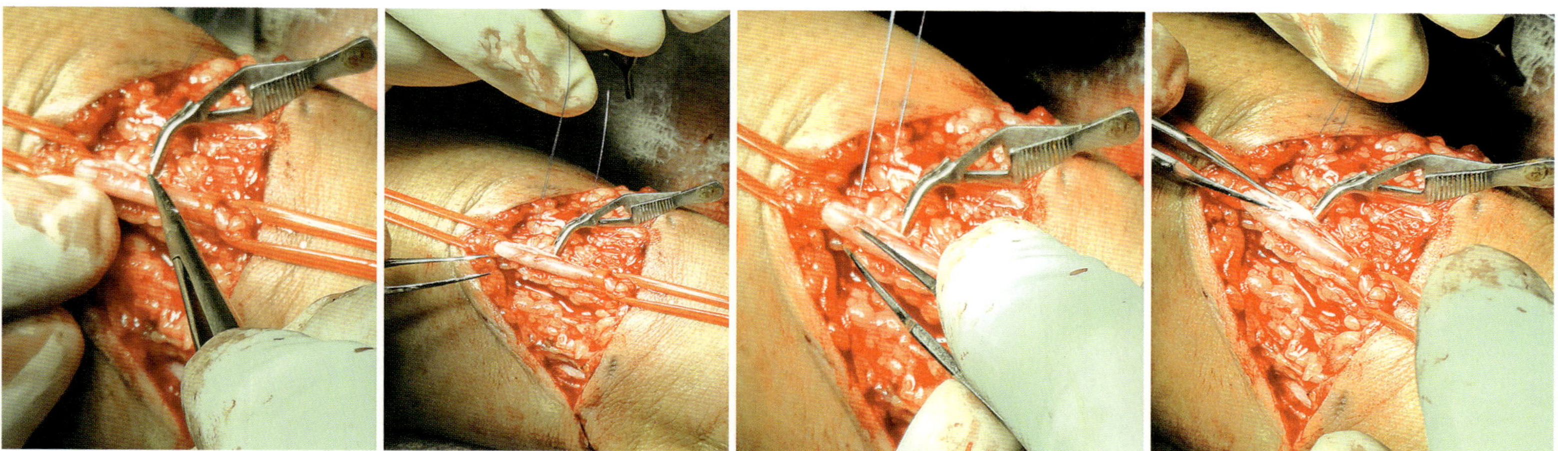

Fig. 11-101: Radiocephalic AV fistula.

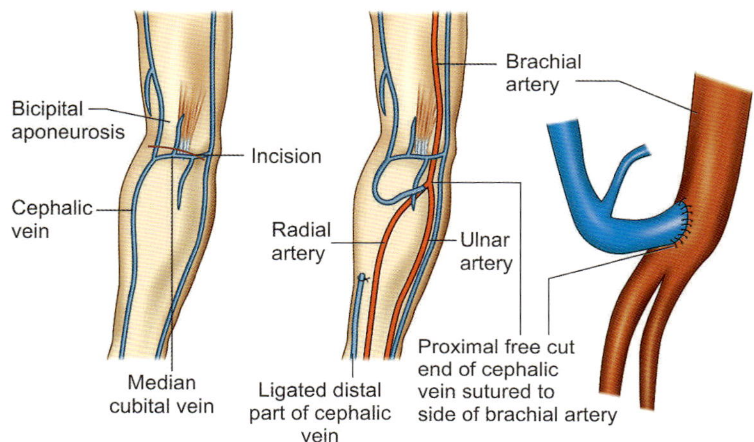

Fig. 11-102: Brachiocephalic AV fistula.

PTFE Graft AV Fistula in Forearm for Haemodialysis Access (Fig. 11-104)

It is done when primary AV fistula is not possible due to inadequate venous length/size/pattern. Graft interposition for creation of fistula between artery and vein is needed. Basilic or cephalic vein can be used. Brachial artery is usually used.

After Doppler venous mapping of the upper limb, under regional anaesthesia, transverse or longitudinal incision is made in the forearm. Brachial artery at the antecubital fossa or just above is dissected for 2-3 cm and isolated with silastic loops. Basilic vein on the medial and upper part of the forearm is dissected for 2–3 cm with ligation of tributaries. PTFE 6 mm graft is used of adequate length. Place where graft crosses the joint should be ringed. Subcutaneous tunneling is done using finger or haemostat or tunneling device.

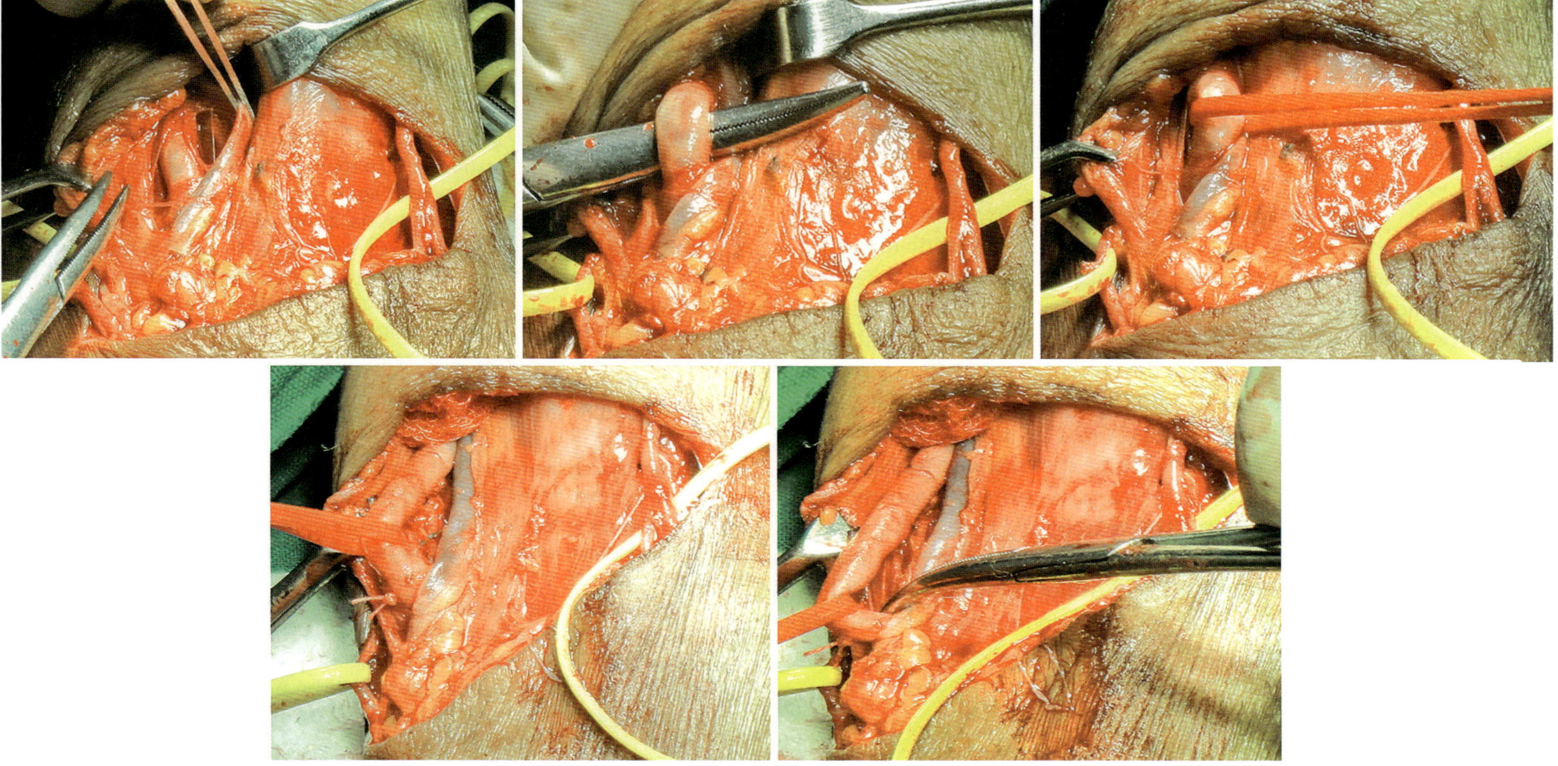

Fig. 11-103: Dissection of vessels for brachiobasilic AV fistula.

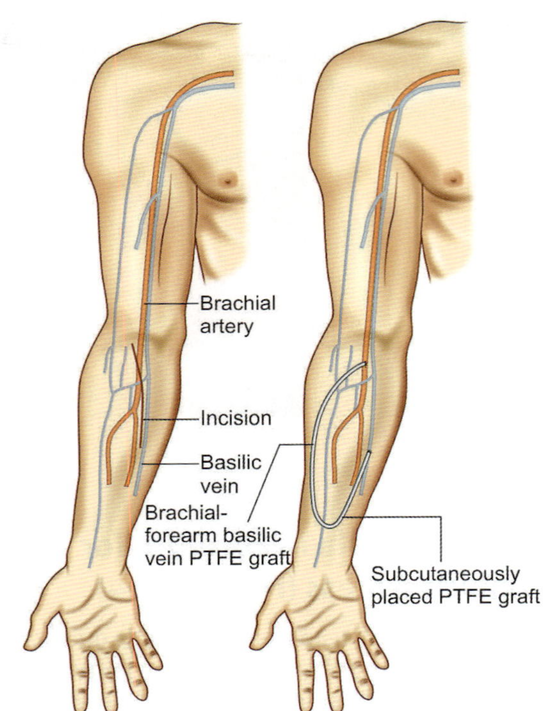

Fig. 11-104: AV fistula in forearm using PTFE graft between brachial artery and basilic vein.

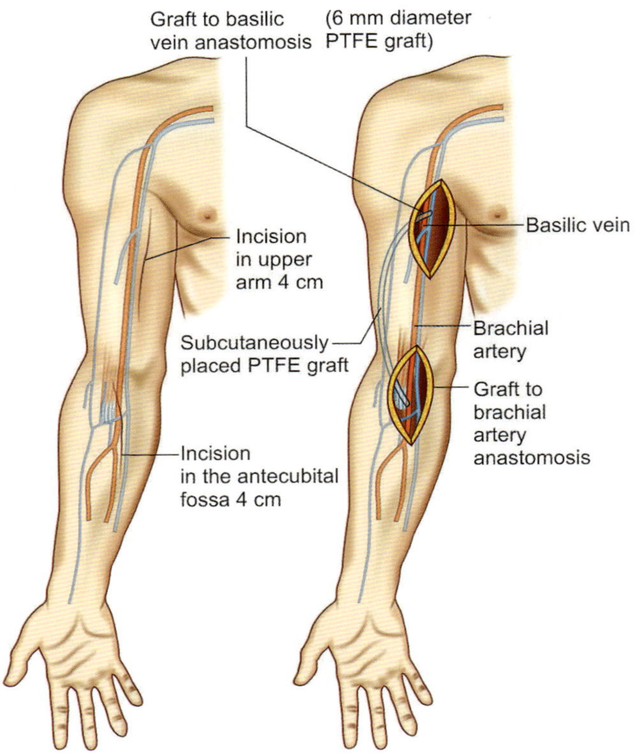

Fig. 11-105: Upper arm prosthetic AV fistula.

Graft is passed through the subcutaneously created tunnel without any kink. IV heparin 3,000 units injected. Arteriotomy and venotomy of 6 mm length is done. Graft is anastomosed to target artery (brachial) and target (basilic) vein as end-to-side using 6-zero polypropylene sutures. First graft to artery anastomosis is done; Graft is palpated ***for thrill***. Adequate distal pulse in radial/ulnar should be confirmed. Venogram may be needed at a later date if stenosis is suspected.

PTFE Graft in Upper Arm Prosthetic AV Fistula Access (Fig. 11-105)

It is done under general or regional anaesthesia. Patient is in supine position with arm at 90°. After cleaning and draping, a 5 cm incision is made on the medial aspect of the upper arm towards axilla. Basilic vein is identified in deeper plane medially and 4 cm length of the vein dissected, isolated circumferentially and silastic loops are placed. Brachial artery is identified and dissected through a 3–5 cm length incision over the antecubital fossa after incising bicipital aponeurosis. 2–3 cm of brachial artery is dissected to place silastic loops. A curved tunnel is created in the subcutaneous plane directed laterally to connect these tow wounds to place the prosthetic graft. Patient is heparinised (with 3,000 units IV). 6 mm arteriotomy is done in brachial artery; 6 mm sized PTFE graft is spatulated to anastomose with arteriotomy as end-to-side using 6-zero polypropylene continuous sutures. Wound and site is irrigated with heparinised saline. Graft is passed through the tunnel to reach the basilic vein proximally. 10 mm venotomy is done; obliquely cut other end of the graft is sutured similarly to the venotomy. Backward bleeding from the venous side and forward bleeding from the graft was done. Thrill in the basilic vein is checked. Radial and ulnar pulses are also checked. Doppler is used to confirm adequacy of flow.

Complications are—sepsis, bleeding, finger ischaemia, nerve injury, fistula thrombosis and block.

Graft Revision after Graft Block

Graft may get blocked by graft thrombosis. Doppler is done to identify the site of block. Incision is made over the graft site extending above and below. Proximal and distal control is obtained. Patient is heparinised. *Balloon thrombectomy* is done through venous side and later through arterial side of the graft. Pulsation is checked after that to confirm the flow over the graft. Fistulogram is done to rule out distal stenosis. If it is present a *jump graft* is placed to bypass stenosis.

Note

- Fistula requires 6 weeks to mature; and 2 weeks in case of graft. Any swelling in the fistulas site after 2nd week should be evaluated for complications. Venous side branches in the fistula may prevent maturation, and so needs proper ligation of side branches.
- If fistula has not matured in 6 weeks, it should be assessed by Doppler study and fistulogram. Rule of 6's criteria in AV fistula if matured are—flow more than 600 mL/min; diameter >6 mm; depth <6 mm.
- Patient should do isometric hand exercise and should do daily self examination of fistula for thrill and features of infection.
- Vein should be checked for distension; non-distensible fistula is sclerotic and will not mature.
- Non-compressible veins are thrombotic.
- While dissecting the major target artery care should be taken not to injure adjacent nerves.
- Steal syndrome is more common when fistula is created above elbow level; when fistula is done with graft than vein; and in diabetic, Steal syndrome may cause gangrene of fingers or entire hand. In such situation access fistula may require to be ligated to save the hand. Otherwise interval ligation of artery distal to fistula level is done with revascularisation of artery distally using another graft from artery above the level of fistula to artery below the level of ligation.
- Possible sites of future access should be preserved and cannulas or venous catheters should be avoided at such sites.
- Proper documentation with a diagram of the fistula is a must in all these patients.

PERITONEAL DIALYSIS ACCESS

Peritoneal dialysis catheter can be placed as an emergency temporary one done in ICU or open placement of the catheter done in operation theatre or laparoscopic assisted catheter placement or totally laparoscopic catheter placement.

In emergency and laparoscopy, trocar placement is blind. So risk of bowel injury should be taken into account.

Tenckhoff or Missouri swan neck catheter (has got intraperitoneal ball deeper to cuff to position underneath the peritoneum whereas cuff comes in front of the peritoneum) is used.

Open Method

With patient in supine position entire abdomen is cleaned and draped. Site for trocar and exit trocar should be marked before making incision by placing the catheter on the abdomen with curl end placing on the pubic symphysis going upward with inflow cuff above the umbilicus on the rectus and exit cuff trocar below the umbilicus lateral to the rectus muscle. Incision is deepened to anterior rectus sheath which is incised vertically and rectus muscle is split. Purse string suture is placed in the posterior fascia which is later incised in the centre of the purse string. Peritoneal dialysis catheter with a guidewire or a stylet is lubricated with jelly. Catheter white line should face anterior upward. Catheter is inserted into the abdominal cavity along the posterior surface of the abdominal wall towards the iliac crest and then towards pubic symphysis. Curl of the catheter is placed in the pelvis just deep to the pubic symphysis close to the abdominal wall. Guidewire is removed; heparinised saline is flushed into the catheter. Fluid should flow without interruption and one should be able to instill, aspirate or siphon the fluid easily if catheter curl is placed properly (Patient is placed in reverse Trendelenburg position). Purse string is tightened around the catheter (Missouri swan neck catheter). A tunnel is created through rectus muscle and subcutaneous tissue to reach exit site. Catheter is passed through this tunnel. Cuff of the exit site of the catheter should be 1 cm proximal to the exit point. Upper wound is closed completely. Suture is placed around catheter at exit wound **(Fig. 11-106)**.

Patient can undertake dialysis at home. Patient cannot go for swimming and bath should be avoided. Shower can be used. Dialysis is done usually 2 weeks afterwards. Initial low volume dialysis is done increasing the volume gradually to therapeutic level.

OMENTOPLASTY

Indications

To improve circulation in peripheral vascular disease, to improve lymphatic drainage from the limb in case of lymphoedema, in revascularisation of the pharynx, cranial cavity.

Surgical Anatomy

Common hepatic artery → Gastroduodenal artery → Right gastroepiploic artery.

Coeliac artery *Omental vessels.*

Splenic artery → Left gastroepiploic artery.

Omentum has got 4 layers of omental arcades with rich lymphatics. By retaining one of the pedicles either right or left gastroepiploic arteries, omentum is mobilised for adequate length to maintain the circulation. It controls the ischaemia, promotes the wound/ulcer healing and reduces the pain. It can also be used in upper limb ischaemia. It can be used in bilateral lower limb diseases as two pedicles. But if patient continues to smoke these omental vessels may acquire the disease (TAO) and recurrence of symptoms can occur.

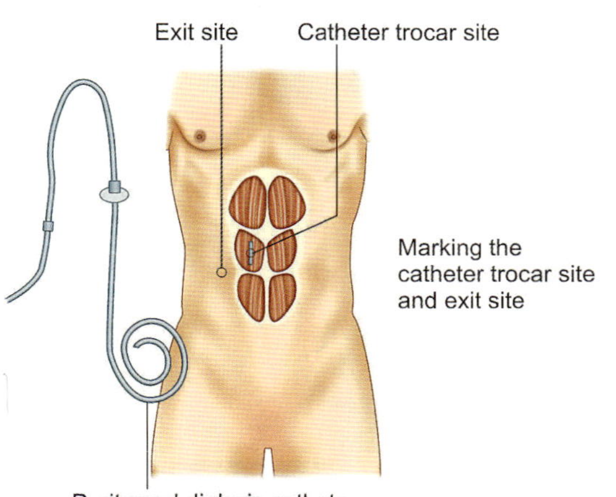

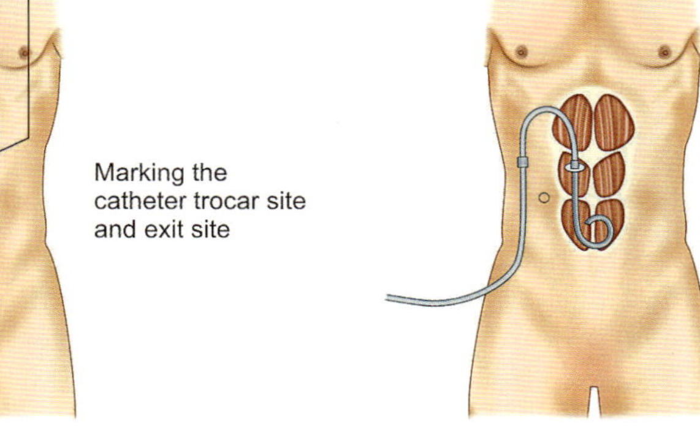

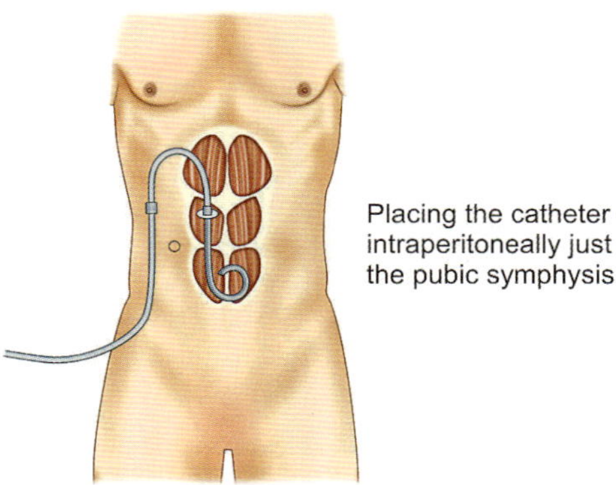

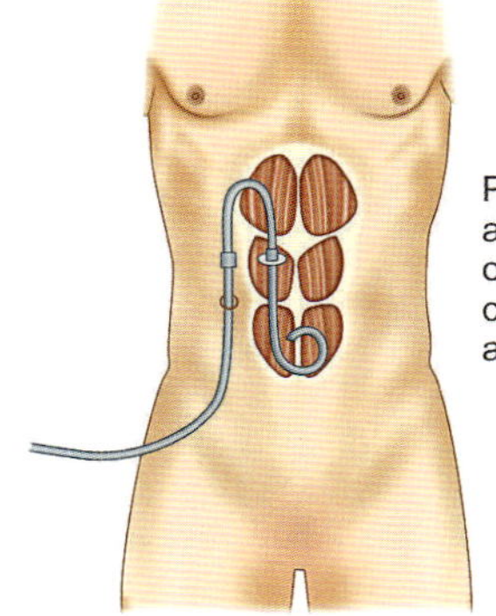

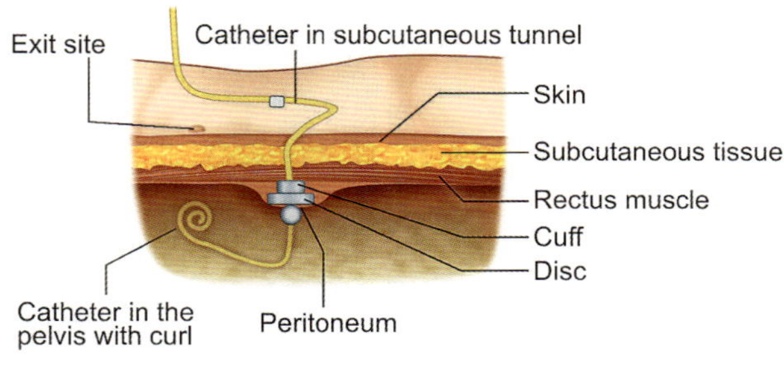

Fig. 11-106: Technique of peritoneal dialysis (open method).

Procedure

Preoperative antibiotic is given. Under general or epidural anaesthesia, entire abdomen and entire lower limb is cleaned and draped. Through upper midline incision abdomen is opened. Omental vessels/arcades are assessed. Omentum is separated from colon through avascular plane. Omentum is also carefully separated from mesocolon through omental bursa. Gastroepiploic arcade along the greater curvature is identified. Branches entering the stomach from gastroepiploic arcade are carefully ligated using 3-zero vicryl. One of the pedicles usually right is retained as pedicle to perfuse the arcade. Omentum is lengthened with careful planning. Bleeding and haematoma formation within omentum should be avoided as much as possible. Cauterisation should be minimum only if at all using bipolar cautery **(Fig. 11-107)**.

Incision is made just above the groin which is deepened across abdominal wall muscles and peritoneum to reach abdominal cavity. Mobilised omentum is brought out of the groin wound into the subcutaneous plane. Multiple transverse incisions are made in the limb downwards to reach the lower part of leg. Subcutaneous tunnels are created to pass the omentum. In the calf/leg deep fascia is opened to bury the tip of the omentum into the muscle. Abdomen is closed in layers. In the limb only skin is sutured without injuring the omental pedicle in the subcutaneous plane.

Patient is kept nil orally for 24 hours.

Doppler study at regular period will reveal the perfusion in the omentum.

Complications

Abdominal sepsis can occur due to removal of omentum from the abdominal cavity. Patient is observed for peritonitis (primary) and septicaemia. It is treated usually with proper antibiotic therapy. Incisional hernia, adhesions, intestinal obstruction can occur. Wound infection in the limb and cellulitis, thrombosis of the omental vessels and failure of the procedure can also occur **(Fig. 11-108)**.

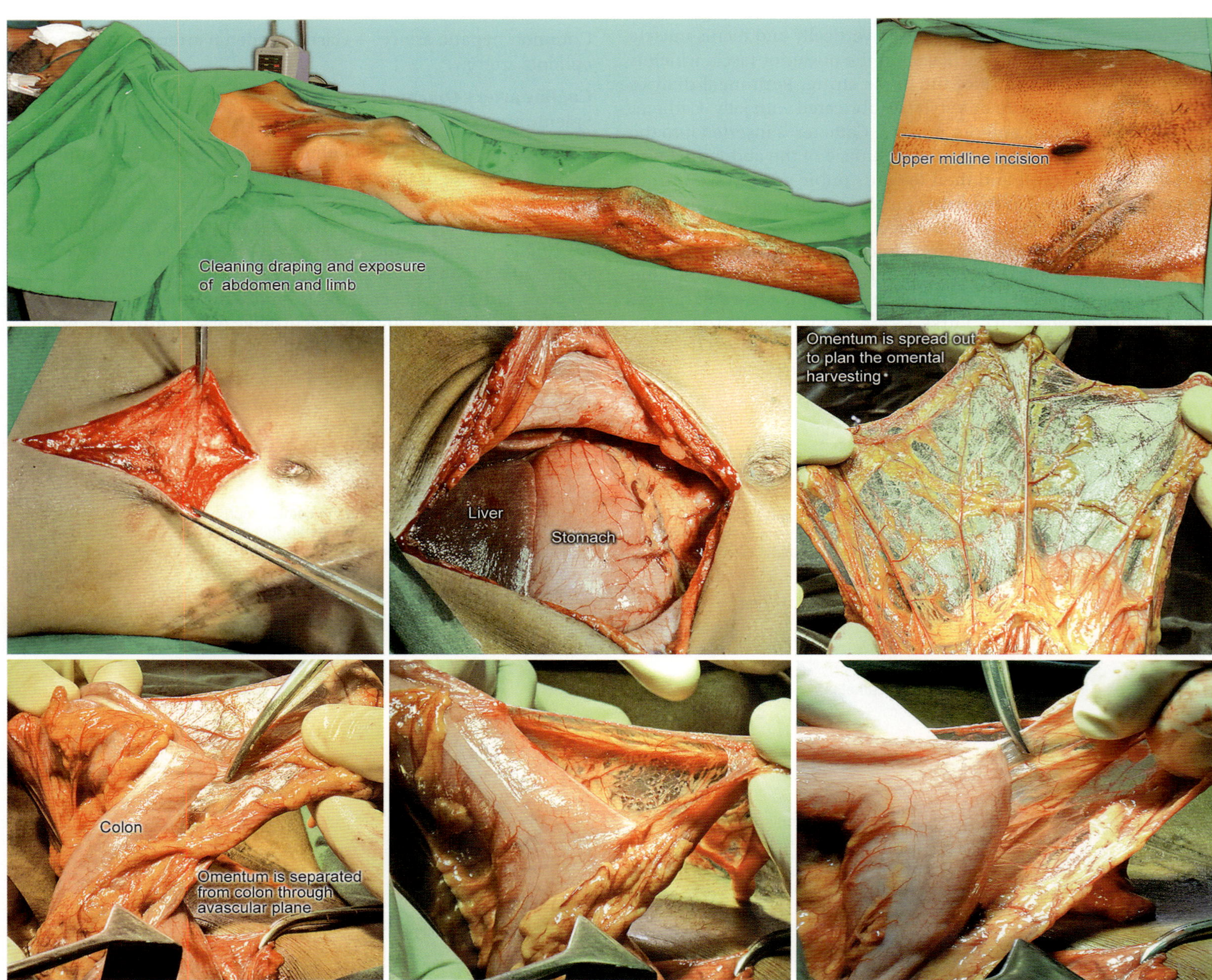

Figs. 11-107(1)

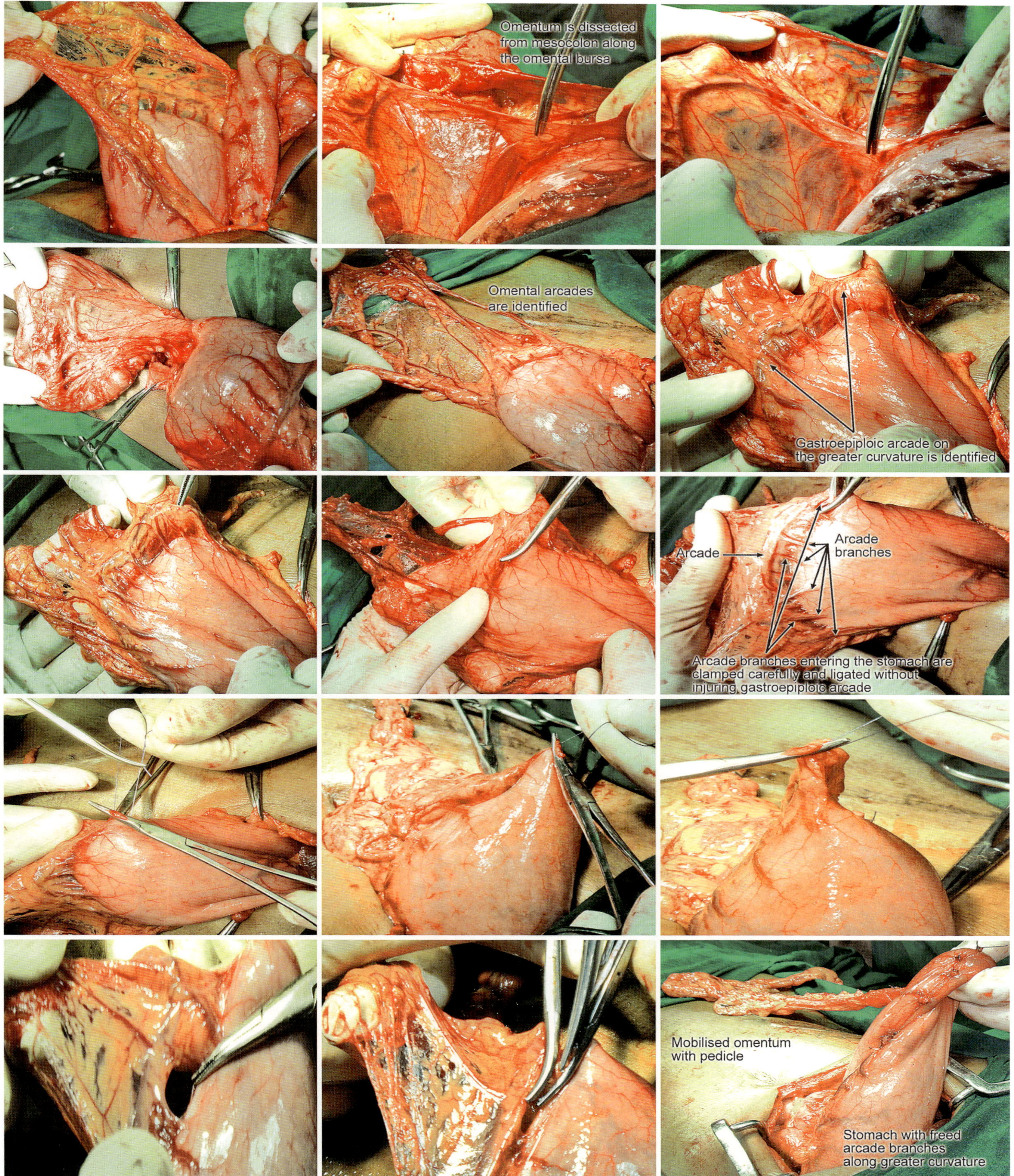
Omentum is dissected from mesocolon along the omental bursa
Omental arcades are identified
Gastroepiploic arcade on the greater curvature is identified
Arcade
Arcade branches
Arcade branches entering the stomach are clamped carefully and ligated without injuring gastroepiploic arcade
Mobilised omentum with pedicle
Stomach with freed arcade branches along greater curvature

Figs. 11-107(2)

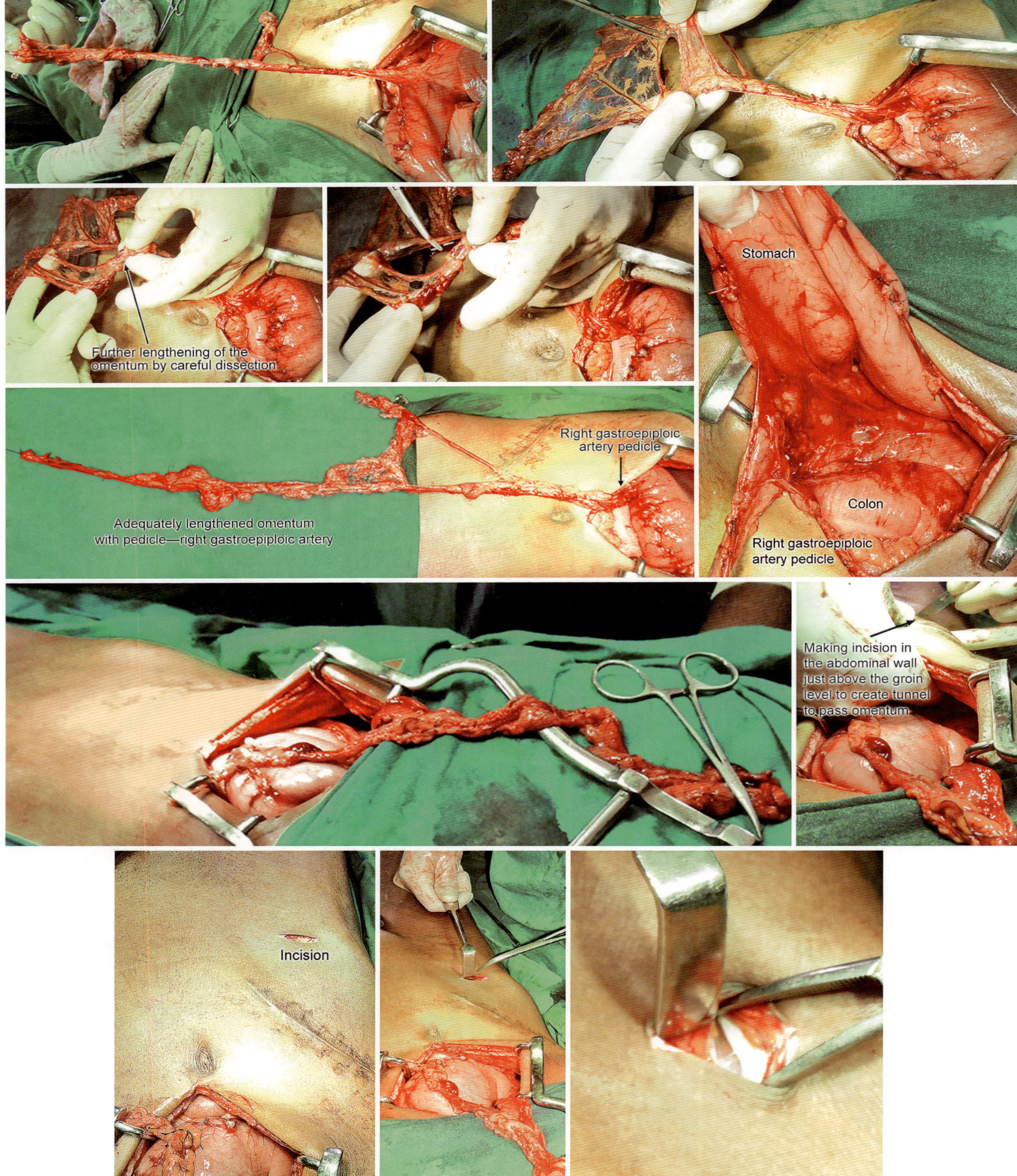
Further lengthening of the omentum by careful dissection
Stomach
Right gastroepiploic artery pedicle
Adequately lengthened omentum with pedicle—right gastroepiploic artery
Colon
Right gastroepiploic artery pedicle
Making incision in the abdominal wall just above the groin level to create tunnel to pass omentum
Incision

Figs. 11-107(3)

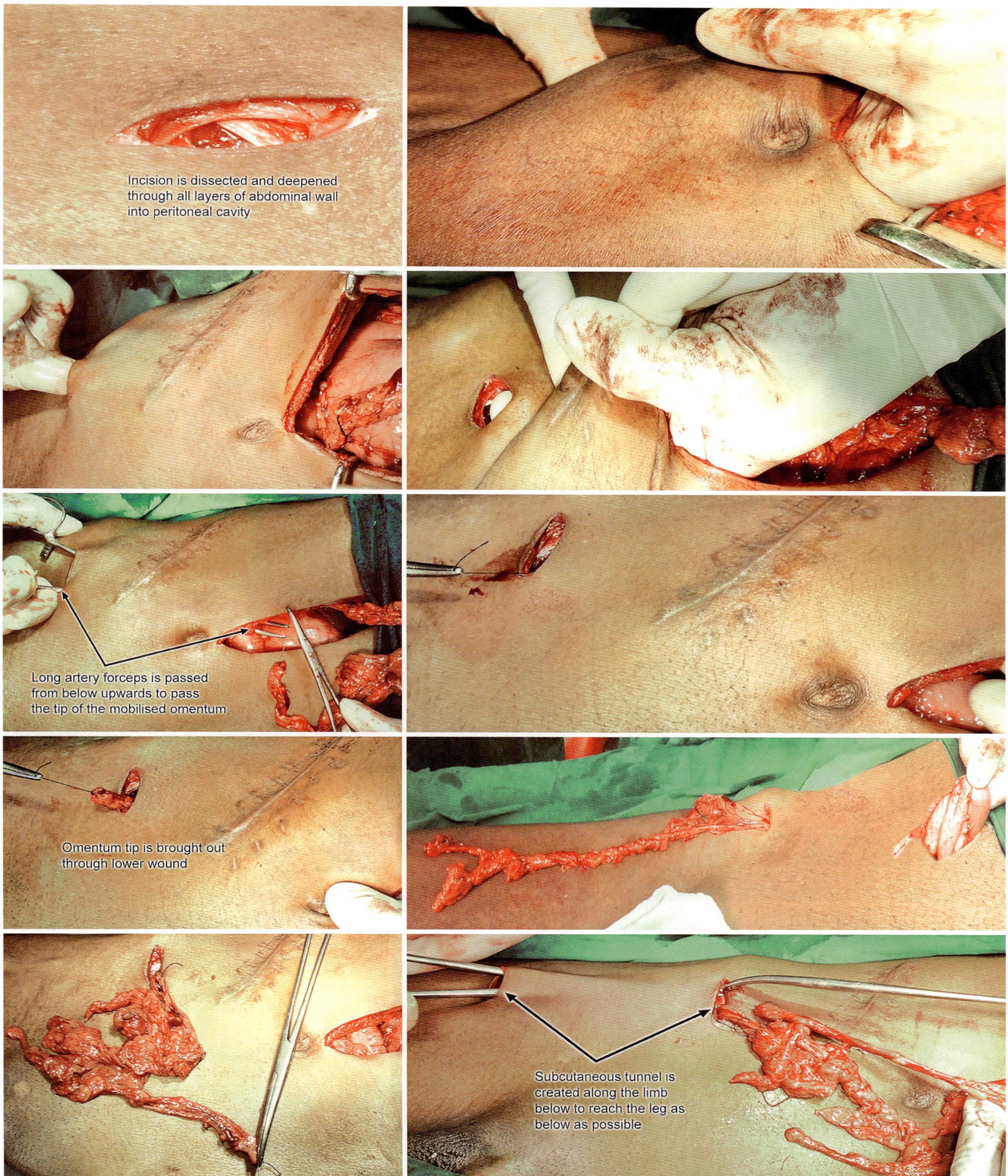
Incision is dissected and deepened through all layers of abdominal wall into peritoneal cavity
Long artery forceps is passed from below upwards to pass the tip of the mobilised omentum
Omentum tip is brought out through lower wound
Subcutaneous tunnel is created along the limb below to reach the leg as below as possible

Figs. 11-107(4)

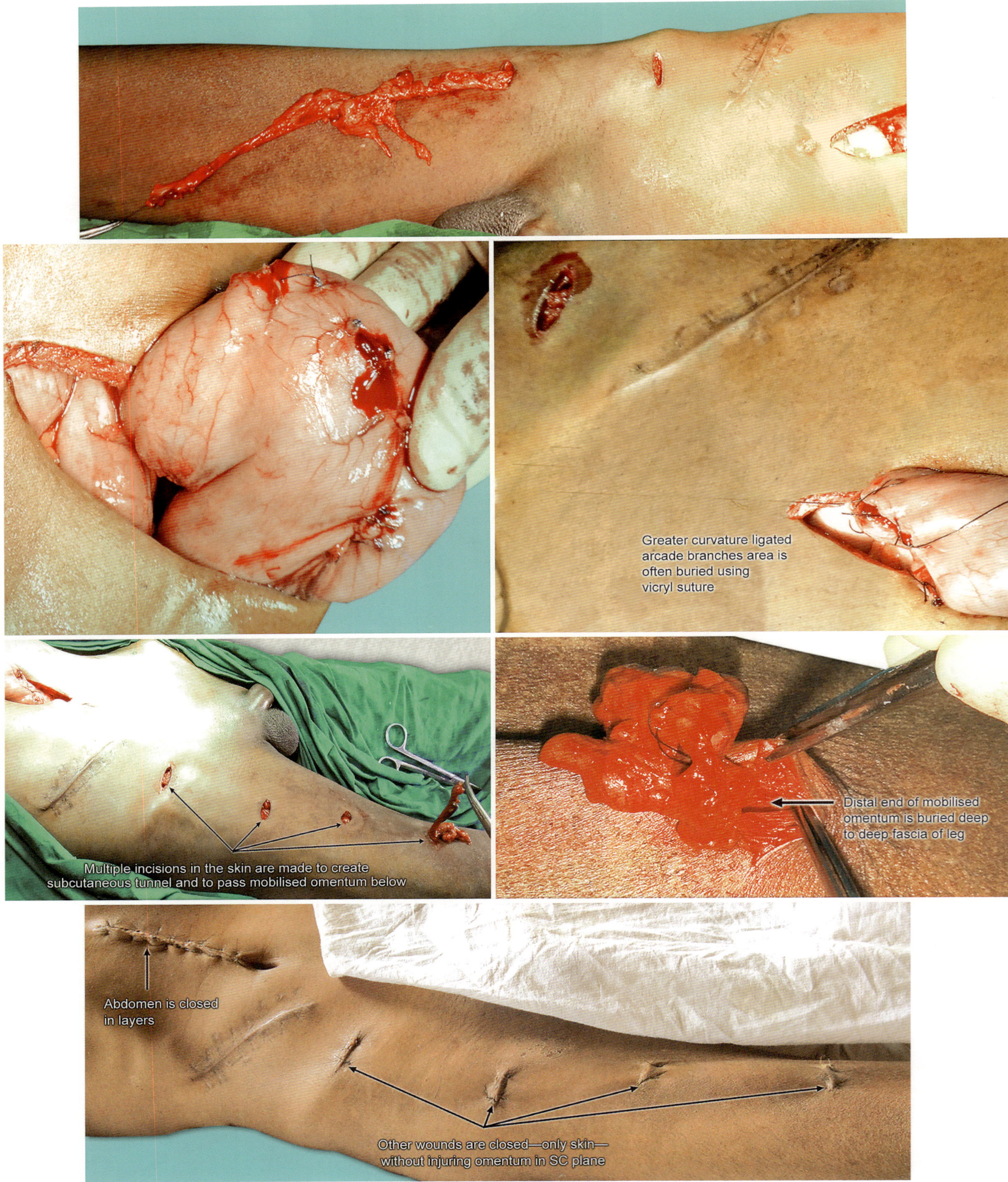

Figs. 11-107(5)

Figs. 11-107(1 to 5): Technique of omentoplasty.

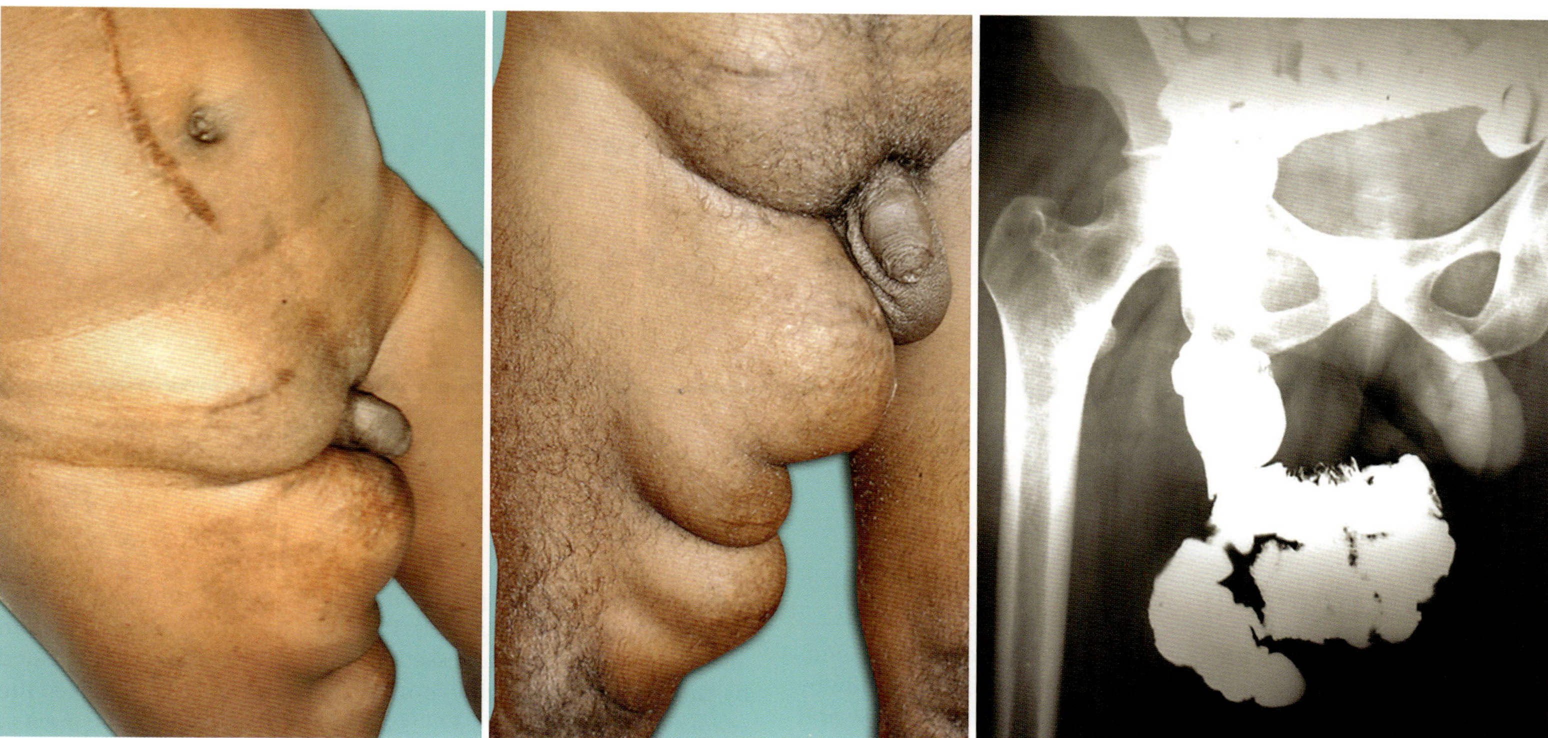

Fig. 11-108: Hernia after omentoplasty along the upper medial part of thigh with colon as content. On percussion it was resonant. Barium enema X-ray showed colon in the hernial sac.

12

CHAPTER

Surgery in Venous and Lymphatic Diseases

VENOUS DOPPLER

With the patient standing; the Doppler probe is placed at saphenofemoral junction (SFJ) and later wherever required. Basically by hearing the changes in sound, venous flow, venous patency, and venous reflux can be very well identified. A *uniphasic signal* means flow is in one direction. A *biphasic signal* means flow in both forward and reverse direction suggesting incompetence. Reversal can often be better appreciated by releasing a tourniquet applied earlier at saphenofemoral junction. An *audible whoosh signal > 0.5 sec* on performing the Valsalva manoeuvre with probe kept at the SFJ suggests incompetence.

Venous Doppler in varicose veins

- To find out DVT—very important.
- To find out saphenofemoral, saphenopopliteal incompetence.
- To find out perforator incompetence.
- Uniphasic signals signify flow in one direction—normal; biphasic flow signifies reversal flow with incompetence.

DUPLEX SCAN

Duplex scan is a highly reliable ultrasound Doppler imaging technique (here high resolution B mode ultrasound imaging and Doppler ultrasound is used) which along with direct visualisation of veins, gives the functional and anatomical information, and also colour map. Examination is done in standing and lying down position and also with *Valsalva manoeuvre*. Hand held Doppler probe is placed over the site and visualised for any block and reversal of flow. DVT is very well identified by this method. All patients with varicose vein should be assessed preoperatively by ultrasound with *proper venous mapping (Venous haemodynamical mapping; VHM; Cartography)*—i.e. marking on the patient's limb manually using permanent marker under ultrasound guidance. All surgeries should be done with on table ultrasound guidance. Post-operatively, all patients should be assessed using ultrasound for result, and for residual venous diseases. VHM is done in standing; in warm room with adequate time **(Figs. 12-1 to 12-4)**.

Air Plethysmography

Patient is initially in supine position with veins emptied by elevation of leg. Air filled plastic pressure bladder (inflatable polyurethane cuff filled with air) is placed on calf to detect volume changes. Minimum volume is recorded. Patient is turned to upright position and venous volume is assessed. Maximum venous volume divided by time required to achieve maximum venous volume gives the *venous filling index (VFI)*. VFI is a measure of reflux. *Ejection fraction* is volume change measured prior and after single tiptoe manoeuvre, which is a measure of calf pump action. *Residual venous fraction* is an index of overall venous function which is venous volume in the leg after ten toetip manoeuvres divided by venous volume prior to manoeuvre. Patients with *increased VFI and diminished ejection fraction will benefit from surgery* **(Fig. 12-5)**.

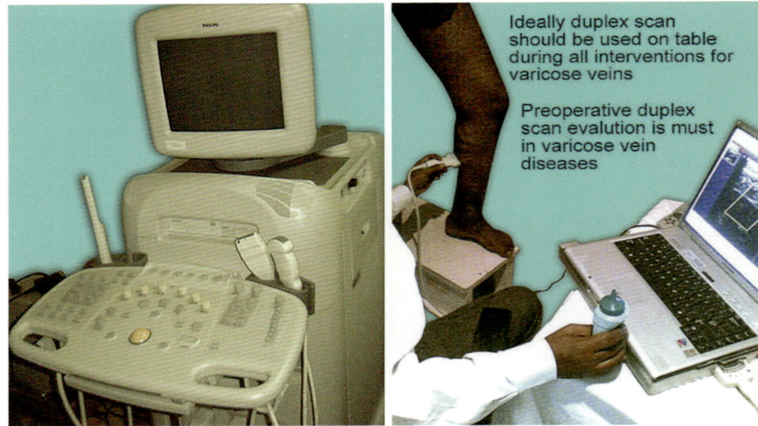

Fig. 12-1: Duplex scan (with Doppler) machine used for varicose veins and DVT. Preoperative duplex scan, marking of veins and on table duplex scan is a must in managing varicose vein diseases.

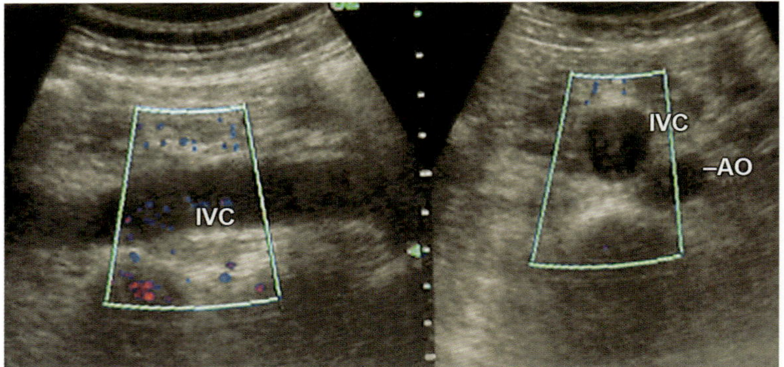

Fig. 12-2: Ultrasound showing IVC thrombosis.

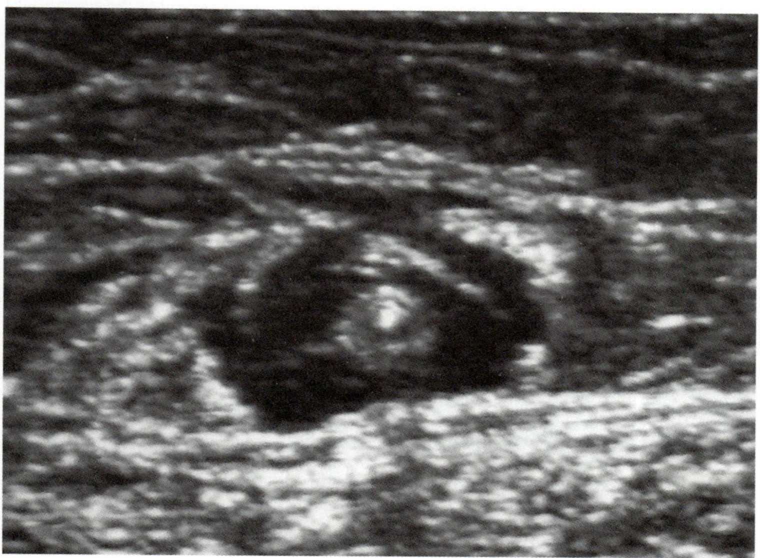

Fig. 12-3: Saphenous eye—as seen in US duplex scan.

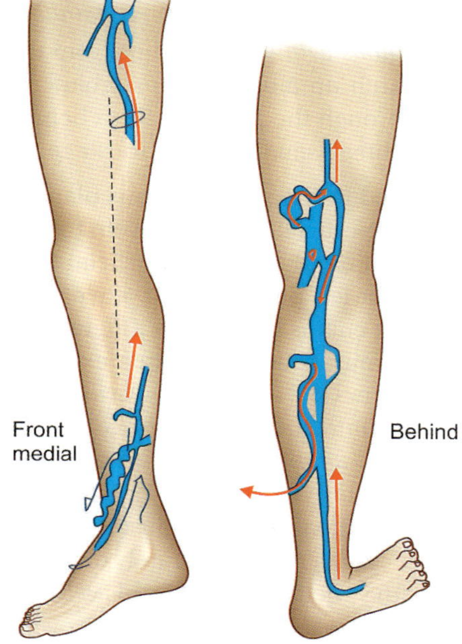

Fig. 12-4: Venous haemodynamic mapping (VHM) of the lower limb.

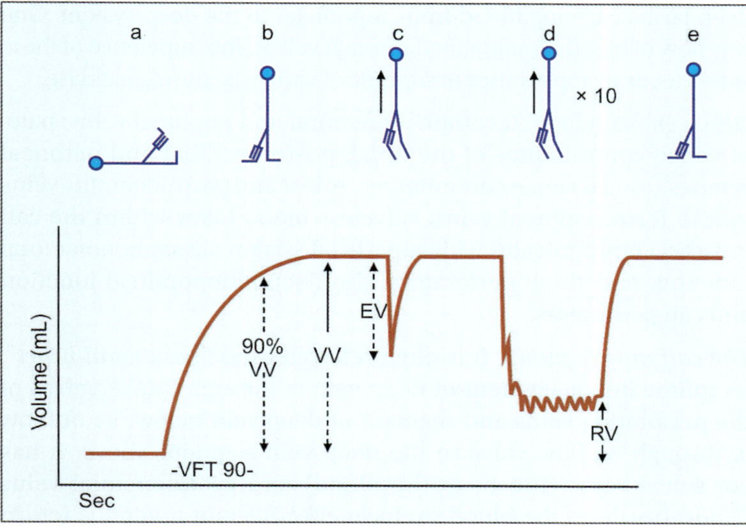

Fig. 12-5: Air plethysmography.

Venography/Phlebography

Ascending venography was a very common investigation done earlier to Doppler period.

A tourniquet is tied above the malleoli and the vein of dorsal venous arch of the foot is cannulated. Water soluble dye injected flows into the deep veins (because the applied tourniquet prevents its flow into superficial veins). X-rays are taken below and above the knee level. Any block in deep veins, its extent, perforator status can be made out by this.

Note:

In the presence of Duplex scan ascending venography is not a necessary investigation. If deep vein thrombosis (DVT) is present, surgery or sclerotherapy are contraindicated.

Descending venogram is done when ascending venogram is not possible and also to visualise incompetent veins. Here contrast material is injected into the femoral vein through a cannula in standing position. X-ray pictures are taken to visualise deep veins and incompetent veins.

Phlebography

- Ascending phlebography defines obstruction.
- Descending phlebography identifies valvular incompetence.
- Regularly not required to be done.

Levels of Investigations

Level I: History, examination with Trendelenburg test, hand held Doppler scanner.

Level II: Non-invasive—Duplex scan, air plethysmography.

Level III: Invasive and complex imaging—descending and ascending venography; venous pressure measurement; CT scan; venous helical scanning; magnetic resonance imaging (MRI).

Note:

Advanced CEAP (continuous positive airway pressure) classification is used now rather than basic CEAP.

VCSS (Venous Clinical Severity Scoring) is also useful **(Table 12-1)**.

Intravenous ultrasound (IVUS) is the new form of assessment of the veins especially inferior vena cava (IVC), iliac and femoral veins **(Figs. 12-6A to C)**.

TABLE 12-1: VCSS system.

	None – 0	*Mild – 1*	*Moderate – 2*	*Severe – 3*
Pain	None	Occasional; no restriction of daily activity	Daily that only interferes with daily activity	Daily pain that prevents from working
Varicose veins	None	Few scattered branch vein varicosities; >5 blue telangiectases on the inner part of foot—ankle flare	Multiple varicosities of calf or thigh	Multiple varicosities of both calf and thigh
Inflammation	None	Perimalleolar area	Lower 1/3rd calf	More than lower 1/3rd of calf
Induration	None	Perimalleolar area	Lower 1/3rd calf	More than lower 1/3rd of calf
Active ulcer duration	No active ulcer	<3 months	3–12 months	>12 months
Other parameters similarly				

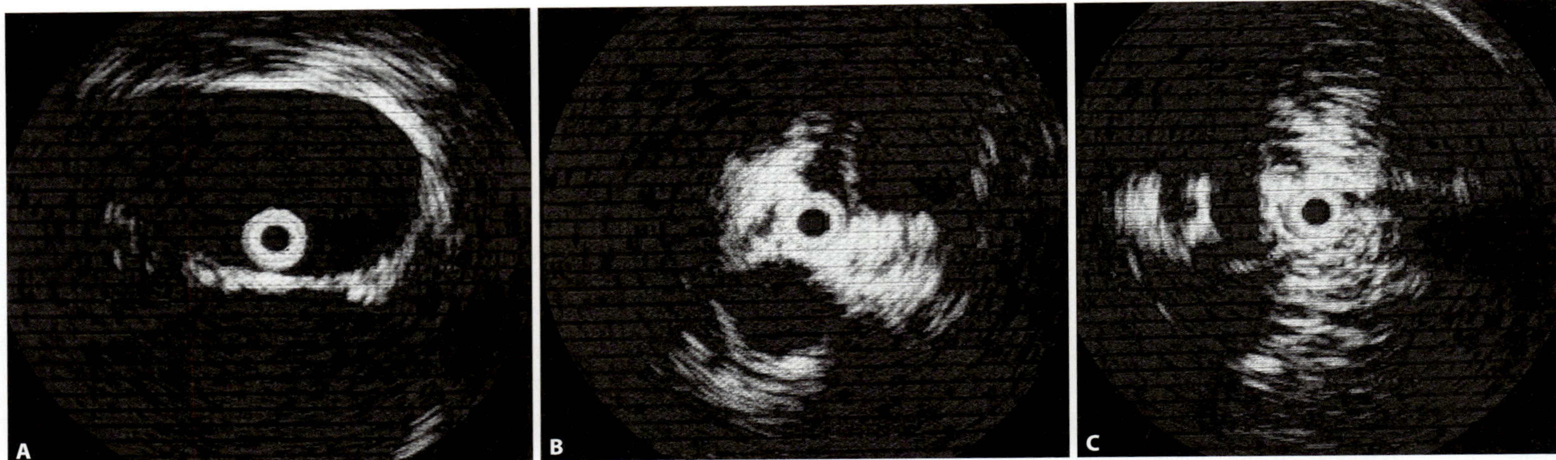

Figs. 12-6A to C: Intravenous ultrasound (IVUS) showing: (A) Inferior vena cava; (B) External iliac vein web; (C) Popliteal vein thrombus.

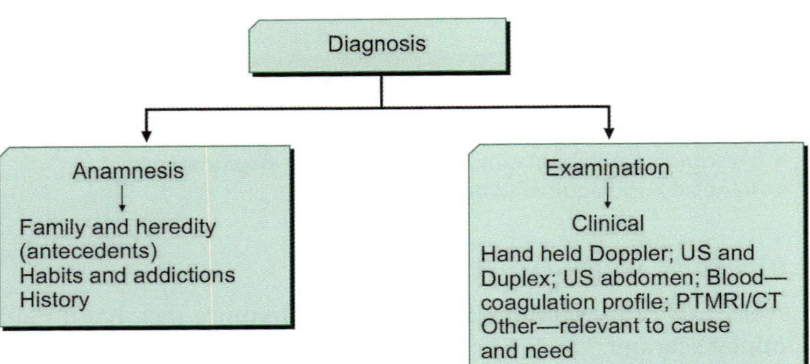

SURGICAL ANATOMY OF LOWER LIMB VEINS (FIG. 12-7)

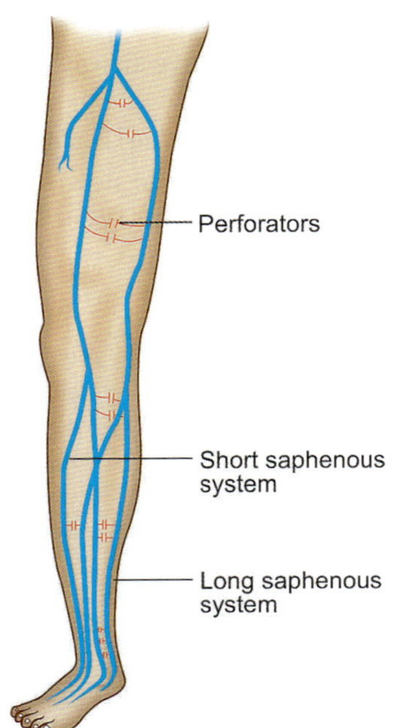

Fig. 12-7: Anatomy of lower limb veins.

Superficial Venous System

It is located in the saphenous compartment which is between subcutaneous plane and deeper aponeurotic plane. GSV and SSV are in this plane.

Great (Long) saphenous vein (GSV): It runs from the medial end of the dorsal venous arch up along the anteromedial aspect of the leg and thigh until it empties into the femoral vein. There is one valve at the junction—is called as *ostial/terminal* valve and reflux through it is called as *ostial reflux*. One more valve proximal to the main junctional tributary veins is called as *preterminal valve*. More than 50% reflux occurs at preterminal valve (*preterminal reflux*).

Small (Short) saphenous vein (SSV): It runs from the lateral end of the dorsal venous arch up along the posterolateral aspect of the calf until it passes through the popliteal fossa behind the knee and empties into the popliteal vein just above the knee.

Tributaries are located in the subcutaneous plane which joins the saphenous system. Superficial circumflex vein (often joins AAGSV), superficial external pudendal vein, superficial inferior epigastric vein, anterior vein of the leg, posterior arch vein of the leg (joins GSV), posterolateral venous chains of leg—are different tributaries. Long intersaphenous communicating vein often exists between cranial extension of SSV to join GSV and can be varicose and pathological and is called as *communicating vein of Giacomini-Cruveilhier*. *Anterior accessory great saphenous vein (AAGSV, Anterolateral vein of thigh)* is communicating vein into the GSV anteriorly and laterally. AAGSV communicates into GSV usually just proximal to preterminal valve (60%); often at confluence (39%); rarely onto femoral vein (1%). In many patients with varicose veins, it is this vein which is diseased than GSV. It often receives superficial circumflex vein before joining the GSV **(Figs. 12-8A and B)**.

Perforator system of veins (communicating veins): They pass through the deep fascia carrying blood from superficial to the deep system. One way flow of blood is maintained through valves. Incompetence of these valves leads to appearance of superficial varicosity during exercise.

Deep venous system: It comprises femoral and popliteal veins; pairs of venae commitantes of the tibial, posterior tibial and peroneal arteries (total 6 venae commitantes, soleal and gastrocnemius veins join to form popliteal vein); valveless blood lakes within the calf muscles communicates with superficial system via saphenofemoral junction, mid-thigh perforators, short saphenopopliteal junction and calf perforators.

The calf muscle pump: It is often referred to as *"peripheral heart"*. Its inflow into a segment of deep vein is through intake valves of the perforating veins and segment of deep vein below. Its outflow is through outflow valve to the deep vein segment above. It has got soleal veins (blush up the blood) and gastrocnemial veins (*Gilot*) (push up the blood) to have effective motor venous return **(Figs. 12-9A to D)**.

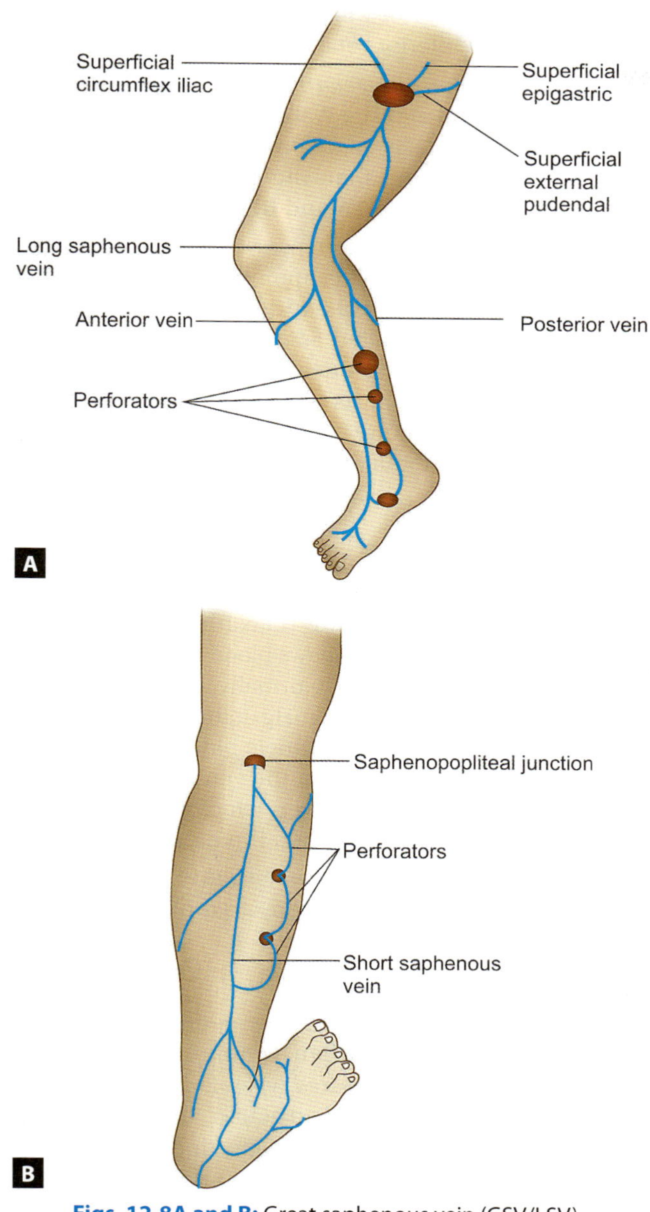

Figs. 12-8A and B: Great saphenous vein (GSV/LSV), small saphenous vein (SSV) and perforators.

DIFFERENT TYPES OF PERFORATORS

Para Achillean *(Bassi)*; **Ankle perforators**; (*May or Kuster*); **Lower leg perforators** between deep veins and posterior arch vein *(Cockett)*: I (posteroinferior to medial malleolus), II (10 cm above the medial malleolus), III (15 cm above medial malleolus); **Gastrocnemius perforators** between GSV and deep veins—upper proximal paratibial *(Boyd)*—below knee; **Lower and medial paratibial** (*Sherman*); *24 cm perforator* between deep veins and GSV; **Mid-thigh perforator** between deep vein and GSV *(Dodd)*; **Hach perforator in the posterior thigh; Hunter's adductor canal perforator** in the thigh **(Fig. 12-10)**.

PHYSIOLOGY OF VENOUS BLOOD FLOW IN LOWER LIMB

Veins are thin walled vessels with collapsible walls that assume an elliptical configuration in collapsed state and circular configuration in the filled state. Venous valves are abundant in the distal lower

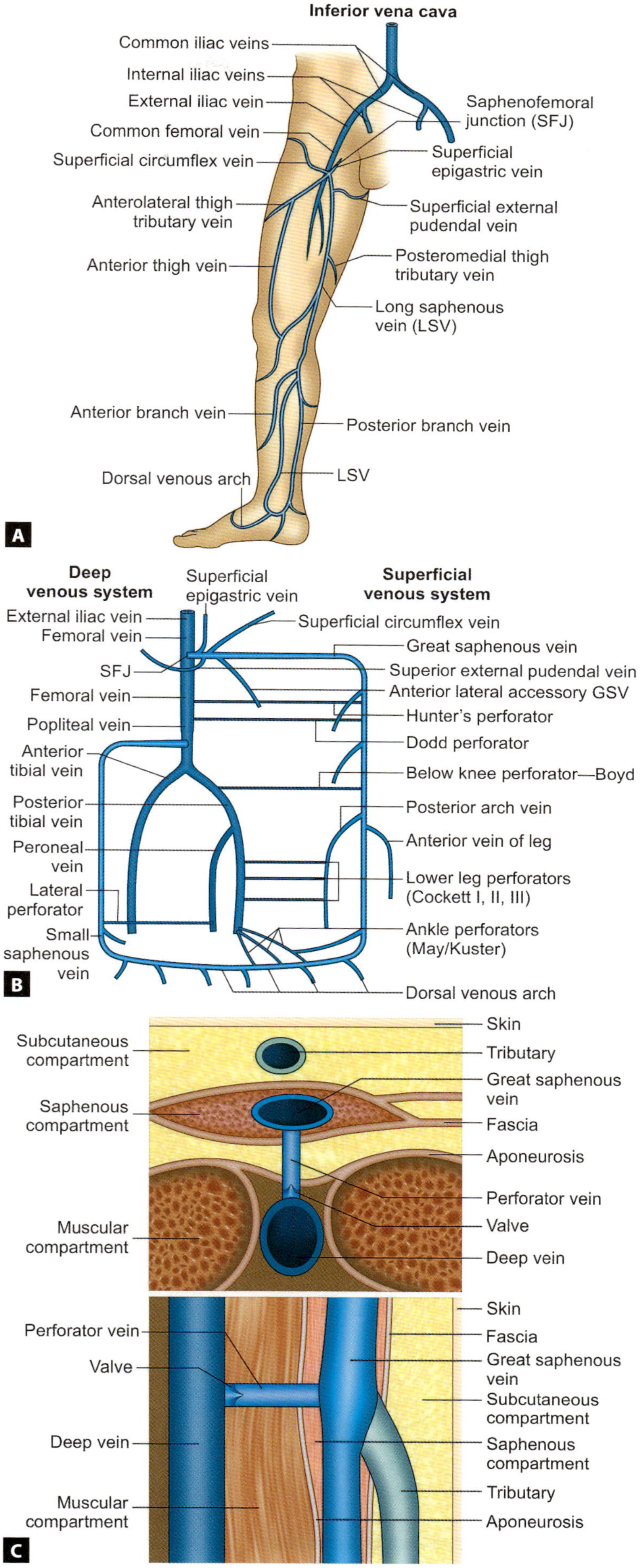

Figs. 12-9A to C

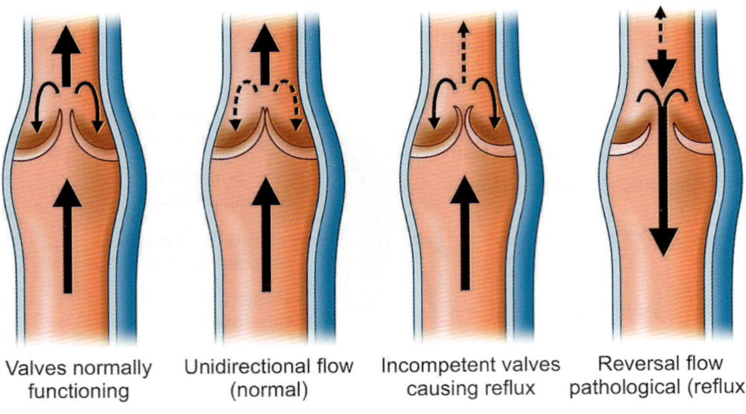

Fig. 12-9D

Figs. 12-9A to D: Diagrams showing venous anatomy of the lower limb. Also note the functioning of the valve in the vein.

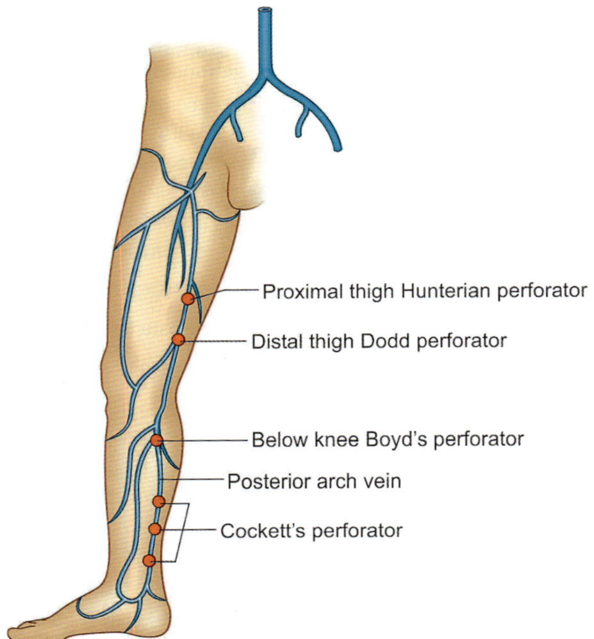

Fig. 12-10: Diagram showing different perforators.

extremity and the number of valves decreases proximally, with no valves in superior and inferior vena cava.

Venous pressure at the ankle with normal legs: Recumbent—10 mmHg; Standing—90 mm Hg; Walking—25-35 mmHg. The effect of calf and ankle pumps takes place only after 7 steps. The elasticity of a vein is 200 times more than the one of an artery; they are capacitance vessels **(Figs. 12-11A and B)**.

Muscular pump in the legs are four types—foot pump (plantar veins); leg pump (soleus muscle); popliteal pump (gastrocnemius muscle); thigh pump (semimembranosus and biceps muscles). Leg and popliteal pumps together called as calf pump which is essential for proper venous haemodynamics and is truly peripheral heart. Soleal veins have got two parts—medioseptal and lateroseptal. Medial gastrocnemius veins are bigger in popliteal pump which has got anterolateral and posterolateral trunks.

Factors affecting venous return are: (a) Arterial pressure across the capillary increases the pumping action of vein; (b) *Calf musculovenous pump:* During contraction phase of walking, pressure in the calf muscles increases to 200–300 mmHg; This pumps the blood towards the heart; During relaxation phase of walking, pressure in the calf falls and so it allows blood to flow from superficial to deep veins through perforators; Normally while walking, pressure in the superficial system is 20–30 mmHg at the level of ankle; During walking, foot pump mechanism propels blood from plantar veins into the leg; (c) Gravity. Pressure in the vena cava where it enters the right atrium is very low (-5 mmHg) which allows rapid filling of vena cava from high pressure peripheral veins.

Factors responsible for venous return: Negative pressure in thorax; Peripheral pump—calf muscle; *Vis-a-tergo* of adjoining muscle; Non-refluxing valves in course of veins.

VENOUS PATHOLOGY

Venous pathology develops when venous return is impaired. It can be of *deep, superficial or mixed types.* It can be due to primary muscle pump failure, venous obstruction, and venous valvular incompetence. It may be segmental or affecting the entire leg. Here venous wall shows increase in collagen and reduction in elastin. *Causes of primary muscle pump failure are*—muscle wasting, neuromuscular disease, deep fasciotomies, local vein valve failure. It leads to non-reduction of postambulatory pressure; causes increased hydrostatic pressure and thus decreased arterial inflow.

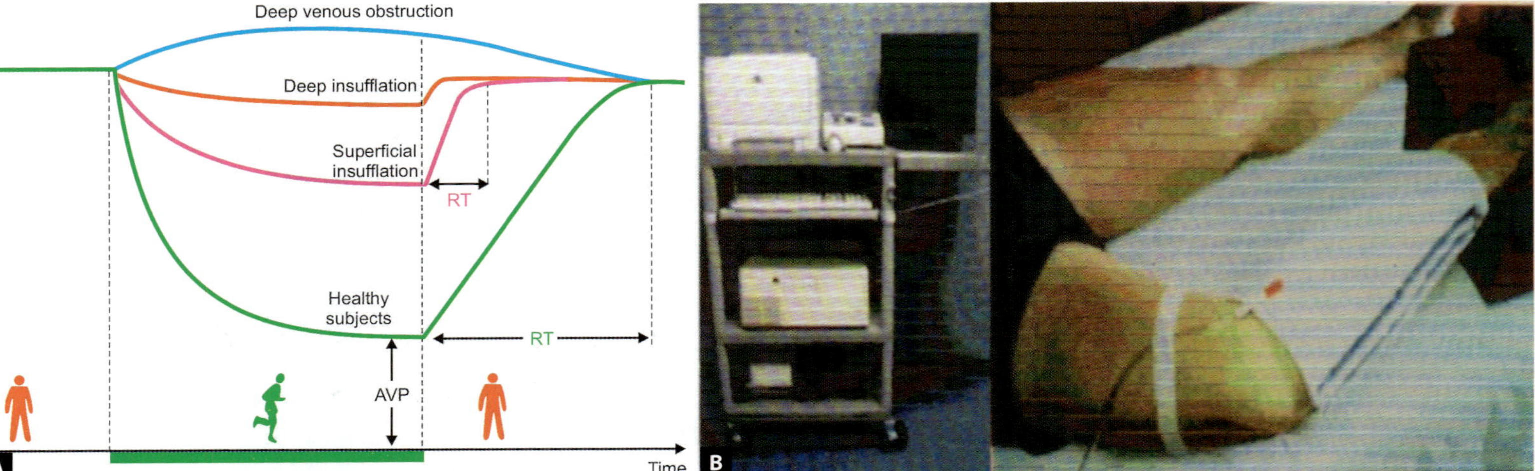

Figs. 12-11A and B: Ambulatory venous pressure is one of the important methods to evaluate venous system.

Present concept is inflammatory pathology of the venous wall and valve. Present theory is a changed concept from top to bottom with segmental pathophysiology. So VHM (venous mapping) is essential prior to surgical intervention.

Incompetence can be of three types—perforator; superficial and deep.

Perforator incompetence is reversal of normal flow across the perforators. Normal flow is from superficial veins to deep veins. Perforator valve failure causes deep to superficial reflux causing congestion and venous hypertension. It causes transmission of extreme high pressure (150–200 mmHg) generated at the deep veins into the superficial veins. This high pressure reflux (*hydrodynamic reflux*) causes distal valvular incompetence of the superficial venous system causing varicosity and its problems. Problems here are more rapid and progressive than just superficial vein incompetence.

Superficial vein incompetence is the most common form of the venous disease. It shows retrograde flow (*hydrostatic reflux*) due to malfunctioning of valves. It is the tributaries which commonly become incompetent and diseased as it is in subcutaneous plane with less support and also has thin muscle layer in the wall. Here effects are slow and gradual.

Deep incompetence may be isolated incompetence of deep veins or may be associated with incompetence of superficial venous system. Here blood pumped out in normal volumes but extremity refill includes normal arterial inflow and also pathological reflux. Venous refill is rapid with normal or elevated ambulatory venous pressure **(Fig. 12-12)**.

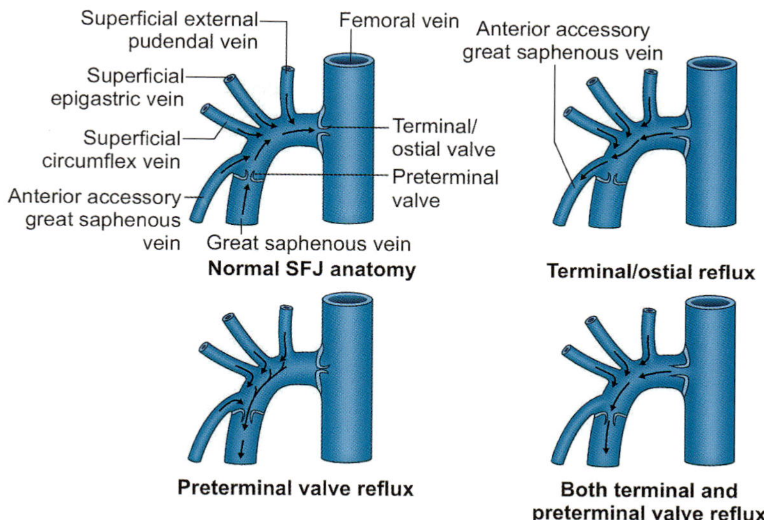

Fig. 12-12: Great saphenous vein anatomy at its saphenofemoral junction showing reflux.

MANAGEMENT OF VARICOSE VEIN DISEASE

One has to remember that varicose vein is a disease with progressive deterioration. Surgeon should not jump to do surgery to every patient with varicose vein. Selection of the case for surgical intervention is very important. It is done to relieve significant symptoms, reverse or reduce skin changes, to promote healing of the ulcers. Cosmesis and treating the asymptomatic uncomplicated varicose veins for prophylaxis are also the mentioned indications, but surgeon should be careful and should clearly discuss with the patient properly the drawbacks of interventions.

Venous mapping *is mandatory* prior to surgery. *Duplex scan with Doppler should be used always during all intervention procedures for varicose veins* **(Figs. 12-13 and 12-14)**.

Venous interventions are required as:

- Superficial vein surgery.
- Venous stenting.
- Deep venous valve reconstruction.
- Venous bypass.
- As compression therapies.

Contraindications for Surgery

DVT is an *absolute contraindication* for surgery.

Pregnancy, females taking contraceptive pills and recent episode of superficial thrombophlebitis are *relative* contraindications.

Indications for interventional procedures:

- **Complaints** which are relevant like pain, discomfort.
- **Complications.**
- **Cosmesis.**

Endovenous ablation can be thermal or chemical. Thermal ablations (TA) are—radiofrequency (RFT) or laser ablation. Chemical are liquid or foam sclerotherapy (FS). Venous mapping is mandatory for all mapping. Presently recommendation is all endovenous therapies should be done under US guidance. FS is simpler than TA. TA and FS both are effective, simple and safe. TA is more effective for vein >5 mm. FS is appropriate for recurrent and complex varicosities.

TRENDELENBURG OPERATION (SAPHENOFEMORAL CROSSECTOMY) AND/OR STRIPPING

It is *juxtafemoral flush ligation* of long saphenous vein (flush with femoral vein) after ligating named (superficial circumflex, superficial external pudendal, and superficial epigastric vein) and unnamed tributaries. Anomalies of great saphenous vein (GSV) should be remembered. Double saphenous vein is the commonest anomaly occurring near SFJ.

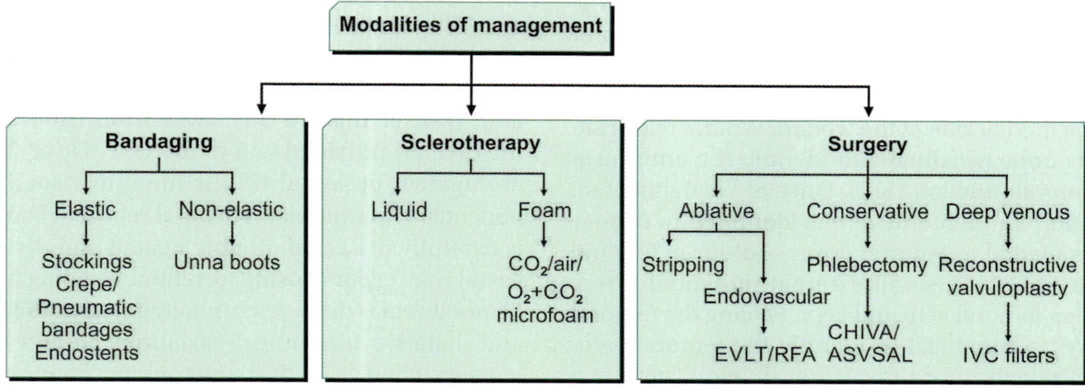

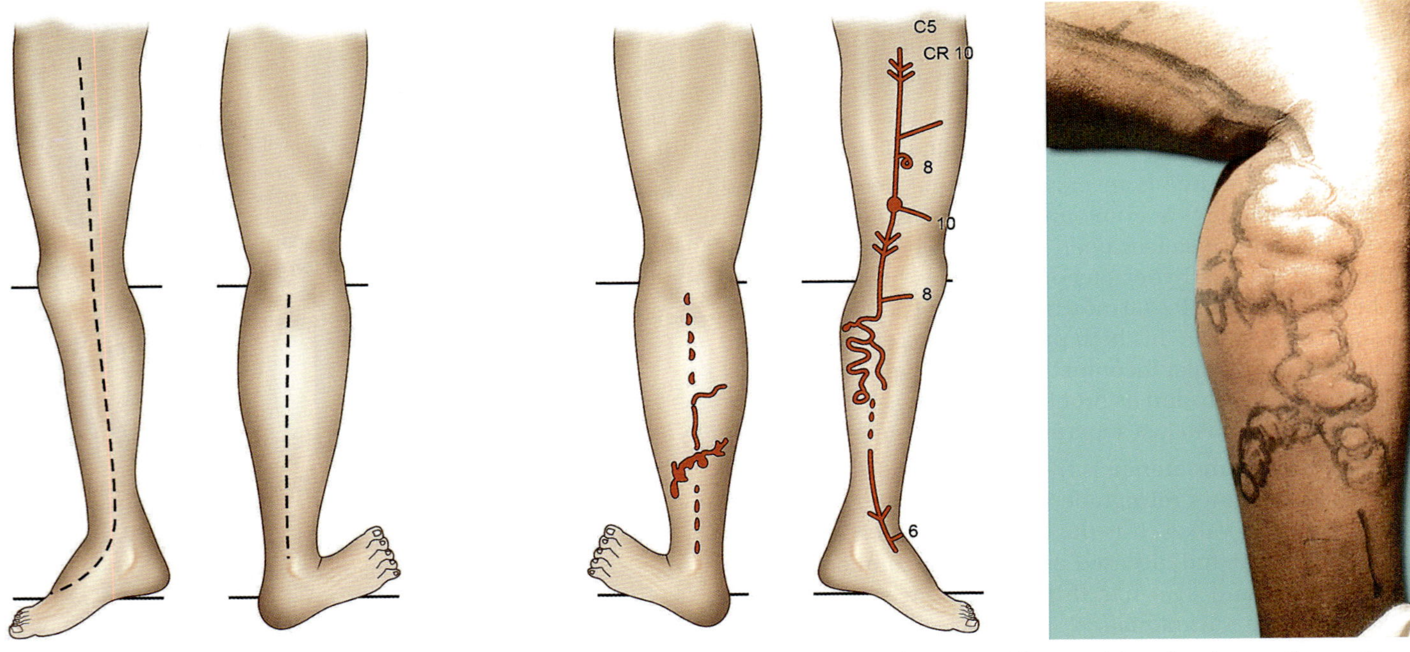

Fig. 12-13: Venous mapping should be done prior to any intervention to varicose veins. It is done using US scan with patient in *standing position*.

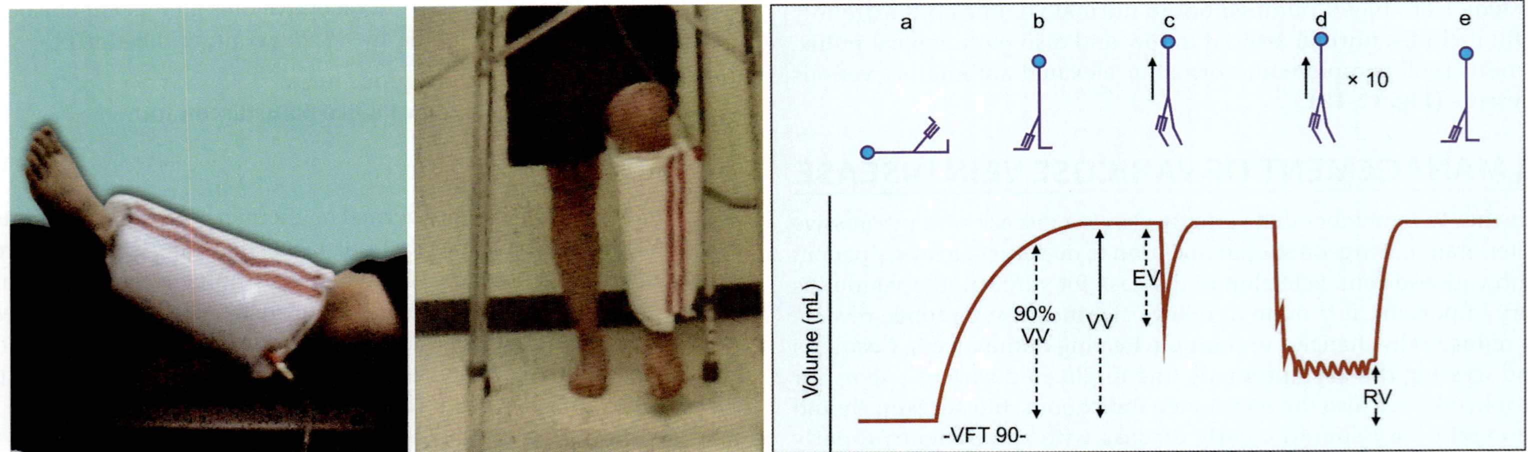

Fig. 12-14: Air plethysmography.

Procedure

It is done under spinal/epidural/general anaesthesia. Just prior to giving anaesthesia all dilated veins and perforators should be marked with proper marker in standing position. Marking can be done using Duplex scan with Doppler. It is ideal to use Doppler with duplex scan during procedure also.

Entire limb, groin and perineum from ankle is cleaned and draped. Patient is placed in supine position with knee slightly flexed and rotated externally. Saphenous opening is marked which is 3–4 cm below and lateral to pubic tubercle. Horizontal incision of 6 cm length is placed at this point at the crease. Subcutaneous fat, membranous layer of superficial fascia (Scarpa's fascia) is incised. GSV is identified on the medial side of the wound. Wound edges are retraced. Dissection is done proximally to identify the cribriform fascia and saphenofemoral junction (SFJ). Once SFJ is delineated, SFJ is dissected all round and femoral vein is identified in deeper plane. Femoral vein is medial to femoral artery. Colour of femoral vein differs from that of GSV. A small external pudendal artery often may cross between femoral vein and GSV. Feeling the femoral arterial pulsation may be beneficial to identify the femoral vein. Care should be taken not to injure the femoral vein. There is a possibility of developing inadvertent tear at SFJ causing severe bleeding. In such situation blind application of the haemostat should be avoided. First head end is lowered to reduce the venous pressure; firm pressure over the site using a mop facilitates proper identification of the site of bleed which is ligated using polypropylene sutures. Superficial external pudendal, superficial external (circumflex) iliac, superficial epigastric veins are identified and dissected until they reach to their further tributaries. These smaller tributaries are dissected individually, ligated and divided. Other unnamed tributaries along the length of 3 cm of GSV from SFJ are also dissected, ligated and divided. All these smaller tributaries are ligated using 3-zero/2-zero vicryl. Finally main named tributaries are ligated. Often it is done after transecting the GSV away from tributaries level and lifting the divided proximal end of the GSV. Once three main tributaries are ligated, proximal GSV is lifted to visualise the deep external pudendal vein which joins femoral vein or SFJ on medial side. This vein is carefully dissected, double ligated and divided. Avulsion of this vessel may occur causing torrential bleeding from the femoral vein. Femoral vein is dissected carefully adjacent to SFJ for 2 cm proximally and distally. Anatomical variations should be considered in all patients while dissecting which are not common **(Figs. 12-15A to J)**.

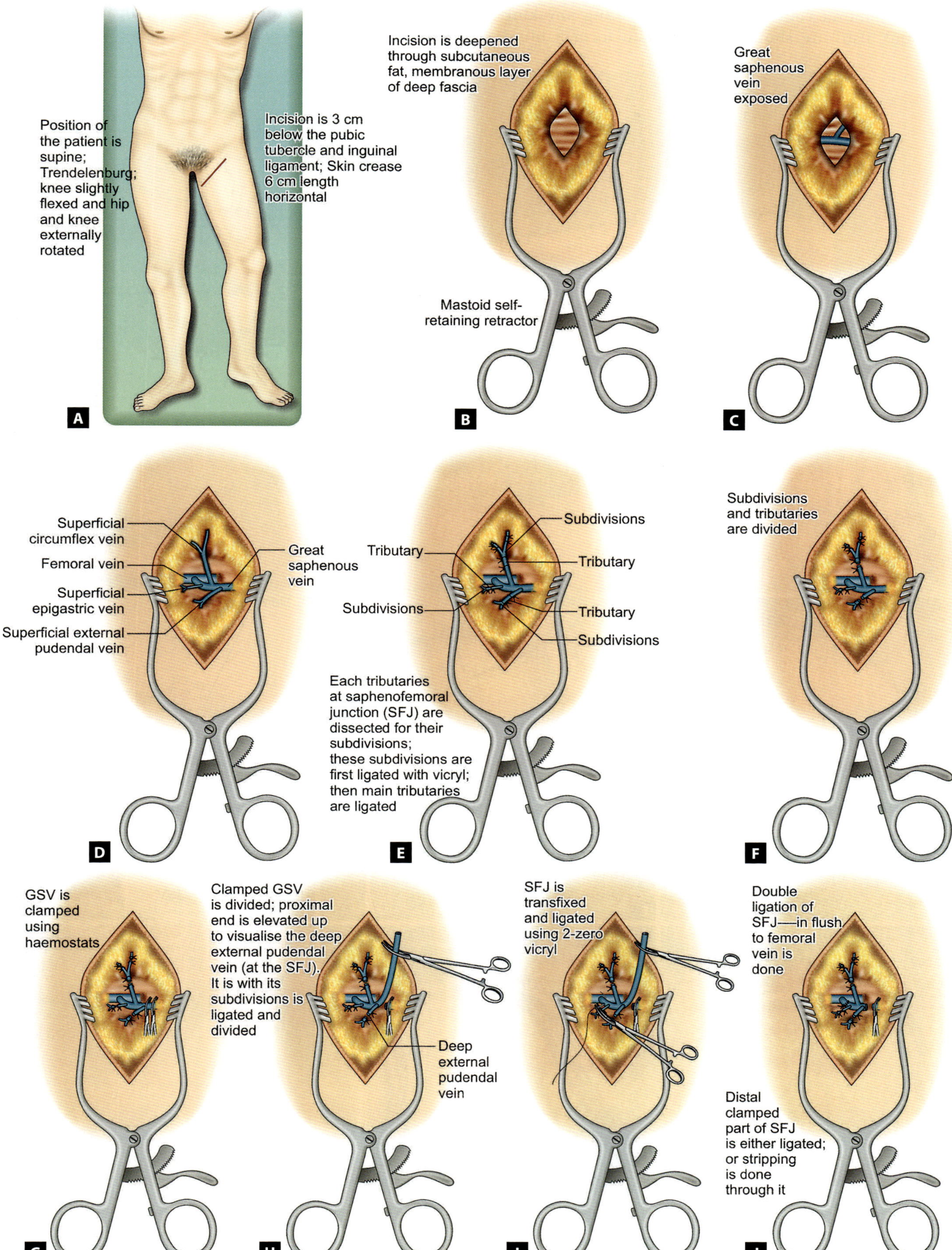

Figs. 12-15A to J: Diagram showing steps of saphenofemoral flush ligation.

GSV is transfixed and ligated using 2-zero vicryl suture on the wall of the femoral vein flush without creating any kink to the vein and also one should not allow to form a blind pouch by doing ligation little distal to the SFJ which may later create *saphena varix*. Additional simple ligature is also placed **(Figs. 12-16A to Y)**.

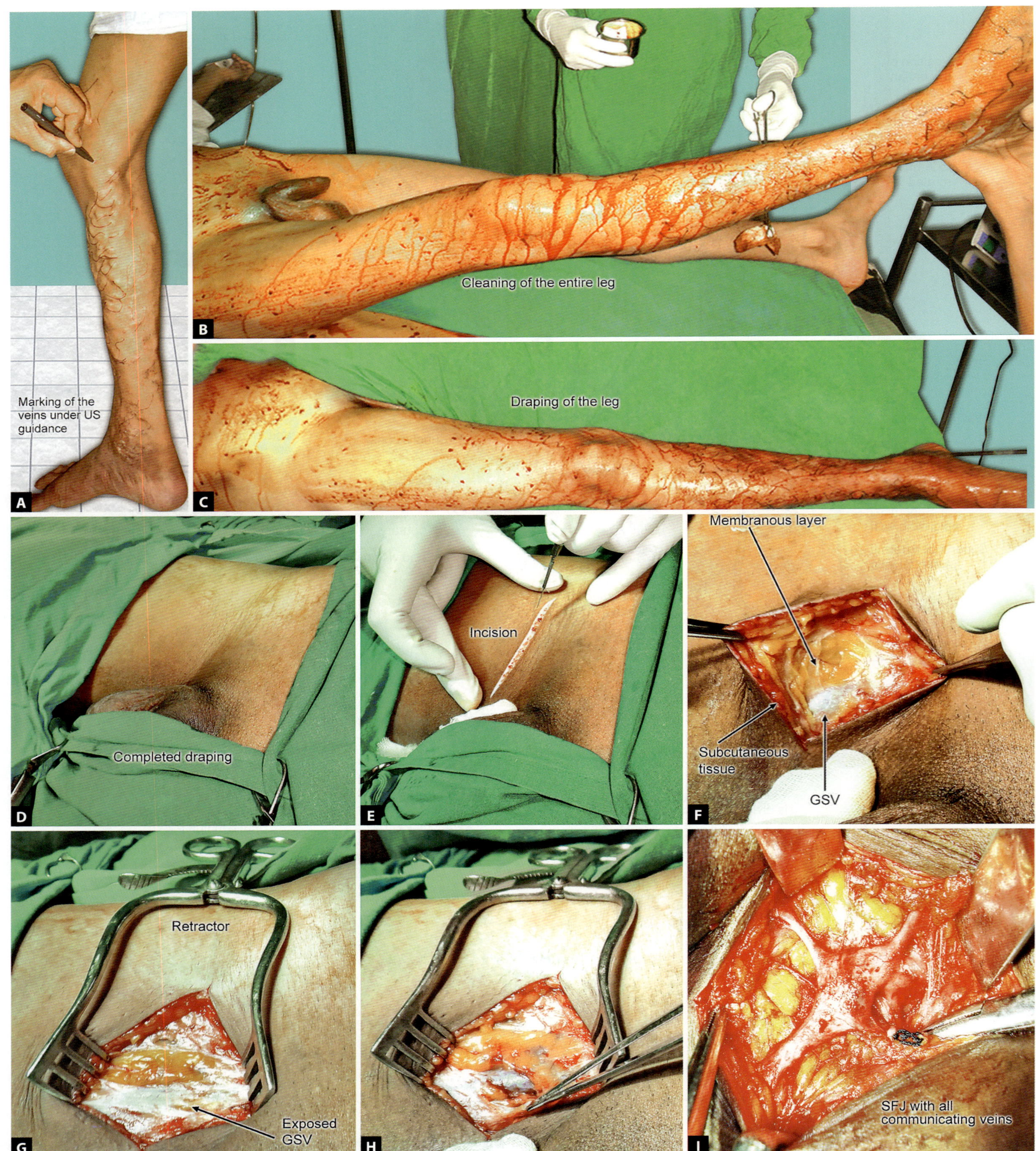

Figs. 12-16A to I

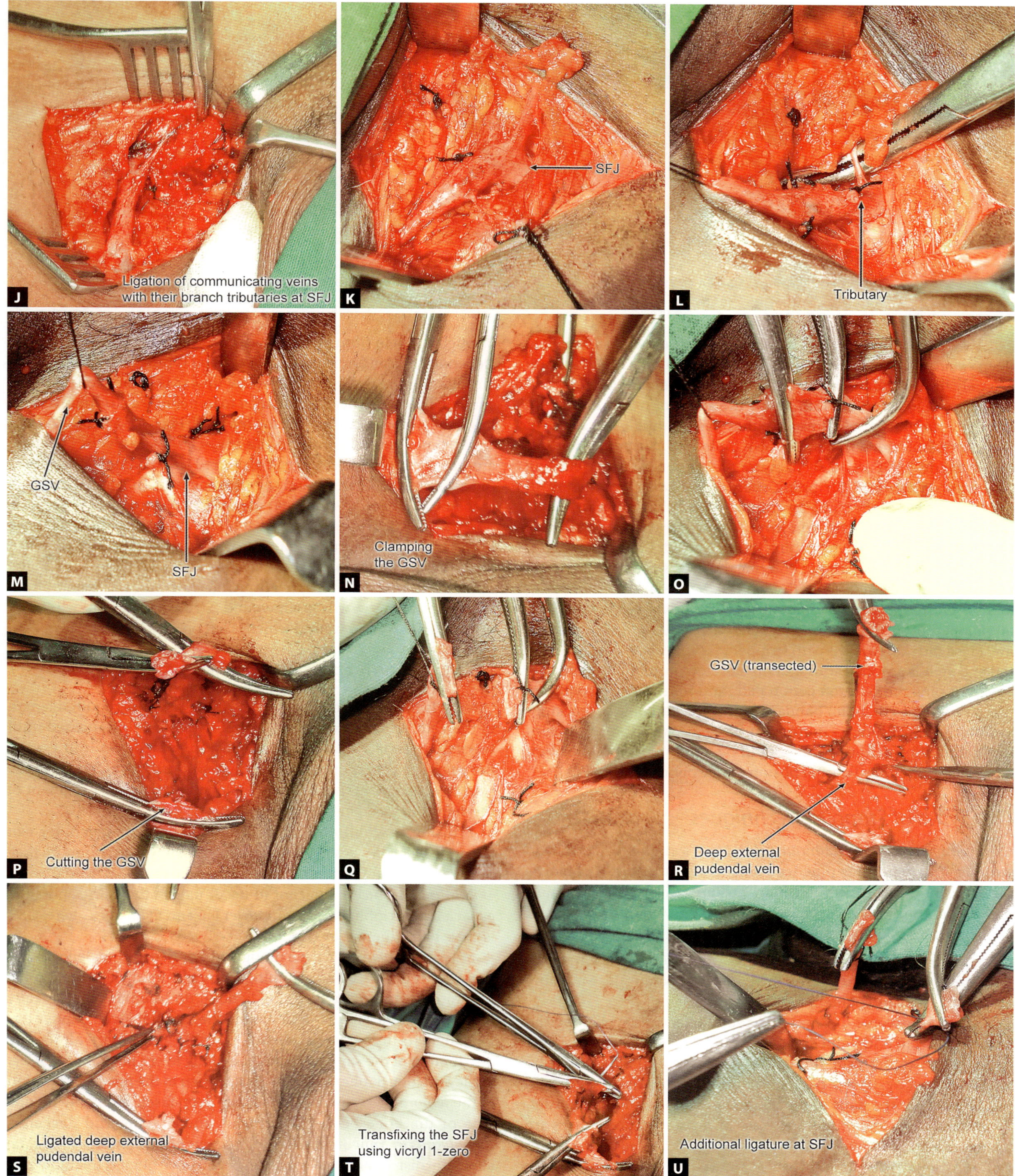

Figs. 12-16J to U

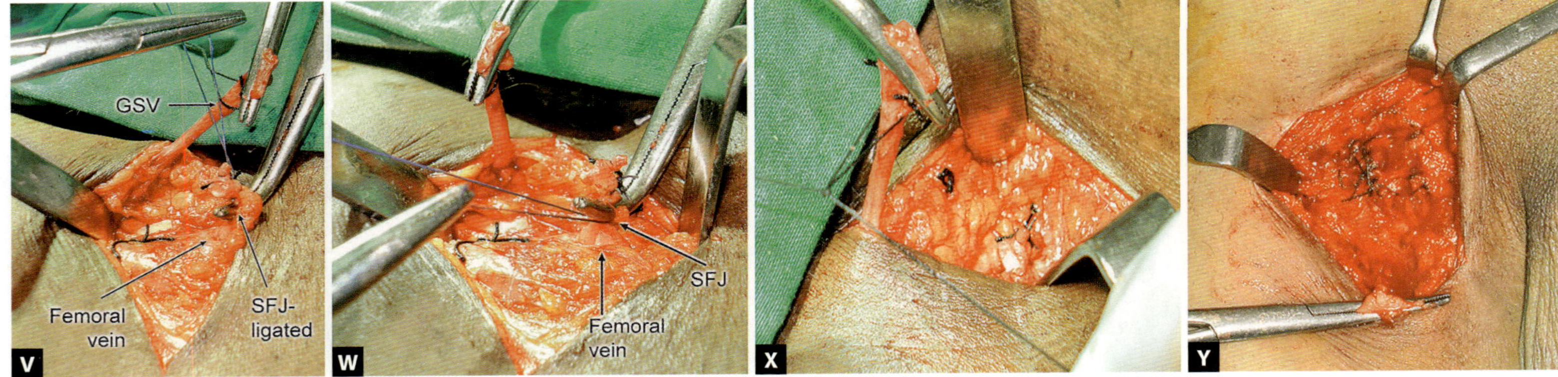

Figs. 12-16V to Y

Figs. 12-16A to Y: Saphenofemoral flush ligation for varicose veins—operative steps.

Lower part of the wound is retracted to expose the posteromedial deep external pudendal vein and other tributaries of GSV which are securely ligated. Remaining tributaries up to the middle of the calf (or up to 4 cm/hand breadth below the knee joint line to include Boyd's perforator) are addressed either by stripping or by series of small incisions along the line of GSV (ablation). Stripping the GSV below the mid-calf will likely to injure the saphenous nerve causing *saphenous neuralgia*. Stripping *should preferably be done* from above downwards after passing stripper from below upwards. *Many advocate* stripping of the vein from below upwards and is said to be technically easier with keeping limb elevated. But here injury to saphenous nerve and stripper entering the deep system are the likely complications to occur even though incidences are low. *Stripping avulses all significant thigh perforators.* It is advisable to complete all planned procedures like foam sclerotherapy/multiple avulsions and close the skin wounds with stripper placed ready for stripping; at the end vein is stripped with limb in elevated position. Immediately after stripping the vein soft cotton pads and roller dressing pads are placed from toes to groin; bandage and crepe bandage or stockings are placed. Stripping is done with limb in elevation to prevent haematoma formation. Limb should be kept in elevated position adequately (3 pillows) during postoperative period.

Two Types of Stripping Techniques

Extraluminal collision technique using Myer's stripper (Acorn head stripper, 73 cm long) is practiced since long time; but it damages the adjacent tissue, causes infection, postoperative pain, discomfort and haematoma along the stripped track with possibility of revascularisation of the track haematoma.

Invagination technique is better with less damage to adjacent tissue. *Codman's stripper* is used for invagination technique. Stripping avulses the vein and obliterates the tributaries.

A small transverse incision is made at mid-calf level along the line of GSV. Vein is identified and dissected. Saphenous nerve which is very close to the vein should be separated and should not be injured. Vicryl ligature is passed to distal part of the isolated vein. After ligating it, the ends of the ligature are lifted using haemostat. Proximal to this, an additional 2-zero or 3-zero vicryl ligatures are passed around and temporarily held with two haemostats without tying. Proximal to ligature vein is held by two haemostats and anterior part of the vein is incised between two haemostats. It is better to place two 3-zero vicryl stitches instead of two haemostats and vein is incised between these two ties. Olive tip of the Myer's stripper is passed through the vein from below upwards towards groin crease wound. Depending on surgeon's choice *acorn head* is threaded into the lower end if stripping is done from below upwards (practiced by many surgeons) or acorn head is threaded to upper end if stripping is done from above downwards (*technically ideal*) **(Figs. 12-17 and 12-18)**.

Proximal vicryl ligature in the mid-calf wound vein is ligated around the threaded acorn head of desired size. Wound is closed over the acorn head. Cleaning and soft dressing pads (roller dressings are placed to the wounds and leg) along with elevation of the limb is done. An elastic crepe bandage is applied from toes to groin up to the level just below the groin wound. Groin wound is also closed in two layers except for the part where stripper end with handle is coming out. With full elevation stripper is pulled with jerky movements from below upwards towards groin wound. Stripper with vein will come out. Part of the groin wound which is left open is sutured.

Problems with SFJ Ligation and/or Stripping

Often it is not possible to pass the stripper to entire required length of the vein. In such occasion stripper with olive tip is passed until resistance develops and a small incision is made on it to expose the vein. The vein is opened and stripper is further guided along the vein or stripping of this segment is done and later next segment of the vein is stripped in 2–3 parts.

Bruising, discomfort, pain, haematoma and oedema of leg can occur. Usually they resolve spontaneously in few days; rarely do they require drainage. Elevation and stockings are essential needs.

Multiple leg ulcers adjacent to lower part of the shin is possible especially if stripping is done in lower leg and at ankle, as here, GSV is close and adherent to skin.

Saphenous neuralgia even though mentioned, its incidence is less than 1%. It occurs when stripping is done from distal to proximal. It is more common if stripping is done up to ankle level. Ideally stripping should not be done below the midcalf level. Saphenous neuralgia is hyperesthesia and burning sensation along the distribution of the saphenous nerve—along lower medial part of leg, ankle and foot. Saphenous nerve is a branch of the posterior division of the *femoral nerve* which pierces the deep fascia along the medial side of the knee between sartorius and gracilis and descends *downwards in front* of the GSV. *Small areas of numbness and tingling* along the distribution are common occurrence but it is tolerable and acceptable to the patient.

DVT after varicose vein surgery and stripping can occur. Elevation and stockings prevent formation of DVT. It is advisable to have

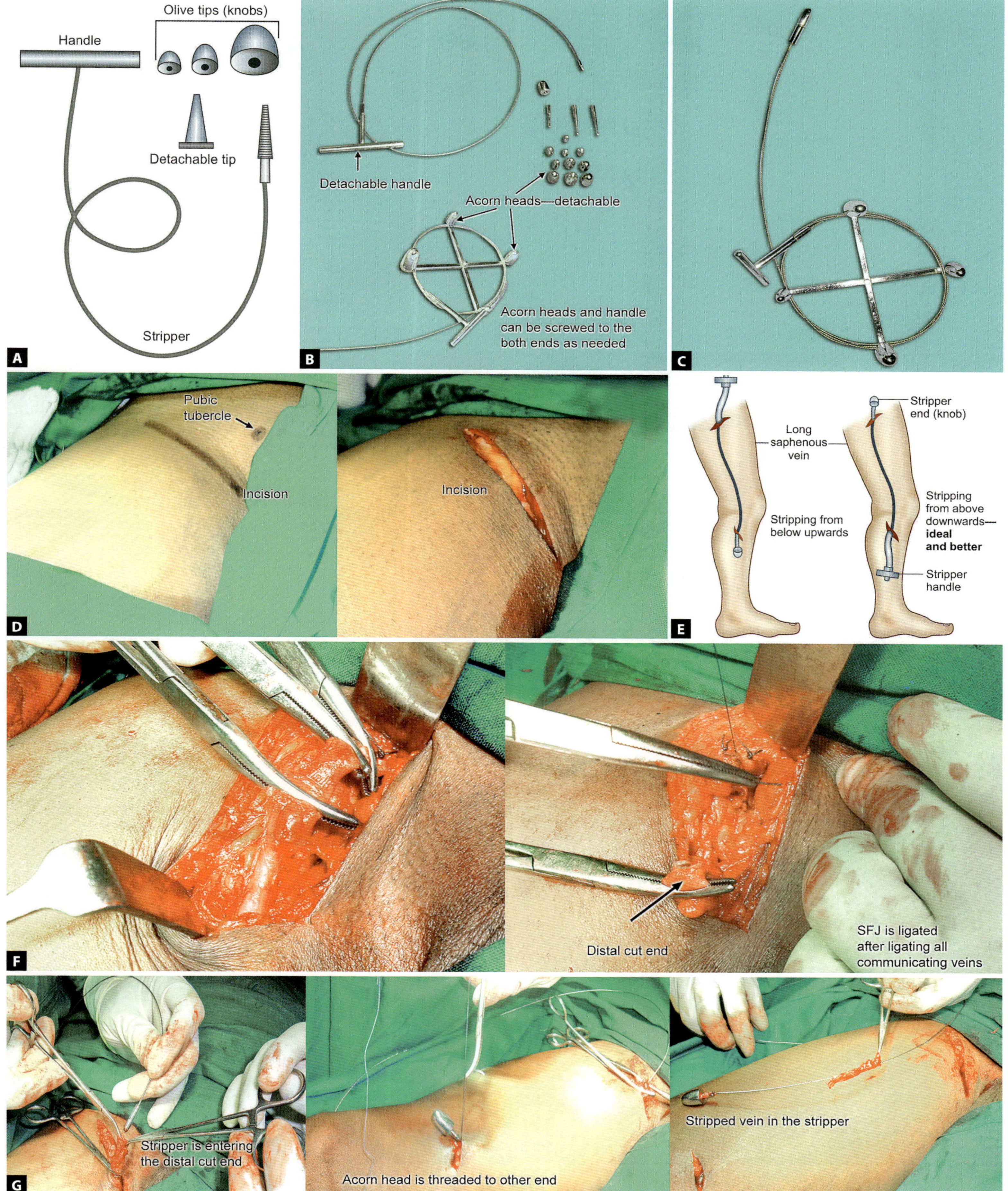

Figs. 12-17A to G: Technique of extraluminal stripping of the varicose vein using Myer's stripper.

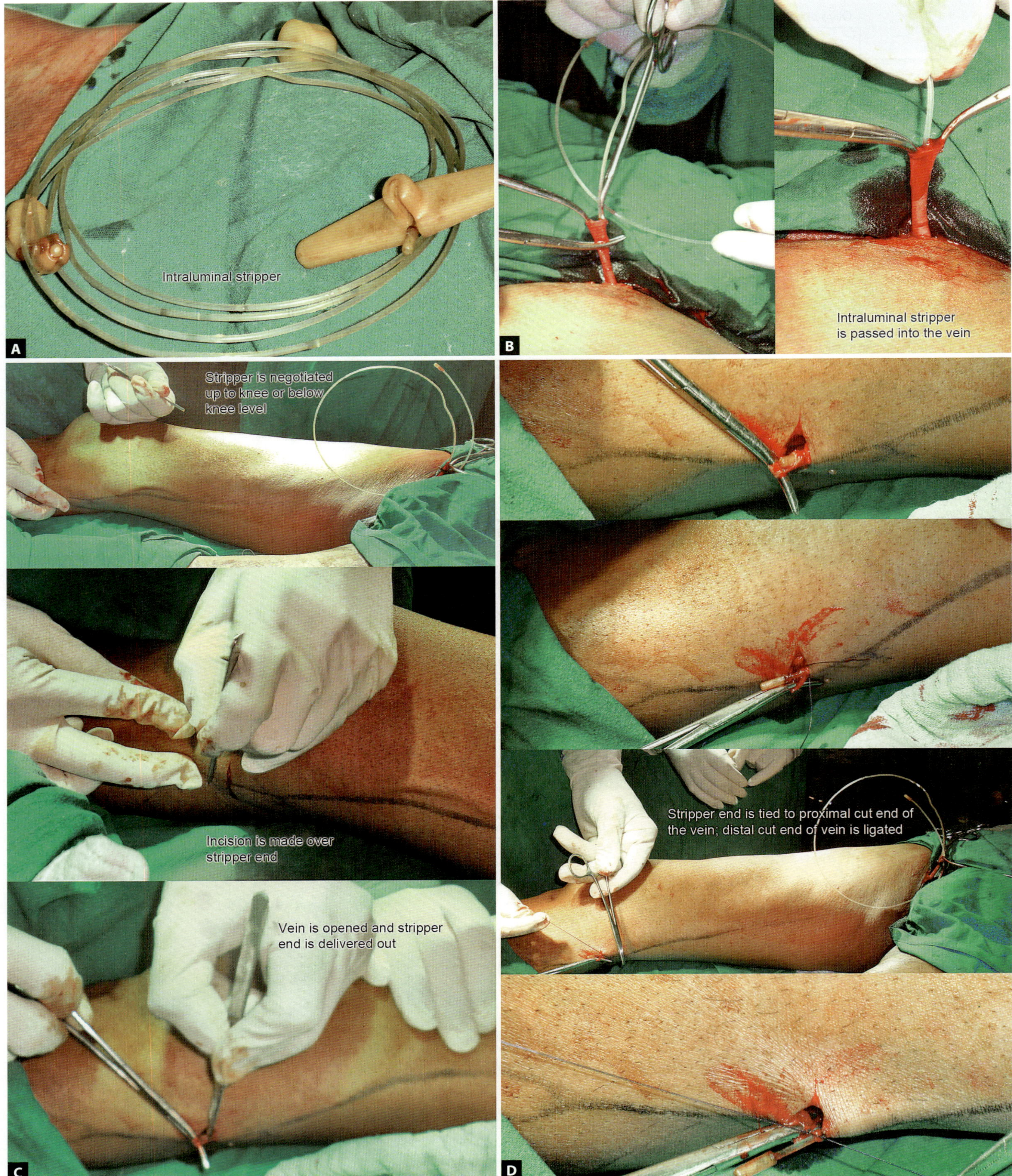

Figs. 12-18A to D

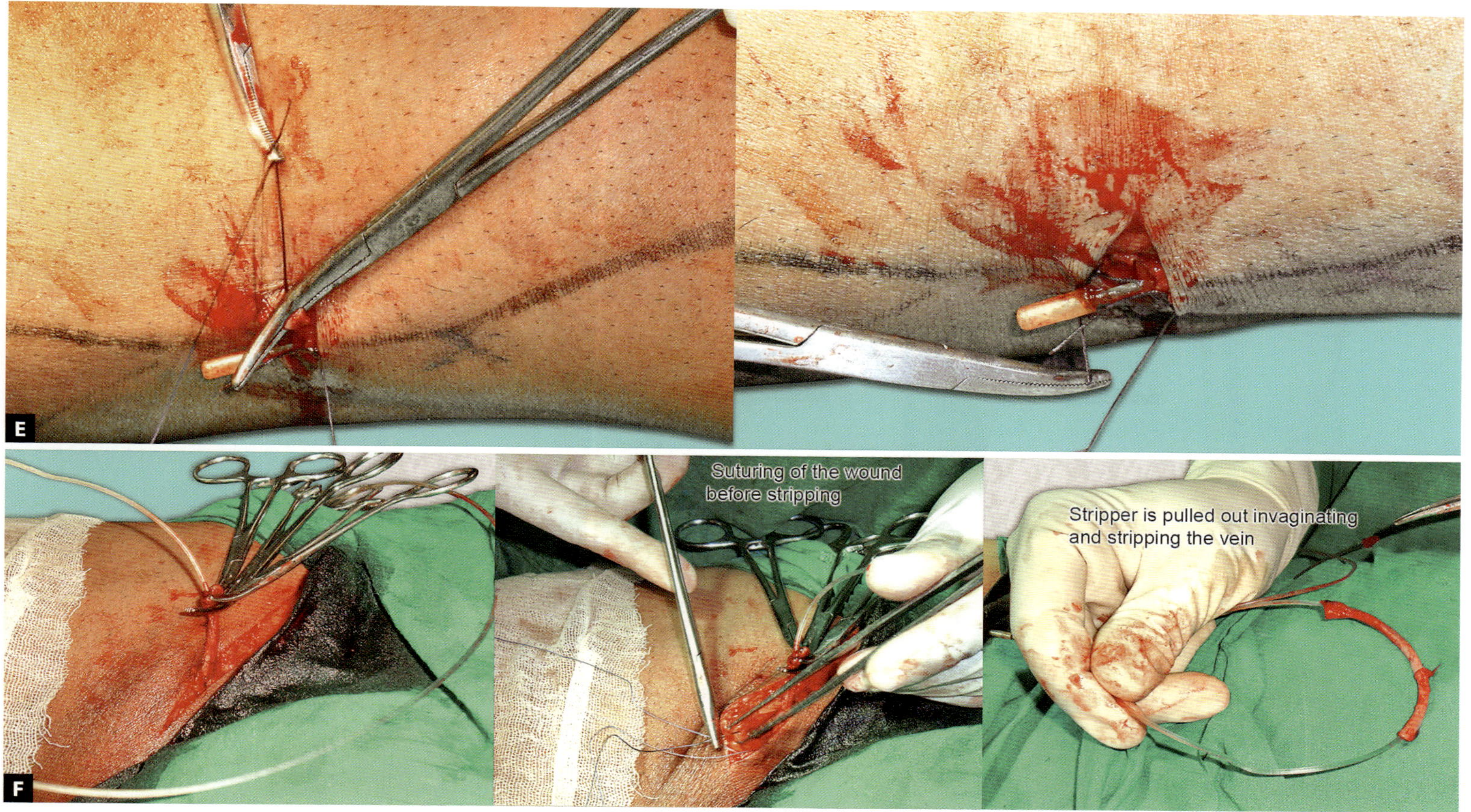

Figs. 12-18E and F

Figs. 12-18A to F: Intraluminal stripping of the varicose vein—operative steps. It is better than extraluminal stripping but chances of neovascularisation are more due to exposure of the endothelium during invagination.

prophylactic heparin therapy 5,000 units subcutaneously 6th hourly especially in patients who are in high-risk group like those who are on oestrogen therapy.

Infection, cellulitis, abscess and limb oedema are other complications which are treated accordingly.

Recurrence of the disease is common (30%). It is not due to any technical default but is due to progression of disease itself by *neoangiogenesis and revascularisation.*

Other complications—injury to femoral vein, inadvertent ligation of femoral vein, thrombosis of femoral vein, haematoma in groin wound are basically technical complications. It can be prevented by proper identification of vein and branches, haemostasis and taking proper care while ligation.

Wound *infection* in groin is common due to close proximity to perineum, more fat in subcutaneous area and lymphatic disruption. Often *lymph ooze* can occur for short periods.

Oesch Pin Stripping

Oesch pin stripping (perforate invaginate) is better as postoperative pain and haematoma formation are less common. But there is a possibility of endothelium getting inverted triggering neoangiogenesis and recurrence. SFJ is dealt as usual. Oesch pin stripper has got a bend near the tip and an eye at proximal end. Bent tip is passed through the vein from above downwards up to midcalf or just below the knee level. Through a small incision tip is brought out through the skin. Thick vicryl (No. 1) is passed through the eye of the stripper. Vicryl is tied around the proximal part of the vein, keeping suture long. Tip of the stripper is pulled down to invert the vein which will be extracted through the lower incision. Wound at SFJ is closed. Steri-strip is placed to lower small incision **(Fig. 12-19)**.

Groin Reoperation for Recurrent Disease

Recurrence after SFJ ligation is due to incomplete disconnection at SFJ and neovascularisation. Recurrence also can occur whenever stripping of the distal part of GSV is not done which may create a new communication between common femoral vein and GSV. Recurrence also can occur through a mid-thigh perforator. If SFJ is not ligated in flush or tributaries in groin are left in situ recurrence reflux at groin can occur. Neovascularisation occurs always in front of the femoral vein and these vessels are adherent and thin walled. Duplex scan and varicography are ideal investigations for assessing recurrent diseases **(Fig. 12-20)**.

Incision for groin SFJ reexploration is done through same transverse scar or through a vertical incision or combination of both. Vertical incision gives better exposure. First femoral artery is identified and then femoral vein is identified. Careful sharp dissection is ideal than blunt dissection as blunt dissection may cause significant obscuring of visibility of the field. Adequate length of the femoral vein is dissected from lateral and medial sides. All tissues with scar are ligated in front of the femoral vein to clear all tributaries and neovascularisation. SFJ is re-ligated flush with femoral vein. If GSV is not stripped in earlier surgery, it should be stripped properly up to mid-calf level.

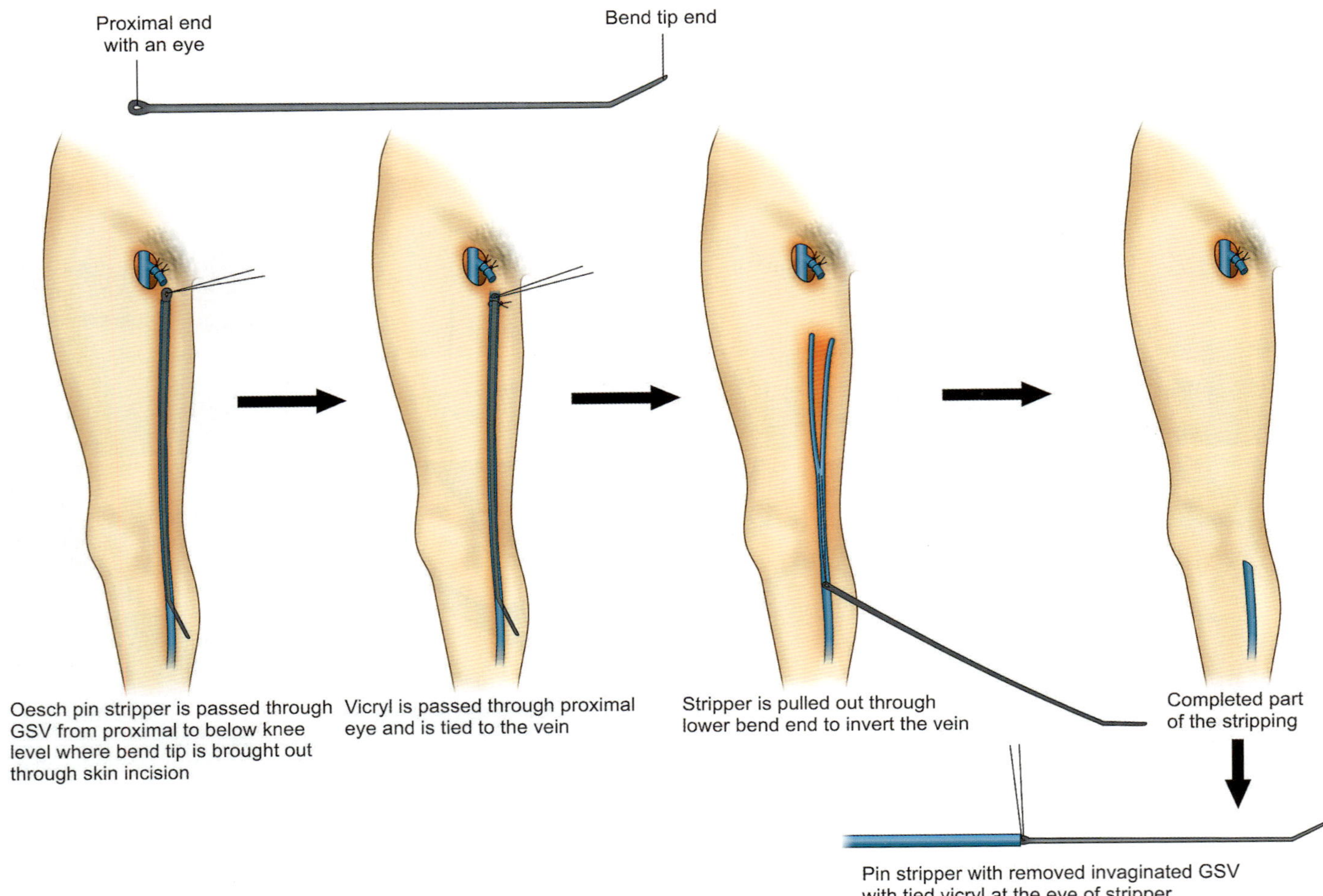

Fig. 12-19: Diagram showing technique of Oesch pin stripping.

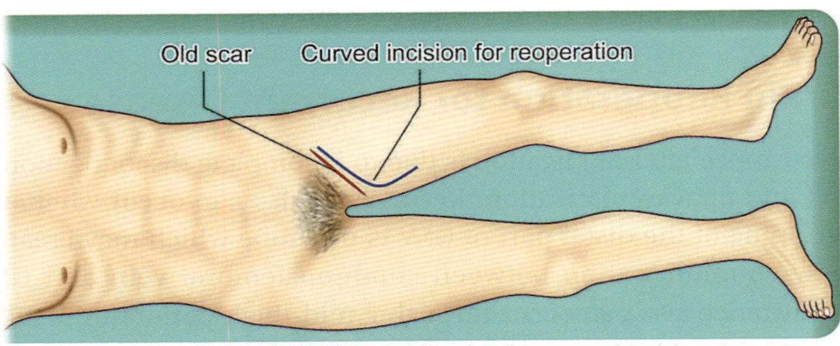

Fig. 12-20: For reoperation at saphenofemoral junction a curved incision placed with vertical part at medial side of thigh.

Complications of reexploration of groin are—haemorrhage, haematoma/seroma formation, lymph ooze, infection, injury to femoral vein and DVT.

LIGATION OF SAPHENOPOPLITEAL JUNCTION AND STRIPPING OF SMALL SAPHENOUS VEIN

It is needed if SSV varicosity is evident. Semiprone or prone position is needed. SPJ should be marked using duplex scan preoperatively. Variation of entering of the small saphenous vein into popliteal vein is common. It may enter high up more proximally above the level of knee joint in 25% of patients. In 15% of patients SSV joins GSV. Transverse incision is placed in the popliteal fossa 2–3 cm above the transverse skin crease. Deep fascia is opened vertically; SSV is identified; one superficial tributary will be present which runs in middle from back of the thigh which often may connect above to posteromedial thigh vein or may connect through a perforator vein into deep femoral vein. SSV entering the fossa is identified. It is accompanied with sural nerve which should be dissected and safeguarded. Sural nerve arises from tibial nerve at middle of the popliteal fossa leaving the fossa at its inferior angle to supply the skin of the lower half of back of leg and entire lateral part of the foot till tip of little toe. SSV is dissected up to the SPJ if there is no variation. It is always ideal to ligate the SPJ at junction. If variation is present it is often difficult to reach SPJ. In such situation many advocate ligation in the popliteal fossa deep to deep fascia to proceed further for stripping of the varicose vein. Gastrocnemius veins instead of normal draining into the popliteal vein may drain into the SSV and in such situation these veins should not be ligated as ligation may cause troublesome venous claudication and discomfort in the calf. Stripping of the SSV is easier. It is ideal to use intraluminal stripper to reduce injury to sural nerve. Stripping is done from above downwards even though many surgeons strip the vein from below upwards. Stripping of the SSV obliterates the midcalf perforator vein which reduces the recurrence.

SUBFASCIAL LIGATION

It is ligation of perforator where it enters the deep fascia (deeper to deep fascia). It is done for perforator incompetence. Perforators are marked prior to procedure using duplex scan. Different approaches are available to tackle perforators **(Fig. 12-21)**.

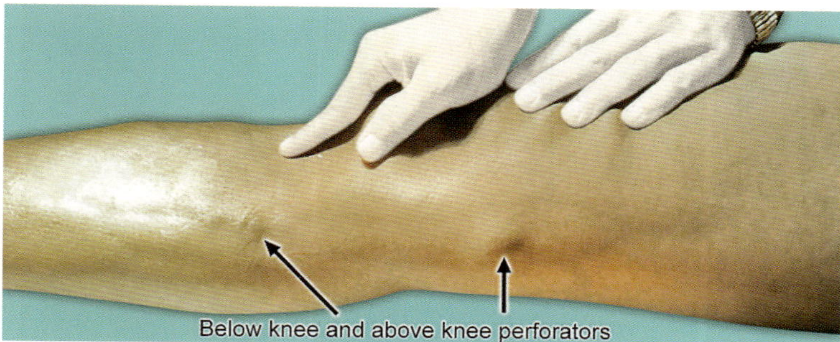

Fig. 12-21: Dodd (mid thigh) and Boyd (below knee) perforators.

Subfascial Ligation of Cockett and Dodd

Perforators are clearly marked prior to surgery by Fegan's clinical method or ideally using duplex Doppler scan. Multiple small transverse incisions are made on the sites of perforators. Perforators are ligated deep to deep fascia using vicryl **(Fig. 12-22)**.

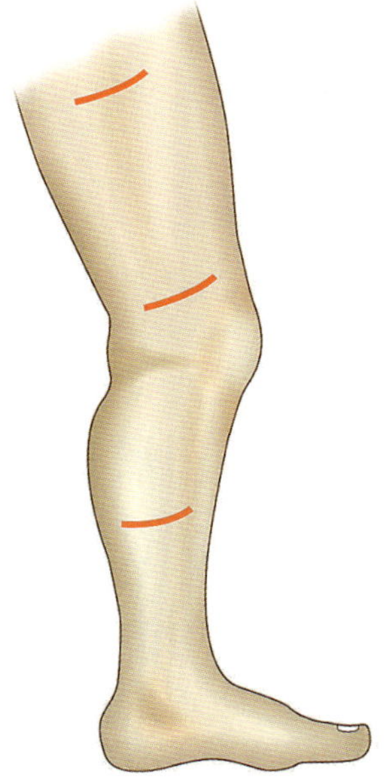

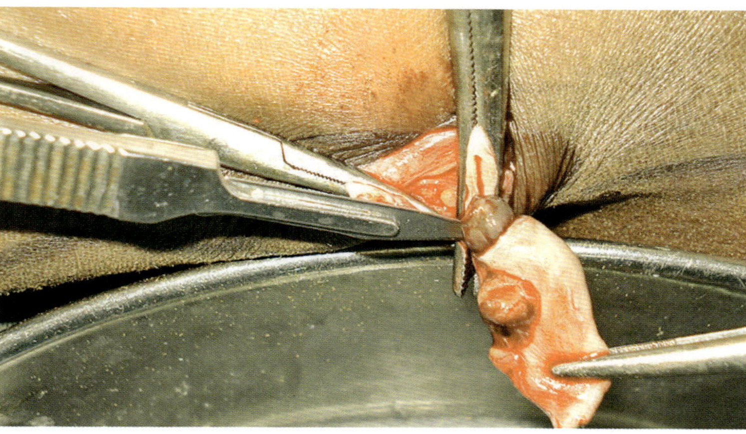

Fig. 12-22: Cockett and Dodd perforator ligation using small multiple transverse incisions.

Subfascial Ligation of all Perforators by Linton's Vertical Approach (1938)

Here vertical incision is made on the medial side of the calf at the anterior margin of the soleus little away from tibia. Often the incision over the ankle is divided like in an inverted 'Y' or a posterior 'stocking seam' incision. Skin, subcutaneous tissue and deep fascia are incised without raising any flaps under the skin. Perforators passing across gastrocnemius and deep fascia will be clearly seen. All perforators are identified, ligated using vicryl and divided. Deep fascia is closed using vicryl. Problem with this procedure is lengthy scar which is cosmetically poor even though wound heals well **(Fig. 12-23)**.

Stab Avulsion of the Perforator (Multiple Phlebectomies)

Multiple *small vertical* incisions are made over all marked varicose veins in the leg. Veins are identified. Using vein hook or mosquito artery forceps vein ends are held and gently avulsed using rotation and pulling movements. Often it needs 50–70 incisions to clear the veins. Usually there is no need to suture the wounds as they get closed naturally. Steri-strip placing is sufficient. Postoperative compression bandage is a must. During hook avulsion of the vein, care should be taken not to injure the common peroneal nerve near the neck of fibula, tibial nerve near medial malleolus, saphenous nerve in medial part of leg, and sural nerve on the lateral part of the calf **(Fig. 12-24)**.

Subfascial Endoscopic Perforator Surgery (SEPS)

A special telescope is introduced deep-to-deep fascia through a single small vertical incision at proximal leg selecting healthy skin. Technique is done under tourniquet. Endoscope is advanced down along the medial border of the tibia. Perforators travelling in subfascial vein are identified and fulgurated using bipolar cautery or clips can be applied into the perforators. It is recommended in chronic venous insufficiency (CVI). But its limitation is difficulty in getting 'lift off' the skin in cases with severe lipodermatosclerosis to identify the perforators (German Surgeon Hauer, 1985).

Complications are—infection, haematoma formation, neuralgia **(Fig. 12-25)**.

AMBULATORY SELECTIVE VARICES ABLATION (ASVA/ASVAL) (Ablation Sélective Des Varices Sous Anésthesie Locale)

It is based on newer haemodynamic concept—antegrade haemodynamic evolution of saphenous vein incompetence from suprafascial compartment to great saphenous vein. Evolution of disease starts in collateral veins and their reflux leads into varicose reservoir. If varicose reservoir is abolished saphenous reflux will stop—a newer concept. Procedure is done under local anaesthesia (Ambulatory Selective Varices Ablation under Local anaesthesia/ ASVAL).

CHIVA: It is one of the methods used to achieve ASVA (Cure Hemodynamique de'l Insufficiency Veineuse en Ambulatoire).

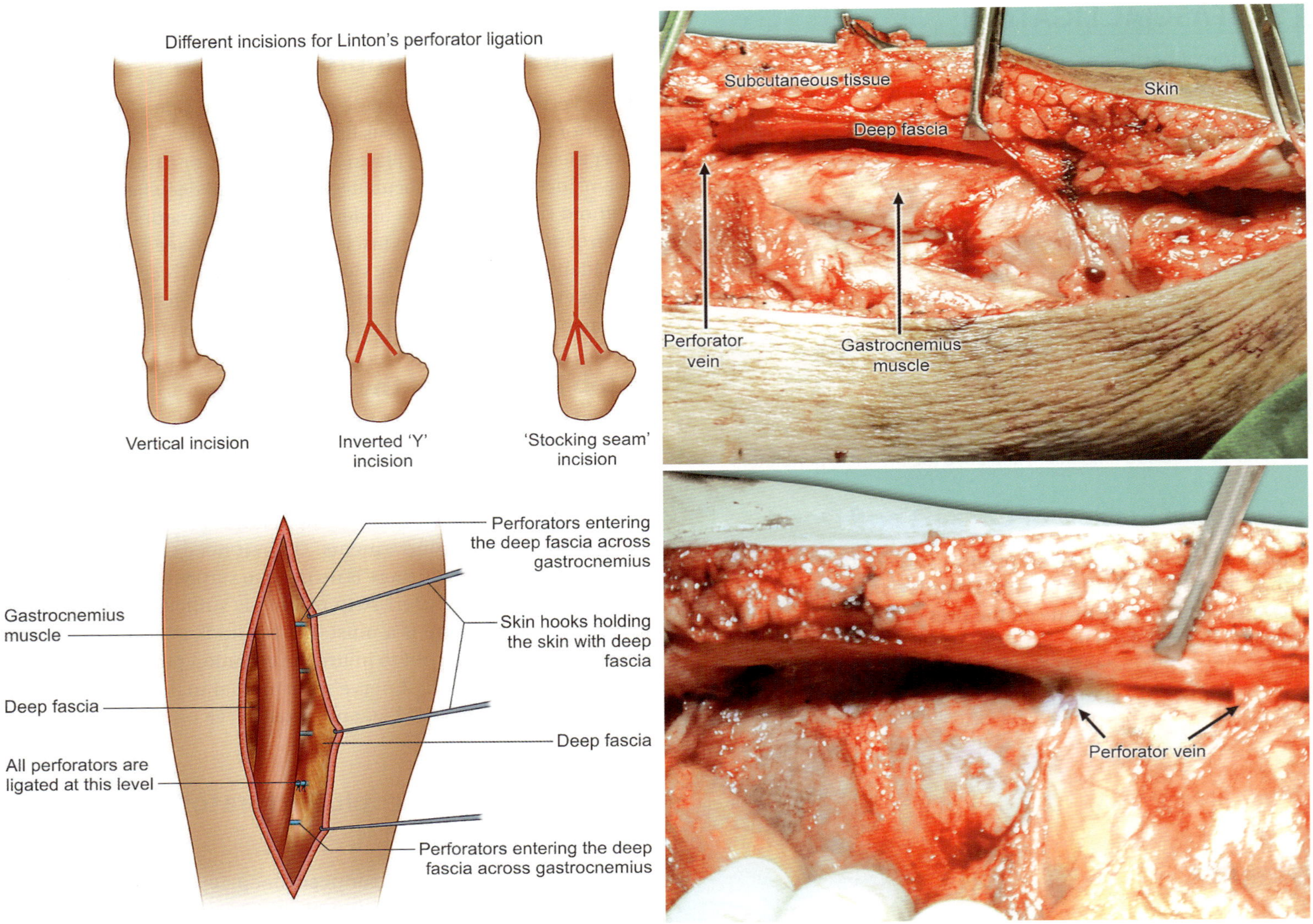

Different incisions for Linton's perforator ligation

Vertical incision

Inverted 'Y' incision

'Stocking seam' incision

Perforators entering the deep fascia across gastrocnemius

Gastrocnemius muscle

Skin hooks holding the skin with deep fascia

Deep fascia

Deep fascia

All perforators are ligated at this level

Perforators entering the deep fascia across gastrocnemius

Subcutaneous tissue

Skin

Deep fascia

Perforator vein

Gastrocnemius muscle

Perforator vein

Fig. 12-23: Linton's vertical approach for subfascial ligation of perforators.

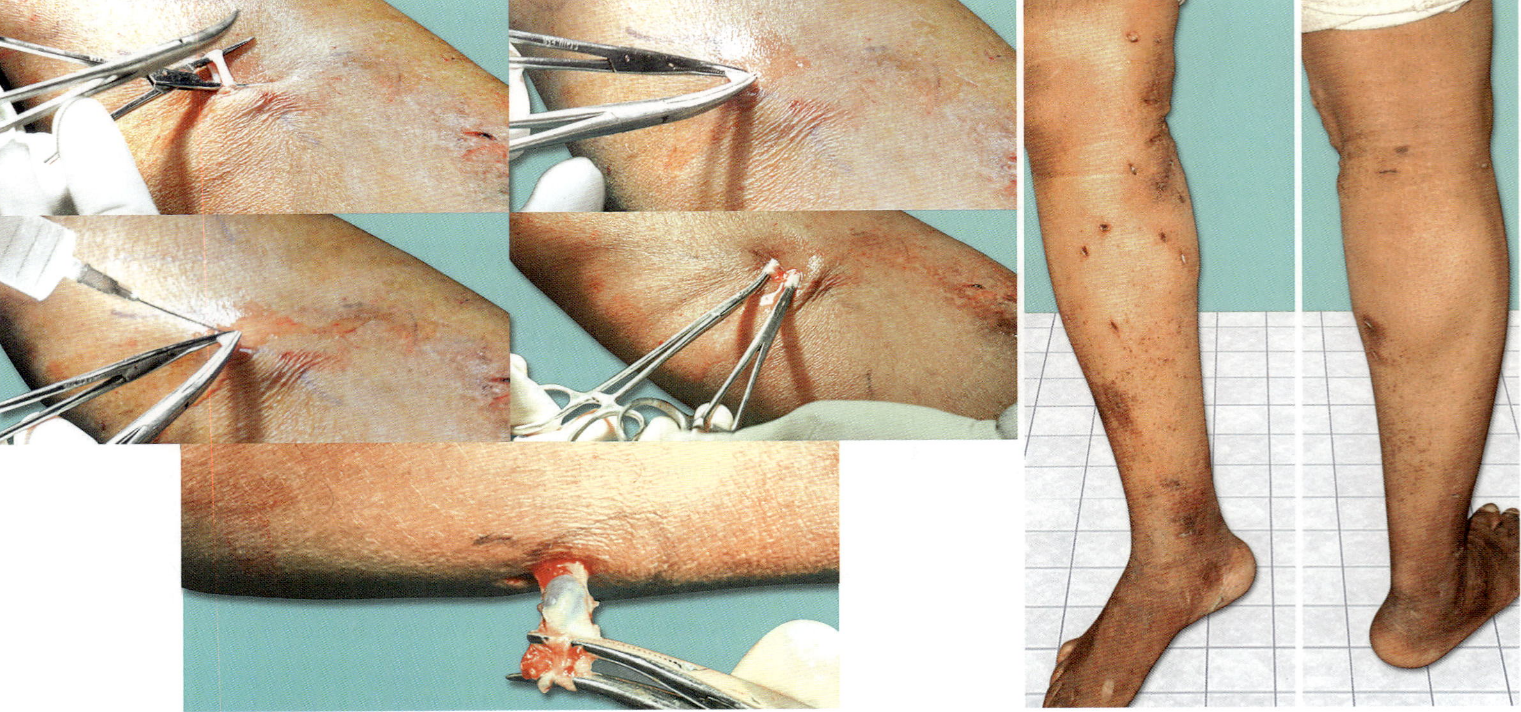

Fig. 12-24: Stab avulsion of the vein and perforators (multiple phlebectomies). It is becoming popular and shows good result.

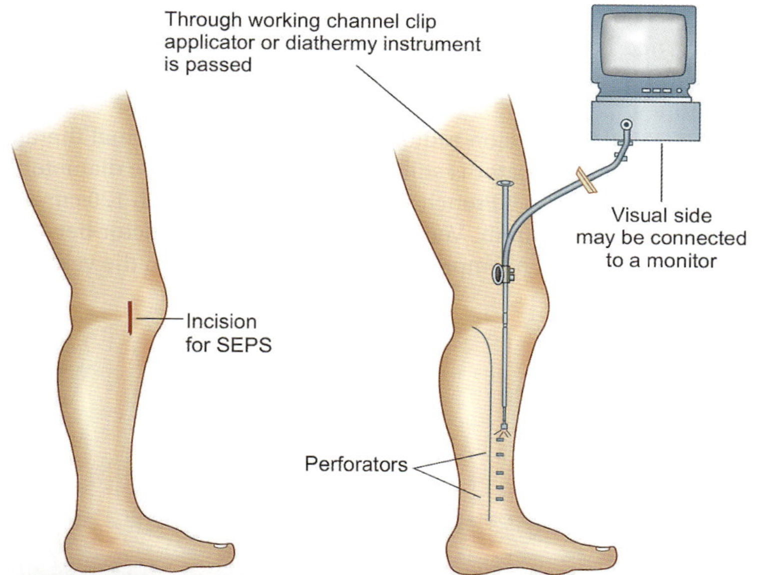

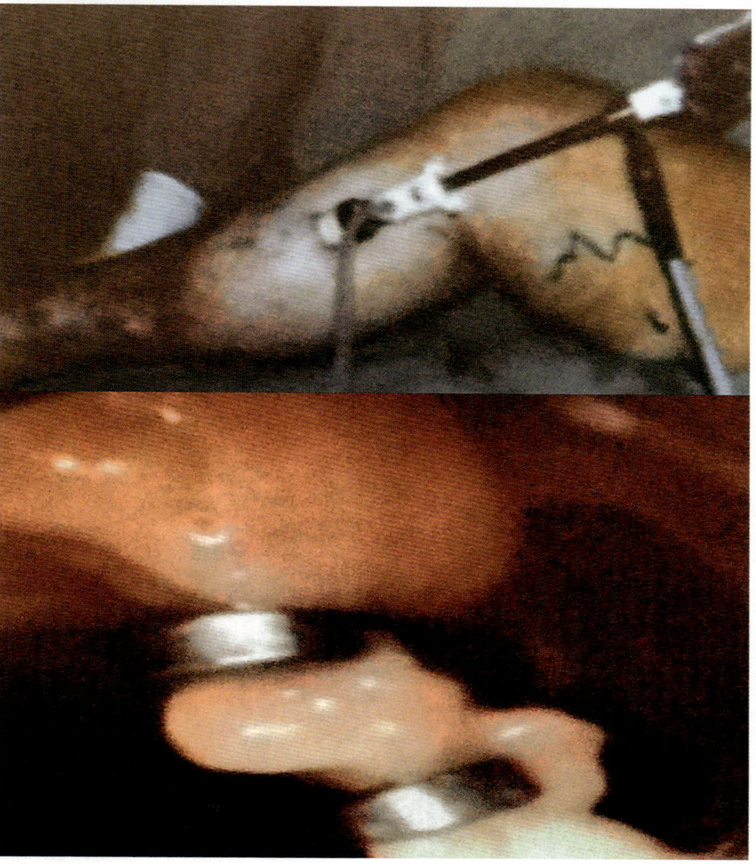

Fig. 12-25: Subfascial endoscopic perforator ligation surgery (SEPS).

Pittaluga technique is used (Dr Paul Pittaluga, A French vascular surgeon, founder of Riviera Vein Institute). Here attention has focused on surgical treatment of tributaries retaining the main trunk—ambulatory conservative haemodynamic management of varicose veins.

Saphenofemoral and saphenopopliteal junctions are identified and marked under US guidance. Individual gastrocnemius, intersaphenous, popliteal area veins are identified and marked; longitudinal 3 mm stabs are made using No. 11 blade; phlebectomy is achieved. Selective targeted diseased veins only are removed with preservation of healthy veins. Minimum pain, minimum haematoma, microincision and so minimum scar **(Fig. 12-26)**.

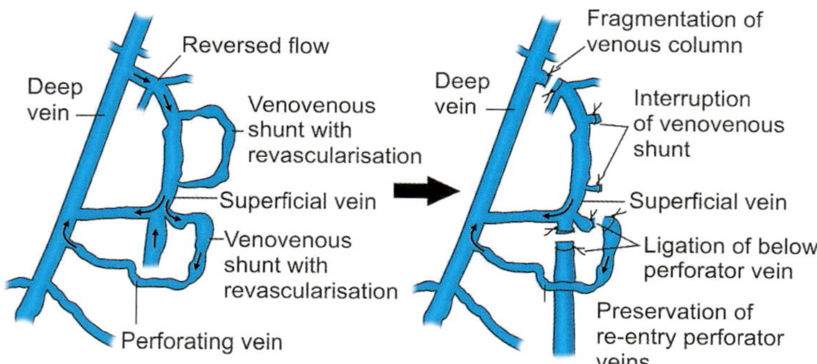

Fig. 12-26: Chiva—Pittaluga technique.

ENDOVENOUS THERMAL ABLATION

Thermal ablation works by generating heat energy within the vein, which inflicts direct thermal damage to inner wall of the vein causing destruction of intima and collagen denaturation of media eventually leading to fibrosis and occlusion. Radiofrequency ablation (RFA) and endovenous laser ablation (EVLA) are two methods used. Thermal ablation is used for varicosities of great, short, accessory saphenous veins, perforating veins as well.

RADIOFREQUENCY ABLATION (RFA) METHOD (VNUS CLOSURE METHOD) (VNUS Medical Technologies Inc; Sunnyvale, CA, USA—By Goldman 2000)

Politowski described this method 50 years ago. Electric energy is converted into heat to denature the collagen tissue in the vein in a bloodless field.

VNUS closure system is the present RFA device used. This procedure is done under general or regional anaesthesia. A RFA catheter is passed into long/short saphenous vein near saphenofemoral or saphenopopliteal junction under US guidance. A special heater probe is inserted into the vein which obliterates 6 cm of vein at a time using 'pull-back' technique. The catheter has a central core for irrigation which prevents coagulum accumulation during the procedure. Temperature of 85°C is used for longer duration of time to cause endothelial damage, collagen denaturation and venous constriction. Phlebectomy is done while withdrawing the catheter. Wall of the vein is destroyed through its full thickness. Vein forms a cord, which gets dissolved by macrophages and immune cells. Procedure is slow one as it will take 25 minutes to obliterate 45 cm vein **(Figs. 12-27 and 12-28)**.

Newer generation device VNUS Closure FAST is used with high temperature of 120°C and can be done under general anaesthesia. In this, 45 cm of vein will be obliterated in 5 minutes. It has got VNUS Closure RFS Stylet to tackle perforator veins. It can be done under local anaesthesia. It is better than pull back technique. 7 cm segment is fired in 20 seconds. Catheter is passed 10 cm below the knee by percutaneous access under US guidance or by venesection. Nitroglycerine (NTG) spray may be used to dilate vein and make it easier to cannulate. RFA catheter is passed into the vein up to 2 cm below the SFJ. Tumescent anaesthesia is infiltrated—10 cc per 1 cm vein length. Vein should be made 1 cm depth from the skin. Tumescent creates thermal buffer around the vein; compresses and empties the vein. Initially patient is in reverse Trendelenburg position (head up) until catheter is passed; then tilted to 15° Trendelenburg position (head down). RF is fired for 20 seconds for 7 cm segment length. During firing compression over the vein is achieved from outside (external pressure) by pressing with the US probe longitudinally and by pressing the vein line distal to the probe using two fingers. Above knee compression bandage (grade II—30-40 mm Hg pressure) is applied for 2 weeks. Patient can walk in 1 hour. Running, jumping, straining and weight lifting are avoided for 2 weeks. Analgesics can be taken. Usually antibiotics and analgesics are not needed. Many use prone position for RFA.

RFA is better in relation to pain, quality, speed of recovery and recurrence compared to open surgery. It is done as outpatient procedure; can resume work early; no hospitalisation; no scar; no sutures.

CELON RFITT—Celon radiofrequency-induced thermal therapy with a bipolar applicator is still newer technique. Probe diameter is 1.8 mm which fits to 6 French sheath with a total length 120 cm and electrode length 15 mm. Vein wall is used as a conductor between both poles to reach a temperature of 650–950°C within the vein wall

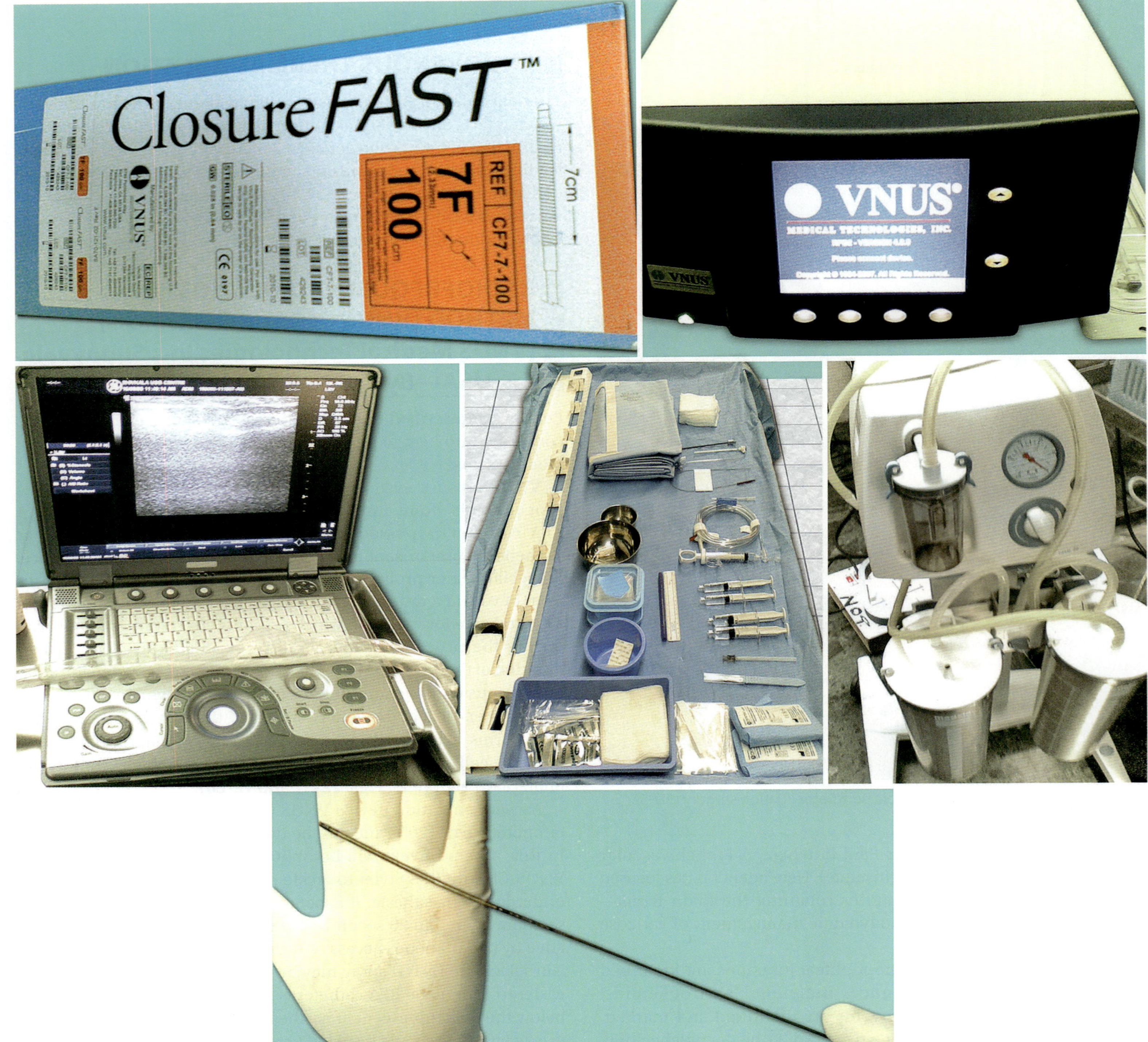

Fig. 12-27: Set up required for radiofrequency ablation of varicose vein (VNUS-RFA).

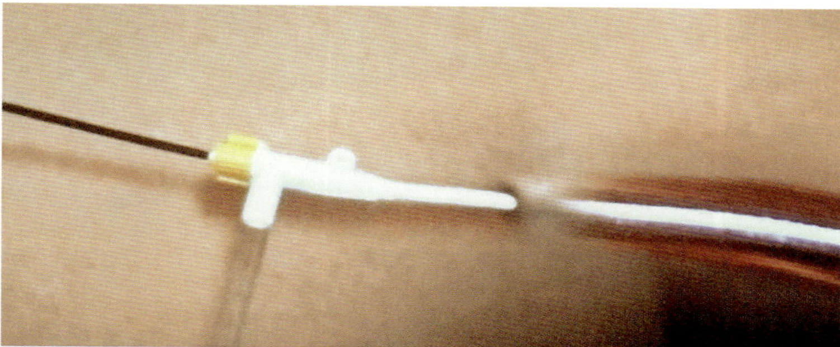

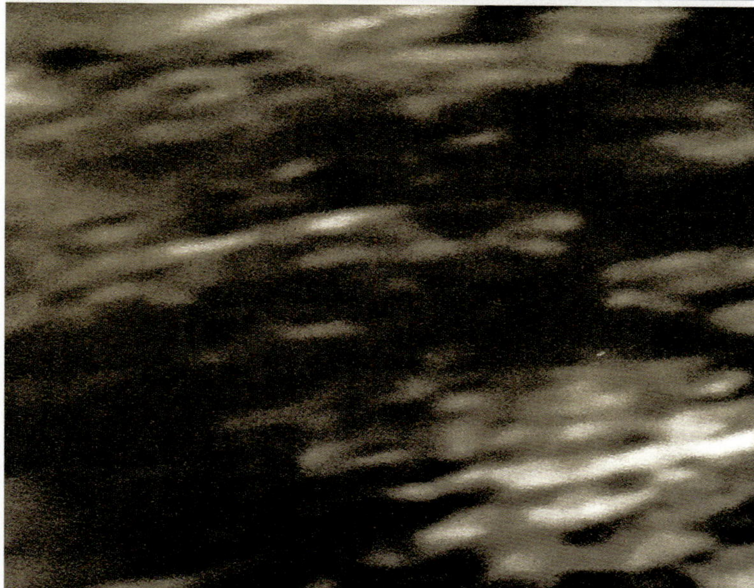

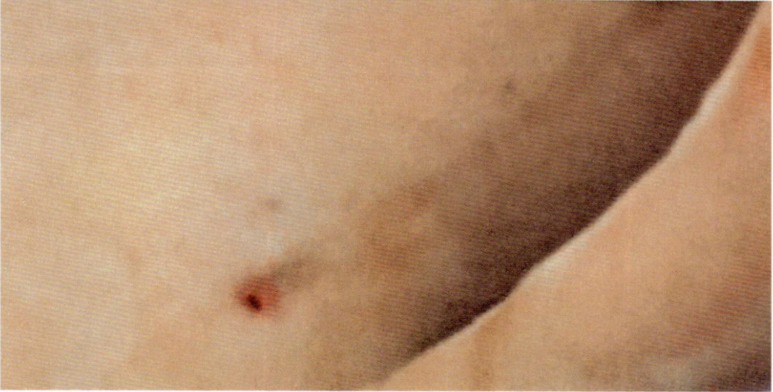

Fig. 12-28: Steps in VNUS-RFA closure therapy.

but applicator remains cold. Power (P) of 18–20 W and an applicator time (T) of ≥1.5 sec/cm is used.

Complication rates are 7% in RFA compared to EVLT (20%) but recurrence rate is more compared to EVLT.

ENDOVENOUS LASER ABLATION/ TREATMENT (EVLA/EVLT)

It causes direct and indirect thermal injury of the venous wall with endothelial denudation, contraction of collagen and fibrosis creating a non-thrombotic occlusion of the vein. EVLA is done for truncal varicosities and large branch veins and tributaries.

EVLA was first described by Bone in 1999. The Diomed 810 nm diode laser received US FDA approval in 2002. It is as effective as surgical stripping but with shorter recovery time and less side effects. Vein wall destruction occurs by conductive and convective heating. Direct contact, steam bubble and carbonisation occur. Thermal energy is absorbed by haemoglobin or water. Bare tipped, radial, jacketed, self-centering tulip fibres are available. Single use/multiple uses fibres are also available. 400/600/1100 microns fibre size are available.

It is done ideally under *local anaesthesia* with US/duplex scan guidance. Spinal/general anaesthesia can be used. Vein should be marked with marker pen. It is done as an outpatient procedure or as day-care surgery. *System* contains endovenous generator with wavelengths of either 810 nm or 1064 nm, laser firing fibre, monitor showing all the needed parameters related to laser foot switch. Diode laser is used. Procedure is done under US guidance. ***Hyper Diode 1470 with atraumatic and 360° optical fibres are also now available for faster precise ablation*** **(Fig. 12-29)**.

Patient lies supine with diseased leg flexed, hip externally rotated and knee flexed. With aseptic precaution, under US guidance LSV is cannulated (18 G cannula) above or just below the knee at the level of Boyd's perforator; needle is removed keeping cannula in place; a 0.035" J guidewire is passed beyond SFJ; 18 G cannula is removed; 5-French introducer catheter/sheath is passed over guidewire; tip is placed 1 cm distal to the junction; guidewire is removed; laser fibre is inserted into the catheter up to the tip of the catheter and catheter is withdrawn for 2 cm and laser fibre protrudes for 2 cm beyond the sheath/catheter. Position of catheter and laser fibre tip are confirmed using US. Vein can be cannulated at ankle also **(Fig. 12-30)**.

Tumescent anaesthesia (500 mL of cold saline, 30–50 mL of 1% xylocaine with adrenaline, 30 mL of 8.4% sodium bicarbonate) is prepared and injected along the entire length of the GSV to be fired. Injection is done manually using 50 cc syringe or tumescence pump or using as drip set. It should form a *cushion* surrounding the vein along its entire length to provide local anaesthesia, to give protection like a 'heat sink' preventing thermal damage of skin and soft tissues, to provide adequate venous compression to create complete apposition of the venous wall and so effective venous obliteration. Tumescent anaesthesia is given under US guidance.

Laser fibre is fired step by step using diode laser, 1–3 mm withdrawal in 2–3 seconds. Introducer sheath/catheter having mm markings on the surface with the laser fibre are slowly withdrawn. Intermittent pulsed mode firing or continuous mode firing set ups are available in the generator. Proximal thigh 14 mm Watts; lower thigh 12 mm Watts; knee and upper leg 10 mm Watts energy are used. Presently ablation of entire great saphenous vein even up to midcalf level is approved and commonly done by surgeons. But thermal injury to saphenous nerve is a possible problem. Once procedure is over, catheter is removed. Total obliteration of the vein should be confirmed using ultrasound. Pressure bandage is applied for 2 weeks **(Fig. 12-31)**.

Heat produced (729°C - 1000°C at tip) by the laser produces steam bubbles with thermal damage of endothelium leading into occlusion of the vein. Laser energy acts on the blood within the vein rather directly through the wall and heats the blood which in turn heats the vein wall.

Advantages of EVLA are—minimally invasive; cosmetically acceptable; no large wounds or scars; done under local anaesthesia; done as day care procedure; easier to do the procedure; rapid recovery and rapid return to work; less chances of neovascularisation and so less chances of recurrence (2% in 2 years) as compared to surgery (30-40%). Technique has got 95% efficacy.

Disadvantages of EVLA are—inability to create flush occlusion allowing tributaries to open up to cause possible recurrence;

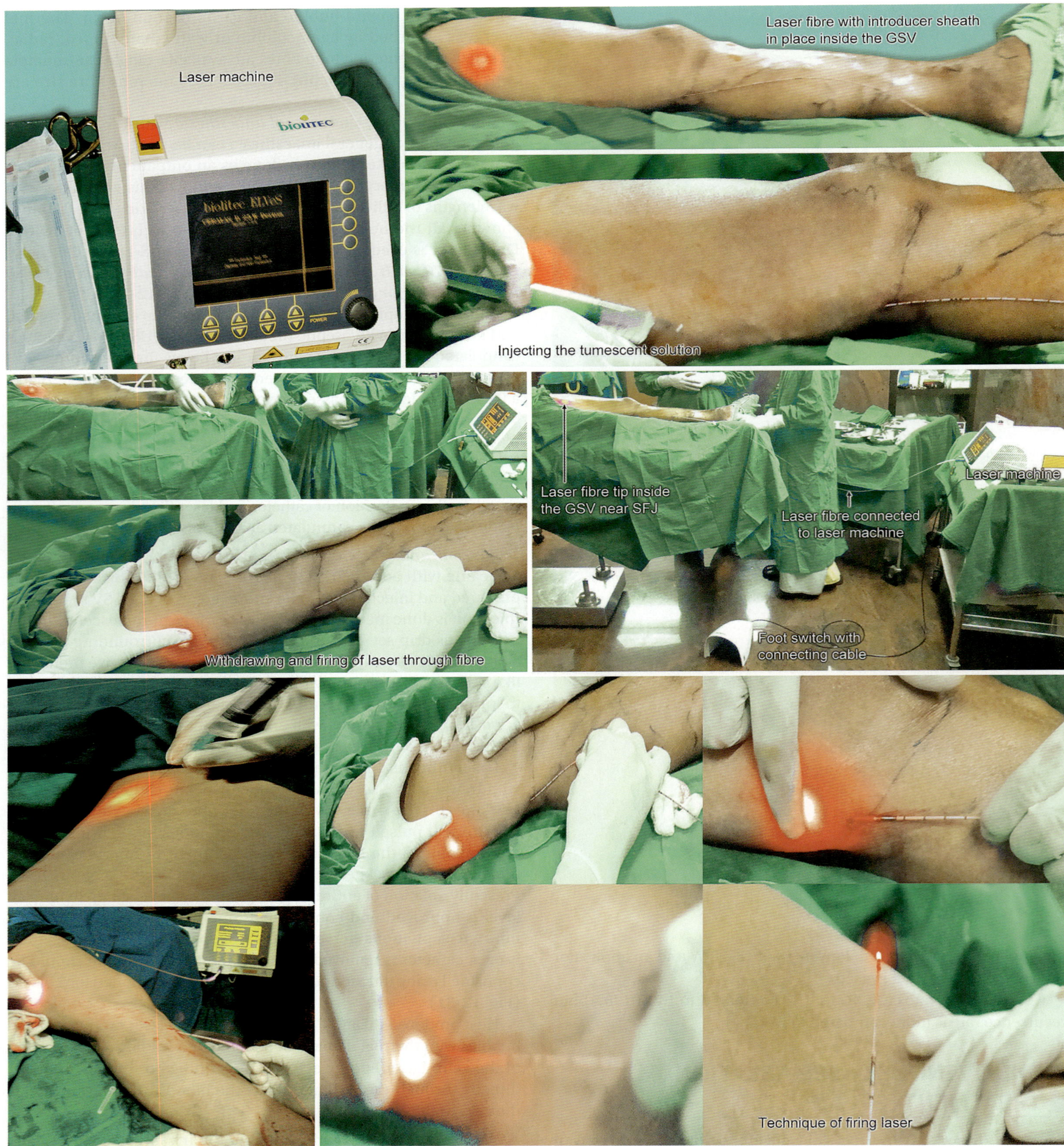

Fig. 12-29: Laser machine and its setting to patient.

cost factor, laser fibre kit is disposable; difficulty in cannulating the vein; multiple punctures often may be needed; need of duplex scan in operation theatre; need of trained surgeons to do venous duplex scan and Doppler. One should remember that it is not totally 'pain free.'

Complications of EVLA are—transient postoperative pain; skin ecchymosis; haematomas; thermal injury of the skin; DVT; residual varicosities; sensory disturbances if 1064 nm generator is used **(Figs. 12-32 and 12-33)**.

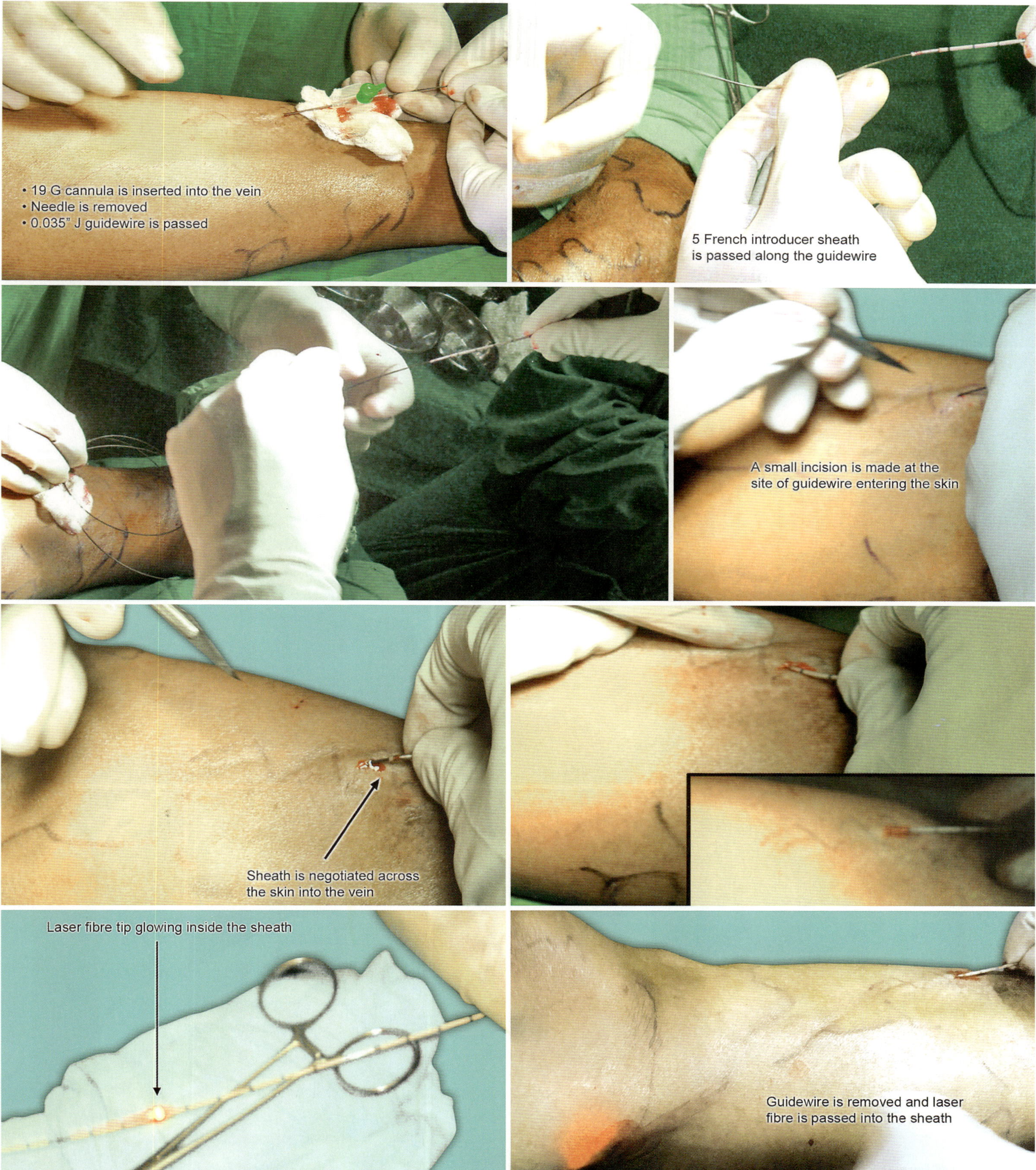

Fig. 12-30: Laser fibre insertion—initial procedure.

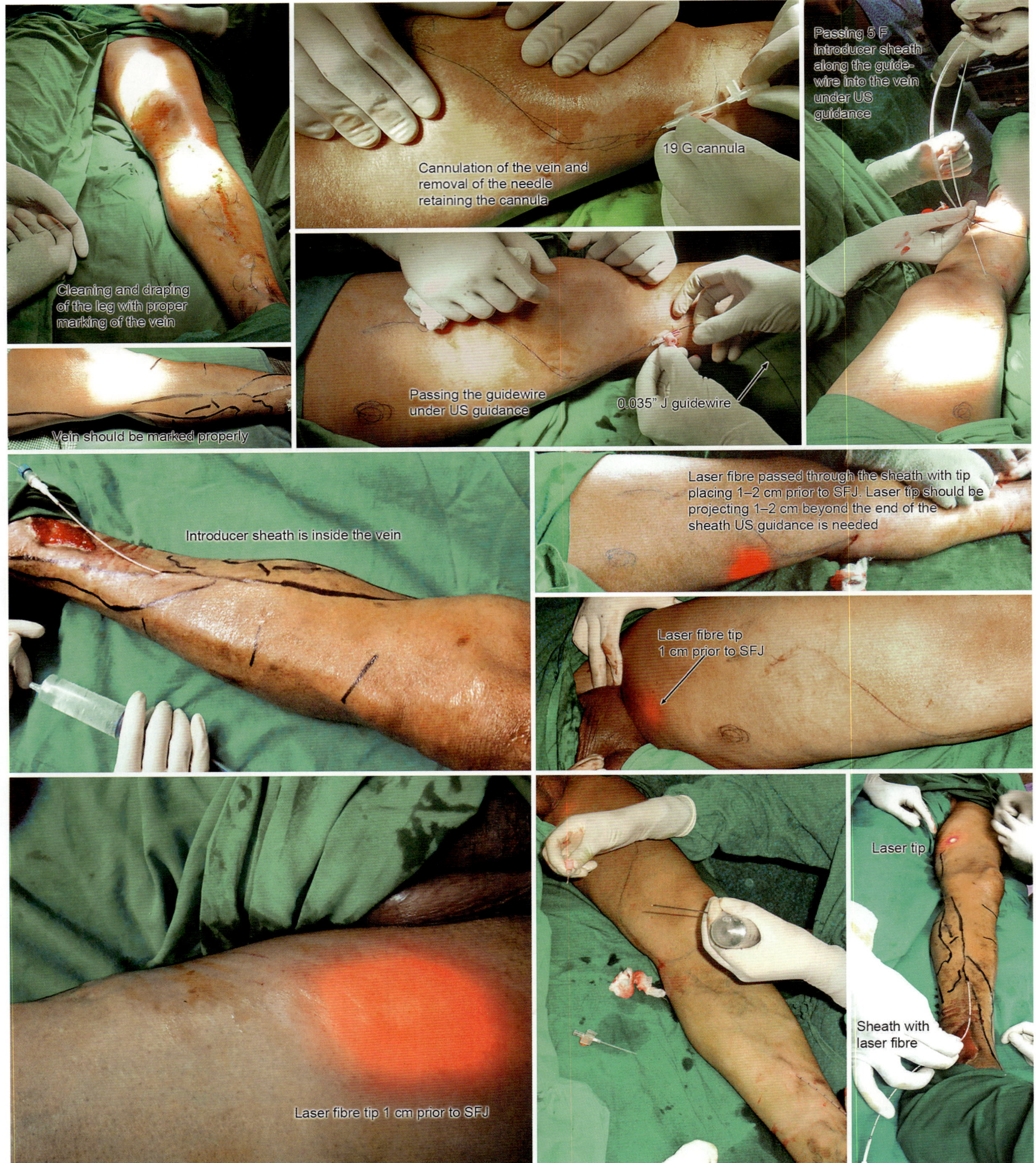
Cleaning and draping of the leg with proper marking of the vein
Cannulation of the vein and removal of the needle retaining the cannula
19 G cannula
Passing 5 F introducer sheath along the guide-wire into the vein under US guidance
Vein should be marked properly
Passing the guidewire under US guidance
0.035" J guidewire
Introducer sheath is inside the vein
Laser fibre passed through the sheath with tip placing 1–2 cm prior to SFJ. Laser tip should be projecting 1–2 cm beyond the end of the sheath US guidance is needed
Laser fibre tip 1 cm prior to SFJ
Laser fibre tip 1 cm prior to SFJ
Laser tip
Sheath with laser fibre

Figs. 12-31(1)

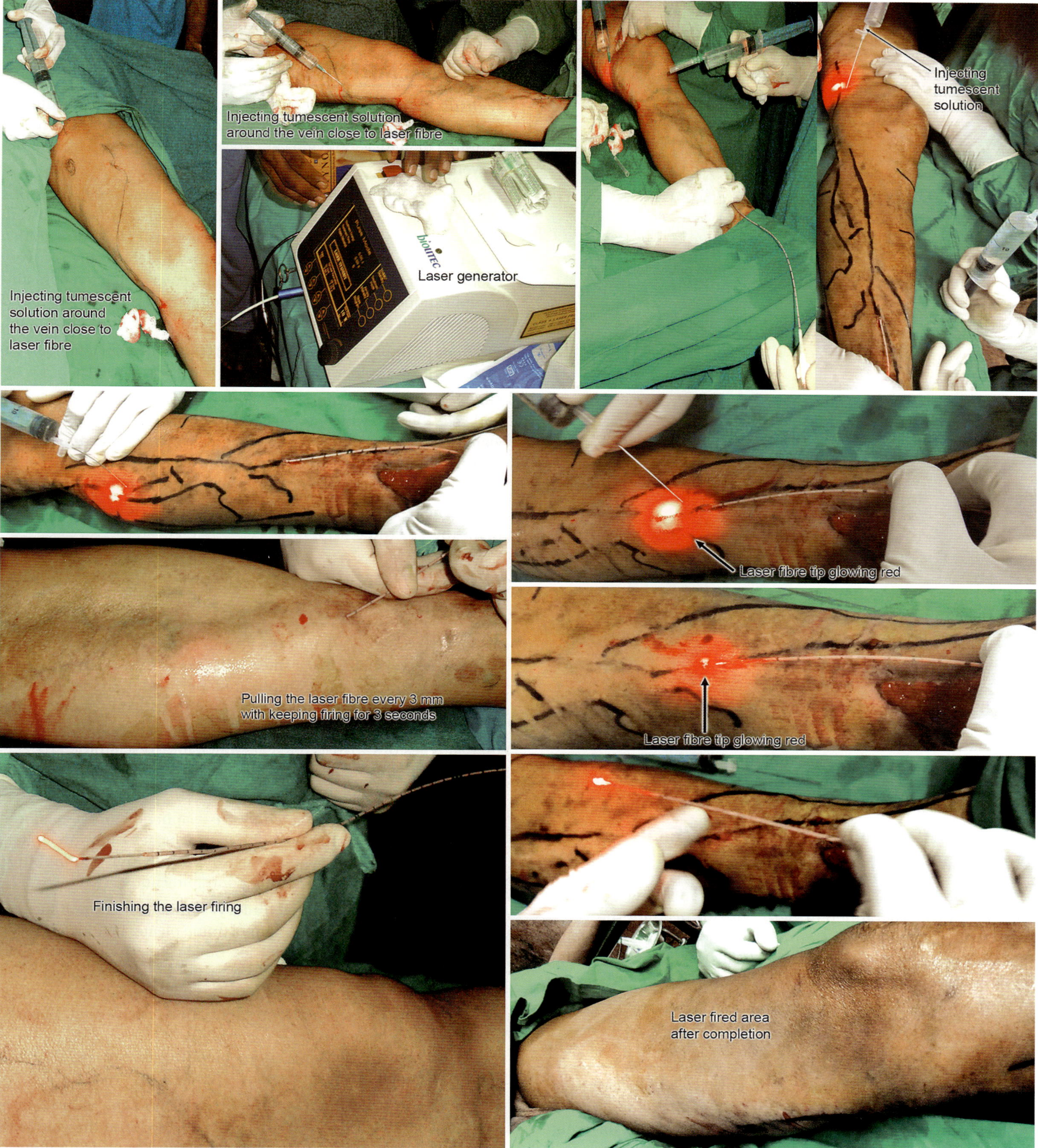

Figs. 12-31(2)

Figs. 12-31(1 and 2): Technique of endovenous laser treatment/ablation.

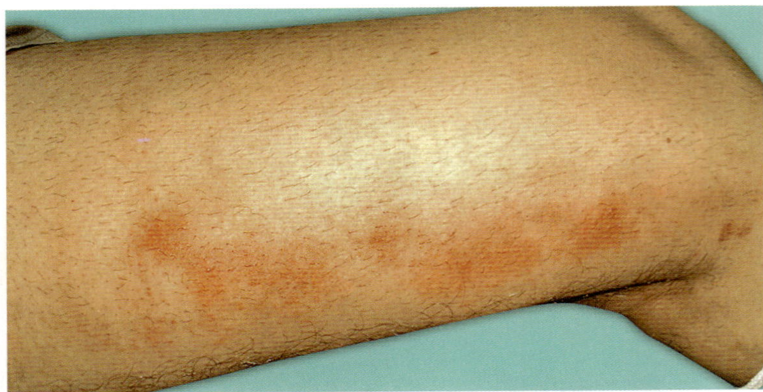

Fig. 12-32: Ecchymosis due to laser ablation of varicose vein.

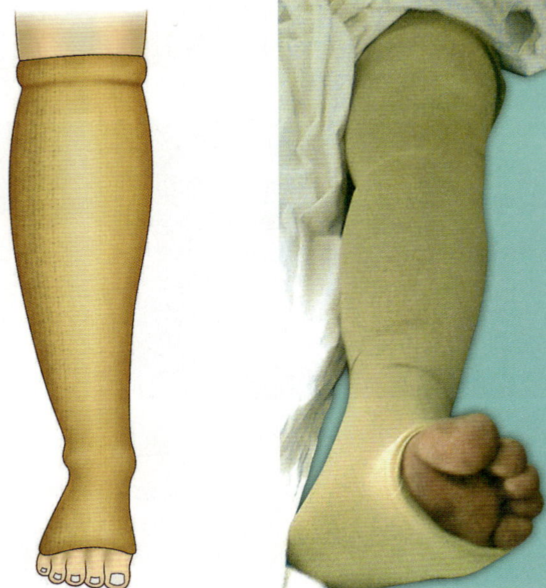

Fig. 12-33: Wearing stocking is very essential after any procedure. Wearing stocking for minimum period of 6 months is needed. It is better to advice to wear stockings during day time for life long to reduce recurrence and neovascularisation.

HEAT ABLATION FOR CLOSURE OF INCOMPETENT PERFORATOR VEIN (ICPV)

Mark Whiteley has invented thermoablation device which is passed into the incompetent perforator to occlude the vein by heat—Transluminal Occlusion of Perforating Veins (TRLOP) or Percutaneous Ablation of Perforators (PAPs). Technique is useful in recalcitrant venous ulcers.

Complications of PAPs are—paraesthesia, DVT, infection.

TRIVEX METHOD

Under subcutaneous illumination and local anaesthesia, a large quantity of fluid is injected percutaneously to identify the underneath superficial veins. Tumescent anaesthesia created causes hydrodissection. Trivex resector and illuminator are placed under the skin. Resector gently extracts veins by suction and morcellation. Further stages of tumescence flushes all blood and delivers vasoconstricting solutions. Solution is passed through 18 gauge needle to clear all blood underneath. Method is cosmetically acceptable; removes all sized veins; achieves good pain relief; with minimal complications like bruising, induration which gets resorbed eventually; can be used when there are venous ulcers.

OTHER METHODS

Transilluminated phlebectomy is done by passing transilluminating light under the skin and passing a rotating blade through another small incision. Veins are grasped and removed by rotating movements.

Ambulatory phlebectomy is done through tiny small incisions using special phlebectomy instruments. *Ramelet's hook* is used. It has sharp harpoons to grip the perivenous collagen of tunica externa of the vein and lift it. Ambulatory phlebectomy is a very useful OP procedure with minimal pain, safety, effectiveness and complications mainly useful in vein collaterals, reticular/perineal/foot and small perforators.

Electrodessication using weak electric current through a fine needle directly into the spider veins (telangiectasis) is also used.

Obliteration of saphenous veins with hyperheated steam is simple and cost effective which is designed by Milleret et al (France). Here water is pressurised at 600 atmospheres which is forced through a narrow tube into the needed vein to cause coagulation and sealing of the vein. Vapour once condenses turns into harmless water.

Cryostripping of the vein is also tried. Cryo probe is used only in part of the therapy while stripping.

INJECTION SCLEROTHERAPY FOR VARICOSE VEINS (FEGAN'S)

Sclerosants are injected into the vein to achieve complete sclerosis of the venous wall. It is used since 100 years as *liquid sclerotherapy.*

It is *indicated* in uncomplicated perforator incompetence; in managing reticular and thread veins; recurrent varicosities; isolated varicosities; in aged and unfit patients. Presently it is said that all types of varicose veins are amenable to sclerotherapy. It is very useful in managing spider veins less than 3 mm. In veins more than 3 mm sclerosant may get washed away.

Contraindications for sclerotherapy are—saphenofemoral incompetence, deep venous thrombosis; huge varicosities—may precipitate DVT; peripheral arterial diseases; hypersensitivity/immobility; pregnancy; venous ulcer—relative contraindication.

Sclerosants used are **sodium tetradecyl sulphate 3% or polidocanal 1%** or sodium morrhuate or ethanolamine oleate. Polidocanal 0.5% or 1% is also used in many countries. But it causes more allergy than sodium tetradecyl sulphate. It is not tried in varicose veins more than 3 mm; it is more useful for reticular veins and telangiectasias.

Sclerosants cause aseptic inflammation, perivenous fibrosis, endothelial obliteration.

Allergy, pregnancy, infection, bleeding disorders, DVT are contraindications for sclerotherapy.

Procedure: A 23 gauge needle is inserted into the vein; vein is emptied; 0.5 to 1.0 mL of sclerosant is injected into the vein with limb in elevated position; immediate compression is applied to prevent thrombosis; complete endothelial apposition and sclerosis is achieved. Injection is started at ankle level and later proceeded upwards. Compression stockings for 6 weeks should be used. Repeated sessions of injections with 2–4 weeks intervals can be given. It is called as *macrosclerotherapy.*

Microsclerotherapy: Very dilute solution of sclerosing agent like STDS, polidocanal is injected into the thread veins and reticular veins followed by application of compression bandage (30 G needle). Dermal flare will disappear well by this method.

Note:
Sclerotherapy can be—liquid or foam. Foam type may be with air or with CO_2.

Foam Sclerotherapy by Tessari

Cabrera introduced foam sclerotherapy using CO_2 in 1997. In 2000, Tessari started creation of foam from liquid sclerosant through three way stopcock and two syringes. It is simple, affordable, safe, efficient and repeatable. Foam fills the vein, stays longer and also causes spasm prolonged contact with the endothelium exposes subendothelium and causes fibrosis of venous wall. Thick consistency of foam makes it easier to treat large and bulging veins.

Foam displaces blood but never dilutes it; foam does not get mixed with blood and so would not get deactivated; causes wider area of chemical ablation of trunk veins. Gas embolism is a rare complication.

STD taken in a syringe is passed rapidly into another syringe which contains air that results in formation of foam. This foam in much larger quantity is injected into the superficial vein. Air gets absorbed between foam and endothelial lining is destroyed. Foam is created by different methods. Entire procedure is done under US guidance even through foam sclerotherapy without US guidance is also accepted method.

One of the methods which is followed by many is as follows—1 mL of STDS is taken in a 5 mL syringe; 4 mL of air is taken in another 5 mL syringe; both syringes are connected through a stopcock; by repeated to and fro movements between two syringes air gets mixed with sclerosant causing soap like foam. Usually 12–15 strokes are needed to create optimum foam. Large quantity of foam can be created by using 20 mL syringe using 4 mL of STDS in one and 16 mL of air in another 20 mL syringe to create 20 mL foam. Maximum sclerosant used is 6 mL for one sitting with 30 mL foam. Response to treatment is assessed by ulcer healing, disappearance of symptoms, US showing disappearance of varices. Leg should be raised during injection to prevent air embolism. Immediate stockings should be applied and should be continued for 6 weeks. Even though DVT can develop, its incidence is less. Foam which is dense gets coaxed into venous wall and so unlikely to flow to distant; so DVT and air embolism usually will not occur **(Fig. 12-34)**.

Foam minimises thrombosis by pushing the blood out of the site of the vessel where action is needed. Polidocanol or sodium tetradecyl sulphate is used for foam sclerotherapy.

It is better to use lowest dose for ankle veins and spider veins than reticular veins.

In small veins, magnifying glasses can be used to cannulate the vein. US guided foam sclerotherapy is standard which makes visualisation of foam and its passage.

Modified microfoam sclerotherapy: 3 mL distilled water and 0.2 mL sclerosant is mixed; foam is created similarly and injected using fine needle with gentle sustained force; it avoids air embolism with equal efficacy. Microfoam sclerotherapy with veinlite is also used. 30 mmHg compression is started immediately. Ambulation immediately, with aerobic exercise is important. One should avoid exposure to sun for 6 weeks. Postoperatively whealing, bruising, discolouration will be there initially **(Fig. 12-35)**.

Pharmaceutical microfoam is available now. It is low density uniform small bubbles of 100 µm. It is generated from O_2/CO_2 gas mixing with low nitrogen and gas gets absorbed in blood faster minimising gas embolism. Incidence of gas embolism is very less with this microfoam compared to manually created air-based foam.

Complications are—anaphylaxis, headache, transient blindness, stroke, air embolism are rare but specific to foam sclerotherapy. Thrombophlebitis, DVT, skin discolouration, skin necrosis are other complications.

Complications of sclerotherapy

Minor	***Major***
◈ Pigmentation	◈ Anaphylaxis
◈ Haematoma	◈ DVT
◈ Bruising	◈ Pulmonary embolism
◈ Ulceration	◈ Thrombophlebitis
◈ Extravasation	◈ Visual disturbances
	◈ Air embolism
	◈ Stroke

Advantages are—cheap, easier, anaesthesia is not needed, done on day care/OPD basis, can be combined with other procedures for varicose veins.

Echosclerotherapy

Sclerotherapy is done under duplex ultrasound image guidance.

Transillumination Microsclerotherapy *(Veinlite)*

It is better to image the veins using light generated by halogen bulb with high quality fibre with uniform illumination over the skin and passing 30 gauge needle for microsclerotherapy.

Catheter Directed Sclerotherapy

It was devised at Miami Vein Clinic, with specific catheter for sclerotherapy. This catheter has got side holes all around the specific length for uniform contact of venous wall with the foam. It also has got a balloon at the tip which after inflation blocks the SFJ thus preventing embolisation of foam. It has got three external ports one for balloon inflation; one for bladder valve port; one for injection. This technique is under trial **(Fig. 12-36)**.

Remember about sclerotherapy

- ◈ Current place of sclerotherapy is mainly for recurrent varicosities and thread/telangiectatic veins.
- ◈ Sodium tetradecyl sulphate (STDS) is most commonly used sclerosant.
- ◈ Hyperpigmentation is common after STDS.
- ◈ Anaphylaxis is common after sodium morrhuate.
- ◈ Anaphylaxis is least with polidocanol.
- ◈ Extravasation (presence of pain/irritation/burning) should be avoided as it will cause skin necrosis.
- ◈ Postsclerotherapy walking immediately after injection for 30 minutes with elastic bandage in place prevents/minimises the chances of DVT.
- ◈ Compression bandage should be worn for minimum period of 6 weeks.
- ◈ Sclerotherapy can be—macrosclerotherapy; microsclerotherapy; echo (ultrasound guided) sclerotherapy; foam sclerotherapy; trans-illuminated sclerotherapy.

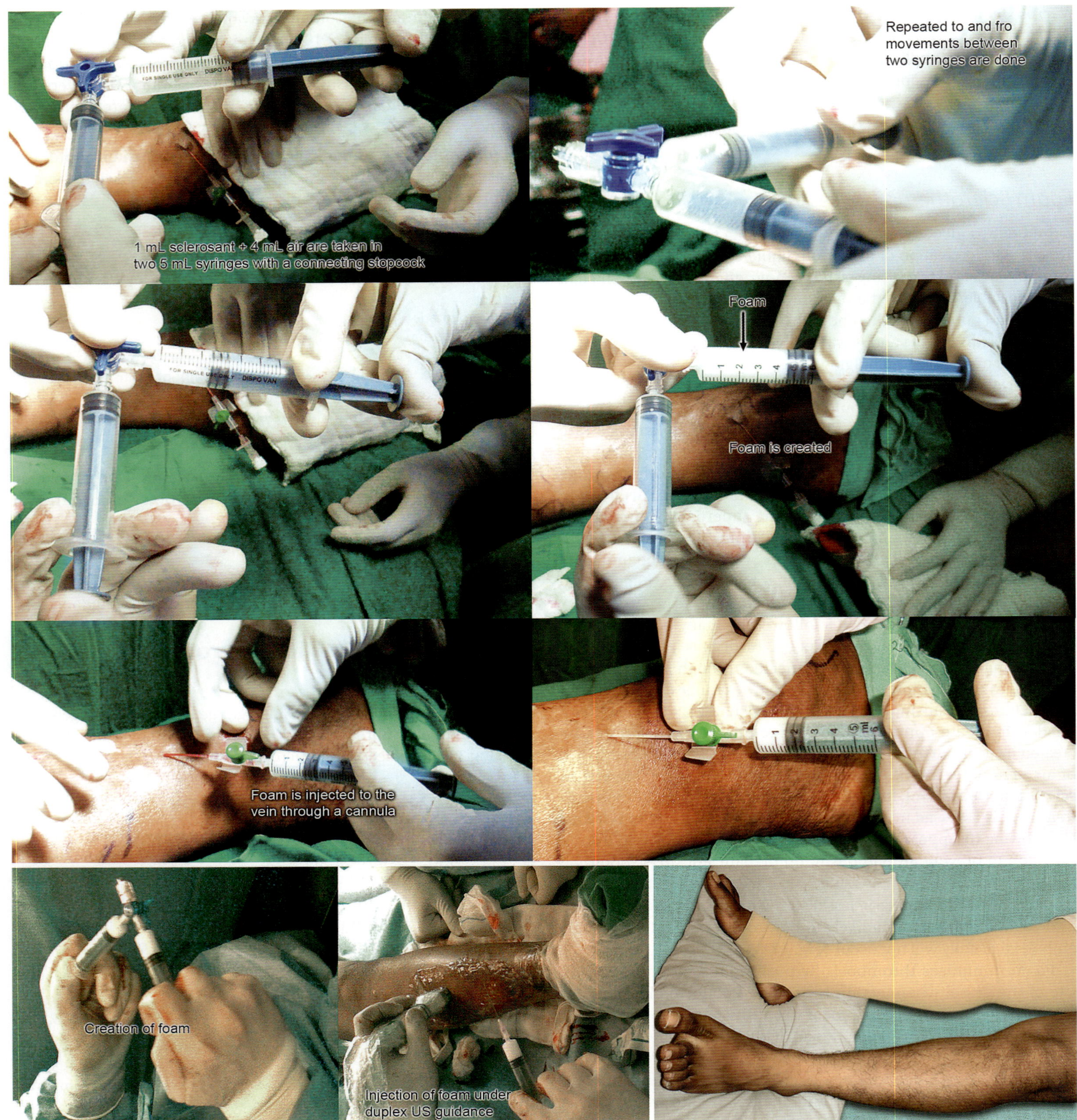

Fig. 12-34: Technique of foam sclerotherapy. Stockings and elevation of the limb is important in post-procedure period.

Steam vein sclerosis (SVS): Endovenous laser treatment with a bare fibre requires high levels of heat and can cause blood carbonisation, or perforation of the venous wall due to thermal damage. But tulip and radial fibres can reduce perforations. So, it was thought that homogeneous wall heating and obliteration could be obtained by injecting steam directly into the veins. The SVS device system (cermaVEIN, Archamps, France) is used to achieve steam ablation. Micropulses of steam are injected into a catheter to deliver the steam into the vein. 16G infusion catheter is placed into the GSV around knee area through a small venotomy. Flexible stainless steel SVS catheter (60 cm), covered with Teflon [diameter of 1.2 mm (cermaVEIN)] is inserted through the infusion catheter and forwarded under ultrasound guidance to a level of 2–3 cm below the SFJ (guidewire is not necessary). Through SVS generator using foot

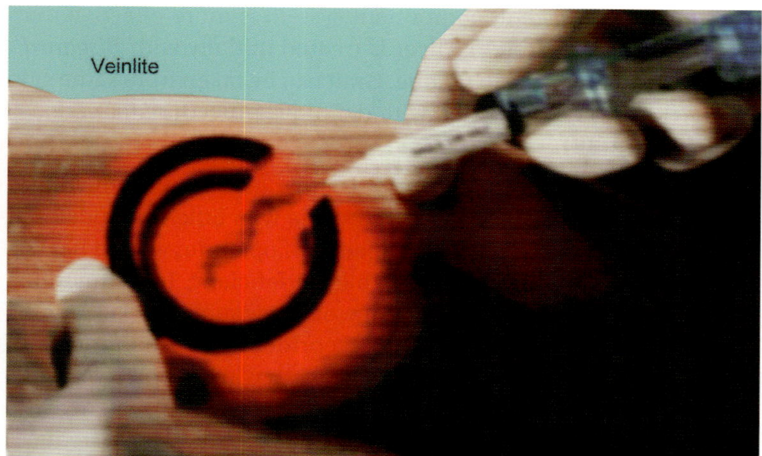

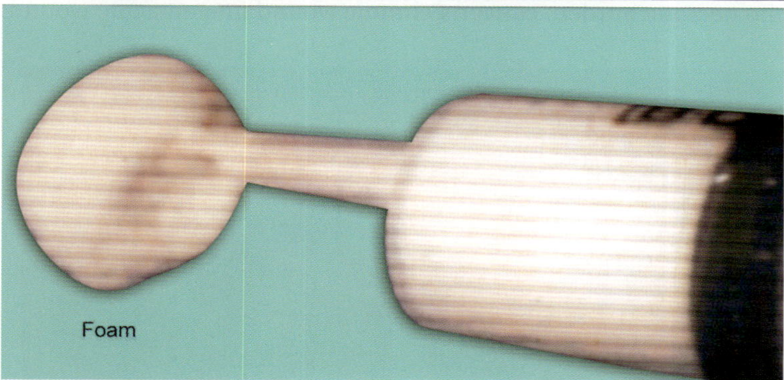

Fig. 12-35: Microfoam sclerotherapy (MFST) using veinlite.

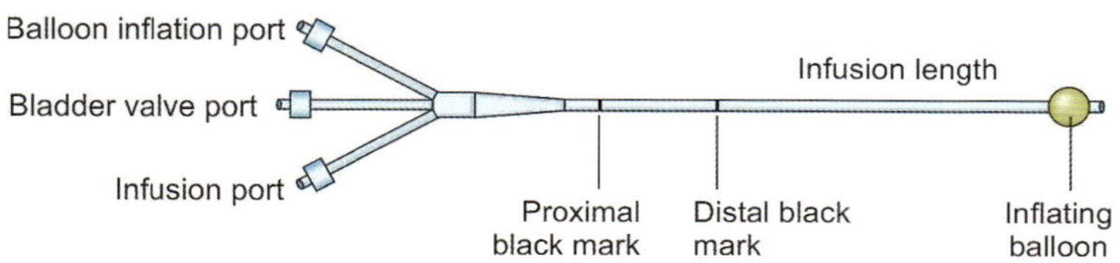

Fig. 12-36: Catheter directed sclerotherapy.

pedal three pulses with one pulse of 1.8 seconds of 60 J energy with 120°C temperature at the tip. (Initially SVS generator activation is done to dispel the condensed water in the catheter by releasing two pulses of steam). Catheter is withdrawn 1 cm to deliver further three pulses. Standard is two pulses for 7 mm vein; three pulses for 7–12 mm vein; four pulses for vein >12 mm. phlebotomies can be added to bulging tributaries. Tumescent solution should be injected along the line of catheter like in EVLA. Compression stockings should be used for 2 weeks postoperatively with limb elevation. Advantages are: No venous perforation or carbonisation; safe; effective; can be done as day care surgery. Disadvantages: Procedure is under trial; smaller veins cannot be treated.

Endovenous microwave ablation (EMWA): It is endovenous therapy for varicose veins using microwave energy. Technique is similar but precautions for laser done in EVLA is not necessary.

Clarivein (Mechanochemical ablation/MOCA): It is endovenous ablation of vein using both mechanical and chemical sclerosants. Here tumescent solution is not required as heat energy is not used. Nerve damage will not occur. It is used in varicose veins below the knee and lower leg and with leg ulcers. Clarivein catheter is placed into the lumen of the vein under ultrasound guidance. Device trigger when pulled catheter tip rotates with 3000 revolutions per minute. Simultaneously sclerosant is injected into the vein through the device. Rotated tip rips the vein wall by making small tunnels and injected sclerosant creates a Swiss Cheese effect into the vein obliterating it. Sodium tetradecyl sulphate is used. Large veins cannot be used **(Fig. 12-37)**.

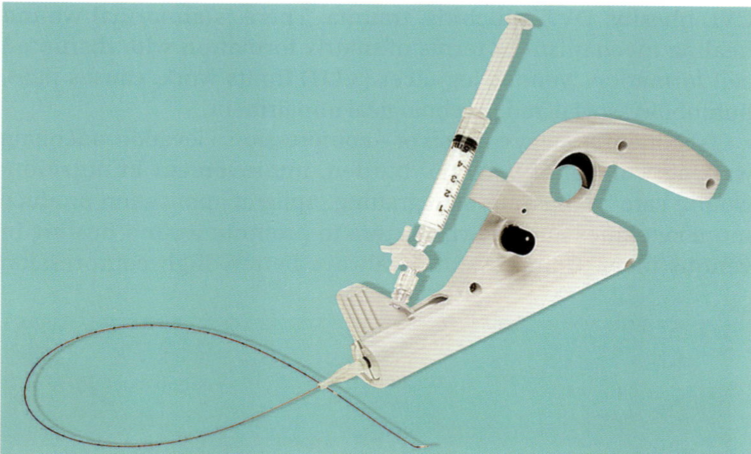

Fig. 12-37: Clarivein catheter for Mechano chemical ablation (MOCA).

Transluminal occlusion of perforators (TRLOP; Mark Whiteley and Judy Holdstock): Usually there are around 150 perforators in leg connecting superficial veins to deep veins with a valve allowing unidirectional blood flow from superficial to deep system. So it is common to have perforator incompetency along with superficial vein incompetency or often only perforator incompetency. Using needle hole in the vein and passing VNUS catheter into the perforator vein, it is occluded with 85°C heat. Procedure is same as PAP (perforator ablative procedure) where laser may be used to occlude the perforator.

Sapheon venaseal/superglue therapy for varicose veins: It is done under ultrasound guidance using specialised superglue injection device.

Sonovein–HD: Echotherapy using high intensity focused ultrasound (HIFU) is 100% non-invasive. Ultrasound is generated in a cone-shaped manner to focus at exactly right point with generation of 90°C at the specific point which ablates the cells to cause sclerosis. It is a non-invasive disruptive technology. Eight seconds to heat the vein is required and 50 seconds to cool the vein afterwards. Often it requires local anaesthesia. But newer devices heat in half to one second which does not require local anaesthesia. It is useful for superficial veins and perforator veins as well. Glue used is cyanoacrylate.

Note

- Non-chromate glycerin is better for sclerotherapy of telangiectatic veins.
- 5 mL syringe should be used.
- Ideally finer needle should be used; 30 gauge is better.
- Light and magnification if used it will be better in telangiectatic sclerotherapy.
- Liquid sclerosant is better for smaller veins less than 3 mm.
- Injection should be felt rather than flash back in hub.
- Injection should be stopped if there is white pallor formation in the skin.
- Leg should be elevated while injecting.
- Larger and deeper veins should be injected first before smaller and superficial veins.
- Trapped blood source should be evacuated.
- 3 way stopcock should be used to create foam.

MANAGEMENT OF VENOUS ULCER

Venous ulcer is a complication of chronic venous hypertension occurring around ankle in *Gaiter's* zone (Gaiter-French—a covering of cloth/leather around ankle and lower leg). 80% of leg ulcers has got venous component. Prevalence of ulcer increase with age and in females. Recurrence of venous ulcer is 60–70%. It is due to CVI, obesity, DVT, phlebitis, trauma. There is abnormal wound healing mechanism in terms of matrix formation with disrupted cell formation. Venous leg ulcer (VLU) limits work, causes pain, immobility, social and psychological impairment.

Treatment strategy consists of—compression; elevation, adequate walking; control of bacterial burden, improvement in nutrition, wound care by dressing; skin grafting. Apligraf application produce more cytokines and growth factors to promote wound healing in venous ulcer. Compression is always better; high compression is better than low; multicomponent system is more effective than single component system. Ulcer is treated initially with *Bisgaard's method*; later by split skin grating. Graft can be taken from same side thigh. It should be combined with definitive procedure for varicose veins **(Fig. 12-38)**.

Ulcer/wound bed preparation: It is creation of optimum wound healing environment by vascularised stable with little/no exudates in the bed. Factors which prevent formation of optimum wound healing environment are—**T**issue non-viable or deficient; **I**nflammation/**I**nfection; **M**oisture imbalance; **E**dge of the wound non-advancing or undermined (***TIME principle***). Debridement is the process of removing devitalised or necrotic tissue often with the foreign body it is harbouring. Debridement is the most important component of the Wound Bed Preparation. It facilitates the therapeutic efficacy, reduces the necrotic burden, converts chronic wound into an acute wound.

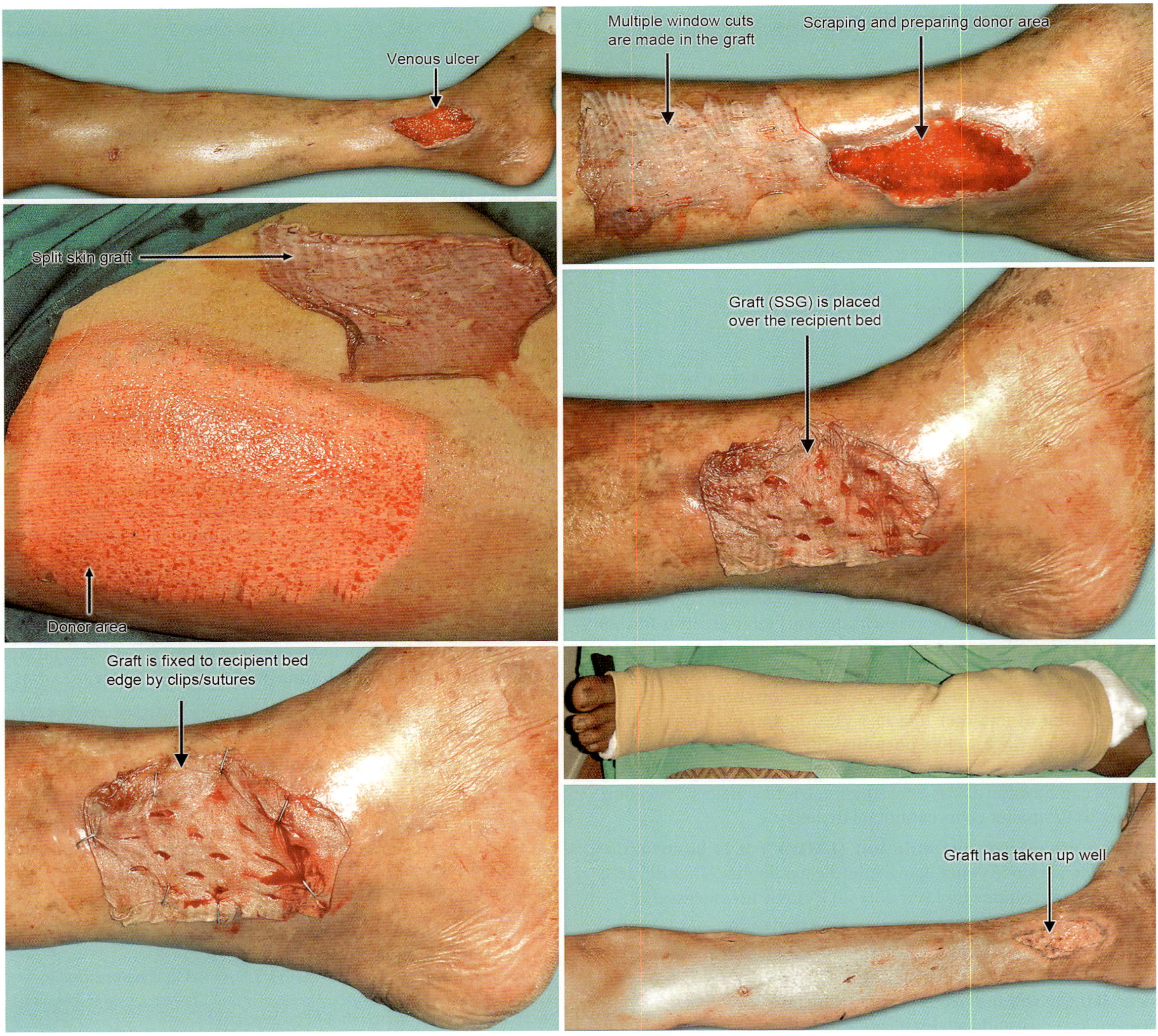

Fig. 12-38: Split skin grafting can be used to cover the venous ulcer after treating the varicose veins.

Different methods of wound debridement are present—surgical, autolytic, enzymatic, mechanical, larval. Surgical debridement is sharp anatomical technique wherein only dead tissue is removed demarcating live tissue to salvage; it is helpful to remove extensive devitalised tissue; it decreases the bacterial burden and removes old senescent cells also. But it may cause often undue bleeding and damage to vital tissues adjacent and so proper anatomical knowledge is essential. In autolytic process endogenous proteolytic enzymes liquefy necrotic material and eschar from healthy tissues. In enzymatic debridement, papain, urea, collagenase, fibrinolysin are used. In mechanical type—wet to dry dressings; irrigations to wound and hydrotherapy; whirlpool technique are used. Larval method (biosurgery) is often beneficial by using Lucila Serricata (green bottlefly) which digest necrotic material and also secretes bactericidal enzymes which is useful MRSA and beta haemolytic streptococci; Phanicia Aericata (blow fly maggots) dissolve necrotic material and biofilm without disturbing normal tissues.

COMPRESSION THERAPY FOR VARICOSE VEINS

Core Indications for Compression Therapy

As conservative therapy for varicose veins; in treating oedema; after interventions for varicose veins; in advanced chronic venous insufficiencies; in treating venous leg ulcers.

- Compression reduces the venous wall tension; prevents reflux; controls the venous over distension; decreases ambulatory venous hypertension; improves microcirculation; improves filtration and exchange dynamics.
- Compression diverts the blood towards deep veins through perforating veins; prevents the outward flow of blood in perforator incompetence; improves the efficacy of calf muscle pump. Compression reduces the oedema and improves the venous and lymphatic drainage; improves venous elasticity; improves the microcirculation and more important is that it prevents further damage of the venous wall.
- Compression may be elastic/inelastic/combination of elastic and inelastic (*Unna boot*)/multilayered (four layered) compression system which can provide sustained high compression for several days—usually up to a week/intermittent pneumatic compression. Unna boot is three layered paste gauze compression dressing containing calamine, zinc oxide, glycerin, sorbitol, gelatin and aluminium silicate which has mainly inelastic inner component with partly elastic outer layer wrap.
- *Inelastic type* is used for continuous use in severe chronic venous disease. *Elastic type* is used as self applied at day time. Elastic types are—short stretch <70%; medium stretch 70–140%; long stretch >140%.
- Recommended pressure in mild varicose veins, pregnancy and postoperative period is 20 mmHg; in symptomatic varicose veins and after sclerotherapy it is 30 mmHg; in venous ulcer and post-phlebitic leg it is 40–45 mmHg; in phlebolymphedema (venous oedema with lymphatic oedema which is more dangerous) it is more than 45 mmHg.
- Skin maceration, excoriation, dryness, infection, ulceration and failure are the complications of compression therapy.
- The efficacy of the compression therapy is more if compression is graduated with more pressure (strongest) at ankle and decreasing proximally.
- Compression therapy should be strong enough to compensate venous hypertension, to prevent/reduce oedema, should regress the pathological consequences occurred in the tissues; but compression therapy is commonly a symptomatic treatment.
- Compression therapy should not be too high to compromise the arterial supply.
- The person should understand the reasons for wearing the compression bandage.
- The person should know how to put and take of the stockings; best time to put stockings is in the morning as first thing prior to development of any limb oedema.
- Correct fit stockings should be worn—either standard sized or custom made.
- While person is off the stockings, application of the emollient is important to avoid skin dryness and irritation.
- If the person is having difficulty in tolerating the level of compression, one should try a lighter compression bandage. If a person is having difficulty in using thigh level stockings, one should use below knee level stockings.
- A stockings application aid may be beneficial to people who are having difficulty in wearing the stockings.
- Bandage <10%—inelastic (cotton bandage); short stretch >10% <100%; long stretch <100%.
- Compression works by pressure (interface pressure—pressure between compression and bandage) and stiffness; low resting pressure for comfort; high working pressure for efficacy. Static stiffness index (SSI = standing pressure – supine pressure); SST <10 means not stiff; >10 means it is stiff. Stiffness enables the higher venous return while working and so more efficacious.
- In venous ulcer high pressure compression is mandatory (>30 mmHg); multilayered bandages or multilayered compression stockings with superimposition are better.
- Short stretch bandages have got 60% stretchability from resting length with low resting pressure and high working pressure. Long stretch bandage has got 140% stretchability with high resting pressure and low working pressure **(Figs. 12-39A and B)**.

Remember

- Compression improves rate of ulcer healing.
- Supplementation of phlebotonic drugs in conjunction with compression therapy is accepted.
- Inelastic compression causes more improvement (reduction) in venous filling index (VFI) than elastic compression. But elastic compression is more commonly used because it is better accepted.
- Multilayered bandage system is most effective.
- Ankle-arm pressure index less than 0.6 is contraindication for compression therapy as it may precipitate ischaemic ulcer formation.
- Exercise may improve the muscle-pump action.

Compression class and compression pressure (Phlebology, 2009)

Standard	*Class I*	*Class II*	*Class III*	*Class IV*
British	14–17	17–24	24–35	NA
International – European	20–30	30–40	40–50	50–60
Draft European	15–21	23–32	34–46	>49
German	18–21	23–32	34–46	>49
French	10–15	15–20	20–36	>36
USA	15–20	20–30	30–40	NA

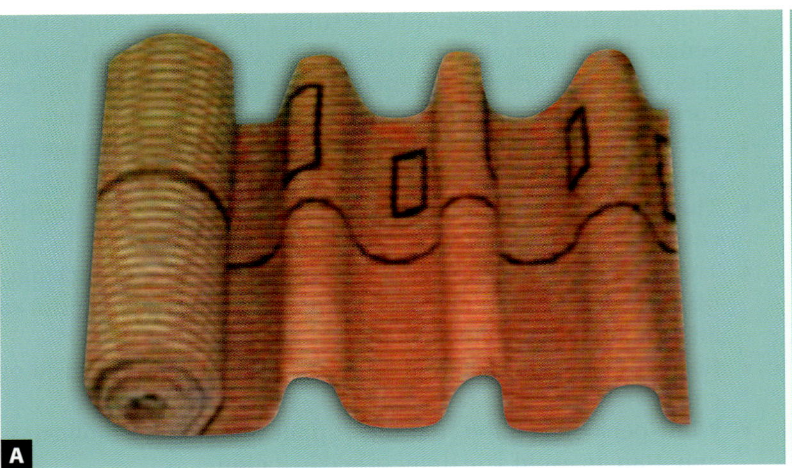

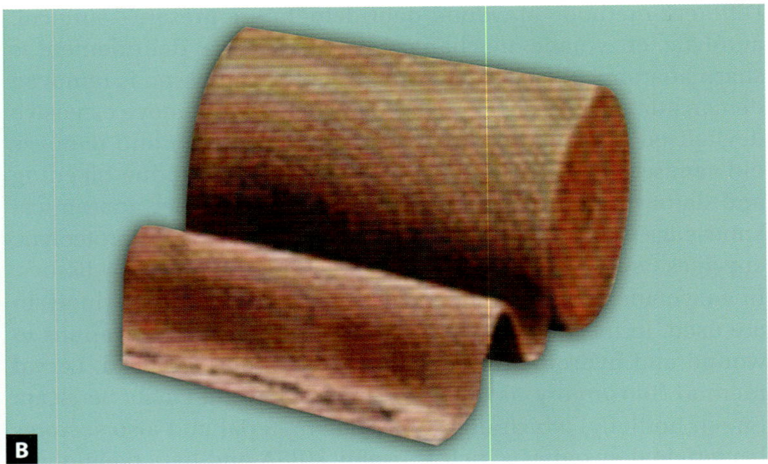

Figs. 12-39A and B: Long and short stretch bandages.

Compression Bandages

- *Type 1:* Light weight confirming stretch bandages. These comprise light weight elastomer with high elasticity but little power. It is used to retain dressings.
- *Type II* (Short stop): Light support bandages. Minimal stretch. Exhibit limited elasticity but tends to lock out on minimal extension. In ambulant patient with CVI they form an essentially inelastic covering to the leg which will exert pressure during calf systole but not during diastole. They are unsuitable for control of oedema.
- *Type III* (Long stop): These are extensible elastic and powerful to a varying degree **(Fig. 12-40)**.

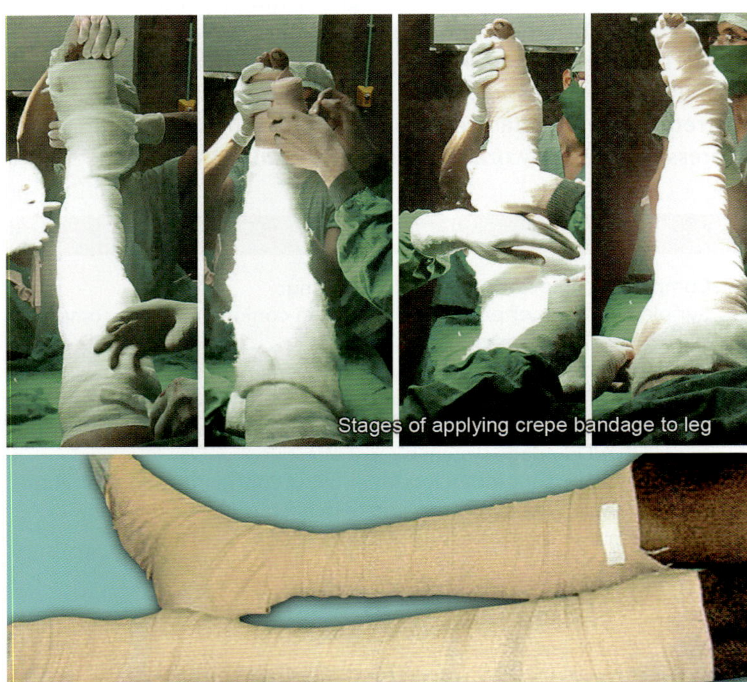

Fig. 12-40: Stages of applying crepe bandage immediately after intervention procedure. Elevation of the limb is also equally important.

CAUSES OF RECURRENT VARICOSE VEINS

Causes are—neovascularisation (55%); pelvic veins (33%); perforator incompetence (32%); missed de novo reflux (30%); inadequate surgery (10%); earlier untreated veins (7%). Pelvic congestion syndrome can be successfully treated by coil embolisation of the pelvic veins.

SURGICAL TREATMENT FOR DEEP VENOUS THROMBOSIS AND VENOUS THROMBOEMBOLISM (VTE)

Palma Operation

In iliofemoral thrombosis, common femoral vein below the block is connected to opposite common femoral vein using opposite great saphenous vein **(Fig. 12-41)**.

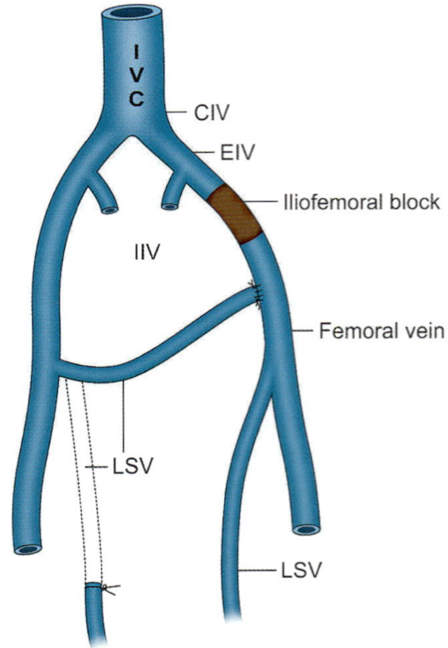

Fig. 12-41: Palma operation for iliofemoral block. Using opposite great saphenous vein femoral vein is connected to other femoral vein. (IVC: inferior vena cava; CIV: common iliac vein; EIV: external iliac vein; IIV: internal iliac vein; LSV: long saphenous vein)

May–Husni Operation

When popliteal vein is blocked popliteal vein below the block is anastomosed to great saphenous vein as end-to-end bypass **(Fig. 12-42)**.

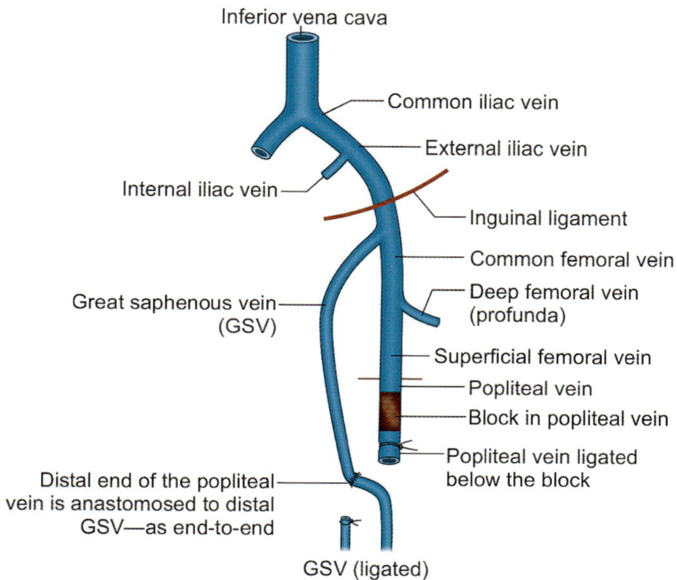

Fig. 12-42: May–Husni operation.

Venous Thromboembolism (VTE)

Incidences in DVT

- 20% of hospitalised patients; 50% of orthopaedic surgery patients; 1% of adult population after 40 years; 40% of patients undergoing abdominal or thoracic surgeries; one out of 100 DVT patients will die of pulmonary embolism.
- 5% of pulmonary embolism forms chronic thromboembolic pulmonary hypertension with right ventricular failure.
- More than 50% of DVT leads into chronic venous insufficiency (CVI).
- 30% DVT recurs 10 years after discontinuation of the anticoagulant therapy.
- Post-thrombotic syndrome (PTS) occurs in 50% of DVT patients with leg oedema, pain, nocturnal cramping, venous claudication, skin pigmentation, dermatitis and ulceration on the medial side of the lower leg.
- VTE can be provoked or unprovoked (idiopathic).

Well's criteria for DVT probability is based on—active ulcer; paralysis/recent immobilisation; bedridden for >3 days; recent surgery within 1 month time; swollen leg; tenderness along deep veins; calf girth difference >3 cm; pitting oedema; others.

SMART tool: Surgical and Medical Assessment of Risks for Thrombosis.

DVT risk can be:

Low risk—<10% (minor surgery in mobile patients); *moderate risk*—10–40% (general; gynaecologic/urologic surgeries)—needs LMWH or mechanical thromboprophylaxis if there is high bleed; *high risk*—40–80% (hip/knee arthroplasty, fractures, major trauma) needs LMWH, mechanical thromboprophylaxis. Dose of LMWH is full dose (5,000 units) 2 hours prior to surgery, then half or full dose for 10 days.

High risk can be brought down to 5% by prevention and prophylaxis.

Calf vein thrombosis is defined as any clot involving the deep veins of the calf that did not extend to the popliteal veins. Calf has got three paired veins—posterior tibial, anterior tibial and peroneal. Calf also has got two unpaired muscular veins—soleal and gastrocnemial. Peroneal veins are commonly involved. Isolated calf muscle vein thrombosis (ICMVT) occurs when thrombosis is confined only to muscular veins; when thrombosis present in paired calf veins, it is called as deep calf vein thrombosis (DCVT). If both paired veins and muscular veins are involved then it is called as isolated distal deep vein thrombosis (IDDVT). Its prevalence is 5–30%. Incidence of propagation of thrombus from deep veins to proximal vein is 5–30%. But post-thrombotic syndrome is not common in IDDVT (calf). Thromboembolism is more common once thrombus extends to proximal vein. Present recommendation is—ultrafraction heparin intravenously or LMWH subcutaneously for 10 days; then vitamin K antagonist (Warfarin) for 3 months. INR should be maintained between 2.0 to 3.0 (2.5). Extended therapy for 6 months may be done depending on the risk factors.

Non-compressible clot in compression ultrasound (duplex) is very useful method of evaluation.

In a confirmed case, thrombectomy may be needed using Fogarty catheter.

Catheter directed thrombolysis (CDT) can be done after cannulating (5F or 6F, US guided, multihole catheter) popliteal vein clot area is reached under ultrasound and also fluorescence guidance and tissue plasminogen activator (tPA) and reteplase are injected into the clot (intraclot). Short saphenous vein or post-tibial veins also can be used.

Catheter directed thrombolysis also can be done by puncturing pedal vein with US guidance and then using 4 F catheter clot is reached to create lysis. High dose of thrombolytics are injected into the thrombus directly with less systemic effects with better patency and success rates. Systemic effects, prolonged infusion of 8 hours, risk of bleeding are problems. US guided EKOS endowave infusion system is better which reduces the infusion period less than 24 hours. Drugs used are—Altepase 0.25–2 mg/hour with 10 mg start and then 1 mg/hour over 24 hours using infusion pump; reteplase 0.75 units/hour; tenecteplase 0.25–0.5 mg/hour. Contraindications are—severe uncontrolled hypertension; uncontrolled clotting disorders; active bleeding; recent CVA; intracranial neoplasm; allergy to drugs.

Mechanical or pharmacomechanical thrombectomy is also useful often in acute thrombus. Suction thrombectomy, Rotarex device, Angiojet **(Fig. 12-43)**, Trellis system are different methods used for the same. Problems with pharmacomechanical thrombectomy are—haemolysis, haemoglobinuria, renal impairment, bradycardia, pulmonary embolism.

Thrombus (DVT) should be classified as suprapopliteal or infrapopliteal. Infrapopliteal DVT initially treated LMWH or warfarin.

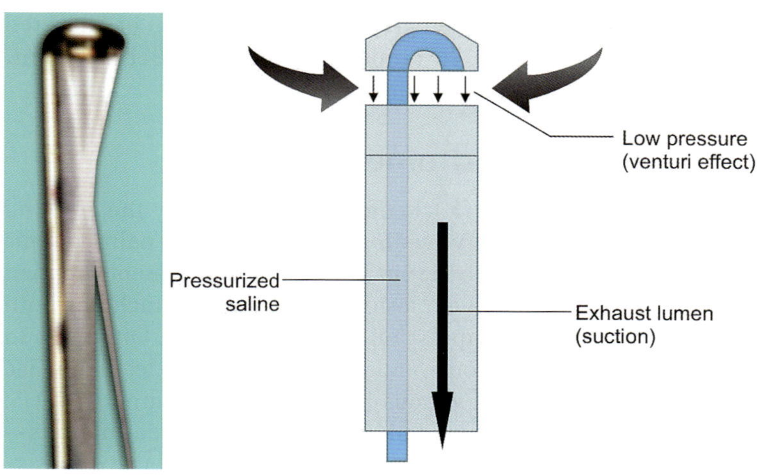

Fig. 12-43: Angiojet.

Suprapopliteal DVT needs evaluation or possible pulmonary embolism or IVC or iliac vein extensions which need catheter directed thrombolysis or pharmacomechanical thrombectomy. Retrievable IVC filters in case of possibility of pulmonary embolism and iliac vein stenting in case of iliac vein stenosis is needed.

IVC filters are used when anticoagulation has failed (recurrent pulmonary embolism), anticoagulation has caused bleeding, and when anticoagulation is contraindicated (intracranial haemorrhage).

Pulmonary embolism causes acute dyspnoea, haemoptysis, chest pain, shock, right ventricular dysfunction, severe respiratory distress and death. Well's and modified Geneva criteria are used. CT angiogram is very useful. Treatment is—heparin, thrombolysis, catheter-directed thrombolysis, surgical embolectomy with cardio-pulmonary bypass.

Leg elevation, stockings and early ambulation are preventive measures. In confirmed DVT cases massage and hot fermentation are contraindicated.

Duration of anticoagulation in isolated calf vein DVT is 6 weeks; in provoked DVT it is 3–6 months with risk factor it is with extended therapy of more than 6 months; unprovoked DVT duration is 3–6 months, if 2nd episode extended therapy for >6 months. For recurrent DVT it is for life long.

In patients with acute proximal DVT of limb, anticoagulant therapy (LMWH) alone is suggested over systemic/catheter-directed thrombolysis or venous thrombectomy.

Thrombolysis is indicated in extensive thrombosis of iliofemoral or proximal sites, threatened limb viability, venous anatomical anomaly.

In pregnancy LMWH is used for DVT. Ultrafraction heparin, vitamin K analogue (warfarin), direct thrombin (dabigatran) inhibitors and anti-Xa (rivaroxaban, apixaban) are not used in pregnancy.

VTE treatment is categorised as—initial; long term; extended.

Chronic DVT

It leads into chronic venous insufficiency (CVI). It presents as non-healing ulcer over malleoli and lower leg; lymphovenous oedema; ankle fibrosis; pigmentation; lipodermatosclerosis of leg; joint osteoarthritis; quadriceps and calf muscle wasting. It is evaluated by discharge culture study, Doppler study, CT/MRI of part; D dimer test; biomarkers P; selectin/CRP.

It is managed by elevation to reduce edema; compression devices; venous stenting; venous valve repair (valvuloplasty).

Venous ulcer is treated by—compression therapy—40 mmHg multilayered (four) sustained graduated compression or 2 layered zinc oxide impregnated 25 mmHg compression; debridement; infection control; colloid silver dressing.

May–Thurner Syndrome

It is compression of the (left) common iliac vein by the crossing right common iliac artery leading into the left leg pain, venous oedema and often iliofemoral vein thrombosis. It is presently termed as non-thrombotic iliac vein lesions (NIVL) which includes both common iliac veins' compression of varying causes. Often due to arterial compression, fibrous venous spur develops to lead into iliac vein thrombosis. Duplex venous Doppler, MR venography, IVUS, coagulation profile is needed investigations. Treatment is—thrombolysis, angioplasty and venous stenting; in extensive disease pharmacomechanical thrombectomy is required.

Nutcracker Syndrome

It is the compression of the left renal vein between abdominal aorta and superior mesenteric artery; it presents with left loin, groin and testicular pain, haematuria, left-sided varicocele. In females it causes pelvic congestion syndrome. It is diagnosed by CT abdomen, left renal venography (gold standard) and MR venogram. Treatment is endovascular stenting or renal vein re-implantation.

Post-thrombotic Syndrome

Post-thrombotic syndrome (PTS) is late effect of DVT. It can occur in iliofemoral or femoropopliteal or calf vein DVT. But iliofemoral DVT is more commonly involved with PTS. Residual thrombus increases the risk. It develops in 50% of DVT patients as late effect usually in 2 years. Around 3% of PTS patients develop venous ulcers (post-phlebitis ulcers). It can occur in a DVT patient in spite of anticoagulation therapy. PTS is measured by Villalta scale and Ginsberg measures are used for the assessment of PTS. CEP, VCCS, Wildmer classification is used for chronic venous insufficiency (CVI) assessment. PTS incidence can be reduced by initial treatment of heparin/LMWH for DVT, Warfarin, and early ambulation with compression stockings. Active thrombus removal (thrombectomy) and thrombolysis should be done. US Duplex scan is diagnostic tool. Near infrared spectroscopy (NIRS) is also useful in early detection **(Fig. 12-44)**.

Villata PTS scale

Patient related symptoms	*Clinical sign assessed by clinician*
♦ Heaviness ♦ Pain, cramps ♦ Pruritus ♦ Paraesthesia	♦ Pretibial oedema ♦ Skin induration ♦ Hyperpigmentation ♦ Venous ectasia, redness ♦ Pain (tenderness) during calf compression
Each symptom and sign should be rated as 0—absent; 1—mild; 2—moderate; 3—severe; Ulcer should be marked as present or absent.	
0–4: Absent of PTS 5–9: Mild PTS 10–14: Moderate PTS >15 or presence of an ulcer: Severe PTS	

Treatment—drugs, elastic bandage and deep venous reflux surgery—valvuloplasty.

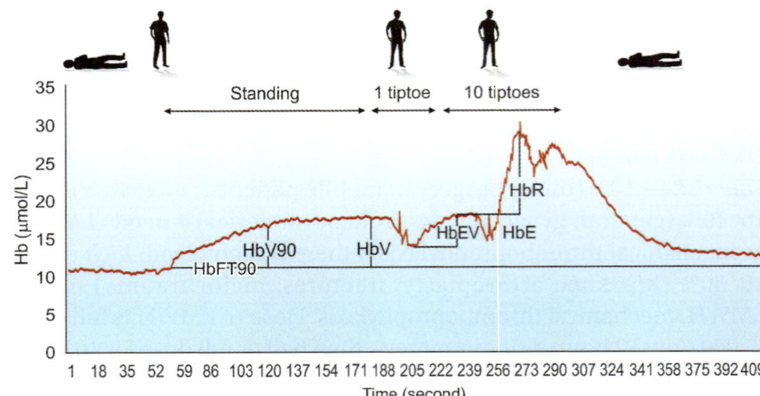

Fig. 12-44: Near infrared spectroscopy.

IVC Filters

IVC filters are used to prevent dislodged thrombus from entering into right atrium. ACP 2012 (American College of Chest Physicians) and ACR-SIR 2010 (American College of Radiologists and Society for Interventional Radiologists) guidelines are used.

Indications for IVC filters	
Absolute	*Relative*
• DVT or pulmonary embolism with a recognised contraindication for anticoagulation • Recurrent pulmonary embolism despite anticoagulation • Bleeding complications requiring discontinuation of anticoagulation • After pulmonary embolectomy	• Large free floating iliofemoral thrombus • Propagation of iliofemoral thrombus despite anticoagulation • Chronic pulmonary embolism with pulmonary hypertension and cor pulmonale • Prior to thrombolysis • Septic venous thromboembolism

IVC filters are used in pulmonary embolism and DVT when anticoagulants are contraindicated and symptomatic pulmonary embolism with thrombotic load in the limb. IVC filters are indicated in recurrent DVT and pulmonary embolism despite therapeutic anticoagulation; may be useful in free floating thrombus in iliofemoral segment or IVC. IVC filter is indicated in pregnancy when anticoagulants are contraindicated and when there is extensive thromboembolism. If patient had recent history of VTE and he has to undergo some other surgery, then IVC filter is indicated. Chronic thromboembolic pulmonary hypertension needs IVC filters. Retrievable IVC filters are placed.

Prophylactic filters may be used in trauma like closed head injuries, spinal cord injuries, and multiple long/pelvic bone injuries. Infrarenal IVC thrombus, duplication of IVC, larger (pelvic mass prior to surgery) if IVC mobilisation is needed, in pregnancy when filters are indicated—suprarenal IVC filters are placed. IVC filters are placed under Duplex US and fluoroscopic guidance **(Fig. 12-45)**.

Retrievable filters are commonly used now. Retrieving is done in 6-12 months or once chances of re DVT have become less. Retrieving is technically easy and safe.

IVC filters are placed percutaneously; highly effective against formation of the pulmonary embolism; it is non-thrombogenic; preserves caval patency. Preplacement venacavagram is a must to detect the presence and location of the clot, to determine the caval diameter, to detect venous anomalies, to determine the location of the renal veins.

Different filters are—Mobin Uddin; Greenfield; Bard, etc.

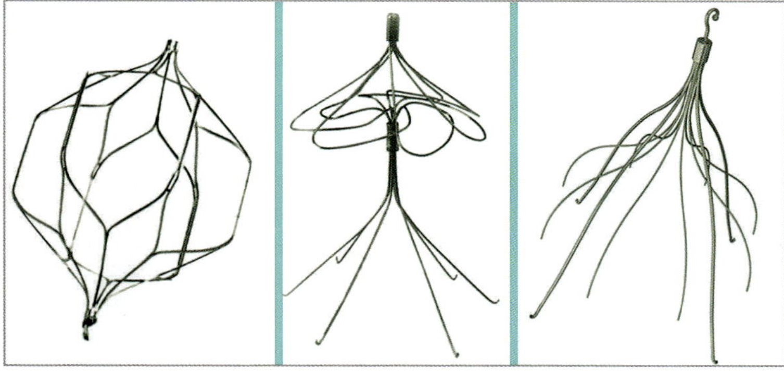

Fig. 12-45: Different IVC filters.

SURGERIES FOR LYMPHOEDEMA

"Lymphoedema cannot be cured but can be endured".

Surgeries or lymphoedema are so many as each one has got us own problems and advantages. From historical surgeries to nodal transplant wide range of surgeries are practiced. Surgeries are grossly classified as excisional wherein lymphoedematous tissues are excised properly; physiological wherein some technique is used to communicate deep and superficial lymphatics so that to improve the drainage through deep lymphatics.

Excisional: • Charle's operation • Modified Charles operation • Homan's operation • Liposuction	**Combined:** • Sistrunk operation • Thompson's operation • Kondoleon's operation
Physiological: • Omentoplasty • Nodovenous shunt • Lymphovenous shunt • Ileal mucosal patch • Lymph node transplant surgery (Vascularised lymph node transfer) • Silicone tube implantation (Waldemar L Olszewski)	**By pass procedures:** • Handley's procedure • Gilles skin bridge across the thigh and abdomen • Nodovenous shunt • Lymphovenous shunt • Ileal mucosal patch (Kimmonth) • Baumiester lymphatic graft • Free lymphatic flap autotransplantation
Limb reduction surgeries: • Sistrunk operation • Homan's operation • Thompson's operation • Kondoleon's operation • Macey's operation • Miller's procedure	

Handley's procedure: Handley in London (1908) did first surgery for lymphoedema by placing silk threads/nylon/polyethylene tubes in the subcutaneous plane from ankle to mid-abdominal level as drainage procedure; such materials are kept in place for one year. This procedure is now of historical interest.

Gilles procedure (Sir Harold Gillies, 1920): He started "waltzing" skin flap containing lymphatic wicks to bridge in obstructed lymphoedema; here skin with subcutaneous tissue is bridged across.

Ileal mucosal patch (Kinmonth): Segment of ileum with pedicle is isolated and opened to expose he mucosa; mucosa is denuded and this mucosa is placed in the thigh as burial to communicate with lymphatics to drain into abdominal lymphatics across ileum.

Vascularised lymph node transfer: Here lymph node with its artery and vein is transferred to the recipient are and placed by anatomosis its artery and vein using fine sutures of polypropylene (7-zero or 8-zero); it needs microscope to suture. It is done usually post-mastectomy upper limb lymphoedema; here groin lymph node is used to transfer. Submental lymph nodes in the neck are alternative nodes which can be used. Often it is done while finishing the modified radical mastectomy in a single sitting; usually along with the lymph node transfer breast reconstruction is also done using deep inferior epigastric perforators (DIEP) flap.

Lymphovenous shunt (O'Brien): It is anastomosing the tiny lymphatics in the drainage area to tiny veins at same place using 11-zero polypropylene suture using supermicrosurgical technique; these lymphatics are very fine of 0.1–0.8 mm in diameter; often they can be anastomosed to the long saphenous vein also. Indigo cyanine green lymphography is used to assess and evaluate the limb for the same.

Nodovenous shunt (Neibulowiz): Here regional lymph node is sutured to the superficial vein in that area. For lower limb lymphoedema, inguinal lymph node is identified; its anterior surface is dissected; capsule is opened at its convex part and is sutured to long saphenous vein using 7-zero polypropylene continuous suture **(Fig. 12-46)**.

Suction-assisted lipectomy (Hakan Brorson, 1987): It is similar to liposuction but is done using specialised vibrating device cannulae, tourniquet and tumescent. Procedure needs further compression therapy to get desirable effect.

Lymphatic vessel grafting (Reudiger Baumeister, 1980): Here free lymphatic vessels usually 3–4 are isolated for 20–30 cm and grafted across the recipient lymphatics; it is done commonly after regional node dissection like MRM or groin dissection.

Low level laser therapy is useful in early lymphoedema. It is said to be useful by stimulating the lymphangiogenesis, activating the macrophages and immune system thereby decreasing the fibrotic evens.

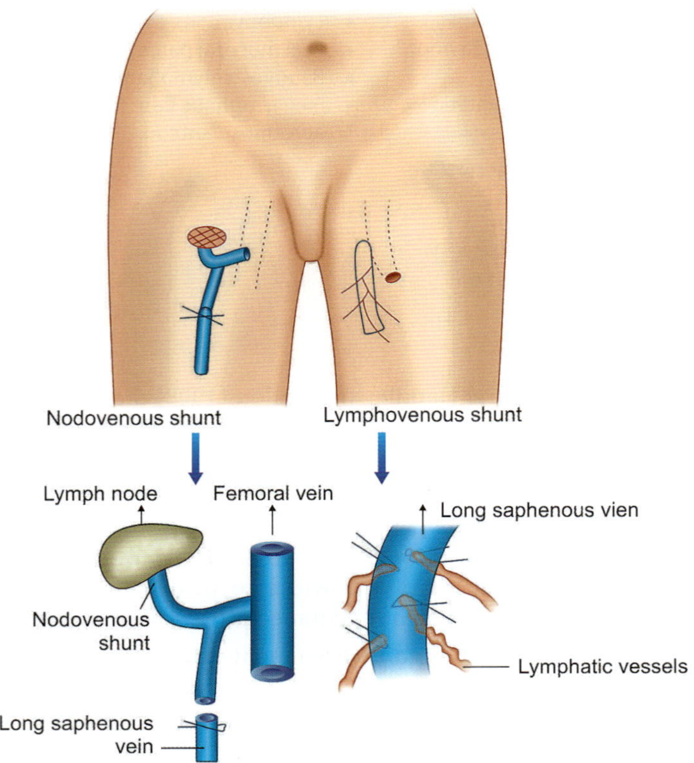

Fig. 12-46: Nodovenous shunt—here lymph node is sutured to vein at its capsule using continuous 7-zero polypropylene sutures. In lympho- venous shunt, fine lymphatics 3–4 are identified by lymphoscintigraphy and are anastomosed to long saphenous vein or to tiny adjacent veins using super microsurgical technique and operating microscope; 11-zero polypropylene sutures are used.

Silicone tube implantation (Waldemar L Olszewski) along the limb is also under trial; it showed decrease in limb circumference by 15% and decrease in tissue stiffness by 50%. It needs intermittent pneumotic compression and elastic support; it also needs prophylactic antibiotic to prevent bacterial colonisation. Silicone tubes are placed in subcutaneous tissue from lower limb to lumbar or hypogastric region. Sterile silicone tubes of 3 mm outer diameter are placed. Three tubes are used which are tied together; multiple holes are made in the tubes at 3 cm interval. 2–3 cm incision is made in lumbar or hypogastric area and using a metal tube of 100 cm in length, blunt dissection is done across downwards along the groin, thigh and calf. 1.5–2 cm incisions are made in these places to pass this blunt metal instrument to create adequate space; once adequate space is created metal tube is removed and prepared silicone tubes are placed in situ across longitudinally; tubes are not fixed to tissues (if needed fixed with only absorbable sutures to deep fascia). As tubes are hydrophobic tissues will never grow inside or around the tubes **(Figs. 12-47A to C)**.

Omentoplasty: Omentum contains plenty of lymphatics; its pedicled transfer is supposedly improve the lymphatic drainage of the limb; technique of omental transfer is similar as to for peripheral vascular disease.

Kondoleon's procedure (1912): Here excision of lymphoedematous tissue is done along with excising the vertical strips of the deep fascia to create the communication between the deep and superficial lymphatics.

Homan's–Miller's procedure (1936): Here thin skin flaps are elevated anteriorly and posteriorly; lymphoedematous tissues are excised; skin flaps are trimmed as per need and sutured back. Both medial and lateral areas of the limb is done using vertical lengthy incisions; usually done in separate incisions with a 4–6 months time gap between medial and lateral area.

Sistrunk's operation (1918): Here lymphoedematous tissue is excised; window cuts are done in the deep fascia to create communications between deep and superficial lymphatics.

Thompson's operation: Here skin flaps are raised; lymphoedematous tissues are excised; epidermis and part of the dermis of one of the skin flaps is shaved using Humby's or skin grafting knife (like split skin graft procedure); this shaved dermal flap is buried under the opposite skin flap into the muscle deep to the deep fascia like a Swiss roll—

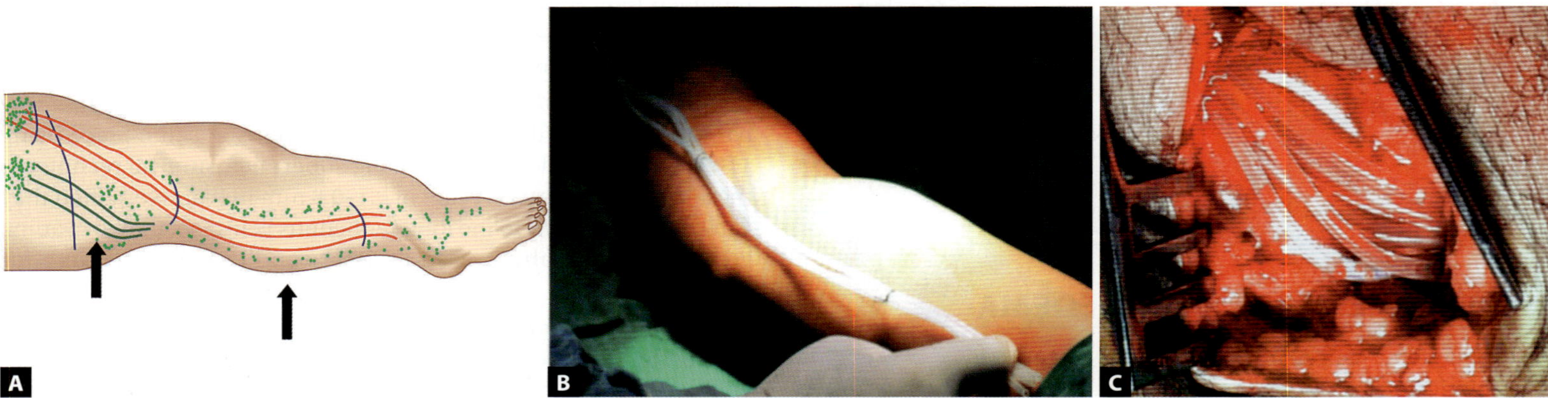

Figs. 12-47A to C: Waldemar L Olszewski method of silicone implantation in subcutaneous plane across the limb.

Swiss roll operation/buried dermal flap operation. Complications here are formation of epidermal cysts and sinus **(Fig. 12-48)**.

Macey's operation: Here skin and subcutaneous tissues are peeled back with deep fascia; split skin graft is done over the denuded area; overlying tissue is sutured back temporarily and is trimmed after 10 days.

Charle's operation [Sir Richard Henry Havelock Charle's, 1912—He actually did the procedure for lymphoedema of the scrotum; but later used by others for lymphoedema (elephantiasis) of the limb]: Here lymphoedematous tissue is excised with skin, subcutaneous tissue and deep fascia. Prior to that or immediately after the procedure split skin graft is taken from the same skin which is placed over the raw recipient muscle bed; graft intake is good as vascular muscle bed is used. Complications are—sepsis, bleeding, graft failure, hyperkeratosis, discharge, dermatitis **(Fig. 12-49)**.

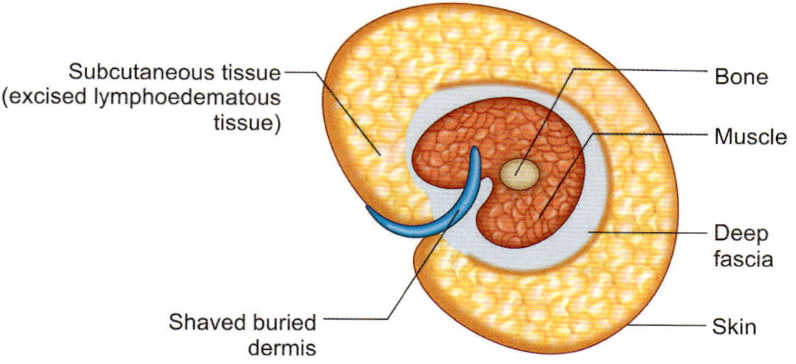

Fig. 12-48: *Thompson's Swiss-roll operation.* Here after removal of lymphoedematous tissue, deep fascia is opened to expose the muscle. Epidermis abraded using skin graft knife. This shaved dermis is buried into the muscle to get communication into the deeper lymphatics.

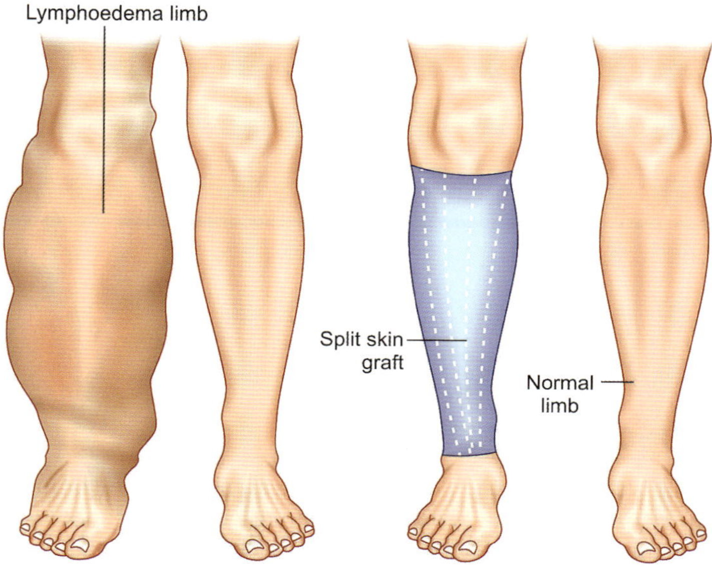

Fig. 12-49: Charle's operation (1912): Here lymphoedematous tissue with skin and deep fascia is excised; split skin graft taken from the same skin which is excised and placed over the raw area to cover the defect.

13 CHAPTER

Surgeries of Nerves, Muscles and Tendons

MUSCLE REPAIR

Longitudinal clean incision of the muscle can be left alone or loose 2-zero vicryl sutures are placed. But deep fascia in front should be sutured, muscle hernia can occur otherwise **(Fig. 13-1)**.

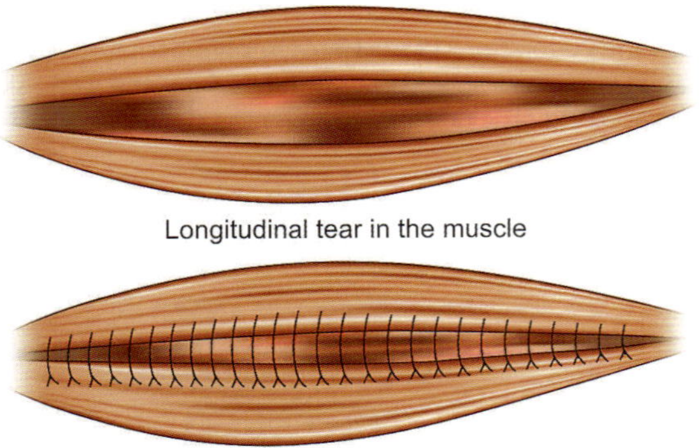

Fig. 13-1: Longitudinal muscle tear is simpler and safer.

It is *the transverse cut/incision* of the muscle which is *more* problematic. It should be sutured with *figure of eight sutures* using vicryl. Direct simple suturing will tear and will not hold. It is often ideal to take the bite of the *adjacent fascia* of the muscle to achieve a proper strength on suturing. Kocher's, horizontal, bucket handle incisions create horizontal cuts in the abdominal muscles. If transverse cut of muscle is not sutured, muscle fibres retract and may atrophy. *Partial transverse cut* may cause hypertrophy of remaining muscle fibres to compensate and function like earlier. Partially cut muscle retracts and forms a '*tumour like' swelling* which should be left alone without any surgical intervention. All *complete transverse cuts* in muscle need proper suturing using vicryl. 6 weeks of splintage is necessary **(Fig. 13-2)**.

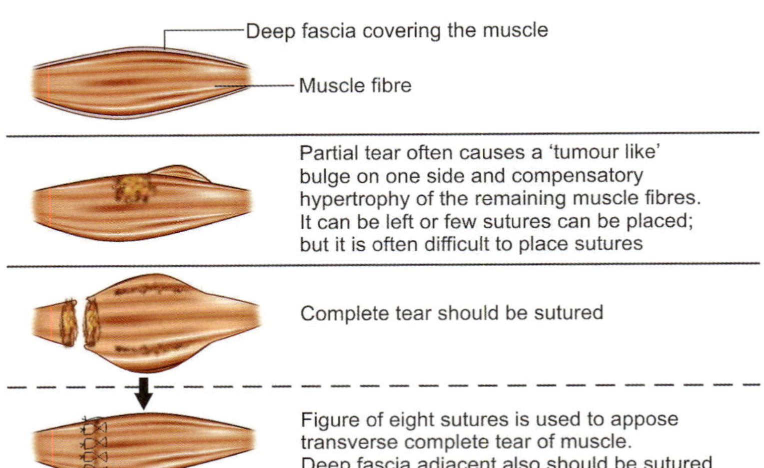

Fig. 13-2: Transverse muscle tear is difficult to manage either partial or complete.

MUSCLE DEBRIDEMENT (MUSCLE EXCISION)

When muscle is dead or badly infected, entire necrosed muscle should be excised until proper bleeding occurs. All unhealthy, pale, lusterless grey muscle tissues should be liberally excised. Excised muscle bed should be thoroughly irrigated and washed with warm normal saline. A corrugated drain should be placed before suturing. Only skin suturing will suffice; if at all loose apposition sutures using interrupted vicryl 2-zero sutures can be used. One should not place continuous sutures in an infected bed. Proper adequate antibiotics, prevention of tetanus or gas gangrene is also important.

COMPARTMENT SYNDROME

It occurs due to oedema, haematoma deep-to-deep fascia, in muscular compartment. It is common after trauma, infection, burns. Fracture of bone with haematoma is also a precipitating cause. Pressure within the compartment increases causing poor perfusion of the tissues locally and distally often by blocking the main artery. It is common in *leg*, forearm, thigh and arm. Early emergency decompression by *fasciotomy* is needed. Pain which gets aggravated on muscle action; pallor; absence of distal pulse are typical features. *Lengthy deep multiple fasciotomy incisions* are needed. It releases the pressure, improves the perfusion, and reduces the oedema. Later secondary suturing is done once wound becomes clean and oedema subsides completely.

Fasciotomy in the Calf

It is done by a deep vertical incision placed behind the medial margin of the tibia to release posterior compartment; another deep vertical incision is placed 4 cm lateral to tibia to release anterior and peroneal compartments **(Fig. 13-3)**.

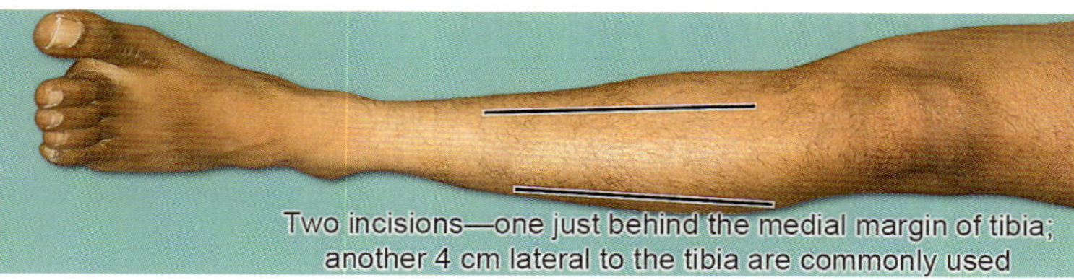

Fig. 13-3: Fasciotomy incision in the leg.

Often *flaps can be raised at the level of deep fascia* through a single lateral incision over the fibula (with elevation of flaps) to reach all four compartments of the leg **(Fig. 13-4)**.

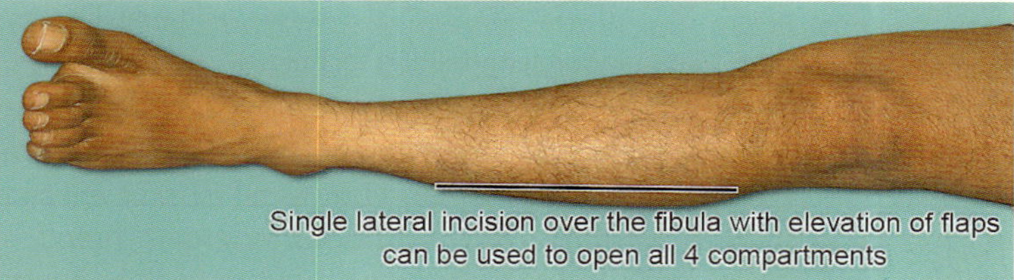

Fig. 13-4: Single lateral incision with elevation of the flap can be used to reach all compartments.

TENDON REPAIR

Tendon heals either by *intrinsic method* when there is no stress to tendon or by *extrinsic method* when there is stress to tendon. Extrinsic healing often causes fibrous mass called *tenoma* which may interfere the tendon gliding.

Tendon injury may be a clean incised injury, or laceration, or tendon rupture due to blunt force or tendon avulsion from the bone.

Flexor and extensor tendons of the fingers are commonly affected. Achilles tendon is commonly injured in the lower limb.

Tendon repair can be primary (within 24 hours); delayed (within a week after 24 hours); secondary (after one week).

Two types of tendon suturing are here.

1. In Kessler method knot stays in the cut part of the tendon.
2. In Goldner method knot comes away from cut ends of the tendon **(Fig. 13-5)**.

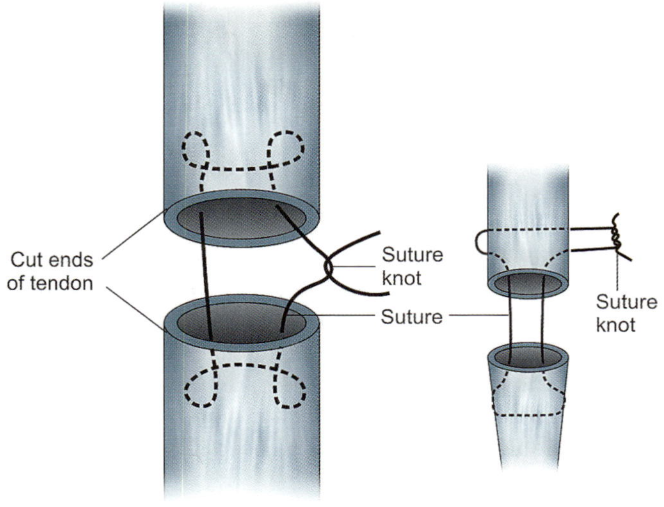

Fig. 13-5: Types of tendon suturing: (1) Kessler method. (2) Goldner method.

Suture material used for tendon repair is *polypropylene with round body needle*. 3-zero or 4-zero suture is used for smaller tendons; 2-zero is used for tendons like Achilles tendon. Absorbable sutures *should not* be used as with suturing, full tensile strength of the tendon is achieved only after 8 months of the injury. Silk is not used because it causes extensive tissue reaction. In olden days strips of fascia were used (now not used). *Continuous suturing* is done.

Postoperative splintage for 4–6 weeks is needed. Later passive and active exercises are started with proper advice of physiotherapy.

Complications are—infection, adhesion, stiffness and failure.

In avulsion injury of tendon, it is attached to bone by drilling holes in the bone through which tendon is passed. Often this tunneled tendon is buttressed with suture and a button which are removed after 4–6 weeks **(Figs. 13-6 and 13-7)**.

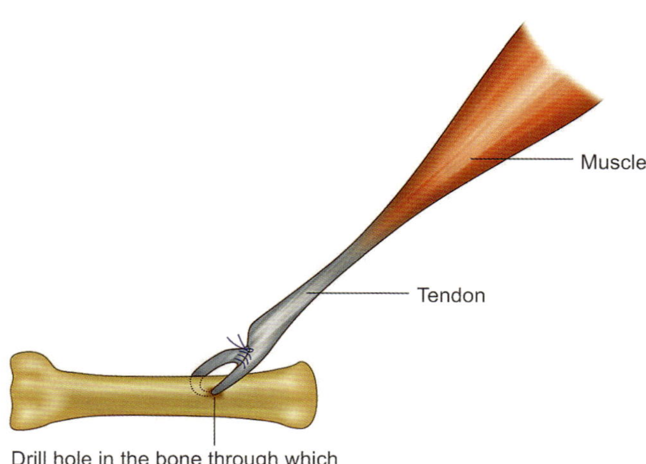

Fig. 13-6: Suturing of the avulsed tendon into the bone is done by passing tendon across the drilled holes in the bone.

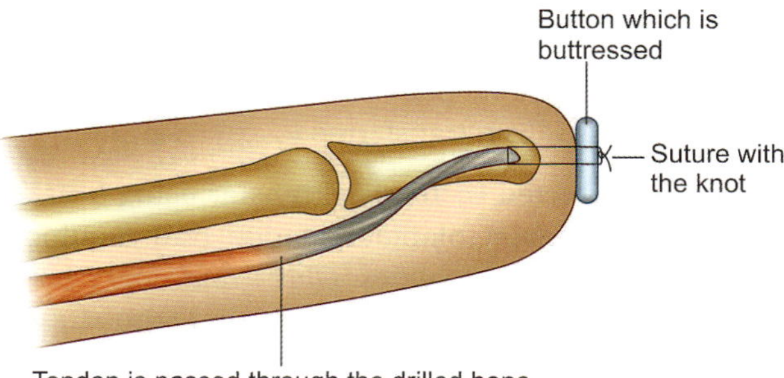

Fig. 13-7: Tendon is passed through the bone and buttressed using a button outside which is removed later.

TENDON RELEASE

It is done for stenosing tenosynovitis of finger (middle or ring) or thumb. Surgical release of the tendon is done, if steroid injection fails. Procedure can be done under local anaesthesia. Release of adjacent soft tissue is often required.

Either transverse or longitudinal incision can be placed over the site just distal to transverse palmar crease.

Similarly tendon release is done for de Quarvain's stenosing tenosynovitis.

TENDON TRANSFER

It is the transfer of one tendon from its existing site to another site where its function is required to have a new function required at the newer site (restore the lost function at the newer site). Function of the transferred tendon should be maintained by other tendons. Tendon should be able to acquire the function at the newer site properly. Tendon should be strong enough to have a newer function and should have adequate amplitude of movements. For example, in ulnar claw hand, flexor digitorum superficialis (FDS of index finger) is transferred to lumbrical canal of the digits to have flexion at MCP joint and extension of proximal IP joint. Extensor indicis tendon can be used to replace extensor pollicis longus tendon **(Fig. 13-8)**.

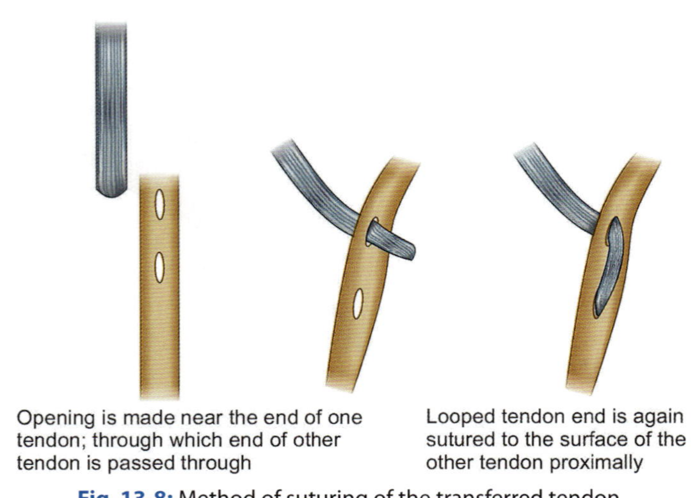

Fig. 13-8: Method of suturing of the transferred tendon.

Examples

Paul Brand's operation is done for claw hand. Here extensor carpi radialis brevis is transferred with a graft to extensor hood through lumbrical canal. Graft is taken from palmaris longus.

Stye Bunnell's operation is done for ulnar claw hand only. Here flexor digitorum superficialis is transferred to extensor hood.

Foot drop is corrected by tendon transfer using tibialis posterior muscle with intervening plantaris tendon graft. Tendon is inserted to cuboid and cuneiform bones. *Ober's and Barr's procedures* are different routes of transfer of the tendon into the cuboid and cuneiform bones.

TENDON GRAFT

When tendon suturing or transfer is not possible because of inadequate length, tendon of a muscle which is not functionally much useful (non-essential tendon) is taken as a graft to obtain required length. ***Common grafts used are*** palmaris tendon in forearm and plantaris tendon in leg.

Example: Extensor carpi radialis brevis (ECRB) is lengthened using tendon graft to transfer to lumbrical canals in claw hand.

Problems in tendon graft: Infection, adhesions, graft failure, stiffness of the part.

TENDON LENGTHENING

It is done when existing tendon is short or has become shortened by trauma/infection. It is commonly used in Achilles tendon, hand, forearm, etc. Tendon is slit like a lengthy 'L' and is sutured with lengthening **(Fig. 13-9)**.

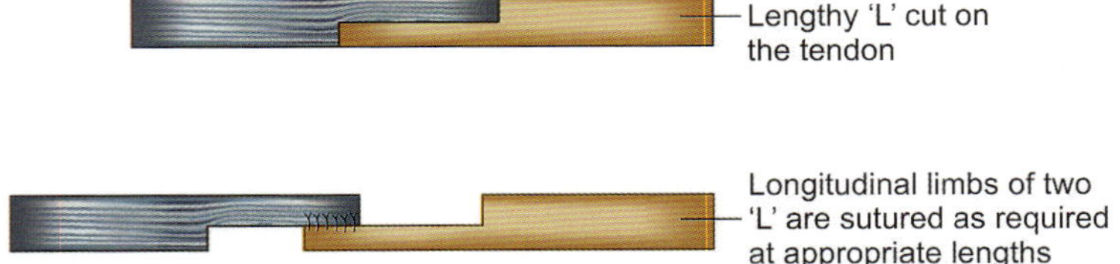

Fig. 13-9: Tendon lengthening technique.

NERVE REPAIRS

Types of Nerve Suturing

Epineurorrhaphy:
Only epineurium is sutured using interrupted sutures. It is commonly used.

Epi-perineurorrhaphy:
Initially perineural sheath and then epineurium is sutured. It is not commonly used.

Repair should be delayed if nerve is lacerated; *marker stitches* (*using silk*) are then placed at the cut end site to identify the nerve for suturing at a later period. Usually microscope or loup is used for nerve suturing **(Fig. 13-10)**.

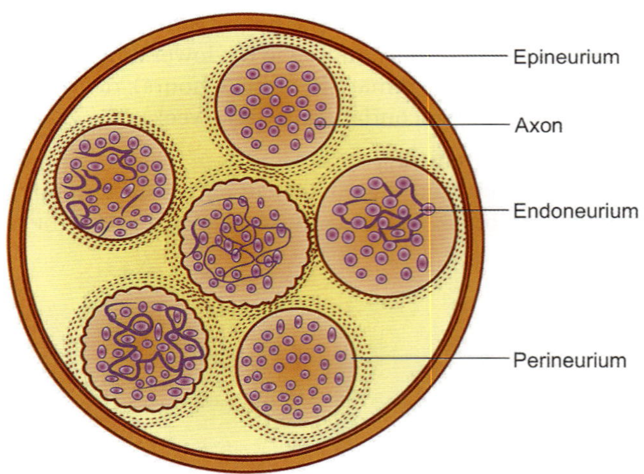

Fig. 13-10: Cross section of a peripheral nerve.

Note:
Incomplete injury usually does not require any suturing. Initial management is conservative. Though incised injury commonly transects the nerve; but possibility of nerve injury in blunt trauma should also be remembered. Proper clinical examination for nerve injury is essential.

All suspected nerve injury should be explored under anaesthesia, general or regional. Tourniquet can be used if there is no evidence of ischaemic injury.

Primary repair is done immediately after injury. Nerve ends are minimally trimmed very close using a blade. All fascicles of the nerve are oriented correctly. Two stay sutures are placed to keep the orientation properly. Usually epineural suturing is done using 8-zero polypropylene interrupted sutures. It needs magnification. 6–8 sutures are placed for large peripheral nerve like median or ulnar nerve. For small nerve like digital nerve, only 2–3 sutures are placed **(Fig. 13-11)**.

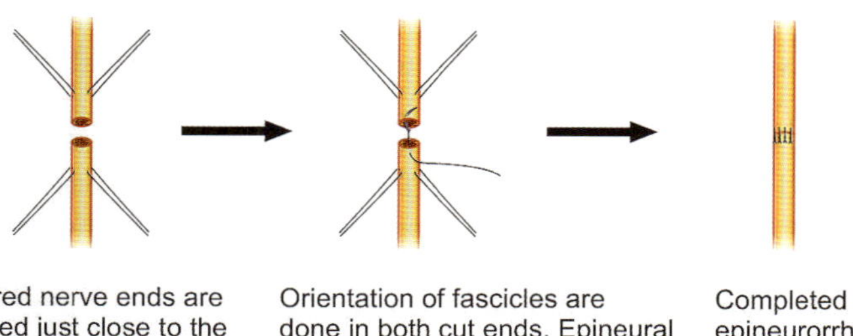

Fig. 13-11: Primary nerve repair.

Secondary repair is done at a later period. It is done in a preexisting scar tissue. Here first nerve ends, both proximal and distal are identified, carefully dissected adequately. Proximal neuroma and distal glioma are trimmed for 1 cm to expose the normal fascicles of the nerve ends. Often guide sutures of silk may be present which were placed earlier during exploration of the trauma. Once nerve ends are clean, it is sutured alike primary suturing with stay sutures, with proper alignment of fascicles, followed by epineural suturing. Here as epineurium is thicker, suturing is easier **(Fig. 13-12)**.

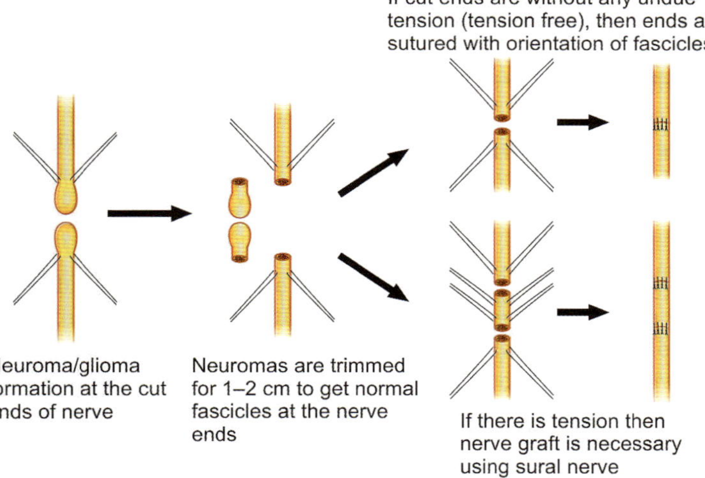

Fig. 13-12: Secondary nerve repair.

All nerve suturing should be done *tension free*. If there is tension, it should be corrected by various methods—relaxing incisions; trans-positioning of the nerve (like of ulnar nerve in elbow joint); shortening of the bone; nerve graft—usually sural nerve is used for nerve graft (often saphenous nerve is used); positioning of the limb; doing initially *neurolysis* (release of the scar tissue adjacent to injury). Nerve graft is needed if gap is more than 2 cm between the cut ends.

Immobilisation of the part is a must for 3–6 weeks. Adjacent joint should be kept in flexed position; later extension is achieved slowly and gradually. Denervated distal part should be taken care of properly as there may be paralysis, loss of sensation, with possible development of contracture.

Prognostic factors in healing of the nerve injury:

Higher the lesion worse the prognosis (more the distance nerve has to grow means less chance of complete recovery); more the gap between the cut ends worse the prognosis; associated injuries alter the prognosis; children do better with nerve injury; type of the injury also decides the prognosis; technical precision also decides the outcome of the surgery.

If nerve suturing fails or cannot be done, then tendon transfer is done at a later period after 4–6 months.

Different Nerve Injuries

Facial nerve injury occurs during parotidectomy. It may be neuropraxia or complete injury. If it is neuropraxia, it is treated conservatively with steroid, tarsorrhaphy. If it is complete injury, it is repaired using nerve graft. Grafts used are great auricular nerve or hypoglossal nerve.

Recurrent laryngeal nerve injury is seen after thyroidectomy, oesophagectomy, tracheal surgery, mediastinal surgery. Its management is discussed in Chapter 15 'Surgery for Thyroid and Parathyroid'.

Radial nerve injury causes wrist drop. Its primary suturing is effective as it is mainly motor. But it takes a year time for recovery. So tendon transfer is often done.

Median and ulnar nerves can be damaged at wrist, forearm or at elbow. They are repaired primarily. If lacerated or crushed, guide stitches are placed and later secondarily repaired. Ulnar nerve when injured at the elbow is sutured in front of the elbow to reduce the tension.

Brachial plexus injury is complicated injury as it may be supraclavicular/infraclavicular; pre-ganglionic or post-ganglionic. It needs a combined, specialised, multidisciplinary approach.

Tibial and common peroneal nerves are also repaired using similar principles. *Sciatic nerve* suturing does not give good result even though it looks technically sound.

Autonomic nerves being non-myelinated, axonal growth will not occur and so nerve repair is not effective.

Classification of Nerve Injuries

Seddon's Classification

Neuropraxia: It is temporary physiological paralysis of nerve conduction. Here recovery is complete. There is no reaction of degeneration.

Axonotmesis: It is division of nerve fibres or axons with intact nerve sheath. There is reaction of degeneration distally with near complete recovery. Patient can present with sensory loss, paralysis of muscles or causalgia.

Neurotmesis: Here complete division of nerve fibres with sheath occurs. Degeneration occurs proximally up to the first node of *Ranvier* as well as distal to the injury. Recovery is incomplete even after nerve suturing. There is complete loss of motor and sensory functions with loss of reflexes. If the nerve is mixed type other than pure motor or sensory recovery is still poorer.

Sunderland's Classification

i. Conduction block—temporary neuronal block.
ii. Axonotmesis but endoneurium is preserved.
iii. Axonotmesis with disruption of endoneurium but perineurium is preserved.
iv. Here disruption of endo and perineurium has occurred but epineurium is intact.
v. Neurotmesis with disruption of endo, peri and epineurium has occurred.

TINEL'S SIGN

It is the clinical sign (*prognostic indicator*) used to assess the level of regeneration. It is elicited 3 weeks after the nerve injury (regeneration begins after the completion of nerve degeneration). Tapping over the course of the nerve is done *from distal to proximal* to elicit a sensation of *'pins and needles' or hyperaesthesia*. If sensation is felt at the site as well as distally along the distribution of the nerve that means *good recovery* can be expected. If sensation is felt only at the site of tapping, then result is *equivocal*. If no sensation is felt it means no recovery.

MANAGEMENT OF NERVE ENTRAPMENT/ COMPRESSION (NERVE RELEASE)

Nerve entrapment and specific nerve injury is commonly due to trauma, constriction bands, fibrosis. It is treated by steroid injections, surgical release of entrapped nerve. Examples are median nerve entrapment in carpal tunnel syndrome, meralgia paraesthetica of thigh, tardy ulnar palsy causing ulnar nerve compression.

Carpal Tunnel Syndrome

It presents with median nerve palsy. Median nerve is deep to flexor retinaculum which gets entrapped under the flexor retinaculum due to causes like trauma (lunate dislocation, malunited Colle's fracture), myxoedema, acromegaly. Flexor retinaculum is also called as *transverse carpal ligament* which extends laterally from trapezium and scaphoid, medially to pisiform and hook of hamate. Flexor retinaculum maintains the concavity of the wrist. It is diagnosed clinically and confirmed by nerve conduction studies. Cervical rib and cervical spondylosis are the differential diagnosis **(Fig. 13-13)**.

Carpal tunnel release is cutting the both layers of the flexor retinaculum/transverse carpal ligament adequately to relieve the compression of the median nerve and so treating the neuropathy. Open or endoscopic minimally access surgery or using needle and thread can be used to release.

Open carpal tunnel release surgery (OCTR): Tourniquet is applied. It is done under local anaesthesia (LA) or Bier's block or brachial block. General anaesthesia (GA) is occasionally used. Incision is along the web space between the mid and ring fingers—3rd web space or inner border of middle finger; distal end of incision ends at *Kaplan's line* **(Fig. 13-14)**. This line is—line drawn on the medial surface of the abducted thumb joining up to the hook of the hamate (from the apex of the skin fold between thumb and index finger to the hook of the hamate). Proximal extension of the incision is up to wrist crease or variable but ideally should not cross the wrist crease. Incision is just medial to the curved crease and straight, longitudinal ideally; even though many advocate slight curved incision with convexity towards ulnar side parallel to the crease line. Palmar cutaneous nerve of the median nerve should be safeguarded; so incision should be medial (towards ulnar side); this nerve arises 4 cm proximal to wrist crease travels along the flexor carpi radialis (FCR) tendon and hence skin incision has to be medial. Double hook retractor or mastoid retractor is used to retract cut skin edges. Deep fascia—palmar aponeurosis is cut longitudinally; Deep dissection once is done, transverse carpal ligament (flexor retinaculum) is identified; origin of thenar muscles are identified to confirm the structure as transverse carpal ligament. After making a small incision in transverse carpal ligament, *Mc Donald retractor* is placed underneath to protect the just underlying median nerve which is whitish shiny stout longitudinal structure. Ligament is cut distally up to visibility of the fat; fat visibility marks the end of the transverse carpal ligament release. *Entire ligament should be cut completely to avoid recurrence.* Proximally deep fascia of the forearm is cut up to 3 cm from the wrist line subcutaneously without extending the skin incision proximally; tourniquet is released. Haemostasis maintained using bipolar cautery or fine ligatures. Skin is used using 3-zero polypropylene sutures using curved cutting needle; dressing is placed; 4″ crepe bandage is applied for few days; sutures removed in 7–10 days. Postoperative exercise is required during recovery period. Cutaneous nerve or median nerve injury; incomplete release; bleeding by injuring arches of the palm; scar and contracture development; wound infection; persistent wrist pain—are complications **(Fig. 13-15)**.

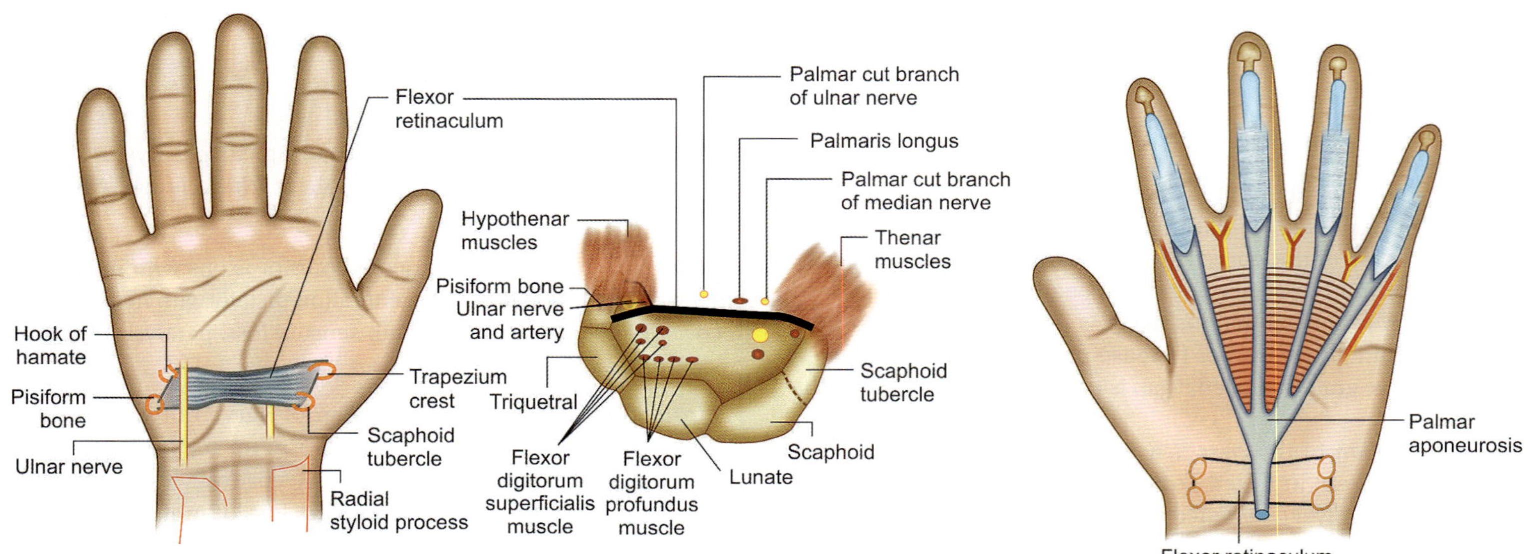

Fig. 13-13: Anatomy of the carpal tunnel and flexor retinaculum.

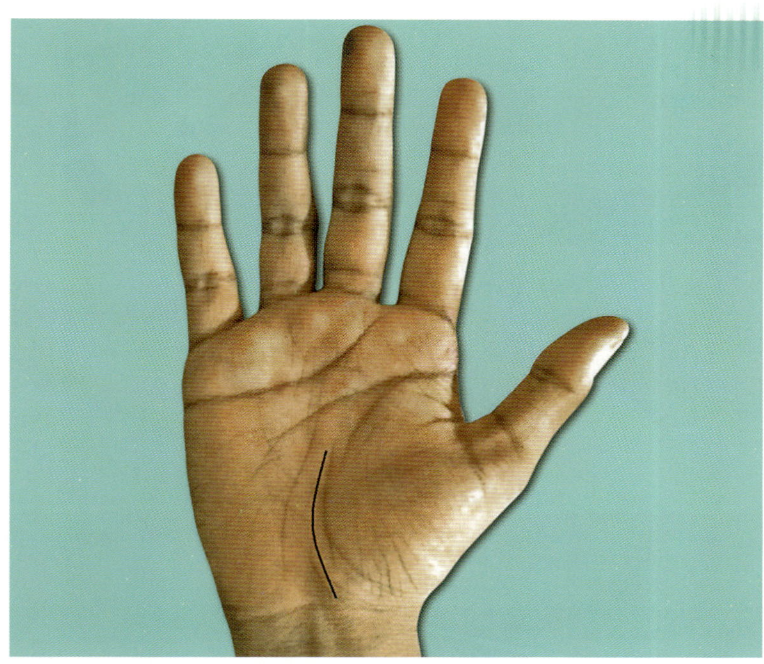

Fig. 13-14: Incision for carpal tunnel syndrome.

In endoscopic carpal tunnel release (ECTR), two ports are placed in the distal forearm one for telescope another for cutting the transverse carpal ligament under vision. Here subcutaneous tissue and deep fascia is not cut; it is minimally invasive method with fast recovery and is also done under LA. But chances of recurrence are slightly higher compared to open transverse carpal ligament release. Chow two portal device or 3 M Agee single portal devices are available for endoscopic release.

Newer method called ***thread carpal tunnel release (TCTR)*** is being advocated. Under LA, under sonological guidance spinal needle is passed underneath the transverse carpal ligament from distal (hand) to proximal (wrist); fine thread is passed through this needle from proximal to distal; needle is removed and reinserted again from distal to proximal but this time in front of the transverse carpal ligament under the skin and subcutaneous tissue; proximal end of the remaining thread is passed through the needle to reach distally so that both ends of the thread will be distal encircling the transverse carpal ligament. Frictional effect of the thread (sawing like) is utilised here to cut the carpal ligament by repetitive sawing motion of the ends of thread; once ligament is cut fully ends of the thread with intact entire thread will come out of the distal needle puncture. Needle puncture site is covered with a tiny plaster.

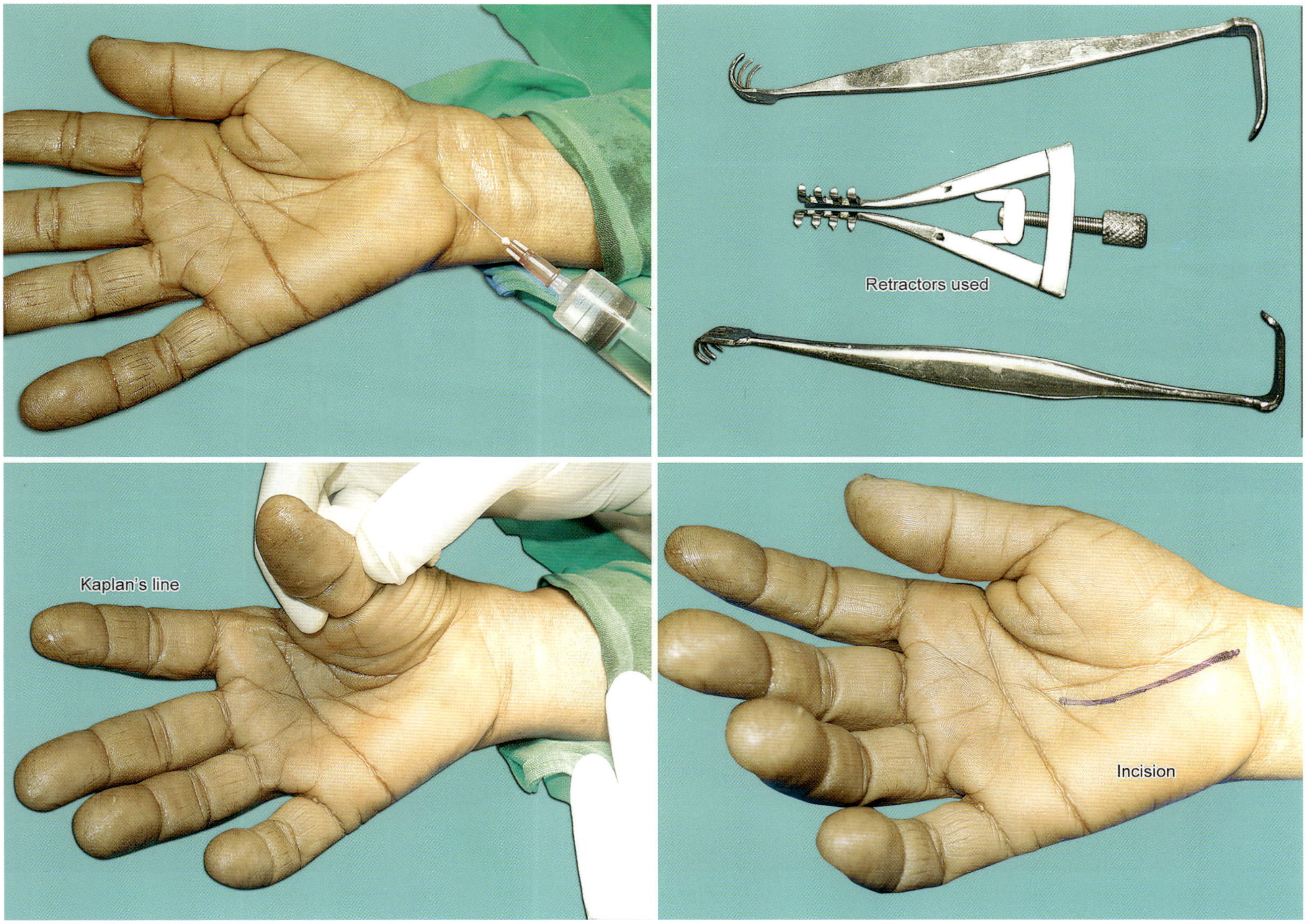

Retractors used

Kaplan's line

Incision

Figs. 13-15(1)

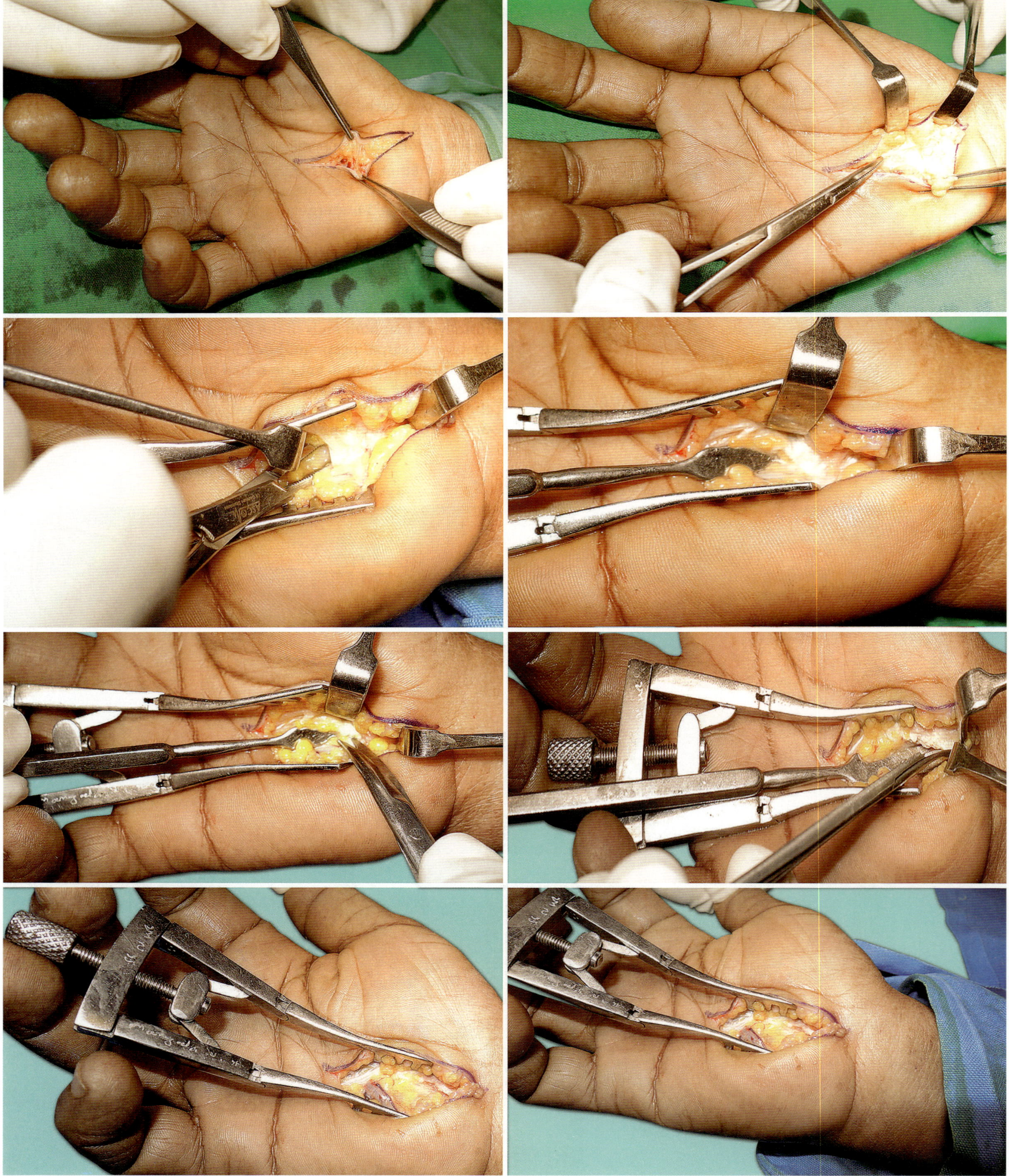

Figs. 13-15(2)

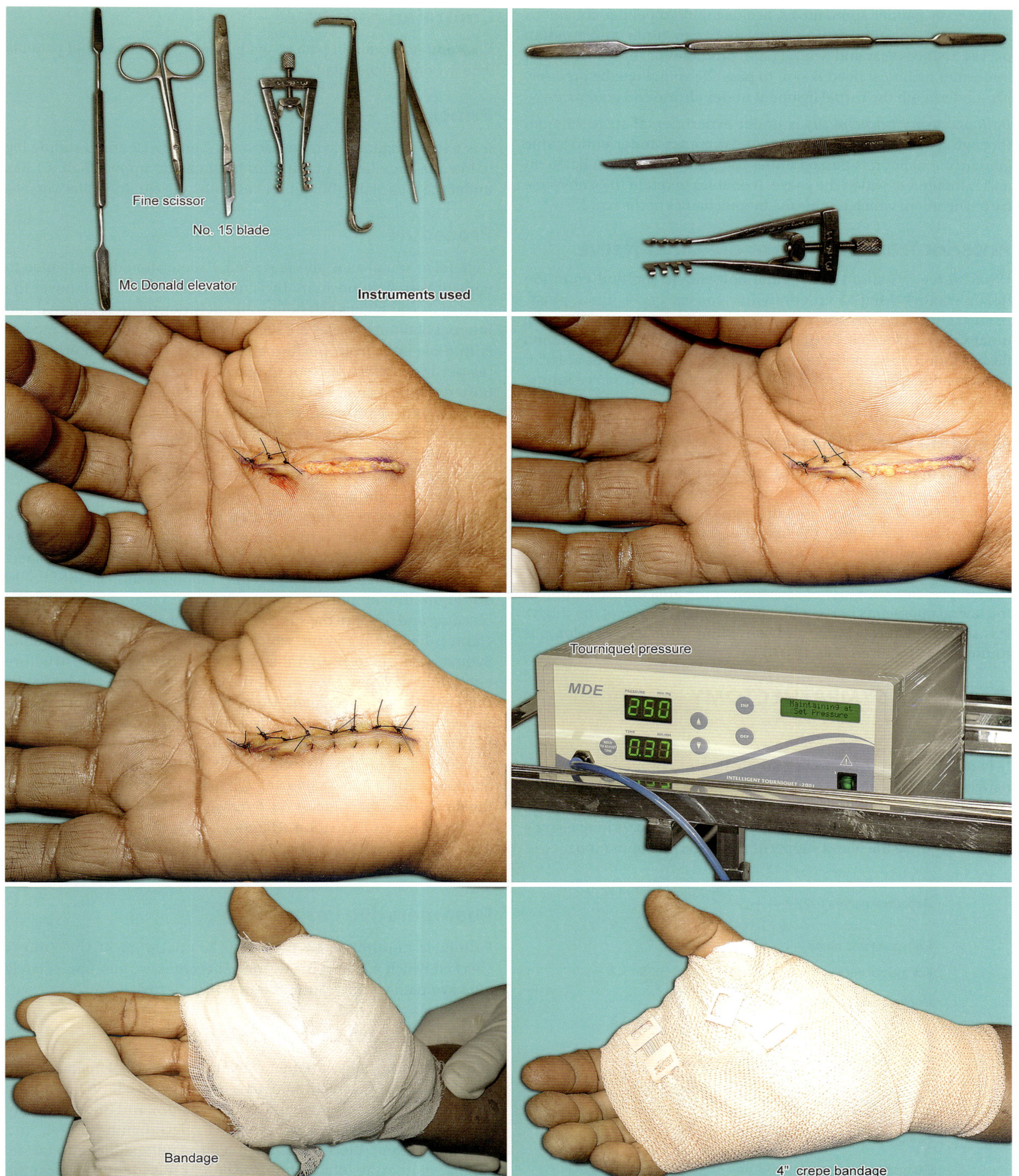

Figs. 13-15(3)

Figs. 13-15(1 to 3): Open carpal tunnel release (OCTR). Other methods are—endoscopic carpal tunnel release (ECTR) and thread carpal tunnel release (TCTR).

It preserves palmar aponeurosis, avoids injury to palmar cutaneous nerves and communicating nerve between ulnar and median nerves, reduces scar and wound pain, promotes faster recovery. But important technical need is skill to pass the spinal needle precisely just underneath the carpal ligament under ultrasound guidance.

Balloon carpal tunnelplasty is under experimental stage wherein through a small incision distal to wrist crease under endoscopic guidance a balloon is passed under the transverse carpal ligament and is inflated to widen the space. It enables to retain the transverse carpal ligament which retains the biomechanics of the hand.

Anterior Transposition of the Ulnar Nerve

Ulnar nerve is behind the medial epicondyle (behind common flexor origin). Medial epicondylitis causes tardy ulnar palsy. In such situation common flexor tendon is released from its origin; ulnar nerve is placed in front of the flexor origin; detached common flexor tendon is reattached to medial condyle. It is called as anterior transposition of ulnar nerve. It is also used in ulnar nerve injury. Elbow is immobilised for 3 weeks.

Meralgia Paraesthetica

It is entrapment neuropathy of lateral cutaneous nerve of thigh under the inguinal ligament. It arises from posterior divisions of lumbar plexus (L2, 3); runs over the quadrates lumborum and iliacus muscles; emerges behind the lateral part of the inguinal ligament; divides into anterior and posterior branches, supplying skin over anterolateral part of the thigh and anterior part of the gluteal region. Patient presents with loss of sensation at the area of distribution of the lateral cutaneous nerve of thigh (upper lateral part of the thigh). It is treated by reassurance and steroid injection. Nerve release is routinely not required **(Fig. 13-16)**.

LUMBAR SYMPATHECTOMY

Indications

It is mainly used to improve the healing of cutaneous ulcers in patients with vascular disease like TAO; in causalgia of lower limb (it is common in upper limb). Its benefits are temporary. It causes cutaneous vasodilatation by sympathetic blockage. It may also be used to improve the blood supply of skin flaps in amputations.

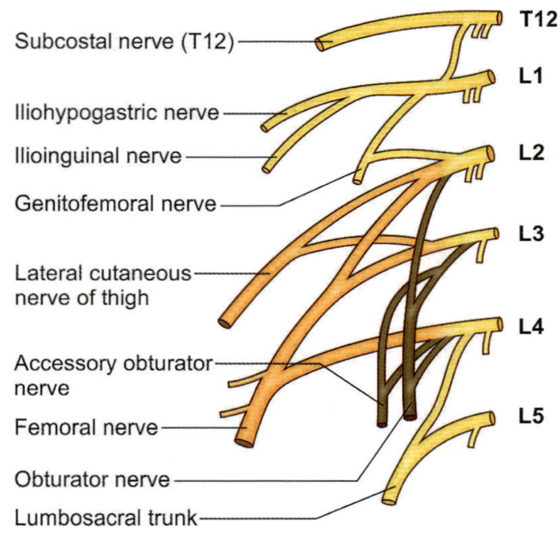

Fig. 13-16: Lumbar plexus showing origin of lateral cutaneous nerve of thigh.

Contraindications

It is contraindicated in patients with bleeding disorders and patients who are on anticoagulants.

Principles

It is a pre-ganglionic sympathectomy. Ganglia L2 and 3 supply leg below the knee level. L1 supplies buttock and upper thigh. L1 lies under the crus of diaphragm. L4 lies under the common iliac vessels.

Procedure

General or spinal anaesthesia is used. Patient should be strapped to table in lateral tilt position. Incision is transverse or oblique at the level of the umbilicus extending obliquely downwards. External and internal oblique muscles are divided; transverse abdominis muscle is initially split from posterior part, then towards anterior part (as peritoneum is adherent to muscle in anterior part but free in posterior aspect and so to avoid opening of the peritoneum it is split from behind). Peritoneum is pushed medially by finger dissection. If peritoneum is opened it is closed using vicryl continuous sutures. It is swept in front of the psoas major muscle towards medially. Genitofemoral nerve and ureter are identified. Ureter along with peritoneum is retracted medially using Deaver's retractor. Additional Deaver retractor is used to tract the upper part of the wound. Self-retaining retractor may be useful at this stage. Inferior vena cava (IVC) is visualised as a bluish structure. Its posterior aspect is gently dissected using peanut and fine dissections. One should not injure the lumbar veins which if injured may cause torrential bleeding and obscure the surgical field. On the left side sympathetic chain is behind the aorta, which is mobilised to reach the chain. Sympathetic chain is identified as stiff vertically placed structure behind the IVC/aorta in front of the vertebrae which can be felt by rolling the finger. *L2 is identified* as it is largest ganglion. L1 is high up behind the diaphragmatic crus and it should not be removed. L2, 3 and 4 are removed. L5 is often below which may or may not be removed. Chain is dissected off the vertebrae using scissor for adequate length and is cut using scissor. It is not necessary to ligate the chain on either side. After removal specimen chain is sent for histology for confirmation. Haemostasis is confirmed. Wound is closed in layers using 1-zero vicryl. Drain is usually not necessary unless there is bleeding **(Fig. 13-17)**.

Postoperative Period

Patient is monitored for bleeding. Temperature of the limb is checked which will become warmer (becomes warmer immediately after sympathectomy). Sutures removed in 7–10 days.

Problems and Complications

Often, reaching the sympathetic chain may be problematic. Injury to IVC (rarely aorta on left side) may be dangerous. If IVC is injured, it should be clamped using Satinsky clamp; and sutured using 4-zero polypropylene suture. Injury to peritoneum, bowel, and ureter can occur. Bleeding lumbar veins is quite difficult to tackle. Bipolar diathermy fulguration is useful. If it is identified it can be ligated gently. Often it is ligated during surgical dissection itself to avoid bleeding. Spasm of spinal cord vessel and spinal cord ischaemia and paraplegia can develop rarely. If L1 ganglia of both

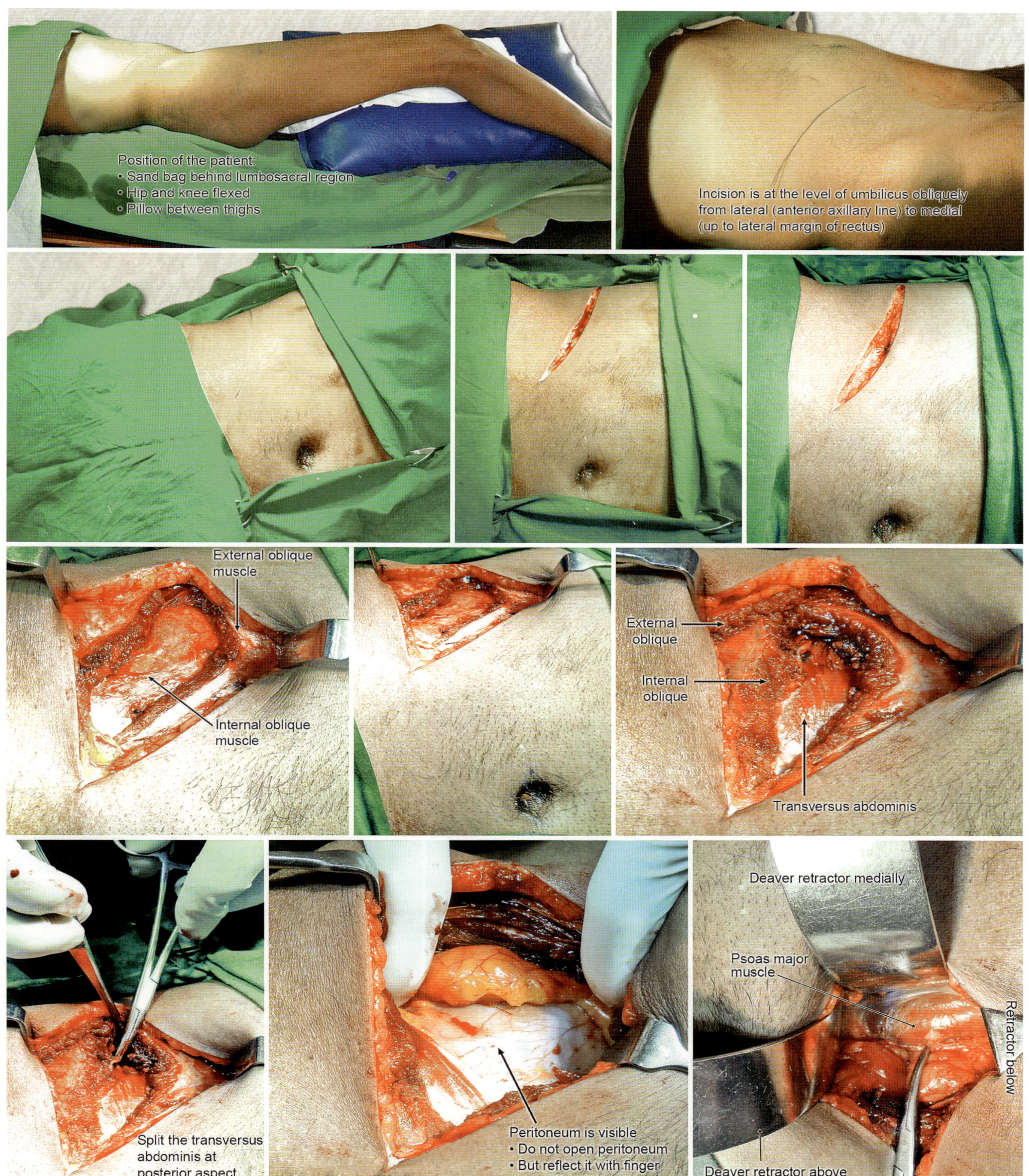

Position of the patient:
• Sand bag behind lumbosacral region
• Hip and knee flexed
• Pillow between thighs
Incision is at the level of umbilicus obliquely from lateral (anterior axillary line) to medial (up to lateral margin of rectus)
External oblique muscle
Internal oblique muscle
External oblique
Internal oblique
Transversus abdominis
Split the transversus abdominis at posterior aspect
Peritoneum is visible
• Do not open peritoneum
• But reflect it with finger dissection/sweeping
Deaver retractor medially
Psoas major muscle
Retractor below
Deaver retractor above

Figs. 13-17(1)

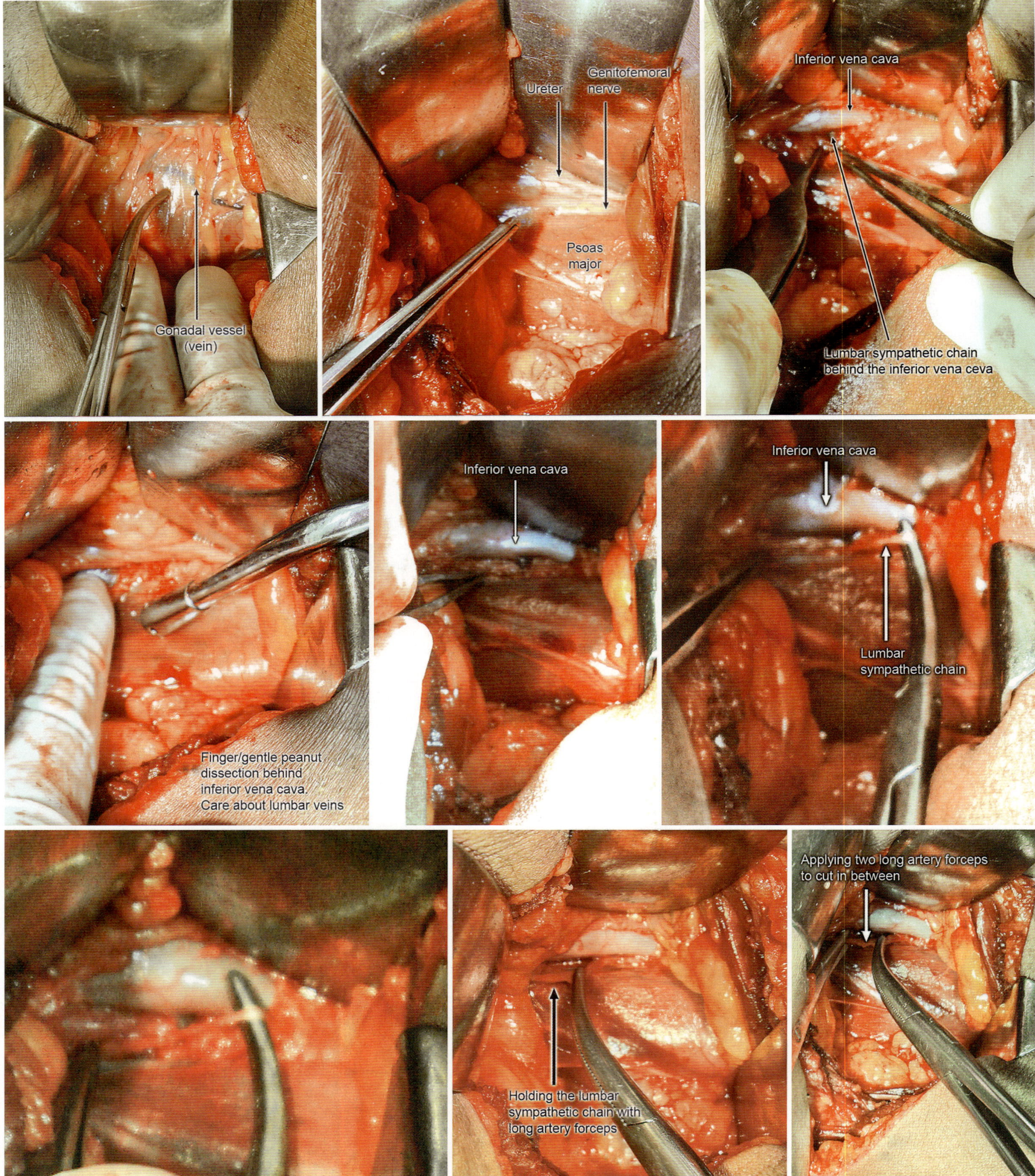
Gonadal vessel (vein)
Ureter
Genitofemoral nerve
Psoas major
Inferior vena cava
Lumbar sympathetic chain behind the inferior vena ceva
Finger/gentle peanut dissection behind inferior vena cava. Care about lumbar veins
Inferior vena cava
Inferior vena cava
Lumbar sympathetic chain
Holding the lumbar sympathetic chain with long artery forceps
Applying two long artery forceps to cut in between

Figs. 13-17(2)

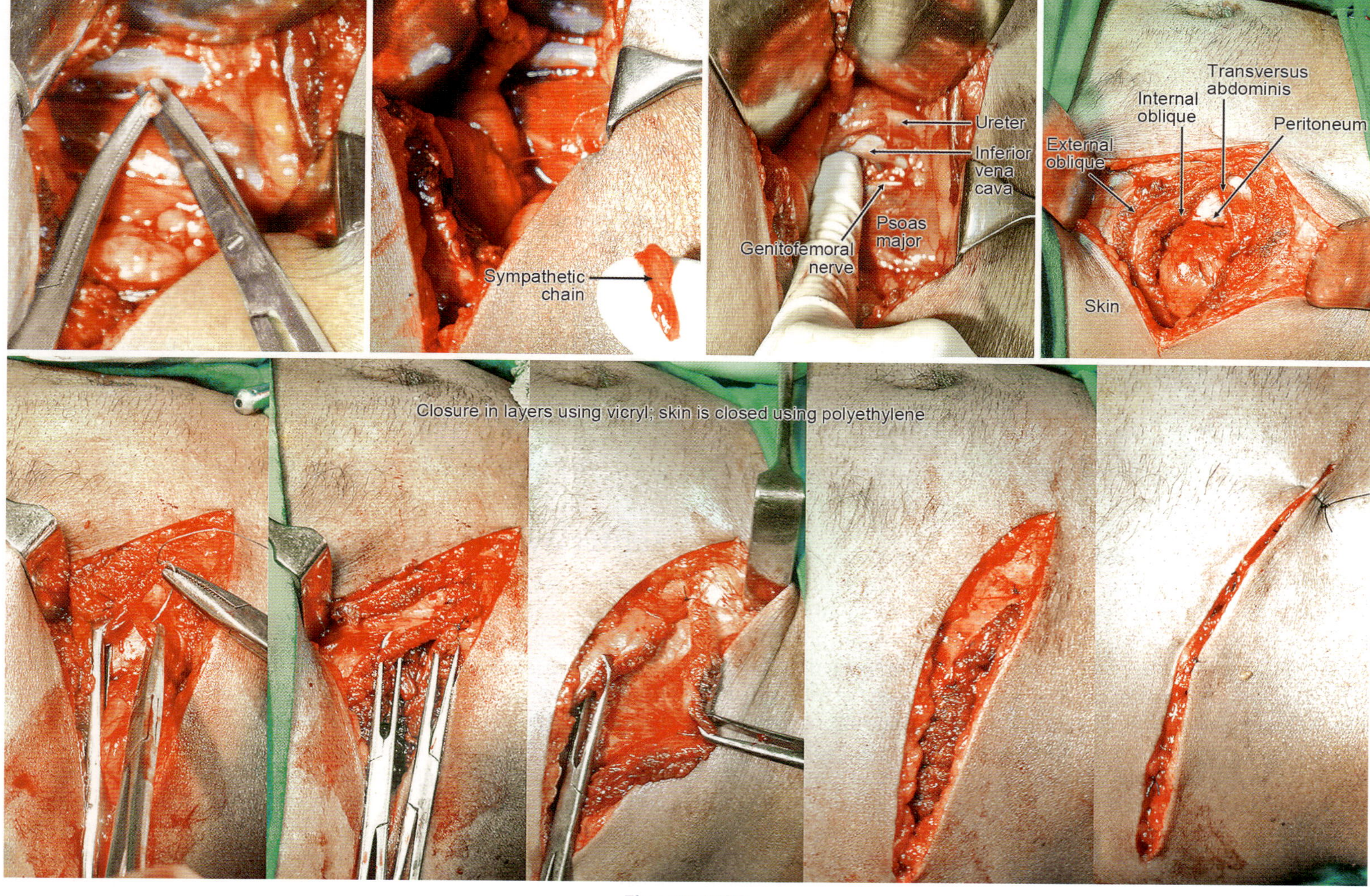

Figs. 13-17(3)

Figs. 13-17(1 to 3): Operative steps in lumbar sympathectomy.

sides are removed, ejaculatory failure can develop (dry ejaculation). Haematoma formation, wound infection are other complications.

Effects of lumbar sympathectomy are *temporary (3–4 weeks)*. By improving the cutaneous blood supply it promotes ulcer healing. But it may reduce the blood supply of deeper muscles (as it is diverted towards skin), and hence claudication is not benefited by lumbar sympathectomy but may get aggravated.

Laparoscopic Retroperitoneal Lumbar Sympathectomy

Lumbar sympathectomy also can be done using laparoscopic retroperitoneal approach with same position by placing three ports. One port is placed at anterior axillary line (10 mm port for camera); two 5 mm ports are placed medially above and below. Dissection is done in front of the psoas major muscle towards medially reflecting the peritoneum, ureter in front. IVC is identified. Dissection is done behind the IVC. Sympathetic chain is identified and removed.

Chemical Sympathectomy

It is done in lateral position using a long spinal needle. Local anaesthesia is infiltrated first. Position of the chain is confirmed under fluoroscopy by injecting dye. 5 mL of phenol in water or absolute alcohol is injected lateral to the vertebral bodies of 4th and 2nd lumbar vertebrae. Needle should not enter the IVC or aorta. Limb becomes warmer immediately. Initial trial injection of the lignocaine to confirm the benefit may be done. Technique should not be done in bleeding disorders and in patients who are on anticoagulants.

CERVICOTHORACIC SYMPATHECTOMY

It is the removal of 2nd and 3rd thoracic ganglia which contain postganglionic fibres supplying the upper limb. Preganglionic white rami communicantes fibres of 2nd and 3rd sympathetic nerves enter thoracic T1 ganglion supplying the head and neck region through upper part of the stellate ganglion. Preganglionic sympathetic nerve entering the 2nd and 3rd ganglia from below supplies sympathetic fibres of upper limb through lower part of the stellate ganglion.

In cervical sympathectomy for upper limb ischaemia, lower part of the stellate ganglion and Kuntz nerve is divided. For head and neck hyperhidrosis entire stellate ganglion is removed which leads to development of Horner's syndrome.

For hyperhidrosis of axillary region stellate ganglion, upper four thoracic ganglia are removed.

Surgical Anatomy

Preganglionic fibres arise from lateral horns of the T_1 to T_{12} segments of spinal cord. T_1 to T_{12} lateral horns → Preganglionic fibres → Ventral roots of spinal cord → Beginning of ventral rami → White rami communicantes (14 on each side)

↓ ↓ ↓ ↓

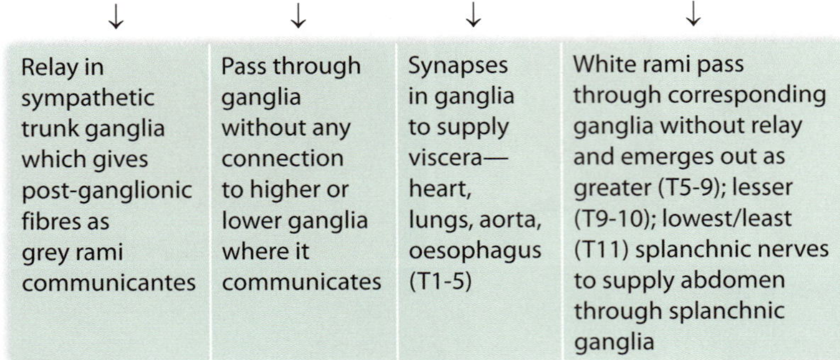

Relay in sympathetic trunk ganglia which gives post-ganglionic fibres as grey rami communicantes	Pass through ganglia without any connection to higher or lower ganglia where it communicates	Synapses in ganglia to supply viscera—heart, lungs, aorta, oesophagus (T1-5)	White rami pass through corresponding ganglia without relay and emerges out as greater (T5-9); lesser (T9-10); lowest/least (T11) splanchnic nerves to supply abdomen through splanchnic ganglia

Ganglia are connected to respective spinal nerves through white rami (from spinal nerve to ganglia) and grey rami (from ganglia to spinal nerves) communicantes.

In the neck there are three cervical sympathetic ganglia—*superior,* at the level of greater cornu of hyoid; *middle,* at the level of cricoid; *inferior,* 3 cm above the sternoclavicular joint. Sympathetic chain here is located behind the carotid sheath in front of the prevertebral fascia. Superior is the largest of the three—2.5 cm; located below the skull opposite 2nd and 3rd cervical vertebrae behind carotid sheath; which actually is fused upper 4 cervical ganglia. It communicates with 9th, 10th, 12th cranial nerves and external and recurrent laryngeal nerves. It sends branches to plexus around external carotid artery (ECA), internal carotid artery (ICA) and other branches in the neck; branches to otic, submandibular, ciliary and pterygopalatine ganglia in neck; to pharynx. Middle cervical ganglion is very small, often it is branched or absent; situated in front of the C6 vertebra above inferior thyroid artery behind the carotid sheath. It is formed by 5th and 6th ganglia; is connected to inferior cervical ganglion through a looped ansa subclavia and also directly. It gives branches to C5 and C6 spinal nerves, thyroid, parathyroid, trachea, oesophagus and middle cervical cardiac branch. Inferior cervical ganglion is formed by 7th and 8th cervical ganglia; often it is fused with 1st thoracic ganglion to form stellate ganglion. It is located between transverse process of C7 vertebra and neck of first rib. It gives branches to C7, C8 ventral nerves, vertebral and subclavian artery plexus, inferior cervical cardiac branch **(Fig. 13-18)**.

Sympathetic outflow to upper limb is from T2 to T9; T1 also may contribute to supply arm in 10% of cases. A direct communication may be present between 2nd and 3rd thoracic ganglia and brachial plexus through *nerve of Kuntz*.

Indications

Hyperhidrosis (very useful), causalgia (very useful), autonomic nerve dystrophies, cervical rib with vascular manifestations (useful), Raynaud's phenomenon (useful), other causes of upper limb ischaemia (useful), acrocyanosis (useful), Sudeck's osteodystrophy (useful). Conditions with vasospasm will get benefited rather than conditions with obliterative digital vessel occlusion.

Approaches

Supraclavicular, transthoracic/axillary approach *(Hedley Atkins),* thoracoscopic approach (better) are the different approaches used.

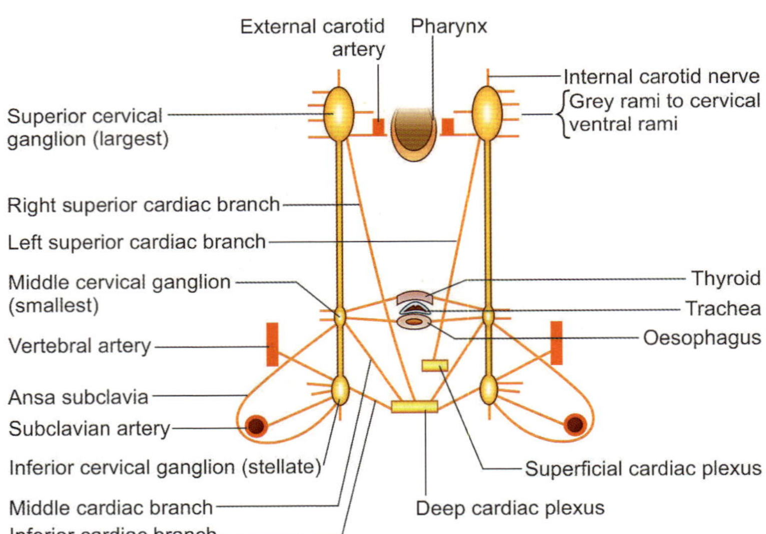

Fig. 13-18: Cervical sympathetic chain—surgical anatomy.

Supraclavicular Approach

It is done under general anaesthesia. Patient is positioned supine with head end of the table elevated by 15° to reduce venous congestion and head is tilted to opposite side; arms are placed on the sides of the patient. Incision is placed a fingerbreadth (1.5 cm) above the clavicle from anterior border of the sternocleidomastoid muscle extending laterally for 7–8 cm. It is usual but not mandatory practice to pull/drag the skin downwards below the clavicle and make incision on the clavicle from medial to lateral; and when pulled skin is released after making incision, incision will be in supraclavicular area. It is said to prevent inadvertent injury to deeper structures. Incision is deepened; Platysma is incised. External jugular vein is divided with ligatures. Supraclavicular nerves are retained. Exposed sternocleidomastoid muscle is identified for its full width. The clavicular head is divided using scissor/cautery/or by piecemeal using fine forceps (used in olden days). Internal jugular vein (IJV) behind the muscle should not be injured. Scalene pad of fat is dissected. Inferior belly of omohyoid muscle is divided. IJV is mobilised and retracted medially. Bipolar cautery dissection is done in front of the scalene muscle. Phrenic nerve is identified in front of the scalenus anterior muscle deep to deep fascia running vertically downwards from lateral to medial side. Phrenic nerve is retracted medially (should not be retracted laterally as it may cause traction injury to upper trunk of brachial plexus). Dissected scalenus anterior muscle is cut layer by layer carefully using scissor/by piecemeal method to protect subclavian artery underneath. Medial part of the brachial plexus is dissected carefully. Subclavian artery is dissected on its summit and pushed downwards. Occasionally thyrocervical trunk may have to be ligated. Often subclavian artery is dissected and slinged upwards; but one should be careful while pulling the sling especially in atherosclerotic vessel. Head light may be better used for further dissection. Subclavian artery is retracted downwards. In the triangle between brachial plexus, subclavian artery and IJV, suprapleural membrane (Sibson's fascia) is felt with index finger which is divided using finger dissection by pushing it downwards against vertebra (*Sibson's fascia* also called as vertebropleural fascia is tent like thickening of the prevertebral fascia extending from transverse process of C7 to first rib). Once it is divided, retropleural space is dissected by pushing the pleura downwards using finger and pleura and Sibson's fascia is retracted downwards. Stellate ganglion is identified at the neck of the first rib. By finger and swab dissection entire ganglion is exposed. Right angle is passed underneath; sympathetic chain below is dissected up to 3rd ganglion. Intercostal veins crossing the chain should be carefully separated or ligated between haemoclips. Entire ganglion is not removed for upper limb diseases as it will cause Horner's syndrome. Lower part of the ganglion, where rami from 1st thoracic nerve enters is divided. Lower end is dissected downwards below the level of thoracic 3rd ganglion and chain is cut again at this level. Chain is sent for histology. Lung is inflated. Wound is closed in layers. Drain is usually not necessary **(Figs. 13-19 and 13-20)**.

Complications

Complications are bleeding; injury to subclavian artery and nerves; pneumothorax and haemothorax; Horner's syndrome presenting as ptosis, miosis, anhydrosis, enophthalmos, loss of ciliospinal reflex. Chest X-ray is taken during postoperative period when suspected to rule out pneumothorax. If pneumothorax is present, intercostal tube should be placed. Left-sided sympathectomy may cause thoracic duct injury. Neuropraxia of brachial plexus is known to occur due to traction during procedure.

Advantages

Postoperative recovery is faster with less duration of hospital stay and less disability.

Disadvantage

Difficult narrow space approach is the limitation.

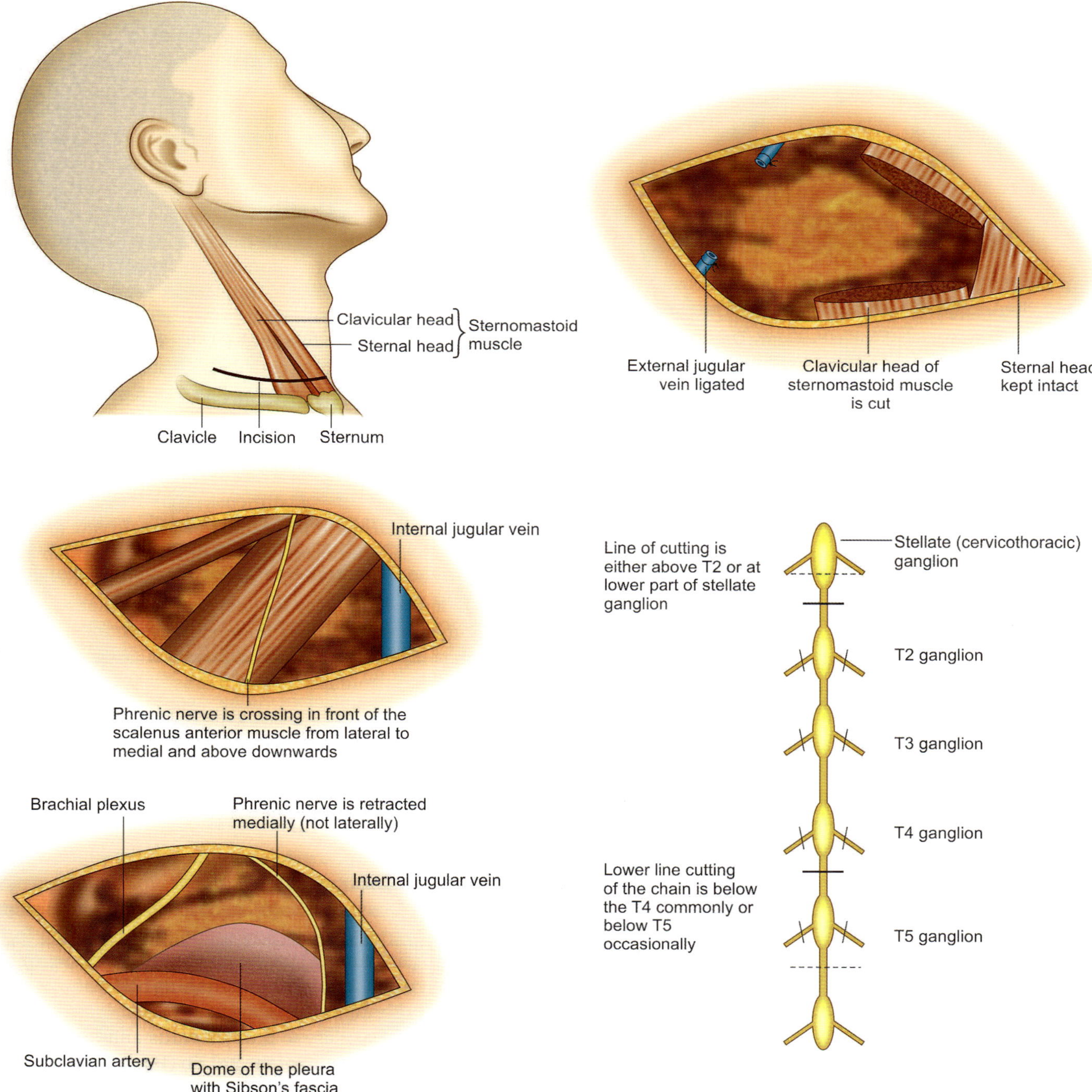

Fig. 13-19: Cervicothoracic sympathectomy—through supraclavicular approach.

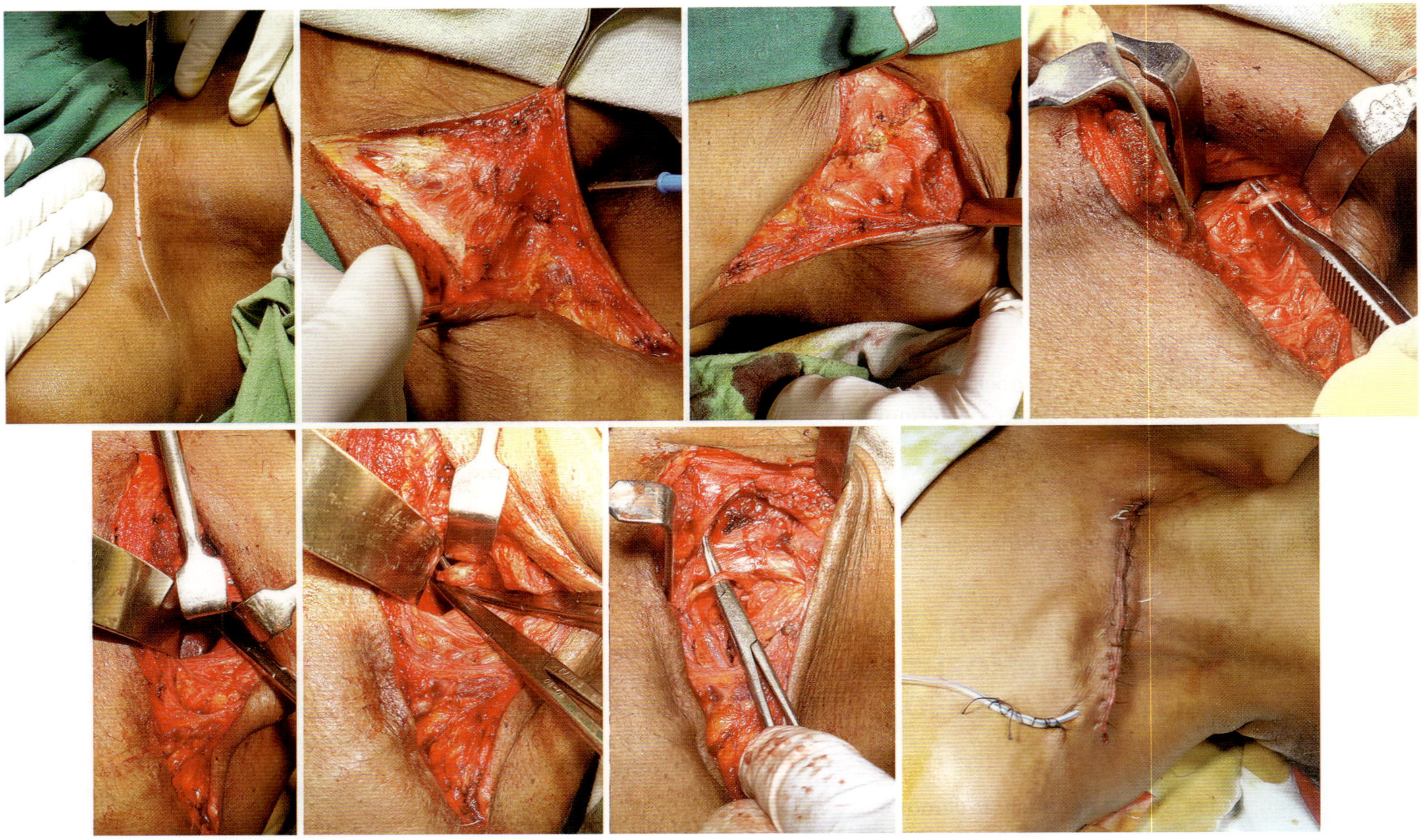

Fig. 13-20: Steps in cervical sympathectomy. One can observe the sternocleidomastoid muscle, thoracic duct, phrenic nerve, scalenus anterior, Sibson's fascia and stellate ganglion.

Transaxillary Approach

It is better approach but needs prolonged hospitalisation and has slow postoperative recovery. Either extrapleural or transpleural approaches are used.

Transaxillary extrapleural approach is done using standard thoracotomy position. Arm of the same side is fully abducted to expose the entire axilla. Arm, chest, back, shoulder area is cleaned and draped. Incision is placed at lower margin of the axillary hair line from margin of pectoralis major in front to margin of latissimus dorsi behind **(Fig. 13-21)**.

Incision is deepened to reach the first rib. Intercostobrachial nerve is divided. A branch from axillary artery is divided. Anterior scalene muscle is divided to expose the superior surface of the first rib. Intercostal muscles are stripped off from the inferior surface of the first rib using periosteal elevator. First rib is excised using bone cutter and end is smoothened using rongeur. Pleural dome is pushed away from the mediastinum using finger dissection. Subclavian vessels are identified. Sympathetic chain is identified between T1 nerve root and subclavian artery. Sympathectomy is done from lower half of the stellate ganglion to lower margin of T 3 ganglion. One should confirm that there is no pleural tear and pneumothorax, if it so chest tube may be placed and wound is closed in layers. Postoperative chest X-ray is a must.

Transaxillary transpleural approach is done through 3rd intercostal space. Position is same as extrapleural approach. Incision of 15 cm in length is made along the line of 3rd rib from posterior axillary

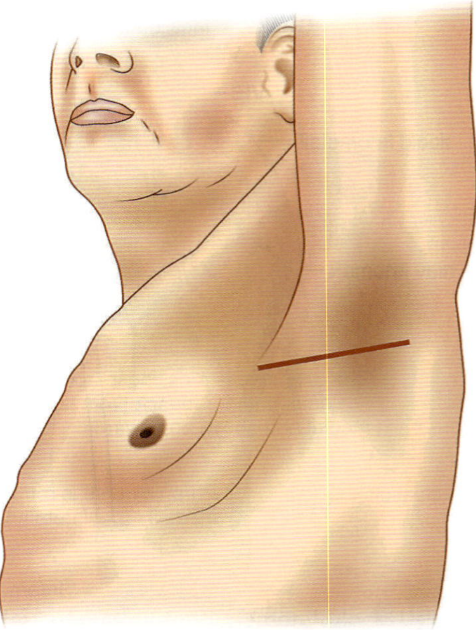

Fig. 13-21: Incision for the transaxillary extrapleural approach: It is in the axilla placed at lower margin of the hairline from pectoralis major to latissimus dorsi muscle along the first rib.

fold to anterior axillary fold downwards and forwards. Incision is deepened to periosteum of the 3rd rib **(Fig. 13-22)**.

Pectori are retracted forward; latissimus dorsi, teres major, subscapularis and long thoracic nerve are retracted backward.

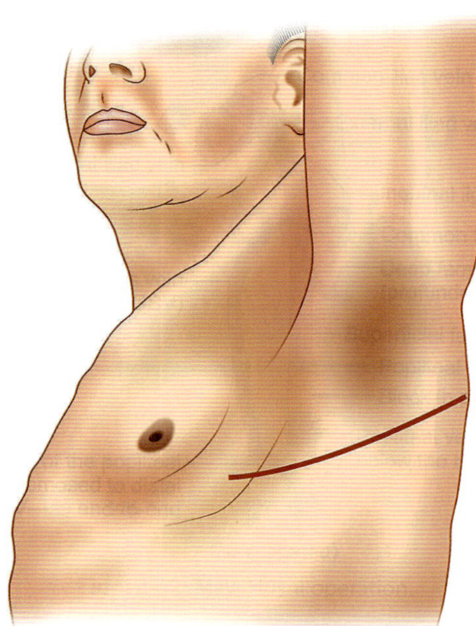

Fig. 13-22: Incision for transaxillary transpleural approach is through 3rd rib.

Lateral thoracic artery near the posterior portion of the wound is divided. Attachment of serratus anterior is removed from 3rd rib. Using cautery, periosteum of the 3rd rib is incised throughout its full length. Often 3rd rib is resected deep to its periosteum. Pleura is opened through the periosteum of the 3rd rib to avoid injury to intercostal neurovascular bundle. Thorax is opened widely using a rib spreader. Lung is deflated to visualise the mediastinum and dome of the pleura. Thoracic vertebrae (upper five) and corresponding ribs are exposed to visualise the mediastinum chain beneath the pleura on the necks of the ribs. Parietal pleura is opened vertically on the sympathetic chain using long fine scissor. Nerve is held with nerve hook below the 4th thoracic ganglion and cut and rami communicantes are divided. Chain above the 2nd or lower half of the stellate ganglion is cut to remove needed segment of the sympathetic chain. Dissection along the chain should be careful and gentle as intercostal vessel bleeding, if occurs, is often difficult to control. If bleeding occurs, bleeding point is carefully identified by proper suction and haemoclips are applied. Bipolar cautery is used for fulguration if needed. Care should be taken not to injure or cauterise the intercostal nerve which will cause troublesome neuralgia. Chest tube is inserted to pleural cavity and wound is closed in layers. Bilateral sympathectomies, if needed, should be done in different sittings.

Thoracoscopic Sympathectomy

It is preferred method than open method as there is better visualisation and identification of the sympathetic chain, faster recovery, and small incisions. Procedure is done under general anaesthesia with open thoracotomy position with operating side of the patient elevated. Double lumen or bronchial blocker is used to facilitate the deflation of the same side of the lung. Zero or 30° telescope is used through 10 mm port at the centre of 4th or 5th intercostal space in anterior or mid-axillary line. Two 5 mm ports are placed side wards above and below the 10 mm port through intercostal spaces which will be in front of the 10 mm camera port to provide adequate triangulation. Lung is deflated by anaesthetist. If not deflated properly then CO_2 insufflation may be used. Sympathetic chain is visualised properly on the necks of the ribs. Overlying pleura is opened using cautery, harmonic scalpel or scissor. Care should be taken not to injure intercostal vessels and nerve. Chain from T4 to T1 is removed. Haemostasis is maintained. Chest tube is placed. Difficulties lie in identifying the chain, lifting the pleura, haemostasis. Advantages are fast recovery, good magnification, and less painful.

14

CHAPTER

Surgeries of Face, Head and Neck

SURGICAL ANATOMY OF NECK

Neck has got anterior and posterior triangles on each side. Skin over the anterior triangle is supplied by anterior cutaneous nerve of neck (C_2, C_3).

Superficial fascia in anterior triangle contains *platysma*, cervical branch of facial nerve, anterior jugular vein and few superficial lymph nodes. Flaps in the neck are usually elevated in *subplatysmal plane*.

Platysma is a wide thin subcutaneous muscle running upwards and medially from *deltoid and pectoral fascia* to the *base of the mandible*. It is supplied by cervical branch of facial nerve. It prevents the skin pressing into superficial veins. Superficial vessels and nerves lie deep to platysma.

Anterior jugular vein is located in superficial fascia which begins below the chin runs vertically downwards 1 cm from the midline; 2.5 cm above the sternum, it pierces the deep fascia to reach suprasternal space where it communicates with opposite anterior jugular vein through jugular venous arch and travels above the clavicle behind the sternocleidomastoid muscle to join external jugular vein.

Structures above the hyoid bone are—anterior belly of digastric, submandibular salivary gland, mylohyoid nerve and vessels, submental branch of facial artery, hyoglossus, intermediate digastric tendon with pulley, stylohyoid muscle tendon, and hypoglossal nerve. *Subhyoid bursa* is located between posterior surface of the body of hyoid bone and thyrohyoid membrane to reduce the friction between the two during swallowing **(Figs. 14-1 and 14-2)**.

Structures below the level of hyoid bone are—infrahyoid muscles [sternohyoid (medial front), omohyoid [lateral in front], sternothyroid (lateral deep, below), thyrohyoid (lateral, deep, above); pretracheal fascia (with thyrohyoid membrane, thyroid cartilage, cricothyroid membrane, cricoid arch, cricothyroid muscle, trachea and carotid sheath).

Anterior triangle of neck is bound by midline, sternocleidomastoid muscle laterally, base of mandible and line joining angle of mandible and mastoid process above. Triangle is divided by digastric muscle and superior belly of omohyoid muscle as muscular, submental, carotid and digastric triangles. Suprahyoid muscles are digastric, mylohyoid, stylohyoid and geniohyoid muscles **(Fig. 14-3)**.

Submental triangle is median in location and is bound by anterior bellies of digastric muscles of both sides with the base on the hyoid bone. Floor is formed by right and left mylohyoid muscles. It contains submental veins and submental lymph nodes (*located in superficial fascia*) which drain from superficial tissues below chin, central part of lower lip, adjacent gum, anterior part of floor of the mouth, and tip of tongue. These lymph nodes drain into submandibular lymph nodes.

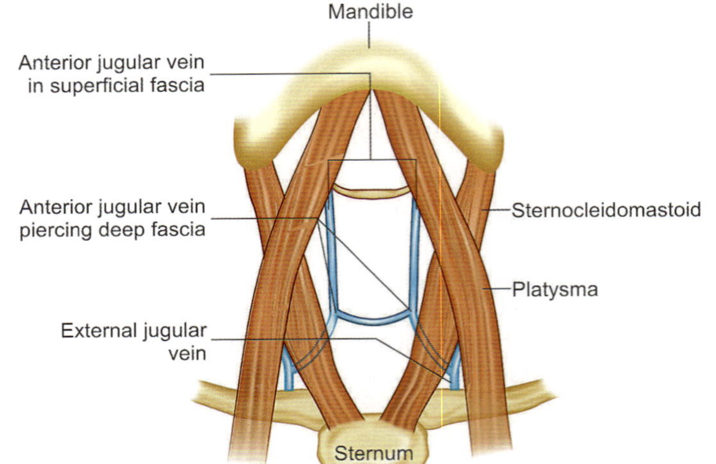

Fig. 14-1: Anatomy of anterior jugular vein and platysma.

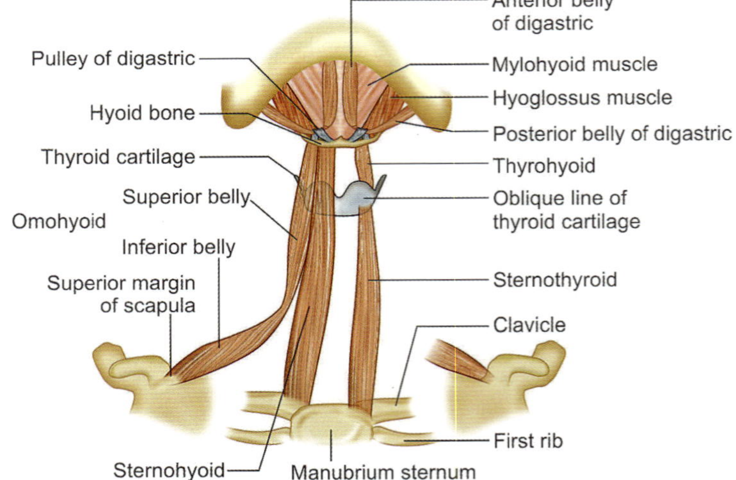

Fig. 14-2: Strap and front muscles of the neck.

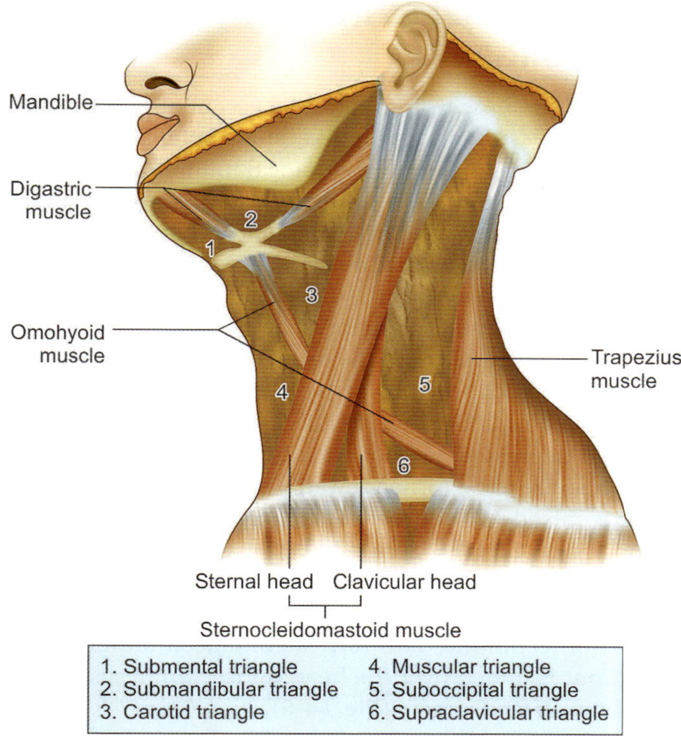

Fig. 14-3: Different triangles in neck.

Digastric triangle is formed by two bellies of digastric muscle, posteriorly also by stylohyoid muscle, base above is by the base of mandible and line joining the angle of mandible and mastoid process. Its roof is formed by skin; superficial fascia with platysma, cervical branch of facial nerve and ascending branch of anterior cutaneous nerve; deep fascia splits to enclose submandibular salivary gland. Its floor is formed by mylohyoid muscle in front, hyoglossus behind and middle constrictor partly. Structures superficial to mylohyoid and hyoglossus are—submandibular salivary gland (superficial part), facial vein, submandibular lymph nodes, submental artery and mylohyoid nerve and vessels, intermediate tendon of the digastric muscle and stylohyoid, hypoglossal nerve. Facial artery is deep to mylohyoid muscle. In the posterior part of digastric triangle lower pole of the parotid and external carotid artery entering the parotid are in superficial location; whereas structures passing between external carotid artery (ECA) and ICA (styloglossus, stylopharyngeus, glossopharyngeal nerve, pharyngeal branch of vagus, styloid process) are in deeper plane. Internal carotid artery (ICA), internal jugular vein (IJV) and vagus are located still in deeper plane. Submandibular lymph glands are located *deep to deep fascia* on the surface of submandibular salivary gland which drains from forehead, nose, frontal, maxillary and ethmoidal air sinuses, inner canthus of eye, upper lip, anterior cheek with adjacent gums and teeth, outer part of lower lip with adjacent teeth and gums except incisors, anterior 2/3rd of tongue except tip of tongue and floor of the mouth, from submental lymph glands. Efferent vessels drain mainly into jugulo-omohyoid lymph nodes.

Carotid triangle is bound above and in front by posterior belly of digastric and stylohyoid muscle; below by superior belly of omohyoid; behind by sternocleidomastoid muscle. Its roof is formed by skin; superficial fascia with platysma, cervical branch of facial nerve and transverse cutaneous nerve; deep fascia. Its floor is formed by thyrohyoid, hyoglossus, and middle and inferior constrictor muscles. It contains—arteries (CCA, ICA, ECA, superior thyroid, facial, ascending pharyngeal, occipital arteries); veins (IJV, common facial vein entering the IJV, pharyngeal vein entering IJV or common facial vein, lingual vein entering the IJV); nerves (vagus, superior laryngeal nerve and its branches, spinal accessory nerve, hypoglossal nerve, ansa cervicalis, sympathetic chain behind carotid sheath); carotid sheath with its contents; lymph nodes (jugulodigastric is below the posterior belly of digastric and jugulo-omohyoid above the inferior belly of digastric).

Investing layer of deep fascia is attached above to external occipital protuberance, superior nuchal line, mastoid process; fascia splits between angle of mandible and mastoid process to enclose parotid. Above the parotid the outer lamina (split part) which is dense and thick gets attached to zygomatic arch. Thin deeper lamina is attached to styloid process, mandible and tympanic plate. Deeper lamina is condensed between angle of mandible and styloid process to form stylomandibular ligament. Below, investing layer is attached to scapular spine, acromion, clavicle, manubrium in front. Behind it is attached to ligamentum nuchae and C_7 spine; in front to symphysis menti and hyoid bone. Investing layer of deep fascia *encloses* trapezius and sternocleidomastoid muscles, parotid and submandibular salivary glands, supraclavicular and suprasternal spaces. Deep fascia forms digastric and omohyoid *pulleys*. Suprasternal *space of Burns* contains tendinous sternal heads of both sternocleidomastoids; jugular venous arch, a lymph node and interclavicular ligament.

Prevertebral fascia is in front of the prevertebral muscles is attached above to the base of skull; below extends into the superior mediastinum to attach to anterior longitudinal ligament and body of T_4 vertebra. In front it is separated from pharynx by retropharyngeal space. Laterally, it merges deep into trapezius. Cervical and brachial plexus of nerves lie behind this fascia. Four cutaneous branches of cervical plexus pierce this fascia. Subclavian artery and brachial plexus runs between scalenus anterior and medius carrying with them prevertebral fascia as *axillary sheath*. Subclavian and axillary veins are away and below this fascia and so are not inside the axillary sheath.

Posterior triangle is the space located between sternocleido-mastoid muscle, trapezius and middle 1/3rd of clavicle. Its *roof* is formed by investing layer of deep fascia. Superficial fascia in posterior triangle contains platysma, external jugular and posterior jugular veins.

External jugular vein is located in superficial fascia deep to platysma; begins at lower part of the parotid by union of posterior auricular vein and posterior division of retromandibular vein; descends downwards in front of the sternocleidomastoid muscle; enters the roof of posterior triangle—investing layer of deep fascia at anteroinferior angle of roof to join subclavian vein. Deep fascia is densely adherent to vein at the point of entering the roof and so external jugular vein when cut, opening cannot be closed, as a result of which air is sucked inside causing air embolism. Before ligating the vein deep fascia should be cut to collapse the vein. Tributaries of external jugular vein are—posterior external jugular vein, transverse cervical vein, suprascapular vein and anterior jugular vein. An oblique jugular vein connects between external jugular vein and IJV at anterior margin of sternocleidomastoid at middle third of the muscle. Surface marking of the vein is from below and behind the angle of the mandible to a point lateral to the posterior border of the sternocleidomastoid near clavicle.

Floor of the posterior triangle is formed by prevertebral fascia over splenius capitis, levator scapulae, scalenus medius, and often scalenus posterior **(Fig. 14-4)**.

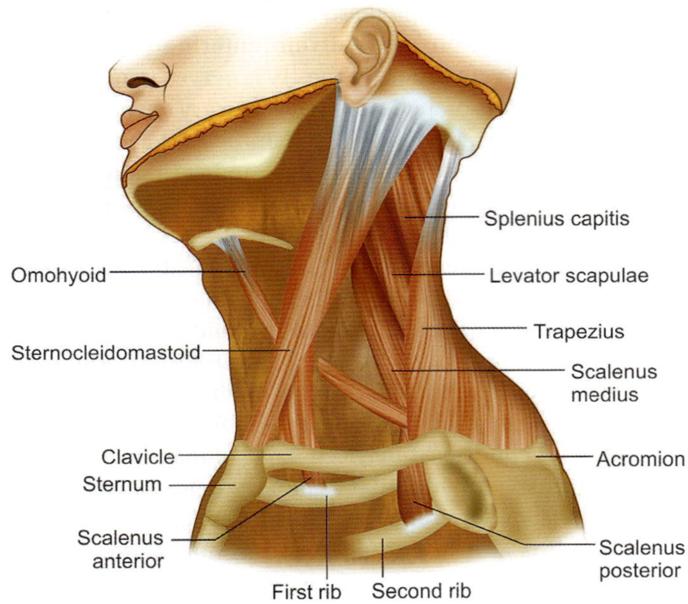

Fig. 14-4: Structures forming the floor of posterior triangle.

Posterior triangle is divided by inferior belly of omohyoid into a *smaller lower supraclavicular*/subclavian triangle and a *larger upper* occipital triangle. *Contents of the posterior triangle* are: The nerves—the spinal accessory nerve; four cutaneous branches of cervical plexus [lesser occipital (C_2), great auricular ($C_{2,3}$), anterior cutaneous nerve of the neck ($C_{2,3}$), supraclavicular nerves ($C_{3,4}$)]; muscular branches to levator scapulae and trapezius ($C_{3,4}$); nerve to rhomboideus (C_5); nerve to serratus anterior ($C_{5,6,7}$); nerve to subclavius ($C_{5,6}$); suprascapular nerve ($C_{5,6}$); three trunks of brachial plexus. Arteries, from above downwards are—occipital artery at the apex of the posterior triangle superficial to splenius capitis, transverse cervical artery, suprascapular artery and subclavian artery. Transverse cervical artery arises from thyrocervical trunk, crosses scalenus anterior, phrenic nerve, upper trunks of brachial plexus, nerve to subclavius, suprascapular nerve, and scalenus medius. It is deep to inferior belly of omohyoid muscle. At the anterior margin of levator scapulae it divides into superficial and deep branches. Posterior triangle also contains many deep lymph nodes of the neck (level V) **(Fig. 14-5)**.

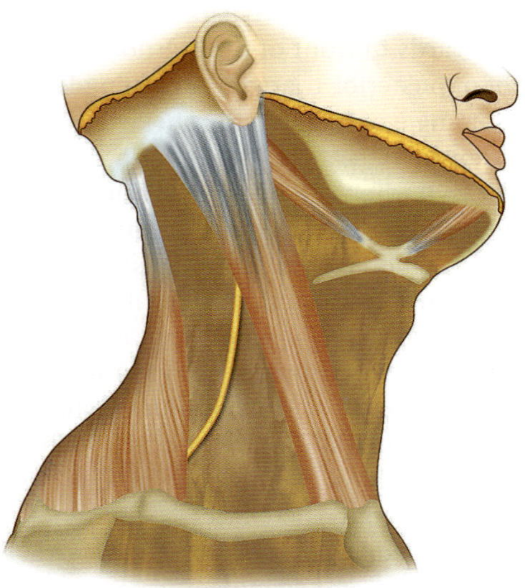

Fig. 14-5: Location of spinal accessory nerve.

BASIC PRINCIPLES IN HEAD AND NECK SURGERY

General anaesthesia with intubation is essential in all head and neck surgeries. Only surgeries like superficial excision (cyst/lipoma excision) can be done under local infiltration anaesthesia. Cervical block is often used by few experts for laryngeal surgeries, carotid endarterectomy, and thyroidectomy. Fitness for prolonged anaesthesia, arranging adequate amount of blood, proper assessment of the lesion by CT scan, usage of different energy sources, need for tracheostomy should all be thought of.

Extension of the head is usually needed in most of the head and neck surgeries which is achieved by placing a sandbag/rolled up towel/round pillow under the shoulder. Arms are pulled down with the shoulder depressed and both hands tugged under the buttock. Neck may require to be turned towards opposite side. Head end of the table is raised 15° in order to reduce venous congestion and bleeding.

Cleaning is done over entire neck in front, face, upper chest up to the nipple line, both shoulder area. Head is draped with sterile double towel technique. Two towels are placed under the head; towel in front is folded over the head up to chin in neck surgery, up to eyebrow in face surgery **(Fig. 14-6)**.

Skin incisions in the neck are usually placed along the lines of natural skin crease which are horizontal in front of the neck, horizontally oblique on the side of the neck. So, most of the neck incisions are horizontally placed to achieve better scar. Vertical incision causes scar contraction, hypertrophy and results in poor scar. Vertical incision is used for major vascular access (for carotids), and in trauma. In such occasions, incision is placed along the anterior border of the sternocleidomastoid muscle or along the anterior border of the trapezius.

Surgical dissection in head and neck is done using 15 number scalpel blade or fine scissor or fine monopolar/blended cautery tip. Skin hooks are used while elevating the skin flaps. Dissection should be perfect with meticulous haemostasis. Proper knowledge of surgical anatomy of neck is essential. Usually subplatysmal plane is raised. Finally closure is also equally important to achieve cosmetically acceptable good healthy scar.

Since neck is a compact area, small incision should be avoided. An adequate incision which will expose the surgical area is essential. Proper haemostasis by ligature/cautery harmonic energy is needed. *Haematoma in the neck under the deep fascia* will compress trachea and can cause life-threatening respiratory arrest. A *suction drain* is usual practice to prevent this. Drain is removed in 48 hours. *Haematoma superficial to deep fascia* also can occur but is not life threatening. It may cause fibrosis and poor scarring. During closure, deep fascia, platysma are closed in layers using absorbable 3-zero vicryl interrupted sutures.

Skin is closed with interrupted sutures (using monofilament non-absorbable suture material) in major surgeries. Skin clips also can be used. Subcuticular absorbable 3-zero vicryl or monocryl or PDS sutures can be placed if there is sure about complete haemostasis. These sutures are not removed. Additional advantage of subcuticular suture over interrupted suture is doubtful. Often it causes troublesome induration and discomfort. Interrupted sutures are removed in 5–7 days.

Surgery of larynx and laryngectomy are beyond the scope of this book as it s a specialised subject as such. But basic anatomy of larynx and principles should be remembered by general surgeon **(Fig. 14-7)**.

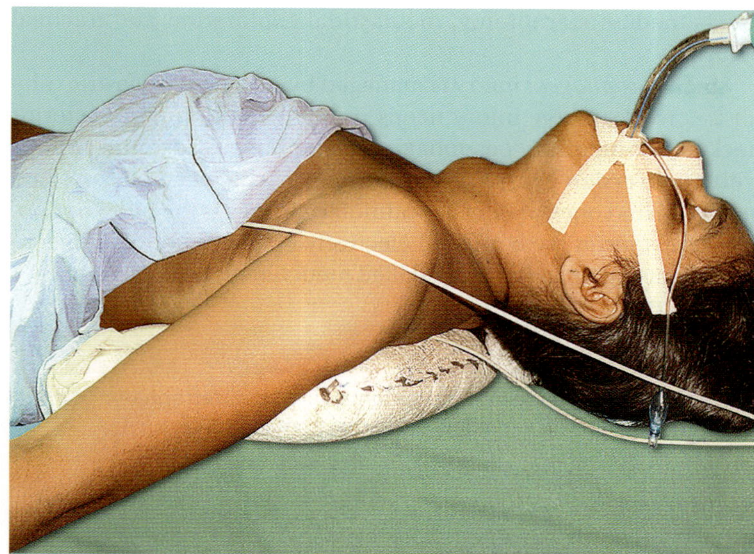

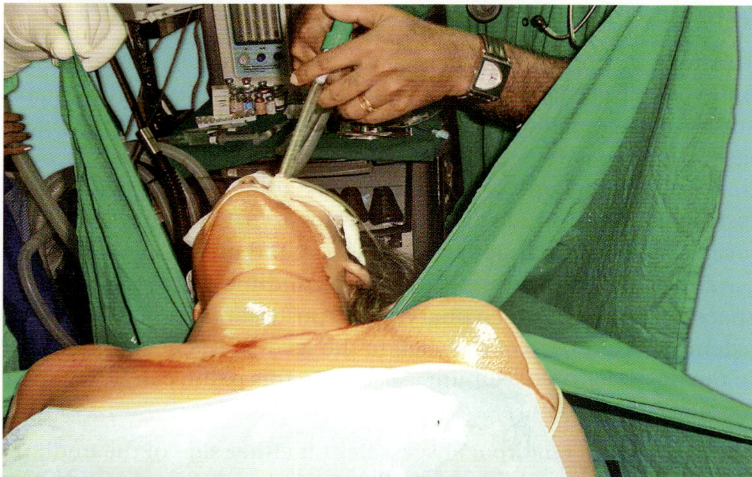

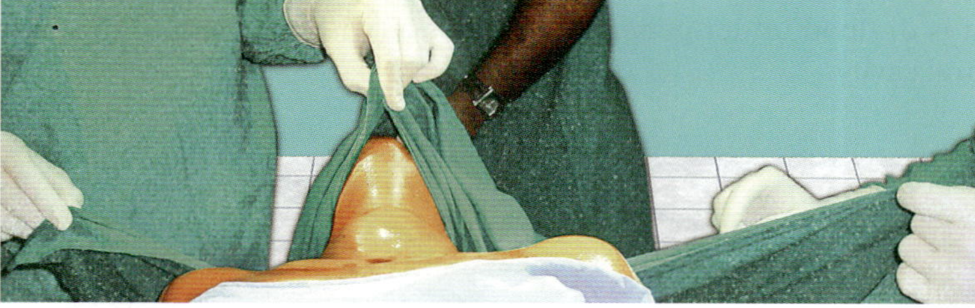

Fig. 14-6: Position, cleaning and draping of the neck for neck surgery.

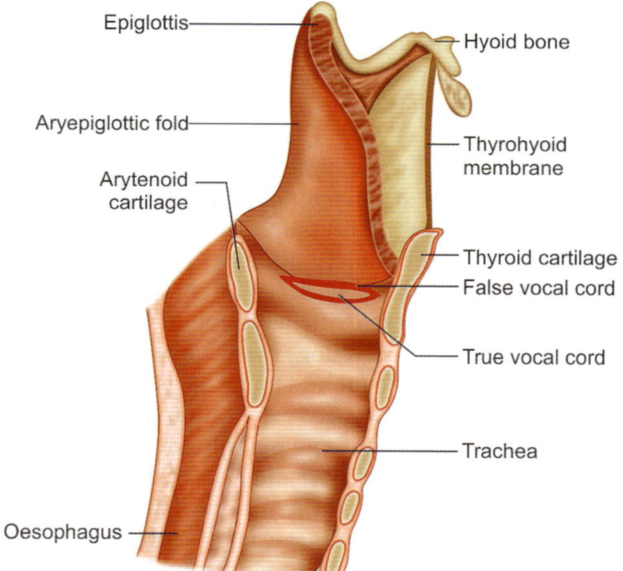

Fig. 14-7: Anatomy of the larynx.

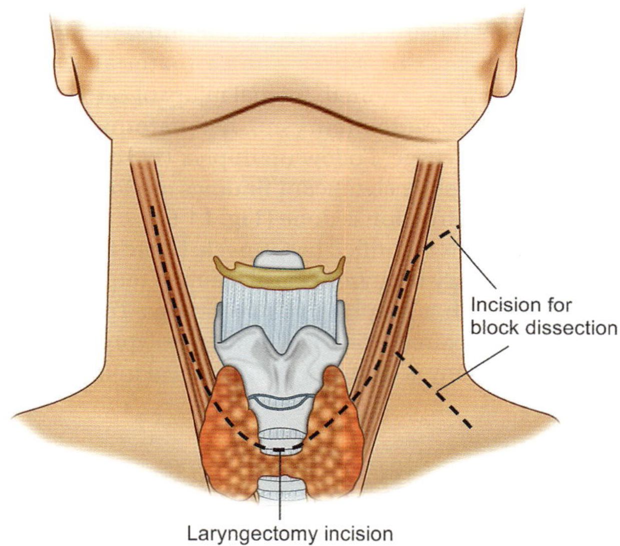

Fig. 14-8: Gluck–Sorenson incision for laryngectomy.

Incision used for laryngectomy, *Gluck–Sorenson's incision* is shown in **Figure 14-8**. Different surgeries are done for laryngeal cancers—partial or total. Neck node dissection also should be done. Permanent tracheostomy is needed. In case of pharyngeal involvement laryngopharyngectomy with tracheostomy, gastric pull up as pharyngo-oesophageal substitute. Speech therapy, tracheostomy care, prevention of respiratory infection are essential postoperative care needed in these patients.

HEAD AND NECK TRAUMA

It can be open trauma or a closed one. Open trauma is usually penetrating. It can be from knife, sickle, and bullet injuries. Injury can occur to major vessels, trachea, oesophagus, soft tissues, thyroid, nerves, cervical and brachial plexus. External wound/stab injury may be small but deeper injury may be extensive.

Closed trauma may be to cervical spine; carotid artery leading to an intimal tear which may cause *carotid blowout* at a later period. Slowly expanding haematoma may be possible with blunt injury to neck. Only external bruising may be evident in such occasion. Unstable fracture of cervical spine may be present; spine should be protected mechanically in such suspected cases.

Injury to oral cavity, pharynx can cause bleeding into the airway causing life-threatening airway block. Maintenance of the airway is a crucial need here.

Major vessel injury can cause torrential bleeding. Digital compression, early exploration and vessel repair is the treatment.

Management of Head and Neck Trauma

General condition should be assessed. Immediate resuscitation by inserting a central venous line, and an airway is done.

Adequate blood should be arranged for transfusion. Other injuries in the body should be looked for—abdomen/thorax/head/limb fractures. Duplex US scan of neck is a good way of assessing the neck injuries. *Assessment* is done as 3 categories—vascular, tracheal, oesophageal injuries.

Airway is maintained by endotracheal intubation or tracheostomy or cricothyroidotomy as an emergency procedure.

Bleeding is controlled by pressure, packing, early exploration, ligation of external jugular vein, IJV, ligation of small vessels. Torrential bleeding in face, and proximal neck can be controlled by ligating the external carotid artery distal to origin of superior thyroid artery. ECA has got branches whereas ICA does not have branches in the neck. Wounds in lower neck zone (zone 1) may be associated with injury to mediastinal major vessels and so exploration of mediastinum with *median sternotomy* is needed. Angiography should be done for all zone 1 penetrating injury. CT chest and neck is also often desirable if patient is stable. Penetrating injuries in zone 3 may include injury to ICA extending onto the intracranial cavity. Neurosurgical approach may be needed in such injury. Lateral injury in zone 2 causes carotid injuries which require wound exploration. Wound should be explored with an adequate lengthy incision. All haematomas are gently evacuated. Suction should be used to identify the bleeding point. Vascular clamps should be used if carotid injury is present. Intraluminal stent is better to maintain the brain circulation until repair is over. Small tear in the carotid is sutured using continuous polypropylene 3-zero or 4-zero suture material. Occasionally venous patch or graft is required. Intimal injury of carotid is observed for formation of pseudoaneurysm, haematoma, late rupture, thrombosis and blockage. Follow up duplex US scan is essential at repeated sittings. If such significant findings are found, exploration and vascular reconstruction is done **(Fig. 14-9)**.

Laryngeal injury is identified by CT neck. Hyoid fracture is treated conservatively. Injury to thyroid cartilage may require repair using wires or plates with a covering tracheostomy. *Tracheal injury* in proximal part is repaired using interrupted polypropylene or vicryl sutures. Tracheostomy is often needed. Tracheal injury in lower neck needs median sternotomy, mediastinal exploration and tracheal suturing.

Small *oesophageal injury* is managed by placing nasogastric tube for 2–3 weeks. Large injury needs proper exploration of posterior neck, suturing of the oesophagus. A feeding gastrostomy with or without diversion oesophagostomy in neck which can be corrected at later period once patient's condition stabilizes is the other option.

Nerve injuries are corrected electively at a later period by nerve suturing using microscope by skilled meticulous method.

Penetrating injury

Incision

Sternomastoid muscle

Incision for zone 1 injury which extends to mediastinum

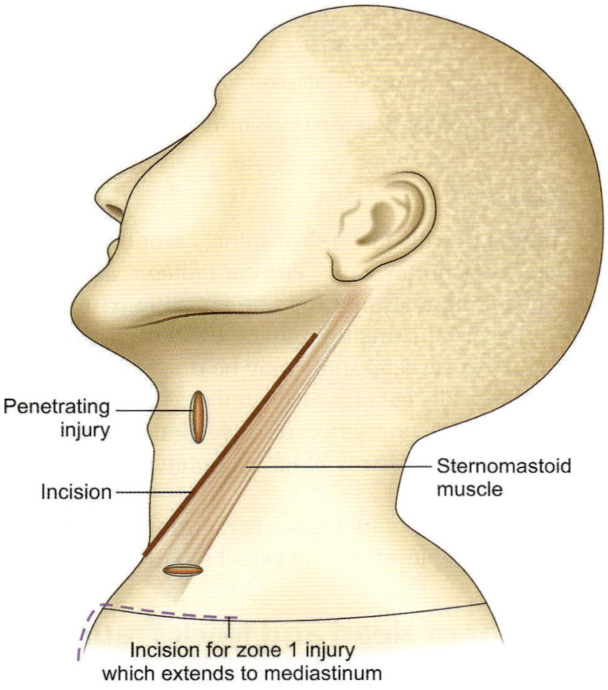

Fig. 14-9: Incisions used in head and neck trauma.

Complications

Airway block, bleeding, haematoma, infection, retropharyngeal or parapharyngeal haematoma or abscess formation.

RETROPHARYNGEAL ABSCESS

Surgical Anatomy

The wall of the pharynx has got 5 layers. Mucosa, submucosa, pharyngobasilar fascia, muscular layer (contains 3 constrictors and stylo, salpingo, palatopharyngeus muscles) and buccopharyngeal fascia that covers outer part of constrictors and extends over buccinator. Buccopharyngeal fascia is adherent to prevertebral fascia posteriorly in the midline. Retropharyngeal lymph nodes are located between buccopharyngeal fascia and prevertebral fascia in paramedian (eccentric) position (not midline). Retropharyngeal space is situated between pharynx and posterior layer of deep fascia, extending from base of the skull to the level of tracheal bifurcation in the posterior mediastinum. Abscess in this plane can be acute or chronic **(Fig. 14-10)**.

Acute is seen in children; abscess lies on either side of the midline. It is due to bacterial infection like staphylococci or streptococci. It is drained under general anaesthesia (with intubation) through oral cavity.

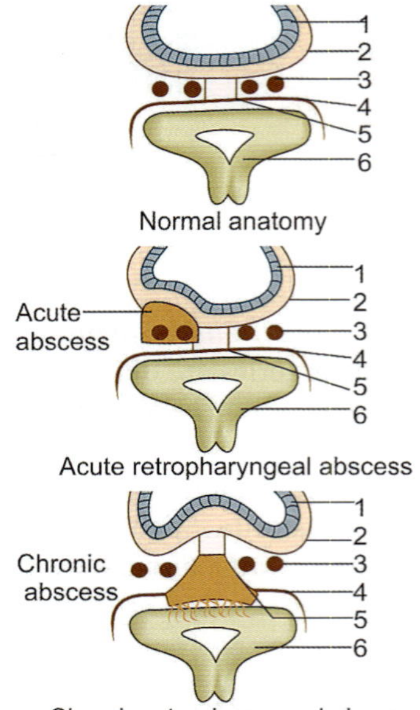

Fig. 14-10: Note acute and chronic retropharyngeal abscess. Normal anatomy is also shown. Acute is eccentric and is due to suppuration of retropharyngeal lymph nodes. Chronic is central, midline and is due to tuberculosis of the cervical vertebra.

Chronic retropharyngeal abscess is usually due to tuberculosis of the cervical spine which is in the midline; confirmed by CT scan; it is drained through neck incision under general anaesthesia. Horizontal incision is made 2 cm below the angle of the jaw. Sternomastoid muscle is separated from tail of the parotid and is retracted behind. Carotid sheath is identified and retracted behind. Superior constrictor is identified; finger is passed behind the muscle to reach retropharyngeal space; pus is drained and collected for culture and acid fast bacilli (AFB) staining. Antituberculous drugs are started.

PARAPHARYNGEAL ABSCESS

Parapharyngeal space is cone-shaped space with its base at base of skull and apex at greater cornu of hyoid bone. Medial wall is formed by superior constrictor; lateral wall by lateral pterygoid, angle of mandible and parotid gland; posteriorly by carotid sheath, below by submandibular salivary gland. Abscess in this region usually is spread from tonsils, infected lower 3rd molar tooth. Thrombosis of internal jugular vein, erosion of ICA and bleeding, and septicemia are the possible complications **(Fig. 14-11)**.

It is drained under general anaesthesia with neck extended and turned to opposite side. Horizontal incision is made over the anterior margin of the sternomastoid muscle 2 cm below the jaw. After retracting the muscle behind, deep fascia is opened to reach the abscess cavity. All loculi are broken using finger. After thorough warm saline irrigation drain is placed and dressing is done. Wound is not closed usually but allowed to heal spontaneously. Often secondary suturing may be required. Causative pathology should be addressed.

TREATMENT OF LUDWIG'S ANGINA

It is an inflammatory oedema of submandibular region and floor of the mouth causing diffuse swelling and brawny oedema of the submandibular region usually due to dental or oral infection. It presents with toxicity, trismus, brawny swelling in upper neck, dysphagia and dyspnoea, putrid halitosis and fever.

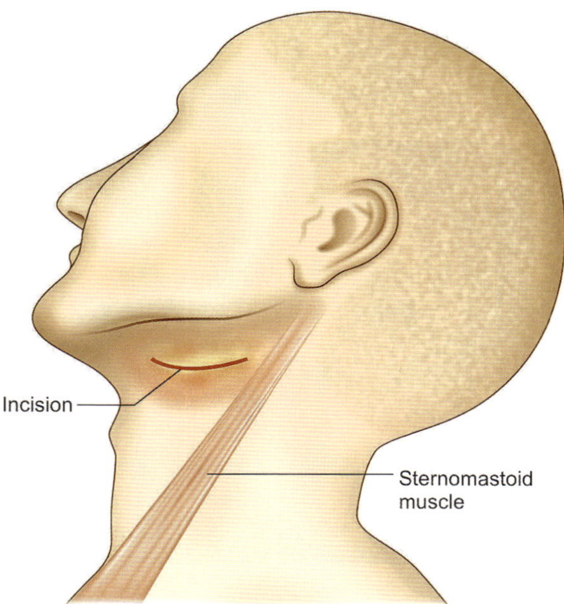

Fig. 14-11: Drainage of parapharyngeal abscess through neck incision.

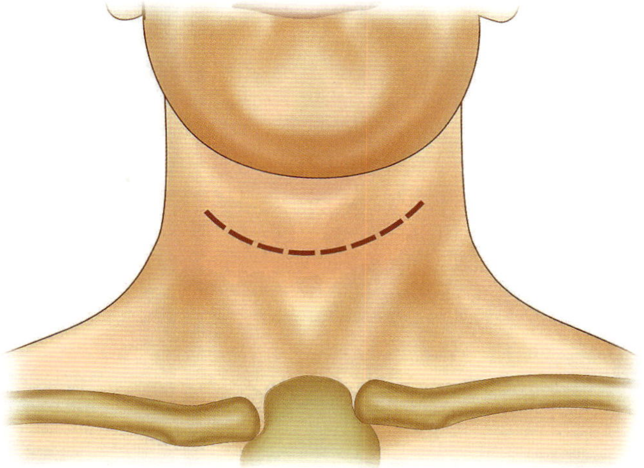

Fig. 14-12: Incision for Ludwig's angina drainage.

It should be drained by making a *transverse skin incision* in submental region; incision is deepened through deep fascia and mylohyoid muscle is cut *vertically*. Wound is left open and delayed suturing is done. Often it is difficult to intubate the patient for anaesthesia due to trismus, and so tracheostomy may be needed **(Fig. 14-12)**.

TREATMENT OF TUBERCULOUS LYMPHADENITIS AND COLD ABSCESS IN THE NECK

In cold abscess, initial *aspiration* is done through a wide bore needle in a non-dependent site using 'Z'/zigzag track (to prevent sinus formation). If aspiration is not effective then *drainage* is done through a non-dependent incision; all caseating material is removed; wound is closed without a drain. *Surgical removal of tuberculous lymphadenitis* is indicated whenever patient is not responding to drugs and in persistence of sinus. It is done by elevating skin flaps and removing all diseased lymph nodes. Due to chronic inflammation adhesions are common. Injury to IJV, nerves can occur. In a *chronic long-standing tuberculous sinus*, treatment is surgical excision of the entire track through an elliptical incision. It is done under general anaesthesia **(Figs. 14-13 and 14-14)**.

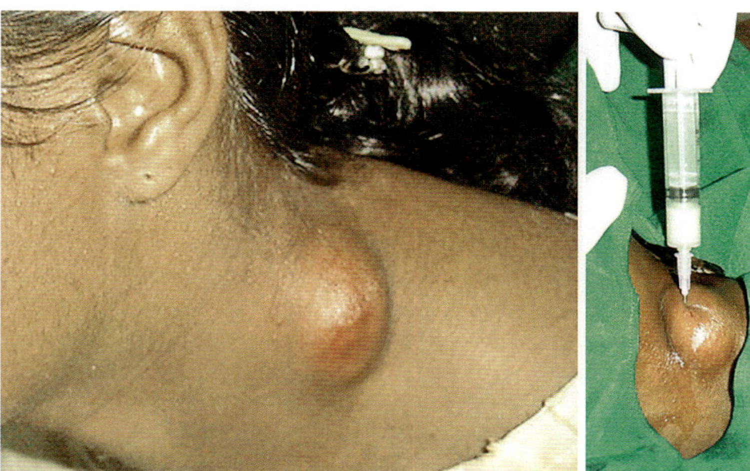

Fig. 14-13: Tuberculous cold abscess and its aspiration.

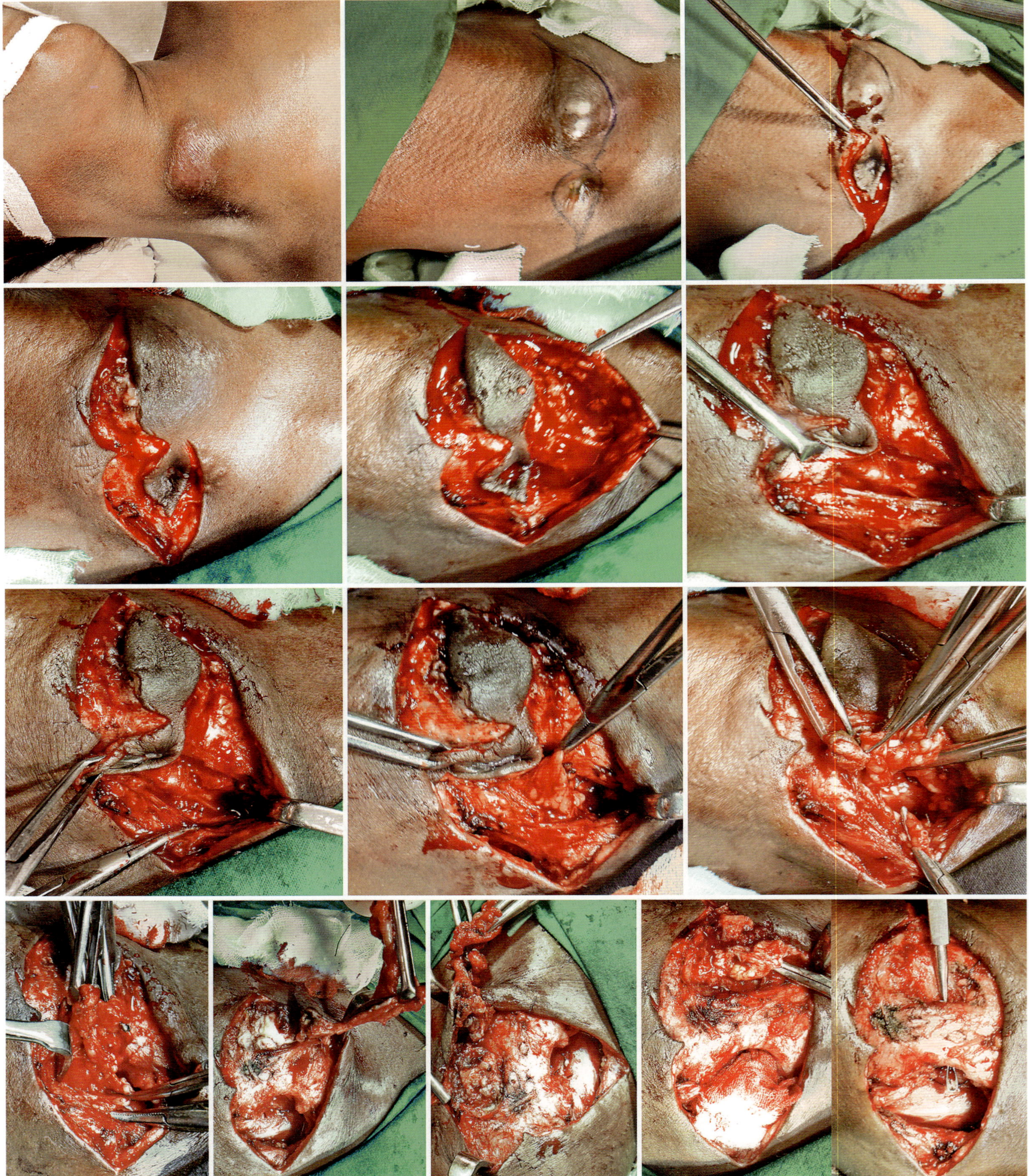

Fig. 14-14: Excision of tuberculous sinus in the neck.

EXCISION OF THE BRANCHIAL CYST AND FISTULA

Branchial Cyst

It is due to remnants of second branchial cleft. Cholesterol crystals are typical. Branchial cyst is situated in the anterior border of the upper third of the sternomastoid muscle. It is seen in adolescent period **(Figs. 14-15 and 14-16)**.

Excision of cyst is done under general anaesthesia. Neck is slightly extended and head turned towards opposite side. After cleaning and draping, horizontal incision is made 2 cm below the mandible; deepened across skin and platysma without elevating the flap to avoid injury to marginal mandibular nerve. Adjacent to anterior margin of the sternomastoid muscle deep fascia is incised carefully to reach the cyst. Cyst is dissected gently and carefully. Often extension of the track between ICA and ECA towards tonsillar fossa will be found which should be dissected carefully using fine scissor and bipolar cautery. Such extended track should be entirely removed. Incomplete removal will lead into fistula formation **(Fig. 14-17)**.

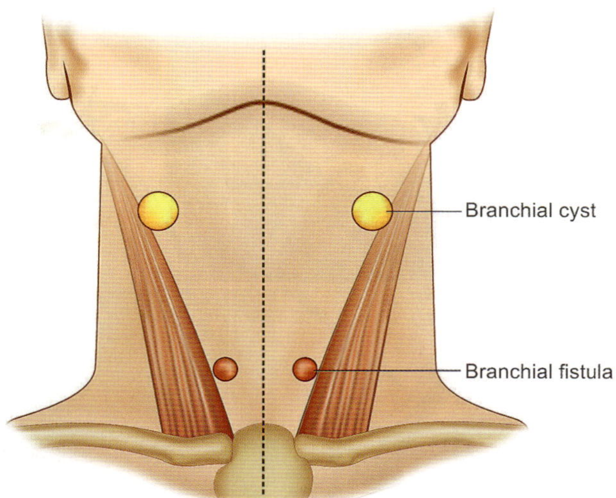

Fig. 14-15: Anatomical location of branchial cyst and fistula.

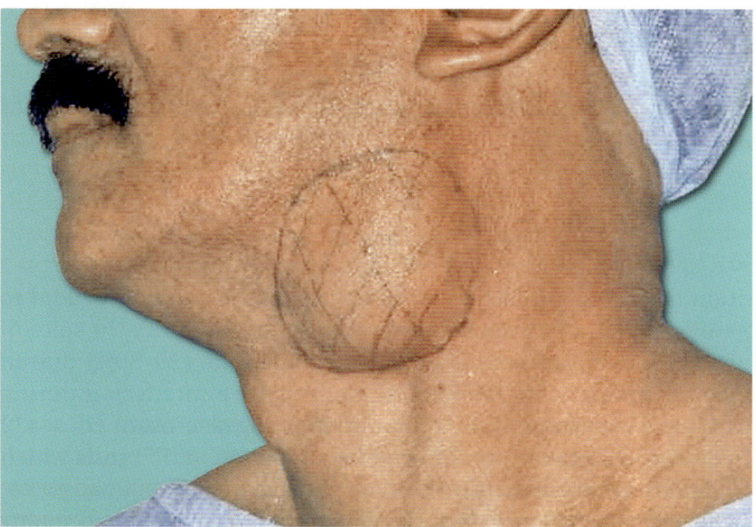

Fig. 14-16: Branchial cyst.

Branchial Fistula

It is usually congenital; its external opening is adjacent to lower third of anterior border of the sternocleidomastoid muscle. Its internal orifice is near posterior pillar of the tonsil. Fistulogram/CT fistulogram and discharge study are the needed investigations. Often it is bilateral **(Fig. 14-18)**.

Stepladder excision: It is excised under general anaesthesia. Position is similar to branchial cyst. An elliptical horizontal incision is placed in the lower neck which includes the external orifice of the fistula. Often methylene blue dye is injected through the external orifice to identify the track during dissection. Track is dissected carefully upwards. Another horizontal incision is made 2 cm below the lower margin of the mandible. Further dissection of the track is done through upper incision. Entire track is dissected up to internal opening at posterior pillar of the tonsil. During dissection, carotids, IJV, hypoglossal, accessory and glossopharyngeal nerves should be taken care of. After excision of the track skin incisions are sutured. Often suction drain may be used. Bilateral fistula can be operated in the same sitting.

Complications are bleeding, incomplete excision of the track, injury to nerves **(Figs. 14-19 and 14-20)**.

PHARYNGEAL POUCH

Progressive symptoms, respiratory distress and dysphagia are definitive indications for surgery **(Fig. 14-21)**.

Procedure

Under general anaesthesia endoscope is passed to identify the opening of the pouch. Pouch is packed with acriflavine soaked gauze for identification. Nasogastric tube is passed into the oesophagus under visualisation. Pouch is approached through neck incision for proper removal. As pouch is usually left sided, left sided lower third horizontal incision is made. Gauze filled pouch sac is felt which is dissected with sharp and finger dissection. Opening of the pouch is located usually behind/on posterior aspect of the oesophagus. Entire pouch is dissected to visualise fundus, neck and junction. Neck is partially opened to identify the nasogastric tube. Traction over the pouch sac stretches the cricopharyngeus. Vertical posterior midline 4 cm myotomy is done to this muscle. Both recurrent laryngeal nerves which are on lateral walls are safeguarded. Sac/pouch at the neck are divided and pouch is removed. Defect in the posterior oesophagus is closed using 2-zero vicryl or silk interrupted sutures. Wound is closed with a drain.

In *Dohlman's operation* pharyngeal pouch is excised endoscopically.

Postoperatively nasogastric tube left in place for 7–10 days. Nasogastric feeding can be started early. Drain is removed in 5–7 days.

Problems and Complications

Often there will be dense adhesions between pouch wall and adjacent structures due to recurrent infection and inflammation which makes dissection difficult. Injury to surrounding structures can occur.

Infection, mediastinitis, pneumonia, lung abscess can occur as often fundus of the pouch may be in the mediastinum. Abscess neck itself can occur postoperatively. Pharyngeal fistula may develop whenever there is sepsis and dense adhesions. Stenosis of oesophagus leading into recurrence is known to occur.

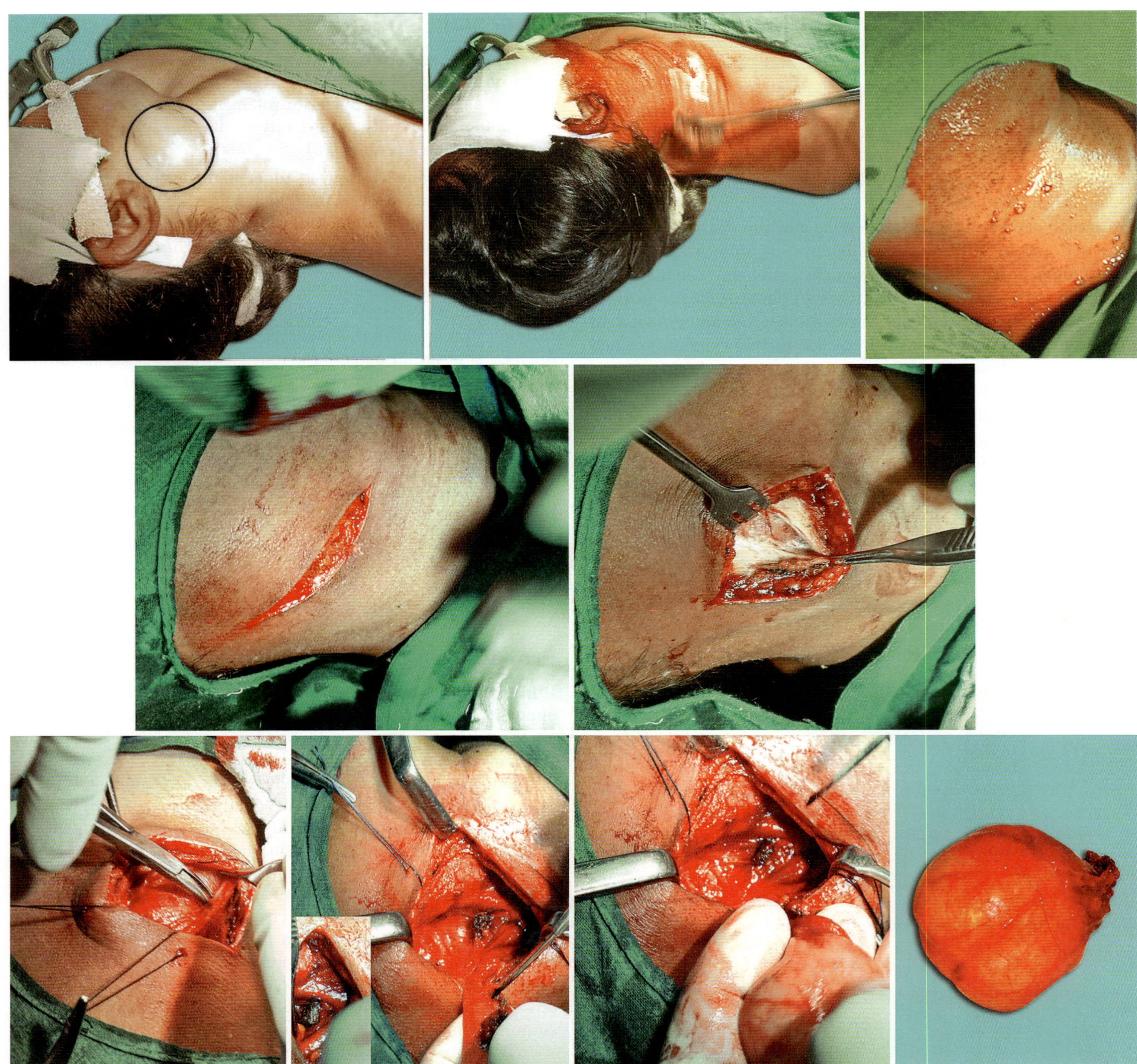

Fig. 14-17: Excision of branchial cyst.

SURGICAL TREATMENT OF CYSTIC HYGROMA

Excision is done under general anaesthesia with neck extended and head turned towards opposite side. Transverse skin incision in the supraclavicular region of adequate length is made. Subplatysmal plane is reached. Circumferential meticulous dissection with slow gradual mobilisation of cyst is done. Cyst does not occupy the natural planes; but encroaches vital neurovascular structures. Often it extends into mediastinum also. After complete excision, drain is placed, antibiotics are given. Higher lesion may extend to parotid region often causing risk of facial nerve injury. In spite of proper dissection there is high recurrence rate (20–30%) due to incomplete excision, inability to identify the entire lesion during excision. Aspiration of the cyst and injecting sclerosant OK - 432 (*picibanil*) will cause pronounced inflammation and fibrosis which facilitates complete excision at a later period.

Staged surgery/repeated surgery/adding superficial parotidectomy are additional things needed to achieve complete cure.

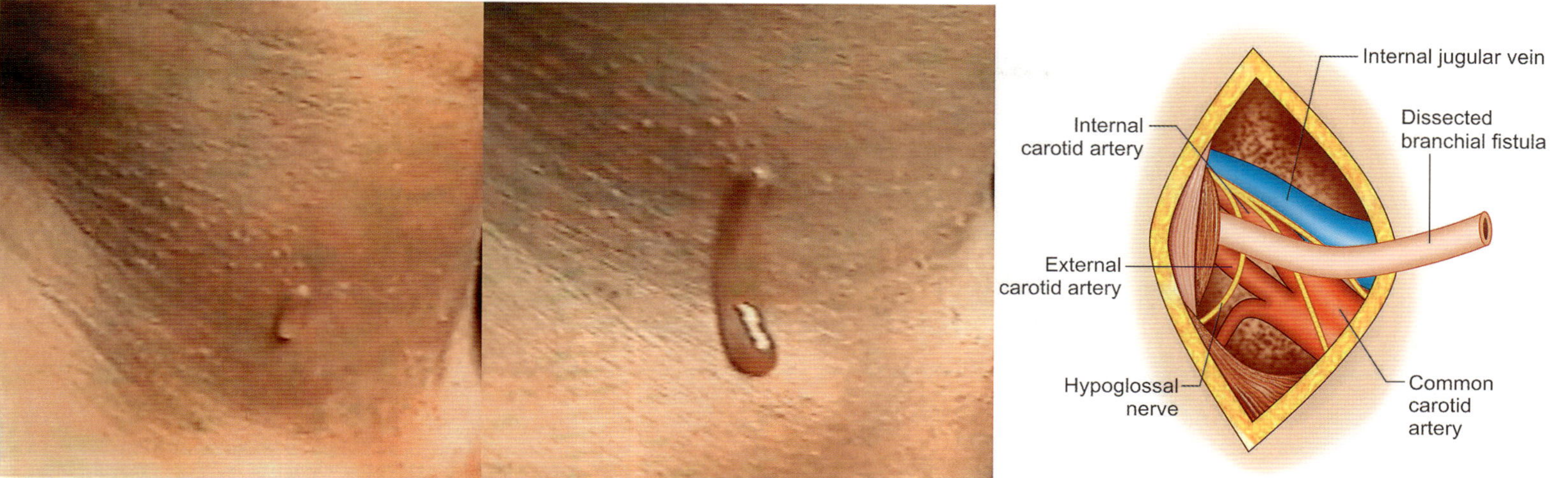

Fig. 14-18: Branchial fistula—photograph and diagram.

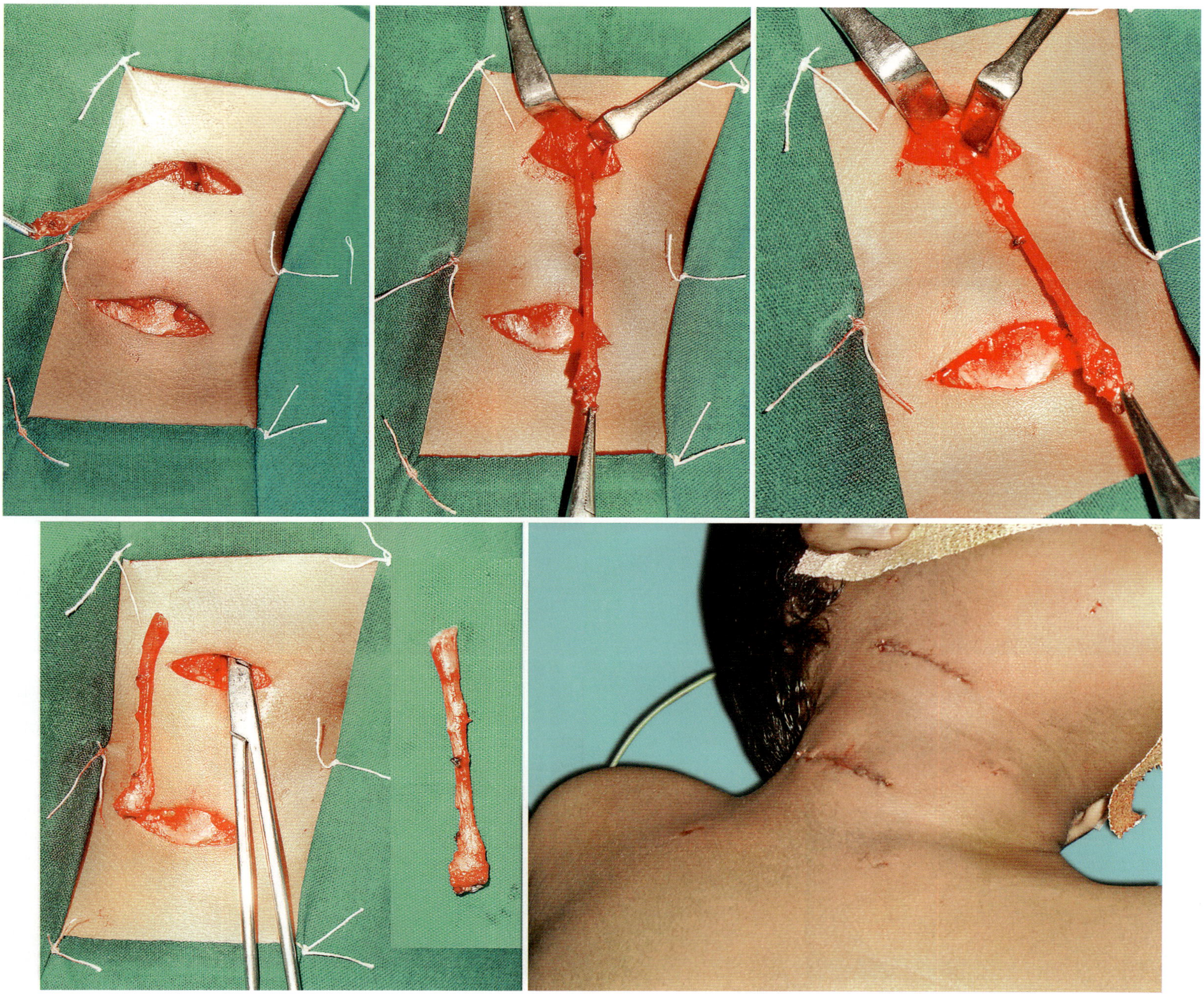

Fig. 14-19: Branchial fistula surgery in a child/boy.

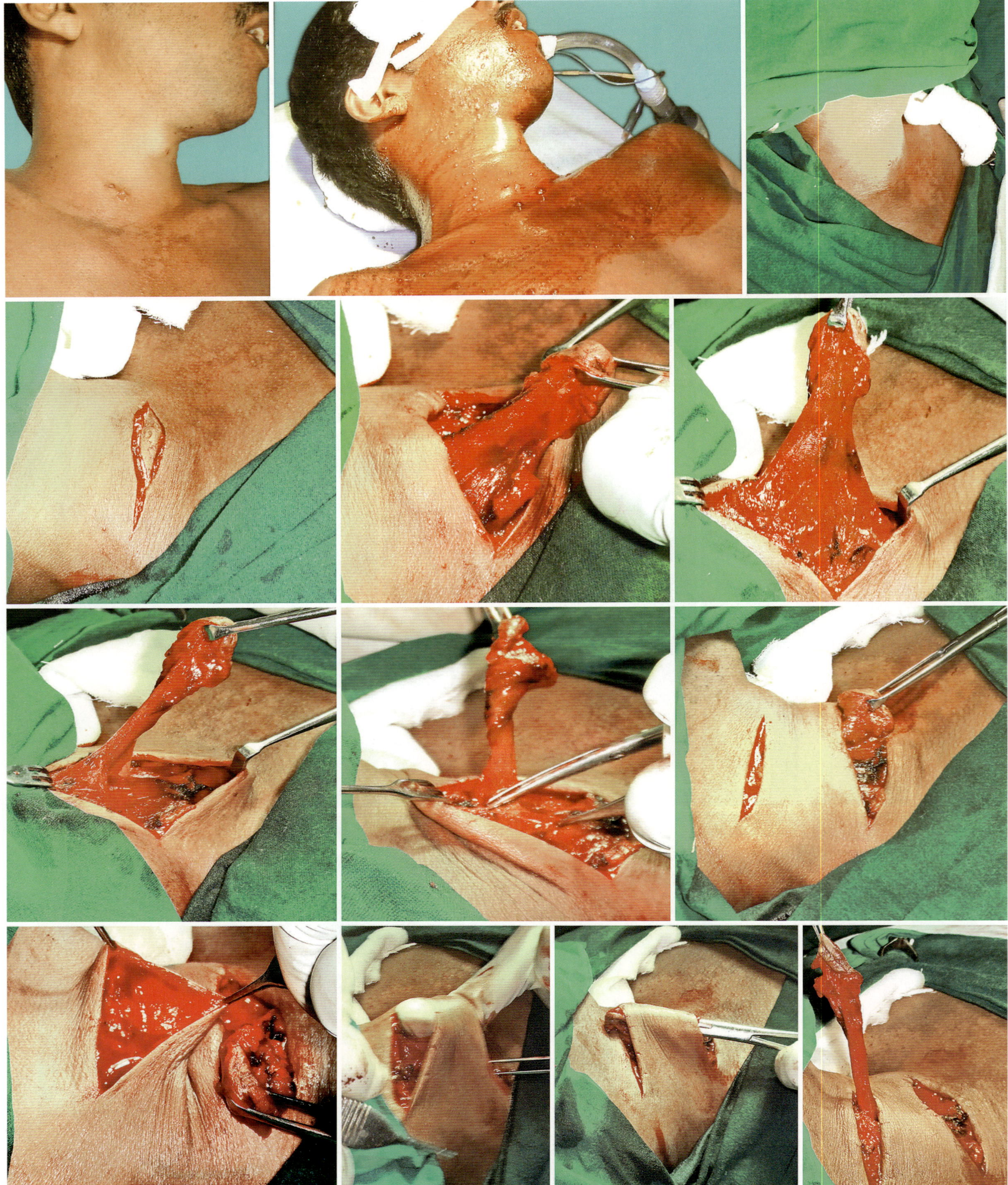

Figs. 14-20(1)

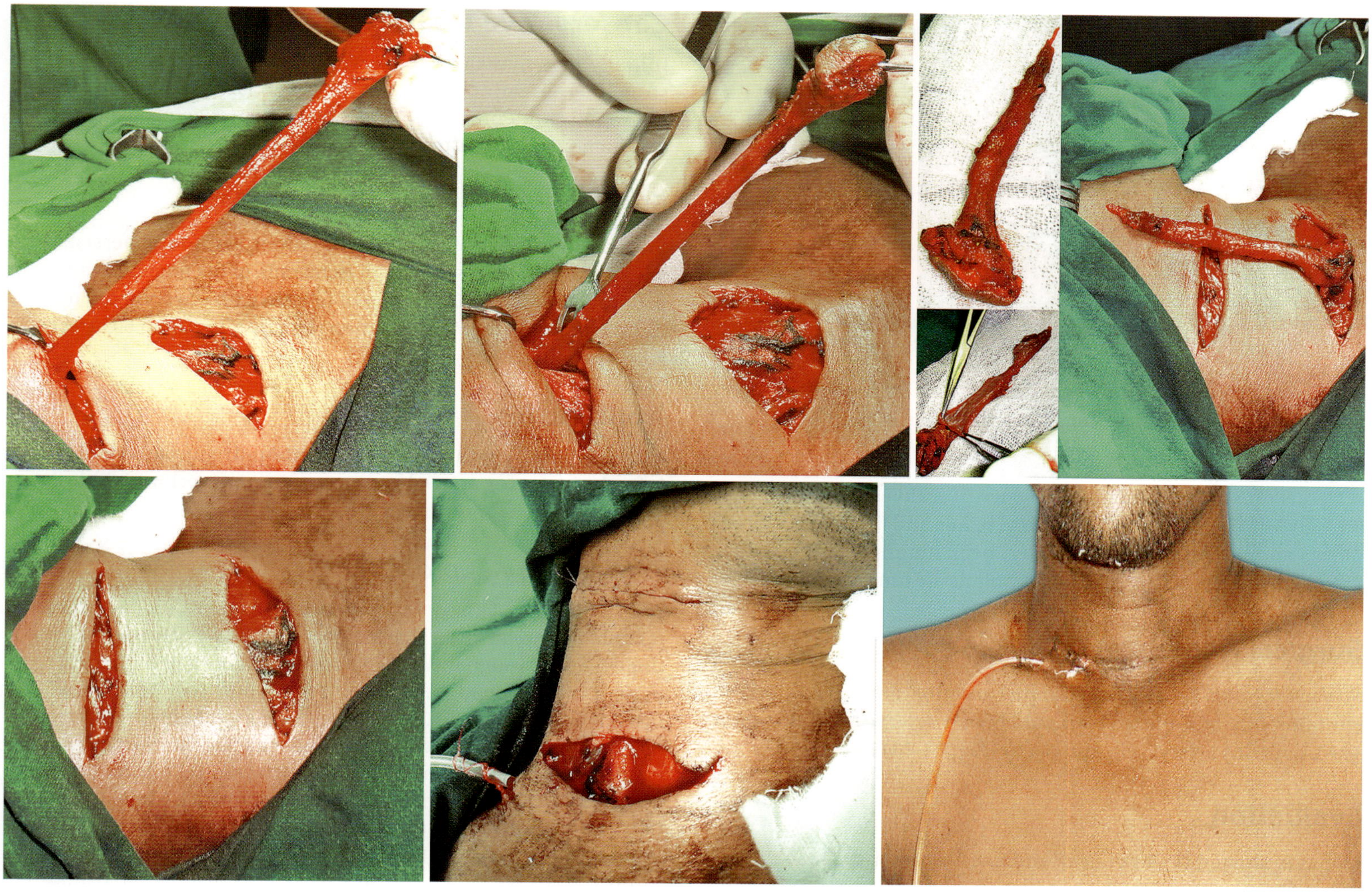

Figs. 14-20(2)

Figs. 14-20(1 and 2): Branchial fistula surgery in an adult.

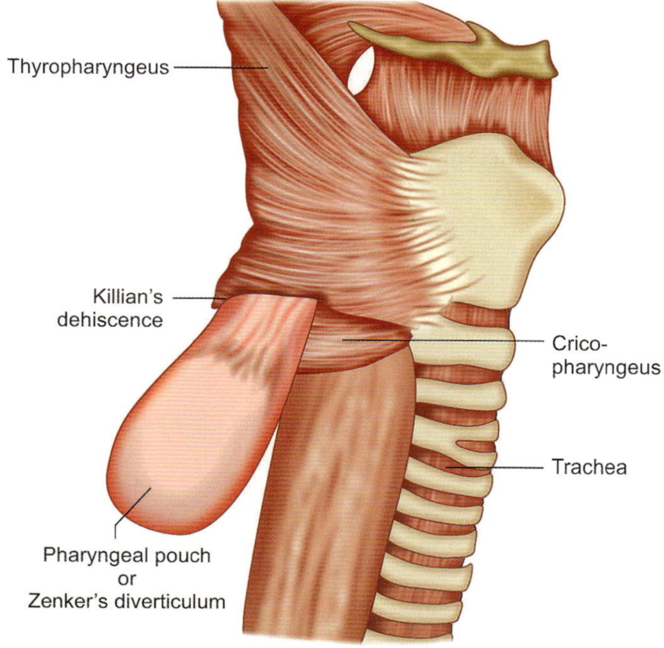

Fig. 14-21: Anatomy of pharyngeal pouch.

TONGUE TIE

It is short, thick fibrous frenum linguae. During protrusion tip and lateral margins of the tongue will be everted with dorsal mid part heaping. It causes difficult in speech and also cleaning the inner part of the lower teeth. It is treated surgically either under local or general (in child) anaesthesia. Stay suture is placed at the tip of tongue to lift it upwards. Fibrous frenum is divided using fine scissor. Linear wound is either left alone or closed longitudinally using fine 4-zero catgut continuous sutures from the tip of the wound towards the margin of the floor of the mouth **(Fig. 14-22)**.

SURGICAL MANAGEMENT OF CERVICAL RIB (THORACIC OUTLET SYNDROME/TOS)

It is done in case of thoracic outlet syndrome (TOS) which is due to cervical rib. Rib compresses the neurovascular bundle causing neurological and vascular manifestations. Arterial TOS is mainly caused by cervical rib or rudimentary first rib. Venous TOS is due to costoclavicular ligament and subclavius muscle compressing subclavian vein. Neurogenic TOS is caused by congenital anatomical factors like cervical rib, long C_7 transverse process, anomalous first rib, anomalous insertion of scalene muscles, split scalenus anterior,

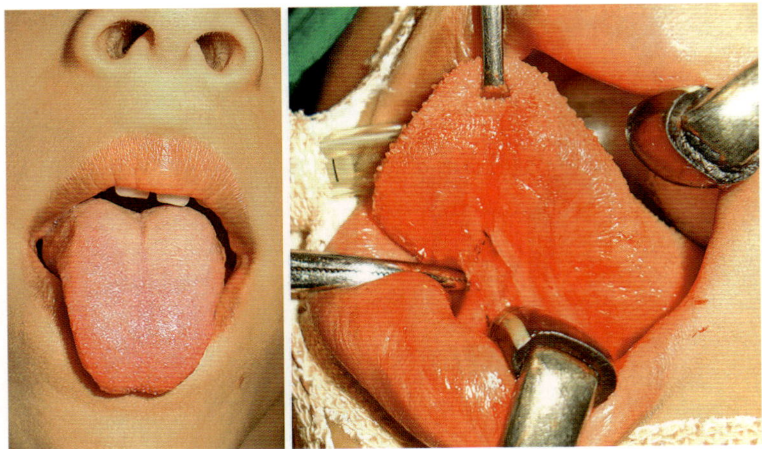

Fig. 14-22: Tongue tie and its release.

scalenus muscle hypertrophy, presence of scalenus intimus muscle (is seen 55% of individuals), abnormal bands and ligaments, brachial plexus anomalies, sagging shoulder; neck trauma (clavicle, callus, first rib, scalene muscles, old scars); soft tissue tumours.

Surgical Anatomy

Scalene triangle is between scalenus anterior, medius and first rib contains brachial plexus and subclavian artery. *Costoclavicular space* contains artery, vein and nerve **(Fig. 14-23)**.

Evaluation

TOS is evaluated by X-ray neck and chest along with X-ray cervical spine; Doppler study, nerve conduction studies, electromyography, CT angiogram, CT neck. Normal nerve conduction velocity is 85 m/second.

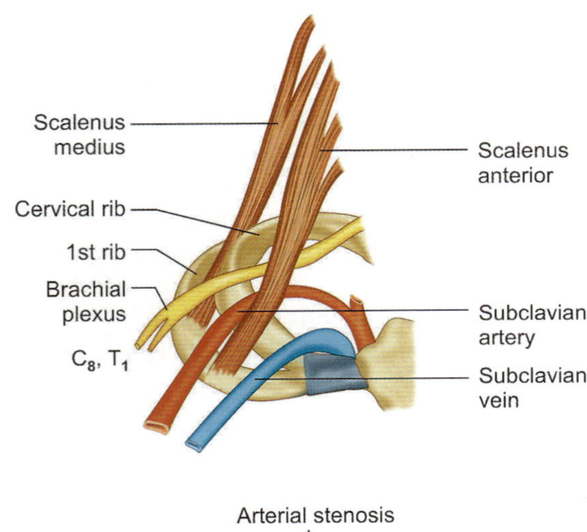

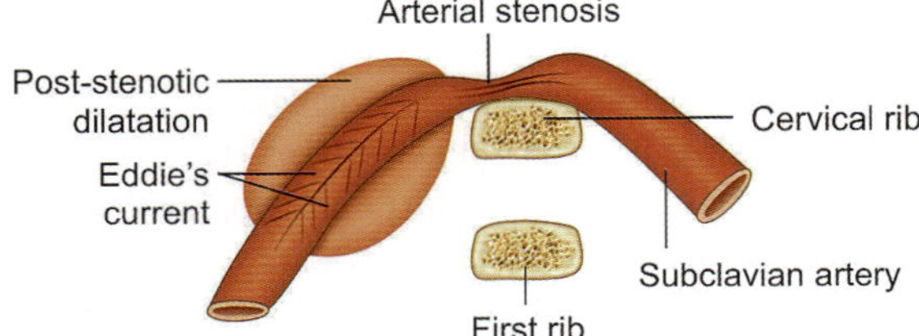

Fig. 14-23: Surgical anatomy of cervical rib.

Conservative Treatment

Initially it is managed conservatively with exercises like—neck stretching, breathing and postural exercises, analgesics, muscle relaxants, antidepressants. Conservative approach is used if nerve conduction velocity is more than 60 m/second.

Surgery

Surgical intervention is required when symptom persists and vascular features are severe with ischaemia of the fingers. Removal of cervical rib and middle portion of first rib with scalenotomy relieves the symptoms. If nerve conduction velocity is less than 60 m/second surgery is indicated.

Approaches

Transaxillary, supraclavicular; combined; supraclavicular and infraclavicular for arterial reconstruction; posterior high thoracoplasty approach for recurrent TOS.

Transaxillary Approach

Roos (1966) popularised this approach. It is mainly used to excise the first rib. Release of lower brachial plexus and vascular compression is done better through this approach. After giving general anaesthesia patient is positioned laterally with arm abducted. Transverse skin incision is made on the 3rd rib level. Axillary tunnel is developed by blunt dissection to reach the first rib and scalenus anterior **(Fig. 14-24)**.

Intercostobrachial nerve is cut. Subclavian vessels and brachial plexus are safeguarded. Vessels are separated by gentle dissection to expose the insertion of the scalenus anterior. Muscle is divided at its attachment. 1–2 cm length of the muscle should be excised to prevent development of fibrosis and recurrence of symptoms. Scalenus medius and intercostal muscles are pushed off the first rib. Subclavius muscle tendon can also be released. C_8 and T_1 nerve roots are identified before dividing posterior part of the first rib behind these nerves. Neurolysis of C_7, C_8 and T_1 is done with fine specialised instruments. Often resection of the costoclavicular ligament is needed.

Supraclavicular Approach

It is used for excision of cervical rib or upper brachial plexus decompression wherein extensive scalenotomy is needed or if there

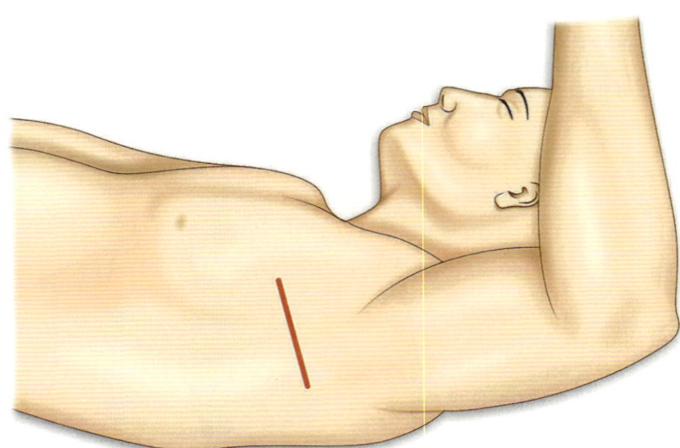

Fig. 14-24: Incision for cervical rib excision through transaxillary approach.

is a need of arterial (subclavian) reconstruction. It is done under general anaesthesia. Patient is positioned supine with head end of the table elevated by 15º to reduce venous congestion and head is tilted to opposite side; arms are placed on the sides of the patient. Incision is placed a fingerbreadth (1.5 cm) above the clavicle from anterior border of the sternocleidomastoid muscle extending laterally for 7–8 cm. It is usual but not mandatory practice to pull/drag the skin downwards below the clavicle and make incision on the clavicle from medial to lateral; and when pulled skin is released after making incision, incision will be in supraclavicular area. It is said to prevent inadvertent injury to deeper structures. Incision is deepened; platysma is incised **(Fig. 14-25)**.

External jugular vein is divided with ligatures. Supraclavicular nerves are retained. Exposed sternocleidomastoid muscle is identified for its full width. The clavicular head is divided using scissor/cautery/or by piecemeal using fine forceps (used in olden days). IJV behind the muscle should not be injured. Scalene pad of fat is dissected. Inferior belly of omohyoid muscle is divided. IJV is mobilised and retracted medially. Bipolar cautery dissection is done in front of the scalene muscle. Phrenic nerve is identified in front of the scalenus anterior muscle deep to deep fascia running vertically downwards from lateral to medial side. Phrenic nerve is retracted medially (should not be retracted laterally as it may cause traction injury to upper trunk of brachial plexus). Dissected scalenus anterior muscle is cut layer by layer carefully using scissor/by piecemeal method to protect subclavian artery underneath. Medial part of the brachial plexus is dissected carefully. Subclavian artery is dissected on its summit and pushed downwards. Scalenus medius is also excised. Cervical (accessory) rib is cleared of scalenus medius with its tendinous attachments to it and first rib. T_1 nerve root is identified carefully to avoid injury. Cervical rib is divided posteriorly in level with its transverse process. Central portion of the 1st rib is also excised. Wound is closed with a suction drain **(Fig. 14-26)**.

Posterior High Thoracoplasty

Vertical high paraspinal incision is made at the level of C_7 to T_4 between medial margin of the scapula and spinous process. Through muscle splitting approach, accessory (cervical) rib and first ribs are identified and resected. Neurolysis of C_7, C_8 and T_1 is done. If needed posterior dorsal sympathectomy is also added **(Fig. 14-27)**.

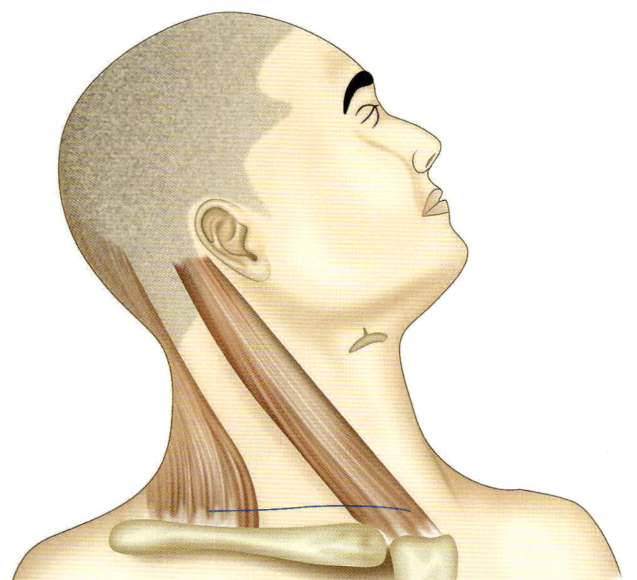

Fig. 14-25: Incision for cervical rib excision through supraclavicular approach.

Complications

- Haemorrhage—due to venous or arterial injury.
- Pain in the wound mainly in transaxillary approach.
- Pleural injury if occurs, ICT should be placed.
- Injury to nerve roots of brachial plexus.
- Fibrosis can cause recurrence of symptoms.

CAROTID BODY TUMOUR

It was first described by *Von Haller* in 1743. *Riegner* in 1880 described the first surgical removal of carotid body tumour. Carotid body is *3–5 mm* in diameter size, reddish brown or tan coloured body found in the adventitia of the common carotid artery at its posteromedial wall at bifurcation with a feeding vessel through *Meyer's ligament*. Its size may be larger in individuals in high altitude. It gets its afferent nerve supply from glossopharyngeal nerve. Cells: *Type I—chief cells* store and release catecholamines; *Type II—sustentacular cells*. Carotid body has got autonomic control over cardiovascular and respiratory systems. Hypoxia, hypercapnia, low pH stimulates chief cells to begin autonomic reflex. It gets stimulated also by raise in body temperature, cyanide and nicotine.

Carotid body tumour is usually 4–6 cm in size, behind the bifurcation of the CCA splaying it and extending along the ICA as it enlarges towards skull base. Its incidence is <0.5% of all neoplasms. It is common in females and in high altitudes. *Presentations* are—neck mass (75%) which shows *transmitted pulsation* and headache, neck pain, dizziness, tinnitus, hoarseness, dysphagia, syncope. It moves sideward but not longitudinally. Thrill and bruit (25%) may be present. Aneurysmal dilatation of the carotids is *not common*. 90% of them are benign; 10% are malignant type, spreads to regional nodes, lungs, liver, kidneys, pancreas, thyroid, heart. *Shamblin classification*: Type I—localised, resectable easily (25%); Type II—adherent, resectable with difficulty (45%); Type III—adherent and surrounds the carotids, difficult resection and needs bypass during procedure and carotid to ICA interposition vein graft. It is diagnosed by angiogram which shows widening of the carotid bifurcation with tumour blush—*Lyre sign*. CT/MR angiogram is useful. Fine needle aspiration cytology (FNAC)/biopsy are contraindicated **(Fig. 14-28)**.

Surgical Treatment

Excision is done under general anaesthesia. *Nasotracheal intubation* is ideal to facilitate better retraction beneath the mandible. Often common carotid artery (CCA) with bifurcation and carotid body tumour area is divided into 3 zones—lower, at the level of CCA bifurcation as zone I; upper front, towards ECA as zone II; upper behind towards ICA as zone III. Vagus, hypoglossal nerve, sympathetic chain will be very close during dissection and should be taken care of.

Whenever high exposure of the carotid is needed, ipsilateral mandible should be subluxated. Thigh and leg should be prepared for harvesting long saphenous vein if interposition vein graft is needed. Carotid shunts should be kept ready if temporary bypass is needed. ECA is usually ligated above the origin of the superior thyroid artery.

In small tumour less than 4 cm, incision is along the anterior margin of the sternocleidomastoid muscle; in large tumour 'T' incision is preferred to have adequate exposure **(Figs. 14-29 and 14-30)**.

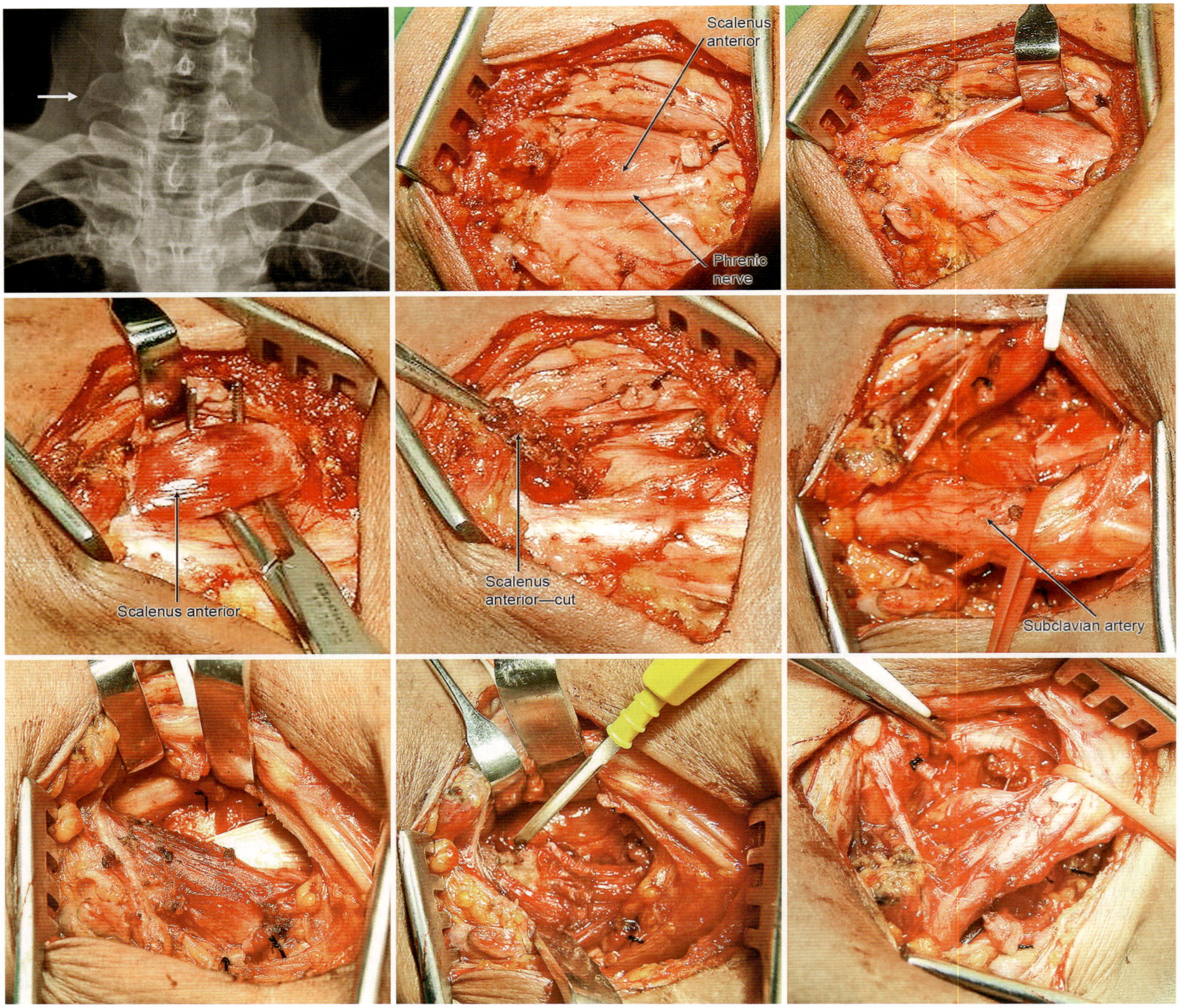

Fig. 14-26: Cervical rib excision through supraclavicular approach.

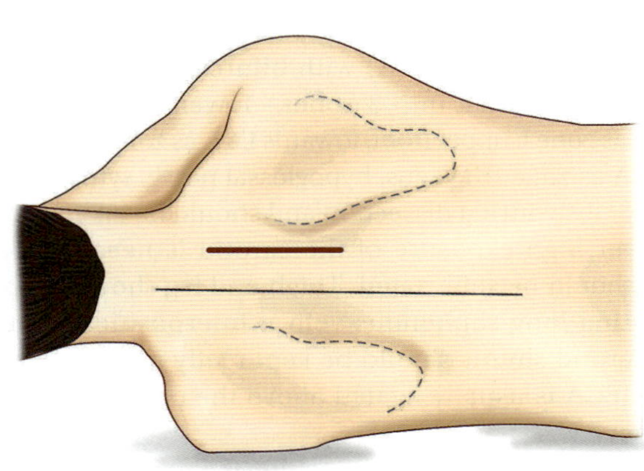

Fig. 14-27: Incision for cervical rib excision through posterior high thoracoplasty approach.

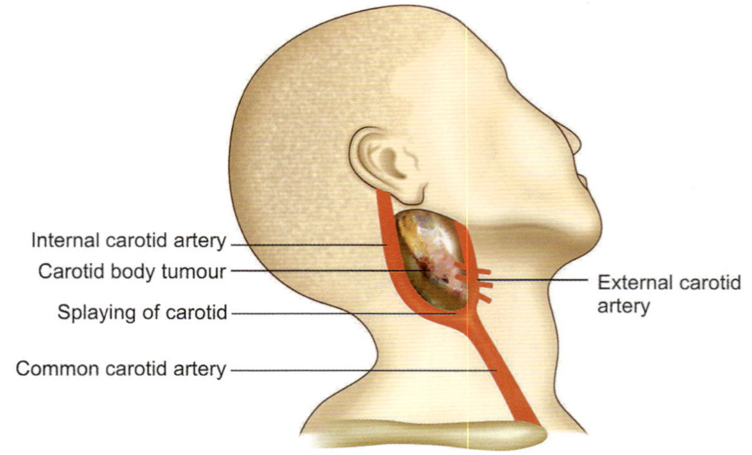

Fig. 14-28: Location of the carotid body tumour.

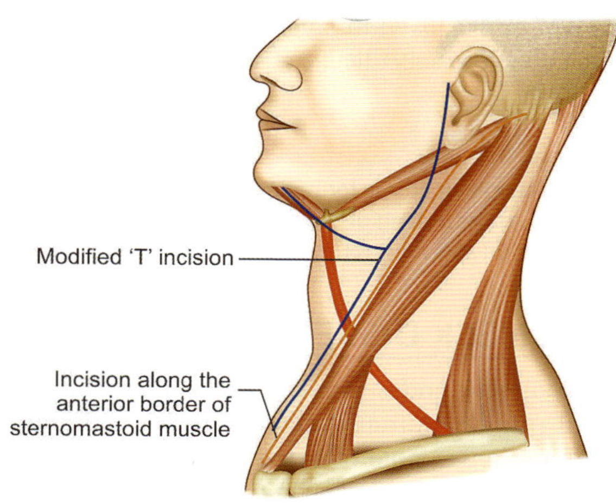

Fig. 14-29: Incision for excision of carotid body tumour.

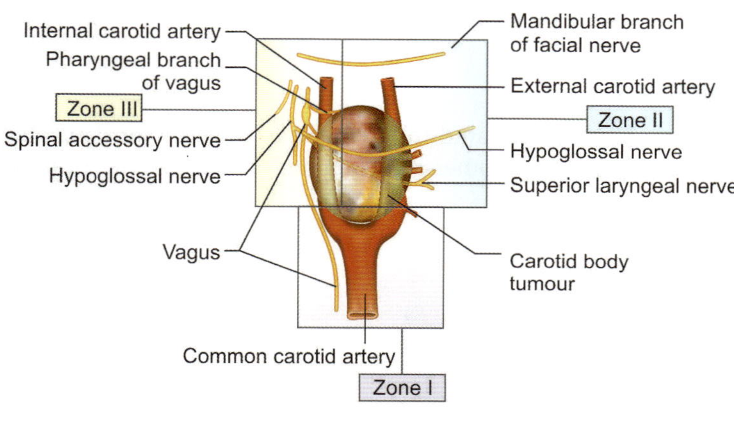

Fig. 14-30: Relations of carotid body tumour.

CCA, ECA, ICA with tumour is dissected and isolated carefully and meticulously with proper haemostasis. Bipolar cautery should be used. Loops/slings are passed around CCA proximally and ECA and ICA distally. Hypoglossal nerve is identified and separated and held using a fine sling gently. *Subadventitial plane* is created to dissect the tumour carefully from the carotid bifurcation from below upwards. All vessels entering the tumour should be individually secured and ligated. Vagus is identified at this stage which is dissected and isolated and held with a sling. ICA should be preserved with care. If injured, it should be repaired. In case of tumour encasement, temporary shunt from CCA below to ICA above is achieved to maintain the cerebral perfusion. Segment of the bifurcation with ICA and ECA with tumour is removed en mass. ECA is doubly ligated using silk above. Great saphenous vein is harvested from the thigh and is interposed as vein graft between CCA below and ICA above.

Complications

- Injury to vagus and hypoglossal nerves (40%).
- Vascular injuries.
- Stroke due to compromised cerebral perfusion (3%).

BIOPSY IN HEAD AND NECK DISEASES

Biopsy in head and neck diseases needs a comprehensive approach as many lesions are easily amenable but many are in deeper places and often not visible.

Lesions which are easily accessible are biopsied with open incision biopsy. Usually more than two biopsies from the edge are taken. Often biopsy site may require suturing using 3-zero vicryl to control bleeding. Cautery is avoided or used only when essential as much as possible (especially in suspected melanoma lesions) to prevent tissue getting desiccated. Suction should always be used during biopsy. Posterior lesions should be biopsied under general anaesthesia with endotracheal intubation.

Nasopharyngoscopy, laryngoscopy, oesophagoscopy are needed to take biopsy from these sites.

CT guided biopsy is done in base skull tumours or deep seated primaries.

Blind biopsy of different suspected areas in the fossa of Rosenmuller, pyriform fossa, lateral wall of pharynx is done in a clinically unknown primary but confirmed secondaries in neck by FNAC.

Maxillary tumour biopsy is done using Caldwell-Luc operation **(Fig. 14-31)**.

Secondaries in neck node are usually confirmed *not by* open biopsy but *by FNAC*. Fungating secondaries can be biopsied by open method.

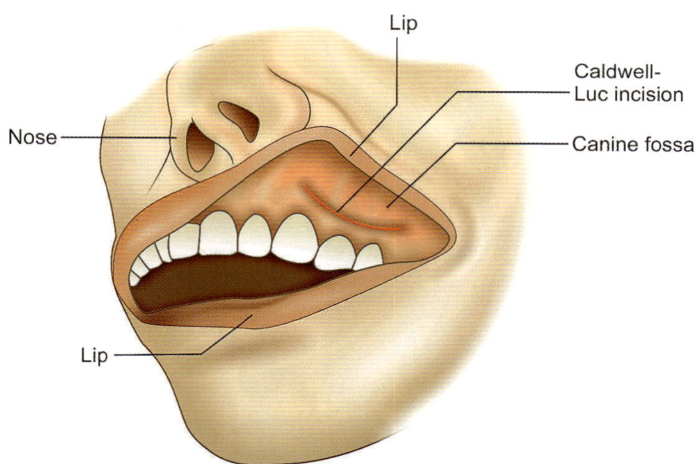

Fig. 14-31: Incision for Caldwell-Luc operation which is used for taking biopsy from maxillary tumour. Incision is not used for definitive therapy for carcinoma maxilla. Incision also used in benign conditions to approach maxillary sinus. Gingivobuccal mucosa is incised and mucoperiosteum is raised. Bone of canine fossa is cut to reach the maxillary antrum.

CERVICAL LYMPH NODE BIOPSY

Indications

Cervical lymph node biopsy is done mainly in patients with suspected lymphoma. Lymph node biopsy is done in patients where FNAC is inconclusive like in tuberculosis, rare lymph node diseases, and chronic inflammation. Staging, grading and histochemistry are needed in lymphoma and so biopsy is mandatory.

Lymph node secondaries are usually not an indication for open biopsy especially in squamous cell carcinoma. Diagnosis is usually done by FNAC. Open biopsy may aggravate the spread to further lymph nodes altering the prognosis and survival.

Malignant supraclavicular lymph nodes are considered as advanced with primary in breast/chest/abdomen. So excision biopsies of these lymph nodes are acceptable as it will not alter the prognosis.

Principles

All nodes in deep cervical and supraclavicular region should be biopsied under general anaesthesia. Biopsy of occipital and posterior triangle nodes can be done under local anaesthesia as these nodes are superficial and no vital structures are present in this region. However, accessory nerve is under risk in this location and should be taken care of while doing excision. Skin incision should be marked prior to injecting local anaesthesia, otherwise node may get masked making it difficult to identify it during surgery. Xylocaine 1% with adrenaline can be used **(Fig. 14-32)**.

Procedure

Position is supine with head turned towards opposite side. After cleaning and draping, an adequate transverse incision is made. Skin and platysma are incised. Sternomastoid is retracted. Deep fascia is incised. Lymph node is held gently using non-toothed forceps. Lymph node is dissected all around. Bipolar cautery may be used to control small bleeders. Earlier surgeons used to cut the node into half to take imprint cytology. Nowadays it is not done. Large adequate '*wedge excision*' of the lymph node is done if lymph node is large, if there are adhesions, if nodes are matted, if node is in close proximity to a vital structure. After removal haemostasis is maintained. Wound is closed in layers. Skin is closed using interrupted non-absorbable or subcuticular absorbable sutures **(Fig. 14-33)**.

Complications

Haemorrhage and haematoma formation can occur which often needs reexploration and controlling of the bleeder. Injury to adjacent nerves can occur. Infection and sinus formation are other complications.

RADICAL NECK DISSECTION (RND)

It is removal of all neck nodes with fat, fascia, internal jugular vein, sternomastoid muscle, spinal accessory nerve, submandibular salivary gland and lower pole of parotid gland with dissection in front of the prevertebral fascia leaving behind structures deep to prevertebral fascia (brachial plexus, cervical nerves, prevertebral muscles); pretracheal fascia; carotid artery; vagus nerve and strap muscles. It is an important oncological clearance surgery in the neck. For operable mobile metastatic neck nodes neck dissection is ideal method. Radiotherapy is not a prime approach whatever the type of primary **(Tables 14-1 and 14-2)**.

Principles

Primary should be treated independently by wide local surgical excision or curative radiotherapy depending on the site of the primary.

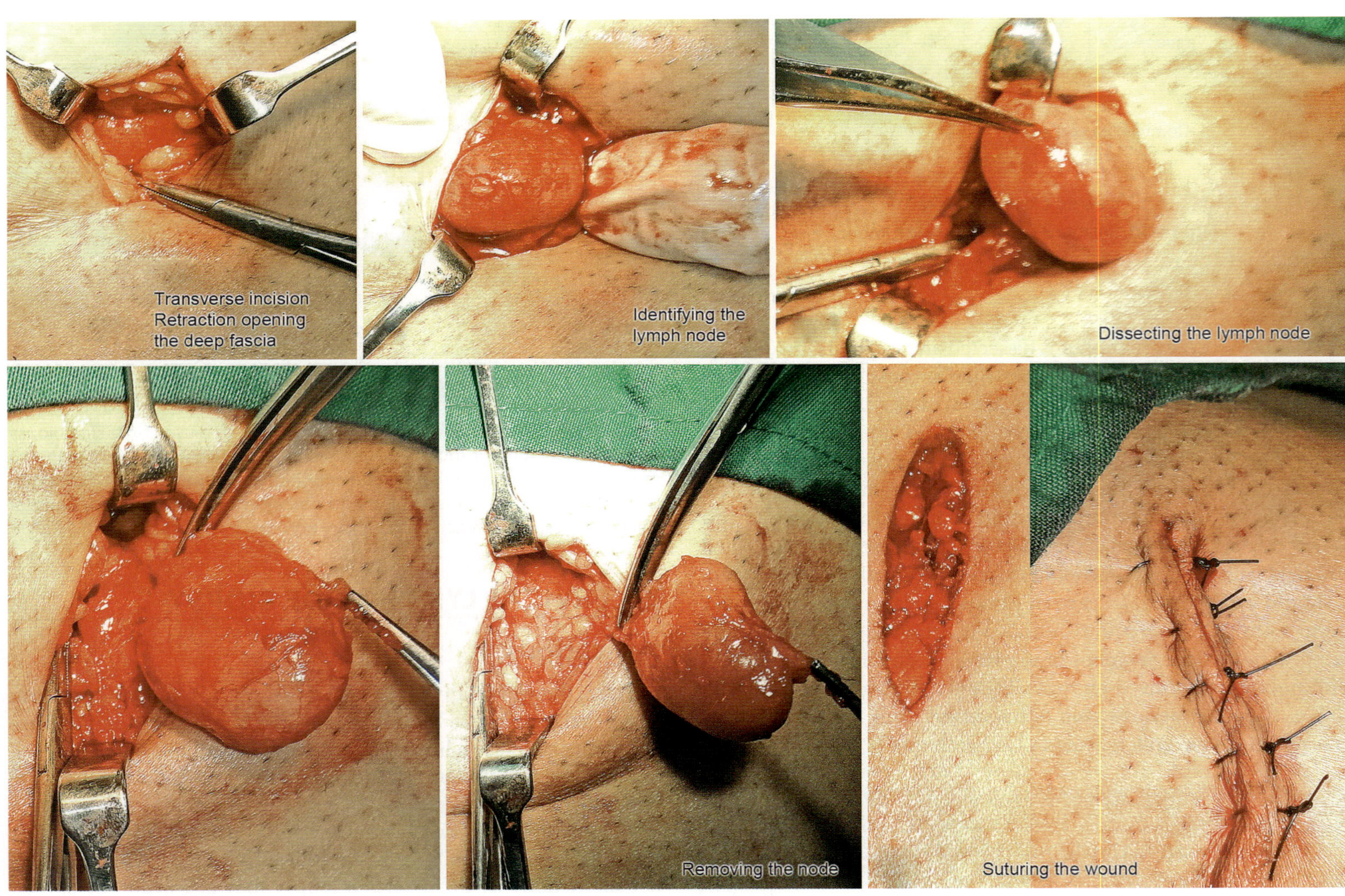

Fig. 14-32: Technique of lymph node biopsy.

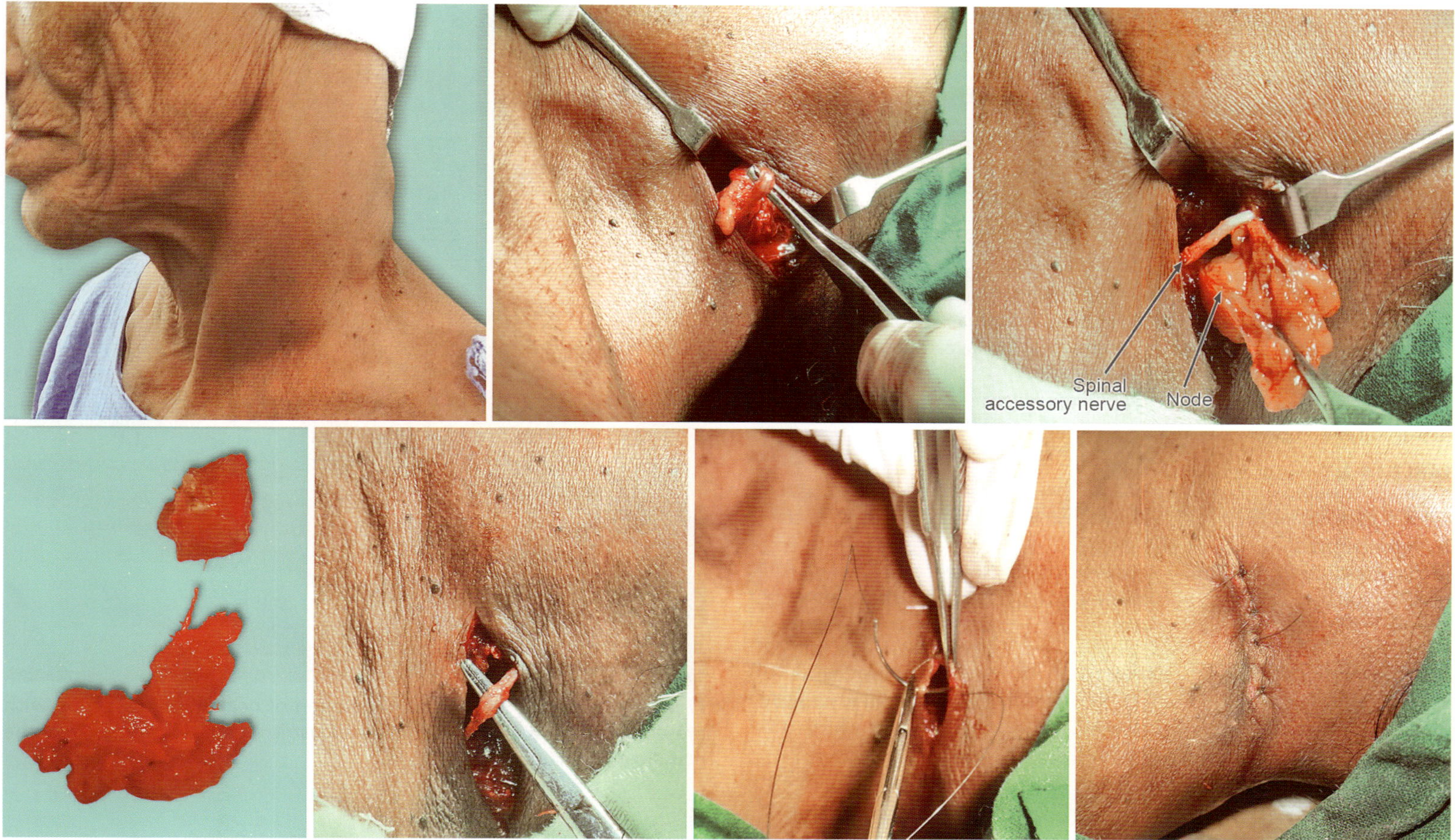

Fig. 14-33: Neck lymph node biopsy. Spinal accessory nerve should be kept intact during nodal biopsy. Biopsy is done under general anaesthesia.

RND or MRND is the choice for all confirmed positive nodes in all oral malignancies.

Supraomohyoid neck dissection (SOHND) is done for oral squamous cell carcinoma with clinically negative nodes. On table frozen section biopsy is needed. If nodes become positive, then MRND I is carried out immediately.

Extended supraomohyoid neck dissection is done when primary is in lateral border of the tongue which also includes level IV, as lateral margin of tongue cancer can cause skip metastasis in the level IV lymph node.

Anterolateral neck dissection is done for laryngeal and pharyngeal cancers (in clinically node negative disease) with level II, III, IV dissection; if primary is in midline, it is done bilaterally.

Posterolateral neck dissection is done for primary cutaneous malignancies of the scalp (posterior aspect) like melanoma or squamous cell carcinoma (SCC).

In thyroid malignancy, total thyroidectomy (MRND type III/ selective neck dissection) with bilateral and central node clearance is done.

Indications

Secondaries in the neck which are mobile (not fixed); common site of primary in head and neck malignancies, thyroid malignancy, malignancy of skin in head and neck region, malignant parotid tumours, etc. Secondaries in the neck with occult primary is initially treated with radical neck dissection; regular follow up is done later, until primary gets revealed; and once primary reveals it is managed accordingly depending on location. Here one cannot wait for primary to reveal as by then metastatic nodes become advanced and inoperable resulting in poor prognosis.

TABLE 14-1: Nodal staging in secondaries in neck.

Nodal stage in secondaries in neck nodes	*Involvement of nodes in different stages*
N_x	Assessment of regional nodes not possible
N_0	Regional nodes not involved by spread
N_1	Spread to ipsilateral single node <3 cm size
N_{2a}	Spread to ipsilateral single node 3–6 cm size
N_{2b}	Spread to ipsilateral multiple nodes, each <6 cm in size
N_{2c}	Spread to bilateral/opposite side nodes, each <6 cm in size
N_3	Spread to any node with size >6 cm

Contraindications for Radical Neck Dissection

Fixity of metastatic nodes, distant spread and advanced uncontrollable primary disease are the contraindications **(Fig. 14-34)**.

Levels in Neck Nodes

(Memorial Sloan-Kettering Cancer Center levelling of neck nodes) **(Figs. 14-35 to 14-37)**.

Structures removed in classical RND:
- All neck nodes
- Fat, fascia
- Internal jugular vein
- Sternomastoid muscle
- Spinal accessory nerve
- Submandibular salivary gland
- Lower pole of parotid gland.

Plane of dissection:
- Anteriorly deep to platysma
- Posteriorly with dissection from the prevertebral fascia leaving behind prevertebral fascia and structures deep to it (brachial plexus, cervical nerves, prevertebral muscles), pretracheal fascia, carotid artery, vagus nerve, and strap muscles.

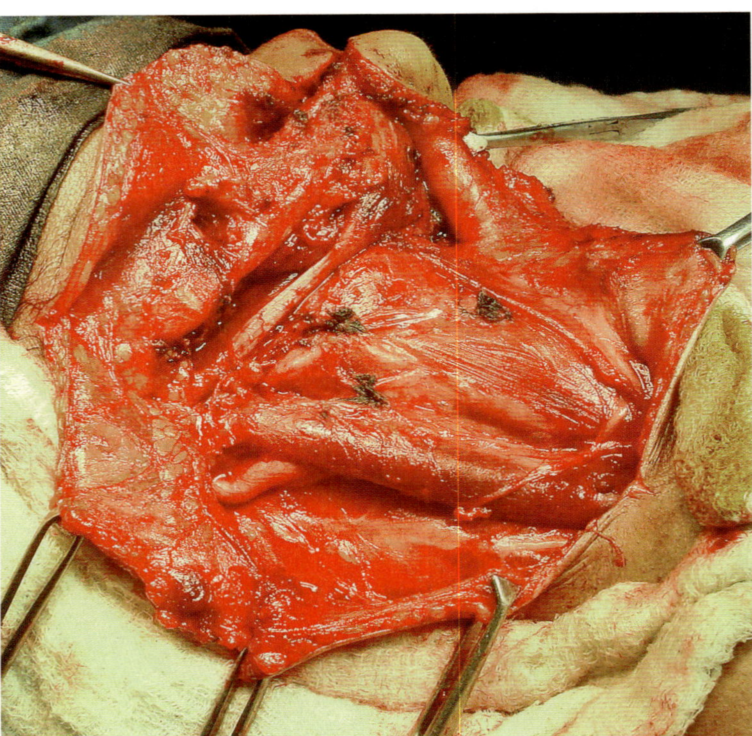

Fig. 14-34: Surgical field after completion of neck node dissection with preservation of the IJV. Carotid artery, digastric muscle, lower margin of the mandible is visualised.

TABLE 14-2: Types of neck dissection.

Type of neck dissection	*Nodes removed*	*Structures preserved*
Comprehensive:		
Radical neck dissection (RND)	Level I-V	None
MRND type I	Level I-V	Spinal accessory nerve
MRND type II	Level I-V	Spinal accessory nerve; sternomastoid muscle
MRND type III	Level I-V	Spinal accessory nerve; sternomastoid muscle; IJV
Bilateral RND	Level I-V (both sides)	
Selective node dissection:		
Supraomohyoid neck dissection (N_0)	Level I-III	Spinal accessory nerve; sternomastoid muscle; IJV
Extended supraomohyoid dissection (N_0)	Level I-IV	Spinal accessory nerve; sternomastoid muscle; IJV
Anterolateral neck dissection (N_0)	Level II-IV	Spinal accessory nerve; sternomastoid muscle; IJV
Posterolateral neck dissection (N_0)	Level II-V with suboccipital, retroauricular nodes	Spinal accessory nerve; sternomastoid muscle; IJV
Anterior/central dissection	Level VI	Spinal accessory nerve; sternomastoid muscle; IJV

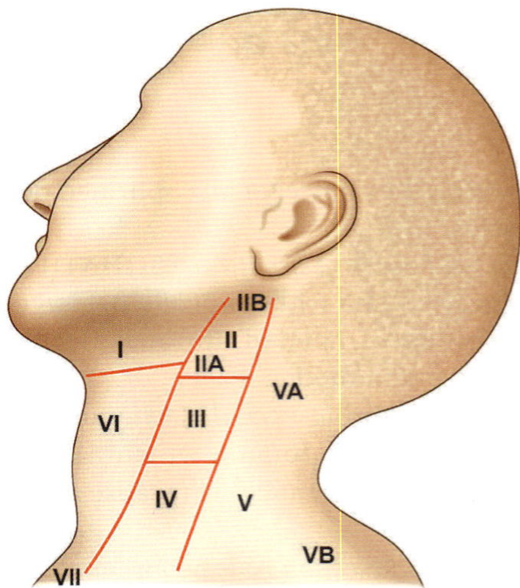

Fig. 14-35: Surgical (oncological) levels of neck lymph nodes.

Level I: Submandibular lymph nodes and submental lymph nodes—from lower border of mandible to hyoid bone and posterior belly of digastric muscle.

Level II: Lymph nodes in upper deep cervical region (It extends from base of skull to hyoid bone and from lateral margin of sternohyoid muscle to posterior margin of sternomastoid muscle).

Level III: Lymph nodes in middle cervical region (from hyoid bone to cricothyroid membrane).

Level IV: Lymph nodes in lower cervical region (from cricothyroid membrane to clavicle).

Level V: Lymph nodes in posterior triangle including supraclavicular region.

Level VI: Lymph nodes in the midline neck—pretracheal and prelaryngeal—from hyoid bone above to suprasternal notch below; laterally medial border of carotid sheath on both sides.

Level VII: Lymph nodes in the mediastinum; from suprasternal notch to inferior mammary artery.

Note: Level II and V are now subdivided into Level IIa/Level IIb and Level Va/Level Vb; depending whether these nodes are above the level (Level IIb/Level Va) of the spinal accessory nerve or below (Level IIa/Level Vb).

Preparation

General assessment for anaemia and nutritional status is done. Cardiac and respiratory assessment; improvement of intraoral hygiene by mouth wash using povidone iodine or hydrogen peroxide is done. When primary is in larynx/pharynx, tracheostomy may be needed. It is done usually on table just prior to surgery. Shaving of the chest, neck and face is done on the day of surgery.

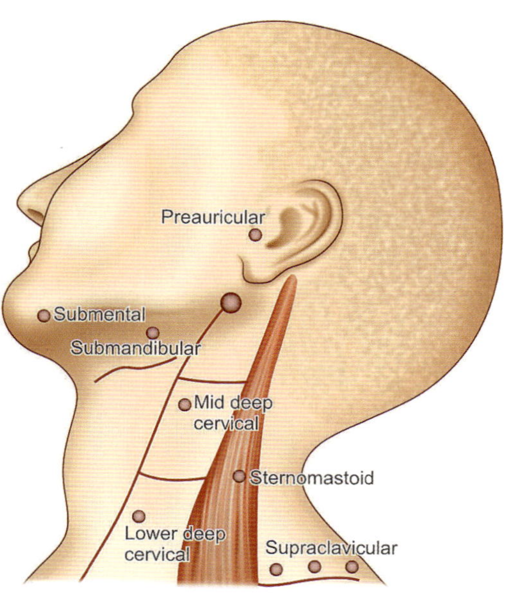

Fig. 14-36: Different lymph nodes in the neck.

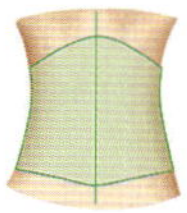	N_0 : Regional nodes involved
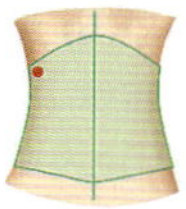	N_1 : Spread to single same side <3 cm sized node
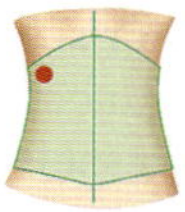	N_{2a} : Spread to single same side 3–6 cm sized node
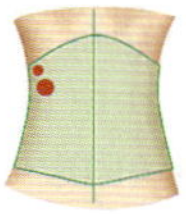	N_{2b} : Spread to multiple same side nodes each <6 cm in size
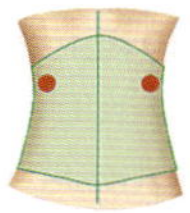 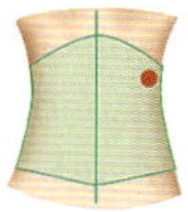	N_{2c} : Spread to bilateral/ opposite side nodes each <6 cm in size
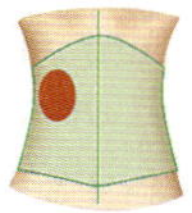	N_3 : Spread to any node with size >6 cm

Fig. 14-37: Staging of neck lymph nodes in secondaries.

If there is need for reconstruction of the wide area of excision of the primary area like cheek, it also should be planned and area should be prepared.

Anaesthesia

General anaesthesia is used with endotracheal intubation. Tracheostomy may be needed depending on the site of primary which is being operated. Some prefer hypotensive anaesthesia. But even though surgical field is clean, postoperative bleeding and haematoma due to eventual bleeding from small vessels, which was not cauterised at the time of surgery, is known to occur.

Position of the Patient

Patient is placed in supine position with hyperextended neck turned to opposite side with sandbags under the shoulder. Head end is elevated to 15° to reduce venous bleeding during surgery. Hands are tucked under the buttock. There should be adequate space near head end to allow assistants and scrub nurse to work on. Anaesthetist and Boyle's apparatus should be on opposite side of the dissecting area.

Incision

Many incisions are used. Modified triradiate incision is commonly used. Mac Fee incision is also used. Selection of incision is of individual surgeon's choice. Centre of the lateral aspect of the neck is the least vascular area for skin flap. One should avoid making incision in this part of the skin **(Figs. 14-38 and 14-39)**.

Technique

Flaps are elevated (*subplatysmal*). Posterior flap, anterior, upper and lower flaps are elevated in subplatysmal plane. Flaps are raised

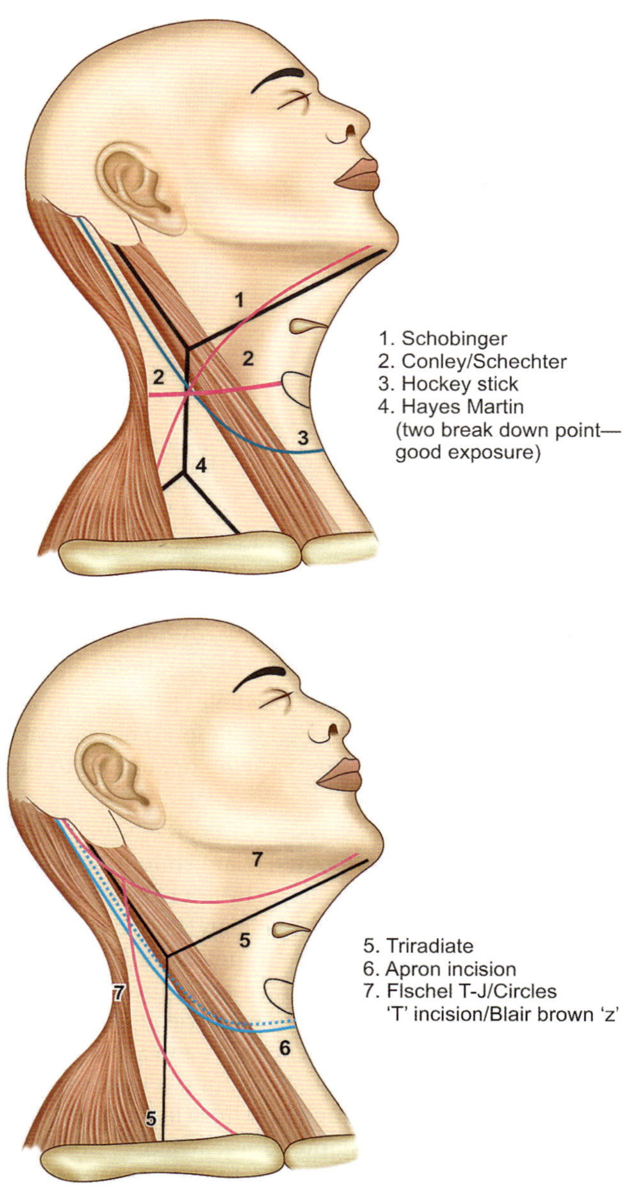

Fig. 14-38: Different incisions used in radical neck dissection.

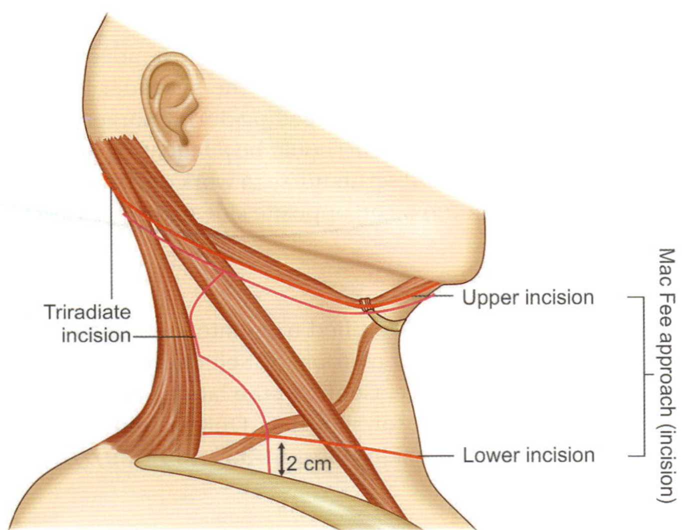

Fig. 14-39: Mac Fee and trifurcate incisions used for radical neck dissection.

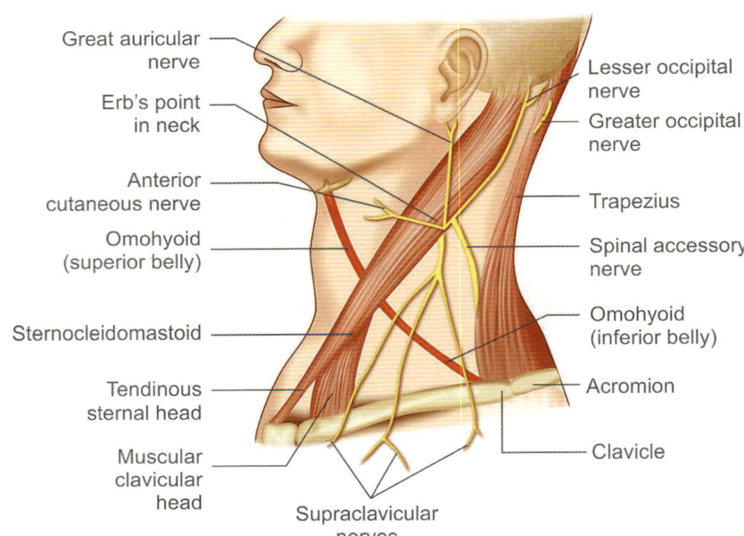

Fig. 14-41: Nerves in relation to posterior triangle which come across during neck dissection.

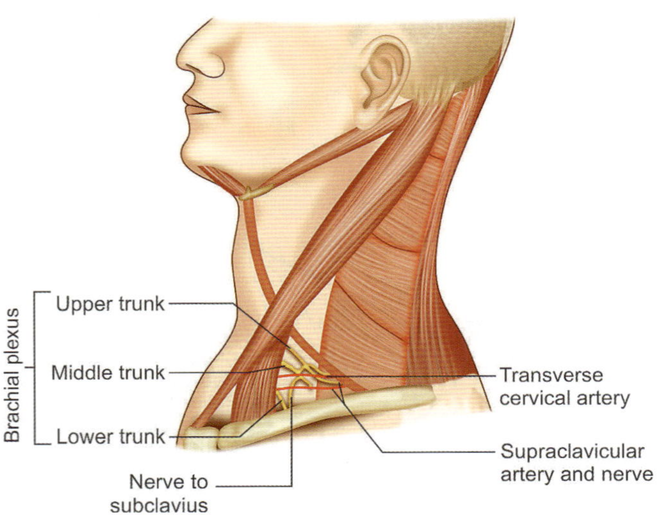

Fig. 14-40: Structures in supraclavicular triangle.

by holding skin hooks. Fine scissor/cautery are used. Trapezius is exposed fully on posterior aspect. While elevating superior flap care should be taken not to injure the marginal mandibular nerve which lies parallel to lower border of the mandible. This nerve crosses the anterior facial vein and vein is ligated. Inferior flap is elevated up to the clavicle. All elevated flaps are retracted or sutured to the drape margin temporarily **(Fig. 14-40)**.

Sternocleidomastoid muscle is cut at its attachments to clavicle (muscular) and sternum (tendinous). Care should be taken not to injure the IJV in the deeper plane. Layer by layer cutting of the muscle is usually practiced. External jugular vein and supraclavicular nerves are divided. Anterior border of the trapezius muscle is dissected to identify the spinal accessory nerve at its lower end. Nerve is traced by careful dissection above towards posterior border of the sternomastoid muscle which is 1 cm above the *Erb's point* or 5 cm below the inferior lobule of the ear. *Erb's point* is located 6 cm below the ear lobule where cutaneous branches (lesser occipital, great auricular, anterior cutaneous and supraclavicular little below) of cervical plexus comes out from posterior border of the sternomastoid muscle. Nerve is dissected upwards through the sternomastoid muscle by cutting the muscle fibres, along the lateral margin of the IJV, behind the posterior belly of the digastric muscle up to a point where it comes out of the skull to skull base through jugular foramen **(Fig. 14-41)**.

Upper attachment of the sternomastoid from mastoid process is detached. It is cut at a line extending from tip of mastoid to angle of jaw. Facial nerve may be existing at higher level in deeper plane. Fibrofatty tissue is dissected off splenius capitis from lateral to medial from splenius capitis, levator scapulae which is passed under the spinal accessory nerve; then dissected off the posterior scalene muscle. Inferior belly of omohyoid muscle is cut from its attachment to upper border of the scapula. Transverse cervical vessels are ligated and divided. Tissues are reflected off the middle and anterior scalene muscles to expose brachial plexus between these two muscles. Phrenic nerve is seen running lateral to medial from above downwards on the anterior surface of the scalenus anterior muscle. Cutaneous cervical nerves are cut adjacent to sternomastoid muscle.

Sternomastoid muscle is dissected off in upward direction to reach carotid sheath. Lateral border of strap muscles are retracted medially to expose carotid sheath from medial side. Carotid sheath is opened to expose CCA, IJV and vagus nerve. IJV is clamped and divided. Ends are doubly ligated and transfixed using 2-zero silk or vicryl. Lymphatics lateral to IJV are ligated using silk and divided. Transverse cervical vessels at its proximal part are also ligated. On left side thoracic duct if encountered is ligated safely to prevent chyle leak.

Fat, fascia, lymphatics with nodes, sternomastoid muscle, ligated IJV are dissected upwards from the carotid and vagus. Middle thyroid vein is identified, ligated and divided. Superior belly of omohyoid is identified, detached from hyoid bone. Superior thyroid vessels are dissected; only superior thyroid vein is ligated retaining the artery **(Fig. 14-42)**.

Upper flap is further elevated deeper to submandibular fascia (fascia in front of submandibular salivary gland) and posterior facial vein. Vein is ligated and retracted along with flap above. Flap is elevated along the lower border of the mandible. Fascia along the margin and angle is cleared. Facial lymph nodes are dissected. Facial artery and facial vein are ligated (at posterosuperior part of submandibular salivary gland). Anterior bellies of same and

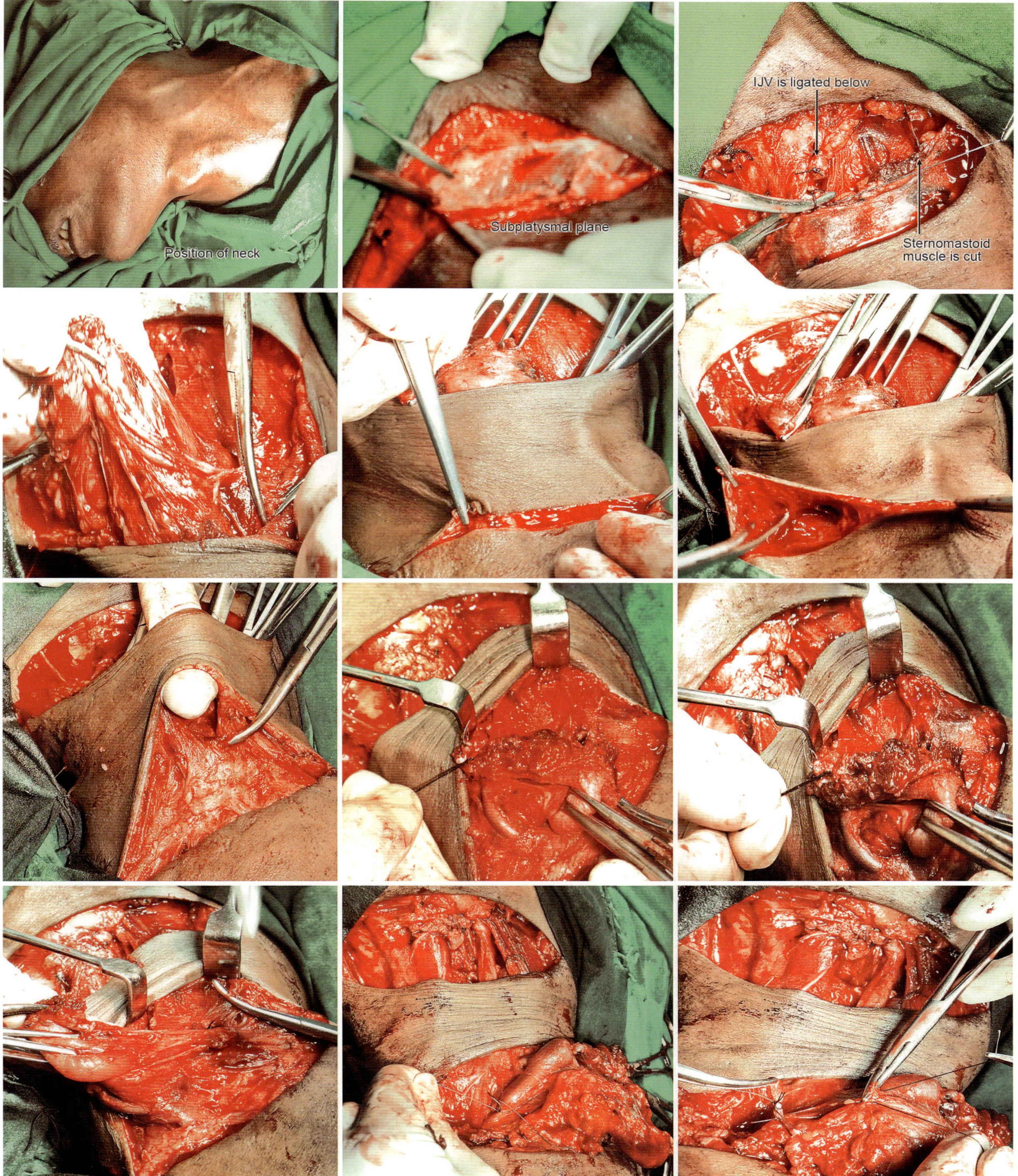
Position of neck
Subplatysmal plane
IJV is ligated below
Sternomastoid
muscle is cut

Figs. 14-42(1)

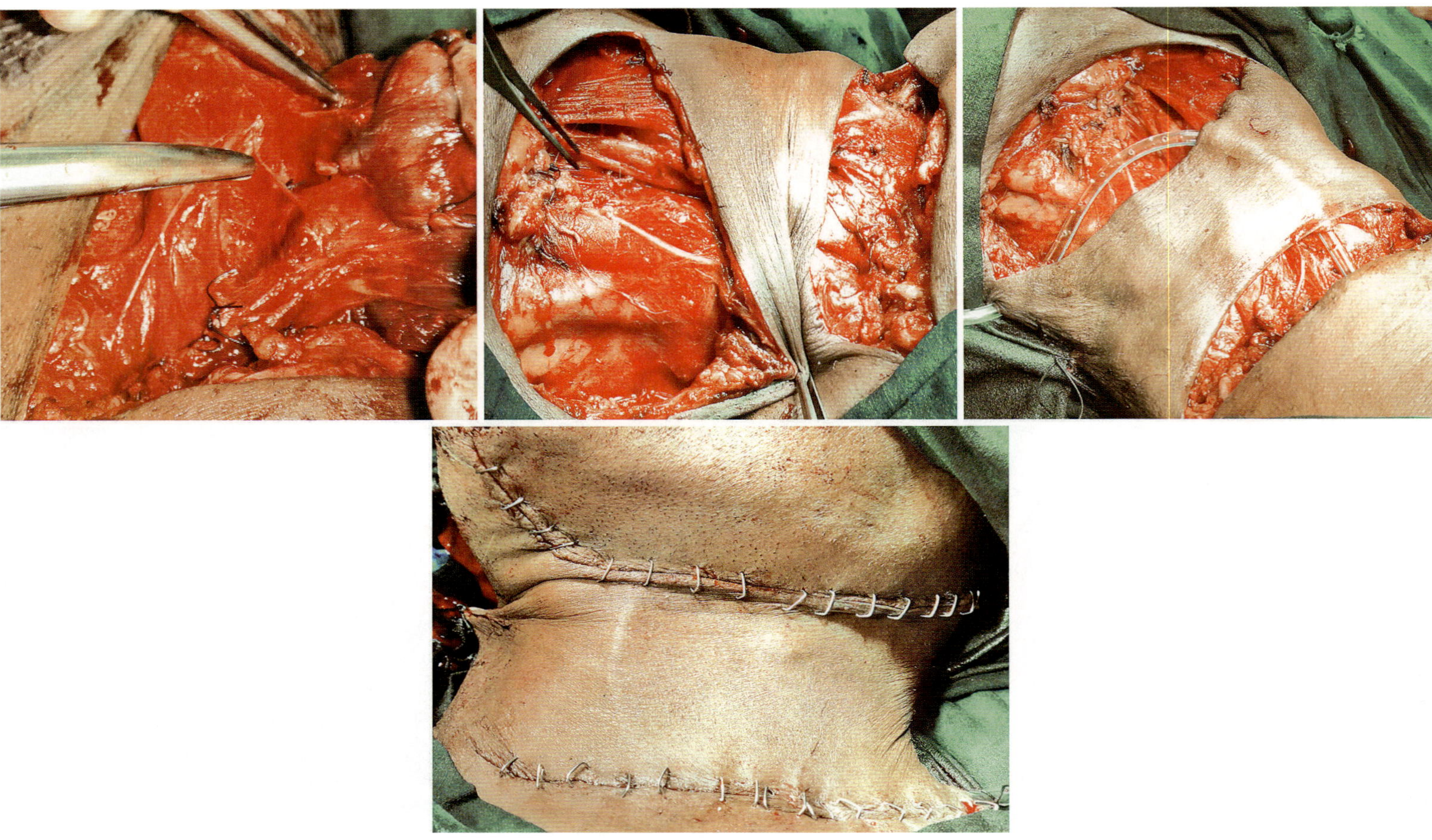

Figs. 14-42(2)

Figs. 14-42(1 and 2): Steps in radical neck node dissection using Mac Fee incision approach.

opposite side digastric muscles are identified and exposed. Nodes in submental triangle are removed. Nodes with tissues are dissected off the submental triangle towards the side to reach and identify mylohyoid neurovascular bundle which is ligated and divided. Gentle traction to submandibular salivary gland is applied using Allis tissue forceps to expose the lingual nerve, secretomotor fibres to submandibular ganglion, submandibular salivary duct. Secretomotor fibres are cut. Duct is cut and often ligated. Fascia over the hyoglossus muscle is kept intact to safeguard the hypoglossal nerve. Submandibular gland is further retracted laterally from posterior belly of the digastric muscle. Proximal part of the facial artery is identified at posteromedial part of the posterior belly of digastric muscle at deeper plane which is doubly ligated using silk and divided. Further retraction of the dissected tissue behind allows ligation of small pharyngeal veins and complete retraction of the posterior belly of digastric muscle. Occipital vessels (artery and vein) are ligated to visualise the upper end of the IJV. Transverse process of atlas can be felt at this level. IJV is dissected around and double ligation is done using 2-zero silk and divided. If upper attachment of sternomastoid muscle is not divided earlier, it is detached now to complete the surgery. Specimen is removed. After proper haemostasis and saline irrigation of the area, suction drains are placed; one in front of trapezius and another along the strap muscle in front of carotid artery. Wound is closed using interrupted 3-zero polypropylene sutures.

Drains are kept for 4–7 days. Sutures are removed in 7–10 days **(Fig. 14-43)**.

Complications

Haemorrhage can occur due to small bleeders, carotid blow out in 7–14 days. Shock, haematoma formation, dyspnoea and compression are the features. Arranging adequate blood and immediate exploration is essential to save the life of the patient. Bleeders are ligated, carotid blow out is treated by ligating carotid artery. Since it is due to infective necrosis of carotid wall, graft reconstruction of the carotid is difficult.

Flap necrosis can occur; if a wide area of flap necrosis develops then some flap reconstruction is done using PMMC flap/deltopectoral cutaneous flap **(Fig. 14-44)**.

Infection, lymph ooze, carotid blow out, seroma formation, frozen shoulder are other complications. Drooping of shoulder can occur due to trapezius muscle paralysis. Pneumothorax and chylous fistula are rare complications.

Note:

To control haemorrhage in head and neck cancers and during head and neck surgeries (like radical parotidectomy, commandos and operation, maxillectomy) ligation of external carotid artery is often required. ***Ligation should be done distal to the origin of the superior thyroid artery***. It should never be ligated below the origin of the superior thyroid artery as this will lead to *eddy current* and thrombus formation at the carotid bifurcation resulting in intracranial embolism through ICA. Ligation of ECA to control bleeding is usually done in continuity **(Fig. 14-45)**.

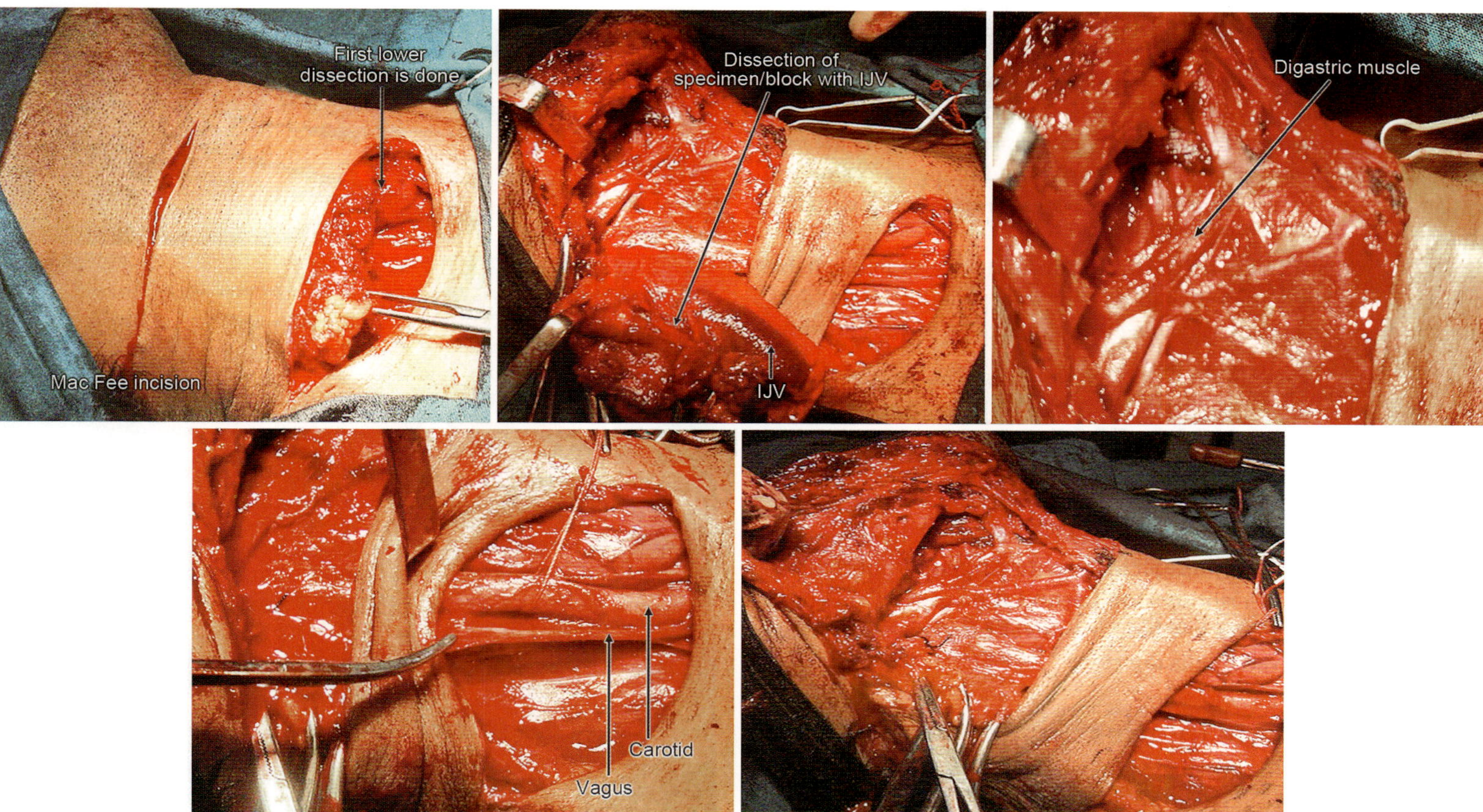

Fig. 14-43: Structures observed in neck node dissection.

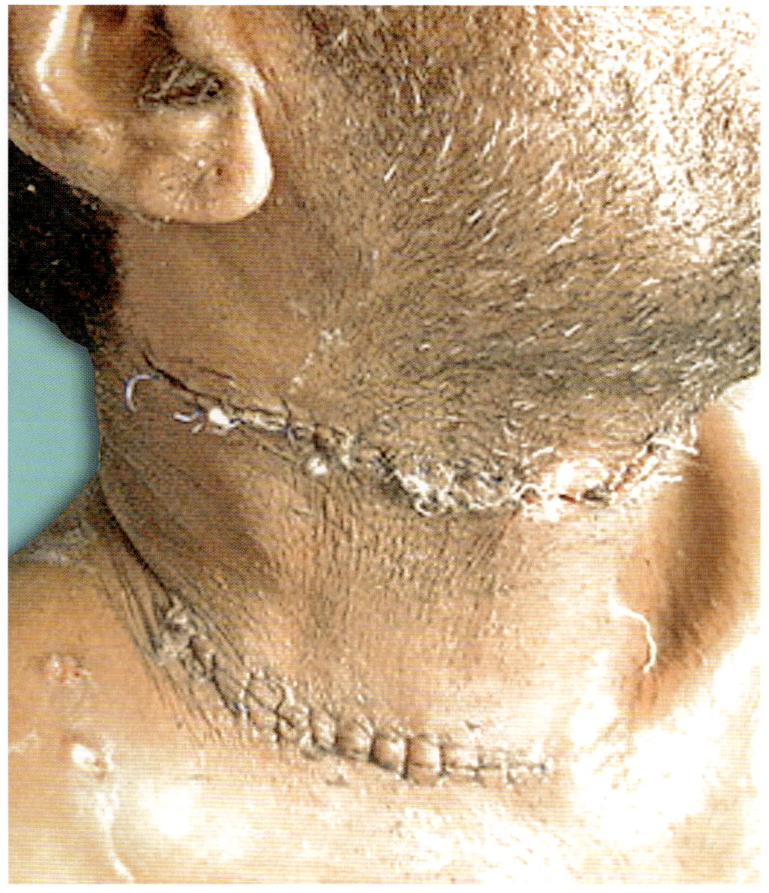

Fig. 14-44: Postoperative look after radical neck dissection.

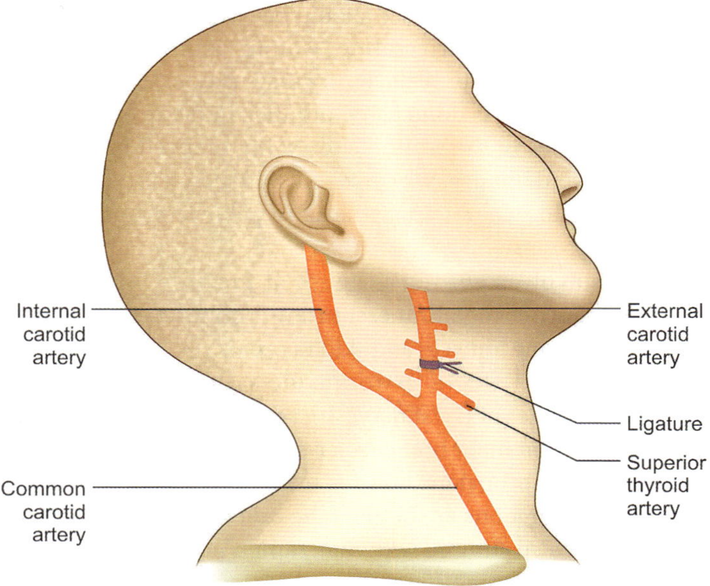

Fig. 14-45: Ligation of external carotid artery should be done when needed distal to the origin of the superior thyroid artery.

Carotid Blow Out

Carotid blow out is most dangerous complication. It is due to sepsis, wound breakdown, arterial adventitious stripping and necrosis and drying of the artery. Ligation of the carotid is done to save the life of the patient but procedure itself has got 20% mortality and 50% morbidity (hemiplegia).

Bilateral Neck Dissection

It is done in carcinoma tongue or pharynx where lesion is in midline. In such case of bilateral neck dissection, internal jugular vein has to be preserved on one side. *Always the side where the vein is preserved is operated first.* Ligation of both the jugular veins will cause cerebral congestion leading to cerebral oedema which is dangerous.

During surgery if both IJV are ligated due to injury as an inevitable consequence, the patient has to be kept in propped position; antibiotics, diuretics and steroids are given; repeated CSF taps are done to control the cerebral oedema.

SURGERY OF HEAD, FACE AND JAW

This is a wide surgical topic which is basically practiced by ENT surgeons/faciomaxillary surgeons/plastic surgeons/ophthalmologists. Extensive descriptions are beyond the scope of this book however basic principles needed for general surgeons or a surgery postgraduate are given in this topic.

Principles in Face Injuries

Initial complete assessment is done like in any polytrauma. Resuscitation should be done accordingly.

Facial wounds retract widely giving false impression of wide area defect. It is due to elastic nature of facial skin and retraction by facial muscles.

All wounds by trauma in face should be cleaned thoroughly using adequate amount of warm saline; wound debridement is done; tissues are apposed layer by layer to create proper acceptable scar. Wound debridement is done using number 15 blade or fine scissor. All foreign bodies in the wound should be removed meticulously. One should avoid unnecessary excision of tissues. It is better to clean and scrub under general anaesthesia to achieve proper thorough cleaning.

If injury involves entire thickness of the face involving skin, muscle and mucous membrane, suturing is done layer by layer from mucous membrane, muscle and skin in order.

Injury to facial nerve, parotid ducts should be identified. If terminal branches of facial nerve are severed, it is not necessary to approximate it. But main branches or trunk should be sutured using fine (6-zero) polypropylene sutures using microscope. Specialised reconstructive surgeons are better to be called to handle such cases. Parotid duct is also sutured with interrupted polypropylene sutures (6-zero) using microscope.

Skin is sutured with interrupted sutures using 5-zero polypropylene sutures. It is placed close to skin edge with deeper fat plane to prevent dead space. Sutures are placed every 5–8 mm gap. Knots should only be adequate to approximate the skin. One should not strangulate the skin.

In the lip, vermillion border should be sutured first to get accurate apposition.

Sutures are removed in 5 days in face. Later wound support may be given using steri strip **(Fig. 14-46)**.

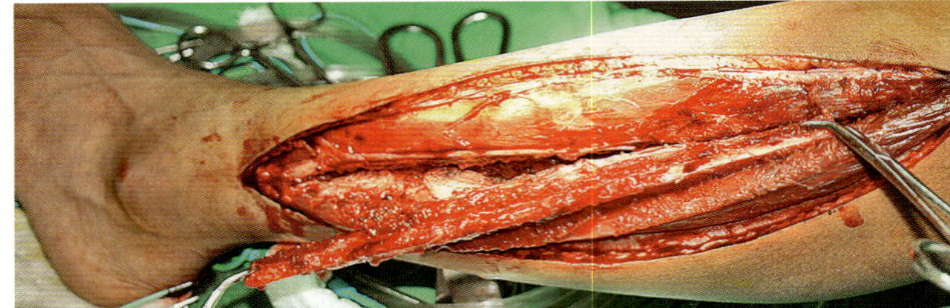

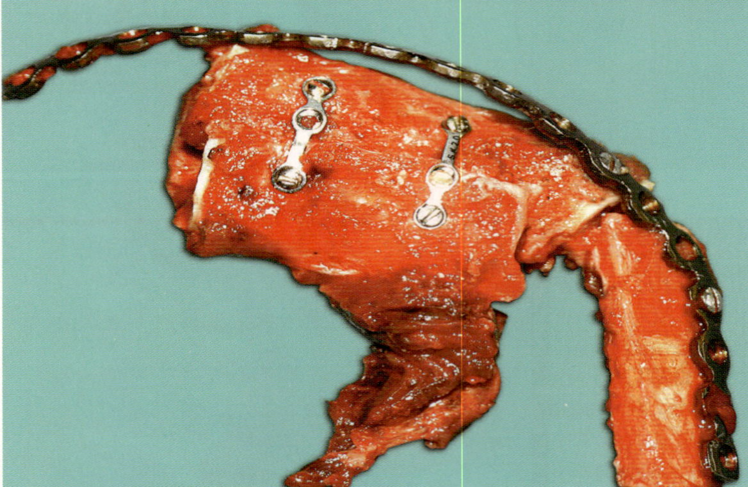

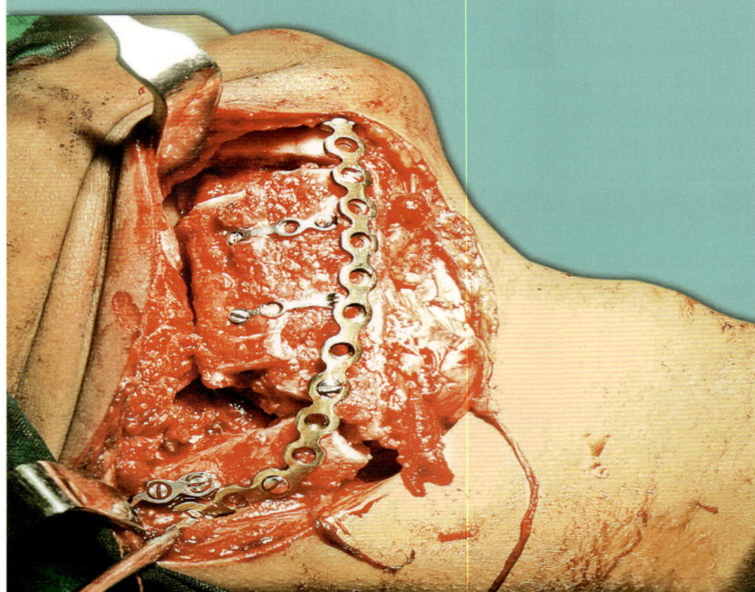

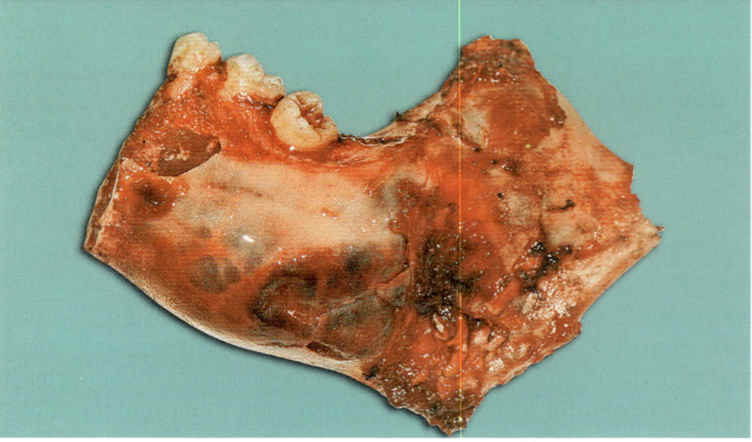

Fig. 14-46: Reconstruction of the mandible after segmental resection of the mandible for ameloblastoma using fibular microvascular flap.

SURGERY OF THE EYELIDS/ORBIT/EYEBALL

Eyelid is sutured accurately using fine interrupted sutures. Grey line of tarsal conjunctiva should be approximated accurately. If it is not accurate 'a step deformity' will develop in the eyelid margin. Tarsal plate should be approximated using fine 5-zero vicryl or PDS sutures (absorbable). If lacrimal canaliculus is injured, a lacrimal probe is passed to assess the injury; then a fine silicone tube is passed across punctum in the lid. Suturing is done over it using magnifying lens. Silicone tube is kept in place for 6 months.

Eyebrows *should never be shaved* in trauma or in any surgeries. If shaved original eyebrow will not come back.

Tarsorrhaphy is a common procedure done as temporary basis. It is done in facial nerve palsy as there is improper closure of eyelids during blinking, trauma, hyperthyroidism with proptosis, burn injury. Lateral 1/3rd of upper and lower eyelid margins are incised between eyelashes and Meibomian glands. Created raw margins are sewed together.

Ectropion is everting of the eyelid due to scarring. It may be due to excision of an infraorbital swelling which causes scarring and ectropion. Scar tissue is released and full thickness (Wolfe) graft is placed.

Entropion is inverting of the eyelid due to conjunctival scarring (trauma, trachoma). Eyelashes get inverted and irritate the cornea. Scarred conjunctiva is excised and full thickness mucosal graft taken from oral cavity is placed on the defect. Deformed tarsal plate should be divided and everted. Radical excision of inverted eyelashes can also be done as a simple procedure. Temporary relief can be achieved by placing everting sutures through skin, tarsal plate and conjunctiva.

Eyelid tumour is excised as a full thickness. If length of excised area is less than 1/4th of the length of the eyelid, then primary suturing of the eyelid can be done. If excised defect is more than 1/4th then proper reconstruction of the defect is needed.

Excision of the external angular dermoid is done under general anaesthesia. Prior X-ray of skull or CT head in suspected intracranial extension is a must. Incision is just below and parallel to the eyebrow. Eyebrow should not be shaved. Incision within the eyebrow should not be done as scarring of hair follicle will cause eyebrow deformity with poor cosmetic outcome. Cautery usage is better during surgery. Two layer closure of the wound is done **(Fig. 14-47)**.

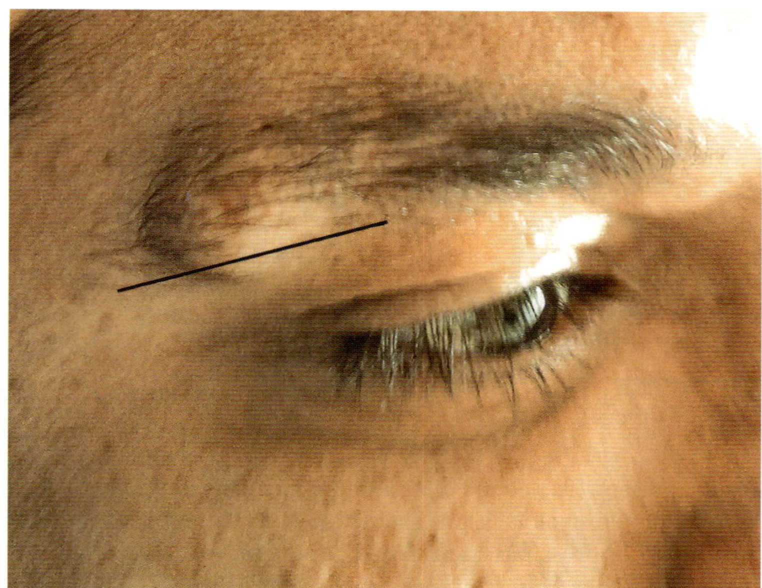

Fig. 14-47: Incision to excise external angular dermoid. Eyebrows should not be shaved.

Periorbital lesion/swelling in the lower eyelid are excised circularly and a full thickness Wolfe graft is placed. Primary closure of the defect can cause ectropion of the lower eyelid with exposure of the lower punctum of the eyelid exteriorly; with its inability to come in contact with eyeball can cause continuous watering of the eye **(Fig. 14-48)**.

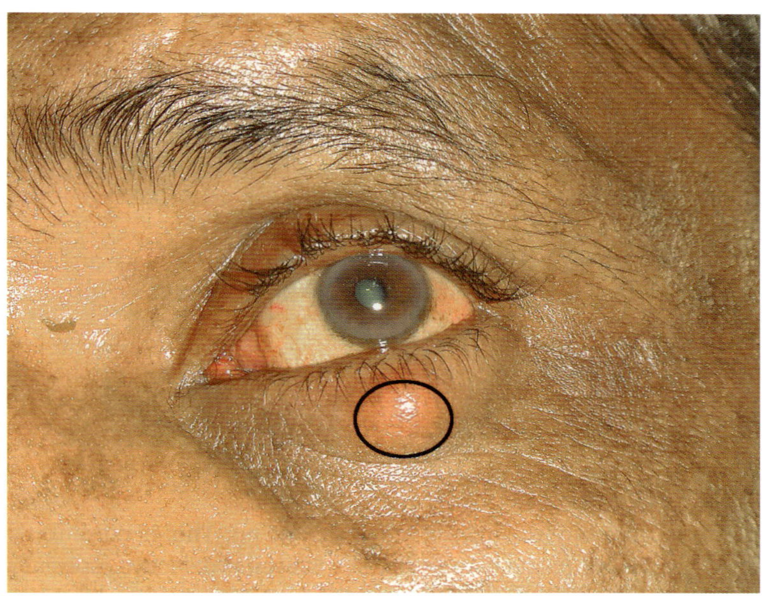

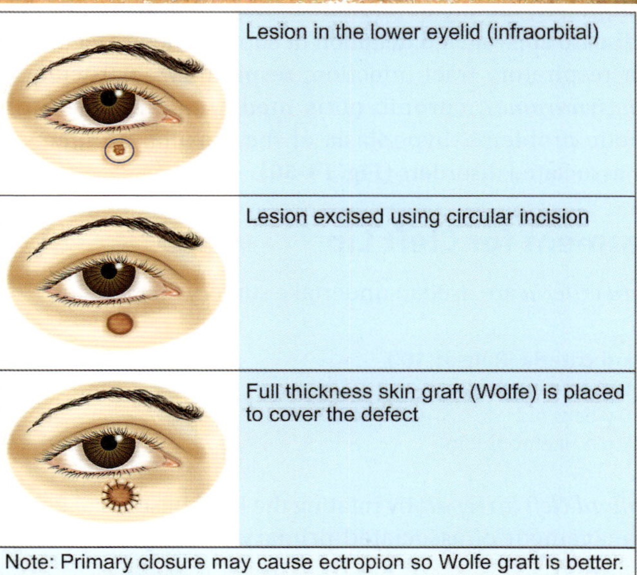

Fig. 14-48: Full thickness Wolfe graft is needed after excision of the periorbital lesion to prevent ectropion.

Evisceration of eye is done to prevent sympathetic ophthalmia (on opposite normal eye). Here cornea is incised and all contents are curetted. All uveal tissues should be removed completely otherwise sympathetic ophthalmia can occur. Evisceration is better to have cosmetic result.

Enucleation is done by removing the entire eyeball. Conjunctiva is incised at the corneal junction. Plane is created around the eyeball. All intrinsic muscles are detached from orbit by hooking forward. At the end optic nerve is cut. Conjunctiva is sutured.

SURGERY OF THE EAR

It is basically done by an ENT surgeon.

Haematoma of the ear is aspirated under aseptic precaution using a syringe and large bore needle. Clot gets slowly organised.

Swelling in the earlobe is excised along with cartilage adjacent

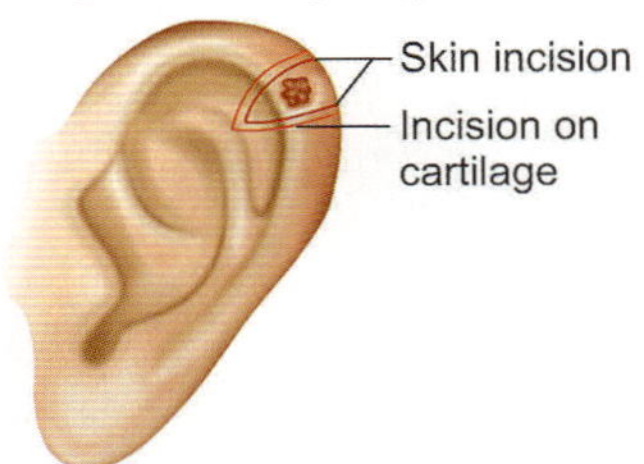

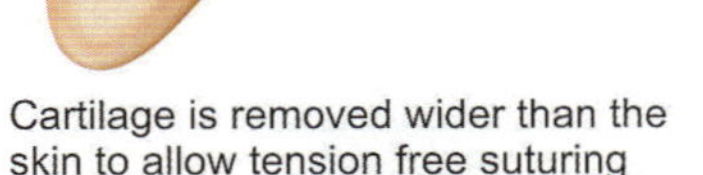

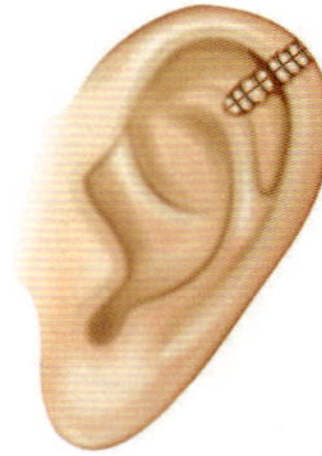

Skin on either side is sutured separately without suturing the cartilage

Fig. 14-49: Excision of benign lesion in the earlobe.

Due to pressure ischaemia of underlying cartilage and necrosis can occur. Multiple small incisions should be made. Repeated aspirations and pressure dressings are needed. Two sterile shirt buttons are placed on either sides of the ear and sutured to achieve adequate compression. *Perichondritis and cartilage necrosis* are dreaded complications. *Cauliflower ear* may develop if not treated properly.

Injury to ear is sutured on both surfaces separately using fine polypropylene sutures (interrupted). Cartilage is not usually sutured. Proper antibiotics (anaerobic infection of cartilage is common) should be given to the patient.

Swellings/tumours in the ear is excised with V shaped incision. Underlying cartilage is excised more widely than skin to facilitate the tension free suturing of the skin on either side. Cartilage is not sutured **(Fig. 14-49)**.

Accessory auricle is excised with its deeper core cartilage and skin is sutured. It is done for cosmetic purpose. *Keloid in the ear* should not be excised.

Earlobe repair is discussed in Chapter 7 (Please refer).

CLEFT LIP AND CLEFT PALATE

Problems in Cleft Lip and Cleft Palate

There is difficulty in sucking and swallowing. This is commonly observed in cleft palate than in cleft lip. Speech is defective especially in cleft palate, mainly to phonate B, D, K, P, T and G. Problems in cleft disease are—altered dentition or supernumerary teeth, recurrent upper respiratory tract infection, respiratory obstruction (*Pierre Robin syndrome*), chronic otitis media, middle ear problems, cosmetic problems, hypoplasia of the maxilla, problems due to other associated disorders **(Fig. 14-50)**.

Treatment for Cleft Lip

Millard criteria are used to undertake surgery for cleft lip.

Millard criteria (Rule of '10')

- 10 pound in weight
- 10 weeks old
- 10 g% haemoglobin

a. *Millard cleft lip repair* by rotating the local nasolabial flaps.
b. Management of associated primary or secondary cleft palate deformity.
c. Proper postoperative management like control of infection, training for sucking, swallowing and speech.

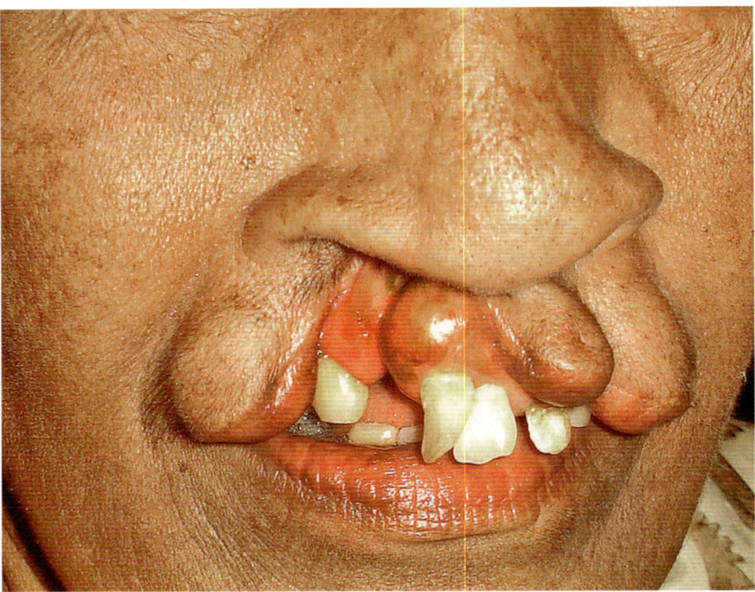

Fig. 14-50: Cleft lip and palate.

d. Tenninson's 'Z' plasty (Tenninson-Randall triangular flap) **(Fig. 14-51)**.

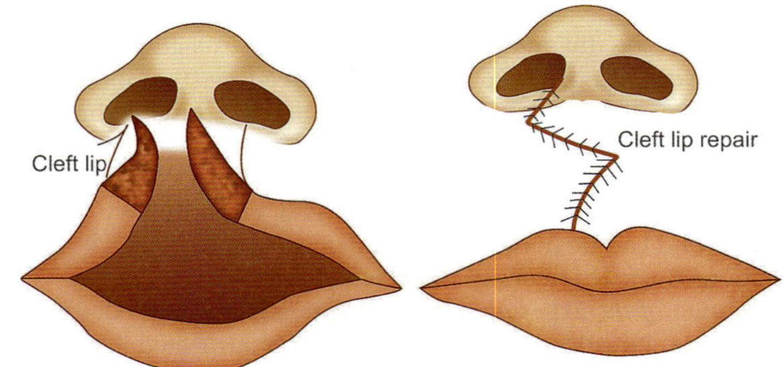

Fig. 14-51: Steps of cleft lip repair.

Principles of cleft lip repair

- 'Rule of 10' should be fulfilled
- It should be operated before 6 months
- Infection should not be present
- Millard advancement flap is commonly used for unilateral cleft lip repair
- Bilateral cleft lip repair can be done either in single or two stages (with 6 months gap between each stage)
- One stage bilateral cleft lip repair is done using Veau III method/Millard's single stage/Black method
- Proper markings are made prior to surgery and incision should be over full thickness lip
- Often 1:2,00,000 adrenaline injection is used to achieve haemostasis
- Three layer lip repair should be done (mucosa, muscle and skin)
- Cupid's bow should be horizontal
- Continuity of white line should be maintained
- Vermilion notching should not be there

Note:

Delaire timing of the cleft surgery: Unilateral/bilateral cleft lip alone, in one stage operation done in 4–6 months. Cleft palate alone involving only soft palate, is one stage surgery done in 6 months. Cleft palate alone but involving both soft and hard palates—

soft palate in 6 months; hard palate in 18 months. In combined cleft lip and palate, unilateral or bilateral, done in two stages—cleft lip and soft palate in 6 months; hard palate in 18 months.

Treatment for Cleft Palate

Criteria for surgery

- 10 kg weight
- 10 months of age (10–18 months)
- 10 g% haemoglobin

Cleft palate is usually repaired in 12–18 months. Early repair causes retarded maxillary growth (probably due to trauma to growth centre and periosteum of the maxilla during surgery if done early). Late repair causes speech defect. Both soft and hard palates are repaired. Abnormal insertion of tensor palati is released. *Mucoperiosteal flaps* are raised in the palate which is sewed together. If maxillary hypoplasia is present then *osteotomy of the maxilla* is done. With help of *orthodontic teeth extraction and alignment* of dentition is done. Regular examination of ear, nose and throat during follow-up period is needed. Postoperative speech therapy is essential. Whenever complicated problems are present, staged surgical procedure is done.

Wardill-Kilner push back operation—here mucoperiosteum flaps based on greater palatine vessels is raised, a better method **(Figs. 14-52 and 14-53)**.

Secondary management: Hearing support using hearing aid is given if defect is present. Control of otitis media when present. Speech problems occur due to velopharyngeal incompetence; articulation problems also can occur—speech therapy is given. It is corrected by pharyngoplasty, veloplasty or speech devices. Dental problems like uneruption, non-alignment are common. They should be corrected in a proper way by a dentist, along with reconstructive surgery. Orthodontic management with alveolar bone graft, maxillary osteotomy—done in 8–11 years of age. Veloplasty, dental implants, rhinoplasty, orthognathic surgeries, etc. are done based on requirement.

Principles of palatoplasty

- Timing is between 10–18 months
- Mucoperiosteum flap is raised
- Palatal defect is closed using 3 layers—nasal, muscle and oral layers
- Hook of pterygoid hamulus is fractured to relax tensor palati muscle to relieve tension on suture line

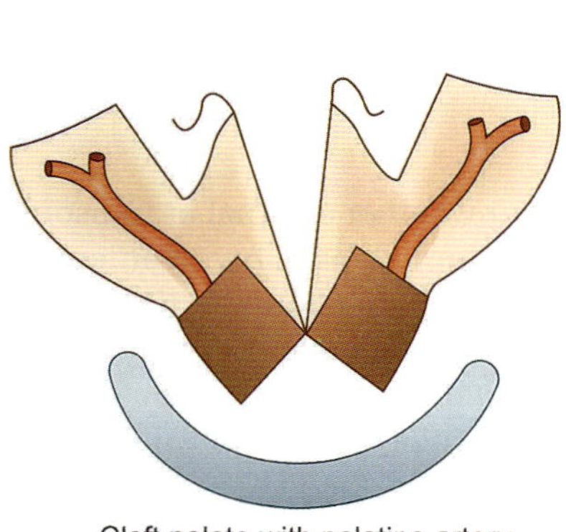

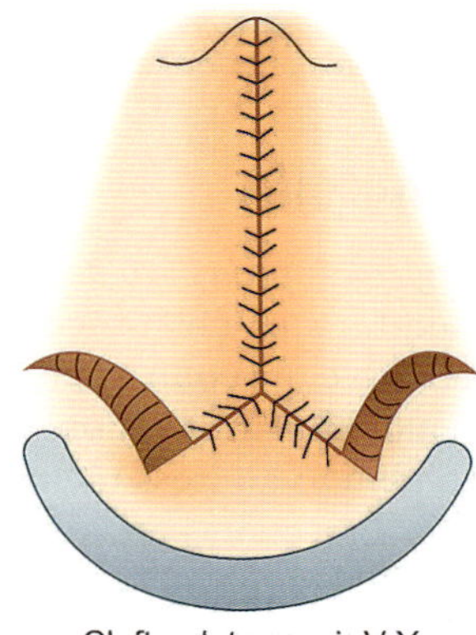

Fig. 14-52: V-Y palatoplasty.

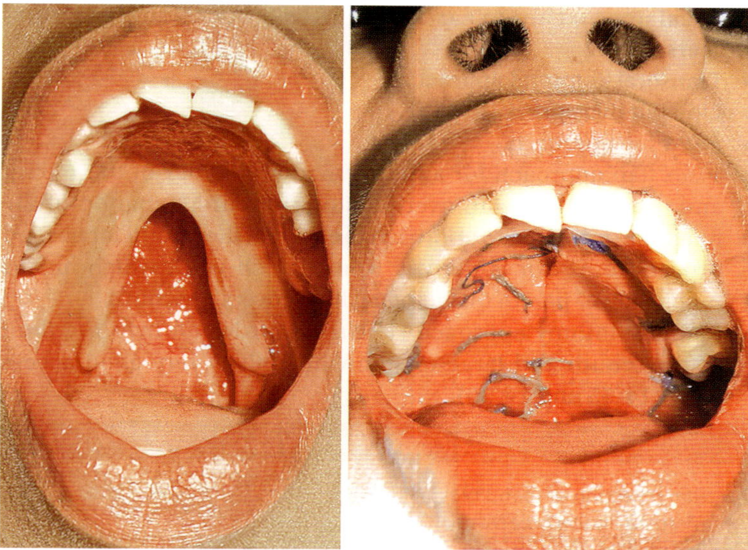

Fig. 14-53: Cleft palate and its repair.

SURGERIES OF THE ORAL CAVITY

Oral surgeries have become a specialty approach. So in detail discussion of each surgery is beyond the scope of this book. However, common procedures and approaches are discussed here. Interested students have to refer specialised books for reference. Laser is often used in oral surgery other than cautery **(Fig. 14-54)**.

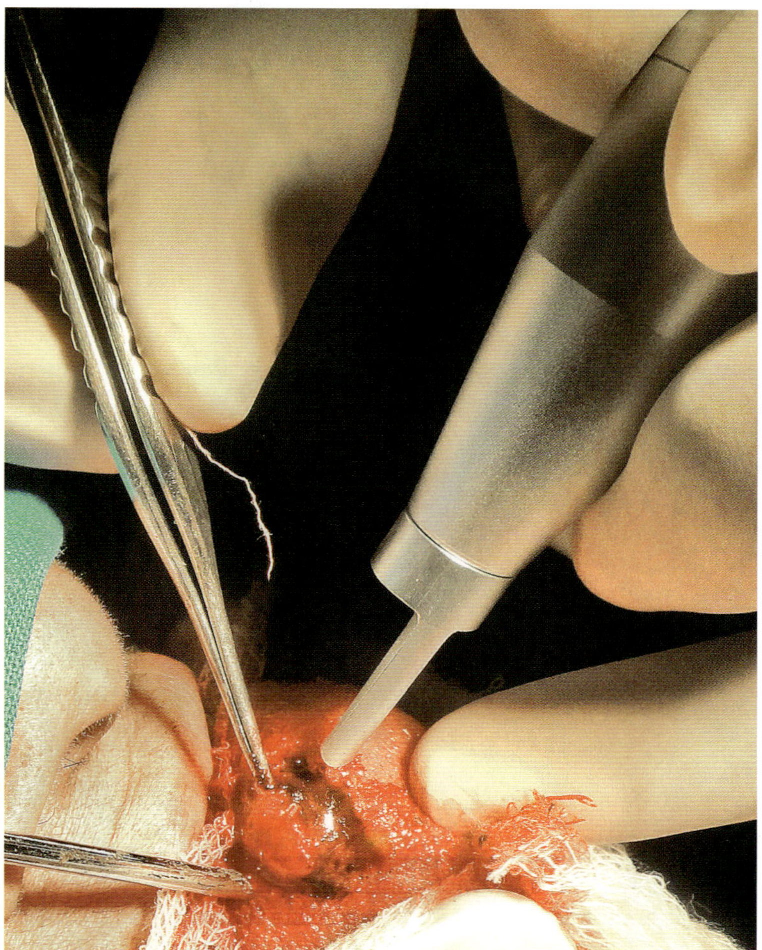

Fig. 14-54: Excision of lesion in the lip using laser.

Surgical approaches to carcinoma cheek (buccal mucosa)/oral cancers:

- Transoral/intraoral approach.
- Lip-split incision.
- *Patterson* approach.
- *Visor* flap approach for anterior mandible, floor of the mouth and tongue. Here skin over the anterior curved margin of the mandible is incised to approach the floor of the mouth for needed procedure. (*Visor* is derived from French word which means mobile lower part of the helmet which covers the chin).
- Mandibulotomy approach (*Kocher's*) for lesion over the floor of the mouth and large tongue which gives very good access **(Figs. 14-55 and 14-56)**.

Different mandibular resections

- Rim resection of mandible
- Marginal mandibulectomy
- Segmental resection
- Partial mandibulectomy
- Hemimandibulectomy
- Resection of the anterior mandible through visor approach

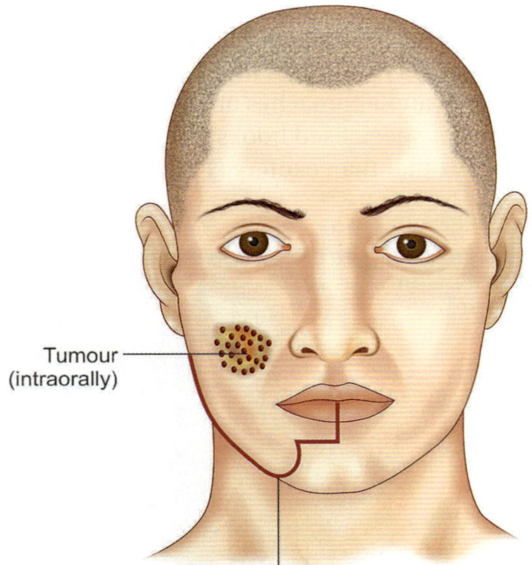

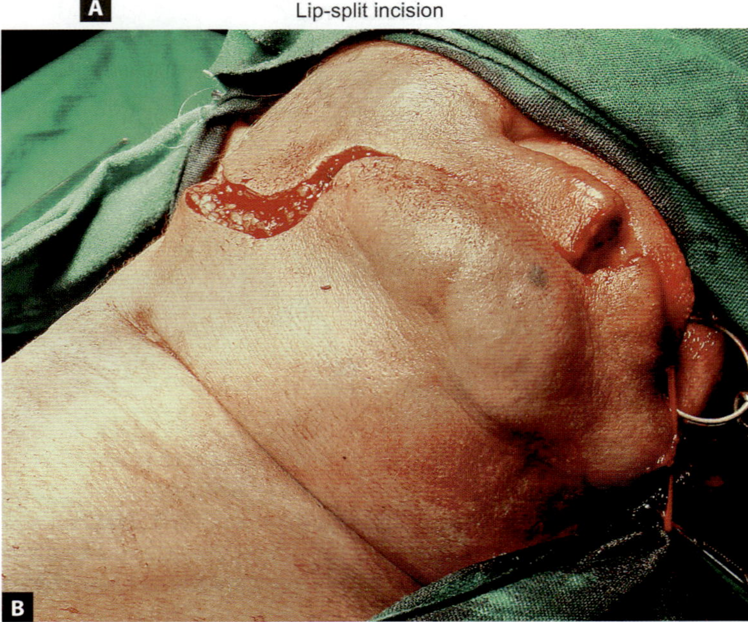

Figs. 14-55A and B

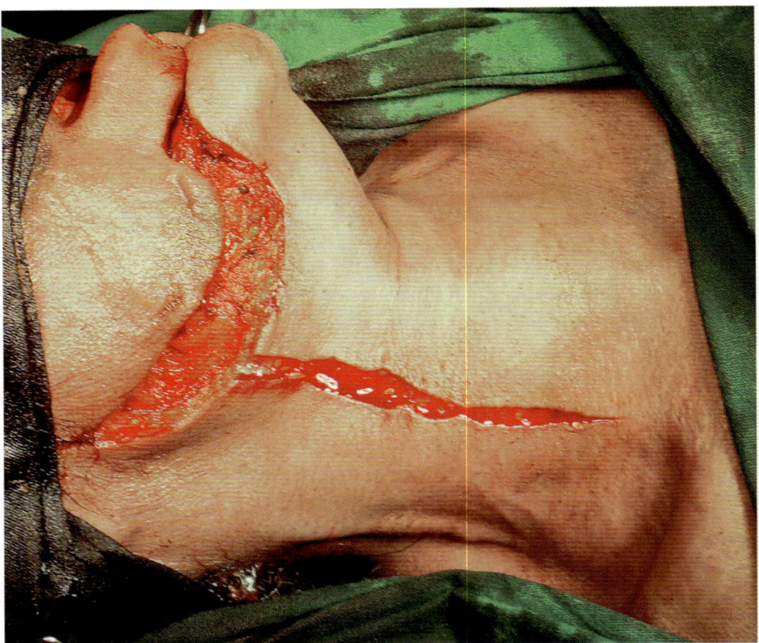

Fig. 14-55C

Figs. 14-55A to C: Lip-split incision is used for wide excision of the carcinoma cheek, hemimandibulectomy, approach to lateral part of the floor of mouth and alveolus.

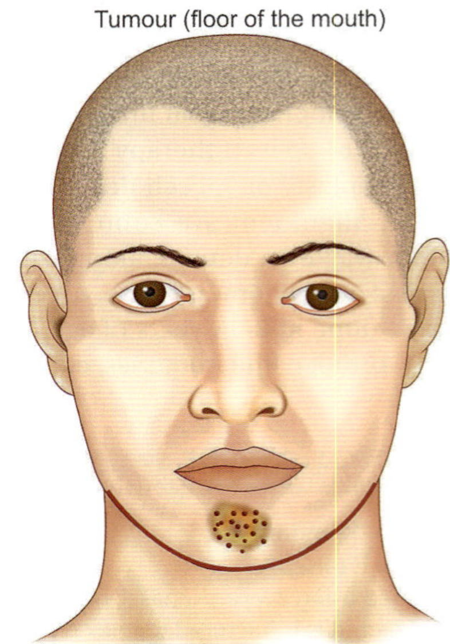

Fig. 14-56: *Visor flap approach* is used for lesions in the floor of the mouth and posterior tongue. Flap necrosis, fistula formation are less, functional results are better in relation to tongue mobility, articulation, swallowing, mastication.

Principles

Surgical approach to primary tumour whether external or transoral; adequacy of clearance in margin and depth; involvement of mandible or requirement of mandibular resection and if so extent of mandibular resection; lymphatic involvement present or not and the plan to address the neck nodes with decision for type of neck node dissection—are to be thought of while approaching the patient with oral cancers. External approaches may be Patterson/lip split/mandibulotomy.

All oral cancers are treated by *multidisciplinary approach*. For surgical treatment it is considered as early and advanced.

Involvement of mandible and nodes are also considered in approaching surgically. Staging of the disease is also essential.

Early superficial oral cancers are treated by wide local excision with 1–2 cm clearance. Frozen section biopsy is essential. Small defect can be closed primarily using 3-zero vicryl continuous sutures. Larger defect can be left alone safely to granulate and heal by secondary intention. Split skin graft (on to underlying buccinators muscle) to a wider area in cheek is useful way of covering the defect. It can be fixed to cheek by passing sutures from outside in and from inside out with knot placing outside which will be removed in 5–7 days **(Fig. 14-57)**.

T_1 and T_2 lesions are approached with wide local excision with supraomohyoid neck node dissection if N_0 OR if nodal status is N_1/N_2 radical or modified radical neck dissection I (MRND I—preservation of spinal accessory nerve) is done with or without mandibular resection depending on whether mandible is involved or not or close proximity of primary tumour to mandible. Type of mandible resection is decided by the extent of the mandible involvement.

T_3 or T_4 lesions are treated probably after initial chemoradiation by surgical wide excision with hemimandibulectomy with neck node dissection (RND). As mucosa, submucosa, buccinators, subcutaneous fat and skin are possibly involved after wide excision a through and through defect will be created. Extension into masseteric space by tumour is common and this area should be cleared meticulously. Reconstruction is essential using free radial forearm flap, rectus abdominis flap, fibular flap, plating, rib flap (opposite 11th rib), etc. Forehead flap may be used for mucosal side with pectoralis major myocutaneous flap for outer coverage. Large PMMF can be split on the skin part after harvesting to fold to cover mucosal as well as cutaneous parts of the defect **(Figs. 14-58 to 14-60)**.

Transoral Approach

It is the best approach for small lesions in the cheek or lesion in the tongue. As there is no incision outside it is cosmetically acceptable. Lesions less than 2 cm can be approached per orally. Larger lesion also can be approached through oral cavity but dissection and reconstruction is difficult. Nasotracheal anaesthesia is ideal. Often endotracheal tube can be placed on the opposite side of the lesion. Neck is turned towards opposite side. Mastoid retractor is used to retract cheek. C retractor is also helpful. Proper suctioning, adequate good light, cautery is essential. Lesion is excised with 1–2 cm clearance. Depth of the clearance also should be adequate. After excision, small defect can be left like that. Larger defect is covered with a quilted split skin graft from inside.

Transfacial—Patterson Operation (Fig. 14-61)

It is used in carcinoma cheek of early stage when only mucosa is involved. Incision is placed over the (lower border) base of mandible or just above the base parallel to it, often extending vertically over the margin of the ramus. Skin flap is elevated adequately upwards. Tumour with 1–2 cm clearance is excised widely. Skin flap is sutured back. Mucosal defect can be closed primarily. Often may require a skin graft inside. Skin is fixed by quilting sutures from outside in and inside out which are removed after 5 days. Skin graft gives the range of movements and prevents mucosal fibrosis and development of postoperative trismus which is distressing. Skin is taken from thigh (Split skin graft). Procedure is technically easier with less complications and faster recovery.

Transfacial Lip Split Incision Approach (Fig. 14-62)

In a wider lesion, transfacial lip split incision is needed to have a wider exposure of the cheek and tumour which facilitates adequate clearance. Inside defect can be reconstructed with forehead flap or SSG; outside, if there is defect, PMMF flap or deltopectoral flap can be used. Hemimandibulectomy or other mandibular resections can be carried out through this incision **(Fig. 14-63)**.

Hemimandibulectomy

Surgical Anatomy of Mandible (Fig. 14-64)

It is the largest and strongest bone of face. It has got horse-shaped body with two rami from its posterior ends projecting upwards. Outer surface of body contains symphysis menti, mental protuberance, mental foramen, oblique line and incisive fossa. Inner surface contains mylohyoid line, submandibular fossa (below), sublingual fossa (above) and genial tubercles. Upper alveolar border bears sockets for teeth. Quadrilateral ramus has got medial and lateral surfaces, anterior, posterior, upper and lower borders and coronoid and condyloid processes. Medial surface of ramus contains mandibular foramen above the centre of the ramus at occlusal surface of teeth (transmits inferior alveolar nerve and vessels across mandibular canal to mental foramen on the outer surface); lingula (bony projection of mandibular foramen gives attachment to sphenomandibular ligament); mylohyoid groove (medial pterygoid is inserted below and medial to this groove). Lateral surface of ramus is flat (attachment of the masseter muscle). Upper border of ramus forms curved mandibular notch; lower border containing angle of mandible is the continuation of the base of mandible. Posterior border of ramus is thick; anterior is thin. Anterior projection is called as *coronoid process* (temporalis is inserted on its apex and medial surface); posterior projection is called as *condyloid process*. Condyloid process is strong with expanded upward head which articulates with temporal bone to form temporomandibular joint. Anterior part of neck of condyloid process has got pterygoid fovea for the insertion of lateral pterygoid muscle. Oblique line on the outer surface of the body gives origin to buccinator; mylohyoid line on the inner surface of body gives origin to mylohyoid and superior constrictor muscles; upper genial tubercle gives origin to genioglossus and lower to geniohyoid; digastric fossa gives origin to anterior belly of digastric muscle. Investing layer of deep fascia and platysma is attached to lower border (base) of the mandible. Masseteric vessels and nerve passes through mandibular notch; mental foramen transmits mental vessels and nerve; inferior alveolar vessels and nerve passes through the mandibular canal; mylohyoid vessels and nerve are related to mylohyoid groove; lingual nerve is related on the medial surface; auriculotemporal nerve is related to medial side of the neck of the mandible. Mandible is the second bone to ossify in the body after clavicle. Ossification centre (*only one centre*) appears in 6th week of intrauterine life, one on each side near mental foramen. Entire *body* ossifies from *membrane* except only near incisor teeth; ramus *above the mandibular foramen* ossifies from *cartilage*. Site at canine socket is weak and is the *commonest site of fracture* which may involve inferior alveolar nerve causing neuralgic pain and loss of sensation over the distribution of mental nerve.

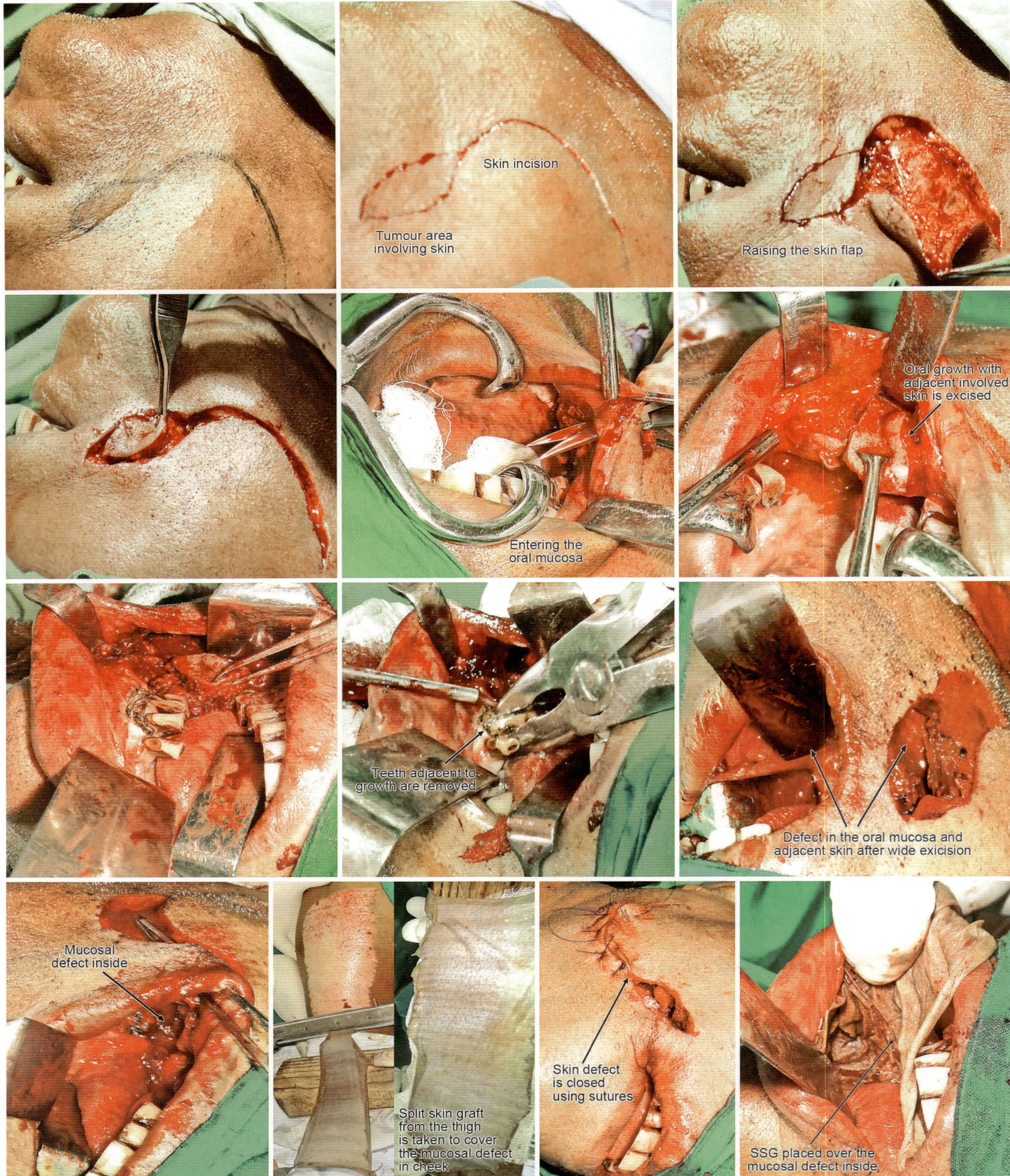
Skin incision
Tumour area involving skin
Raising the skin flap
Entering the oral mucosa
Oral growth with adjacent involved skin is excised
Teeth adjacent to growth are removed
Defect in the oral mucosa and adjacent skin after wide exicision
Mucosal defect inside
Split skin graft from the thigh is taken to cover the mucosal defect in cheek
Skin defect is closed using sutures
SSG placed over the mucosal defect inside

Figs. 14-57(1)

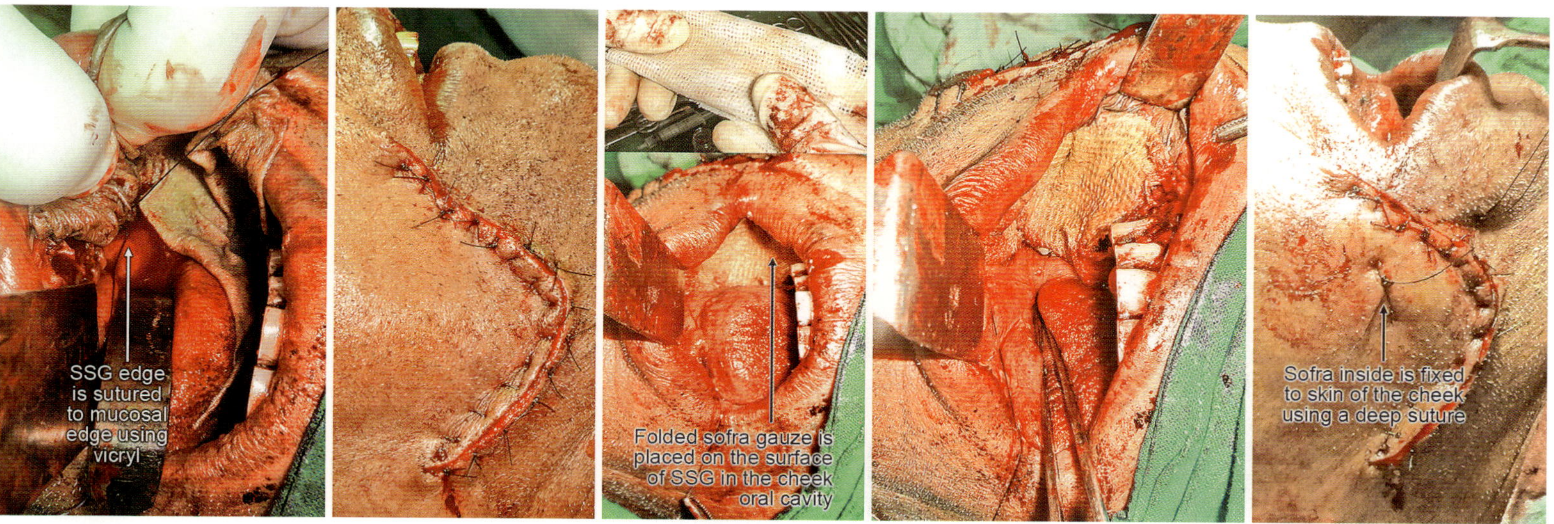

Figs. 14-57(2)

Figs. 14-57(1 and 2): Wide excision of the carcinoma cheek with placement of split skin graft on the mucosal aspect.

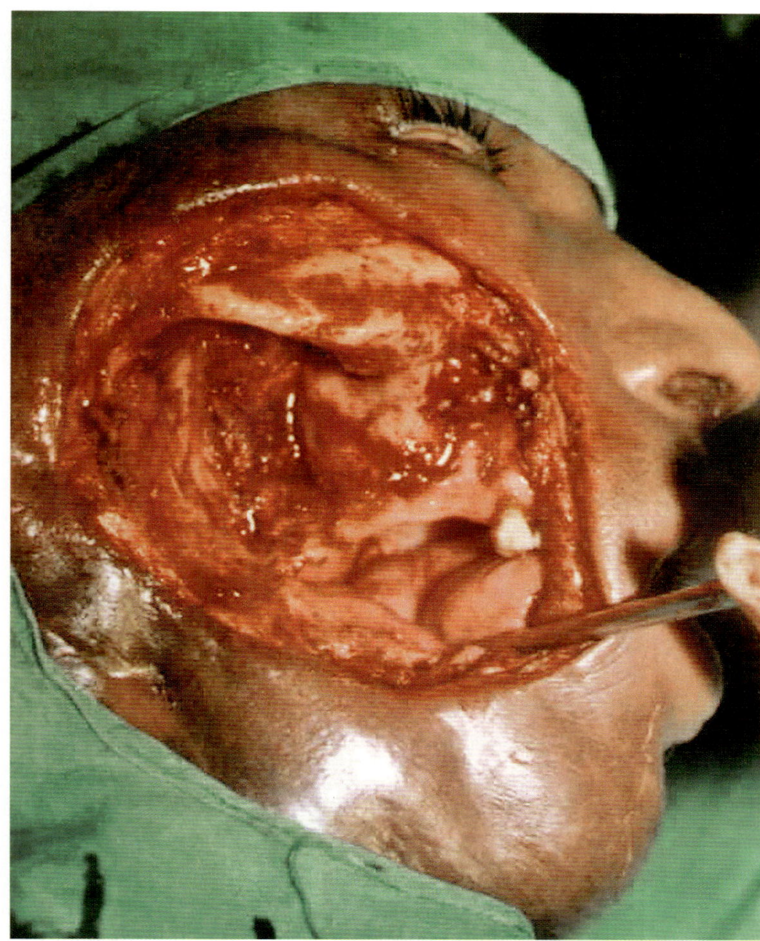

Fig. 14-58: Carcinoma cheek extending into the skin and soft tissues cleared widely. It needs PMMF to cover the defect from outside; split skin grafting or forehead flap to cover from inside.

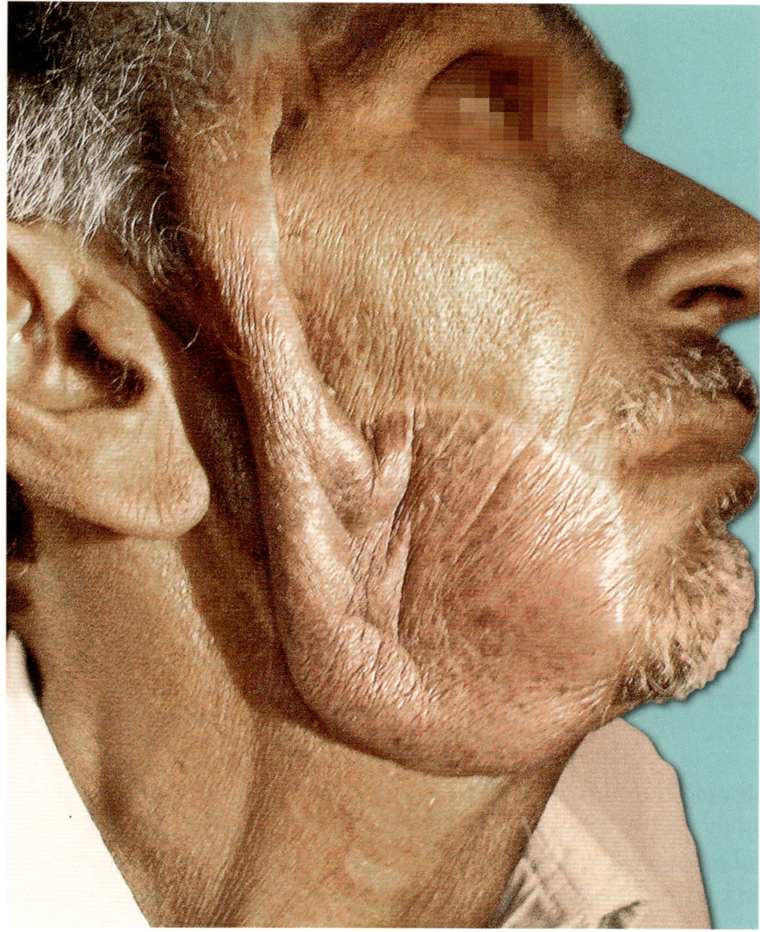

Fig. 14-59: Forehead flap is also often used to cover the defect from outside.

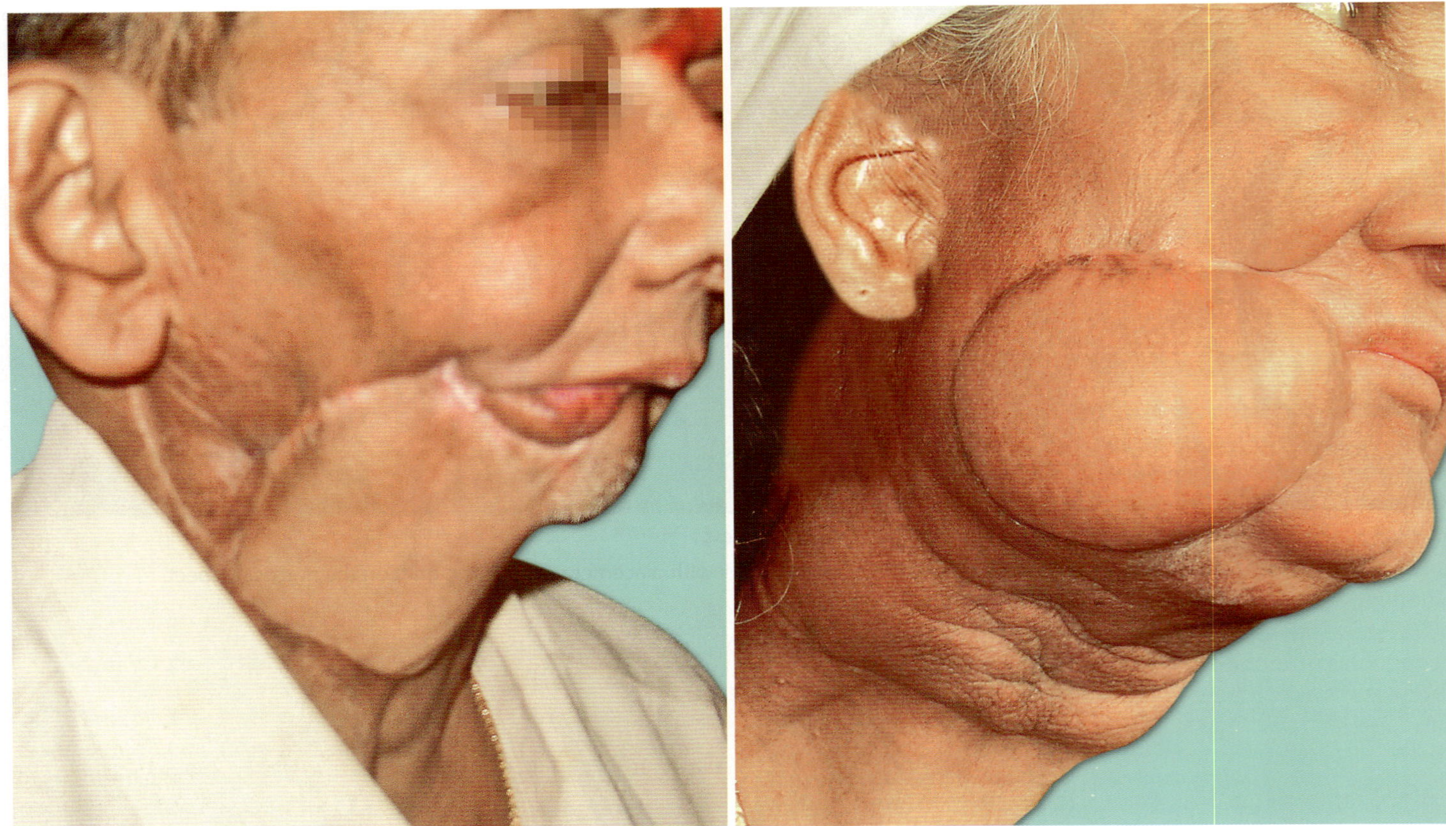

Fig. 14-60: Pectoralis major myocutaneous flap is used commonly to cover the cheek defect.

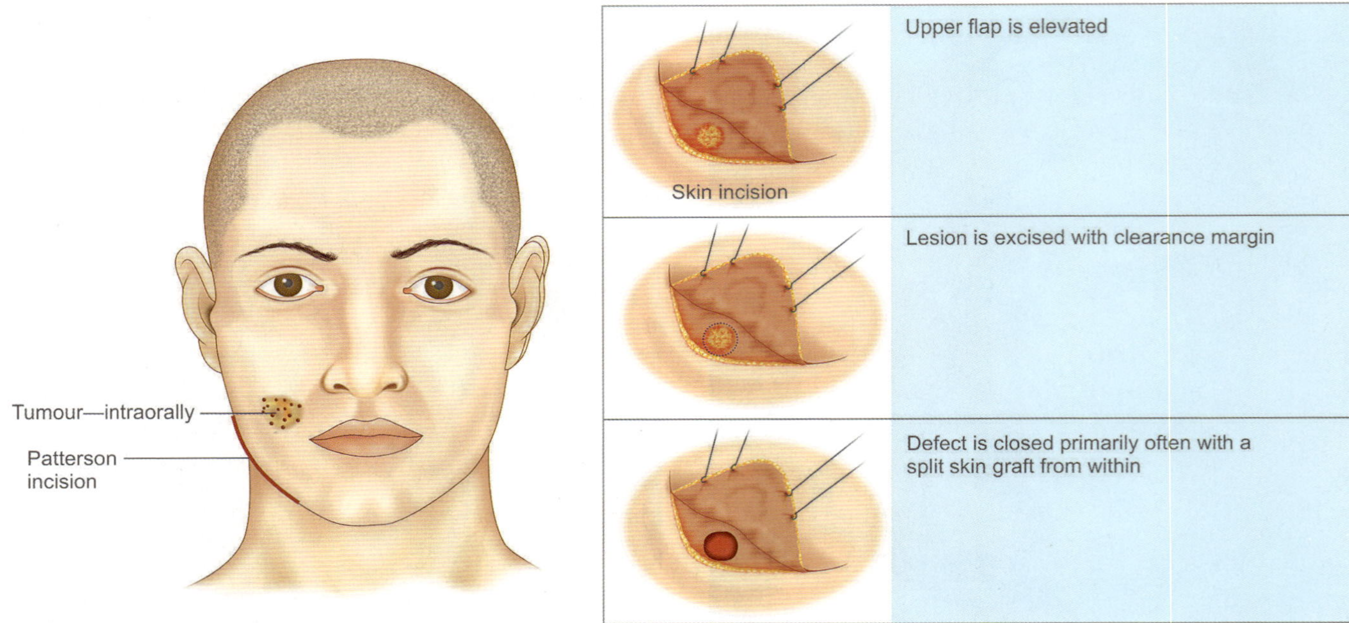

Fig. 14-61: Transfacial—Patterson operation.

Muscles of mastication (derive from mesoderm of 1st branchial arch, supplied by 1st arch nerve—mandibular) are:

1. *Masseter:* A quadrilateral muscle covering outer surface of mandible has got 3 layers—superficial layer arises from anterior 2/3rd of lower margin of zygomatic arch; middle from anterior 2/3rd of deep surface and posterior 1/3rd of lower margin of zygomatic arch; deep layer from deep surface of zygomatic arch. It is inserted into lower, middle and upper part of the ramus of the mandible and coronoid process of mandible. It is supplied by masseteric branch of the anterior division of mandibular nerve. It elevates the mandible **(Fig. 14-65)**.

2. *Medial pterygoid muscle:* It is quadrilateral muscle with superficial and deep heads. Superficial is arising from tuberosity of maxilla; deep head arises from lateral pterygoid plate and adjoining palatine bone. Fibre runs downwards and backwards to reach medial surface and angle of the mandible below and behind the mandibular foramen and mylohyoid groove. It is supplied by nerve to medial pterygoid, a branch from main trunk of mandibular nerve. It elevates

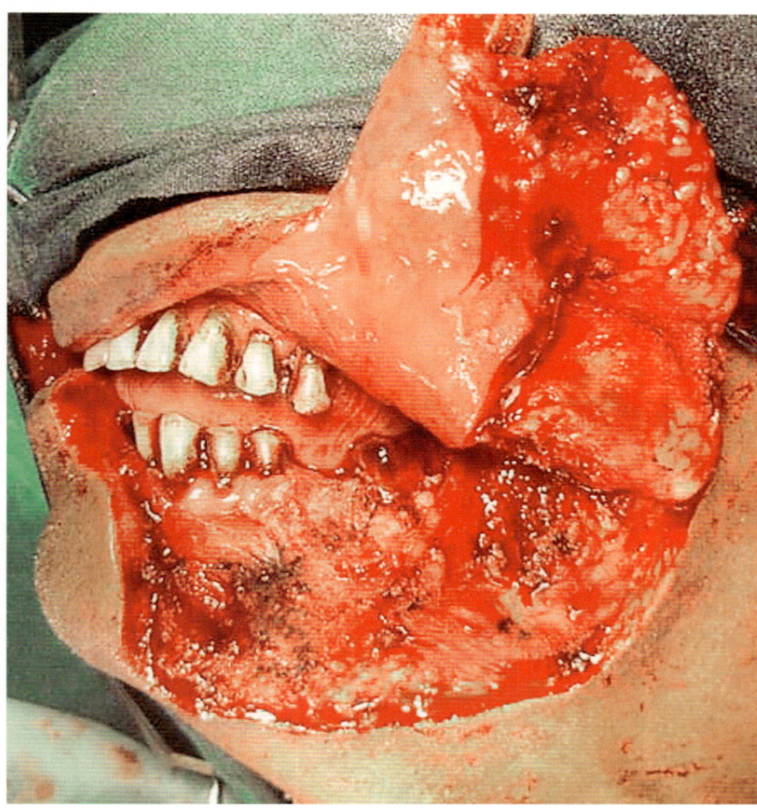

Fig. 14-62: Raising the flap after lip split incision for carcinoma cheek.

and protrudes mandible. Lateral pterygoid plate, lingual and inferior alveolar nerves and lower head of lateral pterygoid lie superficial to the upper part of the muscle; ramus of the mandible, mandibular nerves, maxillary artery and sphenomandibular ligament lie superficial to the lower part of the muscle. Tensor veli palatini, superior constrictor of the pharynx, styloglossus and stylopharyngeus attached to the styloid process are deep to the muscle.

3. *Lateral pterygoid muscle:* It is a short conical muscle with upper and lower heads; upper arises from infratemporal surface and greater wing of sphenoid bone; lower from lateral surface of lateral pterygoid plate. It runs backwards and laterally to insert into pterygoid fovea on the anterior surface of neck of the mandible and anterior margin of articular disc and capsule of temporomandibular joint. It is superficially related to ramus of the mandible, temporalis muscle tendon and maxillary artery. Its deeper relations are mandibular nerve, middle meningeal artery, sphenomandibular ligament and deep head of pterygoid muscle. Deep temporal nerves and masseteric nerve emerges at its upper margin. Maxillary artery passes upwards and buccal nerve passes downwards between the two heads. Two deep temporal arteries run on the outer surface of upper head. Masseteric artery and nerve passes on the surface of lateral pterygoid towards mandibular notch to enter the masseter muscle from its deeper plane. Masseteric artery arises from maxillary artery and nerve from mandibular nerve. Lingual and inferior alveolar nerve descends from deeper plane of lateral pterygoid at its lower border. Middle meningeal artery runs upwards from its lower border at deeper plane **(Figs. 14-66 and 14-67)**.

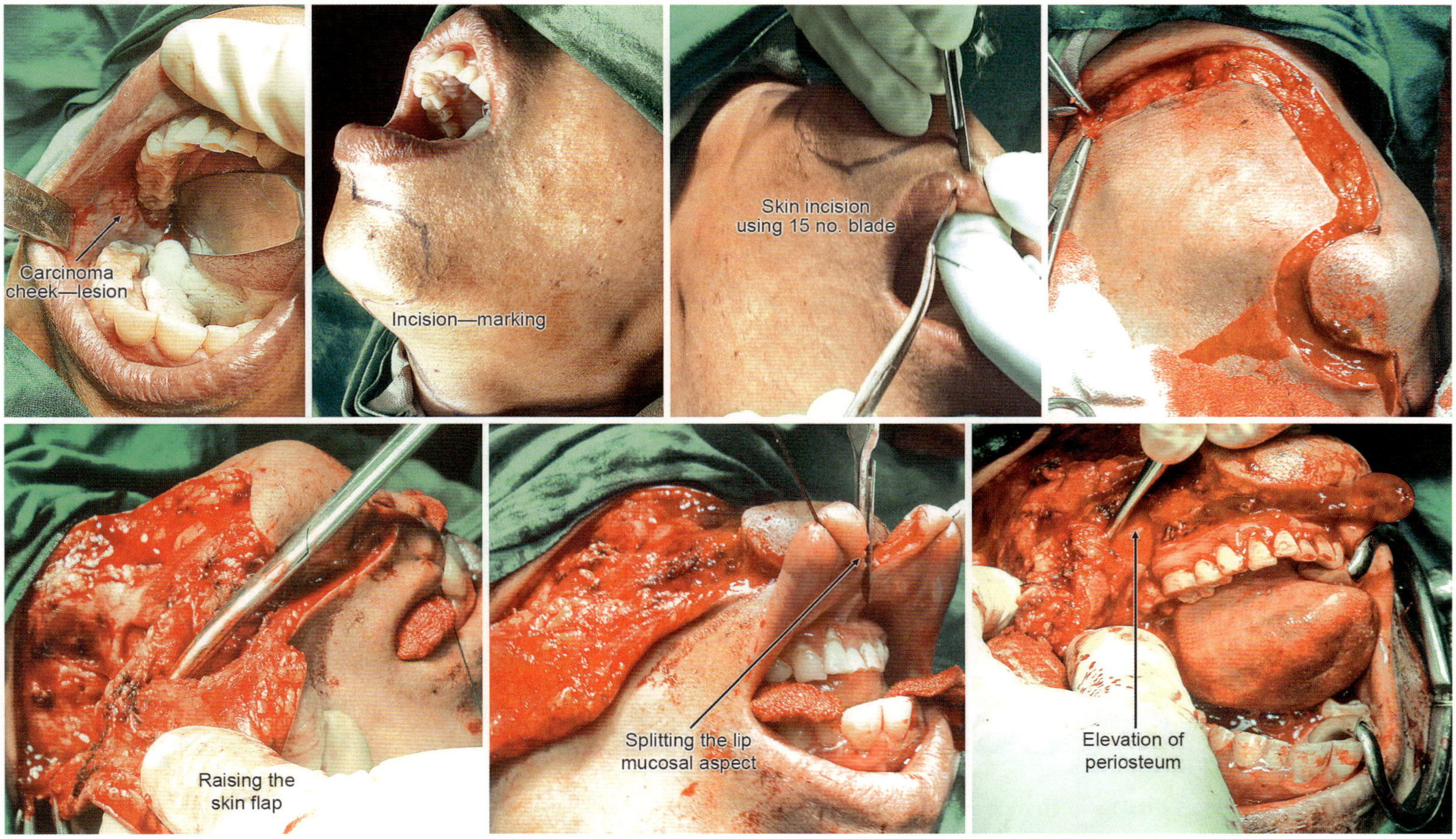

Figs. 14-63(1)

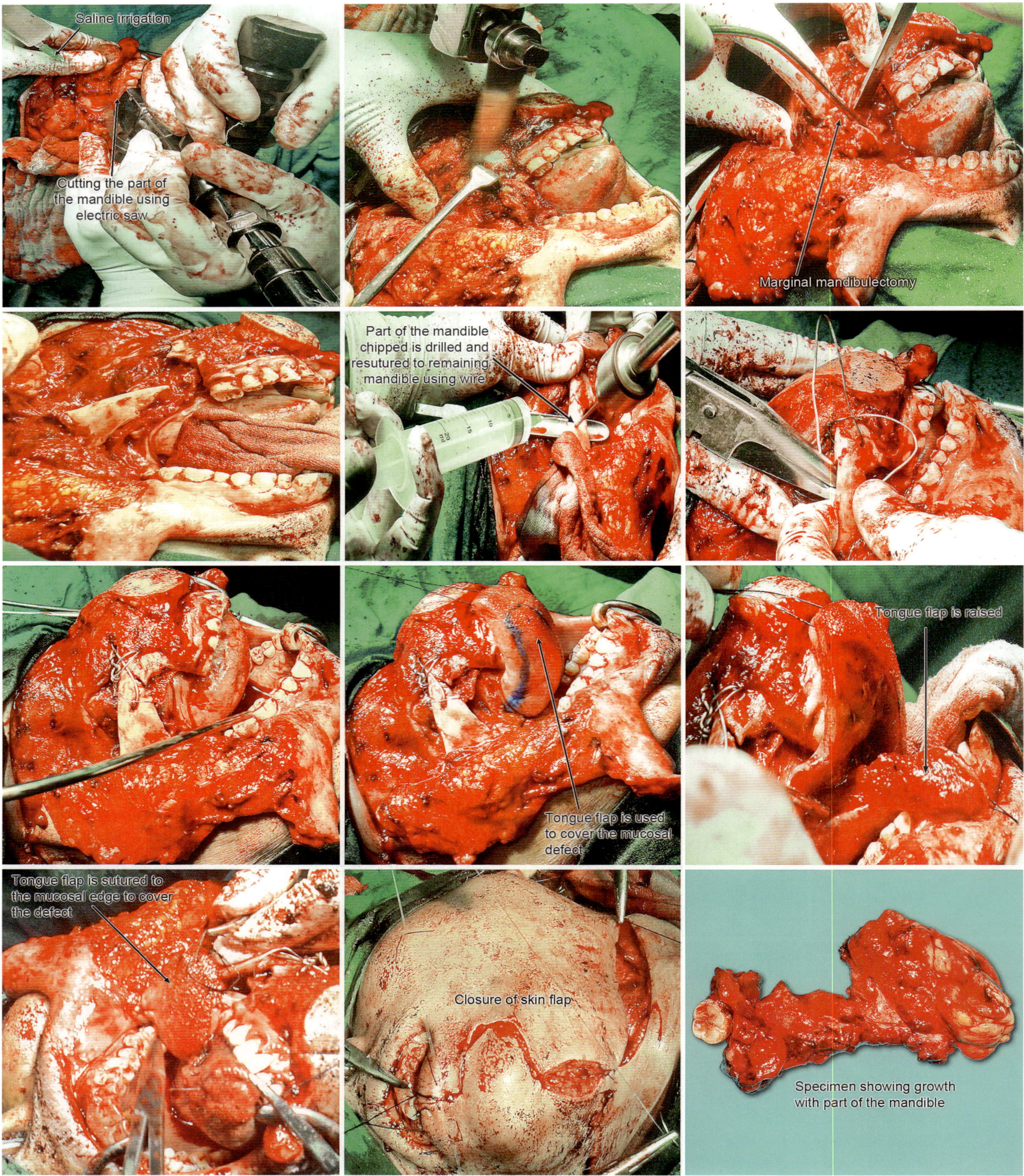

Figs. 14-63(2)

Figs. 14-63(1 and 2): Wide excision with marginal resection of the mandible with bone fixing using steel wires. Mucosal defect is covered using tongue flap based posteriorly.

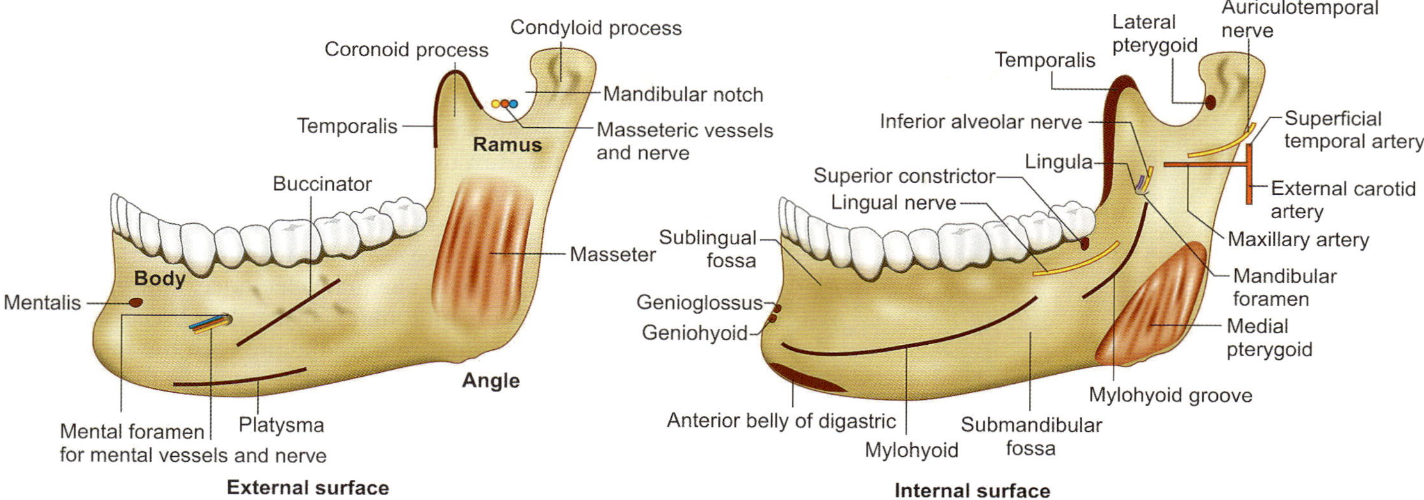

Fig. 14-64: Surgical anatomy of the mandible.

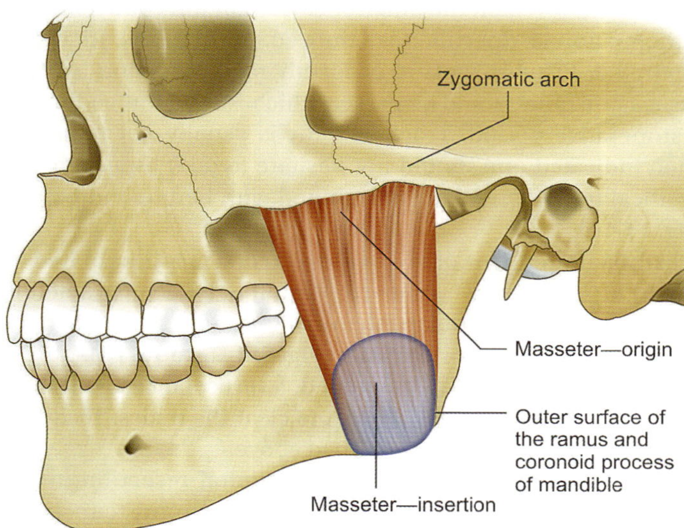

Fig. 14-65: Anatomy of masseter muscle.

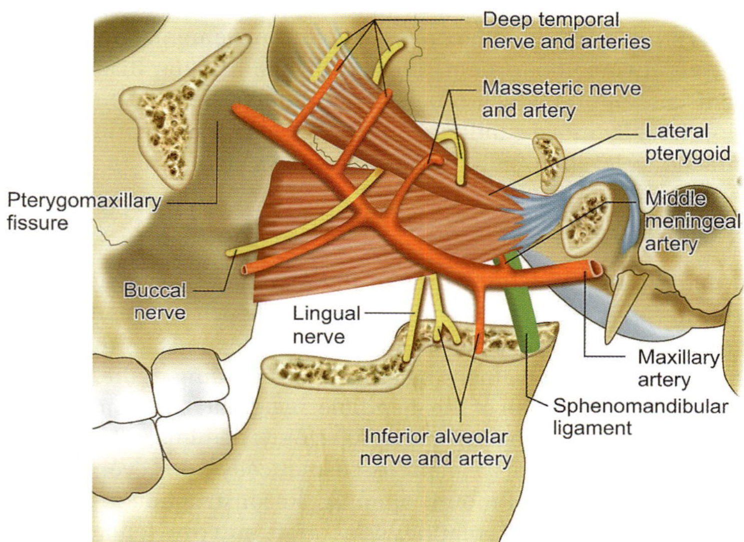

Fig. 14-67: Outer/superficial relations of the lateral pterygoid muscle.

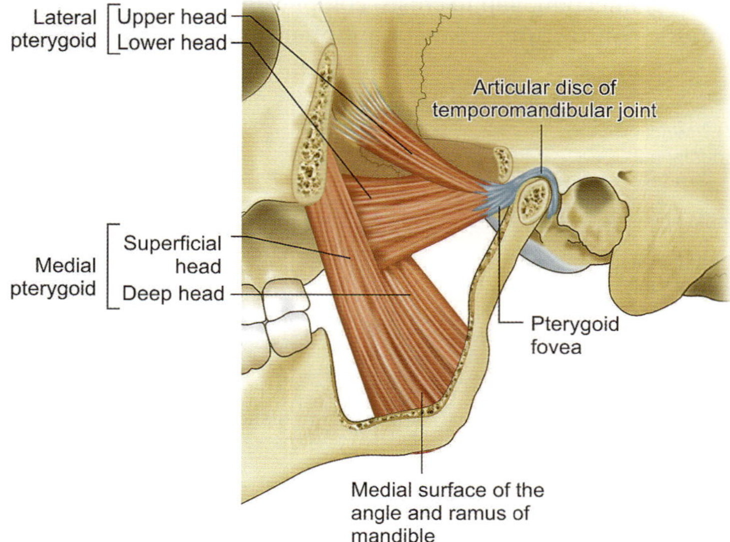

Fig. 14-66: Origin and insertions of the medial and lateral pterygoid muscles.

4. *Temporalis muscle:* It is fan-shaped muscle arising from temporal fossa of temporal bone and temporal fascia passing deep to zygomatic arch towards its insertion at deep surface of coronoid process and anterior ramus of mandible. It is supplied by two deep temporal branches from anterior division of mandibular nerve. It elevates the mandible, retracts the protruded mandible; and facilitates side-to-side mandible movement **(Fig. 14-68)**.

Temporomandibular joint (TM joint): It is synovial condylar joint. Upper part of the articular surface is formed by the temporal bone, articular eminence and anterior part of the mandibular fossa; lower articular surface is formed by the head of the mandible. Joint cavity is divided into upper and lower part by articular disc. *Ligaments of the joint are*—temporomandibular, sphenomandibular and stylomandibular. TM joint is related laterally to skin, fascia, parotid, temporal branches of facial nerve; medially tympanic plate (separates from ICA), spine of sphenoid, upper part of sphenomandibular ligament, auriculotemporal and chorda tympani nerves, middle meningeal artery; posteriorly parotid, external auditory meatus, superficial temporal vessels and auriculotemporal nerve from deep

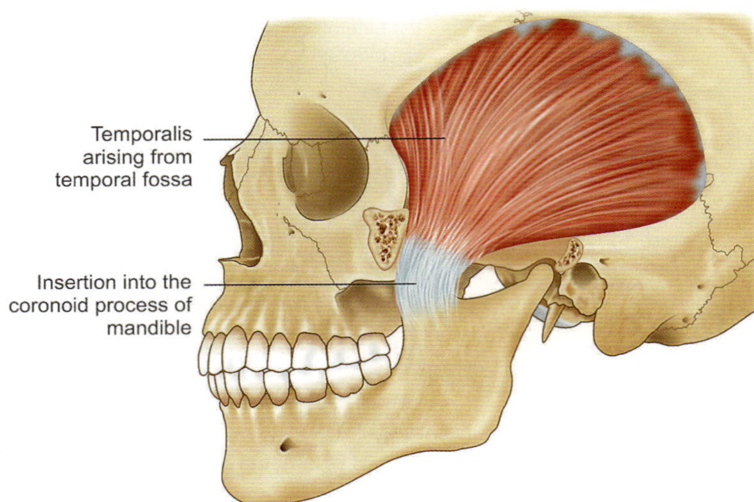

Fig. 14-68: Origin and insertion of the temporalis muscle.

to superficial; superiorly middle cranial fossa and middle meningeal vessels; inferiorly maxillary vessels. Joint movements are divided between two compartments created by the articular disc—upper meniscotemporal, lower meniscomandibular. Both right and left joints usually move simultaneously. *Movements are*—protraction, retraction, elevation, side-to-side movements **(Fig. 14-69)**.

Procedure

In mandibulectomy, growth with the mandible is removed. It is done in carcinoma cheek (oral carcinomas) which is extending into the mandible. Extent of mandible resection depends on the extent of mandibular involvement by growth and grading of the tumour. It may be rim resection of the mandible, marginal mandibulectomy, segmental resection, partial mandibulectomy, hemimandibulectomy (refer figures). Primary closure is cosmetically poor even though it gives good range of mouth opening. Reconstruction is done by various methods—like plating, bone graft, microvascular fibular graft. If there is defect in the skin and soft tissues, then pectoralis major myocutaneous flap (PMMF) or deltopectoral cutaneous flap is used. Mucosal defect if present is covered by simple split skin graft or forehead cutaneous flap. Reconstruction is done with the help of plastic surgeon.

Incision for hemimandibulectomy is 2 cm below the base of the mandible, parallel and extending towards the ear lobule along the ramus of the mandible. Often lip spilt incision is used. Flaps are elevated both upper and lower. Bipolar and monopolar cautery is needed to elevate the flaps. Mandible is transected just adjacent to the mentum towards the side of the lesion using Gigli saw or ideally electric rotary saw. Resected mandible is elevated upwards to facilitate visibility of the soft tissue attachment to the base. Carcinoma lesion can be seen on the mucosal surface of the cheek which is dissected with adequate clearance. Lower flap is elevated to expose the submandibular salivary gland. The submandibular salivary gland in often removed along with the mandible during hemimandibulectomy. Once soft tissue is freed from below, medial pterygoid is cut near its attachment on the inner surface of the mandible. Temporalis is detached from the coronoid process. Small branches of the maxillary artery on the deeper surface of the masseter muscle will be ligated. Masseter muscle is cut from the upper part of its attachment to the mandible. Temporomandibular joint is dissected and lateral pterygoid is detached from its attachment to pterygoid fovea on the anterior surface of the condyloid process of the mandible. Specimen is removed. All bleeders are ligated or fulgurated. Primary closure or ideally reconstruction is planned. Nasogastric tube should be passed which is used for feeding during postoperative period. Tracheostomy is usually not required but when indicated one should not hesitate to do it especially in case if radical neck dissection is combined with hemimandibulectomy **(Fig. 14-70)**.

Flap is sutured. One or two bottles of blood may be required which should be kept ready in theatre. Mandible is reconstructed using cortical bone graft, fibular microvascular flap, synthetic material like, titanium, stainless steel plate **(Figs. 14-71 to 14-73)**.

If radical neck dissection is added, a vertical incision in the neck to the existing incision is sufficient to clear the nodes. Technique of neck dissection is same as described above.

Less aggressive surgeries like segmental resection, marginal mandibulectomy, and partial mandibulectomy can be done depending on the extent of bone involvement **(Figs. 14-74 to 14-78)**.

Complications of Surgeries

Bleeding, infection, flap necrosis, complications of reconstruction, stiffness, contracture, cosmetic problems, swallowing problems

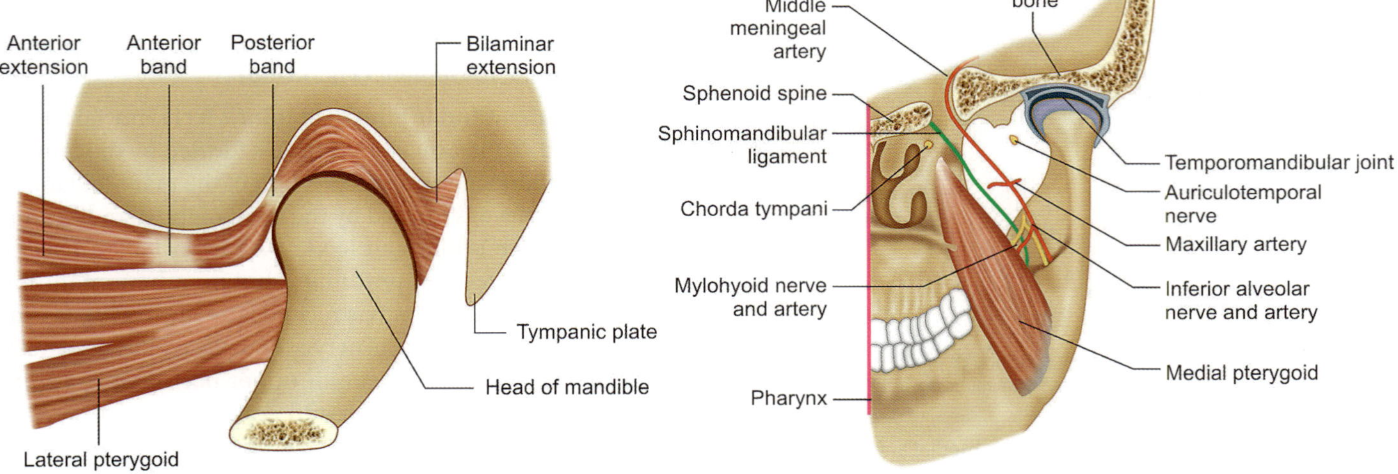

Fig. 14-69: Anatomy and relations of temporomandibular joint.

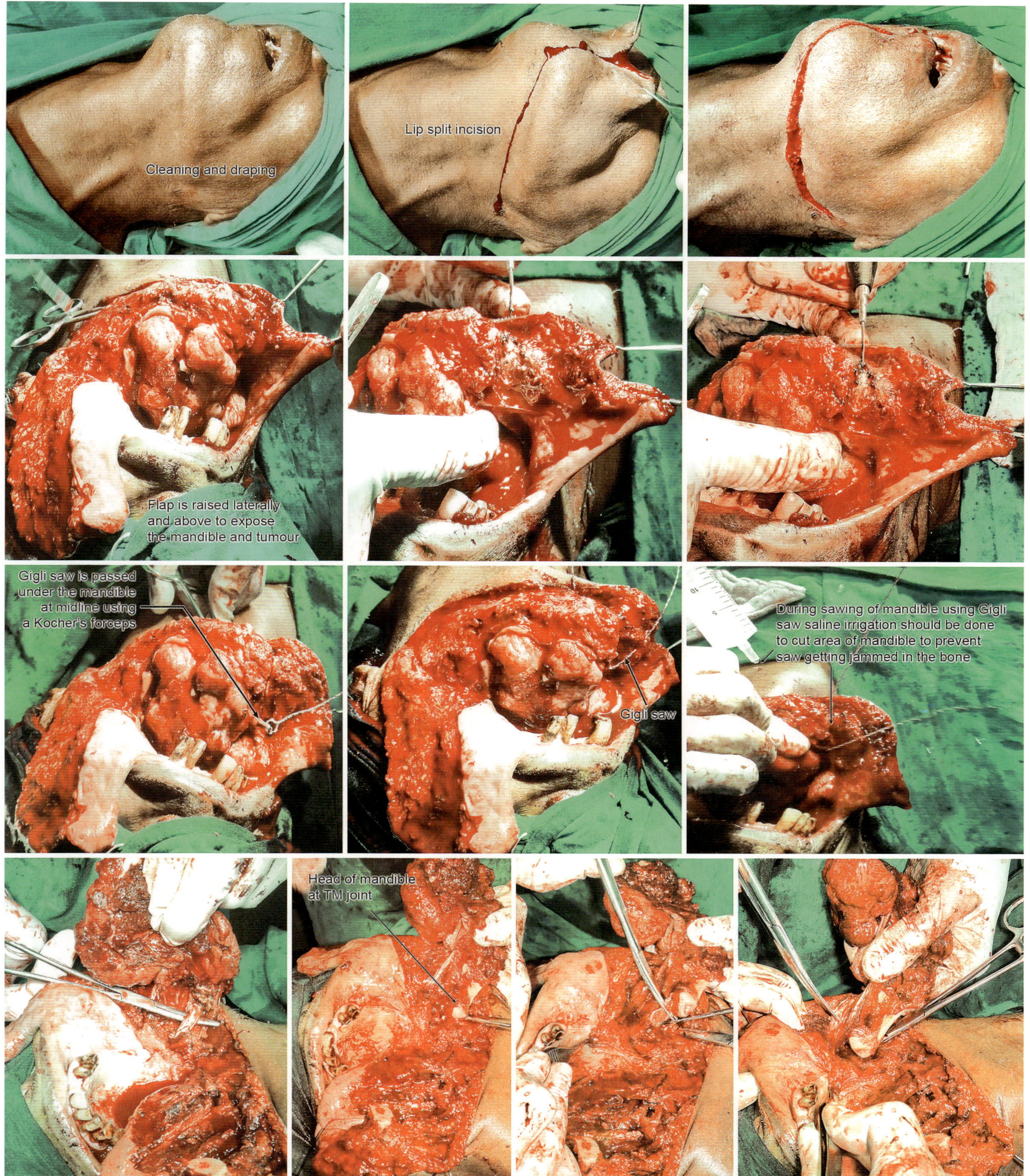
Cleaning and draping
Lip split incision
Flap is raised laterally and above to expose the mandible and tumour
Gigli saw is passed under the mandible at midline using a Kocher's forceps
Gigli saw
During sawing of mandible using Gigli saw saline irrigation should be done to cut area of mandible to prevent saw getting jammed in the bone
Head of mandible at TM joint

Figs. 14-70(1)

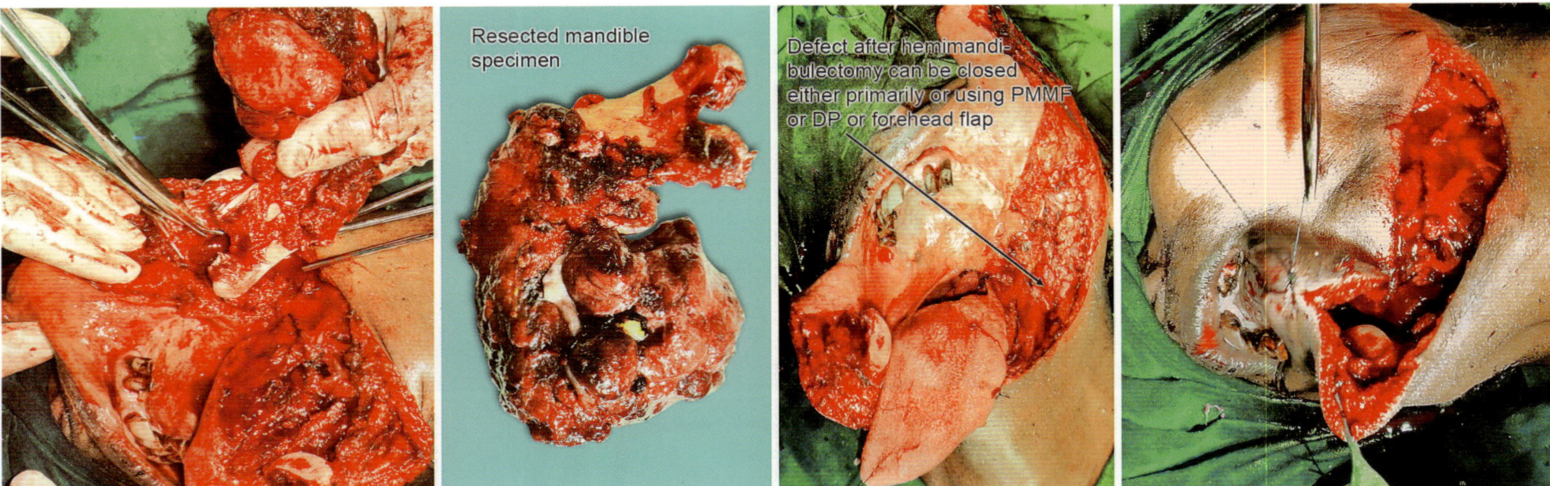

Figs. 14-70(2)

Figs. 14-70(1 and 2): Hemimandibulectomy technique using lip split incision with wide excision of primary tumour in the cheek.

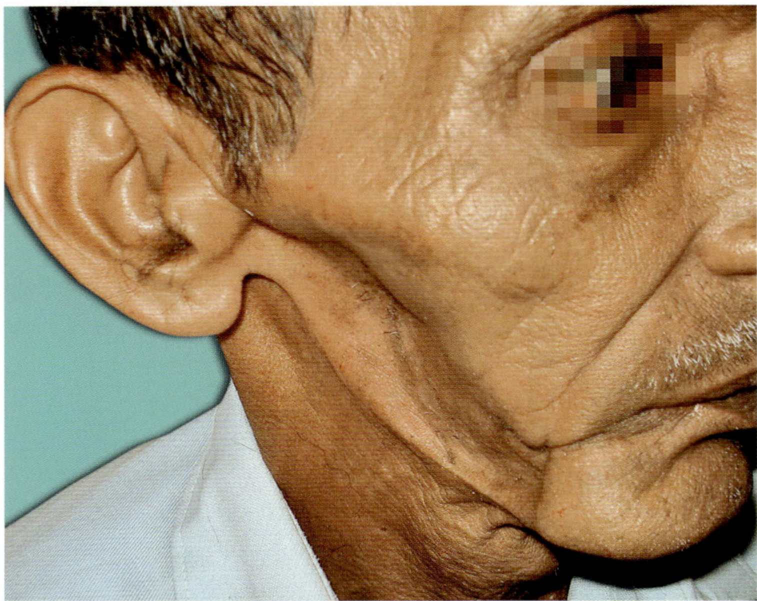

Fig. 14-71: Hemimandibulectomy is done in this patient. Reconstruction is not done in this patient leading into poor cosmetic outcome. But mouth opening and jaw movements will be adequate.

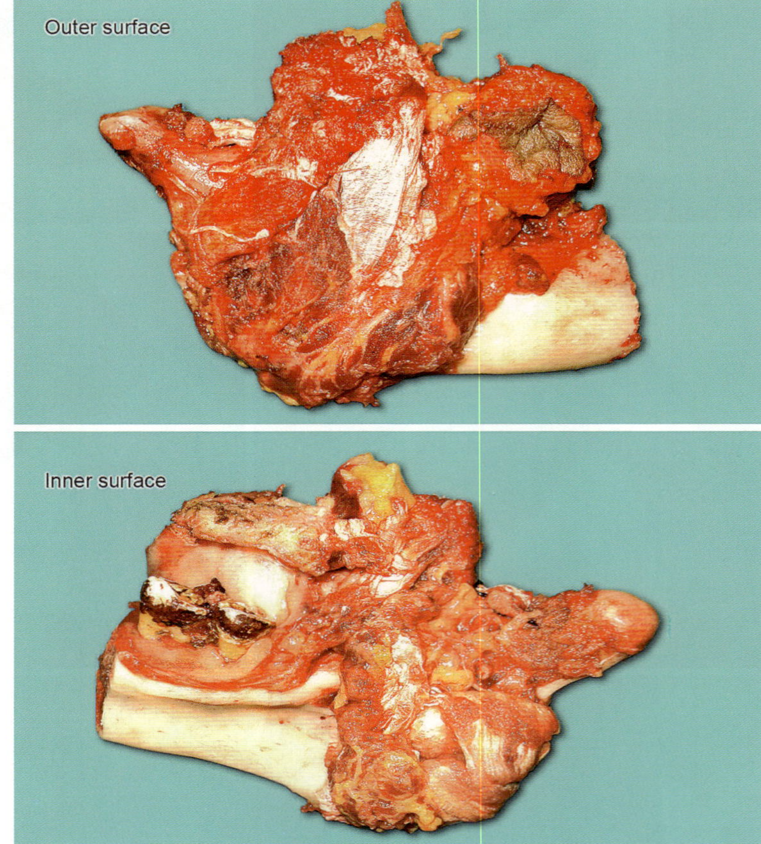

Fig. 14-72: Hemimandibulectomy specimen as viewed both from outer and inner surface.

and speech problems are the complications observed. Respiratory complications like aspiration and bronchopneumonia are often life threatening. Anaesthetic complications and deep venous thrombosis are other complications.

Approach to Floor of the Mouth

Anatomy: It is U shaped area bounded by lower gum and oral tongue. It ends posteriorly at the insertion of anterior tonsillar pillar into the tongue. Sublingual papilla is present on each side of the frenulum; on summit of which is the opening of the duct (*Wharton's*) of submandibular salivary gland. Laterally and behind this papilla, sublingual fold is present which overlies the sublingual gland. Genioglossus and geniohyoid muscles are deeper to it. On either side mylohyoid muscles form the muscular part of the floor of the mouth. It arises from mylohyoid ridge of the mandible extending up to the 3rd molar tooth. Submandibular salivary gland rests on the external surface of mylohyoid muscle; only small deeper part extends into the internal surface. Submandibular salivary duct runs about 5 cm between sublingual gland and genioglossus to end in papilla. Lingual and hypoglossal nerves are closely related to gland and duct. Alveolingual sulcus is valley-shaped space between tongue and mandibular alveolar bone.

In carcinoma floor of the mouth adjacent to ventral part of the tongue, alveolus, submandibular ducts and opposite nodes are involved early. CT scan is a must to assess the stage and plan the therapy.

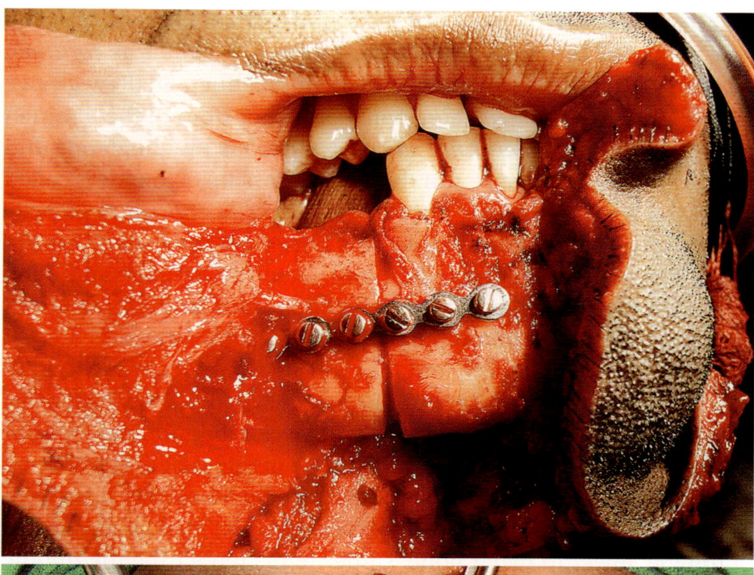

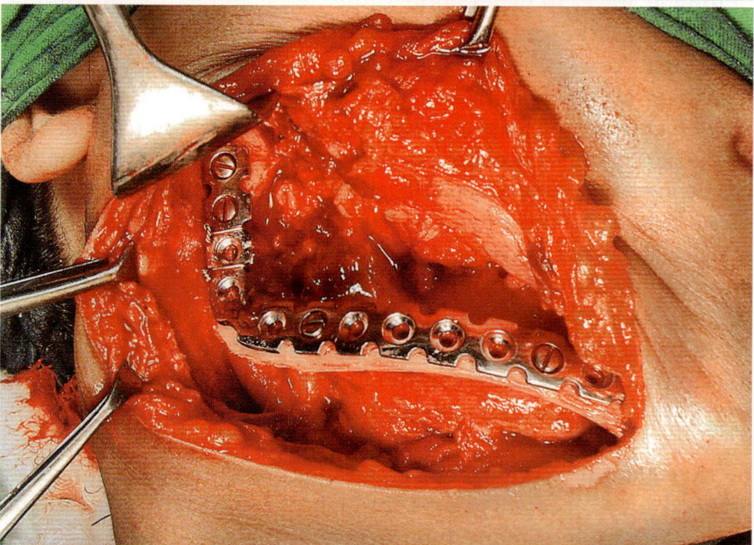

Fig. 14-73: Reconstruction of the mandible is done using plates, screws and bone graft.

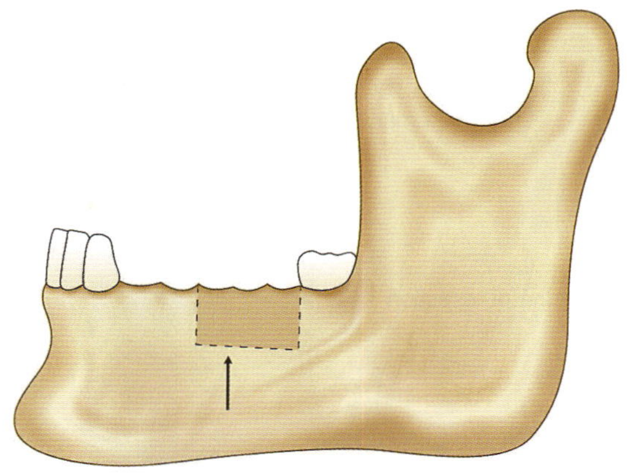

Fig. 14-75: Extent of resection in marginal mandibulectomy.

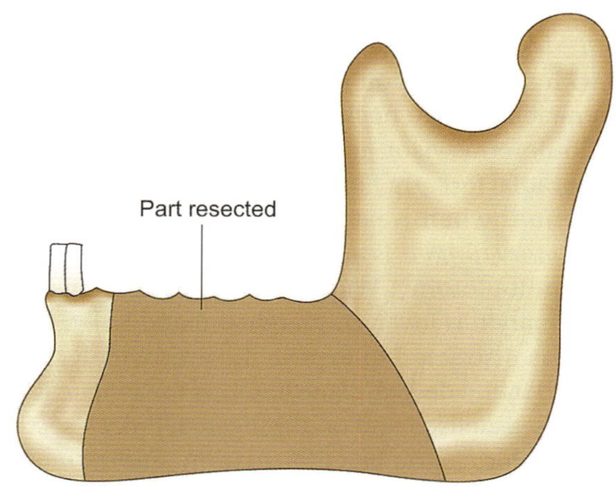

Fig. 14-76: Extent of bone removal in segmental resection of the mandible.

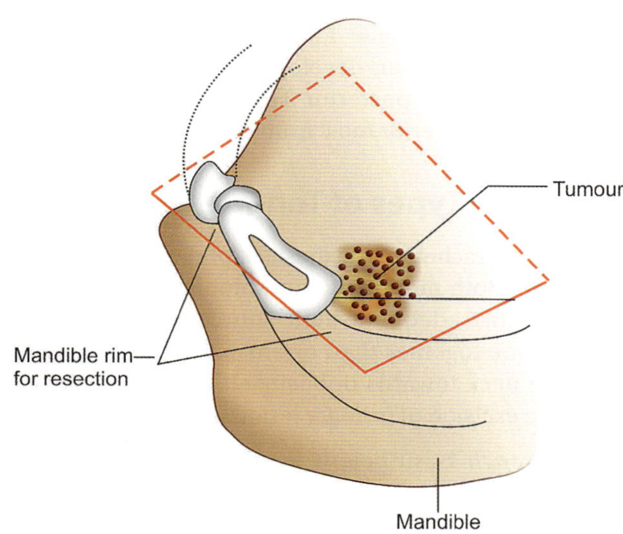

Fig. 14-74: Extent of removal in mandible rim resection.

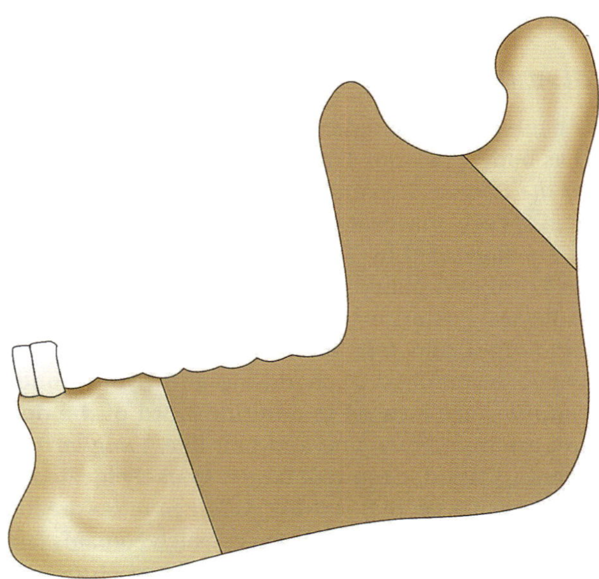

Fig. 14-77: Extent of removal in partial mandibulectomy.

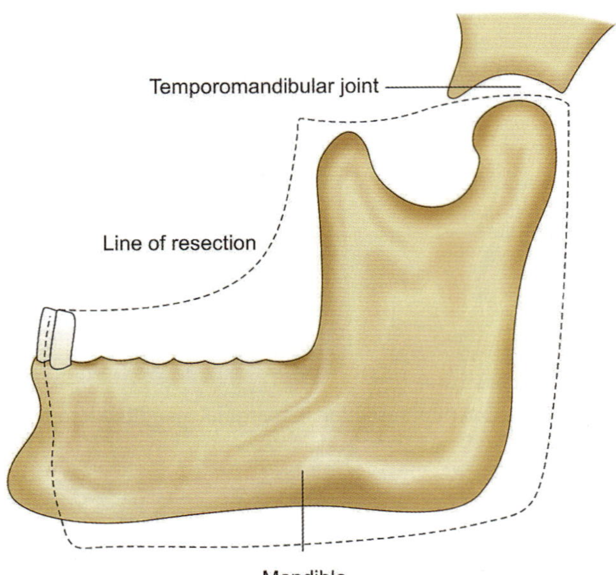

Fig. 14-78: Extent of resection in hemimandibulectomy.

T_1 and T_2 lesions are treated with wide excision with 2 cm clearance with frozen section biopsy confirmation. Lesion deeper than 4 mm needs elective neck node dissection—N_0. Transoral/lip split/mandibulotomy/visor approaches are used. Reconstruction is done using radial forearm flap.

T_3 or T_4 lesions when treated surgically needs a well-planned approach. *Primary tumour* is approached with lip split and anterior stair step mandibulotomy. Wide excision with 2 cm clearance is done. If bone margin is involved marginal mandibulectomy is done. Cut mandible is distracted to expose the area widely. Hypoglossal nerve visualised in the deeper plane entering the tongue is preserved. Lingual artery is visualised and doubly ligated. Frozen section biopsy should be done for clearance confirmation. *Supraomohyoid neck dissection* one side or both in N_0 nodes is done and frozen section biopsy should be done for nodes. If positive, RND should be done. *Tracheostomy is essential* in all patients. *Nasogastric tube insertion* is also essential for later feeding purpose. Often *percutaneous gastrostomy,* if needed, should be done.

Approach to Tongue Cancers

Surgical Anatomy

Tongue is a muscular, glandular, vascular flat organ. Anterior 2/3rd is termed as body; posterior 1/3rd is base/root. Superior surface *is dorsum of the tongue.* It is an essential organ of taste. Tongue is important in speech, mastication and swallowing. Oral and pharyngeal parts are separated by V-shaped sulcus terminalis. Oral part is anterior 2/3rd and pharyngeal part is posterior third which is lymphoid tissue. Posterior tongue is connected to epiglottis by median and right and left lateral glossoepiglottic folds. Root of the tongue is attached to mandible and hyoid bone below. *Filiform papillae* are located in anterior 2/3rd of the dorsum of tongue and are numerous, fine and hair like. *Fungiform papillae* are mushroom shaped, deep red, larger, sparsely located near the tip of the tongue. Large, red, leaf-like *foliate papillae* are located in posterior third of tongue on lateral aspect which contains taste buds. *Circumvallate papillae* are 8–12 in number, mushroom shaped, arranged in large V-shaped row near posterior third of the dorsum tongue and contains plenty of taste buds. Small circular opening just posterior to this V row in the midline is called as *foramen caecum* which is the remnant of thyroglossal duct. Shallow groove just behind the circumvallate papilla on either sides of the foramen caecum is called as *terminal sulcus.* Numerous mucin glands and lymph follicles in the posterior third of the dorsum of tongue is called as lingual tonsil. *Posterior third of the tongue is difficult to inspect;* it needs head light, and spatula. It is better felt than seen. *Ventral surface* is smooth, has a median fold, *frenulum linguae* and deep lingual veins on either side. *Lingual frenulum* is attached about 10–15 mm below the mandibular central incisor tooth.

There are four extrinsic and four intrinsic *muscles of the tongue.* Extrinsic muscles are—genioglossus, hyoglossus, styloglossus, palatoglossus; intrinsic muscles are—superior longitudinal, inferior longitudinal, transverse, and vertical. Genioglossus is fan-shaped muscle arising from the genial tubercle of the mandible. It fans out and backwards. Upper fibres are inserted to tip; middle to dorsum of tongue; lower to hyoid bone. Upper fibres retract the tip; middle fibres depress the tongue; lower fibres by pulling the posterior part of the tongue forward helps in protruding the tongue.

Arterial supply is from lingual artery, a branch of ECA. Tonsillar and ascending pharyngeal arteries supply root of the tongue. Two venae commitantes accompany the lingual artery; one accompanies the hypoglossal nerve. Deep lingual vein is seen on the ventral surface of the tongue. All these veins join together at posterior border of the hyoglossus below the hypoglossal nerve to form lingual vein which enters either the common facial vein or IJV.

Lymphatic drainage—tip is to submental nodes; remaining anterior part to submandibular lymph glands; posterior third to jugulo-omohyoid nodes. Lymphatics in the midline of the tongue freely cross and communicate each other.

Nerve supply—all intrinsic and extrinsic muscles are supplied by hypoglossal nerve except palatoglossus which is supplied by cranial root of accessory nerve through pharyngeal plexus. Lingual nerve, a branch of mandibular nerve supplies general sensation and chorda tympani for taste of the anterior 2/3rd of the tongue except vallate papillae; glossopharyngeal nerve supplies general and taste sensation of posterior third of the tongue; internal laryngeal nerve of vagus supplies posterior most part of the tongue. Taste buds are numerous on the sides of vallate papillae, foliate papillae and posterior third of the tongue; are very less/sparse in fungiform papillae, soft palate, epiglottis, pharynx; are absent in mid-dorsal region of the oral part of the tongue.

Anterior 2/3rd of the tongue develops from two lingual swellings and one tuberculum impar, developed from first branchial arch (lingual nerve supply); posterior 1/3rd from 3rd arch (glossopharyngeal nerve); posterior most from 4th arch (vagus nerve).

Principles and Types of Tongue Cancer Surgery

Anaesthesia: Nasotracheal anaesthesia is preferred. Throat packing should be done. Both monopolar and bipolar cautery and proper suction apparatus, adequate light source are needed. If neck dissection is done together then extension of the neck is needed. Turning of the neck towards opposite side of the RND/MRND is done after wide excision of primary lesion.

Intraoral approach is sufficient for small lesions. Lip split or mandibulotomy may be needed for larger and extensive tumour. Total glossectomy even though possible, it is very morbid and distressing surgery to the patient and so usually not practiced unless proper reconstruction is planned and implemented including voice restoration, and swallowing. Composite excision, commando operation requires tracheostomy, nasogastric intubation, often gastrostomy for feeding purpose.

Small lesion less than 1 cm in the lateral margin is excised widely with 1 cm clearance. Margin and depth clearance should be confirmed by frozen section. Defect is closed *vertically primarily* using 3-zero vicryl or chromic catgut continuous locking sutures or interrupted sutures. Cautery is used for excision. Laser may be used if available. *Vertical closure* maintains the mobility well. *Horizontal closure* is technically easier and practiced by many surgeons but causes tethering of the dorsum of tongue to the floor of mouth restricting the mobility. Interrupted sutures are better as continuous sutures may get torn off from the tissue. Supraomohyoid dissection is added (N_0) in all tongue cancers as they are usually aggressive **(Figs. 14-79 and 14-80)**.

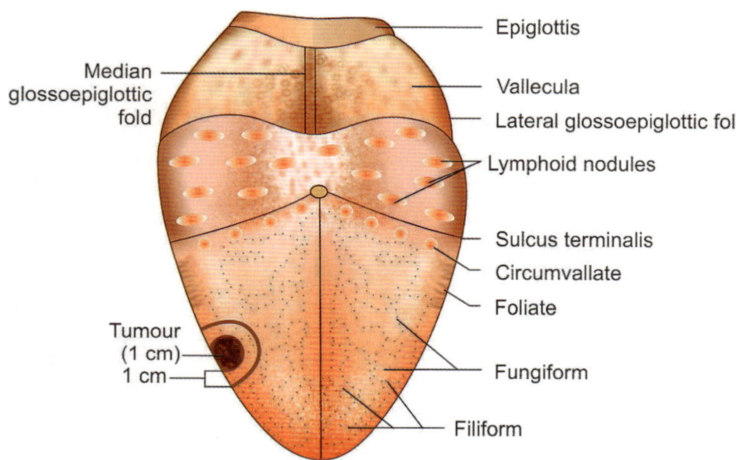

Fig. 14-79: Wide excision of the tongue lesion lesser than 1 cm.

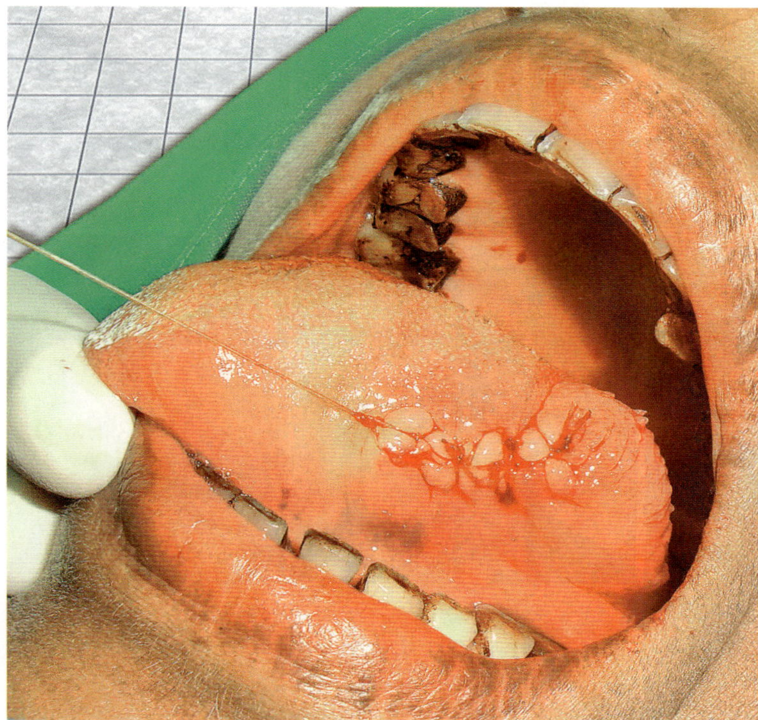

Fig. 14-80: Suturing of the raw area can also be done after excising the lesion.

Lesion in the lateral margin of size 1–2 cm is treated with partial glossectomy with 2 cm clearance. Defect can be sutured primarily or raw area can be left to granulate on its own. Split skin grafting to cover the defect can be done. Supraomohyoid dissection is done for N_0 lesion **(Figs. 14-81 and 14-82)**.

Tumour larger than 2 cm in the lateral margin is treated by hemiglossectomy where anterior 2/3rd of the tongue in front of the sulcus terminalis and lateral to midline one side is removed using cautery. Lingual vessels should be doubly ligated using vicryl or monocryl. Reconstruction is done by cheek flap or simply rotating remaining half of the tongue (retained) over the defect. It gives good range of movements of the tongue. Supraomohyoid dissection (N_0) or MRND I/RND are done if nodes are positive **(Fig. 14-83)**.

If mandible is involved hemimandibulectomy and RND is done along with hemiglossectomy which is often called as *commandos operation*.

Composite resection of the tongue cancer (*Commando operation*) with resection of the mandible with RND is done using lip split incision after elevating the skin flaps above.

Dorsal tongue cancer is not common. It is treated by sagittal resection and closed primarily.

Posterior third of the tongue is approached through lip split and anterior mandibulotomy approach.

Pull through visor flap approach to the tongue is another approach for deep rooted tumour. It needs preliminary tracheostomy, nasogastric intubation, gastrostomy for feeding. Bilateral neck dissection is done. One side RND other side MRND II with retaining IJV is done. Side where IJV should be retained is decided prior and should be operated first. A visor flap of skin is elevated up to the inferior margin of the mandible. Mucosa on the uninvolved side of floor of the mouth is incised and extended to involved tongue side with 2 cm margin. Mylohyoid muscle is cut and anterior and lateral cuts are communicated. Tongue with tumour is delivered under the mandible through an external neck wound. Lesion is excised with 2 cm clearance taking care of clearance in depth. Reconstruction is essential using radial forearm and PMMF flaps. Postoperative speech therapy and training for swallowing are needed.

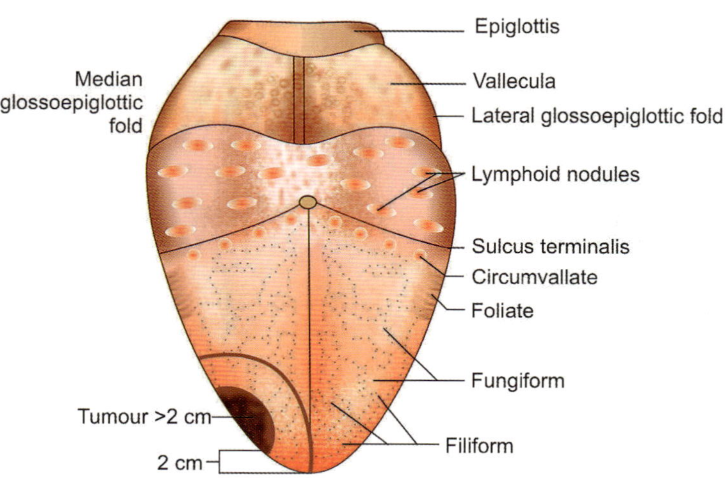

Fig. 14-81: Partial glossectomy is done if lesion is 1–2 cm in size over the lateral margin.

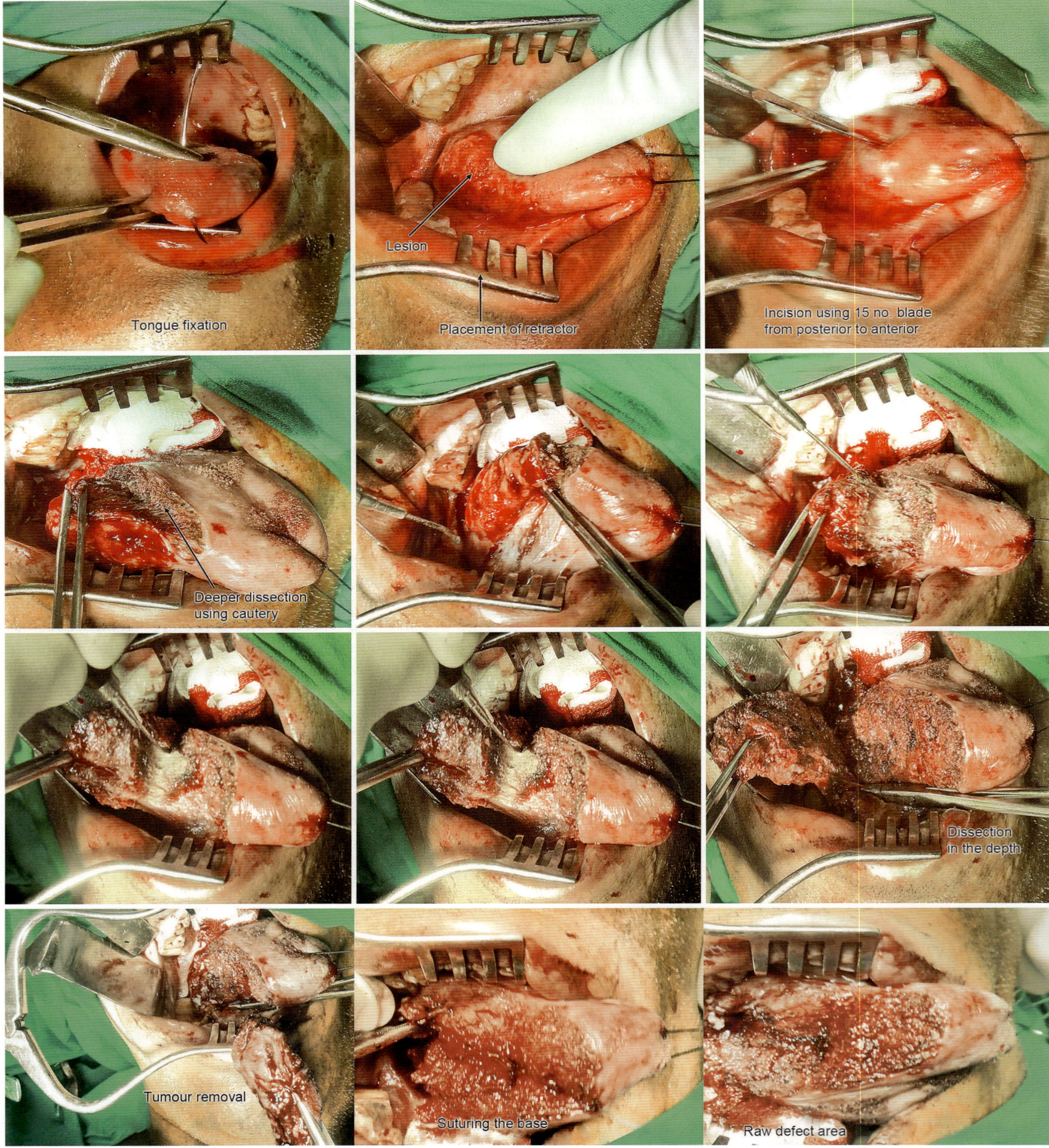
Tongue fixation
Lesion
Placement of retractor
Incision using 15 no. blade
from posterior to anterior
Deeper dissection
using cautery
Dissection
in the depth
Tumour removal
Suturing the base
Raw defect area

Figs. 14-82(1)

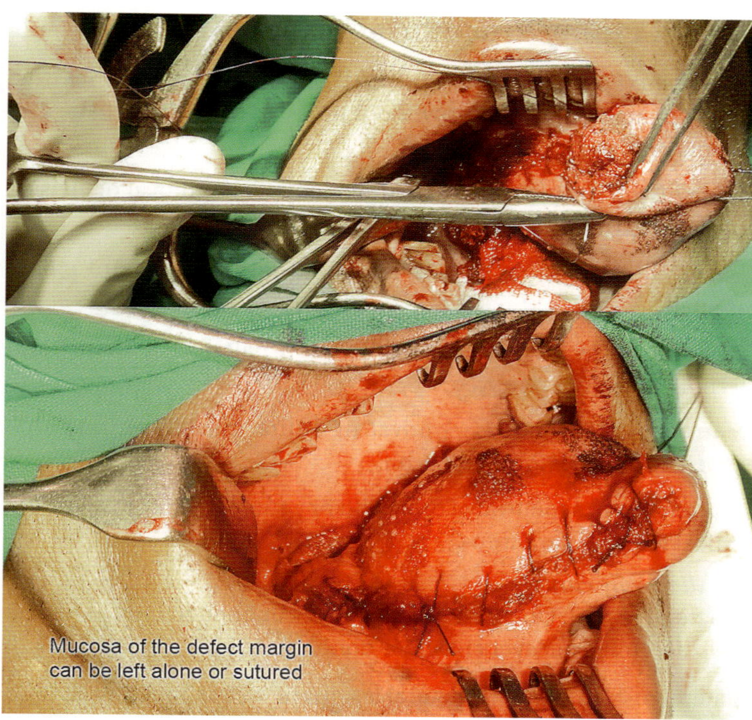

Fig. 14-82(2)

Figs. 14-82(1 and 2): Partial glossectomy technique.

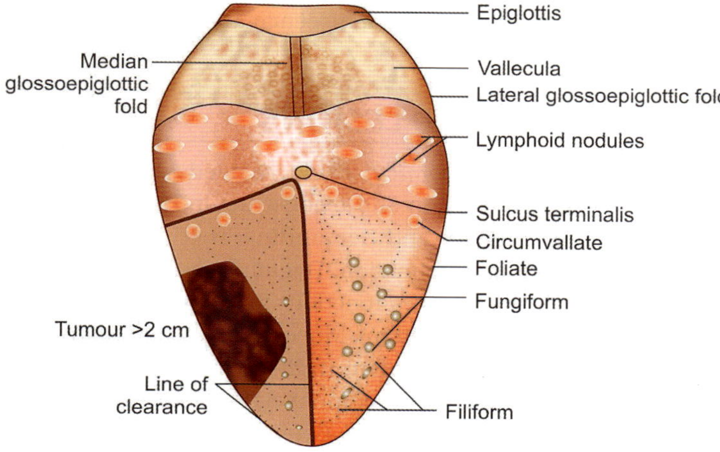

Fig. 14-83: Hemiglossectomy is done if lesion is more than 2 cm in lateral margin.

Approach to Hard Palate Cancers

Surgical Anatomy

Roof of the mouth is formed by hard palate and soft palate. *Hard palate* is firm anterior part of the roof of the mouth ending opposite 3rd molar anterior to fovea palatine. *Soft palate* is mobile posterior part of roof of the mouth. Junction between hard and soft palate is called as *vibrating line*. Small rounded elevation of tissue in the midline behind the central incisors is called as *nasopalatine papilla* which is over incisive foramen through which nasopalatine nerve traverses to supply anterior hard palate. Slightly elevated central line is called as *palatine raphe*. Here mucosa is firmly adherent to underneath periosteum without any fat and so it is harder area of hard palate. Sides of hard palate contain fat and minor salivary glands (there are around 350 minor salivary glands in posterior hard palate). Series of elevations in hard palate are called as *palatine rugae* useful for food positioning and aiding tongue to produce specific sounds. Hard palate is partition between nasal and oral cavity. Anterior 2/3rd is formed by palatine process of maxillae; posterior 1/3rd is by horizontal plates of palatine bones. Anterolateral margins continue with alveolar arches and gums. Posterior margin attaches to soft palate.

Soft palate is redder than hard palate due to its vascularity. There is no bone in soft palate behind vibrating line. Soft palate vibrates or moves. It is mobile muscular fold. It has got anterior and posterior surfaces, superior and inferior margins. Uvula is small fleshy part projecting from centre of the posterior margin of the soft palate. Pair of pits on either side of the centre of the soft palate just behind the vibrating line is called as *fovea palatini* to which palatine mucous glands opens. Side of the uvula has got anterior and posterior folds. Anterior palatoglossal arch contains palatoglossus muscle which ends as anterior pillar of fauces (in front of tonsils). Posterior palatopharyngeal arch contains palatopharyngeus muscle which ends as posterior pillar of fauces (behind tonsils). Soft palate contains mucous glands and taste buds. Soft palate contains following muscles—tensor veli palati; levator veli palati; musculus uvulae; palatoglossus; palatopharyngeus. All muscles except tensor palati are supplied through pharyngeal plexus by cranial part of accessory nerve; tensor palati is supplied by the mandibular nerve. General sensory nerves are derived from middle and posterior palatine nerves which are branches of maxillary nerve and from glossopharyngeal nerve. Gustatory special sensations are carried through lesser palatine nerve → greater petrosal nerve → geniculate ganglion of facial nerve → nucleus of solitary tract. Secretomotor fibres are derived from superior salivatory nucleus through greater palatine nerve and lesser palatine nerves. Paralysis of the soft palate (vagus nerve lesions) causes nasal regurgitation of liquids, nasal twang in voice and flattening of palatal arch.

Maxillectomy

Surgical Anatomy

Maxilla is the 2nd largest bone of the face (after mandible). Two maxillae form upper jaw with formation of face, nose, mouth, orbit infratemporal and pterygopalatine fossae. Maxilla has got a body and 4 processes—frontal, zygomatic, alveolar and palatine. Body is pyramidal in shape with base directed medially towards nasal surface and apex directed laterally at zygomatic process. Anterior surface contains incisive fossa and canine fossa. Above the canine fossa there is infraorbital foramen with infraorbital vessels and nerve. Posterior surface forms the anterior wall of the infratemporal fossa. Posterior superior alveolar nerve and vessels are near the centre of the surface. Posteroinferiorly rounded maxillary tuberosity articulates with pyramidal process of the palatine bone. Maxillary tuberosity gives origin to superficial head of medial pterygoid. Anterior wall of the pterygopalatine fossa is above the maxillary tuberosity and is grooved for maxillary nerve. Superior surface forms the floor of the orbit; its medial border forms nasolacrimal canal with lacrimal bone; its medial border articulates with lacrimal, labyrinth of ethmoid, orbital process of palatine bone; superior surface has got infraorbital groove, canal and foramen to transmit infraorbital nerve and vessels. Medial surface forms lateral wall of the nose; posterosuperiorly there is hiatus for maxillary sinus. Above the hiatus parts of ethmoidal and lacrimal air sinuses are present. Inferior nasal meatus is below the hiatus. Medial surface below the hiatus articulates with perpendicular plate of palatine bone forming greater palatine canal for greater palatine vessels and anterior, middle and posterior palatine nerves. Nasolacrimal groove is present in front of the hiatus to form nasolacrimal canal with the lacrimal bone and inferior nasal concha to transmit nasolacrimal duct to the inferior meatus of the nose. The pyramidal shaped large cavity of 3.5 × 3.5 × 2.5 cm dimension, the maxillary sinus (maxillary antrum) has its base medially and apex laterally. Maxillary sinus opens into the middle nasal meatus with two openings. Roof is formed by the floor of the orbit; floor is formed by alveolar process of maxilla. Floor has got conical elevations by roots of upper molar and premolar teeth. Root of canine tooth projects into the anterolateral wall. Maxilla articulates above to nasal, frontal and lacrimal bones; medially to ethmoid, inferior nasal concha, vomer, palatine bones and opposite maxilla; laterally to zygomatic bone. Maxilla ossifies in membrane from 3 centres—one for maxilla just above the canine fossa during 6th week of intrauterine life; one of the two for premaxilla arise just above the incisive fossa during 7th week of intrauterine life and another at ventral margin of nasal septum during 10th week. Mucosa of the maxillary sinus is lined by squamous epithelium.

Procedure (Fig. 14-84)

Endotracheal general anaesthesia is used. Weber-Ferguson incision is made. Entire thickness of upper lip, cheek and lower eyelid is elevated as a lateral flap. The periosteum on the floor of the orbit is elevated. Orbital contents are protected by placing a spatula between the periosteum and the bone. Ala of the nostril is drawn medially after separating from the bone. Nasal process of maxilla is divided at its junction with the nasal bone. Later it is separated from the lacrimal and ethmoid bones towards inferior orbital fissure. After dividing zygomatic bone, mouth is widely opened with a gag. Alveolus and hard palate are divided in midline and then from pterygoid process. Maxillary artery and nerve are cut; soft tissues are divided. Gauze pack is placed. Cheek flap is placed on the pack and sutured. Often ligation of external carotid artery in continuity is needed to prevent haemorrhage. In olden days, 7 days prior to surgery ECA used to be ligated. With proper prosthesis and obturator cosmetically it sounds good.

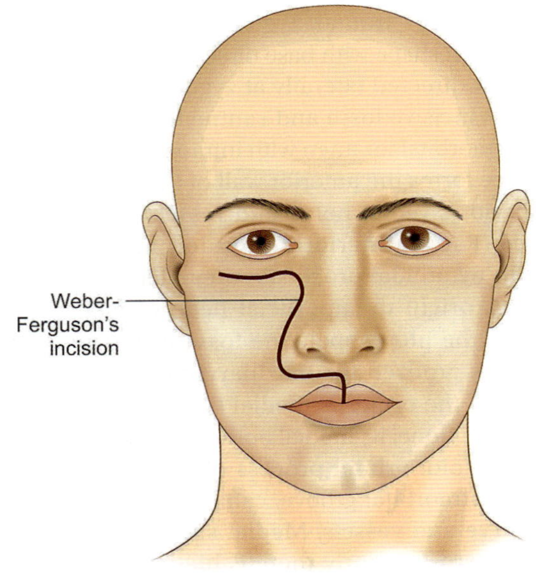

Fig. 14-84: Weber-Ferguson incision for maxillectomy.

Maxillectomy Procedure—Types

Partial maxillectomy: It is removal of portions of maxilla, incisive bone, palatine bone with or without portions of the zygomatic and lacrimal bones.

Premaxillectomy: It is unilateral or bilateral with removal of incisive bone and perhaps rostral maxilla.

Central maxillectomy: Here maxilla and portions of hard palate resected.

Caudal maxillectomy: Here maxilla, hard palate, zygomatic, and lacrimal bones are removed.

Hemimaxillectomy: It is removal of entire maxilla on one side extending dorsally to ventral orbit.

Orbitectomy: It is removal of orbit with or without caudal maxilla and vertical mandibular ramus.

Maxillectomy can be:

Unilateral rostral: Done when lesions are confined to hard palate on one side. Here one layer closure is done.

Bilateral rostral: Done in bilateral lesions of rostral hard palate.

Lateral: Done in laterally placed midmaxillary lesions; it needs viable buccal mucosa for closure of flap.

Bilateral: Done in bilateral palatine lesions. Defect closure needs formal reconstruction. Closure dehiscence and oronasal fistula is common.

SURGERY FOR LIP LESIONS

Lip being a *complex anatomical structure* needs comprehensive approach to excise the lesion and reconstruct it. Upper lip reconstruction is *more difficult* and demanding as it *involves* in oral competence, speech and phonation. Dynamically upper and lower lips are independent. Lower lip functions in many axes. Thickness, location, size of the lip is important. Mucosa, muscle and skin should be approximated separately as an individual layer. Defect <30% can be closed with local advancement flaps; defects >60% need complicated complex approaches. Grafting, local flaps, regional flaps, free flaps are the options. Grafting is not ideal as it creates scarring and poor cosmesis. Contracture, microstomia, adynamic flap in relation to dynamic flap, often need of a second surgery like reconstruction of the commissure are the *problems*.

Simple cyst of the lip derived from mucus gland is excised under local anaesthesia (xylocaine without adrenaline) and sutured primarily using fine absorbable sutures either continuously or intermittently **(Fig. 14-85)**.

Surgical Anatomy of Lip

Lip is the area between the nasolabial folds from the gingivolabial sulcus to the labiomental fold. Vermilion is coverings of lip margin. Its wet part comes into contact with opposite lip; dry part is external lip. Orbicularis oris which origins from modiolus and inserts to philtrum maintains the oral competence. Its horizontal fibres compress the lip; oblique one everts the lip. Elevation of the upper lip is achieved by levator labii superioris, zygomaticus major and levator anguli oris. Lower lip depression is brought about by depressor labii inferioris; movement of commissure below and lateral is brought

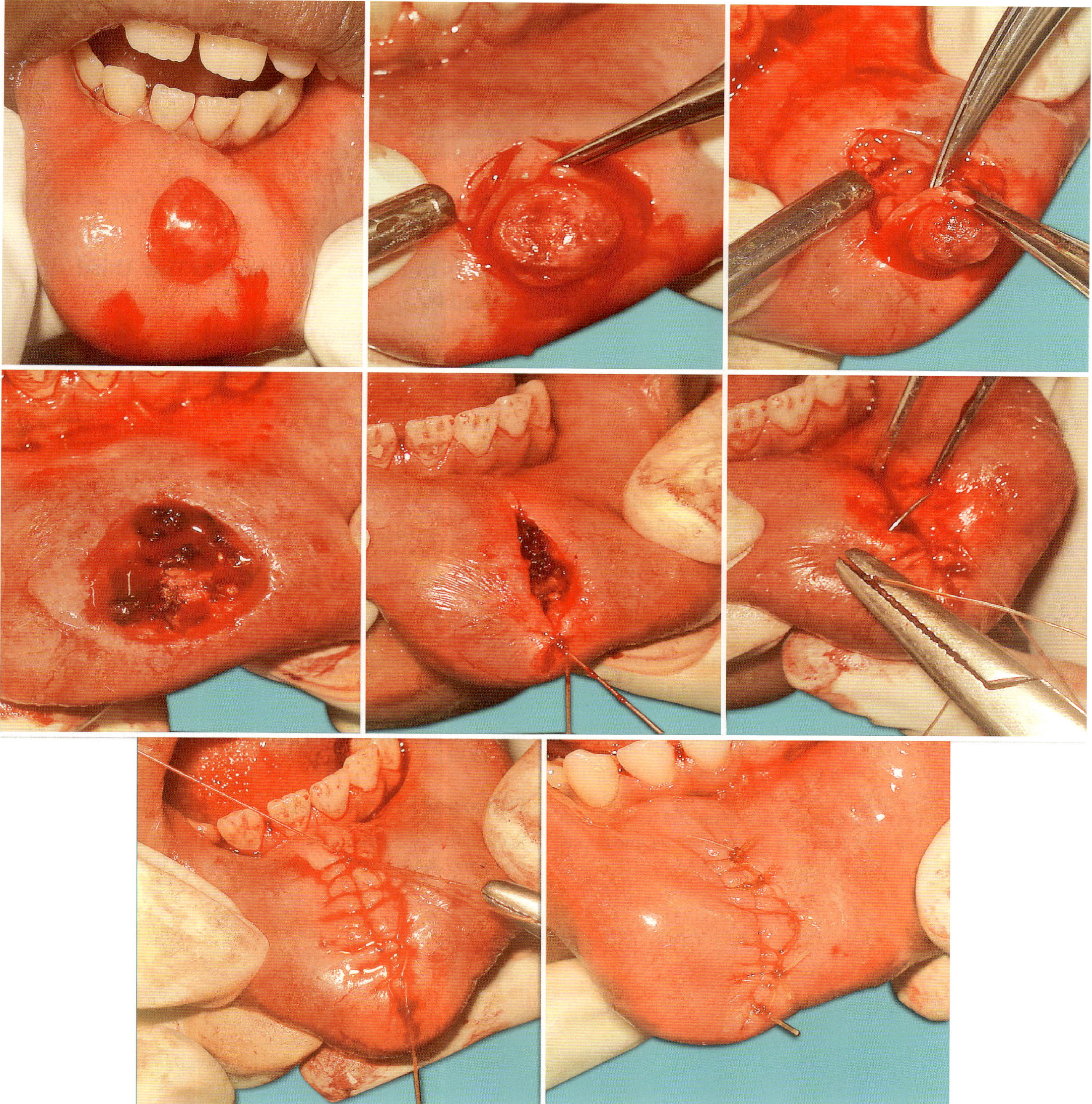

Fig. 14-85: Simple cyst in the lip is excised under local anaesthesia and sutured primarily.

about by depressor anguli oris. Central lip is elevated by mentalis. Muscles around mouth are—orbicularis oris, levator labii superioris, zygomaticus major and minor, levator anguli oris, depressor anguli oris, depressor labii inferioris, mentalis, risorius and buccinators. Motor supply of orbicularis oris is by facial nerve—buccal branch. Depressors are supplied by marginal mandibular branch. Sensory supply of upper lip is infraorbital nerve a branch of ophthalmic division of trigeminal nerve, lower lip is by mental nerve, a branch of mandibular division of trigeminal nerve. Blood supply of lip is by superior and inferior labial arteries, branches of facial artery. Upper and lateral parts of lower lip drain into submandibular lymph nodes; central lower lip drains to submental lymph nodes **(Fig. 14-86)**.

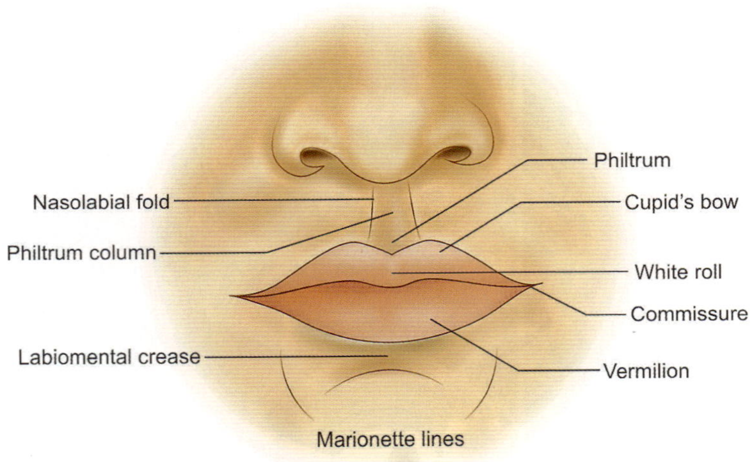

Fig. 14-86: Surgical anatomy of the lip.

Principles in lip surgeries are—restoration of oral competence to achieve control of secretions, drinking, eating and speech; cosmetic achievement of lip; achieving good muscular function; scar placement; prevention of microstomia; creating adequate labial buccal sulcus to prevent drooling. It is impossible to achieve perfect normal lip in texture. Only optimum lip can be achieved by reconstruction.

Indications for lip reconstruction are—carcinoma of lip after wide excision; trauma; dog bite; vasculitis; septic necrosis of lip; congenital anomaly.

Anaesthesia for lip surgery—general or local field block can be used. Upper lip is entirely anaesthetized using bilateral infraorbital nerve block using 26 G needle at a point lateral to alar base and medial to nalolabial fold 7 mm below the infraorbital margin of the medial limbus. This nerve can also be blocked intraorally. Lower lip can be anaesthetised by regional block of mental nerve. Local anaesthetic agent is infiltrated 1 cm lateral to the canines into buccal sulcus.

Defect Less Than One-third of the Lip

Primary Closure

Excision of lower lip up to 1/3rd is sutured primarily without causing any microstomia. Vermilion border of the lip should be kept in opposition. Lip is sutured in layers; deeper layer with 3-zero vicryl; outer layer with 3-zero polypropylene sutures. It is used in upper lip lateral defect and lower lip defects **(Fig. 14-87)**.

Skin grafting, ear composite graft and Abbe flaps are used for upper lip central defects less than 1/3rd.

Defects between One-third to Two-third of the Lip

Here primary closure will cause microstomia, speech, eating and drinking problems. So it should be avoided.

In the upper lip central defect skin grafting, composite graft of ear, Abbe flap, perialar crescent, cheek advancement flaps are used. *In the upper lip lateral defect* Abbe-Estlander flap, perialar crescent, cheek advancement flap, nasolabial flap, reverse Karpandzic flaps are used.

In the lower lip central defect Abbe flap, Schuchardt flap, Webster flaps are used. *Lower lip lateral defect* is covered with Estlander flap, Gillies flap, Karapandzic flap, or McGregor flaps **(Fig. 14-88)**.

Defect More than Two-third of Lip

In upper lip defect: Abbe-Estlander with perialar crescent, cheek advancement flap; nasolabial flap; reverse Karapandzic flap; forehead flap; deltopectoral flap; radial forearm free flap are used **(Fig. 14-89)**.

In lower lip defect: Abbe-Estlander flap, Webster flap; bilateral Gilles flap; deltopectoral or radial forearm flaps are used **(Figs. 14-90 and 14-91)**.

Different Procedures

Estlander's (Abbe-Estlander's) rotation flap of upper lip is based on upper labial artery. It is used when defect is less than half of lip

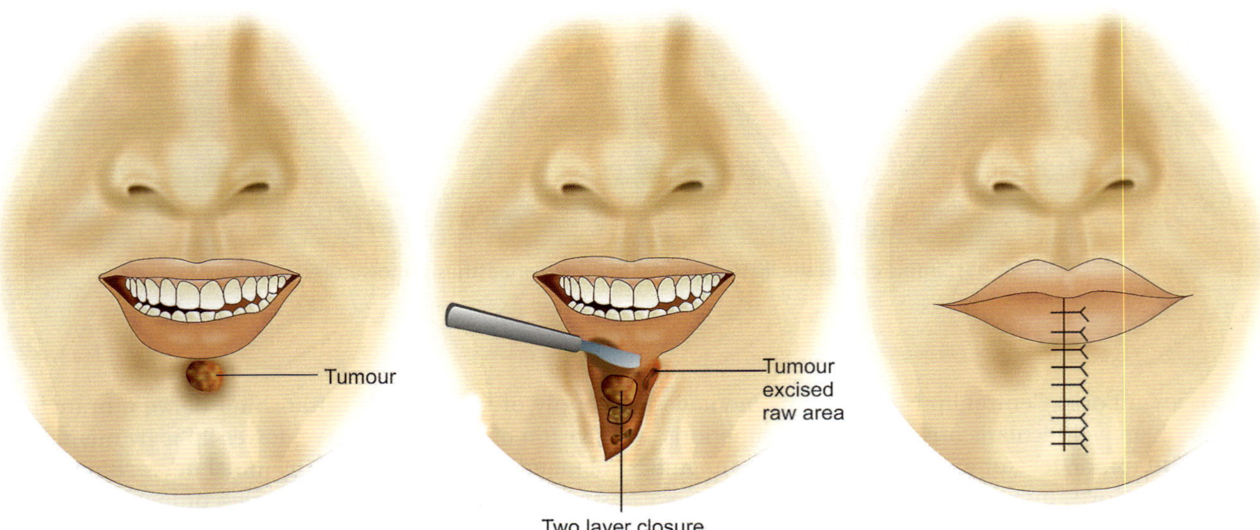

Fig. 14-87: Primary closure of the defect in the lip is possible when defect is less than 1/3rd.

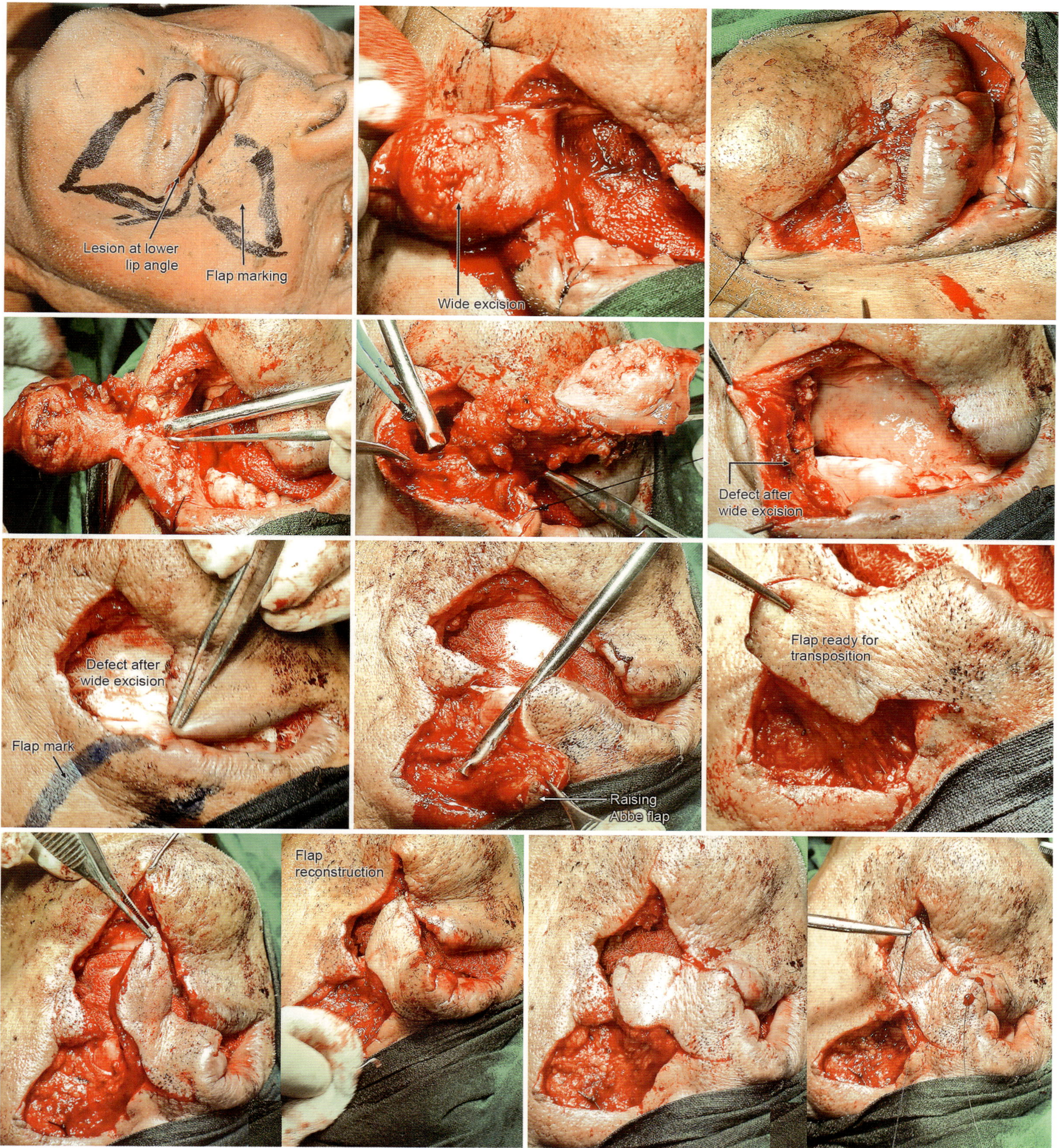
Lesion at lower
lip angle
Flap marking
Wide excision
Defect after
wide excision
Defect after
wide excision
Flap mark
Raising
Abbe flap
Flap ready for
transposition
Flap
reconstruction

Figs. 14-88(1)

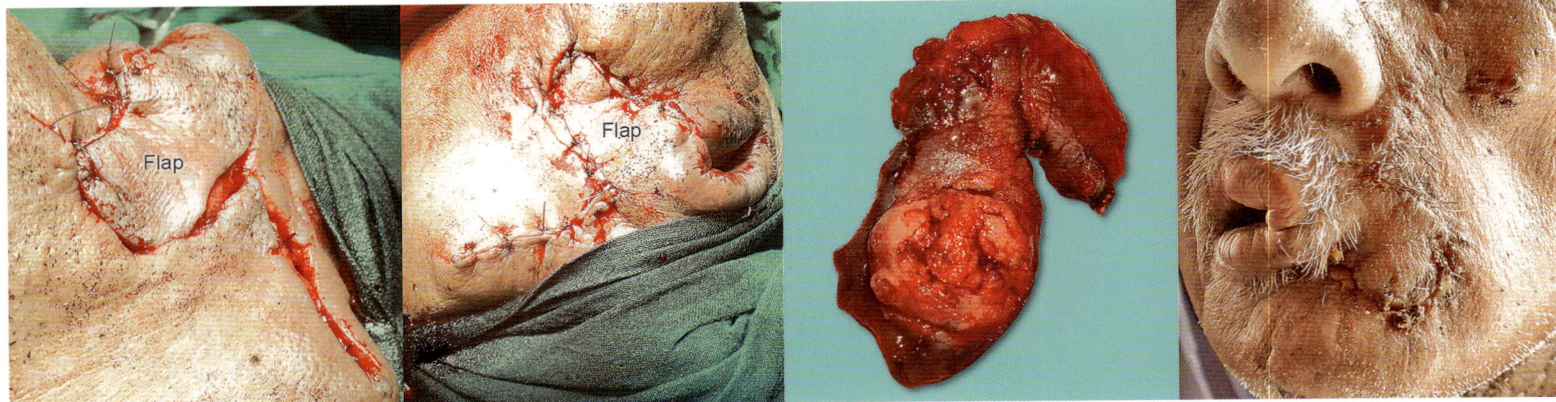

Figs. 14-88(2)

Figs. 14-88(1 and 2): Abbe-Estlander flap—reconstruction of the defect in the lip after wide excision. Here 2nd stage base division is not done.

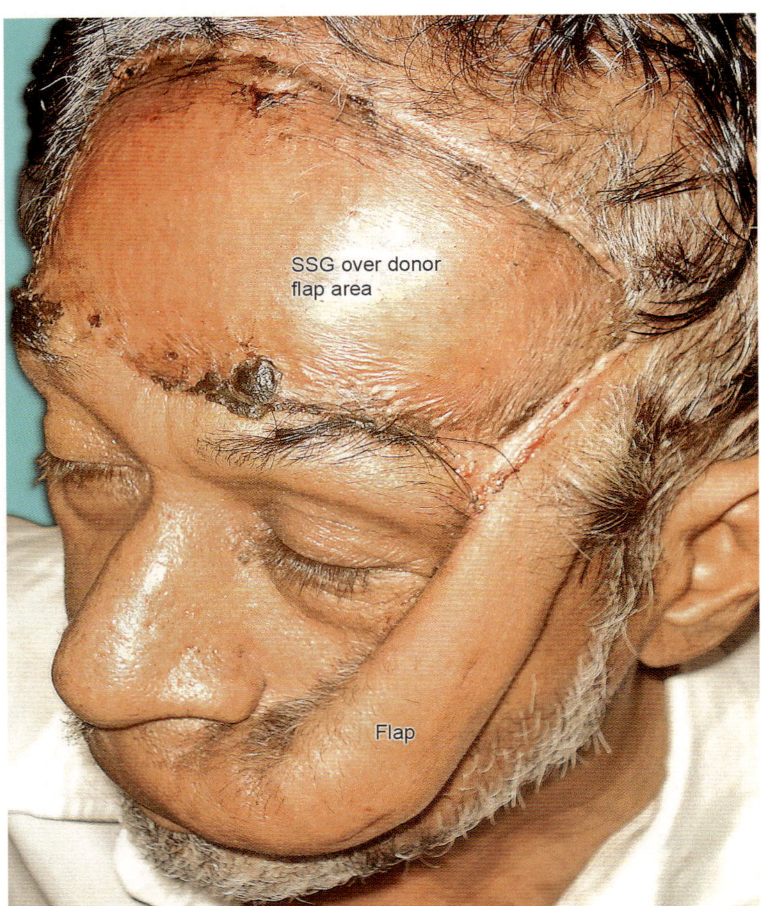

Fig. 14-89: Forehead flap can be used for defect after excision of upper lip lesion of more than 2/3rd in size.

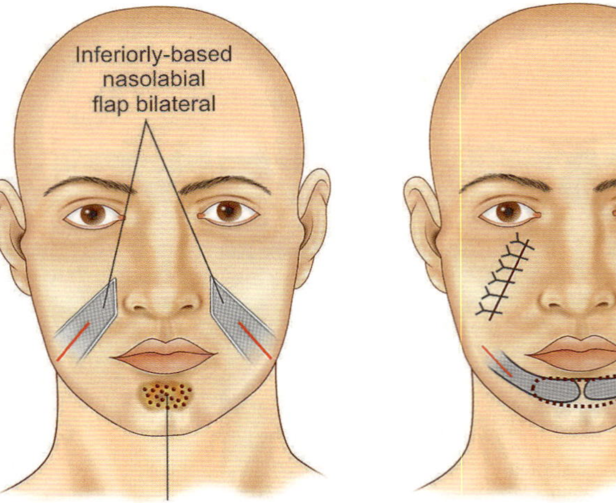

Fig. 14-90: Nasolabial flap can be used in large central defect.

but more than 1/3rd. It is done in lateral lip defects, upper or lower, involving commissure. Flap is denervated and so sensation is absent and drooling of saliva is possible **(Fig. 14-92)**.

Frie's modified Bernard facial flap is done using lateral facial flaps. It is used when defect is more than ½ of lip, midline defect and for commissure reconstruction. Two triangles are excised and cheek flap is rotated and advanced. Vermilion is constructed using advancement of oral mucosa **(Fig. 14-93)**.

Different microvascular flaps are used to cover the defect. Free radial artery flap also can be used.

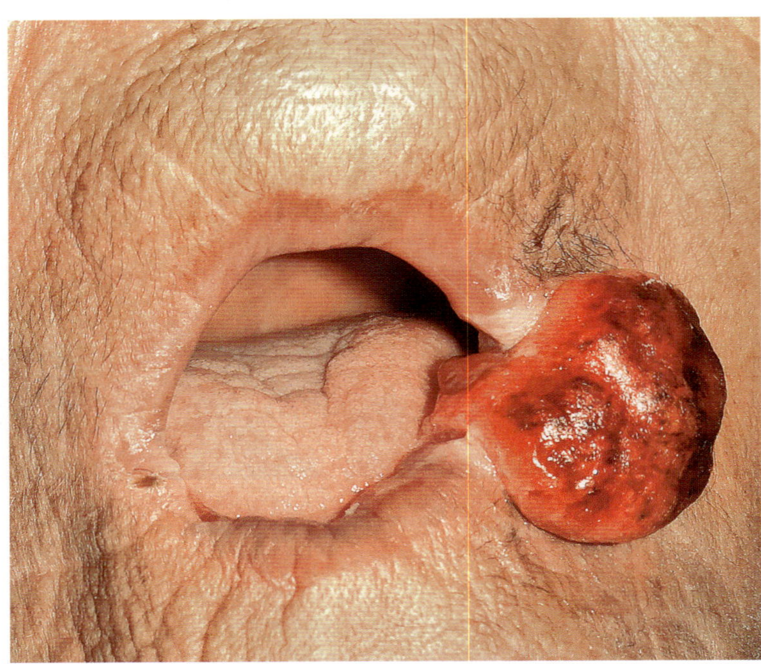

Fig. 14-91A

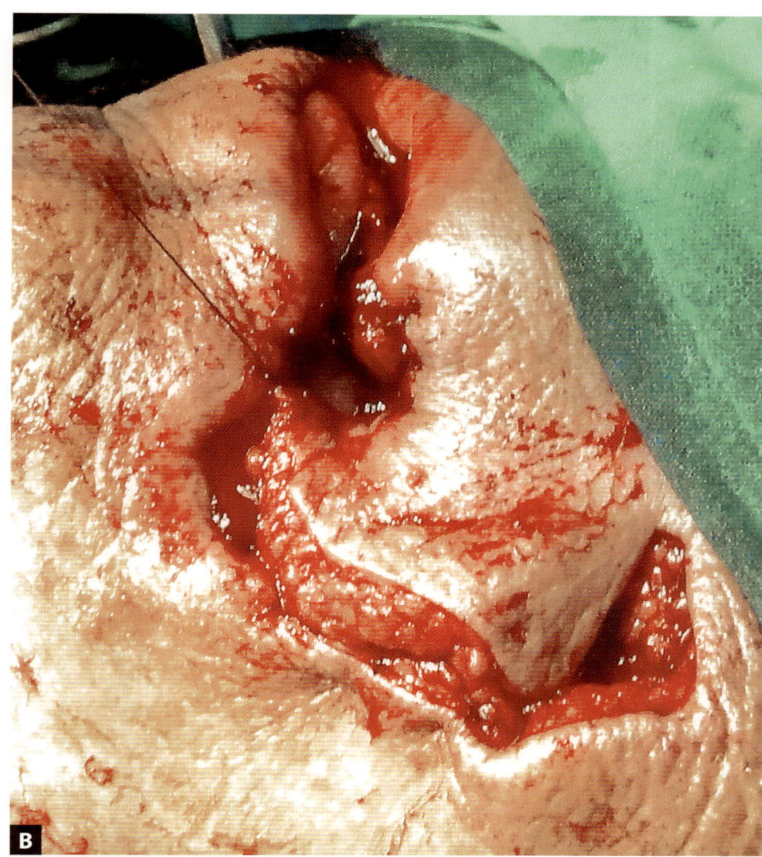

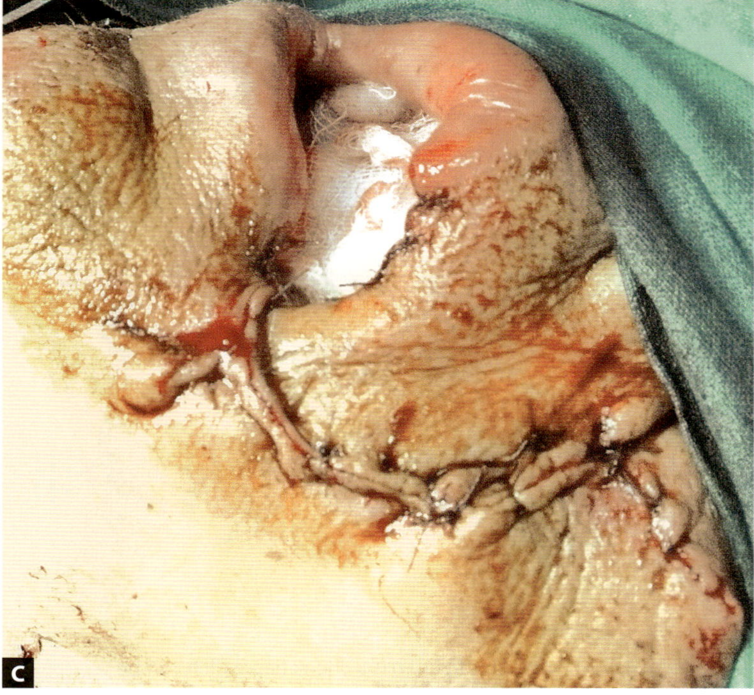

Figs. 14-91B and C
Figs. 14-91A to C: Abbe-Estlander flap.

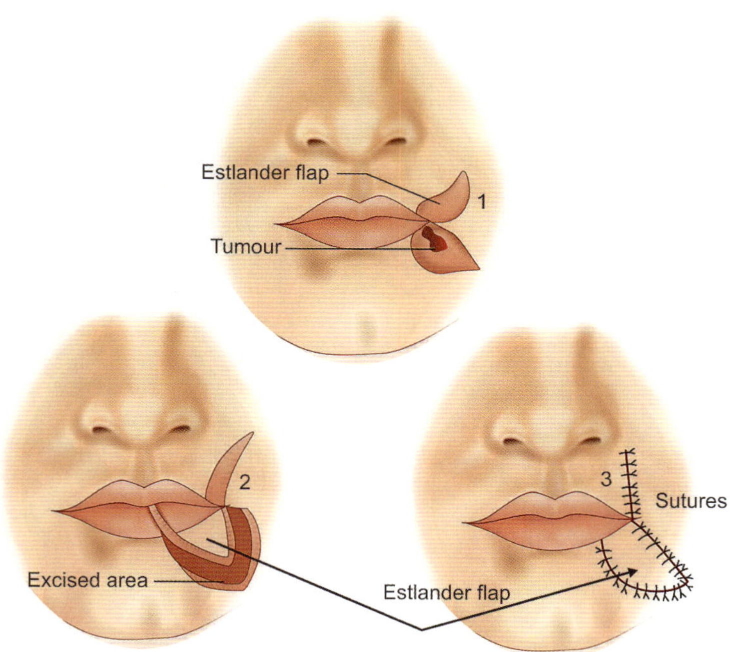

Fig. 14-92: Abbe-Estlander flap for lateral defects in the lip.

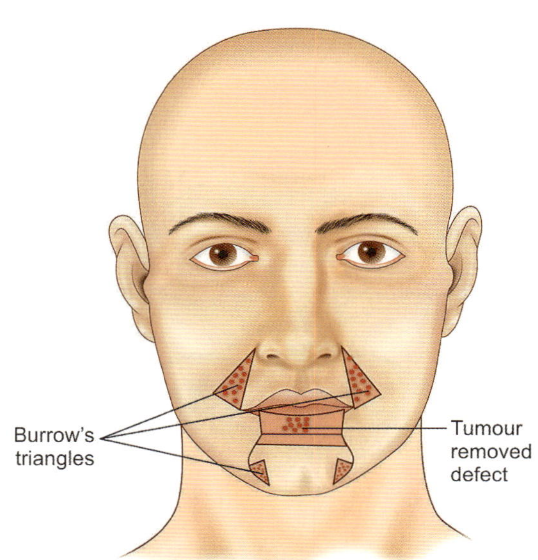

Fig. 14-93: Bernard lateral flaps for central defect.

Nasolabial flap is used when defect is more than ½ of lip and lateral or defect is in the floor of the mouth.

Cheek flap can be rotated when lesion is near the angle of the mouth.

Abbe flap (switch flap) is used in upper/lower lip lesion—central defect. It is taken from lower/upper lip with inferior/superior labial artery as base. It is transfer of myocutaneous lower/upper lip to upper/lower lip in two staged technique. In first stage myocutaneous full thickness lip flap is elevated with labial artery pedicle to suture into the upper/lower lip defect. Pedicle is divided after 2–3 weeks and rotation is completed (switch) with suturing of the further flap **(Fig. 14-94)**.

"W' flap plasty—It is done for lower lip middle tumour which is less than 1/3rd of the lip **(Fig. 14-95)**.

Gillies fan flap—It is a cheek flap usually bilateral but can be unilateral. Incision is full thickness around commissures extending into nasolabial fold and upper lip up to upper lip vermilion border. Flap which is based on labial vessels is advanced towards the defect. Vermilion is reconstructed with tongue mucosal flap which is divided in 3 weeks. Flap is denervated and so sensation is absent and drooling of saliva is possible **(Fig. 14-96)**.

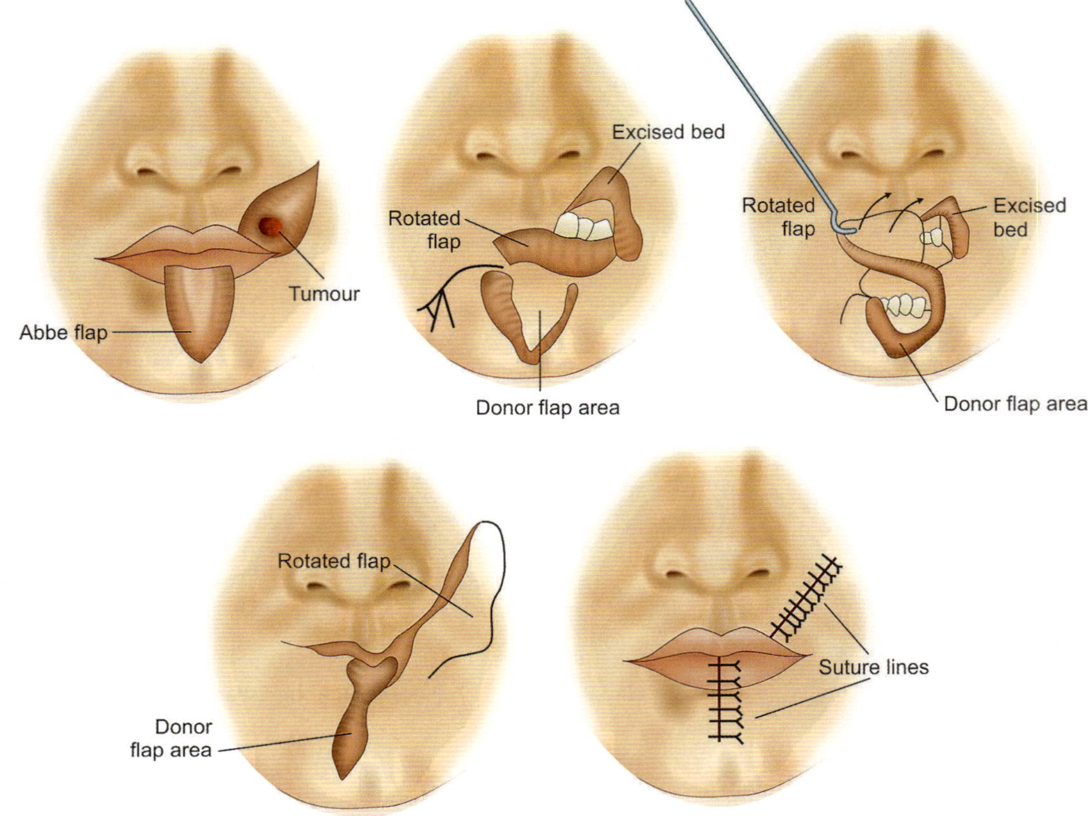

Fig. 14-94: Abbe switch flap.

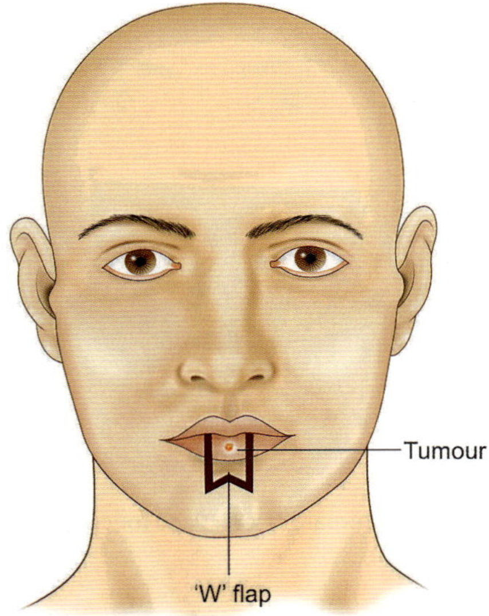

Fig. 14-95: 'W' flap is used for lower lip central defect which is less than 1/3rd of the lip.

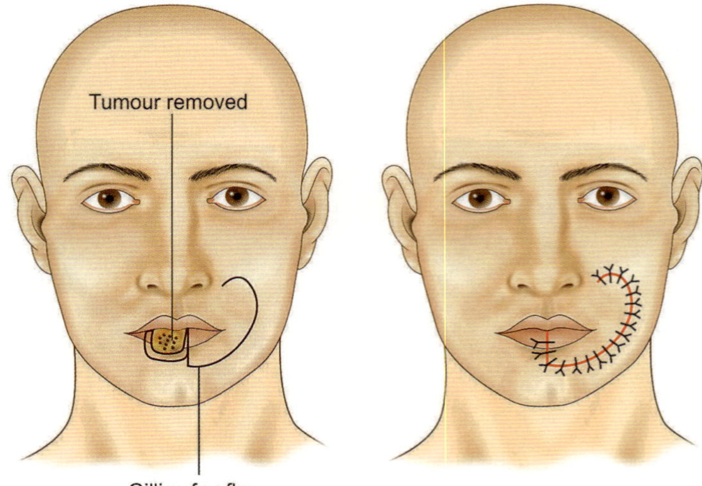

Fig. 14-96: Gillies fan flap is a cheek flap which can be unilateral or bilateral.

Karapandzic flap—It is modified (myocutaneous) version of the Gillies flap used for lower lip defect with less angulation towards upper lip. It preserves motor and sensory supply of flap and so drooling is avoided. Reverse Karapandzic flap is used for upper lip defect.

McGregor and Nakajima flaps modified Gilles flap (denervated) pivot around commissure which prevents microstomia but drooling of saliva can occur.

Zisser technique—Cheek tissue is moved medially after excising two upper and lower triangles later to upper and lower lip. Horizontal incision is made along the commissure to advance de-epithelialised two triangles.

Platz and Wepner method is similar like Zisser's where nasolabial and submental areas are excised triangularly to advance superior and inferior cheek flaps.

Johansen 'step ladder' procedure is used for extensive carcinoma of lower lip.

Cheek advancement with perialar crescent excision is done for wide upper lip defect **(Fig. 14-97)**.

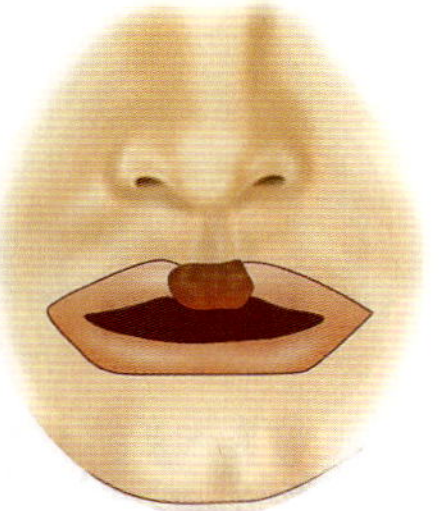

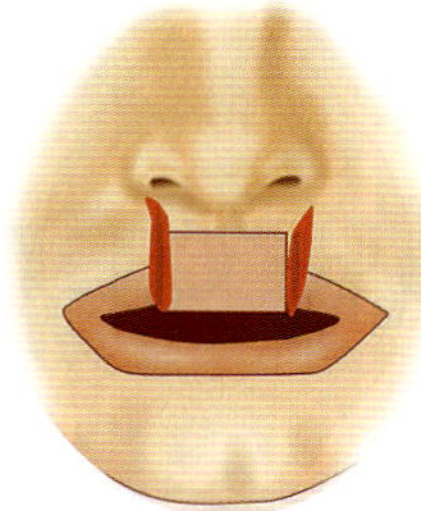

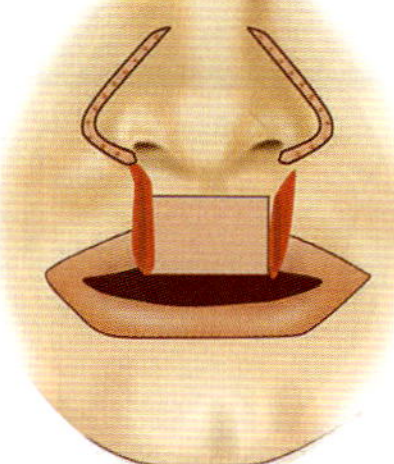

Fig. 14-97: Cheek advancement with perialar crescent excision.

Other regular flaps like forehead flap, deltopectoral flap also can be used.

Upper Lip Reconstruction

Due to presence of philtrum, upper lip reconstruction is more demanding than lower lip. Wound close to philtrum if primarily sutured, will shift the philtrum to the lesion side.

Lateral defect less than 1/3rd is either closed primarily or V-Y flap or nasolabial flap is used. In males nasolabial flap being hairless may be problematic for upper lip.

Central lip defect needs reconstruction of Cupid's bow to prevent flattening. Abbe lip switch flap, skin graft, ear cartilage composite grafts are required to reconstruct Cupid's bow.

Defects between 1/3rd to 2/3rd are corrected using Abbe flap, perialar excision cheek advancement flap.

Defect more than 2/3rd in upper lip is repaired by bilateral reverse Karpandzic flaps, bilateral nasolabial flaps, and forehead flap. First two flaps denervate the lip and may precipitate drooling of saliva. But insensate lower lip is more problematic than insensate upper lip as saliva collects in lower lip and drooling occurs from gravity across the lower lip. Other methods used are perialar crescent excision and cheek advancement; radial forearm free tissue flap with microvascular and nerve anastomosis (anterior cutaneous nerve of forearm to mental nerve).

Lower Lip Reconstruction

It is easier to reconstruct the lower lip than upper as lower lip is devoid of central structure.

Defect less than 1/3rd is closed primarily. One should avoid formation of dog ear or incision crossing the labiomental fold. W flap can be used in central defect less than 1/3rd.

Defect between 1/3rd to 2/3rd is covered using Abbe switch flap from upper lip lateral 1/3rd. 1/4th or 2 cm of upper lip tissue can be transferred. Width of donor lip needed is 1/2 of width of the recipient defect. Recipient site attains pain, temperature, touch and sweating functions in 2 years. Upper lip donor defect can be reconstructed additionally using perialar excision and cheek advancement if needed. *Schuchardt technique* may be used with a modified wedge resection with advancement of the lip contralateral to the lip switch. Webster flap with triangular excisions of skin along the nasolabial crease of the upper lip to mobilise cheek can be used. *Johansen stepwise/stepladder excisions* of 2–4 fold skin around labiomental fold can be used. This avoids microstomia. Unilateral advancement is done for smaller defects; bilateral advancement is done for larger defects.

Defect more than 2/3rd is corrected using bilateral Karpandzic flap or McGregor flap or Webster modification of Bernard burrow flap. Here cheek is advanced medially by triangular excision of skin. Nasolabial fold skin is excised triangularly. Inferiorly based nasolabial Fujimori gate flap, bipedicled tongue flaps, deltopectoral flap and free flaps are other flaps used.

Vermilion Reconstruction

White roll is the mucocutaneous junction. Any defect even of 1 mm size in vermilion is easily seen. White roll should be marked using 25 G needle tip dipped in methylene blue prior to injecting the local anaesthetic drug. One should not place sutures directly on white roll as healing erythema will mask the white roll. Sutures on either side of the white roll should be placed one on vermilion side other on cutaneous side. White roll should cross 90° while placing the incision. Resection of the entire vermilion from the white roll to wet-dry junction of vermilion is called as *lip shave/ total vermilionectomy* which is done for premalignant conditions and actinic lip involvement. Buccal mucosa is advanced above orbicularis oris as bipedicled flap. V-Y advancement of labial or buccal mucosa is commonly used. Mental nerve runs in submucous gland plane and so plane of dissection is between submucous gland plane and orbicularis oris. Lip switch or tongue flaps are also often used. Ventral tongue flap is used in females to facilitate application of the lipstick; dorsal tongue flap is used in males. Full thickness palatal mucosal graft and tattooing are other options for vermilion reconstruction.

Commissure Reconstruction

It is done using Estlander flap, Fries technique, Zisser procedure, or Platz and Wepner technique **(Fig. 14-98)**.

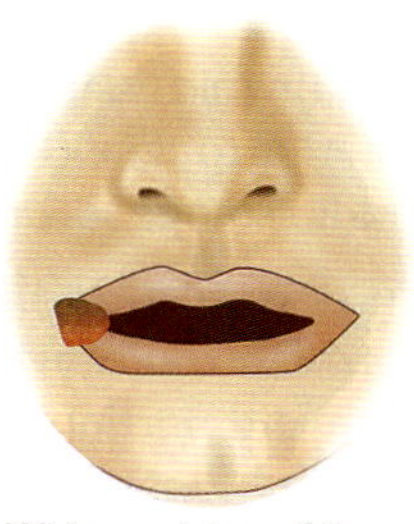

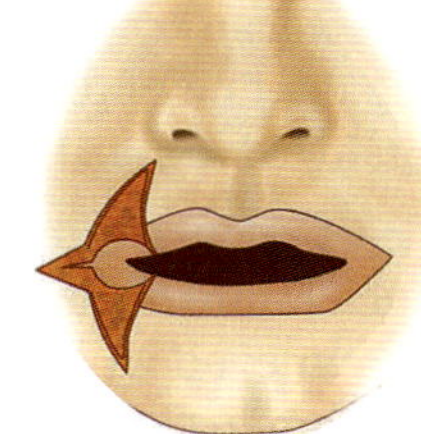

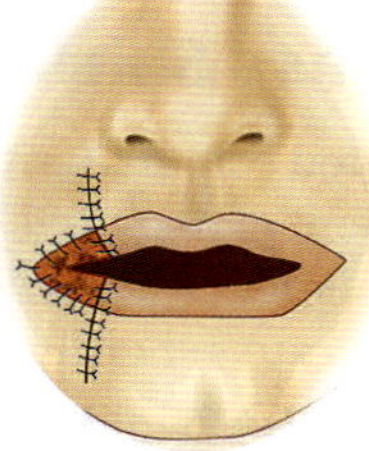

Fig. 14-98: Zisser commissure reconstruction method.

15

CHAPTER

Surgery for Thyroid and Parathyroid

SURGICAL ANATOMY OF THYROID *(THYROID – 'SHIELD LIKE')*

Development

Thyroid gland develops (*origin*) from columnar cells of pharyngeal floor as a median down growth between 1st and 2nd pharyngeal pouches; point which later forms foramen caecum at the base of primitive tongue (*thyroid primordium*). These columnar cells form a tube which gets canalised to form thyroglossal duct. While descending downwards (*by migration*) it gets displaced forward by the developing hyoid bone and below which it descends further slightly towards left side which eventually bifurcates into one on each side to form two lateral lobes. Part present at its junction of bifurcation forms isthmus. Once gland is formed remaining portion of the duct obliterates; part of the duct on left side forms pyramidal lobe.

> Origin → migration → obliteration of duct mostly except lower most part which forms pyramidal lobe → differentiation of the gland, isthmus and pyramidal lobe.
>
> Neural crest → along the ultimobranchial body → incorporation of parafollicular C cells in the thyroid adjacent to follicles.

Ectopic thyroid tissue can occur and may be the only thyroid tissue which is present along the line of the duct in the posterior tongue (lingual thyroid) or suprahyoid region. It is identified by radioisotope scanning.

Thyroglossal cyst occurs due to persistence of a portion of the thyroglossal duct. Entire duct and centre portion of the body of hyoid bone has to be removed with removal of suprahyoid portion of the duct up to the foramen caecum.

Agenesis of one lateral lobe or both can occur. Only the existing one lateral lobe may present as toxic or non-toxic solitary nodule.

Anatomy (Thyroid Means – Shield)

It is a butterfly shaped, brownish red coloured, vital endocrine gland situated in the central compartment of neck. It is located in anterior triangle of neck, 5 (height) × 3 (depth) × 1.5 (width each lobe) cm in size weighing about 20–25 gram (slightly more in women). Gland may get enlarged during menstruation and pregnancy. It has got right and left lateral lobes occupying the thyroid space between trachea and oesophagus medially and carotid sheath laterally extending from middle of thyroid cartilage to 6th tracheal ring. Right lobe is larger than left. Isthmus is connecting part between two lateral lobes extending from 2nd to 4th tracheal rings. Isthmus is around 1.5 ×1.5 cm in size. It is absent in 10% of individuals. Gland extends from C5 to T1 vertebral level behind; from middle of thyroid cartilage to 5th/6th tracheal rings in front. Thyroid space is between trachea and oesophagus medially and carotid sheath laterally. Normal gland is soft and supple. *Pyramidal lobe* is an extension of gland upwards on the surface of the cricoid towards left side which often extends above to the hyoid bone as a fibrous or muscular strand from the junction of isthmus and left lateral lobe. It is present in only 33% (1/3rd) of individuals. Fibromuscular extension to hyoid bone is called as *levator glandulae thyroideae*. Gland is invested by pretracheal fascia. It is supported by a strong condensed vascular connective tissue between lateral lobe and cricoid cartilage on each side called as *Berry's ligament*. True thyroid capsule is peripheral condensed connective tissue and blood vessels are deeper to it. True capsule is covered by false capsule which is derived from pretracheal layer of deep cervical fascia. It is thin in front; thick behind and forms Berry's ligament above and behind. Surgical avascular plane is located between true and false capsule. (In prostate, surgical cleavage plane is located deep to true capsule) **(Figs. 15-1 to 15-5)**.

Each lateral lobe has got lateral, medial and posterolateral surfaces; anterior and posterior borders; apex and base. Lateral surface is covered by sternocleidomastoid, sternohyoid and omohyoid; and sternothyroid in deeper plane. Medial surface is related to trachea, oesophagus, cricothyroid and inferior constrictor; external laryngeal and recurrent laryngeal nerves. Anterior jugular veins run on the anterior surface in front of muscles **(Figs. 15-6A and B)**.

Deep fascia of neck has got four compartments—investing layer; prevertebral fascia; pretracheal fascia; carotid sheath.

Muscles in the anterior aspect of the neck are classified as:

Suprahyoid muscles

- Stylohyoid
- Geniohyoid
- Mylohyoid.

Infrahyoid muscles—strap muscles

- Sternohyoid—in front
- Omohyoid—in front
- Sternothyroid—deep to above muscles
- Thyrohyoid—deep to above muscles

Arterial supply is:

1. ***Superior thyroid artery*** which is a branch of external carotid artery enters the gland near the superior pole as a larger anterior

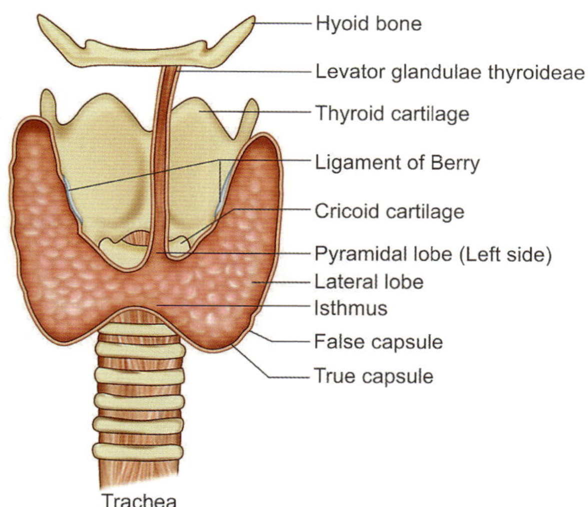

Fig. 15-1: Parts of the thyroid with their locations and relations. Two lateral lobes; one isthmus; one pyramidal lobe.

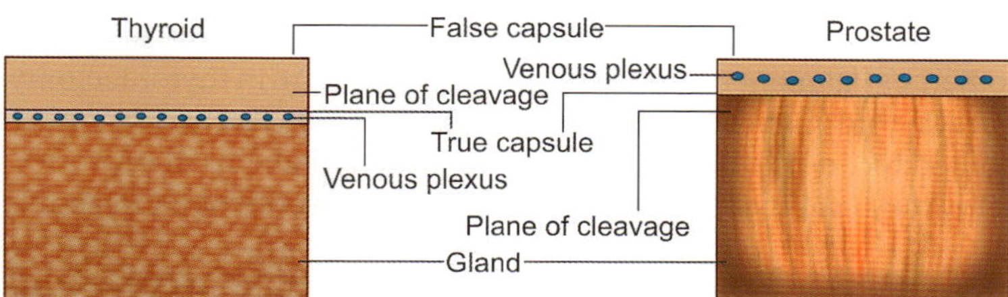

Fig. 15-2: Surgical avascular plane in thyroid is located between true and false capsule. In prostate surgical cleavage plane is located deep to true capsule.

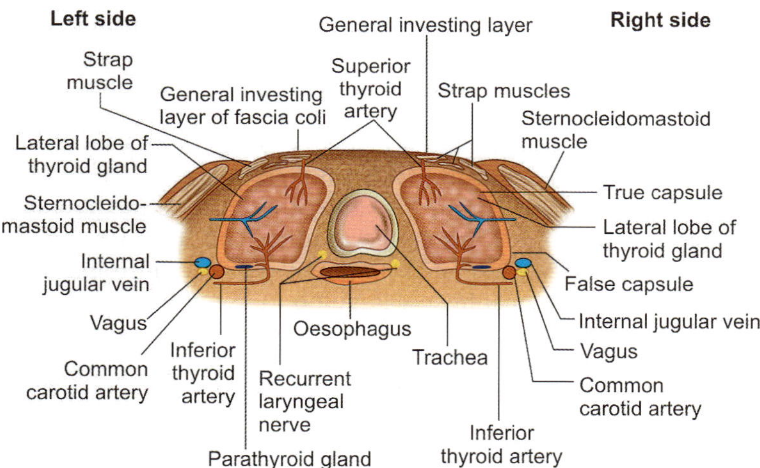

Fig. 15-3: Fascia around thyroid with true and false capsules.

superficial branch and a smaller posterior branch. It is accompanied by external laryngeal nerve, a branch of superior laryngeal nerve (a branch of vagus), which supplies cricothyroid muscle.

2. ***Inferior thyroid artery*** is a branch of thyrocervical trunk of subclavian artery runs upwards, medially then downwards behind the carotid sheath and middle cervical sympathetic ganglion, in front of vertebral vessels divides into 4–5 terminal branches which pierce the pretracheal fascia separately to supply and enter the lower pole of the thyroid. Its ascending branch also supplies the parathyroid glands (both lower and upper).

3. *Thyroidea ima* artery (3–10%) also called as lowest thyroid artery arises from arch of aorta or brachiocephalic artery enters the gland and isthmus.

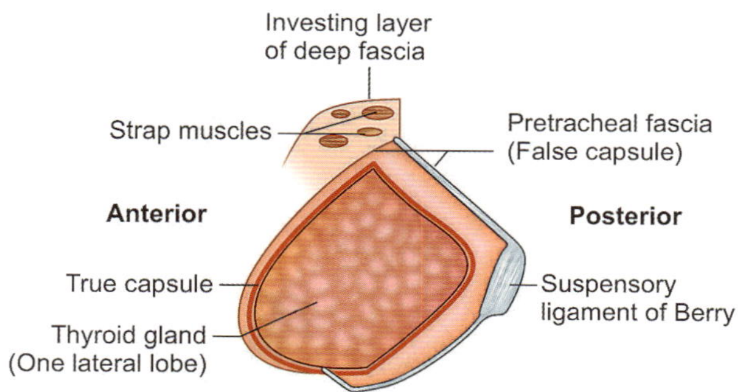

Fig. 15-4: True and false capsules of thyroid and suspensory ligament of Berry.

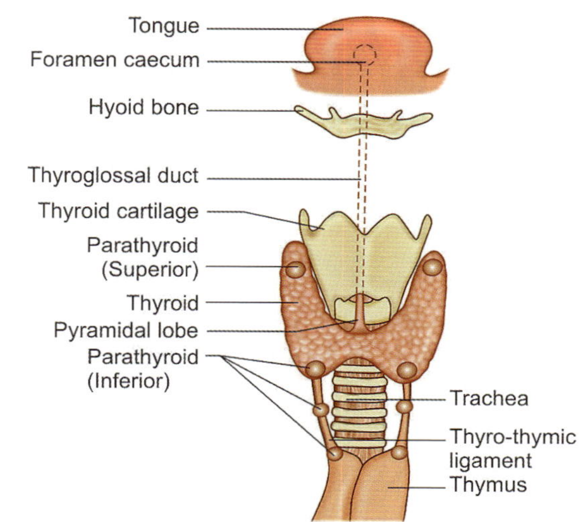

Fig. 15-5: Anatomy of thyroid gland, thyroglossal duct and parathyroids.

4. *Accessory thyroid arteries* arise from tracheal and oesophageal arteries also supply the gland **(Fig. 15-7)**.

Venous supply is by:

1. *Superior thyroid vein* from upper pole accompanying the artery to join IJV or common facial vein.

2. *Middle thyroid vein* is a short, wide, thin walled vein begins from mid-lateral aspect of the lateral lobe running a short distance in front or behind the carotid artery, immediately enters into the internal jugular vein (IJV). Secure ligation of the vein is important and if it tears, it may extend into IJV causing torrential haemorrhage. As it is the one that holds the gland posteriorly, it should be ligated first to mobilise the gland. Occasionally this vein may be absent. One should also remember that there is no middle thyroid artery.

3. *Inferior thyroid veins* begin at lower pole of isthmus form a plexus in front of trachea later joining the respective brachiocephalic vein. These veins are not accompanied with inferior thyroid artery. Occasionally both inferior thyroid veins form a common trunk—thyroidea ima vein which joins left brachiocephalic vein.

4. *Kocher's 4th thyroid vein* may be present occasionally between middle and inferior thyroid vein, joins either IJV or middle thyroid or inferior thyroid vein.

Note:

Anterior jugular vein is a small but variable vein begins at submental region below the chin, descends vertically in superficial fascia 1 cm from midline. At 2.5 cm above the sternum, it pierces the deep investing fascia to enter the suprasternal space. Here it is connected by a communicating vein to opposite side called as jugular venous arch.

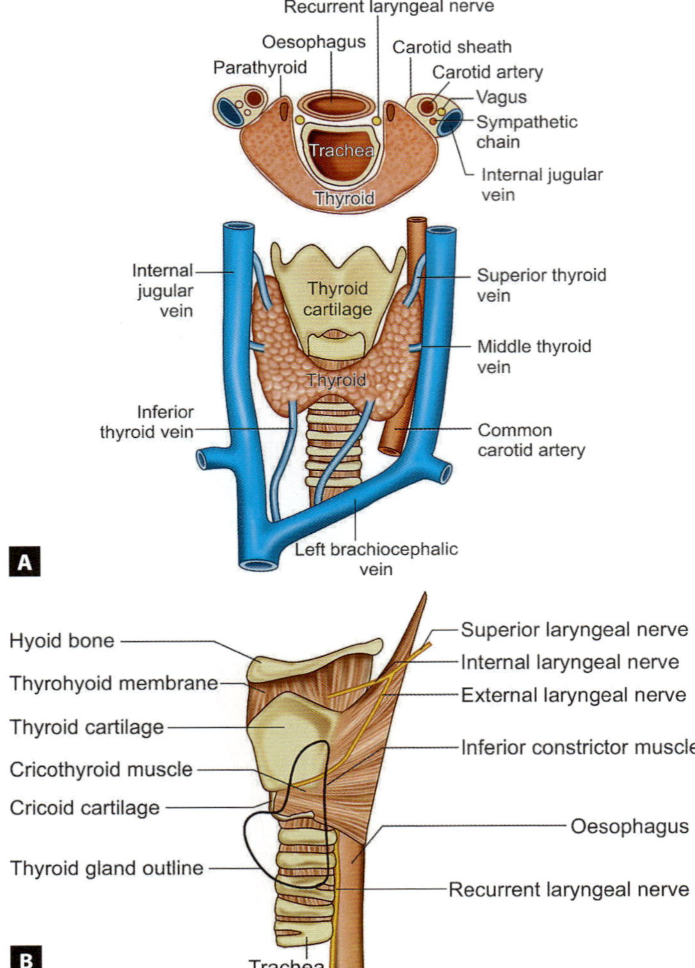

Figs. 15-6A and B: Relations of thyroid gland—diagrammatic look.

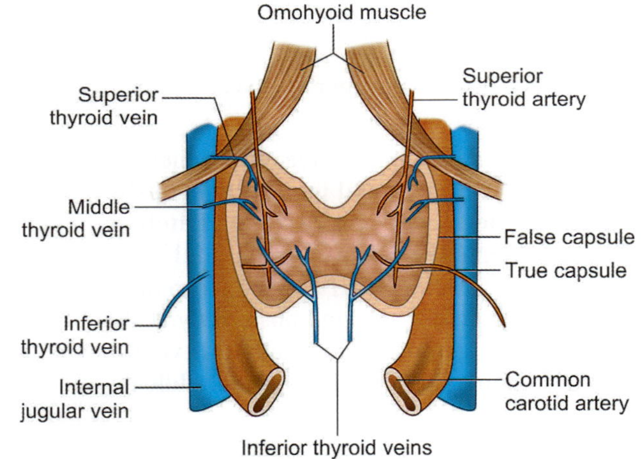

Fig. 15-7: Vessels of the thyroid gland.

Later the vein runs laterally deep to sternocleidomastoid towards its posterior border up to the clavicle to join the external jugular vein. Anterior jugular vein is variable—may be absent; may be in midline; may be quite large drained by common facial vein. This vein is important in thyroid surgeries even though it is not related to venous drainage of thyroid gland **(Fig. 15-8)**.

Nerve Supply

It is mainly from middle cervical ganglion partly from superior and inferior cervical ganglion.

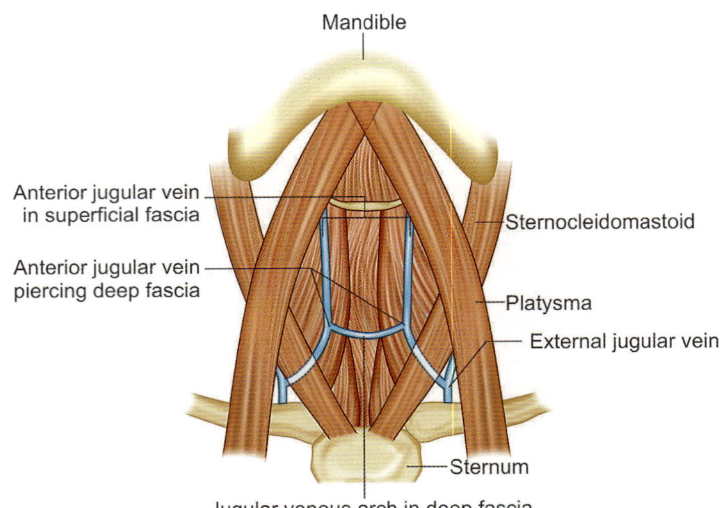

Fig. 15-8: Anatomy of anterior jugular vein.

Note:
Recurrent laryngeal nerve is in tracheo-oesophageal groove in relation to Berry's ligament and is very important structure in thyroidectomy. Parathyroid glands are four in number, two on each side—often embedded in thyroid gland. Removal of all four glands in thyroidectomy may lead into severe hypoparathyroidism and hypocalcaemia.

Lymphatic Drainage of Thyroid

Thyroid drains through primary and secondary lymph nodes. Prelaryngeal or cricothyroid node is also called as *Delphian node* is a node (single node) located anterior to cricothyroid membrane between cricothyroid muscles and is the most important node among level VI nodes. Delphian node receives afferent lymphatics from larynx and from upper anterior parts of the both lobes of the thyroid gland and its isthmus. It has got two efferent lymphatics; one towards paratracheal and lower jugular, other towards pretracheal (sub-Deplhian), mediastinal and supraclavicular lymph nodes **(Fig. 15-9)**. R Randall from Harvard coined the term Delphian (as formerly purpose of this node was uncertain. Delphi is a place in Greece where Pythia, snake women after sulphurous fume inhalation uttered meaningless jargon purpose of it was unclear; it also means that spread to this node predicts the outcome of laryngeal and thyroid cancers in the same way prophecy of Apollo at temple of Delphi foretold the future in the ancient Greece).

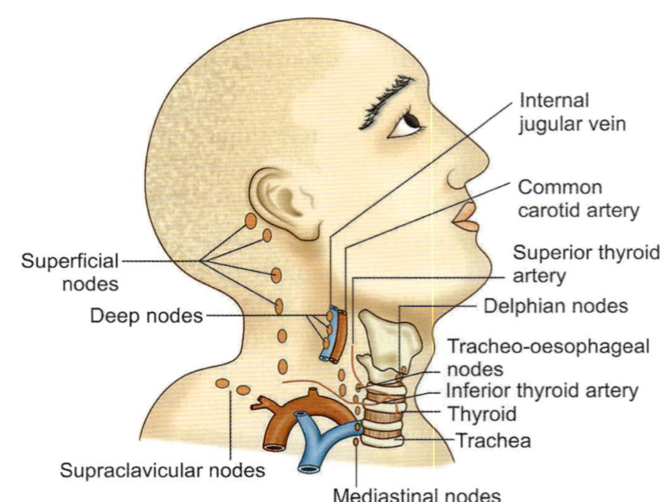

Fig. 15-9: Lymphatic drainage of thyroid gland.

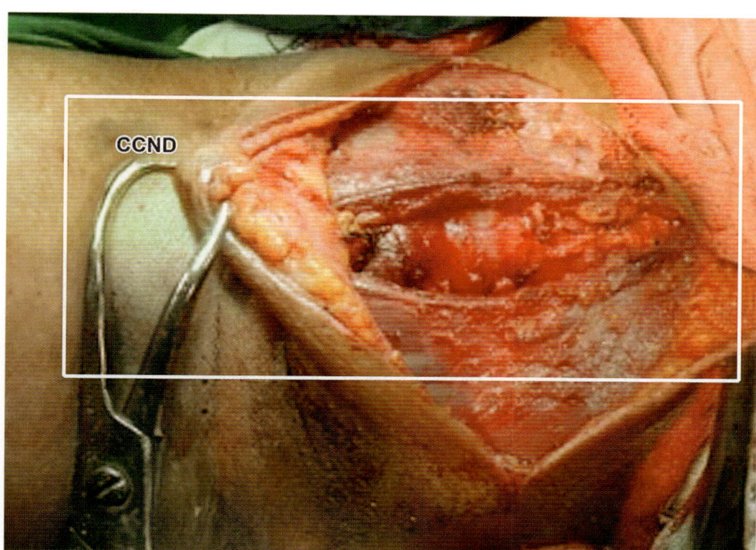

Fig. 15-10: Central cervical node dissection (CCND) area—central compartment dissection area.

Paratracheal (located at lateral wall of the trachea and tracheo-oesophageal groove) *and pretracheal (sub-Delphian nodes* are in front of trachea and isthmus) receive afferents from remaining thyroid and from Delphian node. Its efferents reach lower jugular and mediastinal nodes. *Perithyroidal nodes* are nodes along the superior and inferior thyroid veins which drain into pretracheal, paratracheal nodes. *Mediastinal nodes* up to the level of innominate (brachiocephalic) vessels get the afferent from pretracheal and paratracheal nodes. *Central nodal compartment* includes all nodes from trachea to carotids; nodes from hyoid bone above to innominate artery below with pretracheal nodes. It is level VI and mediastinal nodes above the level of innominate artery.

Secondary nodes are neck nodes—level IIA, III, IV, VB

Central cervical node dissection (CCND) includes the removal of all nodes between trachea and carotid sheath; from the thoracic inlet to hyoid bone above, innominate vein is the lower landmark of the central node dissection. Lateral cervical node dissection (LCND) is removal of level IIA, III, IV, VB. CCND is often done as prophylactic also. LCND is done only as therapeutic when lateral neck nodes are positive either by FNAC or sonologically with typical features **(Fig. 15-10)**.

Anatomy and Relations of Nerves with Thyroid Gland

External Laryngeal Nerve

External laryngeal nerve is a branch of superior laryngeal nerve. Vagus gives superior laryngeal nerve branch from its inferior ganglion of vagus which is at the level of greater cornu of hyoid bone, which in turn, divides into internal laryngeal and external laryngeal nerves. Internal laryngeal nerve pierces the thyrohyoid membrane and gives sensory supply to larynx above the vocal cord and hypopharynx. External laryngeal nerve runs close to superior thyroid vessels to supply cricothyroid muscle which is tensor of vocal cord. It may get injured while ligating superior pedicle causing defective pitch of the voice. So the upper pedicle of thyroid should be ligated close to gland but after identification and dissection of the nerve **(Figs. 15-11A to C)**.

Recurrent Laryngeal Nerve

Recurrent laryngeal nerve (RLN) is a branch of vagus which hooks around *ligamentum arteriosum* on the left with arch of aorta and right subclavian artery on the right side **(Fig. 15-12)**. It runs in the tracheo-oesophageal groove near the posteromedial surface close to thyroid gland. Nerve lies in between branches of inferior thyroid artery. On the right side, the nerve runs between branches of the artery in approximately 50% of patients, anterior to the artery in 25% and posterior in 25%. On the left, the nerve runs posteriorly to the artery in 50% of patients, in 35% the nerve runs between branches, in 15% it is anterior to the artery. So the nerve is always near the artery, but the exact relationship cannot be determined. Hence inferior thyroid artery should be ligated away from the gland (old theory, not practiced now). Anomalies of the nerve should be remembered. In 5% of cases nerve passes through the gland. Nerve may be much more away from the gland. Nerve may be closely adherent to gland posteriorly. Nerve may lie within the ligament of Berry (25%). Redd in 1943 described 28 variations in RLN relation to inferior thyroid artery.

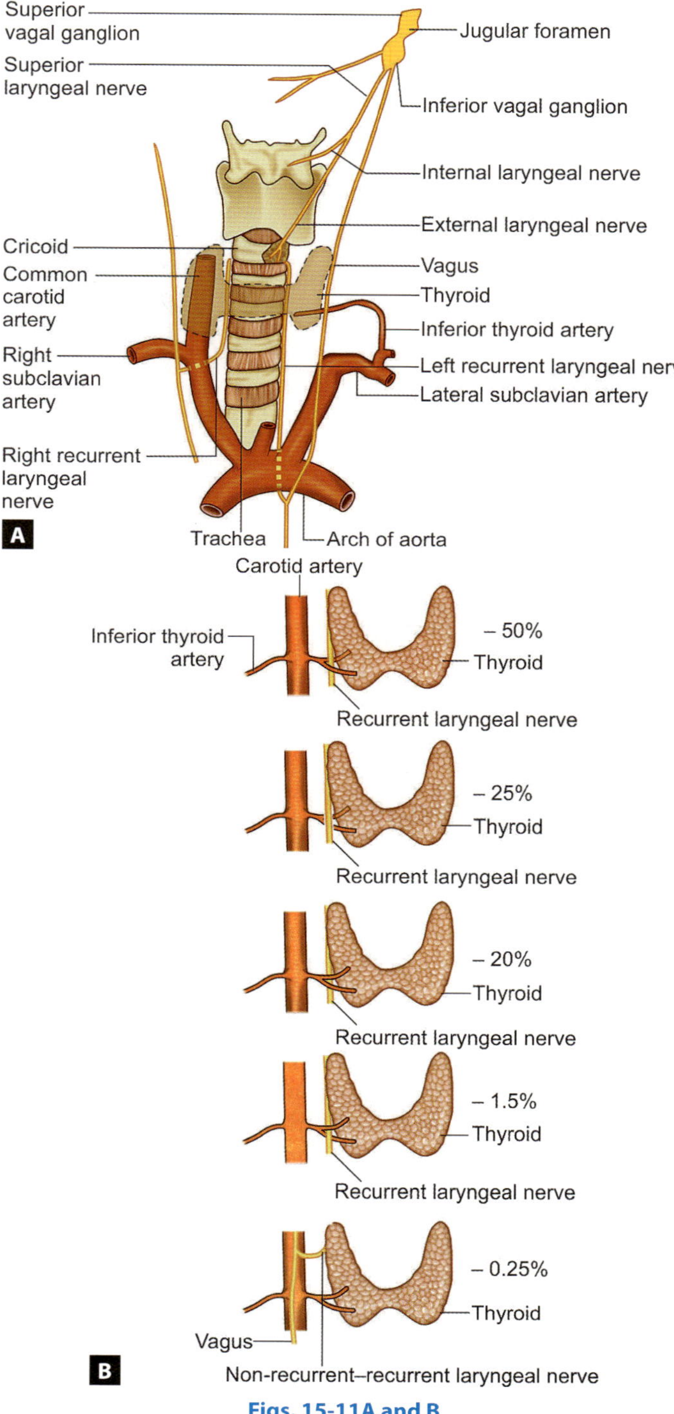

Figs. 15-11A and B

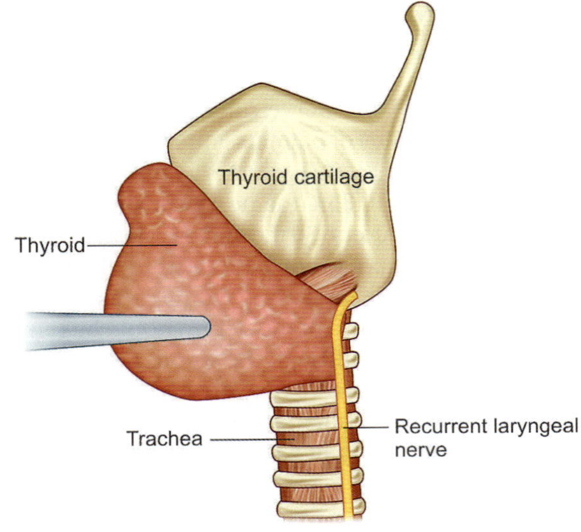

Fig. 15-11C

Figs. 15-11A to C: Anatomy of recurrent laryngeal nerve and external laryngeal nerve.

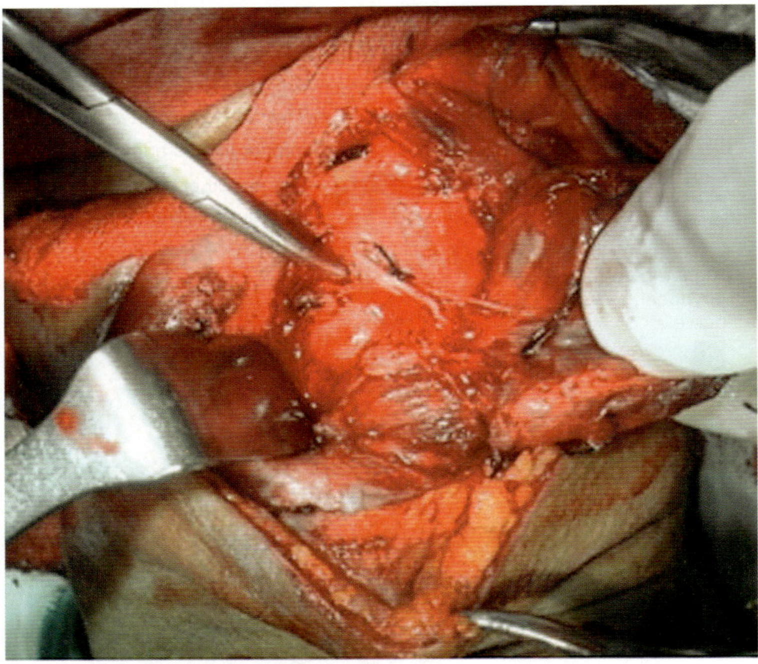

Fig. 15-12: Recurrent laryngeal nerve in thyroidectomy.

In his observation—RLN is deep to artery in 40%; superficial in 20% and in between branches in 35%; only in 17% of cases pattern were same in both sides.

Non-recurrent laryngeal nerve may be present in 1 to 5 in 1,000 cases with a horizontal course. In 5 of 1000 patients, a non-recurrent laryngeal nerve is found on the *right side*. This arrangement occurs when a retro-oesophageal right subclavian artery arises from the dorsal side of the aortic arch. *The non-recurrent laryngeal nerve branches* from the vagus at approximately at the level of the cricoid cartilage and directly enters the larynx without looping around the subclavian artery. A left-sided non-recurrent laryngeal nerve can occur only when a right-sided aortic arch and ligamentum arteriosum are concurrent with a left retro-oesophageal subclavian artery.

Recurrent laryngeal nerve supplies all muscles (abductors, adductors) of the larynx except cricothyroid and also sensory supply of larynx below the vocal cords **(Fig. 15-13)**.

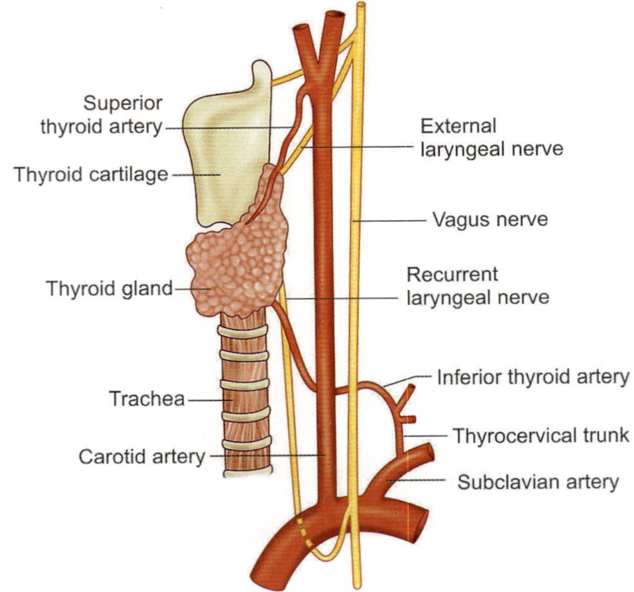

Fig. 15-13: Nerves and arteries related to thyroid gland. External and recurrent laryngeal nerves and superior and inferior thyroid arteries are important structures while doing thyroidectomy. Parathyroid glands are also equally important.

Muscles of the Larynx

- Cricothyroid: It is the only muscle which is located on the external aspect of the larynx. It is supplied by external laryngeal nerve. It is tensor and mild adductor of the vocal cord.
- Abductors of the vocal cord: Posterior cricoarytenoids.
- Adductors of the vocal cord: Lateral cricoarytenoids, transverse arytenoid, thyroarytenoids and cricothyroids.
- Relaxant of vocal cords: Thyroarytenoids and vocalis.
- Muscles which close the laryngeal inlet: Oblique arytenoids and aryepiglottic.
- Muscles which open the laryngeal inlet: Thyroepiglotticus **(Fig. 15-14)**.

  Positions of vocal cord:

  Median; paramedian (1.5 mm); normal; cadaveric/neutral (3.5 mm); gentle abduction (7 mm); completely abducted (9.5 mm).

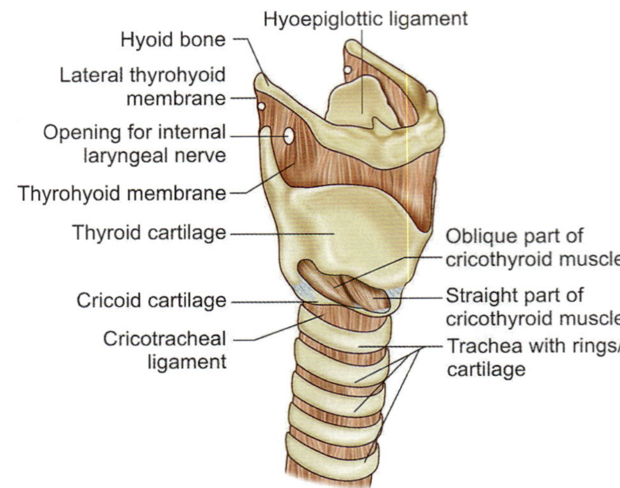

Fig. 15-14: Thyroid and cricothyroid cartilages with cricothyroid muscle. Cricothyroid has got straight and oblique parts. Straight originates from arch of cricoid cartilage to posteroinferior margin of the thyroid lamina. Oblique part runs from cricoid cartilage to inferior horn of thyroid cartilage. Cricothyroid is supplied by external branch of superior laryngeal nerve. Branch is closely associated with superior thyroid vessels.

Assessment of voice change

- Pitch of the voice—whether raised/lowered or pitch locked
- Breath support during speaking is adequate or not
- Ability to alter the rapidity of speech—slow/fast/medium
- Altered laryngeal and neck muscle tension
- *Indirect laryngoscopy (ILS)*—with tongue pulled out using gauze, warmed ILS is introduced into the oral cavity to see vocal cords. Patient is asked to say 'e' to see the vocal cord movements

Rule of '2' in thyroid

- 2 lobes
- 2 origins—thyroglossal duct, C cells neural crest
- 2 capsules—true, false
- 2 arteries
- 2 nerves related deep
- 2 tubes related deep
- 2 muscles related deep
- 2 lymphatic drainage area—central and lateral
- 2 parathyroids each lateral lobe
- 2 triangles—Beahrs; Jolls
- 2 hormones (T3/T4; calcitonin)

Jolls triangle	Beahrs triangle
Formed by midline; strap muscles; superior thyroid pedicle. Its floor is cricothyroid. It contains external laryngeal nerve.	RLN; common carotid artery (CCA); inferior thyroid artery; at antero-medial aspect of the thyroid.

Hyoid Bone

It is U-shaped bone located in the middle of the anterior aspect of the neck between chin and thyroid cartilage. It develops from 2nd and 3rd branchial arches. It is suspended by tips of the styloid processes of two temporal bones by stylohyoid ligament. It lies at the level of base of the mandible in front and 3rd cervical vertebra behind. It provides attachment to tongue and floor of the mouth above; larynx below; epiglottis and pharynx behind. It has got central body and two pairs of greater and lesser cornua.

Anterior surface of the body is convex and is directed forwards and upwards. Posterior surface of body is directed backwards and downwards. There is a transverse ridge in the body which divides the body of the bone into upper and lower parts and deep cervical fascia is attached to it. Geniohyoid, mylohyoid, genioglossus, hyoglossus, sternohyoid, omohyoid and thyrohyoid muscles are attached to body. Thyrohyoid membrane is attached to upper border from behind and below. Pretracheal fascia is attached to lower border. Greater cornua gives origin to middle constrictor medially and hyoglossus laterally; insertion of stylohyoid muscle; attachment of fibrous loop (pulley) of central tendon of the digastric muscle. Two small conical spike like projections lesser cornua give attachments to stylohyoid ligaments one on each side.

Thyroid moves upwards during deglutition:
- During 1st stage of deglutition
  ↓
- Hyoid moves upwards by constrictor action
  ↓
- Pulls pretracheal fascia upwards
  ↓
- Pulls ligament of Berry
  ↓
- Pulls thyroid upwards

Contd...

Contd...

Note:
All structures enclosed in pretracheal fascia will move with deglutition:
- Thyroglossal cyst
- Pretracheal lymph nodes
- Subhyoid bursa

EXCISION OF THYROGLOSSAL CYST

Thyroglossal cyst is due to congenital incomplete regression of the thyroglossal duct along its pathway, persisting as tubulodermoid cystic swelling in the midline towards left which causes a 'tug' like feel while protruding the tongue out and also moves upwards while swallowing. Often gland will be present only in the wall of the cyst with empty thyroid fossa. Ultrasound neck, radioisotope study, T3, T4, thyroid stimulating hormone (TSH) and fine needle aspiration cytology (FNAC) of cyst is needed before surgical removal. Entire track up to the foramen caecum of tongue (at the junction of middle and posterior third of the tongue) should be excised to prevent recurrence or fistula formation **(Figs. 15-15A and B)**.

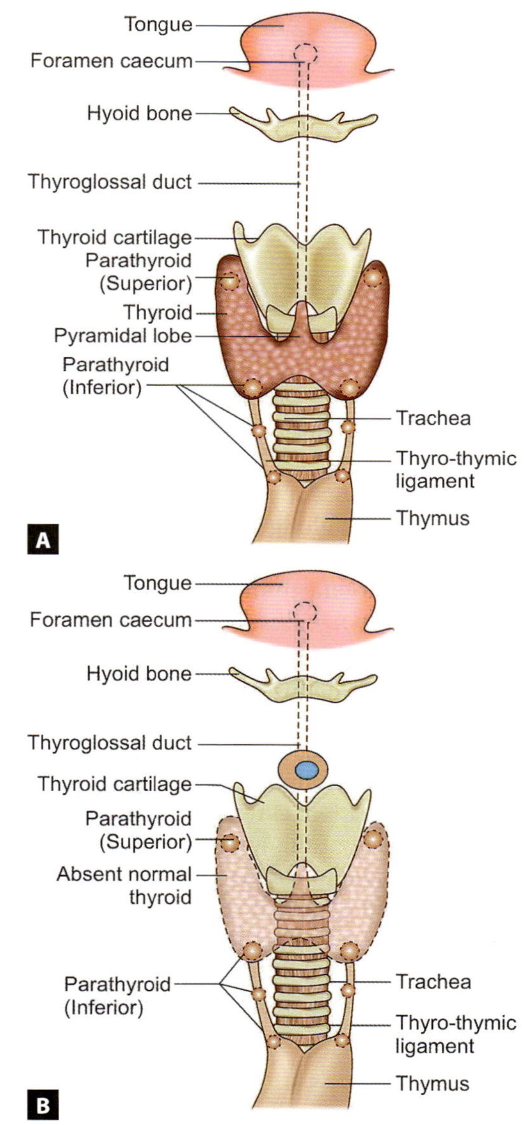

Figs. 15-15A and B: Thyroglossal cyst when present commonly normal lateral lobes will be present. But occasionally normal lateral lobes may be absent and only thyroid tissue existing in these patients will be in the wall of the thyroglossal cyst.

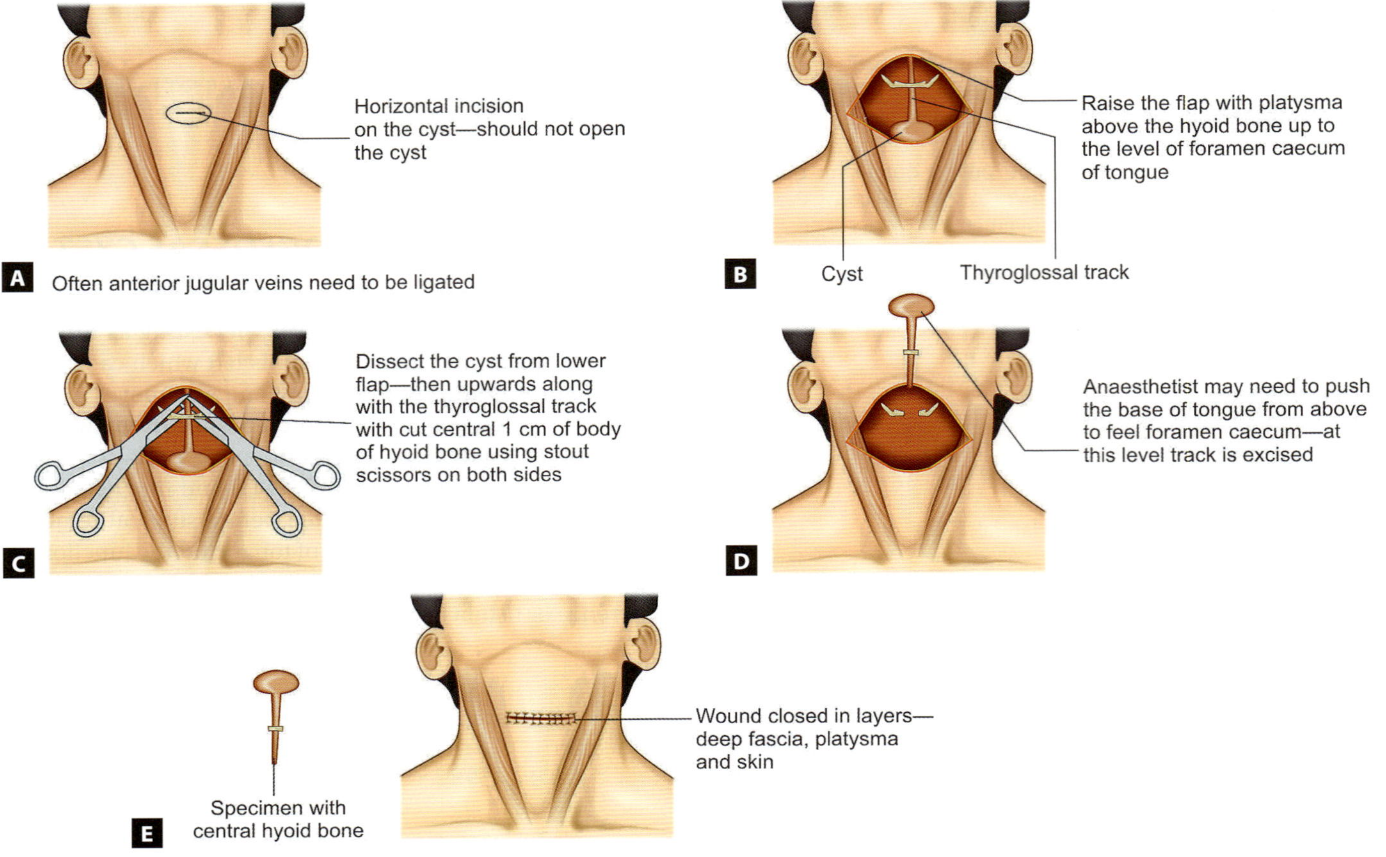

Fig. 15-16: Thyroglossal cyst excision steps—A to E.

Technique (Sistrunk Operation) (Fig. 15-16)

It is done under general anaesthesia. Position is supine with neck extended. Through transverse neck incision placed over the cyst, skin flap is raised above along with platysma. Care should be taken not to open the cyst. Deep fascia is opened vertically in midline. Cyst with surrounding tissues is dissected up to the hyoid bone. Sternohyoid and thyrohyoid muscles are separated and retracted. Cyst is mobilised upwards along with the track. Track is densely adherent to the body of hyoid bone above. Hyoid bone is separated from the thyrohyoid membrane through a clean fascial plane without fear of opening the pharyngeal wall. Geniohyoid and mylohyoid muscles superiorly and sternohyoid inferiorly are divided off from the hyoid. Central 1 cm part of the hyoid bone is resected along with intact track within it. Track with adjacent tissues is dissected above up to the foramen caecum. Adjacent tissues also should be removed because of possibility of multiple tracks which otherwise lead to recurrence or fistula formation. Often anaesthetist is asked to apply digital pressure over base of the tongue near foramen caecum to facilitate the dissection and to confirm the reach up to the foramen caecum. Track is ligated at foramen caecum using 3-zero vicryl and removed. Recurrence rate by removal of only track without central hyoid is 25%. Removal of track with central hyoid reduces the recurrence rate to 5%. Haemostasis is maintained using bipolar cautery. A suction drain is placed.

Complications

Complications are recurrence, thyroglossal fistula formation, haemorrhage/haematoma formation and infection. Occasionally two transverse incisions are needed to allow proper dissection

THYROIDECTOMY

Thyroidectomy is a surgery of *precision, patience and perfection.*

Principles are:

- Absolute haemostasis. Bipolar cautery should be used. Minimise/avoid using monopolar cautery in main dissection as lateral heat may damage RLN or parathyroid blood supply.
- Prevention of injury to recurrent laryngeal nerve and external laryngeal nerve.
- Preservation of parathyroid glands.
- Cosmesis.
- Meticulous technique.
- RLN and external laryngeal nerve (ELN) should be identified during dissection. All vessels should be ligated individually. One should avoid mass ligation even though it is commonly practiced.
- Middle thyroid vein, superior thyroid artery and vein then inferior thyroid vessels are ligated in order.

Preoperative preparation

- Blood grouping, cross matching and required blood should be kept ready.
- Indirect laryngoscopy. Patient is asked to tell 'E' to check the abduction of vocal cord. Indirect laryngoscope (ILS) should be soaked in warm water to prevent fogging and blurring of the IL scope. Videostroboscopy is ideal.
- Serum calcium estimation; T3, T4, TSH; thyroid antibodies, endocrinologist's opinion.
- ECG and cardiac fitness especially in toxic goitre.
- Radioisotope iodine scan; FNAC.

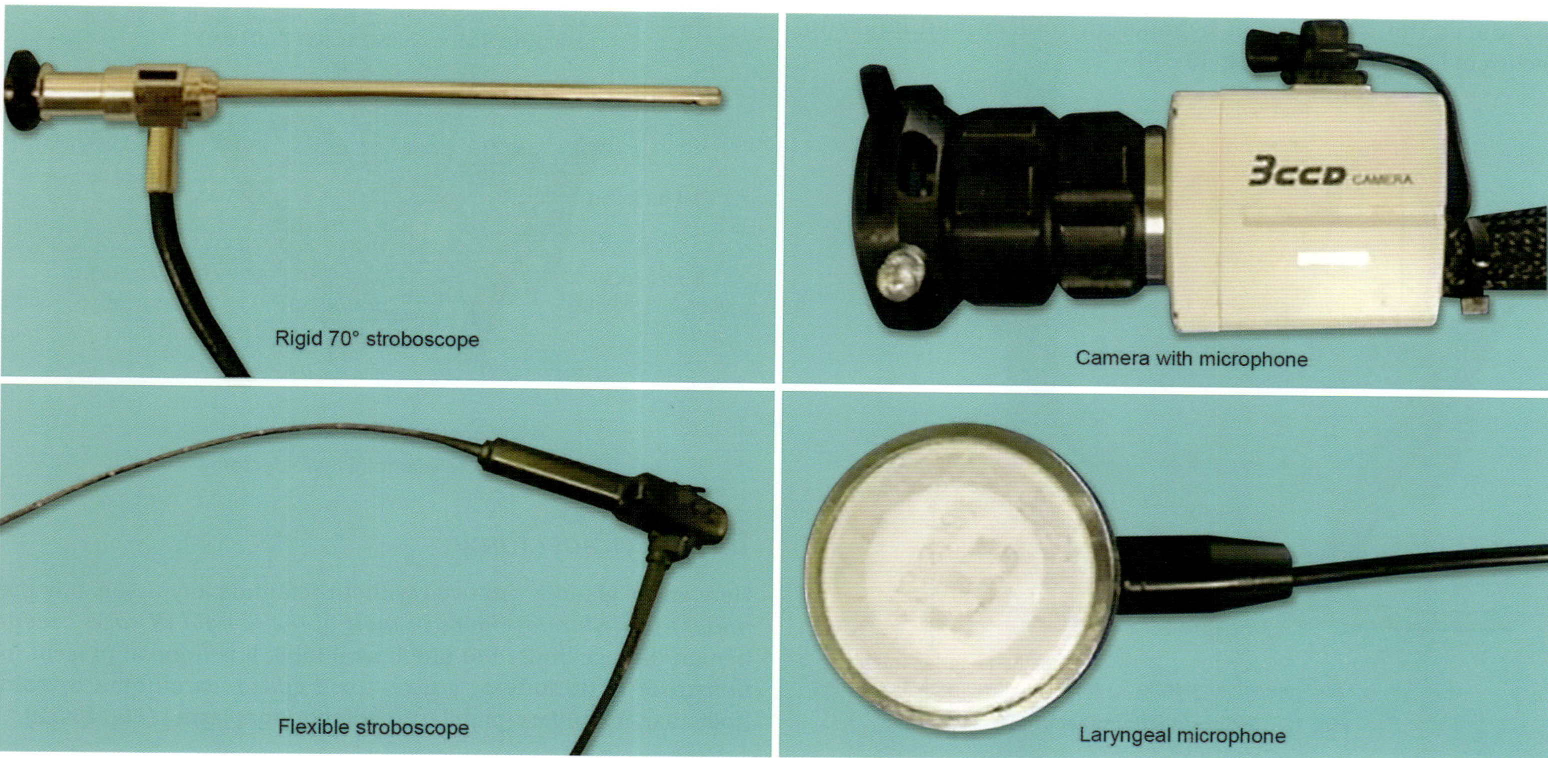

Fig. 15-17: Videostroboscope with parts.

Note:

Videostroboscopy

- ***Videostroboscopy*** is the technique used to have clinical evaluation of viscoelastic properties of phonatory mucosa, i.e. vocal cord mucosa. It assesses the vocal cord motion biomechanics and mucosal vibration and also to detect impact on voice and airway function.
- Here synchronised flashing light passed via flexible or rigid telescope; these flashes of light are synchronised with vocal cord vibration slightly at slower speed which allows clinician to observe during sound production at slow motion. It gives real time information about vibration, vocal pathology and video recording of the same for documentation.
- It visualise the mucosal waves which are actually too fast for human eye to appreciate by slowing the process to visualise the vibration.
- Videostroboscope unit has light source, camera, microphone, endoscope, video recorder. Stroboscopy can be rigid (70°) or flexible. Procedure is done with patient in sitting position. Patient leans forward with neck flexed with head extended at atlo occipital joint (Kirstein position). Xylocaine local topical anaesthetic spray is used. Microphone is calibrated. Scope is dipped in hot water. Vocal folds are focused. Patient is asked to say "EE". Assessment should be done at different frequency pitches—low, mid, and high. Arytenoids, mucosal waves, vocal fold mobility, glottis closure pattern, pliability and any lesions should be assessed **(Fig. 15-17)**.
- Findings also be looked for are—vocal cyst; vocal nodule; vocal polyp; vocal cord movements.

Different Types of Thyroidectomies

Hemithyroidectomy

It is removal of one lateral lobe with entire isthmus. It is done in benign disease involving only one lobe like solitary nodule thyroid either toxic or non-toxic (adenoma/colloid goitre of one lobe/colloid cyst). After hemithyroidectomy, if histology report comes as differentiated malignancy either papillary or follicular then completion thyroidectomy is done immediately within one week. If histology report comes after one week then completion thyroidectomy is done after 3 weeks. Reexploration is not advisable in 2nd and 3rd week **(Fig. 15-18)**.

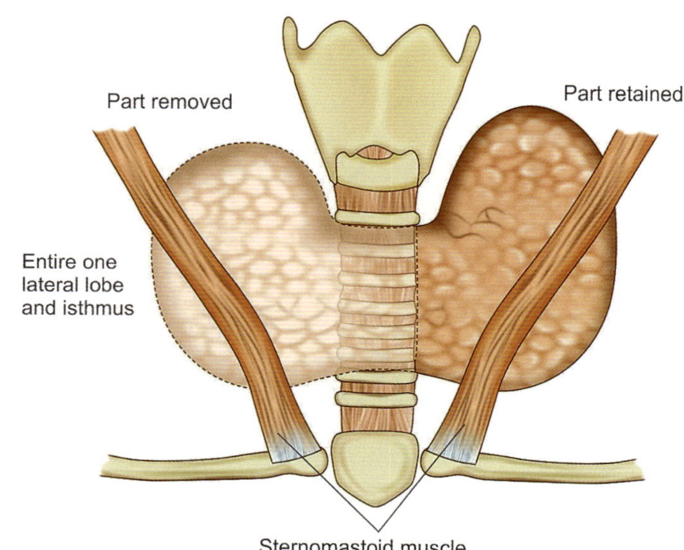

Fig. 15-18: Hemithyroidectomy: Entire one lateral lobe and entire isthmus are removed retaining entire opposite lateral lobe. It is done in solitary nodule/toxic or non-toxic adenoma in one lobe.

Subtotal Thyroidectomy

It is removal of most of both lateral lobes including isthmus, except around 8 gram of tissue (or tissue equal to pulp of little finger) in lower pole. It is done in toxic thyroid and often in non-toxic multinodular goitre.

It reduces the incidence of hypoparathyroidism and injury to recurrent laryngeal nerve **(Fig. 15-19)**.

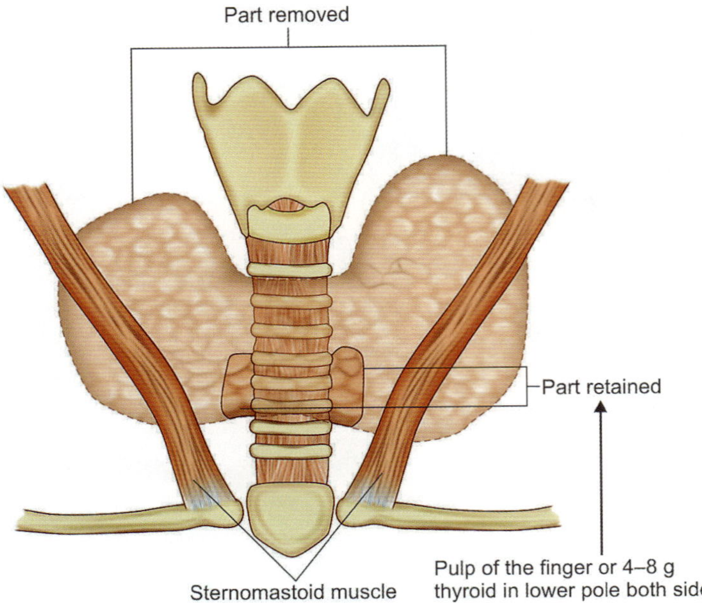

Fig. 15-19: Subtotal thyroidectomy.

Partial Thyroidectomy (Thomas)

It is removal of mobilised gland in front of trachea including entire isthmus. It was the procedure done earlier in non-toxic multinodular goitre. It is at present *not commonly used* **(Fig. 15-20)**.

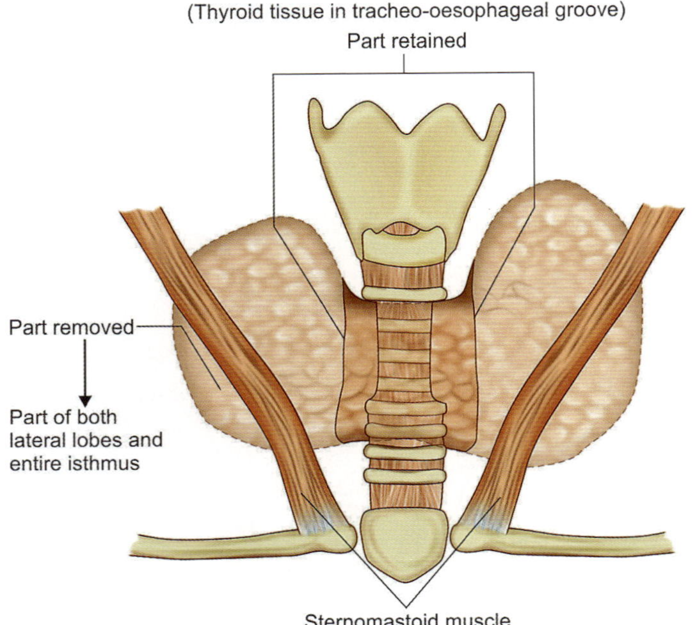

Fig. 15-20: Partial thyroidectomy is removal of mobilised gland in front of the tracheal level. Glands in tracheo-oesophageal grooves are retained. It is not commonly done now.

Near Total Thyroidectomy

Here both lateral lobes except small tissue in lower pole are removed. It is to safeguard the recurrent laryngeal nerve and *parathyroid blood supply*. It is advocated in papillary carcinoma of thyroid (usually in young individuals). Isthmus is entirely removed. Tissue is retained either in one or both sides **(Fig. 15-21)**.

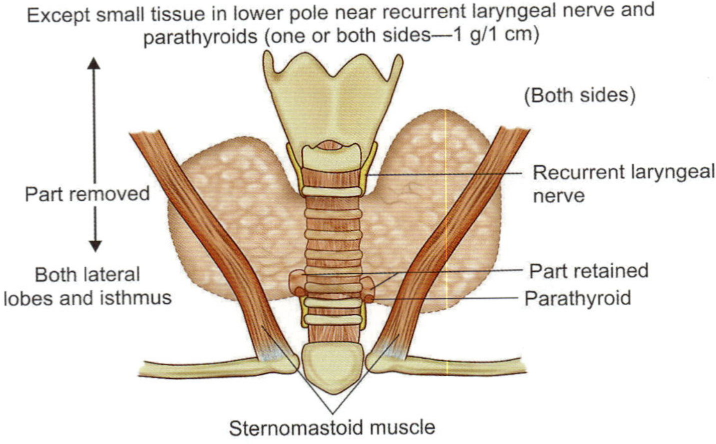

Fig. 15-21: Near total thyroidectomy.

Total Thyroidectomy

Here entire gland is removed without retaining any tissue. It is the *present procedure of choice in most of the thyroid diseases* except benign disease limited to one lateral lobe. It is done at present in non-toxic multinodular goitre, toxic goitre, carcinoma thyroid (follicular/medullary/papillary/operable/anaplastic) **(Fig. 15-22)**.

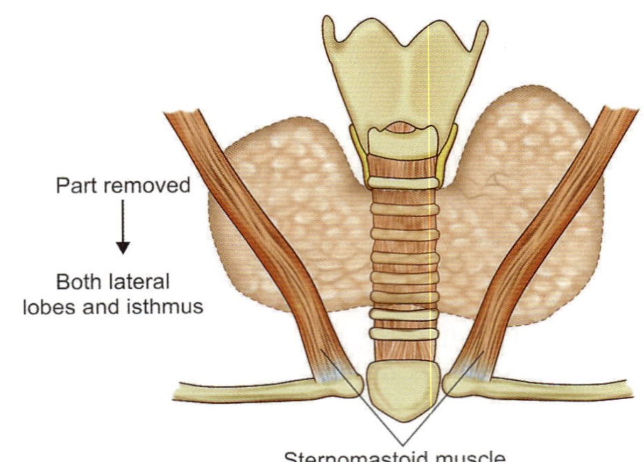

Fig. 15-22: Total thyroidectomy. It is done in follicular carcinoma and medullary carcinoma of thyroid.

Hartley Dunhill Operation

It is removal of one entire lateral lobe, isthmus and partial/subtotal removal of opposite lateral lobe. It is used in non-toxic multinodular goitre **(Fig. 15-23)**.

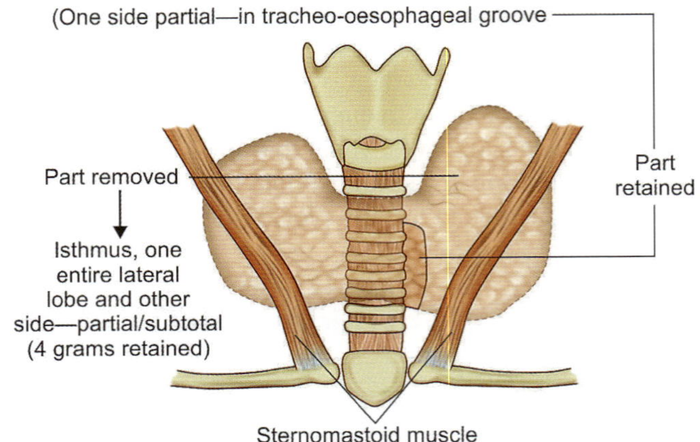

Fig. 15-23: Hartley Dunhill operation.

Isthmectomy

It is done in advanced carcinoma or occasionally in Riedel's thyroiditis to treat severe stridor due to tracheal narrowing.

Note: Isthmus should be removed in entirety in any type of thyroidectomy, and if it is retained partially it gets adherent to wound in front creating a cosmetically poor scar **(Fig. 15-24)**.

Procedure (Fig. 15-24)

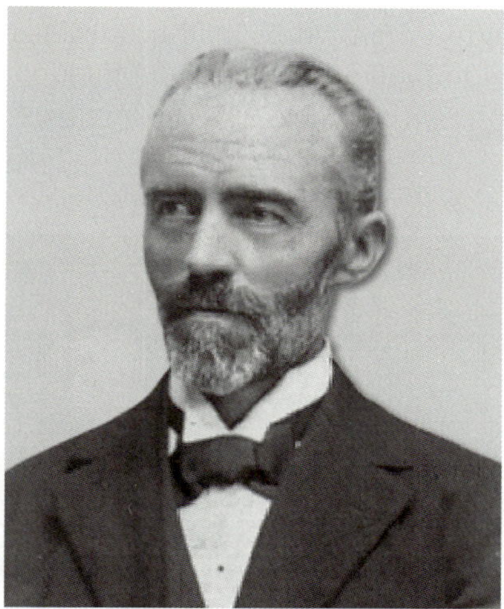

Fig. 15-24: Emil Theodor Kocher—Father of thyroid procedure who described the steps of thyroidectomy procedure.

Anaesthesia

General anaesthesia is used. Occasionally local anaesthesia can be used in patients who are not fit for general anaesthesia. Oesophageal stethoscope often may be required to place in case of retro/para-oesophageal goitres.

Position

Neck is extended by placing sandbag/round bolus/Dunhill pillow/folded sheet/*inflatable thyroid pillow*/inflatable intravenous fluid cuff underneath the shoulder. Ring should be kept under the occiput. Both arms are kept beside patient's body and hands are tugged/tucked under the patient's buttock. Cotton pads are placed under the elbow to prevent ulnar nerve compression. Head end of the table is elevated to 15° to improve venous return so as to reduce venous congestion in the neck and so oozing (reverse Trendelenburg/Rose/Barking dog/Kocher's position). This increases the risk of air embolism due to negative pressure created in neck veins. Veins should be ligated securely and then only cut. Any doubtful air in IJV should be aspirated immediately **(Fig. 15-25)**.

Anaesthetists are on the head end away from the field of surgery with sides kept free for surgeon, assistant and scrub nurse.

Cleaning of the area—neck, face, chest up to nipples is done. Draping is done on all sides. *Double towel* is placed under the head and one of the towels (outer one) is covered over the outer part of the endotracheal tube. Sterile transparent plastic drape is ideal if available. Surgeon stands on right side, assistant on left side and scrub nurse on right side at foot end of the patient. Energy sources like cautery (both unipolar and bipolar)/ligaseal/harmonic, etc. are kept ready. Suction apparatus with fine suction tip is needed **(Fig. 15-26)**.

Incision

Horizontal crease incision is placed two fingerbreadth (2–3 cm) above the sternal notch extending from posterior border of one sternocleidomastoid to opposite side. Incision is marked by placing stretched thread or silk over the skin. It can be marked using marking ink. Often few surgeons use 60 mL of 1 in 400,000 adrenaline saline to inject into the superficial fascia to reduce bleeding while raising the flap. Skin is incised using no. 15 blade. In women with heavy breasts incision is placed slightly at higher level than usual as subsequent scar may be dragged downwards close to sternum creating ugly scar. Platysma is identified and incised slightly at higher level than skin to prevent it getting adherent to scar at a later period **(Fig. 15-27)**.

Raising the Flaps

Upper flap (*subplatysmal flap*) is raised up to thyroid cartilage (platysma is absent in the midline); lower flap up to sternoclavicular joint/clavicular heads and suprasternal notch **(Figs. 15-28 and 15-29)**.

Rising of flap is done either using cautery or no. 15 blade or curved sharp scissor or blunt gauze dissection using finger. All bleeders are fulgurated properly. Care should be taken not to injure anterior jugular veins running on either side of the midline. There may be chance of air embolism if it is injured. In the lower part of the wound near lower flap both anterior jugular veins communicate through a communicating vein which if injured may cause bleeding and air embolism. In such situation anterior jugular veins distal to the communicating vein level should be ligated to prevent air embolism. Later veins are ligated proximally **(Fig. 15-30)**.

Retraction of the Flaps

A self-retaining Joll's thyroid retractor is placed. Silk skin sutures to upper and lower flaps can be placed to retract instead of Joll's retractor. Hamburger–Brennan–Mahorner self-retaining retractor can also be used **(Figs. 15-31 to 15-33)**.

Dissection

Deep fascia is incised vertically in midline/median raphe. Strap muscles are retracted (sternohyoid and omohyoid are in outer plane; sternothyroid is in deeper plane). Midline plane is bloodless field. Incision is done and plane is opened using either cautery or 15 no. blade or fine scissor. Strap muscles are retracted laterally using a deep retractor. If gland is large and if there is difficulty in mobilising gland then strap muscles can be cut between two Kocher's clamps at their upper part (as nerve supply to strap muscles is at lower part through ansa hypoglossi/ansa cervicalis) **(Figs. 15-34 and 15-35)**.

Thyroid fossa lateral and deep to the lateral lobe is dissected using blunt (peanut) and sharp dissection. Lateral lobe of the thyroid is held using gauze or Babcock's forceps to retract medially. Short stout middle thyroid vein is identified and ligated securely (double ligation is better) using 3-zero silk/vicryl. Blind dissection (should be avoided) near middle thyroid vein may tear or avulse it from IJV causing torrential haemorrhage. This allows proper mobilisation of the gland to identify parathyroid glands and recurrent laryngeal nerve **(Fig. 15-36)**.

Gland is now retracted downwards and laterally to expose the superior pole. It is dissected with sharp and peanut dissections.

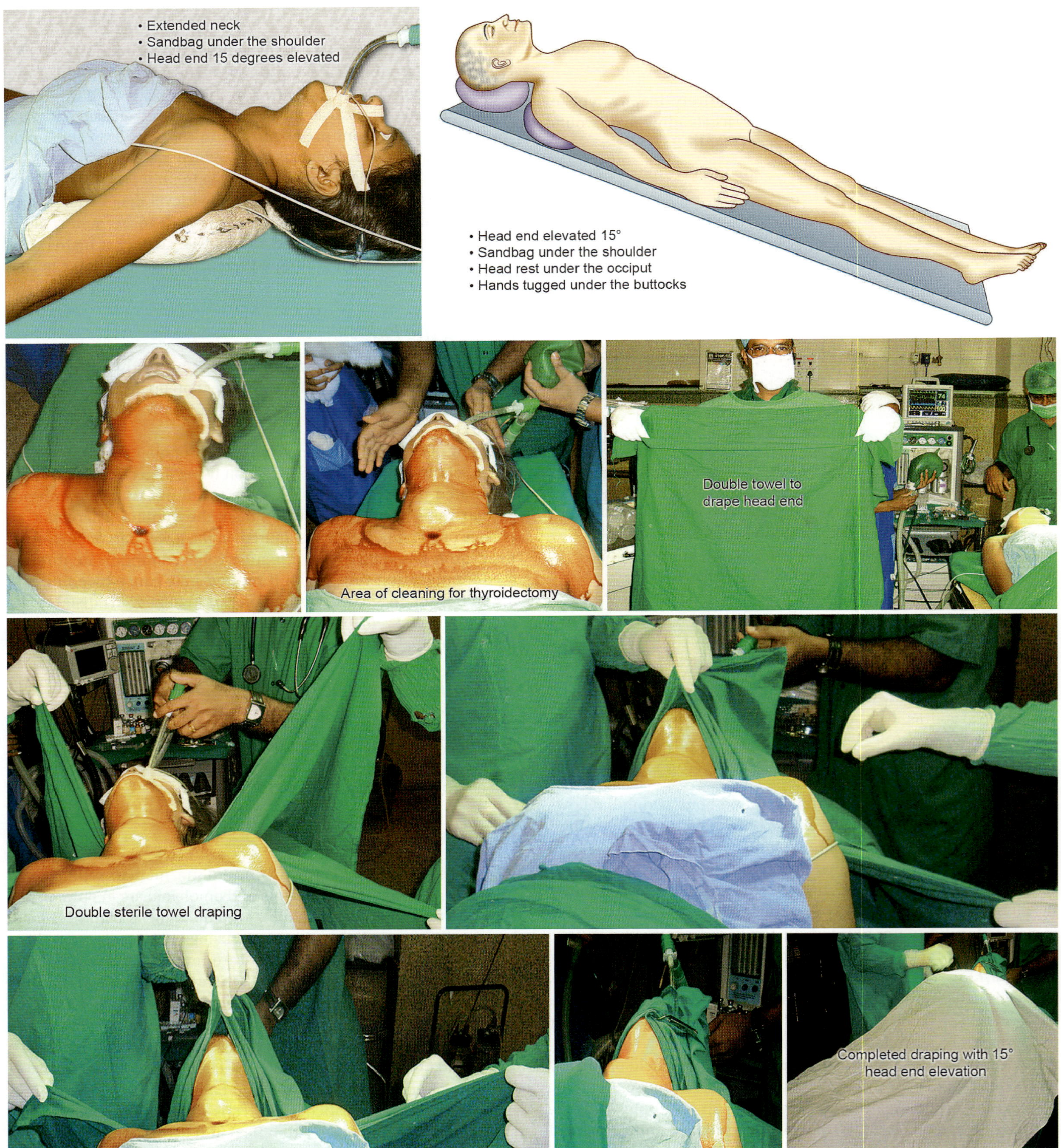
• Extended neck
• Sandbag under the shoulder
• Head end 15 degrees elevated
• Head end elevated 15°
• Sandbag under the shoulder
• Head rest under the occiput
• Hands tugged under the buttocks
Area of cleaning for thyroidectomy
Double towel to drape head end
Double sterile towel draping
Completed draping with 15° head end elevation

Figs. 15-25(1)

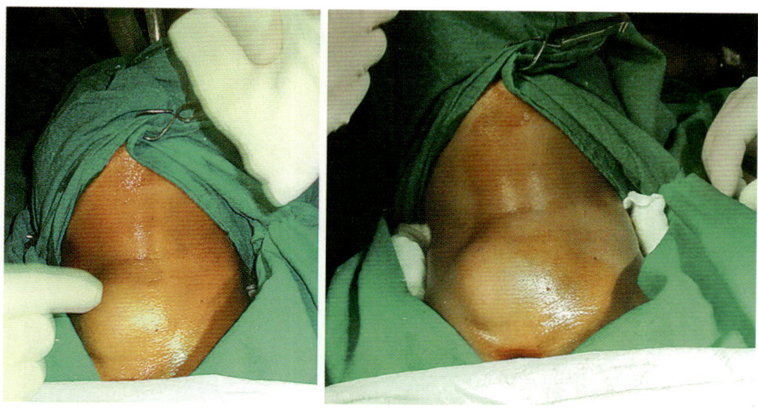

Figs. 15-25(2)

Figs. 15-25(1 and 2): Position of the patient in thyroidectomy. Neck is extended by placing the sandbag under the shoulder. 15° head up position is used. After cleaning, draping is done using double sterile towels to the head.

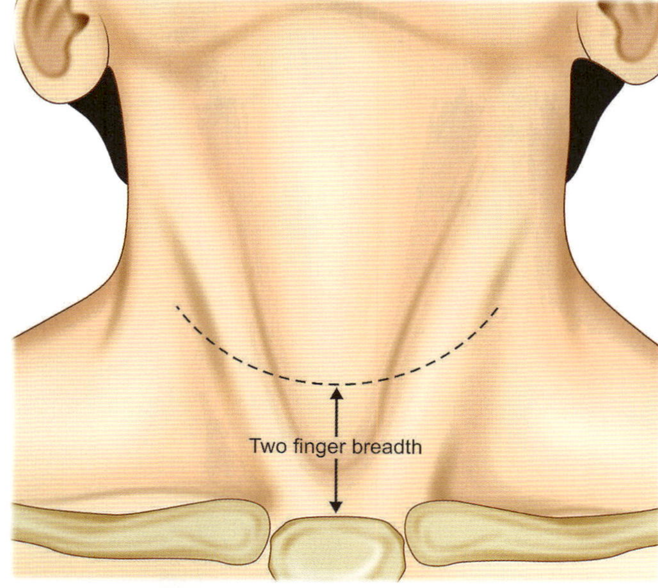

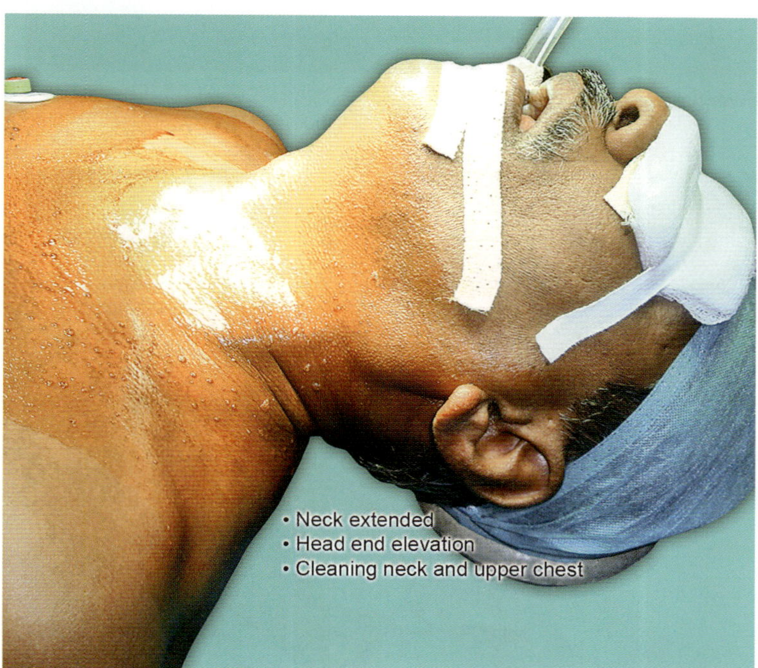

Fig. 15-26: Position and cleaning the area.

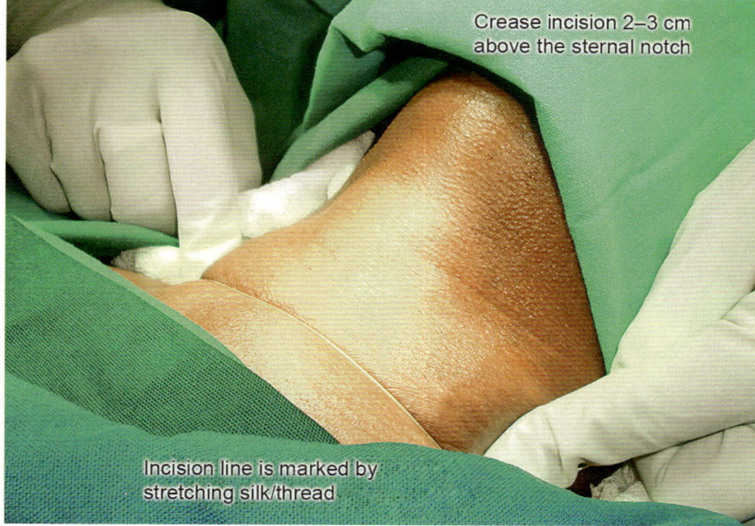

Fig. 15-27: Incision for thyroidectomy.

Superior thyroid artery and vein supplies the gland from superior pole. This space in front of cricothyroid is called as cricothyroid *space of Reeves.* In this space external laryngeal nerve which is just proximal to superior pole deviates towards cricothyroid muscle. Cricothyroid muscle is tensor of vocal cord which maintains the pitch of the voice. This nerve should not be injured. So artery and vein are *individually ligated close to the gland* to avoid injuring the nerve. Individual ligation of artery and vein also prevents rare problem of arteriovenous (AV) fistula. Artery should have 2 or 3 zero vicryl ligatures proximally. Often clips/ligaseal device are used to the vessel. Slipping of the ligature postoperatively can cause life threatening haemorrhage or compressing haematoma. *Often by many,* superior pedicle is ligated en mass. Prior to this Kocher's grooved director when available is passed underneath so that deeper tissues are safeguarded while cutting the pedicle. It is *advisable to identify the external laryngeal nerve* with careful dissection to safeguard it to prevent developing *altered pitch of voice (timber of voice).*

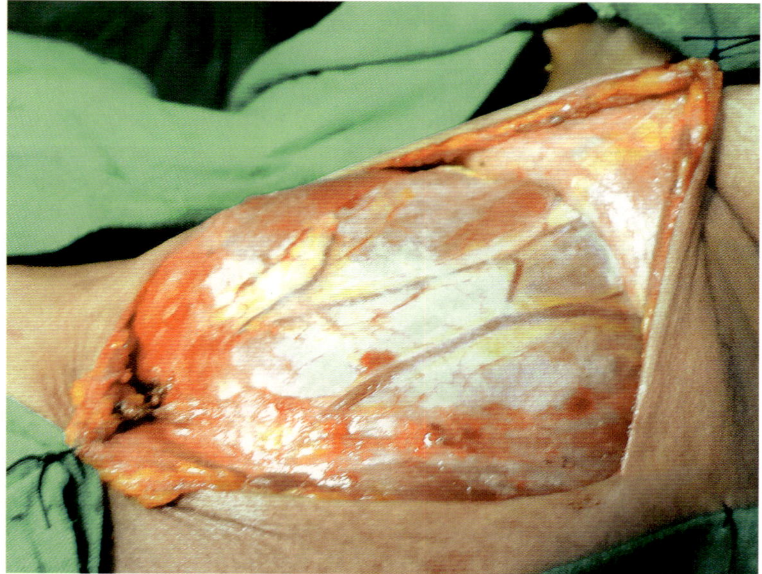

Fig. 15-28: Subplatysmal plane is used while raising the flap in thyroidectomy.

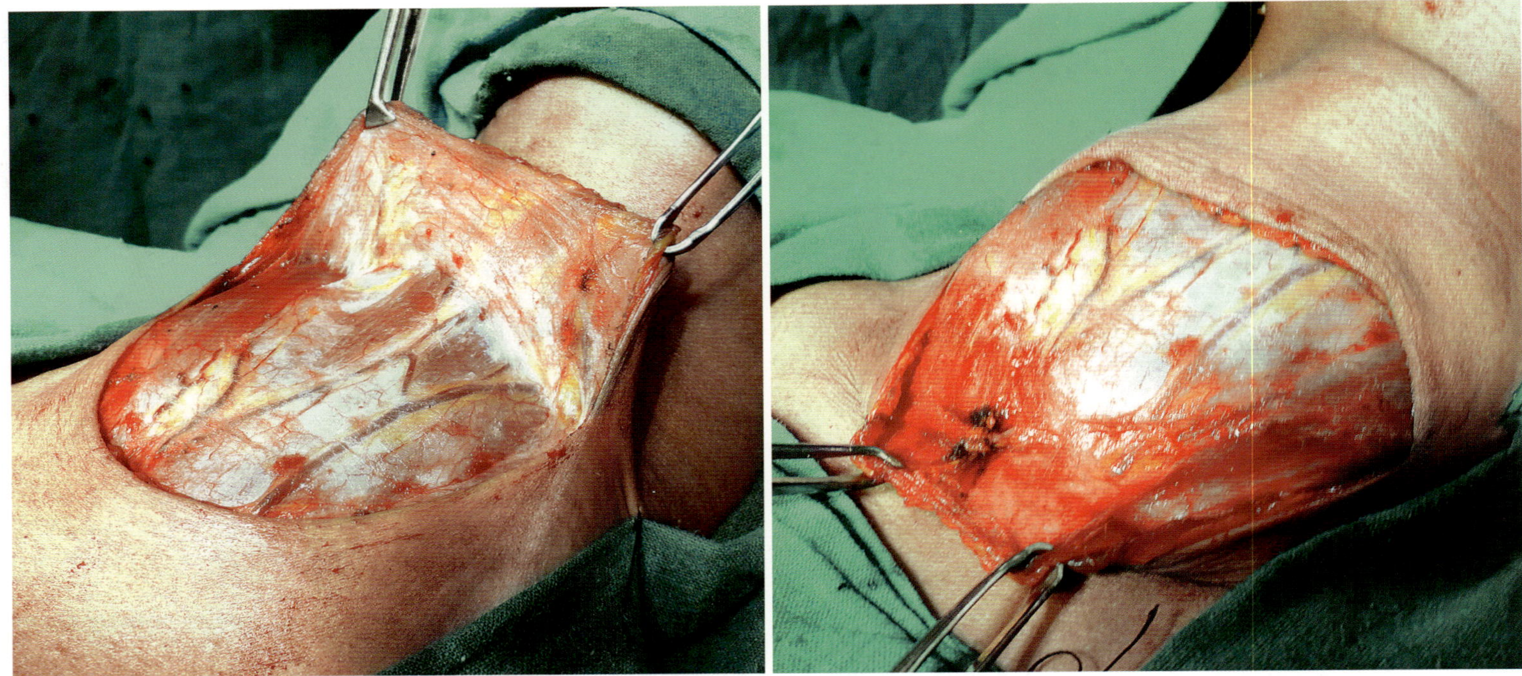

Fig. 15-29: Raising of upper flap and lower flaps in subplatysmal plane.

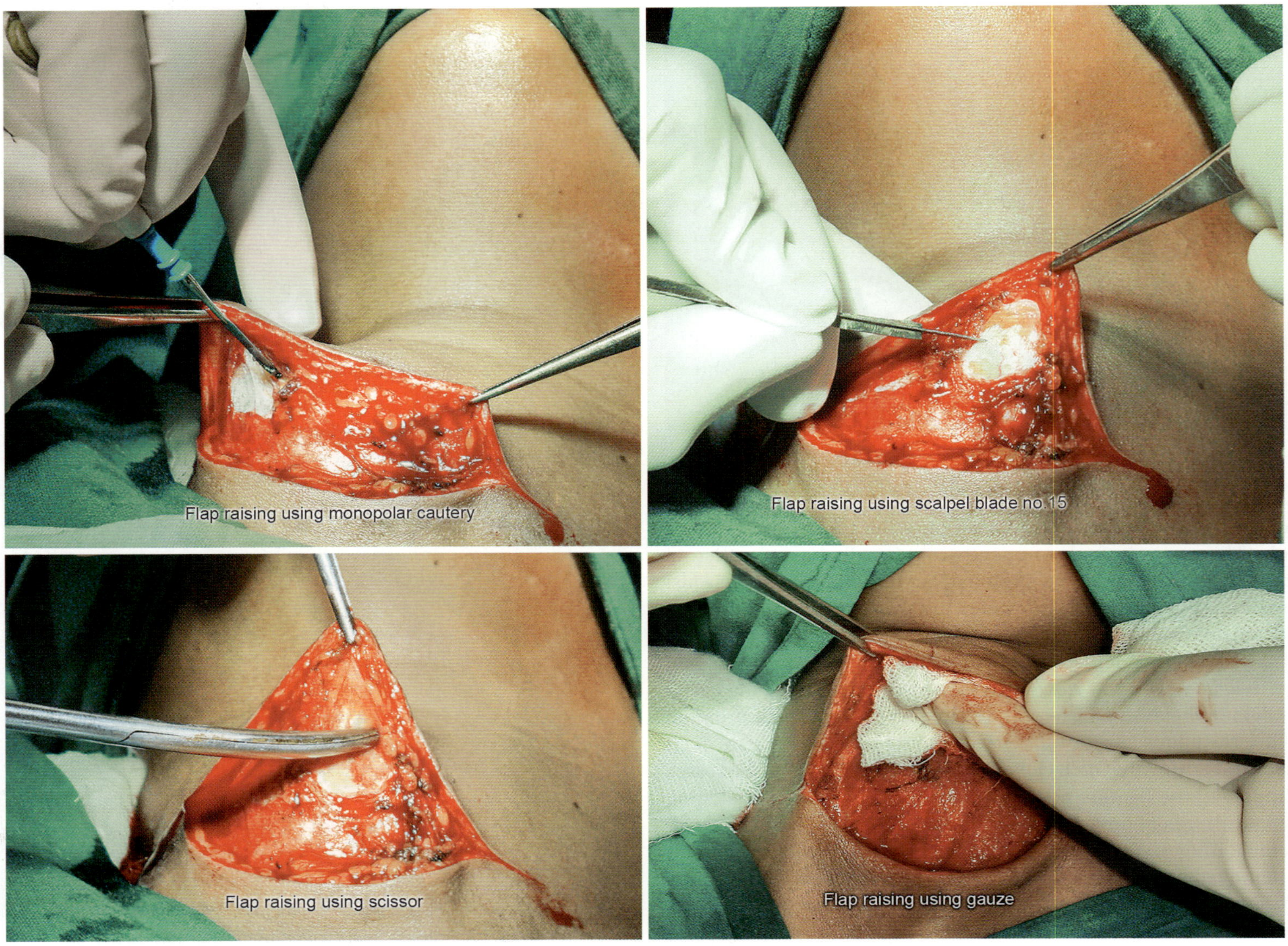

Fig. 15-30: Flaps are raised using monopolar cautery or scissor or gauze or finger dissection.

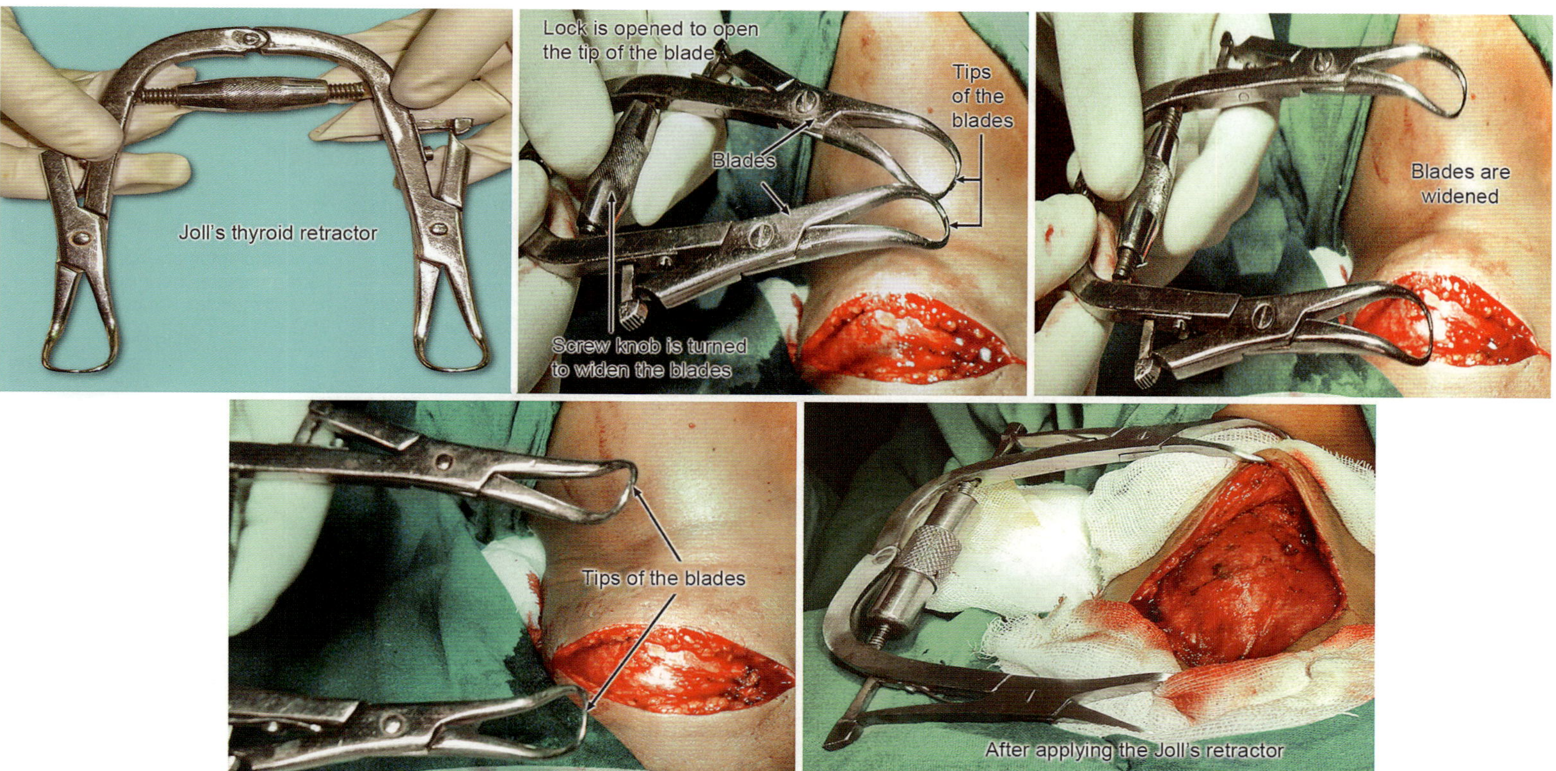

Fig. 15-31: Joll's thyroid retractor is commonly used to retract the upper and lower flaps.

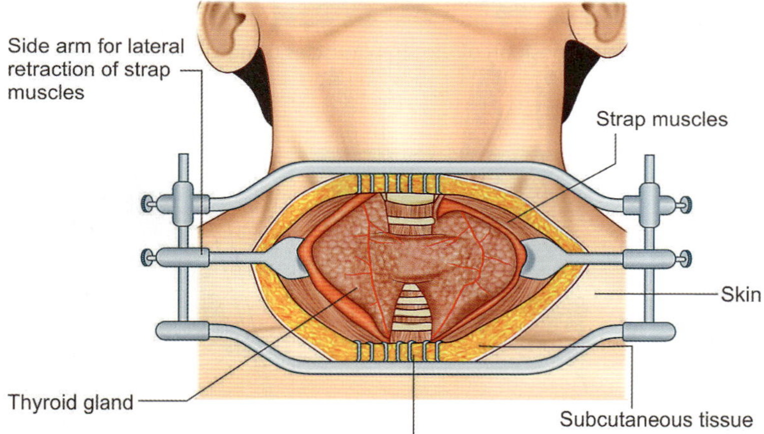

Fig. 15-32: Hamburger–Brennan–Mahorner self-retaining retractor with side arm to retract strap muscles.

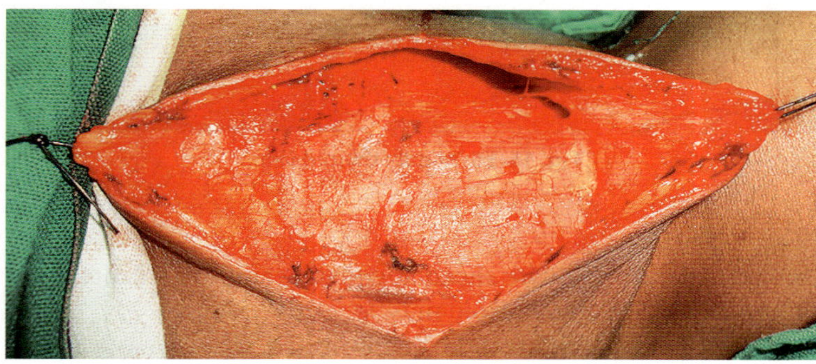

Fig. 15-33: Retraction of the elevated flaps in thyroidectomy using silk sutures.

Inferior pole of the thyroid is exposed and inferior thyroid veins are ligated adjacent to gland. Often thyroid ima venous plexus may be present in front of the trachea in midline which should be ligated properly **(Fig. 15-37)**.

Both blunt and sharp dissection using peanut, fine scissor, mosquito forceps with gentle traction over the gland medially will expose the recurrent laryngeal nerve and parathyroid glands. Recurrent laryngeal nerve passes behind the inferior thyroid artery in tracheo-oesophageal groove. But one should be aware of different variations which can cause nerve injury. Inferior thyroid artery arises from thyrocervical trunk of subclavian artery, running upwards, downwards and then medially under the carotid artery to reach the gland in front of the recurrent laryngeal nerve. To control any bleeders in this region *bipolar cautery* should be used (*never monopolar*). Branches of inferior thyroid artery while entering the gland should be ligated using 3-zero vicryl or silk. Ligating inferior thyroid artery or its branches close to gland avoids injury to the artery of parathyroid from inferior thyroid artery (*capsular dissection or orange peel dissection*). Olden day's classical method of ligating the inferior thyroid artery away from the gland just after crossing behind the carotid artery (ligation in continuity using absorbable suture—catgut) is *not commonly practiced* now **(Figs. 15-38A to C)**.

Berry's ligament which is adherent to thyroid is cut with care to properly mobilise the gland medially as recurrent laryngeal nerve is very close to the Berry's ligament. RLN should be identified unlike older concept ('nerve not seen is not damaged' is *disproved*; present concept is '*nerve not seen is damaged*') **(Fig. 15-39)**.

Parathyroid glands vary in their position on the surface of the gland but can be easily identified by its different colour (golden yellow/caramel like). Glands should be dissected off the thyroid with their blood supply. ⅓ of one gland is sufficient to maintain the function (calcium metabolism by releasing PTH).

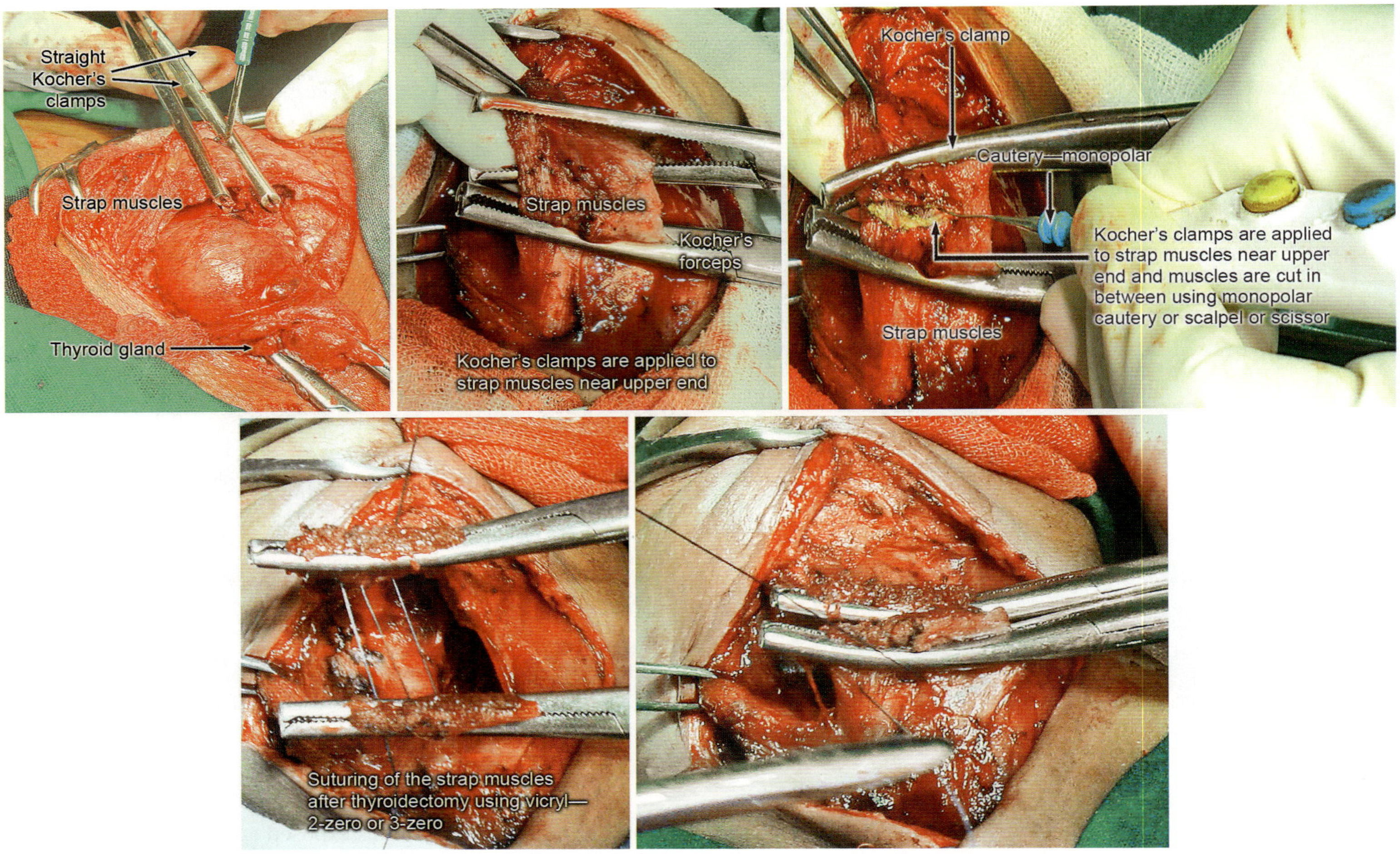

Fig. 15-34: Cutting the strap muscles near upper end and later after thyroidectomy apposition of the strap muscles using vicryl.

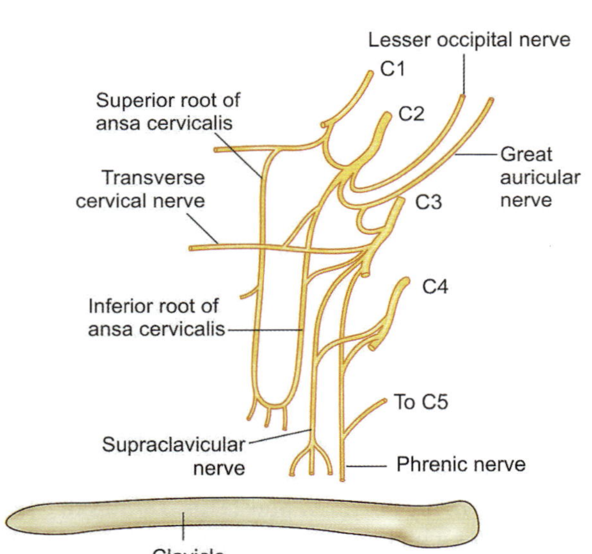

Fig. 15-35: Ansa cervicalis/hypoglossi and other neck nerves.

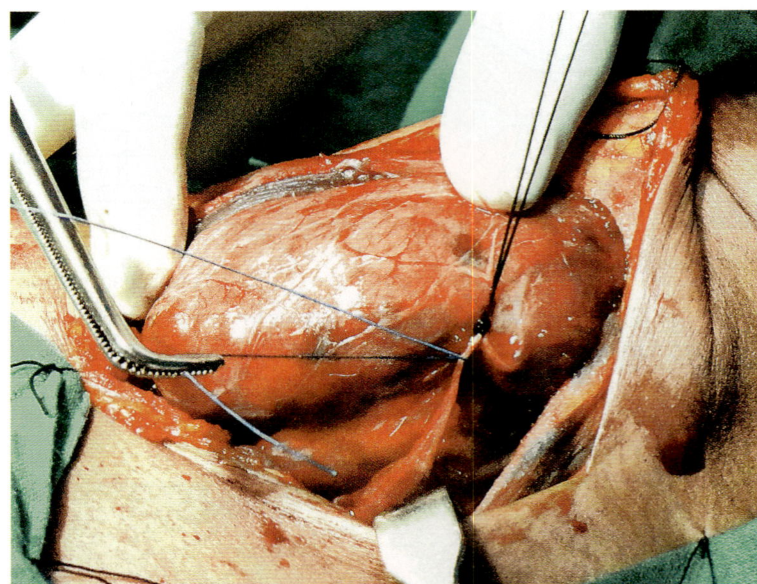

Fig. 15-36: Middle thyroid vein.

Ideally *all four parathyroids should be preserved*. Due to vasospasm of vessels of the parathyroids temporary hypoparathyroidism is common but reversible. Unnecessary handling of parathyroids should be avoided. Handling of the gland makes it congested. Viability of parathyroid can be checked by carefully incising it using fine scalpel. Doubtful gland should be sliced adequately and transplanted into same side sternocleidomastoid muscle.

Inferior pole vessels are individually ligated.

Opposite lateral lobe is also dissected similarly. It is surgeon's choice to decide on which side to stand while dissecting on opposite side.

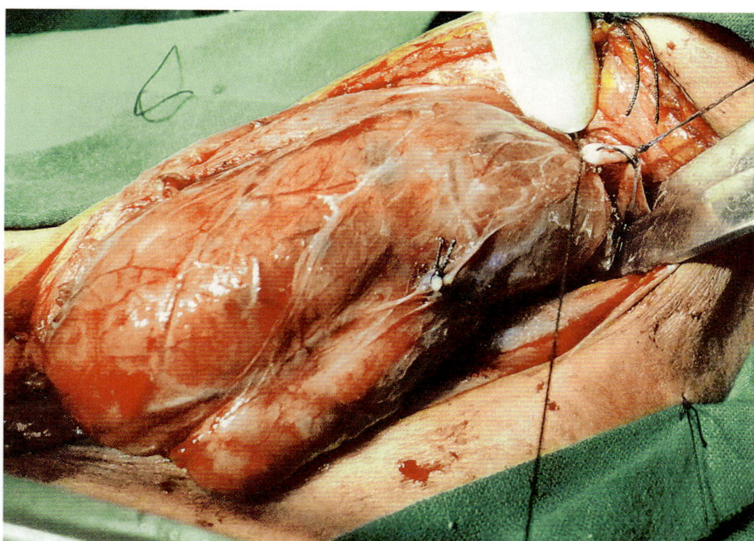

Fig. 15-37: Ligation of superior thyroid artery is done close to the gland individually after identifying the external laryngeal nerve.

In difficult thyroids it is often preferred to go to opposite side and dissect the gland.

Thyroid is dissected from anterior surface of trachea using cautery or fine scissor. If part of the gland is retained in the tracheo-oesophageal groove (subtotal) it should be oversewn using 3-zero vicryl. Fine clamps are placed in series on the thyroid capsule. Gland is transected using no. 15 blade. Retained gland is undersewn using vicryl continuous locking sutures. Anterior part of this retained gland is sutured to trachea **(Fig. 15-40)**.

In hemithyroidectomy, one lateral lobe and entire isthmus is removed. Junction of isthmus and opposite lateral lobe is clamped using haemostat/Kocher's clamp and gland is cut. Clamped retaining gland is under run using vicryl **(Fig. 15-41)**.

Proper haemostasis is done using bipolar cautery. Pedicles are inspected again for their security **(Fig. 15-42)**.

Closure

Sandbag is removed. Again haemostasis is confirmed. Often stretched neck prevents bleeding from small veins but once sandbag is removed they may bleed which should be controlled. Traditionally suction drain is placed which is brought out through a separate stab incision or one of the ends of the main wound. Drain should pass under the strap muscles to reach the thyroid fossa. If proper haemostasis is done drain can be avoided. Controversy still surrounds the use of drains after thyroid surgery. Strap muscles are approximated using interrupted 3-zero vicryl sutures. Platysma is sutured using 3-zero vicryl interrupted sutures. Subcuticular absorbable 3-zero monocryl suture is used for skin. Dressing with pressure using dynaplast is the usual practice. But a dressing that covers the wound *may mask* haematoma formation, delaying its recognition. Placing soft light dressing or without any dressing may be ideal even though it is not practiced by most surgeons **(Fig. 15-43)**.

The *prevention of postoperative bleeding* depends on good intraoperative hemostasis. Hemostasis in thyroid surgery is achieved by means of clamp and tie, surgical clips, diathermy—unipolar initially and bipolar in the depth, ultrasonic coagulating—dissection such as a harmonic scalpel (HS) or electrothermal bipolar vessel sealing systems (EBVSS) **(Figs. 15-44 and 15-45)**.

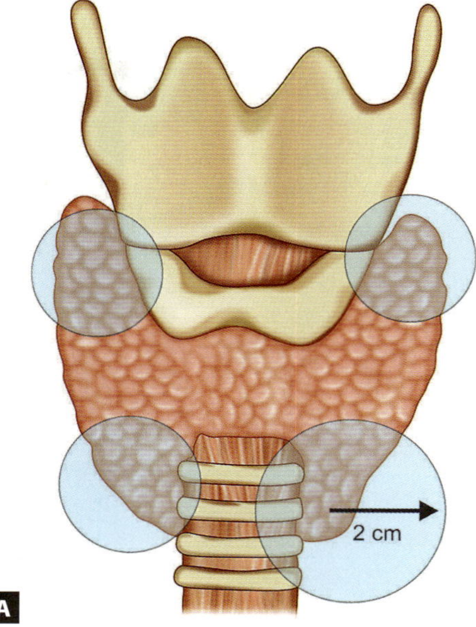

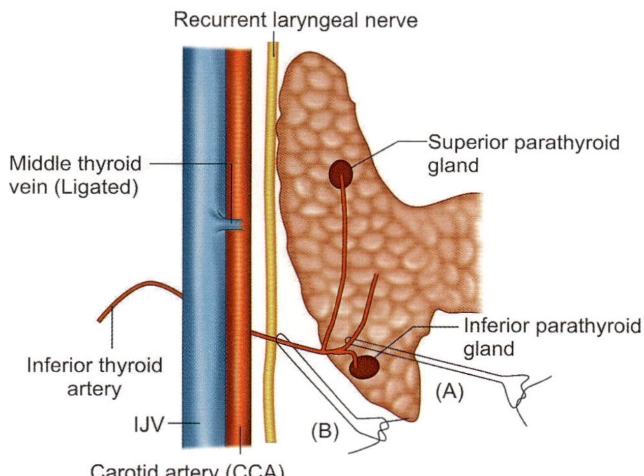

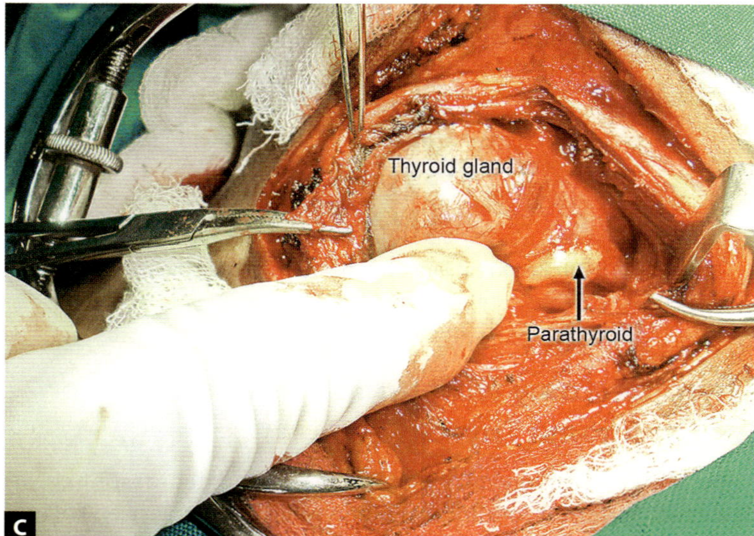

Figs. 15-38A to C: Location of parathyroids and their variations should be remembered. Parathyroids should be retained during thyroidectomy. It is also important to retain their blood supply also.

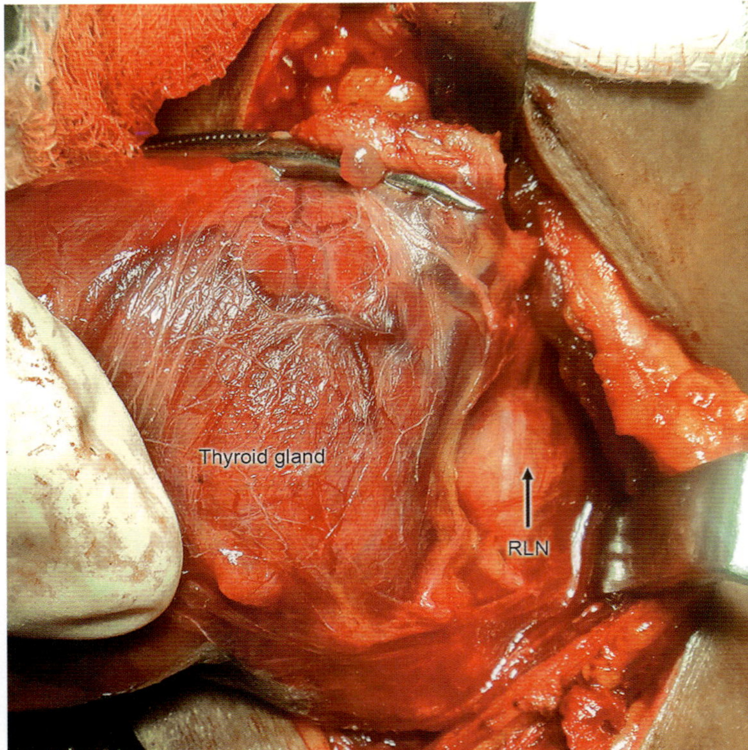

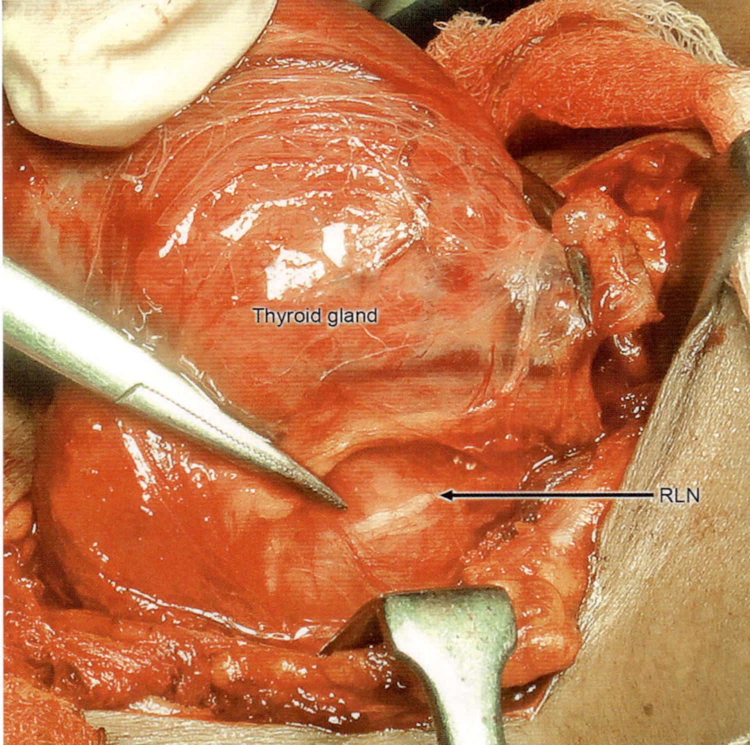

Fig. 15-39: Recurrent laryngeal nerve should be identified in all thyroidectomies.

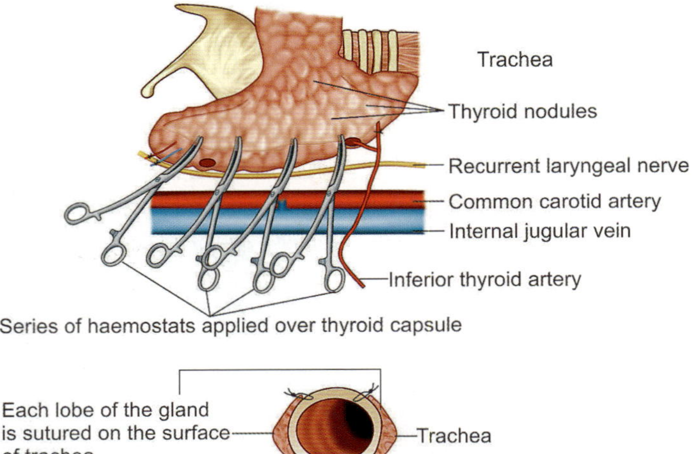

Fig. 15-40: Partial or subtotal thyroidectomy is done by applying series of haemostats on the thyroid capsule to facilitate the removal of the gland in front. Retained gland is under run using vicryl sutures.

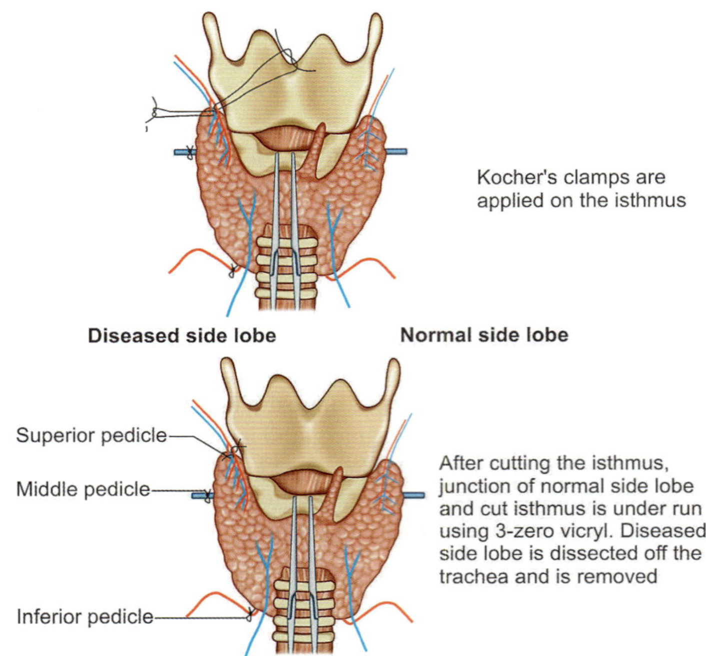

Fig. 15-41: Isthmus at its junction to retaining lobe of the thyroid gland is transected between clamps and retaining cut part of the thyroid tissue is under run using vicryl.

Thyroidectomy with Lymph Node Dissection for Carcinoma Thyroid

Level VI (cervico-central/pretracheal and tracheo-oesophageal) nodes are removed routinely in all thyroid cancers. Frozen section biopsy of level III deep cervical node is done. If it is involved, a modified radical neck dissection preserving IJV, accessory nerve and sternocleidomastoid muscle is done. Same thyroid incision extended laterally and above towards mastoid process is usually sufficient to do additional lymph node dissection. For bilateral neck dissection, incision is extended on both sides. Sympathetic chain and hypoglossal nerve above will come into picture during dissection which should be preserved.

In medullary carcinoma of thyroid, central node dissection, often modified radical neck dissection with dissection of upper mediastinal nodes (level VII) and thymus is done. Meticulous dissection is needed to preserve recurrent laryngeal nerve and parathyroids.

In any malignancy with clinically significant palpable neck nodes confirmed by FNAC modified radical neck dissection is done along with total thyroidectomy.

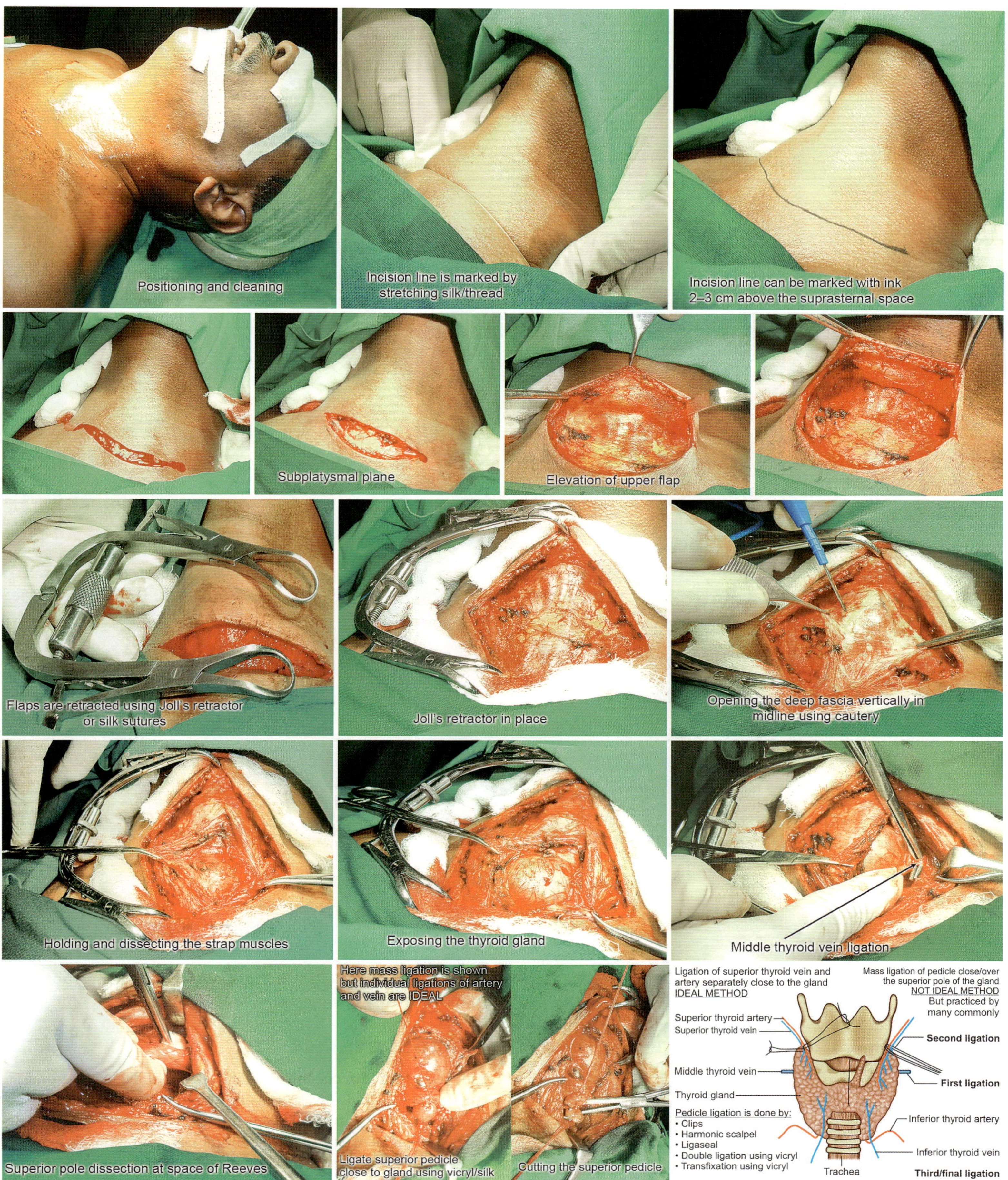
Positioning and cleaning
Incision line is marked by stretching silk/thread
Incision line can be marked with ink 2–3 cm above the suprasternal space
Subplatysmal plane
Elevation of upper flap
Flaps are retracted using Joll's retractor or silk sutures
Joll's retractor in place
Opening the deep fascia vertically in midline using cautery
Holding and dissecting the strap muscles
Exposing the thyroid gland
Middle thyroid vein ligation
Superior pole dissection at space of Reeves
Here mass ligation is shown but individual ligations of artery and vein are IDEAL
Ligate superior pedicle close to gland using vicryl/silk
Cutting the superior pedicle
Ligation of superior thyroid vein and artery separately close to the gland
IDEAL METHOD
Mass ligation of pedicle close/over the superior pole of the gland
NOT IDEAL METHOD
But practiced by many commonly
Superior thyroid artery
Superior thyroid vein
Second ligation
Middle thyroid vein
First ligation
Thyroid gland
Pedicle ligation is done by:
• Clips
• Harmonic scalpel
• Ligaseal
• Double ligation using vicryl
• Transfixation using vicryl
Inferior thyroid artery
Inferior thyroid vein
Trachea
Third/final ligation

Figs. 15-42(1)

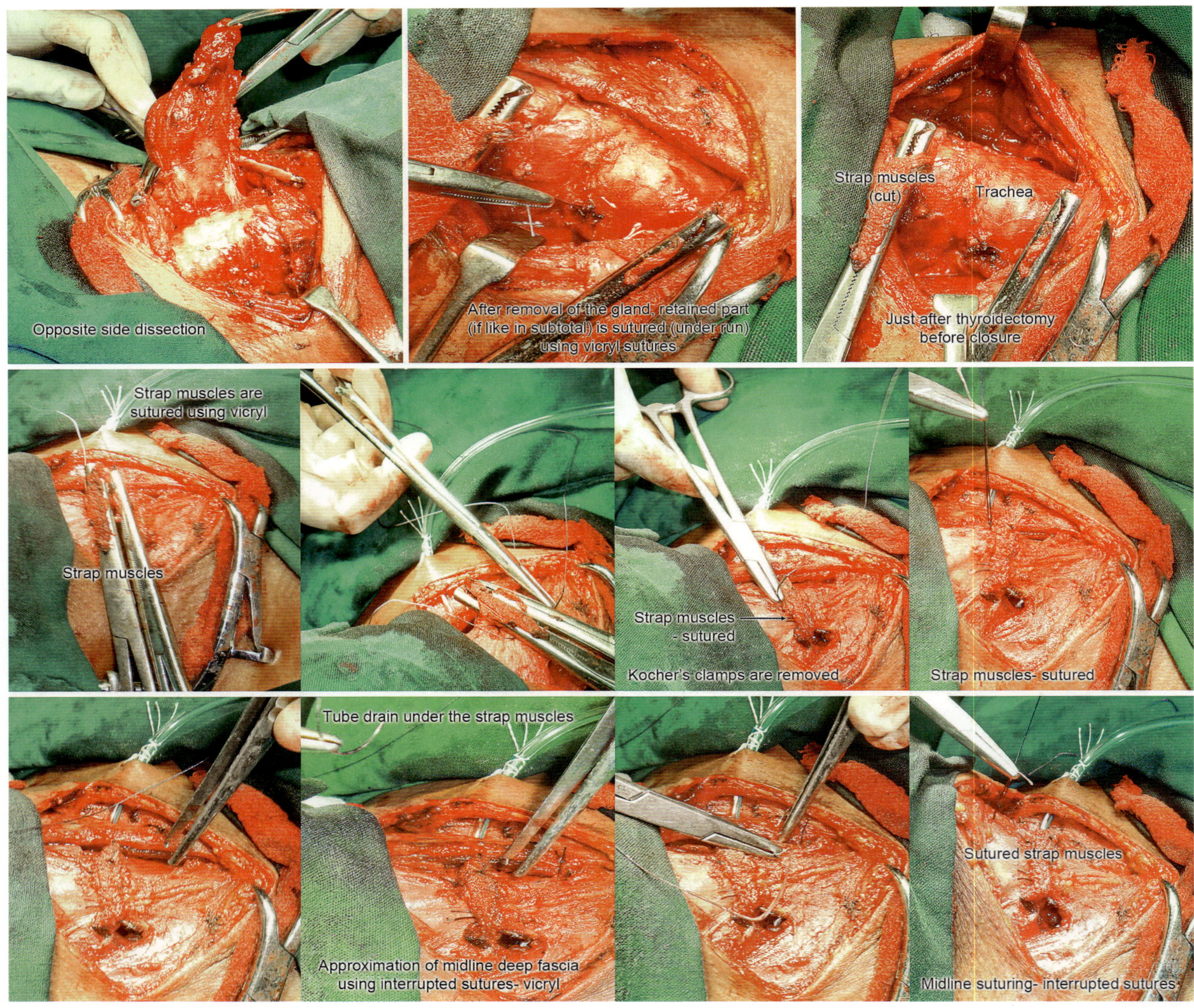

Figs. 15-42(2)

Figs. 15-42(1 and 2): Technique of thyroidectomy.

Lateral Approach Thyroidectomy

Lateral approach is used in large thyroid enlargement/recurrent thyroid disease/often thyroid carcinoma instead of classical neck approach. After lengthy skin incision, plane is created between anterior border of sternomastoid muscle and lateral to strap muscles to proceed with surgery. Often sternocleidomastoid muscle may need to be removed.

Removal of Retrosternal Goitre

Usually there will be enlarged neck thyroid of similar pathology. As retrosternal thyroid receives its blood supply from neck it is usually delivered to thyroid incision of neck with blunt dissection and removed. Occasionally in large/vascular/adherent retrosternal goitre a median sternotomy may be added to remove it.

Postoperative Care

Patient is kept in postoperative room with head end tilted 30° upwards. Once patient is fully awake with normal breathing (in 4–6 hours), patient is shifted to ward. Patient should be observed for bleeding, formation of haematoma, stridor, drop in O_2 saturation, tachycardia or tachypnoea. Tetany may be observed in 3–4 days. *Hungry bone syndrome* can cause severe hypocalcaemia in immediate postoperative period. Drain is removed in 24–48 hours depending on the quantity of collection in drain.

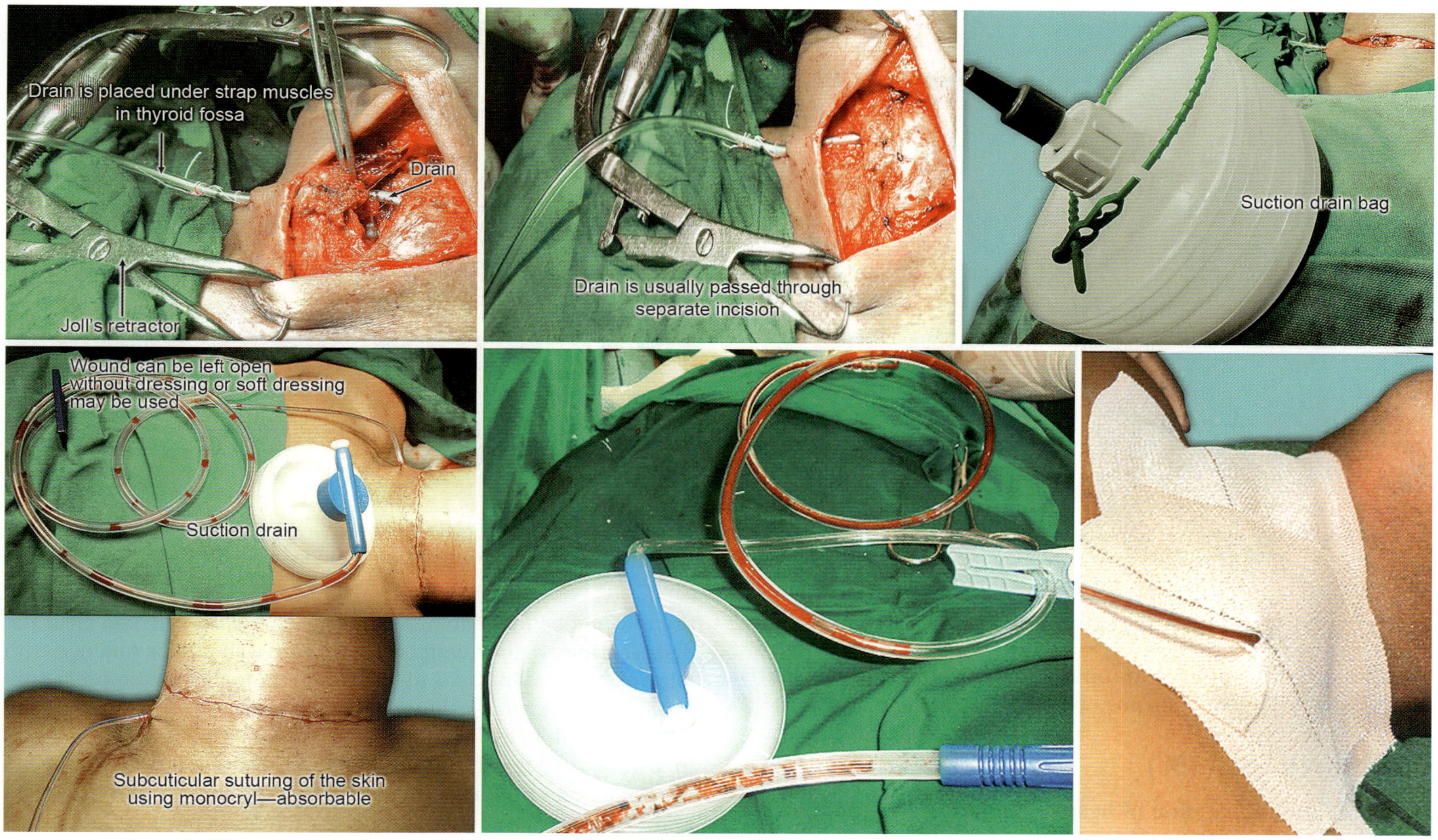

Fig. 15-43: Placing the drain in thyroidectomy. Wound is left open or soft dressing may be placed. Compression dressing is commonly used even though practice is not necessary/ideal.

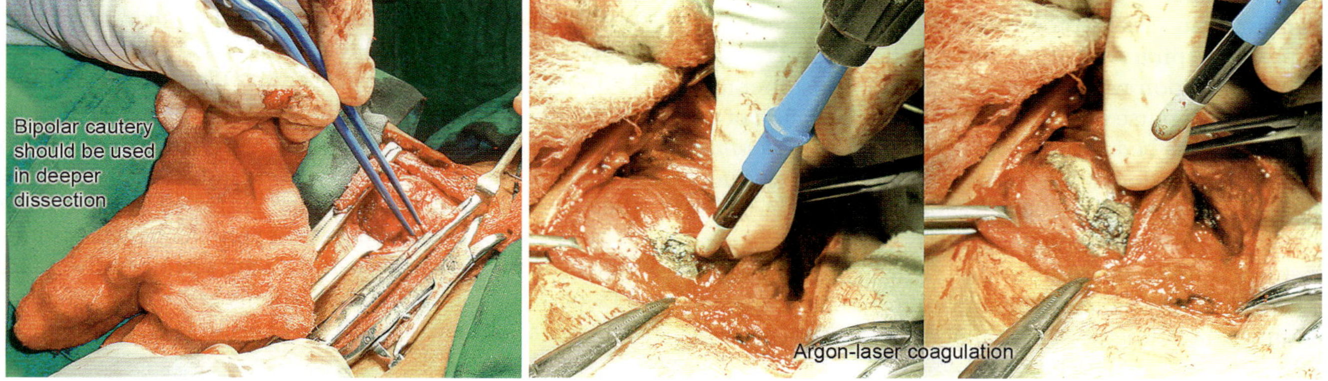

Fig. 15-44: Bipolar cautery is used in deeper dissection. Monopolar cautery is used only during raising flaps and incising the deep fascia in midline. Often argon laser coagulation may be used on the surface.

Remember in thyroidectomy

- Middle thyroid vein is present only in 30% of cases.
- Bipolar cautery or harmonic scalpel (harmonic wave) are better to control bleeding and to prevent injury to RLN
- RLN should be identified in both sides. Variations should be remembered.
- Parathyroids should be retained and also their blood supply.
- Parathyroid autotransplantation may be needed if their blood supply is compromised.
- Rapid influx of serum calcium into bones in immediate postoperative period may cause severe hypocalcaemia—hungry bone syndrome which is initially corrected by IV calcium gluconate—10 mL of 10%. It is more commonly observed in patients with beta blockers. It is due to sudden drop in PTH level after surgery.
- Tension haematoma under strap muscles is very dangerous and should be relieved by removing sutures from the skin and strap muscles. It can be life saving with immediate intervention otherwise it can be life threatening.
- Permanent hypoparathyroidism is rare (0.5–1%) even though temporary hypoparathyroidism and hypocalcaemia is common (25%) which is corrected well with calcium for certain period of 3–6 months.
- External laryngeal nerve injury is more common than RLN injury. There is loss of tension of vocal cords causing reduced power and range in voice (pitch).
- Thyroid insufficiency develops in 25–45% cases. It is confirmed by doing serum T3, T4 and TSH after 2, 3 and 6 months.

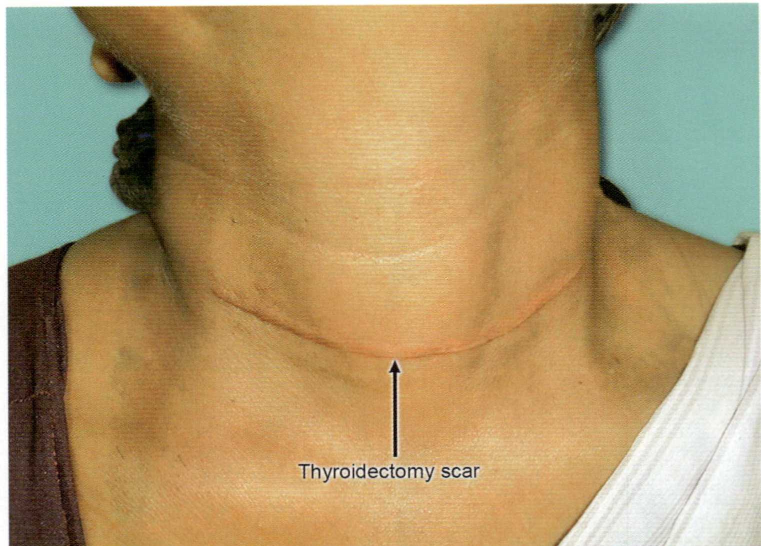

Fig. 15-45: Thin linear scar usually forms after thyroidectomy which is cosmetically acceptable.

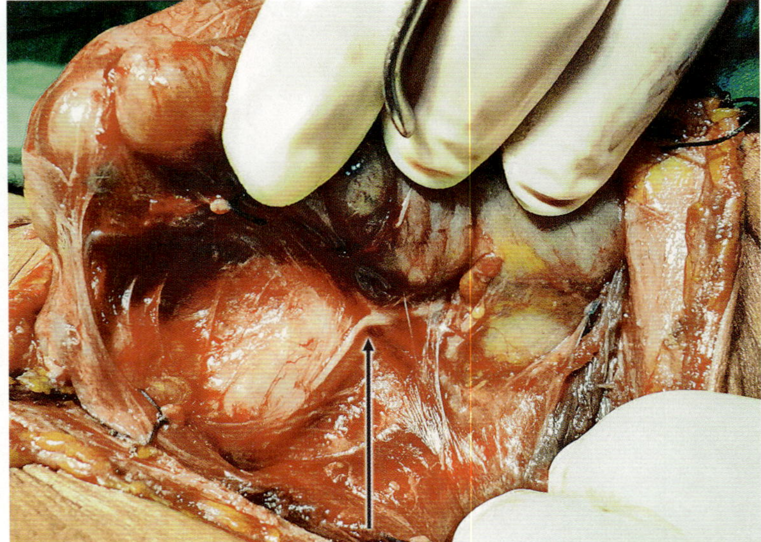

Fig. 15-46: Recurrent laryngeal nerve should be identified in all thyroidectomies and safeguarded.

COMPLICATIONS OF THYROIDECTOMY

Complications can be intraoperative or immediate/in early postoperative period or late postoperative.

Haemorrhage (1%)

It may be due to slipping of ligatures either of superior thyroid artery or other pedicles or of small veins. It is often precipitated by vigorous coughing or retching in postoperative period. It causes tachycardia, hypotension, and breathlessness, tracheal compression due to progressive tension haematoma formation in thyroid fossa under sutured strap muscles causing severe respiratory obstruction, cyanosis, hypoxia, respiratory failure and cardiac arrest. Tension haematoma is a condition which is often missed in postoperative ward by the monitoring nurse or intensivist. Early identification of the problem with immediate bedside removal of skin and *deeper sutures* prevents further compression of the trachea relieving the respiratory obstruction. Ultrasound of neck may be useful but unnecessary time should not be wasted just to do sonology. It is essentially life-saving procedure which is often failed to undertake causing mortality. Later patient is shifted to operation theatre and wound is inspected under anaesthesia; bleeding vessel is caught and securely ligated. Often transfusion of blood is also required.

Respiratory Obstruction

It may be due to haematoma or due to laryngeal oedema or due to tracheomalacia or due to bilateral recurrent laryngeal nerve palsy. Evacuation of clot, emergency tracheostomy is required. *Fiberoptic laryngoscopy* is useful to assess the vocal cord palsy.

Recurrent Laryngeal Nerve Palsy

It can be *transient or permanent*. During extubation anaesthetist should be asked to visualise the movements of vocal cord to confirm that there is no recurrent laryngeal nerve injury. It should be documented both by anaesthetist and surgeon in the case sheet. Distressing change in voice should be assessed and treated by *steroid* (in case of neuropraxia), *speech therapy* and counselling. In malignant condition it is better to inform the patient about voice change as there would be possible need for transecting the nerve to clear the disease. However, in benign diseases, nerve should be retained with all care. If nerve injury is identified on table during the procedure it *should be repaired* using microscope with 9-zero polypropylene sutures. Incidence of transient RLN palsy is 3%. It usually recovers in 3 weeks to 3 months. Permanent palsy is rare but do can occur. RLN palsy can be—unilateral; bilateral; unilateral combined RLN and external laryngeal nerve palsy; bilateral combined RLN and external laryngeal nerve palsy **(Fig. 15-46)**.

Unilateral RLN palsy causes median or paramedian vocal cord position. Here all intrinsic muscles of larynx except cricothyroid on one side are paralysed. Cricothyroid, which is the only retained muscle is a weak adductor of the vocal cord causing median or paramedian position of vocal cords (*Wagner–Grossman hypothesis).* Abductor fibres (nerve supply of posterior cricoarytenoid) of the RLN which are phylogenetically newer are more susceptible and paralysed than adductors (*Semon's law).* It causes change in voice (hoarseness) which gradually gets corrected by compensatory action of opposite vocal cord. Speech therapy will benefit for these patients. Short course of steroid in immediate postoperative period is used. 33% of unilateral RLN palsy patients are asymptomatic. Aspiration and airway obstruction will never occur **(Fig. 15-47)**.

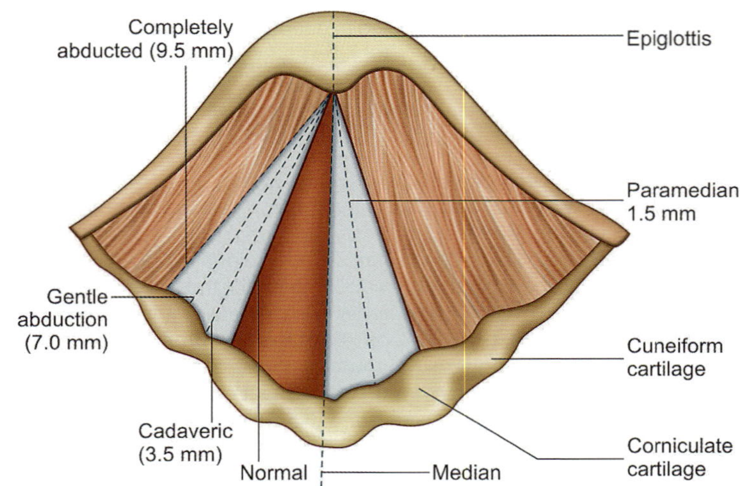

Fig. 15-47: Different vocal cord positions and also RLN palsy.

Unilateral combined RLN and superior laryngeal nerve palsy: All muscles of larynx on one side is paralysed. Vocal cord will be in cadaveric position, 3.5 mm from the midline. It leads into hoarseness of voice, ineffective glottis causing aspiration, ineffective cough and respiratory congestion. Treatment is speech therapy, Teflon injection to paralysed vocal cord, placement of muscle/cartilage implant to paralysed cord, arthrodesis of cricoarytenoid joint.

Bilateral RLN palsy: Both side intrinsic muscles of larynx are paralysed except cricothyroids. Unopposed actions of both cricothyroids cause vocal cord in median/paramedian position. Condition causes voice change, severe dyspnoea, airway block and respiratory arrest. Treatment: Emergency tracheostomy; lateralisation of cord by arytenoidectomy; vocal cord lateralisation, cordectomy by open or laser method; sternohyoid implantation; thyroplasty.

Bilateral combined RLN and superior laryngeal nerve palsy: Here there will be total paralysis of the intrinsic muscles of larynx and total laryngeal anaesthesia, causing aphonia (no voice), severe glottis incompetence causing aspiration, absence of cough, retention of lung secretions leading into severe distress. It is treated by emergency tracheostomy, fixing epiglottis to arytenoids, vocal cord plication and often by total laryngectomy.

Assessing the vocal cord palsy: It is done by indirect laryngoscopy, direct fibreoptic endoscopy, laryngeal electromyography (EMG). EMG may be useful to distinguish vocal fold paralysis from injury to the cricoarytenoid joint secondary to intubation. EMG may help in assessing the prognosis of the patient with RLN injury. Thick connective tissue called the *Berry ligament* attaches the thyroid to the trachea at the level of the second or third tracheal ring. This is the most common site of injury to the RLN. The nerve may run deep to the ligament, pass through it, or even penetrate the gland a short distance at this level. Retraction of the thyroid lobe may result in traction injury and make the nerve susceptible to transection. The path of the nerve must be clearly identified. An endotracheal-tube electrode and an RLN-postcricoid-laryngeal surface electrode may be used in difficult thyroid surgeries to have continuous electrophysiologic monitoring to reveal the location of RLN. Proper identification of the RLN minimises the risk of injury. During thyroidectomy, when the nerve is identified and dissected, the reported RLN injury rate is 0–2.1%; if surgery is repeated (re-thyroidectomy) it is 2–12%; if the nerve is not identified it is 4–6.6%. Intraoperative haemostasis and a thorough understanding of the anatomy are essential for identifying and preserving the nerve.

Bilateral RLN palsy	***Most dangerous.***
Bilateral combined RLN and superior laryngeal N palsy	*Dangerous.*
Unilateral RLN palsy	Not dangerous.
Unilateral combined palsy	Not dangerous.

For unilateral vocal cord paralysis corrective procedures are not done until at least 6 months after thyroidectomy because a reversible injury improves by that time. If the nerve was definitely transected during surgery, treatment for the paralysed fold may be performed sooner than this.

Medialisation of the vocal cords is the most commonly performed. Medialisation of the impaired vocal fold improves contact with the contralateral mobile fold. It is done by injection laryngoplasty or laryngeal framework surgery. Type I thyroplasty is probably the most common procedure. A window in the thyroid cartilage is created at the level of the true vocal fold. An implant is then placed to push the vocal fold medially. Medialisation with an injection of absorbable gelatin sponge may be performed before 6 months. But gelatin sponge gets absorbed after sometime and is a temporary treatment. An implant made of silicone or polytetrafluoroethylene is permanent. The implant may be removed if nerve function recovers later.

Reinnervation procedures are done for permanently injured RLN. These procedures maintain/restore tone of the intrinsic laryngeal muscles. When the true vocal fold atrophies after denervation, it loses contact with the contralateral fold and the voice weakens. By preventing atrophy, reinnervation procedures help to improve the patient's voice.

Primary neurorrhaphy is done immediately to repair the transected RLN.

In bilateral vocal cord paralysis, initial treatment involves obtaining an adequate airway by *emergency tracheotomy*. Often first endotracheal intubation is done; neck is explored to ensure that there are no reversible causes of nerve injury; if RLNs show good preservation, a trial of extubation may be performed after several days. Intravenous steroids are used. If nerve function has not recovered after a second trial of extubation, tracheotomy is certainly needed.

In bilateral vocal cord paralysis in order to improve airway patency, *cordotomy and arytenoidectomy* are the common procedures done. These procedures enlarge the airway and allow de-cannulation of a tracheostomy. However, the patient must be counselled that his or her voice will likely to worsen after surgery.

Intraoperative nerve monitoring (IONM) of recurrent laryngeal nerve: IONM is used to identify accurately RLN during thyroidectomy. Specialised endotracheal tube with electrodes which are connected to power and monitor and stimulator is used in IONM. Electrodes should be in contact with vocal folds. During surgery stimulator is used while dissecting the RLN area. While touching e RLN signal will be sent through electrode sensor placed at on the endotracheal tube which causes graphic wave of the nerve stimulation; nerve stimulation produces electromyographic signal at vocal cords which is detected through electrodes and transmitted to monitor; it also gives audio warning signal also. So, meticulous dissection can be done to safeguard the RLN at the area. Standardisation is important by initial vagal nerve stimulation, visual nerve identification, direct on table stimulation of RLN, and final confirmation of intact RLN function. But system is costly but safer.

Continuous intraoperative nerve monitoring (CIONM) is newer modification wherein temporary implantable electrode is attached to the vagus nerve; it allows real time continuous monitoring with vagus recurrent circuit during dissection **(Figs. 15-48A to D)**.

Hypoparathyroidism—Types

Types		
Temporary	More common (2–50%) average 10%	Usually lasts for 2 months maximum up to 6 months.
Permanent	Less common (0.4–13%) average 1%	Permanent—continues beyond 6 months.
Hungry bone syndrome	Common (5–13%)	Severe, rapid begins in immediate postoperative period.

The parathyroid glands produce parathyroid hormone (PTH), which is involved in the regulation of serum calcium. PTH increases serum calcium levels by causing bone resorption, increasing renal absorption of calcium, and stimulating the synthesis of the biologically active form of vitamin D (1, 25-dihydroxy vitamin D).

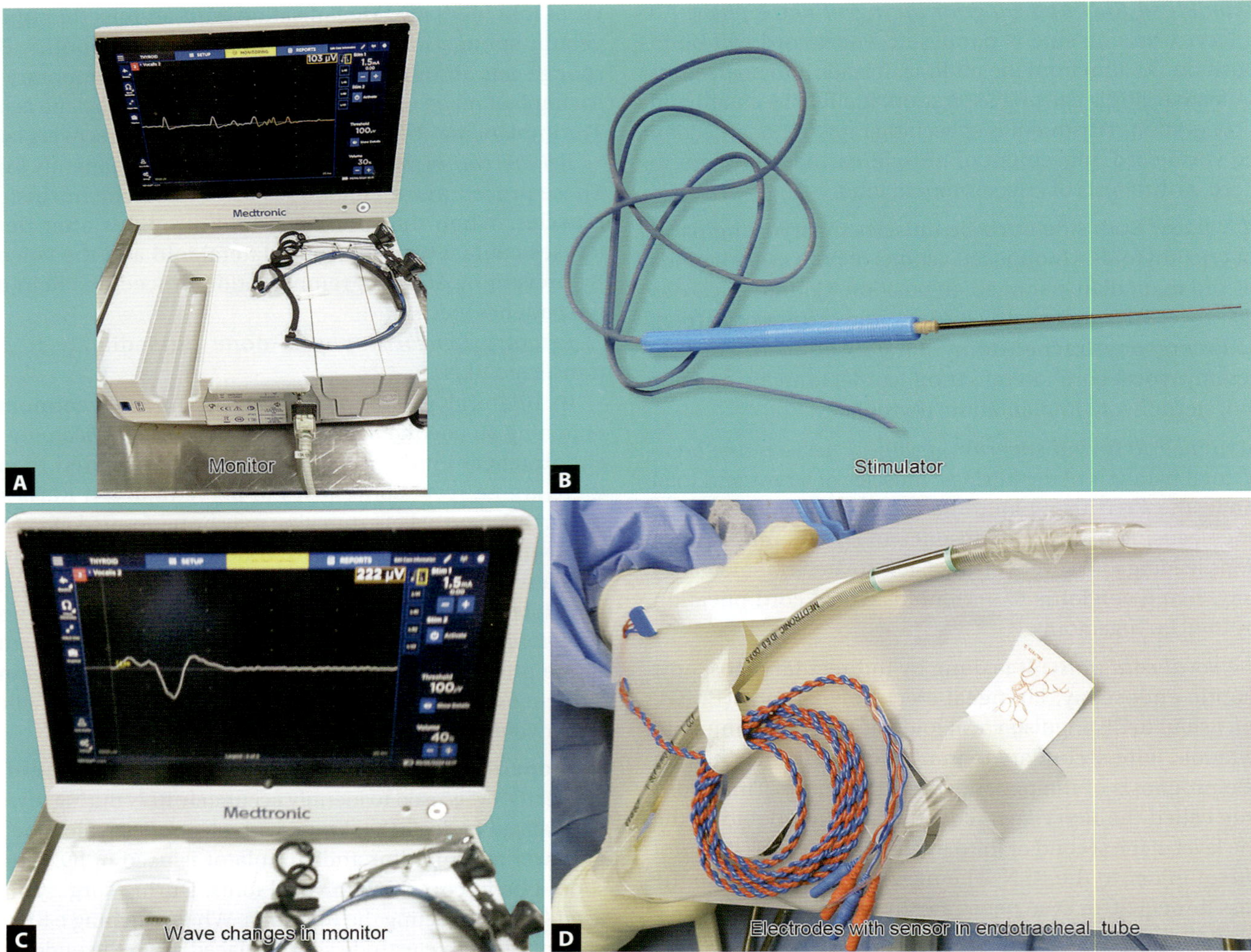

Figs. 15-48A to D: Intraoperative nerve monitor (IONM) with electrode sensor on the endotracheal tube, monitor, stimulator.

1, 25-dihydroxy vitamin D increases serum calcium levels by increasing the intestinal absorption of calcium. PTH also increases renal excretion of phosphorous. Low PTH levels result in high serum phosphorous levels.

Inadequate production of PTH leads to hypocalcaemia. Hypoparathyroidism, and the resulting hypocalcaemia, may be permanent or transient. The rate of permanent hypoparathyroidism is 0.4–13%. Causes are—direct trauma to the parathyroid glands, devascularisation of the glands, or removal of the glands during surgery.

The rate of *temporary hypocalcaemia* is reportedly 2–50%. The cause of transient hypocalcaemia after surgery is due to temporary hypoparathyroidism caused by reversible ischaemia to the parathyroid glands, hypothermia to the glands, or release of endothelin-1. Endothelin-1 is an acute-phase reactant which suppresses PTH production. Other hypothesis is—calcitonin release and hungry-bone syndrome. Calcitonin is produced by the thyroid C cells which inhibits bone breakdown while stimulating renal excretion of calcium (opposite of PTH).

Risk factors for hypocalcaemia after thyroidectomy include Graves disease, malignancy, type of procedure performed (total thyroidectomy, thyroidectomy with neck dissection, repeat thyroidectomy, subtotal thyroidectomy, near-total thyroidectomy).

Initially asymptomatic for 4–5 days, later develop circumoral paresthesia/numbness, change in mental status, tetany, carpopedal spasm, *Chvostek's sign* (tapping the region of the facial nerve in the preauricular area results in facial contractions), *Trousseau's sign* (carpal spasm that is elicited by inflating blood pressure cuff on the upper arm), laryngospasm (stridor), seizures, prolongation of QT on ECG, and cardiac arrest.

An effective method of evaluation of parathyroid function is to assess ionised calcium (or total calcium and albumin) levels in the perioperative period. A normal postoperative PTH level can accurately predict normocalcaemia after thyroid surgery. Immediate postoperative PTH level if <1.5 pmol/L and morning serum calcium <2.0 mmol/L, then patient is at risk of hypocalcaemia. Other causes like renal failure, hypomagnesaemia, medications should also be considered. Serum phosphorous levels are elevated in patients with hypoparathyroidism secondary to decreased renal excretion; this difference may help in distinguishing low PTH levels due to other etiologies of hypocalcaemia. PTH levels may be checked repeatedly till 6 months during the follow-up period. Identifying the glands on table and maintaining their blood supply is essential and also crucial to prevent hypoparathyroidism. 77% of superior parathyroid glands lie at the cricothyroid junction and intimately associated with the RLN; 22% on the posterior surface of the upper lobe of the thyroid; 1% behind the junction of the hypopharynx and upper oesophagus.

Location of the inferior parathyroid glands is variable. 42% are on the anterior or lateral surfaces of the lower lobe of the thyroid, hidden by vessels or creases in the thyroid; 39% are located within the superior tongue of the thymus. 15% extra-thyroidal and lateral to the lower lobe; 2% in the mediastinal thymus; another 2% in other ectopic positions, such as in the carotid sheath.

The inferior parathyroid glands and the thymus both develop from the third branchial pouch, causing close association of these structures. The inferior parathyroid glands receive their blood supply from the inferior thyroid artery. The superior parathyroids also usually receive their blood supply from the inferior thyroid artery. The superior parathyroids may also receive their vascular supply from the superior thyroid artery, the anastomotic loop between the inferior and superior thyroid arteries, or direct branches from the thyroid gland.

The parathyroids should be identified and their blood supply should be preserved by ligating all vessels distal to them. The vessels are ligated as close to the thyroid gland as possible. The parathyroid glands are identified by their *caramel-like* colour and size. When blood supply of parathyroids is lost, they appear darkened. The surgical wound and the excised thyroid gland should be carefully examined for parathyroid tissue. The devascularised gland (pathologically confirmed with frozen-section), should be removed, cut into 1- to 2-mm pieces, and re-implanted into the sternocleidomastoid muscle or strap muscle. The location may be marked with a permanent suture or a metallic hemoclip for easier identification in any future surgeries.

Intraoperative identification of parathyroid glands: Near infrared fluorescence (NIRF) imaging on table with or without fluorescence dye injection is ideal method to identify the parathyroid glands on table during thyroidectomy. Indocyanine green (ICG) is the exogenous fluorescence dye used to identify with exposure to near infrared light wavelength 806 nm. Near infrared autofluorescence (NIRAF) imaging further increase the identification of parathyroid clearly.

Patients who have *asymptomatic hypocalcaemia* in the early postoperative period *should not* be treated with supplemental calcium. The hypocalcaemic state may stimulate the parathyroid glands to produce PTH.

Patients who have *symptomatic hypocalcaemia* in the early postoperative period or whose calcium levels continue to fall rapidly need treatment. In symptomatic patients, intravenous calcium gluconate 10 mL 10% solution (1 g) is administered over 10 minutes. A calcium infusion is started at a rate of 1–2 mg/kg/h if symptoms do not resolve. Rate of infusion is decided by repeated analysis of serum calcium and clinical features. One to two grams of elemental oral calcium should be given each day. Calcium carbonate 1250 mg provides 500 mg of elemental calcium; the patient should take 2500–5000 mg/day. The patient needs vitamin D supplementation with calcitriol 0.25–1 µg/d. The calcium supplementation should be divided 4–5 times per day rather than in a single dose to maximise absorption by the GI tract.

In 2 months, trial weaning of oral calcium can be made to identify whether the hypoparathyroidism is temporary. Need for calcium supplementation longer than 6 months, indicates *permanent* hypoparathyroidism.

Hungry Bone Syndrome

It occurs usually in patients with preoperative hyperthyroidism. They have increased bone breakdown in their hyperthyroid state. When a patient's thyroid hormone level drops acutely after surgery, stimulus to breakdown bone is removed. The bones are now "hungry" for calcium, remove calcium from the plasma rapidly.

It usually occurs after parathyroidectomy; thyroidectomy for toxic thyroid; prostate cancer patients on estrogen therapy. Sudden cessation of existing increased bone breakdown makes bones to absorb calcium, magnesium and phosphorus rapidly. Calcium levels in blood prior to operation cannot predict hungry bone syndrome. Hypocalcaemia, hypophosphataemia, hypomagnesaemia and hyperkalaemia are four typical features in these patients. Estimation and correction of all these four factors is essential. ECG changes can occur. Hyperkalaemia should be treated judicially. Magnesium infusion is needed. There is an unusually high need for calcium, with a low calcium excretion in the urine. Bone-specific alkaline phosphatase (ALP) continues to rise in the first few weeks indicating increased bone reconstruction. Supplementation of vitamin D and elemental calcium is needed during discharge for 6 months. Postoperatively they need calcitriol (gradually increased to 16 mg in 1 month, then gradually can be reduced) with 2 g calcium supplement. Monitoring is done by evaluating serum calcium, albumin, magnesium, and phosphorus and bone-specific alkaline phosphatase.

Thyrotoxic Storm/Crisis

Thyrotoxic storm is an unusual complication of thyroid surgery. This condition may result from manipulation of the thyroid gland during surgery in patients with hyperthyroidism. It can develop preoperatively, intraoperatively, or postoperatively. It is observed in thyrotoxic patients who are inadequately prepared/controlled; it begins due to surgery (thyroidectomy) or any other stress or operations other than thyroidectomy. Thyrotoxic storm is potentially lethal and must be dealt with utmost care. It can be seen in toxic nodule or toxic nodular goitre or more commonly in Grave's disease. Mortality is more than 50%. There is exacerbation of hyperthyroidism with decompensation of organ systems.

Features

Features of thyrotoxic storm in the anaesthetised patient include evidence of increased sympathetic output, such as tachycardia and hyperthermia. In an awake postoperative patient features are nausea, tremor, severe dehydration, circulatory collapse, hypotension, hyperpyrexia, out of proportion tachycardia, cardiac arrhythmias/failure and altered mental status. Cardiac arrest may also occur. If treatment is not adequate, the patient may progress to coma. Prevention is by restoring the thyroid status as close to euthyroid as possible. Morbidity and mortality rates in adequately prepared patient are low.

Intraoperative Management

The first step in managing a thyrotoxic crisis during thyroidectomy is to stop the procedure. Intravenous beta-blockers, propylthiouracil, sodium iodine, and steroids are administered to control sympathetic activity, the release of thyroid hormone and hyperthermia. Cooling blankets and cooled intravenous fluids are used to reduce the patient's body temperature. Oxygen demand increases dramatically during a thyroid storm.

Treatment of thyrotoxic crisis postoperatively

- Injection hydrocortisone 500–1000 mg intravenously.
- Proper fluid therapy to maintain hydration, blood pressure.
- Control of hyperpyrexia by total body sponging, cooling blankets, cooled intravenous fluids, steroids (dexamethasone), antipyretic injections.
- Sedation using chlorpromazine.
- Digoxin and diuretic therapy with monitoring of blood pressure.

Contd...

Contd...

- Intravenous heparin in case of atrial fibrillation.
- Beta blockers—oral propranolol—80 mg 4th to 6th hourly (through nasogastric tube if needed); or oral diltiazem. Heart rate should be kept below 100/minute. Often to achieve this intravenous esmolol may be needed. Refractory cases require reserpine therapy.
- Antithyroid drugs—orally. Propylthiouracil or methimazole or carbimazole is given. Lugol's iodine is given 4 hours after propylthiouracil. Injection propranolol also can be given.
- Plasmapheresis and charcoal plasma perfusion or exchange perfusion is used if patient does not respond in 48 hours.
- Intravenous injection of sodium iodide 1 gram is often used.
- ICU care, oxygen, ventilator support, cardiac monitoring; electrolyte/blood gas/liver and renal function/thyroid hormone estimation at regular intervals is needed.
- Prevention of second episode of crisis by continuing the therapy is needed.

External Laryngeal Nerve Injury

The superior laryngeal nerve has two branches—internal and external. The internal branch provides sensory innervation to the larynx. It enters the larynx through the thyrohyoid membrane and not at risk during thyroidectomy. The external branch supplies cricothyroid muscle after passing through cricothyroid space of *Reeves* and is at risk during thyroidectomy. This muscle causes elongation of the vocal folds (tensor). Injury to this branch causes inability to lengthen the vocal fold and creates a high-pitched sound. The external nerve is probably the nerve most commonly injured in thyroid surgery (0–25%).

Features

Most patients do not notice any change. Patient may present with mild hoarseness or decreased vocal stamina. However, for a singer or a person who professionally relies on his or her voice (teachers), paralysis of this nerve may threaten his or her career. The most damaging consequence is loss of the *upper* register.

Diagnosing an external laryngeal nerve injury with indirect or fibreoptic laryngoscopy is difficult. Posterior glottic rotation towards the paretic side and bowing of the vocal fold on the weak side may be noted. The affected vocal fold may be lower than the normal vocal fold. Use of videostroboscopy and laryngeal EMG will help to diagnose ELN paralysis. Videostroboscopy demonstrates an asymmetric, mucosal traveling wave. EMG demonstrates denervation of cricothyroid muscle.

Prevention and Treatment

The external branch of SLN travels inferiorly along the lateral surface of the inferior constrictor until it terminates at the cricothyroid muscle. This branch is intimately related to the superior thyroid artery, though its exact relation to the artery varies. Study suggests that the nerve may cross the superior thyroid artery more than 1 cm above the upper pole of the thyroid gland (42%), less than 1 cm above the upper pole (30%), or under the upper pole (14%). In some people, the nerve runs dorsal to the artery and crosses only its terminal branches after the artery has ramified (14%). The critical area, 1.5–2 cm from the thyroid capsule is described. In this area, the ELN is most intimately involved with the branches of the superior thyroid artery.

Most surgeons agree that identifying the ELN, in contrast to the RLN, is unnecessary even though by principle it is ideal and must. Instead the terminal branches of the superior thyroid artery are ligated as close to the thyroid capsule as possible to avoid nerve damage. Direct trauma to the cricothyroid muscle can cause fibrosis and poor muscle function, which may result in a presentation similar to that of a patient with an injury to the ELN, even when the nerve is preserved. Therefore, careful dissection near this muscle is advised to avoid damage due to electrocautery. Treatment for ELN palsy is speech therapy.

Hypothyroidism

Systemic thyroid hormone levels are low in hypothyroidism. It may be *primary* due to thyroidectomy/radioactive iodine ablation/primary thyroid diseases or may be *secondary* due to hypopituitarism or *tertiary* due to hypothalamic diseases.

Presentation

Untreated hypothyroidism causes symptoms such as cold intolerance, fatigue, constipation, and muscle cramping, brittle hair, dry skin, sluggishness, hypothermia and weight gain. Cardiovascular system (CVS) manifestations are important which present as bradycardia, hypotension and conduction problems and pericardial effusion. Hypothyroidism secondary to thyroid surgery should never be left untreated long enough to elicit signs and symptoms of myxoedema (e.g. hair loss, large tongue, cardiomegaly). One should suspect, diagnose and promptly treat postoperative hypothyroidism.

Hypothyroidism will worsen the situation of critically ill patient causing severe pulmonary dysfunction, pleural effusion and hypothermia.

Renal insufficiency can occur in hypothyroidism and so renal function tests should be done.

Evaluation

The most useful laboratory test for detecting or monitoring hypothyroidism in a patient who has undergone thyroidectomy is the measurement of thyrotropin, thyroid-stimulating hormone (TSH) levels. Total T4 and T3 levels may be useful to fine-tune the dosing of levothyroxine, but may be unhelpful in the typical postoperative patient. In primary type T4, free T4, free T3 are low; but TSH level is high. In secondary type, free T4 index, free T3 and TSH are all low. *Adrenal insufficiency* is associated with *secondary* type.

Features of myxoedema coma	*Precipitated by*	*Treatment*
• Hypothermia—skin is *deadly cold* like a toad. • Hypotension • Hyponatraemia • Hypoventilation • Hypoglycaemia • Bradycardia • Loss of tendon reflexes • Cardiopulmonary collapse • Coma	• Cold infection, trauma.	• Drug of choice—IV T3 10 μg • Levothyronine 300 μg IV; later 1000 μg orally—large dose. • Glucocorticoids—IV • Antibiotics • Slow warming • Fluid and electrolyte therapy • Monitoring; ICU care; ventilator

Prevention

Hypothyroidism is an expected sequelae of total thyroidectomy. In goitre surgery, the extent of thyroidectomy is controversial. The main goal of surgery is to prevent recurrent hyperthyroidism because recurrent hyperthyroidism after surgery is more difficult to manage than permanent hypothyroidism. Because of this fact, the present authors recommend total thyroidectomy in this setting.

Treatment

Levothyroxine (about 1.7 µg/kg/d) 100–150 µg/daily (single dose, morning) is started. Their thyrotropin level is checked in 4–6 weeks to adjust the dosage. Patients who are to receive postoperative radioiodine therapy with scanning must stop taking levothyroxine before the procedure. In cardiac patients initially 50 µg/day is started; later gradually increased to the required dose.

In myxoedema coma, IV hydrocortisone, IV levothyroxine, IV levothyronine is started.

Types of hypothyroidism
- *Primary:* Thyroidectomy or thyroid diseases like thyroiditis—free T4, T4, and free T3 are low; TSH is high.
- *Secondary:* Hypopituitarism—TSH, free T3 are low.
- *Tertiary:* Hypothalamic diseases.

Presentations
- Asymptomatic.
- Chronic hypothyroidism status.
- Myxoedema coma: Acute presentation with loss of deep tendon refluxes, respiratory problem, cardiac irregularities, coma with 50% mortality.

Causes
- Agenesis or dysgenesis.
- Enzyme deficiency.
- Iodine deficiency.
- Hashimoto's thyroiditis.
- Antithyroid drugs.
- Radioiodine.
- Drugs: Lithium, amiodarone.
- *After thyroidectomy.*

Clinical features
- *General:* Tiredness, weight gain, cold intolerance, goitre, hyperlipidaemia.
- *Cardiovascular:* Bradycardia, angina, cardiac failure, pericardial effusion.
- *Haematological:* Anaemia.
- *Dermatological:* Dry skin, vitiligo, alopecia, erythema.
- *Reproductive:* Infertility, menorrhagia, galactorrhoea.
- *Gastrointestinal:* Constipation, ileus.
- *Developmental:* Growth and mental retardation, delayed puberty.
- *Other features:* Carpal tunnel syndrome, myalgia, hoarseness, deafness, ataxia, depression, psychosis (myxoedema madness).

Infection

Infection is rare due to good aseptic methods. Perioperative antibiotics are used in many centres. Bleeding from vascular thyroids, haematoma, infected suture material are the causes of infection. In large malignant thyroid, during thyroidectomy injury may occur to oesophagus which causes severe localised sepsis in the neck. Gastrografin study, CT scan/magnetic resonance imaging (MRI) may reveal the site and extent of the injury. Pus culture, starting higher generation antibiotics, nasogastric tube insertion, and endoscopic identification of the injured area are needed management in such rare patients. Usually they recover but may need to keep the nasogastric tube (feeding can be done through the tube) for few weeks.

Recurrent Thyrotoxicosis

Recurrent thyrotoxicosis is difficult to manage. It is more common with subtotal thyroidectomy (4–15%) than with total thyroidectomy. So at present, total thyroidectomy is commonly done for toxic thyroid. Management is proper anatomical assessment of the residual thyroid tissue by using radioisotope scan, MRI neck and radioactive iodine ablation of residual thyroid tissue if patient's age is more than 45 years or surgical reexploration and complete removal of residual thyroid tissue on both sides. It carries higher risk of injury to recurrent laryngeal nerve and parathyroids. Meticulous dissection, adequate exposure and proper retraction is needed.

Minor Complications

Small seromas can be left as such to resorb. Large seroma may require repeated aspirations. Wound infection and poor scar are other complications.

Minimally Invasive Video-assisted Thyroidectomy

Minimally invasive video-assisted thyroidectomy (MIVAT) is becoming popular for small nodules and gland without thyroiditis. But it is costly.

The development of videolaparoscopic surgery in the last decade has allowed several operations to be performed with minimally invasive techniques. After the first parathyroidectomy procedure performed endoscopically in 1996, this minimally invasive approach was applied to thyroid surgery. MIVAT was described in 1998. The technique was described using a central access with a 1.5 cm incision and external retraction. Postoperative morbidity rates in patients seem to be equivalent to those of patients who have undergone conventional surgery.

Chao et al (2004) prospectively compared video-assisted thyroid lobectomy and conventional lobectomy in 116 patients with thyroid nodules. Transient RLN palsy occurred in 5 (8.5%) patients who underwent conventional surgery versus 3 (5.8%) patients in the video-assisted group; the difference was not significant. Patients in both groups were discharged home on the second postoperative day.

In a 5-year study, Miccoli et al (2004) selected 579 patients to undergo MIVAT. The operation consisted of total thyroidectomy in 312 patients and lobectomy in 267. The mean operative time was 41 minutes (range, 15–120 min) for lobectomy and 51.6 minutes (range, 30–140 min) for total thyroidectomy. The postoperative hospital stay was 24 hours (overnight discharge) for all patients. Complications included postoperative bleeding (0.1%), recurrent nerve palsy (1.3%), and definitive hypoparathyroidism (0.2%). Some have suggested that pain following VAT is less when compared to conventional thyroidectomy because of limited dissection, retraction, and injury to tissues.

MIVAT provides endoscopic magnification of nerves and vessels, potentially decreasing the risk of injury to these structures. The endoscopic technique cannot be used in nodules larger than 3.5 cm because the specimen is too large to retrieve through the incision. In addition, this technique is not ideal for removing carcinomas in which an intact capsule is desired for oncologic reasons and for accurate histological assessment.

In summary, if the general principles of conventional thyroid surgery are followed, video assistance may help in identifying structures and in minimising the incision. Experienced surgeons may consider using this technique when the equipment and additional surgical staff is available for patients with small follicular nodules/adenomas, or well-differentiated papillary carcinoma, or when prophylactic thyroidectomy is being performed in oncologically needed patients.

Extracervical scar less in the neck endoscopic thyroidectomy (SET): Here endoscopic device approach is used to reach thyroid area to do thyroidectomy. Different approaches are present—(1) BABA (bilateral axillo breast approach); (2) ABA (axillo breast approach); (3) ABBA (axillo bilateral breast approach); (4) Retroauricular facelift approach; (5) Transoral vestibular approach (Transoral endoscopic thyroidectomy vestibular approach/TOETVA); (6) Anterior chest wall approach. BABA with robotic thyroidectomy is more specific and better.

PARATHYROID SURGERY

Surgical Anatomy of Parathyroid

Two pairs of parathyroids are located within the false capsule and posterior border of thyroid gland. Superior parathyroids develop from endoderm of 4th pharyngeal pouch and called as *parathyroid IV*; inferior parathyroids are called as *parathyroid III* (3rd pouch). Each parathyroid is lentiform/pea sized in shape with 6 × 4 × 2 mm in size weighing 50 mg and red brown in colour. Glands lie in close relation to anastomotic branch of superior and inferior parathyroid arteries. *Superior* usually lies in constant position at the middle of posterior border of the thyroid, *behind recurrent laryngeal nerve*. *Inferior* lies in variable positions—within the thyroid capsule below the inferior thyroid artery/outside the thyroid capsule above the inferior thyroid artery/within the thyroid substance in posterior border. Inferior is usually *in front of the recurrent laryngeal nerve*. Inferior parathyroid and thymus develop from 3rd pharyngeal pouch and so can also be occasionally located in mediastinum. Parathyroids receive their blood supply from inferior thyroid artery (80%) and anastomotic artery. Single end artery is the common method of supply **(Fig. 15-49)**.

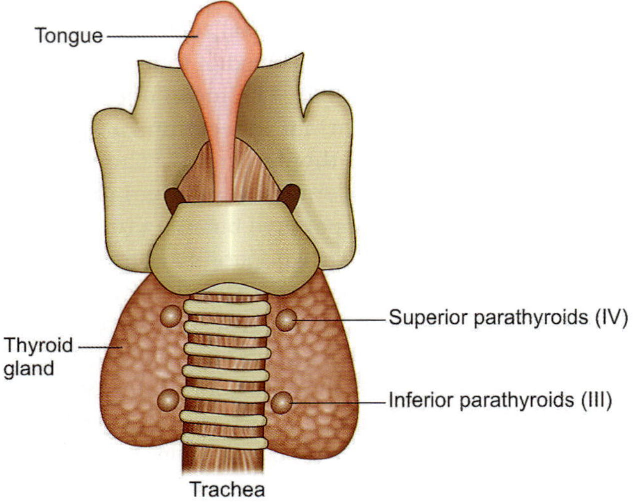

Fig. 15-49: Anatomy of parathyroid glands.

Glands (chief cells) secrete parathormone (PTH) which controls the calcium metabolism.

Parathyroid hormone

- Increases absorption of the calcium from the gut.
- Mobilises calcium from the bone.
- Increases the calcium reabsorption from the renal tubules.
- Half life is 4 minutes.

Indications for Parathyroidectomy

Primary hyperparathyroidism (HPT): Criteria (2002) for surgical intervention are—raise in serum calcium level more than 1 mg/dL of upper limit of the normal calcium range; 24 hour urinary calcium if more than 400 mg; creatinine clearance when reduced more than 30%; bone density greater than two standard deviations below peak bone mass in lumbar spine/hip/lower end of radius; age below 50 years; when medical therapy is not possible.

Common cause for primary HPT is single benign parathyroid adenoma (85%). 95% of such adenomas are single in one gland. 5% cases are having double adenomas each one in two glands. Proliferation causing hyperplasia involving all four glands (15%) also causes primary HPT. This type may be associated with MEN syndrome type I and IIA. Slow growing invasive parathyroid carcinoma accounts for 1% of primary HPT.

Four dimensional CT, PET scan, Technetium 99m sestamibi scintigraphy are the present methods of evaluation in these patients. On table methylene blue injection (5 mg/kg over an hour infusion) will make only the parathyroid gland blue to identify it.

Secondary HPT: It is an indication for removal of all four glands with autotransplantation of parathyroid only in severe cases or with renal osteodystrophy.

Indications for parathyroidectomy

- Severe symptoms.
- Young age group.
- Markedly reduced bone density.
- Serum calcium more than 11 mg%.
- Urinary calculi.
- Neuromuscular presentations.
- Urinary calcium more than 400 mg/24 hours.

Preoperative Preparation

Vocal cords should be assessed by preoperative indirect laryngoscopy.

High calcium levels preoperatively may require treatment with hydration; diuresis; steroids (prednisolone 20 mg TID for 5 days before surgery); 100 mmol phosphate infusion in 6 hours; 200 units calcitonin subcutaneous injection for 5 days twice daily before surgery; diphosphanate—etiodronate disodium 7.5 mg/kg daily as slow IV infusion for 3 days; mithramycin 25 μg/kg as single dose.

Anaesthesia and Position

General anaesthesia is used with neck hyperextended by placing rolled sheet under the shoulder blades. Head is placed on the head—ring; head end of the table is raised to semi-erect position (*Semi-Fowler position)*.

Incision and Dissection

It is same as for thyroidectomy. Flaps are raised in similar way. Strap muscles are separated after opening the deep fascia in the midline. Thyroid gland is mobilised to identify the parathyroid adenoma. Parathyroid having adenoma is mobilised which is close to recurrent laryngeal nerve. End artery of the parathyroid is identified and ligated. Adenoma is separated from adjacent thyroid tissue using gauze dissection. Either on table venous sampling for PTH assay is done or venous sample from cubital vein is done for PTH assay. Reduction in PTH level more than 50% in 10 minutes after parathyroidectomy and more than 85% in 15 minutes suggest adequacy of parathyroidectomy **(Fig. 15-50)**.

Parathyroid may be confirmed by frozen section biopsy or on table aspiration of parathyroid tissue which is analysed for PTH assay which will be more than 1500 pg/mL (confirms removed tissue as parathyroid).

Total parathyroidectomy is done for parathyroid hyperplasia by removing all four glands and ⅓ of one gland is autotransplanted into the forearm muscle (brachioradialis) or sternocleidomastoid muscle with marker stitch. Transplanted gland is sliced into 1 mm pieces and around 18 pieces are embedded in decided muscle with a marker stitch or clip. If in postoperative period patient still presents with feature of primary HPT; then transplanted area is re-explored and further reduction in parathyroid tissue is done.

Wound is closed with proper haemostasis.

Effects of Surgery

Among neuromuscular symptoms of primary HPT, proximal muscle weakness responds better than respiratory muscle weakness by parathyroidectomy.

Among psychiatric illnesses, depression and spatial learning and processing improve well by surgery.

Complications

Haemorrhage, recurrent laryngeal nerve palsy, hypocalcaemia and hungry bone syndrome are known to occur.

Persistent HPT (serum calcium is not normalised immediately after surgery leading total failure) or *recurrent HPT* (serum calcium after surgery becomes normal but in 6–12 months, it again increases) may be a problem.

Hypoparathyroidism with severe hypocalcaemia is a problem when all glands are removed (3½) with bilateral neck exploration. 10 ampoules of calcium gluconate is diluted with 1 liter of normal saline and given as continuous infusion at a rate of 30 mL/hour—initial method of management. Hypomagnesemia should also be corrected.

Migration or inability to identify the transplanted parathyroid is often a problem in autotransplantation of parathyroid.

Bone mineral density in hip and lumbar spine becomes better.

Nephrocalcinosis is improved by surgery; but hypertension and renal excretion will not improve much.

Half life of PTH is 4 minutes. On table serial PTH assays are done at several intervals—before dissection of the gland, during dissection and after dissection. 50% reduction in PTH level from baseline in post- removal sample is a 96% predictor of complete removal.

Operative failure rate is 1.5 to 6%. Intraoperative PTH assay improves the success rate very much (76–94%). Cure rate is defined as normocalcaemia in 6 months postoperative period.

Radio-guided parathyroidectomy using intravenous injection of 20 mCi of 99mTc sestamibi 2 hours before surgery is not routinely practiced but may be useful for removal of adenoma appropriately. Hand held quantitative gamma counter is used intraoperatively on the neck over all parathyroid tissues.

- Primary HPT is commonly sporadic than familial.
- Histological difference between adenoma and hyperplasia is difficult to assess.
- Gross on table look is preferred method.
- Adenoma is usually single. Multiple adenomas occur in elderly.
- Hyperplasia involves all four parathyroids.
- Parathyroid cyst may be developmental/secondary to degeneration of nodule or adenoma. Cyst aspiration shows clear fluid with high PTH level in the content fluid.
- Preoperative IV methylene blue 5 mg/kg in 500 mL dextrose saline which stains parathyroids is often used to localise glands.
- 50 mg of one gland is sufficient to maintain function.
- Persistent HPT is one in which HPT persists immediately even after initial surgery.
- Recurrent HPT (initially after first surgery HPT is corrected but recurs 6–12 months after surgery) is due to parathyromatosis, development of new adenoma, and hyperplasia of transplanted parathyroid. *Parathyromatosis* is due to rupture and spillage of parathyroid tissue in neck, mediastinum and forming functioning nodules there.
- Re-exploration and removal in persistent/recurrent HPT needs on table PTH assay. On table PTH level drop more than 50% of preoperative value indicates the success of surgical removal.
- CT, MRI, PET scan and selective angiography are usually done only for recurrent diseases.

Problems in parathyroidectomy

- Permanent hypoparathyroidism.
- Recurrent hyperparathyroidism—hypercalcaemia 12 months after parathyroidectomy.
- Recurrent laryngeal nerve injury.
- Often needs additional thyroidectomy.
- Variations in positions of the gland especially lower—may be in mediastinum.
- Sudden drop in calcium level after surgery due to increased absorption of calcium by bones—***hungry bone syndrome***.

Approaches

Classic Approach (Traditional Approach)

It is under general anaesthesia exploring bilateral neck to remove parathyroid tissue which is confirmed by frozen section biopsy. It shows 95% cure rate with 2% complication rate.

Minimally Invasive Parathyroidectomy (MIP)

It is done in case of *single adenoma* of parathyroid under regional cervical block anaesthesia usually in ambulatory set up. It is actually unilateral parathyroidectomy with removal of adenoma and involved entire that particular one parathyroid gland using limited neck exploration (small incision of 2–4 cm). Procedure is not useful in multiple adenomas or hyperplasia. Preoperative localisation with sestamibi combined with SPECT is a must. Intraoperative PTH assay is a must to confirm drop in PTH level to required level. Cervical block is given by infiltrating xylocaine (1%) with adrenaline along posterior and deep to sternocleidomastoid muscle and also along the neck incision. Direct field block along the anterior border of the

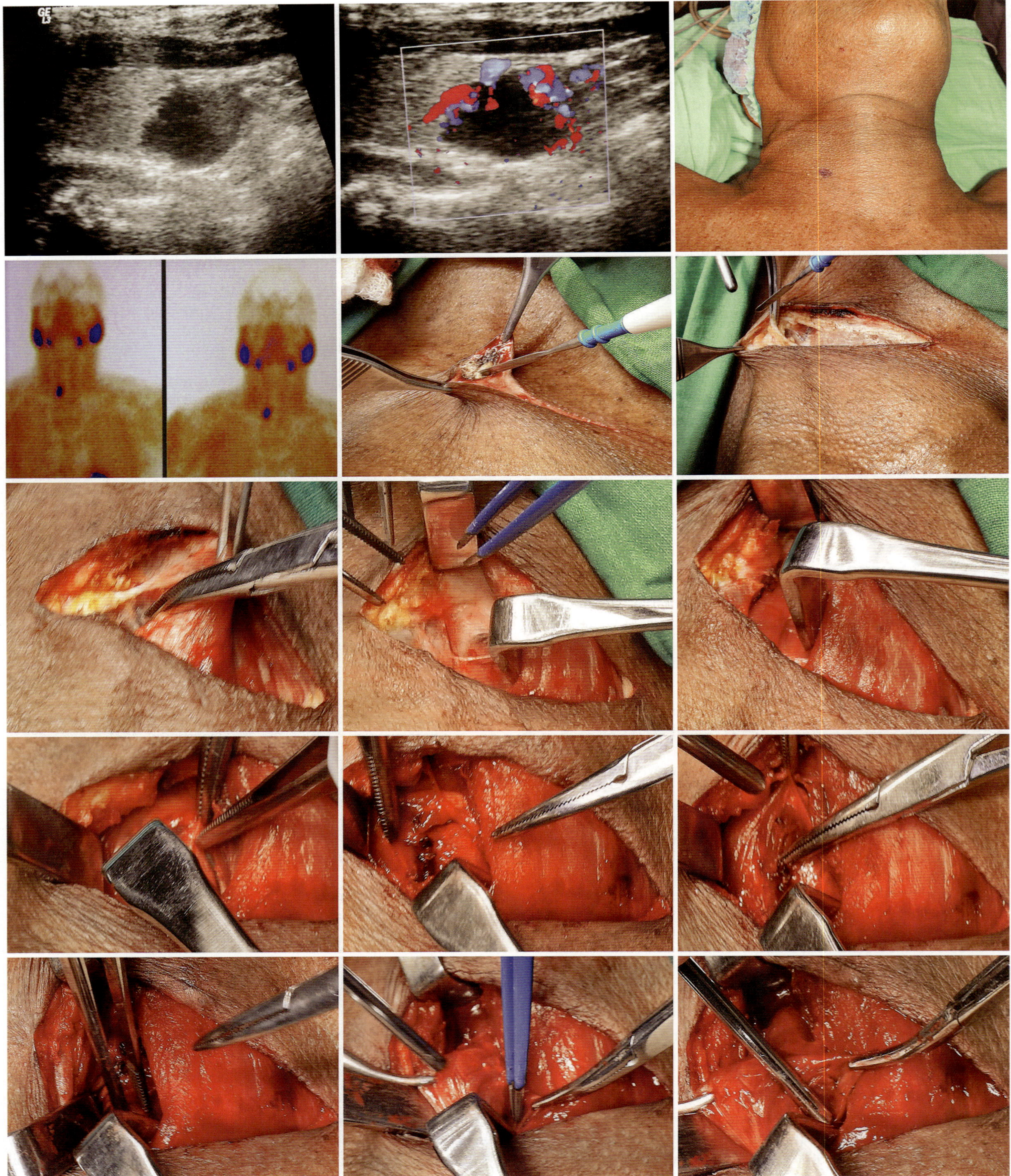

Figs. 15-50(1)

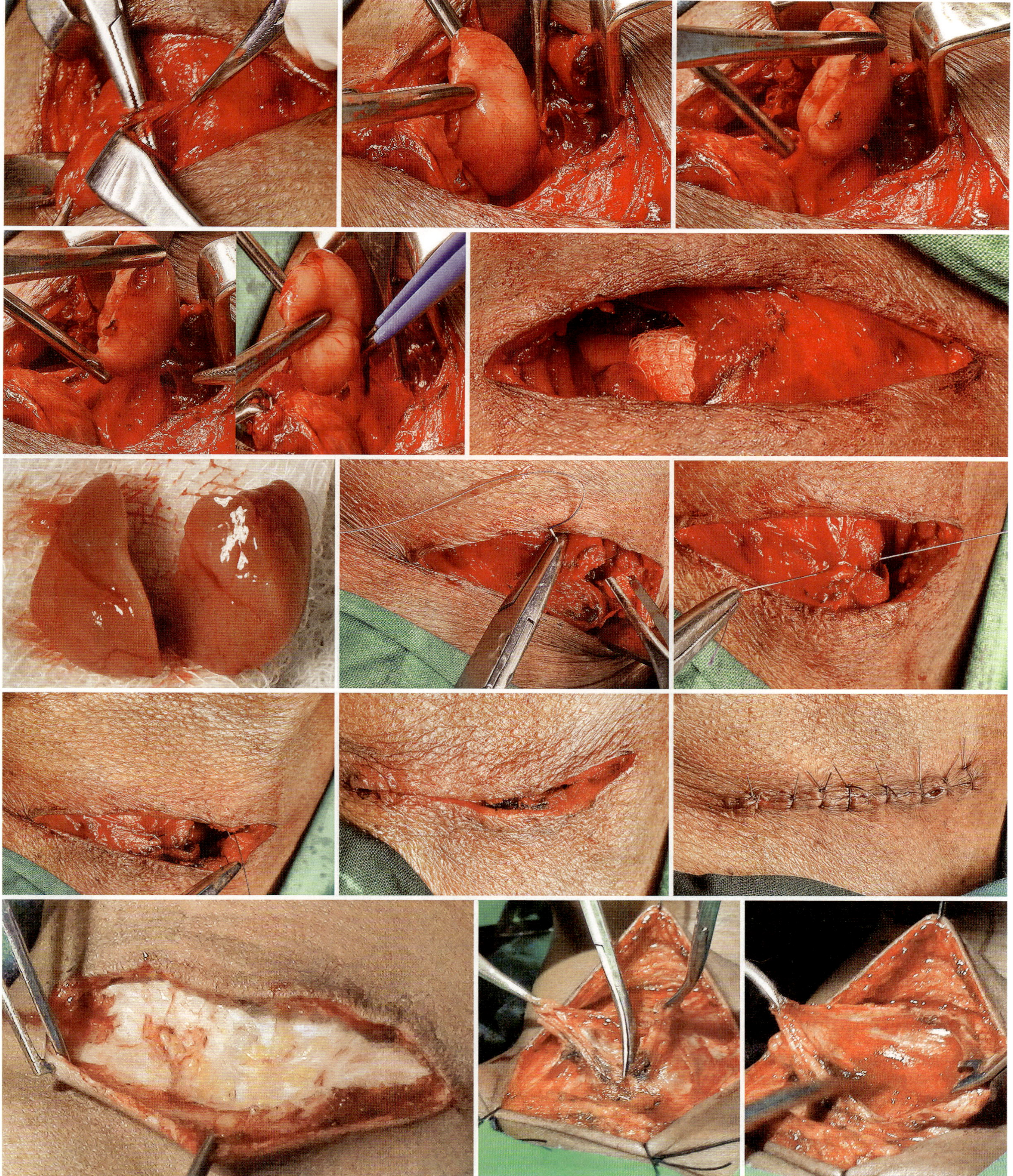

Figs. 15-50(2)

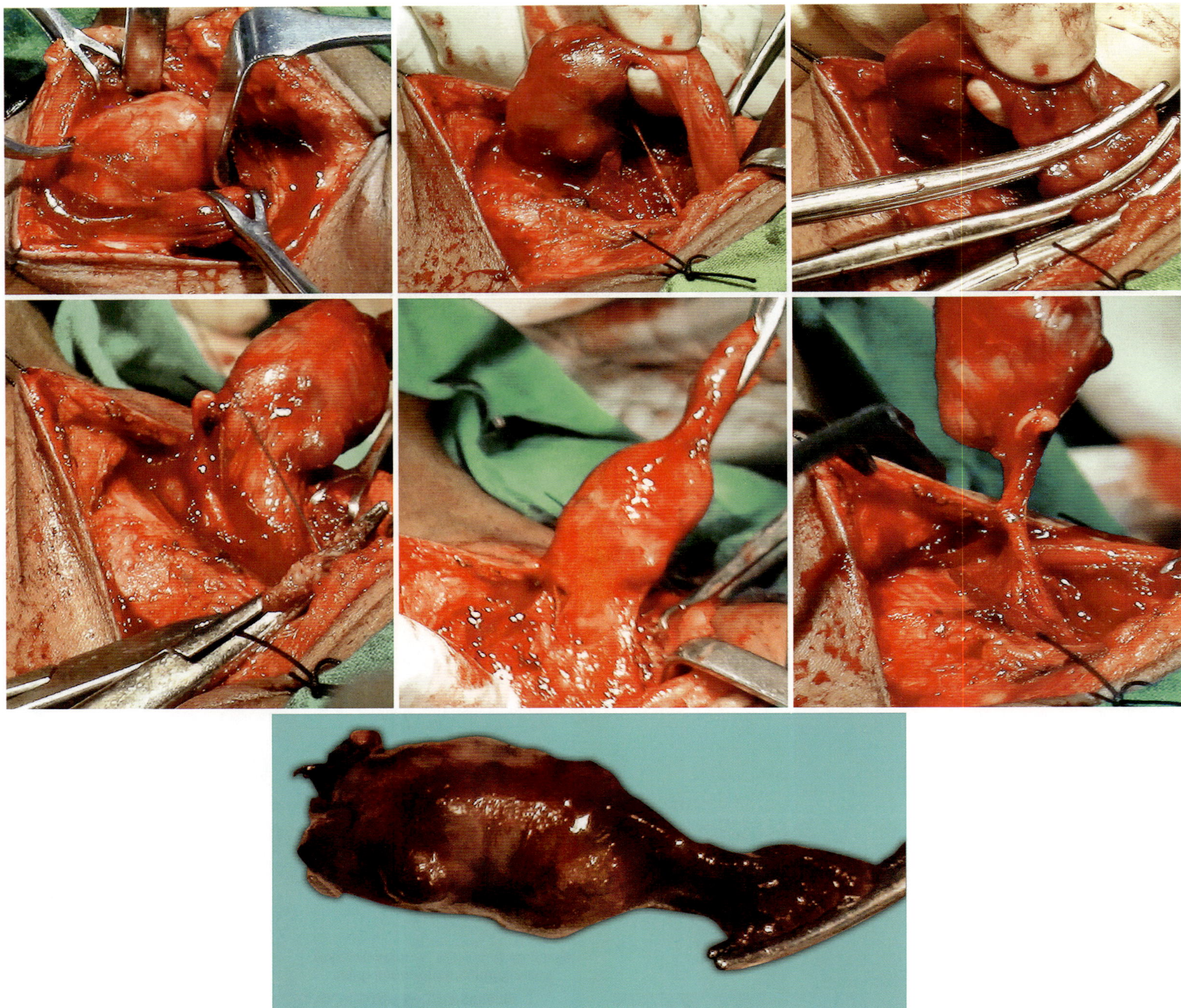

Figs. 15-50(3)

Figs. 15-50(1 to 3): Technique of parathyroidectomy for adenoma in two different patients.

sternocleidomastoid and over the incision is also used. Postoperative serum calcium and PTH level should be assessed until 7th day.

Median Sternotomy (3%) Extension

Median sternotomy is often needed when parathyroid is in anterior mediastinum along with thymus. Often parathyroids may be 5, 6 or 7 in numbers instead of four.

Video-assisted Parathyroidectomy (Paolo Miccoli)

It is done in *localised single adenoma* using multiple ports on one side with intermittent CO_2 insufflation and suction irrigation. 1.5 cm incision 1 cm above the sternal notch helps in tactile assessment and dissection. Strap muscles are retracted laterally and thyroid is retracted medially. Conversion rate is 11%; RLN palsy is 2%.

Endoscopic Parathyroidectomy

Entire parathyroidectomy is done using laparoscopy. It is first used (1994) for a mediastinal parathyroid adenoma. In 1996, it was used for neck parathyroid hyperplasia by Gagner for removing 3½ glands. Now technique is *limited to single adenoma* to remove tumour and gland. Low pressure insufflations with 5 mm four trocars are used. Placement of trocars is dependent on the need of the operating surgeon. Many place trocars on one side only; but few prefer to place working trocars on opposite side.

Remedial Parathyroidectomy

It is done for persistent HPT (serum calcium is not normalised immediately after surgery leading to total failure) or recurrent HPT (serum calcium after surgery becomes normal but in 6–12 months, it again increases). It is done through lateral approach (*Feind*) between anterior margin of sternocleidomastoid and strap muscles so that scar tissues are avoided from initial dissection. On table localisation methods, on table PTH assay are needed. Median sternotomy often may be needed to explore the mediastinum for complete removal of the gland. Parathyroids in such situations may be embedded in the tissue of thyroid or thymus. So removal of these glands also may be a need in such situations.

Subtotal Parathyroidectomy

It is indicated in hyperplasia or secondary HPT wherein 3½ glands are removed, retaining ½ of one gland.

Total Parathyroidectomy with Parathyroid Autotransplantation

It is done alternatively in hyperplasia wherein all four glands are removed; ⅓ or ½ of one gland is transplanted into sternocleidomastoid or brachioradialis muscle with a marker. Disease control will not occur if more part of the gland is transplanted. It is removing of all four glands and 1/2 or 1/3 of one gland is autotransplanted into the forearm muscle (brachioradialis) or sternocleidomastoid muscle with marker stitch. Transplanting gland is sliced into 1 mm pieces and around 18 pieces are embedded in decided muscle with a marker stitch or clip. If postoperatively still patient presents with feature of primary HPT; then transplanted area is re-explored and further reduction in parathyroid tissue is done. Migration or inability to identify the transplanted parathyroid is often a problem in auto-transplantation of parathyroid.

PARATHYROID CARCINOMA

It is rare but shows marked hypercalcaemia (more than 14 mg/dL). Renal and bone complications are more common. Palpable neck swelling, features of hypercalcaemia, high PTH level are typical. Lymph nodes in neck may be involved. Tumour is large grayish white, invasive to adjacent thyroid. Distant spread occurs to lung, liver and bone. *En bloc parathyroid resection, ipsilateral thyroid lobe removal, adjacent soft tissue resection* along with ipsilateral neck lymph node dissection if needed—is the treatment. Simple parathyroidectomy should not be done as it shows high recurrence rate (50%) and spread. Recurrence rate for en bloc removal is 8%. Nodal and distant spread carries poor prognosis. *Cinacalcet* (30–180 mg/day) is used for symptomatic control of hypercalcaemia. Removal of metastatic area may be needed to control severe hypercalcaemia. Chemotherapy is not useful. External radiotherapy may be used to neck and metastatic area; but results are not adequate.

16

CHAPTER

Surgeries for Breast Diseases

SURGICAL ANATOMY OF BREAST

Breast, a *modified sweat gland* lies in superficial fascia in pectoral region with a small extension called as *axillary tail of Spence* into the axilla through *foramen of Langer* in deep fascia. Vertically it extends from 2nd to 6th rib; horizontally from lateral border of sternum to midaxillary line. Deep to breast, structures related are—retromammary space containing loose areolar tissue, pectoral deep fascia, muscles (pectoralis major, serratus anterior, external oblique), chest wall **(Fig. 16-1)**.

Retromammary bursa/space is located between deep layer of superficial fascia and pectoral (deep) fascia allowing free mobility of breast.

Nipple is located at the level of 4th intercostal space just below the centre/summit of the breast. It contains circular and longitudinal muscles to make nipple stiff or flat. It is pierced by 15–20 lactiferous ducts. Each duct independently opens into the nipple. It has rich sensory nerve endings. It also contains modified sweat and sebaceous glands. Nipple is supplied by 4th intercostal nerve.

Areola is circular pigmented area around the nipple. It is rich in modified sebaceous glands which enlarge during pregnancy and lactation as *Montgomery tubercles*. They secrete oily lubricant to nipple and areola. Areola and nipple do not contain hair and fat beneath.

Breast parenchyma contains 15–20 lobes. Each lobe contains alveoli, lactiferous sinus and lactiferous duct. Alveolus is lined by cuboidal (in rest) and columnar (in lactation); smaller duct is by single layer columnar; larger ducts by many layered columnar; lactiferous duct (2–4 mm in diameter) is by stratified squamous epithelium. *Myoepithelial cells* lie between epithelium and basement membrane from alveoli to duct. *Stroma* contains fibrous tissue and fat. Fibrous stromal septa, anchoring from skin to pectoral fascia, is called as *suspensory ligament of Cooper*. Fat is distributed all over the breast *except* under nipple and areola **(Fig. 16-2)**.

Arterial Supply

It is by—internal thoracic (mammary) artery (60%), branch of subclavian artery through its perforators; lateral thoracic (30%), superior thoracic and acromiothoracic branches of axillary artery;

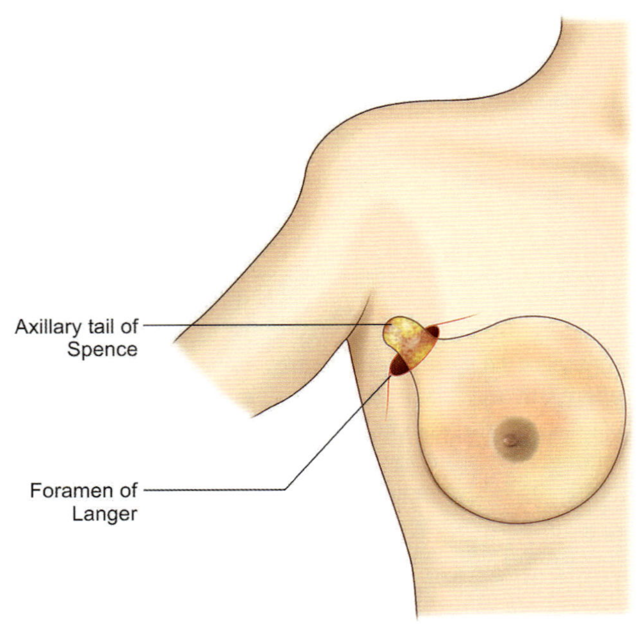

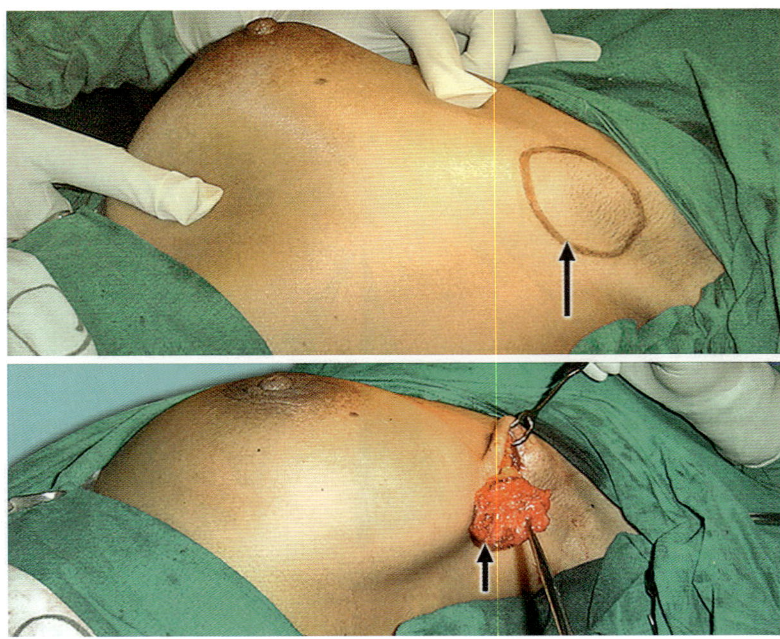

Fig. 16-1: Axillary tail of Spence, located deep to deep fascia, is an extension of main breast from superficial fascia through foramen of Langer.

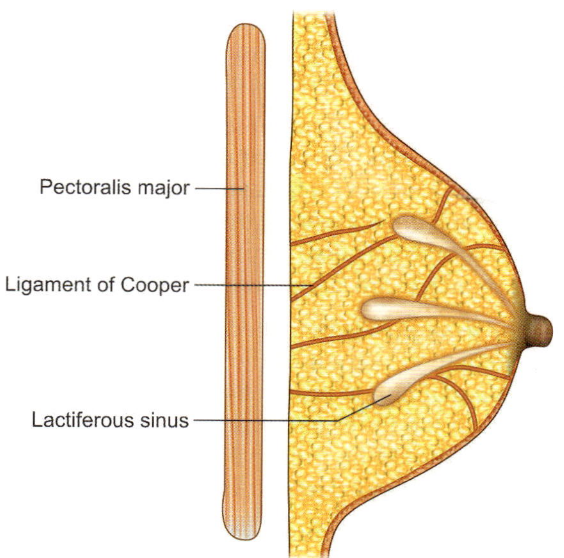

Fig. 16-2: Cooper's ligament.

lateral branches of posterior intercostal arteries. Thoracodorsal branch of subscapular artery is not supplying the breast but its location and pathway is important because it is very close to central and scapular (posterior) axillary lymph nodes. So during lymph node dissection injury of this vessel can cause significant damage; and it is essential to retain this branch, if at all LD flap is needed at a later period **(Fig. 16-3)**.

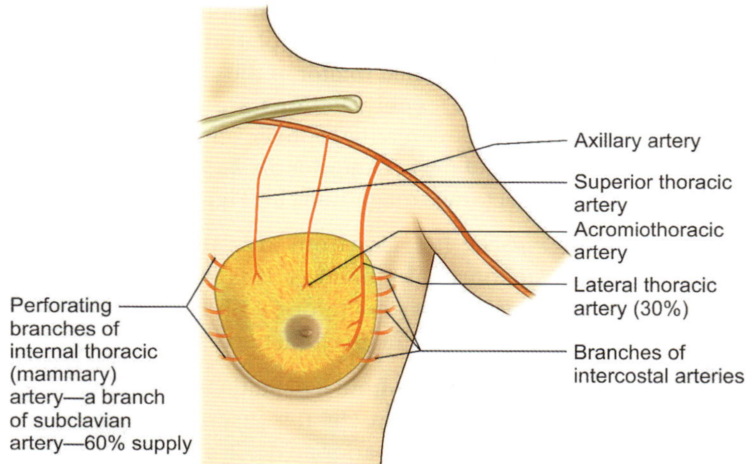

Fig. 16-3: Arterial supply of breast.

Venous return is by: Posterior intercostals with perforating branches which is also in continuity with Batson's vertebral plexus; axillary vein (primary); internal mammary vein. Venous network form an anastomotic venous circle near base of the nipple which eventually sets into superficial and deep veins. Superficial veins drain into internal thoracic vein; deep into internal thoracic, axillary and posterior intercostal veins.

Nerve supply of breast is from anterior and lateral cutaneous branches of the 4th to 6th intercostal nerves. They supply skin, smooth muscles, and blood vessels. They do not control milk secretion. Nipple is supplied by 4th intercostal nerve.

Milk secretion is controlled by prolactin.

Lymphatic drainage of breast: Superficial lymphatics drain skin over the breast except nipple and areola. Deep lymphatics drain parenchyma, nipple and areola. 75% drain into axillary nodes; 20% into internal mammary nodes (parasternal—along internal thoracic vessels deep to the costal cartilage); 5% to posterior intercostal nodes. In axilla, lymphatics mainly drain to pectoral nodes (anterior/external mammary along the lateral thoracic vessels); then to posterior (along subscapular vessels), lateral (along axillary vein), central (in the fat in centre of the axilla) and apical (subclavicular/*Halsted)* nodes (along pectoralis minor tendon). Supraclavicular, deltopectoral (cephalic), posterior intercostal nodes, subdiaphragmatic lymph plexus are other drainage areas. Sappey's subareolar lymphatic plexus drains into pectoral group of lymph nodes. Central group is the *most properly clinically palpable* axillary node. *Internal mammary nodes* are located in retrosternal intercostal spaces 1–2 cm lateral to the sternal margin; it is vertically placed parallel to internal mammary vessels in relation to endothoracic fascia; its efferent ends in subclavicular nodes.

Intercostal lymph nodes are located posteriorly in intercostal spaces near the origin of ribs. Its efferent drains into the right lymphatic duct or thoracic duct.

Diaphragmatic nodes are located on the thoracic surface of the diaphragm. Anterior prepericardial nodes are located under xiphoid process; lateral one is located on each side, right side near inferior vena cava (IVC), left side near oesophageal hiatus; posterior group is located near crura of diaphragm.

Axillary reverse mapping (ARM): Here blue dye is injected on inner aspect of upper part of the arm to achieve a mapping of axillary lymphatic drainage **(Fig. 16-4)**.

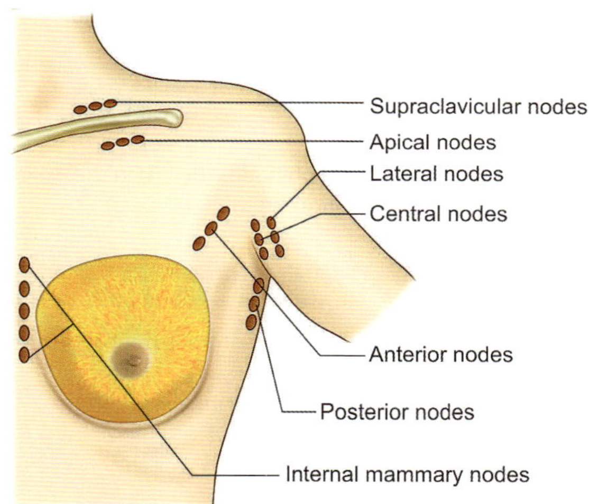

- 75% of lymph from breast drain to axillary nodes
- 20% into internal mammary nodes
- 5% to posterior intercostal nodes
- Internal mammary drains not only from inner but also from outer quadrant
- Lymphatics from deep part of breast pass through pectoralis major muscle and clavipectoral fascia to reach apical nodes and internal mammary nodes
- Lymphatics from lower inner quadrant of the breast communicate with subdiaphragmatic and peritoneal lymphatics across costal margin and linea alba

Fig. 16-4: Lymphatic drainage of the breast.

Axilla

Axilla is pyramidal in shape with apex, base and four walls—anterior, posterior, medial and lateral. Apex (*cervicoaxillary canal*) is bound by clavicle, scapula and outer border of first rib. Anterior wall is formed by pectoralis major, clavipectoral fascia; posterior wall by subscapularis, teres major and latissimus dorsi; medial wall by upper four ribs with intercostal muscles, upper part of serratus anterior muscle; lateral wall by shaft of humerus, coracobrachialis, short head of biceps. It contains axillary artery with its branches, axillary vein with its tributaries, axillary groups of lymph nodes, and long thoracic nerve of Bell to serratus anterior, intercostobrachial nerve, fat and fascia. Subscapular vessels run along the lower border of the subscapularis with its nerve and thoracodorsal nerve. Medial wall is related to long thoracic nerve and intercostobrachial nerve. Anterior/pectoral group of lymph nodes lie along the lower border of pectoralis minor on lateral thoracic vessels. Lateral group of nodes lie posteromedial to axillary vein. Central group lies in the fat of the axilla towards medial side. Apical nodes lie behind, above the pectoralis minor, medial to axillary vein. *Axillary sheath* covers axillary artery and brachial plexus *but not* axillary vein.

Note: A communicating vein between cephalic vein and external jugular vein (neck) is present which runs across the clavicle. It is important in draining the upper limb in axillary vein removal (in carcinoma breast, segment may be removed)/blockage **(Fig. 16-5)**.

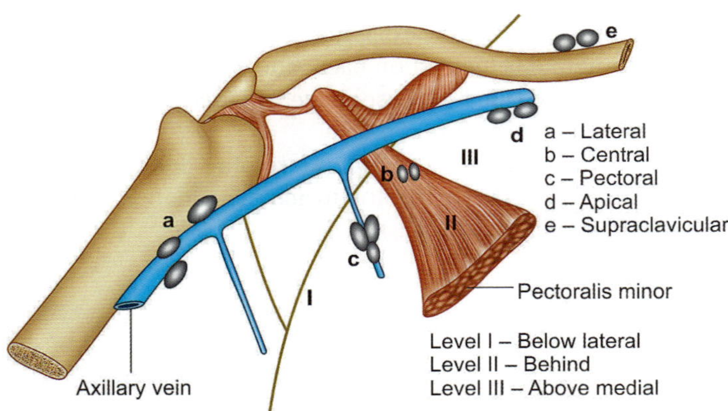

Fig. 16-5: Surgical levels of lymph nodes (Berg's) in the axilla draining from breast.

Levels of the axillary nodes (Berg's)

- Level I—Below and lateral to the pectoralis minor muscle—anterior, lateral, posterior.
- Level II—Behind the pectoralis minor muscle—central.
- Level III—Above and medial to pectoralis minor muscle—apical—Halsted's node.

Note in carcinoma breast

- Spread restricted to Level I nodes carries better prognosis.
- Spread to Level II has poor prognosis.
- Spread to Level III indicates worst prognosis.

Nerves Related to Axillary Dissection

Long thoracic nerve arises from C5, 6, 7 nerve roots of brachial plexus, enters the axilla running on the lateral surface of the serratus anterior muscle invested by serratus fascia and supplies serratus anterior which on division during axillary dissection causes *winged scapula* with inability to fix the shoulder.

Thoracodorsal nerve arises from posterior cord of brachial plexus runs posteriorly downwards to supply latissimus dorsi muscle. Its division may cause difficult in extending the shoulder but more importantly reconstruction with latissimus dorsi myocutaneous flap (LD flap) after mastectomy is not possible.

Intercostobrachial nerve is communicating nerve between lateral cutaneous branch of 2nd intercostal nerve and medial cutaneous nerve of arm, denervation of this nerve causes sensory loss of skin of upper medial and inner aspect of the arm, apex and lateral axilla. Second intercostobrachial nerve may be present occasionally arising from anterior branch of 3rd lateral cutaneous nerve.

Medial pectoral nerve arising from medial cord of the brachial plexus runs along the lateral margin of the pectoralis minor supplying pectoralis minor mainly and pectoralis major muscle partly. It often may pass through the fibres of the pectoralis minor muscle at its lateral aspect. It should be preserved during axillary dissection otherwise atrophy of pectoral muscles occur.

Lateral pectoral nerve arises from lateral cord of the brachial plexus after running on the medial aspect, supplies the medial part of the pectoralis major muscle (Lateral pectoral nerve is medial; medial pectoral nerve is lateral. They are not named on anatomical location but on their origin of cord).

Muscles Related to Breast/Breast Surgery

Pectoralis major muscle: It arises from medial half of clavicle (clavicular fibres), anterior part of manubrium and sternum up to 6th costal cartilages (sternal fibres), 2nd to 6th costal cartilages (costal fibres). It is inserted as bilaminar tendon into lateral lip of bicipital groove of the upper end of humerus. It is supplied by lateral and medial pectoral nerves. Fibres are mainly placed as *transverse* and oblique. It is adductor and medial rotator of the shoulder; clavicular fibres flex the arm also. Deeper relations are pectoralis minor, clavipectoral fascia which is pierced by cephalic vein, thoracoacromial artery and lateral pectoral nerve. Anterior axillary fold is formed by twisted fibres of the pectoralis major muscle **(Fig. 16-6)**.

Pectoralis minor muscle: It arises from 3rd, 4th and 5th costal cartilages near costochondral junctions. It is inserted to medial upper part of the coracoid process (along with coracobrachialis). It is supplied by medial and lateral pectoral nerves **(Fig. 16-7)**.

Serratus anterior muscle: It arises from 8 digitations from upper eight ribs and intervening intercostal fascia. It is inserted into the costal surface of the scapula; first to superior angle; 2–4 to medial margin of the scapula; last 4 into inferior angle of the scapula. It is supplied by long thoracic nerve to serratus anterior (*of Bell*)—C5, 6 and 7. Muscle pulls the scapula forward in pushing and punching movement; it rotates the scapula forward; it helps in raising the arm above the head; it steadies the scapula during weight carrying. Its paralysis causes inferior angle and medial border of the scapula to become more prominent during the pushing movement causing '*winging of the scapula*'.

Latissimus dorsi (LD) muscle: It arises from posterior third of outer lip of iliac crest; lumbar fascia; T7 to T12 spines; lower four ribs; inferior angle of scapula. It forms posterior fold of the axilla, with twisted tendon inserted into the floor of the intertubercular sulcus of the upper end of the humerus. It is supplied by thoracodorsal nerve (C6, 7 and 8). It causes adduction, extension and medial rotation of the shoulder. It is a muscle of climbing, swimming and rowing. Muscle is important in mastectomy while creating the LD myocutaneous flap.

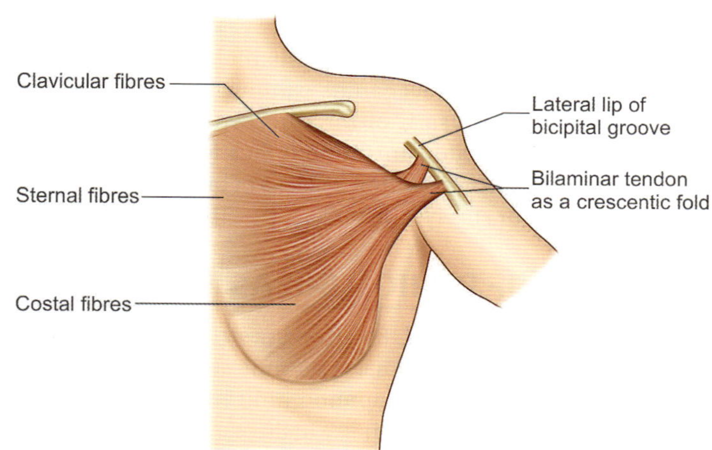

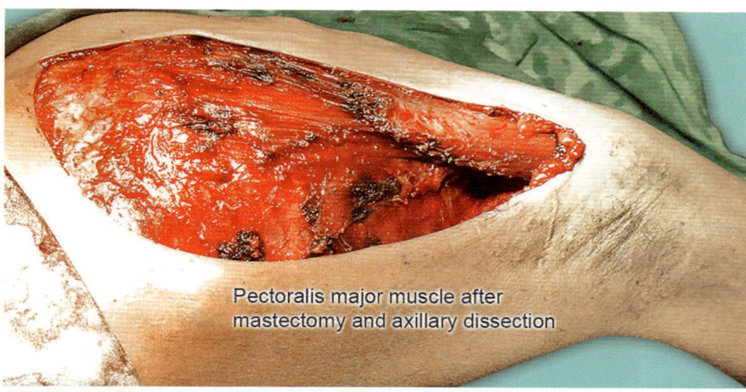

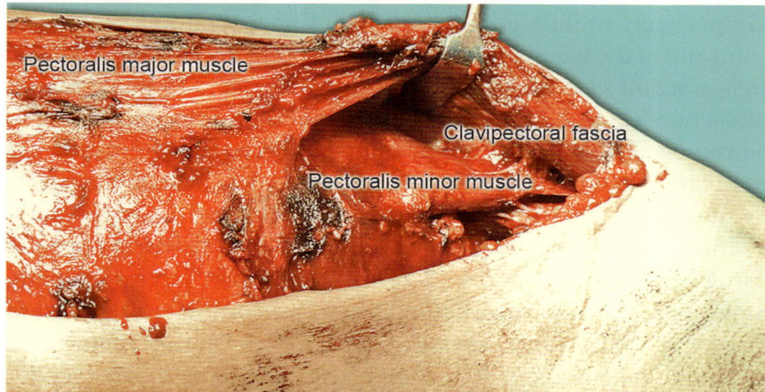

Fig. 16-6: Pectoralis major muscle.

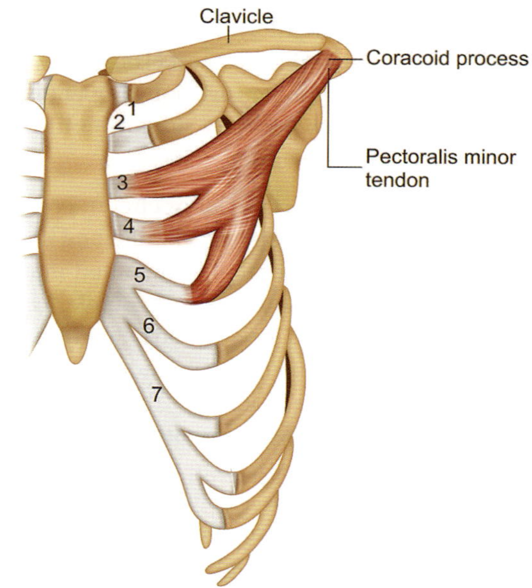

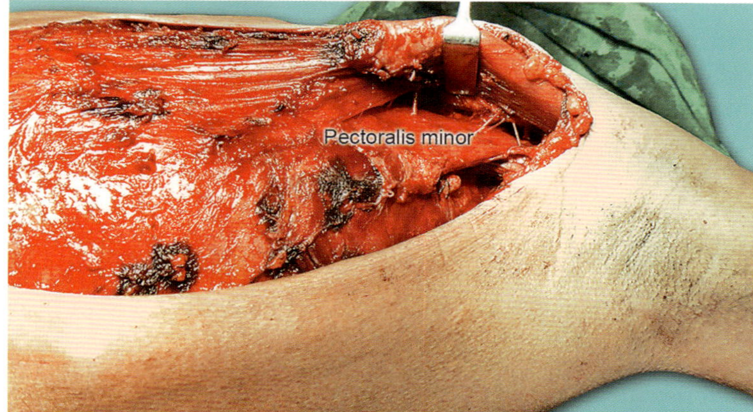

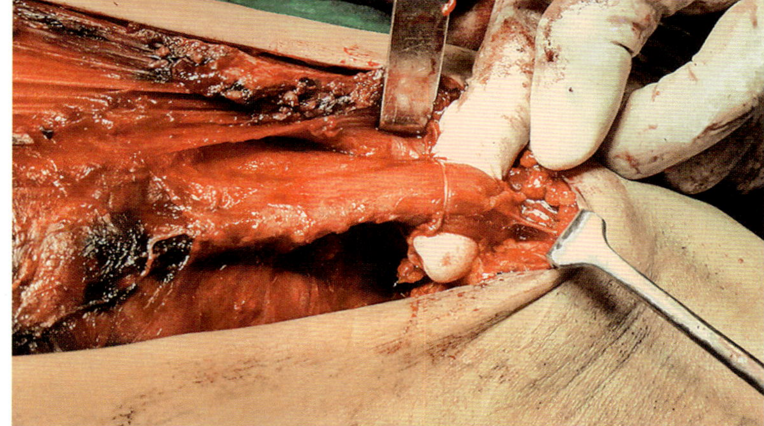

Fig. 16-7: Pectoralis minor muscle.

Fine Needle Aspiration Cytology (FNAC)

Often, 22 gauge needle with 20 mL syringe with syringe holder (aspiration gun) is used. Two syringes are usually required. After cleaning the area, needle is passed into the required tissue/mass obliquely; - 40 cm of H_2O suction is created into the syringe. Needle is manoeuvred at different angles at same site to allow cells to enter the needle. Cells should fill the needle not the syringe. Before removal of the needle from the tissue suction is released. Needle is withdrawn; contents are carefully expressed into glass slides. 5 mm drop of contents are placed over the slides, smear is created by rubbing another slide over it. One slide is air dried; other slides are fixed with 95% ethanol. Remaining cells in the needle can be used for culture, cytocentrifugation. Complications of fine needle aspiration cytology (FNAC) of breast are rare. Rarely pneumothorax, haemothorax, haematoma and acute mastitis can develop. Sensitivity is 98%. Specificity and positive predictive value is near 100%.

OPEN BIOPSY OF BREAST LESION

Indications: Lesions with atypia; lobular carcinoma in situ (LCIS); radial scar; atypical papillary lesions; high-risk group with suspected lesions; radiologic-pathologic discordance; phyllodes tumour; inadequate tissue harvesting; negative FNAC/core biopsy but doubtful lesion; failure of infection to subside in spite of proper treatment plan; mammographically suspected lesion.

Anaesthesia: Xylocaine 1% local (plain) anaesthetic agent is used (with adrenaline may cause epidermolysis). Infiltration is done deep into retromammary space. General anaesthesia is used when mass is not palpable or deeply placed; apprehensive non-cooperative patient; if one stage procedure (biopsy—frozen section confirmation—definitive surgical procedure) is planned.

Procedure: Incision is placed as periareolar or circumferential along the Langer lines which is cosmetically acceptable and should able to include the specimen of the eventual anticipated mastectomy. Sharp dissection is preferred method in biopsy. Bipolar cautery can be used (unipolar cautery should be avoided). Surrounding 1 cm margin of normal breast parenchyma is included with the lump. A 'figure of eight' suture may be placed on the mass to facilitate the dissection around. Holding the mass with crushing/damaging instruments should be avoided. Skin edge is retracted using hook retractor. After excision, haemostasis is achieved by bipolar cautery. Wound is irrigated with saline and drain is placed if required. Skin is sutured with subcuticular or interrupted sutures. Specimen should be oriented with marker stitches **(Figs. 16-8 and 16-9)**.

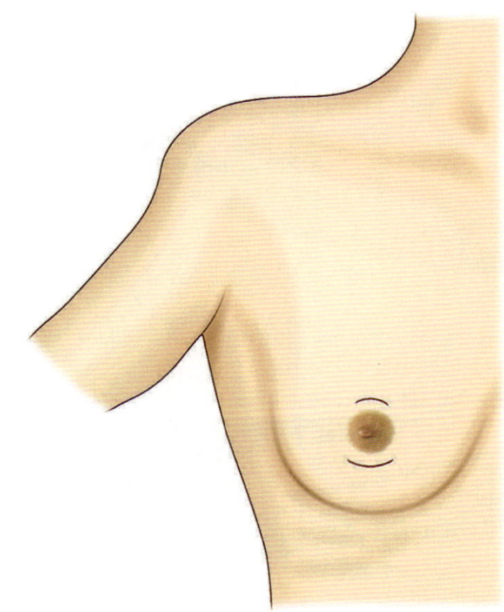

Fig. 16-8: Circumferential incision is preferred in breast biopsy.

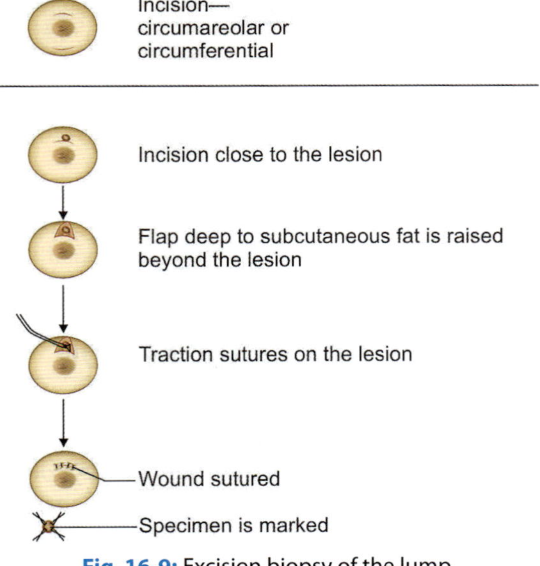

Fig. 16-9: Excision biopsy of the lump.

Incision biopsy instead of excision biopsy is done when tumour is more than 4 cm in size.

When there is nipple discharge suspicious of malignancy without any mass lesion, duct can be cannulated with a fine probe and circumferential excision of the duct with the lobe is done. Haematoma (10%), infection are the complications of breast biopsy.

Definitive surgery if done within 2 weeks of biopsy, it will not alter the recurrence rate or survival benefit.

EXCISION OF BENIGN BREAST LUMP

Palpable cyst can be aspirated. Recurrent cysts, solid benign masses need to be excised. Fibroadenoma, cysts, indicated fibrocystadenosis, traumatic fat necrosis are the common indications. Circumareolar, circumferential, lateral submammary incisions are commonly used. Smaller lesions are excised using circumareolar incision *(Webster's);* larger lesion is excised using submammary incision (*Gaillard Thomas incision*). Type of incision is decided on individual patient basis. Superomedial incision is usually avoided as scar may become hypertrophic **(Figs. 16-10 to 16-13)**.

Procedure

General anaesthesia is usually used. Patient is placed in supine position, cleaning and draping is done. Both monopolar and bipolar cautery can be used. Incision is made depending on the location and size of the lump. In *circumareolar incision*, dissection under the nipple should be done in deeper plane otherwise areolar necrosis may occur. Fine scissor and cautery dissection is done around the lump. Freely mobile and encapsulated fibroadenoma will easily come out of the wound with dissection around the capsule. *Figure of eight traction suture* on the swelling is beneficial to facilitate proper dissection around. It prevents destruction of the swelling/tissue to be removed by multiple applications of forceps. When cautery is used for excision, it should be wider to prevent coagulation artifacts in the specimen surface. Haemostasis achieved using cautery. Suction drain is placed. Deeper subcutaneous tissue is apposed using absorbable sutures (3-zero vicryl). Skin is closed using monofilament non-absorbable (3-zero polypropylene) or 3-zero monocryl. Compression dressings are applied. Drain is removed in 48 hours. Specimen should be sent for histology after making proper markings. Special sports bra is used in postoperative period until recovery occurs. An icepack over the breast may be useful to relieve the pain in immediate postoperative period **(Fig. 16-14)**.

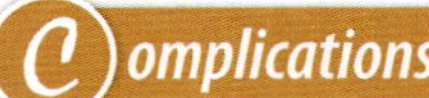

Complications

Seroma, haematoma, areolar necrosis, nipple deformity, asymmetry of breasts.

Subcutaneous Mastectomy

It is removal of entire breast with retaining skin over the breast, areola and nipple. It is done through a submammary *Gaillard Thomas incision*. Adequate skin flap is raised with flap containing subcutaneous fat which maintains the blood supply of the flap and prevents flap necrosis. Entire breast is removed using fine scissor dissection or cautery dissection. It is done in gynaecomastia, as a prophylactic mastectomy in high-risk patients. After haemostasis drain is placed. Breast implant can be placed in subcutaneous/submuscular plane either immediately or as delayed reconstruction.

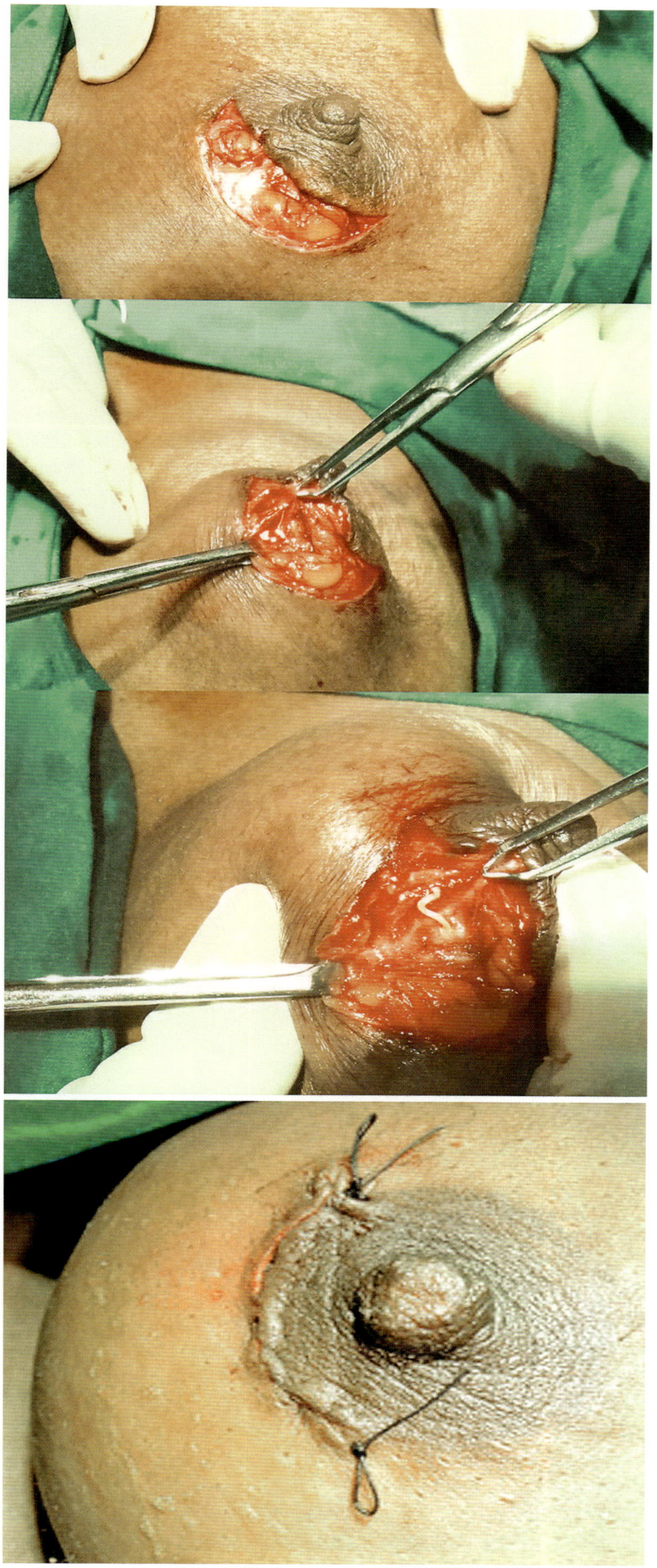

Fig. 16-10: Circumareolar (Webster's) incision. Areolar flap is raised carefully in deeper plane otherwise areolar necrosis can occur.

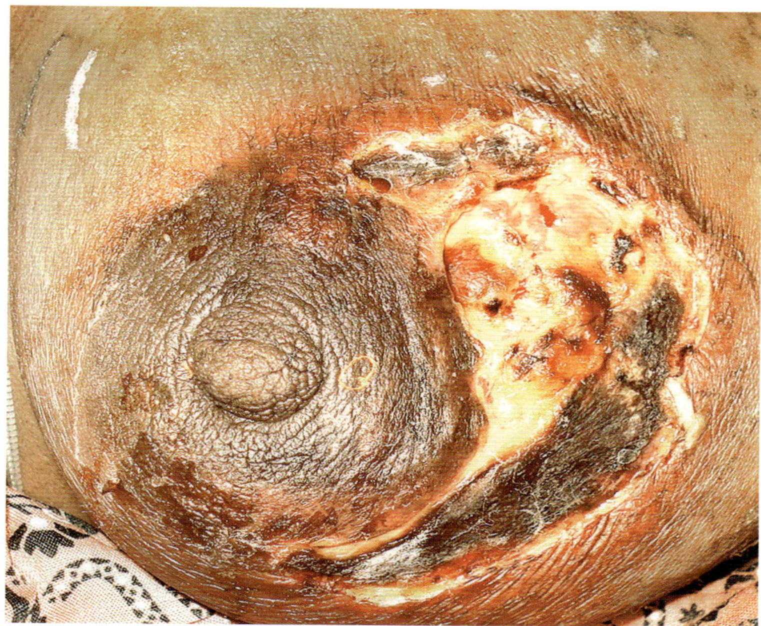

Fig. 16-11: Areolar necrosis developed after circumareolar incision.

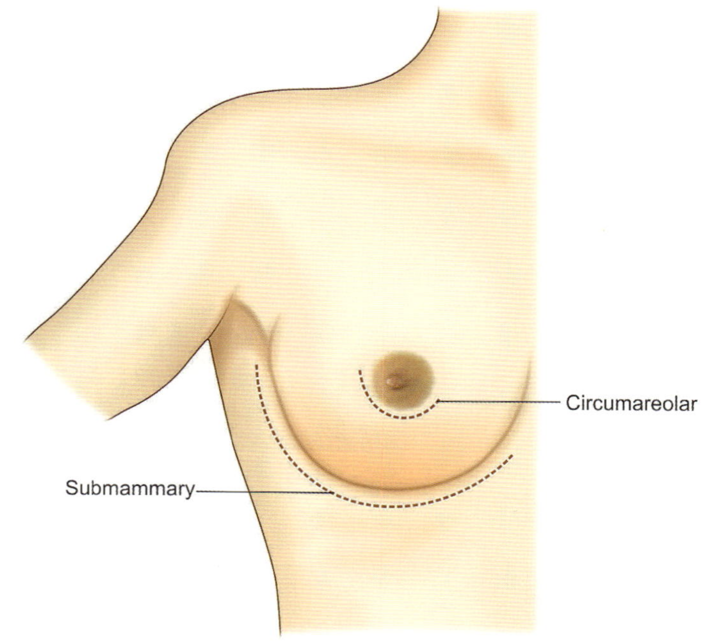

Fig. 16-12: Incisions used for breast lump excision. Circumareolar (*Webster's*) incision is cosmetically better and is used for small lumps. *Gaillard Thomas* submammary incision is used for excision of the large lump.

Indications for subcutaneous mastectomy are—fibrocystadenosis with epitheliosis, sclerosing adenosis, persistent nodules, gynaecomastia and ductal carcinoma in situ (DCIS). Breast implants (silastic) are placed in the subcutaneous/submuscular plane **(Fig. 16-15)**.

Complications

Nipple/areolar ischaemia, nipple distortion, saucer deformity of nipple, haematoma, seroma, wound infection, skin necrosis, asymmetry of breasts.

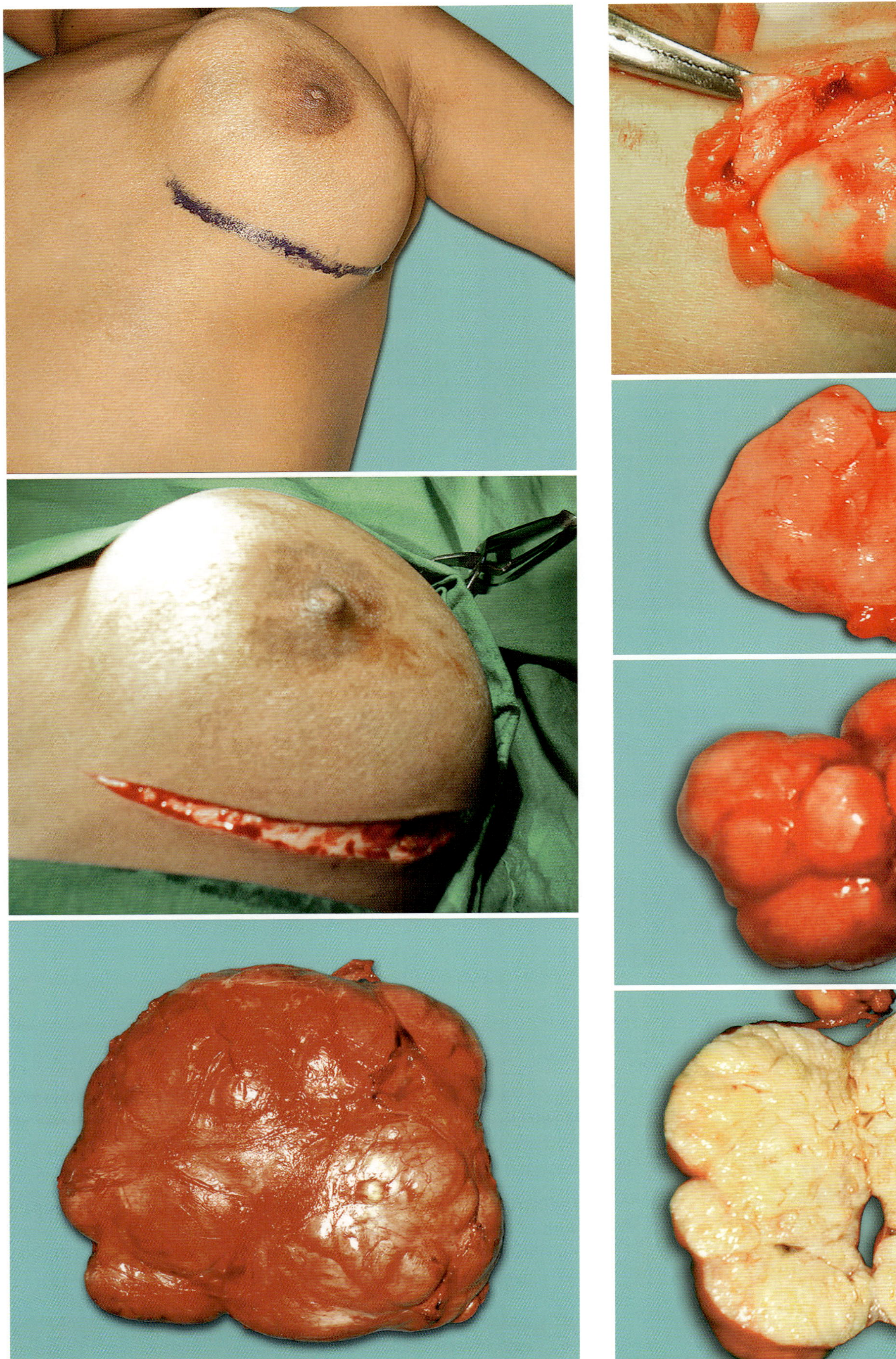

Fig. 16-13: Submammary incision is used to remove large benign swelling like fibroadenoma.

Fig. 16-14: Fibroadenoma is well capsulated and so easier to excise/enucleate. Circumareolar incision is used for small fibroadenomas. Submammary incision is used for large/multiple fibroadenomas.

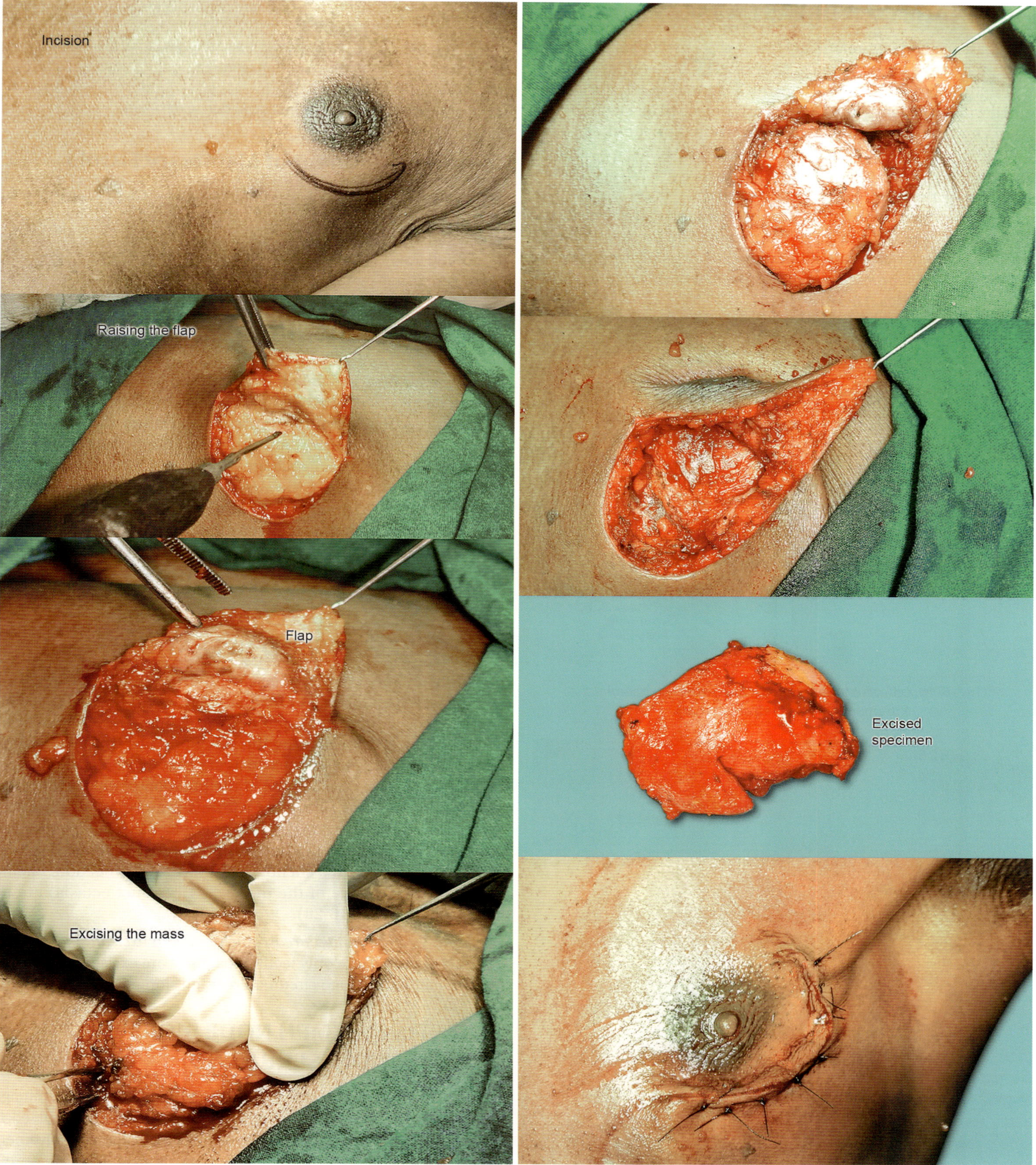

Fig. 16-15: Excision of gynaecomastia—steps. Drain may be placed if needed.

DRAINAGE OF A BREAST ABSCESS

Both subareolar and intramammary breast abscess should be drained. Drainage is done under general anaesthesia. Subareolar abscess is drained with a subareolar incision. Intramammary abscess is drained with a deep incision. Once cavity is reached all loculi should be broken using a sinus forceps/finger/scoop. Pus should be sent for culture. *Counter incision* is often needed to achieve complete drainage of the abscess cavity. Corrugated drain is placed for 72 hours or more or as required. Since intramammary abscess is common in lactating women, milk fistula may be a sequelae. It is often very difficult to manage such case. Milk from opposite breast should be expressed at regular intervals either manually or using breast pump. Only occasionally suppression of milk is needed using bromocryptine 2.5 mg for 5 days **(Figs. 16-16 to 16-18)**.

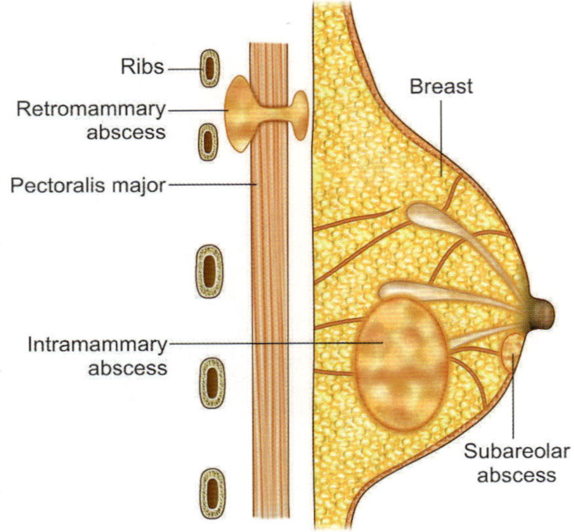

Fig. 16-16: Different types of breast abscesses—subareolar, intramammary and retromammary.

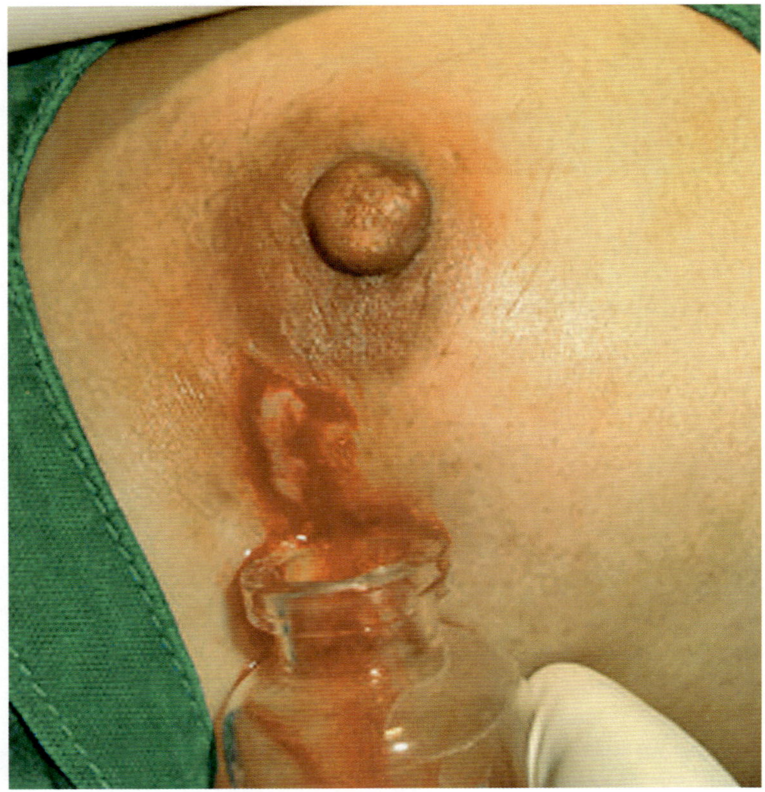

Fig. 16-17: Drainage of subareolar breast abscess.

Indications for drainage in mastitis/breast abscess

- Mastitis not resolving with antibiotics in 48 hours.
- Persistent fever and progression of mastitis.
- Brawny induration.

Do not wait for abscess to form (fluctuation to develop).

Surgical Treatment of Mammary Fistula

Mammary fistula develops in a chronic abscess cavity at the drainage site or where abscess has pointed and opened. A probe is passed through the fistula towards the apex of the nipple. Track is laid open by cutting tissues along the probe. Opened wound is left to granulate. Often it requires major duct excision **(Fig. 16-19)**.

MICRODOCHECTOMY

It is excision of the entire lactiferous duct (single duct disease). It is done for duct papilloma. In a duct papilloma when there is no palpable mass, duct is expressed to see the discharge. A fine probe/stiff nylon suture (as a probe) is passed gently into the duct. Probe is fixed to nipple skin using silk sutures so that it will not displace during procedure. A triangular area is cut 1 mm away from the probe using fine scissor to raise the skin flaps. The duct with the probe is excised with the skin flap for 5 cm till the papilloma is identified. Papilloma will be always situated within 5 cm from the duct orifice. Wound is closed without a drain. Compression bandage is applied. It is ideal to rule out DCIS by frozen section biopsy.

MAJOR DUCT EXCISION (ADAIR-HADFIELD OPERATION)

It is done mainly for duct ectasia with involvement of many ducts or multiple papillomas. A circumareolar incision is made usually along lower half of the areola not exceeding more than 3/5th of circumference. After incising the subcutaneous tissue, with blunt dissection terminal lactiferous ducts are circumferentially dissected. All dissected ducts are divided at the junction of nipple. A cone of tissue of 4 cm depth and 2 cm width is removed with base deep in the breast parenchyma. Excised entire lactiferous ducts are sent for histology. Cavity in the breast is obliterated with vicryl sutures. Wound is closed with a suction drain. Bruising, infection, haematoma and recurrence of the disease—15% (duct ectasia) are the complications **(Fig. 16-20)**.

Melhem Novel modified breast ductal system excision is also done for duct ectasia. Here only lactiferous ducts are excised after raising the areolar flap through circumareolar incision.

SENTINEL LYMPH NODE BIOPSY/ DISSECTION (SLNB/SLND)

The first axillary (SLN) node draining the breast (by direct drainage) is designated as the *sentinel node*. SLN is first node involved by tumour cells and presence or absence of its histological involvement, when assessed will give a predictive idea about the further spread of tumour to other nodes. The incidence of involvement of other nodes without SLN is less than 3% and so if SLNB is negative nodal dissection can be avoided but regular follow up is needed. SLNB is done in all cases of early breast cancers, T1 and T2 *without clinically palpable node*. It is not done in clinically palpable axillary node as there is already distortion of lymphatic flow due to tumour.

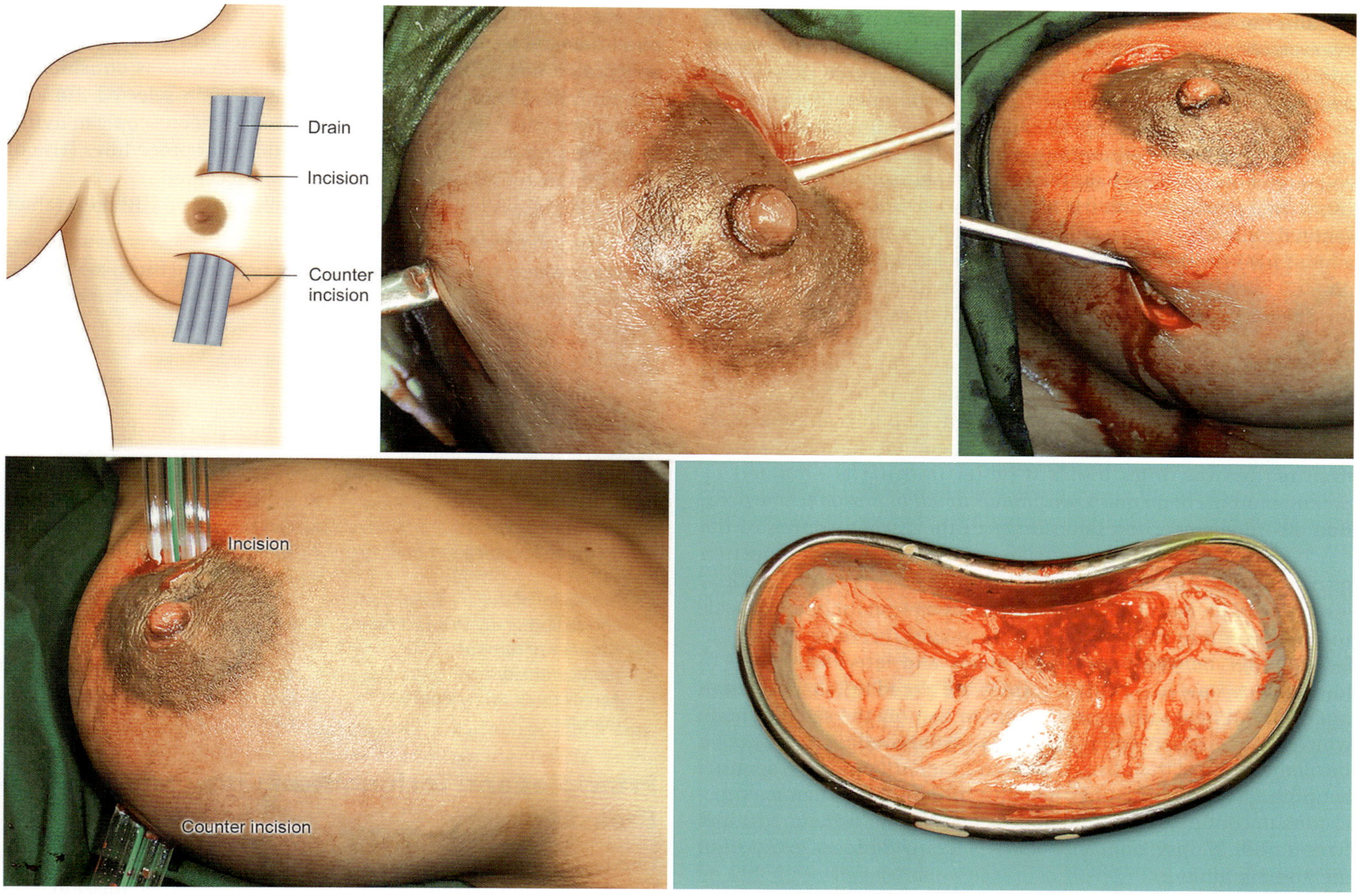

Fig. 16-18: Drainage of intramammary breast abscess. Incision and counter incision is used commonly to prevent cavity getting closed early which may cause recurrence.

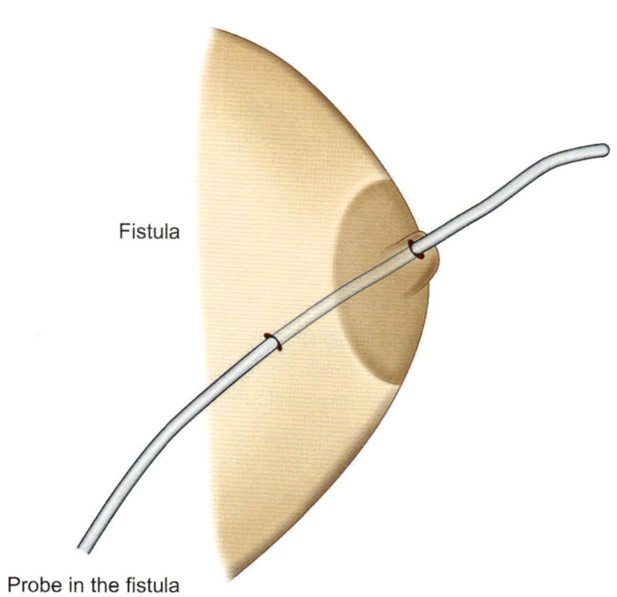

Fig. 16-19: Mammary fistula excision.

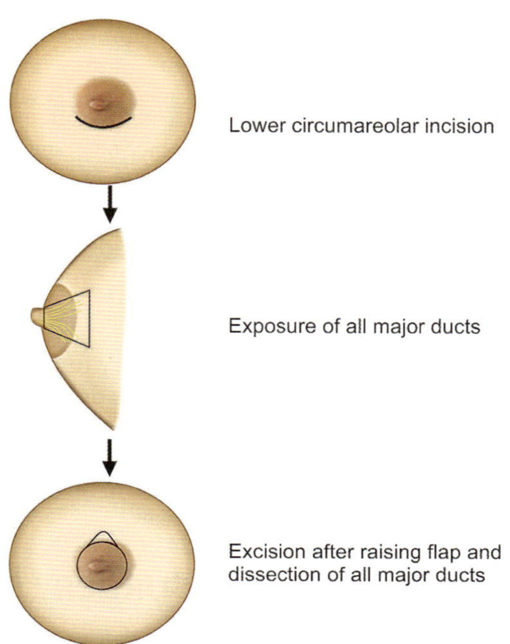

Fig. 16-20: Adair–Hadfield major duct excision.

It is also not done in multifocal and multicentric tumours, as there is involvement of many lymphatic trunks from different places of breast, and chances of false negative is high. Sentinel node is localised by preoperative (within 12 hours prior) or peroperative injection of patent blue (Isosulfan vital blue dye 2.5–7.5 mL) or 99m TC radioisotope labelled albumin (one mCi on previous day)/sulphur colloid (6 hours before) near the tumour (peritumour area) or over subdermal plexus around the nipple. Marker will pass through the sentinel node which can be detected visually as blue staining or with a hand held gamma camera; and is biopsied with a small incision directly over it. Frozen section biopsy or touch imprint cytology is done for presence of malignant cells. If there is no involvement of sentinel node by tumour then further axillary dissection is not required as *skip lesions* (skipping sentinel node) occur only in less than 3% cases. Detection rate of sentinel node for blue dye and radioisotope is 90% and 98% respectively. Subdermal/subareolar injection of radioisotope *has got better* sentinel node localisation than peritumour injection. But better imaging is obtained by peritumour injection and so *peritumour injection is usually* practiced. Radioisotope tracer injection done in the early morning of the day of surgery into peritumour area and perioperative injection of patent blue dye in subareolar region—as a *combined method* is often used in many centres. After injection of patent blue, breast is massaged continuously to enhance the uptake. *Incision* is made after 5–7 minutes between pectoralis major and latissimus dorsi to identify blue stained lymphatics which are traced to 2–3 blue lymph nodes. Hand held radioprobe is used to identify the sentinel node which is later excised. Often 2–3 nodes are removed. *Paraffin section histology is better* than frozen section to identify positive sentinel lymph node. If report comes negative immunohistochemistry test is done to confirm that lymph node is negative for tumour. Sentinel lymph node biopsy *should be done before* wide local excision of the primary tumour.

Wide local excision of the primary tumour is done after SLNB in the same sitting.

SLNB is *less invasive* than axillary dissection. It is ideal in early invasive carcinoma. Positive SLNB is again classified as macrometastasis (>2 mm) or micrometastasis (<2 mm).

SLNB is *contraindicated* in patients who are allergic to vital blue dye or radio-colloid, in pregnancy and in inflammatory carcinoma of breast.

Complications

Complications of SLNB are rare. They are—blue tattooing of skin which gradually fades; blue—green urine and stool for short periods; allergic reactions; anaphylaxis (0.1%); seroma formation. Blue dye binds to oxyhaemoglobin artificially registers in oximeter as hypoxaemia

Axillary Sampling

It is done before wide local excision of primary tumour. Incision is made between pectoralis major and latissimus dorsi muscles. Deep fascia is opened. 10–15 nodes of level I are dissected and removed. Often this procedure is done along with sentinel lymph node biopsy. Occasionally when level I nodes are not found, level II or III nodes are removed to identify 3–5% skip metastases.

BREAST CONSERVATIVE SURGERY (BCS)

In early breast cancer, breast conservative surgeries like quadrantectomy, axillary dissection (level I and II) and postoperative radiotherapy (to the breast) are used which prevents the disfigurement and psychological trauma of mastectomy to the patient. It is very well acceptable cosmetically. When disease outcome is considered, it is equivalent to mastectomy if patient is carefully selected. Tumour is removed with a rim of 1 cm normal tissue (macroscopic margin). Wide excision and QUART therapy are different procedures (Use of word lumpectomy is a debate and not well accepted).

Tumour size is *better* estimated by ultrasound or MRI breast than by clinical examination or mammography.

Breast conservative surgery

Indications	*Contraindications*
◈ Lump ≤ 4cm ◈ Clinically negative axillary nodes ◈ Mammographically detected lesion ◈ Well differentiated tumour with low S phase ◈ Adequate sized breast to allow proper RT to breast ◈ Breast of adequate size and volume ◈ Feasibility of axillary dissection and radiotherapy to intact breast ◈ Absence of tumour multicentricity ◈ Achieving tumour negative margin	◈ Tumour > 4 cm ◈ Positive axillary nodes > N1 ◈ Tumour margin is not free of tumour after breast conservative surgery ◈ Poorly differentiated tumor ◈ Multicentric tumour ◈ Earlier breast irradiation ◈ Tumour/breast size ratio is more ◈ Tumour beneath the nipple/ central tumour ◈ Extensive intraductal carcinoma ◈ Existing collagen vascular disease as RT may be problematic ◈ Strong family history of breast cancer

Principles and Technique of Conservative Breast Surgery

Curvilinear *non-radial incision* (radial incision should not be placed, if there is a need to convert into total mastectomy, then incision plan may be difficult) is used to remove primary tumour. Separate incision is used for axillary dissection. Undermining of the skin flap must be avoided. Tumour clearance should be confirmed by frozen section. It may be often difficult and so tumour is cut and only margin which is close and doubtful is advocated for frozen section. Radiotherapy is a must to breast and chest wall region (locally). Consent for total mastectomy should be taken in case if need arises **(Fig. 16-21)**.

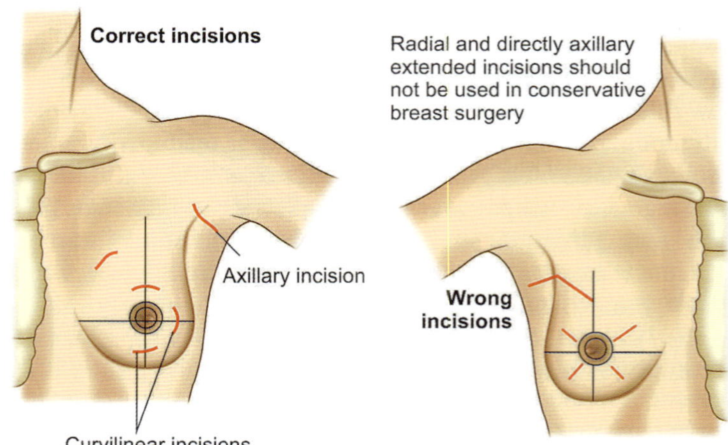

Fig. 16-21: Curvilinear incision should be placed in conservative breast surgeries. Never place wrong radial incisions. If conversion to total mastectomy is needed, it will be difficult in placing incision if radial incision is placed. In conservative breast surgery for axillary dissection separate incision in the axilla should be placed.

Ultrasound is good way of assessing the size of the tumour. If mammography shows calcification, this calcification should be localised using hook wires. Impalpable lesions are localised pre-operatively by blue dye injection, hook wires, radioisotope markers. Intraoperative ultrasound also can be used. By mammography or ultrasound controlled injection of technetium labelled human serum albumin or sulphur colloid into the tumour and using hand held gamma probe lesion is located intraoperatively and excised.

Quadrantectomy and wide local excision are two types of BCS. Breast is distributed into segments with each segment draining into one major duct. Removal of *one entire segment with ductal system with 2 cm clearance* is *quadrantectomy* which is much wider and extensive removal than wide local excision. But presently quadrantectomy is not advocated as it is cosmetically poorer and there is no difference in outcome between quadrantectomy and ***wide local excision***.

Incision over the breast should be circumferential along the *Langer's line* or parallel to the lines of maximum resting skin tension in the breast (*dynamic lines of Kraisl*) **(Fig. 16-22)**.

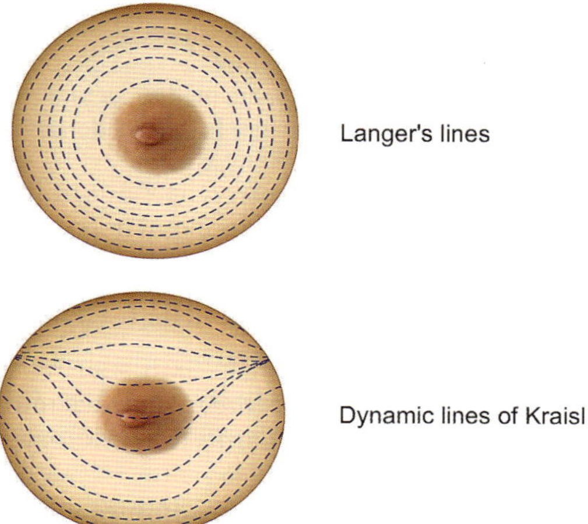

Fig. 16-22: Langer lines and dynamic lines of Kraisl.

If there is previous open biopsy scar, it should be included in the specimen as 'en bloc'. *Mexican hat incision* of the preexisting scar gives better scar. Otherwise routine skin excision is *not* done **(Fig. 16-23)**.

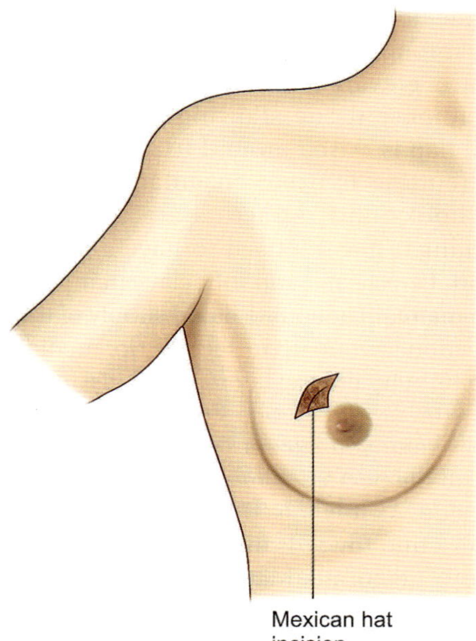

Fig. 16-23: Mexican hat incision is used to include previous scar area.

Skin flaps are deepened straight up to 1–2 cm beyond the lump margin. Only rising skin flaps is *not* advised. Skin with subcutaneous tissue can be raised judiciously.

Dissection is done around the tumour with a volume of normal breast tissue all around. Pectoral fascia *should not* be opened in deeper plane. Tumour with surrounding normal clearance tissue is lifted off the pectoralis fascia and breast tissue in deeper plane can be dissected off the fascia. Bipolar cautery is better than monopolar cautery. After removal of the specimen, it is properly marked using coloured markers or paints as superior, inferior, medial, lateral, anterior and posterior for identification of the clearance margins and *orientation*. Entire specimen is coated in India ink. Specimen should be inspected properly for tumour relation to margins. All marked surfaces and margin which is close to the tumour should undergo frozen section biopsy for confirmation of clearance. Doing *specimen mammography* is often better. Specimen may be kept in an *orientation—grid* and mammography of the specimen is taken. If few margins are close to the tumour, then re-resection at that particular margin is sufficient which again should be confirmed by frozen biopsy. Achieving margin clearance all around the tumour is essential but *width of cleared margin is not important*. Once confirmed, specimen is sent for receptor/molecular/cellular/biochemical study. Wound is closed without a drain. *Small defect* in the breast tissue (tumour area) less than 10% of volume can be left alone; *larger defect* in breast more than 10% of breast volume should be apposed by proper sutures. If many margins are invaded or very close to tumour, then total mastectomy should be planned **(Fig. 16-24)**.

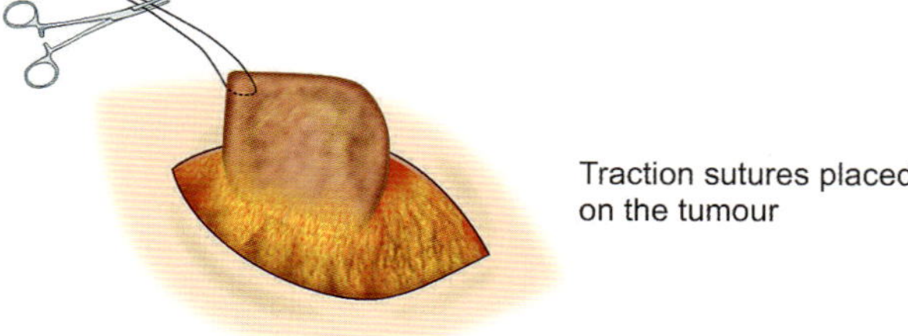

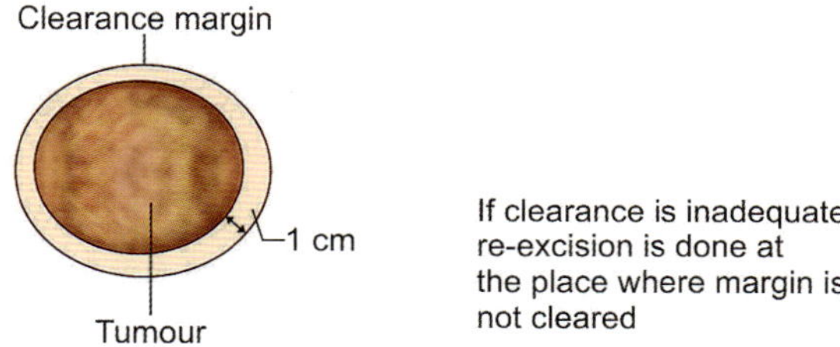

Fig. 16-24: Technique of wide local excision.

Complications of wide local excision are—haematoma (2%); seroma; infection (5%); incomplete excision (15%); poor scar.

Recurrence after BCS is usually at primary site. Young age, family history, small volume breast are the patient related factors for recurrence. Grading of the tumour, lymphatic or vascular invasion (two times more), extensive in situ component (4 times more), multifocal tumours are the *tumour factors* for recurrence of the tumour. Delay in radiotherapy to breast area, further chemotherapy and hormone therapy also influence the local recurrence rate. Radiotherapy to breast is a *must* after BCS. Recurrence is treated by total mastectomy.

Microscopic disease free margin is defined as at least 1 mm rim of normal tissue around the tumour in all directions. Area lesser than 1 mm is considered as inadequate clearance and such area should be re-excised and confirmed for clearance. It is done either through same scar or modified elliptical incision which includes the scar—'*Mexican hat incision*'.

QUART Therapy

It is quadrantectomy, axillary dissection of level I and II nodes with separate axillary incision and postoperative radiotherapy to breast (5000 cGy) and axilla (1000 cGy). First it was started by Umberto Veronesi from Milan.

Axillary dissection is done to identify the nodal involvement of the disease which is an indicator of metastatic breast disease. It is also done for staging of malignancy. Number and level of nodes involved are independent predictors of outcome of the disease. Therapeutic benefit of axillary dissection is a debate. It is done basically for infiltrating carcinoma of breast. In situ carcinomas do not require axillary dissection as incidence of nodal spread in situ carcinoma is less than 2%. Axillary flaps are elevated superiorly and inferiorly. Level I and II nodes are removed with fat and fascia. External mammary, lateral, subscapular and central nodes are removed. A minimum of 10 nodes should be removed. Wound is closed with a suction drain.

AXILLARY DISSECTION

It is done under general anaesthesia. Sandbag is placed under the shoulder to elevate the axilla. Arm, axilla, shoulder and same side chest wall is cleaned and draped. Forearm and hand are draped to facilitate holding and moving it as needed.

Incision is along the crease just below the hair bearing area of axilla. A lazy S incision between pectoralis major and latissimus dorsi muscle or an incision along the anterior axillary fold also can be used **(Fig. 16-25)**.

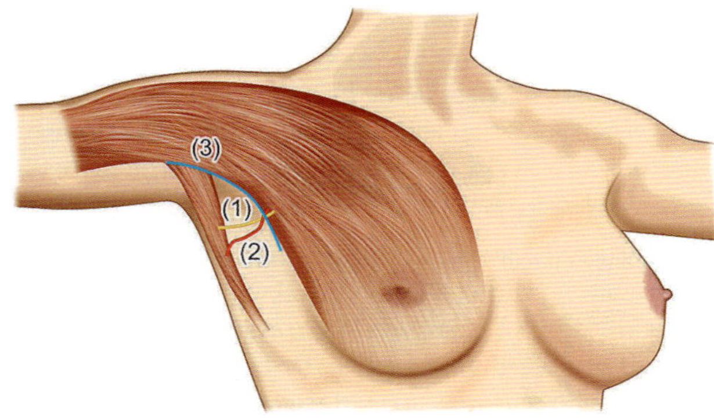

(1) Skin crease incision distal to hair bearing skin of the axilla.
(2) Lazy S incision between pectoralis major and latissimus dorsi.
(3) Anterior axillary fold incision.

Fig. 16-25: Different incisions for axillary dissection.

Skin flap is elevated behind up to the edge of latissimus dorsi muscle. Upper skin flap is raised. Medial part of the dissection is done by identifying the pectoral muscles. Medial pectoral nerve which winds the lateral margin of the pectoralis minor muscle is identified. One must remember that medial pectoral nerve arises from the medial cord of the brachial plexus and often passes through the fibres of the lateral part of the pectoralis minor muscle. Medial margin of the pectoralis minor is reached above to identify the part of clavipectoral fascia which contains few lymph nodes. It is upper medial limit of the dissection. Axillary vein meets the subclavius muscle here. When required pectoralis muscle should be divided from its insertion to coracoid process; index finger is passed around the insertion of the pectoralis minor tendon and muscle is traced towards coracoid process and is divided. Axillary vein is dissected to clear adipose tissue and lymph nodes on it. Now dissection should be done from lateral to medial using sharp and blunt dissection. Apex of the axilla should be cleared. Blood supply to pectoralis major muscle should be retained. Lower flap is dissected further to identify the serratus anterior muscle. Intercostobrachial nerve is identified and is preserved. Long thoracic nerve of Bell is 2 cm posterior to intercostobrachial nerve. It is in the serratus fascia. It should be identified and preserved. Further dissection exposes the thoracodorsal nerve (nerve to latissimus dorsi). Thoracodorsal vein is first identified; thoracodorsal nerve is most medial in thoracodorsal neurovascular bundle. This entire neurovascular bundle should be preserved if latissimus dorsi flap is needed at later period to patient. Dissection is continued laterally and behind to remove all the tissues up to the axillary tail. Specimen is removed. Its directions are marked. Single suction drain is placed. Skin flap is sutured from its deeper plane to chest wall as quilting to prevent seroma formation. Wound is closed in layers. Pressure dressing is placed.

Complications

Seroma formation, prolonged drainage through the drain for many days often weeks, frozen shoulder, lymphoedema of upper limb (10%), pectoral muscle atrophy due to injury to medial pectoral nerve, atrophy of latissimus dorsi muscle due to injury to thoracodorsal nerve, *winged scapula* is due to damage to long thoracic nerve.

Seroma formation is more common in obesity, when axillary nodes are positive, extensive mobilisation.

SKIN SPARING MASTECTOMY (SSM)

It is like a key-hole surgery of breast. Skin sparing/limited skin excision (5–10%) will not alter/affect the recurrence rate.

Indications are—central tumour/multicentric/extensive intraductal/T1/not feasible for breast conservation.

It includes excision of nipple-areola complex with very limited skin removal; marginal skin excision over the tumour/biopsy site; total glandular mastectomy; axillary dissection using either same (extension of SSM incision) or separate incision in the axilla.

Incision is either periareolar/tennis racquet/modified elliptical. Tennis racquet has got lateral extension to axilla. Reduction mammoplasty incision is also used with a periareolar incision extending vertically into an inframammary horizontal incision. Prior biopsy site should be included in the mastectomy incision or should be removed widely through a separate elliptical incision **(Fig. 16-26)**.

Skin flaps are elevated between breast parenchyma and subcutaneous adipose tissue allowing 5–10 mm thick skin flap. Circumferential flap is raised around using scissor/no. 15 scalpel blade/cautery (cutting is used; coagulation can cause cautery artifact). Skin hooks and retractors are used to facilitate the dissection. Headlight may be used to have a better visualisation during dissection. Parasternal and infraclavicular perforating vessels are preserved to maintain adequate blood supply of the retained skin. Superiorly dissection is done up to second rib; medially to sternum; below to inframammary crease; laterally to latissimus dorsi muscle. Entire breast tissue, nipple areolar complex are removed. Usually pectoral fascia is removed except in case of superficial tumours. Breast is raised off the pectoralis major muscle from the medial end towards lateral side. As it is raised it is delivered out of the wound to reach the dissection towards axillary tail. Axillary tail of Spence is separated from pectoralis major, minor and serratus anterior muscles. Junction of axillary tail and axillary tissue is clamped, ligated and cut. Axillary dissection may be added as decided. Wound is closed with a suction drain.

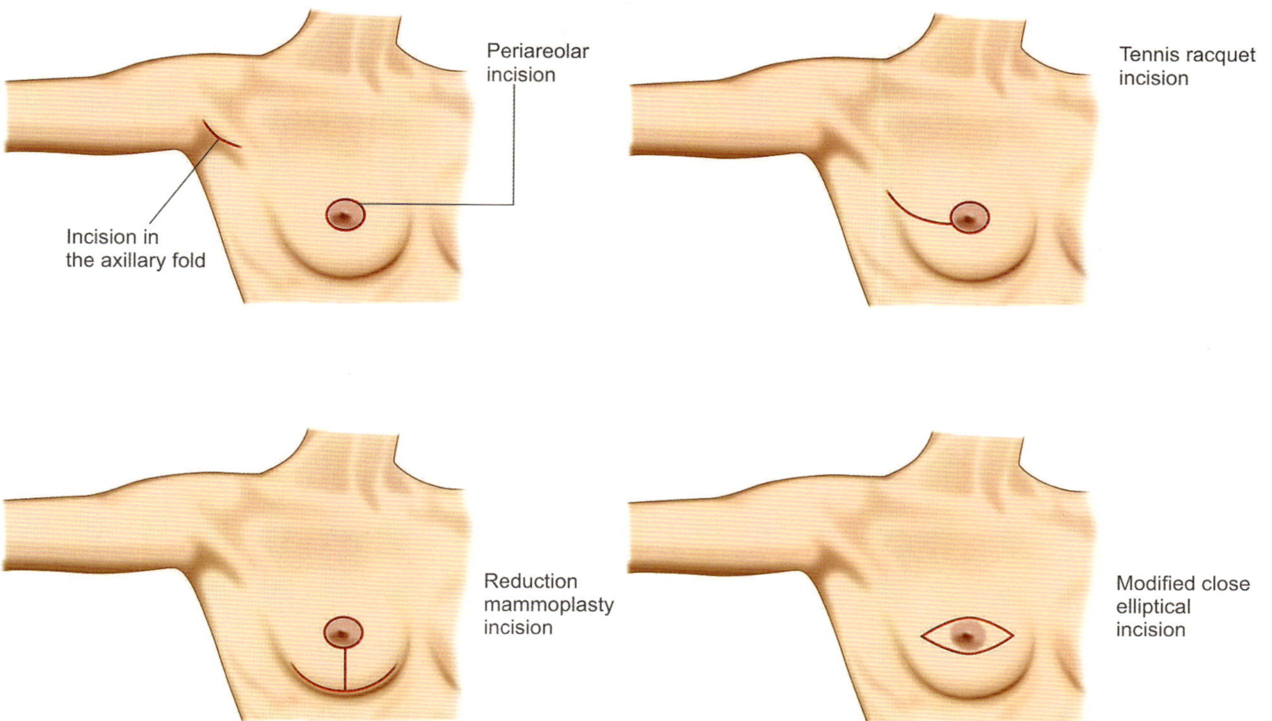

Fig. 16-26: Incisions used for skin sparing mastectomy (SSM).

Immediate reconstruction with latissimus dorsi or TRAM flap is done with tissue expanders placed underneath the subcutaneous or submuscular plane.

Problems with SSM are—difficulty in raising flaps, haematoma/seroma formation, infection **(Figs. 16-27 and 16-28)**.

NIPPLE SPARING MASTECTOMY (NSM)

It is doing mastectomy with saving nipple areolar complex (NAC). It is done in selected breast cancer (therapeutic) and in prophylactic mastectomy (risk prevention mastectomy).

Criteria for NSM are—tumour less than 3 cm; tumour 2 cm away from the nipple; clinically negative axilla; negative sentinel node; no inflammatory carcinoma or Paget's disease; MRI confirmation of no involvement of the NAC. It is avoided in excessively large or excessively ptotic breasts. Intraoperative frozen section biopsy and permanent pathology should be negative for the tissue biopsy taken from the underneath of the NAC. NAC should be adequately perfused; it should be adequately positioned.

Technique: Preoperative markings of both breasts are important for comparison and cosmesis. Lateral and radial incisions are best. NAC flap is raised; mastectomy is done. Proper external retractor to retract flap is essential. Single port device endoscopic, robotic assistance are also helpful to do better dissection in NSM.

Complications: Partial or complete nipple loss; malposition of the nipple; delayed involvement of the NAC by the tumour.

INDICATIONS FOR TOTAL MASTECTOMY/ MODIFIED RADICAL MASTECTOMY IN BREAST CANCER

- When tumour is more than 4 cm.
- Multicentric tumour.
- Poorly differentiated tumour.
- Tumour margin is not clear of tumour after breast conservative surgery.
- Recurrence after BCS.
- Prior radiotherapy to breast.
- Scleroderma or association with other collagen disease.
- Stage I invasive/Stage II, III diseases.

MODIFIED RADICAL MASTECTOMY (MRM)

In MRM, breast tissue, nipple areolar complex, skin over the breast tissue are removed along with axillary clearance with or without removal of pectoralis minor.

Patey's operation: It is total mastectomy with clearance of all levels of axillary lymph nodes with removal of pectoralis minor muscle.

Scanlon operation: Here along with total mastectomy, pectoralis minor is not removed but incised to reach level III lymph nodes.

Auchincloss operation: It is total mastectomy with axillary clearance (level I and II) keeping pectoralis minor intact. It is commonly advocated now.

Patey's operation: It is total mastectomy along with clearance of all levels of axillary nodes and removal of pectoralis minor muscle. It is *en bloc* dissection of breast and axilla.

General anaesthesia is used for the procedure. Patient lies in *supine position* with sandbag under the same side thorax and shoulder. Side of the chest wall, breast area, axilla, neck and sides are cleaned and draped. Same side entire arm and forearm is cleaned and is covered with drape and stockings. Shoulder should have free movement as needed during dissection of the axilla. Shoulder is kept in abducted and extended position. Surgeon stands on the side; first assistant near the shoulder on the same side; second assistant on opposite side; scrub nurse stands next to the surgeon near the leg side.

Different incisions are used as shown in **Figures 16-29 to 16-35**. *Classic elliptical Stewart incision* is commonly used. Incision is decided by the surgeon who is operating.

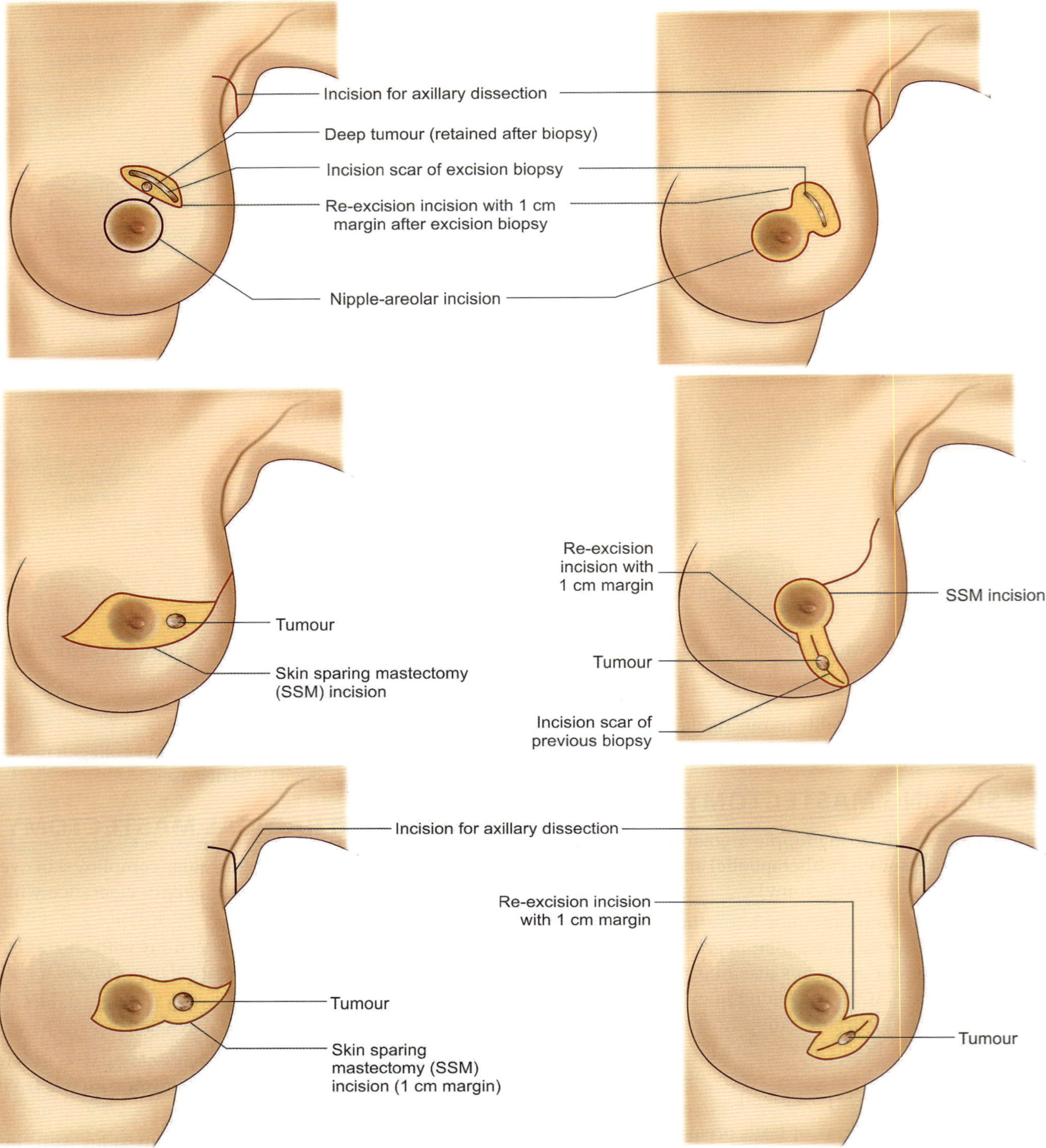

Fig. 16-27: Skin sparing mastectomy for carcinoma breast—different approaches. Skin sparing mastectomy (SSM) does not affect the recurrence rate.

An elliptical incision is made from medial aspect of the second and third intercostals space enclosing the nipple, areola and tumour extending laterally into the axilla along the anterior axillary fold. Upper and lower skin flaps are raised. Flap is raised mainly using scissor/scalpel/cutting cautery along with blunt gauze dissection in between. It extends medially up to the midline on the sternum; laterally to anterior margin of the latissimus dorsi muscle; above up to second rib/subclavius muscle; below 3 cm down the inframammary fold. Skin with subcutaneous fat is dissected off while raising the flap. Breast with tumour is raised from the medial aspect of the pectoral major muscle with pectoral fascia by making a deep incision close to midline, adjacent to sternum. Dissection is proceeded laterally ligating perforating vessels derived from lateral thoracic and anterior intercostal arteries. Once dissection reaches axilla, lateral border of pectoralis major muscle and pectoralis minor is exposed in deeper plane. Medial pectoral nerve (is lateral arises from medial cord of brachial plexus) which supplies lateral part of the pectoralis major muscle is identified here and preserved.

Axillary lymph node dissection is now started in continuity with mastectomy. Investing layer of deep fascia is divided. Fascia in front of the axillary vein is dissected to expose the vein in front. Small tributaries are ligated. Pectoralis major is retracted supero-medially. Finger is swept between the two pectori to clear the Rotter's nodes. Lateral pectoral nerve is identified and preserved

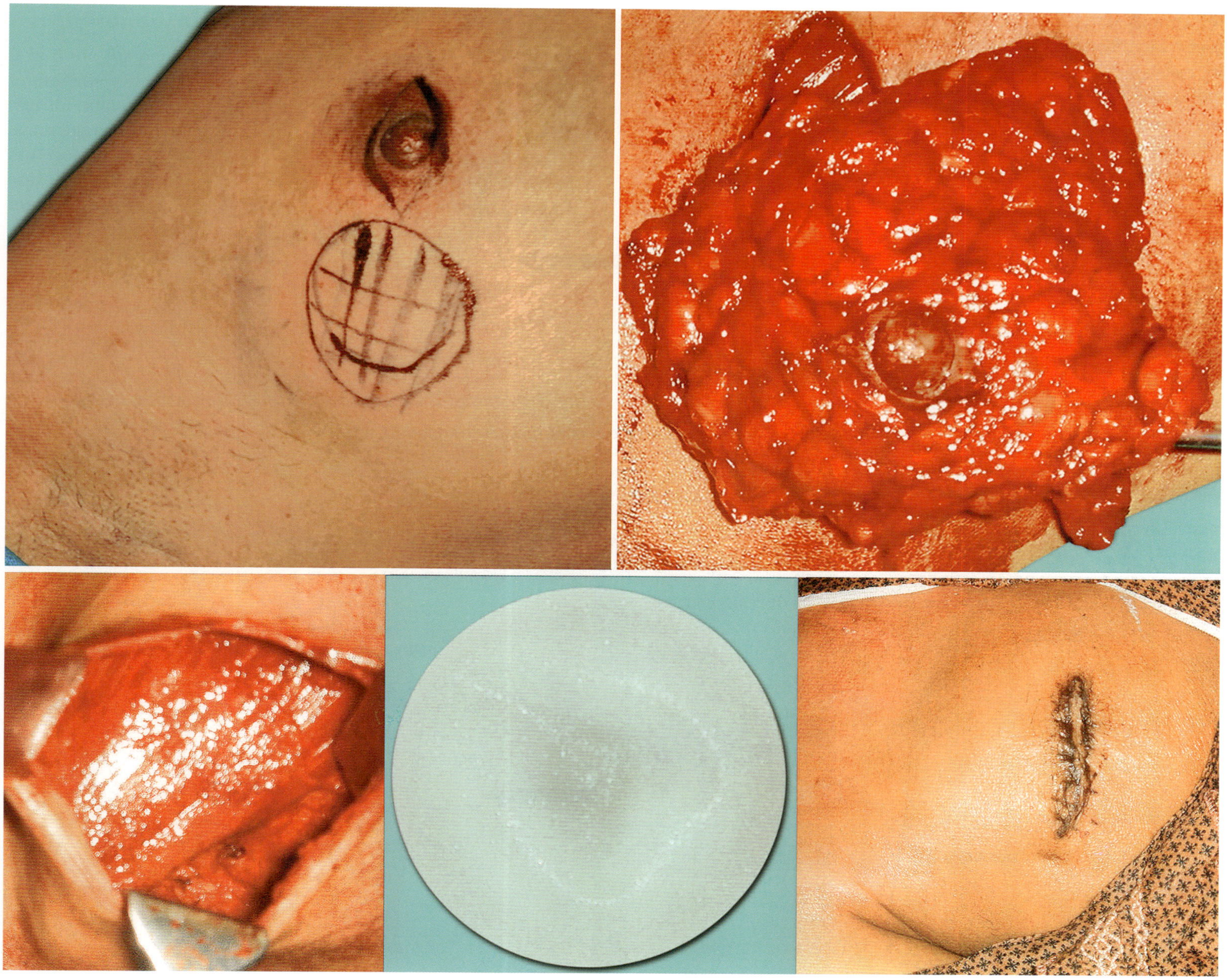

Fig. 16-28: Skin sparing mastectomy incision with prosthesis implant for placement.

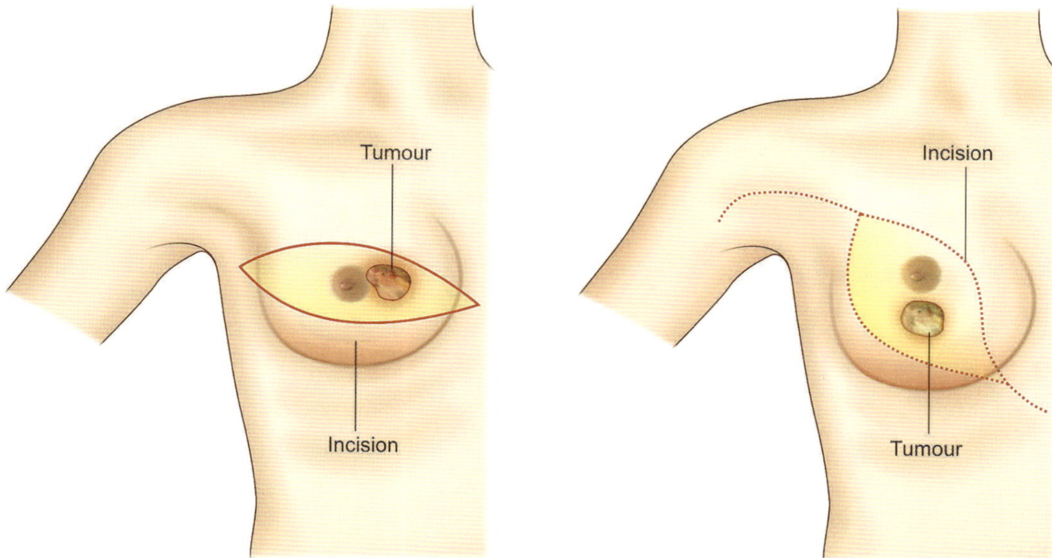

Fig. 16-29: A horizontal or oblique incision is commonly used for total mastectomy or modified radical mastectomy.

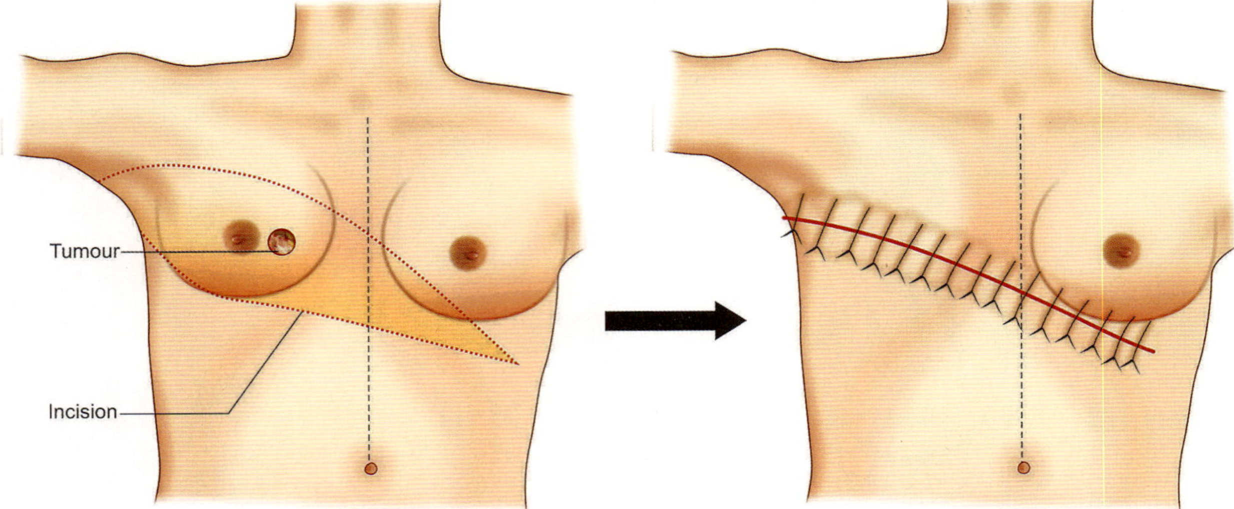

Fig. 16-30: Gray incision crosses the midline towards the opposite side.

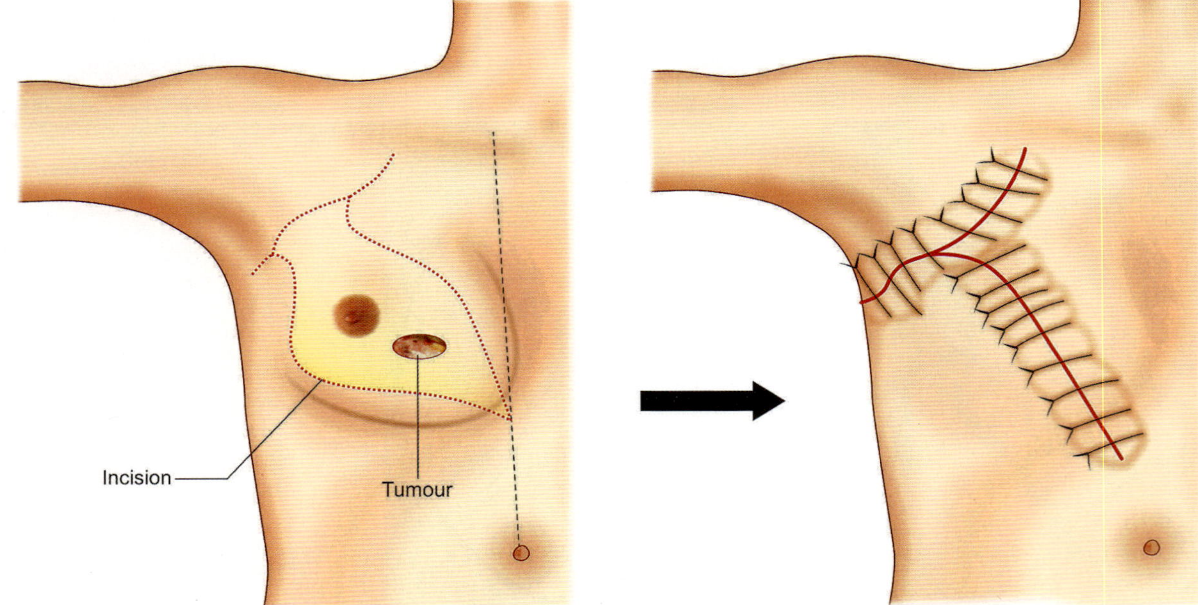

Fig. 16-31: Greenough incision.

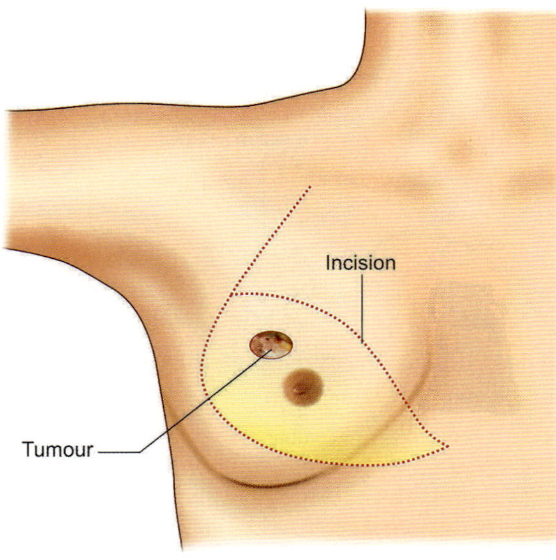

Fig. 16-32: Kocher's incision for mastectomy.

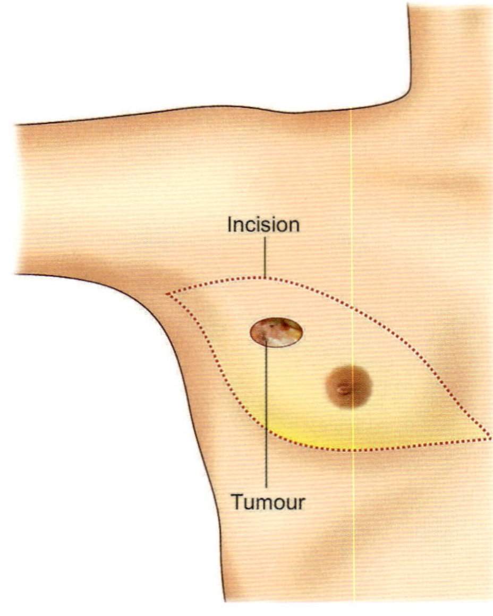

Fig. 16-33: Orr incision for mastectomy.

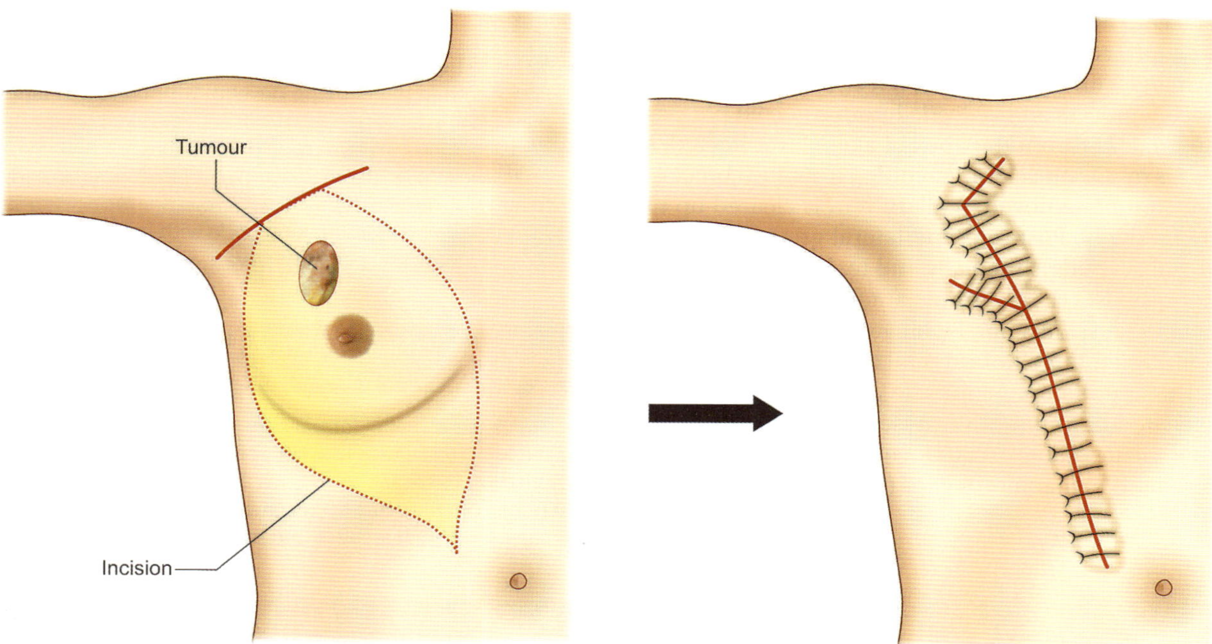

Fig. 16-34: Rodman incision for mastectomy with two branches in the final wound.

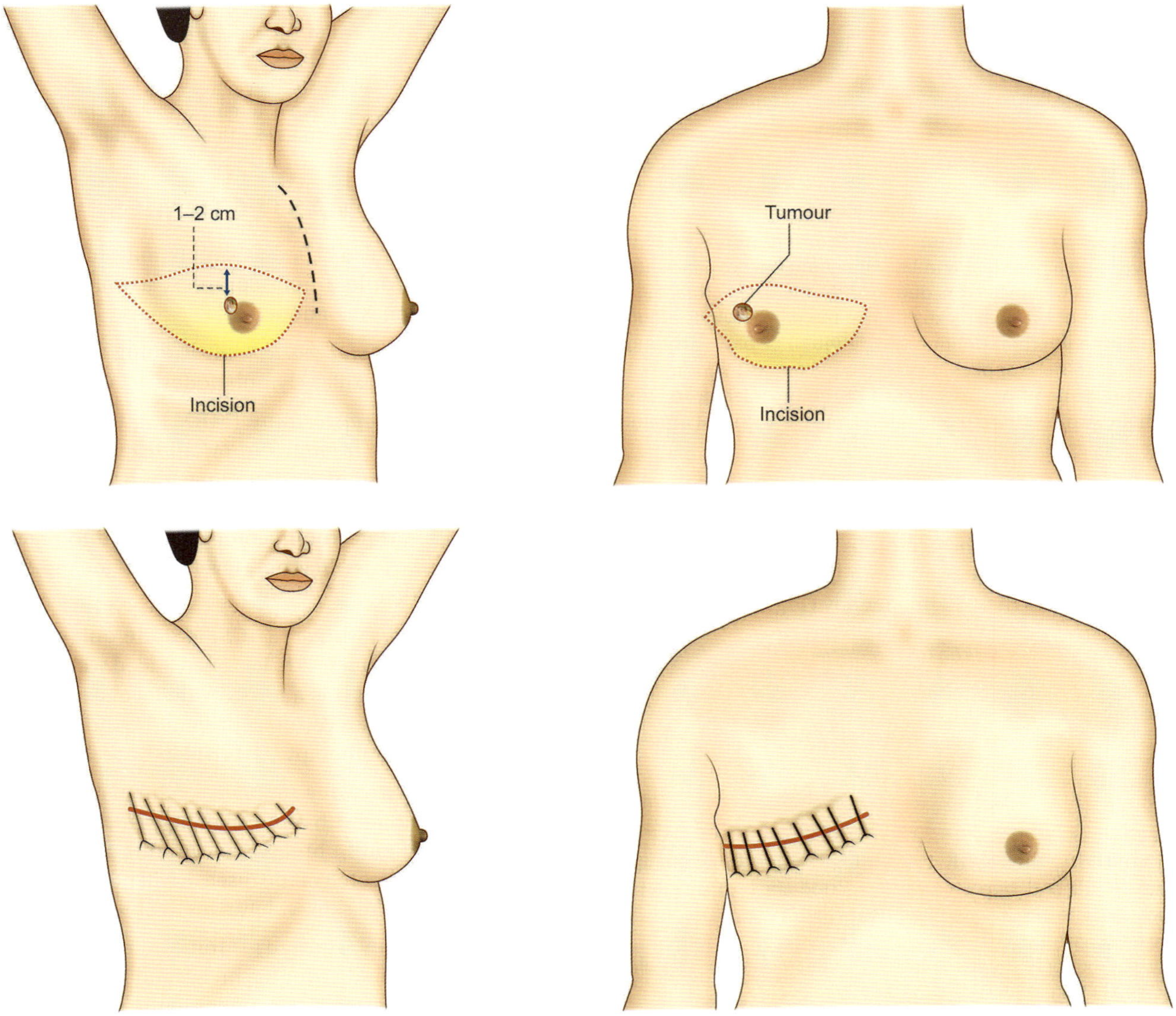

1–2 cm
Incision
Tumour
Incision

Fig. 16-35: Classical Stewart incision for mastectomy.

(it arises from lateral cord and is located medially supplies the medial part of pectoralis major). Attachment of pectoralis minor tendon is felt with index finger and with finger dissection it is hooked round the finger close to coracoid process and is divided from coracoid process to clear level II nodes. Later from the apex of axilla level III nodes are cleared. Pectoralis minor muscle, after cutting from the coracoid process may or may not be removed. Axillary vein is cleared up to subclavius muscle medially. Posterior and lateral group of lymph nodes are cleared. Subscapularis medially and teres major laterally are exposed posteriorly. Nerve to serratus anterior (long thoracic nerve of Bell), nerve to latissimus dorsi with vessels (thoracodorsal neurovascular bundle), intercostobrachial nerve, axillary vein, cephalic vein and pectoralis major muscle are preserved. Long thoracic nerve is located in front of the subscapularis medially on the chest wall within the investing fascia. Once specimen is removed it is marked with orientation markers or clips **(Figs. 16-36 to 16-38)**.

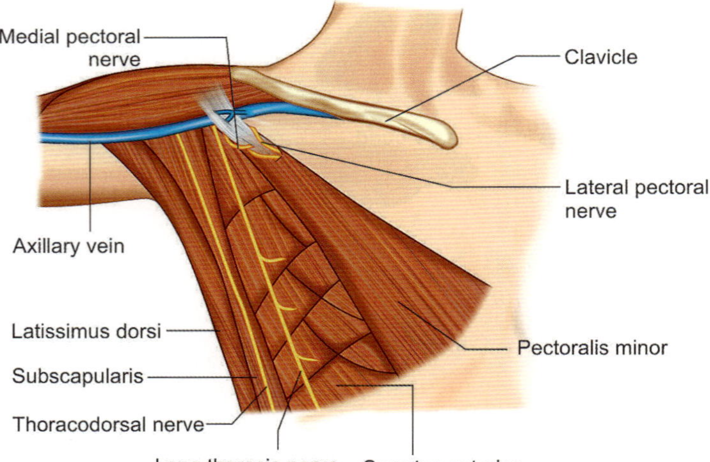

Fig. 16-36: Nerve to serratus anterior (long thoracic nerve of Bell), thoracodorsal nerve, medial pectoral and lateral pectoral nerves and intercostobrachial nerves usually come across during MRM. Medial pectoral nerve arising from medial cord of brachial plexus (hence the name) winds around the lateral margin of the pectoralis minor muscle (40%) or passes through its lateral part of fibres (60%), supplies part of the pectoralis major muscle. Lateral pectoral nerve arising from lateral cord of the brachial plexus runs close to the medial margin of pectoralis minor muscle to supply mainly pectoralis major muscle as its dominant nerve.

Wound is washed with saline. Haemostasis is maintained. *Two silastic suction drains* are placed, one laterally adjacent to latissimus dorsi muscle; another in front of the pectoralis major muscle. Wound is closed with a suction drain. Suction drain is kept for 5–7 days or until drainage becomes less than 30 mL per day **(Fig. 16-39)**.

Complications of MRM/mastectomy

- Injury/thrombosis of axillary vein.
- *Seroma* (50%): It should be aspirated repeatedly supported with compression dressing.
- Shoulder dysfunction (10%).
- Pain (30%) and numbness (70%).
- *Flap necrosis*/infection.
- Haematoma formation: If large needs drainage under general anaesthesia.
- Lymphoedema (15%) and its problems: Dissection above the axillary vein level increases the incidence of lymphoedema.
- Axillary hyperesthesia (0.5–1%).
- *Winged scapula:* Prominent medial border and inferior angle of scapula during punching action.

Contd...

Contd...

- *Stewart–Treves syndrome* is development of lymphangiosarcoma of upper limb in patient who develop lymphoedema (after 5 years) after mastectomy.
- *Weakened shoulder adduction* due to injury to thoracodorsal nerve.
- Anaesthesia over the medial aspect of the upper arm (dysesthesia) due to injury to intercostobrachial nerve.
- Atrophy of pectoralis major muscle with loss of chest wall contour due to injury to medial pectoral nerve.

Mastectomy specimen should be carefully inspected and sent to pathology department

- Specimen is sent in formalin for histology.
- It is sent in saline in low temperature for ER/PR/Her 2 neu status study (histochemistry).
- Tumor grading, tumor clearance, nodal involvement—its number and capsular breach are assessed histopathologically.

Points to be remembered

- Subcutaneous fat is included while elevating the flap of the breast skin; but it should be removed in axillary flaps.
- Dissection in the axilla should be kept below the level of axillary vein.
- All nerves in the axilla which will come across should be preserved as much as possible.
- Subscapular/thoracodorsal vessels should be retained if latissimus dorsi flap is planned.
- Proper haemostasis is essential.
- Double tube silastic drain is a must. Drain is removed when only the discharge drained becomes less than 30 mL/day for 2 days.

DIFFERENT MASTECTOMIES

Total mastectomy also called as simple mastectomy—here tumour, entire breast, nipple areola complex, axillary tail are removed. Axillary dissection is not done.

Extended total (simple) mastectomy is doing total mastectomy with clearance of level I axillary lymph nodes.

Modified radical mastectomy (MRM) is total mastectomy with axillary clearance. In *Patey's MRM* all levels of axillary nodes are cleared with division of tendon of pectoralis minor muscle close to coracoid process with or without removal of the pectoralis muscle. In *Scanlon's MRM* pectoralis minor is incised to reach the level III nodes. In *Auchincloss MRM* only level I and II are removed, pectoralis minor is left intact.

Breast conservative surgery (BCS) is done only when indications mentioned earlier is met with. It is often added with axillary dissection. Radiotherapy to breast is a must. Wide local excision is the commonly done procedure. Veronesi designed quadrantectomy, axillary dissection and radiotherapy (QUART) in BCS.

Skin sparing mastectomy (SSM) is keyhole surgery in which total mastectomy is done with removal of nipple areolar complex, earlier biopsy scar and entire breast and tumour. Skin over the breast is retained as the outcome of the disease will not be altered by removal or not removal of the skin widely over the breast.

Radical mastectomy (Halsted) is removal of tumour, entire breast, nipple, areola, and skin over the breast and tumour, pectoralis major and minor muscles, fat, fascia, nodes in the axilla. Axillary vein, long thoracic nerve and cephalic vein are retained **(Fig. 16-40)**.

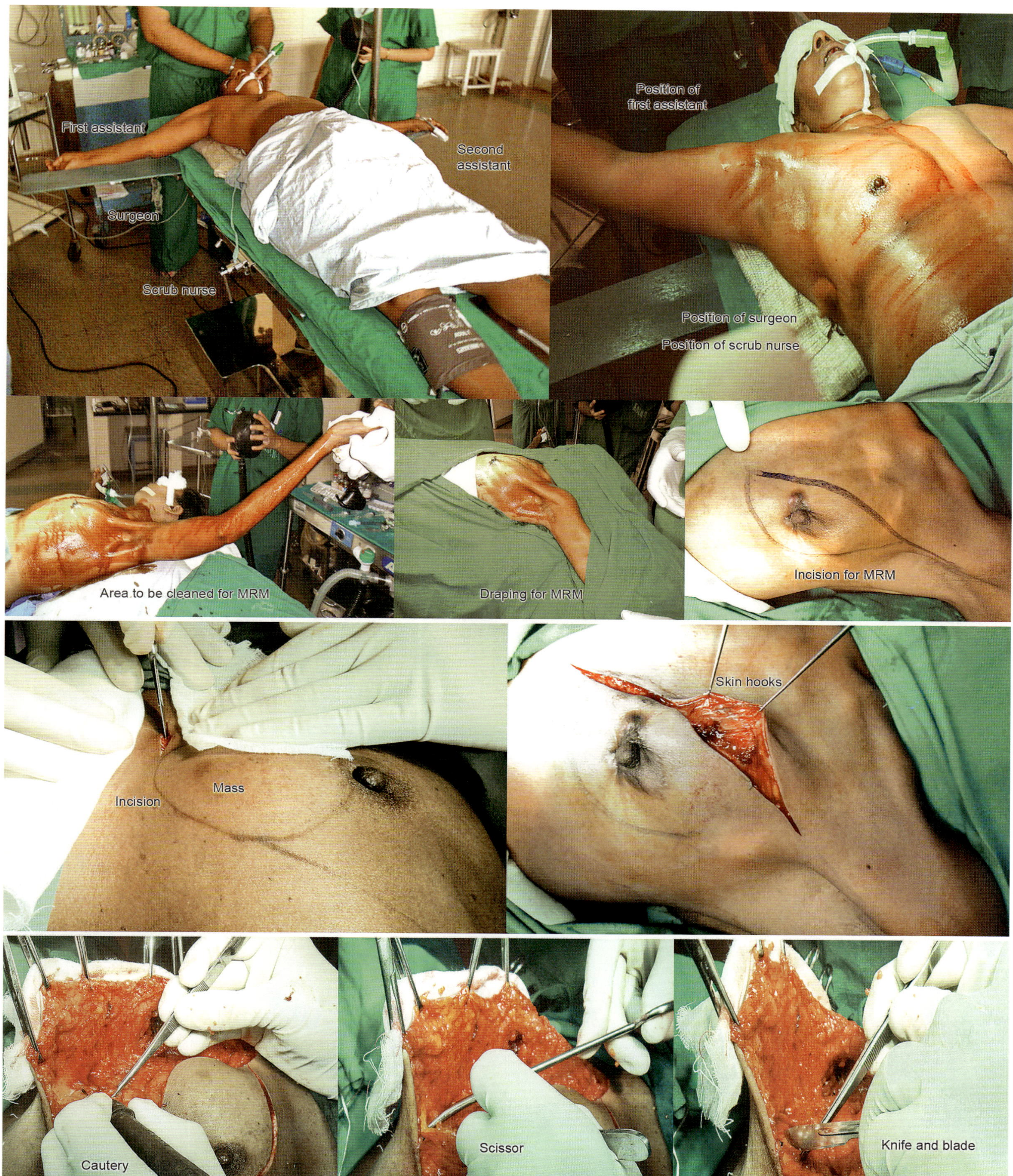
First assistant
Second assistant
Surgeon
Scrub nurse
Position of first assistant
Position of surgeon
Position of scrub nurse
Area to be cleaned for MRM
Draping for MRM
Incision for MRM
Incision
Mass
Skin hooks
Cautery
Scissor
Knife and blade

Figs. 16-37(1)

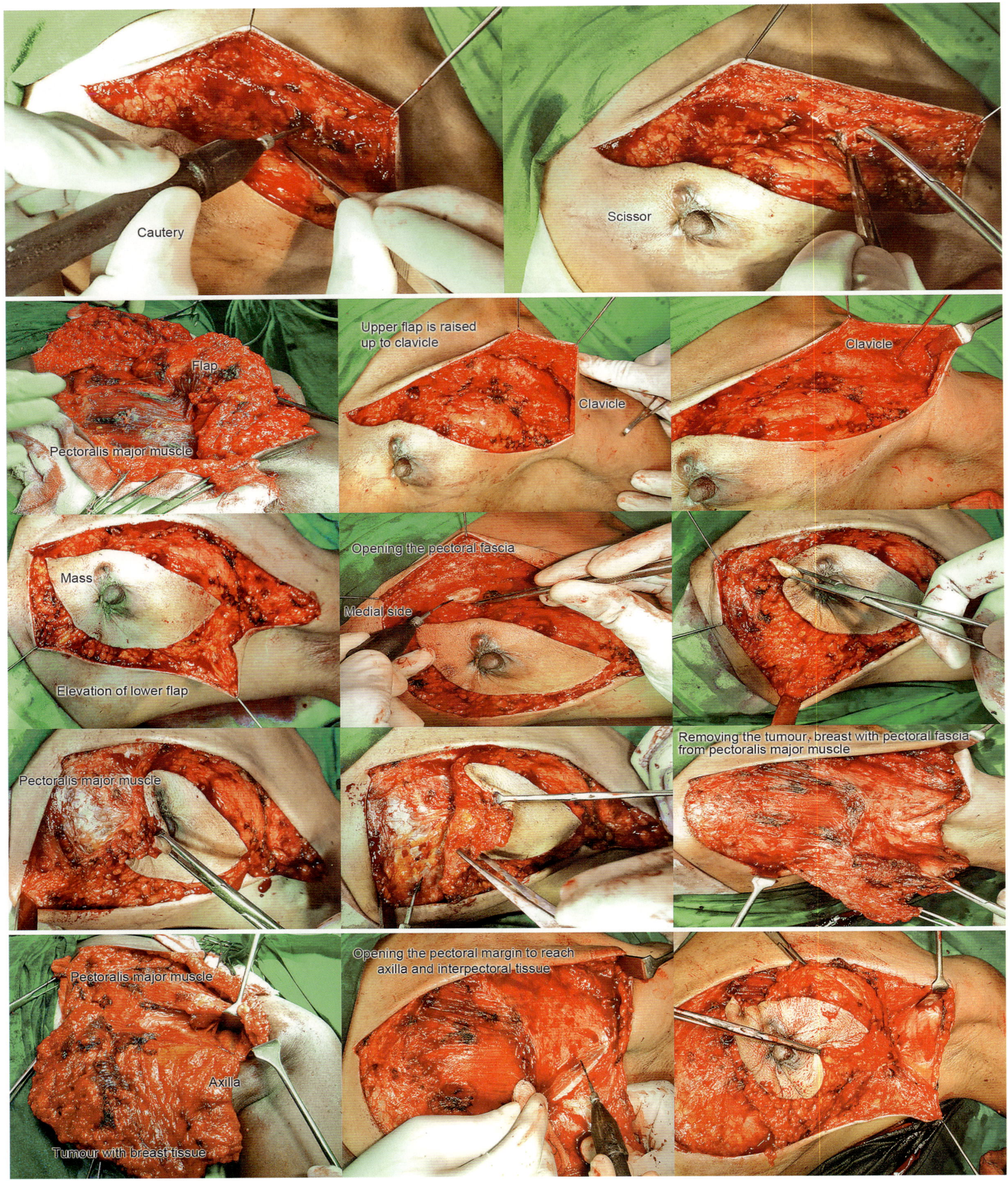
Cautery
Scissor
Flap
Pectoralis major muscle
Upper flap is raised up to clavicle
Clavicle
Clavicle
Mass
Elevation of lower flap
Opening the pectoral fascia
Medial side
Pectoralis major muscle
Removing the tumour, breast with pectoral fascia from pectoralis major muscle
Pectoralis major muscle
Axilla
Tumour with breast tissue
Opening the pectoral margin to reach axilla and interpectoral tissue

Figs. 16-37(2)

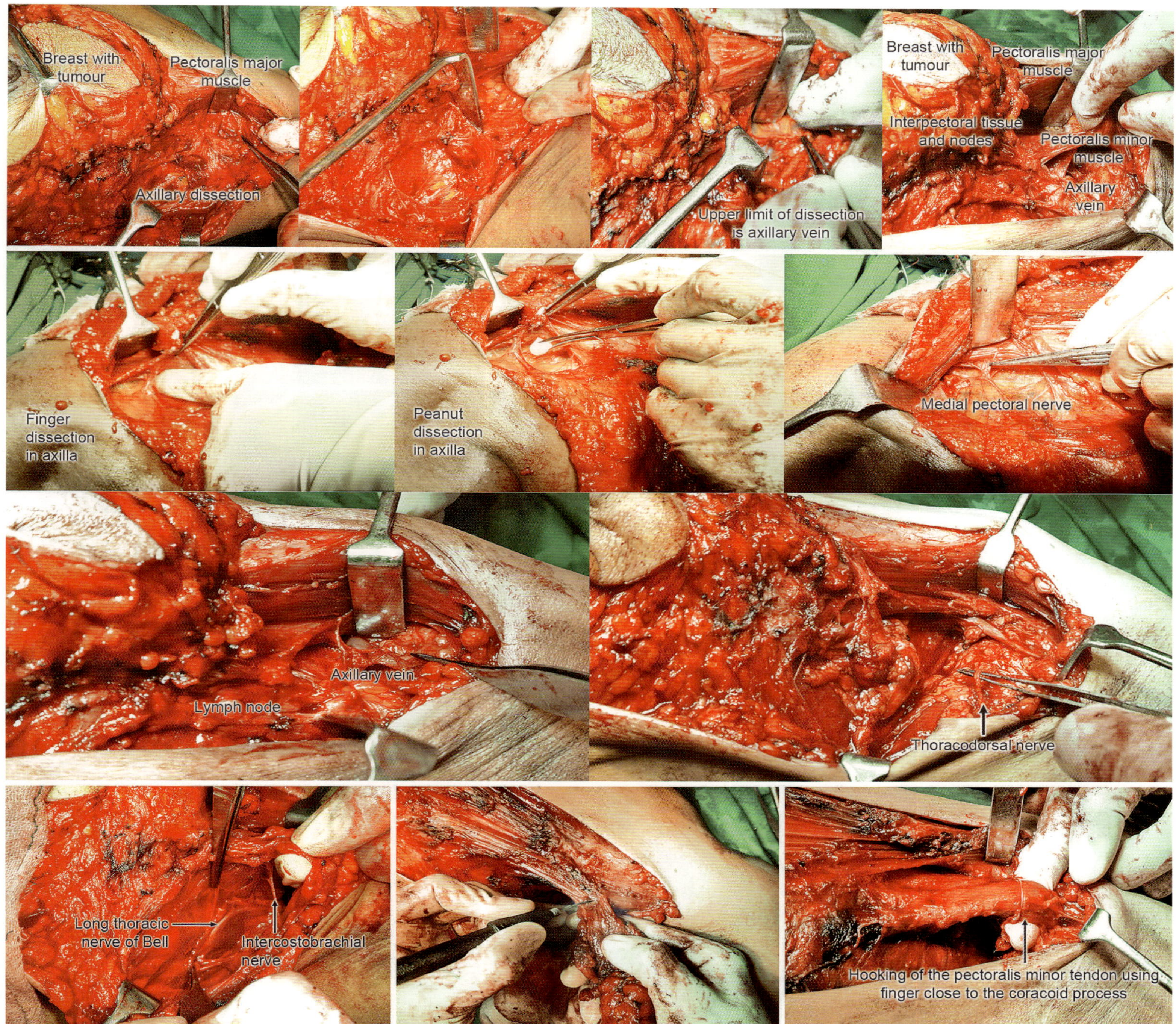

Figs. 16-37(3)

Figs. 16-37(1 to 3): *Technique of modified radical mastectomy (MRM).* Skin over the breast, whole of ipsilateral chest wall, axilla, shoulder, supraclavicular region with neck, part of abdomen and part of opposite chest wall are prepared with antiseptic solution. Slight head up (Fowler's) position with same side tilting of the table upwards often with a sandbag under the shoulder region is used. Hand and forearm is often covered with a sterile towel so that to achieve a free movement of the arm and shoulder during axillary dissection. Incision placed depends on the need, either transverse or oblique which will be 5 cm beyond the tumour margin as an elliptical type. Upper flap is elevated first usually up to the level of clavicle above; up to sternum medially. Lower flap is elevated up to rectus sheath and costal margin below. Lateral flap is elevated up to the margin of latissimus dorsi muscle. Flaps are elevated using either cautery or scissor or scalpel or often with gauze dissection. In axillary region, subcutaneous tissue and fat is also cleared. Fascia on the lateral margin of pectoralis major is incised to expose the pectoralis minor. Deeper part of the pectoralis minor is dissected to expose the axillary vein beyond the subscapular vessels. Clavipectoral fascia is incised to clear the nodes, taking care not to injure the medial pectoral nerve which passes through the pectoralis minor (60%) or its lateral margin (40%) to supply pectoralis major muscle. Main supply of pectoralis major is lateral pectoral nerve which passes medial to the pectoralis minor close to acromiothoracic artery. Pectoralis minor is retracted to clear the apical nodes. Often pectoralis minor tendon is detached from its insertion to coracoid process (Patey's). The fascia over serratus anterior is cleared without injuring long thoracic nerve. Intercostobrachial nerve, if possible, is saved. Posteriorly dissection is continued over subscapular muscle preserving the subscapular vessels and thoracodorsal nerve. At the end specimen is freed from latissimus dorsi.

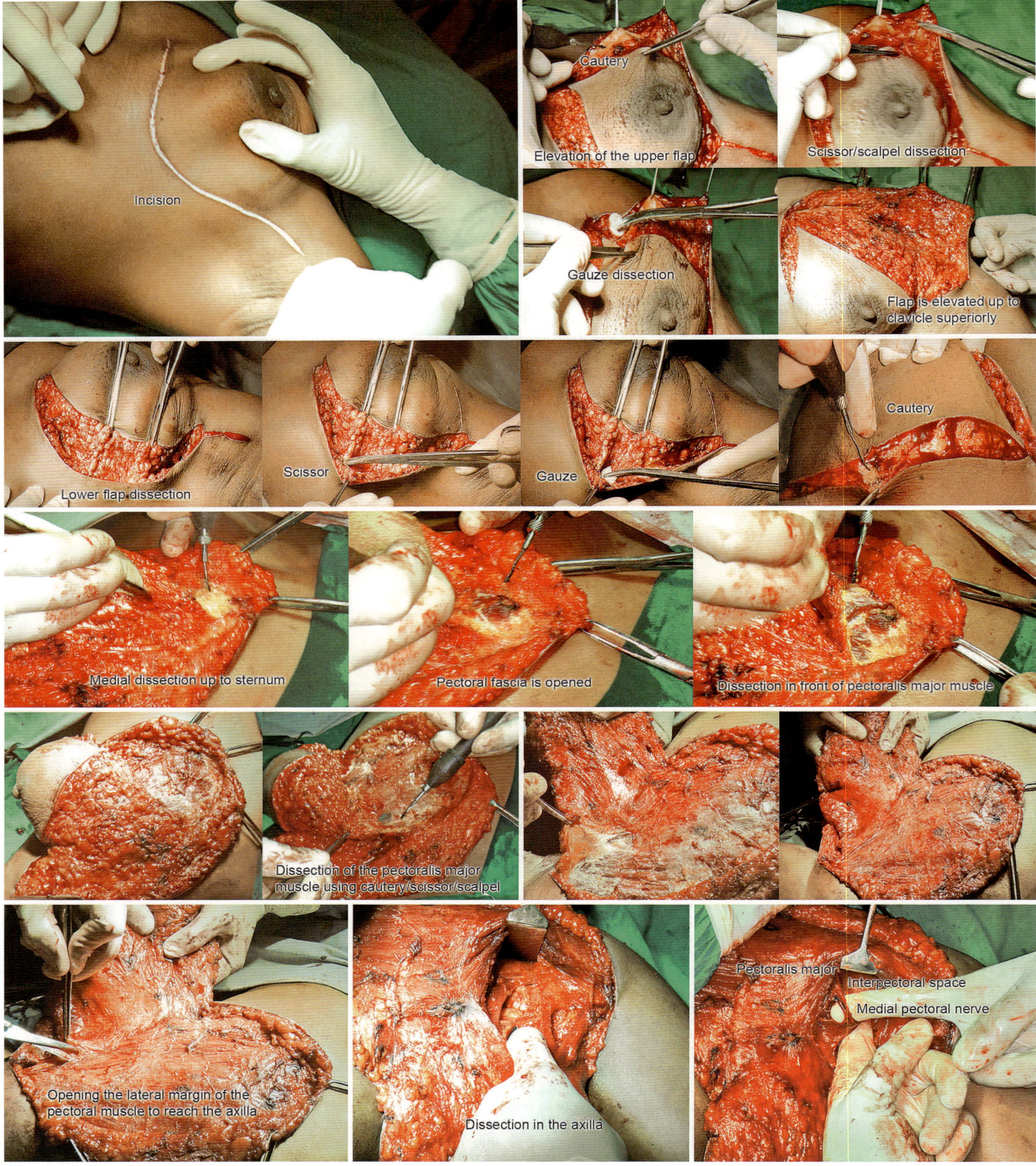
Incision
Cautery
Elevation of the upper flap
Scissor/scalpel dissection
Gauze dissection
Flap is elevated up to clavicle superiorly
Lower flap dissection
Scissor
Gauze
Cautery
Medial dissection up to sternum
Pectoral fascia is opened
Dissection in front of pectoralis major muscle
Dissection of the pectoralis major muscle using cautery/scissor/scalpel
Opening the lateral margin of the pectoral muscle to reach the axilla
Dissection in the axilla
Pectoralis major
Interpectoral space
Medial pectoral nerve

Figs. 16-38(1)

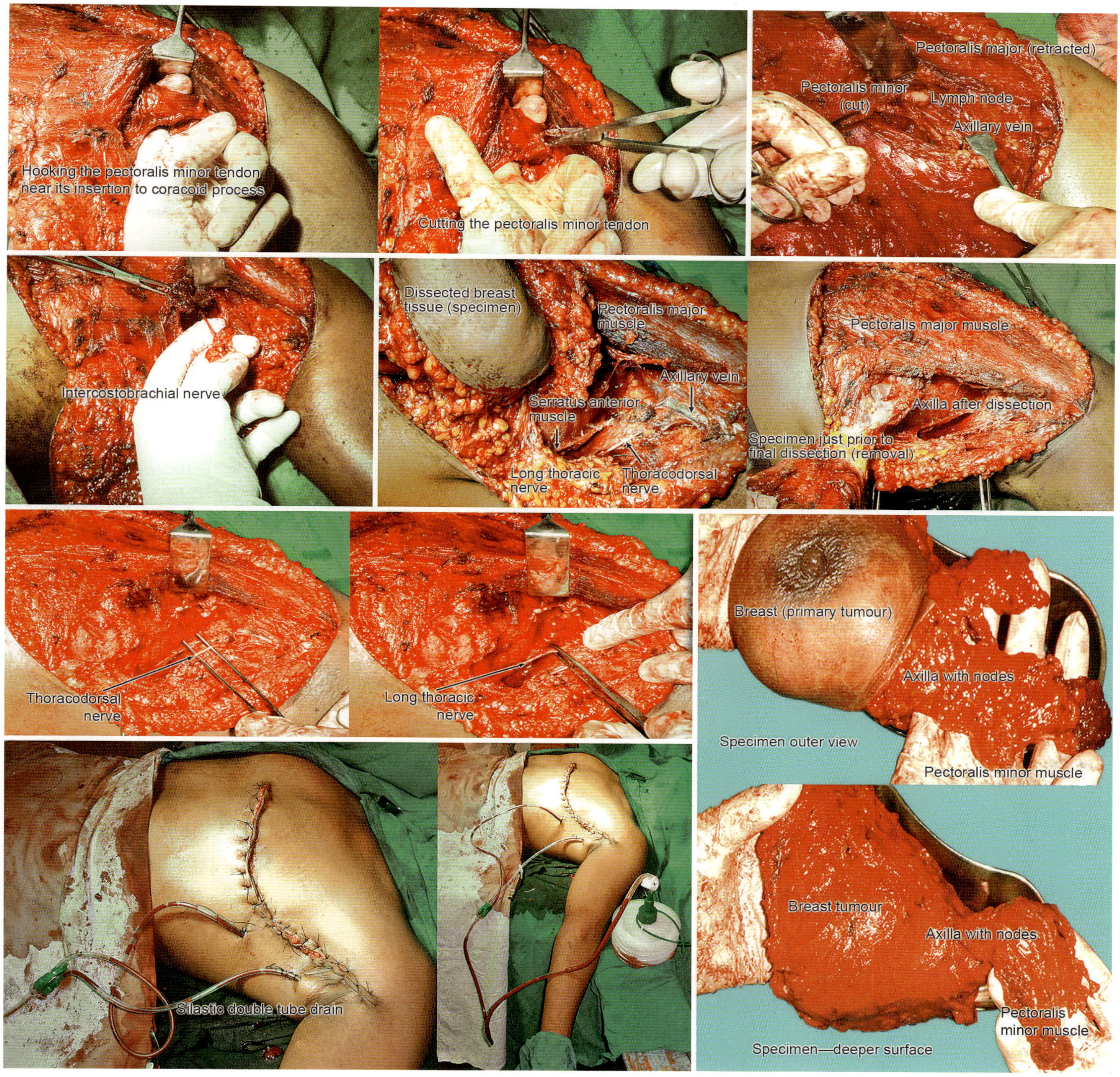

Figs. 16-38(2)

Figs. 16-38(1 and 2): *Patey's modified radical mastectomy*. Here pectoralis minor tendon is detached from coracoid process. It achieves better approach and clearance of apical nodes.

Toilet mastectomy is done in locally advanced tumour with removal of tumour and possible breast tissue to prevent fungation.

Extended radical mastectomy is doing radical mastectomy with removal of internal mammary nodes of same side or opposite side. It is not practiced.

Nipple sparing mastectomy is done with preservation of nipple and areola.

Areola sparing mastectomy is done preserving areola with resection of the nipple.

RECONSTRUCTION OF THE BREAST

Breast reconstruction is done either as *immediate or delayed procedure*. Immediate reconstruction is done in early breast cancer or after prophylactic mastectomy. Reconstruction is delayed for 6 months in advanced cases.

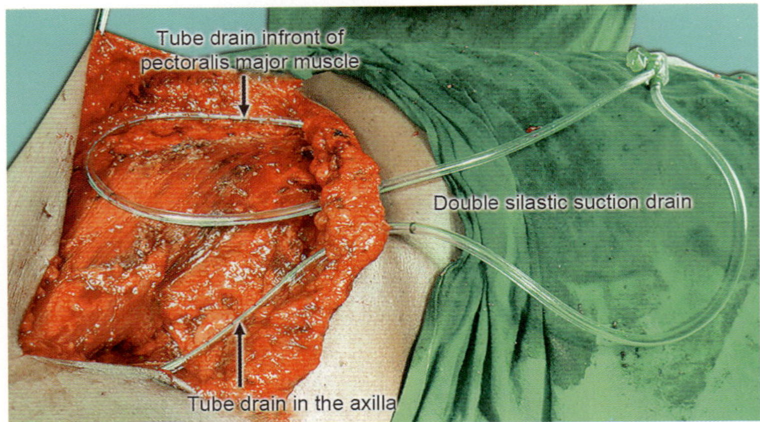

Fig. 16-39: Double tube silastic drain is kept. One tube is in front of the pectoralis major muscle; other in the axilla. Bulky dressings with elastic bandage support are usually used. Drain is removed once drainage is less than 30 mL per day for two consecutive days.

Skin is closed primarily as wound closure. If skin is removed widely and apposition is not possible then *skin graft* is ideal as it will tolerate radiotherapy very well **(Fig. 16-41)**.

Implant is placed under the pectoralis major, serratus anterior, external oblique and rectus abdominis myofascial plane **(Fig. 16-42)**.

Myocutaneous flap with or without breast implant in submuscular plane is good reconstructive approach. Latissimus dorsi myocutaneous flap (LD FLAP) or transverse abdominis myocutaneous flaps (TRAM flap) are used with or without implants. Latissimus dorsi (LD) flap usually needs implant. TRAM flap dose not require implant usually.

Silicone gel implant under pectoralis major muscle or expandable saline prosthesis may be used. Placement of implants is technically easier. One should take care to achieve symmetry. *Complications* of implants are pain, rupture, displacement, infection and capsular contracture.

Breast implant has got outer cover called as implant shell which is usually made up of silicone. Implant is filled with saline or silicone gel. There is slight increase in the chances of formation of anaplastic large cell lymphoma after silicone implant. Often initial tissue expander is used to create space for implant (saline expander). It has got a valve through which saline is infused gradually at regular intervals over the period of 2–6 months to create adequate space. Later tissue expander is replaced by silicone implant. Two types of silicone implants are available—saline filed or silicone gel filled; outer part of the implant

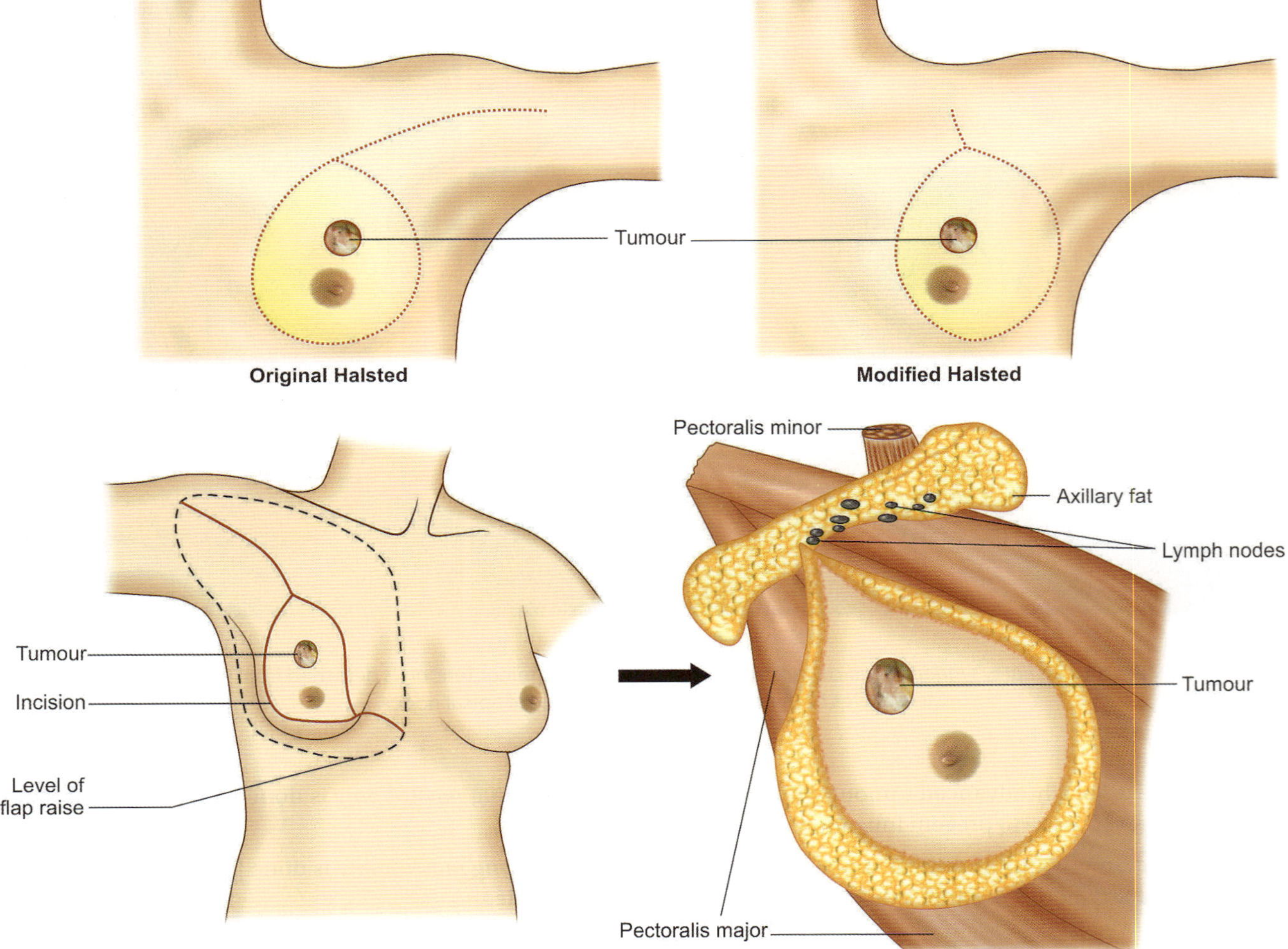

Fig. 16-40: *Halsted radical mastectomy*. It is not used now. Here entire breast with tumour, skin over the breast both pectoralis major and minor muscles, axillary fat, lymph nodes and fascia are removed. Axillary vein, nerve to serratus anterior (Bell's) and cephalic vein are retained.

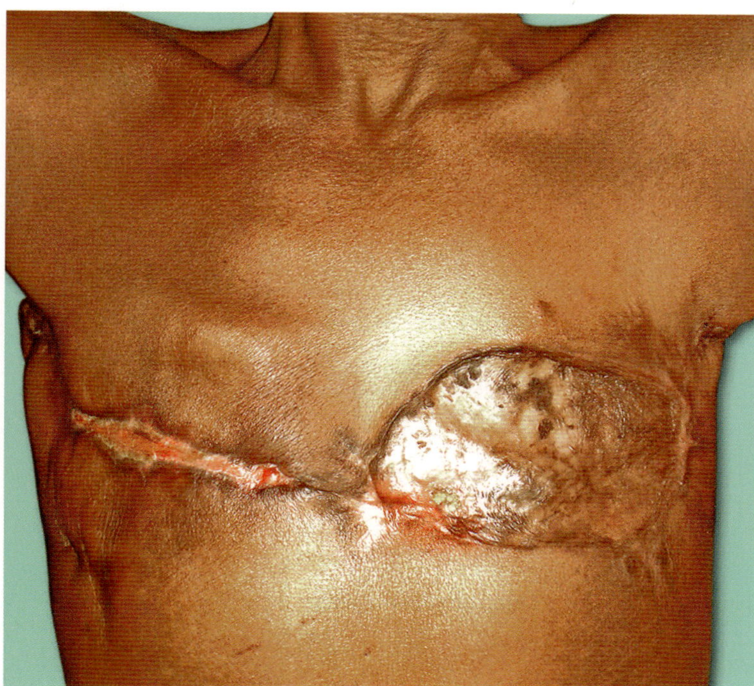

Fig. 16-41: Split skin graft is done after mastectomy on one side. Other side primary closure was done. It was a bilateral carcinoma of breast.

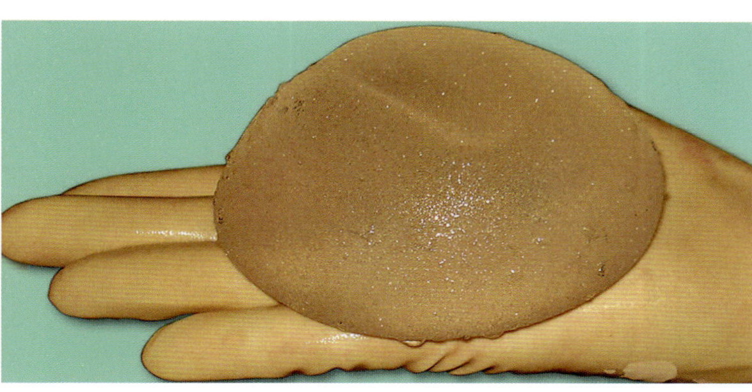

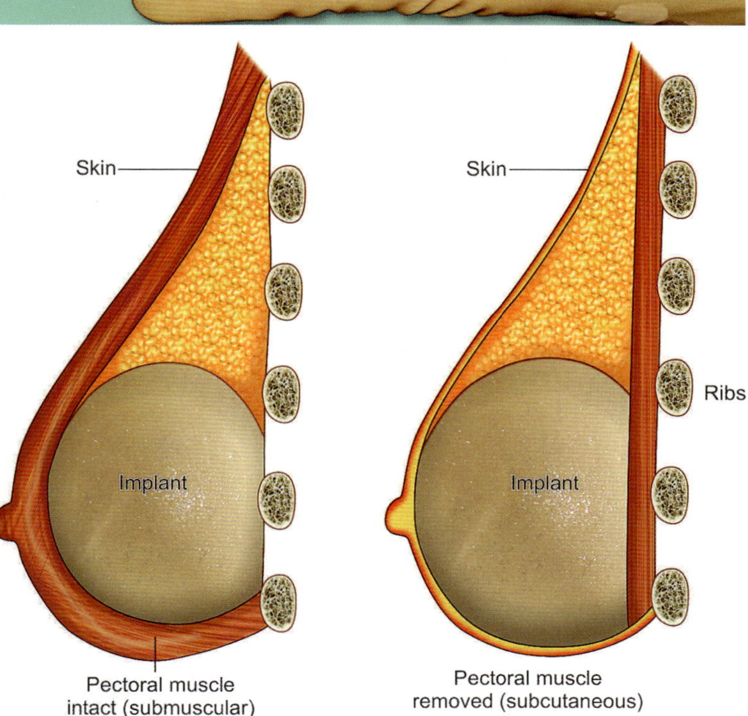

Fig. 16-42: Breast implant used for reconstruction. It is placed either subcutaneous or submuscular plane.

is called as implant shell and is always made up of silicone. Silicone gel filled implant more feels like a natural breast with less uneven surface compared to saline filled. Rupture of the filled material needs replacement of the implant; however, saline filled implant after rupture collapses completely whereas silicone gel filled implant after rupture will not collapse completely. Durability of the implant is around 10 years and may require replacement after that whether it is saline or silicone gel filled. Acellular dermal matrix (hammock) derived from human skin (skin with removed cells) is used to expand the tissue plane initially. Later it is replaced by implant.

TRAM flap can be standard lower TRAM or upper TRAM. Vertical RAM flap is also used as variation. Contralateral submammary flap is also used.

Factors deciding the reconstruction are—amount of skin retained; stage of carcinoma; need of radiotherapy or earlier radiotherapy; need for implant.

Standard lower abdominal TRAM flap is placed horizontally with upper incision at the level of umbilicus; lower incision below suprapubic region with an ellipse. Even though theoretically opposite TRAM flap is better, it is technically not practicable and so ipsilateral TRAM is commonly used. Bilateral TRAM flaps are used to reconstruct both breast areas. Upper incision is deepened through subcutaneous and superficial fascia. Flap is raised often in front of the anterior rectus sheath up to the costal margin and xiphisternum. Anterior rectus sheath protects the muscle. Many advocate the cutting of the anterior rectus sheath and flap is raised in front of the muscle carefully. Small branches of intercostal vessels are ligated. Lower flap is deepened through the rectus muscle which is cut just below the semicircular line. Inferior epigastric vessels are identified which are securely ligated. Muscle with skin is raised from deeper plane above towards xiphisternum as myocutaneous flap. Tunnel for the passage of mobilised flap is done along the midline above. Muscle need not be cut above but can be done so if needed. Skin part of the flap on same side moves towards the axilla and skin part of the flap on opposite side moves towards lower medial part of the defect. Defect is sutured to flap. Suction drains are placed under the flap. Abdominal defect is closed meticulously in layers often placing a synthetic mesh underneath **(Figs. 16-43 and 16-44)**.

Vertical RAM/upper TRAM/contralateral submammary flap are variations of the same, depending on the need. Free TRAM flap can be used to revascularise through internal mammary artery. *Deep inferior epigastric perforator flap (DIEP)* is used as a free flap in breast reconstruction. Revascularisation is done using internal mammary or thoracodorsal vessels **(Figs. 16-45 and 16-46)**.

Other natural tissue reconstruction methods are: Superficial inferior epigastric artery flap reconstruction (SIEA flap), deep inferior epigastric artery (DIEA) flap, superior gluteal artery perforator (cutaneous) flap (S-GAP) and inferior gluteal artery perforator (cutaneous) flap (I-GAP), transverse upper gracilis (myocutaneous) flap (TUG) reconstruction. These flaps need microvascular procedure.

Latissimus dorsi muscle/myocutaneous flap: It is based on thoracodorsal artery, a branch of subscapular artery. Skin over the upper and anterior border of the muscle is used for transfer. It is commonly used to cover the defect after mastectomy. But it does not give the bulk. It is technically easier. It can be used as muscle flap also. It helps as skin cover. Prosthesis (submuscular silicone) is needed to place underneath to provide bulk in postmastectomy defect.

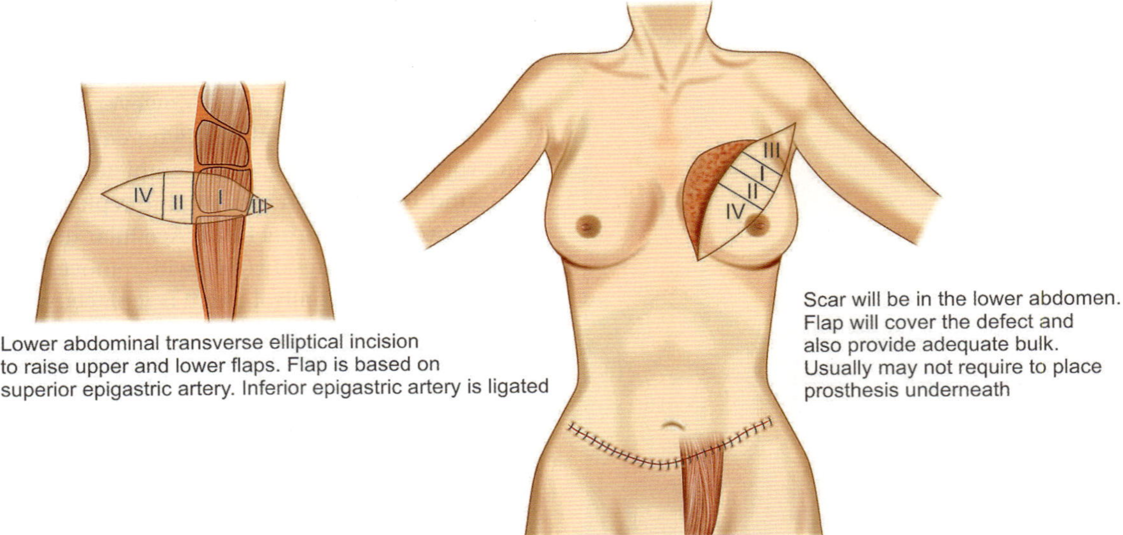

Fig. 16-43: Standard TRAM flap is used from ipsilateral side. It is infraumbilical and is based on superior epigastric artery.

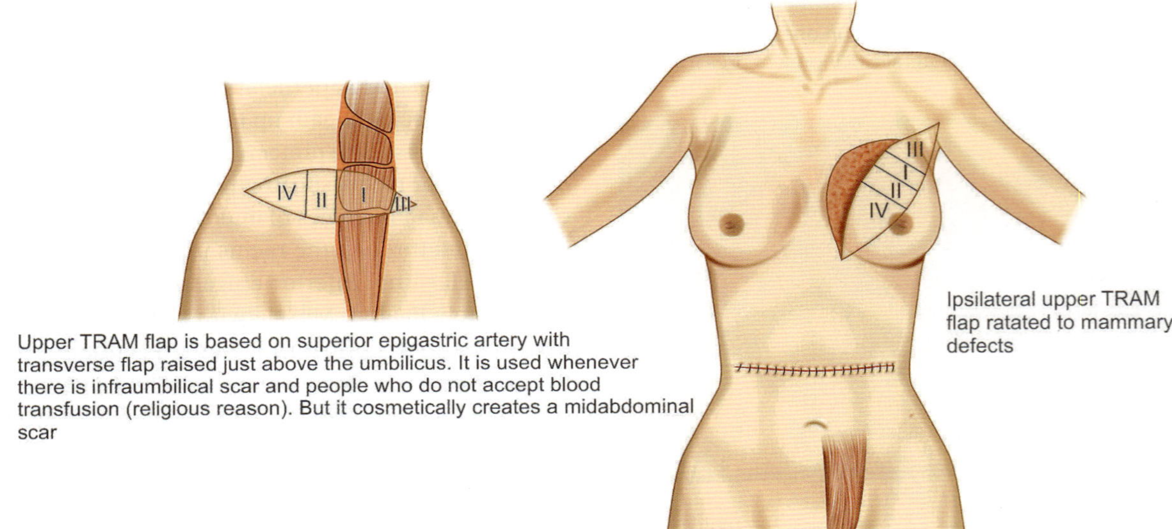

Fig. 16-44: Upper TRAM flap is often used with flap incision in upper abdomen—horizontal.

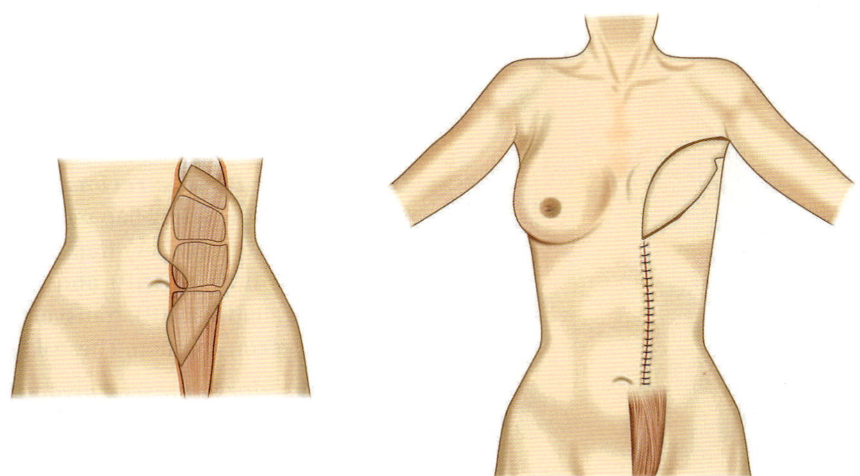

Fig. 16-45: Vertical rectus abdominis myocutaneous flap.

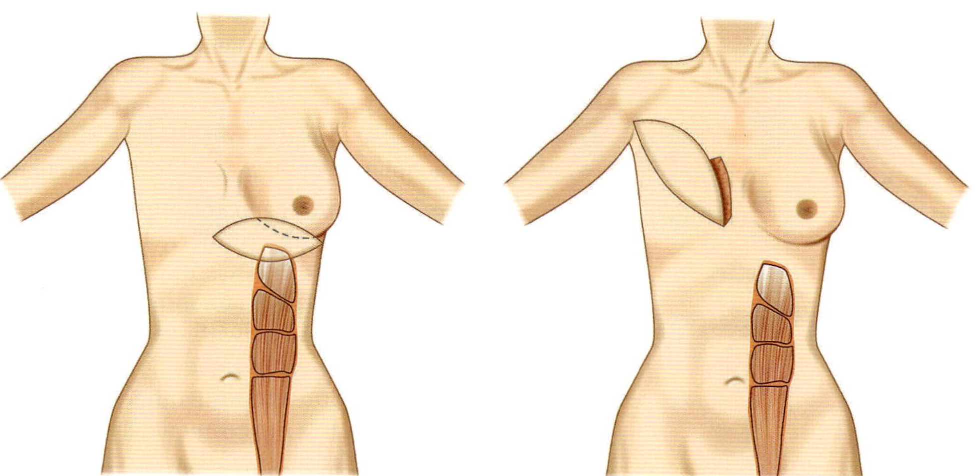

It is cosmetically acceptable contralateral flap with superior epigastric artery as base taking upper most part of rectus abdominis muscle with sufficient skin. Arc of rotation towards opposite side is short and so often needs removal of one or two costal cartilages. It needs implant for size. It provides inframammary scar; useful in young/small breasts

Fig. 16-46: Submammary TRAM flap is used from opposite side with least scar.

Muscle arises from iliac crest upwards to midthoracic spine. Muscle is like a fan below forming tendinous fibres above to insert into humeral shaft. Subscapular artery a largest branch is derived from 3 part of axillary artery runs along posterior wall of the axilla giving circumflex scapular vessels at 4 cm distance and later continues as thoracodorsal artery for about 6 cm, enters the muscle giving many branches. Flap is usually taken as myocutaneous flap with elliptical skin on the surface. Skin part is either horizontal ellipse when taken from upper margin of the muscle or vertical when taken from the anterior margin of the muscle. Point of origin of the subscapular artery is the pivot point of the flap. Artery is accompanied by the vein. While raising the flap after islanding it with skin, only pedicle can be retained cutting muscle above to attain extra length (but commonly anterior attachment is retained) and flap is rotated to the needed area. Donor area can be sutured primarily or covered with a split skin graft. *Often* in LD flap nerve is not retained (if retained it causes *unpleasant muscle contractions* and so it will not maintain the bulk but gives good coverage of the defect). Flap harvesting is done in lateral position. Subscapular vessels maintain the adequate length and caliber and so it is often used as *free flap* based on subscapular vessels **(Fig. 16-47)**.

LD flap	*TRAM flap*
◈ Myocutaneous flap based on subscapular artery. ◈ Easy to perform. ◈ Reliable flap, well vascularised. ◈ Can be placed over prosthesis. ◈ Low complication rate, but causes unsightly donor area on the back.	◈ Transverse rectus abdominis myocutaneous flap based on superior epigastric artery. Ipsilateral or contralateral TRAM flap is used. ◈ It gives the bulk needed for reconstruction and so implant is not needed. ◈ Donor site morbidity and fat necrosis can occur. ◈ Free TRAM flap into internal mammary/ thoracodorsal axis can be done. ◈ Limitations to position, shape and rotate; needs mesh placement in the abdomen wound to prevent the formation of incisional hernia.

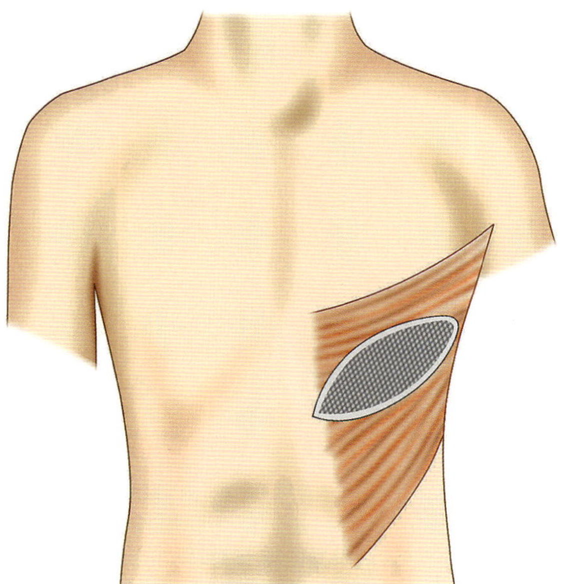

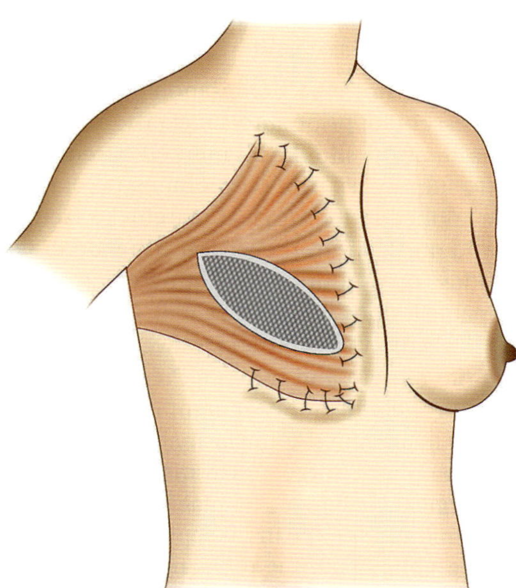

Figs. 16-47(1)

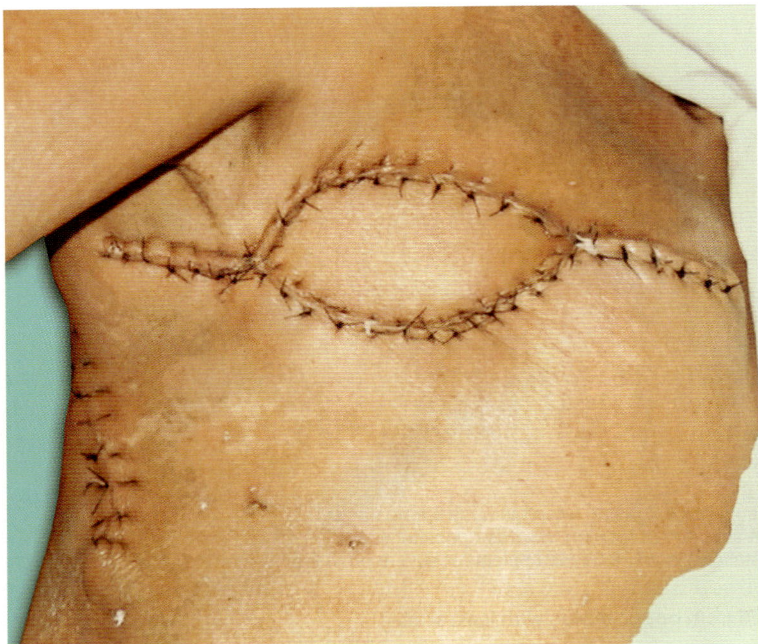

Figs. 16-47(2)

Figs. 16-47(1 and 2): Latissimus dorsi myocutaneous flap.

Nipple is created using—local breast flaps, 3 months after breast reconstruction; nipple sharing from contralateral nipple using composite graft; *skate flap*: local flap with de-epithelialised donor site around the periphery over which a full thickness graft is applied; nipple prosthesis.

Areola pigmentation is created using (*it is done 3 weeks after nipple creation*)—full thickness skin graft from non-hairy skin lateral to *labia majora,* as the pigmentation of this graft matches that of the areola; from contralateral areola if reduction mammoplasty is done on that side; *tattooing*—colour tends to fade with time and may need to be repeated; split skin graft from retroauricular area or from thigh.

Oncoplasty in Breast Conservation

Oncoplasty is multidisciplinay approach with involving breast surgeon, radiologist, pathologist, radiotherapist, oncologist, psychologist, etc. It is the breast conservation with adequate optimum cure with best cosmesis target.

Principles in oncoplastic surgery: Mobilisation and redistribution of the breast tissue essential; prior surgical excision if needed for diagnostic purpose incision should be marked carefully so that eventual oncoplatic surgery will not be problematic. Radiopaque markers should be applied to the surgical margins to facilitate the radiotherapy area identification, reexcision if needed, eventual mammographic follow up. Multiple bracketing wires are used in indistinct or impalpable lesions at crania, caudal, medial and lateral margins and superficial area. Use of intraoperative ultrasound is very helpful to confirm the margin and tumour. Preoperative contrast enhanced breast MRI is helpful. Surgical drain is better considered in oncoplastic surgery to prevent seroma formation which may alter the outcome of the oncoplastic surgery in terms of cosmesis. Proper orientation of the surgical specimen (by placing in an orientation grid), pathologist opinion in the theatre, keeping preoperative and postoperative photographs, retaining the sensation of the NAC—are other important factors to be considered in breast oncoplasty. Selection of the patient is important depends on the tumour size, location, type and grade, breast size, volume. Advancement flap, clearance margin, maintaining the flap blood supply, preventing fat necrosis—are basic technical essentialities. Retained glandular tissue should be approximated meticulously to achieve proper cosmetic result. Both breasts should be marked always in all oncoplastic surgeries to achieve and plan for symmetrical outcome.

Radial ellipse segmentectomy: Here elliptical incision is made on the skin over the properly localised tumour; skin is undermined carefully using fine scissor and bipolar cautery; proper retractors are used; pectoral fascia underneath part is also incised to include in the specimen; tumour with clearance margin, with skin with pectoral fascia is removed together. Drain is placed; wound is closed in layers. This procedure is only in outer quadrants; upper inner quadrant this incision scar is not cosmetically acceptable **(Fig. 16-48)**.

Segmental resection using circumareolar approach: Circumareolar incision is made not more than half circle. Skin flap is raised; undermining is done both medially and laterally adequately to achieve required clearance margin. Tumour is excised with margin with pectoral fascia underneath; subcutaneous tissue is sutured; skin incision is also used as circumareolar fashion. If larger incision is required then donut—round block mastopexy technique is used **(Fig. 16-49)**.

Crescent mastopexy resection: It is done in central quadrant tumour in the superior part without involving MAC; ideally tumour between 10 and 1 o'clock position is removed by this technique. Curved C elliptical incision is made to involve the crescent shaped skin above the areola over the tumour; after elevating medial and lateral flaps tumour with pectoral fascia is removed; breast tissue, subcutaneous tissue and skin are closed after haemostasis and drain placement **(Fig. 16-50)**.

Batwing resection: Here upper central quadrant tumour is removed with clearance margin which is not involving the NAC; batwing shaped superior incision is made as shown in the diagram; flaps are raised; tumour with batwing skin is removed with pectoral fascia; skin is sutured with wings on both sides **(Fig. 16-51)**.

Hemibatwing resection: It is done similarly but smaller tumour at 9–10 o'clock position on the tight side or 2–3 o'clock position on the left side. Otherwise it is similar like batwing resection but one sided **(Fig. 16-52)**.

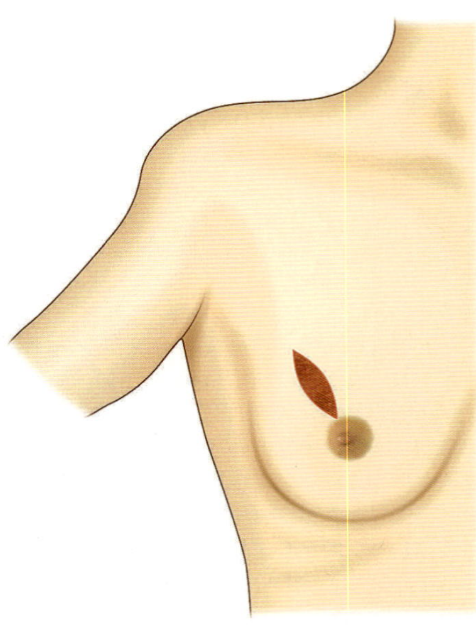

Fig. 16-48: Radial elliptical segmentectomy incision.

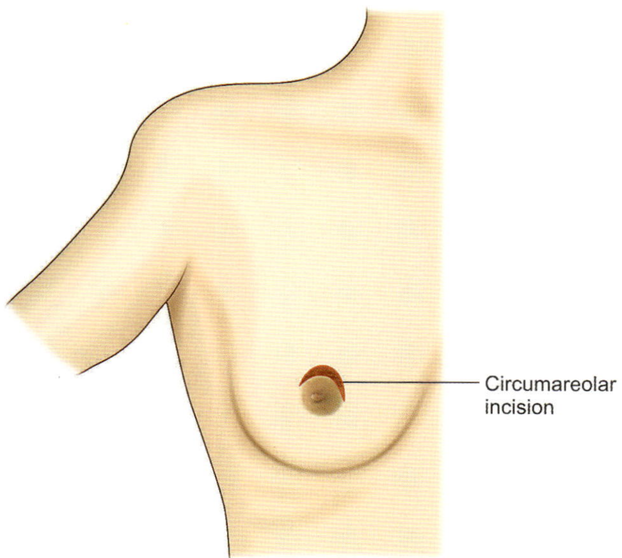

Fig. 16-49: Circumareolar approach for segmental resection; flap should be elevated both medially and laterally; tumour is resected with clearance margin; underneath pectoral fascia is removed; drain is placed after haemostasis. Wound is closed in layers.

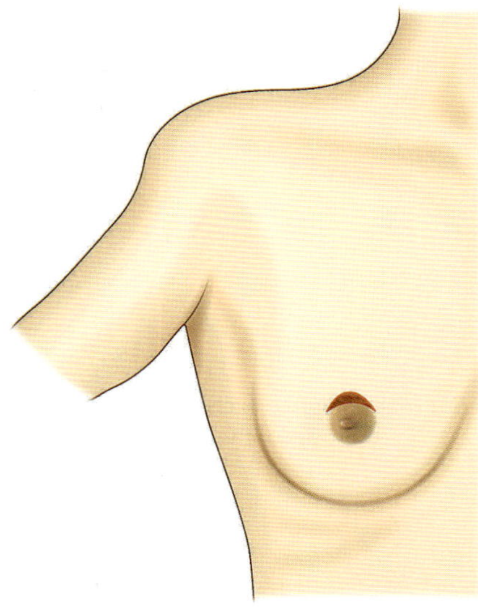

Fig. 16-50: Crescent incision for central tumour in superior area without involving the NAC.

Donut mastopexy resection (round block technique): It is used for any quadrant tumour wherein NAC is not involved. Two concentric circumareolar incisions are made; first incision is around the areola; second incision is parallel to first circumferentially with 1 cm radius. Intervening skin between two is removed. Tissue places are created by elevating flaps circumferentially without compromising the blood supply of the NAC which is derived from the glandular tissue. After wide excision of the tumour with pectoral fascia, glandular tissue is sutured precisely and NAC complex is sutured circumferentially to the skin of the breast after placing a drain **(Fig. 16-53)**.

Grisotti B flap mastopexy: B flap resection is done in central breast tumour with involvement of the NAC. There should be adequate breast volume with moderate breast ptosis of >8 cm from nipple to inframammary skin fold. 'B' shaped incision is placed; upper part of the B covers the NAC which is resected along with the underneath tumour with pectoral fascia with clearance margin. Lower part of the B is a circular skin of areolar size with pedicle which is transposed to the central area to replace the previously existing NAC as a part of

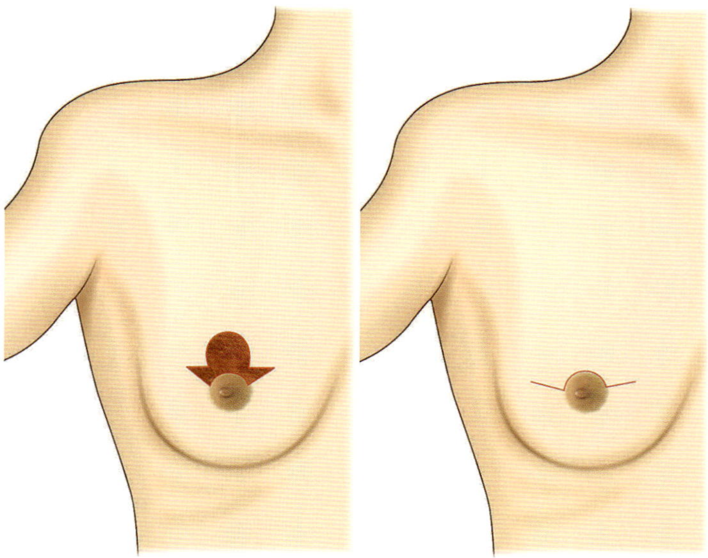

Fig. 16-51: Batwing incision for superior central tumours.

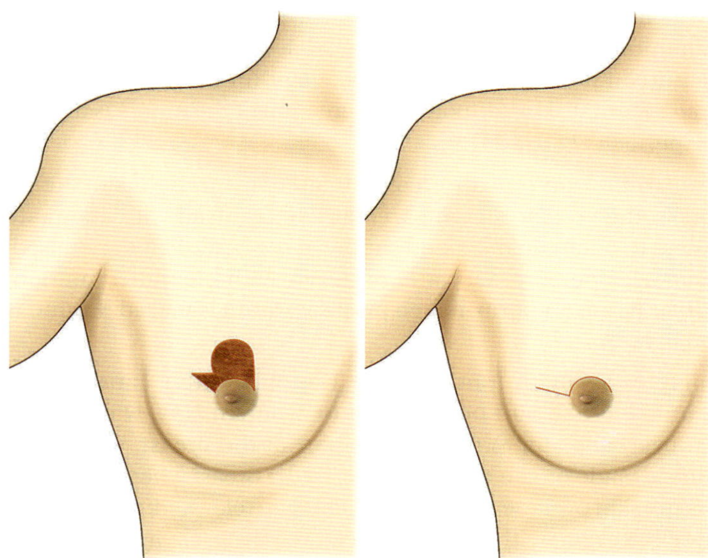

Fig. 16-52: Hemibatwing incision for one sided tumour at 9–10 or 2–3 o'clock positions.

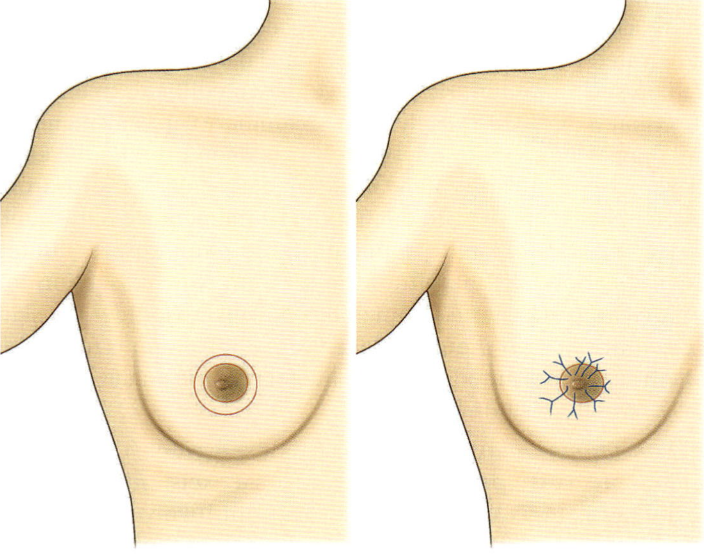

Fig. 16-53: Incision for donut round block resection oncoplasty.

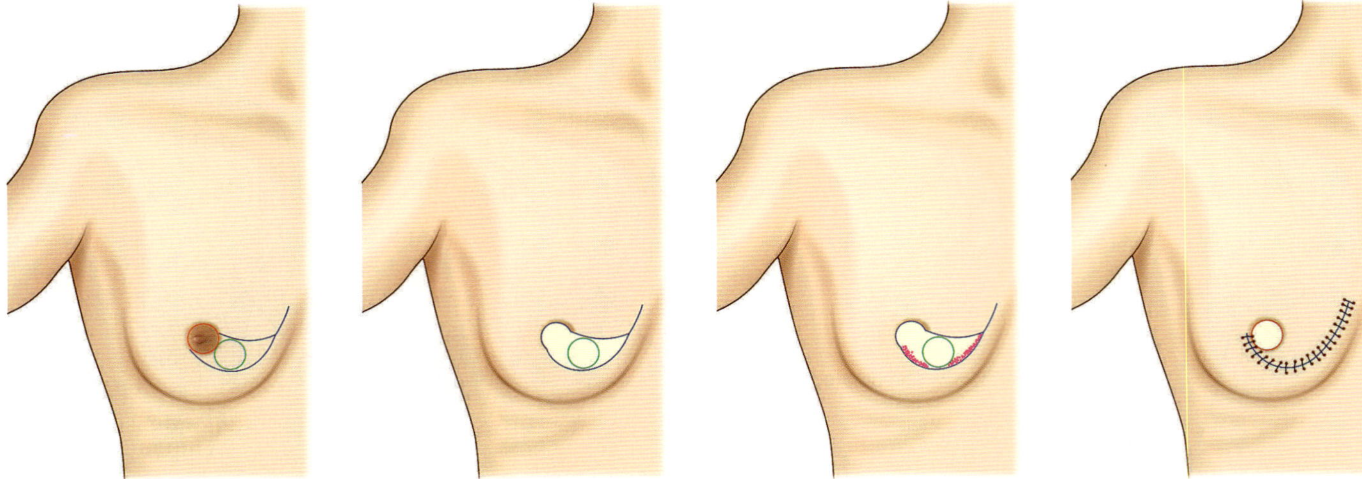

Fig. 16-54: Grisotti B flap resection.

oncoplasty procedure. Initially NAC with tumour is resected; then inframammary incision is made along with pedicled circular disc of skin which is transposed to as new areola. Skin of the (lower margin) inframammary incision is deepithelialised which can be buried and sutured into the glandular tissue. Later transposed skin disc is sutured to breast skin; tattooing and creation of the nipple is done at a later period **(Fig. 16-54)**.

Central quadrantectomy: Here circumareolar incision is made up to 50% of the areolar margin; areolar flap is raised with adequate thickness to maintain the blood supply of the NAC. Flaps are raised; tumour with pectoral fascia is removed with clearance margin; glandular tissue is approximated properly; drain is placed; wound is closed in layers.

Triangle excision: Inframammary tumours often cause lot of disfigurement like bird beak deformity wherein NAC with central breast overhangs on to the inferior part of the breast. Triangular incision is made on the inferior aspect of the breast wherein triangle covers the skin over the tumour area. Flaps are elevated; tumour with clearance margin, with pectoral fascia, rectus fascia and if needed part of the serratus anterior fibers are removed. After placing markers and achieving haemostasis, flaps are sutured like reverse 'T' which prevents the deformity **(Fig. 16-55)**.

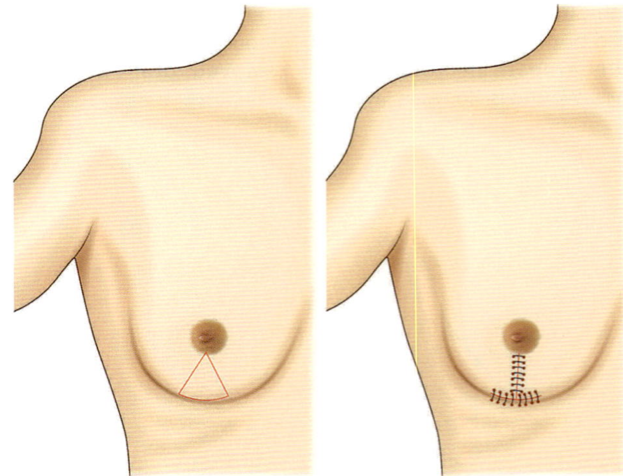

Fig. 16-55: Triangular flap excision for inframammary tumours of the breast.

Inframammary resection: It is done when tumour is located in the posterior aspect of the breast or in the caudal part. This approach is not advocated when tumour is in superficial part of the breast tissue as while resection anteriorly clearance may be difficult to achieve. Skin incision is made adequately at inframammary flap; subcutaneous tissue, deeper tissues are incised towards deeper plane to reach retromammary plane; this plane is elevated carefully upwards from behind to reach 3 cm beyond the tumour; intraoperative ultrasound and wire localisation and proper on table palpation facilitates the identification and margin of the tumour. Now dissection for anterior clearance is started from above downwards under the skin flap; clearance margin should be taken care off. Tumour is removed; glandular tissue is sutured properly; haemostasis is achieved; drain is placed; wound is sutured in layers.

Reduction mammoplasty resection: It is used when the tumour with large breast is operated with wide local excision with breast reduction surgery. NAC is retained if it is not involved; if NAC is involved it is removed along with wide excision of the tumour with later reconstruction of the NAC. 'Wise' incision (keyhole incision) is paced; wile local excision is done with removal of the fat and skin overlying; glandular tissue is sutured; wound is closed in layers with a drain. Reduction mammoplasty should be done on the opposite side also to achieve symmetry **(Fig. 16-56)**.

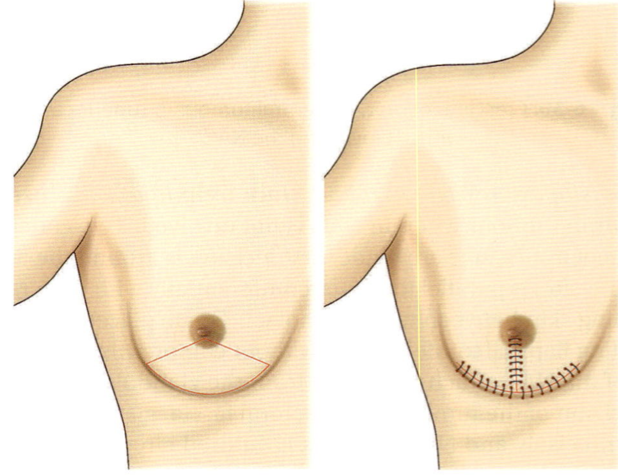

Fig. 16-56: Reduction mammoplasty.

Problems with oncoplasty—areolar necrosis, seroma, haematoma, incomplete clearance, asymmetry.

17 CHAPTER

Surgeries of Salivary Glands

SURGICAL ANATOMY OF PAROTID (PARA – AROUND; OTIC – EAR) GLAND

Parotid, *pyramid* shaped largest of salivary glands (15 gram) is located below the external acoustic meatus, between ramus of the mandible and the sternomastoid. Gland overlaps these structures and masseter muscle. Gland is of ectodermal origin.

Surface marking of the gland: Line joining from a point at upper margin of mandibular head; along a point at the center of the masseter muscle; to a point at posteroinferior angle of the mandible and at a point at upper part of anterior margin of the mastoid process. *Parotid duct* is marked in the middle third of a line joining the lower border of tragus to a point which is at the middle of the line joining the nasal ala to margin of upper lip. *Facial nerve* is marked from a point at middle of the anterior border of mastoid process (stylomastoid foramen lies 2 cm deep to this point) to a point behind the neck of the mandible **(Fig. 17-1)**.

Investing layer of deep fascia of neck splits at the lower posterior margin of the gland into two layers, as a thick adherent superficial lamina, and a thin deep lamina. Superficial part is attached to zygomatic arch above. *Parotid capsule* otherwise the superficial lamina is thick, inelastic and unstretchable. Deep lamina is attached to styloid process, mandible, and forms thick *stylomandibular ligament* to separate it from submandibular salivary gland **(Fig. 17-2)**.

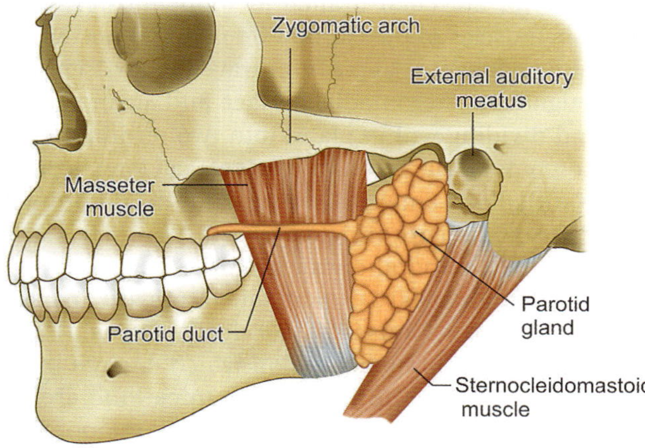

Fig. 17-1: Location of the parotid in relation to masseter muscle.

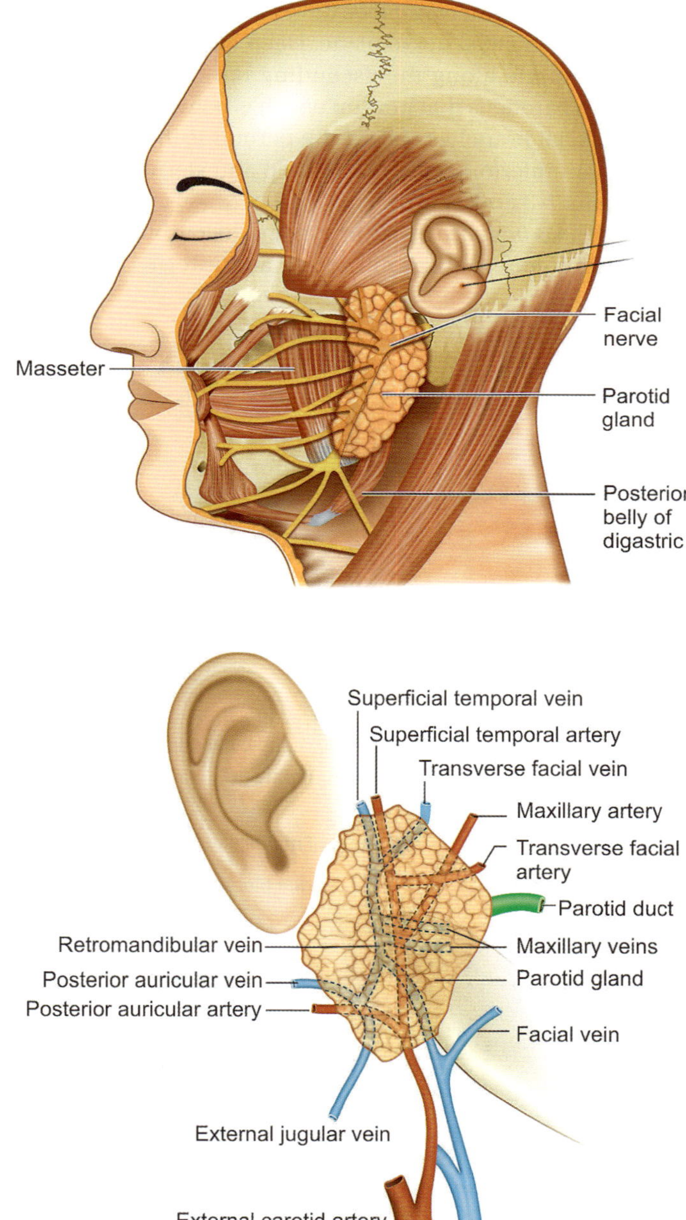

Fig. 17-2: Anatomy of parotid and structures passing through it.

Parotid gland has *4 surfaces*—superior/base; superficial; anteromedial; posteromedial. *Apex* is directed downwards; *3 borders* are—anterior, posterior and medial. Apex lies on the posterior belly of digastric and partly extends into the carotid triangle. Cervical branch of facial nerve and divisions of retromandibular vein emerges at the apex. Upper small concave superior surface is related to auriculotemporal nerve, superficial temporal vessels, temporomandibular joint (posterior part), and cartilaginous part of external acoustic meatus. Largest superficial surface is related to skin, superficial fascia, preauricular/superficial parotid lymph nodes, platysma, risorius, and parotid fascia. Anteromedial surface is related to masseter, lateral part of temporomandibular joint, posterior margin of the mandibular ramus, medial pterygoid, branches of facial nerve. Posteromedial surface is related to mastoid process, sternomastoid, posterior belly of digastric muscle, styloid process. External carotid artery enters the gland through this surface. Internal carotid artery is deep to styloid process.

Parotid gland is divided conventionally into two lobes—*superficial lobe* (80%) is also called as *exofacial lobe* which is outer to facial (7th cranial) nerve plane; *deep lobe* (20%) is also called as *endofacial* which is deeper to facial nerve plane. Deep lobe is located adjacent to masseter muscle along the ascending ramus of the mandible. *Isthmus* of the parotid is that portion which is between temporofacial and cervicofacial branches. Tail of the parotid is the portion which extends posteroinferiorly over mastoid tip and sternocleidomastoid muscle **(Figs. 17-3 and 17-4)**.

Parotid gland is *bounded* above by zygoma, below by styloid process, styloid muscles, internal carotid artery and internal jugular vein,

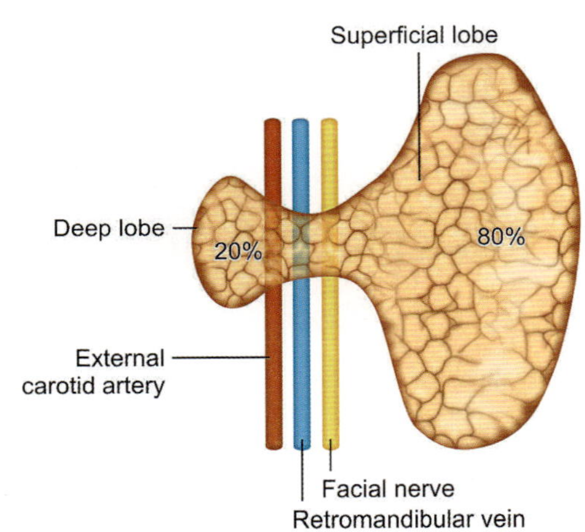

Fig. 17-3: Lobes of parotid.

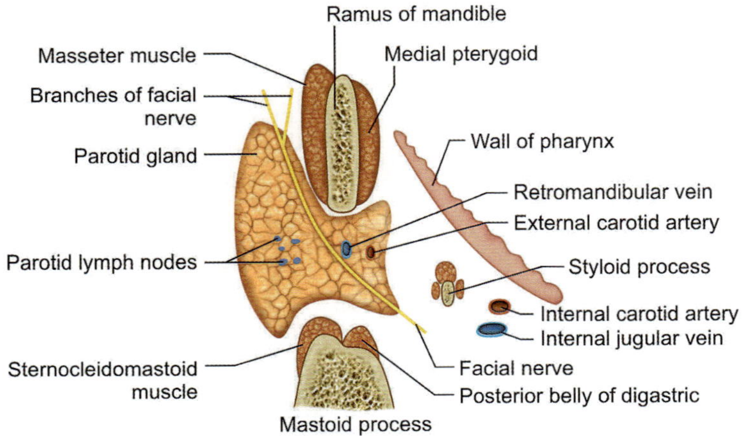

Fig. 17-4: Relations of the parotid gland.

behind by external auditory canal. Fascia deep to deep lobe is extension of the fascia from deeper part of the digastric muscle and is called as *stylomandibular membrane* which occupies between mandible in front, styloid process behind and stylomandibular ligament below. This membrane separates parotid from submandibular salivary gland. Deep lobe tumour extends to parapharyngeal space through this membrane.

Superficial Muscular Aponeurotic System (SMAS): SMAS is a fibrous network that invests the facial muscles and connects them with the dermis with platysma inferiorly, zygomatic arch superiorly and parotid fascia; facial nerve courses deep to the SMAS and the platysma.

Structures passing through the anterior margin are: parotid duct, facial nerve branches and transverse facial vessels.

Structures within the parotid gland are: **Arteries** (deepest)—external carotid artery (ECA) enters the gland through posteromedial surface of the gland; maxillary artery (begins at neck of the condylar process of mandible) leaves the gland through anteromedial surface medial to gland to reach infratemporal fossa; superficial temporal artery comes out through superior surface passing between external acoustic meatus and temporomandibular (TM) joint to reach temporal fossa where it is accompanied by auriculotemporal nerve. Transverse facial artery arises from superficial temporal artery runs horizontally above the parotid duct. Posterior auricular artery arises from ECA passing posteriorly deeper and at upper margin of the posterior belly of digastric to reach posterior auricular region. Posterior auricular artery gives stylomastoid branch which runs in front and along the facial nerve to enter the stylomastoid foramen to supply tympanic cavity, mastoid air cells and semicircular canals. **Veins** (outer to arteries)—superficial temporal vein and maxillary vein (formed by pterygoid venous plexus at lateral pterygoid muscle) joins to form retromandibular vein (posterior facial vein/temporomaxillary vein) within the gland which descend and divides into anterior and posterior divisions which emerge at apex of the gland; anterior division after emerging joins facial vein to form common facial vein which runs superficial to digastric to reach internal jugular vein (IJV); posterior division joins the posterior auricular vein to form external jugular vein which runs downwards in front of posterior belly of digastric muscle, sternocleidomastoid, great auricular nerve to reach subclavian vein. *Patey's faciovenous plane* is important during surgical dissection. **Facial nerve** (outer to venous plane)—comes out of stylomastoid foramen where it is accompanied with stylomastoid branch (in front of facial nerve) of posterior auricular artery (artery enters, nerve comes out). Here it gives posterior auricular branch to supply posterior auricular and intrinsic muscles of the ear and branches to posterior belly of digastric and stylohyoid. Nerve after traveling for 1 cm enters the gland through its posteromedial surface and again runs for 1 cm in the gland dividing within gland into two terminal branches—zygomaticotemporal (larger) and cervicofacial (smaller). Terminal temporal (auricularis anterior and superior part of frontalis) and zygomatic (frontalis and orbicularis oculi) branches arise from larger zygomaticotemporal division. Upper buccal, lower buccal (buccinator, orbicularis oris and elevators of lip), marginal mandibular (lower lip muscles), cervical (platysma) arise from smaller cervicofacial branch/division which emerge through the anteromedial surface. Multiple communications are common between branches especially in zygomatic and temporal branches (*pes anserinus/goose foot*). They supply muscles of facial expression and platysma. **Deep parotid lymph glands**—they are embedded in

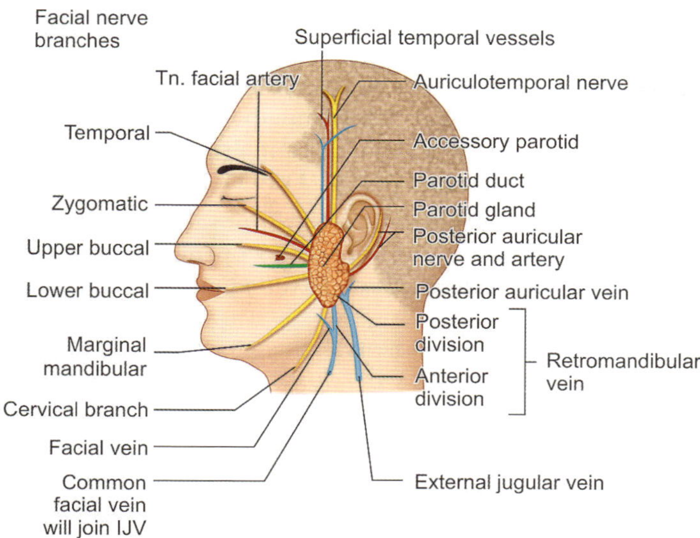

Fig. 17-5: Structures passing out of the parotid gland.

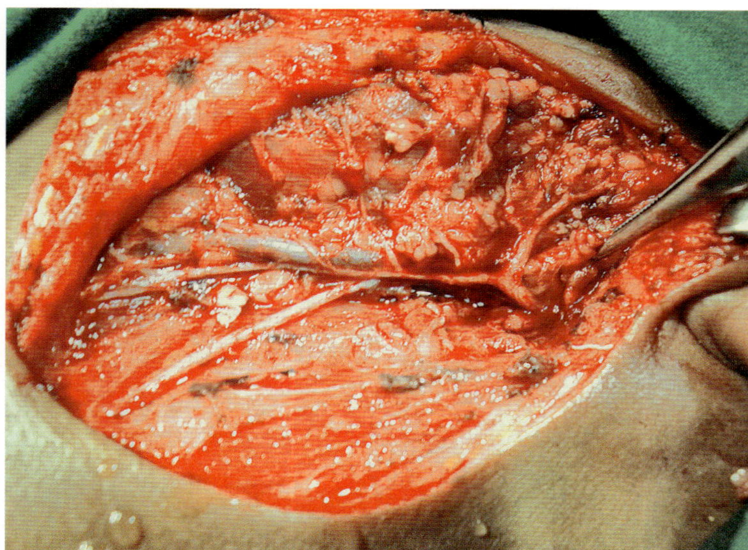

Fig. 17-6: Patey's faciovenous plane.

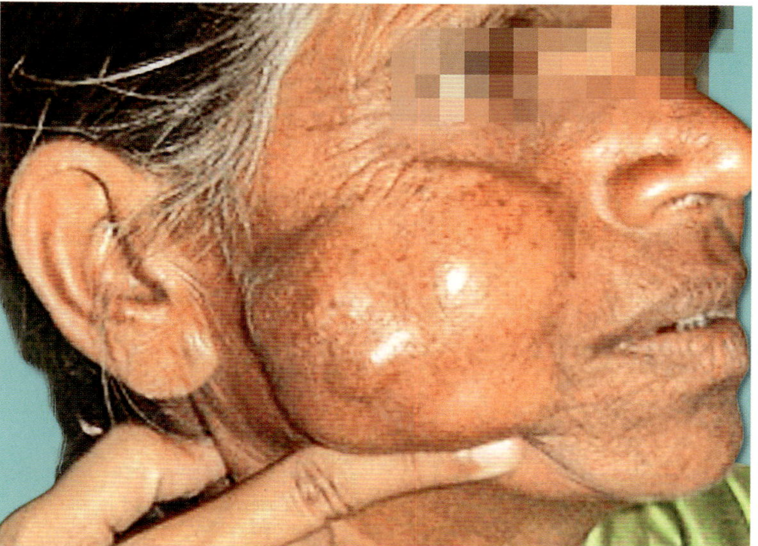

Fig. 17-7: Accessory parotid gland is above the parotid duct.

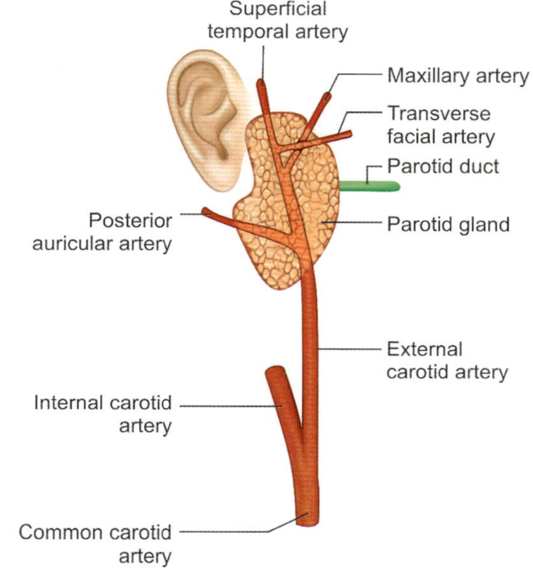

Fig. 17-8: Arterial supply of parotid gland and arteries related to parotid.

the superficial lobe of the gland. *Faciovenous plane of Patey* is a plane where vein and facial nerve branches lie within the parotid with nerve lying superficial to vein in this plane **(Figs. 17-5 and 17-6)**.

Parotid duct (Niels *Stenson's—Anatomist Copenhagen; father of geology)* is 5 cm in length (2–3 mm diameter) with thick wall which after beginning deep behind the angle of mandible runs forwards 1.5 cm below the zygoma emerges from the anterior border of the gland running forward and downward on the masseter muscle up to its anterior margin where it pierces obliquely the buccal pad of fat, buccopharyngeal fascia, buccinator muscle and opens into the vestibule of the mouth opposite the crown of 2nd upper molar tooth. During its course it receives interlobular duct from above and one duct from accessory parotid gland. Above it is related to *accessory parotid gland*, upper buccal branch of facial nerve, transverse facial vessels; below to lower buccal branch of the facial nerve **(Fig. 17-7)**.

Blood Supply

Parotid is supplied by ECA through its direct branches and also branches of ECA in the parotid region; venous drainage is into the external jugular vein **(Figs. 17-8 and 17-9)**.

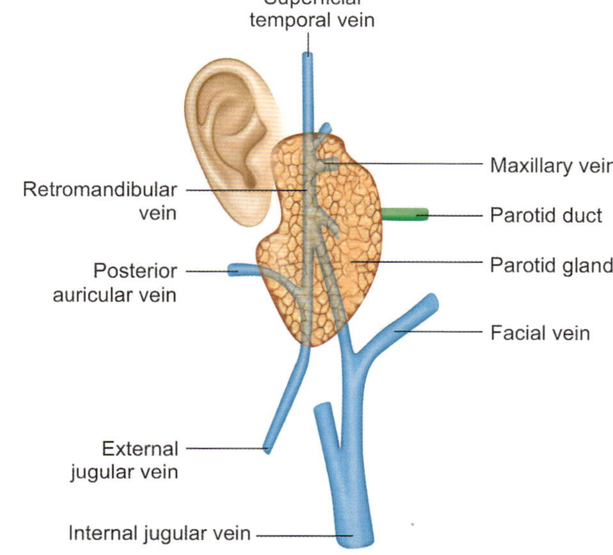

Fig. 17-9: Venous drainage and veins related to parotid.

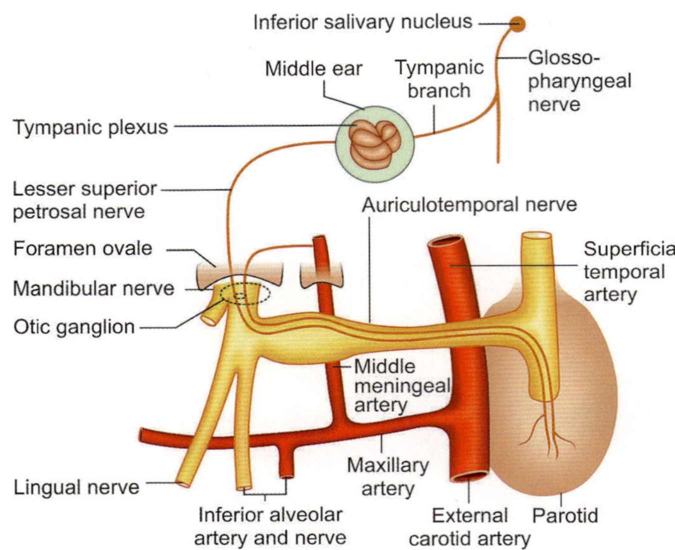

Fig. 17-10: Parasympathetic supply of parotid gland.

Lymphatic Drainage

Superficial parotid lymph glands lie outer to parotid (deep fascia); *deep parotid lymph glands* are located deep to parotid sheath in *superficial* lobe. Drainage area are—temple, side of the scalp, lateral part of ear, external acoustic meatus, middle ear, parotid gland, upper part of cheek, eyelids partly, orbit. Efferent from these nodes drain into upper deep neck nodes.

Nerve Supply

Parotid fascia sheath is supplied by great auricular nerve (C2); *sensory supply* to gland is through auriculotemporal nerve; *sympathetic* vasomotor fibres are from plexus around ECA; *parasympathetic supply* is through otic ganglion with complex pathway. Inferior salivatory nucleus → preganglionic fibres → glossopharyngeal nerve → tympanic branch → tympanic plexus → lesser petrosal nerve → otic ganglion → post-ganglionic fibres → through auriculotemporal branch of mandibular division of trigeminal nerve → parotid gland **(Fig. 17-10)**.

FACIAL NERVE

It is 7th cranial nerve (2nd branchial arch). It is the '*queen of the face*'. It arises from 4 nuclei at lower pons. Sensory (nervus intermedius) and motor roots run along with 8th cranial vestibulocochlear nerve to enter the internal acoustic meatus with labyrinthine vessels. In the meatus two roots join to lie in the petrous temporal bone. In the canal it has got 2 bends. First bend is called as *genu* which is related to geniculate ganglion. Nerve leaves the skull through stylomastoid foramen. *Stylomastoid foramen* is located medial to mastoid tip and lateral to styloid process. Stylomastoid branch of posterior auricular artery (branch of ECA) is just in front of the facial nerve trunk which also enters the stylomastoid foramen. Here facial nerve runs lateral to styloid process to enter the parotid gland; divides into branches behind the neck of the mandible. ***Branches**—in the canal* are greater petrosal, nerve to stapedius, chorda tympani; branches immediately *after coming out of stylomastoid foramen*—are posterior auricular (to post-auricular muscles), digastric (to posterior belly) and stylohyoid; *terminal* branches are—temporal, zygomatic, buccal, marginal mandibular and cervical. Buccal branch is in relation to the parotid duct; marginal mandibular branch crosses over the anterior facial vein. *Chorda tympani* originates from facial nerve 6 mm above the stylomastoid foramen; enters middle ear close to tympanic membrane, then petrotympanic fissure to reach infratemporal fossa where it joins lingual nerve to distribute secretomotor fibres to submandibular ganglion (parasympathetic secretomotor) and submandibular and sublingual glands. It also gives taste fibres to anterior 2/3rd of the tongue **(Figs. 17-11 to 17-14)**.

Greater petrosal nerve pathway is—superior salivatory nucleus → facial nerve → greater petrosal nerve → opening in the petrous temporal bone for greater petrosal nerve → joins sympathetic deep

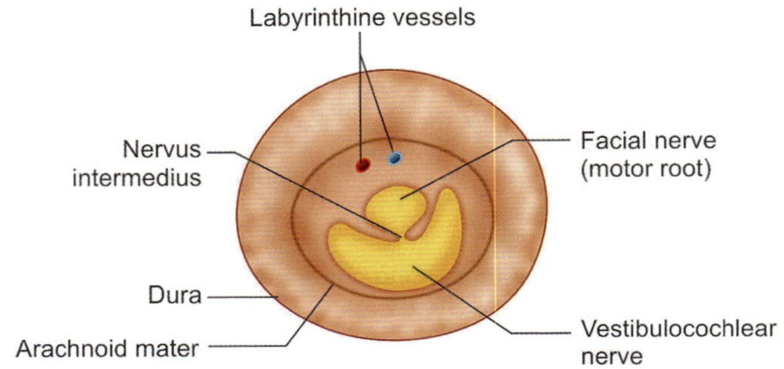

Fig. 17-11: Structures in the internal meatus (left).

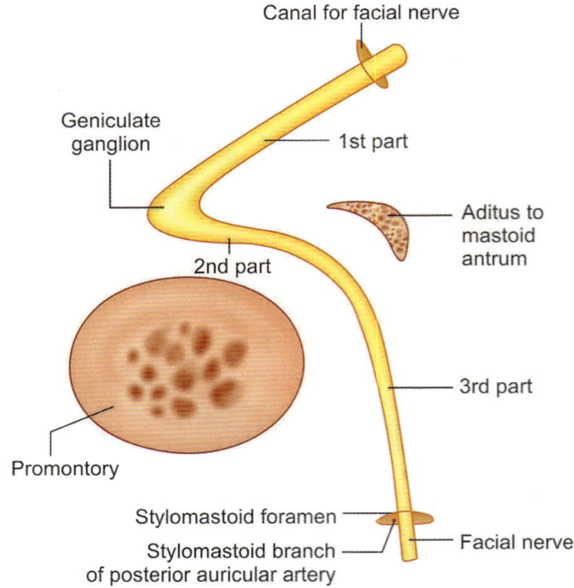

Fig. 17-12: Course of facial nerve to reach face.

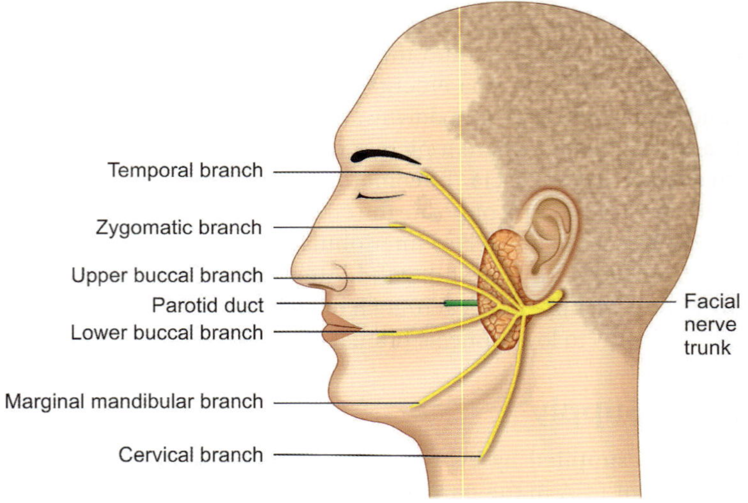

Fig. 17-13: Facial nerve and its branches.

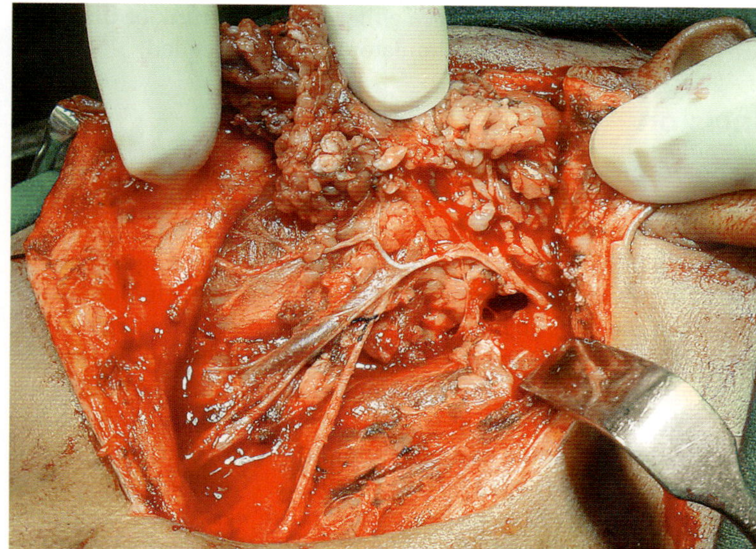

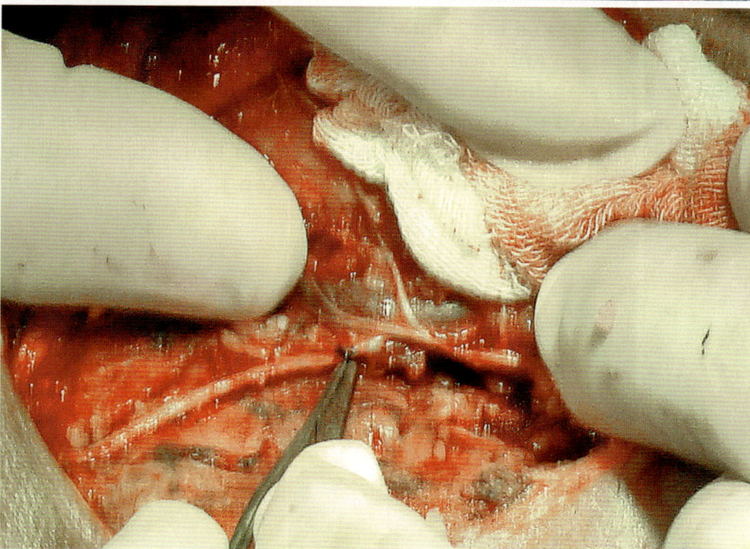

Fig. 17-14: Facial nerve—on table look.

petrosal nerve to form nerve of the pterygoid canal → through canal reaches pterygopalatine ganglion (largest peripheral parasympathetic ganglion) → postganglionic fibres supply lacrimal gland and mucous glands of nose, sinuses, palate and pharynx.

Levels of the parotid (European Salivary Gland Society/ESGS): Five levels are identified by ESGS. (I) Lateral superior; (II) Lateral inferior; (III) Deep inferior; (IV) Deep superior; (V) Accessory **(Fig. 17-15)**.

PAROTIDECTOMY

Indications

Parotidectomy is done in benign/malignant tumours of parotid including adenolymphoma of parotid. Superficial parotidectomy is done only in benign tumours of superficial lobe. In tumours (benign) involving both superficial or deep lobe and only deep lobe total conservative parotidectomy is done. In malignant tumour invading facial nerve radical parotidectomy is done. Presently even in malignant parotid tumours, sacrificing only the involved/infiltrated branches of facial nerve and retaining uninvolved branches, with wide clearance and neck dissection is contemplated; as evidence suggests that there is no survival benefit between removing

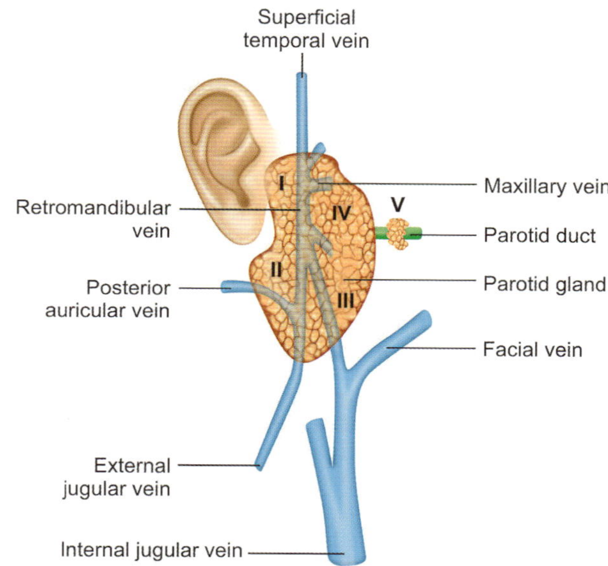

Fig. 17-15: Levels in parotid as per European Salivary Gland Society (ESGS): (I) lateral superior; (II) lateral inferior; (III) deep inferior; (IV) deep superior; (V) accessory lobe.

all branches and removing only the involved branches. In aggressive tumour radical parotidectomy is done sacrificing the trunk of facial nerve with nerve graft.

Occasionally superficial parotidectomy is added as part of radical neck dissection in case if primary tumour is in head and neck region and in skin malignancies of face and scalp. First branchial cleft cyst excision involves removal of the parotid. Type I first branchial cyst is located in the external auditory canal in relation to angle of the mandible and parotid.

Some surgeons even though not well accepted advocate total parotidectomy for chronic parotitis, sialorrhoea, fistula, refractory parotid stones.

Types of Parotidectomy

Superficial/lateral parotidectomy (Patey): It is removal of superficial lobe of the parotid in front of the faciovenous plane of Patey.

Partial (functional) parotidectomy: It involves resection of parotid pathology with normal parotid tissue, done in benign pathology and low grade malignancies. Here main facial nerve trunk is identified but there is no need to dissect the branches.

Total conservative parotidectomy: Here both superficial and deep lobes of the parotid are removed preserving the facial nerve. Dissection along the faciovenous plane is carried out to identify the branches of the facial nerve retaining the isthmus/tumour-bearing area. Nerve branches are retracted aside to reach the deep lobe which is removed entirely by dissecting off the branches of facial nerve carefully without injuring them. This is the right technique even though many advocate removing superficial lobe initially then deep lobe separately. Retromandibular vein is ligated here.

Radical parotidectomy: Involves removal of both lobes of parotid with facial nerve, fat, fascia, masseter, pterygoid, buccinator along with neck lymph node dissection. Facial nerve is sacrificed. Its branches whenever possible can be saved as additional advantage of survival not thereby removing uninvolved branches. On table frozen section biopsy of cut ends of nerve are needed. Ends of the cut nerve branches are tagged by fine sutures for eventual nerve grafting using great auricular nerve or sural nerve. Often radical parotidectomy is combined with removal of temporomandibular joint, mastoid process and external auditory meatus with less additional benefit. Mastoidectomy is done to visualise the clear proximal part of the facial nerve. Reconstruction of the main trunk, marginal mandibular, temporal and buccal branches are done to maintain eye closure and good oral competence.

Extended total parotidectomy: Removal of the superficial and deep parotid gland also may be extended to involve adjacent structures.

Suprafacial parotidectomy: It is done for benign tumour at lower pole wherein all branches of facial nerve need not be dissected.

Newer classifications of parotidectomy

Snow's classification:

Formal parotidectomy
- Superficial parotidectomy
- Total parotidectomy

Limited operations
- Partial superficial parotidectomy
- Selective deep lobe parotidectomy
- Extracapsular dissection (ECD)

Note: Capsular dissection (CD) is not advocated except may be in Warthin's tumour; here minimal extracapsular dissection is also advocated (MECD).

Tweedie and Jacob's classification:
- Total parotidectomy ± Facial nerve resection
- Complete superficial parotidectomy ± Facial nerve resection
- Partial superficial parotidectomy
  - Upper segment ± Deep lobe dissection
  - Middle segment ± Deep lobe dissection
  - Lower segment ± Deep lobe dissection
- Selective deep lobe parotidectomy
- Extracapsular dissection

ESGS proposal of newer parotidectomy classification:
- Parotidectomy I–IV (VII): Total parotidectomy with facial nerve resection
- Parotidectomy I–IV: Total parotidectomy with facial nerve preservation
- Parotidectomy I–IV (VII, S, MM): Extended total parotidectomy with facial nerve resection plus skin and masseter muscle resection
- Parotidectomy I–II: Superficial parotidectomy
- Parotidectomy III–IV: Deep lobe parotidectomy
- Parotidectomy I: Partial superficial parotidectomy
- Parotidectomy II: Partial superficial parotidectomy
- Parotidectomy I–II–III: Superficial parotidectomy extended to the inferior deep lobe
- Parotidectomy V: Accessory lobe removal
- ECD I: Extracapsular dissection with tumour in level I
- ECD II: Extracapsular dissection with tumour in level II
- ECD V: Extracapsular dissection with tumour in level V

TECHNIQUE OF PAROTIDECTOMY

Position and Anaesthesia

Procedure is done under general anaesthesia. Paralytic agents used for intubation purpose are of short acting only as during surgery, facial nerve branches are identified and confirmed by stimulation to achieve contraction of facial muscles. Neck is extended by placing a sandbag under the shoulder with a head support using a ring. After cleaning, draping is done to expose the face and eyelids to see the contractions of muscles whenever needed. Head is extended with face turning to opposite side. Head end of the table is elevated 15° to reduce venous congestion. In many centres of China procedure is done under local anaesthesia also. Nerve monitor device is used. Its electrode tips are placed into orbicularis oculi and orbicularis oris muscles. Nerve either the main trunk or branches are stimulated using nerve stimulator whenever needed.

Incision

Standard incision is '*Lazy S*' incision (*modified Blair/Sistrunk* incision). It begins in front of tragus closely running vertically to the ear lobule; curving on the margin of the ear lobule towards middle of the mastoid (mastoid tip) along postauricular part; again curving back downwards along the margin of the sternocleidomastoid muscle in the superior cervical crease 2 cm below the angle of the mandible. *Inverted T and modified Y incisions* are also used. '*Face lift' incision'* can be used in benign tumours of the tail or middle part of the parotid. It begins at tragus running vertically downwards curving the ear lobule and extending in the postauricular region along the hair line **(Figs. 17-16 to 17-19)**.

Usual plane used is *subplatysmal* in the *neck* area. Incidence of Frey's syndrome and flap necrosis are higher if flap is raised in front of the platysma. Ear lobule is held under traction with suture. Skin flap is raised anteriorly superficial to parotid fascia in *face* by holding with skin hooks up to the anterior margin of the parotid with visualisation of the masseter muscle. While elevating the flap anteriorly close to the masseter, branches of facial nerve will be close to skin flap and care should be taken not to injure them.

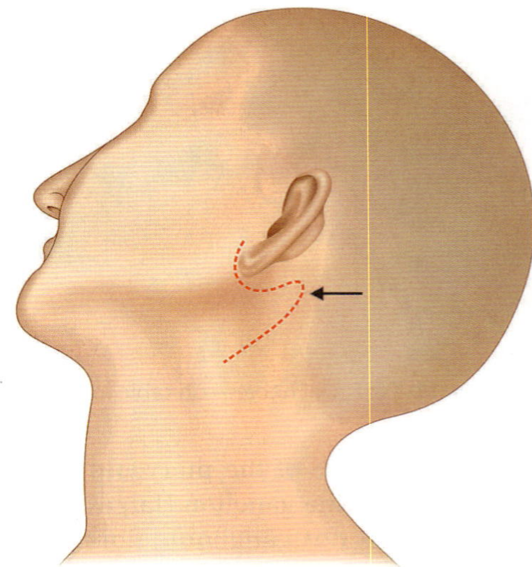

Fig. 17-16: Modified Blair incision for parotidectomy.

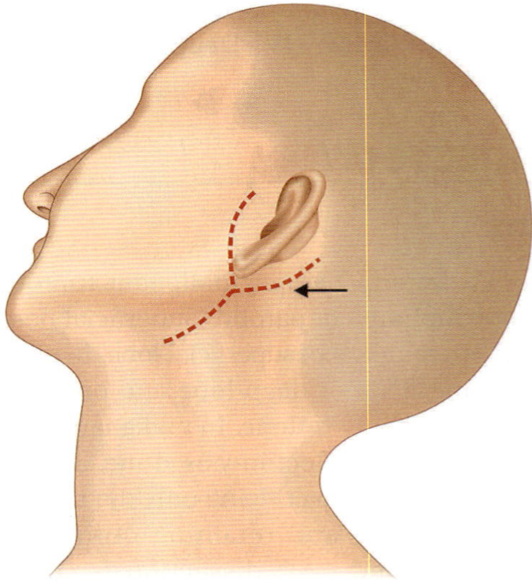

Fig. 17-17: Inverted 'T' incision for parotidectomy.

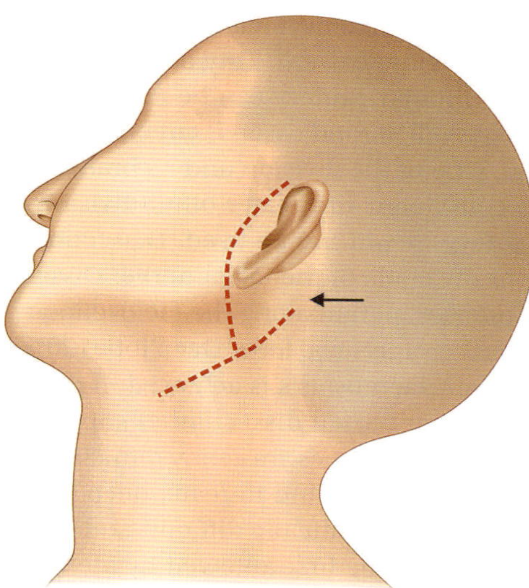

Fig. 17-18: Modified Y incision for parotidectomy.

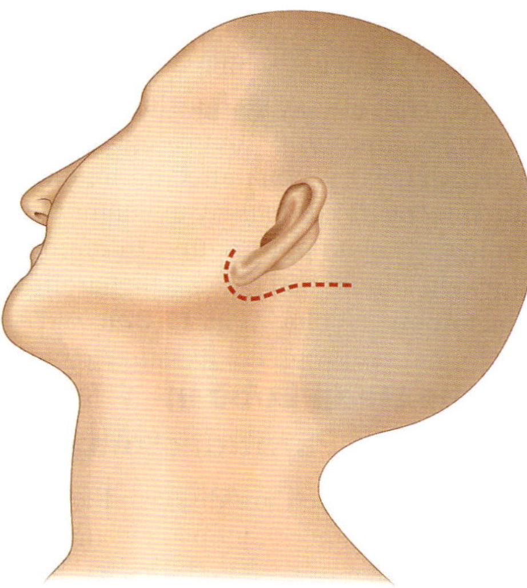

Fig. 17-19: Face lift incision for parotidectomy.

Posterior skin flap is raised to expose the anterior border of the sternocleidomastoid muscle and mastoid process **(Fig. 17-20)**.

Even though *great/greater auricular nerve* has to be cut, it is cut close to the parotid gland or after it gives the posterior branch (it is the largest branch of cervical plexus). Adequate length of the great auricular nerve is dissected for the possible need of nerve graft in case of facial nerve injury. *External jugular vein* with its tributaries is visible which can be retained or transected. Fascia along the anterior border of the sternocleidomastoid muscle is incised to expose the upper part of the muscle. After retracting sternocleidomastoid, once posterior belly of digastric muscle is identified; both muscles are retracted; dissection is done in front of the mastoid along the tragal cartilage. Dissection begins from the posterior part of the gland near tail of the parotid. Gland is freed of the fibrous attachments and with blunt dissection bony cartilaginous junction of the auditory canal, tympanomastoid suture/fissure (groove between mastoid tip and tympanic portion of the temporal bone) and tragal pointer is felt and identified. Parotid tissue between superior border of posterior belly of digastric muscle and tympanomastoid fissure is dissected and separated carefully layer by layer by blunt and sharp dissection. Temporoparotid fascia from tympanomastoid fissure to parotid is cut to visualise facial nerve. Facial nerve is 1 cm below and medial (or *anterior and inferior*) to tip of the tragal cartilage **(Fig. 17-21)**.

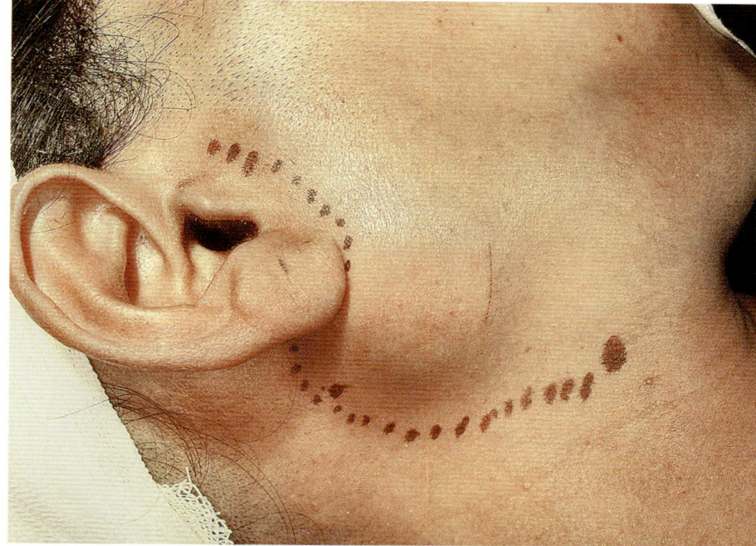

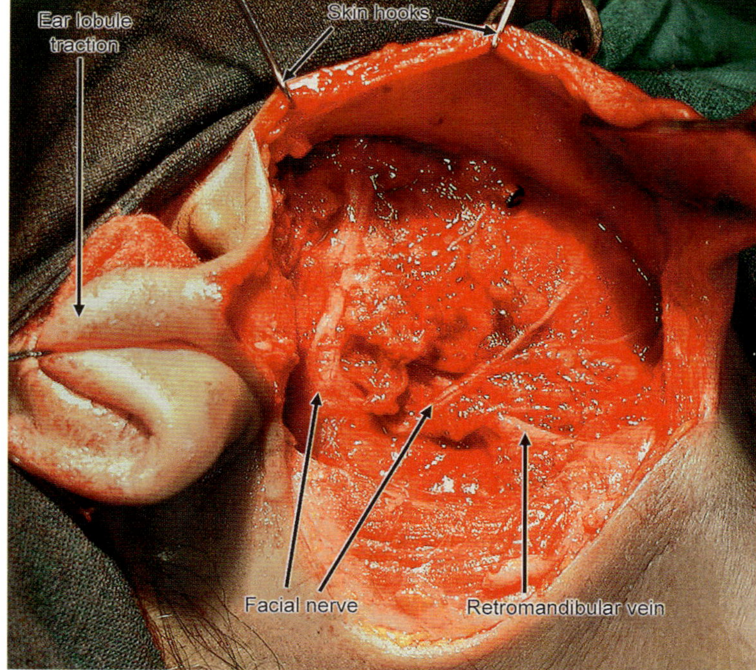

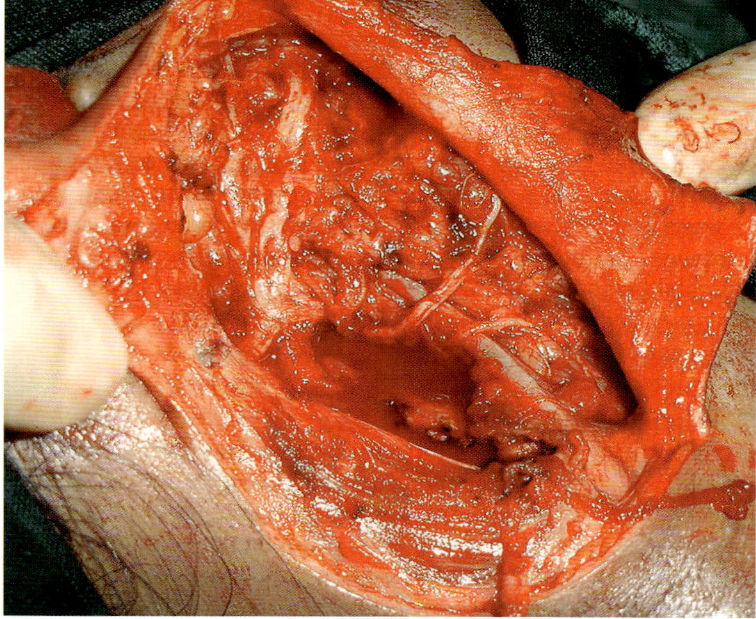

Fig. 17-20: Incision and subplatysmal plane for parotidectomy.

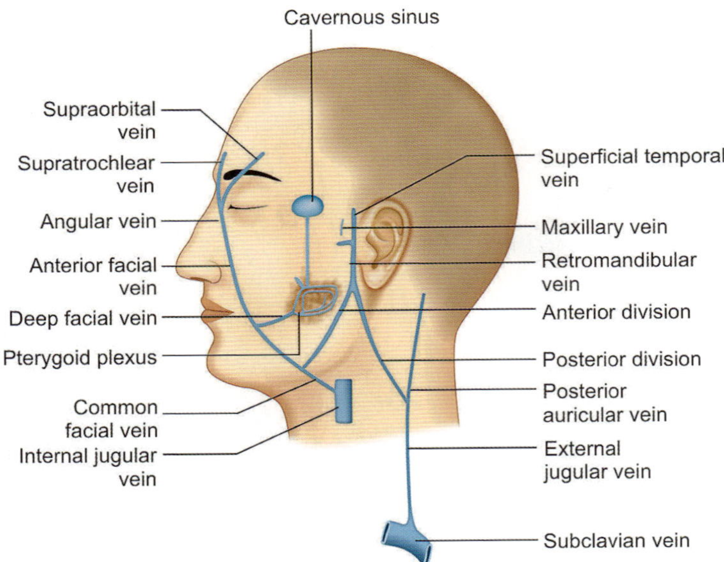

Fig. 17-21: Venous anatomy of face is important in parotidectomy.

Identification of Facial Nerve

Facial nerve trunk is identified by different techniques: (1) Facial nerve is 5–10 mm deep and below from the tip of the cartilaginous canal—*Conley's point.* (2) Sternocleidomastoid muscle is retracted behind, gland is retracted front; posterior belly of digastric is identified where the nerve is anterior to this. (3) Nerve is lateral to styloid process. (4) Tracing branch from distal to proximal—*Hamilton-Bailey* technique through buccal branch or marginal mandibular branch. (5) Using Faradic or mechanical stimulation (pinching tissues) muscle movements/twitching can be observed. (6) Stylomastoid branch of posterior auricular artery lies just in front of the facial nerve trunk which also enters the stylomastoid foramen. Facial nerve after coming out of stylomastoid foramen travels for 1 cm forward and below between mastoid process and membranous portion of external auditory canal and divides into temporofacial/temporozygomatic and cervicofacial branches behind the neck of the mandible. This bifurcation may be often distal or often proximal before coming out of the stylomastoid foramen. Cervicofacial branch divides into cervical (for platysma) and marginal mandibular branch which runs below the horizontal ramus of the mandible within the platysma muscle to supply the lower lip. This branch *does not have any communicating* branch unlike other branches of facial nerve. This branch is more often superficial to posterior facial vein. Buccal and zygomatic branches have numerous communications which supply periorbital and upper lip muscles. Temporal branch supplies frontalis muscle but does not have cross communications and has got weak regenerative power and so often paralysis of frontalis stands permanent in facial nerve palsy. Buccal branch is situated close to parotid duct and so if duct is identified it is easier to look for buccal branch. Dissection from distal to proximal is more difficult than dissection from proximal to distal.

Separation of Gland off the Facial Nerve Branches

It requires patience and fine dissection. There are two methods to dissect the facial nerve. (1) Forward/*antegrade* technique—dissection from main trunk of facial nerve; (2) *Retrograde* technique—dissection from branches towards main trunk (it is followed in many centres in China).

Dissection using fine haemostat and fine scissor is ideal with tip of the instrument facing forward. Tiny oozing points need ligation using fine vicryl. Bipolar cautery can be used carefully away from the nerve branches. All parotid tissue is cut only with visualisation of nerve branches. One of the division and its branches are separated and dissected completely first; later other division and branches. Monopolar cautery *should not* be used. Dissection is first started along the upper divisions of the facial nerve. Dissection is carried out up to the anterior margin along the faciovenous plane of Patey to remove the entire superficial lobe. Deep lobe (20% of total gland) is nicely visualised. Haemostasis is achieved. If deep lobe needs to be removed then after partial dissection of superficial gland from facial nerve branches, branches are gently retracted to dissect beside the isthmus of the parotid gland to reach deep lobe which can be removed. Often this is technically difficult and so many advocate removal of superficial lobe first followed by identification of deep lobe; facial nerve branches are retracted and deep lobe is dissected and removed. Parotid duct is located in relation to deep lobe. Upper buccal branch is above the duct which is larger than lower buccal branch. Ideally all the branches should be identified and dissected. In malignant parotid, branches which are invaded are sacrificed. Main trunk if divided then nerve graft is done using great auricular nerve or sural nerve. Operating microscope is needed for nerve suturing. Even though nerve is not injured postoperative neuropraxia is common which recovers completely at a later period. Many use short-term steroid therapy to prevent this. In removal of deep lobe retromandibular vein should be ligated. The parotidectomy should be done with the tumour 'en bloc' **(Fig. 17-22)**.

Removal of the Deep Lobe in Total Conservative Parotidectomy

Branches of facial nerve which are dissected are gently retracted away using nerve hook or smooth loops to visualise the deep lobe. Parotid duct is transected at its anterior part and ligated. One should not injure upper buccal branch of facial nerve. Duct may be dissected up to the mucosa through buccinator if needed before ligation. Deep lobe is separated from nerve branches from its deeper plane. Often it is required to ligate the retromandibular vein to facilitate easy dissection and reduce bleeding. Deeper part of the deep lobe is dissected of the stylopharyngeus and stylohyoid muscles by blunt dissection while retracting the deep lobe. Superficial temporal vessels, maxillary artery deep to ramus of mandible, the occipital artery, posterior auricular artery and pterygoid venous plexus are deep to deep lobe. Deep lobe can be extirpated superior/inferior/in between nerve branches. Haemostasis should be achieved using bipolar cautery.

Main trunk of the facial nerve is stimulated with electrical probe 0.5 mA to confirm the anatomical and physiological integrity of the branches of the facial nerve.

Points to be remembered are:
Dissection of the facial nerve should be done just superficial to the nerve to expose it clearly. Dissection deep to the nerve is inadvisable. The sheath of the facial nerve should not be opened to avoid damage to the nerve fibres.

Using *wet gauze* is better than dry gauze for haemostasis. Clearing of blood from the operative field should be done by mild pressure absorption of the blood rather than scrubbing. The dissected nerve should be covered by wet gauze to avoid dryness following exposure to air.

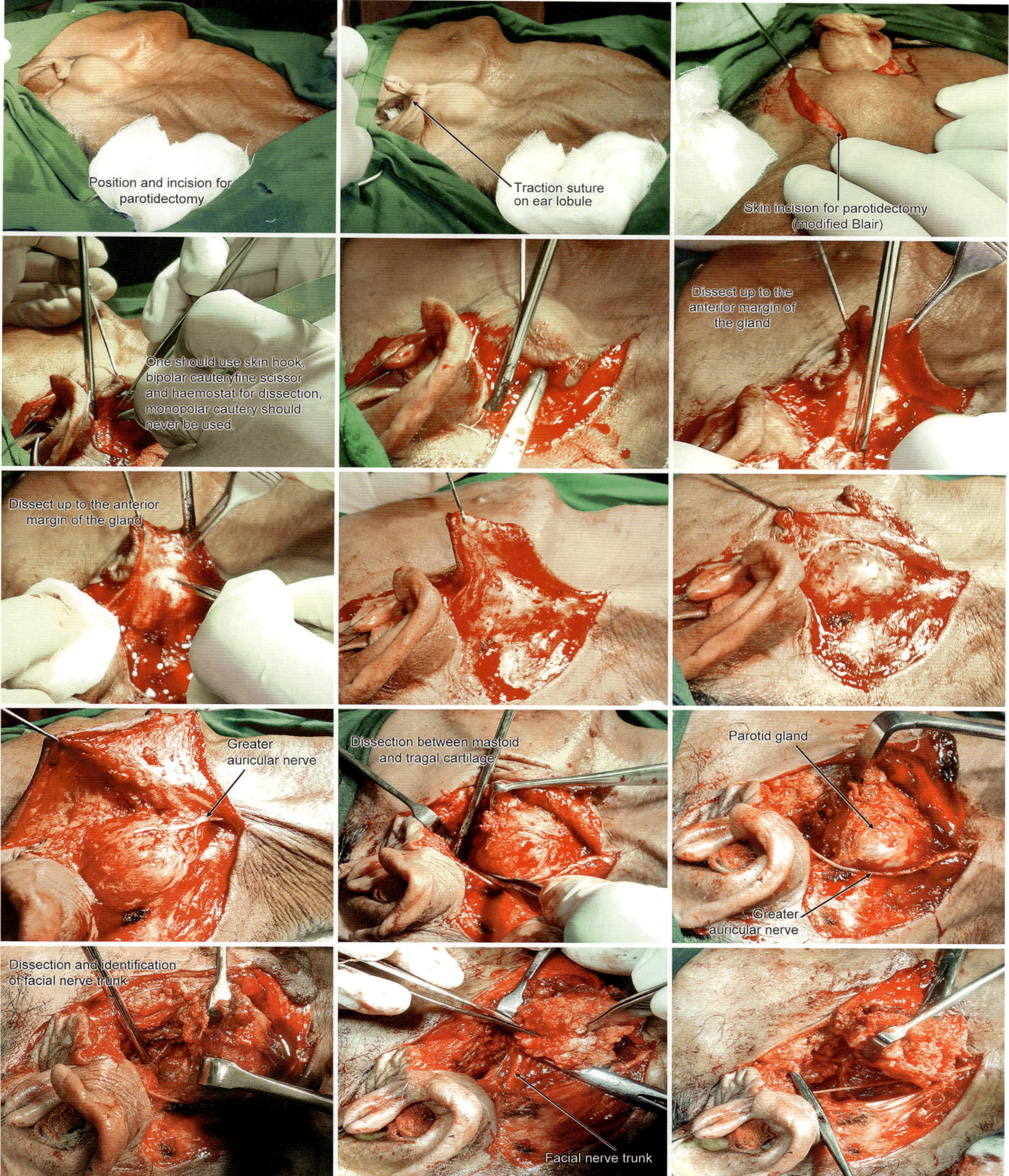
Position and incision for parotidectomy
Traction suture on ear lobule
Skin incision for parotidectomy (modified Blair)
One should use skin hook, bipolar cautery fine scissor and haemostat for dissection, monopolar cautery should never be used.
Dissect up to the anterior margin of the gland
Dissect up to the anterior margin of the gland
Greater auricular nerve
Dissection between mastoid and tragal cartilage
Parotid gland
Greater auricular nerve
Dissection and identification of facial nerve trunk
Facial nerve trunk

Figs. 17-22(1)

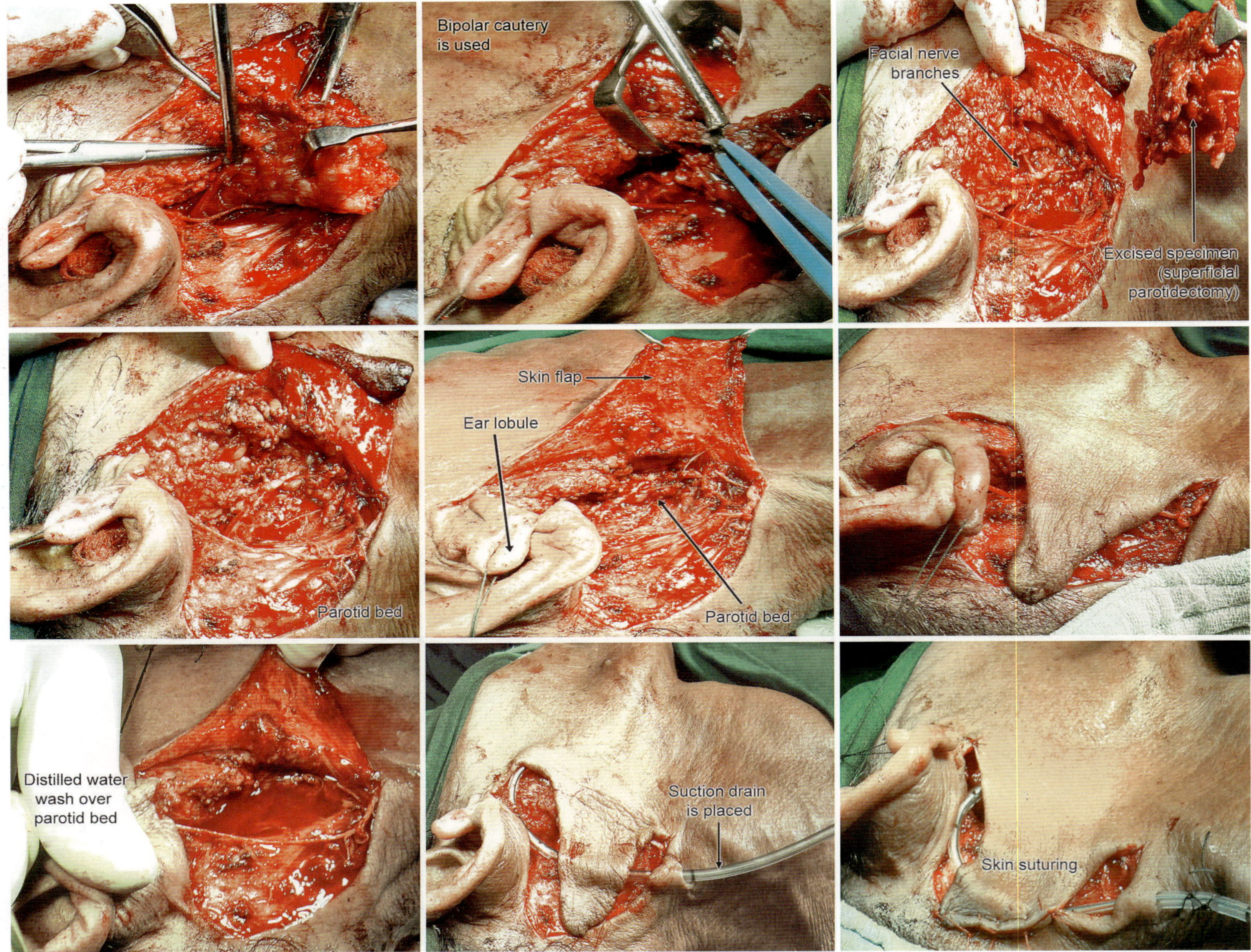

Figs. 17-22(2)

Figs. 17-22(1 and 2): Technique of parotidectomy.

Bleeding from capillary vessels should be stopped by the pressure of wet gauze, as some blood vessels are distributed along with the nerve. The facial nerve is readily damaged if artery forceps are used for haemostasis. The dissection is continued in the other areas of the gland while attaining this haemostasis.

The bifurcation of the nerve is close to the retromandibular vein, and its fine branches should be ligated. Suction is used to achieve a clear surgical field. Any bleeding vessel should be carefully clipped or ligated.

The branching ducts of the gland must be distinguished from the facial nerve. The nerve is *white and shiny,* while the duct is *grey and dull.*

The parotid duct if ligated like done by many, in traditional superficial parotidectomy, then remaining deep lobe of parotid atrophies spontaneously. But it is possible to preserve the duct so that the saliva secreted from the parotid remnant will be made to extrude into mouth. So that partial function of the retained gland is achieved. It is important to ligate the interlobular ducts identified during the dissection carefully to prevent the formation of salivary fistula.

After parotidectomy, even though not practiced widely, parotid remnant is often sutured by absorbable sutures to achieve proper haemostasis and to prevent formation of salivary fistula. If the duct and function of the parotid remnant are to be preserved, deep sutures should be avoided in order to prevent ductal ligation.

The wound is irrigated with hypertonic saline/distilled water probably to destroy the spilled tumour cells. The integrity of the facial nerve is checked by finger pinch or nerve stimulator. If the nerve has been disrupted, an end to end anastomosis of the nerve is carried out or with suitable graft immediately.

Closed suction drainage is used with suction tube placed away from the dissected facial nerve to prevent damage to the nerve. Compression bandage is kept often for 3 days.

Deep lobe mass may appear as lateral oropharyngeal masses. Tail of the parotid mass mimics cervical lymph node. Common site of the parotid tumour is tail of the parotid.

Only FNAC and imaging (CT scan) are the investigations done for parotid tumour. Open biopsy is not done in parotid tumour.

Enucleation of the parotid tumour should not be done. This increases the risk of facial nerve injury, risk of tumour recurrence.

Loupe or microscope is useful in dissecting the branches especially in reoperation.

Nerve stimulator should be used judiciously otherwise it itself can cause neuropraxia.

Concepts in parotidectomy

Operating microscope increases the clarity of facial nerve dissection. ***Three dimensional exoscopes*** which is very popular in ENT surgery would be very useful in dissecting the parotid from facial nerve as it gives higher resolution three dimensional images with more degree of freedom of movement facilitating the proper identification and preservation of branches of facial nerve.
Bipolar is used for haemostasis; avoid monopolar.
Wet gauze to apply pressure over the field.
Avoid pressure and unnecessary handling of the nerve.
Nerve monitoring can be done by asking a dedicated assistant to watch the face for twitches.
Intraoperative electrophysiological facial nerve monitor and/or hand-held nerve locator is useful.
Whenever nerve integrity monitor (NIM) is used, four electrodes are placed in the area of the temporal, zygomatic, buccal and marginal mandibular branches.
Nerve monitoring decreases the rate of immediate facial weakness; helps to localise the facial nerve; it is essential in extracapsular dissection (ECD) where facial nerve is not identified; decreases the chances of permanent postoperative facial nerve palsy.

Closure

Proper haemostasis is achieved using fine vicryl ligatures or bipolar cautery. Often it is of practice to pour distilled water in the parotid bed and keep it for few minutes to kill spilled tumour cells from the capsule. *Digastric flap* is often used to cover the area of facial nerve. Posterior belly of digastric is detached from its hyoid/pulley attachment and rotated upwards over the facial nerve and attached to zygoma. An *acellular dermal matrix graft* can be placed into the wound prior to the skin closure to cover the facial nerve trunk and auriculotemporal nerve area to prevent scar adhesion into the facial nerve trunk and formation of Frey's gustatory sweating. Suction drain is placed before closure which is removed in 3 days. Drain should not come into contact with the facial nerve main trunk. Skin is closed with interrupted polypropylene or polyethylene 4-zero or 3-zero sutures. Slight pressure dressing is often used **(Fig. 17-23)**.

Postoperative Care

Drain is removed in 48 hours. Facial expressions are observed for features of facial palsy. Temporary facial nerve paralysis is common in the postoperative period for which the surgeon should not worry. If closure of eyes is inadequate due to neuropraxia, repeated saline drops to eye and eye cover is needed to prevent exposure keratitis. Neuropraxia recovers in 4 weeks.

COMPLICATIONS OF PAROTIDECTOMY

Haemorrhage

It is rare, usually of venous origin and ooze from the bed. Major arterial injury is rare. When once haematoma develops, patient presents with swelling, pain, distress with blood in the drain.

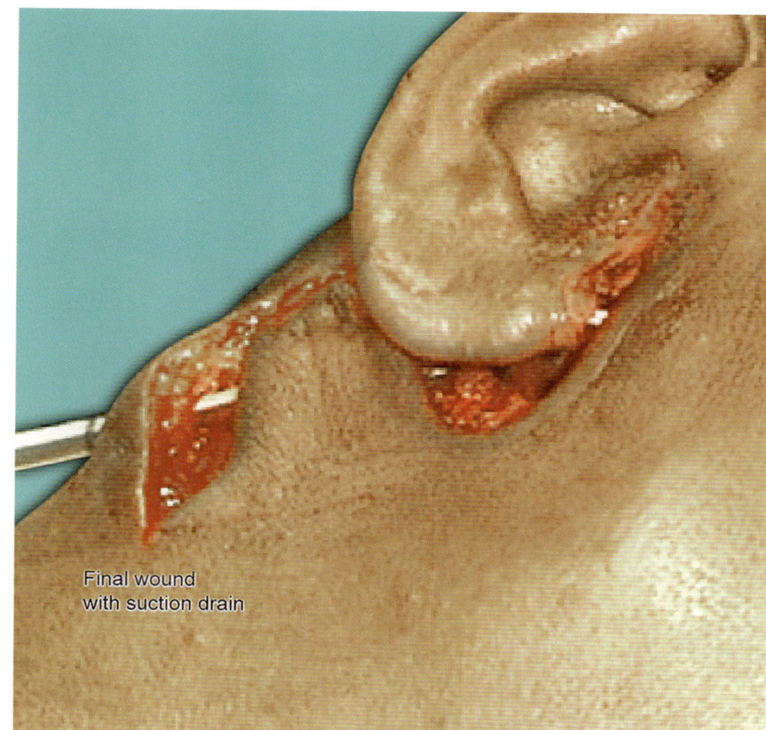

Fig. 17-23: Suction drain is placed after parotidectomy.

It is usually due to bleed from retromandibular vein or its tributaries. If haematoma is progressive then wound is reopened under general anaesthesia. Retromandibular vein is ligated both proximally and distally. Ligation of this vein causes ipsilateral facial oedema which gradually subsides in few weeks.

Facial Nerve Injury

It is the most important, common and worried complication. It may be a simple neuropraxia due to handling during dissection or nerve injury at various levels either of the main trunk in case of neoplastic conditions or few of branches. *Incidence* of temporary facial nerve palsy due to neuropraxia is 40%; whereas permanent palsy is 4%. *Features* are—inability to close the eyelid, difficulty in blowing and clenching; drooping of angle of the mouth; obliteration of nasolabial fold; loss of forehead wrinkles; wide palpebral fissure and epiphora. Effects of temporary facial nerve injury/neuropraxia will recover in few days to few weeks (12 weeks). Oral or intravenous steroids with vitamin B_1 and B_{12} injection are often tried. Permanent facial nerve injury needs specialised methods to correct the deformity. Nerve grafting is done using greater auricular, sural, lateral cutaneous or hypoglossal nerves. It needs operating microscope and is done using 6-zero polypropylene sutures. Angle of mouth can be suspended to zygomatic bone using temporal facial sling. Corneal ulceration is prevented using lateral tarsorrhaphy. Epiphora is controlled by reconstruction of medial canthus. Dynamic surgery like neurovascular muscle graft can also be used **(Fig. 17-24)**.

The House–Brackmann Score

It is a score to grade the degree of nerve damage in facial nerve palsy. The measurement is done by measuring the upward movement of the middle portion of the top of the eyebrow, and the outward movement of the angle of the mouth. Each reference point scores 1 point for each 0.25 cm movement, up to a maximum of 1 cm.

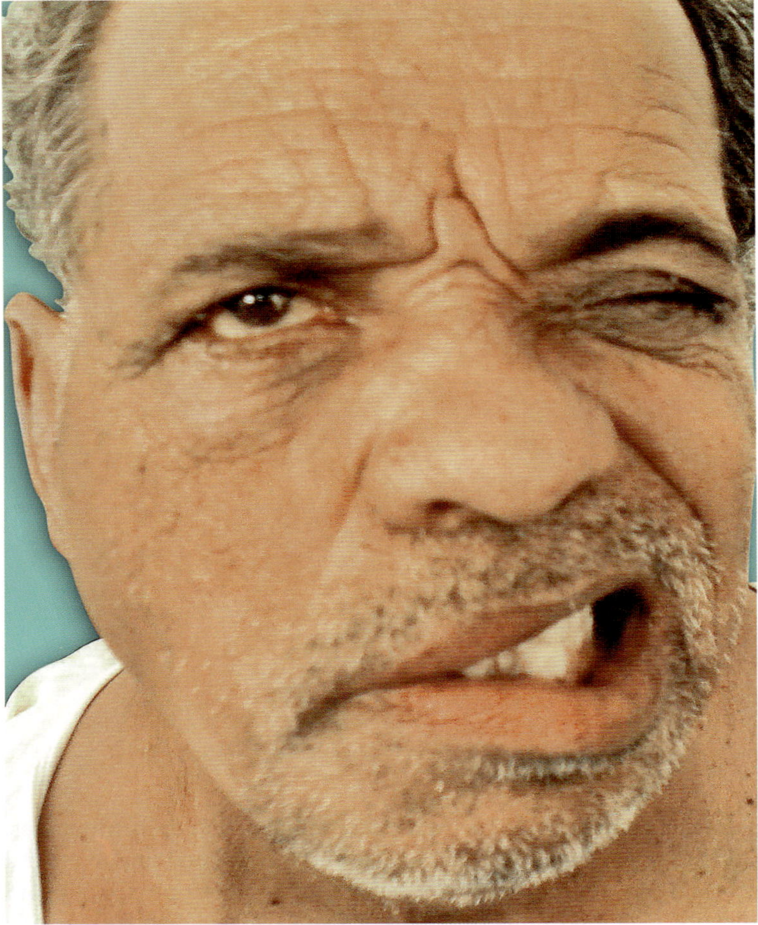

Fig. 17-24: Facial nerve palsy after parotidectomy.

The scores are then added together, to give a number out of 8. It is a measure of the range of intentional movement of the patient's facial muscles. It is based largely on the observations of the physician as a subjective scale. So there may be discrepancies between assessments by different clinicians. But overall reliability is good and is the most commonly used scale. Electroneuronography is the other method used **(Fig. 17-25)**.

Grade	*Description*	*Measurement*	*Function %*	*Estimated function %*
I	Normal	8/8	100	100
II	Slight	7/8	76–99	80
III	Moderate	5/8–6/8	51–75	60
IV	Moderately severe	3/8–4/8	26–50	40
V	Severe	1/8–2/8	1–25	20
VI	Total	0/8	0	0

Surgeries for facial nerve palsy

- Static
  - Suspension surgeries using temporal fascia
  - Correction of medial canthus
  - Lateral tarsorrhaphy to prevent exposure keratitis
  - Upper lid gold weights to protect cornea.
- Dynamic
  - Muscle transfer—temporal to masseter
  - Free muscle graft like gracilis muscle neurovascular transfer
  - Cross facial nerve transplant from opposite facial nerve to injured facial nerve using sural nerve
  - Nerve grafts.

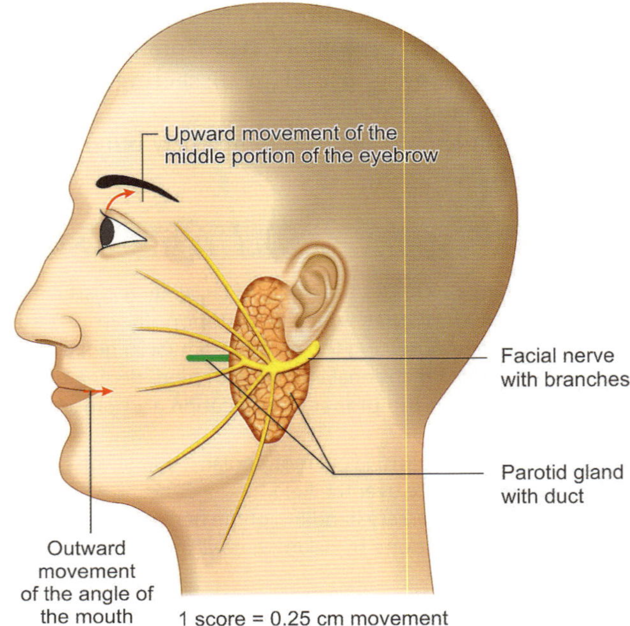

Fig. 17-25: Diagram showing how to look for House–Brackmann score.

Local Accumulation of Saliva under the Wound and Salivary Fistula Formation

It can occur in superficial parotidectomy as deep lobe is retained. This often subsides on itself. Aspiration of collected saliva and compression dressing is usually sufficient. Atropine is useful. Avoidance of spicy and acidic food; injection atropine 0.3 mg 30 minutes prior to food intake is helpful. Repair or reinsertion of duct into the oral mucosa can be done. *Newman-Seabrock's operation*—a probe is passed into the parotid duct through the opening in the mouth. Another probe is passed through the fistula. Duct and fistula are dissected over the probe. After removal of the fistula track severed duct ends are identified; and ends are trimmed. Probes are removed. A tantalum wire is passed into the duct across the severed ends and duct is sutured over it using 4-zero vicryl. Tantalum stent is removed after 3 weeks. If still persists, auriculotemporal nerve which supplies secretomotor component of parotid is cut. If there is stenosis at the orifice of the Stenson's duct, papillotomy at the orifice may help. Total conservative parotidectomy is done in failed cases.

Loss of Sensation of Ear Lobule

It is due to cutting of the great auricular nerve. Numbness of ear lobule causes difficulty in wearing earring. It slowly subsides and ear lobule gains its sensation in 1½ to 2 years. It can be prevented by preserving greater auricular nerve or its posterior branch.

Flap Necrosis

It is not uncommon. It usually heals on its own.

Frey's Syndrome

It is also called as *auriculotemporal syndrome or gustatory sweating (Lucie Frey—Polish Surgeon, 1923)*. It is probably due to injury to auriculotemporal nerve wherein postganglionic parasympathetic fibres from the otic ganglion become united to sympathetic nerves from the superior cervical ganglion creating pseudosynapsis.

Auriculotemporal nerve has got two branches. Auricular branch supplies external acoustic meatus, tympanic membrane surface, skin of auricle above external acoustic meatus. Temporal branch supplies hairy skin of the temple. Sweating and hyperaesthesia occurs in this area of skin. Whenever salivation is stimulated or during mastication, flushing, sweating, pain and hyperaesthesia occur in this area of skin. Involved skin is painted with iodine and dried. Dry starch applied over this area will turn blue in Frey's syndrome due to more sweat (*Minor's starch iodine test*). It is usually treated with conservative treatment with reassurance, drugs like antiperspirants like aluminium chloride, injection of botulinum toxin to skin, topical scopolamine. 10% of such patients later need surgical intervention. Tympanic branch of glossopharyngeal nerve below the round window of middle ear is cut—*intratympanic parasympathetic neurectomy (Jacobsen)*. Condition can be prevented by raising skin flap deep to platysma or deep to parotid fascia or by placing sterno-cleidomastoid/posterior belly of digastric or temporal fascia or artificial membranes over parotid bed.

Other Complications

First bite syndrome: Painful spasm of parotid region during first bite of meals. It slowly subsides but sometimes may persist to certain extent. It is mainly occurs in deep lobe dissection in parapharyngeal space causing sympathetic denervation of the parotid. Carbamazepine may help.

Amputation neuroma at transacted site of great auricular nerve; it is excised if symptomatic like pain, tender swelling.

Trismus can occur which is self-limiting; it is due to inflammatory masseter spasm; anti-inflammatory drugs are helpful.

Surgical site depression often recovers in due course of time; but autologous fat graft can be beneficial.

DRAINAGE OF PAROTID ABSCESS

Parotid abscess being within the tense parotid fascia will not show fluctuation and fluctuations should not be awaited. Brawny induration with tenderness over the parotid is diagnostic; often with trismus.

It is drained followed by under *general anaesthesia* (intubation may be difficult if there is trismus) with a small *vertical* skin incision in front of the tragus with a *transverse* incision/*split* on the parotid fascia to allow pus to drain. Sinus forceps is used to break the loculi; pus should be sent for culture. Facial nerve should not be injured. Irrigation of the cavity with normal saline and packing is needed. Facial nerve palsy and salivary fistula are the *complications* **(Fig. 17-26)**.

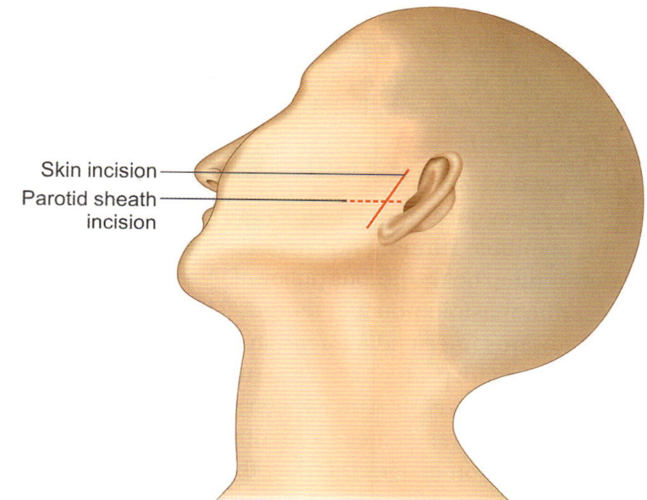

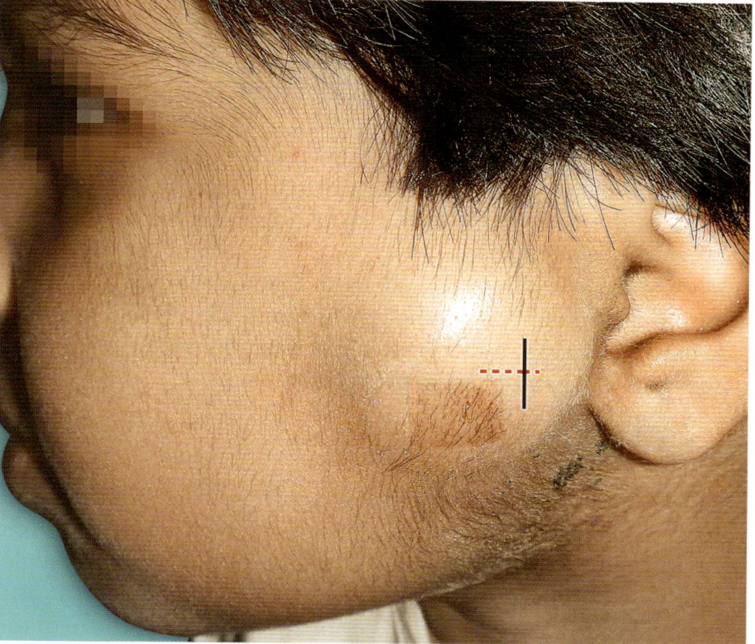

Fig. 17-26: Incision for parotid abscess. Vertical skin incision and horizontal parotid sheath incision.

SUBMANDIBULAR SALIVARY GLAND

It is J shaped salivary gland situated in the anterior part of the digastric triangle which is indented by posterior border of the mylohyoid with larger part located superficial to it and smaller part deep to it.

Submandibular region extends 1.5 cm above the base of the mandible and below to the greater cornu of the hyoid bone. Gland is marked outside as an oval area over posterior half of the base of the mandible and posterior border of the ramus.

Superficial lobe fills the digastric triangle extending above to mylohyoid line deep to mandible. Superficial lobe is covered by superficial and deep lamina of deep fascia of neck; deep lamina is attached to mylohyoid line; superficial lamina is attached to base of the mandible. Inferior surface is covered with skin, platysma, cervical branch of facial nerve, deep fascia, facial vein and submandibular lymph glands. Medial surface is related to mylohyoid muscle, vessels and nerve anteriorly; hyoglossus, styloglossus, lingual nerve, submandibular ganglion and hypoglossal nerve in the middle; styloglossus, stylohyoid ligament, 9th (glossopharyngeal) nerve and wall of pharynx.

Smaller deep lobe lies deep to mylohyoid and superficial to hyoglossus and styloglossus, continuing posteriorly with superficial part after winding round the posterior border of mylohyoid muscle. Anterior end of deep lobe is close to sublingual gland.

Wharton's submandibular salivary gland duct is 5 cm long with thin wall begins at the anterior end of deep part of the gland running over hyoglossus muscle between lingual and hypoglossal nerves. Duct is crossed by lingual nerve at the anterior border of the hyoglossus muscle; it later opens on the floor of the mouth on the side of frenulum of tongue on the summit of the sublingual papilla.

Secretomotor fibres of submandibular salivary gland: Preganglionic fibres from *superior salivary nucleus* → facial nerve → chorda tympani nerve → lingual nerve → *Langley's* submandibular ganglion → postganglionic fibres → submandibular and sublingual salivary glands **(Figs. 17-27 to 17-29)**.

Suprahyoid muscles are:

Digastric muscle has got anterior belly which arises from the digastric fossa of the mandible running downwards and backwards towards intermediate tendon on the fibrous pulley of the hyoid bone; posterior belly arises from mastoid notch of temporal bone runs forward and downwards towards intermediate tendon. Anterior belly is supplied by nerve to mylohyoid; posterior belly is supplied by facial nerve.

Stylohyoid muscle arises from posterior surface of the styloid process to insert into the greater cornu of hyoid bone at its junction to the body. Its tendon is perforated by the tendon of the posterior belly of digastric muscle. It is supplied by facial nerve.

Mylohyoid is triangular muscle arising from mylohyoid line of mandible runs medially downwards to get inserted to body of hyoid bone and median raphe in the midline, connecting to opposite mylohyoid muscle, forms floor of the mouth. It is supplied by nerve to mylohyoid.

Geniohyoid muscle arises from genial tubercles/inferior mental spine runs backwards and downwards to insert on the anterior surface of the body of the hyoid bone. It is supplied by C1 nerve through hypoglossal nerve.

Hyoglossus arises from entire length of greater cornua and lateral part of the hyoid bone running upwards and forwards to attach to side of tongue between styloglossus and inferior longitudinal muscle of the tongue. It is supplied by hypoglossal nerve.

Facial Artery

It was earlier called as *external maxillary artery* arises from external carotid artery just above the tip of greater cornu of hyoid bone (just above the origin of the lingual artery) in the carotid triangle. It shows tortuous course running beneath the digastric and stylohyoid muscles, grooving posterior surface of the groove of the submandibular salivary gland in front of hypoglossal nerve. It curves over the body of the mandible at anteroinferior angle of the masseter muscle, running across the cheek to the angle of the mouth, side of the nose, medial commissure of the eye to end as angular artery. Its tortuosity in neck and face allows movements of pharynx, mandible, cheek and lips. In the neck it lies on middle and superior constrictors of pharynx. In the face it is deep to platysma, risorius, and zygomaticus major but superficial to buccinator and levator labii superioris. Anterior facial vein is posterolateral to the facial artery in the face; but anterior to facial artery in neck. It communicates with dorsal nasal artery of internal carotid artery.

Branches of facial artery are—*in the neck:* ascending palatine artery, tonsillar artery, submental artery, glandular branches; *in the face*: inferior and superior labial arteries, lateral nasal branch (to nasalis) and terminal *angular* artery. Most of the facial muscles are supplied by facial artery.

One has to remember that *transverse facial artery* is a branch of *superficial temporal artery* (not from facial artery) while in the parotid gland. It runs horizontally in the substance of parotid gland, between parotid duct and lower border of zygomatic arch resting on the masseter to supply parotid gland and duct and anastomose with facial, masseteric, buccinator and infraorbital arteries.

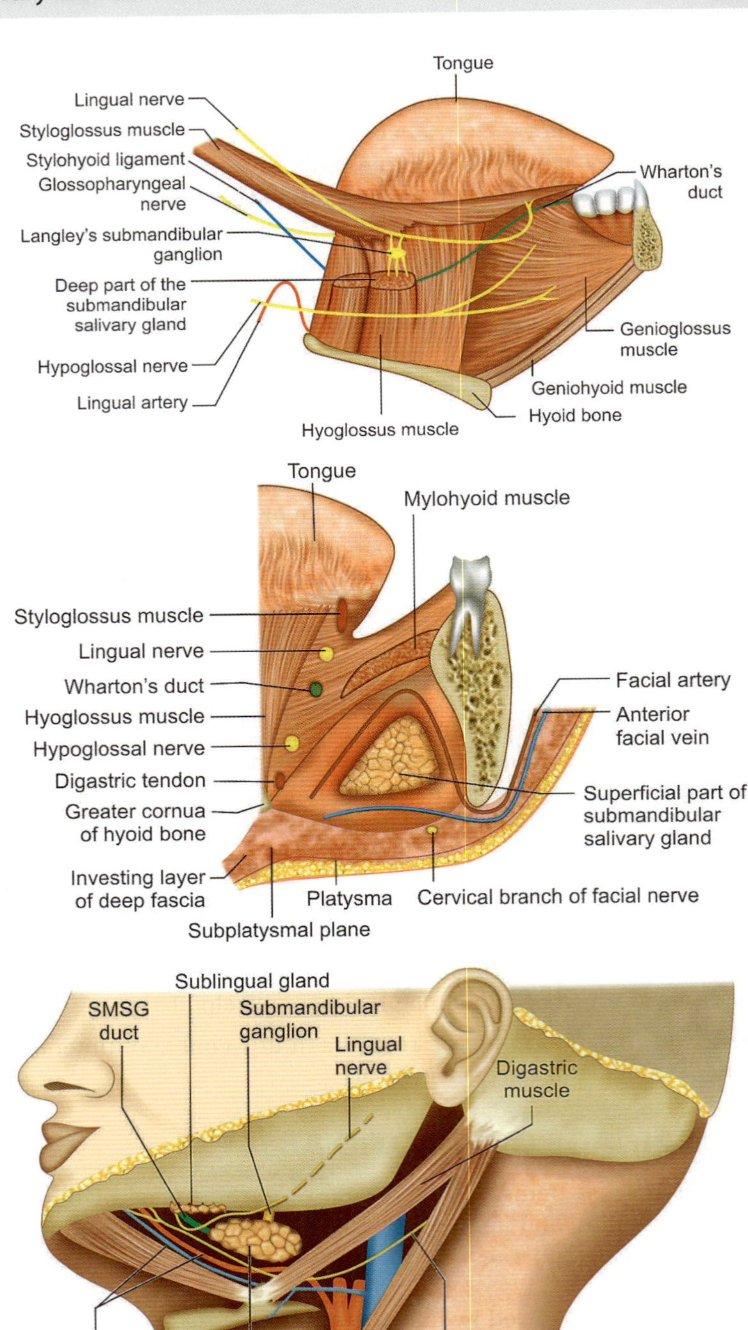

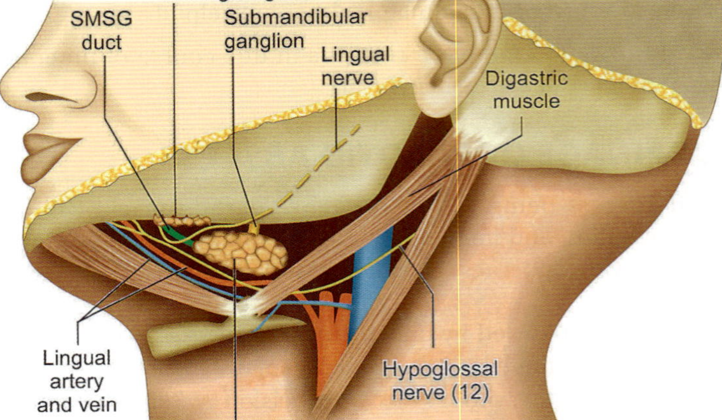

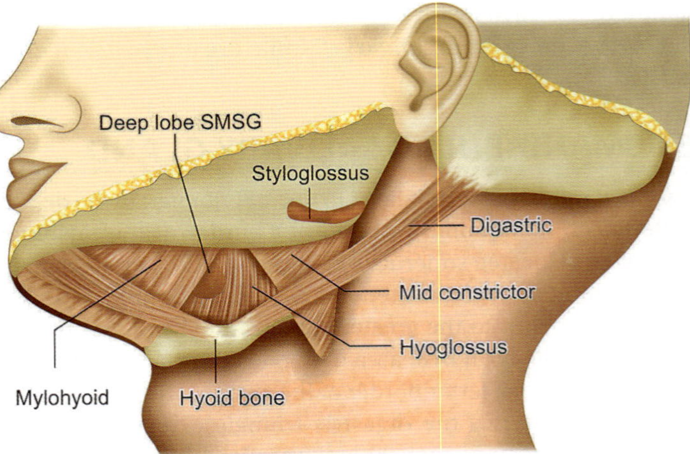

Fig. 17-27: Surgical anatomy of submandibular salivary gland (SMSG).

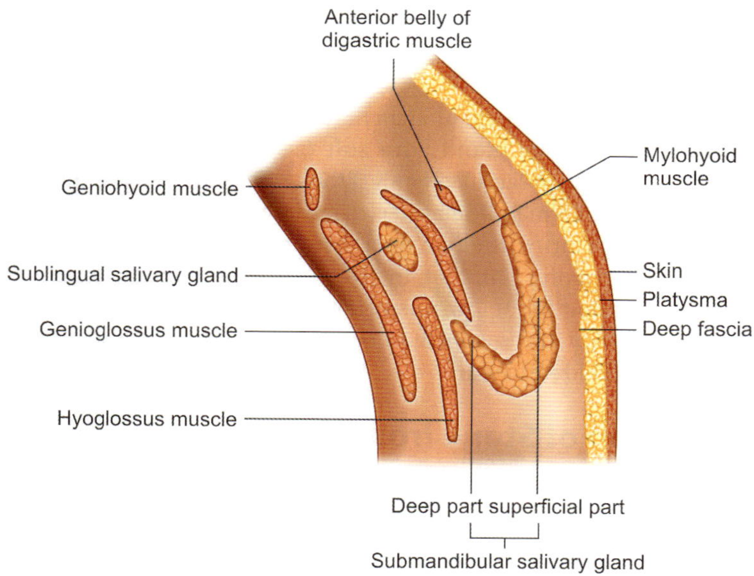

Fig. 17-28: Relations of the submandibular salivary gland.

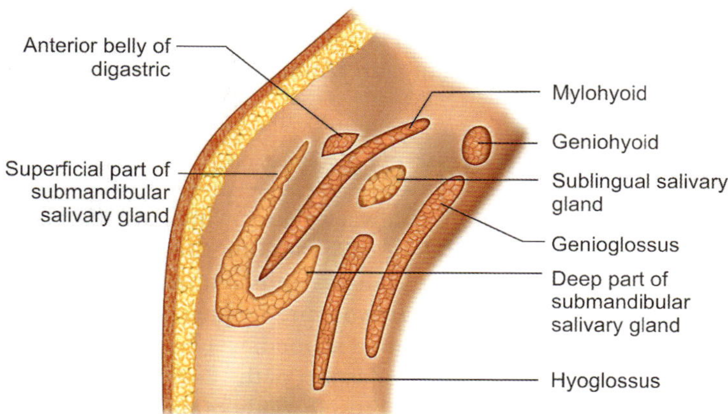

Fig. 17-29: Submandibular and sublingual salivary glands and their muscular relations.

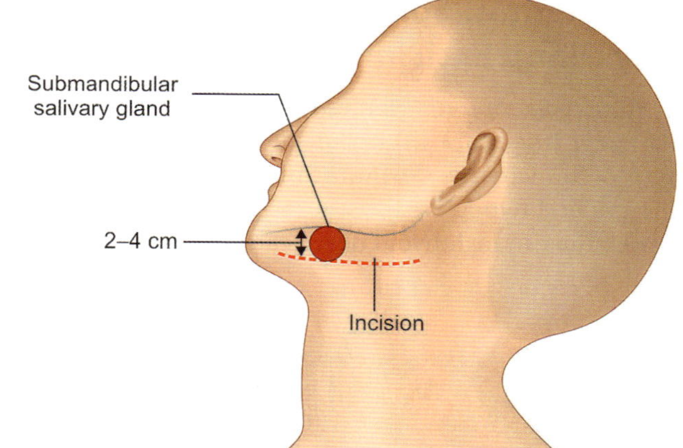

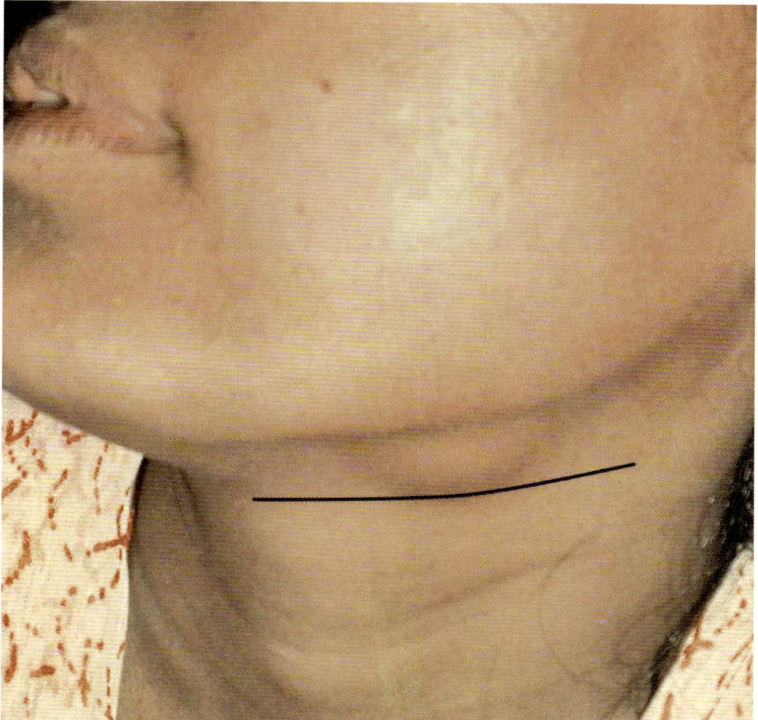

Fig. 17-30: Incision for submandibular salivary gland excision.

Excision of the Submandibular Salivary Gland

It is done under *general* anaesthesia. Neck should be *extended* with chin towards opposite side. *Incision* of 6–8 cm length is made 2–4 cm below and parallel to margin of the mandible **(Fig. 17-30)**.

Marginal mandibular nerve is in subplatysmal plane in neck; incision should be deepened *across* deep fascia *without* raising subplatysmal plane to avoid injury to this nerve. *Anterior facial vein (facial vein anterior tributary of common facial vein)* crossing the superficial part of the gland is ligated using silk or vicryl. Superficial lobe of the gland is exposed fully in *digastric triangle* between two bellies of digastric and stylohyoid muscles below and margin of the mandible above with gland overlapping over mylohyoid muscle medially. Deep fascia of neck covering the gland is visible. Common facial vein with its anterior (facial vein) and posterior (anterior division of retromandibular vein) tributaries are visible deep to deep fascia in close relation to sternocleidomastoid muscle. Few lymph nodes may be present outer to deep fascia also. Dissection begins at the lower end of the gland by incising the fascia just above the digastric muscle. Superficial lobe of the gland is mobilised upwards. *Facial artery* lies in the groove on the deeper aspect of the gland, often either embedding in the gland or runs around the gland with a variable course and so artery has to be ligated twice above anteriorly and below posteriorly. Posterior part of the artery is ligated first using silk or vicryl ligatures. While reflecting the gland upwards from posterior surface hyoglossus with *hypoglossal nerve* is seen and nerve is safeguarded. Hypoglossal nerve at lower part which lies very close to the digastric tendon which is accompanied with lingual vein (*lingual vein* should be ligated) and *lingual nerve* at upper part is identified and safeguarded. Mylohyoid muscle is retracted so as to remove the deep portion of the gland which is in front of the hyoglossus and mylohyoid. Submandibular ganglion is often seen just above the gland which can be sacrificed. Identification of Wharton's duct and ligation is done. Dissection is done using fine scissor and monopolar cautery. Closer to nerves, it is better to use bipolar cautery instead of monopolar especially whenever there is lot of adhesions due to chronic inflammation. *Chronic inflammation* with fibrosis makes dissection difficult risking the injury of hypoglossal and lingual nerves. *Structures in view* after elevation of the submandibular salivary gland are—lingual nerve, chorda tympani, submandibular ganglion and Wharton's duct above; hypoglossal nerve, digastric and stylohyoid muscles below **(Fig. 17-31)**.

Complications of Submandibular Salivary Gland Excision

Complications of submandibular salivary gland excision include: Haemorrhage; infection; injury to marginal mandibular nerve (drooping of saliva with deviation of the angle of the mouth), lingual nerve and hypoglossal nerve (deviation of tongue towards same side); injury to mylohyoid nerve causing anaesthesia over the submental skin.

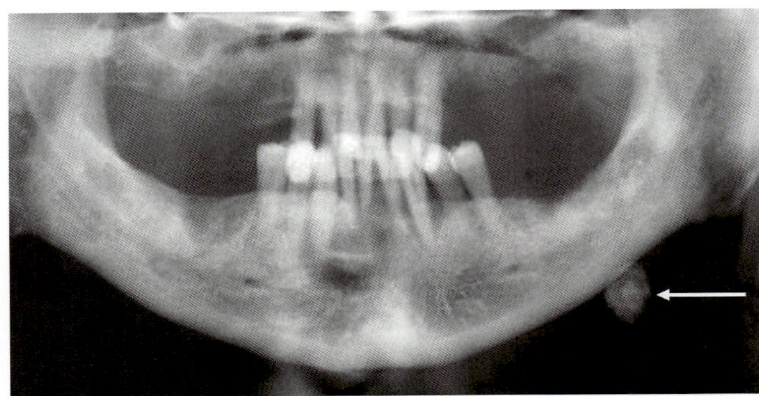

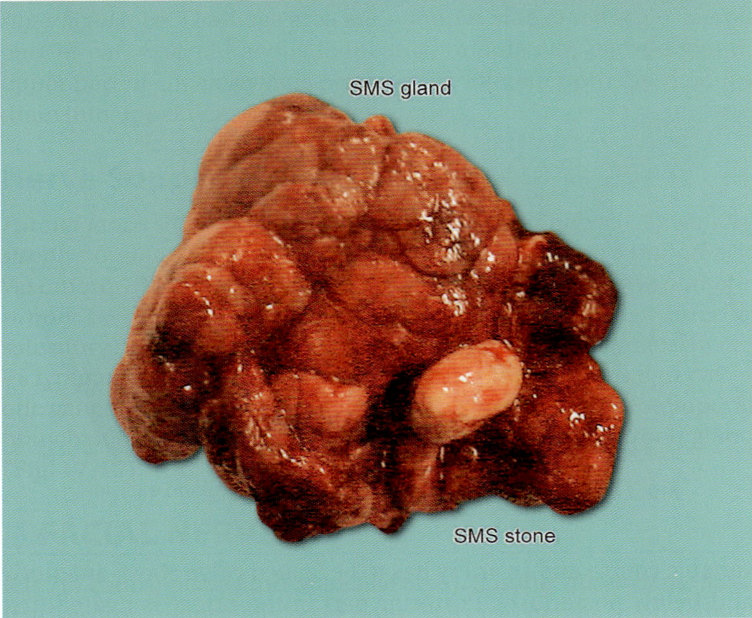

Fig. 17-31: Submandibular salivary (SMS) gland stone on X-ray and gross specimen after excision. Here excision of the gland through external approach is the treatment.

Radical Excision of Submandibular Salivary Gland

Radical excision is done in malignant tumours of the submandibular salivary gland. Here gland with soft tissues aound is removed. However, nerves are sacrificed only if they are infiltrated. It is difficult to retain marginal mandibular nerve in these patients as oncological clearance is priority. Radical neck lymph node dissection is also usually added along with that. Incision is same but much lengthier; it is often extended below posteriorly on the anterior margin of the trapezius or in the centre of the incision if neck dissection is additional added procedure.

Extraction of Stone from the Submandibular Salivary Duct (Wharton's)

Stone in the Wharton's duct is removed per orally under local anaesthesia. Intraoral X-ray or orthopantomogram is done prior to that. Stay suture using 4-zero vicryl is placed on the duct proximal to the stone. A fine dilator or probe is inserted into the duct opening. Longitudinal incision is placed on the duct over the stone. Stone is extracted using fine haemostat. Saline wash is used to clean the duct and clear any debris. Duct is not sutured instead left open into the oral cavity. Patient is sent with antibiotic coverage **(Figs. 17-32 and 17-33)**.

MINOR SALIVARY GLANDS

There are around 450 minor salivary glands which are distributed in lips, cheeks, palate and floor of the mouth. Glands also may be present in oropharynx, larynx, trachea and paranasal sinuses. They contribute to 10% of total salivary volume. *Sublingual salivary glands* are minor salivary glands (almond shaped, weighs 4 gram) one on each side; located in the anterior aspect of the floor of the mouth in relation to mucosa, mylohyoid muscle, body of the mandible near mental symphysis, lateral to genioglossus muscle. Gland drains directly into mucosa through small ducts around or through a duct which drains into submandibular duct. This duct is called as *Bartholin duct.* Mikulicz's disease is common in sublingual salivary gland. Minor salivary glands are *not present* in gingivae and anterior portion of the hard palate.

Incision biopsy of minor salivary gland tumour is done under general anaesthesia if it is posterior. Wide excision of minor salivary gland tumour is done under general anaesthesia with nasal intubation. Wide mouth gag is placed to oral cavity for retraction of jaws. Lesion is excised with 1 cm clearance up to the mucoperiosteum

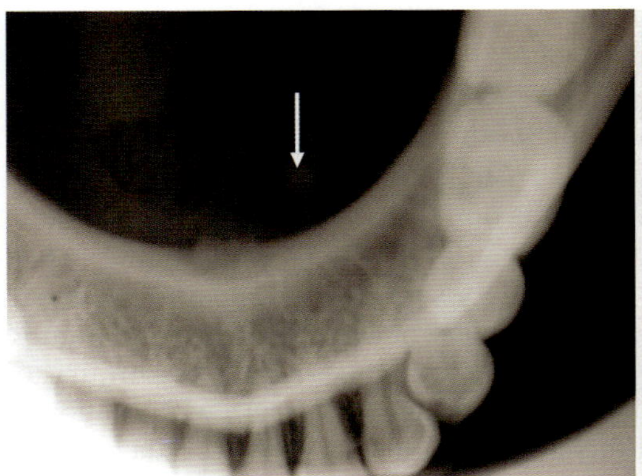

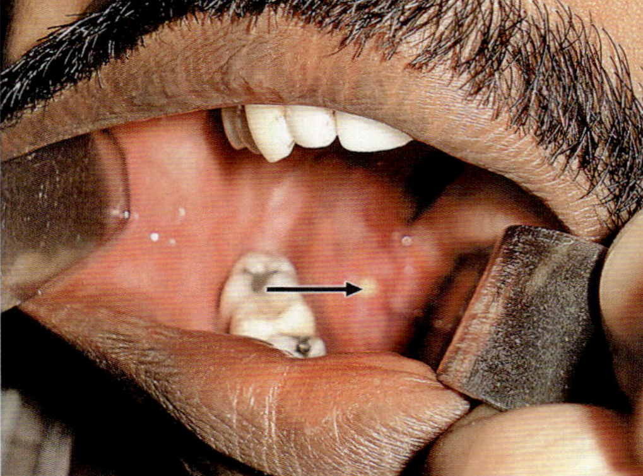

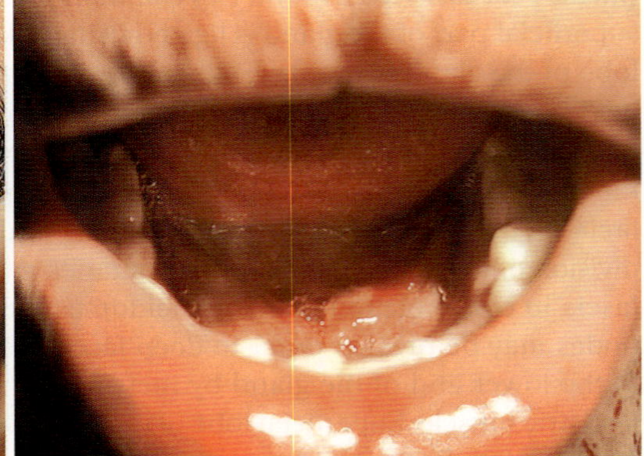

Fig. 17-32: Submandibular salivary duct (Wharton's) stone on X-ray and on clinical examination.

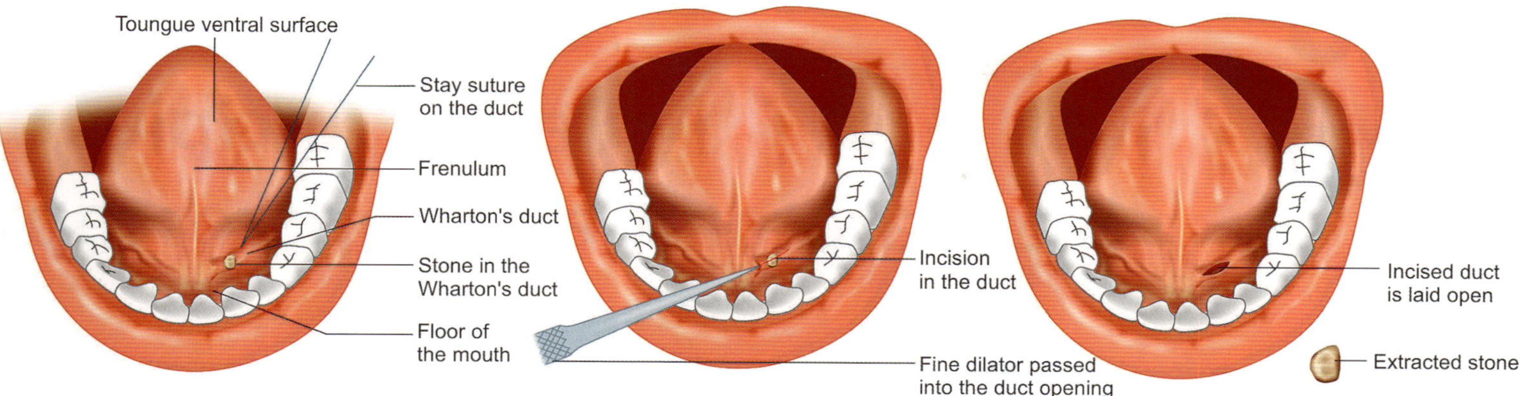

Fig. 17-33: Technique of extraction of submandibular salivary duct (Wharton's) stone extraction.

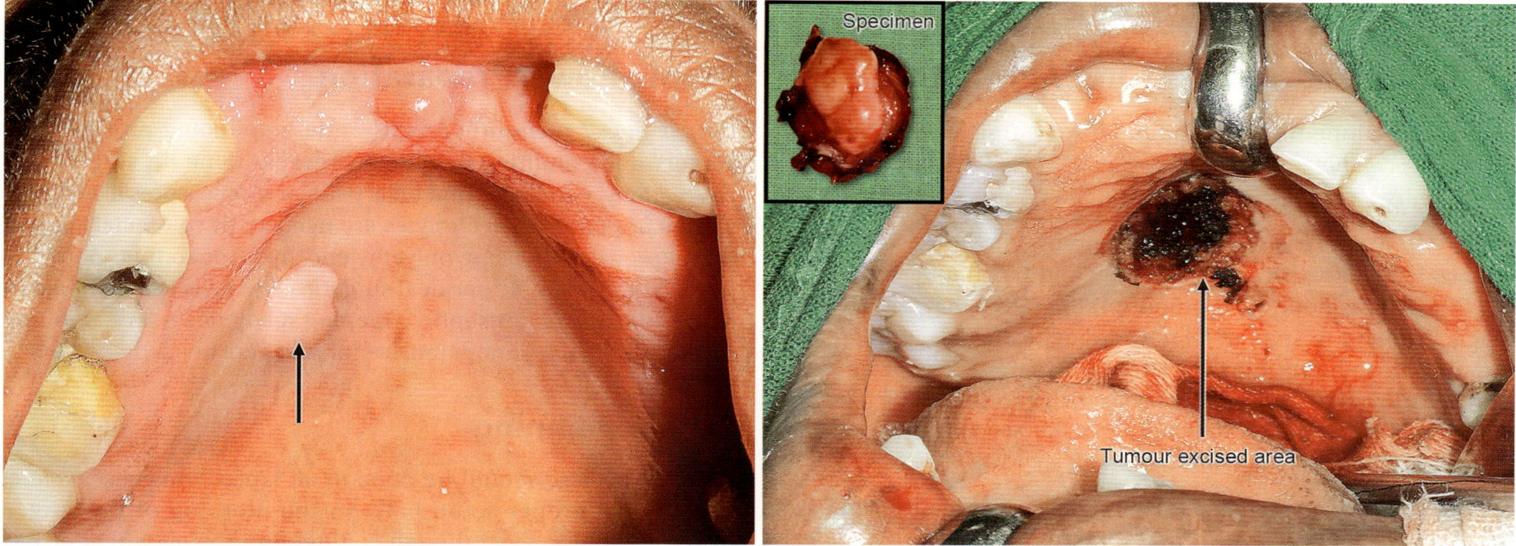

Fig. 17-34: Minor salivary gland tumour. It needs incision biopsy. It is excised as—wide excision under general anaesthesia. Raw area usually granulates and heals by epithelialisation. Larger defect needs reconstruction. Deeper infiltrating tumours need maxillectomy.

when lesion is in the palate. Raw area is allowed to granulate and heal. If palate is involved by disease, palate is excised. Later proper reconstruction is done with the help of reconstructive surgeon **(Fig. 17-34)**.

ECTOPIC SALIVARY GLAND

Ectopic salivary gland also called as aberrant salivary gland/migrant salivary gland is nothing but ectopic lobe of the juxtaposed salivary gland. It is commonly seen in relation to submandibular salivary gland. Commonest ectopic salivary tissue is *Stafne bone cyst*. It is invagination of the juxtaposed submandibular salivary gland into the mandible bone on its lingual aspect. X-ray shows radiolucent area due to the cyst below the angle of the mandible, lower to inferior dental vessels and nerve. Jaws, eyelids, middle ear, paranasal sinus, nose, rarely skin of face and neck are other sites wherein ectopic salivary tissue can be demonstrated.

18

CHAPTER

Basic Principles in Laparotomy and Laparoscopy

GENERAL PRINCIPLES IN LAPAROTOMY

Laparotomy is opening the abdomen for surgical intervention. Laparotomy can be:

1. *Elective laparotomy*

Elective laparotomy wherein proper preoperative diagnosis has been established with various imaging and biochemical analysis. Even though it is done with proper preoperative diagnosis, being a magic box, and in spite of all newer diagnostic aids, finding and diagnosis on opening may be entirely different from what was thought during evaluation. At that stage surgeon should be ready to alter the treatment strategy depending on the need.

2. *Emergency laparotomy*

It is done in trauma and acute abdomen like peritonitis. Even here basic investigations like USG/CT abdomen and haematological assessment are done to proceed with laparotomy at the earliest. Midline vertical incision centred on the umbilicus with curve at umbilicus towards left side is done. This incision is called as *incision of indecision/registrar's incision*. It can be extended above or below easily depending on the need. It also can be extended horizontally if needed **(Figs. 18-1 and 18-2)**.

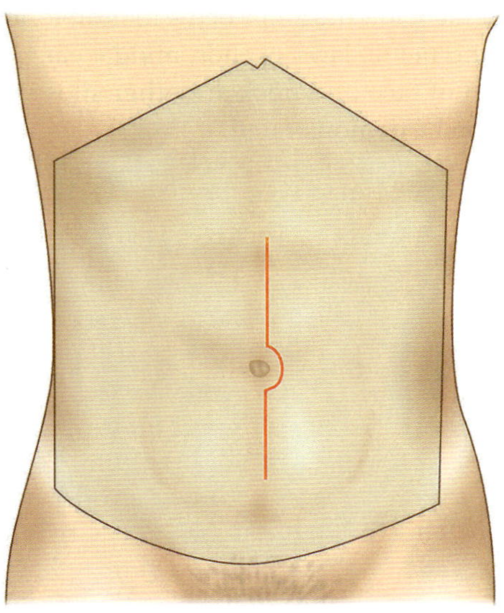

Fig. 18-1: Incision of indecision/registrar's incision.

Proper Bowel Preparation

Proper bowel preparation is essential depending on the type of surgery and condition to which surgery is done. In surgeries like gastrectomy, pancreatic and biliary surgeries, measures like stomach wash, correction of electrolytes are needed; in colorectal surgeries bowel preparation using polyethylene glycol or sodium phosphate is needed. For simple perineal surgeries enema is sufficient. Proper hydration, bowel antiseptics, keeping ready necessary amount of blood for surgery, perioperative antibiotics are needed.

Proper Planning

Proper planning should be done in all laparotomy cases. Patient should take proper scrub bath on the morning of the surgery. Skin preparation even though is done on previous night or early morning of the day of surgery, evidence suggests that it should be done on table.

Anaesthesia: General anaesthesia is required. Epidural supplement may be used. Spinal or epidural anaesthesia is sufficient for lower abdominal surgeries.

Position of the Patient

Position of the patient in laparotomy is very important. It may be—*supine*; supine with *one side tilt*; *lateral position* (for kidney/adrenal); *lithotomy position* (for APR/LAR/AR/perineal surgeries/cystoscopic procedures, etc); position for *thoracoabdominal* approach (in Ivor Lewis operation/diaphragmatic surgery/liver surgeries, etc). Head down position is needed in colorectal surgeries to keep small bowel away from surgical dissection field. For upper abdominal surgeries like cholecystectomy head up position is needed often with right up tilt. Strapping of the pelvis and chest wall to the table is needed in patients who need steep head down position.

Other Essential Needs and Principles

Nasogastric tube, urinary catheterisation, central venous line and often an arterial line (radial) is needed in major procedures. Often two or three venous lines are needed in major surgery and trauma patients. *Stockings* to both legs from foot to proximal thigh are essential to reduce the incidence of deep vein thrombosis (DVT).

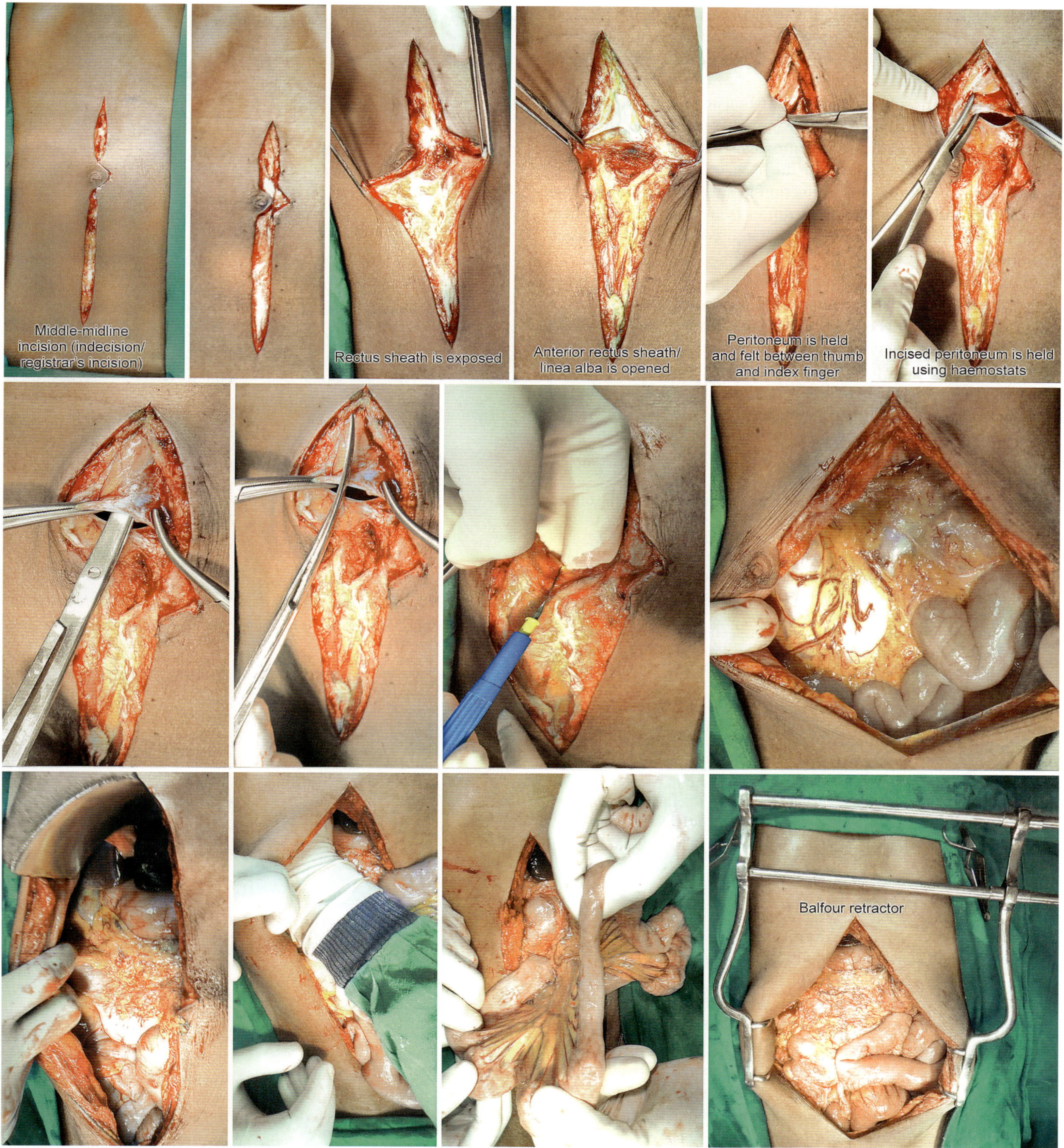

Fig. 18-2: Emergency laparotomy is done using middle-midline incision which can be extended above or below depending on need.

Right selection of the procedure; right way executing it with right principles at right time is important. Selection; execution; timing; implementing; skill are the essential features of successive surgery with best outcome.

Selection of incision; adequacy of incision; good retraction; exposure of the surgical field; proper dissection; no touch or minimum touch technique; haemostasis; on table decision in relation to surgical principles—are the basic need.

Anticipation of problems; perfection in surgical anatomy; tissue touch are important. Live anatomy differs from cadaveric or clinical anatomy (live anatomy bleeds and gets injured; cadaveric anatomy does not bleed).

In present era speedy surgery is not important; perfect proper surgery is more crucial. But then undue slowness should not be there, as it causes unnecessary increase in the anaesthesia and field exposure time. Accuracy is more important than speed in surgery.

Proper light; proper position; adequate height of the table; good assistants; avoiding repetitive movements; clean bloodless surgical field; knowing the next step—are needed.

Holding the instrument: Fingertip pressure (finger grip) is better to hold instruments than vise grip.
Incision is made using scalpel belly while keeping two fingers of the other hand apart.
Depth of the incision is assessed by feel and by vision.
During dissection traction by surgeon's other hand and counter traction by assistant's hand helps rapid separation/creation of the tissue planes.
Dissection can be done using scalpel, scissor, and cautery. It is done using cutting cautery. But cutting cautery may not be haemostatic. Haemostasis is achieved using coagulation cautery. Dissection using coagulation cautery will be haemostatic but causes boiling of fat, more tissue trauma leading into wound infection. Over coagulation of tissues during cautery dissection ideally should be avoided.
Tissues are held using forceps by gentle manoeuvre. Skin and tough structures are held using toothed forceps; soft, smooth, delicate structures should be held using non-toothed forceps.
Needle holder should be held between thumb and ring fingers to achieve rotation movement using wrist (not pushing movement). Index and middle fingers are used to steady the handle. Needle is laced at the junction of proximal 2/3rd and distal 1/3rd of the distal jaws **(Figs. 18-3 and 18-4)**.

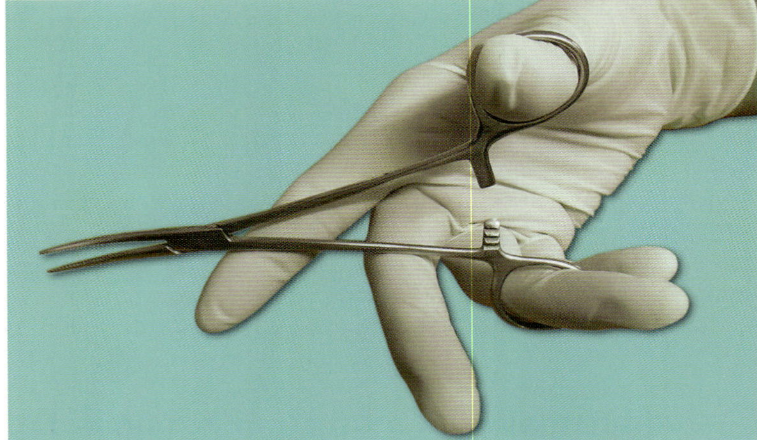

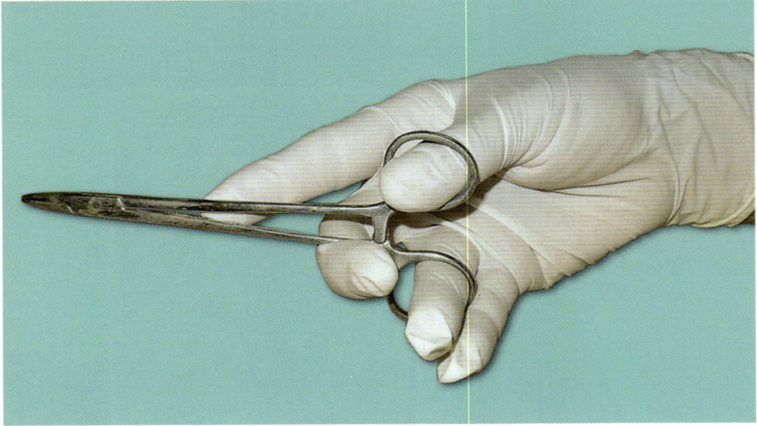

Fig. 18-3: Finger grip holding is better to hold the instrument than vise grip.

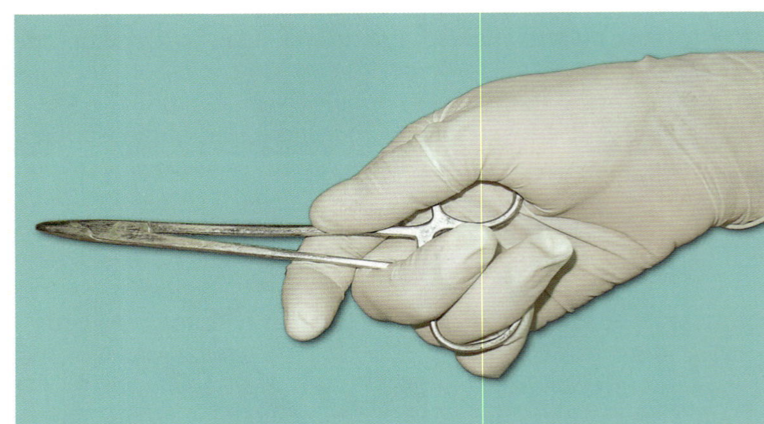

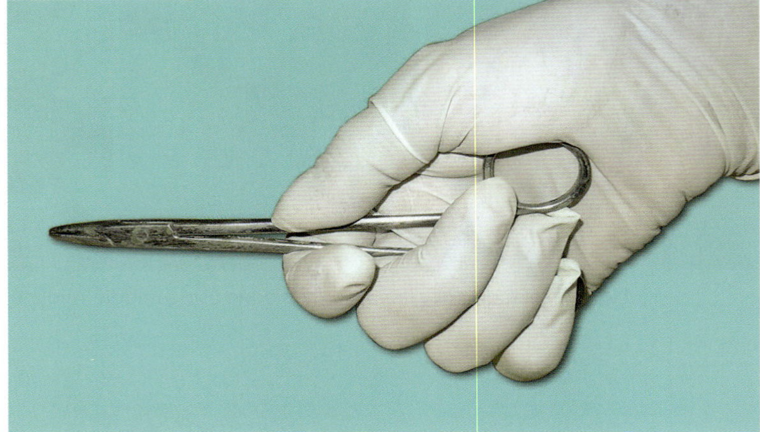

Fig. 18-4: Vise grip to hold the instrument. It is used when extra power is needed while using the instrument.

Cleaning and Draping

Cleaning is done using povidone iodine. Solution is collected in a sterile small bowl, sterile folded/rolled gauze or sponge with Rampley's sponge holding forceps is used to clean the abdomen. In perineal surgery after placing the patient in lithotomy position cleaning with proper scrubbing should be done by OT technician prior to formal cleaning by surgeon. Draping is done using sterile green towel. Often sterile plastic sheet (ioban sheet/plastic surgical adhesive drape/plastic incisive drape) is used on the abdomen over the green cloth drape and incision is made through it. Many studies show that plastic adhesive drape reduces the bacterial contamination of the wound and deeper part compared to cloth drape. There is controversy about pricking the towel clip into the skin of that particular corner point or placing interrupted skin sutures over the drape margins to fix it. It may break the barrier into the deeper plane away from the surgical site incision and it is not much confirmed that such fixation will reduce/prevent the bacterial contamination across **(Fig. 18-5)**.

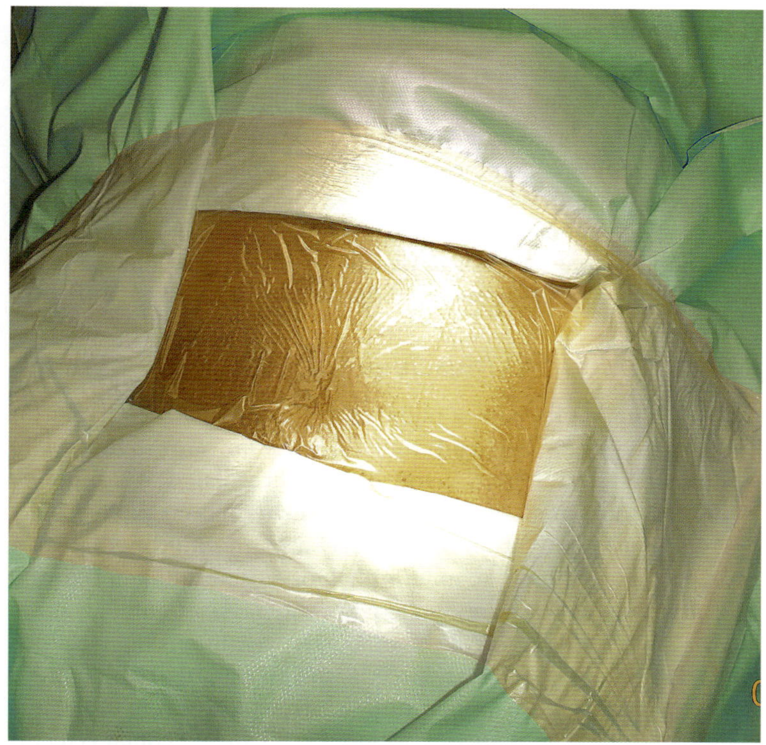

Fig. 18-5: Draping the surgical site using sterile towels.

Incision

Type of incision; possible need for extension of incision, direction of extension—all to be thought of prior to starting the incision.

Principles in abdominal surgery

- Adequate incision: Incision should be long enough for a good exposure.
- Splitting the muscle is better than cutting, except rectus muscle.
- Avoid cutting nerves and vessels in the abdominal wall.
- Adequate retraction: Retract muscle, abdominal organs towards the neurovascular supply.
- Adequate exposure of surgical site and surrounding field.
- Adequate meticulous dissection.
- Adequate haemostasis.
- Adequate proper closure; if required with a drain (tube). Insert a drainage tube through a separate incision.
- Transverse incisions are better than vertical incisions.

Requirements

- Accessibility.
- Extensibility.
- Security.

Surgical Anatomy of Abdominal Wall

Anterior Abdominal Wall

The anterior abdominal wall is a musculofascial dynamic structure which maintains intra-abdominal pressure for various physiological functions. It has got three paired flat muscles, two recti abdominis muscles and linea alba in midline. These are anteriorly related to skin, subcutaneous tissue and superficial fascia; posteriorly related to transversalis fascia and peritoneum. *External oblique fascia* (external layer of the fascia of external oblique muscle is also called as *innominate fascia of Gallaudet*) is thin fascial covering of external oblique muscle and fascia which forms intercrural fibres of the superficial inguinal ring; and it extends below into the scrotum as external spermatic fascia. *Anterior abdominal wall* has got anterolateral part which consists of external and internal oblique and transversus abdominis muscles; and a midline part containing rectus abdominis and pyramidalis muscles **(Fig. 18-6)**.

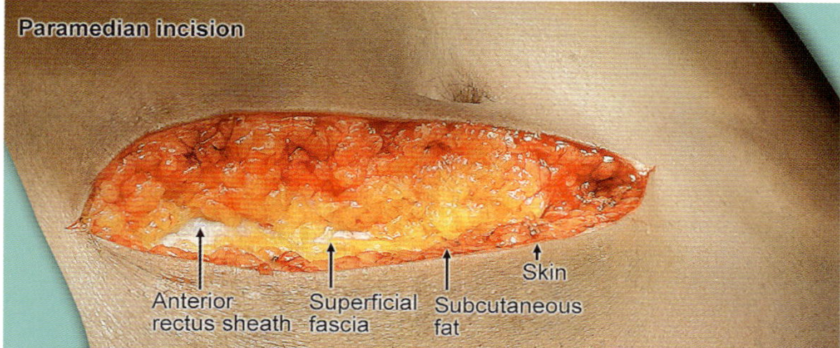

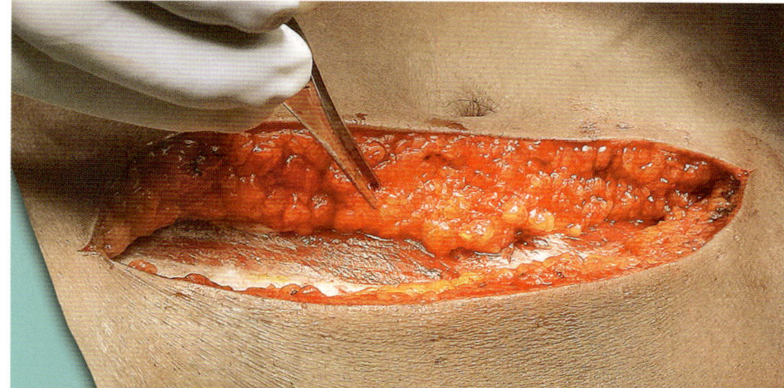

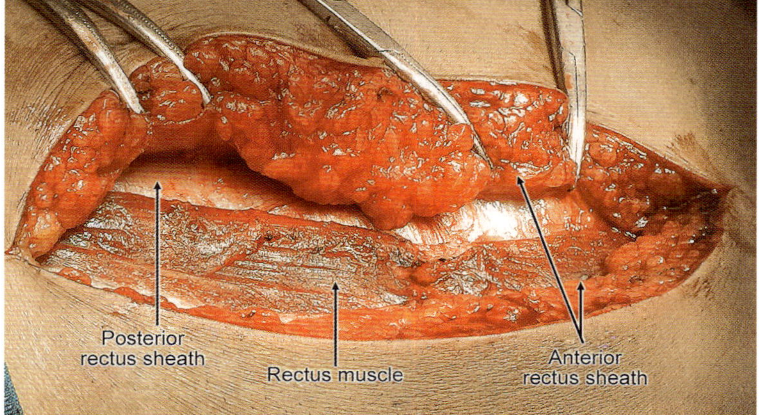

Fig. 18-6: Layers of the abdominal wall—as seen in paramedian incision.

External Oblique Muscle

It arises from middle of body of lower eight ribs running below/downwards, front/forwards and medially inserting into xiphoid process, linea alba, pubic symphysis, pubic crest, pectineal line of pubis and anterior 2/3rd of outer lip of the iliac crest. It is supplied by lower 6 thoracic nerves. Lower free border of the external oblique aponeurosis forms inguinal ligament. Triangular opening in its aponeurosis above the pubic crest is called as superficial inguinal ring **(Fig. 18-7)**.

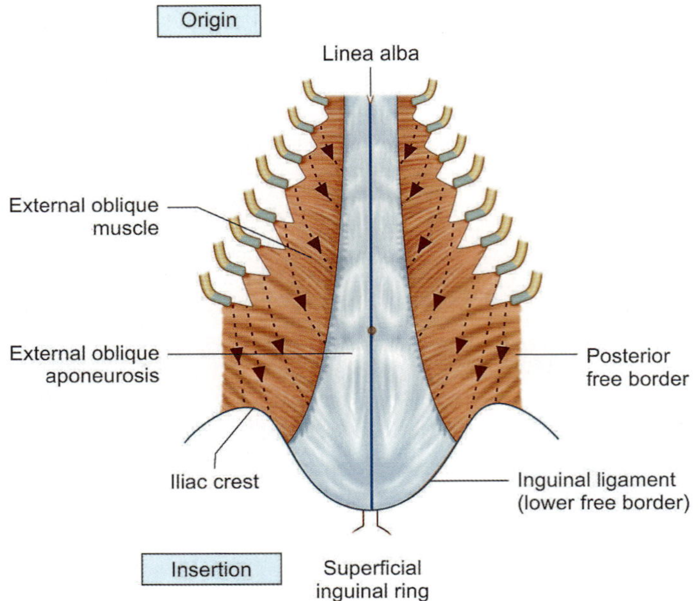

Fig. 18-7: External oblique muscle.

Internal Oblique Muscle

It arises from lateral 2/3rd of inguinal ligament, anterior 2/3rd of intermediate part of iliac crest, thoracolumbar fascia; runs upwards, forwards and medially to insert into lower 4 ribs and cartilages, xiphoid process, pubic crest, pectineal line of pubis. It is supplied by lower 6 thoracic nerves, 1st lumbar nerve. Aponeurosis below the level of umbilicus remains as a single layer forming the anterior rectus sheath and lineal alba. Above aponeurosis splits into anterior lamina which passes medially in front of rectus abdominis and posterior lamina which passes behind rectus abdominis which ends below midway between umbilicus and pubic symphysis as linea *semicircularis of Douglas* (arcuate line). *Semilunar line of Spieghel* lies in lateral border of the rectus sheath from pubic tubercle to the tip of the costal cartilage of 9th rib **(Fig. 18-8)**.

Transverse Abdominis Muscle

It originates from lateral 1/3rd of inguinal ligament, anterior 2/3rd of inner lip of iliac crest, thoracolumbar fascia, lower 6 cartilages with fibres running horizontally forwards inserting into an aponeurosis extending from xiphoid process, linea alba, pubic crest, pectineal line of pubis. Lowest fibres fuse with lowest fibres of internal oblique to form conjoined/conjoint tendon. It is supplied by lower 6 thoracic and first lumbar nerves. Neurovascular plane of abdomen lies between internal oblique and transverse abdominis muscles **(Fig. 18-9)**.

Rectus Abdominis Muscle

It arises from lateral part of pubic crest (lateral head) and anterior pubic ligament (medial head) runs vertically upwards to insert into xiphoid process and 7th, 6th and 5th costal cartilages. It is supplied by lower 6 thoracic nerves. There are three tendinous intersections one at xiphoid, one at umbilicus level and another one between two which are adherent to anterior half of muscle and anterior wall of rectus sheath. They are due to embryologic segmental origin of muscle which adds to the power of muscle. Tendinous intersections *do not extend* into the posterior rectus sheath **(Fig. 18-10)**.

Rectus sheath is an aponeurotic sheath which covers the rectus abdominis muscle in front and behind. Rectus sheath contains rectus abdominis muscle and pyramidalis in its lower part. Pyramidalis lies in front of the lower part of the rectus muscle. Superior epigastric artery enters the sheath by passing between the costal and xiphoid origins of the diaphragm crossing upper margin of transversus abdominis muscle behind the 7th costal cartilage running behind the rectus muscle in front of the posterior rectus sheath to anastomose with the inferior epigastric artery. Inferior epigastric artery enters the sheath behind the muscle by passing across the arcuate line. Superior and inferior epigastric veins also accompany the arteries. Terminal branches of the lower 5 intercostal nerves and subcostal nerve enter the sheath after piercing the posterior rectus sheath at its lateral part running in front of the epigastric vessels to pierce the rectus muscle.

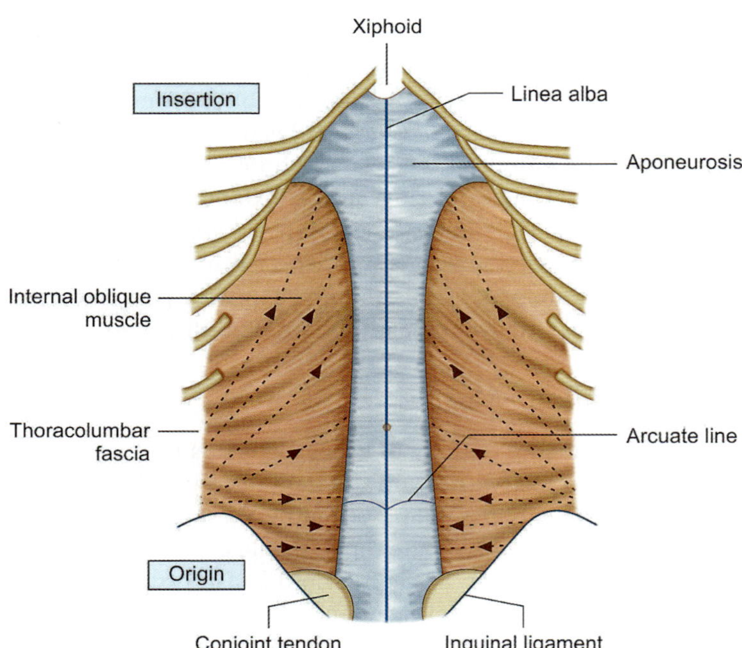

Fig. 18-8: Internal oblique muscle.

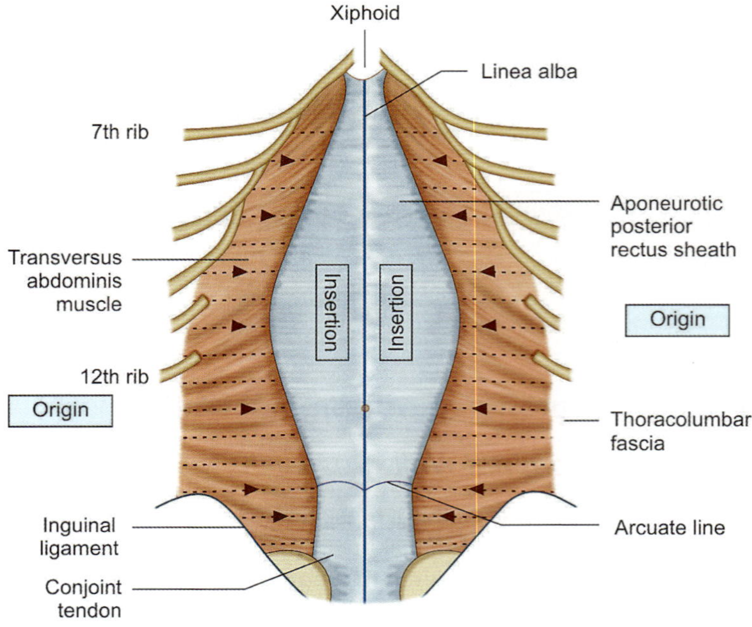

Fig. 18-9: Transverse abdominis muscle.

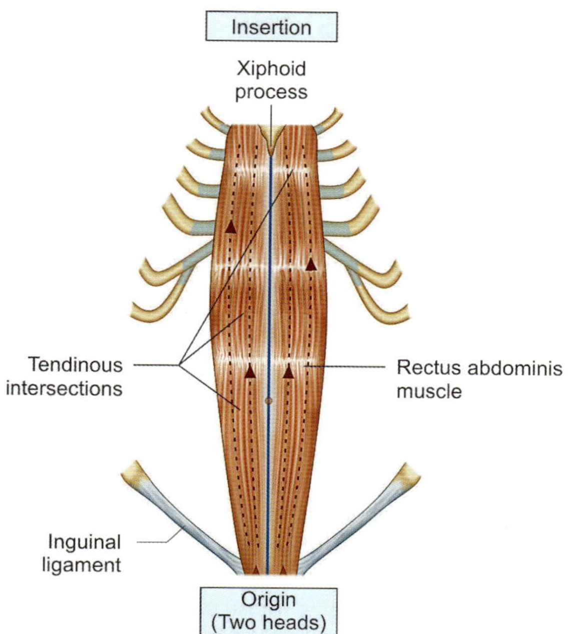

Fig. 18-10: Rectus abdominis muscle.

Anterior rectus sheath is complete covering rectus entirely from origin to insertion. Its upper 3/4th is formed by external oblique aponeurosis and anterior lamina of internal oblique. Its lower 1/4th is formed by all three aponeurosis. In this part aponeurosis of transversus and internal oblique muscles are fused; aponeurosis of external oblique remains separate.

Posterior rectus sheath is deficient above the costal margin and below the arcuate line. Between the costal margin and arcuate line it is formed by posterior lamina of internal oblique aponeurosis and transversus abdominis aponeurosis. Midway between the umbilicus and pubic symphysis posterior rectus sheath ends as arcuate line/linea semicircularis/fold of Douglas which is concave downwards.

In upper 3/4th of the abdominal wall—right and left recti are separated; both anterior and posterior rectus sheaths are present; anterior rectus sheath is formed by external oblique aponeurosis and anterior lamina of internal oblique; posterior rectus sheath is formed by posterior lamina of internal oblique aponeurosis and transversus abdominis aponeurosis; linea alba is well developed; external oblique aponeurosis and fascia is weak.

In the lower 1/4th of the anterior abdominal wall—right and left recti are very close to each other; only anterior rectus sheath is present which is formed by all 3 muscular aponeurosis; posterior rectus sheath is absent; external oblique fascia is stronger; lineal alba is not well developed.

Muscles of the Posterior Abdominal Wall

They are psoas major, psoas minor, quadrates lumborum and iliacus.

Psoas major arises from body and transverse processes of all lumbar vertebrae to insert into the tip and medial part of the lesser trochanter of the femur after passing behind the inguinal ligament along with the iliacus tendon (lateral part of the lesser trochanter). It is supplied by L_2, L_3, L_4 spinal nerves.

Psoas minor is small muscle in front of the psoas major arises from bodies of T_{12} and L_1 vertebrae to insert into the pectin pubis and iliopubic eminence. It is supplied by L_1. *Iliacus* arises from upper 2/3rd of inner aspect of fossa of ilium, upper lateral part of the sacrum to insert into lateral part of the lesser trochanter along with psoas major. It is supplied by femoral nerve.

Quadratus lumborum arises from transverse process of L_5 vertebra and inner lip of iliac crest to insert into medial part of the anterior surface of 12th rib and transverse processes of upper 4 lumbar vertebrae. It is supplied by spinal nerves T_{12} to L_4.

Fascia Transversalis (Cooper's Fascia)

It is the fascia that lines the inner surface of the transversus abdominis muscle separated from the peritoneum by extraperitoneal connective tissue. In front it is adherent to linea alba above the umbilicus; behind merges with anterior layer of thoracolumbar fascia and renal fascia; above with diaphragmatic fascia; below it is attached to inner lip of iliac crest, inguinal ligament; medially it is attached to pubic tubercle, pubic crest and pectineal line which prolongs down as anterior layer of femoral sheath. It also forms internal spermatic fascia around the cord. Deep inguinal ring is U/lambda/oval-shaped opening 1.25 cm above the midinguinal point (between pubic symphysis and anterior superior iliac spine) which is lateral to inferior epigastric artery, transmits spermatic cord in males and round ligament in females. In the inguinal area transversalis fascia is *bilaminar* enclosing the inferior epigastric vessels. *Space of Bogros* is extension of the retropubic *space of Retzius* which is located beneath the posterior lamina of transversalis fascia and in front of the peritoneum. Inlay preperitoneal mesh repair is done by placing mesh in this space. Thickening of the transversalis fascia at medial side of the internal ring and in front of the inferior epigastric vessels is called as *interfoveolar Hesselbach's ligament*.

Endoabdominal Fascia

Endoabdominal fascia is connective tissue that lines inner aspect of the entire abdominal musculature. Part in relation to transversus abdominis is called as fascia transversalis. It forms iliac, diaphragmatic and renal fascia.

Transversalis fascia is a thin aponeurotic fascia between parietal peritoneum and transverse abdominis; it is part of endoabdominal fascia. It continues as iliac fascia and pelvic fasciae below. Below it extends as anterior part of the femoral sheath along the femoral vessels. In the inguinal region posterior wall of the inguinal canal is formed by transversalis fascia; here it is thick and double layered. Behind the inguinal ligament it is strengthened by fibrous tissue which is loosely attached to the inguinal ligament and is called as iliopubic tract. It has got an opening called deep ring through which spermatic cord in male and round ligament in females passes through. Transversalis fascia extends downwards into the scrotum as internal spermatic fascia **(Fig. 18-11)**.

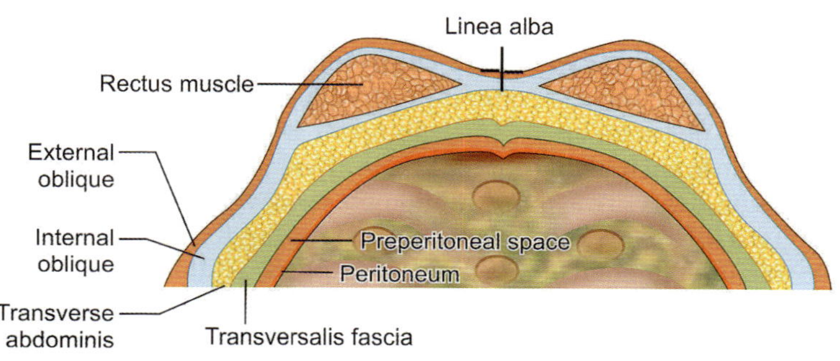

Fig. 18-11: Transversalis fascia.

Deep Nerves of the Abdominal Wall

Lower 5 intercostal and subcostal (Lower 6 thoracic primary rami) nerves and iliohypogastric and ilioinguinal nerves supply the anterior abdominal wall. *Lower 5 intercostal nerves* pass through the slips of origin of transversus abdominis muscles; run between transversus abdominis and internal oblique; pierce the posterior lamina of internal oblique aponeurosis to reach rectus sheath; then pass behind the rectus sheath in front of the epigastric vessels, pierce the rectus muscle to continue as anterior cutaneous nerve. Before piercing it supplies the anterior rectus sheath, transversus abdominis, internal oblique, external oblique and rectus abdominis. During its course it also gives lateral cutaneous nerve of the abdominal wall through flat abdominal muscles. *Battle's incision* which is pararectal incision will injure these nerves causing weakening of the rectus muscle and so is avoided.

Subcostal nerve, anterior primary ramus of 12th thoracic nerve after traveling behind the lateral arcuate ligament of diaphragm, passes in front of the quadrates lumborum and then pierces the transversus abdominis to run like other intercostal nerves. It supplies pyramidalis muscle and gluteal region as lateral cutaneous branch.

Note: There are 11 intercostal nerves and one subcostal nerve.

Blood Supply of Abdominal Wall

It is divided into superficial and deep vessels.

Superficial vessels are superficial epigastric, superficial circumflex iliac and superficial external pudendal arteries—are branches of femoral artery. They travel towards umbilicus in subcutaneous plane. Superficial epigastric artery communicates with opposite superficial epigastric artery and all three communicate with deep arteries.

Deep arteries are posterior intercostal arteries (10, 11), anterior branches of 4 lumbar and subcostal arteries and deep circumflex iliac artery. Deep arteries travel between transversus abdominis and internal oblique muscles. Rectus sheath is supplied by superior and inferior epigastric arteries. *Superior epigastric artery* is one of the two terminal branches of the internal thoracic/mammary artery. It originates at 6th intercostal space enters the abdomen between costal and xiphoid origin of the diaphragm, enters the rectus sheath from above behind the 7th costal cartilage. It descends downwards communicating with inferior epigastric artery behind the rectus muscle. Branches are muscular, cutaneous, hepatic along the falciform ligament and anastomotic to opposite side artery.

Inferior epigastric artery (IEA) originates from external iliac artery just above the inguinal ligament runs upwards and medially in the extraperitoneal connective tissue between peritoneum and posterior lamina of transversalis fascia initially medial to internal ring; pierces the transversalis fascia at the lateral border of the rectus muscle; runs in front of the arcuate line supplying the rectus and ends by anastomosing with superior epigastric artery. Branches are—muscular, cremasteric, pubic, and cutaneous. *Cremasteric branch* after travelling laterally towards deep ring supplies cremaster and runs along the spermatic cord. Pubic branch runs medially along the pubic bone to communicate with pubic branch of anterior division of obturator artery. Often obturator artery may be replaced by this pubic branch of inferior epigastric artery as abnormal/aberrant obturator artery. This pubic branch crosses over femoral ring and Cooper's ligament. This may be injured during fixation of mesh in TEP repair or femoral hernia repair causing torrential bleeding from both cut ends. As medial cut end retracts deep into the obturator fat and fascia it is difficult to control bleeding. This area is often called as *circle of death*. Inferior epigastric vein is medial to IEA.

ABDOMINAL INCISIONS

Principles in Abdominal Incision

- Incision should give adequate proper *access* to the surgical site in the abdomen—well planned; with adequate exposure of adequate length. Patient should lie symmetrical on the operation theatre table.
- It should be amenable for *extension* as needed. Muscle should be split as much as possible, not cut in vertical and oblique incisions.
- Incision should be planned such a way so as to have proper accessibility, extensibility, safeguarding of function, cosmetically acceptable and with possible least complications like dehiscence and incisional hernia.
- Care should be taken while opening the peritoneum. Abdominal contents should not be injured especially bowel. This is more important aspect in previous laparotomy patients. Peritoneum should be incised using fine scissor or scalpel after feeling the site of incision using fingers for any adherent bowel or omentum. One should not use cautery to incise peritoneum.
- If there is previous incision scar (re-laparotomy), care should be taken not to injure bowel while opening the peritoneum; it is better to open the peritoneum at a new site.
- Layer by layer incision should be done.
- Extension across umbilicus is done from left side of the umbilicus.
- Further cutting of the peritoneum after incising should be done under vision with two fingers underneath the peritoneum to prevent injury to bowel.
- Wound dehiscence is less in transverse incision than vertical incision.
- Drain should be kept through a separate incision; not through the main wound. If drain is passed through the main wound it will prejudice the strength of the final scar.
- Proper anaesthetic relaxation is essential before closure of the abdomen otherwise closure will be troublesome.

Exploratory Laparotomy

All opened abdomen should be explored by putting hand inside (right hand usually)—it is done through a proper method called as *laparotomy circuit*.

Outer laparotomy circuit	*Inner laparotomy circuit*
Begins at oesophagogastric junction ↓ *Anticlockwise* Stomach duodenum, liver, gallbladder ↓ Right colon, caecum, pelvis ↓ Sigmoid colon, descending colon, splenic flexure ↓ Spleen, left kidney, pancreas, aorta and transverse colon ↓ ***Completion of outer circuit.***	Ligament of Treitz ↓ Oblique from left to right Small bowel—jejunum and ileum with their mesentery ↓ To reach Ileocaecal junction ↓ ***Completion of inner circuit.***

Complications of Abdominal Incision

- Wound infection.
- Surgical site infection (SSI).

- *Fascial dehiscence* (Burst abdomen): Dehiscence is due to infection, severe cough and vomiting and sudden raise in intra-abdominal pressure. Initially sudden severe pain occurs; feeling of giving way with serosanguineous discharge is common. Abdominal viscera (bowel) will be visible through the given away wound. Occasionally evisceration occurs with intestine coming out of the abdominal wound. Patient is shifted to operation theatre. Under general anaesthesia, bowel contents are placed inside the abdominal cavity. All layer through and through monofilament interrupted sutures are placed after a through wash. Previously retention (tension) sutures are practiced. Usually patient recovers well unless there is bowel injury. *LE Hughes double near and far suture* or *modified Smead-Jones* single layer sutures are better in such situation.
- *Incisional hernia:* It is due to wound sepsis, peritoneal cavity infection, malnutrition and deficiencies, nerve injuries, weak rectus, obesity, precipitating causes like cough, straining, urinary problem and constipation.
- Injury to bowel during laparotomy.
- Fistula formation. Gastrointestinal fistula may be biliary, faecal or pancreatic. It may be end or lateral; high or low output.
- *Nerve injury:* Wound pain. Nerve injury can occur in muscle cutting incisions, lateral incisions, laparoscopic dissection. Ilioinguinal nerve may get injured after appendicectomy causing right sided direct inguinal hernia. Open inguinal hernioplasty may cause inguinodynia postoperatively. Intercostal nerves may get injured in Kocher's subcostal incision or thoracoabdominal incision. Pfannenstiel incision may injure hypogastric nerve.
- Adhesion and its complications.
- *Paralytic ileus:* It is common after 12–24 hours; but depends on the type and condition for which surgery is done. Causes like electrolyte imbalance, sepsis should be ruled out. Often nasogastric aspiration and flatus tube insertion may be required.

Abdominal Incisions may be:

- Vertical or transverse. Vertical may be midline or paramedian. Horizontal incisions are better.

Factors affecting the strength of the scar

- Type of surgery (acute abdomen, surgery for malignancy, major surgery)
- Obesity
- Pregnancy
- Straining
- Cough
- Ascites
- Nutrition
- Diabetes
- Immunosuppression
- Type of incision

- Incision may be with extension or without extension.
- Incision may be upper or lower. Upper incisions are better.
- Muscle retraction or muscle splitting or muscle cutting **(Fig. 18-12)**.

Different Abdominal Incisions (Figs. 18-13 to 18-15)

- Upper midline.
- Upper right paramedian.
- Upper left paramedian.
- Kocher's incision (right subcostal).
- Left subcostal.
- Bucket handle.
- Upper horizontal.
- Thoracoabdominal.
- Umbilical crease incision.
- Subumbilical.
- Incision for lumbar sympathectomy.
- Lower midline.
- Lower right or left paramedian.
- Incisions for appendicectomy—McBurney's, Rutherford Morison's, Lanz, laparoscopic.
- Pfannenstiel incision.
- Lower horizontal.

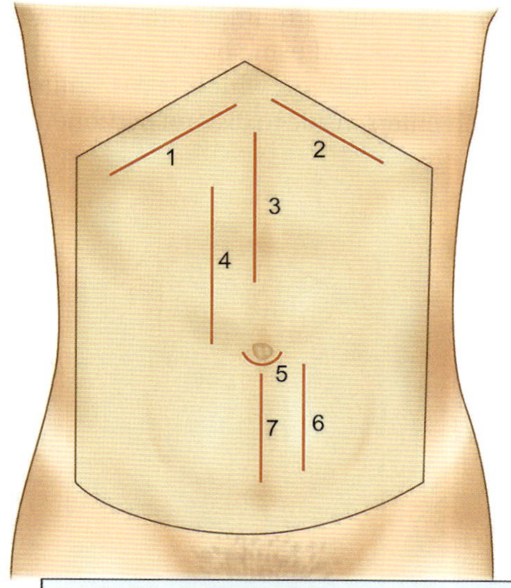

1. Right subcostal incision
2. Left subcostal incision
3. Upper midline
4. Right upper paramedian
5. Subumbilical
6. Left lower paramedian
7. Lower midline
8. Left thoracoabdominal
9. Rooftop (Chevron) incision
10. Upper horizontal
11. Left lumbar sympathectomy incision
12. Lower horizontal
13. Lanz incision
14. McBurney's incision
15. Pfannenstiel incision
16. Incision for inguinal hernia

Fig. 18-12: Different abdominal incisions.

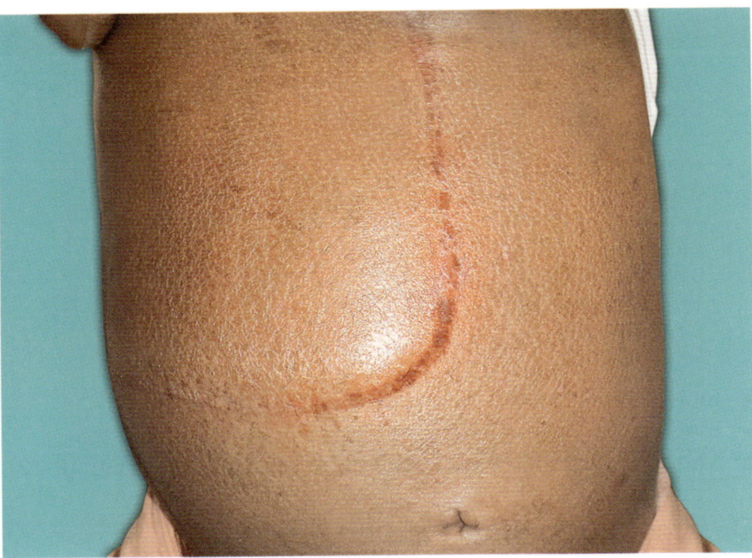

Fig. 18-13: Incision for liver resection.

Classification of abdominal incisions

Vertical incision
- *Midline incision*—upper, lower or entire length from xiphoid to pubis
- *Paramedian incisions*—right, left, upper, middle, lower. Muscle retracting/muscle splitting/pararectal (Battle's)

Transverse incisions
- *Upper abdominal* transverse—one or both sides
- *Lower abdominal* transverse
  - Transverse muscle dividing lower abdominal incision
  - Maylards incision
  - Joel Cohen's incision
  - Pfannenstiel incision
  - Cherney's incision
  - Kustner's incision
  - Turner Warwick's incision
  - Subumbilical incision

Oblique incisions
- *Kocher's* subcostal incision
  - Classical rectus muscle cutting
  - Modified rectus muscle retracting
  - Mini lap Kocher's incision
- Chevron (Roof top modification) incision

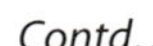

Contd...

Contd...

- Mercedes Benz modification
- Appendicectomy incisions
  - *McBurney's*/Mac Arthur's Grid iron muscle splitting incision
  - *Rutherford Morrison's* muscle cutting (laterally upwards) incision
  - *Rocky Davis or Elliot's* muscle cutting (medially and downwards) incision
  - *Lanz crease* (interspinous crease) line incision
  - Oblique iliac incision (*Abbernethy's*), muscle cutting incision

Abdominothoracic incisions

MIDLINE INCISION

It is commonly advocated incision. It can be upper midline/lower midline or both upper and lower lengthy midline incision. Midline incision is easier to reach across linea alba with rapid access, minimum blood loss, and also quicker and easier to close. Extension above or below will be easier and faster. In emergency surgeries and common elective surgeries midline incision is better. Midline incision gives excellent adequate exposure of the abdomen. It can be extended below, above, horizontally or obliquely or as thoracoabdominal when needed. Gastrectomy, pancreaticojejunostomy, hiatus hernia repair, pseudocyst surgery, exposure of aorta, colectomy and biliary tract surgeries can be done with midline incision **(Figs. 18-16 to 18-19)**.

Upper Midline Incision

Skin is incised vertically in midline from xiphoid to umbilicus. Superficial fascia, external oblique fascia is incised. Whitish crisscross tough linea alba is visible. It is incised using monopolar cautery or 22 no. blade. Once incised in full depth linea alba separates away to visualise the extraperitoneal pad of fat and peritoneum. Extraperitoneal pad of fat is separated of the peritoneum gently. Peritoneum appears like a shiny whitish thin structure. It is carefully held using a haemostat during expiration phase. One should be sure not to hold the deeper contents. Another haemostat is applied 5–10 mm away on the peritoneum horizontally so that peritoneum fold is lifted properly. Lifted fold of peritoneum is gently moved to make any content if at all to get dislodged and fold is pinched between the thumb and fingers to confirm that no content is felt. Peritoneum is incised using blade obliquely or using scissor towards just left of the midline which is avascular. Once peritoneum is opened air enters inside to distend peritoneum and content fall deep.

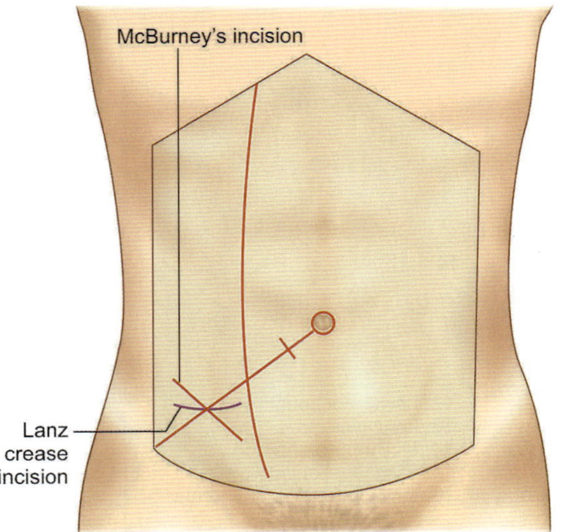

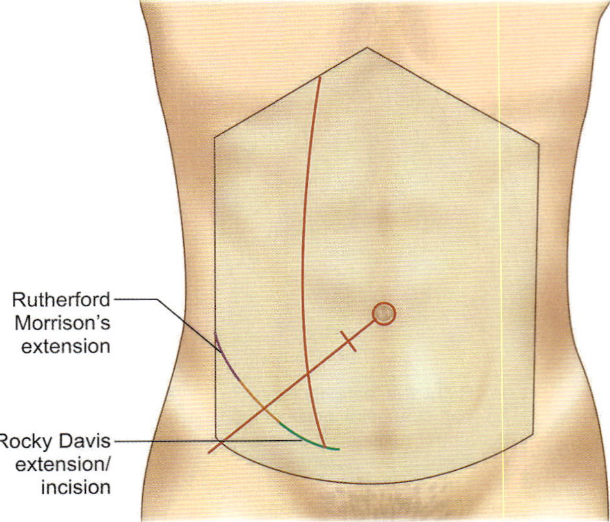

Fig. 18-14: Incisions used for open appendicectomy.

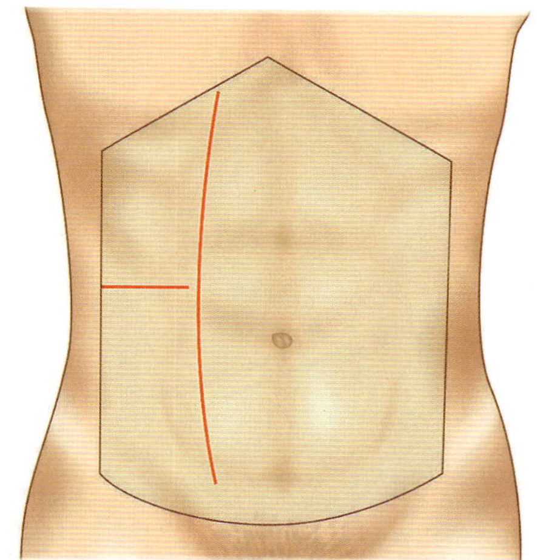

Fig. 18-15: Horizontal incision at umbilical level.

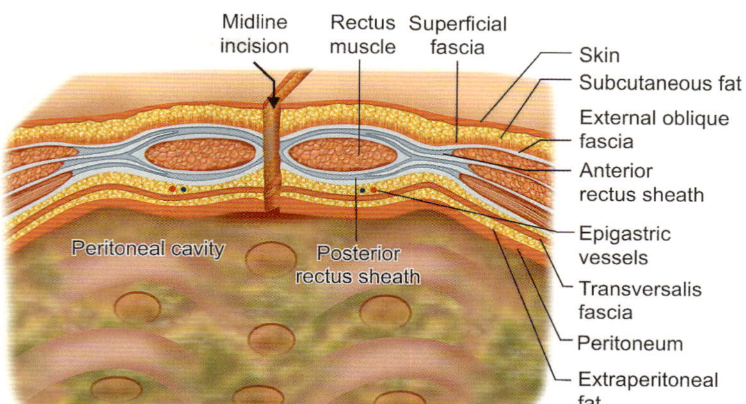

Fig. 18-16: Layers which will come across while making the midline incision.

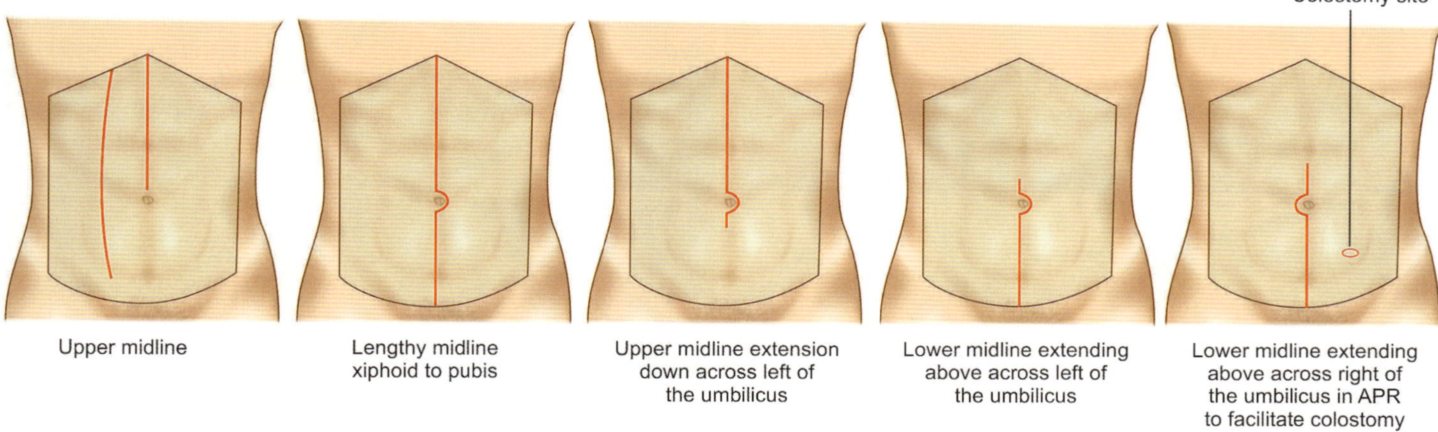

Fig. 18-17: Different types of midline incisions.

Both haemostats are reapplied to cut edges of the peritoneum. Using scissor peritoneum is cut above and below under vision or by placing fingers under the peritoneum to guard the contents with forward lift of the abdominal wall. One should be careful about the adhesions in the peritoneum doing the line of cut. Downward extension is done by curving the incision to left side of the umbilicus. Right side of umbilicus is vascular and falciform ligament is attached towards right side hence incision is curved to the left side of the umbilicus. Few advocate incision vertically through the umbilical midline. Only in abdominoperineal resection (APR) for carcinoma rectum, incision is extended above from right side of the umbilicus as permanent colostomy is placed on the left side in left iliac fossa. Occasionally when approach to the oesophagogastric (OG) junction is inadequate proximal extension is done by cutting the xiphoid process. Care must be taken not to injure terminal branches of internal mammary artery which can cause bleeding **(Fig. 18-20)**.

Lower Midline Incision

In the lower midline incision posterior rectus sheath is deficient, so care is taken while extending the incision downwards as urinary bladder may get injured. Prevesical fat should not be incised. This fat cannot be separated of the deeper bladder. Bladder should be emptied before giving anaesthesia or an indwelling urinary catheter may be needed.

Midline Incision Closure

It is done using non-absorbable monofilament suture material *no. 0 or 1*. Polyethylene/polypropylene/nylon/PDS (polydioxanone) is used. Silk and catgut are not used. Many advocate delayed absorbable suture material like no. 0 or 1 vicryl; but it is not as ideal as non-absorbable monofilament suture material. *Continuous mass closure* is sufficient. Often locking sutures are placed. Peritoneum bite is not always necessary/compulsory as it will appose naturally when anterior layers are sutured. During continuous suturing supporting knots are placed in between at few points to prevent loosening and giving way of the suture line. Minimum distance to be kept between each bite is 1 cm; each bite should be taken 1 cm away from the cut margin. Linea alba/anterior rectus sheath may retract after incision; and often bite is taken only from external oblique fascia of Gallaudet's instead of rectus sheath especially in the lower abdomen. This fascia is not strong and so will eventually dehisce to cause incisional hernia. One should maintain adequate uniform tension on the suture material. Over pulling may cause tissue strangulation. Length of the suture material required is 3 times the length of the abdominal wound. One should be careful while closing incision close to pubis due to close proximity of bladder. Inadvertent bite of the urinary bladder should be avoided. Similarly closing incision adjacent to umbilicus should be perfect otherwise defect may be left leading to incisional hernia at that site **(Figs. 18-21 to 18-23)**.

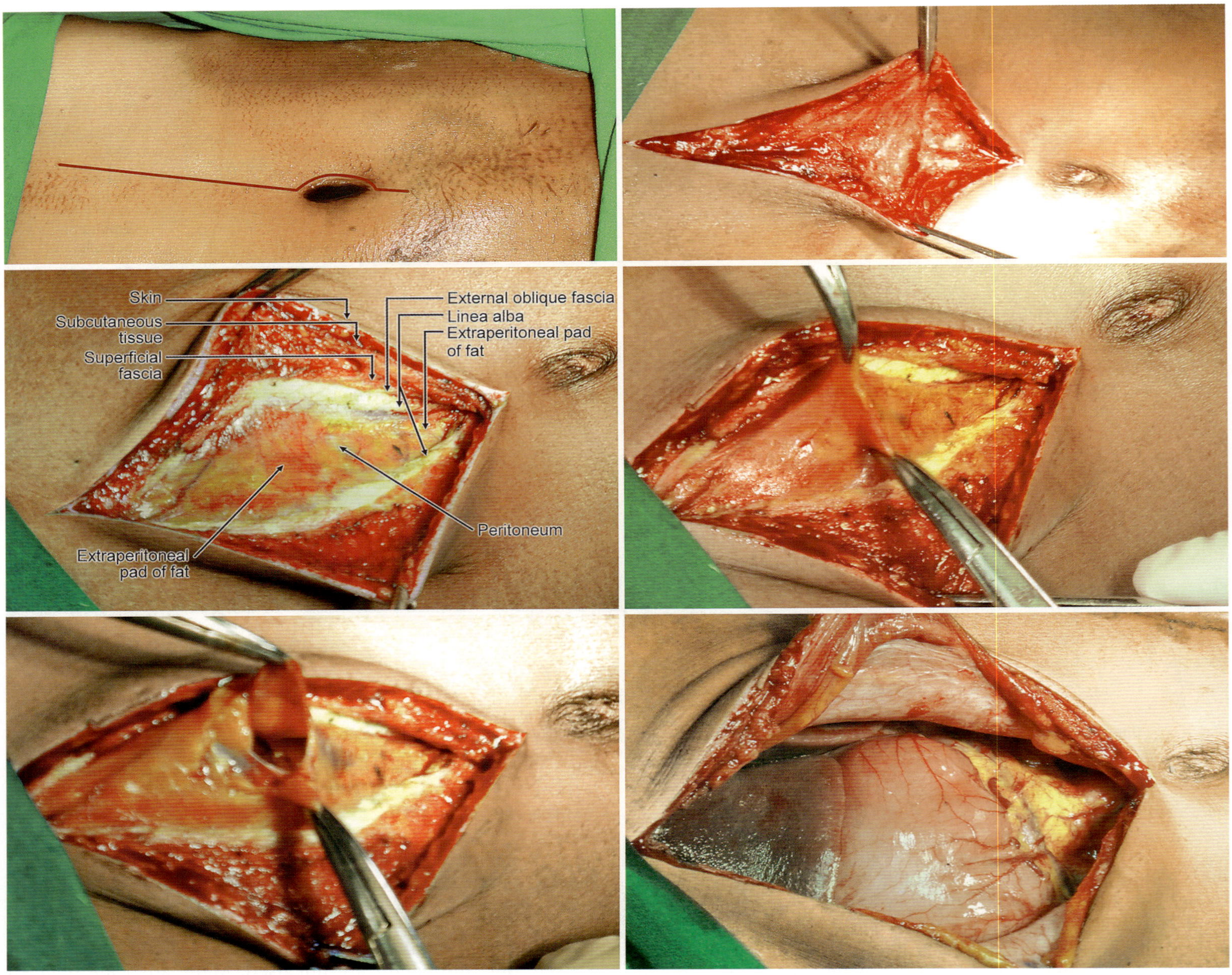

Fig. 18-18: Upper midline incision. It can be extended downwards from left of the umbilicus.

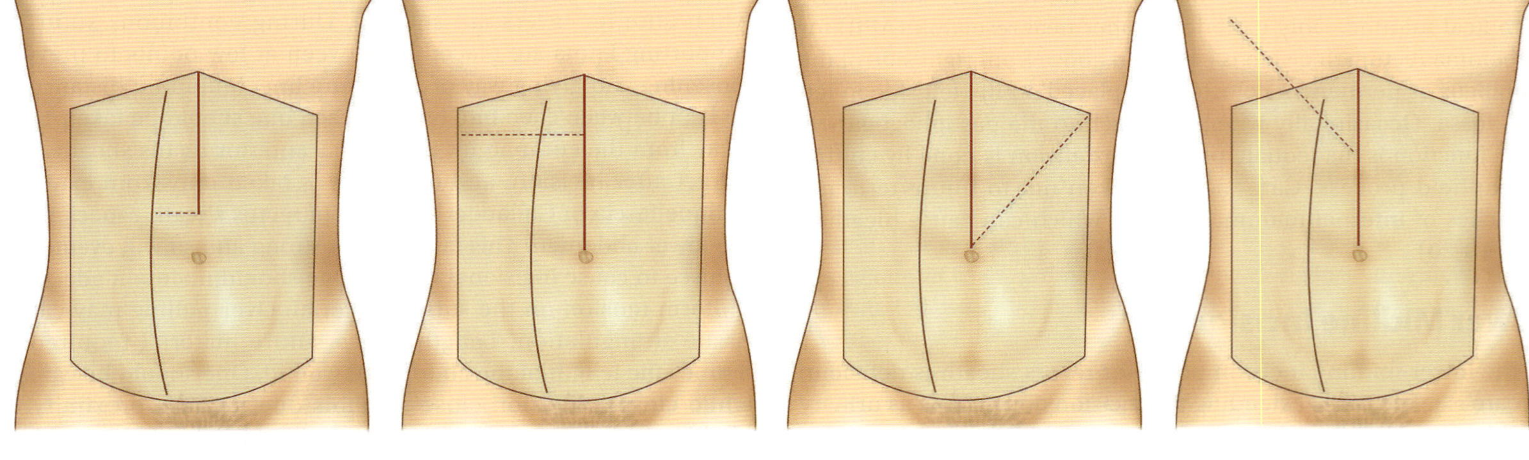

Fig. 18-19: Extension of midline incision in different ways—horizontally, obliquely, or as thoracoabdominal.

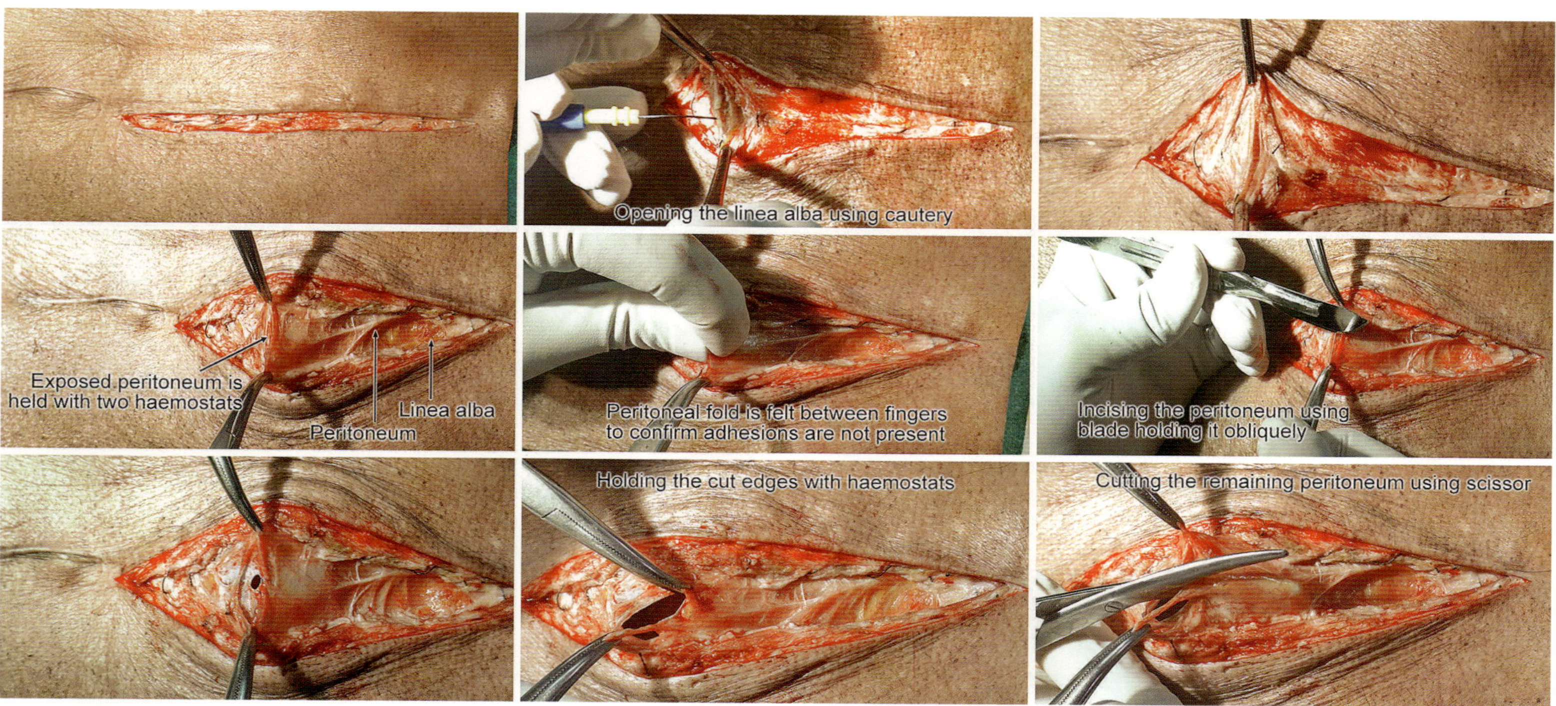

Fig. 18-20: Midline incision approach to peritoneal cavity.

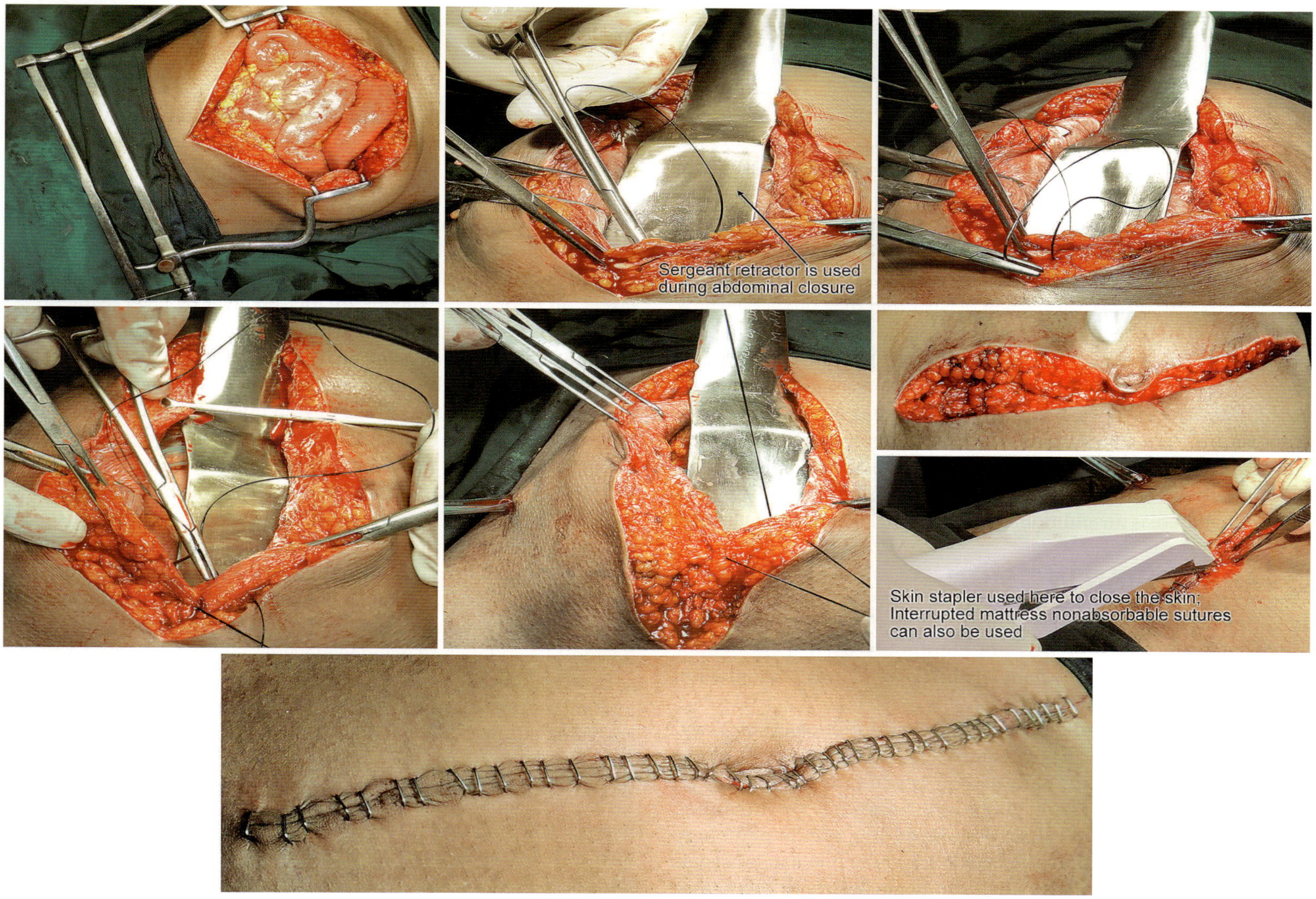

Sergeant retractor is used
during abdominal closure

Skin stapler used here to close the skin;
Interrupted mattress nonabsorbable sutures
can also be used

Fig. 18-21: Technique of closure of the midline.

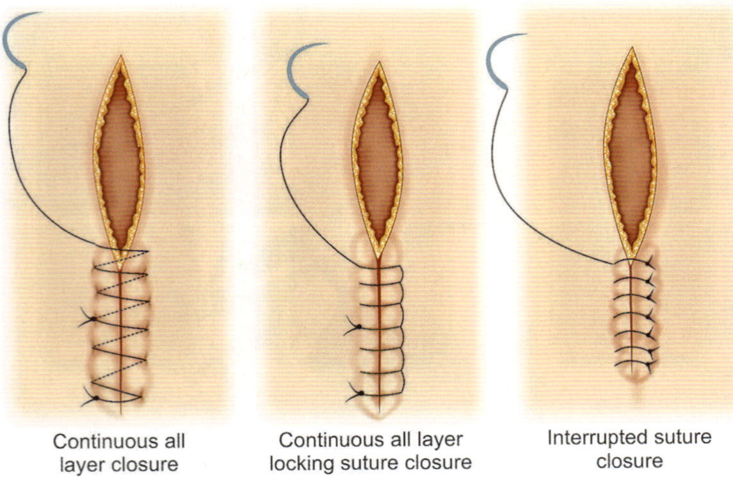

Fig. 18-22: Different methods to close the midline.

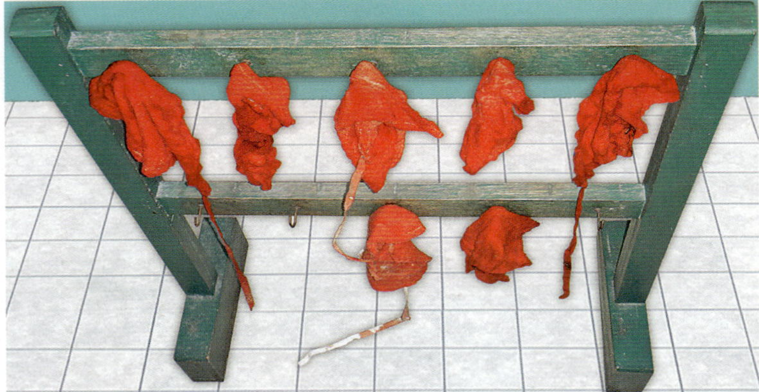

Fig. 18-23: Counting mops properly is very important prior to closure. Number of mops taken to theatre table should be written in the theatre board.

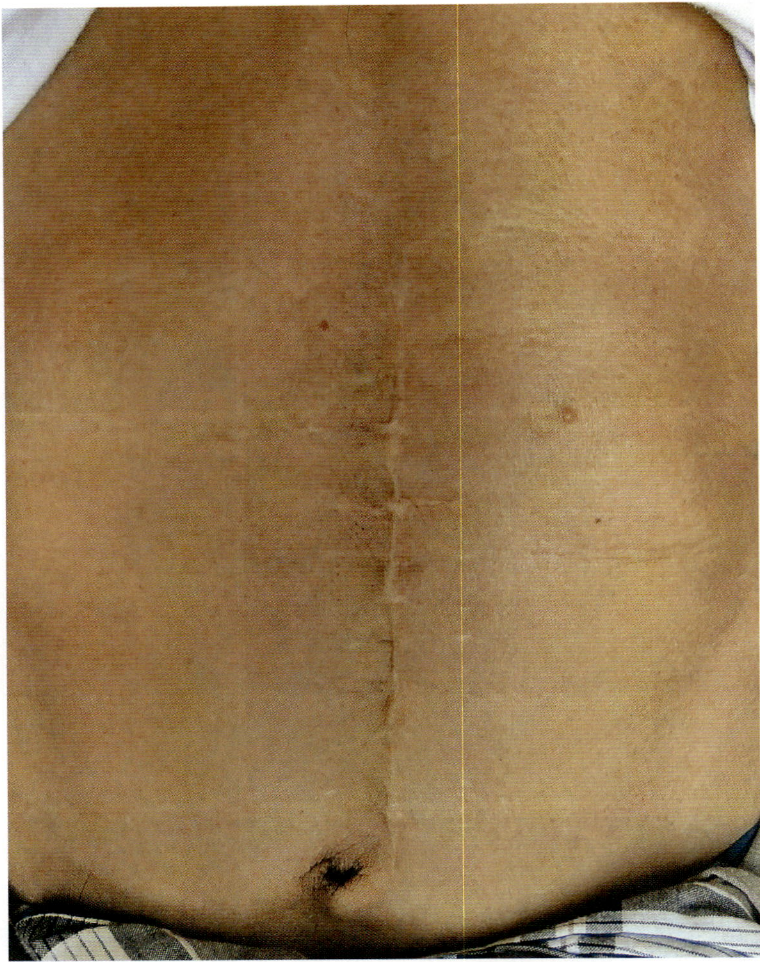

Fig. 18-24: Left paramedian incision scar.

Ending of the continuous suture is done using needle holder by knotting to the previous bite loop. It is better and stronger. At least 4–5 knots should be placed to make it stronger. Knot of the non-absorbable suture material will persists and may project towards skin causing pain in the overlying skin later and so knot should always be buried under the rectus sheath. Many use Aberdeen knot at the end in continuous suture. Interrupted single layer mass closure using non-absorbable suture material is also used with each suture 1 cm apart. Again often peritoneum is closed first by continuous suturing using 2-zero vicryl and rectus sheath is closed by continuous or interrupted (*layer by layer*) suturing. But it is now proved that there is no additional advantage in layer by layer closure.

PARAMEDIAN INCISION

In olden days paramedian incision was the most commonly advocated one; but now it is not commonly used. Paramedian incision is placed vertically parallel and 2.5 cm away from midline. It can extend from costal margin to pubis.

Right upper paramedian incision is used for cholecystectomy, biliary surgery, pyloroplasty, approach to right adrenal gland and liver cyst. Right mid-paramedian is used for laparotomy in doubtful/unknown/unsure diagnosis, approach to intestines and this approach is later extended depending on the pathology found after opening the abdomen. Right lower paramedian is used in burst appendicitis with peritonitis, right hemicolectomy. Left upper paramedian incision is used in vagotomy, gastrectomy, hiatus hernia repair and splenectomy. Left lower paramedian incision is used in left hemicolectomy **(Fig. 18-24)**.

Skin, subcutaneous tissue, superficial fascia, external oblique fascia, anterior rectus sheath are incised layer by layer using no. 22 blade with no. 4 knife handle. Medial edge of the anterior rectus sheath is held upwards using series of haemostats. Rectus muscle is retracted laterally. In the upper part anterior rectus sheath is adherent to muscle on the medial part through tendinous intersections. These intersections should be released using monopolar cautery or sharp dissection. Posterior rectus sheath is visible behind rectus muscle. Vessels and nerves are in the middle level of the rectus muscle. Vessels run vertically. Segmental nerves after piercing posterior rectus sheath run laterally in front of the vessels and enter the muscle at same level just lateral to the middle of the rectus muscle. Posterior rectus sheath is deficient below the arcuate line. Fascia transversalis and extraperitoneal fat is incised; peritoneum is held using two haemostats and incised using blade after confirming that no content is present; cut edges are held using haemostats and by guarding abdominal contents using two fingers peritoneum is opened at both ends along its entire length of incision **(Figs. 18-25 to 18-28)**.

Modifications of Paramedian Incision

Rectus muscle may be split in the line of incision on the medial part of the muscle bulk to avoid injury to nerves and also be used for quick access.

Battle's incision which is pararectal incision will injure these nerves causing weakening of the rectus muscle and so is avoided.

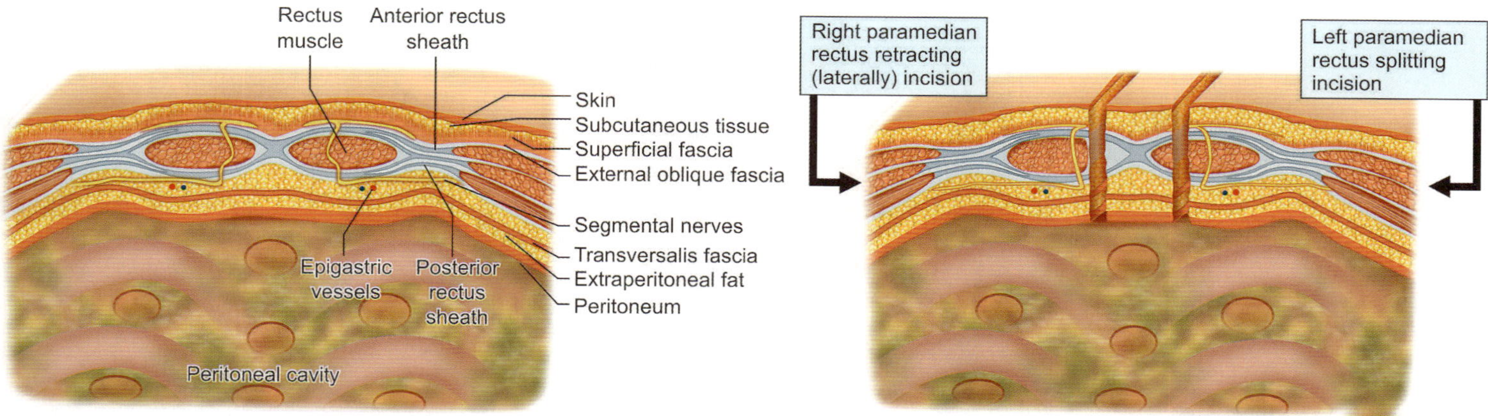

Fig. 18-25: Layers in paramedian incision approach.

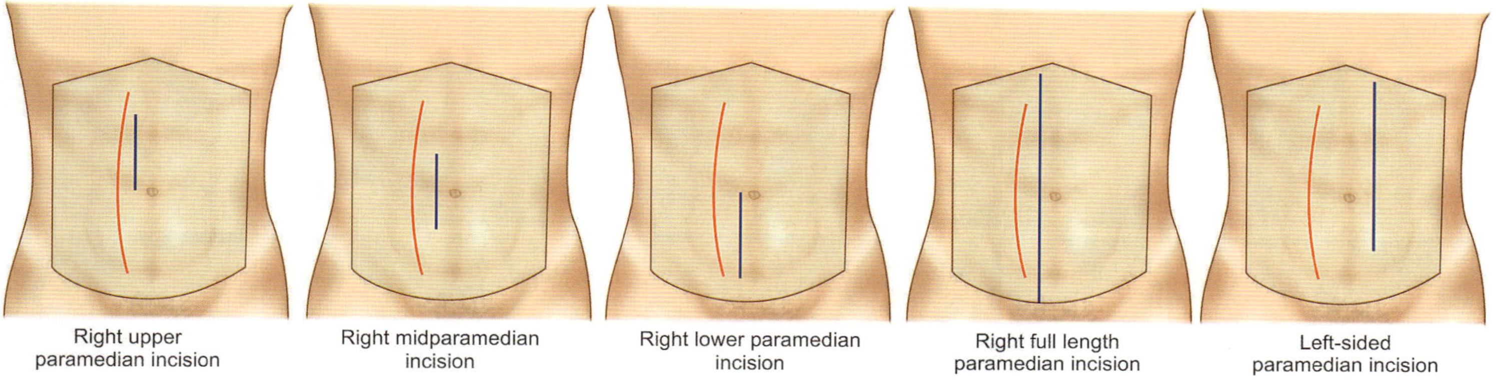

Fig. 18-26: Different types of paramedian incision.

Mayo-Robson incision: Right upper paramedian incision may extend upwards towards xiphoid process in midline as Mayo-Robson incision. One should ensure that in such extension, superior epigastric artery is not injured or otherwise should be securely ligated to prevent troublesome haemorrhage.

Paramedian incision can be extended into the thorax whenever needed as thoracoabdominal incision **(Fig. 18-29)**.

Closure of Paramedian Incision

Paramedian incision is closed in layers. First posterior rectus sheath with peritoneum is closed using monofilament non-absorbable or *delayed absorbable* like vicryl suture material. Anterior rectus sheath is closed using *monofilament non-absorbable suture* no. 0 polyethylene or polypropylene or nylon as continuous sutures.

Advantages

Paramedian incision is safe without cutting the muscle. It creates strong scar with 'trap door' effect.

Disadvantages

Rectus muscle is exposed and dissected and so there are chances of muscle getting atrophied. Incision is laborious and time consuming and difficult to extend above and below which invariably damages muscle and often nerves. Access to the contralateral abdomen is usually inadequate.

TRANSVERSE INCISIONS

It may be upper transverse or lower transverse incision. It is the incision used in infants and early childhood. It is muscle cutting incision. Muscle is cut in line of incision.

Upper Transverse Abdominal Incision

It is placed at transpyloric plane or midway between xiphoid and umbilicus. It is muscle cutting incision. Rectus muscle is cut; but its nerve supply is not interfered as it has got segmental nerve supply. Rectus muscle in upper abdomen after cutting will not retract due to tendinous intersections. It extends from anterior axillary line on one side to other side; but length depends on the side of the pathology which can be variable as needed. Skin, subcutaneous tissue, fascia, superficial fascia, anterior rectus sheath on both sides, recti on both sides, external and internal oblique muscles on both sides, transverse abdominis muscles on both sides are cut. Vessels deeper to rectus muscle are ligated securely. Posterior rectus sheath and transversalis fascia are incised. Peritoneum is held with two haemostats and incised. It is cut in the line of incision transversely. Muscles are cut using monopolar cautery. Postoperative pain is less and chances of wound dehiscence and incisional hernia are rare.

In infants and early childhood, costal angle is obtuse, abdomen is small and wide, muscles are thin, and pelvis is not yet developed and so not deep. Approach to entire abdomen is possible; contracture will not occur compared to vertical scar; cosmetically better. Umbilical vein in falciform ligament may be patent and so requires firm ligation.

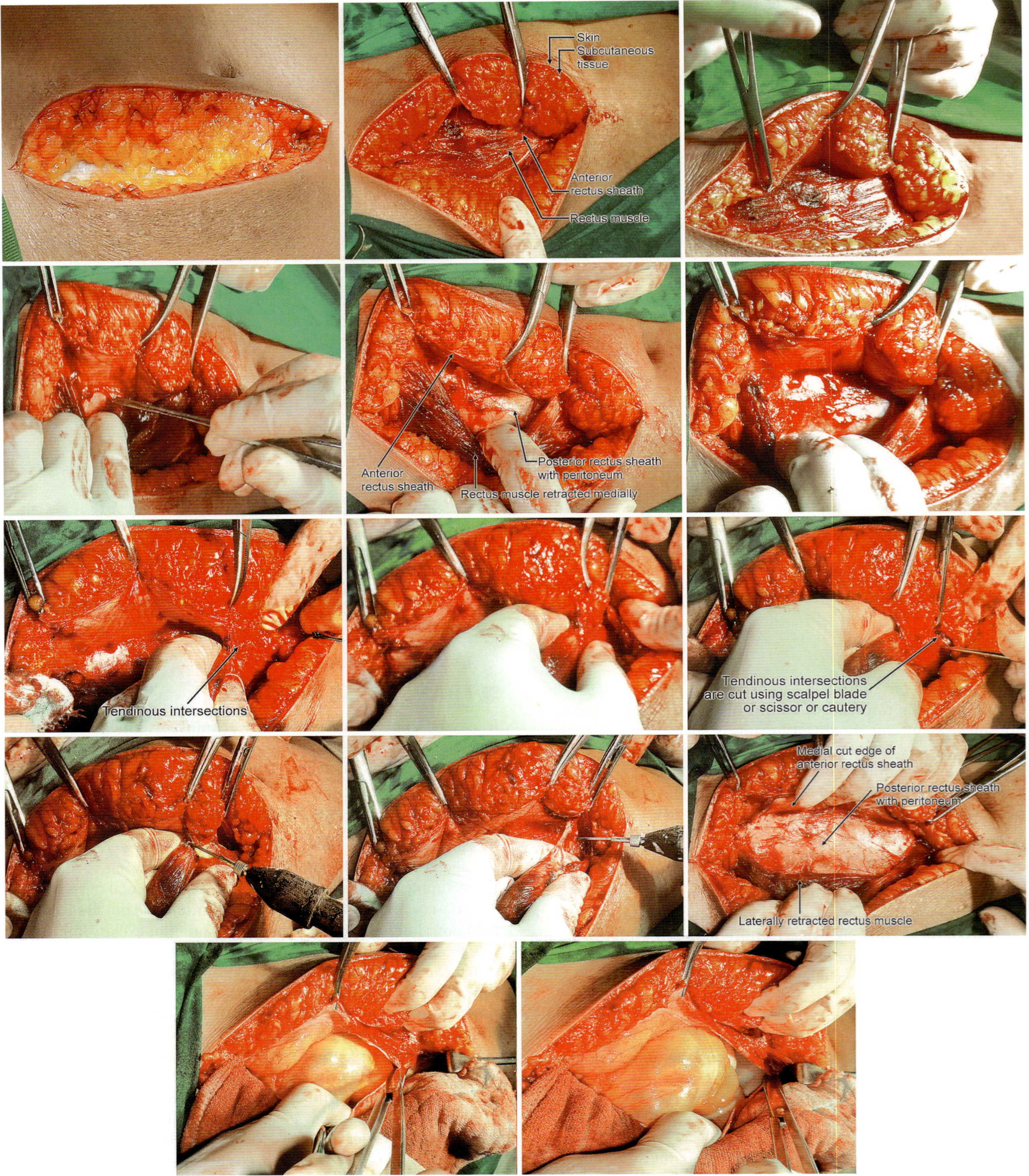

Fig. 18-27: Technique of paramedian incision.

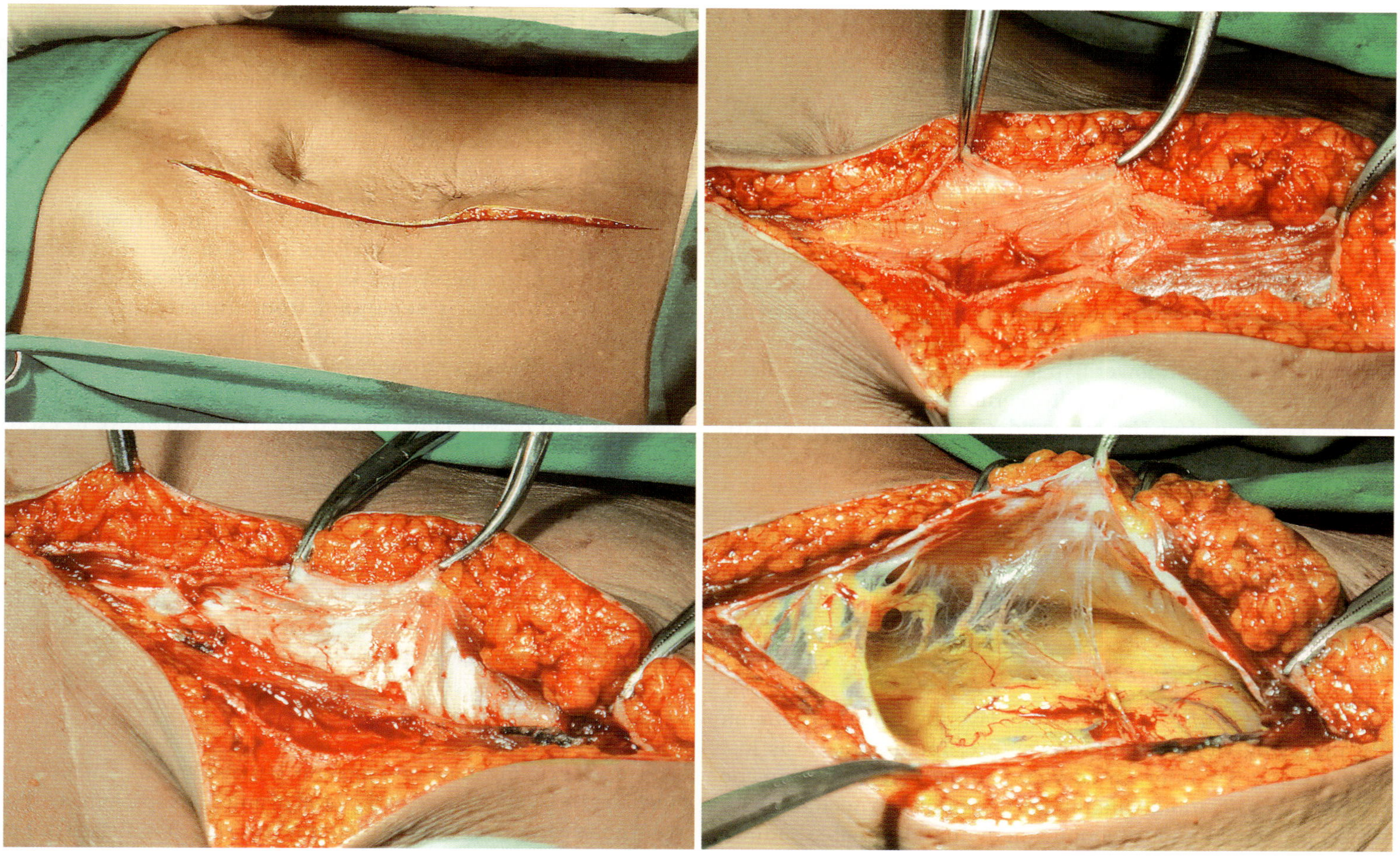

Fig. 18-28: Right paramedian incision.

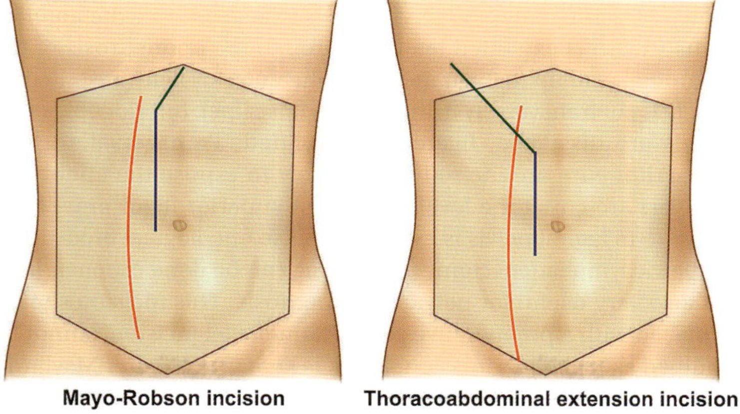

Fig. 18-29: Extensions which can be done in paramedian incision.

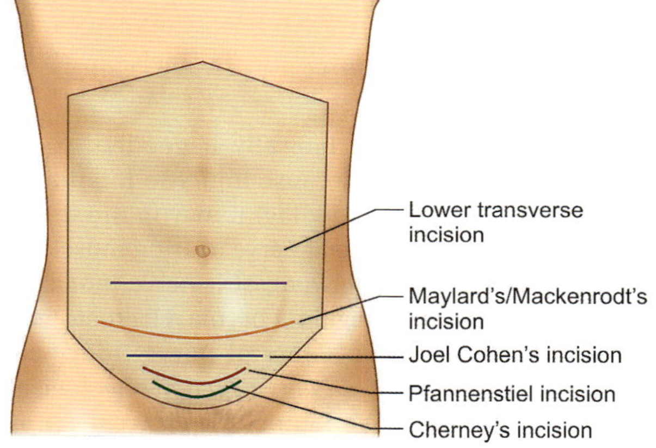

Fig. 18-30: Different types of lower abdomen transverse incisions.

(In infants while putting infraumbilical transverse incision, one has to be aware of that two umbilical arteries in paramedian positions on either side may be patent and so needs ligation).

Closure of upper transverse incision is done either as layer by layer using vicryl; or lateral muscles are closed as mass closure with suturing posterior rectus sheath, rectus muscle and anterior rectus sheath.

Advantages

It gives good exposure of the upper abdomen. Healing is supported by muscle contraction which pulls it transversely. Segmental nerve supply is preserved. Scar contracture is less here compared to vertical.

Disadvantages

Bleeding from epigastric and muscular vessels is troublesome. It takes long time to complete the incision.

Lower Transverse Abdominal Incisions

It is not commonly used; instead Pfannenstiel incision is used. Lower infraumbilical transverse incision is often used in infants and children; here posterior rectus sheath is not formed; recti muscles will retract as there are no tendinous intersections; and so often cause difficulty in apposing the recti firmly. Layers are closed in similar fashion as upper transverse incision **(Fig. 18-30)**.

Pfannenstiel Incision (Pfannenstiel Hermann Johann 1862–1909; German Gynaecologist)

It is rectus *muscle separating/retracting* transverse incision. It is used to approach pelvis. It is commonly used in gynaecological surgery like caesarean section or hysterectomy. The incision is also used in urology procedures like in retropubic urethroplasty.

Incision is placed in suprapubic region 1 cm above the pubis with slight convexity downwards. Laterally incision extends beyond outer margin of the rectus muscle. Skin, subcutaneous tissue and superficial fascia are incised. Anterior rectus sheath is incised in the line of incision; upper flap of the sheath is raised upwards towards umbilicus using scissor; lower flap is raised up to the pubis. Recti are separated from midline laterally. Peritoneum is visualised with extraperitoneal pad of fat. Urinary bladder is visible in the lower part. Peritoneum is held with two haemostats in the upper part midline. It is incised and opened vertically in both directions above and below. Below it is incised until the dome of the urinary bladder. One should be careful below not to incise urinary bladder. Head down position with self-retaining retractor facilitates further operative steps **(Figs. 18-31 and 18-32)**.

Closure of Pfannenstiel Incision

Closure of Pfannenstiel incision is done layer by layer; peritoneum vertically using vicryl continuous suture; rectus muscle is just apposed using few interrupted vicryl sutures (it should not be very tight so as to strangulate the muscle); anterior rectus sheath is closed using continuous monofilament non-absorbable sutures. Subcutaneous tissue is closed using interrupted 3-zero vicryl; skin is closed using subcuticular suture.

Advantages

It is cosmetically better; less painful; heals rapidly; less chance of incisional hernia compared to lower midline incision.

Disadvantages

It is difficult to extend more laterally if needed in case large gynaecological tumours. It may cause injury to inferior epigastric vessels causing troublesome bleeding. It may injure the T_{11} nerve, iliohypogastric nerve and subcostal nerve causing muscle weakness. Entrapment of ilioinguinal or iliohypogastric nerve can occur. Lateral extension may predispose to inguinal hernia. Haematoma, seroma, abscess formation can occur. Femoral nerve injury can occur occasionally. This incision *should not be used* in oncological surgery as there is limited access to lymph node clearance. Its proximity to infected area (perineum) may predispose sepsis.

Joel Cohen's Straight Transverse Lower Abdominal Incision

It is used for caesarean section delivery. It is a straight transverse incision through skin only, 3 cm below the level of the anterior superior iliac spines (higher than the Pfannenstiel incision). The subcutaneous tissue is opened only in the middle 3 cm. The fascia is incised transversely in the midline then extended laterally with blunt finger dissection. Finger dissection is used to separate the rectus muscles vertically and outwards laterally and to open the peritoneum. All the layers of the abdominal wall are stretched manually to the extent of the skin incision. The urinary bladder is pushed below by gentle blunt finger dissection. The uterine muscle is incised transversely in the midline but not to breach the amniotic sac, then opened and extended laterally with finger dissection. It is found that this approach for caesarean section delivery reduces the operating time, blood loss and postoperative hospital stay.

Cherney's Incision

Incision is like Pfannenstiel but still lower than it with *tendon detaching approach*. After incising the skin and subcutaneous tissue above the pubic symphysis, anterior rectus sheath is incised transversely which is separated from underlying rectus and pyramidalis muscles above and below. Posteriorly these muscles are separated from the urinary bladder by blunt finger dissection. Tendons of these muscles are cut 5 mm above the pubic symphysis. Muscles with tendons are retraced and reflected above to expose the peritoneum which is incised transversely. Cherney's incision provides excellent access and exposure to the retropubic space of Retzius for retropubic urethropexy and paravaginal repair. Exposure is the main advantage to Cherney's incision. It is more time consuming due to the dissection required to separate the muscles and tendons from the underlying tissues. Injury to inferior epigastric arteries is a possibility. Reattachment of the tendons to the pubic symphysis is a must during closure which is tedious.

Maylard's Incision

It is muscle cutting transverse incision. It is also called as *Mackenrodt incision.* Incision is placed at the level of anterior superior iliac spine with convexity downwards. Anterior rectus sheath is incised but not separated from the rectus muscle to prevent it from getting retracted on either sides (often after cutting the rectus muscle, its edge is sutured to the cut edge of the anterior rectus sheath to prevent retraction using mattress vicryl sutures). Incision over the anterior rectus sheath is extended laterally through the aponeurosis of the abdominal wall up to 2 cm medial to the anterior iliac crest. Rectus muscle is cut transversely using cautery or scalpel. Inferior epigastric vessels are dissected, ligated and divided. Transversalis fascia and peritoneum are incised transversely to expose the abdomen. All layers are cut at the level of anterior superior iliac spine. Here exposure to lateral pelvis is excellent and so oncological procedures like pelvic lymphadenectomy and staging can be done exponentially. It is also very useful for pelvic endometriosis. This incision should be placed with a preoperative plan. Pfannenstiel incision cannot be modified as Maylard's incision. Drain is kept usually after Maylard's exposure as oozing and collection is common in this incision.

Disadvantages: Haemorrhage, haematoma, seroma formation and infection can occur. Injury to ilioinguinal and iliohypogastric nerves or their entrapment during closure can occur. Lateral femoral cutaneous, genitofemoral and femoral nerves can get compressed during retraction causing neuropraxia.

Kustner's Incision

A transverse incision is made 5 cm above the symphysis pubis and below the anterior iliac spine. The subcutaneous tissue is then separated in the midline to expose the linea alba. A vertical midline incision is made through the linea alba. Superficial epigastric vessels are ligated. This incision is not commonly used as there are no advantages over Pfannenstiel incision and it limits in adequate exposure and cannot extend if needed also.

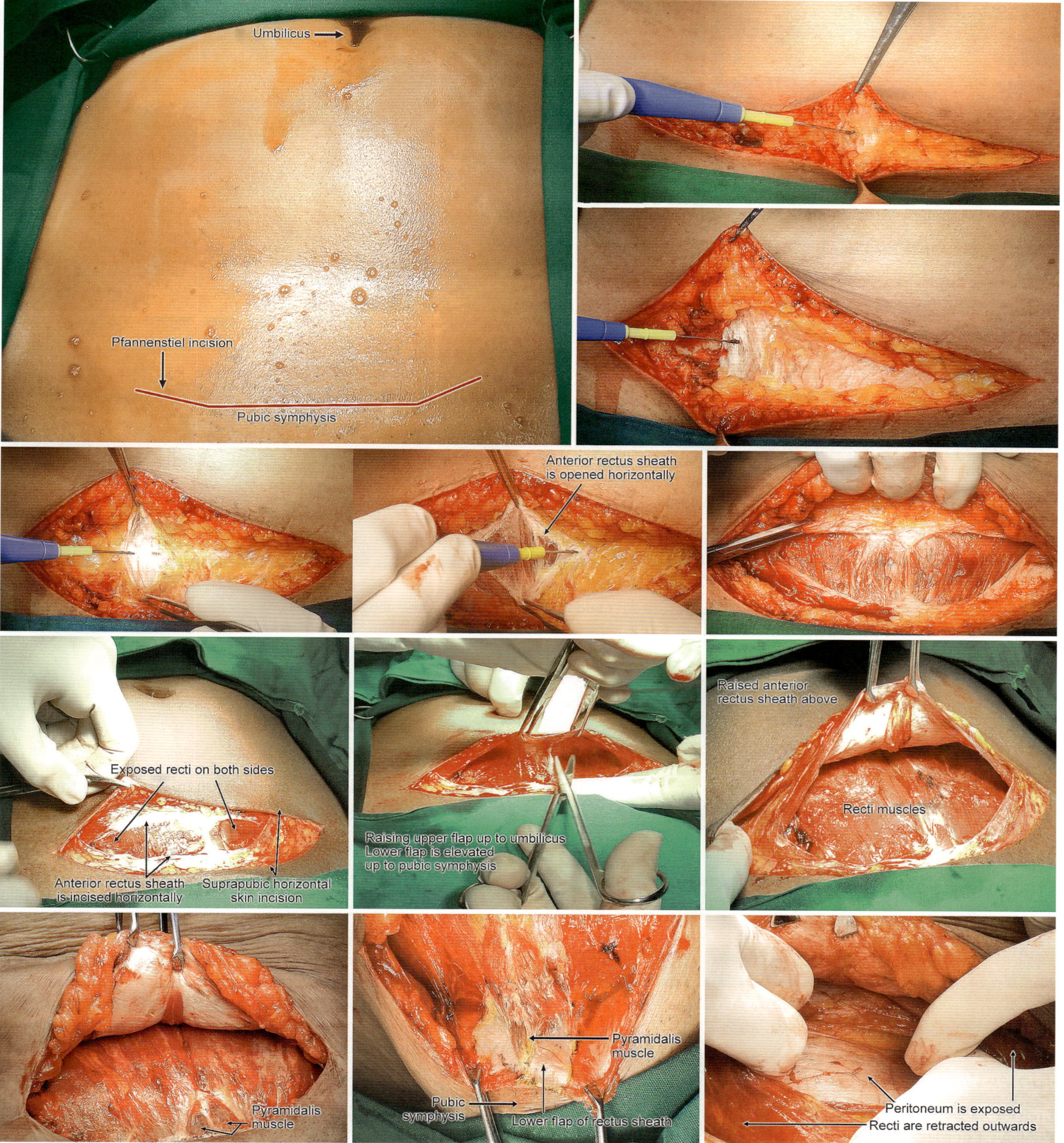
Umbilicus
Pfannenstiel incision
Pubic symphysis
Anterior rectus sheath is opened horizontally
Exposed recti on both sides
Anterior rectus sheath is incised horizontally
Suprapubic horizontal skin incision
Raising upper flap up to umbilicus
Lower flap is elevated up to pubic symphysis
Raised anterior rectus sheath above
Recti muscles
Pyramidalis muscle
Pyramidalis muscle
Pubic symphysis
Lower flap of rectus sheath
Peritoneum is exposed
Recti are retracted outwards

Figs. 18-31(1)

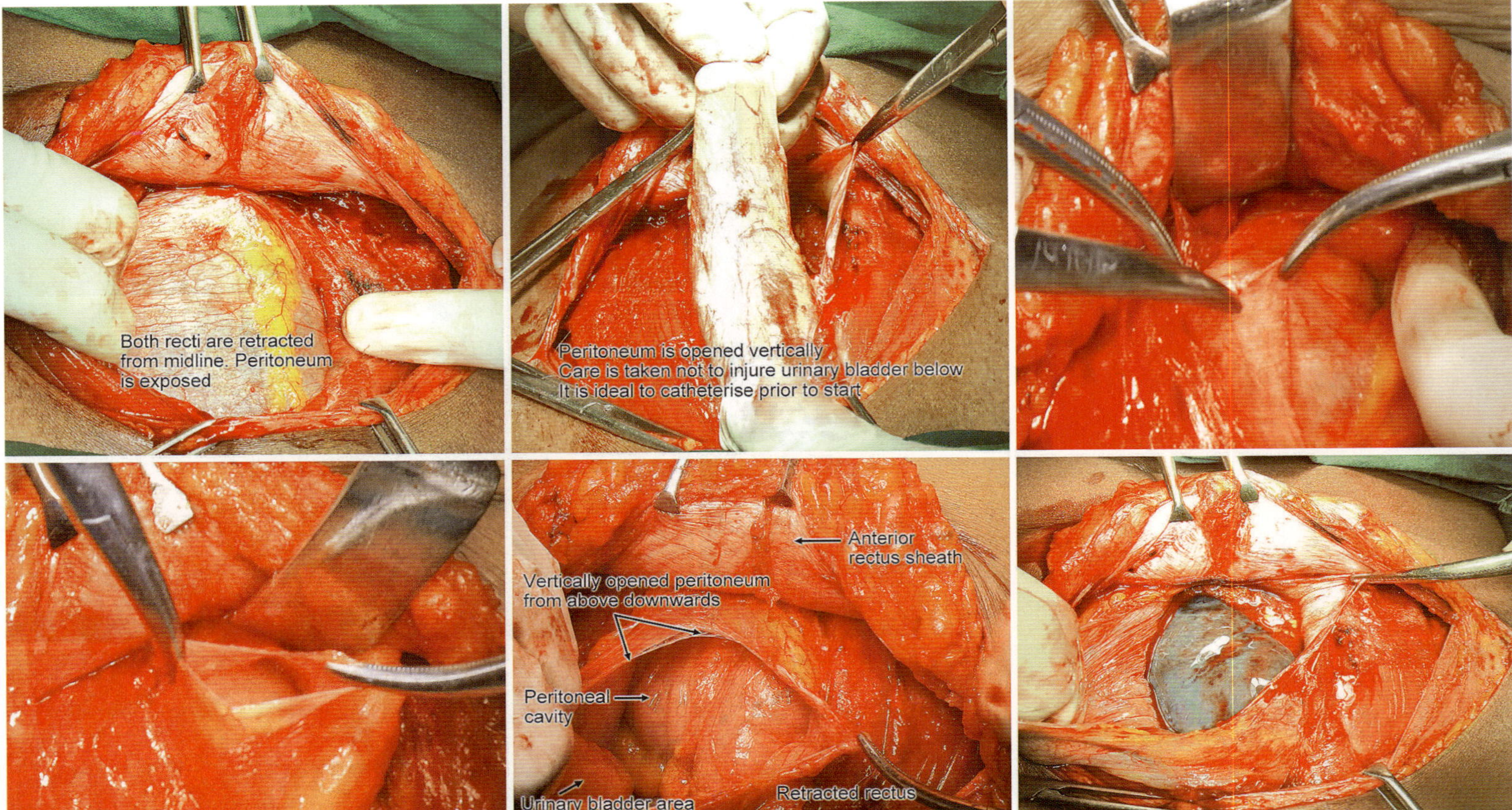

Figs. 18-31(2)

Figs. 18-31(1 and 2): Pfannenstiel incision—steps.

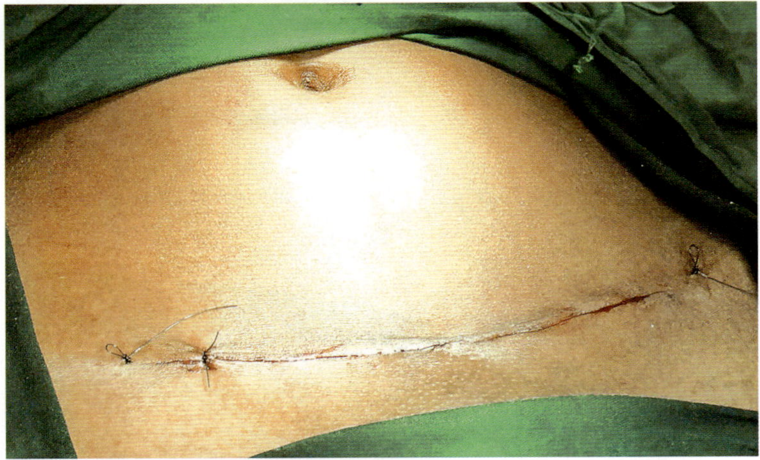

Fig. 18-32: Pfannenstiel incision closure.

Turner-Warwick's Incision

Incision is placed 2 cm above the symphysis pubis and within the lateral borders of the rectus muscles. The sheath overlying the rectus muscles at the symphysis pubis is released for about 4 cm transversely, and the incision angled up to the lateral borders of the rectus muscles. The lateral edges of the incision remain medial to the internal oblique muscles. The recti are separated and the incision is made in the midline. This type of incision is good for the exposure of the retropubic space. Pelvis and abdomen is not exposed adequately in this incision.

OBLIQUE INCISIONS

Kocher's Subcostal Incision (Emil Theodor Kocher)

Right subcostal incision is used for open cholecystectomy and to approach biliary system and liver. Incision extends from anterior axillary line towards xiphisternum up to midline 2–2.5 cm below the costal margin. Skin, subcutaneous tissue, superficial fascia, anterior rectus sheath, rectus muscle, external and internal oblique muscles and transverse abdominis muscle are cut using monopolar cautery. Anterior rectus sheath once cut in front of the rectus muscle, long haemostat (artery forceps) is passed behind the rectus muscle and lifted forward to cut the muscle horizontally using cautery. Superior epigastric vessels deep to rectus muscle are ligated securely. 8th thoracic nerve which is smaller is cut. It is ideal to identify larger 9th thoracic nerve and preserve it to prevent weakening of abdominal muscles. Peritoneum is incised in the line of incision. Large bowel will be very close to this incision and so care should be taken not to injure it inadvertently while opening the peritoneum.

Incision is often *modified* by not cutting the rectus muscle but retracting it after incising the anterior rectus sheath **(Figs. 18-33 and 18-34)**.

Smaller subcostal incision <10 cm in length is used by many surgeon as *mini lap cholecystectomy* without incising the rectus sheath. It causes less postoperative pain, early recovery and good cosmesis. But Calot's dissection is difficult and often is done blindly. Advent of laparoscopic cholecystectomy as standard approach made this a surgical legacy.

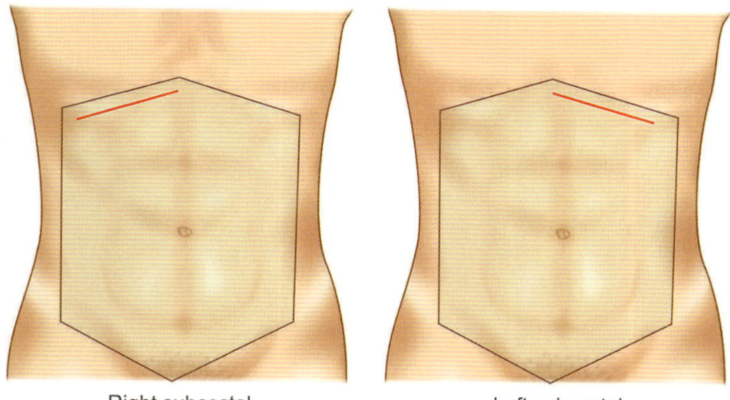

Fig. 18-33: Right and left subcostal incision.

Closure of Kocher's incision is done by closing posterior and rectus sheaths separately and rectus muscle with vicryl sutures. Rectus has got segmental nerve supply and due to its upper tendinous intersections it will not retract and fibrous scar itself causes additional support to the muscle.

Advantages: It gives very good exposure to Calot's and biliary system. It can be extended towards opposite side if needed.

Disadvantages: Injury to 9th thoracic nerve causes muscle weakness and loss of sensation below the scar. Hernia if develops in Kocher's incision is difficult to manage **(Fig. 18-35)**.

Left Subcostal Incision

Left subcostal incision is used for splenectomy, distal pancreatectomy.

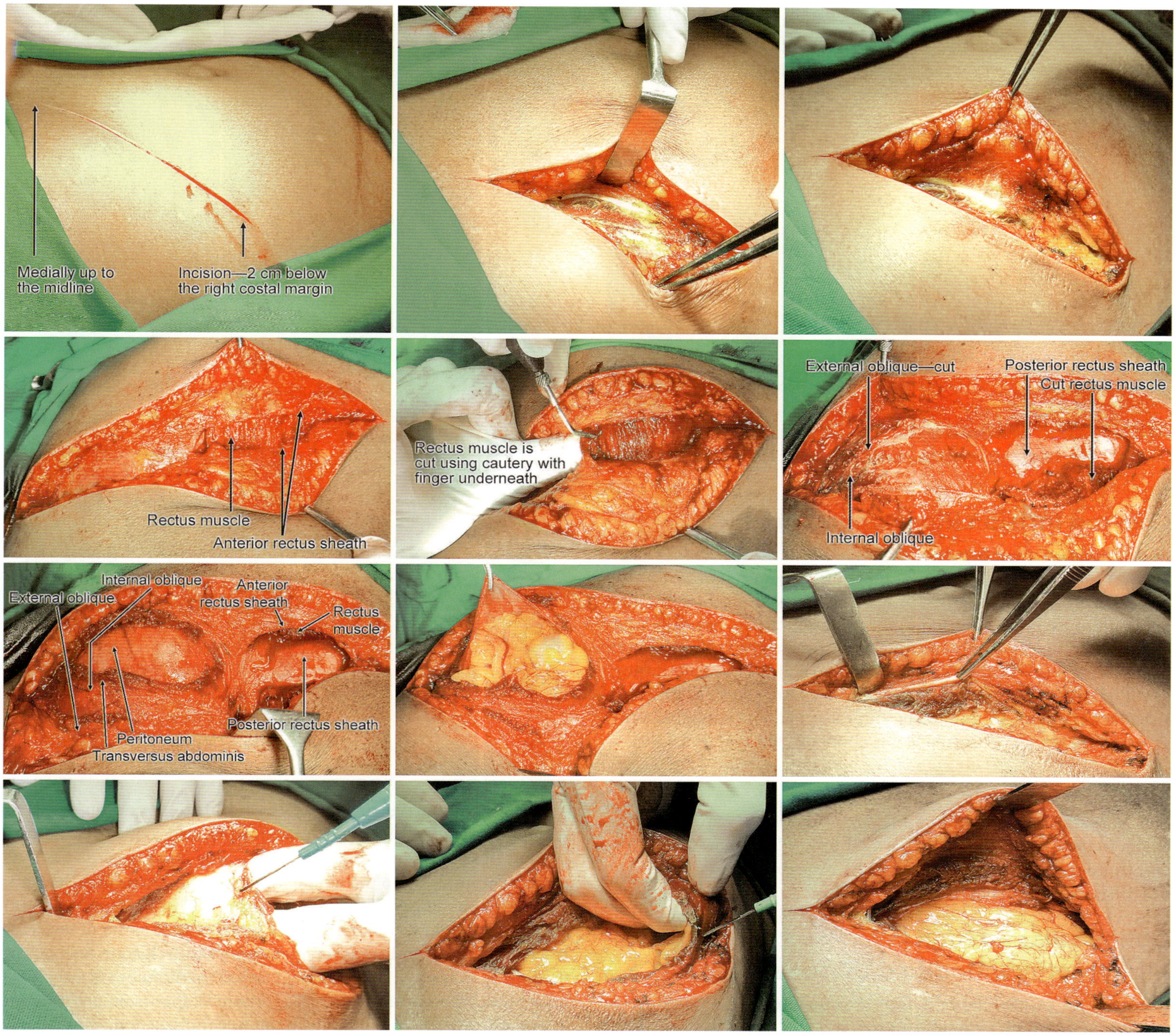

Figs. 18-34(1)

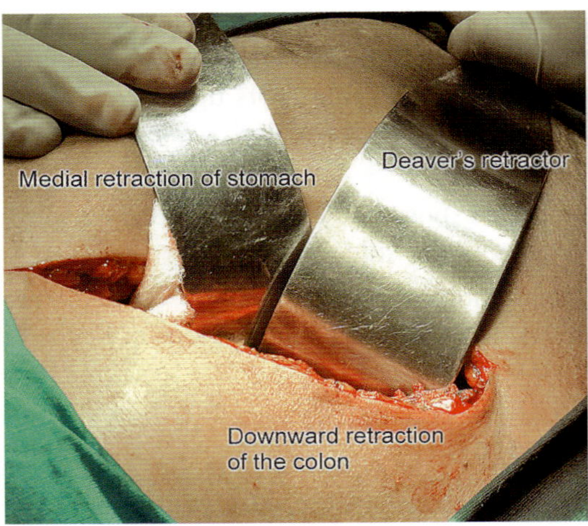

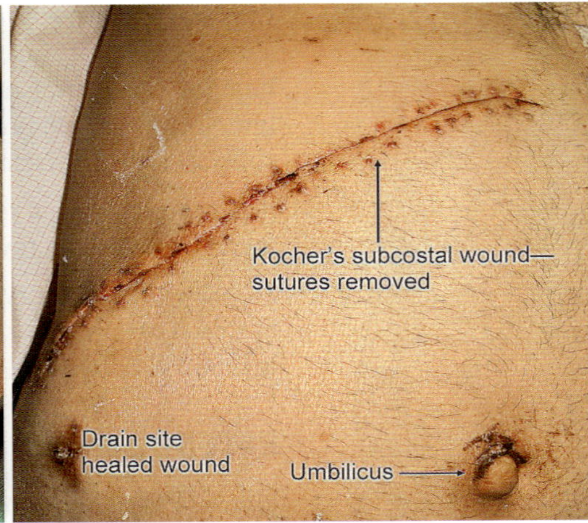

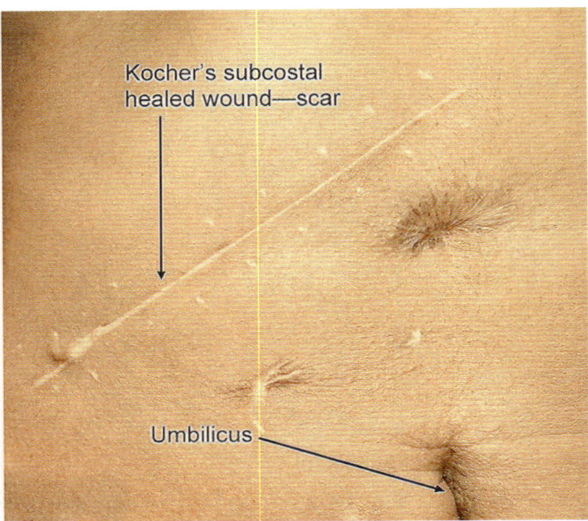

Figs. 18-34(2)

Figs. 18-34(1 and 2): Typical right subcostal Kocher's incision and scar.

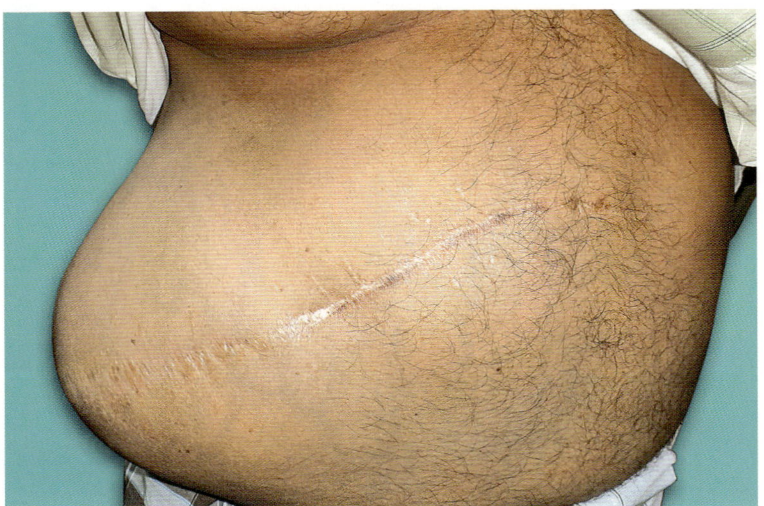

Fig. 18-35: Incisional hernia along Kocher's incision scar.

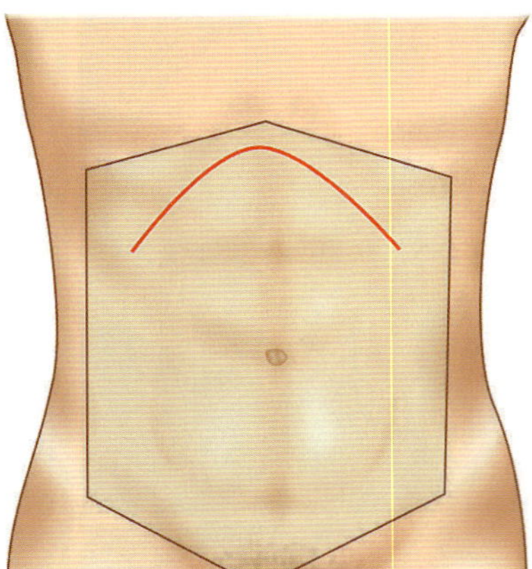

Fig. 18-36: Rooftop incision.

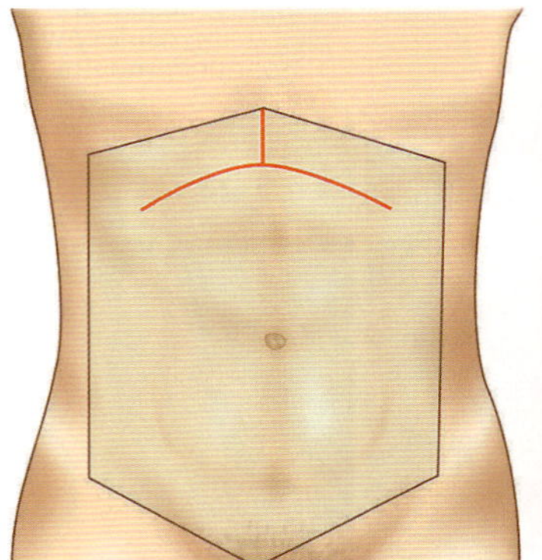

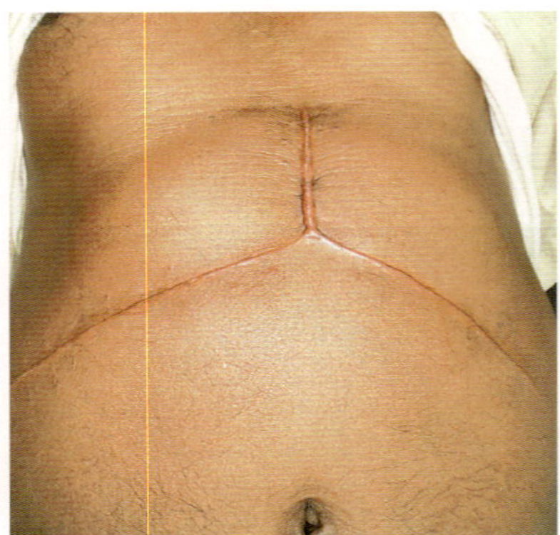

Fig. 18-37: Mercedez Benz incision.

Chevron Incision (Rooftop Incision)

In this incision a cut is made on the abdomen below the rib cage. It is actually bilateral subcostal incision. The cut starts from the mid-axillary line below the ribs on the right side of the abdomen and continues all the way across the abdomen to the opposite mid-axillary line leading into cutting of entire width of the abdomen providing access to the liver for liver resection/transplantation, oesophagogastric junction for oesophagectomy, surgery for reno-vascular hypertension, pancreatic surgeries, bilateral adrenalectomy. The average length of the incision is about 60–80 cm **(Fig. 18-36)**.

Mercedes Benz Incision

It is bilateral lower Kocher's incision (about 3–5 cm below the costal margin) with a middle vertical upper limb passes towards and through the xiphisternum. It gives very good exposure to liver, oesophageal hiatus **(Fig. 18-37)**.

Oblique Iliac Incision (Abbernethy's/Modified Gibson's)

It is used for *extraperitoneal approach* for ureteric stone, urinary bladder and lumbar sympathectomy. It is muscle cutting incision. It can be used as transperitoneal also **(Figs. 18-38 and 18-39)**.

Position is partial or complete lateral, depends on the side surgery is needed. Incision is placed from mid-axillary line at the level of the umbilicus directing downwards and forwards towards pubic symphysis up to the lateral margin of the rectus muscle. Skin, subcutaneous fat, superficial fascia, external oblique muscle and aponeurosis below are incised layer by layer in the line of incision. Internal oblique and transverse abdomen muscles are also cut in the line of incision. Extraperitoneal fat and peritoneum is visualised under transversalis fascia. In extraperitoneal approach, peritoneum is swept forward from behind by blunt finger dissection. Psoas major muscle, genitofemoral nerve and inferior vena cava are identified.

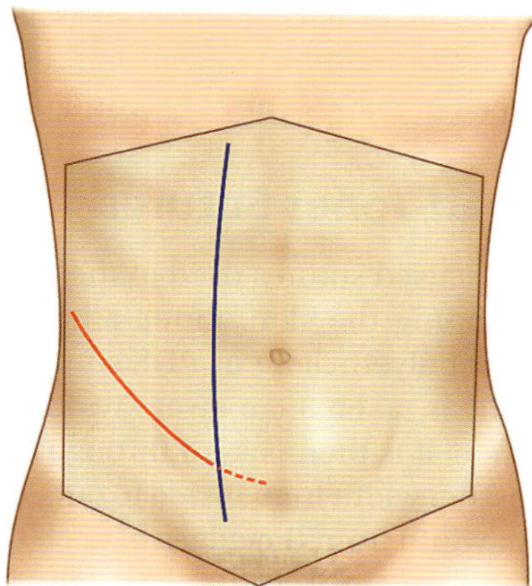

Fig. 18-38: Oblique iliac incision.

Ureter with its typical look and peristalsis is also identified. Depending on the type of surgery further procedure is undertaken. Muscle is retracted using self-retaining retractor. Peritoneum if inadvertently opened, it can be sutured using 2-zero vicryl.

LOIN INCISIONS

It is mainly used to approach kidney, adrenal and retroperitoneum. Patient is placed in loin position. Patient is put in full lateral position with kidney bridge raise with flexion of the knee of the leg which is on the theatre table. Flat wide pillow should be kept between legs. Arm facing upwards is positioned near head end with a support. Patient is strapped firmly to prevent tilting or changing the position during surgery. Back support is often needed. Mayo's table is placed on the leg side after draping which facilitates to keep instruments safely. After cleaning and draping, incision begins posteriorly behind the posterior axillary line in posterior subcostal line extending forward towards the outer margin of the rectus muscle. Rectus is usually not cut. Skin, subcutaneous tissue and superficial fascia are cut. Posteriorly latissimus dorsi, serratus posterior inferior and quadratus lumborum are cut; anteriorly external and internal oblique muscles are cut. Usually 12th or 11th rib is cut. Rib is identified. Incision is made over its periosteum. Periosteum is reflected using periosteal elevator. Care should be taken to avoid injury to vessels underneath which often need proper ligation. Rib after mobilisation, is cut using bone cutter. Cut end is often smoothened using bone file. Pleura lies very close to the rib which should not be opened. If opened pneumothorax develops; which is usually managed by placing vicryl sutures to pleura while anaesthetist is ventilating the lung with adequate expansion. Usually intercostal tube is not necessary. Postoperative chest X-ray is needed to check for the evidence of pneumothorax. Transverse abdominis muscle is usually split from posterior to anterior. Peritoneum is adherent to the abdominal wall in front. So care should be taken not to tear on the anterior aspect. Peritoneum is swept forward to reach the Gerota's fascia **(Fig. 18-40)**.

Closure of the Loin Wound Approach

It is done in two layers. Transversus abdominis and internal oblique muscles are closed using continuous vicryl suture as inner layer. External oblique is closed using non-absorbable or delayed absorbable continuous suture as outer layer. Covering fascia should be included in the bite which is stronger than muscle itself.

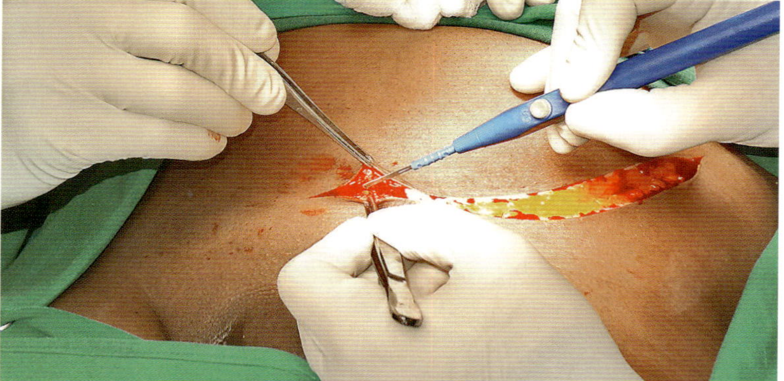

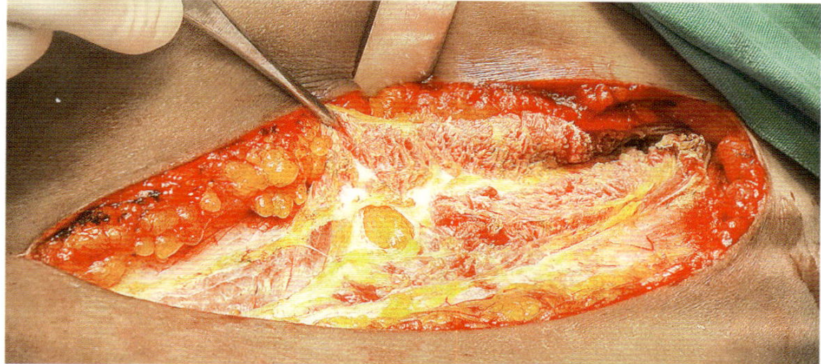

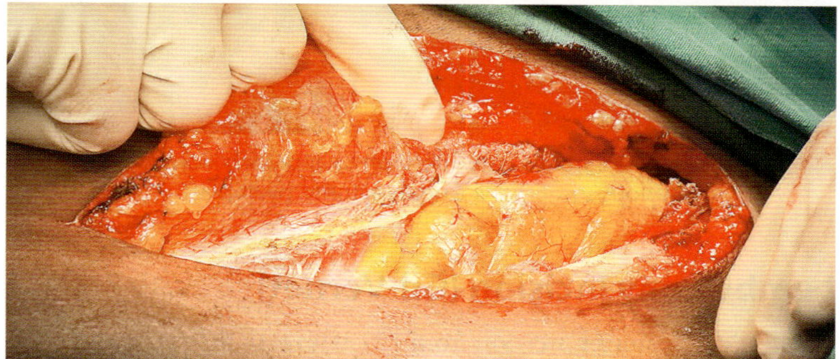

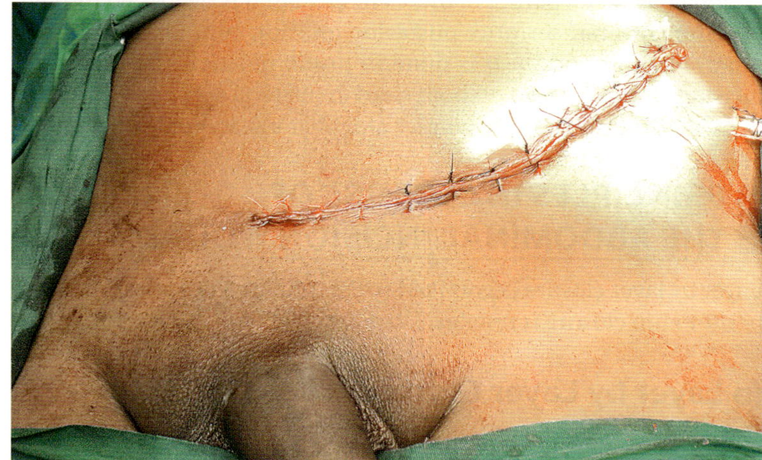

Fig. 18-39: Oblique iliac incision and closed wound also.

Drain when needed should be kept below the lower margin of the wound and on the anterior aspect in front of the level of anterior superior iliac spine; through a separate stab incision.

Incision can be extended into the thorax or into the peritoneal cavity as needed.

High 11th rib excision approach is called as *Nagamatsu approach* which is used in approaching renal cell carcinoma (RCC) in upper pole of kidney.

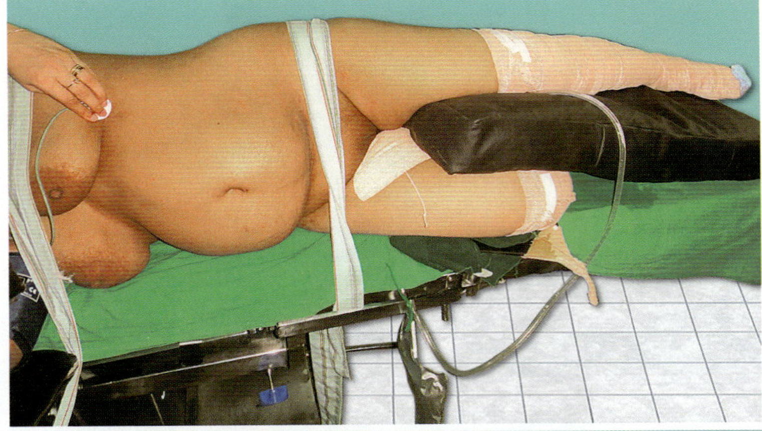

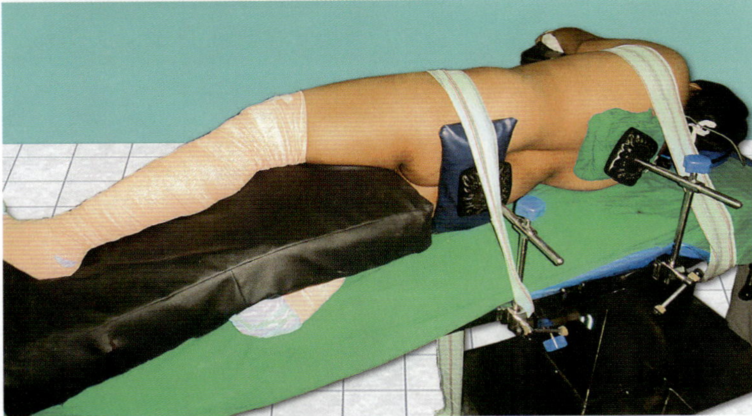

Fig. 18-40: Lateral kidney position to approach kidney for various surgeries like nephrectomy, pyeloplasty.

Lumbotomy Incision (Gil-Vernet)

It is vertical posterior incision from 12 rib level to iliac crest. Incision is along the lateral border of the sacrospinalis. It is deepened through latissimus dorsi, serratus posterior inferior, lumbosacral fascia, quadratus lumborum. It is done in prone position. Two separate incisions can be placed on both sides in bilateral approach. It is used in bilateral partial nephrectomies and bilateral adrenalectomies.

PRINCIPLES IN CLOSURE OF THE ABDOMINAL INCISION WOUND

Layer by layer closure is good old standard. But it is now proved that peritoneum closure is not necessary.

In Layer by Layer Closures

Peritoneum is closed using vicryl or polypropylene; rectus sheath is closed with continuous locking monofilament non-absorbable sutures; (interrupted sutures may be better if there is sepsis); subcutaneous tissue is closed using 3-zero rapid vicryl (ideal) or plain catgut; skin closed using interrupted mattress sutures. Skin stapler can be used as it is quicker and easy to remove; but it is not haemostatic, bleeding may occur from skin edge.

Single Layer

Mass closure is also used. It is also equally good; rapid. Usually continuous suture is placed; but interrupted sutures also can be used. Skin is apposed separately.

Retention sutures, used earlier after an emergency surgery, is more often replaced by modified Smead-Jones sutures. Retention suture is still practiced in many centres of world.

Modified Smead-Jones Sutures

It is interrupted specialised sutures used in the closure of abdomen as single layer excluding the skin. Linea alba is held with Allis' forceps. *Number one* polyethylene or PDS suture material is used. First bite on one side is taken 3 cm away (width) from the margin from outside to inside; it is then passed through the corresponding opposite edge with 3 cm width from inside to outside; later again one small loop of 5 mm width from the edges of each side of the wound from first bite site to second bite site is taken; suture is knotted on the free edge of the first bite side. Full thickness bite holds the suture and maintains the tension in the wound. Smaller loop keeps the linea alba in apposed place. Large curved *Ferguson needle* is better to place these sutures. Each suture is placed at 2 cm interval. This is the type of suturing used at present in acute abdominal conditions instead of the retention sutures. Here also it is better to place all sutures under proper vision and knotting is done at the end. At least four knots should be placed. Excessive tension should be avoided. In upper abdomen peritoneum need not be included in the bite; but in lower abdomen as linea alba is indistinct, peritoneum is included in this **(Fig. 18-41)**.

LE Hughes Double Near and Far Suture

It is similar with same indications as Smead-Jones, with double near and far sutures placed to have a strong loop with knot on one side **(Fig. 18-42)**.

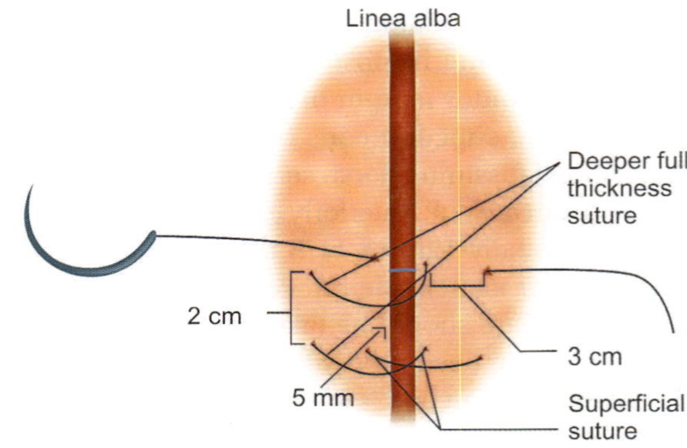

Fig. 18-41: Modified Smead-Jones sutures. These sutures are better than placing retention sutures.

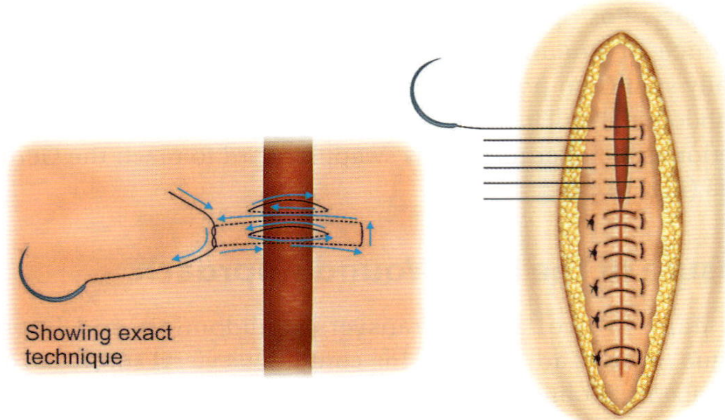

Fig. 18-42: LE Hughes double near and far suture.

While taking bite from the peritoneum, care should be taken not to take bites from bowel; if inadvertently taken leads to dangerous faecal fistula. Guarding the bowel using finger lift or using mop or using sergeant retractor is a must. Before finishing the final bites it is ideal to place index finger under the sutured peritoneum to confirm that suture line is perfect and without any bowel entangling.

Drain if needed to be placed should be away from the main incision; usually along the anterior axillary line; side and site (upper or lower) is decided depending on the type and area of surgery. Often double drains are placed on the same or both sides.

Retention Sutures

In this suturing all the abdominal layers are held together without tension; the sutures take the tension off the wound edges.

Uses

It is used for patients who are debilitated (malnutrition, old age, immune deficiency or advanced cancer); patients suffering from conditions associated with raised intra-abdominal pressure like obesity, asthma or chronic cough; those with impaired healing; burst abdomen.

Material used

Monofilament non-absorbable suture material no. 1 (nylon/polyethylene/polypropylene) is used **(Fig. 18-43)**.

Technique

Retention sutures are inserted through the entire thickness of the abdominal wall leaving them untied in the beginning. All sutures are passed first. Sutures are passed through and through all layers from skin, rectus sheath, rectus muscle and peritoneum on one side and back on the opposite edge with a sufficient gap of 1.5–2 cm from the edges of the wound. Sutures may be simple or mattress. Later peritoneum is closed with continuous vicryl sutures and then anterior rectus sheath with continuous or interrupted followed by subcutaneous tissue and skin (interrupted).

After completion of skin suture, each untied retention suture is threaded with (sleeve) 1–2 cm length of plastic or rubber tubes/sleeves. Plastic sleeves can be placed earlier itself; often it is of practice to place two tubes/sleeves on either sides of the wound to complete the vertical mattress sutures. Now sutures are apposed and tied but without any tension. Undue tension may compromise the blood supply of the tissues at wound edges. Horizontal mattress retention sutures are also used by many.

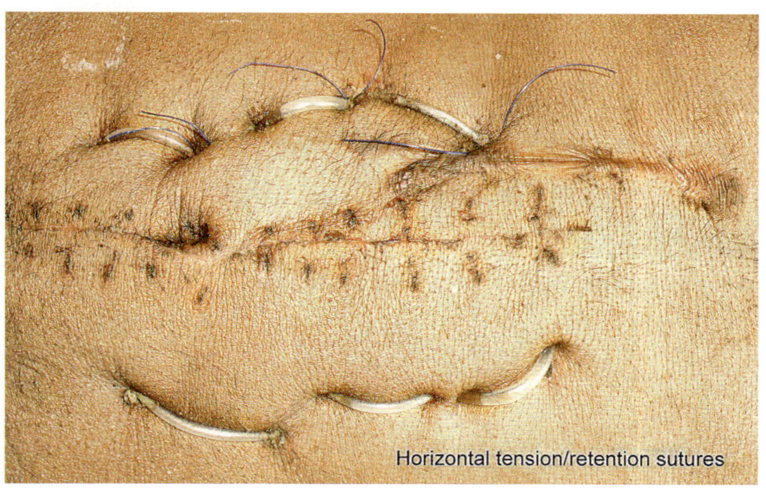

Fig. 18-43: Retention sutures—horizontal.

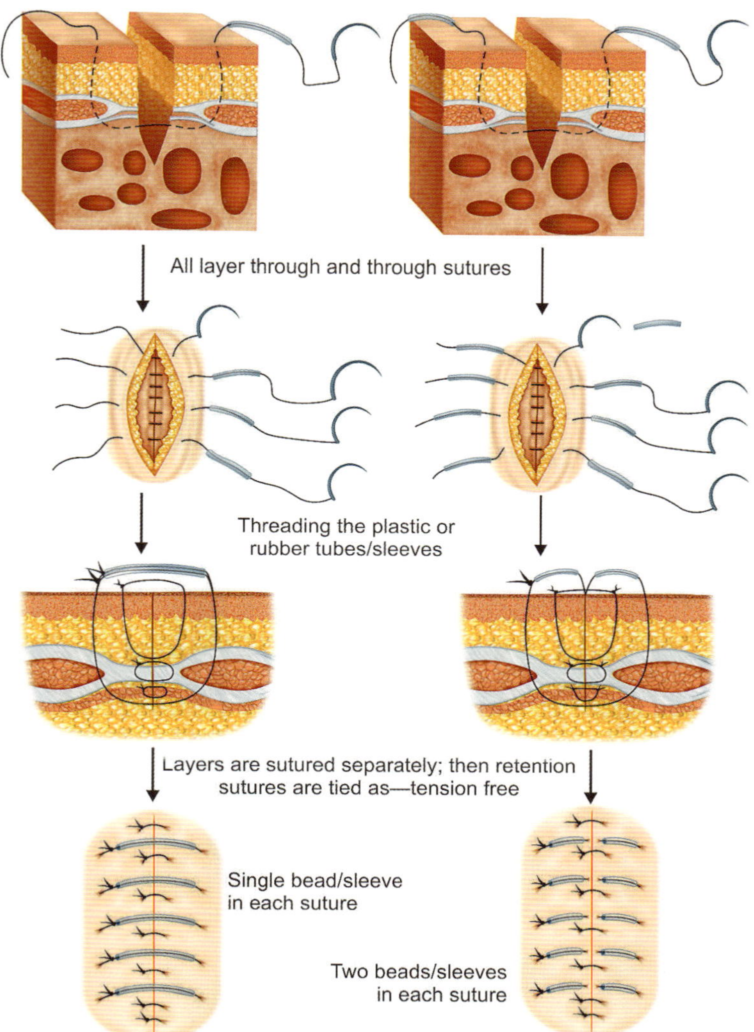

Fig. 18-44: Retention sutures.

Retention sutures are left in place for 14 days.

Many surgeons advocate closure only by placing retention sutures with skin sutures without placing any apposition sutures on peritoneum and rectus sheath **(Fig. 18-44)**.

Controversy

Presently use of retention sutures is controversial. Hughes far and near sutures or Smead-Jones sutures are said to be better. However, retention sutures are still used worldwide even now **(Fig. 18-45)**.

Note

Continuous sutures are started from far point of the wound towards surgeon.

Forehand suturing is better during closure which gives less strain to shoulder, arm and wrist allowing surgeon to do more precise, firm strong sutures at specified sites. Here forearm moves from pronated to supinated position.

In *backhand suturing*, supinated hand rotates to pronated position; here needle should be directed towards surgeon's right foot (right hand surgeon). Scalpel incision and dissection needs backhand movement.

Proper foot positioning is important in various levels of suturing to make suturing easier and perfect.

During scissor dissection, scissor tip should be directed towards surgeon's left foot.

Contd...

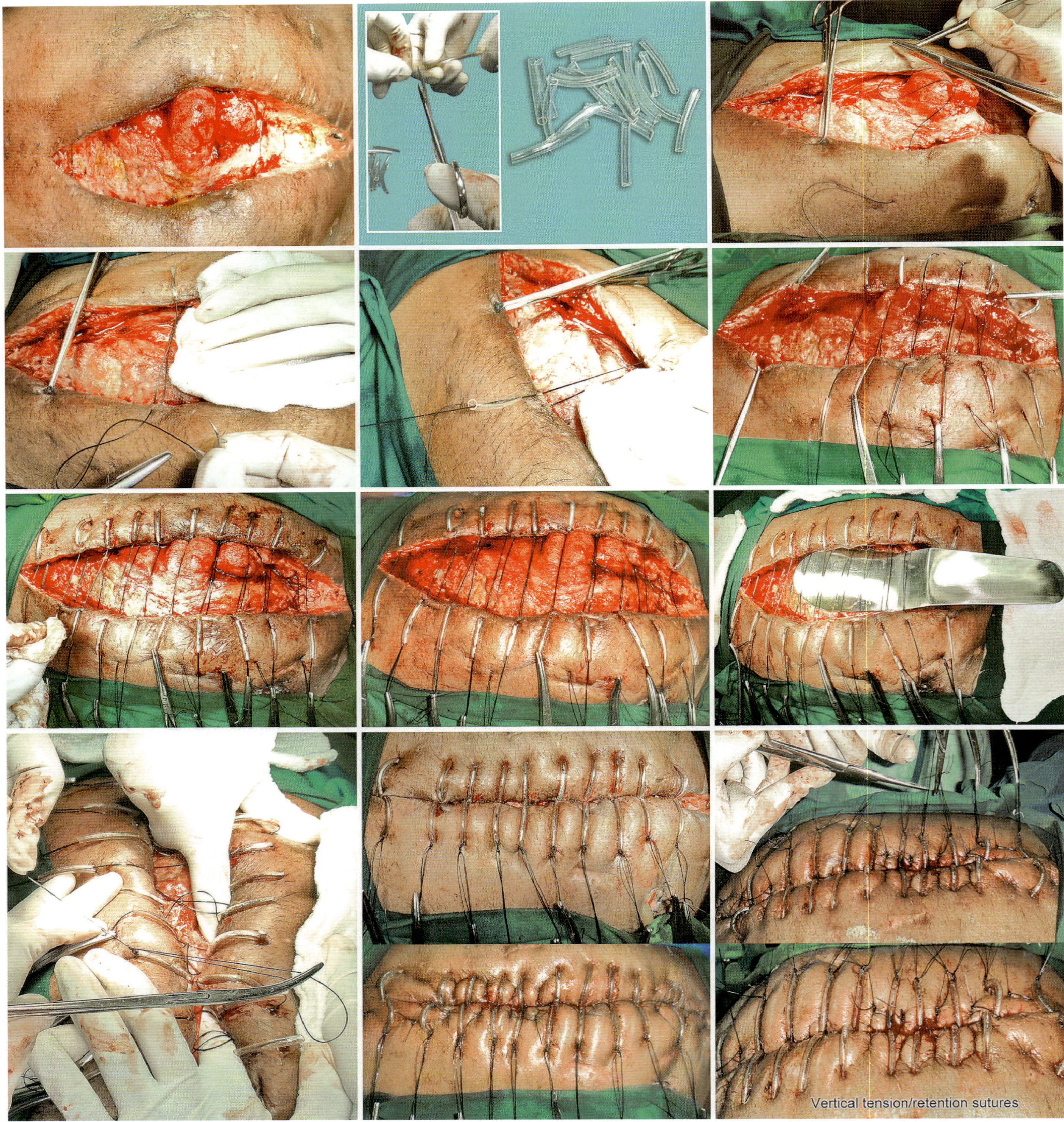

Fig. 18-45: Burst abdomen—placing retention/tension sutures using monofilament non-absorbable sutures.

Contd...

By changing the body and foot position in perpendicular direction (parallel to table) forehand movement can be used in all forehand suturing.
Left foot of the surgeon should be more close to the operating table; right foot should be more lateral.
All instruments should be held in fingertip position.
Instruments should be held with finger grip rather than tight vise grip.
Relaxed wrist movements are essential to avoid wrist tremors.
When suturing comes towards the end of the abdominal wound; last few sutures should not be tied if they are interrupted or last few bites and their loops is kept loose until last bite is taken to avoid injury to deeper structures (bowel).
Suture bite and stitch should not be taken blindly without seeing the tip (point) of the needle at all the time.
Optimum tension should only be used; excessive tension should be avoided.

ABDOMINAL RETRACTORS

Retractors are essential for all abdominal surgeries. Simple Langenbeck to complex self-retaining chain retractors are used in various procedures. Retraction facilitates the surgery in the deeper plane.

Self-retaining or Manual Retractors

Manual retractor is held by assistant constantly. It fatigues the assistant in lengthy procedures and retraction varies depends on the assistant who holds the retractor. But retractor can be temporarily relaxed when not needed so that tissues underneath (muscle) can be allowed to relax in between to reduce crushing effects on the muscle mass. Its position is adjustable in time to time.

Self-retaining retractors are either fixed through its own beams or bars or through a specialised devices strong chain or handle to the side beam of the operation table. They are continuous non-altering (in-position) mechanical retractors. These self-retaining retractors allow assistant's hands to be free for other works like suctioning, passing ligatures, cauterising, etc. But self-retaining retractors may cause more damage to the muscle as retraction is persistent and constant for long period. *Upper hand retractor* is often used with a steel bridge which is attached to both sides of the operating table crossing across the sternum at 5–10 cm height. Retractor blades are placed and fixed on to this steel bridge to facilitate the retraction at the operating site **(Figs. 18-46 to 18-48)**.

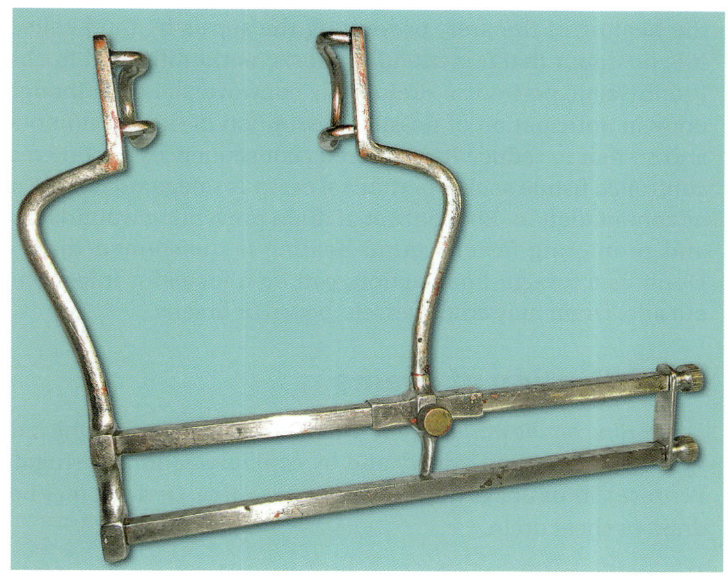
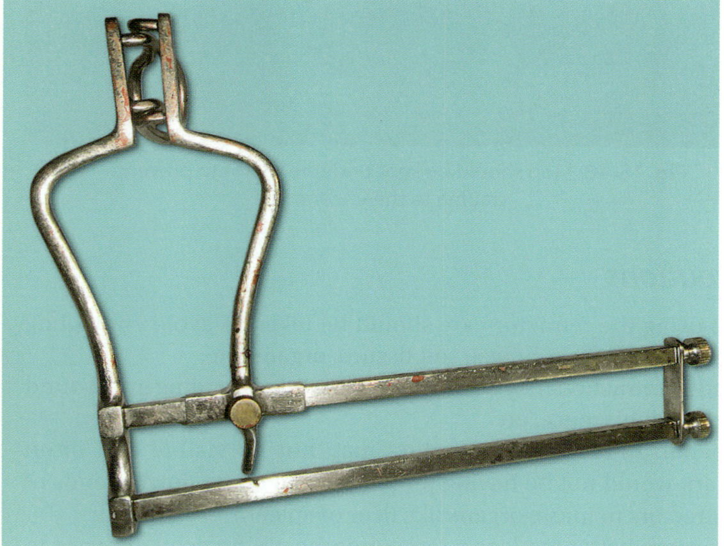

Fig. 18-46: Balfour's self-retaining retractor.

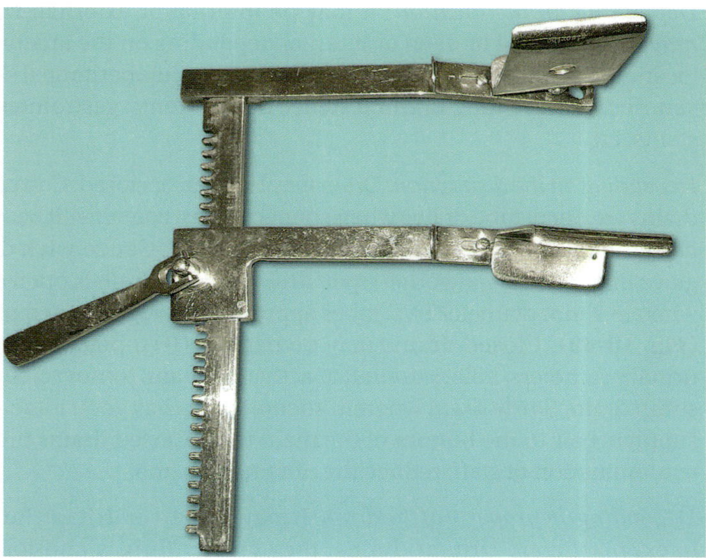
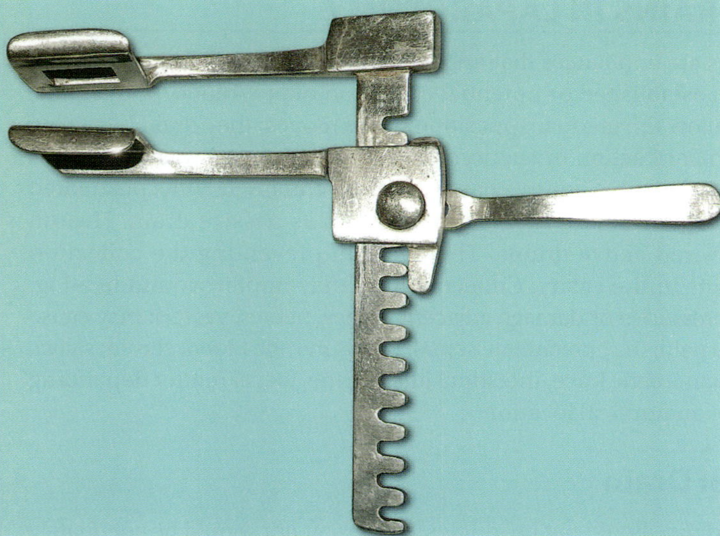

Fig. 18-47: Finochietto retractor.

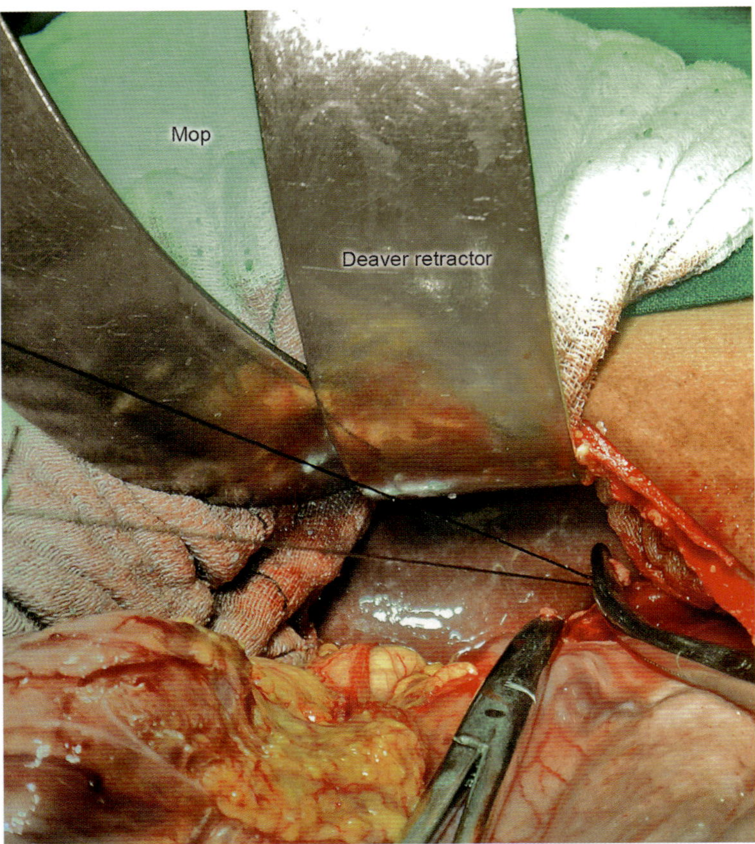

Fig. 18-48: Mop should be kept under retractor to prevent trauma to the viscera.

Precautions

While using the retractor care should be taken to avoid entangling of the vital structures bowel, soft tissues, organs, etc.

Undue retraction may injure the wound edges leading into wound infection, dehiscence, etc.

Deeper ends of the retractors may not be visible and often assistant would not be having proper control on it allowing ends of the retractors to injure organs like liver or spleen.

It is often better to place a mop underneath the deep retractor to avoid injury to organs underneath.

DRAINS IN LAPAROTOMY

Drains are appliances that are deliberately created channels through which established or potential collection of pus/blood/body fluids; they allow the gradual apposition of the tissues; they drain by gravity or capillary action or suction method. Hippocrates was using glass tube/metal tube/bone as passive drain. Leonard da Vinci postulated capillary attraction in small bore tubes as passive drain. Heaton discovered active drains. They help in preventing the collection of fluids in the cavity. Collected fluid may impair wound healing; may pressurise or damage adjacent tissues, nerves, vessels; may cause severe pain; may precipitate sepsis. Fluids may be blood, serum, saliva, bile, pancreatic juice, intestinal juice, urine, faecal matter depending on the anatomical location.

Ideal Drain

Ideal drain should not be too rigid or too soft but should be adequately firm; it should be smooth to avoid fibrin adherence on its surface; material should be resistant or disintegration; drain should be wide and patent; should not get blocked; should function adequately; should be non-electrolytic, non-carcinogenic, non-thrombogenic.

Indications for Usage of the Drain

It may be therapeutic (abscess drainage, VP shunt, urinary catheterisation), prophylactic (postoperative drains in elective cases—thyroid, breast, thoracic, abdominal surgeries), palliative (VP shunt, VA shunt, stenting of the GI malignancies), diagnostic (T tube cholangiogram), monitor purpose (urinary catheter).

Even though advantages are under *debate and controversial*, drain is used to prevent the collection in dead space; to allow the escape of fluid or air from the cavities; to prevent infection; to promote healing.

When there is an abscess or pus in the peritoneal cavity, drain is a must. Here it is therapeutic. Drains commonly advocated are tube drains which are connected outside to a sterile bag or container. Drains placed in other situations are rather prophylactic.

Drain is placed to allow escape of bile, pancreatic and intestinal juices, lymph, serum, blood and pus from peritoneal cavity. Drain creates a track and walls off the leaking/infected site from peritoneal cavity and so prevents the spread of infection. This is said to promote the healing of the area, preventing the sepsis by fluid collection. It is no doubt that it is useful in sepsis, peritonitis, and in abscess. Prophylactic peritoneal drainage is controversial even though it is done in anticipation of possible disruption of the anastomotic site and so that to reduce its dangerous consequences. Drain creates a controlled fistula so that peritoneal cavity is safeguarded from sepsis or contamination. But concept of drain preventing wound infection and promoting faster wound healing is questioned/disproved? Drain as a foreign body action, can be a focus for infection from outside. Drain may erode vessels, bowel or organs.

Classification of Drains

Depending on the nature of the drain: Drain may be flat which drains by dependency and gravity and by capillary action (corrugated or Penrose); its drainage depends on surface area. Or drain may be tube drain or sheet drain.

Depending on the mechanism of action: Drain may be passive or active.

Depending on the location: It may be internal or external. *Drains may be* superficial or deep or internal depending on the anatomical location. Examples of internal drain are—ventriculoperitoneal shunt; ventriculoatrial shunt, urethral stents, biliary stents, gastrointestinal stents, etc.

Depending on the disposition: Drain may be open or closed. Corrugated drains are open; tube drains when connected to a container it becomes closed and if not connected it becomes open. Gauze wick drain, glove finger drain—are other open drains. *Yeates drain* is open drain wherein 2 mm diameter PVC tubes approximated together and placed **(Fig. 18-49)**. Closed drains may be passive (ICT, pigtail catheter, urinary catheters, biliary drains) or active (JP drain, romovac, suction sump drain, *Shirly drain* wherein suction drain has got n intact tube supplying air to the bottom of the main tube. Closed drains prevent contamination of staff; reduce the nursing time too.

Depending on property of the drain: It may be inert or irritant. Rubber, latex, plastic are irritant drains; they create fibrosis and forms a track to achieve controlled fistula (example in biliary system).

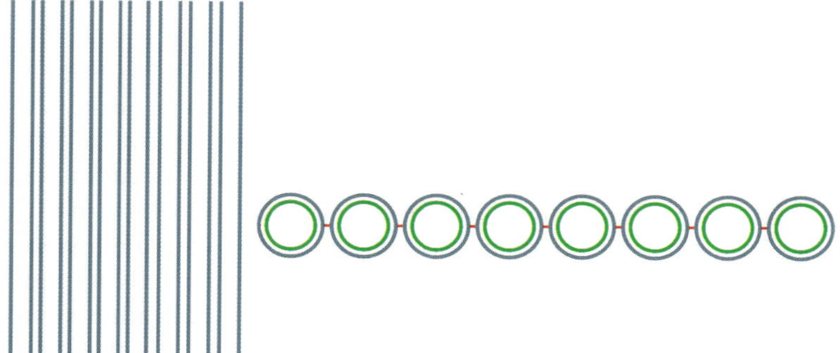

Fig. 18-49: Yeates drain—multiple tubes are approximated each other, each made up of 2 mm PVC.

Poly vinyl chloride (PVC), silastic and silicone are inert materials; they are useful where irritation should be minimal like in urethra.

Deepening on the material it is made up off: Rubber or silicone or latex or plastic or PVC or others.

The efficiency of a drain depends on the diameter and length of the drain; type, viscosity and consistency of the fluid; whether positive or negative pressure area. ***Passive drains*** are used when draining fluid is too viscous and cannot pass through the tube drains; they drain by positive pressure. Drain exit site should be dependent. Bulky absorbable dressing is needed over the drain. Examples of passive drains are—corrugated drain, penrose drain and sump drain. Here it is difficult to assess the quantity of the drain; excoriation is common; discomfort to patient is usual. It may carry infection inside (retrograde infection) the cavity from outside. Tissue apposition may be inadequate and so recollection of the fluid may be possible. Pressure necrosis is low and obstruction is not common. Tube drains are connected outside to a bag quantity of which is measurable; excoriation is not common; but displacement can occur; patient has to carry the tube with bag while mobilising. ***Active drains*** are drained by suction as negative pressure. It may be low continuous/low intermittent or high pressure. Quantity of content can be measured appropriately; there is no tissue trauma; skin excoriation does not occur; infection chances are less; but regular activation of the reservoir is needed. Dependency in position of the drain is not necessary. Retrograde infection is less common. But blockage of the tube is more likely and is the drawback. Multiple holes are made towards inner end to reduce the chances of blockage. Pressure necrosis is also higher. Setting a certain pressure depending on the anatomical location is important. It is usually radiopaque.

Drains may be passive or active. *Passive drain* like Penrose or corrugate function depending on the pressure difference between inside and outside abdominal cavity and high pressure inside forces the fluid outside. *Active drains* use low or high negative pressure (suction) to remove accumulated fluid from a wound. Active drains require some special device and maintenance. The collection reservoir of an active drain expands as fluid is collected by exchanging negative pressure for fluid; if the vacuum is lost, the drain will lose its effectiveness. The fluid collection reservoir is either a manually activated, or through bulb evacuator or a spring-loaded device that has variable preset suction levels.

Drains may be *closed or open system*. Drains may be allowed to function naturally by gravity or by capillary action (corrugated drain) or by suction device. It may be connected to wall suction to have continuous or intermittent vacuum suction in wounds.

Drain should be observed daily for its nature and volume of content accurately. Depending on the quantity of the drain, duration of keeping the drain in situ is decided. Open drains like Penrose and corrugated should have protective dressings over it. Amount of soiling should be assessed for possible quantity of drainage and type—bile/faecal/serous/serosanguineous/purulent/gastric.

Passive Drains

Passive drains even though used by many surgeons, are not very suitable as their efficacy is inadequate and complications are more. Penrose drain and corrugated rubber drains are commonly used. Tube drains like Malecot's/Foley's catheters/nasogastric tubes are also often used for this purpose. Flat drains outside are covered by dressing pads. Tube drains are connected to sterile container (urosac bag) or sterile glove outside. Tube drains are better than flat drains **(Figs. 18-50 to 18-52)**.

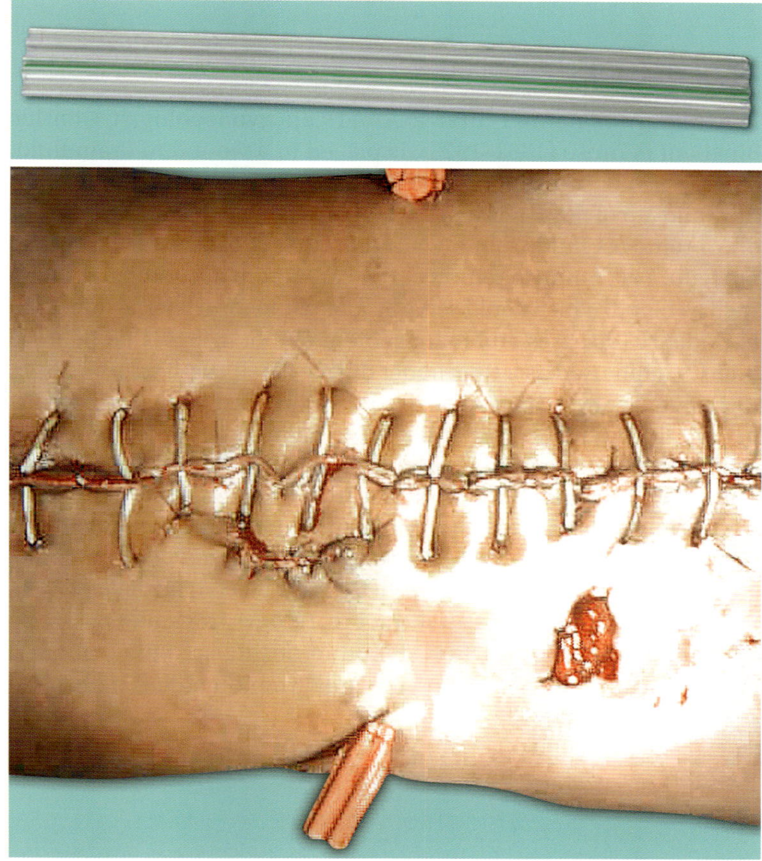

Fig. 18-50: Corrugated drain is a passive drain which drains by gravity and capillary action. It is rather an overflow.

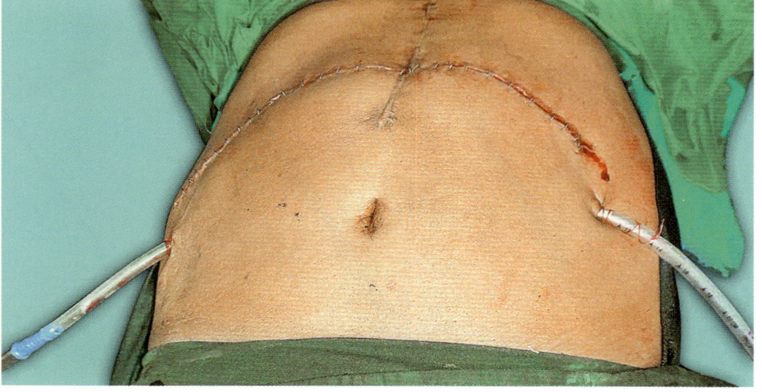

Fig. 18-51: Tube drains placed in the peritoneal cavity.

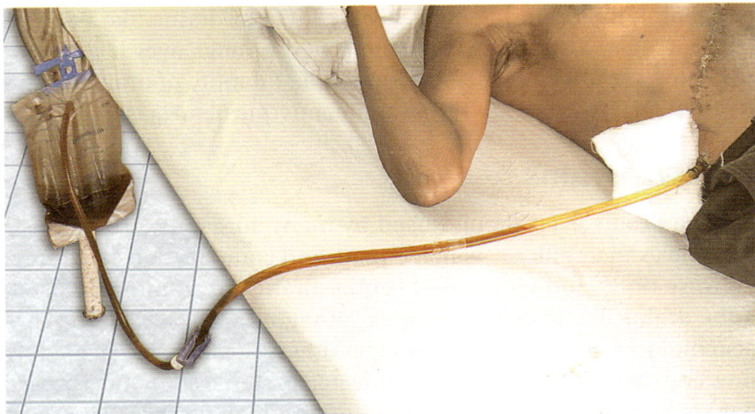

Fig. 18-52: Tube drain placed in biliary surgery. Note the bile collected in the reservoir bag (urosac).

Penrose Drain

Penrose drain named after a American gynaecologist Charles Bingham Penrose (1862–1925), is placed in a wound to drain fluid. It consists of a soft rubber tube placed in a wound area, to prevent the build-up of fluid. It is a passive open drainage system. A Penrose drain removes fluid from a wound area. It is used after a surgical procedure is complete to prevent the area from accumulating fluid, such as blood, which could serve as a medium for bacterial infection. In podiatry (diseases and management of foot diseases), a Penrose drain is often used as a tourniquet during a nail excision or ingrown toenail excision. It can also be used to drain CSF in a hydrocephalus patient. It is a quadrangular flat tube made up of radiopaque thin rubber sheet. It is available as prepacked sterile drain with a safety pin. Safety pin prevents drain getting retracted into the wound while in use. Head of the safety pin should be crimped and closed to prevent injuring the patient's skin. Different sized Penrose drains are available. Multiple Penrose tubes can be placed. It is inexpensive and creates fibrosis to form a tract in 10 days. It drains passively by mere gravity and overflow. Blood in oozing area may clot and block the drain. Infection into the area from outside is a possible drawback **(Fig. 18-53)**.

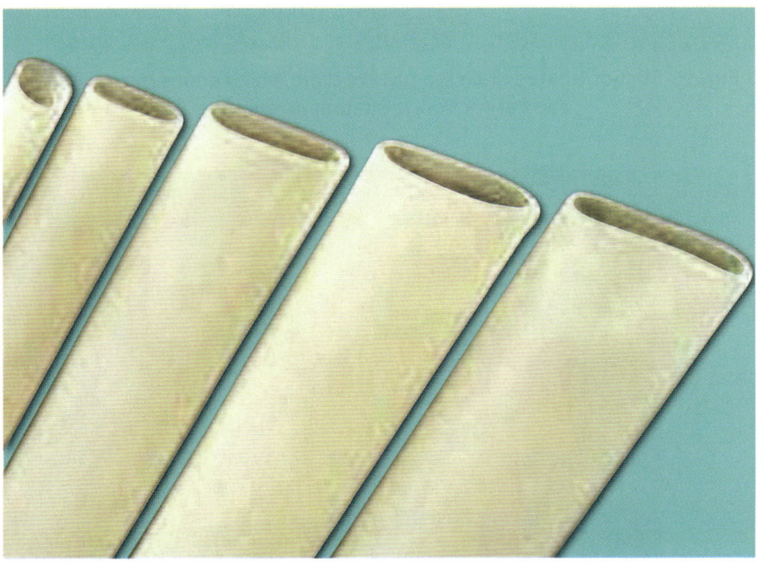

Fig. 18-53: Penrose drain.

Active (Negative Pressure) Drains

Negative pressure causes—continuous wound cleaning thereby decrease the bacterial burden in the wound, remove substances that inhibit wound healing; promotes continuous removal of fluid like exudates so that the mechanical compression by accumulated exudates into the capillaries at the site is prevented which in turn restricts the flow of blood into wound site; causes wound retraction and approximation of wound edges; creates externally applied mechanical stress in the tissues stimulating matrix synthesis and cell proliferation; promotes healthy granulation tissue formation; decreases interstitial oedema which improves the blood flow.

Davol drain: This is a closed wound suction system which is soft, inert silicone drains with X-ray opaque stripe for easy placement identification. Evacuators provide constant suction and feature a dependable anti-reflux valve to inhibit backflow. Evacuators are easy to activate and measure and empty **(Fig. 18-54)**.

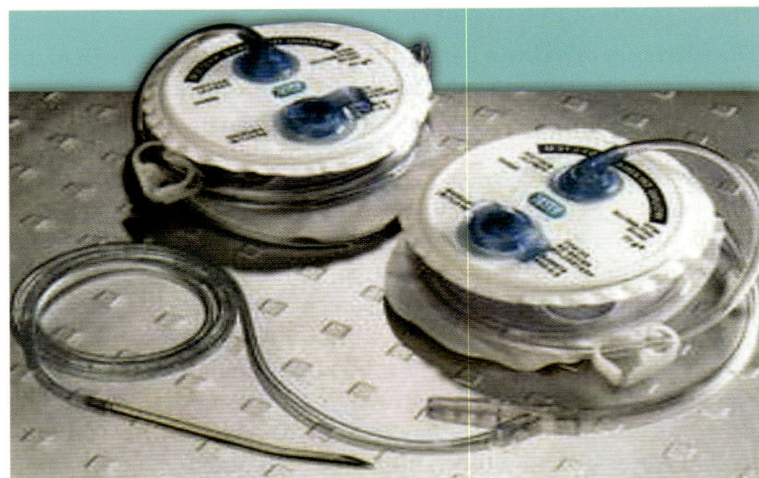

Fig. 18-54: Davol drain. It is closed wound suction drain system.

Negative Pressure Wound Therapy

It is used in infected wounds often in abdominal wall. It creates continuous or intermittent suction of the wound content to keep the wound surface drain which promotes formation of healthy granulation tissue and so wound healing.

Low Pressure Vacuum Drain

Low-pressure vacuum drains have a plastic bulb-shaped reservoir or spring reservoir and a drainage tube (Jackson-Pratt or Romovac), with multiple side holes in the end of the tubing that is inserted into the wound. When the bulb is compressed, air is forced out, which creates low negative pressure to evacuate excess fluid and air gently **(Fig. 18-55)**.

Jackson-Pratt Drain

It is often called as *JP drain*/bulb drain is a flexible plastic tube which connects to an internal plastic drainage tube; it drains excess fluid by constant low suctioning. Due to low pressure vacuum system, intra-abdominal contents like omentum and bowel will not get sucked through the drain thus preventing the possibility of ischaemia of bowel and perforation. Air pressure within the drainage system is removed by removing the plug and squeezing the bulb. Drain is kept folded during uncapping and recapping **(Fig. 18-56)**.

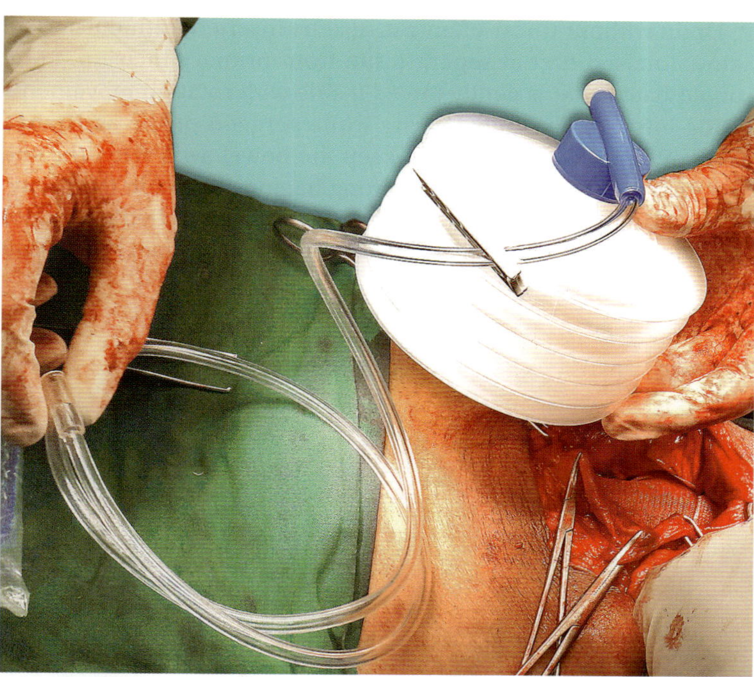

Fig. 18-55: Low suction drain.

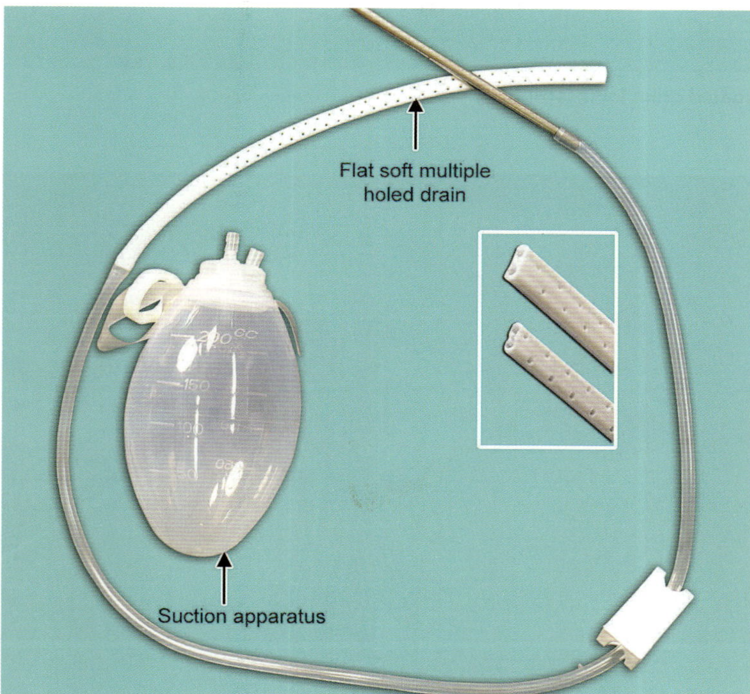

Fig. 18-56: Jackson-Pratt drain; it is bulb-shaped suction device with flat perforated flat soft tube. One end of the tube is placed inside body during surgery. The other end comes out through a small stab wound in the skin. The bulb is connected to this end. The JP drain is used as negative pressure vacuum which removes fluids by creating suction in the tube. The bulb is squeezed flat and connected to the end of the tube. The bulb expands as it fills with fluid. It is used in surgeries of breast, abdomen, thyroid, thorax, etc.

High Negative Pressure Vacuum Drains

They are sealed, closed circuit drain systems (bottled vacuum system) that are easily monitored and allow safe disposal of the drainage. This type of system consists of a clear, plastic/bottled reservoir with a rubber cap and indicator wings that monitor the presence of vacuum pressure and an opening in which the drainage tube connects. When a vacuum is present in the system, the wings on the rubber cap are close together; when the vacuum is lost, the wings are apart. The end of the drainage tube inserted in the wound has numerous openings to evacuate fluid from the wound. The wound should be closed before opening the clamps on the drain; otherwise the vacuum will be lost as the tube pulls in atmospheric air. Bottled vacuum drains are available **(Fig. 18-57)**.

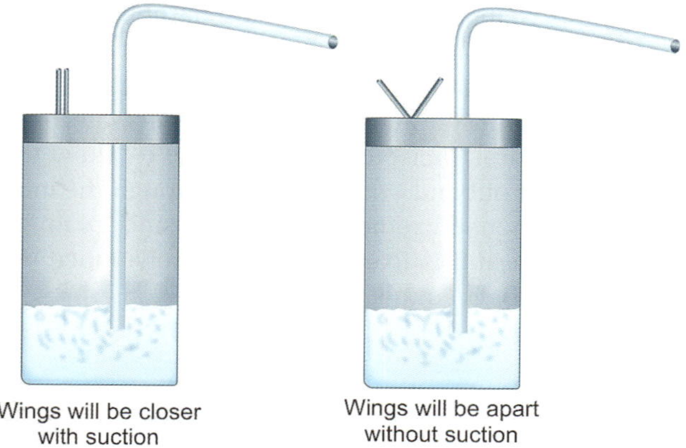

Fig. 18-57: High vacuum suction device. When vacuum is present, wings will be closer together; when vacuum is not present wings will be apart.

Drain Insertion

Technique of insertion of drain is important. When a drain is required, it is inserted at the end of the surgical procedure just prior to closure of the wound. Drain is inserted through a separate stab wound, which is created a few centimeters away from the primary incision which reduces the risk of a postoperative wound infection and dehiscence. Skin incision for drain is usually made at anterior axillary line. Incision is usually within 1 cm in length, transversely placed. Drain should not be inserted towards posterior side as supine position of the patient may be difficult and also drain may get kinked preventing its function.

Drain insertion

It is done in two methods. When there is in-built trocar is not present, long artery forceps is pushed from inside out across peritoneum and abdominal wall muscles; skin is incised using a scalpel; proper track is created by repetitive movements of the jaw of the haemostat. Drain is held with the forceps and pulled inside the abdominal cavity or any other areas/cavities. Drain is securely fixed using shoe lace sutures. When in built trocar is present in the drain (usually suction drains), trocar is passed from inside out across the cavity or abdominal wall and tube is pulled out adequately under observation; trocar is removed from the tube; tube is secured to the skin using stitch (*Roman Garter technique*—using silk). Care should be taken that sharp end of the trocar will not injure the patient or surgical team. So its cap should be reapplied again immediately.

Drain should come out through a shortest, safest, deepest and most dependent route. Drain should be brought out always through a separate stab wound not through main surgical wound with certain exceptions. Incision made to bring out the drain should be larger than drain width (drain should be lesser sized than the stab incision). Drain should not get kinked or migrated from the actual location.

Drain has a sharp trocar attached to the tube is inserted by piercing the trocar to the skin from inside the wound/peritoneal cavity at the desired site; the attached tube is then pulled out through the stab wound; the inner end of the tube is placed at the required site and the trocar is detached. Drain is secured to the skin with proper suture (shoe lace suture). Once the wound is closed, tube is connected to the reservoir; suction is attached to facilitate the drainage.

Drains that do not have an attached trocar is placed by passing a long opened haemostat across the abdominal wall from inside out and skin over it is incised using a scalpel to allow tip of the haemostat to come out and drain is passed through the incision by holding with the opened haemostat towards inside. Drain is placed in desired location and is fixed to skin securely. Once wound is closed, the drain tube is connected to a reservoir.

Drain without trocar often can also be inserted from outside in. Skin is incised first at separate site from primary incision. Long curved haemostat is gently forced inside with rotation movements inside into the peritoneal cavity while surgeon or the assistant's using one of the hands should keep the bowel away from the site of puncture and guide the tip of long haemostat inside the cavity. Once peritoneum is punctured drain is held and pulled out under vision to prevent entangling of any content into the drain site wound **(Figs. 18-58 to 18-60)**.

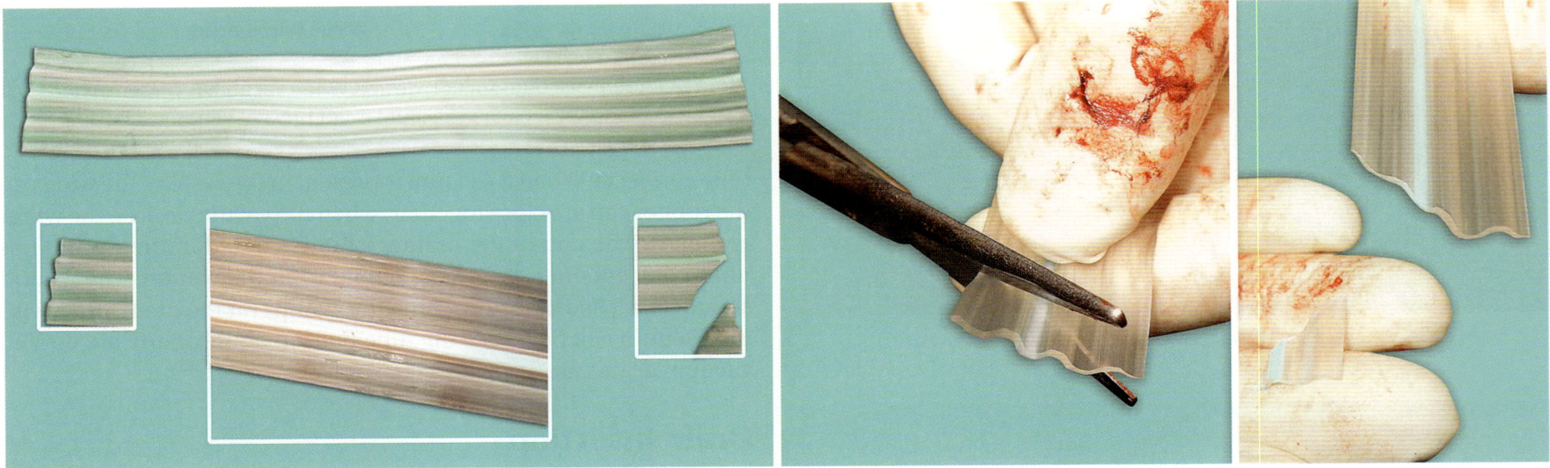

Fig. 18-58: Preparation of corrugated drain for insertion.

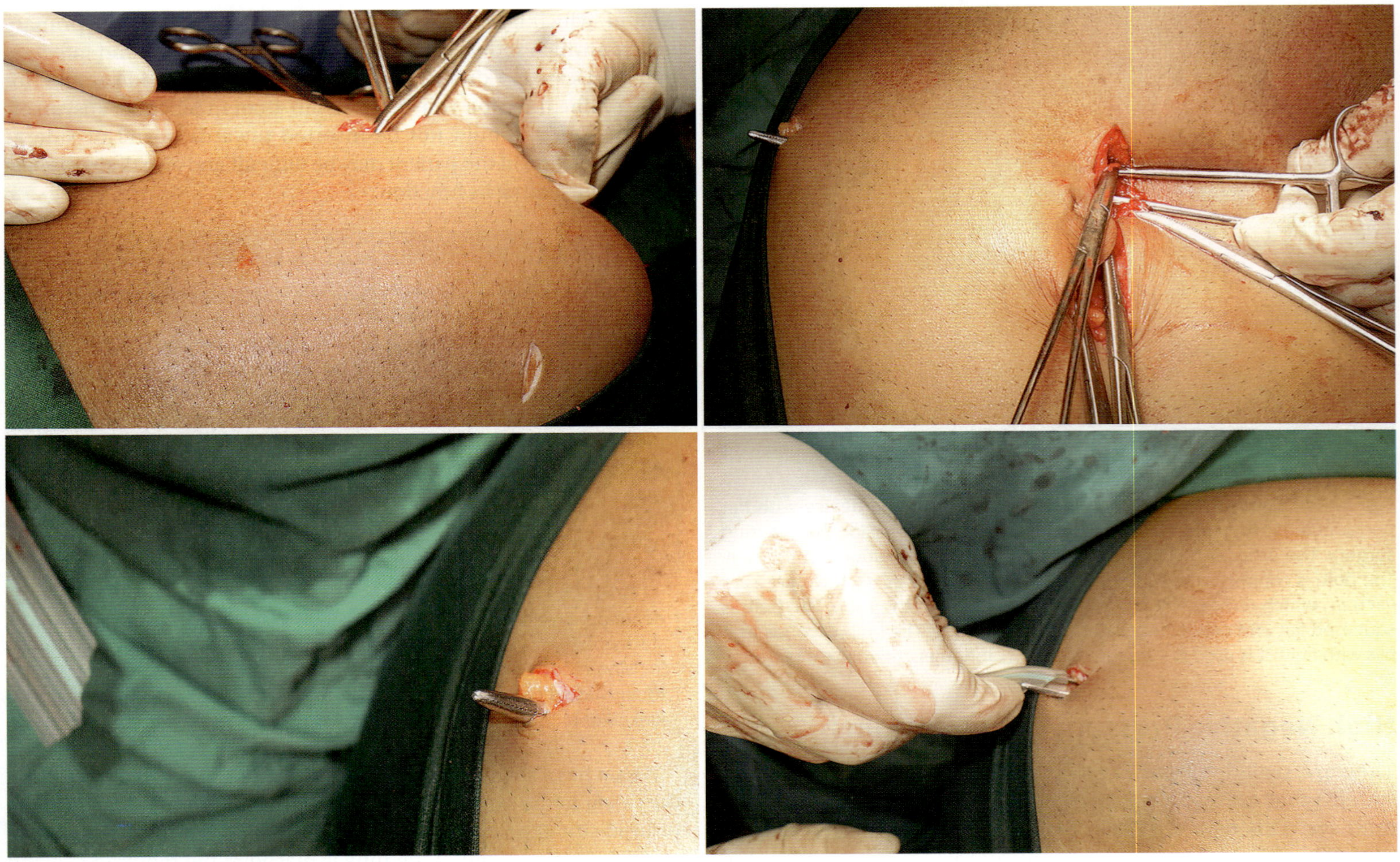

Figs. 18-59(1)

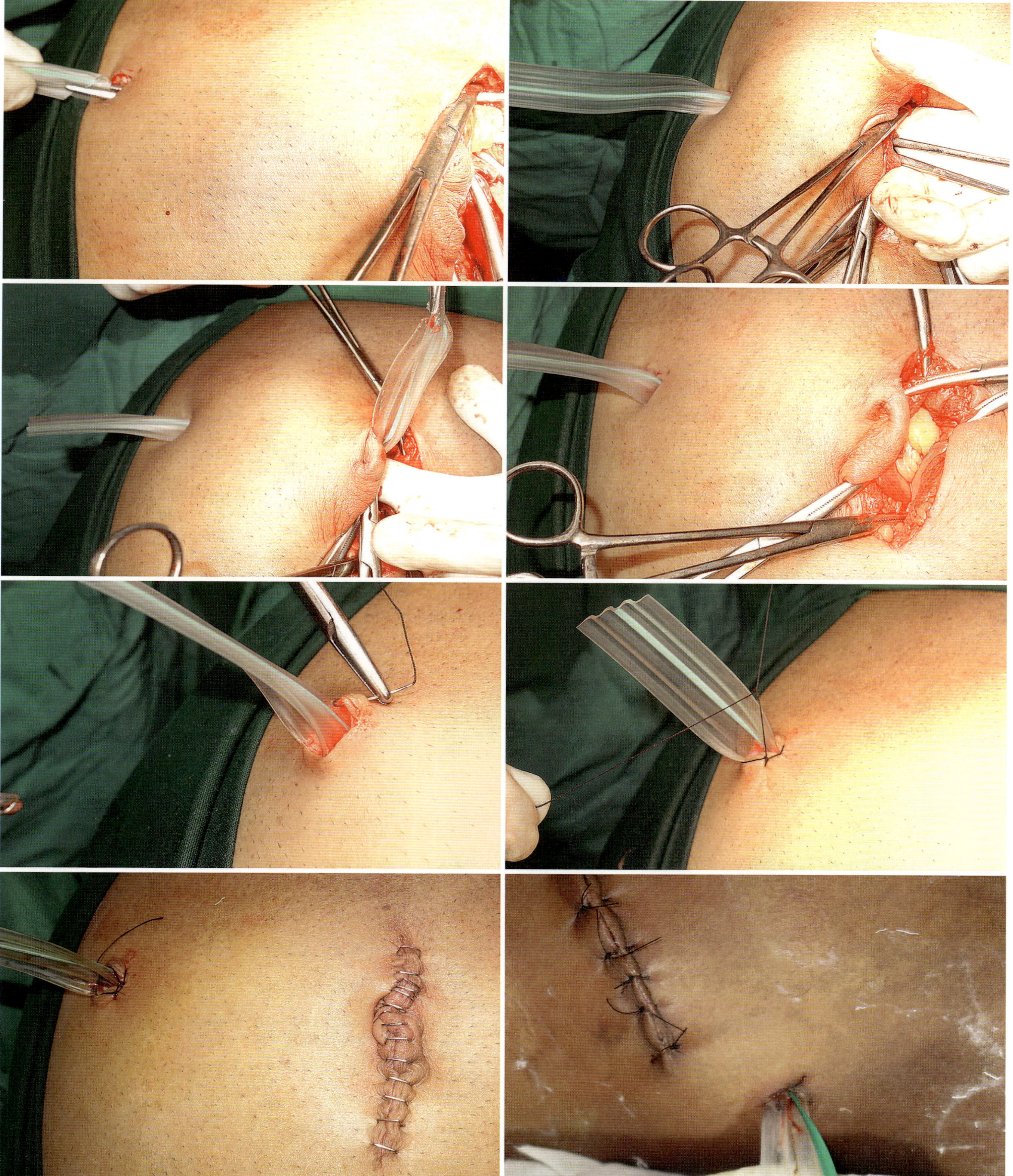

Figs. 18-59(2)

Figs. 18-59(1 and 2): Technique of insertion of corrugated drain.

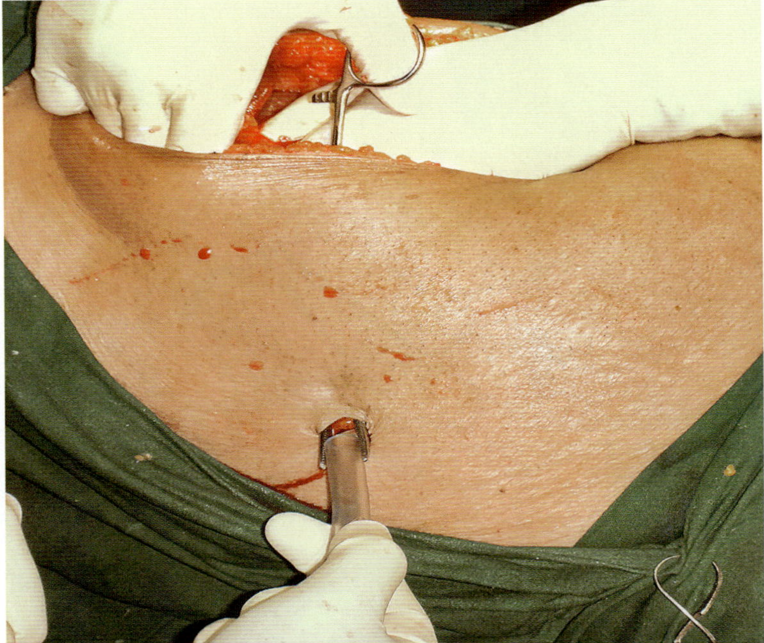

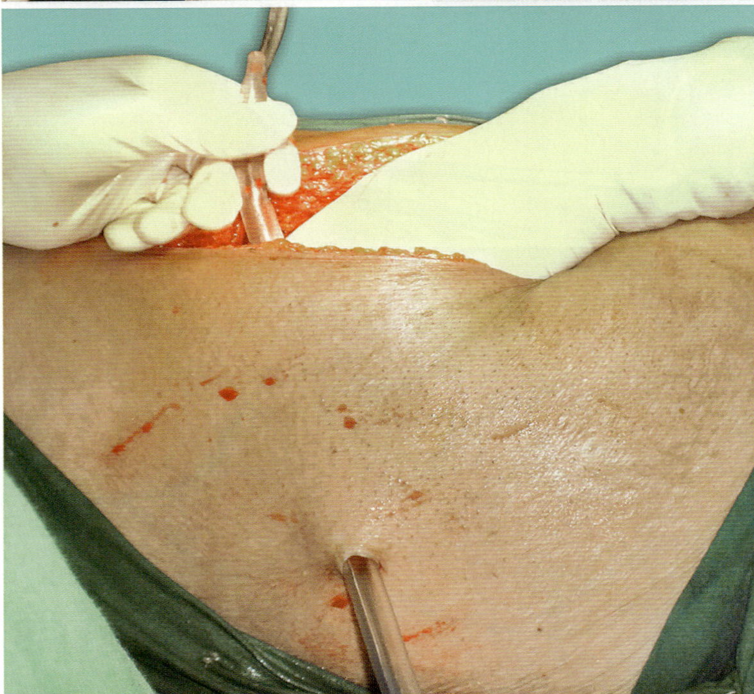

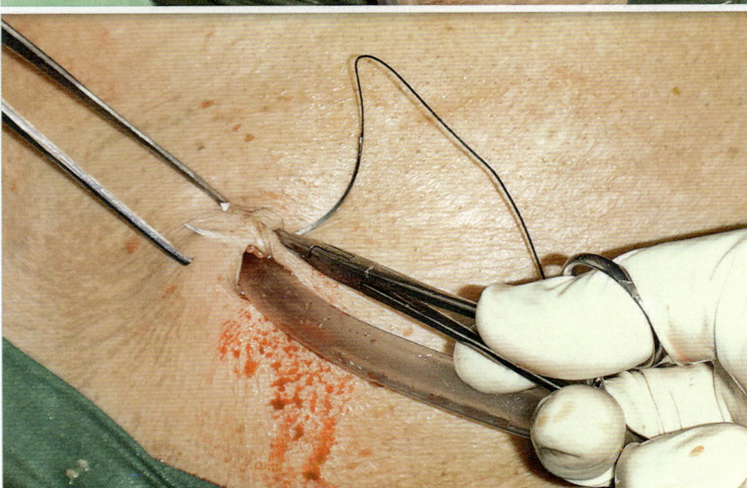

Fig. 18-60: Insertion of drainage tube (without trocar) into the peritoneal cavity.

Complications of the Drain

Drain may cause retrograde bacterial contamination of the abdominal cavity. Drain may erode into the bowel or vessels. Drain acts as a foreign body. Suction drain may suck the bowel or omentum. Drain site after removal forms a puckered scar due to healing by secondary intention. Breakage of drain can occur and inner broken part may be left inside which can cause sepsis. Breakage usually occurs only if drain used is already damaged due to nick by scissor or scalpel. Damaged drain should never be used.

While inserting the drain, injury to bowel or vessel can occur and so care should be taken.

Drain may get blocked giving false impression of healing inside. Blocked drain when suspected should be checked properly either by irrigating the tube with saline or changing the position of the drain. Drain tube can be gently squeezed and released at different points to remove small clogging. If it is presumed that already track is formed then drain can be removed and a newer blunt tipped (Foley's) tube drain can be gently replaced with care along the same tract.

Pain and discomfort at the drain site is common which often hinders the early mobilisation of the patient.

Infection can occur through drain itself; ascending infection from outside is not uncommon. Drain should be removed in such situation; drain tip should be sent for culture and sensitivity and appropriate antibiotics should be given.

Inadvertent removal may be worrisome to surgeon; it often occurs by loosening of the stitch, pulling by the patient. Inadvertent removal may injure the structures along and worry may be that collection or leak can occur at a later period.

Difficulty in removal is another problem; drain should be gently pulled out in such situation or else may require exploration under short anaesthesia to remove the drain entirely and safely.

Drain site often causes ugly scar as it commonly heals by secondary intention. Proper suturing and proper placing of the incision of the drain site may reduce the chances of ugly scar.

Occasionally situation may arise that drain may not be able to removal by all methods; it may be due to long-term drain in position or tissue entanglement or internal suture inadvertently getting entangled. It may require guided reexploration or laparoscopic or endoscopic approach to retrieve the entire drain properly with minimum tissue trauma.

Problems in drain

Mechanical:

- Trauma to tissues.
- Erosion of anatomical structures—vessel (haemorrhage), bowel (fistula), bladder, etc.
- Ugly scar of drain site.
- Drain site herniation.

Physiological:

- Fluid and electrolyte imbalance.
- Pneumothorax.
- Restriction of function—disability temporarily.
- Pain and discomfort at drain site.
- Bacterial ingrow.

Drain related:

- Blockage.
- Displacement.
- Breakage, partial retrieval.
- Leaking from side.
- Improper fixation.
- Retraction of the drain.
- Non-functioning of the drain.
- Inability to removal of the drain—a dangerous situation.

Drain may fall of on its own either by insecure fixation or by pulling out by the patient himself. In such situation first thing to be checked is whether drain has come out completely or not. If part of the drain is left inside, then formal exploration of drain site wound into the deeper plane is needed to remove the retained part of the drain.

Inadvertent pulling of drain while transferring the patient or by entangling into linen or clothes or by patient himself may cause bleeding and pain.

Skin around drain site may get excoriated with redness and pain. Often leak occurs on the side of the drain. In such situation skin around the drain should be dressed using zinc oxide cream.

When drain is kept for long time removal may be difficult due to adhesions and entrapment into the tissue. In such situation exploration at the site may be required to remove the drain.

Drainage may suddenly stop or suddenly increase which should be assessed seriously for the proper cause. It may be more leak or blockage or erosion. Noting the change in colour and odour after more drainage is also important. Nowadays drains commonly used are radiopaque, X-ray of part or ultrasound helps in finding out the cause, site of drain or any collection. Often contrast CT imaging may be required to reassess the situation.

Since drain is passed across the fascial plane, drain site hernia can occur. If pathology in the deeper plane or distal obstruction persists then leak at the drain site may occur.

Removal of Drains

Drains should be removed once purpose is served. Drain placed to cover preoperative bleeding is removed in 48 hours; to drain serous collections it is removed in 2–5 days; in intestinal anastomosis it is removed in 7 days; T tube is removed in 10–14 days. If leak persists it is kept until leak stops after confirmation that source is cleared by imaging method. Drains are removed when draining is of negligible amount (less than 25 mL per day; less than 1 mL per hour).

Skin suture (stay suture) is cut using sterile scissor and drain is gently pulled using continuous constant traction. Drain wound is covered with sterile dressing. Wound usually heals fast without any problem. If drain wound site shows large quantity of drainage then stoma bag can be placed until drainage of fluid stops.

Drain can be shortened gradually—2 cm/day to allow gradual healing of the tissues from within to allow complete removal.

BASIC LAPAROSCOPY

In laparoscopic surgery the prime difference of indirect access to the internal structures means that we have to acquire different set of skills to tackle the given surgical problem. Since there is no open access to the viscera it is very important to have the right kind of instrumentation before we embark on doing laparoscopic surgery. As the most versatile of all the working instruments, the surgeons "hand" is out of bound. Knowing about few technical details about laparoscopic instrumentation helps in long way as often in the operating room the surgeon knows best about electronic equipment. This also ensures proper handling of the expensive equipment and prolongs the life of the same.

History of Laparoscopic Surgery

First laparoscopic cholecystectomy was done by Muhe of Germany in 1985 and by Mouret in Lyon in 1987. McKeran and Saye performed the first laparoscopic cholecystectomy in USA in 1988. First laparoscopic appendicectomy was done by Semm as prophylaxis. First laparoscopic appendicectomy for acute appendicitis was done by Schreiber in 1987. Semm changed 75% open gynaecological surgeries into laparoscopic surgeries.

Prof TE Udwadia, Mumbai did first laparoscopic cholecystectomy in India.

Advantages of Laparoscopic Surgery

It is relatively less painful compared to open surgery. Trauma of access is very less. Shorter hospital stay and early return to work; faster postoperative recovery; better visualisation of the anatomy, i.e. better approach for dissection and visualisation of other parts of abdomen for any other pathology; instrumental access to different abdominal locations is many times better compared to open method and minimal scar on the abdomen—makes laparoscopy more acceptable than open method. Trauma of dissection is also less. Bowel manipulation and exposure is less. Less postoperative ileus facilitates early feeding. Need for intravenous infusion and analgesic is lesser.

LAPAROSCOPIC SET

The most basic to the best equipment shall be briefly described for the reader to get overall picture of equipment. The laparoscopy set up consists of 5 important components.

1. Laparoscopy camera and telescope.
2. Light source and cable.
3. Carbon dioxide insufflator.
4. Monitor.
5. Hand instruments **(Fig. 18-61)**.

Instruments Used

- *Zero* degree laparoscope is commonly used. Side viewing scopes are also used to have better visualisation 30°.
- Cold lights source either halogen lamp or Xenon lamp is used. Halogen lamp is used commonly and is cheaper. Xenon lamp gives high visualisation.
- Camera: 3 chip camera is commonly used with high resolution.
- Video-monitor to display images.
- CO_2 insufflator.
- Long fine dissectors like in open surgical techniques.
- Hooks and spatulas are used along with cautery for dissection.
- Clip applicators.
- Needle holders.
- Endostaplers.
- Veress needle.
- Suction-irrigation apparatus.
- Trocars of different sizes—10 mm, 5 mm.
- Reducers to negotiate smaller instruments through larger parts.

Laparoscopy Camera and Telescope

The laparoscopic camera is like the retina for perception of images during surgery. Without a good camera it is dangerous to embark upon laparoscopic surgery as there cannot be safe surgery without clear vision of the structure on which you operate. The laparoscopic camera has three different components.

a. Camera head
b. Coupler
c. Connector

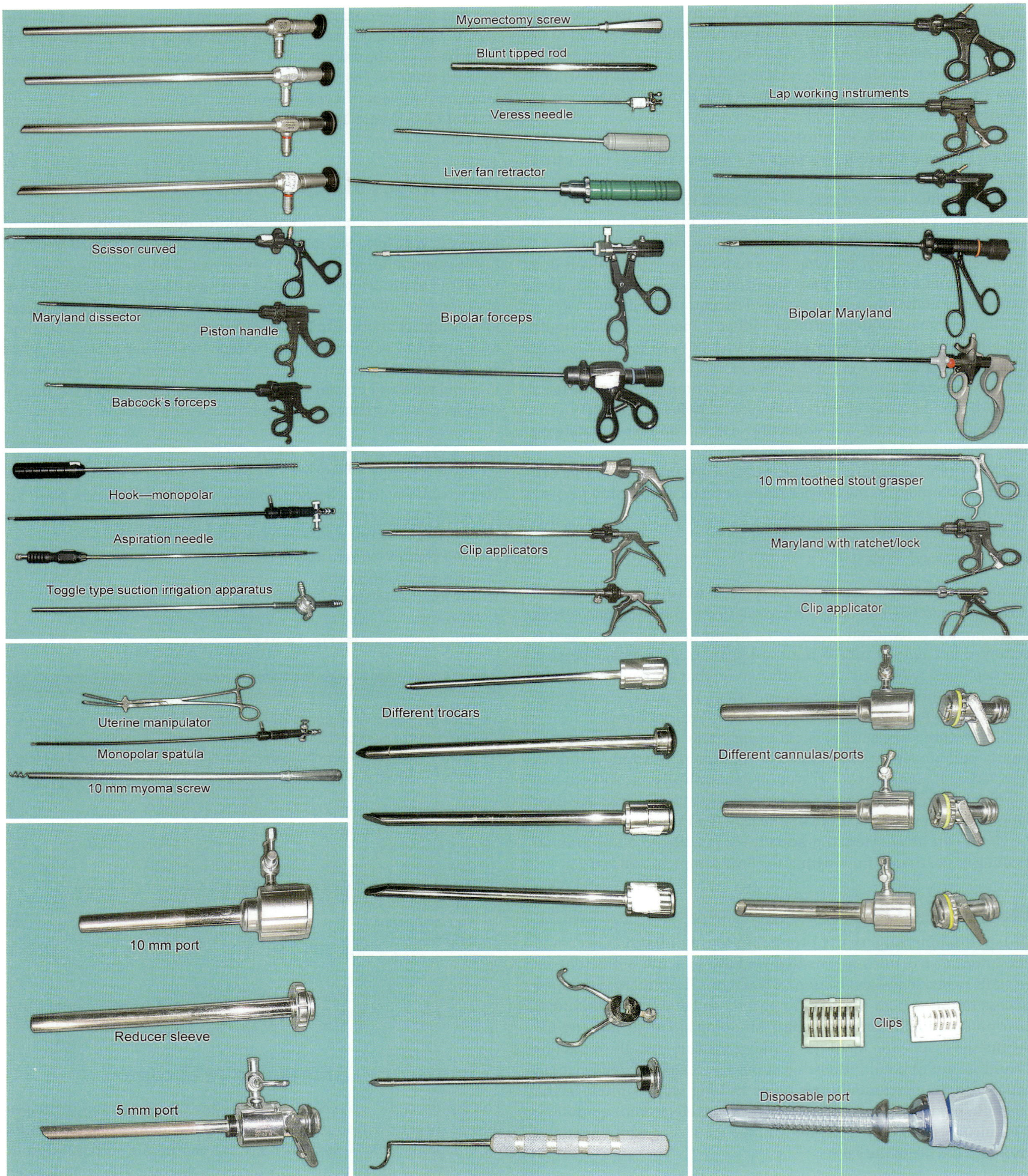

Myomectomy screw
Blunt tipped rod
Veress needle
Liver fan retractor
Lap working instruments
Scissor curved
Maryland dissector
Piston handle
Babcock's forceps
Bipolar forceps
Bipolar Maryland
Hook—monopolar
Aspiration needle
Toggle type suction irrigation apparatus
Clip applicators
10 mm toothed stout grasper
Maryland with ratchet/lock
Clip applicator
Uterine manipulator
Monopolar spatula
10 mm myoma screw
Different trocars
Different cannulas/ports
10 mm port
Reducer sleeve
5 mm port
Clips
Disposable port

Figs. 18-61(1)

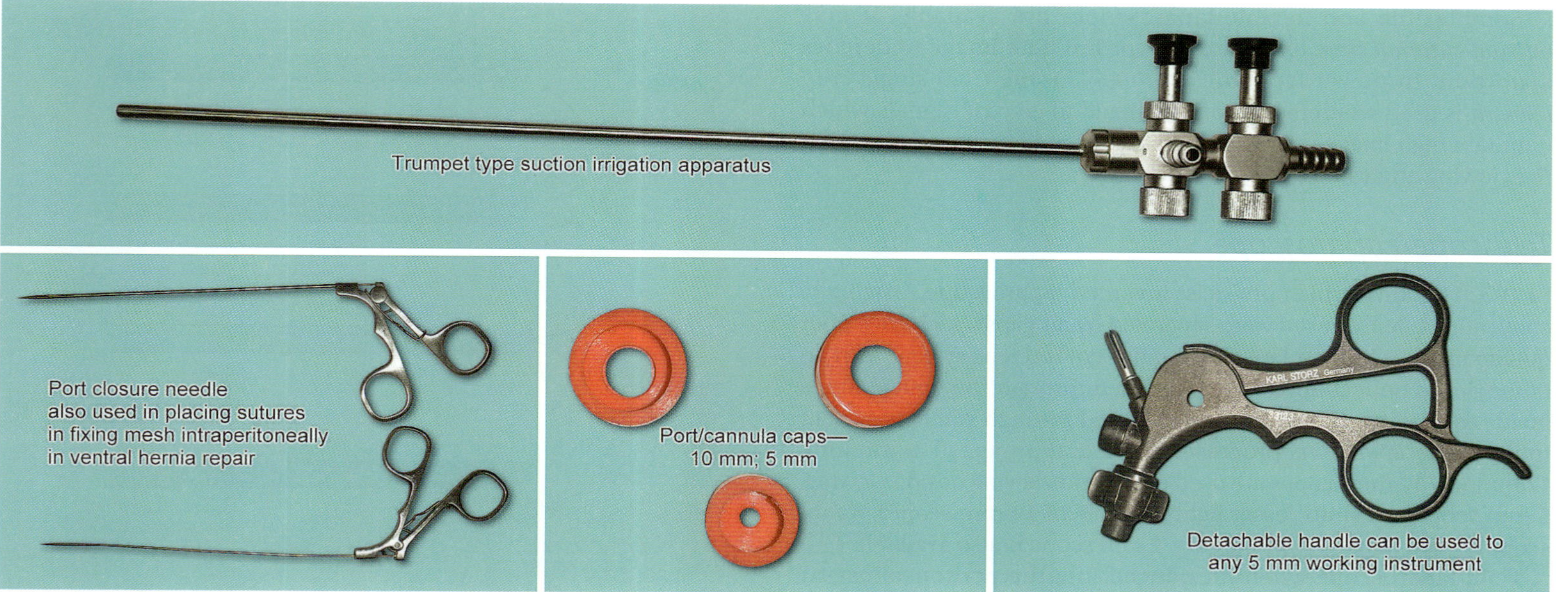

Figs. 18-61(2)

Figs. 18-61(1 and 2): Different instruments used in laparoscopic surgery.

Camera Head

As mentioned already the camera is the most important component of the equipment which makes the procedure comfortable for the surgeon and safe for the patient. The camera is responsible for production of quality pictures in all dimensions such as clarity, colour reproduction and contrast. The light reflected from the viscera is captured by the camera head and is transmitted to the console via the connecting cable. The camera head contains what is termed as charged coupled device or CCD. This chip perceives light and converts the signal into digital form. The basic cameras contain only a single chip or CCD which perceives light as a whole without dividing it into its component red, green and blue light like in a 3 CCD *(Charged Coupled Device)* camera. The resolution of a 3 chip camera is better because the 3 chips individually produce pixels thus increasing the resolution from 470 lines (single chip) to up to 1080 lines which is HD (high definition) quality. Single monochrome CCD chip creates alternate red, green and blue illumination to form a colour image; 3 chip camera has got three separate colour filters which create high quality image with better resolution. Higher resolution can make a difference between a good surgery and a great one only in the hands of an expert with sufficient skills and while performing advanced procedures. For day-to-day practice and for small set ups latest generation single chip camera is adequate. Karl Storz single chip camera and Stryker single chip cameras are the more popular ones but there are always other makes available.

Monitor resolution needs 400–600 lines. White balancing should be done before introduction of the camera into the abdominal cavity. With light source on, camera with telescope is focused on a white gauze and white balance button in the camera source is pressed until 'white balancing is complete' sentence appears on the monitor. Zoom adjustment also can be done in the camera **(Fig. 18-62)**.

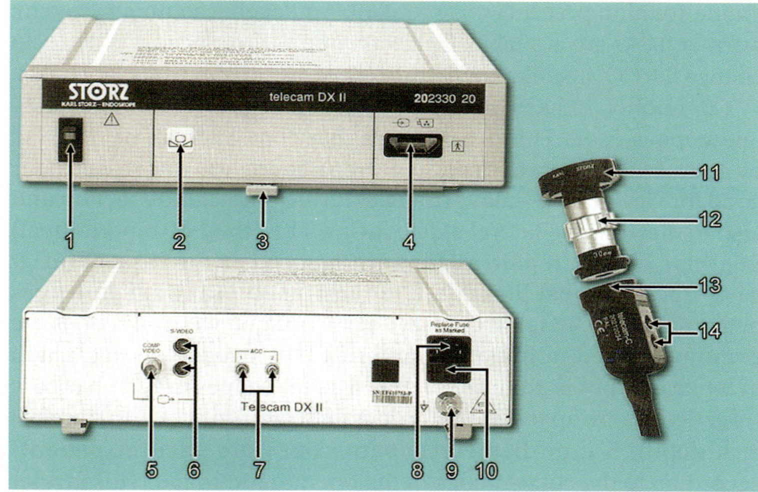

Fig. 18-62: Single Chip camera Karl Storz.

1. Power switch.
2. Automatic white balance.
3. Abridged instructions.
4. Camera cable receptacle.
5. BNC video output connector.
6. S-Video output connector.
7. Accessory control outputs.
8. Power cord receptacle.
9. Potential equalisation connector.
10. Power fuse holder.
11. Grasping mechanism.
12. Focusing ring.
13. C-Mount connection.
14. User control buttons.

A good camera is always complemented by a good telescope/ laparoscope. This is akin to the lens of the eye. The clearer the optics of the lens of the telescope better is the vision. A poor telescope with improper optics makes the picture look bad and the illumination is inadequate. The telescope incorporates the Hopkins rod lens system where in the sheath of the telescope is packed with series of glass lens with air pockets intervening to produce magnified images at the opposite end. The rod lens system is surrounded by optic fibres carrying light from the camera end to the tip of the telescope. If these optical fibres are damaged then the illumination produced at the distal end is poor. Telescopes are available in a variety of diameters and in different forward viewing angles.

Semiflexible and flexible laparoscopes are available. It may be *conventional fibre optic flexible type* but here image undergoes distortion. In newer type, *digital monochrome CCD single chip camera* is used wherein image is changed to electric signals which maintain high image quality. It increases vision four ways improving the viewing angles.

Telescope/Laparoscope

In 1952 Hopkins British physicist invented laparoscope. Originally conventional lenses used were separated by air gaps which gave poor quality images. Present laparoscope has got rod lens system with an outer rim of optical fibre. Light is passed through the optical fibres inside the cavity and image is transmitted through rod lens system to the camera which is processed there and projected at monitor. Commonly 10 mm scopes are used either end viewing or side viewing. 5 mm scope transmits lesser light (10–30% of 10 mm scope). 3 mm scope is used in paediatric surgery. 2 mm scope is also available.

Cold laparoscope when introduced into the peritoneal cavity, *fogging* of the lens of the telescope occurs (it is also due to passage of the cold CO_2 through camera port) which is prevented by dipping the tip of the telescope into warm saline kept in a thermo flask. Cleaning the tip using gauze soaked in warm saline and povidone iodine solution prevents this problem. Antifogging solutions, electric warmer flasks are available. Once other ports are placed it is better to change the CO_2 insufflation tube to one of the other ports **(Fig. 18-63)**.

Commonly, in basic surgeries 10 mm 0 degree (end on viewing) telescope is used. This is a versatile telescope and can be handled by a scrub nurse as well. The 30 degree oblique viewing telescope is good for viewing the Calot's triangle during posterior dissection and also in viewing the lateral sides during TEP (total extraperitoneal) inguinal hernia repairs. They are also used for dissection at gastro-oesophageal junction and rectal mobilisation. Suturing is better aided by 30° telescope. 45 degree oblique viewing scopes are commonly used in bariatric surgeries. The usual working length of the telescopes is around 330 mm. The telescopes used in bariatric surgeries can be up to 450 mm in length to provide access to stomach at a depth. 5 mm diameter laparoscopes are used in patients according to the convenience of the operating surgeon. This further reduces the size of the umbilical incision. Although the light transmitted via the 5 mm telescope is only 10% of that transmitted by a 10 mm telescope, a good camera and suitable monitor can provide a clear operating field. A 3 *CCD (Charged Coupled Device)* camera and xenon light source are good enough to produce clear pictures even in a 2 mm needle scope. These scopes are used for entry site port in paediatric cases and in patients with previous laparotomy wounds.

Light Source and Cable

Having a good light source is a priority as the entire surgery is dependent on the images received on the monitor. It is an important component of the triad of camera, light source and monitor. For performing safe surgery visualisation of structures in its best colour contrast is essential. For this white light produced by a *xenon light source is best.* The light source is composed of replaceable bulb, a heat filter (as the light is condensed by a lens before output, the temperature generated at the tip can be as high as 6,000 K in xenon lamps) and an intensity control. Depending on the make of the light source the intensity of the light can be either manually or automatically controlled. The average life of the xenon bulb is around 500 hours and some light sources even track the life of the bulb.

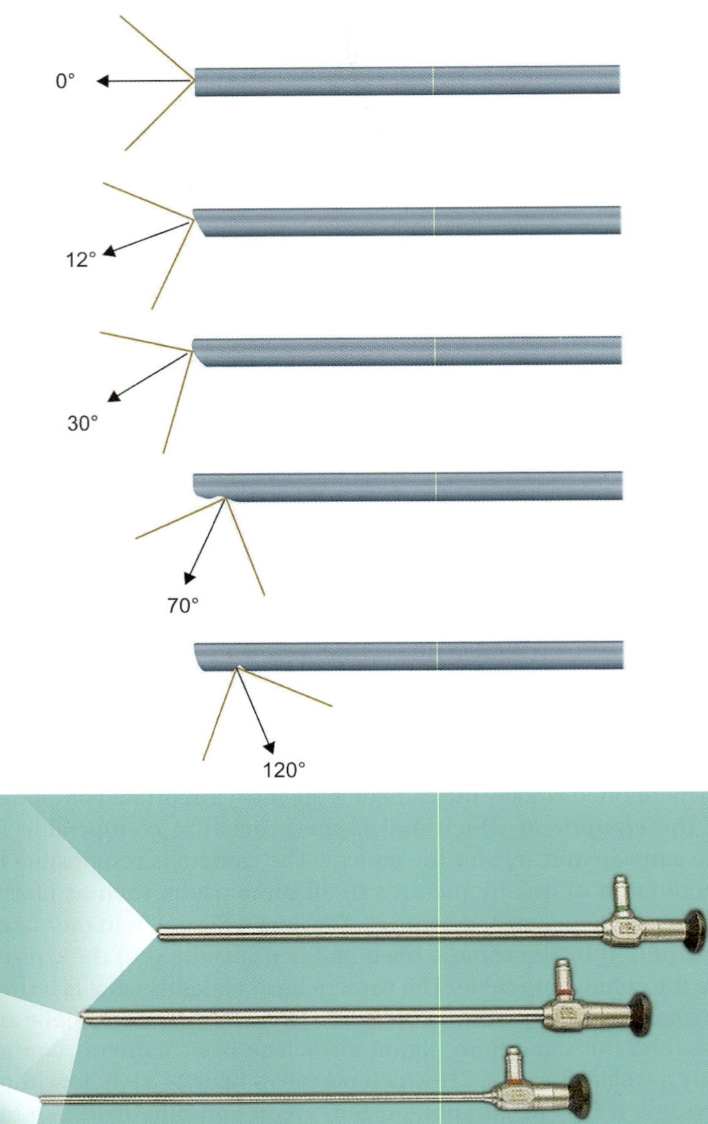

Fig. 18-63: Telescopes of various diameters and viewing angles.

Xenon lamps are of either 175 or 300 Watts. 300 Watts is ideal and standard. Even though xenon light source is cold light source it produces significant heat at the tip of the telescope. Hence tip should not touch bowel, vessels, and skin as burn injury and its dangerous consequences can occur. *Halogen light sources* are country cousins of xenon sources. They are inexpensive and can be acquired for a fraction of the cost. The main disadvantage is the yellow colour of the light that is produced. The field appears yellow and the distinction of vessels becomes difficult in surgery such as cholecystectomy. Besides this the intensity of the light is less compares to xenon and the peripheries of the visual field are much darker making identification of structures difficult. Halogen light sources can be used for performing diagnostic laparoscopy and laparoscopic appendectomies but xenon light source is recommended for doing cholecystectomies and inguinal hernia repairs **(Fig. 18-64)**.

Transmission of the light from the source to the telescope is equally important. Two types of light cables are available for use:

1. Fibre optic cable.
2. Fluid filled/gel filled cable.

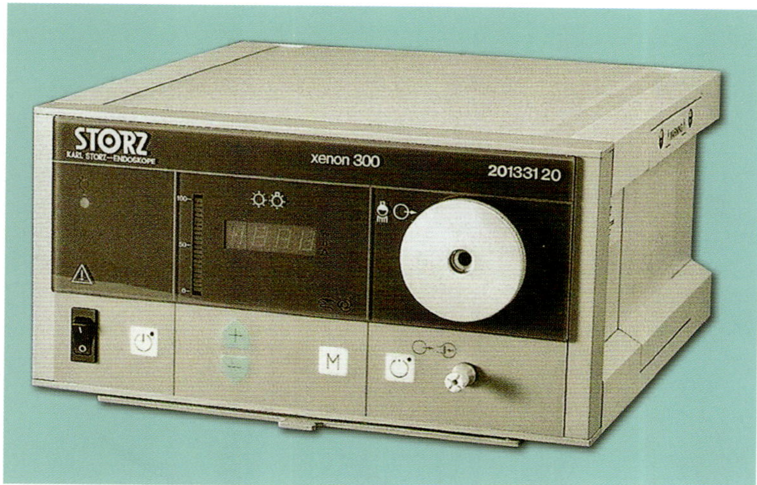

Fig. 18-64: Karl Storz Xenon light source.

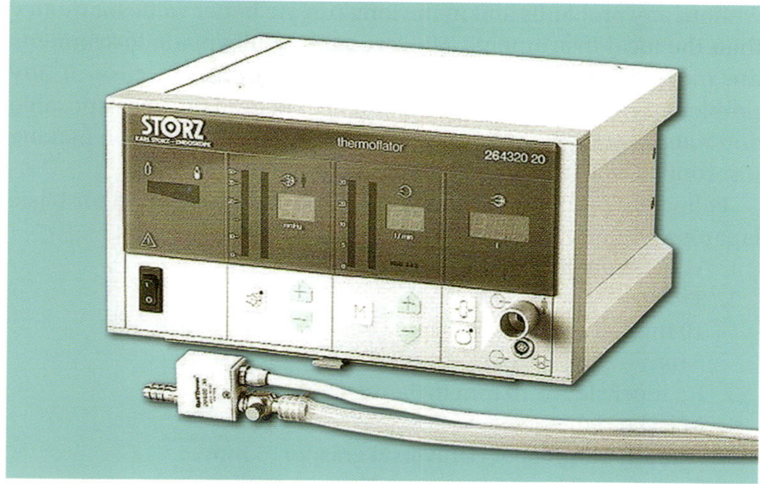

Fig. 18-65: Karl Storz Thermoflator.

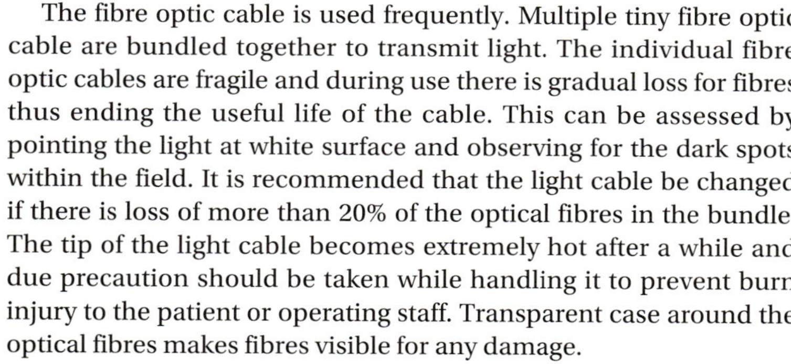

The fibre optic cable is used frequently. Multiple tiny fibre optic cable are bundled together to transmit light. The individual fibre optic cables are fragile and during use there is gradual loss for fibres thus ending the useful life of the cable. This can be assessed by pointing the light at white surface and observing for the dark spots within the field. It is recommended that the light cable be changed if there is loss of more than 20% of the optical fibres in the bundle. The tip of the light cable becomes extremely hot after a while and due precaution should be taken while handling it to prevent burn injury to the patient or operating staff. Transparent case around the optical fibres makes fibres visible for any damage.

The fluid or gel filled cable transmits more light than the fibre optic cable but also has the disadvantage of transmitting more heat and being more fragile makes it difficult to handle than the fibre optic cable. It is also more expensive than the fibre optic cable. It cannot be sterilised by autoclave; it shows poor flexibility and is fragile and so causes difficulty in manoeuvring the camera.

Carbon Dioxide Insufflator

Creation of pneumoperitoneum is the first step in any laparoscopic surgery. Although gasless laparoscopy can be performed, pneumoperitoneum causes fewer traumas and the equipment is easily available and easy to use. Carbon dioxide is ideally suited as it is non-combustible, absorbed by the body, inexpensive and easily available. Air insufflators have been used by many and is still being used by few but carbon dioxide insufflators are safer for the patient when compared to air insufflators wherein as there is risk of air embolism if there is any injury to vascular structures during the procedure. The standard insufflators has an indicator for the amount of CO_2 present in the cylinder. It is wise to know the stock of your CO_2 cylinder before proceeding as it avoids the embarrassing situation where the case has to be converted to open surgery due to empty CO_2 cylinder **(Fig. 18-65)**.

There are three indicators in the console. First one denotes the intra-abdominal pressure with setting. This can be set from 0 to 25 mmHg in most insufflators. The usual intra-abdominal setting used is of 12 mmHg. Higher pressure setting may be used in case of TEP hernia repair to maintain the pre-peritoneal space. The calibration of the instruments is required for patient's safety point of view as the cut off flow of CO_2 at set pressure is important. The second indicator is for the flow rate. The flow rate can be set from 0 to 16, 25, or even 40 with high flow insufflators. For routine procedures a 16 L/min insufflator is adequate although some prefer high flow insufflator for TEP hernia repair, but one can manage to successfully perform the surgery with 16 L/min insufflator. The third indicator is for the total amount of CO_2 used for the particular case. In addition to these standard indicators some newer insufflators has come with additional feature of warming the carbon dioxide to body temperature before it enters the abdomen. This reduces the temperature difference when the telescope is introduced into the abdomen thus preventing fogging of the telescope.

Monitors

The final picture emerging out of a good telescope and camera is complemented by a suitable medical monitor. For a single chip camera which produces images of resolution of around 470 lines, a standard monitor of resolution around 400 lines and above is required. This can easily be substituted by use of our regular television sets. Although a 14 inch colour television is adequate, a 21 inch flat television increases comfort level of the surgeon and the team. For the 3CCD cameras; however, the television monitor is not adequate as the camera produces up to 1,080 lines (HD) and the picture would not translate well on ordinary television. A HD television or a HD monitor is required for a three chip camera to produce best results with a resolution of >1,600 lines. Various types of output signals are delivered out of the camera console. There are RGB out, Y/C out, S video out, composite out and some camera consoles even have a USB out so they can be directly connected to a computer or laptop. Commonly used are composite or RGB out for connecting a television monitor and S video out to connect to a medical monitor. Presence of a USB out can make digital recording of the surgical procedure very simple and inexpensive. A parallel out to the computer allows for recording in the computer thus eliminating the need for a separate recording device.

Hand Instruments

Once the main consoles of the laparoscopy set are arranged we turn out attention to hand instruments. They are available in various makes and qualities. Imported as well as locally manufactured indigenous instruments are available. Imported instruments such as those provided by Karl Storz although expensive lasts very long without any problems and in the long run are better value for money than the local instruments. However, the locally made instruments are inexpensive and can be replaced with ease in case of any problem. Trocars and often instruments are available as disposable and reusable. Disposable trocars are single use precise one making insertion of trocar very easy, quick and perfect.

Following is an indicative list of instruments suggested for basic laparoscopic surgeries:

1. Veress needle.
2. Trocars
   10 mm—2 in number
   5 mm—2 in number
3. Reducer sleeve 10 mm to 5 mm.
4. Maryland dissector.
5. Atraumatic grasper (Universal grasper) 5 mm.
6. Traumatic (Toothed) grasper 5 mm.
7. Gallbladder extracting forceps 10 mm.
8. Curved scissors 5 mm.
9. Suction irrigation system 5 mm/10 mm.
10. Clip applicator for LT300/ LT400.
11. Monopolar hook and spatula.
12. Aspiration needle.
13. Bipolar forceps.
14. Knot pusher.
15. Port closure needle (Optional).

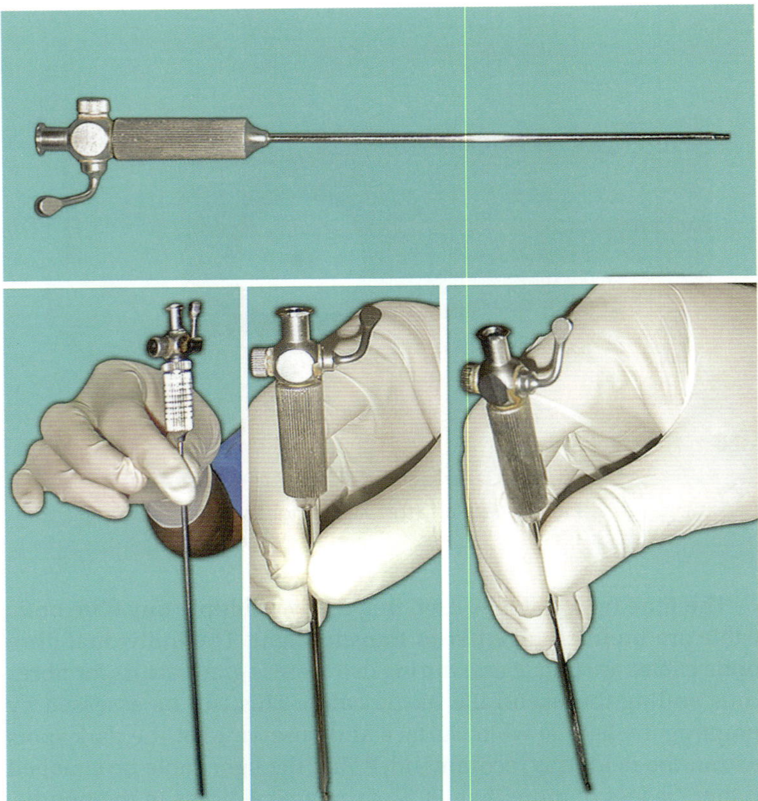

Fig. 18-66: Veress needle and methods of holding it.

Veress Needle

Veress needle was first developed in 1932 by *Janos Veress*, a Hungarian internist working with tuberculosis patients. At that time, one of the mainstays of treatment was to collapse an infected lung and allow the lesions to heal. The needle was introduced as a safer technique to give patients such pneumothoraces. It was in 1938, he published his invention in the German literature. Veress needle is a spring locked needle with a cutting sheath and a blunt tip. It is 2 mm in external diameter and 12–15 cm in length usually. The outer cannula consists of a beveled needle point for cutting through tissues of the abdominal wall. A spring-loaded, inner stylet is positioned within the outer cannula. This inner stylet has a dull tip to protect any viscera from injury by the sharp, outer cannula. Direct pressure on the tip, when penetrating through tissues, pushes the blunt stylet into the shaft of the outer cannula. When the tip of the needle enters a space such as the peritoneal cavity, the blunt, inner stylet springs forward. *Parts are*—beveled needle; stylet; spring action part; lock for valve; head or knob proximally. Instrument should be held below the lock at proximal part of the needle as—guard position. Central sheath has got connector which connects to insufflation tube. Veress needle is available at various diameters and lengths. It may be disposable or reusable **(Fig. 18-66)**.

It is used in closed method to access peritoneal cavity for laparoscopic procedure. Before using the Veress needle its patency should be checked by flushing it with saline. Spring mechanism has to be checked before every use. The spring action in the blunt tip prevents the sheath from injuring the viscera once it enters the peritoneal cavity. Lock for the valve should be in open position. Patient is laid in supine position as in this position bowel will be uniformly spread inside the peritoneal cavity (Many use Trendelenburg position with 15° tilt; but often it is presumed that bowel may come close to umbilicus in this position). After making the umbilical crease incision, Veress needle is passed inside, across the abdominal wall by holding it in slightly oblique position with other hand the abdominal wall is held forward to act initially as counter pressure. Abdominal wall should be held at the level of the umbilicus laterally (not very close to umbilicus) either one side or both sides or below. Assistant can help in holding the abdominal wall. Abdominal wall is held firmly using thenar eminence and fingers of the hand. Length of the needle needed is often assessed by finding the thickness of abdominal wall fat (thickness in cm + 4 cm conventionally). Veress needle should be held below the knob (*gurading position*), not at the head/knob. Initially needle is passed inside at 90° direction; later tilted obliquely. Often 45° oblique angle towards anus is also used to avoid injury to the major vessels. Passing through the layers of the abdominal wall—rectus sheath, transversalis fascia and peritoneum can be felt while pushing the needle. Once peritoneum is reached resistance is lost and blunt tip springs forward thus preventing injury to viscera and vessels. Two click sounds can be heard (if there is no noise in theatre) and felt; one during passage of the rectus sheath and other during forward springing of the blunt tip. Initially with 5 mL syringe, aspiration through the needle is done to check for any blood or bowel contents. Then normal saline is flown under pressure using syringe into the needle and aspirated; if saline does not return then it is in the peritoneal cavity; if saline returns back that means needle tip is not inside the peritoneal cavity. Again drop wise saline is allowed to enter the proximal part of the Veress needle to confirm free entry of the saline into the peritoneal cavity (water/saline drop test; hanging drop test). Saline filled syringe can be connected to the Veress needle knob to observe free flow of the saline into the peritoneal cavity. Veress is connected to CO_2 insufflator tube to create pneumoperitoneum. Veress needle will not allow insufflation flow more than 2.5 litre of CO_2/minute. Veress needle should not be passed in close vicinity of any previous scar.

Confirmation of proper positioning of the Veress needle

- Two click sounds are heard and/or felt.
- Irrigation–aspiration method.
- Hanging drop test.
- Free flow of saline through a syringe.
- Distension of abdomen is observed while gas is on flow and confirmed by the resonant note all over the abdomen.

Note:
81% gynaecologists use Veress needle to create pneumoperitoneum (due to lax abdomen in females); whereas only 48% of surgeons use the same.

Veress needle can be used for port closure also. It is also used to pass stay suture to retract internal organs like in gallbladder in single incision laparoscopic surgery (SILS) or two port laparoscopic surgery **(Fig. 18-67)**.

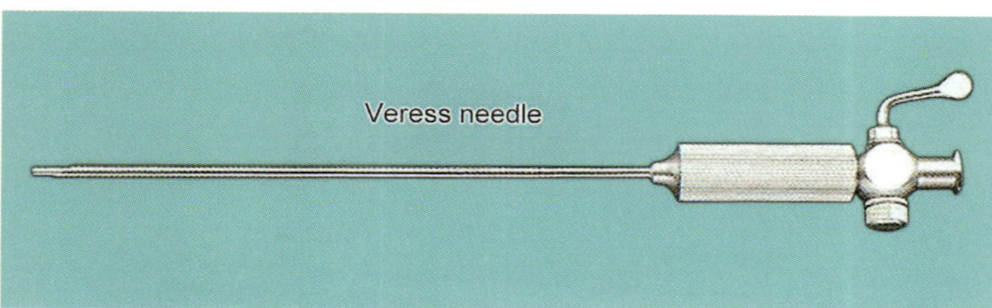

Fig. 18-67: Veress needle available in 120 mm and 150 mm lengths.

Trocars

Trocars are needed to access the peritoneal cavity during the surgery and for maintaining pneumoperitoneum when the instruments are exchanged. Various types of trocars are now available. Commonly used are reusable trocars which can be autoclaved. The disposable ones are convenient to use but the cost factor has to be borne in mind. The trocar has an obturator with pyramidal cutting tip which pierces the sheath and muscle during entry. Bladeless trocars are available in disposable type which cause minimum damage to the muscle and leave a minimum defect on removal. Trocars are available in various sizes with outer diameter of 11 mm, 5.5 mm ones being used frequently in most procedures. Special devices such as endo GI staplers are introduced into abdomen through 13 mm trocars. Tip of trocars may be conical or pyramidal. Pyramidal tip penetrates the wall by sharp dissection and thus reducing the insertion force. Optical view trocars are passed under visual guidance by passing laparoscope into the trocar. Electrosurgical trocars are available wherein thermal energy is used to create track rather than conventional physical force. There are plastic tip trocars with a diathermy loop on the tip. Similarly ultrasonically activated trocars are also available in the market.

Hasson's trocar and cannula is used as an alternate for open method instead of Veress needle approach. It contains three parts—a cone shaped sleeve; plastic or a metal sheath with a trumpet or flat valve; blunt tip obturator. On the sheath or sleeve two struts are present to fix fascial sutures tightly around so that trocar is fixed firmly and also prevents gas leak. Skin is incised subumbilically. Rectus is incised vertically. With haemostat open dissection is done to reach peritoneum which is opened under vision and Hasson's cannula with blunt obturator is passed. Obturator is removed. Hasson's cannula can be passed and used as an outer sheath with other 10 mm cannulas also. Incidence of vessel injury is very much less in Hasson's cannula; but bowel injury can occur if bowel is adherent to the port insertion site. But overall injury rate is less compared to Veress needle method **(Fig. 18-68)**.

Hasson's cannula technique (Open access for primary port—Harry Hasson, Chicago 1974)
Periumbilical vertical/horizontal incision → With retraction, rectus sheath is identified → Two 2-zero vicryl stay sutures are placed in the rectus sheath on either side of the planned vertical incision → Rectus sheath/fascia is incised vertically using 15/11 no. blade → Extraperitoneal tissues are dissected using haemostat → Peritoneum is held with haemostat or forceps and opened using 15 no. blade or scissor → Blunt finger dissection is done under the peritoneum circumferentially to release any adhesions → Hasson's cannula is placed into the peritoneal cavity and 2-zero vicryl sutures are wrapped around the cannula hub to secure it in place firmly → The camera with telescope is passed through the Hasson's cannula to confirm that cannula tip is inside the peritoneal cavity → CO_2 pneumoperitoneum is created.

Contraindications
Previous prosthetic mesh; previous surgery with dense adhesions.

Problems and Complications
- Bowel injury.
- Vessel injury—very rare.
- Difficulty in keeping cannula in place.
- Repeated gas leak.

Special trocar and cannulas are used while using endo GI staplers, morcellator and laparoscopic ultrasound. Radiolucent disposable trocars are available in situation where obstruction of the vision needs to be avoided like intraoperative cholangiogram.

Valve design: In *trumpet valve*, outer knob is pressed fully to release the block to allow passage of the instrument. It may damage insulation of the instrument and is very crude to use. In *flap valve*, spring loaded device is utilised as a seal and is manually controllable. But it is difficult to control the instrument from outside while passing and removing the instruments. Tissues may get caught in the valve making its sealing ineffective and also causes gas leak. In *passive valves*, valves open and close automatically with passage of instruments. In disposable type, plastic or rubber sleeves are used. Magnetic flap valve, multifunctional valve systems are also available. Integrity of valve is checked by pressing it and releasing it to get a sound; if sound is heard rubber like it is good; if it is metallic like then valve is improper.

Note:
Reusable metal cannula/port with pyramidal trocar with flap/passive valve is commonly used in laparoscopic surgical practice.

Fascial sheaths of all 10 mm and above ports should be sutured using 2-zero vicryl. Different closure techniques are available—direct vision closure; using different port closure devices; using Veress needle also. If these layers are not closed properly incidence of port site hernia is very high—2–3% for 10 mm; 4–10% for 12 mm; >40% for 15 mm port site **(Fig. 18-69)**.

Working Instruments

Other instruments are the working instruments which are the miniature versions of hand instruments used in open surgery. Surgical principles of using various instruments are the same as in open surgery. 5 mm sized working instruments are used. They are long (usual one is 33 cm), well insulated and articulated.

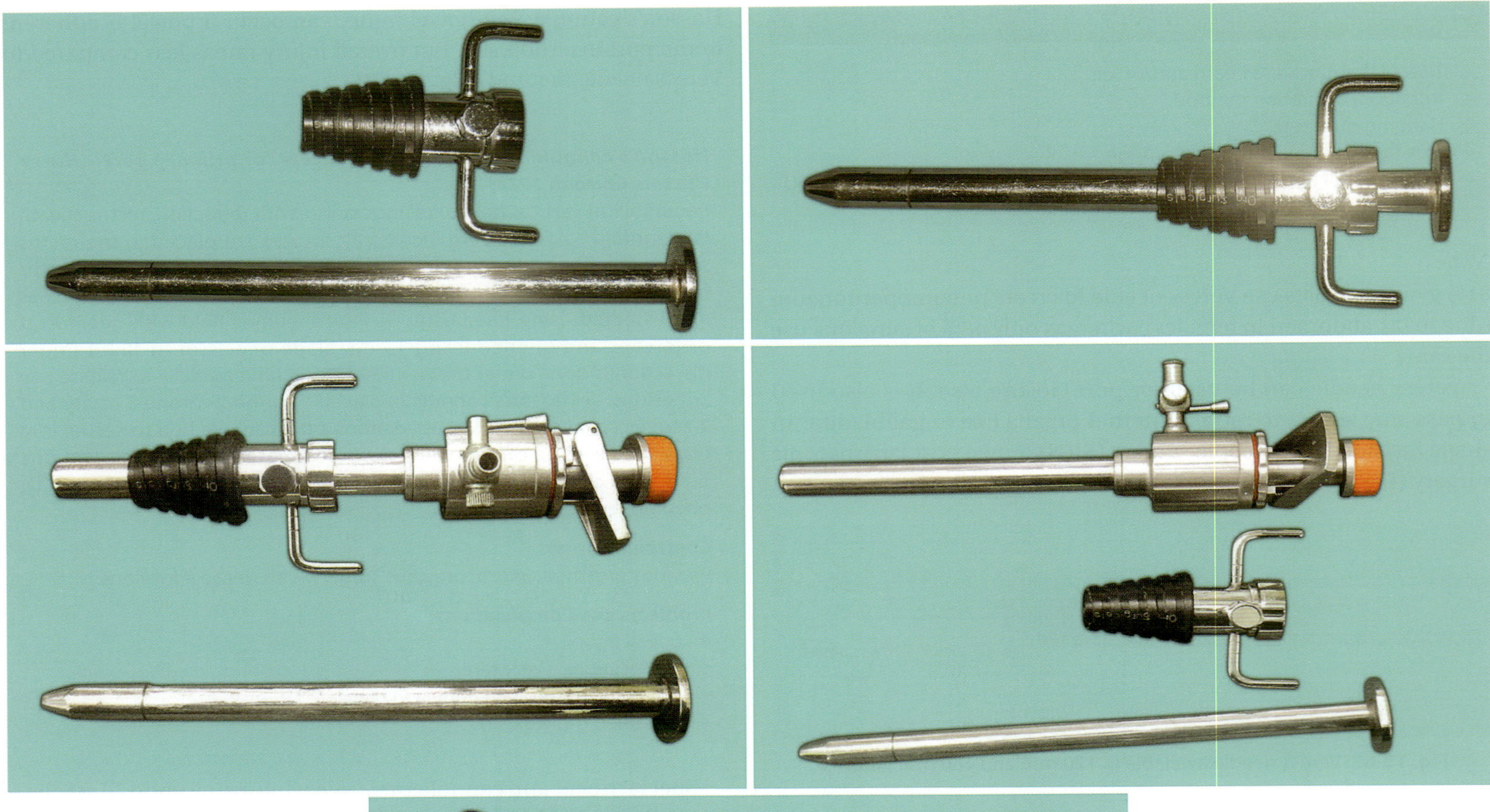

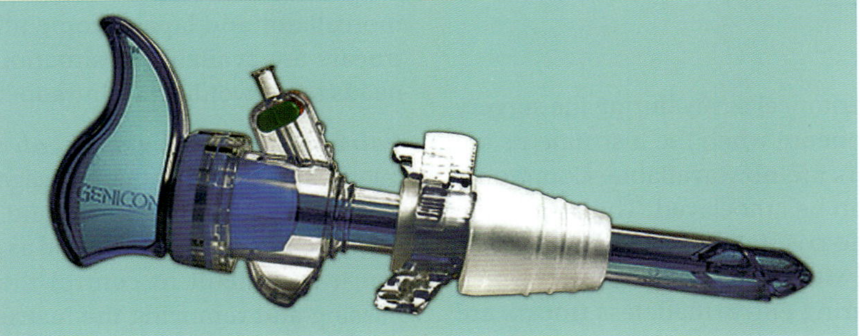

Fig. 18-68: Hasson's cannula used for open method to get pneumoperitoneum and to achieve primary port insertion during laparoscopic surgery.

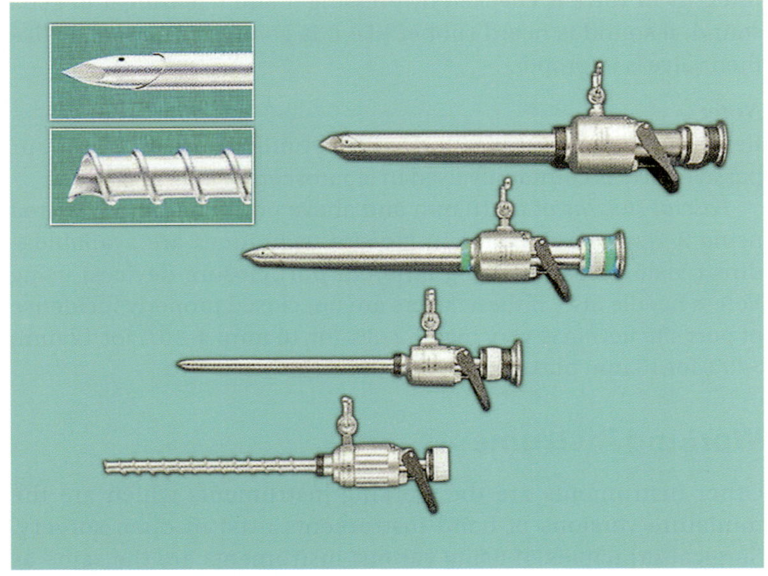

Fig. 18-69: Trocars of various sizes are available in 11 mm, 7 mm and 5.5 mm outer diameter.

Insulation should be perfect as any damage in insulation can cause electrosurgical hazards while performing laparoscopic surgery.

Hand instruments are available as reusable or disposable ones. Both have advantages and disadvantages. Disposable ones are expensive but work well every time. Reusable ones are more suited for our practice as they are cost effective. Instruments such as scissors and Maryland dissectors should be in top working condition before taking up a case for surgery. They are also available in 3 mm diameter. These are not required for performing cases in adults and all instruments of 5 mm diameter are used.

Instruments with locks are used for retraction, suturing and tissue holding. Instruments without lock are used for dissection and cutting (scissors). *Hand grip* may be ring, shank and piston types. Ring and handle may be in line (coaxial) or in an angle (radial) with the shaft. Commonly working instruments are having radial handles with an angle of 70°–90° to the shaft line.

Dissecting instruments can be curved or straight with rotating shaft. Curved Maryland dissector is commonly used. Rotating shaft allows easy dissection with lesser strain to surgeon's wrist.

Scissors must be sharp and insulated. When cautery is used in scissor blades should be opened to prevent blunting of the scissor. Straight scissor is used to cut the suture material. Straight suture cutting scissor is often non-insulated. Microscissor and hook scissors are also used. Bipolar scissor is also available.

Non-toothed, toothed graspers, curved long blade dissectors, blunt dissector, right angle dissector, short and long bowel holding forceps, Allis and Babcock's forceps and claw forceps are other instruments used.

Hook is an insulated instrument which is used for dissection. It is connected to monopolar cautery. Bipolar hook is also available. *Spatula* is used again for dissection, coagulation by connecting to monopolar cautery. Its shaft is insulated.

Stone holding forceps, liver retractor, hydatid trocar, needle holders, clip applicators, loop applicators, clips, endostaplers, and endosutures are other specialised instruments used. Needle holder can be 5 mm or 3 mm; can be straight or curved; can be having coaxial or radial handles.

Suction irrigation apparatus is essential to wash and clean the surgical field using warm normal saline. Two types are available—*trumpet type* where suction and irrigation is done using trumpet like action. *Toggle mode type* where suction and irrigation is done through levering bolt in the system. *Toggle mode is commonly used.* 5 mm and 10 mm apparatus are available. 5 mm is better as it does not cause sudden complete loss of pneumoperitoneum obscuring the field. Here with high flow rate of CO_2 gas pneumoperitoneum can be maintained and so image will be visible in spite of suctioning. 10 mm apparatus even though causes rapid suction and not gets blocked by blood clots easily, it causes rapid loss of pneumoperitoneum leading to loss of image causing discomfort to surgeon. Few surgeons use heparinised saline for irrigation to prevent clotting and thereby preventing clot block in the suction apparatus; but it is not that essential.

Newer instruments like auto endosuturing instrument, tackers and fixation devices are available. Usually tackers and anchors are 5 mm devices. They are used in hernia repair to fix the mesh in position **(Figs. 18-70 to 18-72)**.

Instruments are devised to carry cautery current to the tissue and are available in either unipolar or bipolar mode. Cautery in unipolar mode is used for coagulating bleeders and for dissection of gallbladder from its bed. Bipolar current is used to coagulate mesoappendicular vessels while doing an appendicectomy as we need to minimise lateral thermal damage.

The instruments are insulated over its entire length except the tip and the insulation needs to be checked from time to time as any damage to it can produce leakage of current at that point and inadvertent damage to surrounding structures. The instruments are available in metal or plastic handle. The handles come with or without ratchets. Instruments like the dissector have handles without ratchets allow free movements; toothed graspers are usually with ratchets **(Figs. 18-73 and 18-74)**.

Needle holders are available with curved or straight tip and angled or straight handles. Using needle holder is essential for developing skills and going on to the next step in laparoscopic surgery.

Physiologic Changes due to Pneumoperitoneum

CO_2 causes hypercarbia, acidosis and hypoxia. Pneumoperitoneum exerts pressure on the inferior vena cava (IVC), decreases the venous return and so the cardiac output. It increases the arterial pressure also. It compromises the respiratory function by compressing over the diaphragm impairing the pulmonary compliance.

Respiratory changes are due to—pneumoperitoneum, head down (Trendelenburg) position, increased intra-abdominal pressure reducing cardiac output, reduced venous return (even though CVP in raised).

Raise in intra-abdominal pressure causes reduction in perfusion of spleen, mesentery, and bowel mucosa. So bowel function recovery delays and also renal blood flow.

Intraoperative hypothermia (for 50 L gas flow 0.30°C reduction of body temperature) and prolonged warming using warmer is needed. Warming of insufflation gas will be helpful.

ACCESS TO THE PERITONEAL CAVITY

Access is the key for success—in laparoscopic surgery. Access for camera telescope is for primary trocar which is usually at umbilicus. Access for working trocars are called as secondary trocars which are either 10 mm or 5 mm. Secondary trocars are passed *always* under direct vision **(Fig. 18-75)**.

The first step in a laparoscopic procedure is to access the peritoneal cavity in order to establish pneumoperitoneum. It is done by one of the following two methods.

Closed Technique (Using Veress Needle)

After nasogastric suction and drainage of the urinary bladder, a stab incision is made at the umbilicus, followed by the blind passing of a Veress into the abdominal cavity. *Umbilical incision* may be horizontal supra/infraumbilical or superior crease/inferior crease

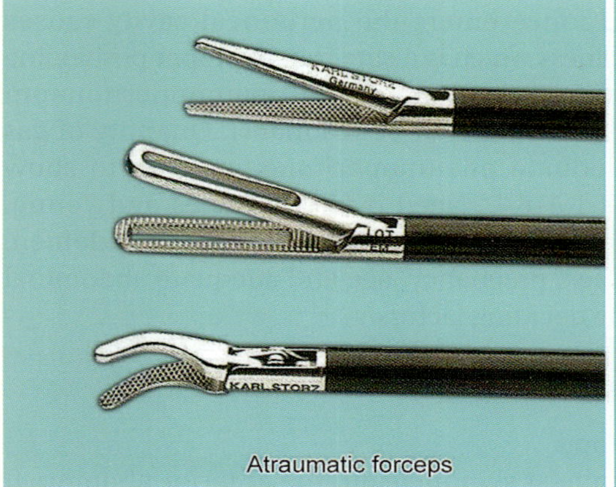

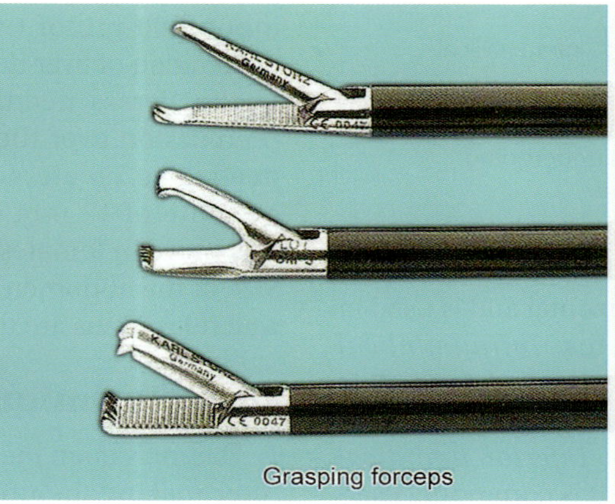

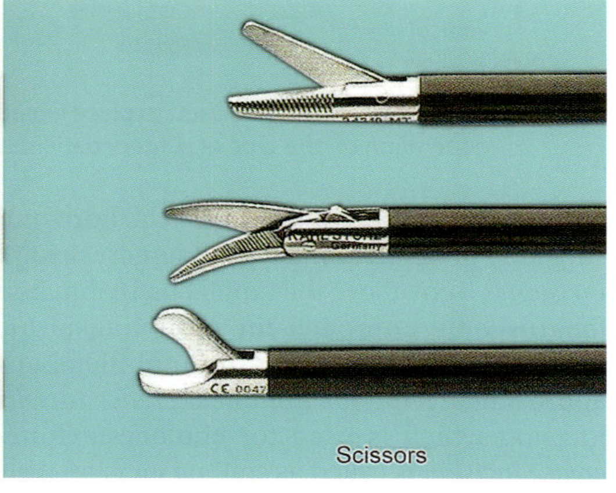

Fig. 18-70: Atraumatic (dissector, bowel holding, Maryland forceps); traumatic forceps and scissors.

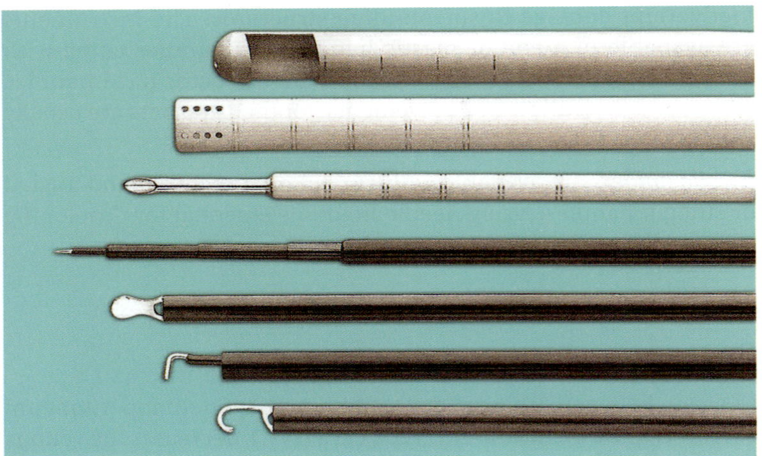

Fig. 18-71: Various needles, electrodes (spatula, hook monopolar and bipolar) and suction irrigation cannula set.

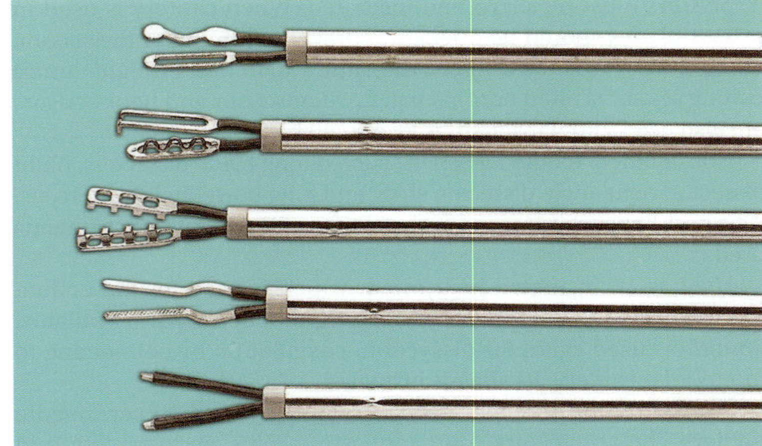

Fig. 18-72: Bipolar forceps of different types.

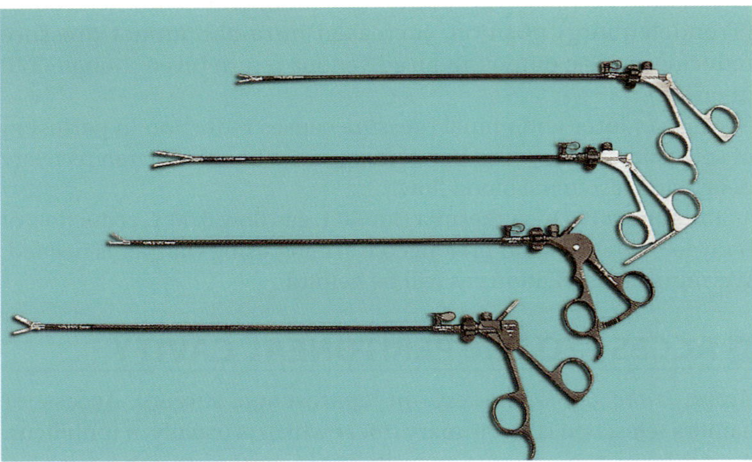

Fig. 18-73: Various common handles with and without ratchets in both plastic and metal handles.

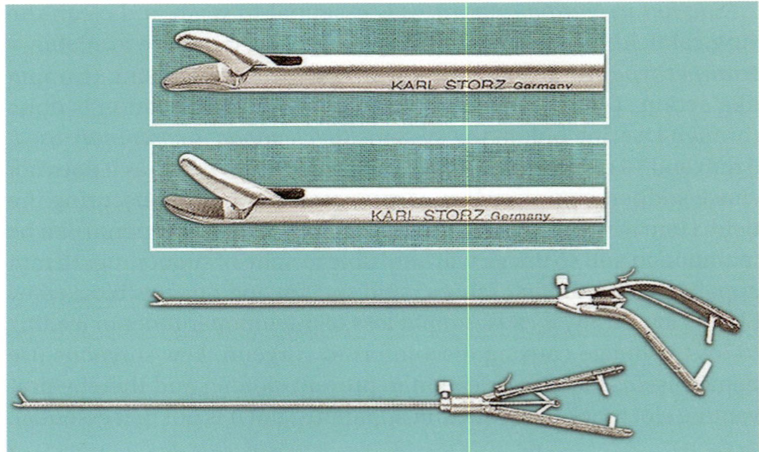

Fig. 18-74: Needle holders with curved and straight tip. Handles are either straight or angled.

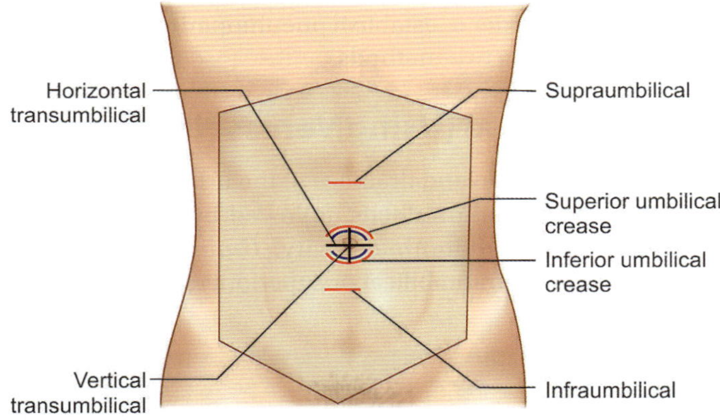

Fig. 18-75: Different incisions used to place laparoscopic primary port depending on the type of surgery patient is undergoing.

umbilical or transumbilical vertical/horizontal depending on the surgeon's preference and type of surgery being done. *Supraumbilical incision* is 5 cm above the umbilicus 10 mm horizontal and is used in laparoscopic approach for oesophageal hiatus. *Infraumbilical incision* is 3-5 cm below the umbilicus and is used for pelvic approaches. *Superior umbilical crease incision* is called as crying incision which is used for cholecystectomy. *Inferior umbilical crease incision* is called as smiling incision which is commonly used access incision. Infection rate and bleeding is less common in inferior crease incision. *Transumbilical transverse or vertical incision* is also used. Position of the needle within the peritoneal cavity can be confirmed by aspiration through a water filled syringe and by the water drop test. Once the surgeon is comfortable that the needle is in the peritoneal cavity, pneumoperitoneum is established and trocars are inserted. Flow rate used for initial creation of pneumoperitoneum in 1 litre/minute (maximum 2.5 L/min). Quadro manometry in the insufflator machine is used to check this. Preset pressure should not be more than 18 mm. Usual pressure created is 12 mm. Peritoneal cavity is distended slowly not rapidly. Rapid creation of pneumoperitoneum may compress IVC causing decreased cardiac input. 200 mL of CO_2 once enters the peritoneal cavity causes obliteration of liver dullness which is a sure sign of proper positioning of the Veress needle and creation of the pneumoperitoneum (Percussion over the abdomen will be resonant). Quantity of gas needed to create adequate pneumoperitoneum so as to show pressure of 12 mm is 1.5-6 L. Need is less in males and young. It is more in females (multipara) and elderly due to lax abdomen. Size of the abdomen, sex, pregnancy, age and adequate abdominal wall relaxations are the deciding factors.

Open Technique

1. Hasson's open method

After making the umbilical skin incision, the anterior abdominal fascia is incised and the peritoneum is identified under direct vision which is opened carefully using scissor or no. 11 blade. Any adhesions prior to insertion of the first trocar is appreciated and released with blunt dissection. The fascia close around the trocar can be sutured to prevent gas leak which is more common in open method than closed method. The wedge-shaped Hasson trocar can be used to establish a seal in order to allow and maintain the pneumoperitoneum.

2. Scandinavian technique

Here small incision is made directly into the scar tissue of the umbilicus and this is dilated using blunt conical tip trocar and cannula to enter into the peritoneal cavity.

3. *Direct layer by layer dissection* method with sub-umbilical crease incision

Here after making sub-umbilical incision, using deep retractors layer by layer dissection is done; rectus sheath is incised horizontally at the junction of the rectus and umbilical fold; peritoneum is adherent to umbilical fold and so can directly enter the peritoneal cavity. Blunt tipped instrument is passed through which 10 mm cannula is passed. Blunt instrument is removed. Cannula is connected to CO_2 insufflator **(Figs. 18-76 to 18-81)**.

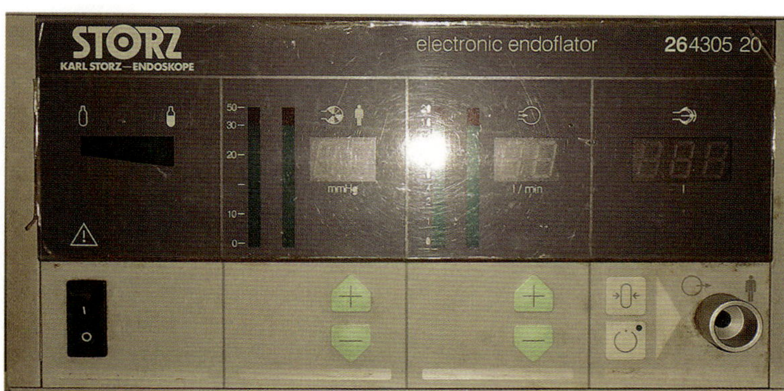

Fig. 18-76: CO_2 insufflator used for laparoscopic surgery to create and to monitor pneumoperitoneum.

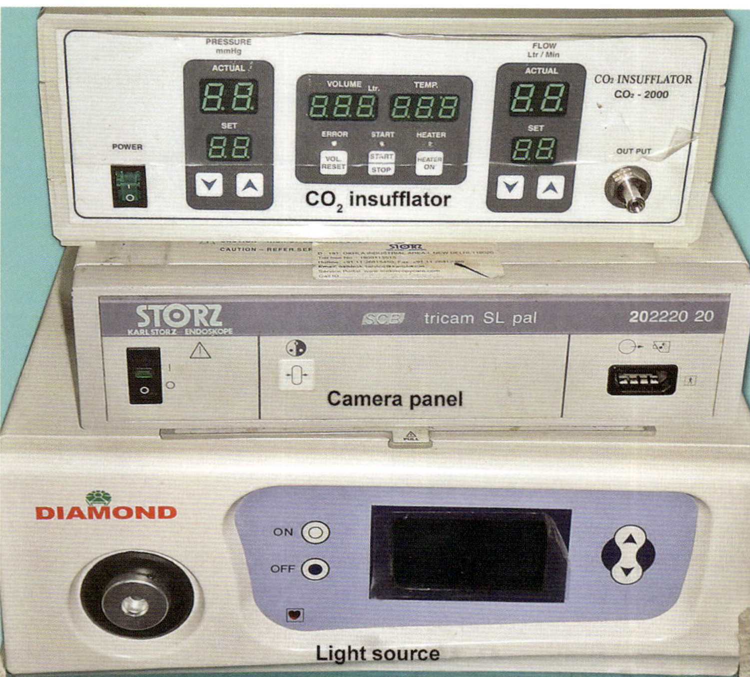

Fig. 18-77: Light source, camera panel and CO_2 insufflator used for laparoscopy.

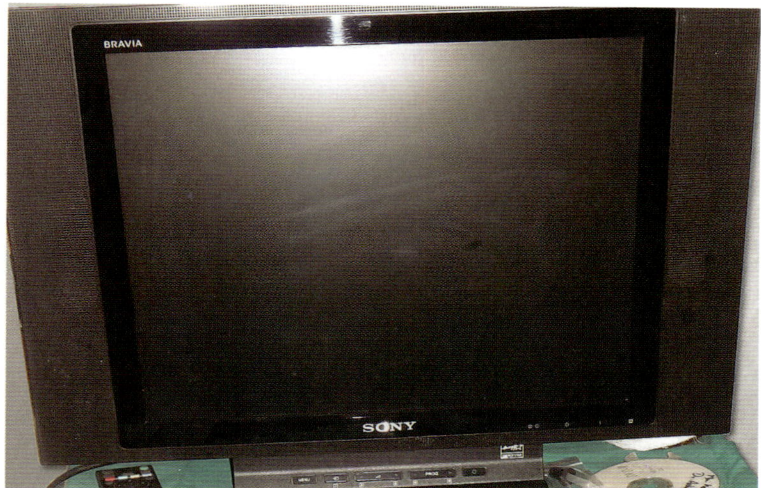

Fig. 18-78: Laparoscopic monitor. Good monitor is essential; flat/medical monitors will give clear images.

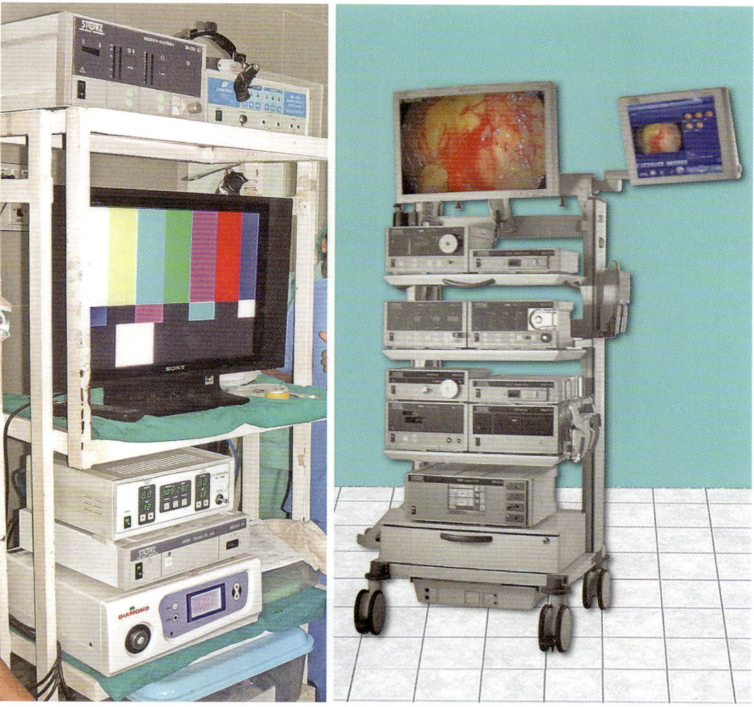

Fig. 18-79: Laparoscopic set trolley used during procedure.

CO_2 is commonly used to create pneumoperitoneum as:
- It is readily available.
- It is cheaper.
- It suppresses the combustion.
- It is easily absorbed by tissues.
- It has a high diffusion coefficient.
- It is quickly released via respiration.

Other gases used are:

Air, nitrous oxide, helium, argon.

Pneumoperitoneum is created up to a pressure of 15 mmHg which distends the abdominal cavity adequately to have proper visualisation of the abdominal contents.

Note:

Stomach and bladder should be empty prior to trocar insertion.

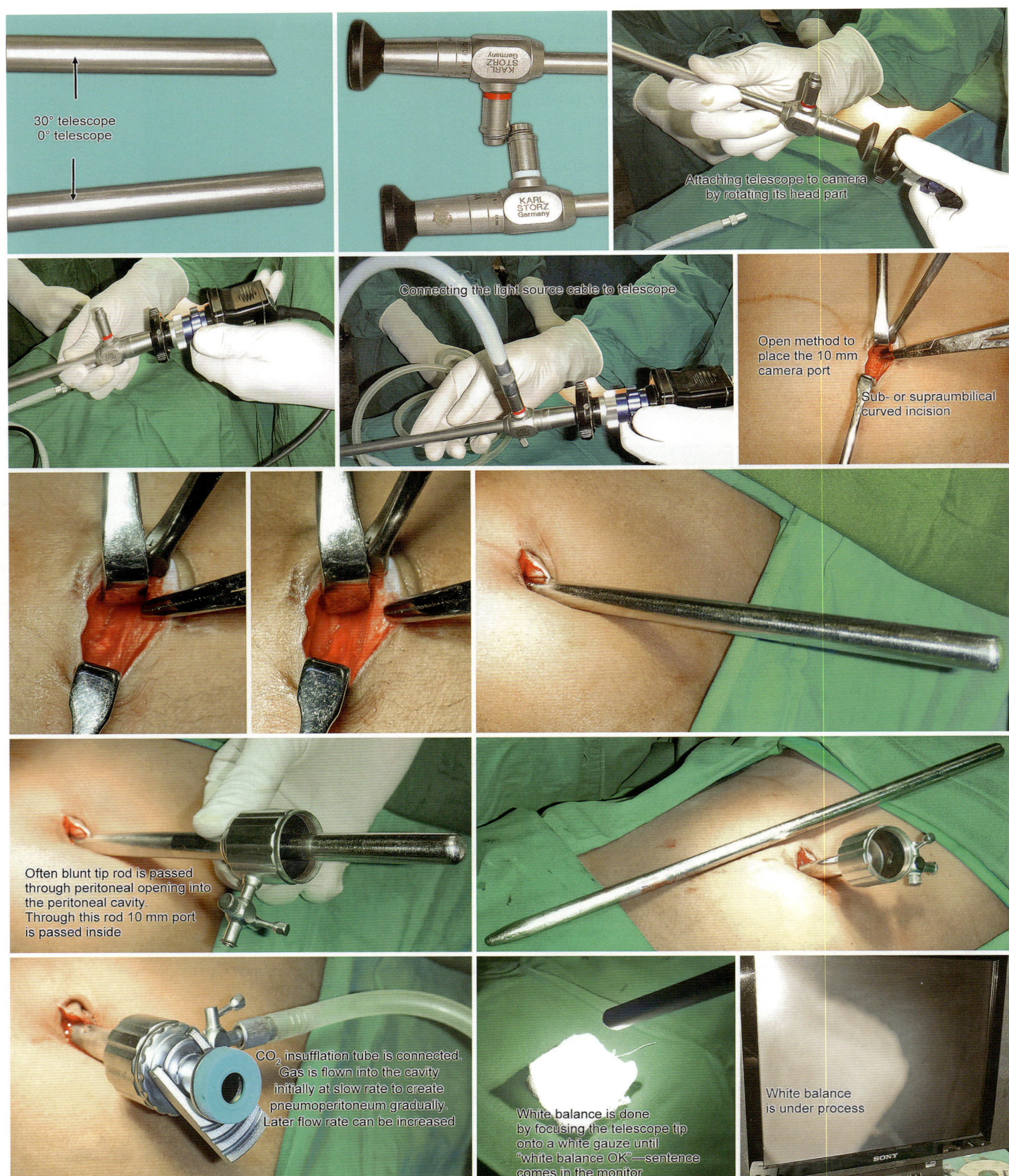
30° telescope
0° telescope
KARL STORZ Germany
KARL STORZ Germany
Attaching telescope to camera by rotating its head part
Connecting the light source cable to telescope
Open method to place the 10 mm camera port
Sub- or supraumbilical curved incision
Often blunt tip rod is passed through peritoneal opening into the peritoneal cavity. Through this rod 10 mm port is passed inside
CO2 insufflation tube is connected. Gas is flown into the cavity initially at slow rate to create pneumoperitoneum gradually. Later flow rate can be increased
White balance is done by focusing the telescope tip onto a white gauze until "white balance OK"—sentence comes in the monitor
White balance is under process
SONY

Figs. 18-80(1)

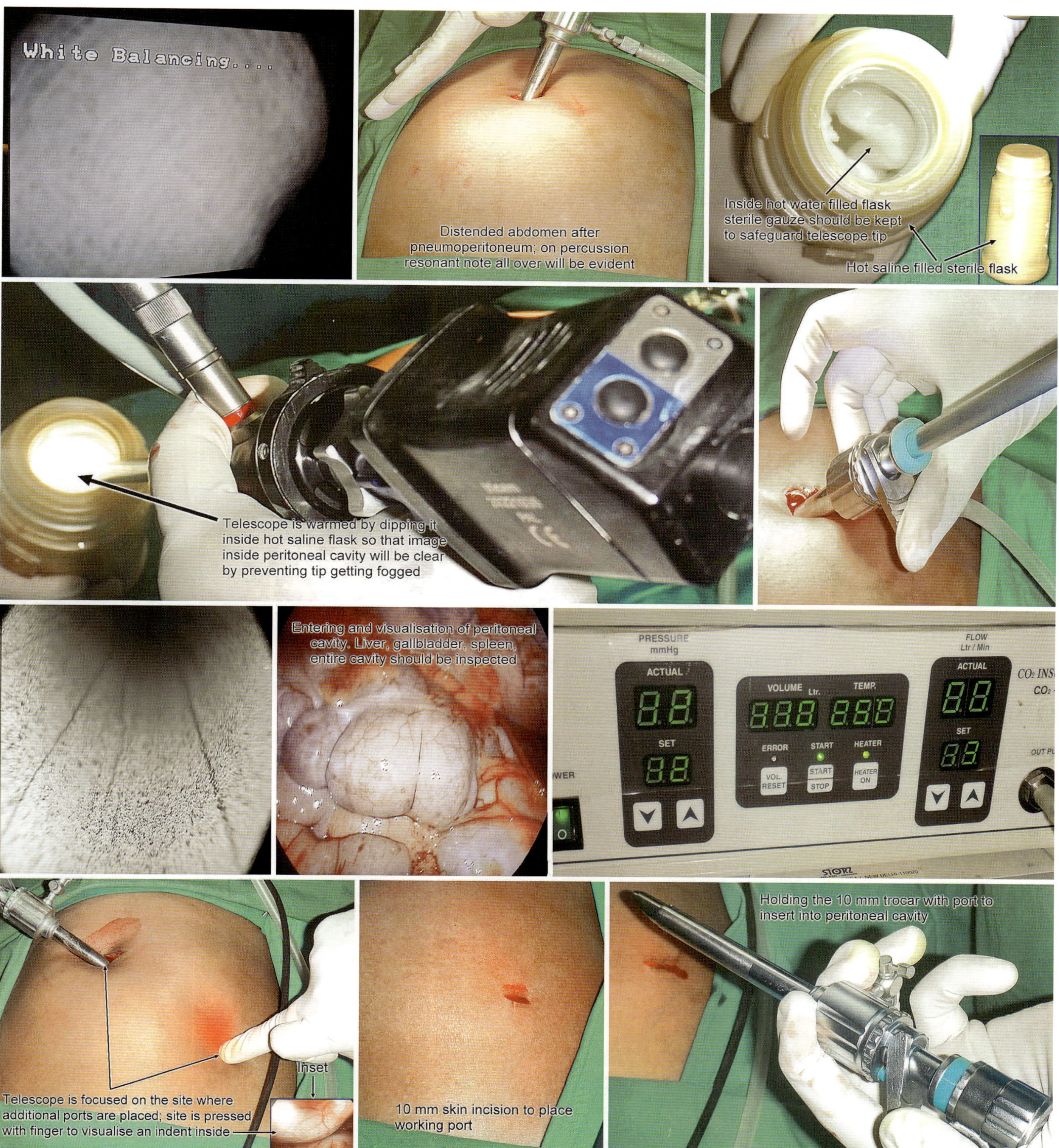
White Balancing....
Distended abdomen after pneumoperitoneum; on percussion resonant note all over will be evident
Inside hot water filled flask sterile gauze should be kept to safeguard telescope tip
Hot saline filled sterile flask
Telescope is warmed by dipping it inside hot saline flask so that image inside peritoneal cavity will be clear by preventing tip getting fogged
Entering and visualisation of peritoneal cavity. Liver, gallbladder, spleen, entire cavity should be inspected
PRESSURE mmHg
ACTUAL
SET
VOLUME Ltr.
TEMP.
ERROR
START
HEATER
VOL. RESET
START STOP
HEATER ON
FLOW Ltr / Min
ACTUAL
SET
STORZ
Telescope is focused on the site where additional ports are placed; site is pressed with finger to visualise an indent inside
Inset
10 mm skin incision to place working port
Holding the 10 mm trocar with port to insert into peritoneal cavity

Figs. 18-80(2)

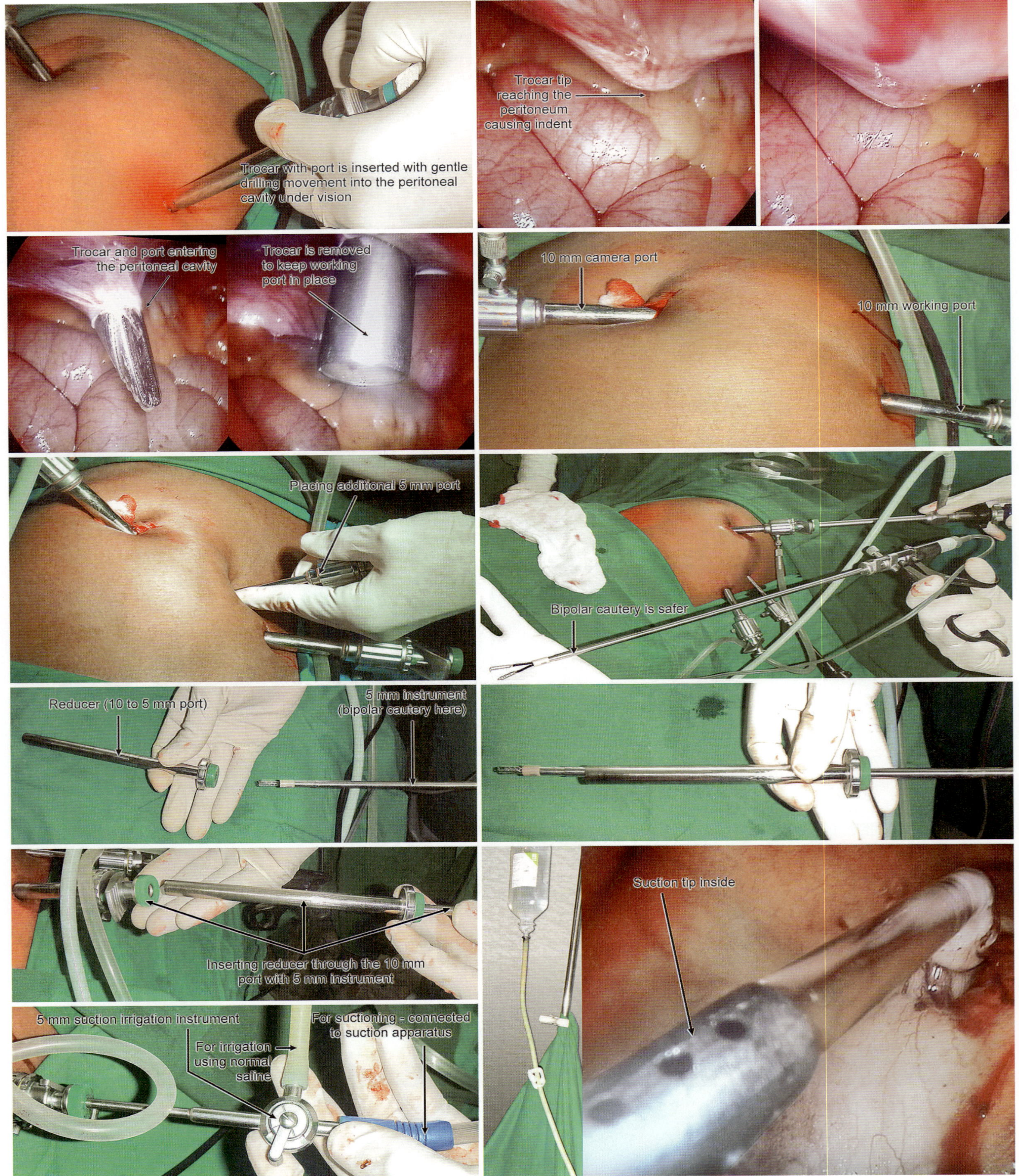

Figs. 18-80(3)

Figs. 18-80(1 to 3): Laparoscopic access technique—steps.

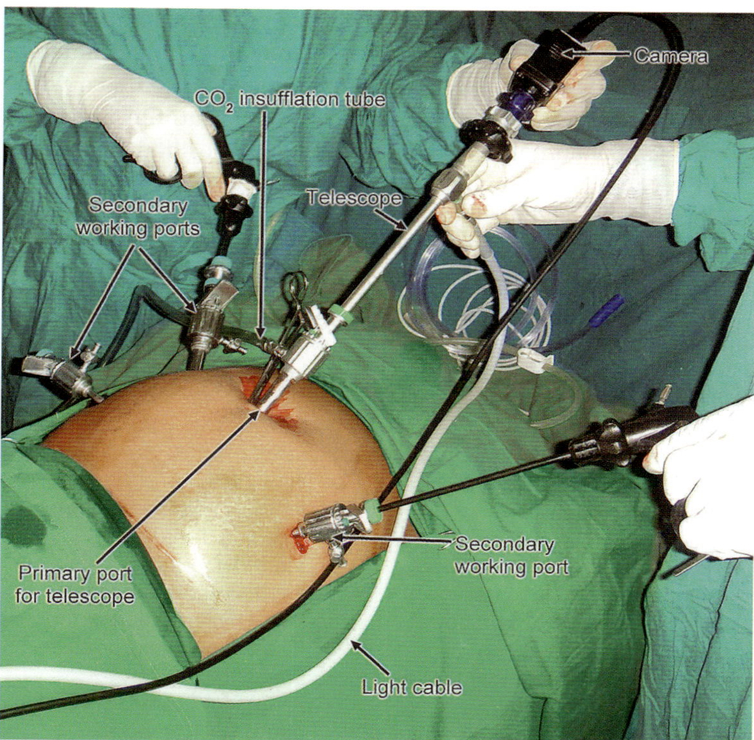

Fig. 18-81: After completion of placing primary and secondary ports, ready for needed surgical technique.

Gas leak: Gas leak may be from the wound site of the trocar or from the faulty valve of the trocar. Carefully if observed, sound of leaking gas can be appreciated. If saline is poured at the suspected site air bubbles can be seen. To confirm whether leak is from valve or wound, all instruments including telescope are removed from the ports. Respective trocars of the cannulas are partially passed again. If leak stops then it is due to leak from one of the valves of the cannulas. Suspected cannula trocar is kept and other trocars are removed which will maintain the pneumoperitoneum. Once it is confirmed that particular port cannula should be changed. If even after placing trocars of all cannulas in place gas leak continues that means it is from wound site. That particular trocar wound is identified and deep non-absorbable temporary stitches are placed to prevent leak. Often Allis' forceps is placed to that particular wound edge. Often 10 mm to 5 mm reducers are used to pass 5 mm instruments. As reducers are valveless, if rubber cap on the reducer is damaged, leak can occur. Cap should be changed immediately.

Open access for primary port is usually done through umbilical incision. But it is often *contraindicated* in previous midline scar; portal hypertension with cirrhosis as umbilical artery may be recanalised; congenital umbilical abnormalities like urachal diseases, vitellointestinal diseases.

Secondary working ports are placed on direct vision. These working ports are usually on right and left sides of the camera (primary) port. It should be at adequate distance from camera port to prevent instrument touching the telescope leading to blockage of free movements of the working instruments. Smaller diameter trocar is usually placed at surgeon's dominant hand side to allow proper wrist movements and also to avoid tremor during procedure. Initially site is pressed with finger on the abdominal wall while visualising the indentation in the monitor. Skin incision must be 1½ times larger than size of the trocar. Dermis should be cut adequately using no. 11 blade stab incision. Trocar is held with the palm of the hand and thumb and index finger. Middle finger is extended along the shaft of the cannula/trocar towards the tip to achieve good control of the trocar while piercing the abdominal wall and also to prevent sudden rapid entry into the peritoneal cavity. Trocar is pierced with rotating and screwing movements (not by pushing), at 90° to skin; once it reaches the peritoneal surface it is angled 45° obliquely while entering the peritoneal cavity. Entire procedure should be done under vision in monitor.

Other Approaches to Access Peritoneal Cavity

Approach Using Visiport

Access can be done under direct vision *using visiport* wherein telescope is passed through it. Tip of the visiport contains fine retractile blade which on firing makes small fine incisions in the tissue allowing movement of the port under vision towards the peritoneal cavity. It is very useful in accessing the peritoneal cavity with previous surgery and also in obese patient **(Fig. 18-82)**.

Left Palmer Point Approach

In abdomen with previous history of surgeries especially for incisional hernia and adhesiolysis, *left Palmer point* (left subcostal point) is used as direct method to access the peritoneal cavity.

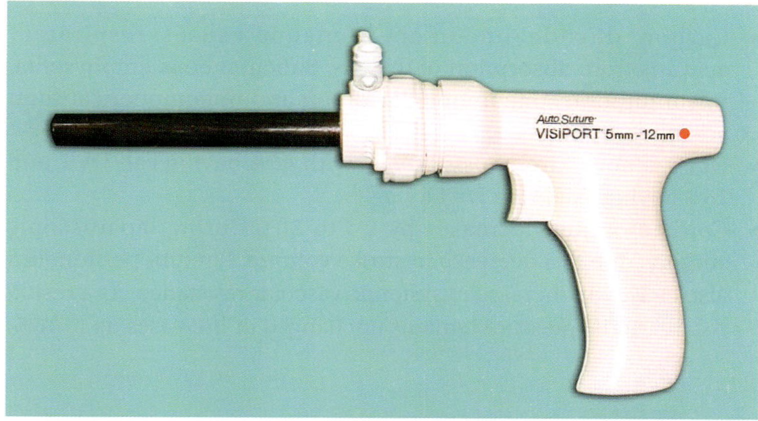

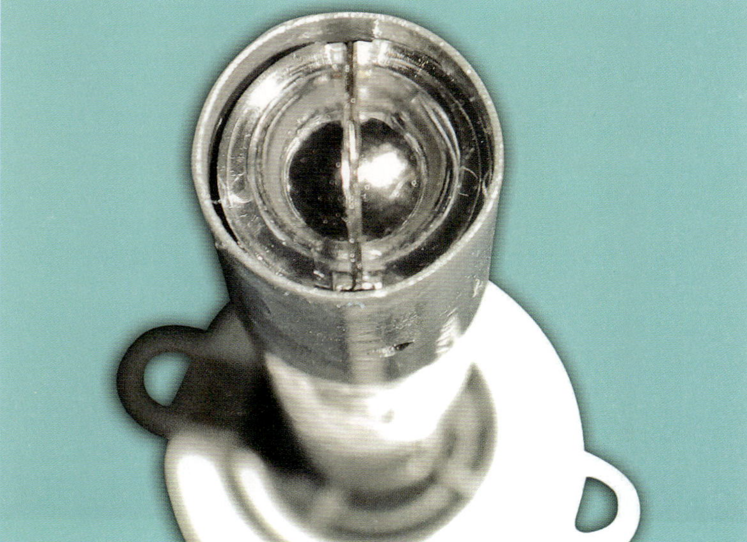

Fig. 18-82: Visiport can be used to pass primary port.

COMPLICATIONS IN LAPAROSCOPY

Complications of Access

The rate of complication associated with Veress needle or trocar insertion is approximately 0.3%. They are—injuries to major retroperitoneal vessels and to bowel (0.2%), which are associated with significant morbidity and mortality; abdominal wall haematoma (2%); wound infection (1.2%); fascial dehiscence and herniation (port site/umbilical—1.5%). Open technique leads to less frequent wound complications in laparoscopic surgery. Though major vascular injuries and bowel injuries with trocar placement are quite rare, use of the open technique may decrease the incidence of these dangerous complications **(Fig. 18-83)**.

Physiologic Complications of Pneumoperitoneum

Pneumoperitoneum causes several local and systemic effects, as reviewed by *Hackam* and *Rotstein*. The majority of these effects are beneficial for patient recovery, such as an observed decrease in postoperative pain and metabolic stress response, as measured by serum glucose and insulin levels and the hepatic catabolic response, measured by functional hepatic nitrogen clearance.

Physiologic Complications of Laparoscopic Surgery

- Carbon dioxide pneumoperitoneum causes respiratory acidosis from absorption of the gas. Subcutaneous emphysema, pneumothorax, pneumomediastinum and pneumopericardium are other problems.
- Deep venous thrombosis (DVT—with 40% having calf DVT and 15% having axial vein DVT).
- Cardiac output decreases by up to 30% during laparoscopic surgery, due to a decrease in stroke volume. Pneumoperitoneum also causes an increase in systemic vascular resistance. As a result, mean arterial pressure remains unchanged or increases up to 16%. Patients with marginal cardiac performance may warrant invasive cardiac monitoring to assure they tolerate pneumoperitoneum. This is partly due to intravascular volume status, and could be ameliorated by preloading patients with isotonic fluid and achieving pneumoperitoneum in the supine position rather than the reverse-Trendelenburg position. Treating these patients with clonidine blunted the increase in mean arterial pressure, systemic vascular resistance and the release of catecholamines. Cardiac arrhythmias (more common if halothane is used) are most common cardiac complication.

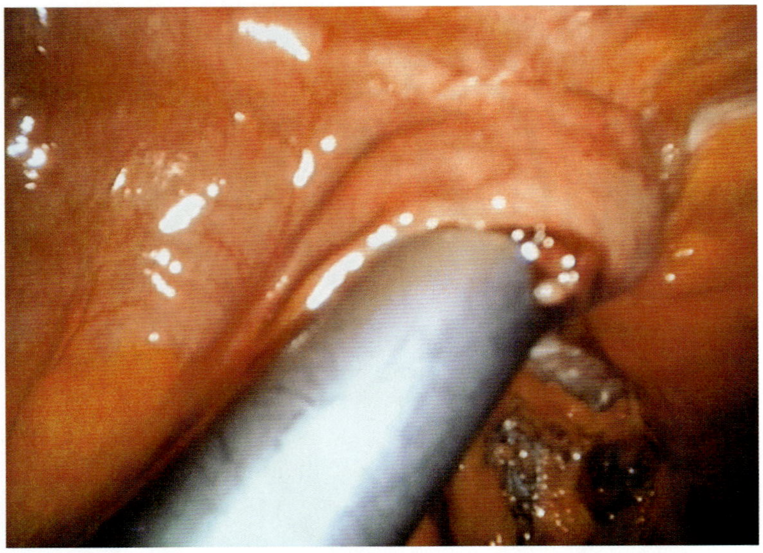

Complications of laparoscopic surgery	*Relative contraindications*
♦ CO_2 narcosis and hypoxia. ♦ Sepsis—subphrenic abscess, pelvic abscess, septicaemia. ♦ IVC compression. ♦ Bleeding. ♦ Leak from the site, e.g. bile leak. ♦ Organ injury during insertion of ports, e.g. major vessels, bowel, mesentery, liver. ♦ Subcutaneous emphysema and pneumomediastinum. ♦ Gas emboli, though is rare but fatal. ♦ Gastric content aspiration. ♦ Hypothermia. ♦ Postoperative shoulder pain due to irritation of diaphragm. ♦ Hyperabduction of arm can cause stretching of the brachial plexus and neuropraxia. ♦ Trendelenburg position can cause common peritoneal nerve injury. ♦ Cardiac dysfunction due to decreased venous return. ♦ Injury to the abdominal wall vessels and nerves. ♦ Cautery burn to abdominal structures. ♦ Abdominal wall hernias—port site hernias. ♦ Wound infection. ♦ Mortality—0.5%.	♦ Patients with compromised cardiac status. ♦ Peritonitis. ♦ Previous abdominal surgeries. ♦ Bleeding disorders. ♦ Morbid obesity. ♦ Third trimester pregnancy. ♦ Portal hypertension, cirrhosis. ♦ Raised intracranial pressure. ♦ Glaucoma. ♦ Peritoneo-jugular, ventriculo-peritoneal shunts. **Limitations** Lack of tactile sensation; tissue feel is absent. Only eye-hand coordination is the method.

Fig. 18-83: Primary port which has passed through small bowel which was adherent abdominal wall due to previous surgery.

- *Gas embolism:* It can occur (but very rare) by direct entry of CO_2 through inadvertent injury by Veress needle or trocar; when small gas bubbles enter the injured vein; absorption of large quantity of gas into the portal system which forms bubbles that get trapped in the portal system as well as in the pulmonary circulation at a later period. Smaller bubbles block pulmonary circulation; larger one causes gas lock in IVC and right atrium (may cause sudden death). On table patient develops tachycardia, hypotension, arrhythmias, convulsions, metallic/*mill wheel* murmur (heard through precordial or oesophageal stethoscope). Foaming of blood in CVP catheter, precordial Doppler (detects passage of even 2 mL of gas), oesophageal Doppler (detects even 0.5 mL of gas). $P_{ET}CO_2$ raises in *capnometry* which is the most valuable non-invasive method to detect gas embolism. 20% of such patients during recovery may show blindness. Once on table gas embolism is diagnosed, immediately pneumoperitoneum is stopped and gas is released; patient is kept in steep head down and left up position; hyperventilation; CVP catheter gas aspirations are done. Nitrous oxide should be stopped.

DIAGNOSTIC LAPAROSCOPY

With the availability of diagnostic modalities like helical CT and MRI scans the role of laparoscope in diagnosing occult abdominal pathologies has greatly reduced. Most often the laparoscope is used as confirmatory investigation before the pre-planned procedure such as appendicectomy or adhesiolysis for subacute intestinal obstruction. The other area where the laparoscope is helpful is to ascertain the anatomical origin of masses in the right iliac fossa in women of reproductive age where there is suspicion of tubo-ovarian pathology. Even abdominal tuberculosis can be now diagnosed with ancillary investigations such as PCR for tubercular DNA. Laparoscopy is now a precursor to appendicectomy or adhesiolysis in case of chronic vague abdominal pain where other investigations have not yielded a diagnosis **(Figs. 18-84 to 18-86)**.

Preparation

- It is done always under general anaesthesia. It can be done under local anaesthesia also but it is cumbersome and painful to the patient. Other preparations are same as for open method.
- Pressure bandages are applied to both legs to improve the venous return and to decrease the stasis.
- Head end of the table is lowered to have easier insertion of Veress needle and scope.
- Ryle's tube and Foley's catheter are essential before insertion of the trocars.
- Pneumoperitoneum is created using Veress needle through umbilical incision. Access can be achieved by open method through an umbilical incision.

Procedure

Peritoneal access is gained by either open or closed method. Before proceeding to place accessory ports attention is given to the suspected pathology. Placement of working port is generally guided by the proposed site of the pathology and also the planned procedure. Lower abdominal pathology demands ports placed on either side of the rectus muscle at or just below the umbilicus. If pathology is anticipated or seen in stomach, liver, spleen on preliminary screening then the ports should be placed above the umbilical level in suitable position. Bowel should be inspected along its entire length by alternately moving the working instruments on the bowel and both sides should be inspected for pathology. The method of inspection is similar to that of exploratory laparotomy. Laparoscopy gives great advantage when inspecting the diaphragm and the pelvic structures. The procedure is converted to a definitive procedure when the pathology is identified. Routinely the procedure culminates in an appendicectomy even when no other obvious pathology is evident as it prevents diagnostic difficulties at later date **(Figs. 18-87 to 18-89)**.

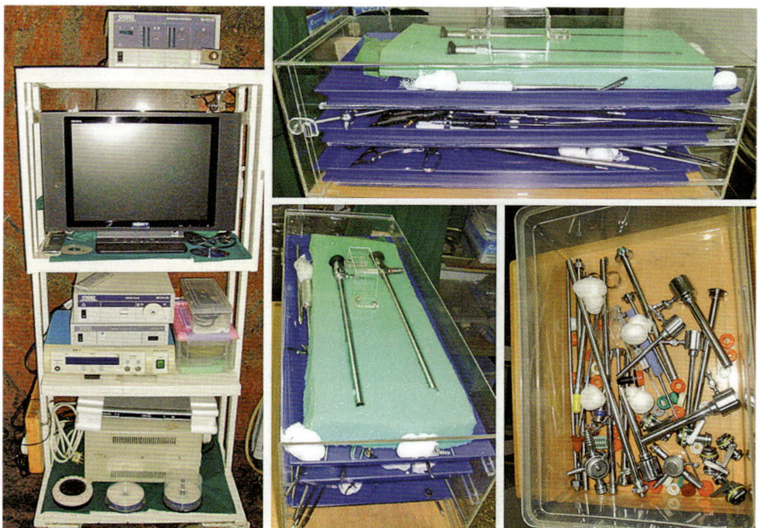

Fig. 18-84: Laparoscopic set showing trolley, telescope and monitor instruments.

Note

- Instruments should be checked prior to procedure for proper functioning.
- Cardiac, respiratory fitness should be assessed.
- Position, preparation is a must.
- Adequate pneumoperitoneum should be created; gas leak should be prevented or tackled effectively.
- Telescope should be warmed before insertion to prevent fogging.
- Tip of light cable is very hot and should not touch drapes or patients' skin. It may cause deep burn injury.
- Camera operator should hold the camera firm and strong to have good view of surgical site.
- Telescope tip can be cleared by obscuring blood by touching her tip to omentum or abdominal wall or solid organ like liver. Otherwise it should be removed and cleaned with savlon and warm saline. Tip of telescope should never be touched to the bowel as it may injure the bowel.
- Insufflation gas inlet can be changed to working port instead to camera port to prevent undue fogging.

LAPAROSCOPIC ULTRASOUND

Fukuda in 1981 used laparoscopic ultrasound. Transducer in ultrasound is made up of piezoelectric cells. USG flexible probes are used which are 7 cm in length and 12 mm in diameter. Two monitors are required; one for laparoscope other for ultrasound. Now single monitor is available where both laparoscope and ultrasound images are seen which allows better hand-eye coordination.

Laparoscopic USG probes are sterilised by glutaraldehyde or through ethylene oxide.

Laparoscopic USG is useful in assessing the liver tumours, biliary tree, hepatic nodal status, pancreas, lymph nodes in different areas of the abdomen, spleen, kidneys and adrenals. Laparoscopic ultrasound is very useful in assessing the solid organs, its use is not very much in assessing the small bowel and colon because of the gas in the bowel. It is used to identify the lesions accurately with its size, vasculature; to stage the disease; to assess the resectability of tumour; to identify the vessels and its relations to the organs like hepatic veins in liver resection.

Laparoscopic USG can be used in different therapeutic purposes in liver like radiofrequency ablation and deroofing of the liver cyst. Laparoscopic USG is very useful in identifying biliary stones and is better than intraoperative cholangiogram. Endocrine pancreatic tumours are well identified by laparoscopic USG. Identification of pancreatic duct during pancreaticojejunostomy is better with laparoscopic USG. Laparoscopic-guided biopsy is even though done, but it is controversial. Laparoscopic FNAC is a good diagnostic tool. Three-dimensional (3D) ultrasound is now available with better clarity of images **(Fig. 18-90)**.

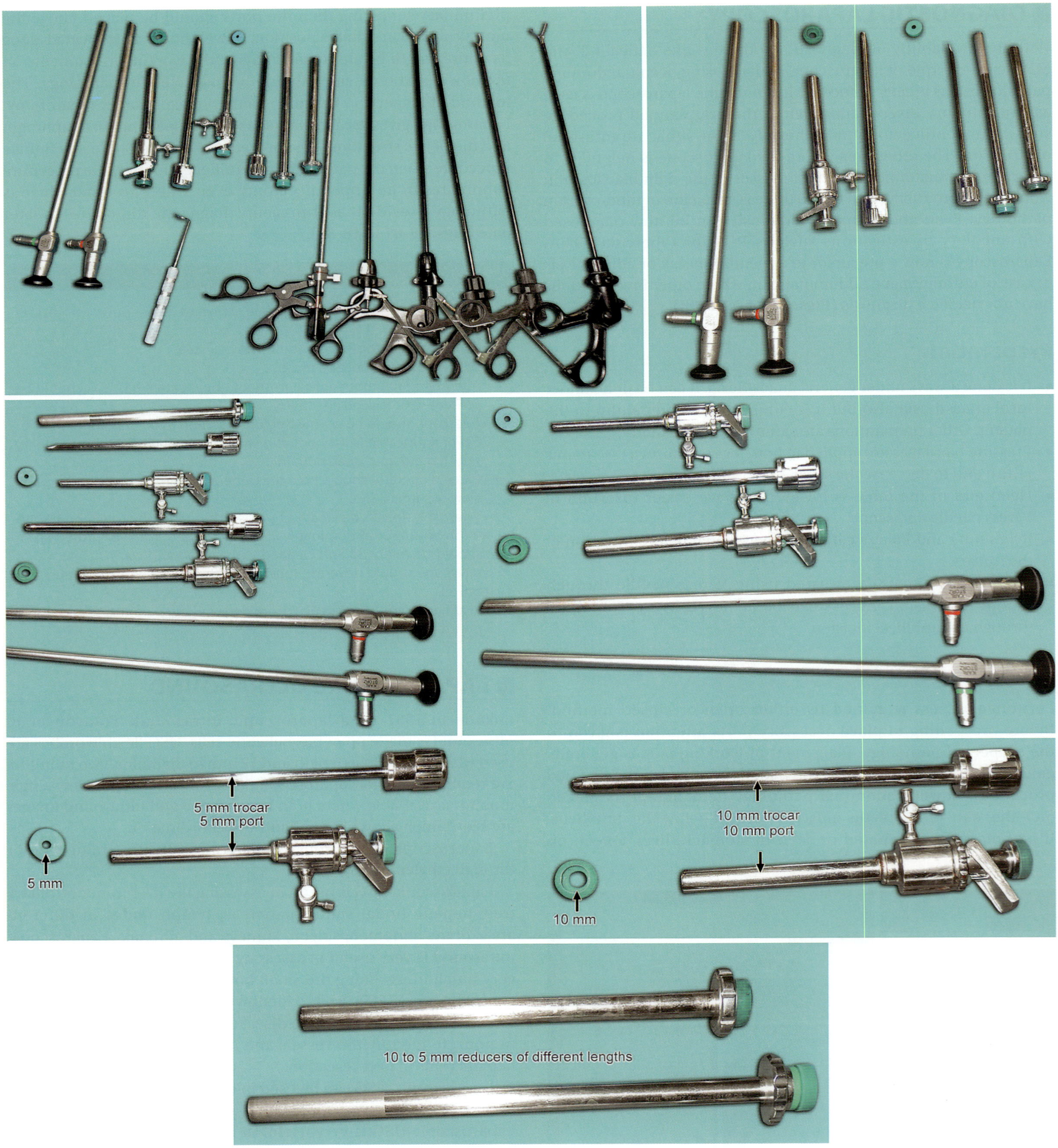

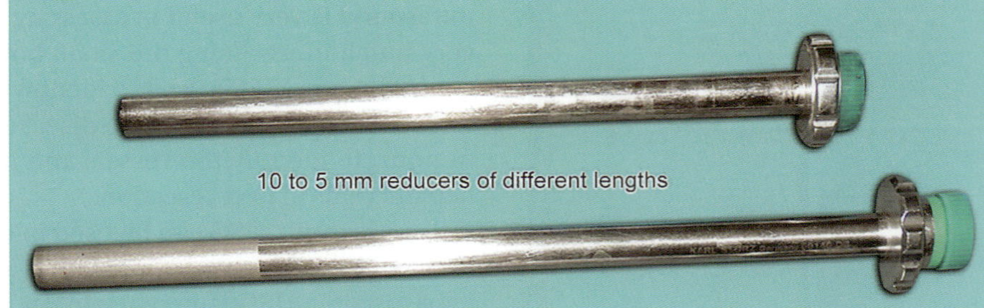

Fig. 18-85: Different instruments used for diagnostic laparoscopy.

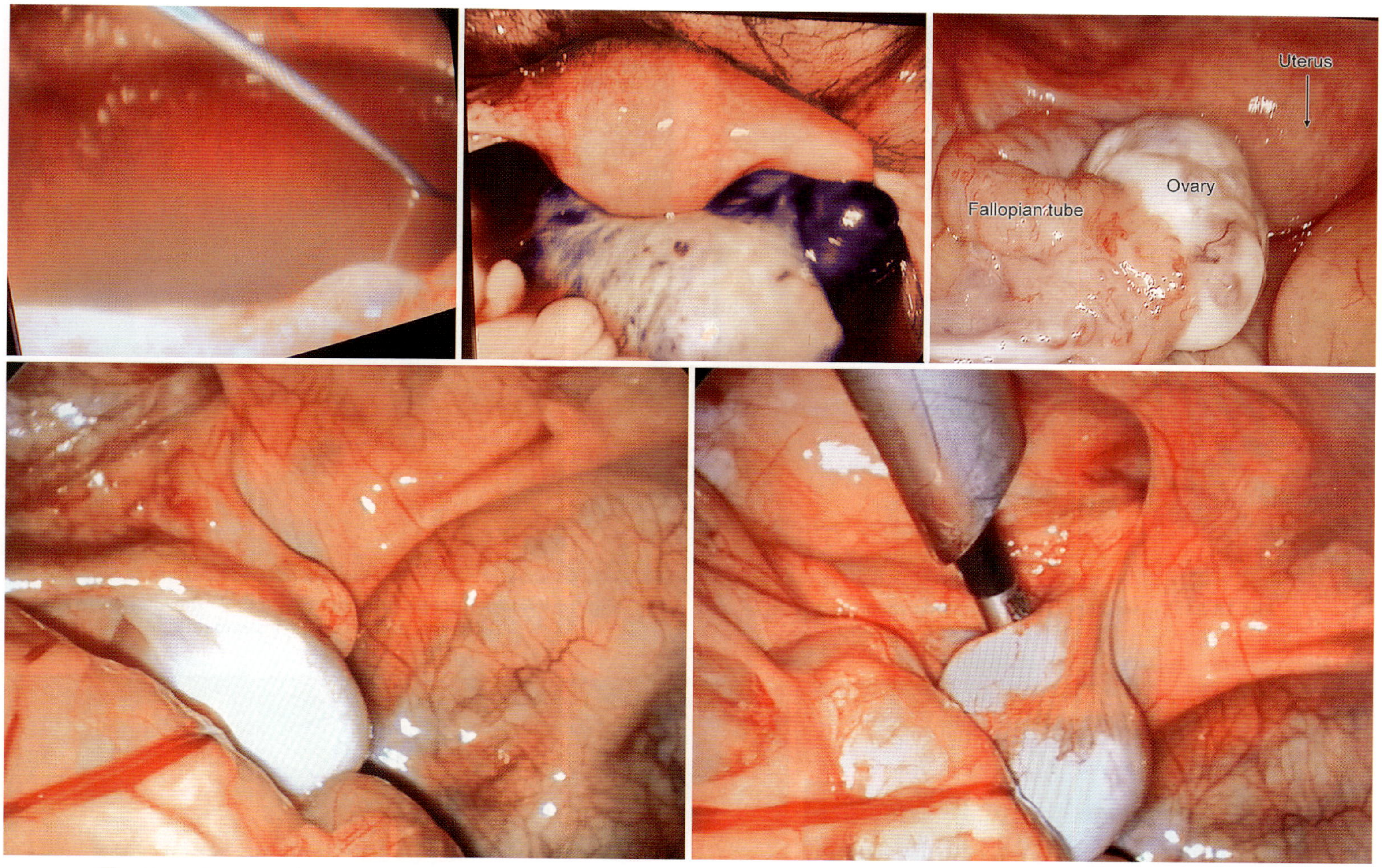

Fig. 18-86: Diagnostic laparoscopic view in ascites (tuberculosis); twisted ovarian cyst, ovary and Fallopian tube; undescended testis with inguinal hernial opening at internal ring.

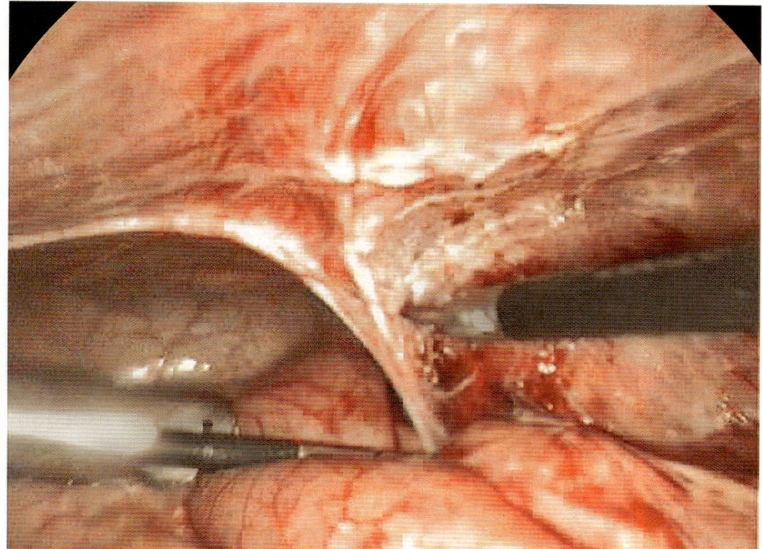

Fig. 18-87: Adhesiolysis.

THREE-DIMENSIONAL LAPAROSCOPY

Three-dimensional (3D) laparoscopy is now available with more clarity and three-dimensional look. 3D camera available at present is heavy (1 kg). It is often difficult for cameraman to hold it and negotiate. Suturing and image quality is good in this but it is costly.

There is marked and significant improvement in operative time with a stereoscopic 3D laparoscopic view of the operative field. As procedure is performed with identical mechanical instrumentation like in two-dimensional (2D) laparoscopic instruments the difference attributable is only to the changes in depth perception obtained with the 3D laparoscope. This skill obtained with this finally will be beneficial in advanced procedures like laparoscopic radical prostatectomy, laparoscopic pyeloplasty, or other complex reconstructive procedures. One of the biggest challenges in laparoscopic surgical training is adaptation to a 2D flat view of the surgical field. 3D laparoscopic visual systems have been developed to augment laparoscopic skills. Suturing skill will be much more precise and accurate and also will be faster.

SINGLE INCISION LAPAROSCOPIC SURGERY

Single incision laparoscopic surgery (SILS) is an advanced minimally invasive surgical procedure wherein surgeon operate exclusively through a single umbilical entry port. It is also called as single port access surgery (SPA), one port umbilical surgery (OPUS), and single-port incisionless conventional equipment-utilising surgery (SPICES), natural orifice transumbilical surgery (NOTUS).

It is used in cholecystectomy, appendicectomy, gynaecologic procedures, hernia surgery and other selected procedures.

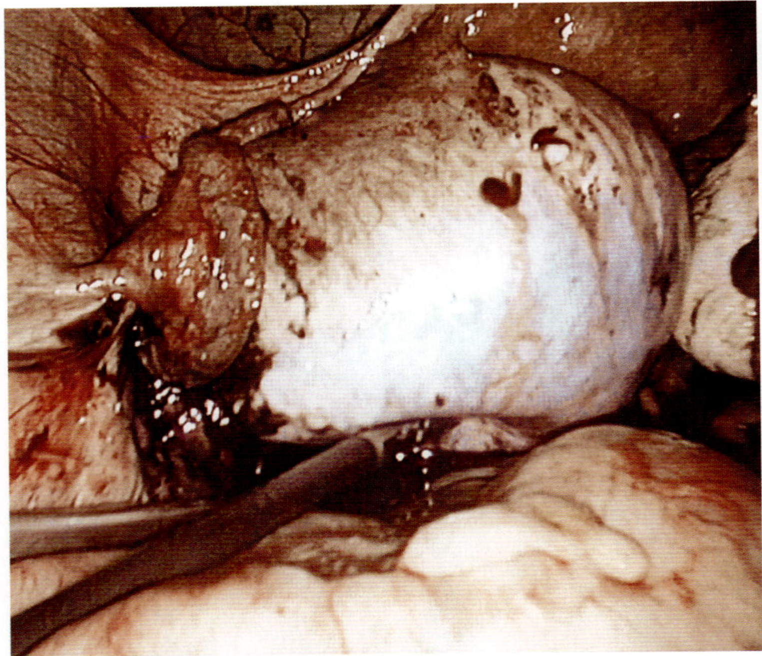

Fig. 18-88: Laparoscopic view of twisted ovarian cyst.

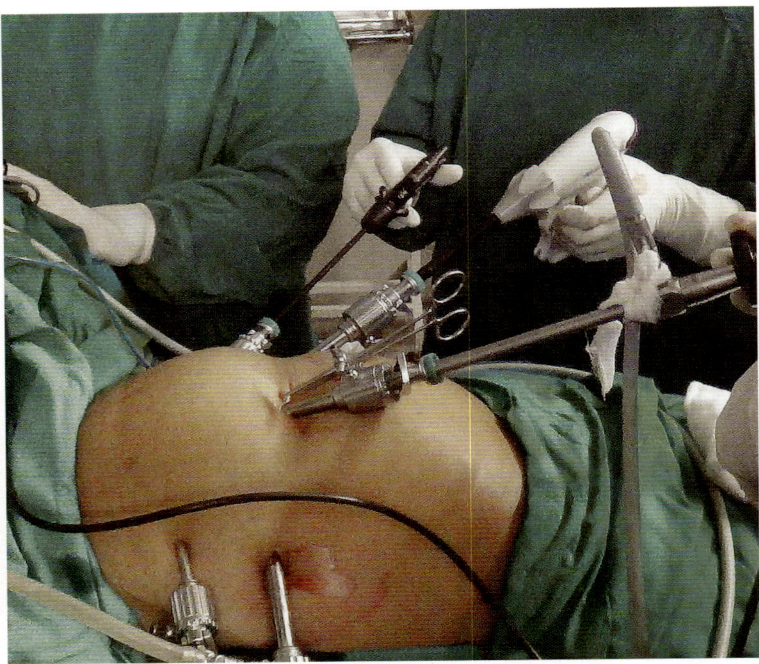

Fig. 18-89: Laparoscopic procedure in progress showing camera, telescope, ports, working instruments.

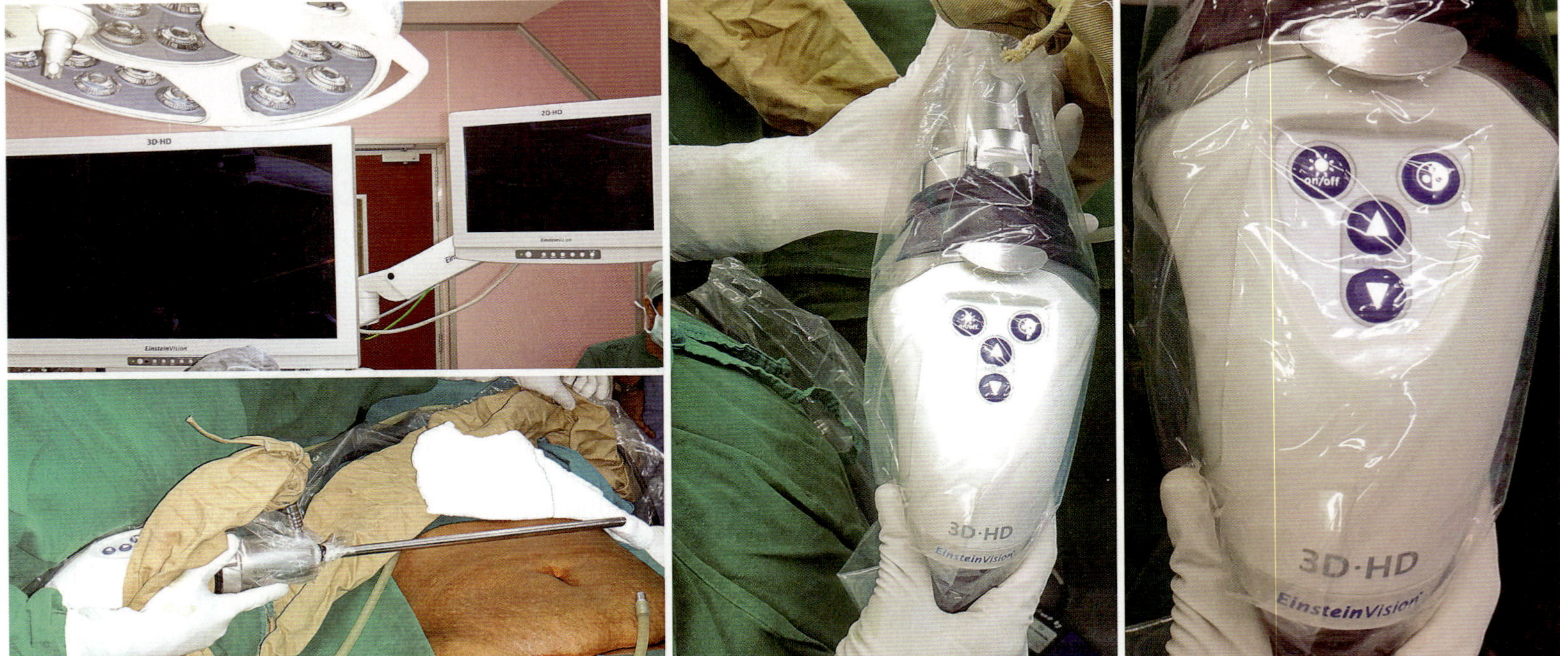

Fig. 18-90: Three-dimensional (3D) laparoscopy camera and monitor. Present 3D camera is heavy weight—nearly one kilogram in weight.

It needs general anaesthesia, specialised umbilical large trocars which accommodates working instruments also, flexible laparoscope, rotatable instruments, articulating handles, harmonic scalpel.

Here through a large 2.5 cm umbilical vertical incision dissection is done by open method to reach peritoneal cavity. Through this is passed a specialised port where one can pass 10 mm telescope and two 5 mm instruments for laparoscopic work. Instruments are angled and flexible to meet the ergonomic principles to certain extent. Dissection of gallbladder is done in similar fashion like four port technique. Specimen is easily retrieved through umbilical port as it is wider enough. If difficulty arises any time one can add additional ports as required.

SILS is now used in appendicectomy, ovarian cyst excision, selected cases in hernia and other procedures also.

Advantages

- There is no visible scar like a traditional multiport.
- Faster recovery time, early return to work.
- Cosmetically better **(Fig. 18-91)**.

Disadvantages

- Expensive trocars and instruments.
- Skilled work, learning curve.
- Dissection against normal surgical ergonomics.

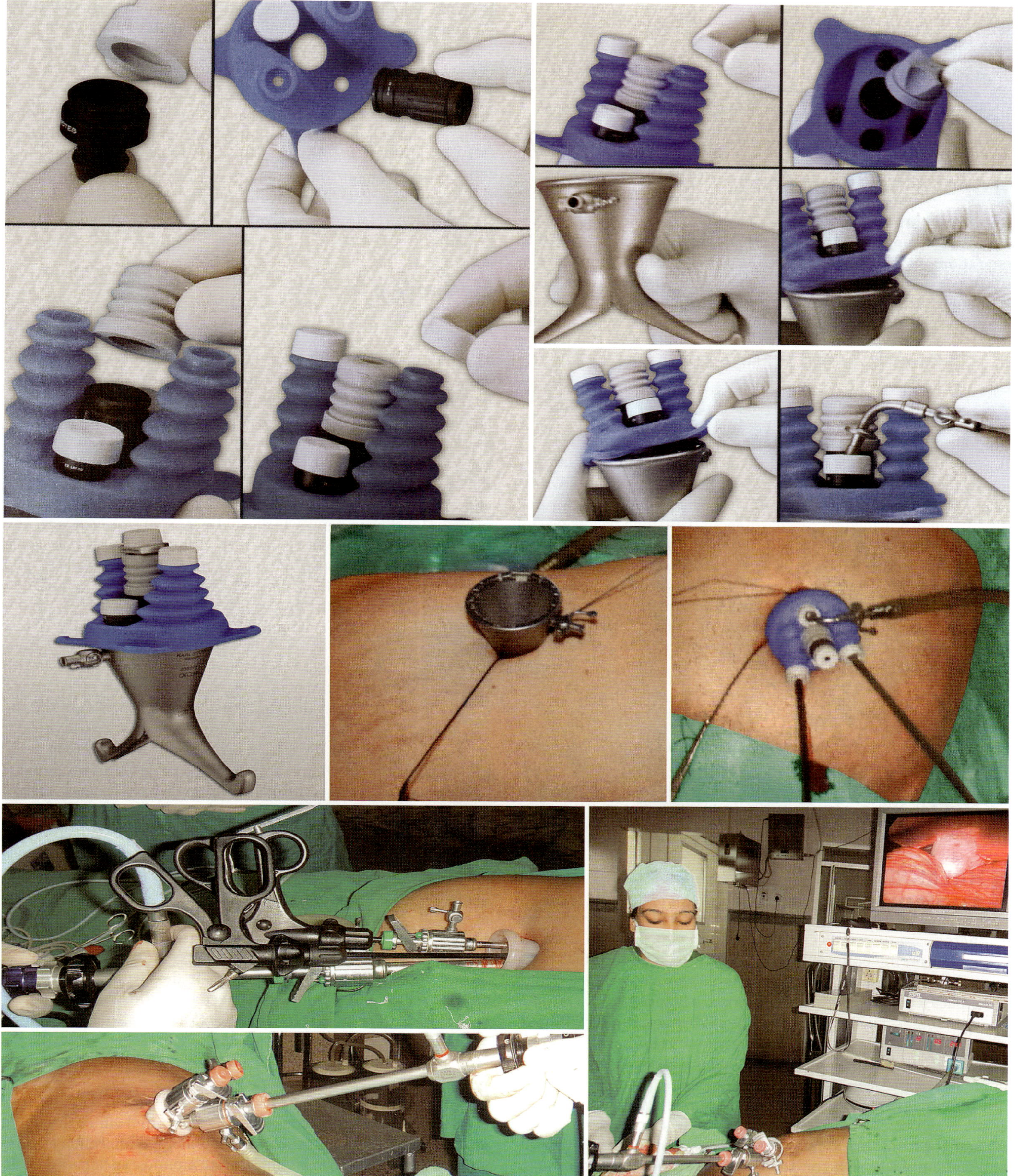

Fig. 18-91: Single incision laparoscopic surgery (SILS) for cholecystectomy/appendicectomy and also for other procedures.

Complications

- Umbilical wound pain, infection.
- Umbilical hernia.
- Time consuming because of limited visibility.
- During learning curve complications of cholecystectomy or other procedures and conversion rate may be more.

GASLESS LAPAROSCOPY (LAPAROLIFT)

Dan Kruschinski is the *Preceptor of Gasless Lift-Laparoscopy* since 1991 with an ongoing process of establishing excellent vision with new abdominal lift devices to ensure a cost-effective laparoscopic start-up system.

It is forward retraction of the anterior abdominal wall so as to create the effective working cavity inside the peritoneum to facilitate the dissection. It may be useful for pelvic and lower abdominal surgeries (APR/ovarian surgeries), appendicectomy, etc.

Advantages

Complications of CO_2 pneumoperitoneum are not present. It can be done under regional anaesthesia. It provides appropriateness, equity, accessibility, availability, affordability to the rural people wherein cost is also a main factor. In developing countries 80% rural population is provided by 20% of surgeons. Laparolift will be useful to these patients considering their need (as they need to return their work earlier) and economy. Valveless trocars can be used. Suction usage can be unlimited. Conventional instruments can be used when need arises. During induction of anaesthesia increased ventilator pressure is not needed. It shows less infection rate; equally cosmetic; less postoperative pain; early faster recovery; shoulder pain will not be present; safer and precise.

Disadvantages

Movement of the viscera during inspiration causes difficulty in targeting the proper dissection unlike in dissection with pneumoperitoneum which is motionless. Technique even though is used in many places, is less popular due to difficulties in developing adequate lift.

HAEMOSTASIS IN LAPAROSCOPIC AND OPEN PROCEDURES

As there is no direct access to the bleeders, it is often difficult to control the bleeding during haemostasis. Often difficulty in controlling the bleeding becomes an indication for conversion into open at least during learning curve period. It is better to have an idea about different haemostasis methods during laparoscopy. Proper ergonomics and triangulations are very important in laparoscopy. One should able to grasp and coagulate the bleeding point in the tissue properly. Meantime blood from bleeding point if spills over the laparoscope tip, it will blur the image and a panic situation is created as bleeding point/area is not visualised. Surgeon should console the cameraman and ask him to stay steadily on the site of bleeding until it is well controlled. While achieving haemostasis, it is also important not to injure the adjacent structures either with clip or energy source. In cholecystectomy with cystic artery bleed, clips may be applied in a hurry to control bleeding over the common bile duct thereby partially injuring it; cautery when used, especially monopolar cautery may cause lateral thermal damage to closely existing common bile duct wall which eventually leads to necrosis of its wall causing disastrous bile leak.

Laparoscopic haemostasis may be achieved by different means.

a. **Mechanical devices:** Clips, lineal stapling devices, pretied suture loops (endoloop/loop done in theatre table as extracorporeal knot which is pushed towards the site as ligature), intracorporeal ligature placement, transfixation suturing intracorporeally.
b. **Energy sources:** Electrocautery, ligasure, laser, ultrasonic dissection (Harmonic), cavitron ultrasonic surgical aspirator (CUSA).

Mechanical Devices

Mechanical Clips

They are made up of titanium inert, least reactive clips available which are applied through 10 mm clip applicator. Clips are available in 7 mm (medium), 9 mm (medium large) and 11 mm (large) size. Medium size is usually used. Size required is decided by the surgeons as per the need. Same clip applicator can be adjusted for different size clips placement by adjusting the applicator gap at the end. Reusable clip applicator is commonly used even though preloaded clip applicator is available. Preloaded disposable clip applicator contains 20 clips in a row which can be applied consecutively, one after other which makes surgery faster. Absorbable clips are available mainly to apply onto the continuous suture intraperitoneally to hold it at the beginning and at the end. Usually two clips are applied proximally close to each other. Third distal clip is applied at 3–5 mm gap. Tissue is cut between proximal two clips and distal clip. While applying the clip, both ends of the clip should encroach the tissue/duct/vessel completely and clip should be applied under vision with confirmation that it is not entangling any other tissues and ends are clearly seen before compressing the clip firmly. While cutting the tissue, gap should be kept distal to proximal two clips to prevent slipping of the clip. At least 5 mm of tissue should be present freely proximal to proximal clips to prevent clip migration (example—while applying clips in cystic duct). Clip applicator is usually straight but angled one is also available. Even though it is of practice that application of ligature along with or after applying the clip; it will loosen the clip due to tissue distortion. In such situation suture ligature should be finished first and then clip should be applied at needed place **(Figs. 18-92 to 18-94)**.

Linear Stapling Devices

Linear stapling devices are very useful to deal with splenic, renal, inferior mesenteric vessels in respective laparoscopic surgeries. Different sizes are available—2.5 mm vascular; 3.5 mm intestinal; 4.5 mm intestinal/colonic **(Fig. 18-95)**.

Pretied Loops

Pretied loops are available as such manufactured which are made up of chromic catgut. It is mainly used in appendicectomy. Same loop can also be used in passing ligature around a specified bleeder. Bleeder is held using a Maryland instrument through a working port; pretied loop is passed through another 10 mm working port through a reducer. Instrument which was holding the bleeder is once released

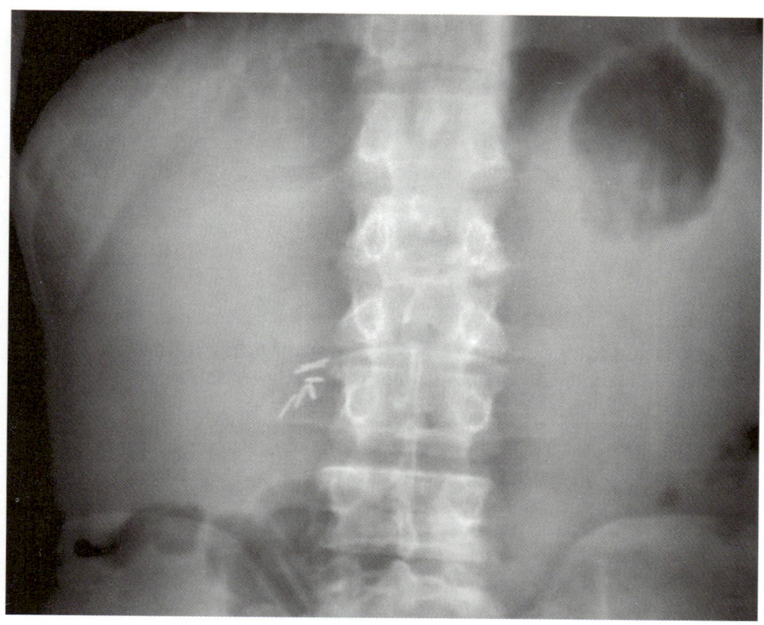

Fig. 18-92: Plain X-ray abdomen showing clips of laparoscopic cholecystectomy.

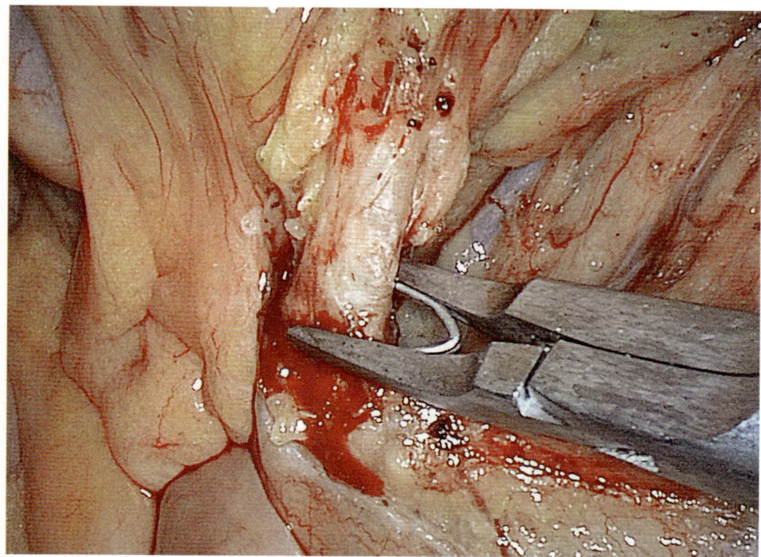

Fig. 18-93: Applying clip for a vessel in the abdominal surgery.

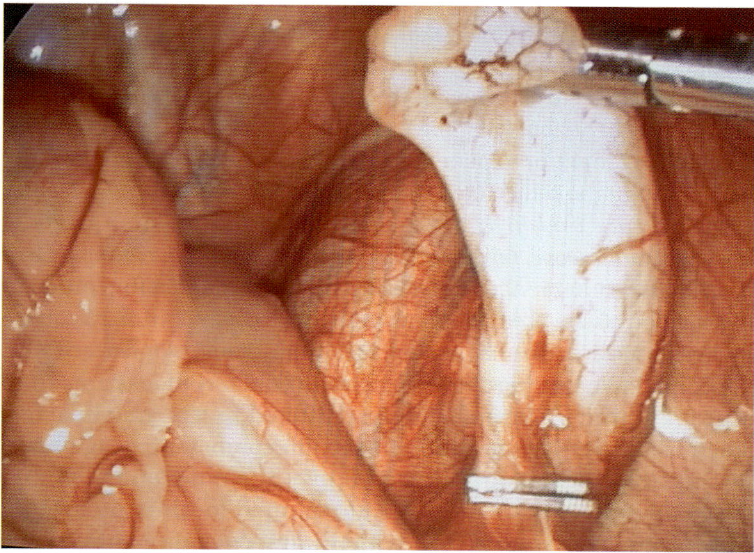

Fig. 18-94: Clip applied for appendicectomy.

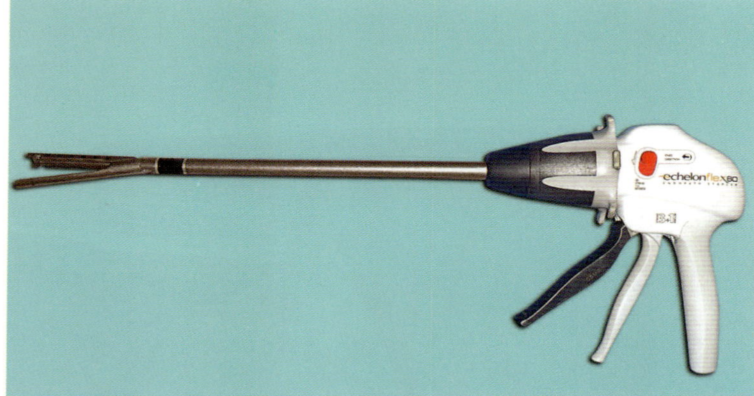

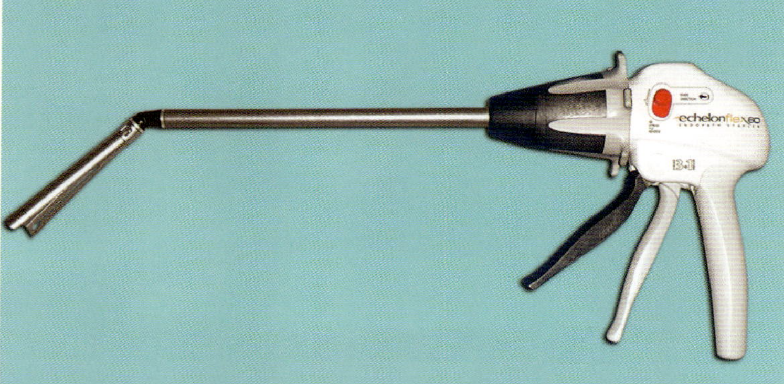

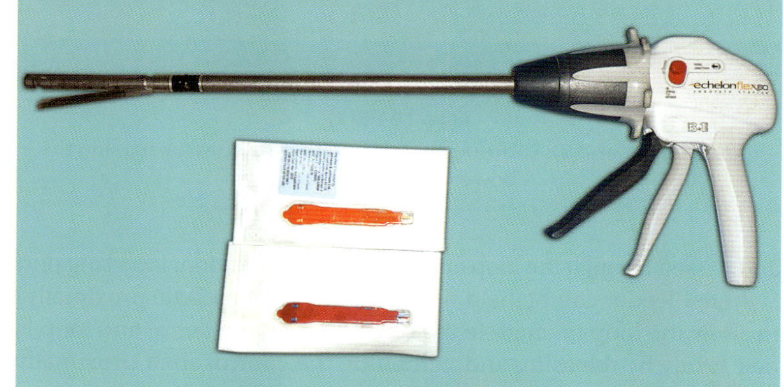

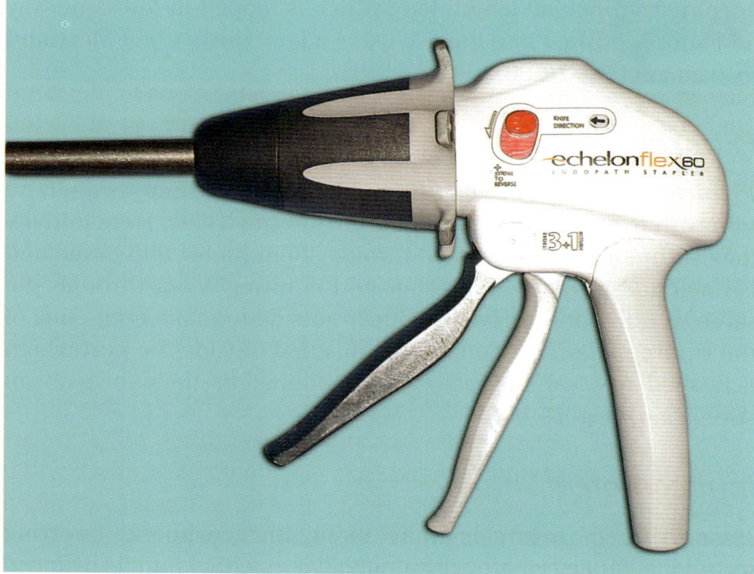

Figs. 18-95(1)

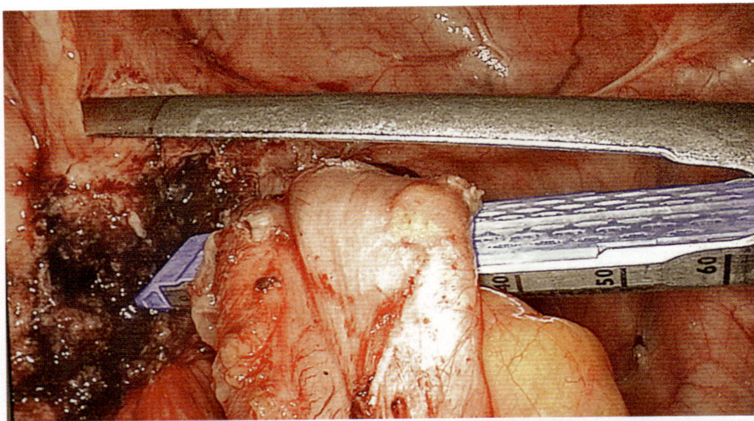

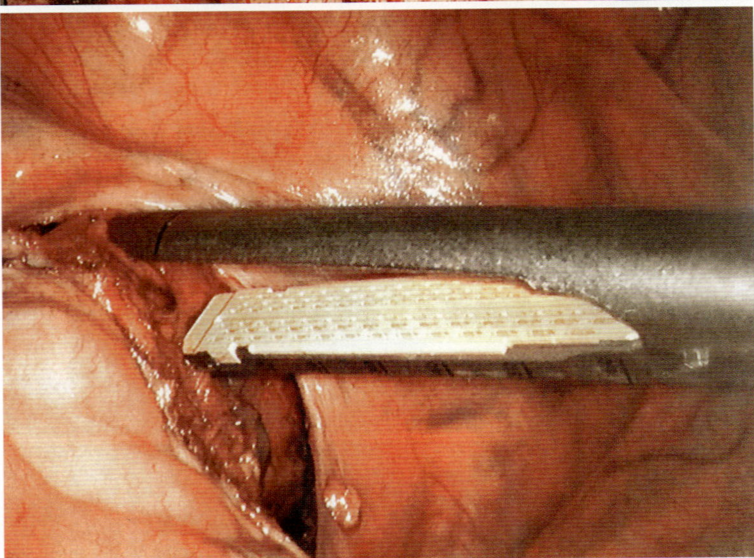

Figs. 18-95(2)

Figs. 18-95(1 and 2): Endostapler device with cartridges for stapling the bowel during resection.

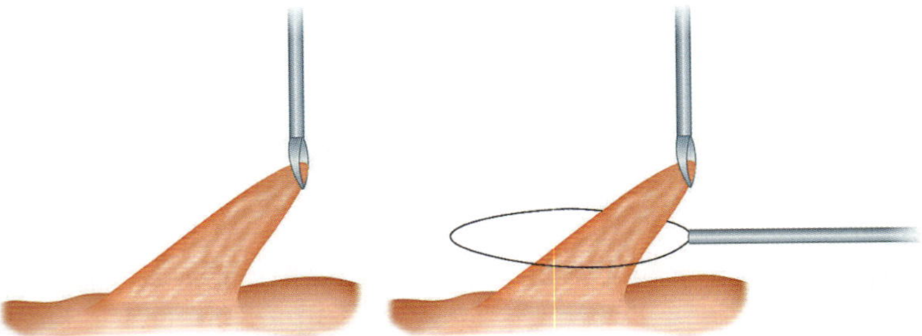

Fig. 18-96: Endoloop is often used to pass a ligature. It may be pre-ttied endoloop (chromic catgut) or endoloop is made using Roeder's knot with vicryl.

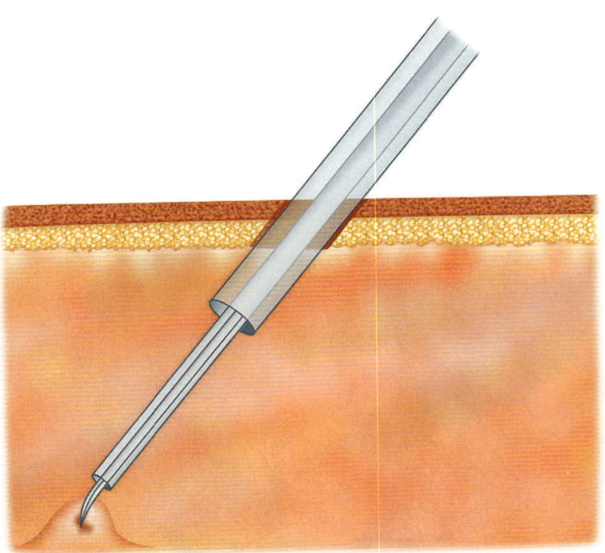

Fig. 18-97: Bleeder is held using a Maryland which can be later fulgurated using cautery.

and passed through the loop and held again (if additional working port is there bleeder can be held using another grasper little proximally) to allow the loop to encircle the bleeder/bleeding tissue and loop is tied firmly by releasing and tightening the control shaft proximally outside. Often Roeder's knot can be made outside using vicryl suture keeping its proximal length long which is looped in the same way and knot is pushed into the site using a knot pusher or a Maryland instrument **(Fig. 18-96)**.

Extracorporeal Ligature

Extracorporeal ligature can be made and is pushed through 10 mm working port through a reducer into the tissue. Here initially long suture material is passed through 10 mm port into tissue and is encircled properly and other end is brought out through the same working port through reducer outside to make both ends of the suture material is outside. Knot is tied outside the port which is pushed across the reducer into the looped tissue to form a firm strong knot **(Fig. 18-97)**.

Intracorporeal Suture

Intracorporeal suture is done using intracorporeal knotting technique. It needs a proper training. It is essential for all advanced laparoscopic surgical procedure.

Energy Sources

Diathermy (Electrosurgery)

Electrosurgical units (ESU) used in operating rooms convert standard electrical frequencies from the wall outlet, which are 50 to 60 Hz, to much higher frequencies, 500,000 to 3,000,000 Hz. This is important to minimise nerve and muscle stimulation, which occurs at electrical currents below 10,000 Hz. High frequency (3 lakh to 6 lakh Hz) current, is allowed to pass through the tissue to create conduction heat achieving haemostasis. *In monopolar type*, current flows from generator to patient through active electrode and returns back through the return electrode to the generator. It is *pulsed wave, low frequency and high voltage* current for *coagulation cautery*. It is *continuous wave, high frequency and low voltage in cutting* type of monopolar cautery. Active electrode passes through a fine probe to the needed tissue area; whereas return electrode is with 22 square inches of surface area flat plate placed under muscular surface with gel conductive coating. Active electrode contacts in less area than return electrode. Current gets concentrated in less area in active electrode to achieve needed effects. Effects may be coagulation or cutting. Coagulation is achieved by protein denaturation and coagulation necrosis. Cutting is due to rapid focal tissue heating causing tissue disintegration without any coagulation necrosis. So cutting cannot cause coagulation. Coagulation at the tip of probe can cause cutting but with more charring. *In laparoscopy mainly coagulation monopolar cautery is used.* Coagulation in hook or spatula can cause cutting by proper holding and positioning the instrument while creating the contact with tissues. Cutting cautery has got limited role. Pulsed coagulation in blend mode is better. During laparoscopic usage of monopolar cautery, one should be careful as instrument which has cautery cable attached is visible at its distal 10%. During usage, one should always confirm that proximal insulation is visible. Instrument should have proper insulation without any damage otherwise severe burns of the abdominal wall at port site or damage to adjacent tissues or bowel perforation or injury to great vessels can occur. Often it may be life threatening. Direct coupling and capacitance coupling can occur. Lateral thermal damage is equally dangerous. Lateral thermal injury can occur up to 8 mm of tissues beyond. In pedicle coagulation, thermal injury and vessel spasm can occur at the base of that particular pedicle **(Figs. 18-98 and 18-99)**.

In bipolar cautery active and return electrodes are separated by few mm passing through the hand probe, not through the body. So conduction (earthing) plate is not needed in bipolar. Bipolar reduces the adjacent tissue damage. It has got less lateral thermal heat. Bipolar can be used only for coagulation but not cutting. Bipolar is very important in laparoscopic surgery as it reduces inadvertent vital structure injury **(Figs. 18-100 and 18-101)**.

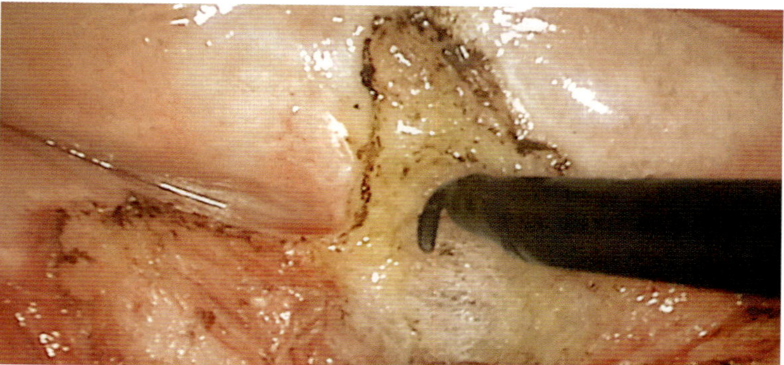

Fig. 18-98: Monopolar hook is commonly used in dissecting the peritoneum, creating the plane, dissecting the gallbladder from its bed. Bipolar hook is also available. It is biflanged.

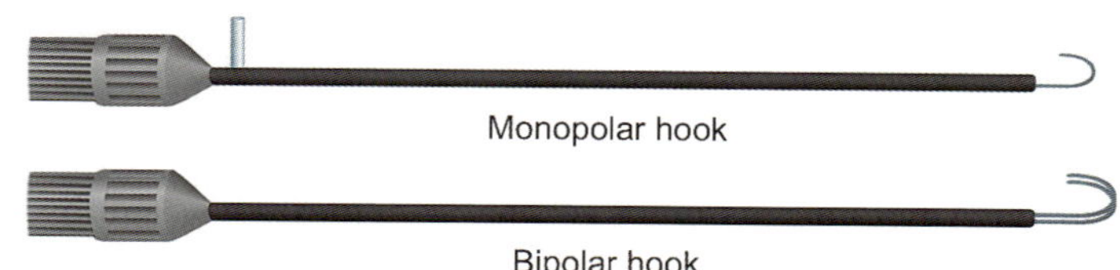

Fig. 18-99: Monopolar cautery is used for dissection as well as coagulation. Bipolar is mainly used for coagulation; but dissection is also possible.

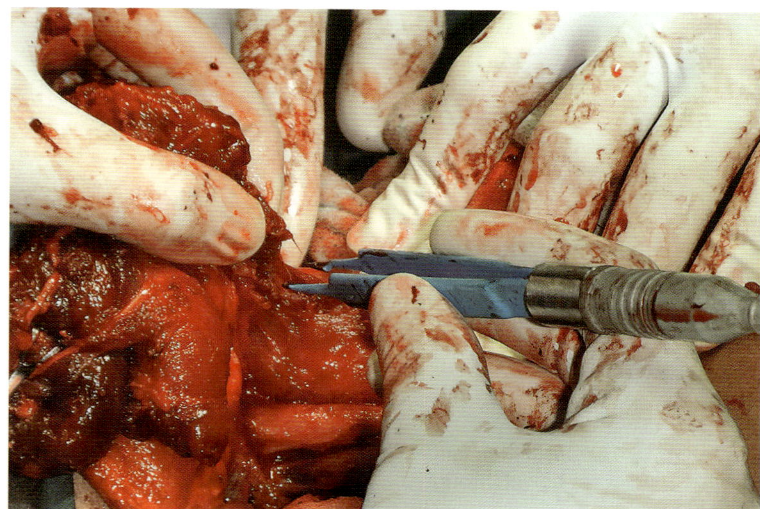

Fig. 18-100: Bipolar cautery in use. Here active and return electrodes are very close by.

Problems and Complications of Cautery

Injury to bowel due to heat, direct or lateral, may be unnoticed or not obvious which may later be able to cause full thickness ischaemic necrosis and perforation with peritonitis. This can occur often as late as 10 days also.

Direct injury of major vessels and vital structures through cautery can occur while instrument touches these structures and cautery gets on inadvertently by the assistant or the scrub nurse or the surgeon himself. Ideal is to disconnect the cable from the instrument when not in use.

Insulation failure can occur as the result of damage to the insulation and damaged part may come in direct contact with bowel. Prior checking the instrument for its insulation and function is essential always **(Fig. 18-102)**.

Direct coupling can occur when instrument which is connected to cautery (e.g. Maryland) touches instrument in the port which is not insulated like laparoscope which is passed through a plastic cannula as plastic port cannula prevents passage of current into return electrode. Current is directed into different tissues which get fulgurated as injury **(Fig. 18-103)**.

Capacitive coupling injury can occur if cautery is activated before the instrument tip makes contact with the tissue with a metal cannula and plastic sleeve which prevents return current to reach return electrode across body causing bowel injury. Capacitor is two conductors separated by an insulator. Electrosurgical device is one conductor; metal cannula is another conductor; with insulator sleeve.

If return electrode is inadequate (inadequate surface area in plating) then return current will pass through other surface metals causing severe surface burns.

If bowel injury occurs and suspected it is better to convert into open to identify proper site of heat injury which needs excision with adequate margin and proper re-suturing using interrupted silk or vicryl sutures.

Ultrasonic Dissector

The *Harmonic scalpel* is a high frequency ultrasonic transducer. The active titanium blade vibrates at 55,000 cycles per second. Electric power is applied into a device which contains piezoelectric crystal to create high frequency vibration waves. From this crystal vibration is carried to a rod to the instrument tip to move along its long axis. Induction of mechanical vibration at cellular level using high frequency waves more than 55,000 Hz leads into friction and shear injury leading to the needed effects. When applied to tissue it causes protein denaturation and coagulum formation at lower temperature (up to 80°C). It seals and cuts the tissues including vessels up to 2–5 mm. There is no risk of electric burn or lateral thermal injury. Charring is less here compared to electrocautery and so less smoke in comparison. Field is clean and bloodless.

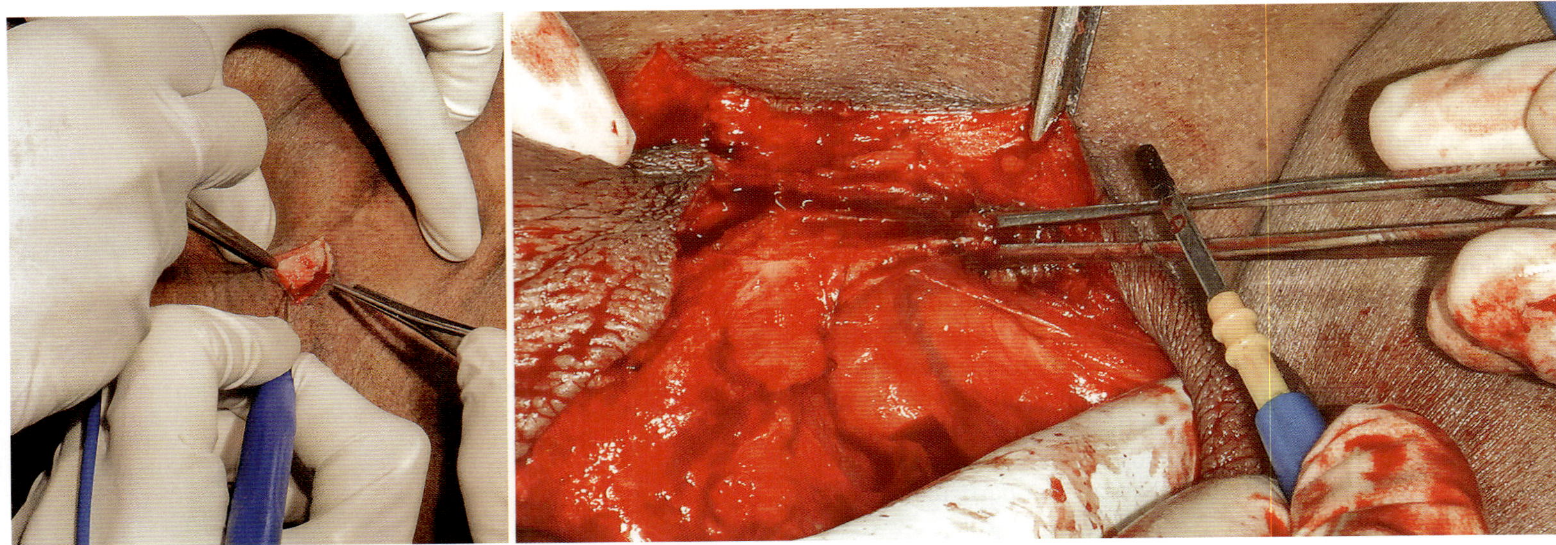

Fig. 18-101: Monopolar cautery used for haemostasis by coagulation current and for cutting by cutting current.

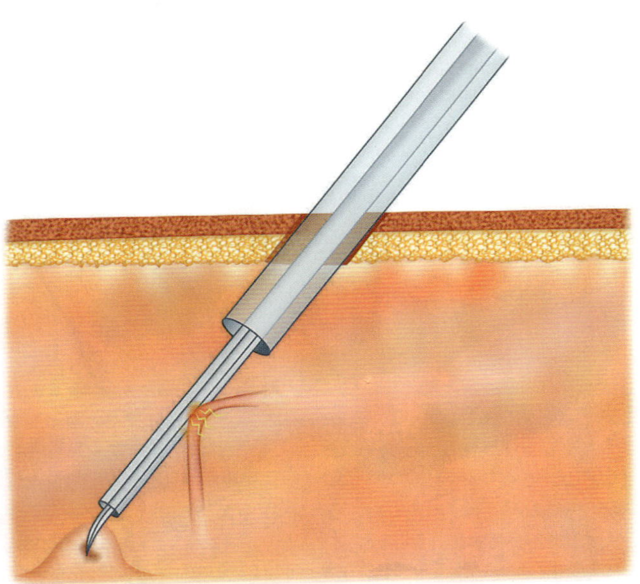

Fig. 18-102: Insulation failure causing direct diathermy injury to adjacent bowel through the 5 mm working instrument.

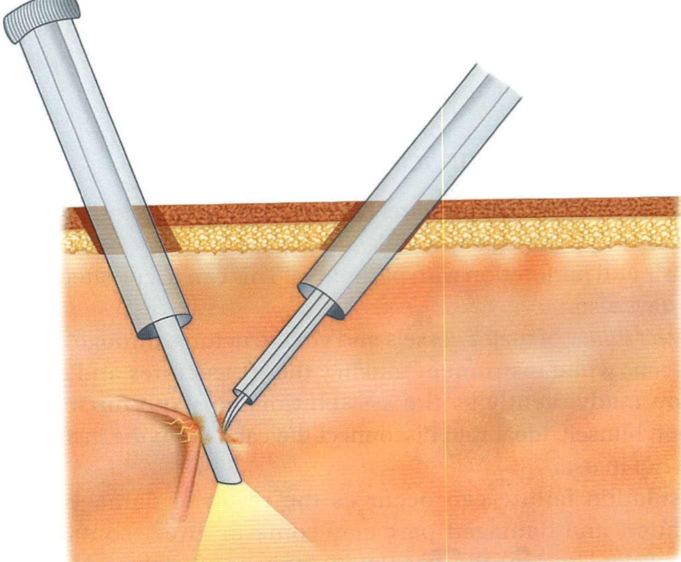

Fig. 18-103: Direct coupling.

Hand instruments are available in 10 mm and 5 mm size in harmonic scalpel. 5 mm harmonic probe is commonly used now even though initially only 10 mm probes were available. It can be used as a grasper, coagulator, dissector and cutting instrument so that exchange of many instruments is minimised leading to faster, cleaner and better surgery. Hand instrument contains an ultrasonically activated blade which can be rotated as sharp/round/flat edges. Non-activated pad opposes this active blade to hold the tissue to create friction and shearing. Power level setting is needed in the instrument to create appropriate action. Level 1—coagulation only; level 5—cutting only; median power of 2–3 is usually used; usually rounded blade is used. Device is very useful in many dissections like mesoappendix in appendicectomy, cystic artery and Calot's dissection in cholecystectomy. Prior using the instrument activation is essential each time **(Fig. 18-104)**.

Harmonic ace is a modified 5 mm harmonic probe with more transection speed and haemostasis and vessel sealing capacity with additional hand activating system. 5 mm blade is available as a hook, straight and curved electrodes. Versatile curved blade is commonly used. As compared to the other devices listed, the Harmonic Scalpel is FDA approved to seal vessels up to 5 mm.

Precaution: Harmonic scalpel is very safe instrument; but integrity of instrument should be touched at the active blade; its sheathing (Teflon pad) should be adequate. While operating tip should not touch other instruments or metallic parts as tip may blast by short circuiting.

Ligasure (Valleylab)

This bipolar electrosurgical device delivers high current, low voltage along with pressure from the jaws to tissues. It can seal vessels up to 7 mm in size. This differs from the high voltage, low current energy used in standard monopolar and bipolar cautery. The system monitors the energy expended while denaturing the collagen and

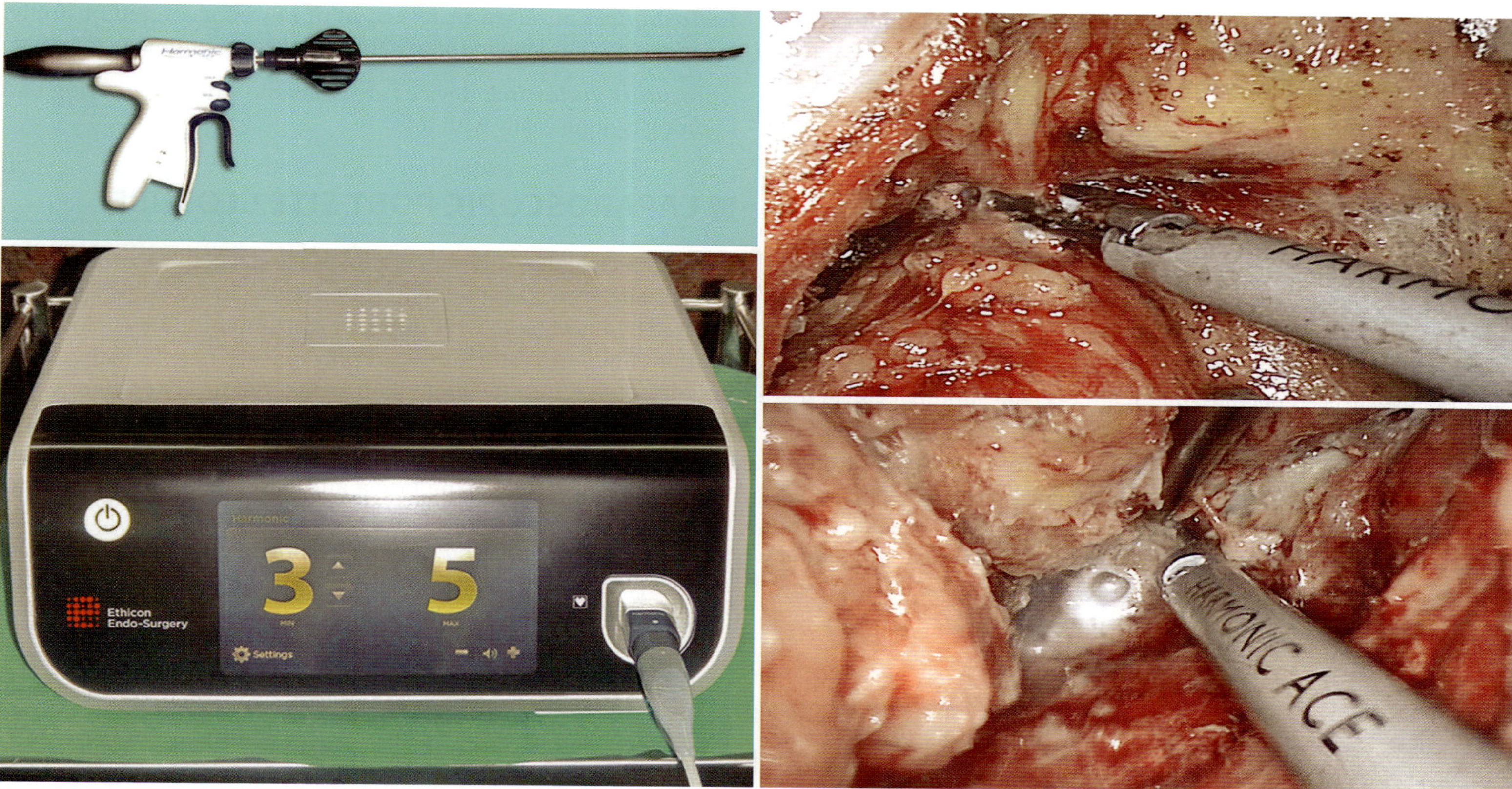

Fig. 18-104: Harmonic scalpel with its use.

elastin within the vessels walls. During the cooling phase of the cycle, cross-linking reoccurs creating a new seal. The instrument is available in 5 or 10 mm sizes. Tissue sensing technology in the Ligasure makes use of a computer algorithm to adjust the current and voltage based on real-time measures of tissue impedance. This results in a constant delivery of voltage over a broad range of tissue types. Grounding pad is not needed. Power comes from electrosurgical generator. Through hand set it reaches the blade. Sealing capacity is more here. It has got the highest burst pressure, low thermal spread, fast sealing time, and low smoke production. But smoke production is more than harmonic scalpel and instrument is not as fine as harmonic. Tissue is held with blades and is locked in handle. Foot switch is pressed to activate ligaseal. Generator gives an audible tone at the completion of cooling period. After that there is a blade in the jaw which moves to cut the tissue through a system in the handle. After that blades are unlocked. Lateral thermal spread is only up to 1.5 mm of adjacent tissues. Open seal instruments are also available for haemorrhoidectomy, thyroidectomy, open GI surgeries. It is useful to seal uterine, splenic, inferior mesenteric arteries **(Fig. 18-105)** safely.

Problems: It cannot be used for dissection; takes more time; after repeated use it becomes sticky, opening the jaw after sealing often becomes difficult and forcible opening results in tissue tear and bleeding.

LAPAROSCOPIC TISSUE APPROXIMATION

Laparoscopic suturing is discussed in Chapter 3. Other methods of tissue apposition are briefed here.

Laparoscopic suturing: Coaxial handled needle holder is better than piston handled for intracorporeal suturing and knotting.

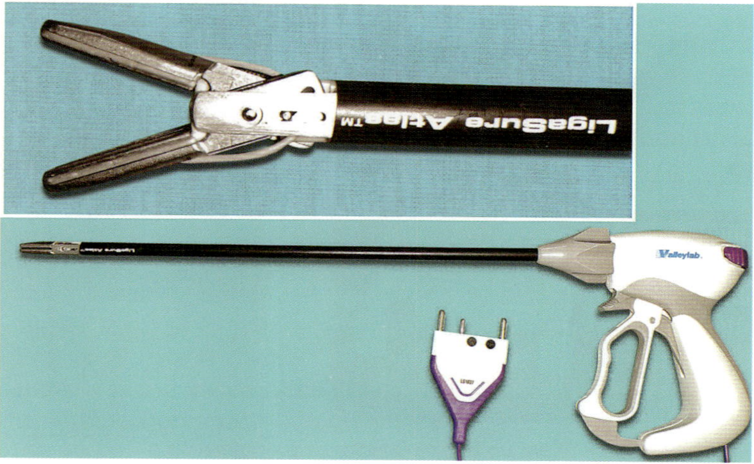

Fig. 18-105: Ligasure instrument.

Needle holder is held in dominant hand; supporting grasper (5 mm atraumatic, without ratchet) is held with non-dominant hand. Length of the suture material is 10 cm for first suture bite and knot with 2 cm for additional each needed suture. Lengthy suture material creates problem in manipulation inside the peritoneal cavity. Usually 2-zero vicryl is used. Needle often needs some bending (straightening) to allow it to pass through the reducer of 10 mm port; otherwise it can be pierced directly across the abdominal wall into the peritoneal cavity under direct vision. 3-zero vicryl is used to suture in pyeloplasty or in bile duct suturing. Triangulation and proper ergonomics are very important for proper endosuturing. Two instruments should meet at 60° angulation. Additional trocars should be placed to create triangulation to prevent sword fighting and crowding. 30° angled camera is better. Zoom in is done while taking bite; zoom out is done while knotting. 3D laparoscope may be much more useful.

Needle is passed into the peritoneal cavity through 10 mm port across reducer. Thread 1 cm away from the needle is held in a grasper or Maryland or needle holder which is already passed across the reducer; needle is pulled into the reducer sleeve; reducer is passed across the port into the peritoneal cavity; needle is released into the place under vision. Needle can be directly punctured separately across the abdominal wall under direct vision in thin individual and children. Needle is also can be passed across the 5 mm port wound after removing the 5 mm port temporarily through a 5 mm instrument needle holder or Maryland in which suture material of the needle is held 1 cm away from needle. Holding the needle at proper site in the needle holder, needle bite taking across tissue, putting a tight proper knot is an art in intracorporeal suturing. Learning curve, dedication and concentration is needed to this technique. Eye-hand coordination is important. Creation of C loop and passing the opposite instrument and pulling the end thread is initial technique to create first knot. Similarly further 2 knots are placed. Roeder's knot, extracorporeal knot creations are all other knotting techniques used.

Endostaplers are used in resection of bowel, gastrojejunostomy, anterior resection, stapling of vessels in splenectomy, nephrectomy, etc.

Autosuture endostitch devices are available wherein suturing and knotting is done easily with this.

LAPAROSCOPIC PORT SITE CLOSURE

Port site is closed by different methods. Fascial plane at any port site more than 5 mm size should be closed using 2-zero vicryl. Different methods are available with different instruments. Direct closure is also possible. Curved stout eyed port closure needle with a stout handle is often used wherein suture material is passed into its eye which is pierced across the both edges of the fascia and later tied. Fine long straight specialised port closure needle is also available which is pierced across the fascia and peritoneum into the cavity under laparoscopic vision; when its fine jaws are opened vicryl suture material which is passed across the port is grasped and pulled out; similarly it is repeated on other side and later knot is placed **(Fig. 18-106)**.

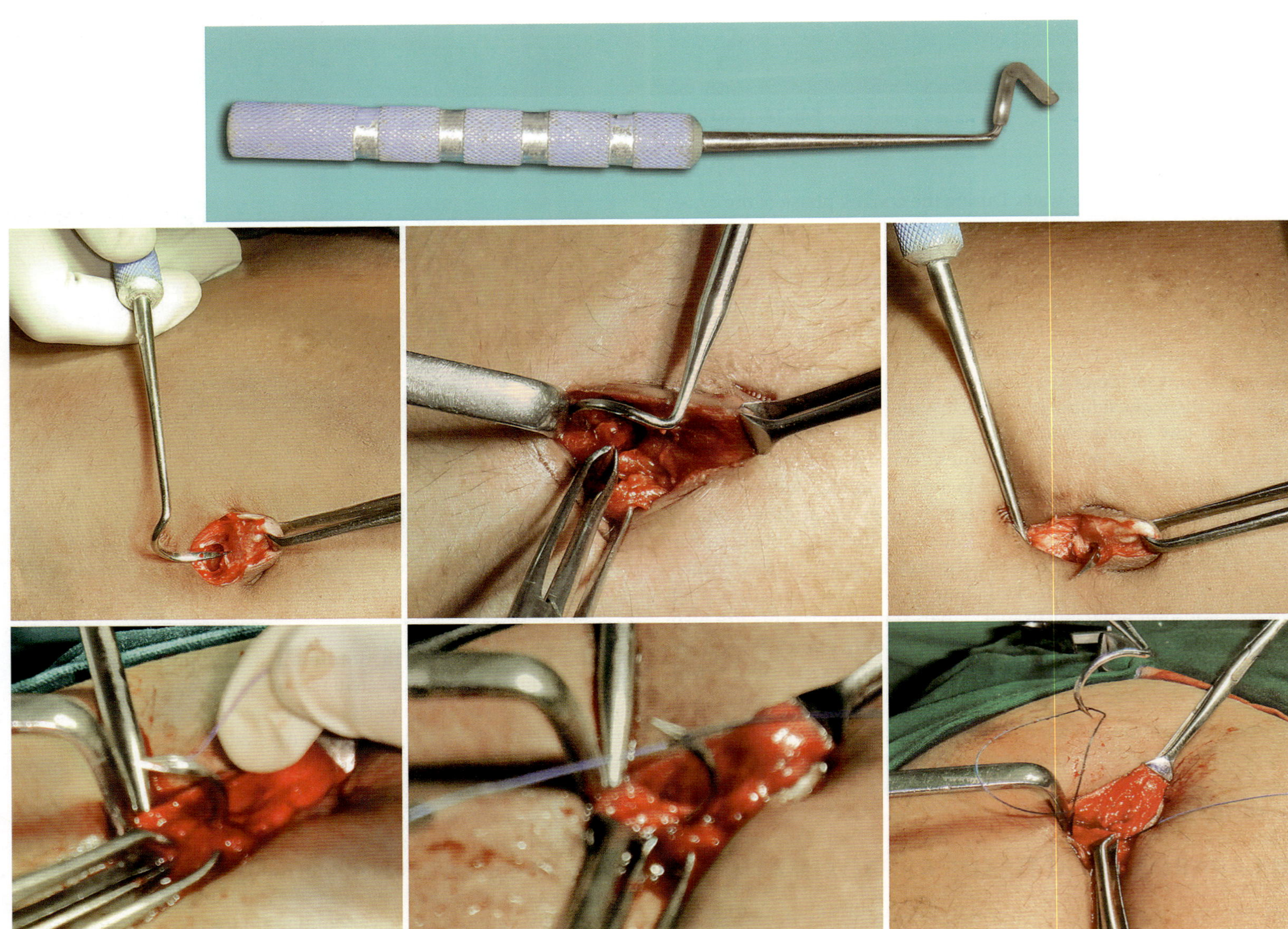

Fig. 18-106: One of the methods of port closure technique.

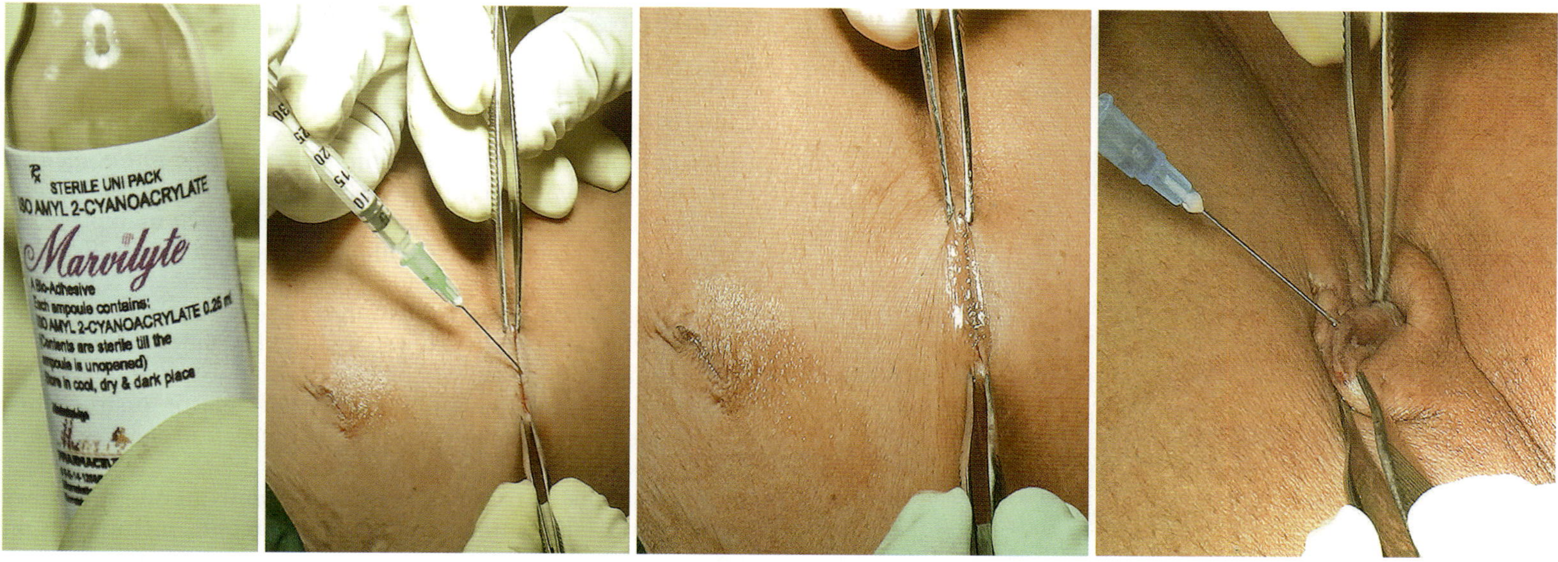

Fig. 18-107: Cyanocrylate glueing to close the skin.

Skin is sutured with absorbable subcuticular suture (monocryl) or clips or interrupted monofilament sutures or cyanocrylate glueing **(Fig. 18-107)**.

STERILISATION/DISINFECTION OF LAPAROSCOPIC INSTRUMENTS

Laparoscopic Instruments are complexly designed, delicate, has increase bioburden in crevices, and difficult to clean. They are used in complex laparoscopic procedures. It is difficult to clean, sterilise or maintain these instruments.

Sterilisation is a process that destroys all forms of microbial life (including spores) absolutely by physical/chemical methods; steam under pressure (autoclave), dry heat, ETO, gas plasma; liquid chemicals. Some disinfectants on prolonged exposure can destroy spores.

Disinfection is a process that destroys many or all pathogenic bacteria but not their spores; used on inanimate objects; use of liquid chemicals (disinfectants).

Splauding Classification of Objects and Level of Sterilisation

Critical	*Semicritical*	*Non-critical*
Entry or penetration into sterile tissue, cavity or bloodstream	Entry to mucous membrane or non-intact skin	Entry to intact skin Non-critical patient care Non-critical environmental surfaces
Surgical instruments, cardiac/urinary catheters, implant, USG probes	Laparoscopes, Endoscopes, respirator and anaesthesia equipment	Bed pans, blood pressure cuffs, furniture, bedside table, utensils
Sterility required	Objects to be free of all microorganisms but not spores	Objects to be clean

DISINFECTION

Disinfection may be:

High Level Disinfection (HLD)

At same concentration as chemical sterilants, but shorter exposure, the same disinfectant can kill only the microorganisms and ***not*** spores, e.g. glutaraldehyde, OPA, per acetic acid, hydrogen peroxide.

Intermediate Level Disinfection

Can kill mycobacteria, vegetative bacteria, most viruses, most fungi but ***not*** the spores, e.g. ethyl/isopropyl alcohol, sodium hypochlorite, iodophors, phenolic compounds.

Low Level Disinfection

Can kill most vegetative bacteria, some fungi, and some viruses within 10 minutes. Same as above and quaternary ammonium compounds.

For laparoscopic instruments high level disinfection may be sufficient. *Reasons are*—only a limited number of organisms (usually ≤10) are introduced into the peritoneal cavity during laparoscopy; minimal damage is done to inner abdominal structures with little devitalised tissue; peritoneal cavity tolerates small numbers of spore forming bacteria; these equipment are easier to clean and disinfect; natural bioburden on rigid lumen devices is low. There are no evidence exists that high-level disinfection instead of sterilisation increases the risk for infection.

But sterilisation is proposed by many. *Reasons are*—degree of tissue damage and bacterial contamination is greater; possibility of transmitting infection by spore-forming organisms; increased bioburden due to complex design; risk of bio film formation.

Choice whether sterilisation or disinfection is needed depends on—type of instrument material; intended use and function; instrument design; compatibility with various sterilisation processes.

Disinfectant/ sterilant	*Advantages*	*Disadvantages*
Glutaraldehyde	♦ Relatively inexpensive ♦ Excellent materials compatibility	♦ Respiratory irritation from vapour ♦ Pungent and irritating odour ♦ Relatively slow mycobactericidal activity ♦ Coagulates blood and fixes tissue to surfaces ♦ Allergic contact dermatitis ♦ Glutaraldehyde vapour monitoring
Ortho-phthalaldehyde (OPA)—0.55%	♦ Fast acting high-level disinfectant ♦ No activation or mixing is required ♦ Odour not significant ♦ Excellent materials compatibility claimed ♦ Good mycobactericidal activity ♦ 20 minutes soak time at room temperature for reprocessing	♦ Stains skin, mucous membranes, clothing, and environmental surfaces ♦ Repeated exposure may result in hypersensitivity in some patients with bladder cancer ♦ More expensive than glutaraldehyde ♦ Eye irritation with contact ♦ Slow sporicidal activity
Per acetic acid (Per oxygen compounds)	♦ Rapid sterilisation cycle time (30–45 minutes) ♦ Low temperature (50–55°C) liquid immersion sterilisation ♦ Environmental friendly by-products ♦ It is bactericidal, fungicidal, virucidal, sporicidal and tuberculocidal ♦ It is highly corrosive and corrosion inhibitor should be used in the formulation	♦ Potential material incompatibility (e.g. aluminium anodised coating becomes dull) ♦ Used for immersible instruments only ♦ Serious eye and skin damage (concentrated solution) with contact ♦ Point-of-use system, no sterile storage
Hydrogen peroxide	♦ No activation required ♦ Removal of organic matter and organisms ♦ No disposal issues ♦ No odour or irritation issues ♦ Does not coagulate blood or fix tissues to surfaces ♦ Inactivates *Cryptosporidium*	♦ Material compatibility concerns (brass, zinc, copper, and nickel/silver plating) both cosmetic and functional ♦ Serious eye damage with contact
Superoxide saline	♦ It is hypochlorous acid derived from salt through electrolysis. It is sporicidal, mycobactericidal until there is no soiling	

Note:

- *CDC Guidelines States:* Laparoscopes, arthroscopes, and other scopes that enter normally sterile tissue should be sterilised before each use; if this is not feasible, they should receive at least high-level disinfection. Objective should be free of microorganisms.

Technique of Achieving Sterilisation/ Disinfection

Cleaning

Cleaning of instruments is the main and important initial method of all disinfection or sterilisation. Cleaning is removal of visible soil—organic/inorganic by manual or mechanical method using soap/detergents/enzymatic solutions; is essential presterilisation/ predisinfection procedure.

Cleaning should begin during surgery itself or immediately after finishing the surgery. Instruments should never be allowed to dry; instrument is rinsed with sterile distilled water on the sterile field itself especially channel and lumen-bearing instruments. It facilitates removal of blood from joints, hinges and crevices. *Saline should not be used.*

After use, the instruments are placed gently in a basin; heavy instruments at the bottom; delicate and fibreoptic instruments on top or preferably in another container. Coils to be loosely wound. Sharp end instruments should be kept separately so that personnel handling them are not injured.

Cleaning process is done in a methodical way: Pre-cleaning → Soaking in enzymatic detergent → Washing → Rinsing → Drying.

Precleaning is done immediately after the procedure.
The instrument is wiped with a disposable cloth dampened in an enzymatic detergent solution. Enzymatic detergent solution is aspirated through the suction/biopsy channels with alternate suctioning of fluid and air which prevents drying of organic and inorganic debris on lumen surfaces and assists in the removal of large numbers of micro-organisms and also dislodges debris from internal lumens. Air/water channels are purged. Removable components are detached. All valves/buttons/caps are removed and soaked in enzymatic detergent solution. Instruments are transported to the cleaning area in a container (without water).

Manual cleaning: It is done using brush and detergent. It is used for fragile instruments, mechanical cleaners are not available. But instruments may get degraded/blunt; it is time consuming and causes friction and fluidics. Nylon brushes of different types and sizes are used. Ports, accessories should be cleaned with brush **(Fig. 18-108)**.

Mechanical cleaning: It is done by—ultrasonic cleaning, washer decontaminator, washer-steriliser. **Ultrasonic cleaner is a mechanical cleaning device** highly efficient on surfaces with crevices, locks, serrations but should be used only after the debris is removed. Solution should be changed frequently as endotoxin contamination of solution can occur. It is unsuitable for plastic as ultrasound waves are absorbed by plastic. It may produce infective aerosols. Instruments of dissimilar metals should not be used together and instruments should not be overloaded.

Laparoscopic instruments require both manual and mechanical cleaning **(Figs. 18-109A to C)**.

Soaking in Enzymatic Detergent

Enzymatic detergents are good to clean all debris. Single or multi-enzymes can be used. Formation of foam, pH of the detergents are deciding factors. Thorough washing is essential. Fast-acting enzymatic cleaning agent (ENZOL) which has mild pH and low foaming feature (contains proteolytic enzymes) can be used in automated equipment: endoscope reprocessors, ultrasonic cleaners, and washer-sterilisers/decontaminators. Minimum 1 minute soak time is sufficient. One-step process reduces the need for mechanical cleaning which may reduce exposure to contaminated equipment. Mild pH reduces likelihood of corrosion of equipment.

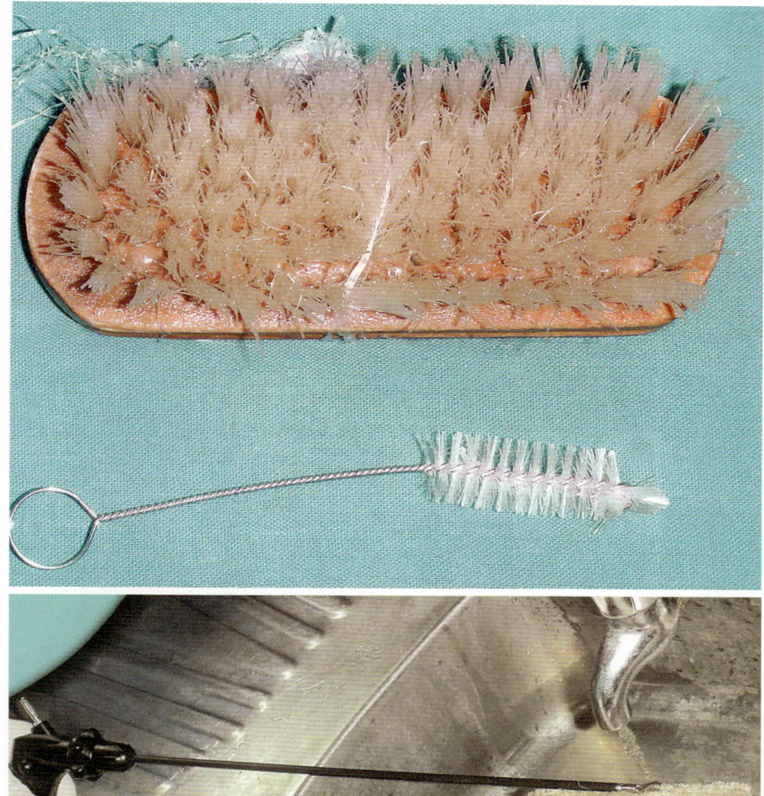

Fig. 18-108: Cleaning with brush is very important part in precleaning process.

Water Rinse

Outer surfaces of the instrument and all removable parts are rinsed with water; all channels are flushed thoroughly with water (water jet); clean running water should be used to remove all traces of detergent prior to disinfection and limit cross infection.

Drying

External/outer surfaces of the instrument is dried with a soft, lint-free disposable cloth. All internal channels are purged with air to remove rinsing water. Removing water from all channels and the exterior of the instrument prevents dilution of the biocide used for disinfection. This process can be completed using a syringe or compressed air.

Decontamination

It is removal of all visible soil, tissue, blood and foreign particle causing reduction of bioburden (microbial load and endotoxins); protects instruments against corrosion; allows safe movement of equipment and materials. It results in reduction in pathogenic bacteria from objects so as to make it safe to handle, use or discard. Cleaning reduces bioburden very significantly.

High Level Disinfection (HLD)

Disinfection clears or reduces the number of microorganisms in the instruments but bacterial spores are not completely killed even though it reduces spore numbers. Adequacy of disinfection depends on number of microorganisms in the instrument;

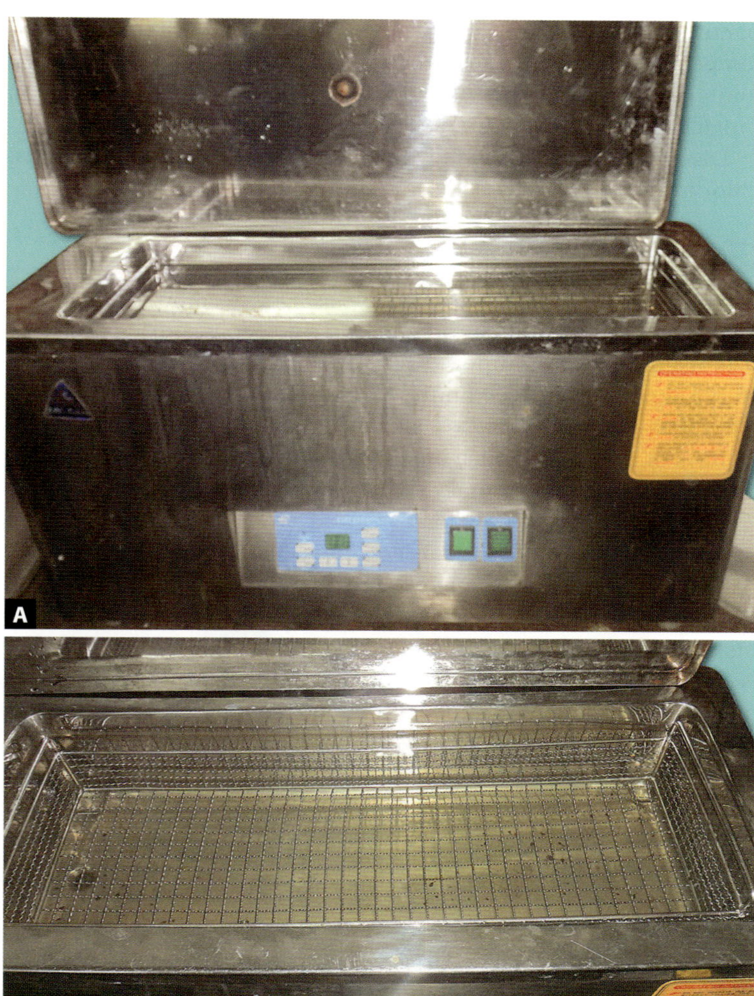

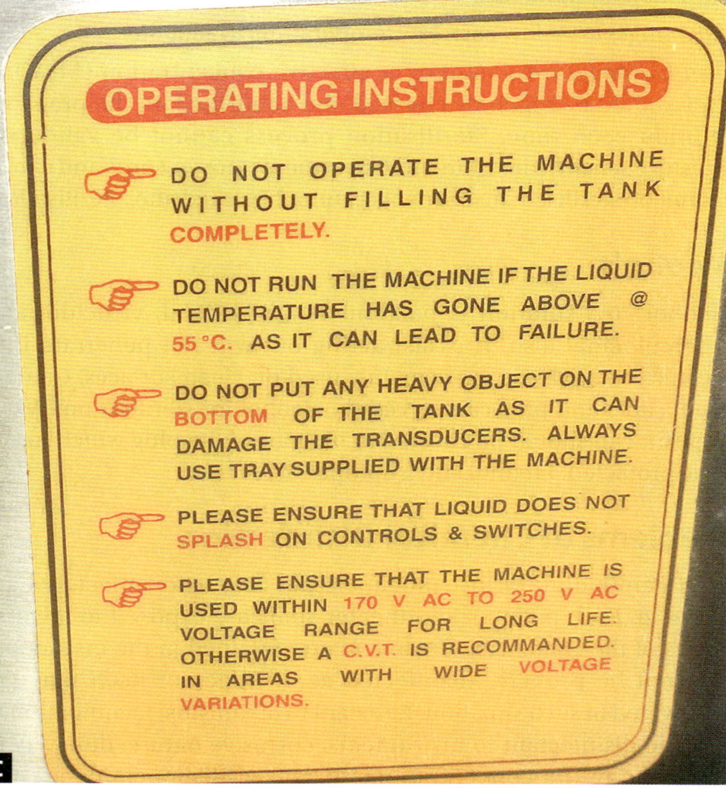

Figs. 18-109A to C: Ultrasonic cleaning device.

bactericidal property of the disinfectant; concentration, pH and temperature at the site; type and design of the instrument (hinges/joints). HLD reduces the bioburden significantly with bactericidal, fungicidal, virucidal and partly sporicidal features.

Disinfectants may be aldehydes; alcohols; per oxide compounds; chlorine dioxide; super-oxidised saline solutions.

Glutaraldehyde

It is non-corrosive aldehyde available as 2.4% alkaline solution. It is bactericidal, fungicidal, virucidal and only slow sporicidal agent. It is used at room temperature. HLD occurs in 45 minutes and sterilisation occurs in 10 hours. It has got 14 days maximum reuse life (Cidex). *Cidex plus* is 3.4% alkaline glutaraldehyde which has got 28 days of maximum reuse life. Entire activator (a rust inhibitor) is added to the solution to make colour of the solution green. Activated solution can be used only for 14 days. Date of activation and date of expiration should be recorded. After cleaning, with detergent, rinsing and drying, instrument is dipped in prepared glutaraldehyde solution; time is 20 minutes for high level disinfection (HLD). Hollow instruments should be dismantled and immersed. Immersion time is 10 hours for sterilisation with container being properly covered to prevent evaporation. Disinfectant should touch and soak all parts of the instrument properly. Instruments should never be placed on the top of the other. After specified time immersed instrument is removed by wearing sterile gloves and rinsed with sterile water for three times and kept in the case table. Water which is boiled for 20 minutes and filtered and cooled can also be used instead of sterile water. Final rinsing can be done using 60–90% ethyl or isopropyl alcohol **(Fig. 18-110).**

Hazards: It can cause on inhalation cough, headache, wheezing and nausea. It can cause skin redness, redness and pain in eyes. Prevention is—proper ventilation, fresh air, wearing gloves and goggles while working on glutaraldehyde. Room should have vapour extraction equipment.

Advantages are—low cost; low temperature; availability.

Disadvantages are—minimum effective concentration (MEC) of 1.5% should be regularly checked and confirmed on the prepared solution each time. Sterilisation process cannot be validated. Moisture sensitive instruments like cameras, power cords and cables cannot be sterilised. Instruments cannot be stored after sterilisation.

Alcohols

Alcohol 70% solution is bactericidal, fungicidal, virucidal and tuberculocidal also. It is fast acting but will not penetrate into organic materials and so is mainly used on clean surfaces. Camera head, cable and plug can be kept in alcohol for sterilisation. Water resistant cap should be covered to the part of the plug which needs to be protected. Ethanol and isopropanol are used.

Problems of Chemical Disinfection

Recontamination of instruments is possible as disinfectants are reusable. Both patients and theater staffs are exposed to adverse effects of the chemicals. Organic matter retained in the instrument may not be properly disinfected as disinfectant itself may get inactivated in such situation. Resistant to organisms; incompatibility of some disinfectant to instruments, corrosive nature; difficulty in determining the concentrations in reused disinfectants are the further problems.

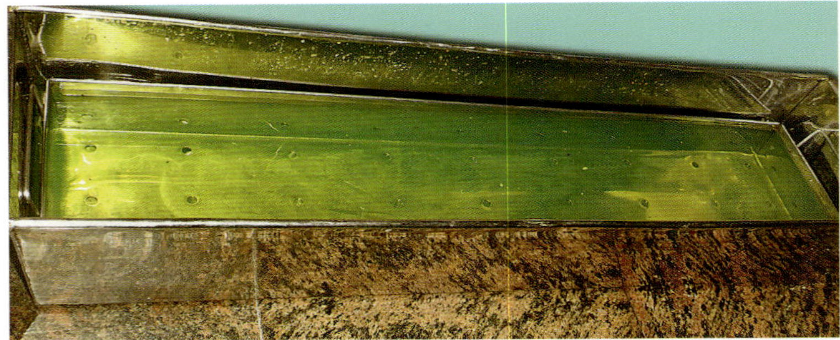

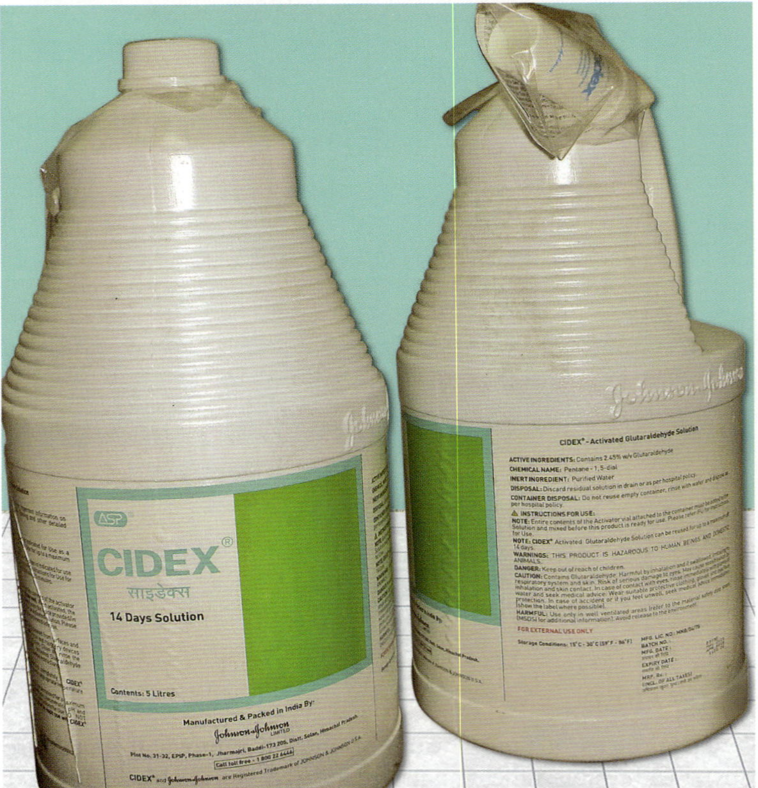

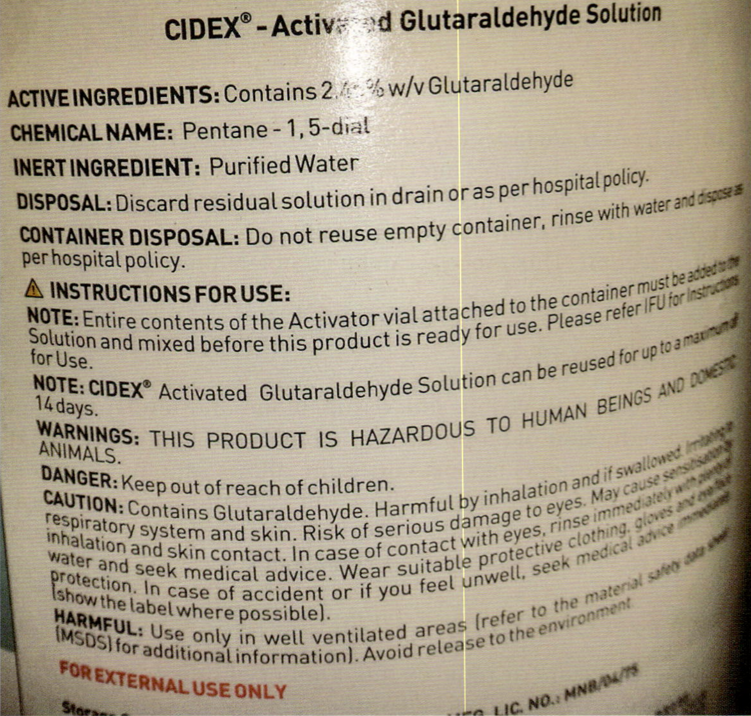

Fig. 18-110: 2.45% glutaraldehyde w/v contains pentane—1, 5 dial. Glutaraldehyde tray having activated solution.

Disinfection of Endoscopic Instruments

High level disinfection is commonly used in endoscopes/laparoscopes. Immediately after use telescopes, light source, cable, tubes are cleaned and wiped gently using 90% ethyl or isopropyl alcohol soaked cloth. Alcohol kills HIV, HBsAg viruses. All equipment are dismantled completely which are placed in a basin of water with non-abrasive soap. Instruments are washed gently using cotton cloth. Channels of the instruments are cleaned using specified brushes with circular movements to clear all organic materials. All instruments and their parts are rinsed with running water properly. Soap should be cleared completely while rinsing with water; brush may be useful while final rinsing with water to clear the retained soap. Instruments are dried with dry cloth or air dry. While cleaning lenses, it should not be touched with fingers; they are cleaned after removing the plastic covers/eyepieces using acetone or 90% alcohol; lenses should be cleaned weekly even if not in use.

Autoclave and boiling the laparoscopes is not advisable. During autoclave each instrument should be wrapped separately with clothing and kept, otherwise touching of each instrument with one another will cause damage to instruments or their insulation. Chemical sterilisation is the best. ETO, gas plasma sterilisation can also be done. After disinfection rinsing with sterile water or cooled boiled water 3 times is essential otherwise instrument may get stuck due to retained chemical. While handling the instruments sterile gloves should be used not forceps which may damage the laparoscope. Only one telescope should be held at one time; holding in groups should be avoided. *Savlon should not be used* as it will cause clouding and it will not cause HLD.

Storage of Laparoscopic Instruments

Instruments are cleaned; washed; decontaminated; dried and stored in a padded container in a cool dry place. When needed for use, stored instruments should be cleaned, sterilised or disinfected (HLD) then used.

STERILISATION

Steam Sterilisation

It kills by denaturation and coagulation of protein in the cells. Autoclave is sterilisation using steam under pressure. It is done with either 135°C for 5 minutes or 121°C for 15 minutes with 15 pounds pressure. There are flash and vacuum types. All instruments that are insulated, all silicone tubing, all cables and cords should be wrapped in double lined lining (double cloth wrapped).

Advantages: It is economical, fast, age old practice for sterilisation of linen and metallic instruments, very effective, and is well monitored. Non-plastic materials, instruments which will not lose their temper are autoclaved. It is ideal for reusable instruments.

Disadvantages: Sharp instruments may get blunt by autoclaving. Heat and moisture sensitive instruments (glass syringes) cannot be sterilised. Rigid endoscopes can be sterilised by porous loaded autoclaves. Instruments with narrow lumen should be sterilised using porous loaded autoclave. Endoscopes/telescopes sterilised by autoclave should not be cooled rapidly as it may cause stress damage to the instruments. It cannot be used for heat sensitive instruments and wet surfaces **(Fig. 18-111)**.

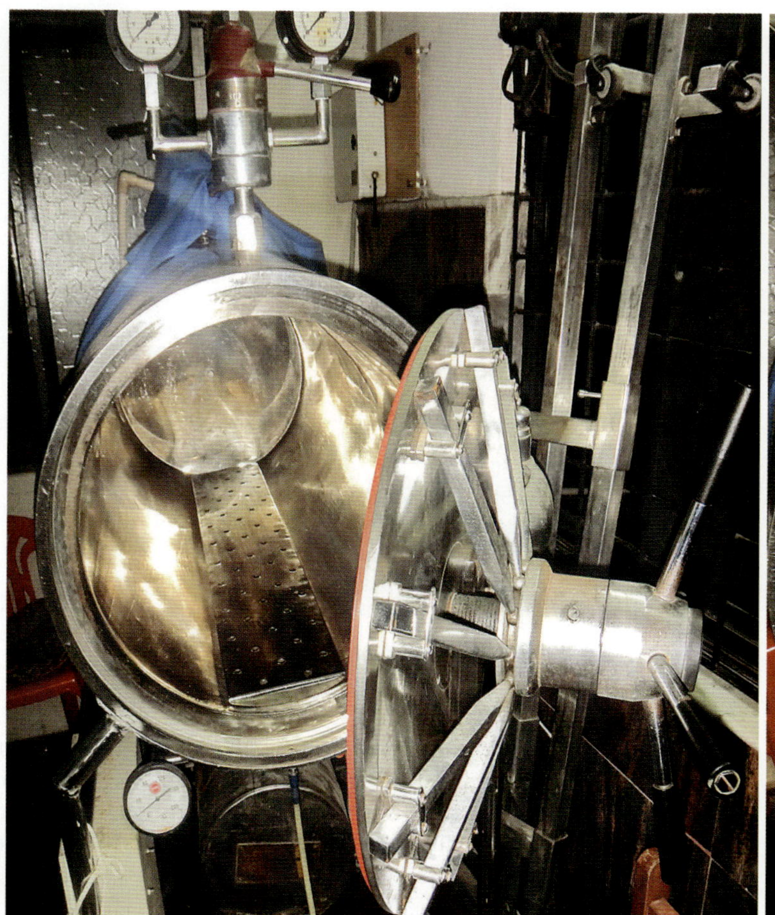
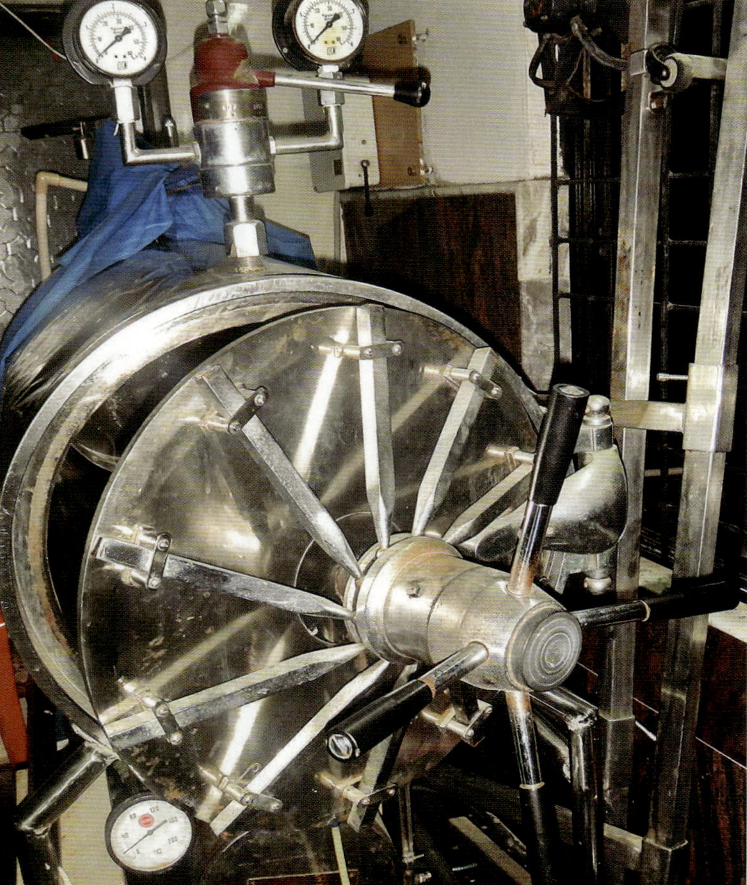

Fig. 18-111: Autoclave for sterilisation.

Ethylene Oxide Sterilisation (EO/ETO)

It kills by alkylation—interfering with the metabolism and reproductive process of cells. Sterilisation temperature is 37–55°C; sterilisation time 3–5 hours; aeration time 12–16 hours **(Fig. 18-112)**.

Technique: Initial chamber evacuation, humidification and ethylene oxide charging phase → dwell sterilisation phase → chamber evacuation phase with aeration. It is commonly sterilised at 54.4°C for 3 hours. Heat sensitised instruments are sterilised at much lower temperature of 37.8°C for 5 hours. After sterilisation, trapped or absorbed gas is removed by aeration using aeration chamber in the set. Aeration is done by continuous flow of warm air at 50–60°C for 12 hours. Personnel should take utmost care to avoid exposure toxicity.

Advantages: It is low temperature sterilisation, can sterilise all kinds of instruments. It does not corrode instruments. It is suitable for all disposable instruments, insulated hand instruments and tubes used for gas, suction and irrigation. Cold or warm ETO is possible. It is material compatible, especially optics.

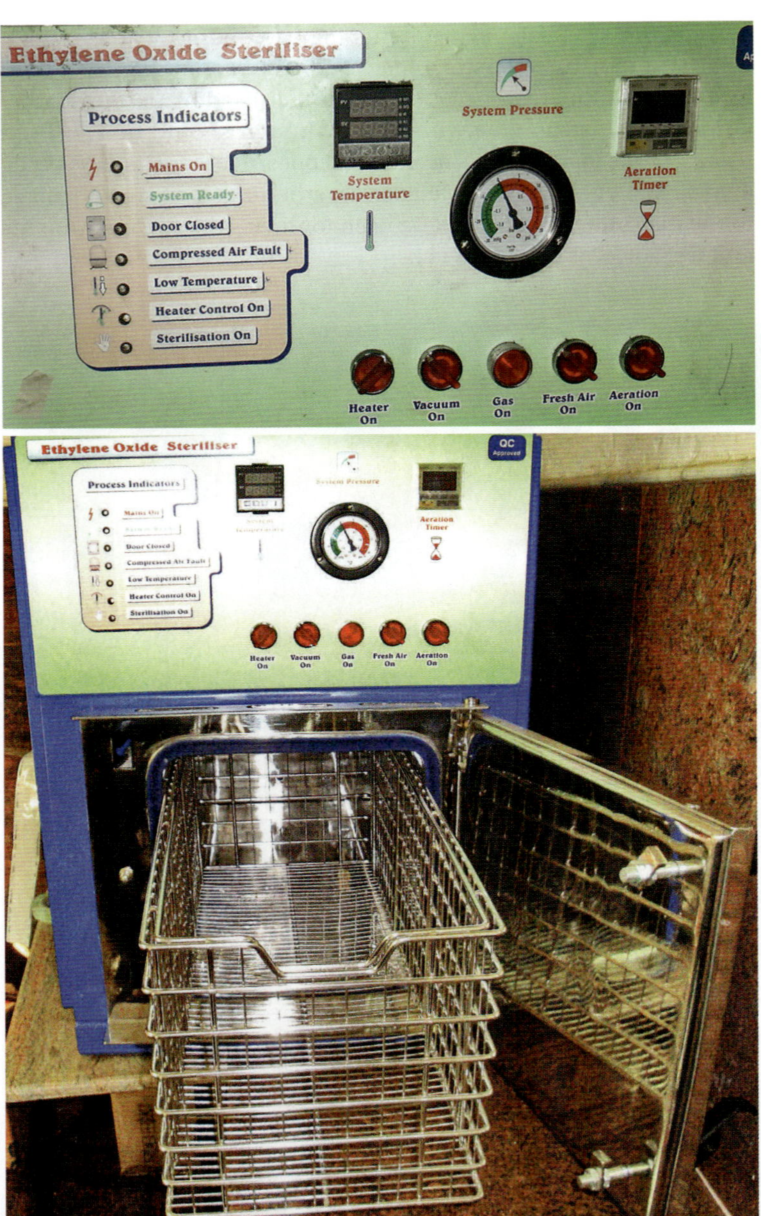

Fig. 18-112: Ethylene oxide sterilisation device.

Disadvantages: It needs aeration and is toxic and carcinogen. Prolonged aeration periods impact instrument availability at right time for surgeries. It is costly. It causes exposure of theatre staff to toxic ethylene oxide gas. Presence of water droplets on the instruments during ethylene oxide sterilisation would form toxic chemical called ethylene glycol. Set is not mobile.

Hazards: Inhalation of ethylene oxide vapour (1000 ppm exposure) can cause pulmonary oedema and respiratory distress; damage to eyes (burns, conjunctivitis, cataract); headache, recurrent vomiting; muscle weakness; neurological manifestations (rare). Direct contact to skin can also cause similar effects by absorption but slowly. It also can cause skin irritations, redness, frostbite like burns (if contaminated shoes or gloves are used), and dermatitis.

Gas Plasma Sterilisation

It is killing of microorganisms using highly active gas ions and free radicals. It uses hydrogen peroxide and plasma which is generated by radiofrequency/ MW (Vapour phase hydrogen peroxide/VHP). It causes generation of free radicals; uses low temperature; by products are safe; aeration is not necessary; short sterilisation cycle even though vary depends on H_2O_2 concentration; good material compatibility; ready to use/store always; requires only an electrical hook up **(Fig. 18-113)**.

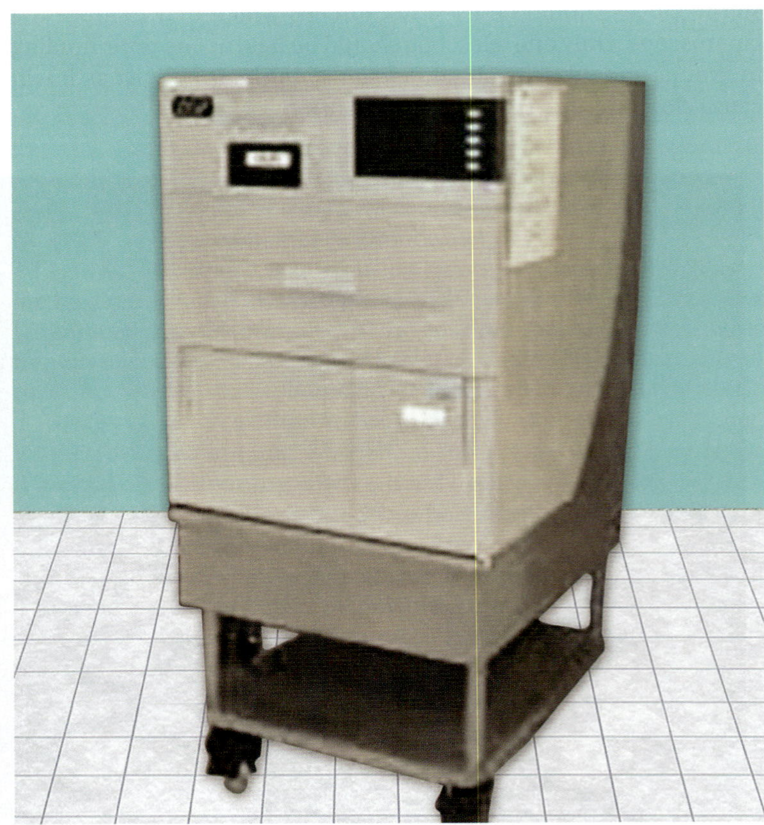

Fig. 18-113: Gas plasma sterilisation device.

Advantages: It is economical; can sterilise all kinds of instruments including the heat and moisture sensitive instruments; it is fast and helps in inventory reduction; it is safe for environment, healthcare workers and patients. It does not require monitoring. It is mobile, simple for installation.

Disadvantages: It cannot sterilise cellulose materials like linen, wood, powders and liquids.

19

CHAPTER

Surgeries in Hernia

Surgical Anatomy of Inguinal Canal

Superficial inguinal ring is a triangular opening in the external oblique aponeurosis and is 1.25 cm above the pubic tubercle. The ring is bound by a superomedial and inferolateral crus. Normally the ring does not admit the tip of little finger.

Deep inguinal ring is a U-shaped (or *Lambda* shaped) condensation of the transversalis fascia, lies 1.25 cm above the inguinal ligament midway between the symphysis pubis and the anterior superior iliac spine (mid-inguinal point).

Inguinal canal: In infants both superficial and deep rings are superimposed without any obliquity of the inguinal canal. In adults it is 3.75 cm long, directed downwards and medially from the deep to superficial ring.

In males inguinal canal transmits the spermatic cord, ilioinguinal nerve (outside the cord within the inguinal canal) and genital branch of the genitofemoral nerve (within the cord). Cord is covered by cremaster muscle which is a continuation of internal oblique muscle, internal spermatic fascia which is a continuation of transversalis fascia. Cord contains testicular artery, artery of vas (a branch of superior vesical artery which is derived from the anterior division of internal iliac artery), cremasteric artery, pampiniform plexus of veins, genital branch of genitofemoral nerve, sympathetic plexus and lymphatics. In females, inguinal canal contains round ligament, indistinct sparse cremaster, cremasteric vessels, ilioinguinal nerve, and genital branch of genitofemoral nerve. Inguinal canal in female is called as *canal of Nuck*. Round ligament (in females) is much more intimately adherent to peritoneum than spermatic cord (in males) **(Figs. 19-1 and 19-2)**.

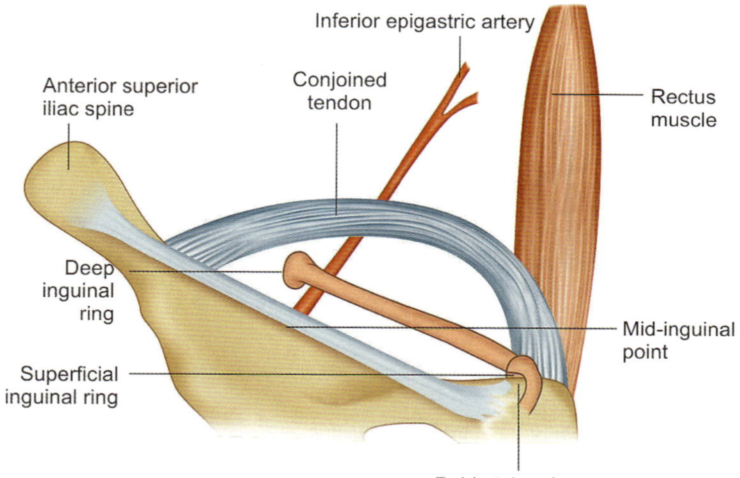

Fig. 19-1: Surgical anatomy of inguinal canal.

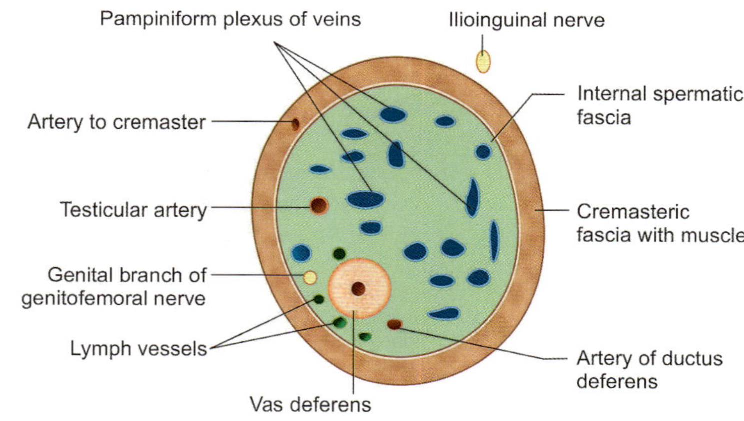

Fig. 19-2: Contents of spermatic cord.

Boundaries of Inguinal Canal

In front: External oblique aponeurosis and conjoined muscle laterally.

Behind: Inferior epigastric artery, fascia transversalis and conjoined tendon medially.

Above: Conjoined muscle (arched fibres of internal oblique).

Below: Inguinal ligament (*Poupart's*) and lacunar ligament (*Gimbernat*).

External ring is a triangular opening in the external oblique aponeurosis lying 1.25 cm above the pubic tubercle. Its superomedial crus is formed by external oblique aponeurosis and inferolateral crus by inguinal ligament.

Internal ring is a normal opening in the transversalis fascia and transverses aponeurosis which is U shaped or lambda (λ) shaped; it is 1.25 cm above the mid inguinal point (between anterior superior iliac spine to pubic symphysis).

An indirect inguinal hernia (hernia though deep ring) travels down the canal on the lateral and anterior aspect of the spermatic cord; whereas the direct hernia pops out directly forward through the posterior wall of the inguinal canal. Neck of the indirect sac is lateral to inferior epigastric vessels but direct sac emerges medial to the inferior epigastric vessels with a wide neck. Saddle-bag or pantaloon hernial sac has got both medial and lateral component. Inguinal hernia is above and medial to the pubic tubercle. Femoral hernia is below and lateral to pubic tubercle **(Figs. 19-3 and 19-4)**.

Direct hernia occurs through *Hesselbach's* (1814) triangle which is bound by inferior epigastric artery laterally, lateral border of rectus muscle medially, inguinal ligament below. It is divided into medial and lateral halves by obliterated umbilical artery (medial umbilical ligament). So direct hernia is classified as *medial or lateral depending on which part of the Hesselbach's triangle, it is arising from.* Lateral umbilical ligament is formed by inferior epigastric arteries. Medial type actually is called as *external supravesical hernia* and this fossa is called as *external supravesical fossa* **(Fig. 19-5)**.

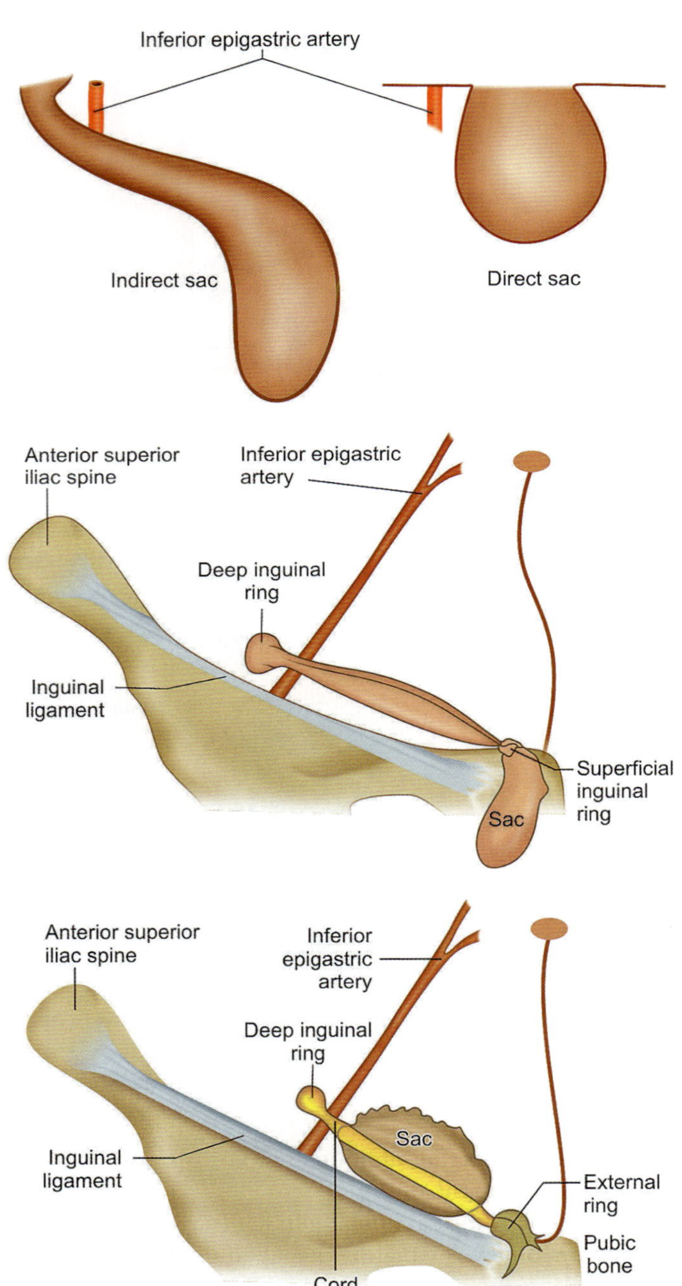

Fig. 19-3: Surgical anatomy of direct and indirect inguinal hernia sac.

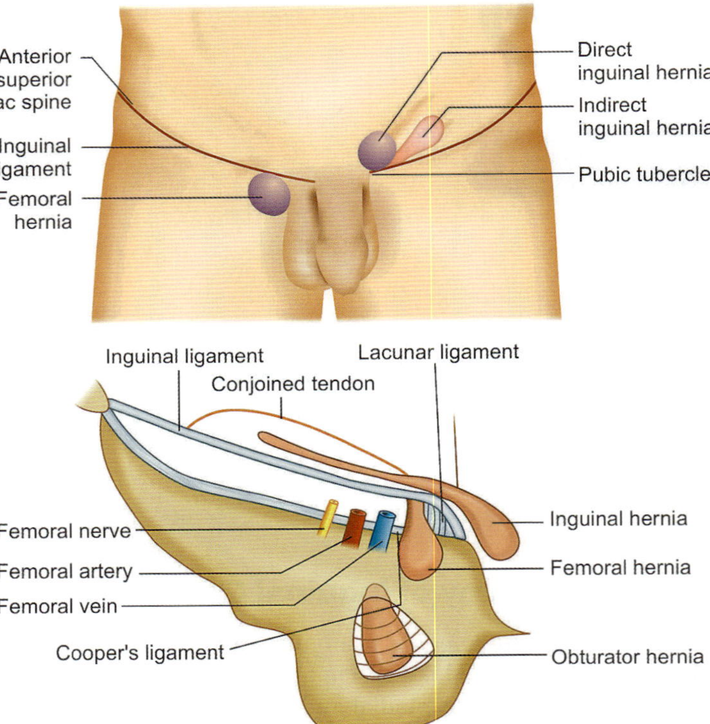

Fig. 19-4: Anatomical relations and locations of the inguinal, femoral and obturator hernias.

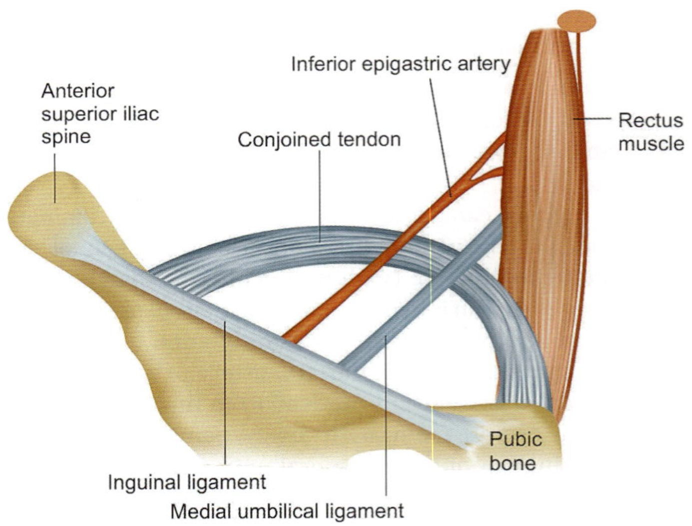

Fig. 19-5: Surgical anatomy of Hesselbach's triangle.

Inguinal Defense Mechanisms

Obliquity of inguinal canal creates flap valve mechanism by approximating anterior and posterior walls of the canal. Cooper described external oblique aponeurosis as outer barrier of the inguinal canal causing step down effect for the spermatic cord.

Shutter mechanism of internal oblique forms anterior, roof and posterior wall of the inguinal canal. Roof apposes to floor like a shutter.

External ring is *guarded* by conjoined tendon behind and reflected part of inguinal ligament in front. Internal ring is *guarded* by fleshy internal oblique. Contraction of external oblique aponeurosis causes *pinch cock/slit valve* effect by approximation of two crura of external ring.

Cremaster muscle on contraction helps cord to plug the external ring—*ball valve mechanism.*

Hormones also play a role to maintain inguinal muscles.

Anatomy of Abdominal Wall

Anterior Abdominal Wall

The anterior abdominal wall is a musculofascial dynamic structure which maintains intra-abdominal pressure for various physiological functions. It has got three paired flat muscles, two recti abdominis muscles and linea alba in midline. These are anteriorly related to skin, subcutaneous tissue and superficial fascia; posteriorly related to transversalis fascia and peritoneum. *External oblique fascia* (external layer of the fascia of external oblique muscle is also called as *innominate fascia of Gallaudet*) is thin fascial covering of external oblique muscle and fascia which forms intercrural fibers of the superficial inguinal ring; and it extends below into the scrotum as external spermatic fascia.

External oblique muscle arises from middle of body of lower eight ribs running below, front and medially inserting into xiphoid process, linea alba, pubic symphysis, pubic crest, pectineal line of pubis and anterior 2/3rd of outer lip of the iliac crest. It is supplied by lower six thoracic nerves. Lower free border of the external oblique aponeurosis forms inguinal ligament. Triangular opening in its aponeurosis above the pubic crest is called as superficial inguinal ring **(Fig. 19-6)**.

Internal oblique muscle arises from lateral 2/3rd of inguinal ligament, anterior 2/3rd of intermediate part of iliac crest, thoracolumbar fascia; runs upwards, forwards and medially to insert into lower four ribs and cartilages, xiphoid process, pubic crest, pectineal line of pubis. It is supplied by lower six thoracic nerves, 1st lumbar nerve. Aponeurosis below the level of umbilicus remains as a single layer forming the anterior rectus sheath and linea alba. Above aponeurosis splits into anterior lamina which passes medially in front of rectus abdominis and posterior lamina which passes behind rectus abdominis which ends below midway between umbilicus and pubic symphysis as linea *semicircularis of Douglas* (arcuate line). *Semilunar line of Spieghel* lies in lateral border of the rectus sheath from pubic tubercle to the tip of the costal cartilage of 9th rib **(Fig. 19-7)**.

Transverse abdominis muscle originates from lateral 1/3rd of inguinal ligament, anterior 2/3rd of inner lip of iliac crest, thoracolumbar fascia, lower six cartilages with fibres running horizontally forwards inserting into an aponeurosis extending from xiphoid process, linea alba, pubic crest, pectineal line of pubis. Lowest fibres fuse with lowest fibres of internal oblique to form conjoined/conjoint tendon. It is supplied by lower six thoracic and first lumbar nerves. Neurovascular plane of abdomen lies between internal oblique and transverse abdominis muscles **(Fig. 19-8)**.

Rectus abdominis muscle arises from lateral part of pubic crest (lateral head) and anterior pubic ligament (medial head) running vertically upwards to insert into xiphoid process and 7th, 6th and 5th costal cartilages. It is supplied by lower six thoracic nerves. There are three tendinous intersections; one at xiphoid, one at umbilicus, one between two which are adherent to anterior half of muscle and anterior wall of rectus sheath. They are due to embryologic segmental origin of muscle which adds to the power of muscle **(Figs. 19-9 and 19-10)**.

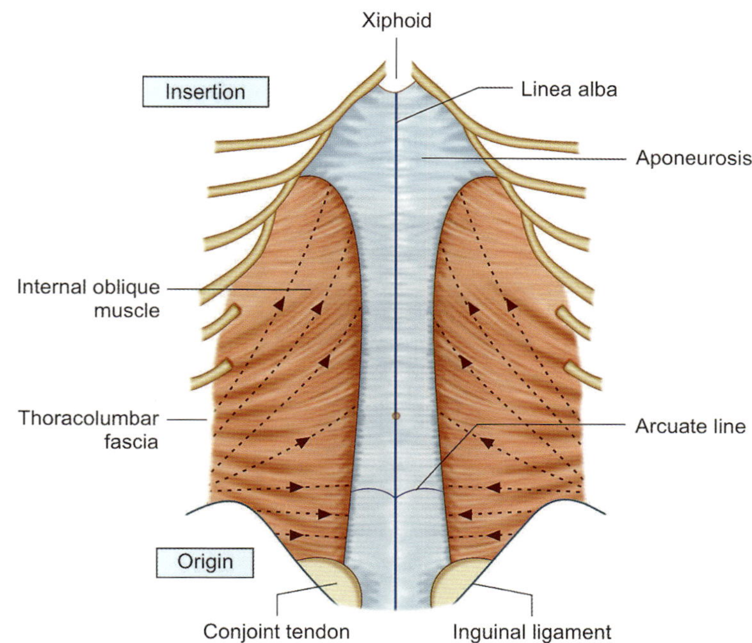

Fig. 19-7: Internal oblique muscle.

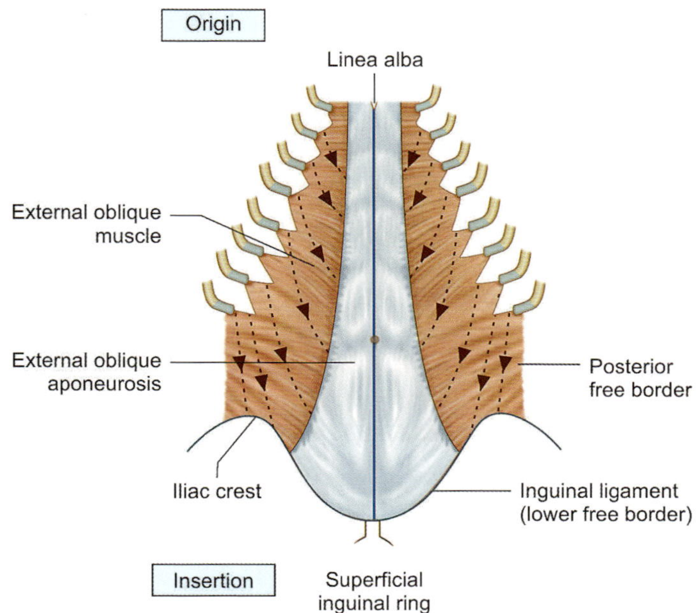

Fig. 19-6: External oblique muscle.

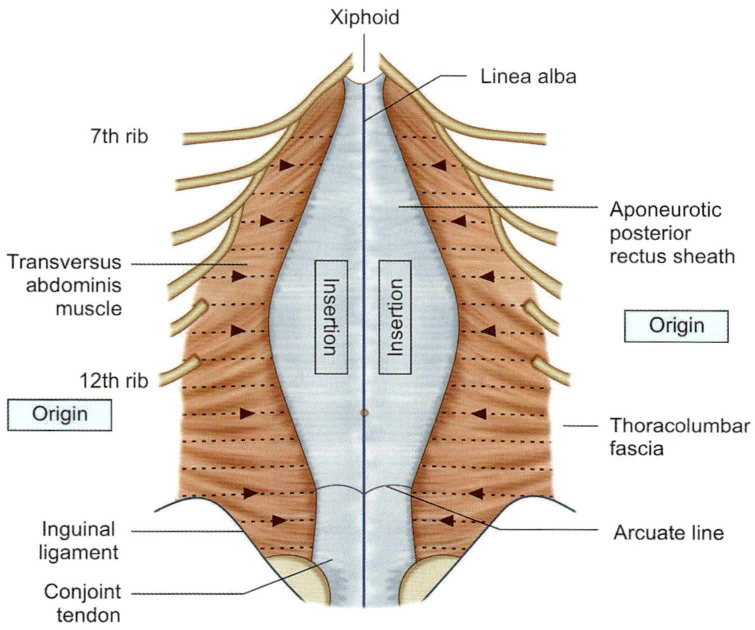

Fig. 19-8: Transverse abdominis muscle.

Inguinal ligament is formed by thickened posteriorly folded lower border of the external oblique aponeurosis extending from anterior superior iliac spine to pubic tubercle; lateral ½ is oblique and rounded and medial ½ is horizontal and grooved. The pectineal part of the inguinal ligament (lacunar) (triangular) is related in front to medial end of the inguinal ligament behind to pectin pubis; apex is attached to pubic tubercle; base directing laterally forms medial wall of femoral ring. Cooper's pectineal ligament is thickened pectineal fascia which is attached to the pectin pubis lateral to the base of the lacunar ligament. Aponeurotic fibres from the inferior crus of the external ring passing superomedially to linea alba is called as *Colles' reflected part of the inguinal ligament*.

Cremaster muscle is muscle fascicule embedded in cremaster fascia *(Scarpa's sheath)* which are attached to inguinal ligament laterally, internal oblique, transverse abdominis and conjoint tendon, pubic tubercle and pubic crest medially. It is seen properly only in males; sparse in females. It is supplied by genital branch of genitofemoral nerve (L1). It suspends the testis in elevated position. It closes when these raise in intra-abdominal pressure; it protects nerves of the inguinal canal. During hernioplasty if cremaster is excised, testis may hang like clapper bell due to loss of suspensory and retractile function of the cremaster. So if cremaster is excised, medial cut end should be sutured to inguinal ligament or pubic tubercle. Stroking medial aspect of upper thigh will cause reflex contraction of cremaster with elevation and retraction of testis—*cremasteric reflex* which is absent in upper motor neuron disease. Reflex is through femoral branch (stroking of medial thigh) of genitofemoral nerve to genital branch of genitofemoral nerve (cremaster muscle) through spinal cord.

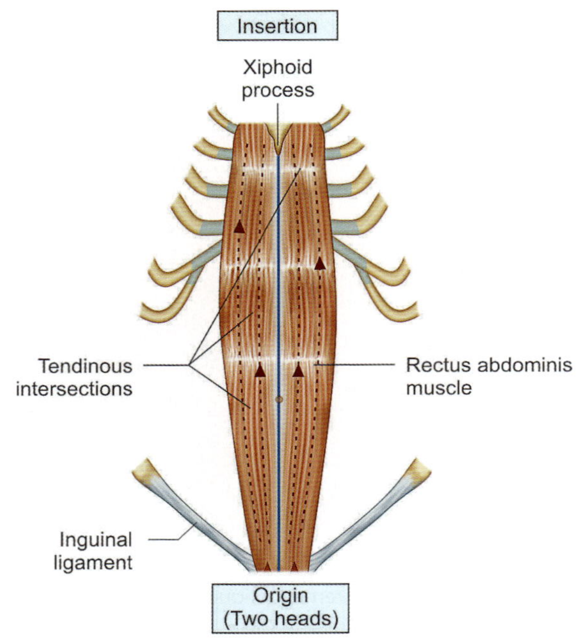

Fig. 19-9: Rectus abdominis muscle.

Pyramidalis is a small triangular rudimentary muscle arising from anterior surface of body of pubis running upwards and medially in front of the rectus abdominis to insert into linea alba; which is supplied by T12 subcostal nerve which is tensor of linea alba **(Fig. 19-11)**.

Deep Nerves of the Abdominal Wall

Lower five intercostal and subcostal (lower six thoracic) nerves and iliohypogastric and ilioinguinal nerves supply the anterior abdominal wall. *Lower five intercostal nerves* pass through the slips of origin of transversus abdominis muscles; runs between transversus abdominis and internal oblique; pierces the posterior lamina of internal oblique aponeurosis to reach rectus sheath; then passes behind the rectus sheath in front of the epigastric vessels, pierces the rectus muscle to continue as anterior cutaneous nerve. Before piercing it supplies the anterior rectus sheath transversus abdominis, internal oblique, external oblique and rectus abdominis. During its course it also gives lateral cutaneous nerve of the abdominal wall through flat abdominal muscles. *Battle's incision* which is pararectal incision will injure these nerves causing weakening of the rectus muscle and so is avoided.

Subcostal nerve, anterior primary ramus of 12th thoracic nerve after travelling behind the diaphragmatic lateral arcuate ligament, passes in front of the quadratus lumborum and then pierces the transversus abdominis to run like other intercostal nerves. It supplies pyramidalis muscle and gluteal region as lateral cutaneous branch.

Iliohypogastric nerve arises from the anterior division of L1 nerve runs away from lateral margin of psoas major muscle in front of quadratus lumborum behind kidney and colon to pierce transversus abdominis just above the iliac crest; runs between transversus abdominis and internal oblique; pierces the internal oblique 2.5 cm above the anterior superior iliac spine, run between internal oblique

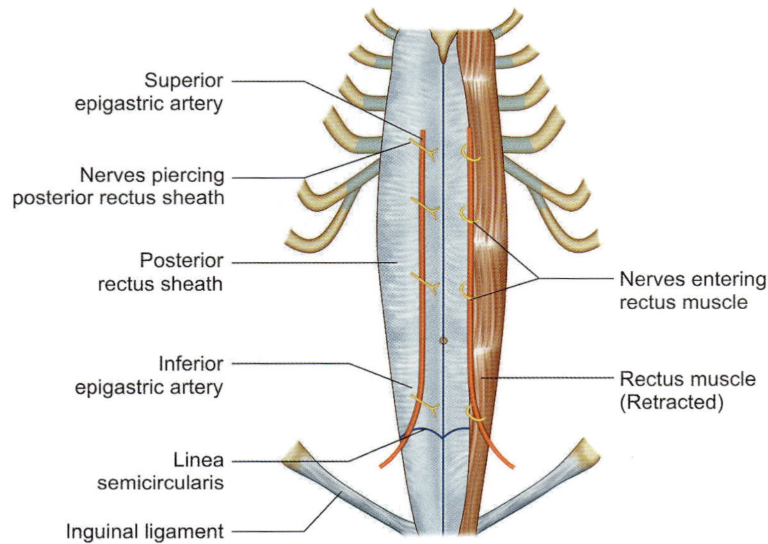

Fig. 19-10: Abdominal wall anatomy behind the rectus muscle.

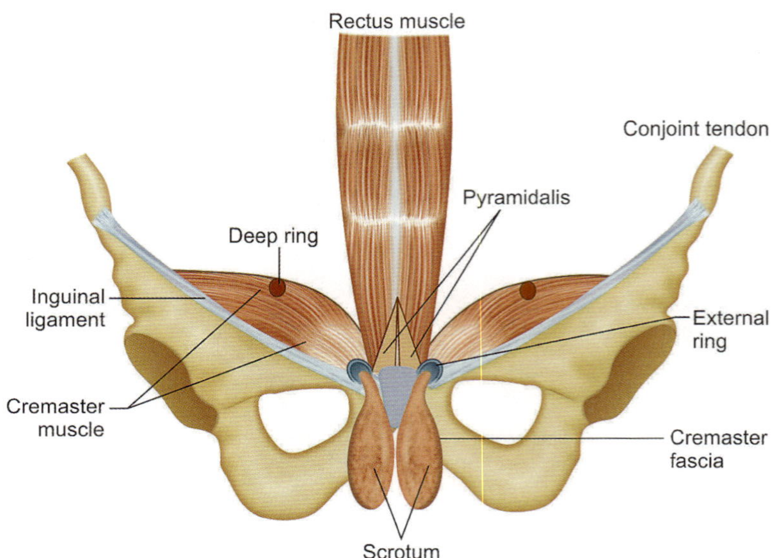

Fig. 19-11: Anatomy of pyramidalis and cremaster.

and external oblique to reach 2.5 cm above the superficial inguinal ring where it pierces the external oblique aponeurosis to supply skin around the area.

Ilioinguinal nerve also arises from anterior division of L1 nerve, runs over the quadratus lumborum, iliac crest before piercing the transversus abdominis 3.5 cm medial to anterior superior iliac spine; runs between transversus abdominis and internal oblique for a short distance, pierces internal oblique just below and medial to iliohypogastric nerve lateral to deep inguinal ring; runs in inguinal canal outside the cord in males or round ligament in females, passes through superficial inguinal ring; runs in front of the scrotum to supply anterior part of the scrotum. While piercing the internal oblique it distributes fibres (motor branches) internal oblique and transverse abdominis.

The genitofemoral nerve arises from ventral divisions of L1, L2 nerves; passes through the medial part of the psoas major muscle running below in front of the muscle; just above the deep ring it divides into medial genital and lateral femoral branches. Genital branch after piercing the psoas sheath runs in front of the external iliac artery and passes through deep ring to enter the inguinal canal within the spermatic cord in males or round ligament in females. It supplies cremaster muscle, runs in the cord to reach anterolateral aspect of the scrotum and supplies that part. In females it gives sensory branches to round ligament and labium majus. Femoral branch passes along with the femoral artery to supply skin over the femoral triangle.

Lateral cutaneous nerve of thigh (lateral femoral cutaneous nerve) arises from dorsal divisions of L2, L3 of lumbar plexus comes out at lateral border of the psoas major muscle passing on the inner lower short part of the quadratus lumborum to run on the main bulk of the iliacus muscle downwards and laterally; pierces the transversus abdominis, internal oblique and external oblique through and through (without travelling in between these muscles); passes behind the lateral part of the inguinal ligament 2–2.5 cm medial to anterior superior iliac spine. It supplies the skin over upper lateral part of the thigh and anterior part of the gluteal region after dividing into anterior and posterior branches **(Figs. 19-12 to 19-14)**.

Femoral nerve arises from dorsal divisions of L2, L3, L4 nerves of lumbar plexus, runs in the lower lateral border of the psoas major muscle in a groove between psoas major and iliacus muscles to reach the thigh along the lateral most compartment of the femoral canal. It supplies the iliacus muscle.

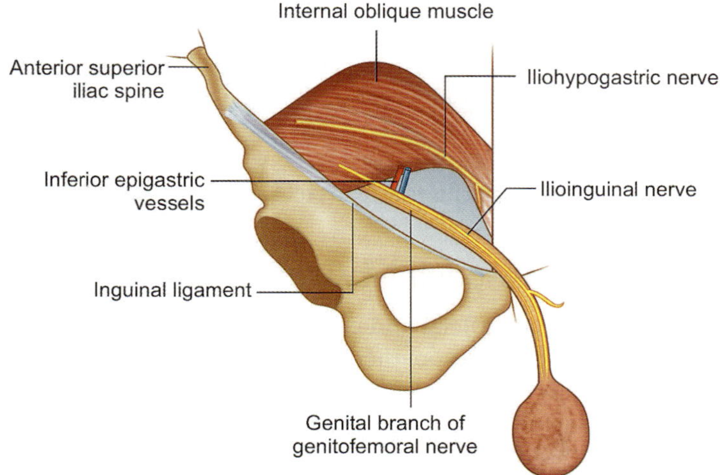

Fig. 19-12: Nerves in the groin. Ilioinguinal, iliohypogastric and genital branch of genitofemoral nerves are important three nerves which surgeon will come across during the open inguinal hernia surgery.

Obturator nerve arises from ventral divisions of L1, L2, L3 nerves of lumbar plexus runs on the medial aspect of the psoas major muscle; passes forwards and below into the pelvic brim where it is crossed by internal iliac artery and ureter to enter the obturator canal. In the canal it divides into anterior and posterior divisions. Anterior division supplies pectineus, adductor longus, gracilis and often adductor brevis muscles and hip joint. Posterior division supplies obturator externus, adductor magnus and often adductor brevis muscles, and through genicular branch which runs in adductor canal, popliteal fossa, pierces oblique popliteal ligament the supplies and knee joint. This genicular branch often gets compressed in obturator hernia to cause referred pain in knee joint (*Howship Romberg sign*).

Muscles of the Posterior Abdominal Wall

They are psoas major, psoas minor, quadratus lumborum and iliacus. *Psoas major* arises from body and transverse processes of all lumbar vertebrae to insert into the tip and medial part of the lesser trochanter of the femur after passing behind the inguinal ligament along with the iliacus tendon (lateral part of the lesser trochanter). It is supplied by L2, L3, L4 spinal nerves. *Psoas minor* is small muscle in front of the psoas major arises from bodies of T12 and L1 vertebrae to insert into the pectin pubis and iliopubic eminence. It is supplied by L1. *Iliacus* arises from upper 2/3rd of inner aspect of fossa of ilium, upper lateral part of the sacrum to insert into lateral part of the lesser trochanter along with psoas major. It is supplied by femoral nerve. *Quadratus lumborum* arises from transverse process of L5 vertebra and inner lip of iliac crest to insert into medial part of the anterior surface of 12th rib and transverse processes of upper four lumbar vertebrae. It is supplied by spinal nerves T12 to L4.

Fascia Transversalis (Cooper's Fascia)

It is the fascia that lines the inner surface of the transversus abdominis muscle separated from the peritoneum by extraperitoneal connective tissue. In front it is adherent to linea alba above the umbilicus; behind merges with anterior layer of thoracolumbar fascia and renal fascia; above with diaphragmatic fascia; below it is attached to inner lip of iliac crest, inguinal ligament; medially it is attached to pubic tubercle, pubic crest and pectineal line which prolongs down as anterior layer of femoral sheath. It also forms internal spermatic fascia around the cord. Deep inguinal ring is U/lambda/oval shaped opening 1.25 cm above the mid-inguinal point (between pubic symphysis and anterior superior iliac spine) which is lateral to inferior epigastric artery, transmits spermatic cord in males and round ligament in females. In the inguinal area transversalis fascia is *bilaminar* enclosing the inferior epigastric vessels. *Space of Bogros* is extension of the retropubic *space of Retzius* which is located beneath the posterior lamina of transversalis fascia and in front of the peritoneum. Unduly preperitoneal mesh repair is done by placing mesh in this space. Thickening of the transversalis fascia at the medial side of the internal ring and in front of the inferior epigastric vessels is called as *interfoveolar Hesselbach's ligament*.

Transversalis fascia is a thin aponeurotic fascia between parietal peritoneum and transverse abdominis; it is part of endoabdominal fascia. It continues as iliac fascia and pelvic fasciae below. Below it extends as anterior part of the femoral sheath along the femoral vessels. In the inguinal region posterior wall of the inguinal canal is formed by transversalis fascia; here it is thick and double layered. Behind the inguinal ligament it is strengthened by fibrous tissue which is loosely attached to the inguinal ligament and is called as ***iliopubic tract***. It has got an opening called deep ring through which spermatic cord in male and round ligament in females passes through. Transversalis fascia extends downwards into the scrotum as internal spermatic fascia **(Fig. 19-15)**.

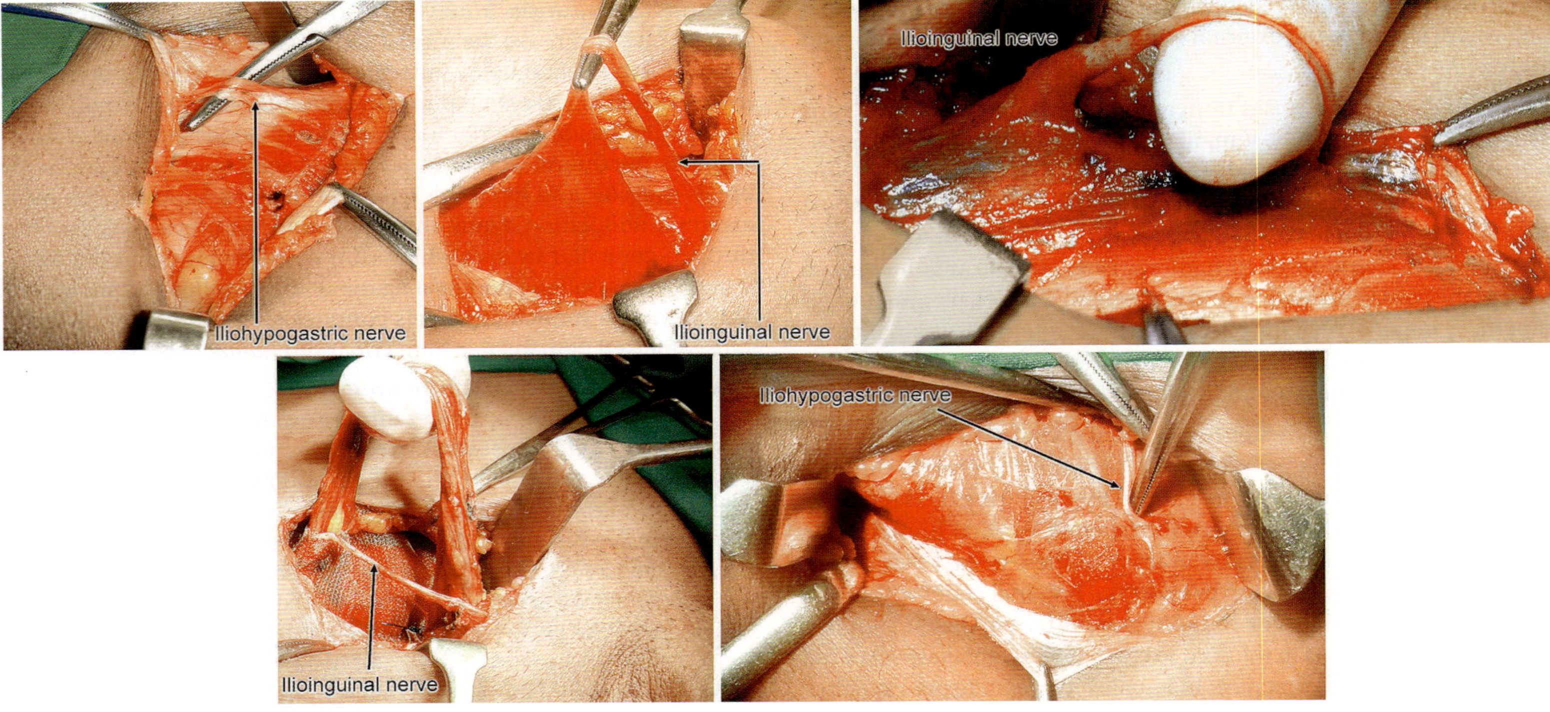

Fig. 19-13: Ilioinguinal nerve and iliohypogastric nerves.

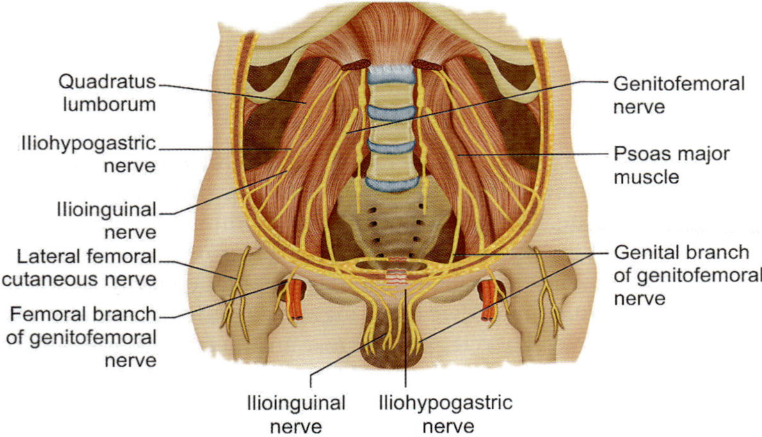

Fig. 19-14: Anatomy of different nerves in relation to groin hernia.

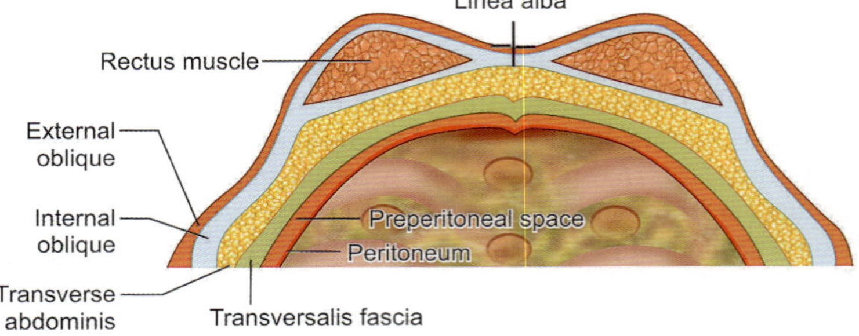

Fig. 19-15: Transversalis fascia.

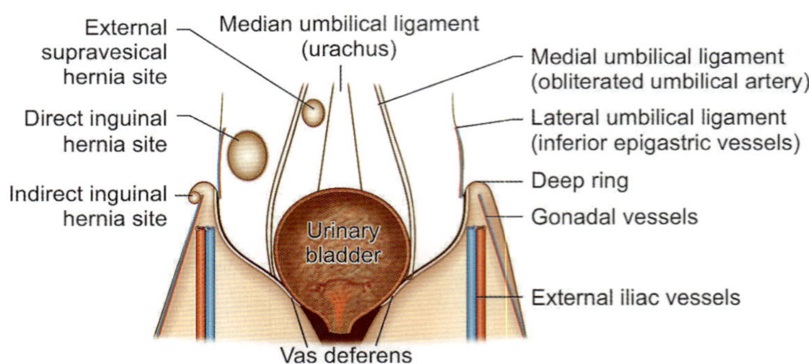

Fig. 19-16: Ligaments related to groin and hernia surgery.

Endoabdominal Fascia

Endoabdominal fascia is connective tissue that lines inner aspect of the entire abdominal musculature. Part in relation to transversus abdominis is called as fascia transversalis. It forms iliac, diaphragmatic and renal fascia.

Iliopubic Tract (Bandelette of Thomson)

Iliopubic tract is confused with inguinal ligament. It is an aponeurotic band extending from iliopectineal arch (thickened medial part of the iliopsoas fascia) and anterior superior iliac spine to superior ramus of the pubis forming deep musculoaponeurotic layer with transversus abdominis muscle, aponeurosis and transversalis fascia; it runs medially along inferior margin of the deep ring, anterior margin of the external iliac vessels, femoral sheath to attach to the pectineal ligament of Cooper **(Fig. 19-16)**.

Blood Supply of Abdominal Wall

It is divided into superficial and deep vessels. ***Superficial vessels*** are superficial epigastric, superficial circumflex iliac and superficial external pudendal arteries—are branches of femoral artery. They travel towards umbilicus in subcutaneous plane. Superficial epigastric artery communicates with opposite superficial epigastric artery and all three communicate with deep arteries.

Deep arteries are posterior intercostal arteries (10, 11), anterior branches of four lumbar and subcostal arteries and deep circumflex iliac artery. Deep arteries travel between transversus abdominis and internal oblique muscles. Recti are supplied by superior and inferior epigastric arteries. *Superior epigastric artery* is one of the two terminal branches of the internal thoracic/mammary artery. It originates at 6th intercostal space enters the abdomen between costal and xiphoid origin of the diaphragm, enters the rectus sheath from above, behind the 7th costal cartilage. It descends downwards communicating with inferior epigastric artery behind the rectus muscle. Branches are muscular, cutaneous, hepatic along the falciform ligament and anastomotic to opposite side artery.

Inferior epigastric artery (IEA) originates from external iliac artery just above the inguinal ligament, runs upwards and medially in the extraperitoneal connective tissue between peritoneum and posterior lamina of transversalis fascia initially medial to internal ring; pierces the transversalis fascia at the lateral border of the rectus muscle; runs in front of the arcuate line supplying the rectus and ends by anastomosing with superior epigastric artery. Branches are—muscular, cremasteric, pubic, and cutaneous. *Cremasteric branch* after travelling laterally towards deep ring supplies cremaster and runs along the spermatic cord. Pubic branch runs medially along the pubic bone to communicate with pubic branch of anterior division of obturator artery. Often obturator artery may be replaced by this pubic branch of inferior epigastric artery as abnormal/aberrant obturator artery. This pubic branch crosses over femoral ring and Cooper's ligament. This may be injured during fixation of mesh in TEP repair or femoral hernia repair causing torrential bleeding from both cut ends. As medial cut end retracts deep into the obturator fat and fascia it is difficult to control bleeding. This area is often called as *circle of death*. Inferior epigastric vein is medial to IEA **(Fig. 19-17)**.

Deep circumflex iliac artery arises from lateral side of the external iliac artery behind the inguinal ligament which after piercing the transversalis fascia runs along the iliac crest; at its middle it again pierces the transversus abdominis and internal oblique to reach adjacent to anterior superior iliac spine where it anastomoses with superior gluteal, superficial circumflex iliac, lateral circumflex femoral arteries. Here it also gives ascending branch which runs in abdominal wall which may be injured in TEP causing large haematoma.

Bendavid circle: It is the circle where venous network is situated in *space of Bogros* formed by branches of inferior epigastric, iliopubic, suprapubic, and retropubic veins. They communicate with aberrant obturator vein which is commonly existing (70%). During laparoscopy (TEP/TAPP) veins will collapse due to high insufflation pressure and will not bleed during dissection but bleeds later in postoperative period.

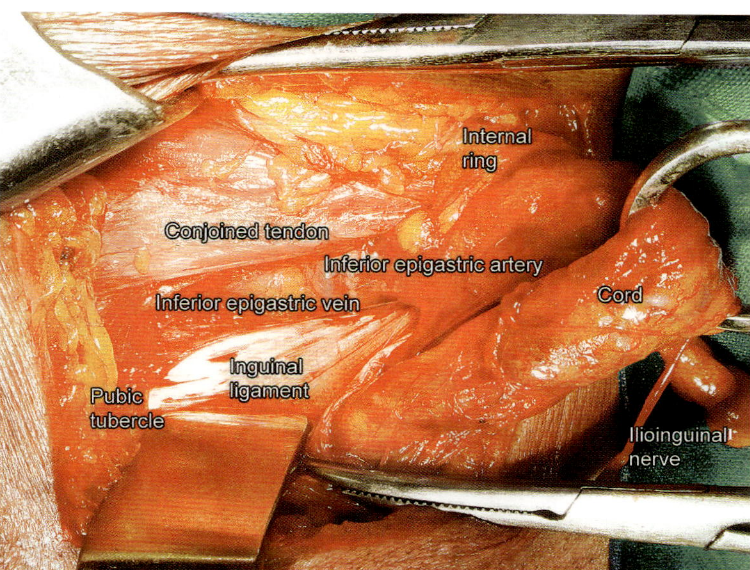

Fig. 19-17: Inferior epigastric vessels—on table look.

Triangle of doom is observed in laparoscopic hernia procedure. It is a triangle formed medially by vas deferens, laterally by testicular vessels and peritoneal reflection below with the apex at internal ring. External iliac vessels lie in this triangle and so extreme care should be taken while dissecting the hernial sac in this triangle.

Preperitoneal Space of Nyhus

It is the space between transversalis fascia and peritoneum. Medially, it is in front of the urinary bladder and behind pubic bone as retropubic space of Retzius (1858). Laterally it continues as space of Bogros (1823). Below it is limited at iliopubic tract; laterally to anterior superior iliac spine and iliopsoas fascia. Iliopubic tract is analogue of the inguinal ligament, extends from Cooper's ligament to anterior superior iliac spine which divides endoscopic view of pre-peritoneal space into *superior compartment* [contains inferior epigastric artery, Hesselbach's triangle, cord structures and is site of inguinal hernia) and *inferior compartment* [contains femoral canal, iliac vessels (vein medially and artery laterally), iliopsoas muscle, genitofemoral nerve, lateral femoral cutaneous nerve]. External iliac vessels lie in a triangle formed by gonadal vessels laterally, vas deferens medially and peritoneal reflection inferiorly (*triangle of doom*). Aberrant obturator artery which is an occasional branch of inferior epigastric artery replacing its pubic branch travels across Cooper's ligament, which during fixation of mesh can cause torrential haemorrhage—*circle of death. Triangle of pain* is formed by gonadal vessels medially, iliopubic tract laterally and peritoneal reflection below. Genitofemoral nerve and lateral cutaneous nerve of thigh traverse this triangle. Injury to these nerves either by dissection or by tacks causes severe postoperative pain. Tacks/staplers should not be placed in this triangle.

Endoscopic hernia repair needs dissection and exposure of the entire myopectineal orifice from midline to anterior superior iliac spine.

Fruchaud's (French Surgeon) Myopectineal Orifice (MPO)

It is an osseo-myo-aponeurotic tunnel. *It is through this tunnel that all groin hernias occur.* It is bound medially by lateral border of rectus sheath; above by the arched fibres of internal oblique and transverse abdominis muscle; laterally by the iliopsoas muscle; below by the pectin pubis and fascia covering it **(Fig. 19-18)**.

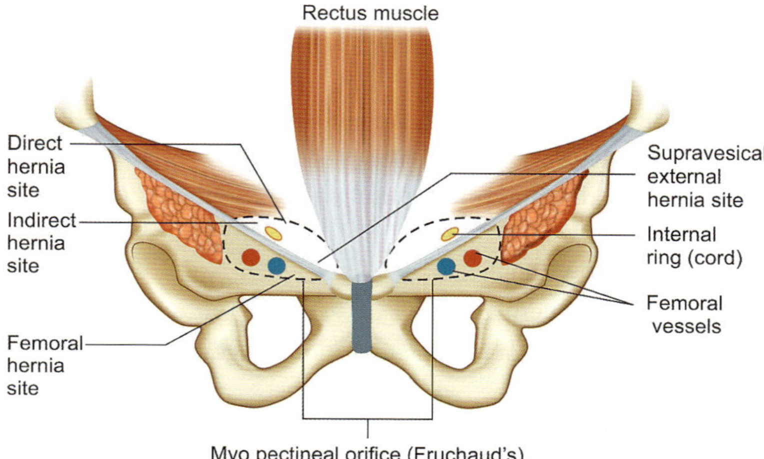

Fig. 19-18: Myopectineal orifice (MPO) of Fruchaud's.

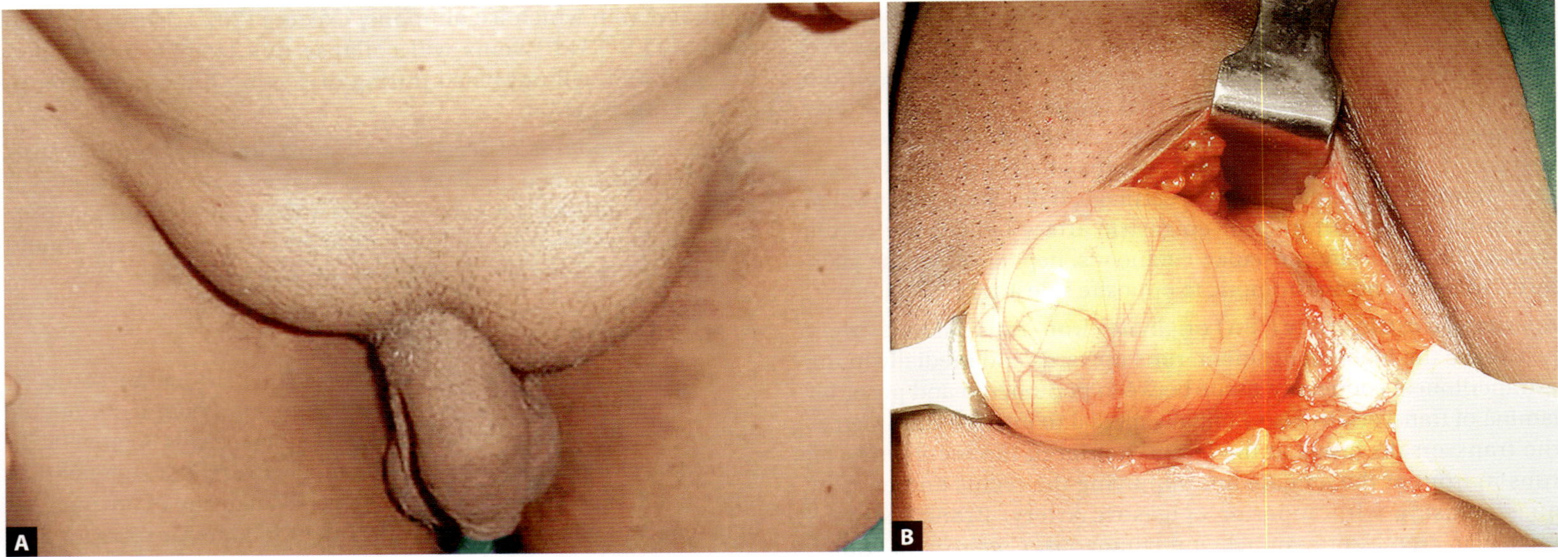

Figs. 19-19A and B: Bilateral direct hernia.

Fossae of the Anterior Abdominal Wall

There are three fossae on the inner surface of the anterior abdominal wall above the ligament and below the umbilicus. *Lateral fossa* is lateral to lateral umbilical ligament (which contains inferior epigastric artery) which is the site of indirect inguinal hernia. Lateral fossa contains deep inguinal ring. *Medial fossa* is between lateral and medial umbilical ligament (obliterated umbilical artery). Here direct hernia develops. *Supravesical fossa* is between medial and median (obliterated urachus) umbilical ligament which is the site of external supravesical hernia. Internal supravesical hernia develops in relation to urinary bladder directly, as anterior prevesical, posterior retrovesical and lateral paravesical.

NEWER CLASSIFICATIONS OF GROIN HERNIA

Gilbert Classification

Type I: Hernia has got snug internal ring through which a peritoneal sac passes out as indirect sac.

Type II: Hernia has a moderately enlarged internal ring which admits one finger but is lesser than two fingerbreadth. Once reduced it protrude during coughing or straining.

Type III: Hernia has got large internal ring with defect more than two fingerbreadth. Hernia descends into the scrotum or with sliding hernia. Once reduced it immediately protrudes out without any straining.

Type IV: It is direct hernia with large full blow out of the posterior wall of the inguinal canal. The internal ring is intact.

Type V: It is a direct hernia protruding out through punched out hole/defect in the transversalis fascia. The internal ring is intact.

Type VI: Pantaloon/double hernia.

Type VII: Femoral hernia.

Types VI and VII are Robbin's modifications **(Figs. 19-19A and B)**.

NYHUS Classification

It is based on size of the internal ring and posterior wall weakness.

Type I: Indirect hernia with normal deep ring.

Type II: Indirect hernia with dilated/widened deep ring.

Type III: Posterior wall defect.

a. Direct.
b. Pantaloon hernia: Indirect with posterior wall weakness.
c. Femoral hernia.

Type IV: Recurrent hernia.

BENDAVID Classification

Type I: Anterolateral defect (indirect).
Type II: Anteromedial (direct).
Type III: Posteromedial (femoral).
Type IV: Posterior prevascular hernia.
Type V: Anteroposterior defect: Inguinofemoral hernia.

INDIRECT (OBLIQUE) INGUINAL HERNIA (FIG. 19-20)

This is the most common type of hernia. It is more common in younger age group as compared to direct inguinal hernia which is more common in elderly. It is more common on right side in 1st decade but in 2nd decade the incidence is equal on both sides.

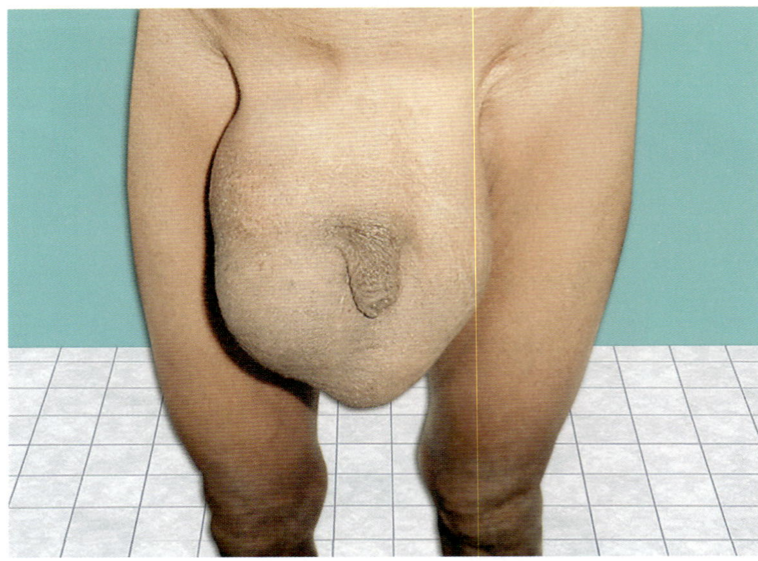

Fig. 19-20: Complete indirect hernia.

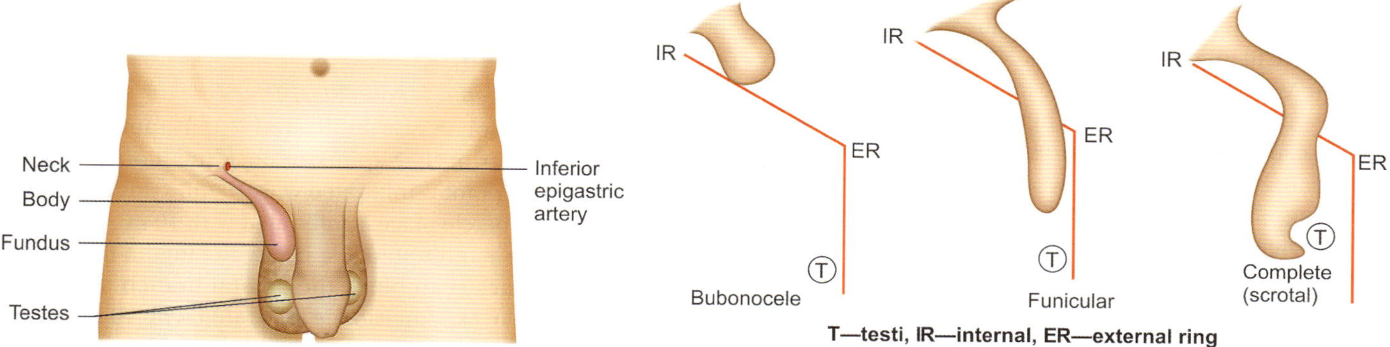

Fig. 19-21: Surgical anatomy of indirect hernia and types of indirect inguinal hernia.

Hernia is bilateral in 30% of cases. Sac is thin in indirect type. Neck is narrow and, lies lateral to inferior epigastric vessels **(Fig. 19-21)**.

Types: (1) *Bubonocele*, where the hernia is limited to inguinal canal; (2) *Funicular* where processus vaginalis is closed just above the epididymis. Contents of the sac can be felt separately from testis, which lies below the hernia; (3) *Complete (Scrotal)* where testis appears to lie within the lower part of hernia. It can occur in any age group. It occurs in a congenital preformed sac (*processus vaginalis*). More commonly contents descend into the pre-existing sac only when there are precipitating causes which force the content down **(Figs. 19-22 to 19-24)**.

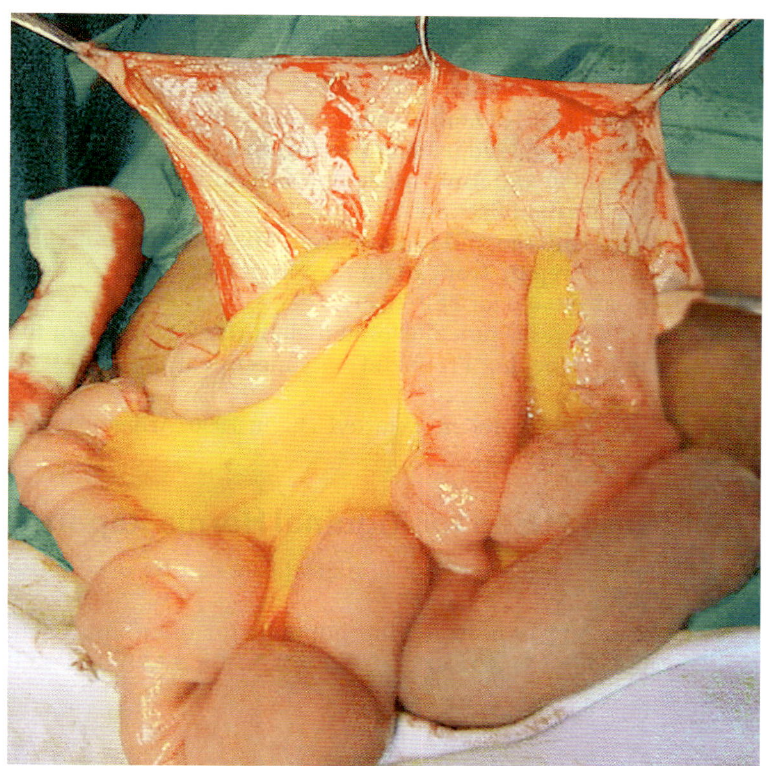

Fig. 19-23: Enterocele in a hernial sac.

SURGERIES FOR INGUINAL HERNIA

History of Hernia Surgery

Original Eduardo Bassini (Padua, 1889) repair is though an anterior approach. He opened posterior wall of inguinal canal and did a sutured three layered repair. In modified Bassini repair transverse arch is sutured to the shelving edge of inguinal ligament as single layered interrupted sutures.

De Chauliac differentiated inguinal from femoral hernias (1363). Kaspar Stromayr differentiated direct and indirect hernias in 1559. Ambroise Pare (1550) used trusses in hernia. John Hunter, Astley Paston Cooper (1841) Franz Hesselbach, Antonio Scarpa (1832),

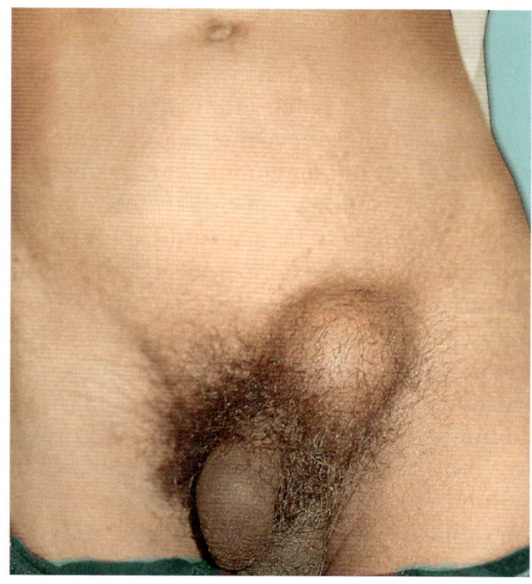

Fig. 19-22: Bubonocele.

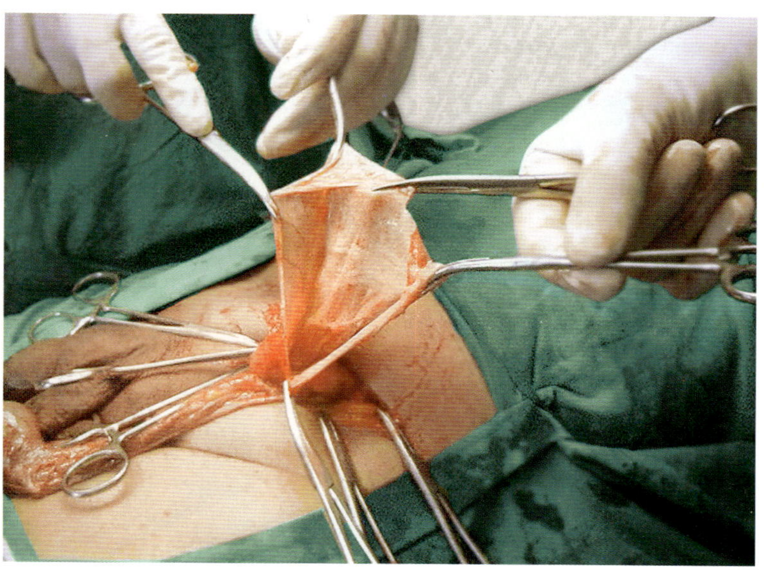

Fig. 19-24: Indirect hernial sac.

Pieter Camper, Jules Germain Cloquet (1883), Bogros, Retzius contributed in understanding anatomy of the groin.

La Roque, GL Cheatle, JP Hoguet, AK, Henry, McVay, McEvedy, Lotheissen, McArthur (used strips of external oblique aponeurosis to approximate conjoined tendon to inguinal ligament), Kirschner (used thigh fascial grafts), Gallie (used strips of fascia lata for repair using his specialised needle *Gallie's needle*), Handley (used silk with staylace darning), Meick (used first multifilament Nylon), Haxton (used monofilament Nylon), Moloney (Nylon darn procedure, 1948) are the others who contributed to hernia surgery.

Halsted (John Hopkins Baltimore) did four layered repair shifting cord anterior to the external oblique aponeurosis thus bringing superficial and deep ring to lie very close causing higher chances of recurrence.

EE Shouldice (1945) of Toronto did repair of transversalis fascia under local anaesthesia as a tension free 4/6 layered tissue repair.

Usher from Texas in 1958 first used Marlex mesh in posterior wall for repair as tension eliminating.

Lichtenstein (1970) did rolled plug mesh repair of femoral hernia. Newman (New Jersey) did tension-free inguinal hernia onlay mesh repair. Lichtenstein and Amid made this technique popular worldwide with certain modifications.

Nyhus from Chicago and Condon from Milwaukee popularised open posterior repair from higher approach. Their technique probably became basis for TEP/TAPP.

Stoppa and Rives (France) evoluted giant reinforcement of the visceral sac by blocking Fruchaud's myopectineal orifice (MPO) bilaterally.

EH Phillips and JB McKeran started TEP in 1990. Arregui started TAPP in 1992 **(Fig. 19-25)**.

Anaesthesia Used for Inguinal Hernia Repair

General/spinal/epidural or local anaesthesia can be used to do inguinal hernia repair.

Local anaesthesia is becoming popular; for open approach. General anaesthesia is needed in children, for TAPP and TEP procedures.

Technique of Local Anaesthesia

Around 50–60 mL of xylocaine 0.5% is used. Plain xylocaine 0.5% or xylocaine 0.5% with adrenaline can be used. Plain xylocaine—dose is 2 mg/kg body weight. Xylocaine with adrenaline—dose is 7 mg/kg body weight **(Fig. 19-26)**.

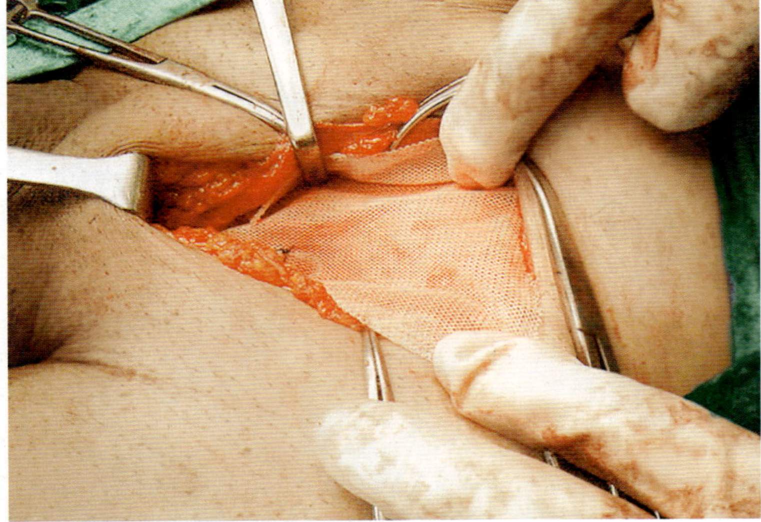

Fig. 19-25: Mesh plasty has become standard now.

Two Methods are Used

1. *Nerve block method (Point block)*
   10 mL of xylocaine is infiltrated 2 cm above and medial to anterior superior iliac spine to block the iliohypogastric nerve. Midinguinal point is infiltrated with 10 mL xylocaine. Area around the pubic tubercle place is infiltrated with 10 mL xylocaine. 10 mL of xylocaine is infiltrated just below the inguinal ligament lateral to femoral artery to block the genital branch of genitofemoral artery. Line of skin incision is infiltrated with 10 mL of xylocaine. Later neck of the hernial sac is infiltrated with 10 mL of xylocaine.
2. *Field block method (Shouldice method)*
   Skin of around 4 cm wide area is infiltrated including the subcutaneous plane as first layer from anterior superior iliac spine to pubic symphysis. Skin, subcutaneous and two layers of superficial fascia (Camper and Scarpa's) are incised. Area deep to external oblique aponeurosis is infiltrated with 10 mL of xylocaine. External oblique aponeurosis is incised. Exposed inguinal canal and hernial sac is infiltrated with 10 mL of xylocaine to continue with the dissection.

Different Surgeries (Fig. 19-27)

Herniotomy in Infants

In infants, whether it is hernia or hydrocele, *only herniotomy* is done through inguinal approach (*Michaelis plank operation*). High ligation is the procedure of choice. Few advocated bilateral inguinal herniotomy in all children with unilateral/bilateral inguinal hernias. Hernia here is due to patent processus vaginalis and always indirect. It is common in boys (9:1); common on right side; 15% bilateral. Often presentation is like hydrocele. It is often associated with undescended testis. Incarceration of bowel is very high in male infants with inguinal hernia. It is near 30% in premature or child less than 1 year. From 1 year to 18 years age group incarceration is around 15%. In girls, ovary and Fallopian tubes are common content; strangulation of ovary is common. Conservative treatment should not be done in childhood inguinal hernia **(Figs. 19-28 to 19-30)**.

Inguinal canal approach: Technique is same as in adults but more care and meticulous technique is needed. Superficial inguinal ring should not be opened to avoid the scarring of the superficial inguinal ring. Vas deferens should not be held with haemostat or forceps. Fine non-toothed Adson's forceps can be used if only needed. Whenever sac is complete distal part is left alone after transecting the sac; proximal part is ligated high above the level of the deep ring. Before ligating one should ensure that contents are pushed properly into the peritoneal cavity. Usually hydrocele is due to infantile hernial sac and so there is no need to do a separate incision for hydrocele; instead distal part of the sac is opened for an adequate length, followed by removal of fluid content and later sac is left open like that. Separate hydrocele or encysted hydrocele if present, should be dealt through same incision. Repair is not needed along the floor of the inguinal canal; as it will disturb the shutter mechanism. Transversalis fascia should not be injured. *Very rarely* when direct sac is present posterior wall may be repaired by suturing conjoined tendon to inguinal ligament using 3 interrupted polypropylene sutures. But a surgeon should remember that *in children there is no repair in inguinal hernia*. Wound is closed in layers. Contralateral exploration is often advocated by many as a routine practice.

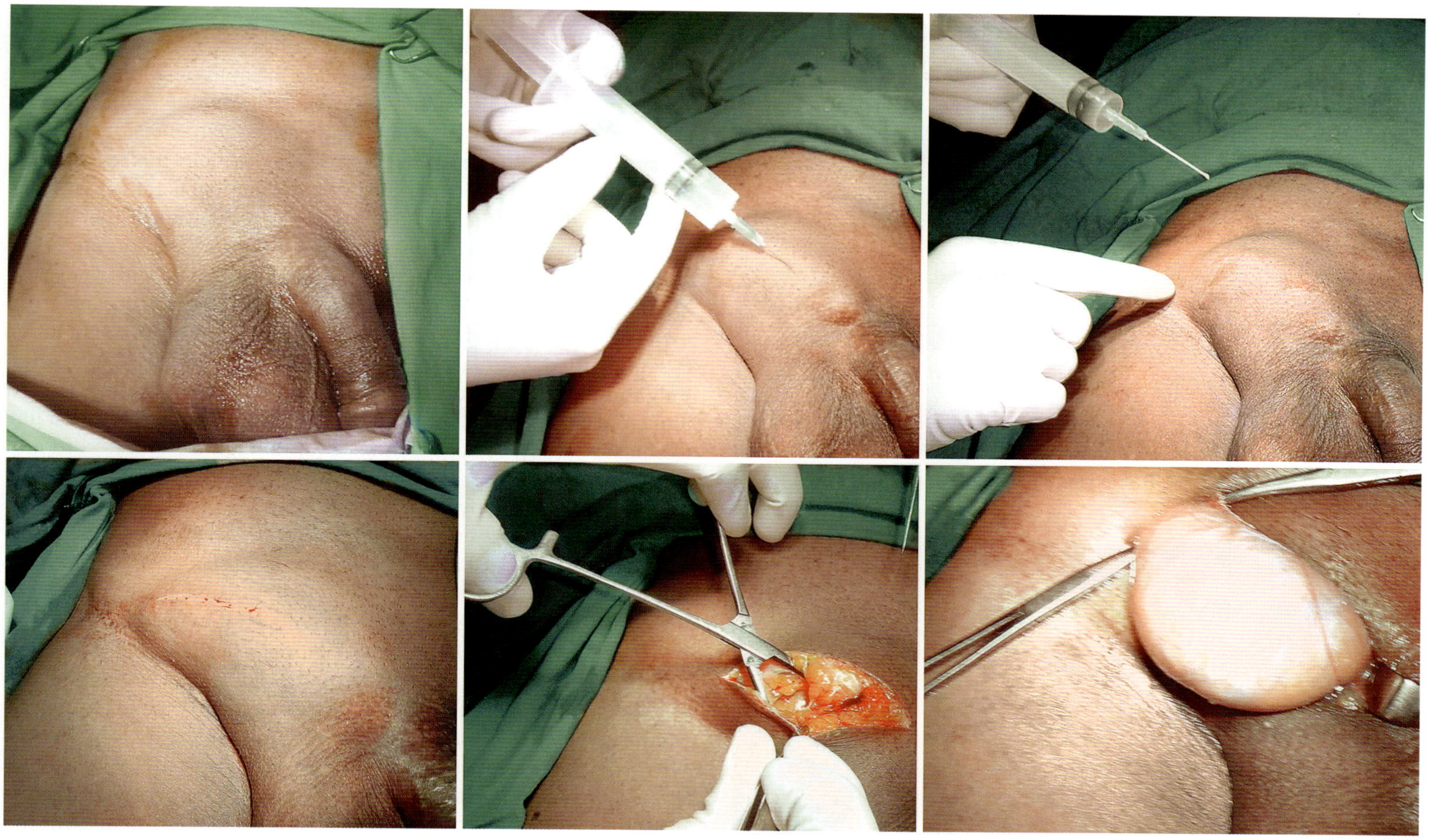

Fig. 19-26: Open inguinal surgery is commonly done under local anaesthesia.

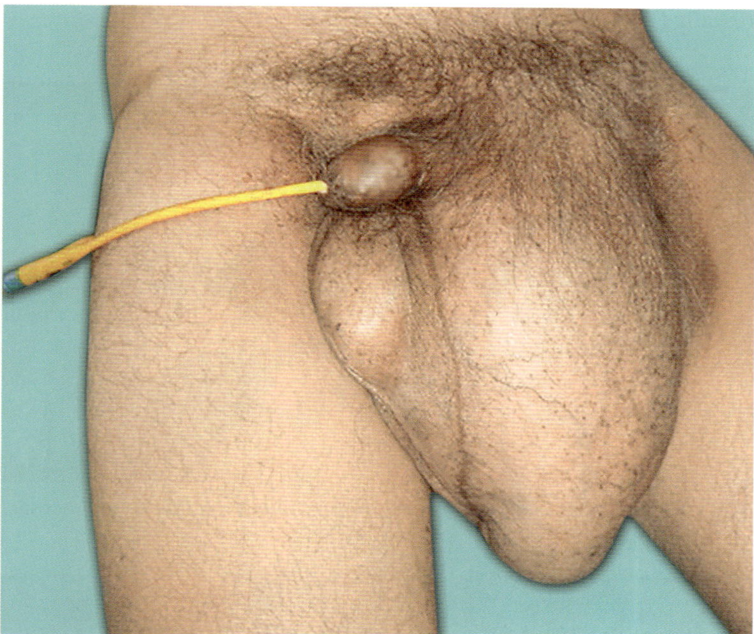

Fig. 19-27: Large hernia needs catheterisation before surgery.

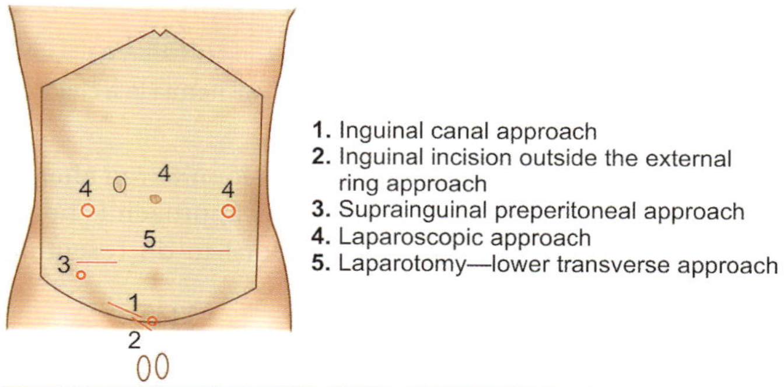

Inguinal incision without opening the inguinal canal approach: In infants variation in approach can be undertaken but with difficulty. Here medial inguinal incision is made. Cord structures coming out of the superficial inguinal ring is identified without opening the superficial inguinal ring and external oblique aponeurosis. Inguinal canal in infants is very short with superficial and deep rings lying at same level. Sac once identified by careful meticulous dissection and

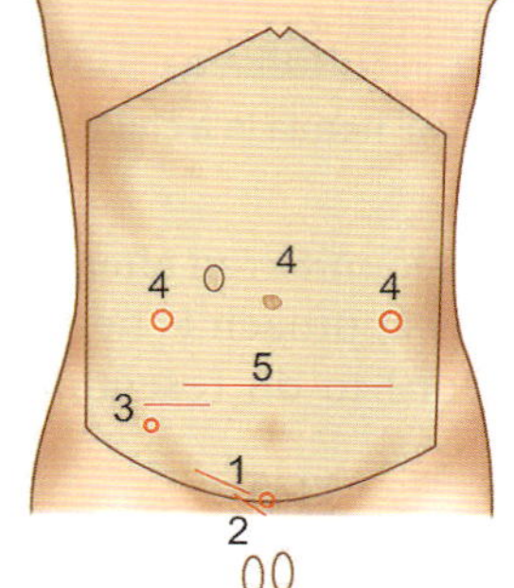

1. Inguinal canal approach
2. Inguinal incision outside the external ring approach
3. Suprainguinal preperitoneal approach
4. Laparoscopic approach
5. Laparotomy—lower transverse approach

Note:
- Superficial ring should never be cut
- Inguinal repair should never be done
- Distal part of the sac should not be ligated
- Separate exploration of hydrocele is not needed

Fig. 19-28: Different approaches for herniotomy in infants and children.

traction, can be reached up to deep ring. Proximal sac is ligated with transfixation. Distal sac is left open. One should avoid injuring vas, testicular veins in the cord as they are very fine in infants. Use of bipolar cautery (not monopolar) is essential. Wound is closed in layers.

Suprainguinal preperitoneal open approach is also used. External oblique, internal oblique and transverse abdominis are split after skin and subcutaneous layer incision. Transversalis fascia is incised. Preperitoneal space is entered to identify the indirect sac which is dissected. Proximal part of the sac is ligated and distal part is cut and left open to retract below.

Transperitoneal laparoscopic approach is present alternative where the hernial sac is ligated proximal to deep ring by placing polypropylene purse string sutures on both sides.

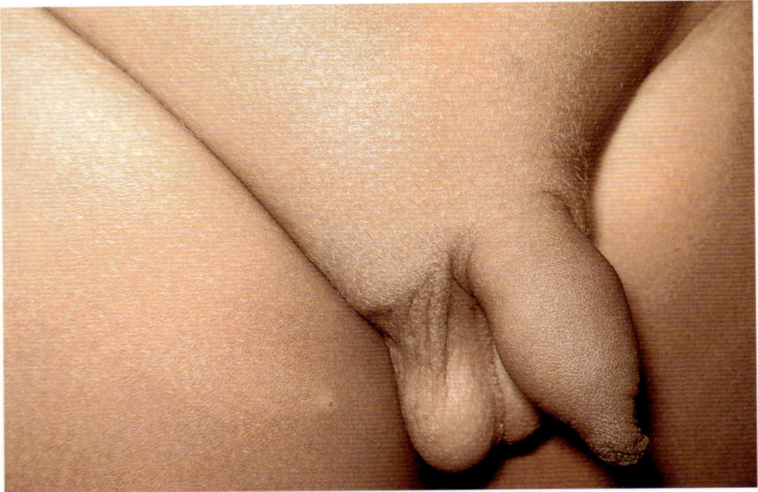

Fig. 19-29: Right sided inguinal hernia in a child.

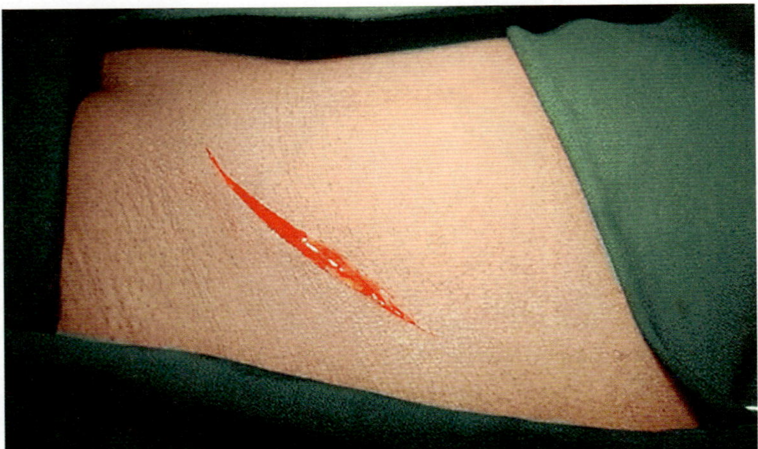

Fig. 19-30: Incision for right sided inguinal hernia in a child.

In incarcerated hernia if strangulation is found even after release of the constriction band, then laparotomy approach is better and safer (lower abdomen horizontal incision) to do resection and anastomosis of the bowel.

Complications

Recurrence (<1%), haematoma, seroma, injury to vas, post-herniotomy hydrocele, testicular atrophy. Recurrence is due to injury to transversalis fascia (leads into direct hernia later), missed sac, improper ligation of the sac, sepsis, connective tissue disorders. As vas deferens and testicular vessels are very fine structures in infants and children injury may occur which should be avoided. If injury to vas occurs it should be repaired using 8-zero polypropylene sutures using microscope.

In Adults

It includes *herniotomy, i.e.* excision of hernial sac and ***herniorrhaphy or hernioplasty*** (strengthening of the posterior wall of inguinal canal either by repair or mesh).

Herniotomy

Anaesthesia: Spinal or general anaesthesia or local anaesthesia.

Procedure

After cleaning and draping, skin is incised 1.25 cm above and parallel to the medial two-third of inguinal ligament. Two layers of superficial fascia (outer Camper's fascia and inner Scarpa's fascia) are incised. Superficial pudendal and superficial epigastric vessels are ligated with catgut or cauterised. Self-retaining mastoid or similar retractor is placed to retract the skin edges. External oblique aponeurosis is incised along its long axis parallel to the line of skin incision. Incision is extended on either ends of the incision; medially it is extended to cut the margins of the superficial ring. Upper leaf is reflected above and held with haemostat; using peanut dissection upper leaf is raised adequately to visualise conjoined tendon and lateral rectus sheath. Lower leaf is reflected downwards to visualise and expose the inguinal ligament. Entire inguinal ligament is dissected medially and exposed with its shelving edge and iliopubic tract. Ilioinguinal nerve is safeguarded. Cremasteric muscle (box) with its fascia is opened longitudinally as medial and lateral flaps. Cremaster vessel is ligated and cremaster muscle is excised after ligating proximally and distally. Cremasterectomy is not essential. Even though it exposes cord and posterior inguinal wall; it causes hanging testis without support (*clapper in bell*). Many advocate stitching the distal sutured part to pubic tubercle after cremasterectomy, so that it will give support to testis partially. It is not mandatory to excise entire cremaster. If there is a lipoma of the cord *it should be* excised; but normal fat in the cord should not be removed. If removed it may cause testicular oedema and hydrocele. Cord structures are dissected. Sac lying anterior and lateral to cord is identified as it is pearly white in colour. Dissection is usually started from the fundus and extended towards the neck which is identified by the extraperitoneal fat. The neck is narrow and is lateral to inferior epigastric artery. *High dissection beyond the deep ring* is done. Sac is opened at the fundus. Finger is passed to release any adhesions. Sac is twisted so as to prevent the content from coming back. It is transfixed using absorbable suture material (chromic catgut 2-0 or vicryl) and is excised (redundant sac) distally **(Figs. 19-31 to 19-35)**.

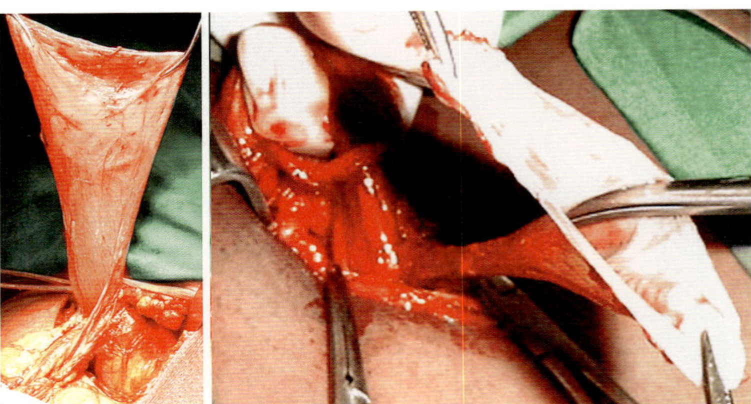

Fig. 19-31: High dissection above the internal ring is required in indirect sac.

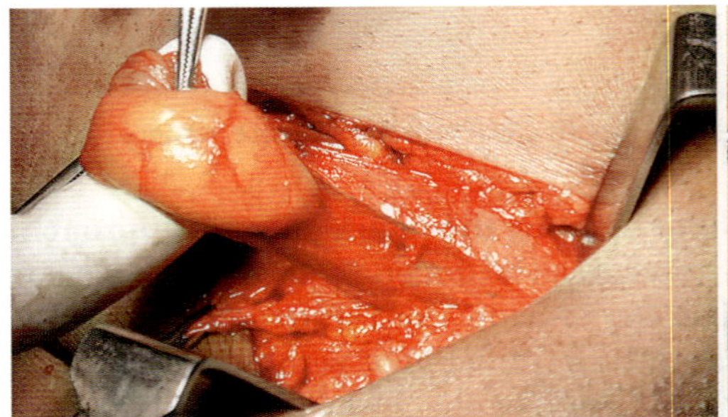

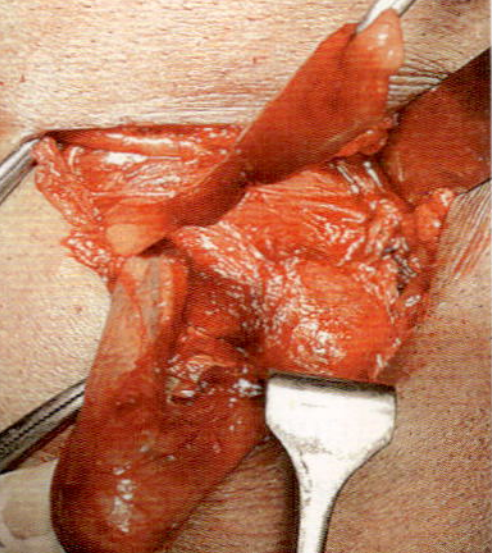

Fig. 19-32: Lipoma of the cord is a common entity; when present it should be excised.

Hernia Repair

Repair may be
- *Pure tissue repair:* Shouldice, Mac Vay (still very useful repair) and modified Bassini, Deserda tension free repair.
- *Prosthetic repair:* Lichtenstein, Rives, Gilbert, Stoppa, TEP, TAPP.

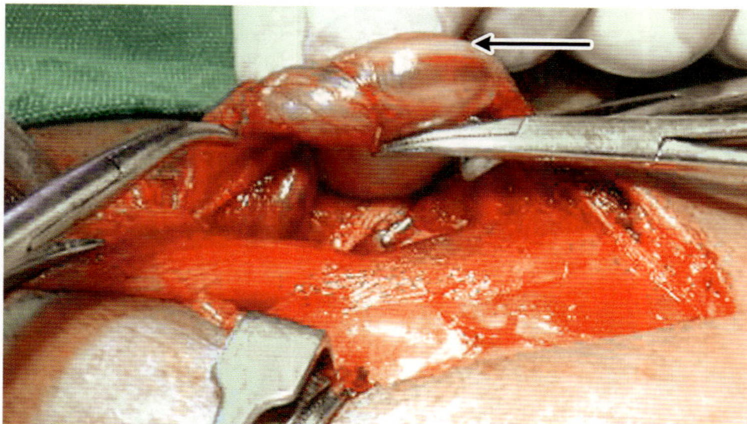

Fig. 19-33: Vas deferens should be identified and safeguarded especially in children.

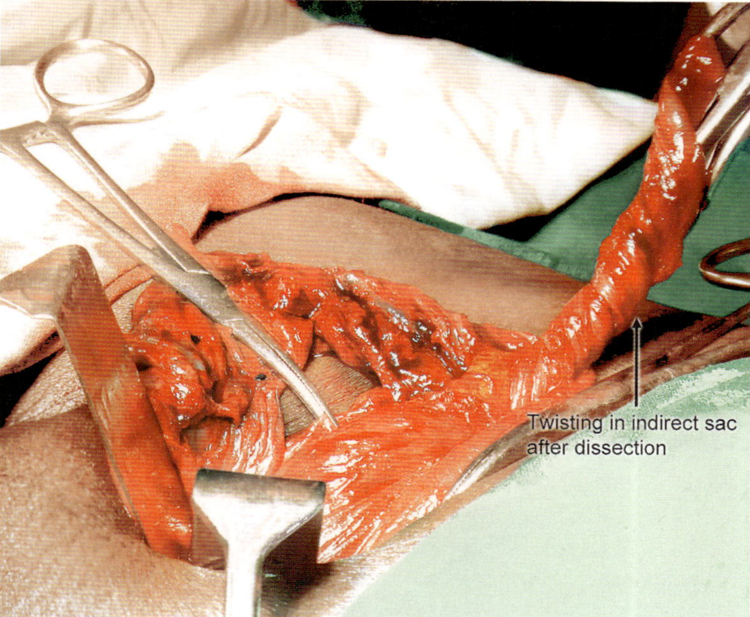

Fig. 19-34: Indirect sac after opening at the fundus is twisted to avoid contents getting entangled prior to transfixation.

It means repair or strengthening of the posterior wall of the inguinal canal. By principle defective first layer which is transversalis fascia should be used in repair. Strengthening can be done by tissue or prosthetic repair. Strengthening by tissue repair has got various approaches where transversalis fascia or tendinous fascioaponeurotic upper part is approximated to iliopubic tract or Cooper's ligament or shelved edge of the inguinal ligament. Upper leaf taken for repair should be tendinous fascioaponeurotic layer not fleshy red muscle. Non-absorbable monofilament sutures like polypropylene should be used ideally. In few centres delayed absorbable sutures are used but it is not considered to be ideal. Prosthetic repair is done by placing mesh or prosthesis by onlay/inlay/sublay/sublay intraperitoneal method. Tissue prosthesis like tensor fascia lata or temporal fascia are not used now. Polypropylene mesh is commonly used with different modifications. Approach for repair may be ***anterior*** through inguinal canal (for tissue repair and mesh repair either onlay or sublay) or ***posterior*** through high suprainguinal preperitoneal.

Modified Bassini's Herniorrhaphy

Conjoined tendon and inguinal ligament are approximated using interrupted non-absorbable monofilament sutures (polypropylene); medial most stitch is taken from the periosteum of pubic tubercle (*called as key or Bassini's stitch)*; external oblique is closed and other layers are closed. Bassini originally used silk suture for the repair (1887). He also used triple layer of upper leaf which contains transversalis fascia, transversus abdominis and internal oblique muscles in this repair. Care should be taken not to injure iliac vessels (mainly vein) while taking bite from inguinal ligament. It is often practiced to take bites in inguinal ligament at different levels to prevent tearing of the fibers of inguinal ligament. Laterally repair is done beyond the line of internal ring. Few advocate horizontal mattress sutures starting from conjoined tendon to inguinal ligament and from inguinal ligament to conjoined tendon **(Figs. 19-36 to 19-38)**.

Complications of herniorrhaphy

- Haemorrhage.
- Haematoma.
- Infection (5%).
- Haematocele.
- Post-herniorrhaphy hydrocele, lymphocele.
- Hyperaesthesia over the medial side of inguinal canal due to injury to ilioinguinal or iliohypogastric nerve.
- Recurrence.
- Osteitis pubis.
- Injury to urinary bladder/bowel.
- Testicular atrophy, penile oedema rarely can occur.

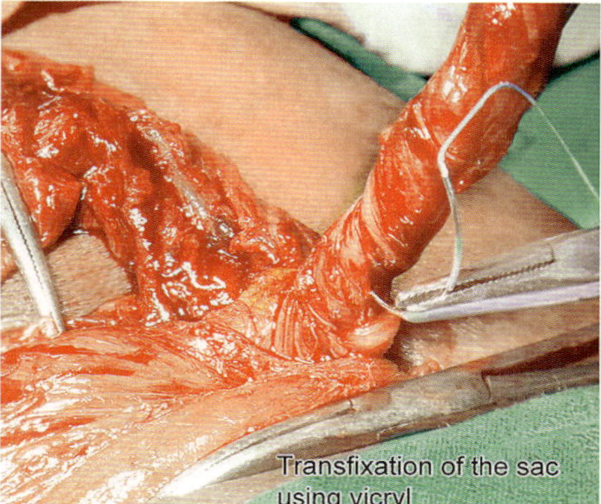

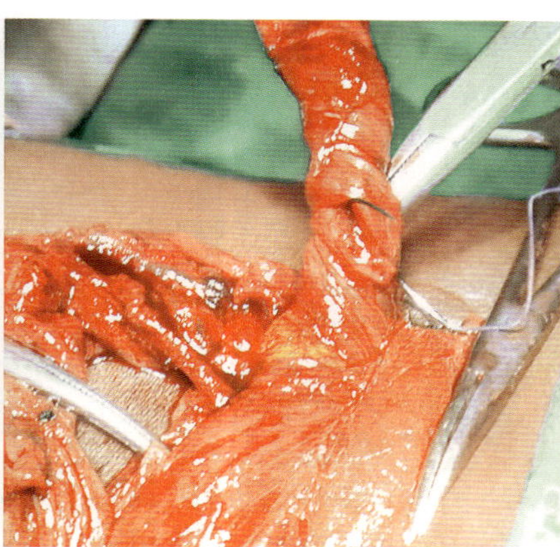

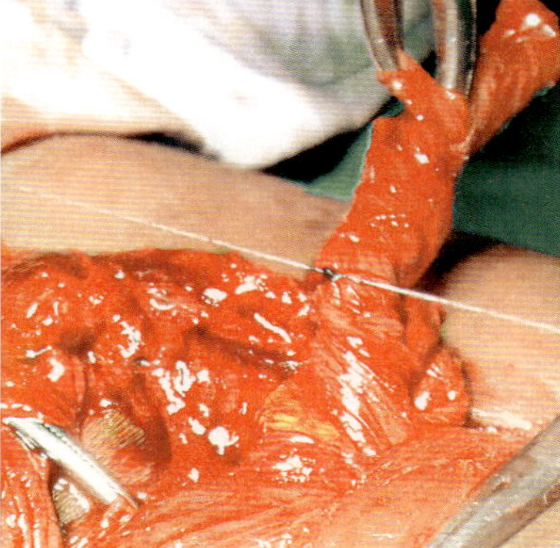

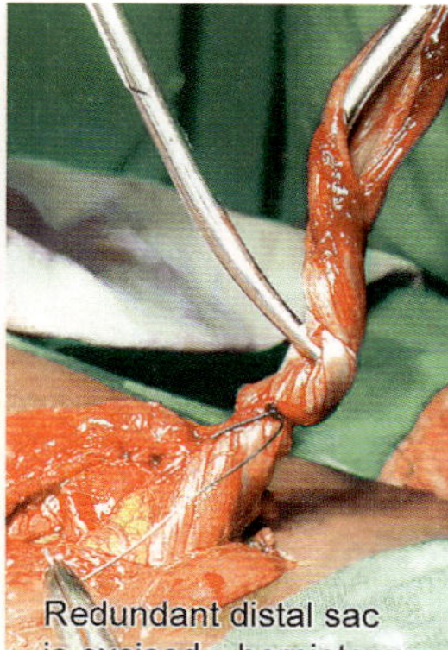

Fig. 19-35: Technique of transfixation of the sac.

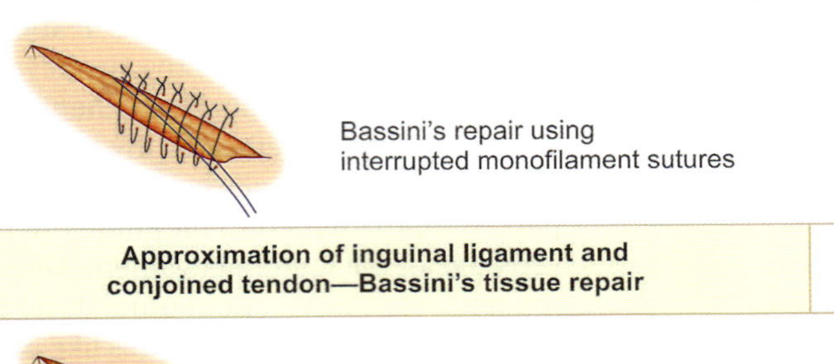

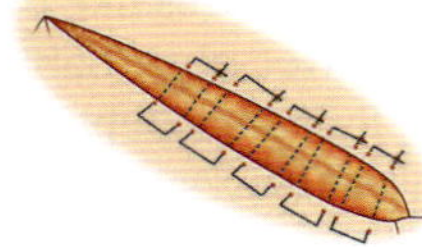

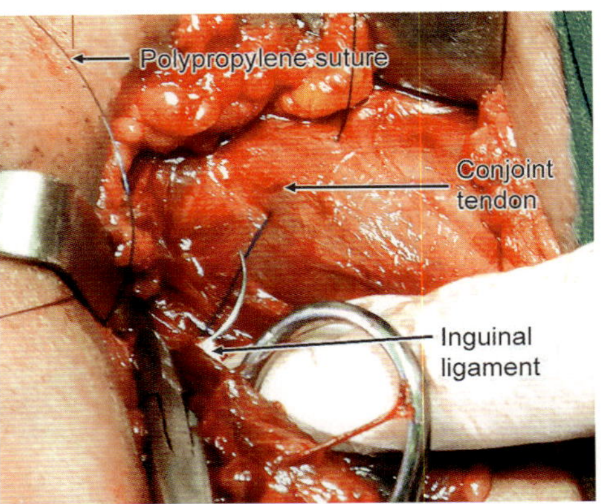

Fig. 19-36: Bassini's tissue repair. It is not commonly used now; it is useful in strangulated inguinal hernia or when there is infection where mesh is contraindicated.

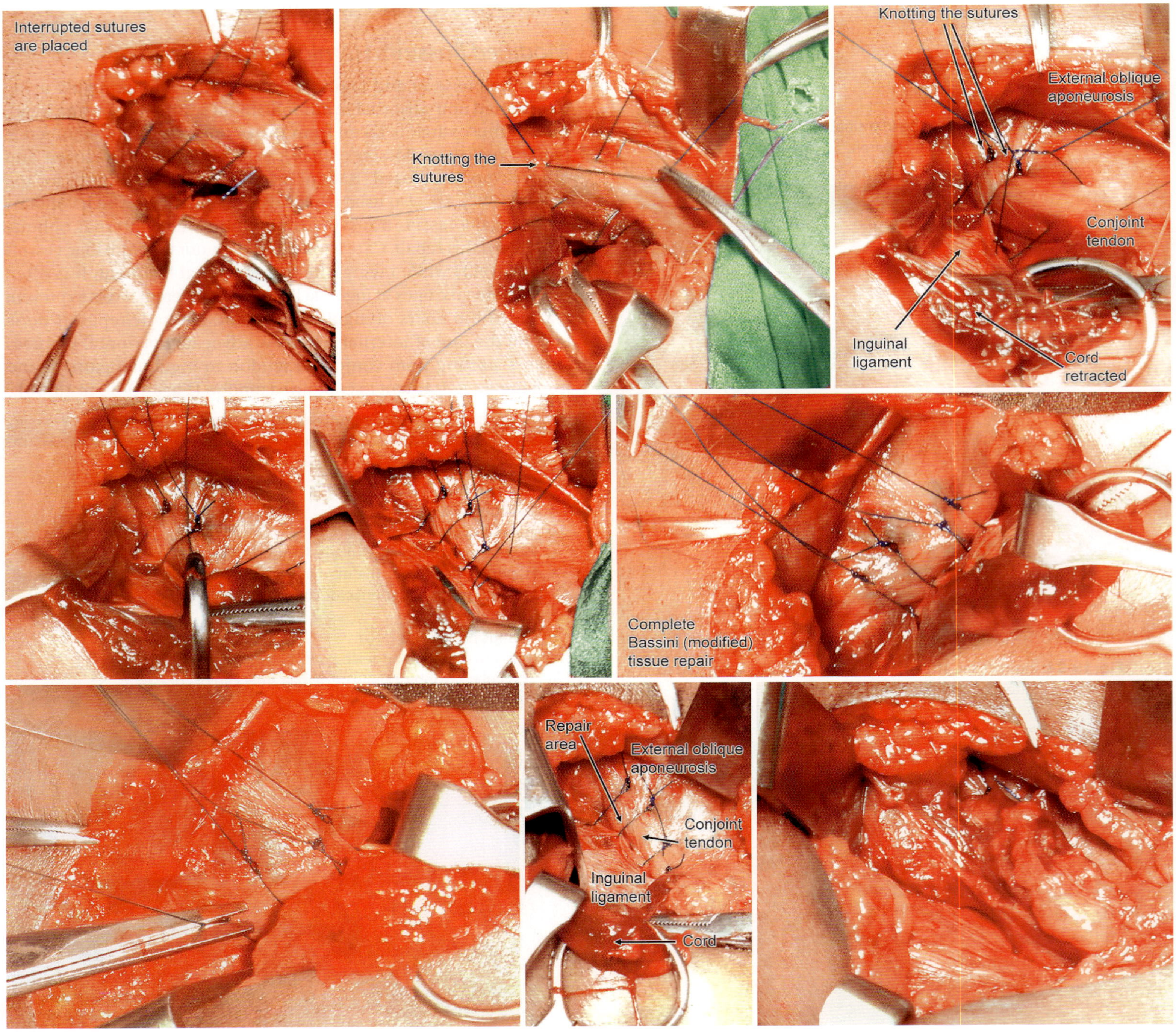

Fig. 19-37: Bassini's repair. It is a type of tissue repair.

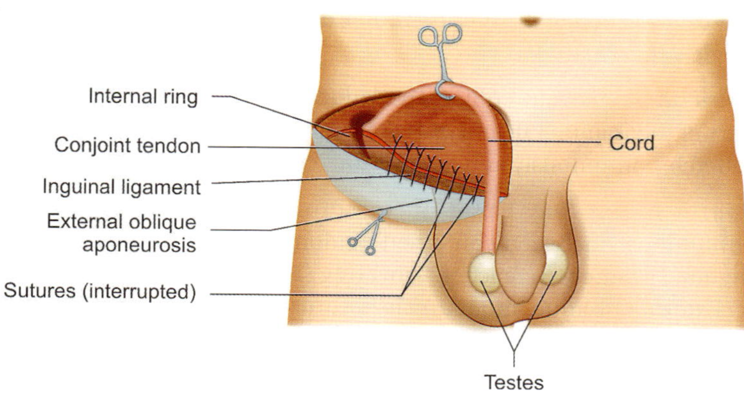

Fig. 19-38: Modified Bassini repair.

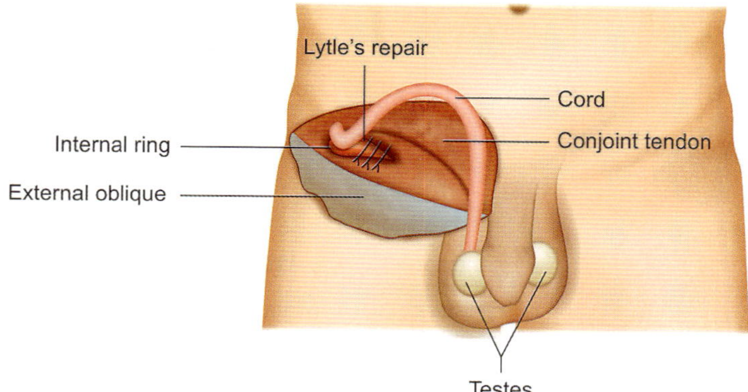

Fig. 19-39: Lytle's repair is narrowing the internal ring.

Lytle's Repair (William James Lytle)

Often internal ring is narrowed by placing interrupted sutures over the medial side of the ring to the transversalis fascia using either silk or polypropylene (to narrow the ring and push the cord laterally) **(Fig. 19-39)**.

Halsted (USA)—Tanner (London) Slide Operation

To reduce the tension in the repair area, relaxing incision is placed over the lower rectus sheath so that conjoined tendon is allowed to slide downwards **(Fig. 19-40)**.

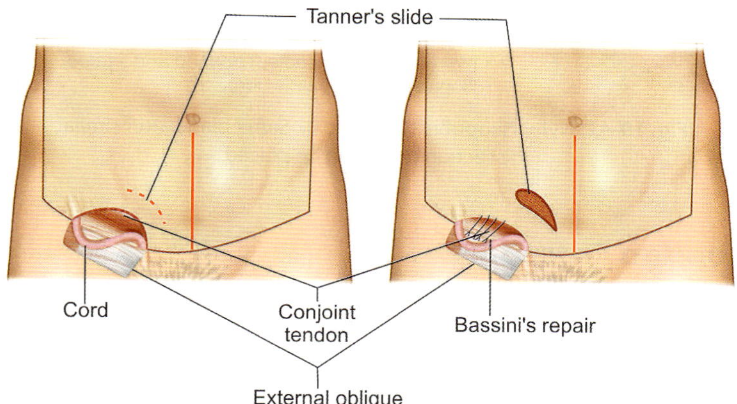

Fig. 19-40: Tanner slide operation.

Abrahamson Nylon Darning

Continuous intervening network of non-absorbable sutures are placed between conjoined tendon and inguinal ligament to give good support to posterior inguinal wall **(Fig. 19-41)**.

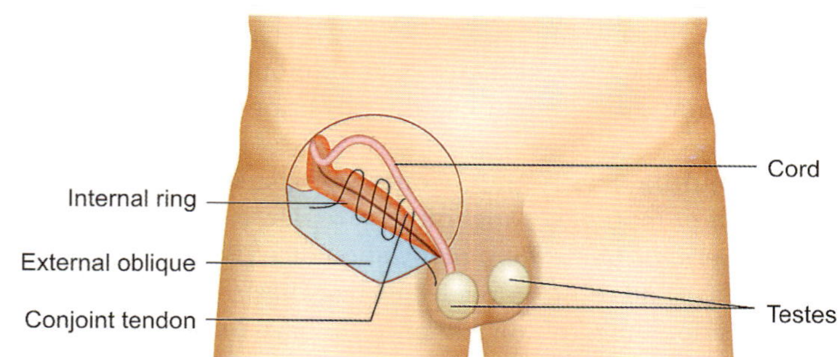

Fig. 19-41: Darning in inguinal hernia.

Koontz Operation (Koontz AR—New York, 1963)

In old people after taking consent, orchidectomy is done along with removal of full cord, testis and total closure of posterior inguinal wall by repair so as to reduce the recurrence.

Removal of Cord in the Inguinal Canal

Cord is removed from the inguinal canal by ligating both at external and internal ring. But testis is retained (for psychological reason) and closure of inguinal canal by repair is done.

Mc Vay Operation—1940 (Cooper's Ligament Repair)

It is repaired by placing interrupted sutures between the edge of transversus abdominis to Copper's ligament starting from pubic tubercle medially towards femoral sheath and later continued as suture repair between transversus abdominis and iliopubic tract laterally up to the entrance of cord. It is a pure tissue repair. It requires relaxing vertical/curvilinear oblique incision at the lateral border of the anterior rectus sheath from pubic tubercle to a point superiorly for 4 cm. It covers all three groin defects (myopectineal orifice)—indirect, direct and femoral.

Nyhus (Original) Iliopubic Repair

To have a suprainguinal approach, a transverse incision is made two fingerbreadths above the pubic symphysis to expose the rectus sheath. Left index finger is passed into the external ring; level of internal ring is confirmed. Anterior rectus sheath is incised horizontally above the level of the deep ring; lateral part of lower end of the rectus is retracted. Posterior rectus sheath is opened. External oblique, internal oblique and transversus abdominis muscles are cut along the length of the incision. Transversalis fascia is cut to reach the preperitoneal space. If it is direct sac it is dissected without opening and isolated. Sac is inverted using absorbable purse string suture. If it is an indirect sac, it is dissected proximally high up, opened and ligated. Transaponeurotic arch (transverse abdominis muscle and transversalis fascia) is sutured below to Copper's ligament and iliopubic tract. Nyhus mesh repair is done similarly through this approach by placing mesh and suturing to Cooper's ligament **(Fig. 19-42)**.

Andrew's Operation

It is overlapping of the external oblique aponeurosis.

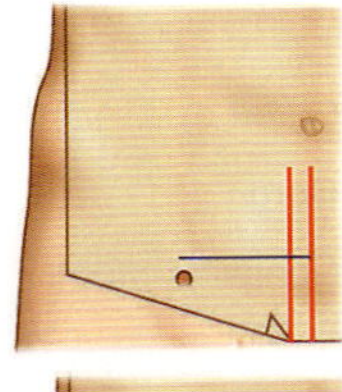

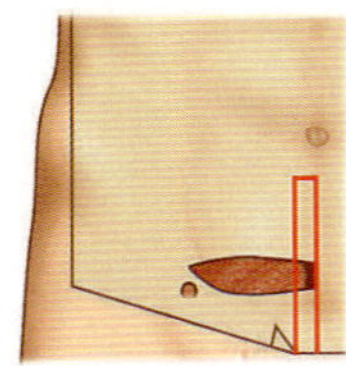

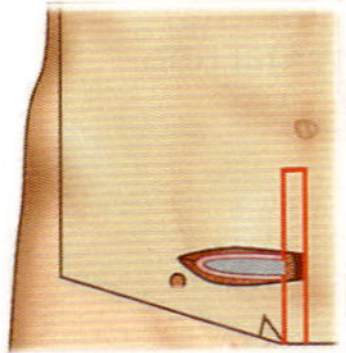

Fig. 19-42: Nyhus iliopubic tissue repair. Same plane after similar dissection mesh can be placed.

Condon Procedure

It is anterior iliopubic tract repair wherein the transversus abdominis is sutured to iliopubic tract from pubic tubercle to deep ring; then extending lateral to the cord. In direct sac relaxing incision is made on the lower rectus before tying all placed sutures.

Shouldice Repair

Even though transversalis fascia is thin, it is a tough layer and so double breasting of this fascia using continuous sutures (with non-absorbable material) strengthens the posterior wall of the inguinal canal.

It is a multilayered repair. Continuous sutures provide *even distribution of tension* throughout the repair. It was originated at *Shouldice hernia clinic in Toronto* by Shouldice (EE Shouldice, 1930) where it was usually done under local anaesthesia. Often cremasteric resection is done in Shouldice in order to have proper revelation of the posterior inguinal wall. Cremasteric vessels (located at lateral part of the cord along with genital branch of genitofemoral nerve) need ligation during cremasterectomy. After doing herniotomy as in any other inguinal hernia, transversalis fascia is incised along the line of the wound from deep ring to pubic tubercle. Upper medial flap is elevated without elevating lower lateral flap. If there is redundant part of the transversalis fascia it should be excised to leave adequate amount of clean cut edges. Superior pubic vein is located on the deeper surface of the iliopubic tract which should not be injured while operating. Cribriform fascia of thigh is incised deep to the inguinal ligament to free the lateral flap of external oblique aponeurosis and also to visualise femoral opening.

First suture line: Lower lateral flap of fascia is sutured to posterior deep part of the elevated upper flap using continuous sutures from pubic tubercle to internal ring which is tied at deep ring without cutting/ending.

Second suture line: Using same suture which is not cut, free margin of upper flap is sutured to the shelving edge of the inguinal ligament from deep ring towards pubic tubercle. It causes double-breasting of the transversalis fascia. Knot is placed at the end over the pubic tubercle. First and second line sutures are done using a single suture material.

Third suture line: The conjoined tendon and anterior to the shelving part of the inguinal ligament is sutured from internal ring to pubic tubercle continuously and tied without cutting.

Fourth suture line: Same uncut suture is again sutured back continuously between conjoined tendon and anterior fibres of the inguinal ligament to reach internal ring **(Figs. 19-43A to J)**.

External oblique aponeurosis is sutured in two layers (5th and 6th suture lines; double-breasting) in front of the cord in original Shouldice repair. Hence this original Shouldice repair is 6 layered procedure. First two layers of transversalis fascia, next two layers of conjoined tendon and last two layers of external oblique aponeurosis. Suture material used here is 34 gauge fine steel wire (in original Shouldice repair) or polypropylene or polyethylene. Nowadays external oblique is sutured as a single layer. Often it is difficult to close external oblique aponeurosis. Medial part of the cut end of the cremaster is sutured to pubic bone or inguinal ligament to prevent drooping of the testis. Recurrence rate in Shouldice repair is 1%.

Berliner modified Shouldice repair: It involves double-breasting of the transversalis fascia like in Shouldice repair and single layer closure of the external oblique aponeurosis without any additional two-layered repair of conjoined tendon to inguinal ligament.

Desarda Tension Free Tissue Repair

Desarda no mesh tension free tissue repair (Professor Mohan Desarda, Pune, India): It is live external oblique tissue flap reconstruction of the posterior wall of the inguinal canal. He proposed that strength of the inguinal canal depends on the aponeurotic extensions from the transverse abdominis aponeurotic arch normally which is physiologically dynamic and strong and his repair supports this effectively with least complications and recurrence. Inguinal canal is approached like usual hernia repair surgery. Indirect sac is dissected and ligated high using vicryl. Direct sac is not opened but buried by placing purse string sutures or interrupted mattress sutures over the transversalis fascia. Edge of upper leaf of the cut external oblique aponeurosis is sutured to the inguinal ligament below using continuous or interrupted polypropylene sutures. Cord should be outside this suture line. Upper leaf of sutured external oblique aponeurosis is incised horizontally around 1.5 cm above the sutured line; this incision extends laterally up to the internal ring level and medially up to the rectus sheath near midline. Lower edge of this newly cut part of the upper leaf of the external oblique is sutured to the conjoined tendon underneath using interrupted polypropylene sutures adequately. New upper cut part of the upper leaf of the external oblique is sutured to the edge of the original lower leaf in front of the cord structure. So live transposed external oblique acts as natural tissue prosthesis to support the posterior part of the inguinal canal. This technique said to have low recurrence rate with avoiding the placement of mesh (foreign body) with minimal complications **(Figs. 19-44 to 19-47)**.

Repair of Sliding Hernia

In *LaRoque repair* deep ring is incised above and below; reefing of the sigmoid colon mesentery is done which forms the posterior wall of the inguinal canal so that entire sigmoid is replaced into

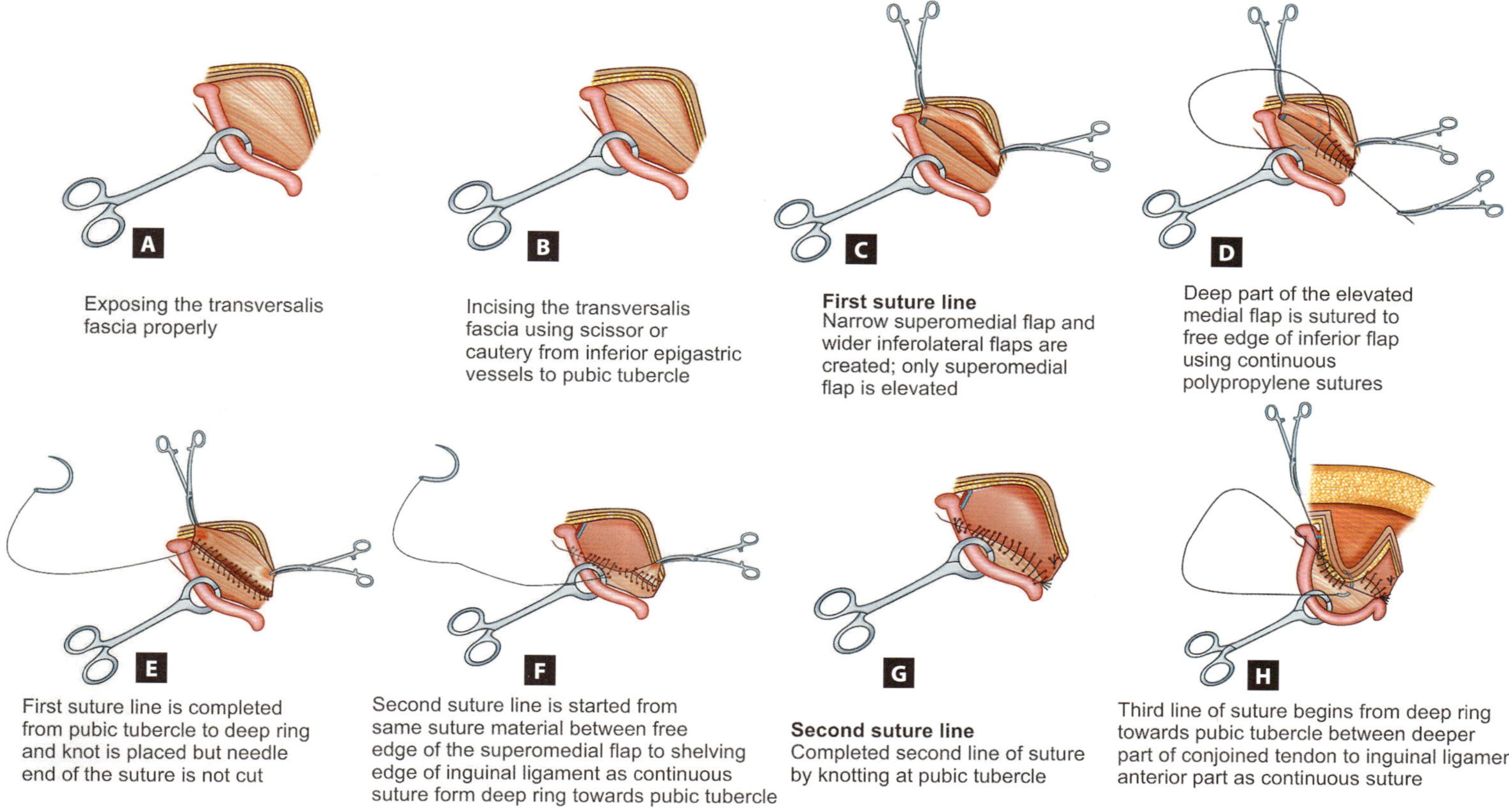

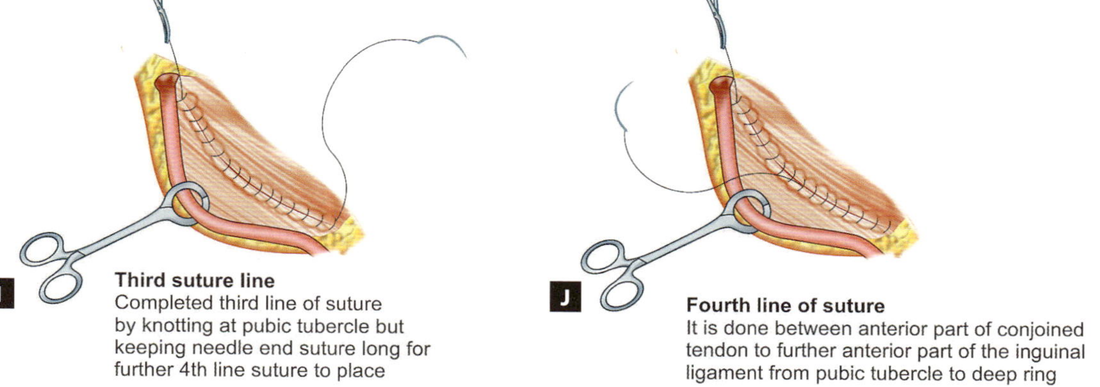

Figs. 19-43A to J: Technique of Shouldice repair.

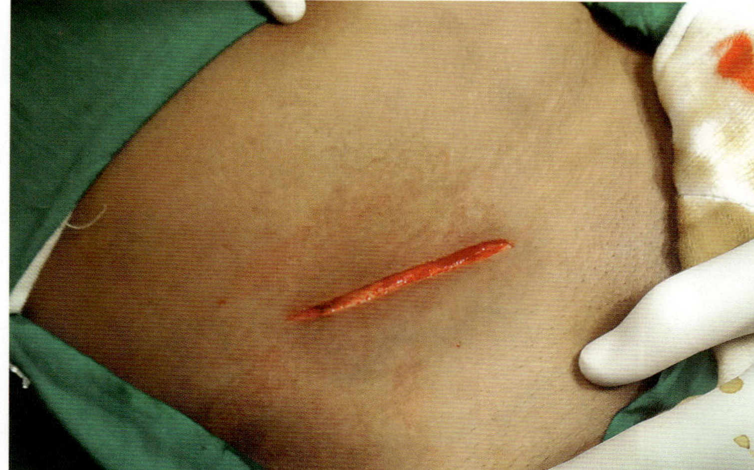

Fig. 19-44: Incision for Desarda technique is similar as other anterior open inguinal approach.

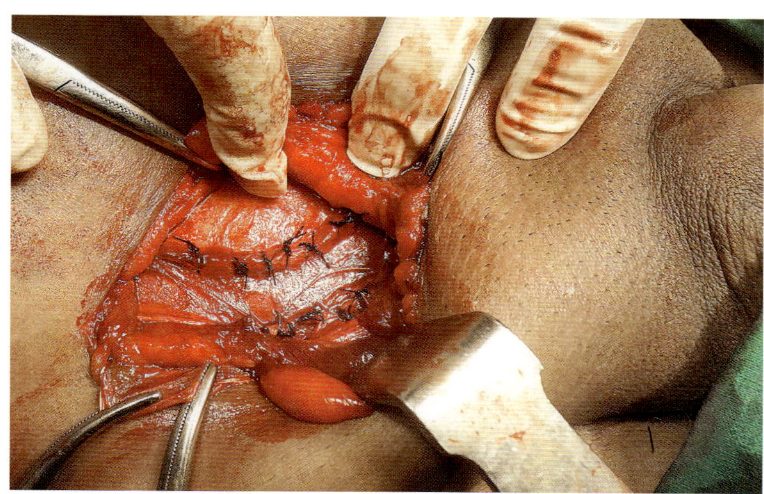

Fig. 19-45: Final look of Desarda—no mesh tension free tissue repair for inguinal hernia.

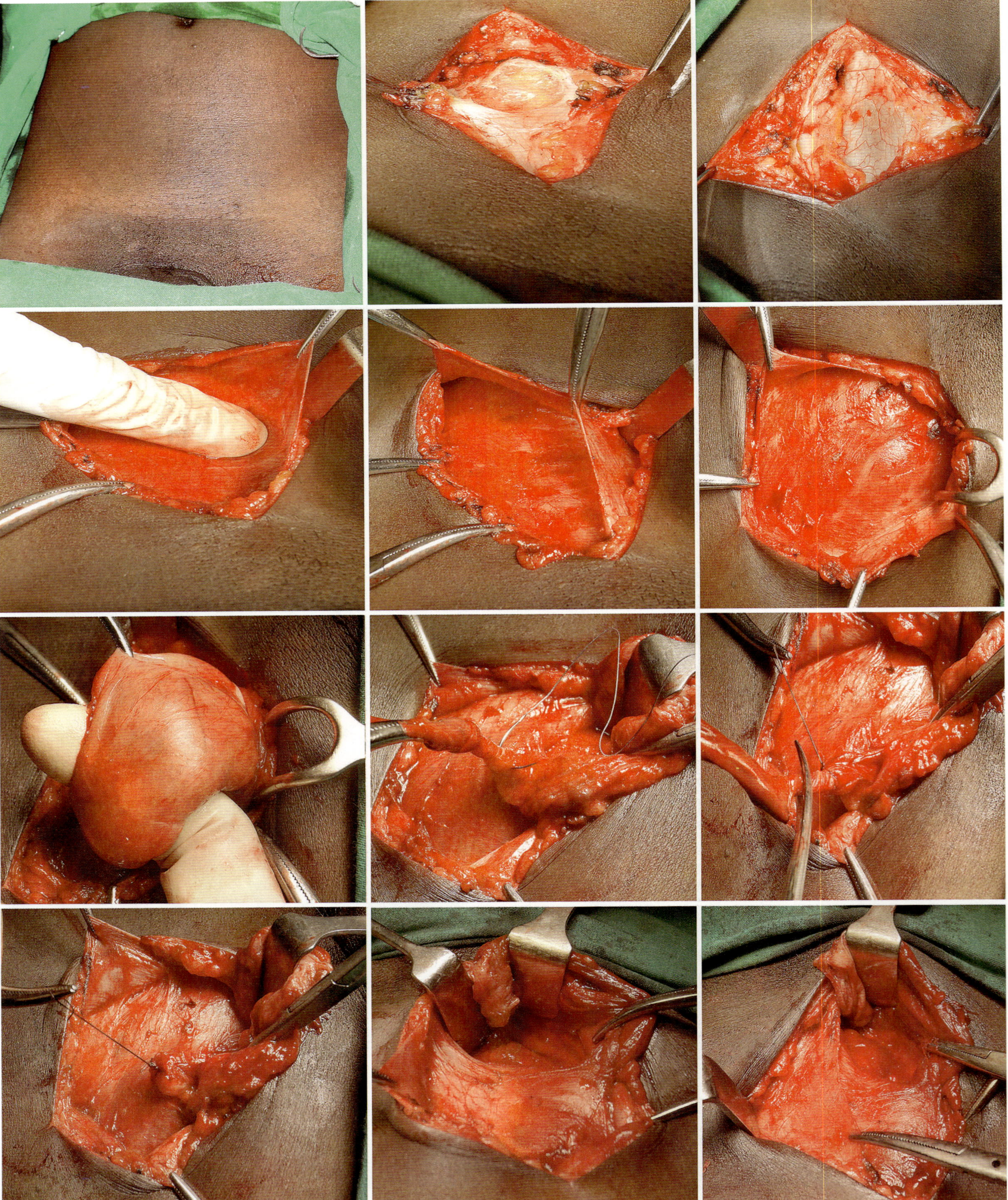

Figs. 19-46(1)

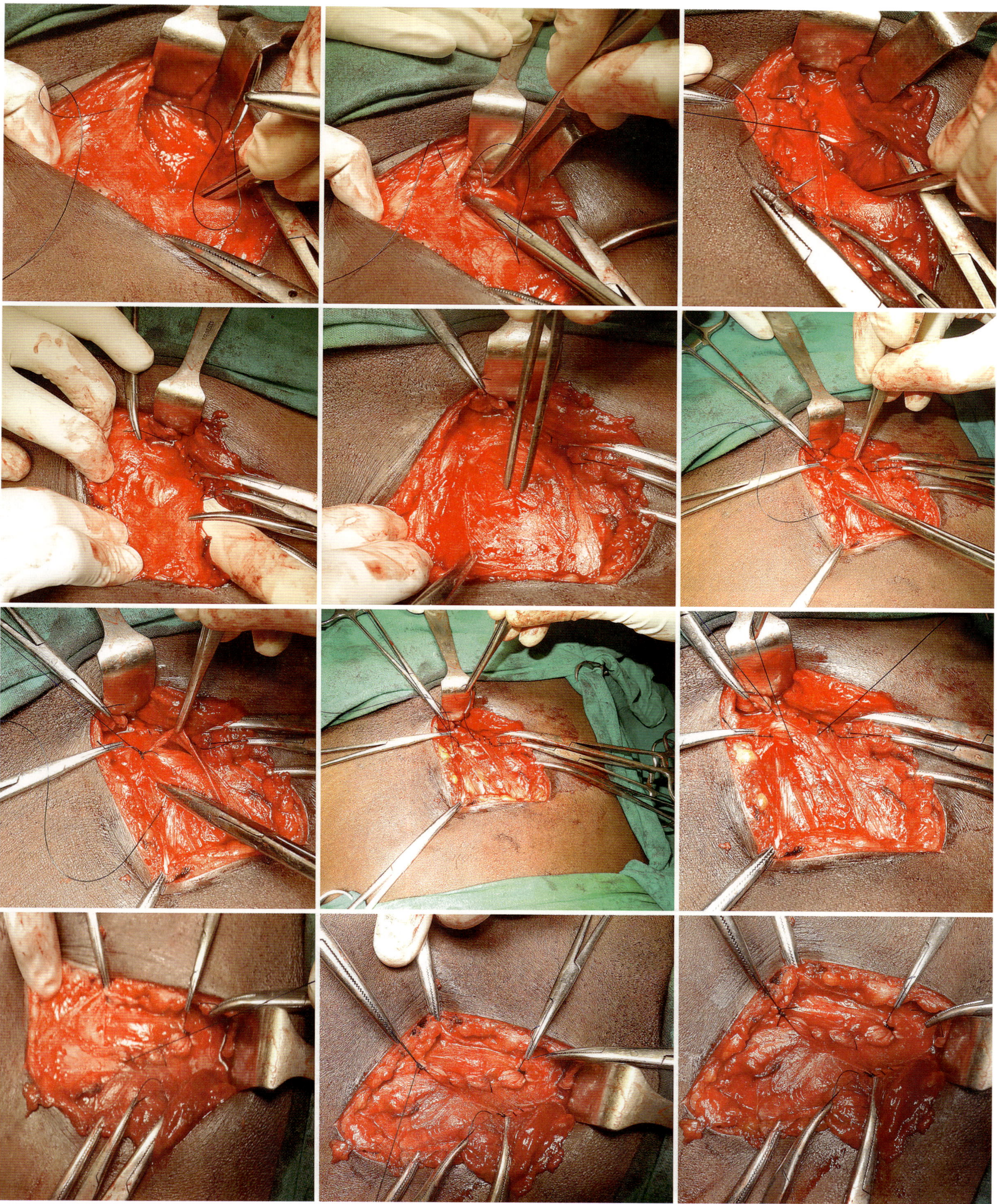

Figs. 19-46(2)

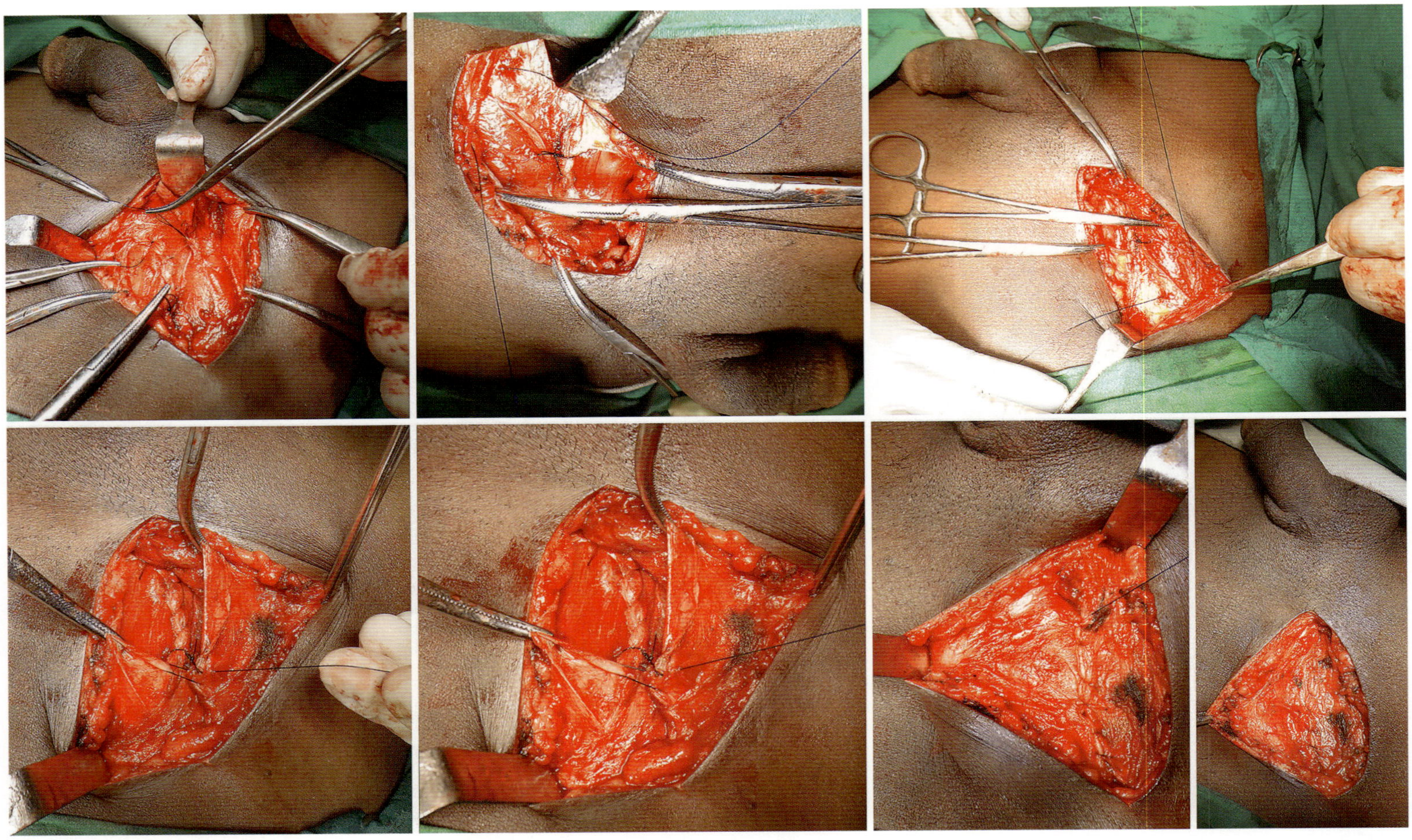

Figs. 19-46(3)

Figs. 19-46(1 to 3): Technique of Desarda repair in an indirect inguinal hernia repair. Here continuous suture is placed on both edges.

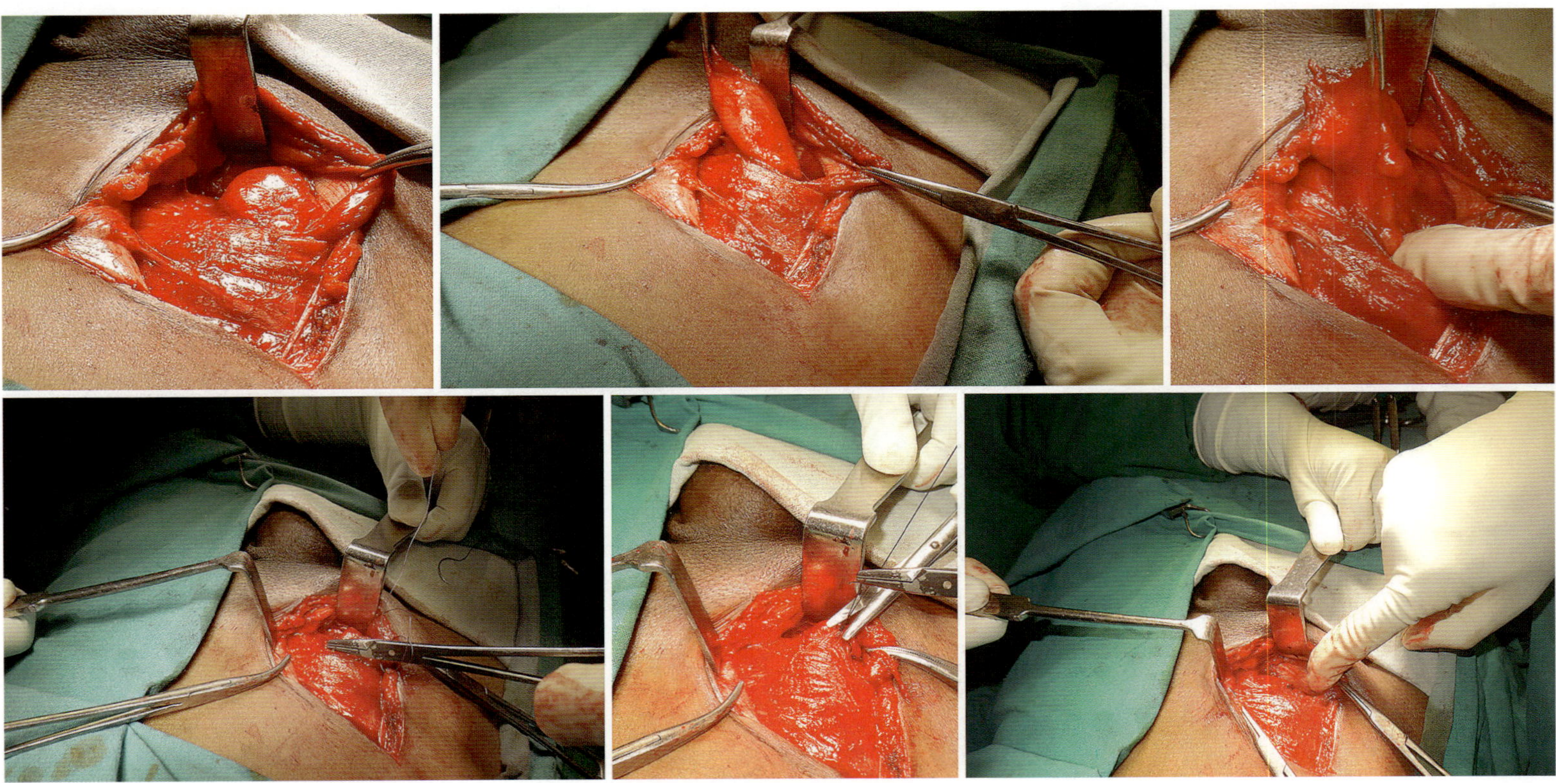

Figs. 19-47(1)

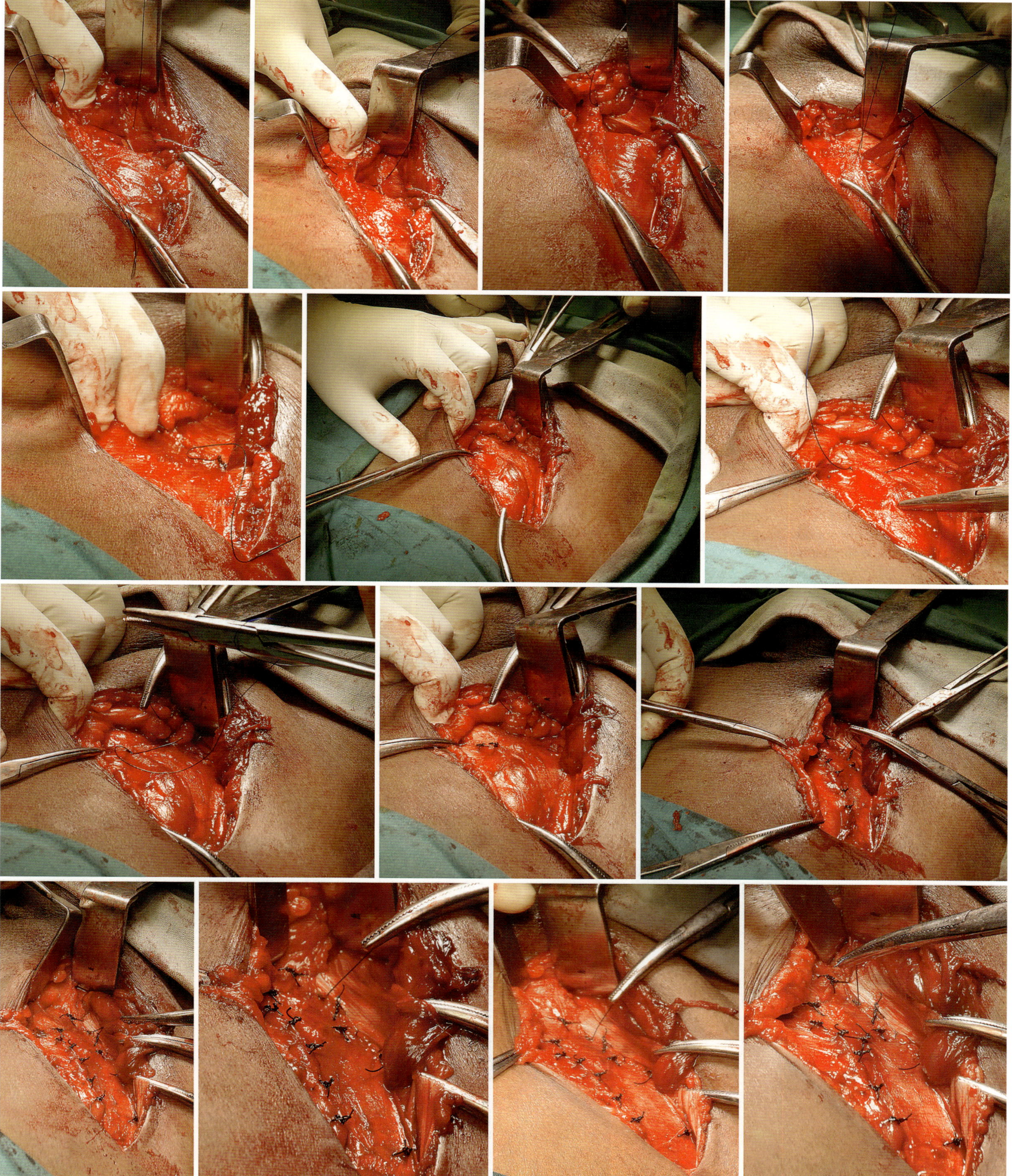

Figs. 19-47(2)

Figs. 19-47(1 and 2): Desarda technique in a direct inguinal hernia repair; here interrupted sutures are placed in the upper part—suturing to the conjoint tendon.

the peritoneal cavity. Posterior wall of the sac should not be separated from large bowel or bladder. If tried it may lead to faecal or urinary fistulas. Often sac can be excised partially; this partially excised sac can be pushed into peritoneal cavity. Right sided sliding hernia will have caecum and appendix in its posterior wall; caecum should not be separated from posterior wall of the sac which may otherwise create faecal fistula. Appendix should not be removed as it may precipitate sepsis. Appendices epiploicae from sigmoid colon should not be removed as there are chances that they may contain small colonic diverticula which may get opened to contaminate the field. Bladder will be present on medial side of the sac and sac should not be separated; if bladder injury occurs it should be sutured in two layers of vicryl. Inside out purse string suture on the opened sac is applied and the sac with its posterior wall is pushed into the abdominal cavity. Urinary catheterisation is a must **(Figs. 19-48 and 19-49)**.

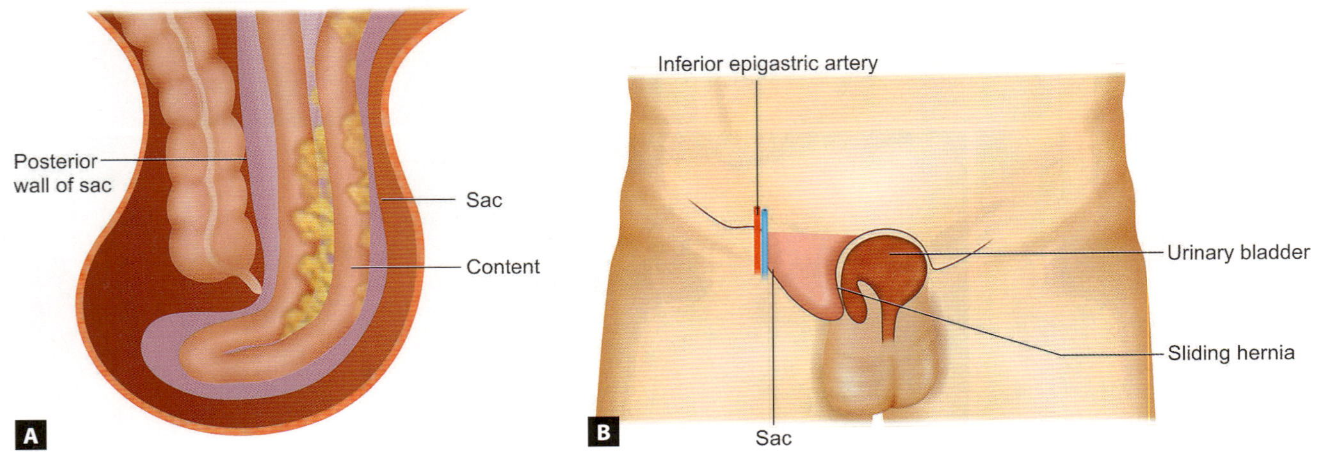

Figs. 19-48A and B: Sliding hernia is common in left side; exclusively seen in males. Posterior wall of the sac should not be separated in sliding hernia; if done will injure the colon or urinary bladder. Insertion of urinary catheter is a must prior to surgery. It is usually indirect type; huge hernia which is often irreducible is typical. Posterior wall is formed by sigmoid colon or urinary bladder. Contents are small bowel and omentum.

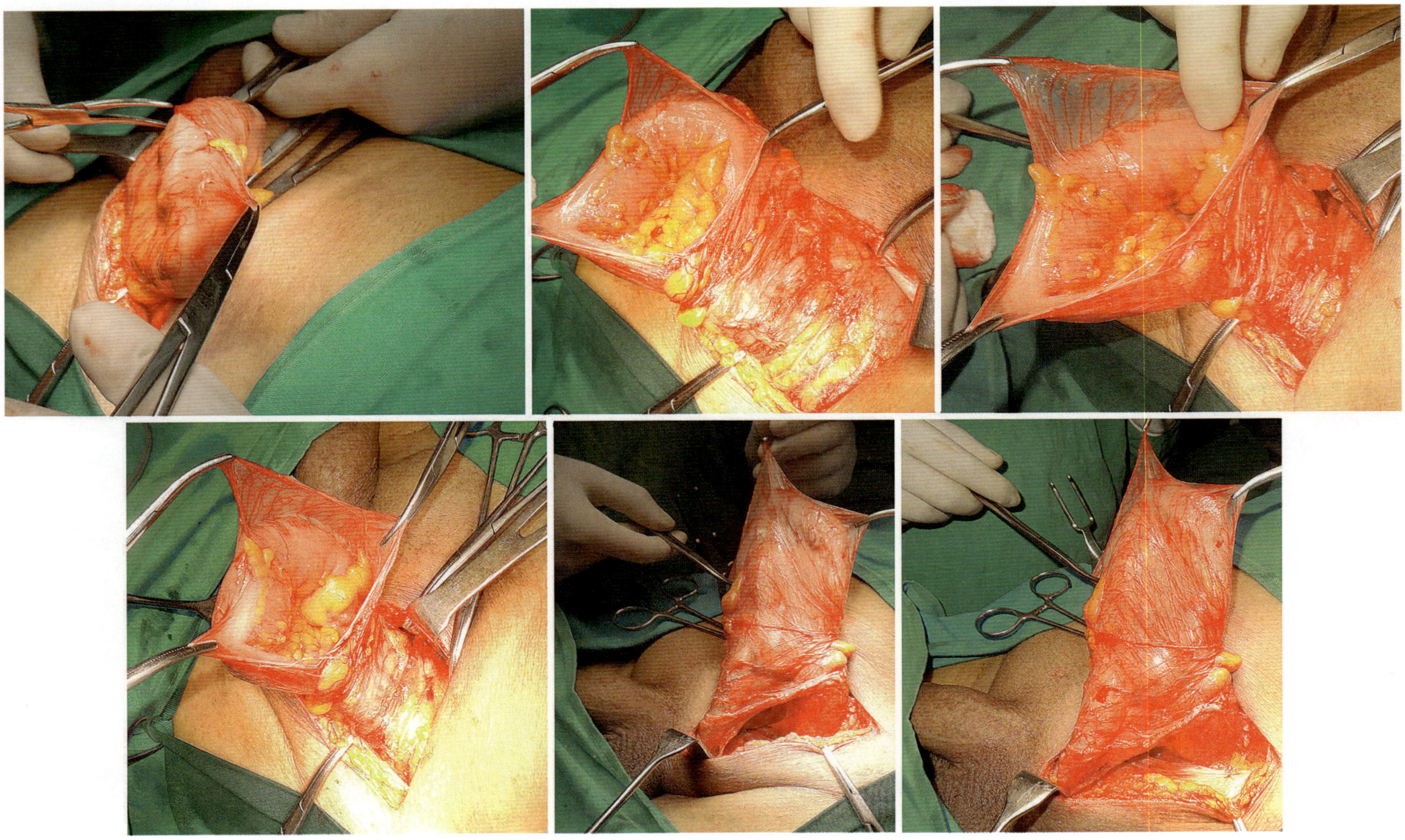

Fig. 19-49: Sliding hernia—on table.

Hernioplasty (Figs. 19-50 and 19-51)

Approach to preperitoneal space

Anterior transinguinal approach (Anandale)
- Condon approach.
- Rive's repair.

Posterior approach
- Suprainguinal (Nyhus).
- Grid iron (Kugel's).
- Midline: Cheatle-Henry's-Stoppa's GPRVS.
- McEvedy's: Oblique incision (rectus sheath).
- Laparoscopic: TEP (Dulucq); TAPP (Arrigue/Dion and Morin).

Advantages of preperitoneal approach are: **Less chance of** damage to nerves, spermatic cord and testicular atrophy. It is most tension free approach. Entire MPO in Bogros space is covered with prosthesis beyond the pubic symphysis (beyond 2.5 cm) and anterior superior iliac spine (2.5 cm). Coverage should be 2/3rd over anterior abdominal wall; 1/3rd beyond and below Cooper's ligament.

Disadvantages are: It involves more extensive dissection of preperitoneal space; requires larger mesh reinforcement; it makes future entry for surgical approach difficult (especially for uro/vascular surgeries). Risk of damage to major vessel (iliac vein), bowel and bladder, extraperitoneal haematoma are high.

Selection for posterior approach: All recurrences after anterior/onlay repairs; all Nyhus type 3 and 4 hernias; incarceration; TEPP to open conversion. It is *avoided* in patients who are unfit for regional anaesthesia, bleeding tendency, concurrently with TURP/bladder surgery, known malignancy.

Technical tips and requirements are: good visibility and retraction, regional/ideally general anaesthesia, exact full knowledge of preperitoneal anatomy (both for operating surgeon and camera man/assistant). Larger mesh (15 x 15/15 x 10 cm) is needed; two point fixation to Cooper's ligament.

Complications are: haematoma (avoid in patients taking aspirin/clopidogrel); seroma—in inguinal/scrotal space—aspiration is done.

Recurrences are due to: inadequate creation of space, inadequate mesh overlap, mesh migration—(fixation to Cooper's ligament is needed mainly in direct defect).

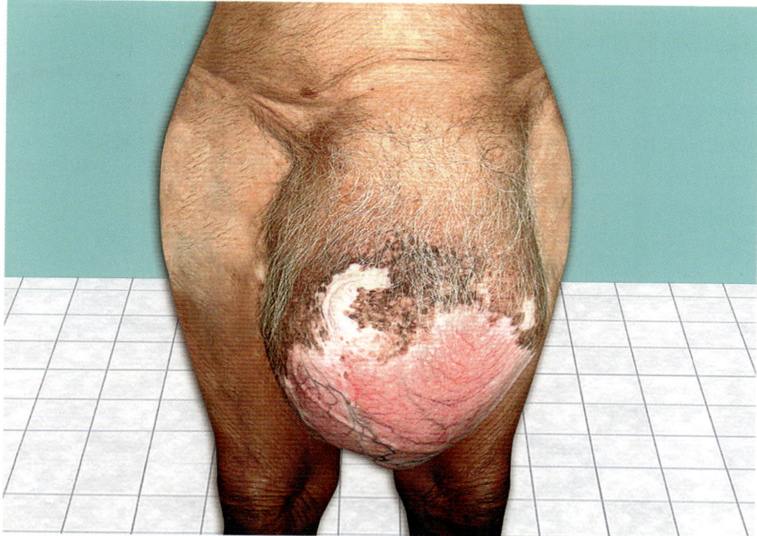

Fig. 19-50: Giant inguinal hernia. It requires open hernioplasty.

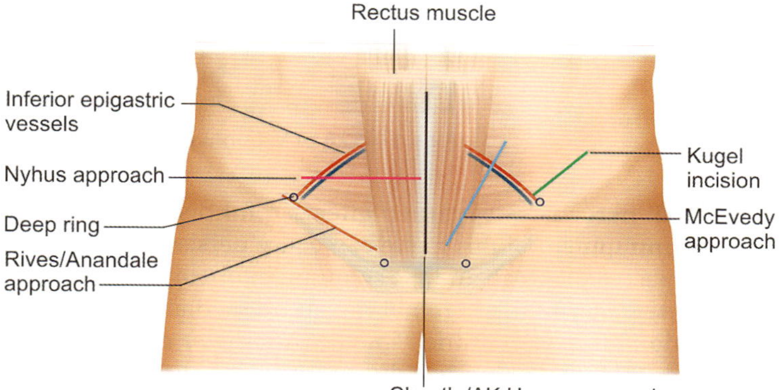

Fig. 19-51: Different approaches for preperitoneal inguinal hernia (groin hernia) surgeries.

Lichtenstein's Inguinal Hernia Mesh Repair Under Local Anaesthesia

20 mL of xylocaine 2% mixed with 10 mL of bupivacaine 0.5%, 50 mL of normal saline, 1 mL of 1:1000 adrenaline solution with hyalase solution is used for local anaesthesia. Different combinations are in use. 50:50 of xylocaine 1% with 0.5% bupivacaine with 1 in 2,00,000 epinephrine in normal saline is also used. 45–50 mL of this prepared solution is sufficient. Propofol sedation with intravenous drip may be added. Anaesthetic agent is injected layer by layer. 5 mL is injected into subdermal plane along the line of incision using 25 G long needle; 3 mL is injected intradermally; 10–20 mL is injected deep subcutaneously. After skin and subcutaneous incision, subaponeurotic injection of anaesthetic agent is done (10 mL) first at lateral end of the incision to anaesthetise all three nerves of the inguinal canal; then along the line of the incision up to the pubic tubercle.

Procedure

After cleaning and draping, line of skin incision is marked using marking pen at 1.25 cm above and parallel to the medial 2/3rd of inguinal ligament. Using 24 G or 26 G long spinal needle, prepared anaesthetic agent is injected into the skin underneath along the marked line of incision and into the subcutaneous plane below and above. Skin is incised. Using cautery or scalpel blade skin incision is deepened. Two layers of superficial fascia, outer Camper and inner Scarpa's fascia are incised. Often these superficial epigastric, superficial circumflex, superficial external pudendal veins are ligated using fine absorbable sutures (3-zero vicryl/catgut). External oblique aponeurosis is identified by its shining fibres. It is exposed above, below up to inguinal ligament and medially up to pubic tubercle and midline. Around 20 mL of local anaesthetic solution is injected underneath the external oblique aponeurosis medially and laterally. External oblique aponeurosis is incised using no. 15 scalpel blade or cautery. Cut edges of the aponeurosis are held with artery forceps. Aponeurosis is incised medially and laterally along the line of the incision. Medially it is extended often up to the external ring to open it. Two leaves of the aponeurosis are elevated above to visualise the conjoined tendon and below to visualize the shining inguinal ligament (Poupart's). Self-retaining mastoid retractor can be used to expose the canal clearly. Iliohypogastric nerve is identified above and medially which after piercing the internal oblique enters the external oblique. In the inguinal canal cord is covered by cremasteric muscle and internal spermatic fascia; external spermatic fascia covers the cord below the level of the superficial inguinal ring. Ilioinguinal nerve is in the inguinal canal outside the cord which enters the canal through a gap between external and internal oblique muscles, passes through superficial inguinal ring. Genital branch of genitofemoral nerve passes through the cord structures. Both nerves supply the (L1) anterior 1/3rd of the scrotum and penis. Posterior 2/3rd of the scrotum is supplied by the posterior scrotal nerves and perineal branch of the posterior cutaneous nerve of the thigh (S3).

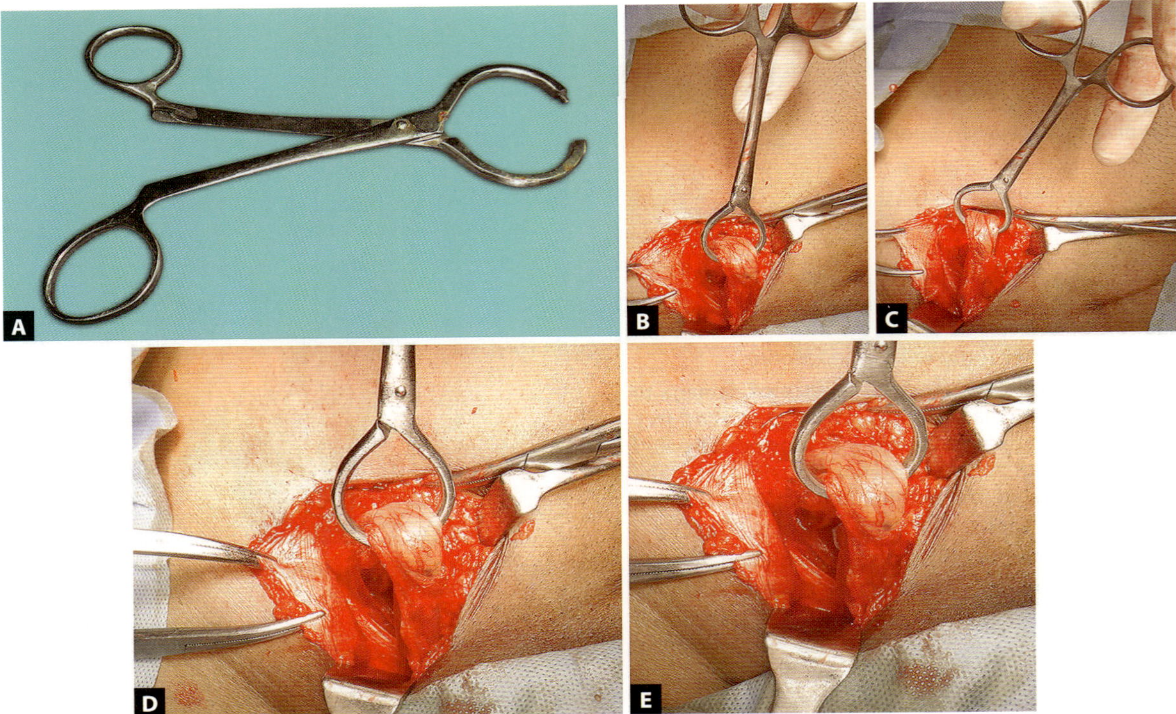

Figs. 19-52A to E: Cunnigham's cord holding forceps—it is used in open inguinal hernia repair.

Ilioinguinal nerve is safeguarded after careful dissection. Partial injury or entrapment of this nerve can cause persistent pain in the medial aspect of the thigh and the scrotum. Injury to iliohypogastric nerve causes pain in the inguinal region on medial aspect and in lower abdomen near midline. This *inguinodynia* may be due to entrapment by suture or mesh or due to partial injury of these nerves. Complete transection of the nerve can cause anaesthesia of skin of this region **(Figs. 19-52 and 19-53)**.

Cremaster muscle (cremaster box) is opened. Many advocate excision of cremaster to achieve good repair but it causes loss of support to cord and testis causing *"clapper in bell"* like problem due to hanging testis. Chances of inguinodynia are increased as the protection to genital nerve and paravasal nerves is removed. Even though it is not proved it is thought that one of the causes of distressing dysejaculation could be due to cremaster dysfunction after cremasterectomy. Medial dissection is done beyond the pubic tubercle. Hernial sac is identified. Sac is pearly white in colour which is anterolateral in position with respect to cord in case of indirect sac. Fundus, body and neck of the sac are dissected using scissor or cautery. Cord is held using hernia ring (Collingwood Stewart) or thin gauze or penrose drain and kept aside (usually below the inguinal ligament). Cord is dissected 2 cm beyond the pubic tubercle. Neck of the sac is identified by its narrow area, being lateral to inferior epigastric vessels and by presence of extraperitoneal pad of fat. Sac is dissected *high up above* the level of the internal ring ***(high dissection)***; sac is opened on the summit of the fundus; held with two artery forceps; finger is passed into the sac to confirm that all contents are reduced; if not, by finger dissection adhesions are released and contents are reduced completely; sac is twisted adequately so that no contents will return back to the sac during ligation; sac is transfixed high above the internal ring using 3 zero vicryl or monocryl and ligated. Presently it is thought that high dissection is more important than high ligation; but usually it is common to advocate high ligation of the sac. Redundant sac is excised to complete the herniotomy. There is presently a debate on ligation of sac as ligation of sac increases the chances of postoperative pain due to mechanical pressure, ischaemia and irritation of somatic peritoneal nerve. It is also found that without ligation of indirect sac will not increase the chances of recurrence **(Fig. 19-54)**.

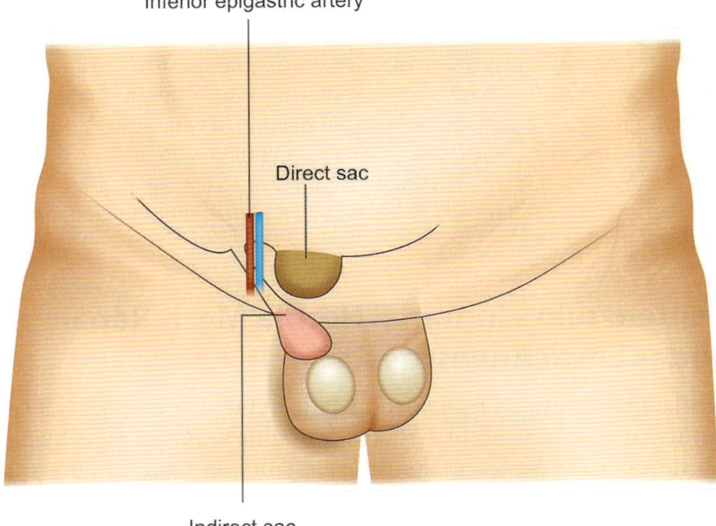

Fig. 19-53: In case of direct sac, always one should dissect the cord and look for indirect sac (pantaloon hernia); otherwise if present and missed recurrence can occur.

If sac is extending into the scrotum as complete type and if there is difficulty in dissecting such sac from scrotum, then distal part of the sac is left in situ open after transecting at superficial ring level. Important aspect here is distal part of the sac should not be ligated *(Wantz technique)* and if ligated it will lead into hydrocele. In direct hernia, sac is medial to inferior epigastric vessels and is usually not opened unless there is obstruction. Direct sac is pushed underneath. Transversalis fascia is identified and cut along the line of incision obliquely as medial lower and lateral upper flaps. It is common to do plication of this fascia even though it is not mandatory (using continuous non-absorbable monofilament polypropylene sutures) **(Figs. 19-55 and 19-56)**.

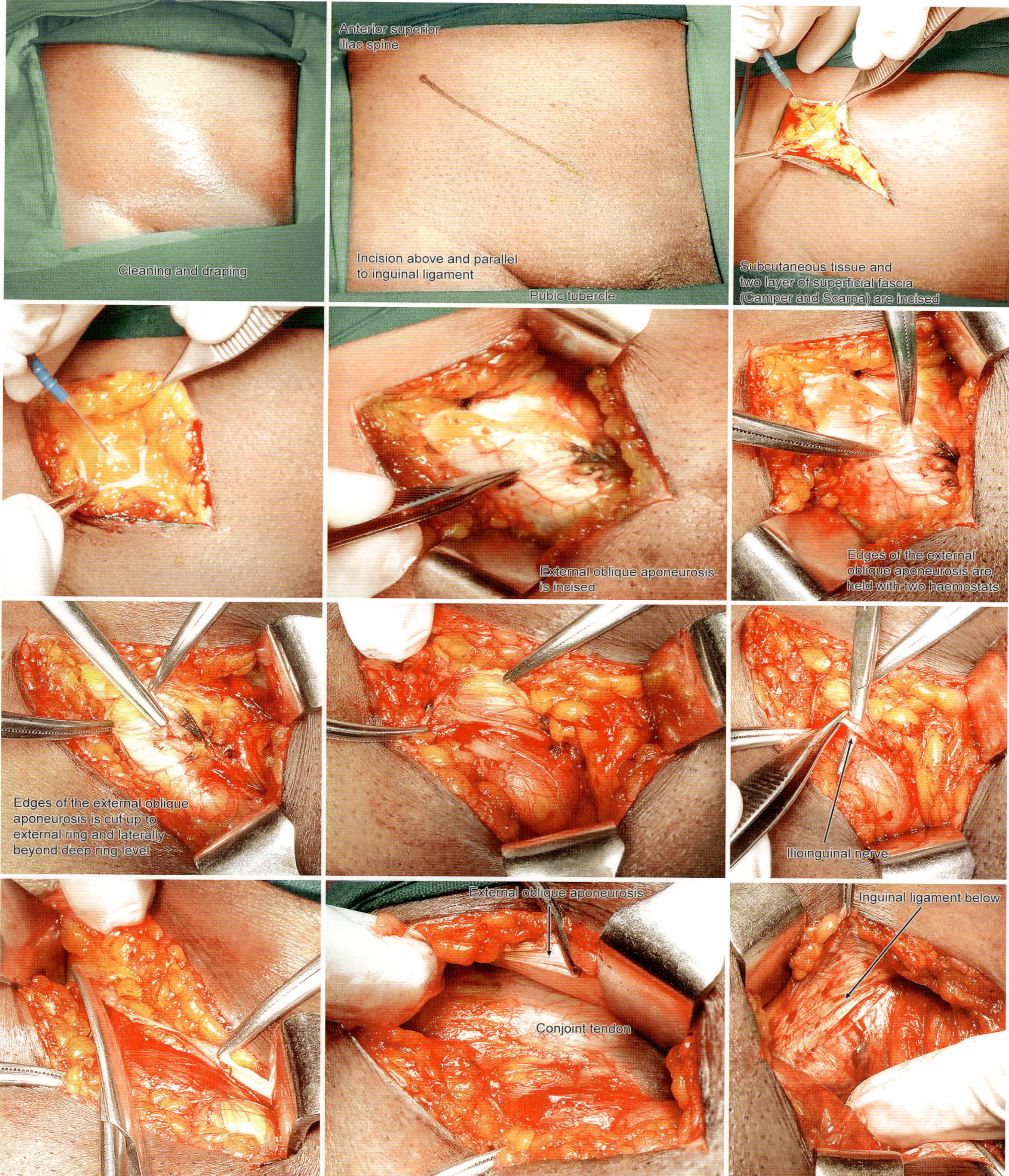
Cleaning and draping
Anterior superior iliac spine
Incision above and parallel to inguinal ligament
Pubic tubercle
Subcutaneous tissue and two layer of superficial fascia (Camper and Scarpa) are incised
External oblique aponeurosis is incised
Edges of the external oblique aponeurosis are held with two haemostats
Edges of the external oblique aponeurosis is cut up to external ring and laterally beyond deep ring level
Ilioinguinal nerve
External oblique aponeurosis
Conjoint tendon
Inguinal ligament below

Figs. 19-54(1)

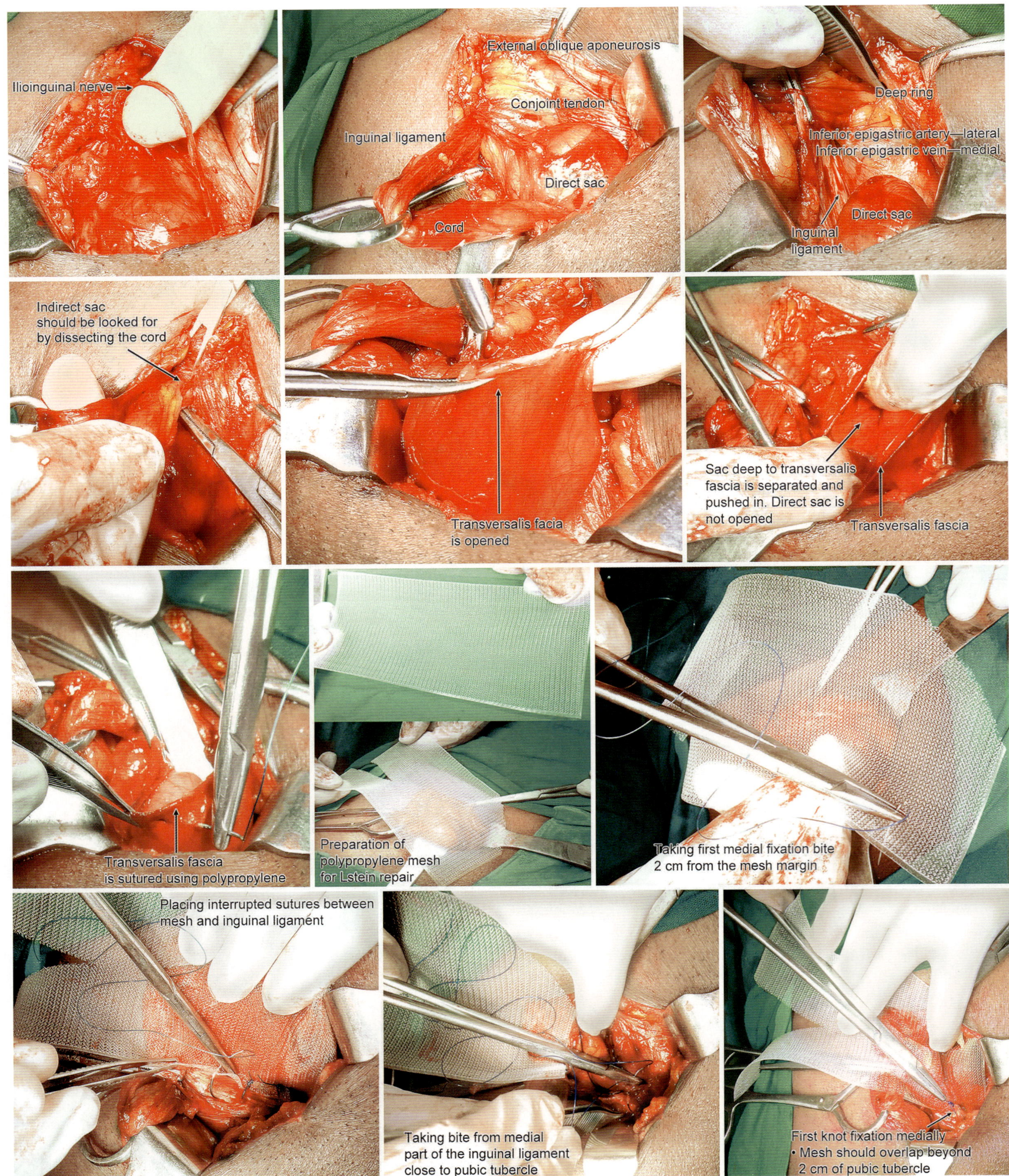
Ilioinguinal nerve
External oblique aponeurosis
Conjoint tendon
Inguinal ligament
Direct sac
Cord
Deep ring
Inferior epigastric artery—lateral
Inferior epigastric vein—medial
Direct sac
Inguinal ligament
Indirect sac should be looked for by dissecting the cord
Transversalis facia is opened
Sac deep to transversalis fascia is separated and pushed in. Direct sac is not opened
Transversalis fascia
Transversalis fascia is sutured using polypropylene
Preparation of polypropylene mesh for Lstein repair
Taking first medial fixation bite 2 cm from the mesh margin
Placing interrupted sutures between mesh and inguinal ligament
Taking bite from medial part of the inguinal ligament close to pubic tubercle
First knot fixation medially
• Mesh should overlap beyond 2 cm of pubic tubercle

Figs. 19-54(2)

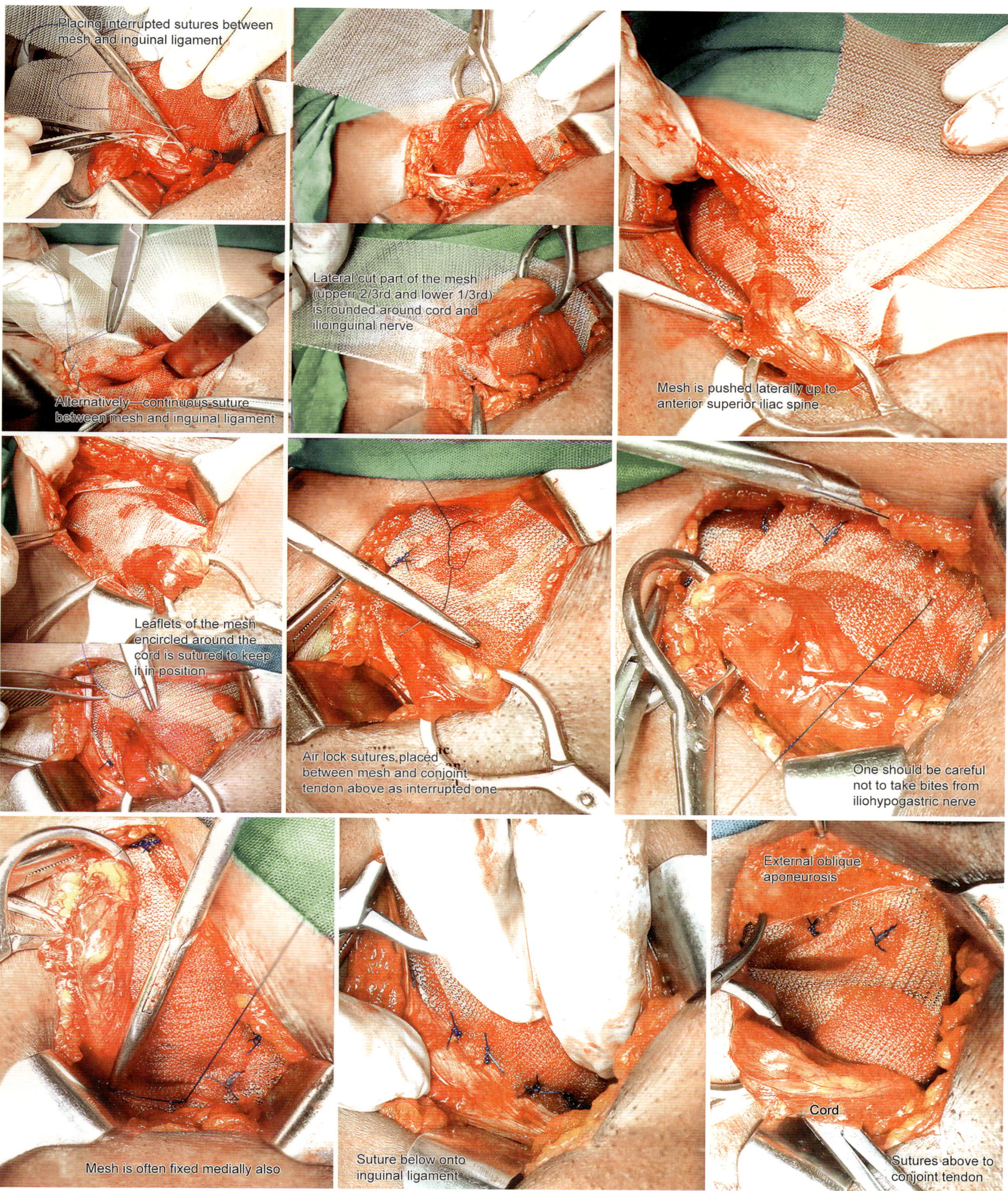
Placing interrupted sutures between mesh and inguinal ligament
Alternatively—continuous suture between mesh and inguinal ligament
Lateral cut part of the mesh (upperr 2/3rd and lower 1/3rd) is rounded around cord and ilioinguinal nerve
Mesh is pushed laterally up to anterior superior iliac spine
Leaflets of the mesh encircled around the cord is sutured to keep it in position
Air lock sutures placed between mesh and conjoint tendon above as interrupted one
One should be careful not to take bites from iliohypogastric nerve
Mesh is often fixed medially also
Suture below onto inguinal ligament
External oblique aponeurosis
Cord
Sutures above to conjoint tendon

Figs. 19-54(3)

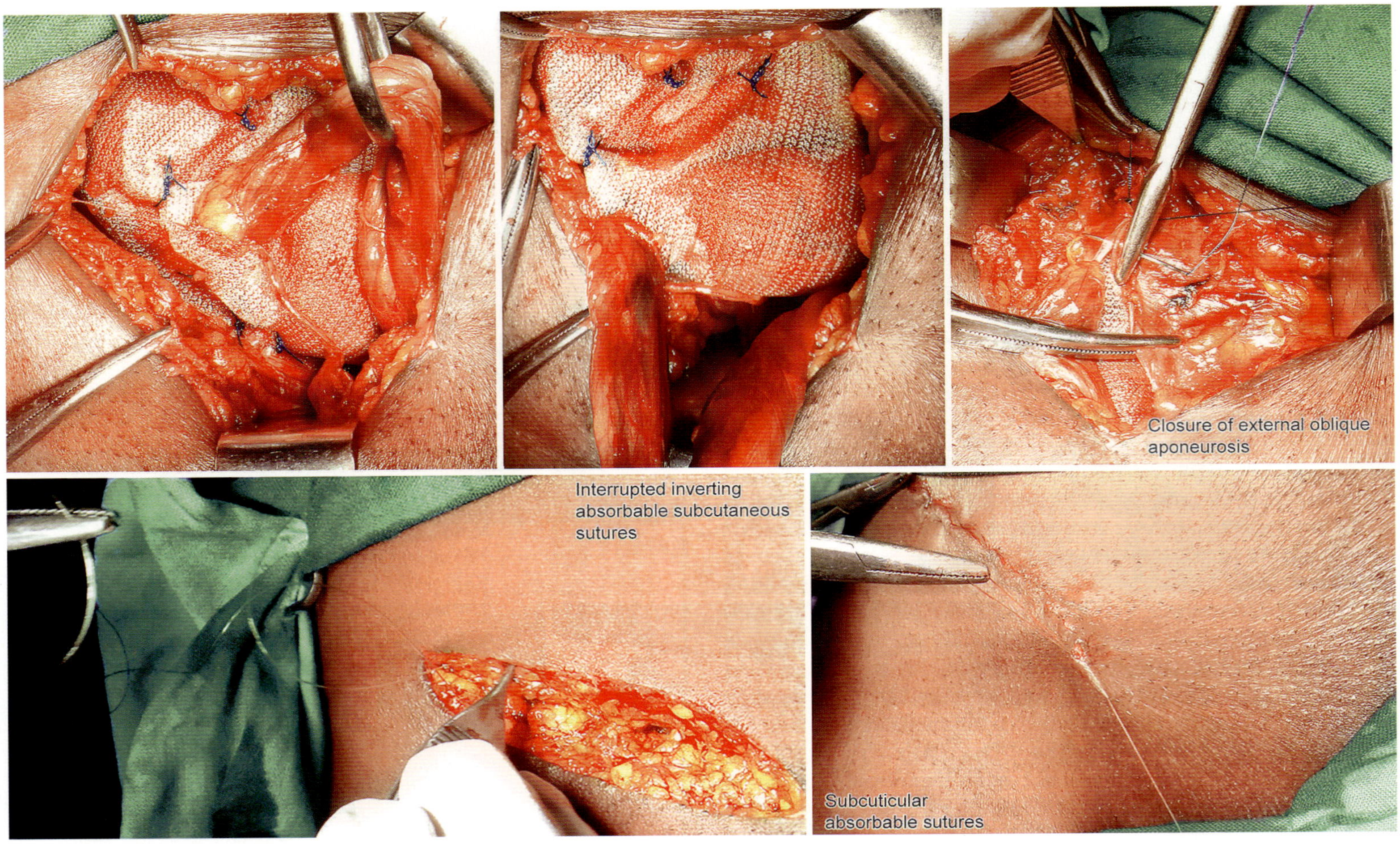

Figs. 19-54(4)

Figs. 19-54(1 to 4): Lichtenstein hernioplasty—mesh repair.

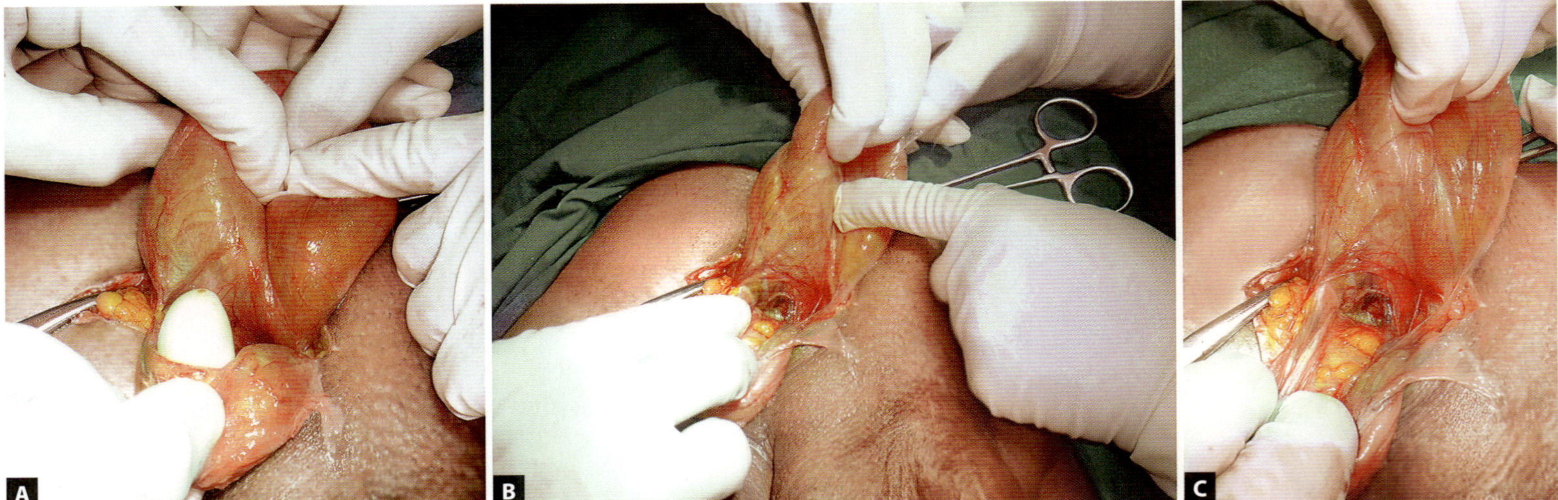

Figs. 19-55A to C: Direct sac—inguinal hernia.

Inguinal canal is exposed well using Langenbeck retractor above and Czerny's retractor below and medially. Cord is kept away below. Polypropylene mesh is used for repair (15 × 7.5 cm size); size is decided based on the width of the defect; adequate sized mesh covering 2.0 cm above and medially should be used. Often mesh of required size is cut. Mesh is sutured below to the inguinal ligament; medial most suture is taken from a point very close to the pubic tubercle. One should be sure that mesh covers well medial to the pubic tubercle (2 cm beyond). Size of the mesh used is usually 15 × 7.5 cm. Size should accommodate defect well beyond pubic tubercle (2 cm), superior margin (4 cm) and deep ring (6 cm) laterally. Presently it is thought that light weight large pore combined absorbable and non-absorbable mesh is better than only non-absorbable mesh. As part of the mesh gets absorbed in 120 days; support by mesh is well achieved with very less incidence of distressing mesh inguinodynia (due to ilioinguinal and iliohypogastric nerves getting adherent to the mesh). Suturing of mesh is done using interrupted non-absorbable monofilament polypropylene or polyethylene sutures below to inguinal ligament. Continuous sutures also can be used while suturing lower flap of mesh to inguinal ligament. Mesh is sutured below

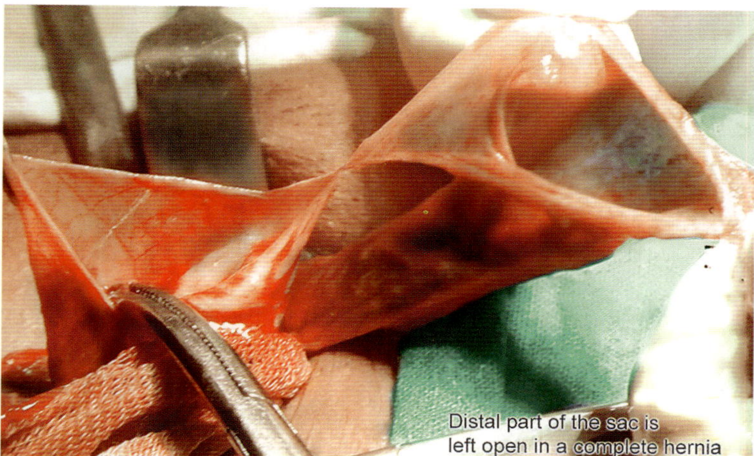

Fig. 19-56: Distal part of the sac should not be ligated; it is left open probably by giving slit on its wall. If ligated, distal part forms a cavity where fluid may collect forming hydrocele.

to inguinal ligament up to the level of deep ring not beyond (if so femoral nerve may occasionally get injured). It is important to keep needle facing forward to avoid taking inadvertent bite of femoral/iliac vessels (mainly vein) especially in thin individuals. Even though it happens rarely, in such situation without get panicked on seeing the sudden torrential bleed from the site of needle bite, one should gently pull out the suture without allowing further tear of the bitten tissue and sufficient pressure should be applied using a mop to stop the bleeding. Knot tying in such situation would not be correct as tying may further tear the vessel. Occasionally, further exposure of the major vessel may be needed to control the bleeding using 4-zero vascular continuous suture. Laterally mesh is partially cut horizontally (3 cm upper flap × 2 cm lower flap) so as to enclose the cord and ilioinguinal nerve; lower flap of the cut part is narrower than upper flap. Often few surgeons excise a circular piece of mesh to accommodate cord and remaining tails of the mesh is crossed laterally and sutured. It is important to place lateral tails beyond the incision area (6 cm from deep ring) under the external oblique up to the level of anterior superior iliac spine. Lastly upper end of the mesh is sutured to the conjoined tendon in front with loose sutures (*air lock sutures*) just to keep mesh in place. It is often of practice to use absorbable sutures in these upper part so that nerve entrapment in case if occurs (iliohypogastric nerve) will get corrected or may not cause much problem; for same reason only loose sutures are used just to keep mesh in place (air lock). It is also allowed to place continuous sutures below to inguinal ligament. But it is not ideal to place continuous sutures above. Mesh should be sutured with relaxation to bear the forward protrusion pressure of the transversalis fascia during standing. Pressure difference between intra-abdominal area and abdominal wall in lying down position is 8 cm of water; which rises to 80 cm in standing position. Mesh placed should bear this pressure change effectively to prevent recurrence of hernia **(Figs. 19-57A and C)**.

Cord and ilioinguinal nerve is placed back in the inguinal canal. External oblique is sutured using absorbable vicryl sutures. Subcutaneous interrupted sutures are placed. Skin is closed with continuous subcuticular monocryl 3-zero sutures or monofilament 3-zero interrupted sutures. Waterproof dressing is placed.

Postoperatively patient is asked to take normal diet. Intraoperative intravenous antibiotic is given. Patient is asked to take analgesics and oral antibiotics for 3–5 days.

Procedure can be done as a day care surgery unless the patient is elderly, with cardiac or respiratory problems. Dressing is changed and wound is observed in 5–7 days. Sutures if non-absorbable are removed in 7 days.

Different Types of Hernioplasty

Onlay mesh repair is placing mesh in front: It is sutured above to conjoined tendon and below to inguinal ligament using monofilament non-absorbable suture material.

Inlay mesh repair is done by placing mesh deep to conjoined tendon at par with muscular or aponeurotic plane (*bridging).*

Lichtenstein tension free onlay mesh repair (1984) where the cord is encircled with mesh which is often done under local anaesthesia. Suturing of mesh is done similar to onlay mesh repair. It has got less recurrence rate.

Nyhus preperitoneal mesh repair (sublay)

It is done through *suprainguinal* horizontal incision (*posterior approach)* above the pubic symphysis and internal ring. Preperitoneum is approached through lateral border of the lower part of rectus muscle by making an opening in the posterior rectus sheath. Mesh is placed in the preperitoneal space deep to the cord, conjoined tendon, and transversalis fascia. Below, it is folded deep to the iliopectineal ligament of Cooper and sutured to it using two or three interrupted non-absorbable sutures. It is sutured to transverse abdominis above and transversalis fascia from deep.

Modified Rives preperitoneal mesh repair (Read-Rives—Sublay)

It is preperitoneal mesh repair through *transinguinal approach (anterior approach)*. Direct sac is inverted with sutures. For indirect sac a *high dissection and ligation* is done. Here mesh is placed in preperitoneal space, folded and sutured below to iliopectineal ligament, above to the transverse abdominis in deeper plane. Often transversalis fascia opened earlier is sutured back using non-absorbable suture material in front of the placed mesh **(Figs. 19-58 and 19-59)**.

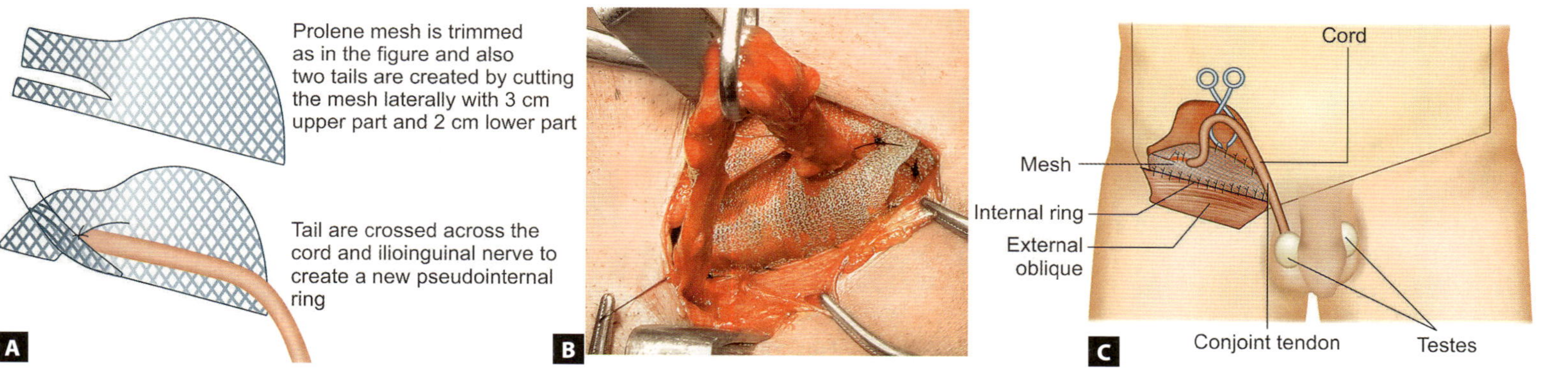

Figs. 19-57A to C: Lichtenstein mesh repair—polypropylene is used; often mesh is trimmed.

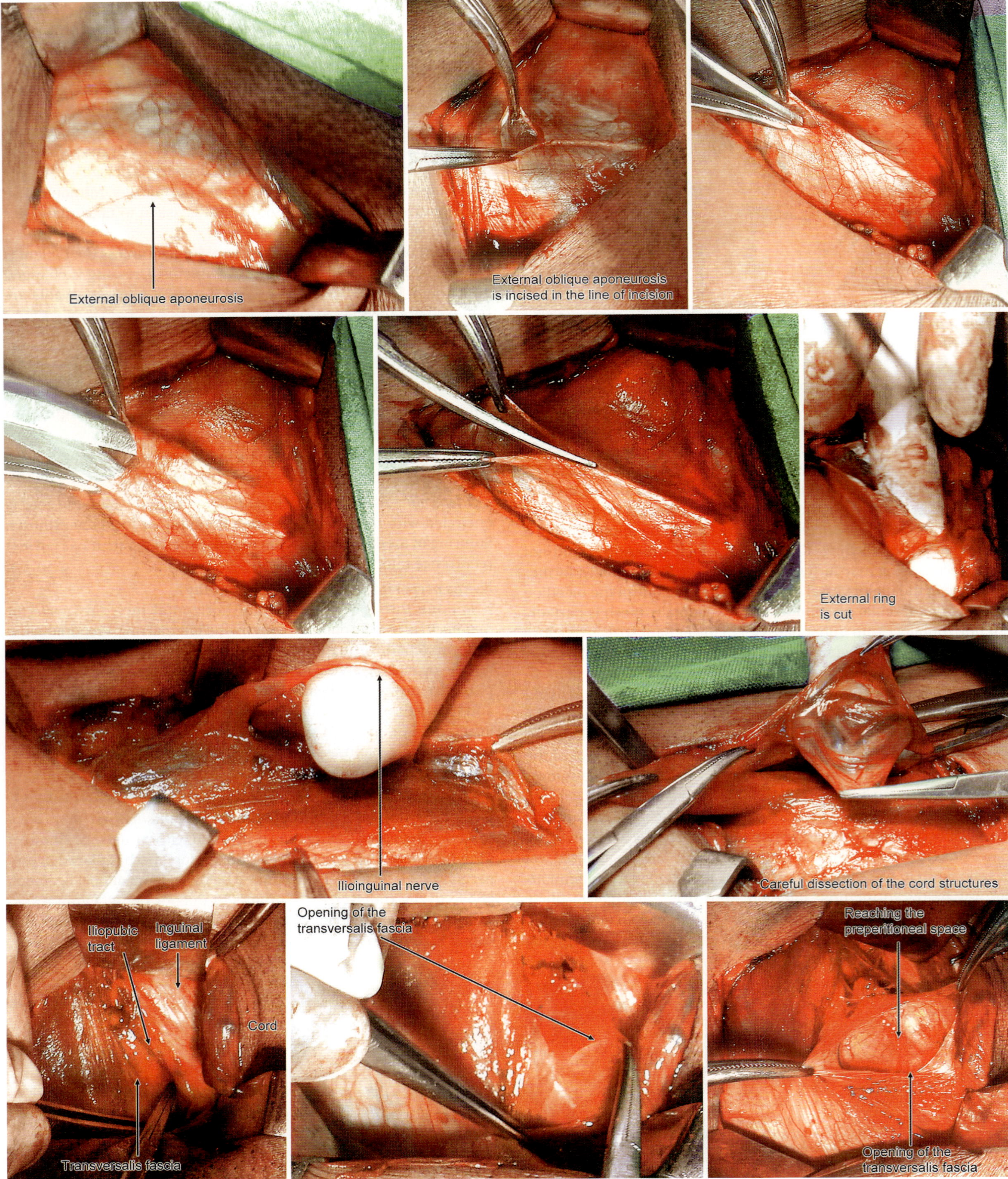
External oblique aponeurosis
External oblique aponeurosis
is incised in the line of incision
External ring
is cut
Ilioinguinal nerve
Careful dissection of the cord structures
Iliopubic
tract
Inguinal
ligament
Cord
Transversalis fascia
Opening of the
transversalis fascia
Reaching the
preperitioneal space
Opening of the
transversalis fascia

Figs. 19-58(1)

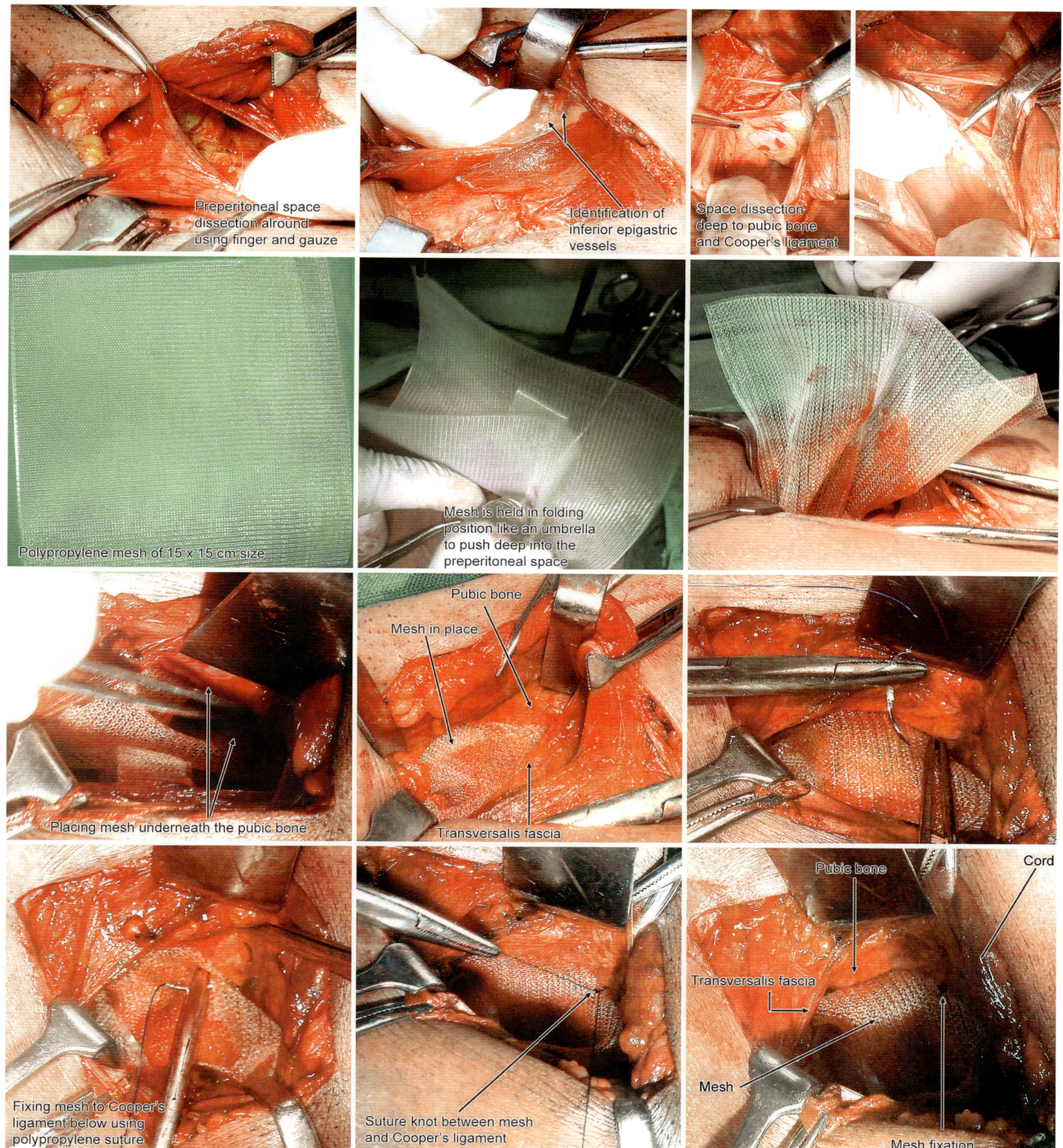
Preperitoneal space dissection alround using finger and gauze
Identification of inferior epigastric vessels
Space dissection deep to pubic bone and Cooper's ligament
Polypropylene mesh of 15 x 15 cm size
Mesh is held in folding position like an umbrella to push deep into the preperitoneal space
Placing mesh underneath the pubic bone
Pubic bone
Mesh in place
Transversalis fascia
Fixing mesh to Cooper's ligament below using polypropylene suture
Suture knot between mesh and Cooper's ligament
Pubic bone
Cord
Transversalis fascia
Mesh
Mesh fixation

Figs. 19-58(2)

Inguinal ligament
Closure of transversalis fascia using polypropylene suture
Closed transversalis fascia

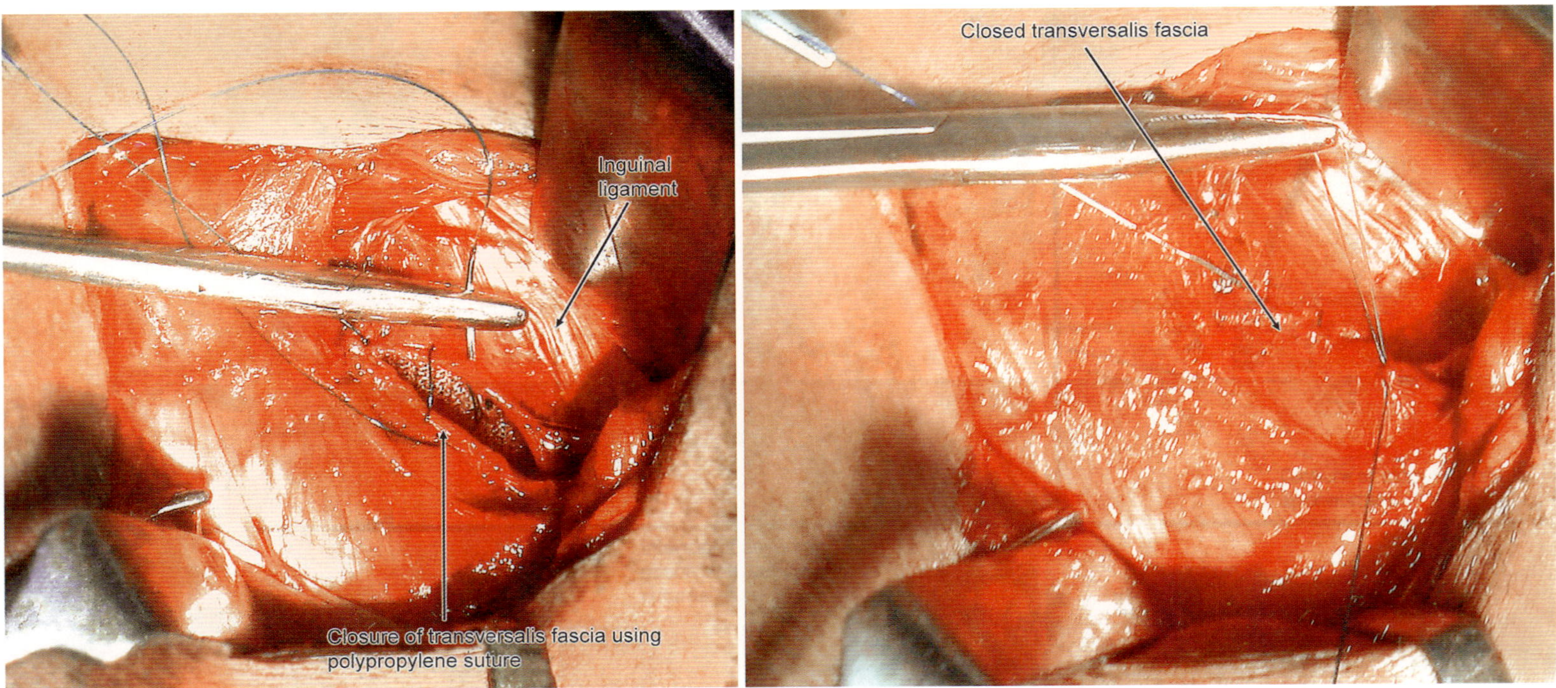

Figs. 19-58(3)

Figs. 19-58(1 to 3): Rives transinguinal preperitoneal mesh repair.

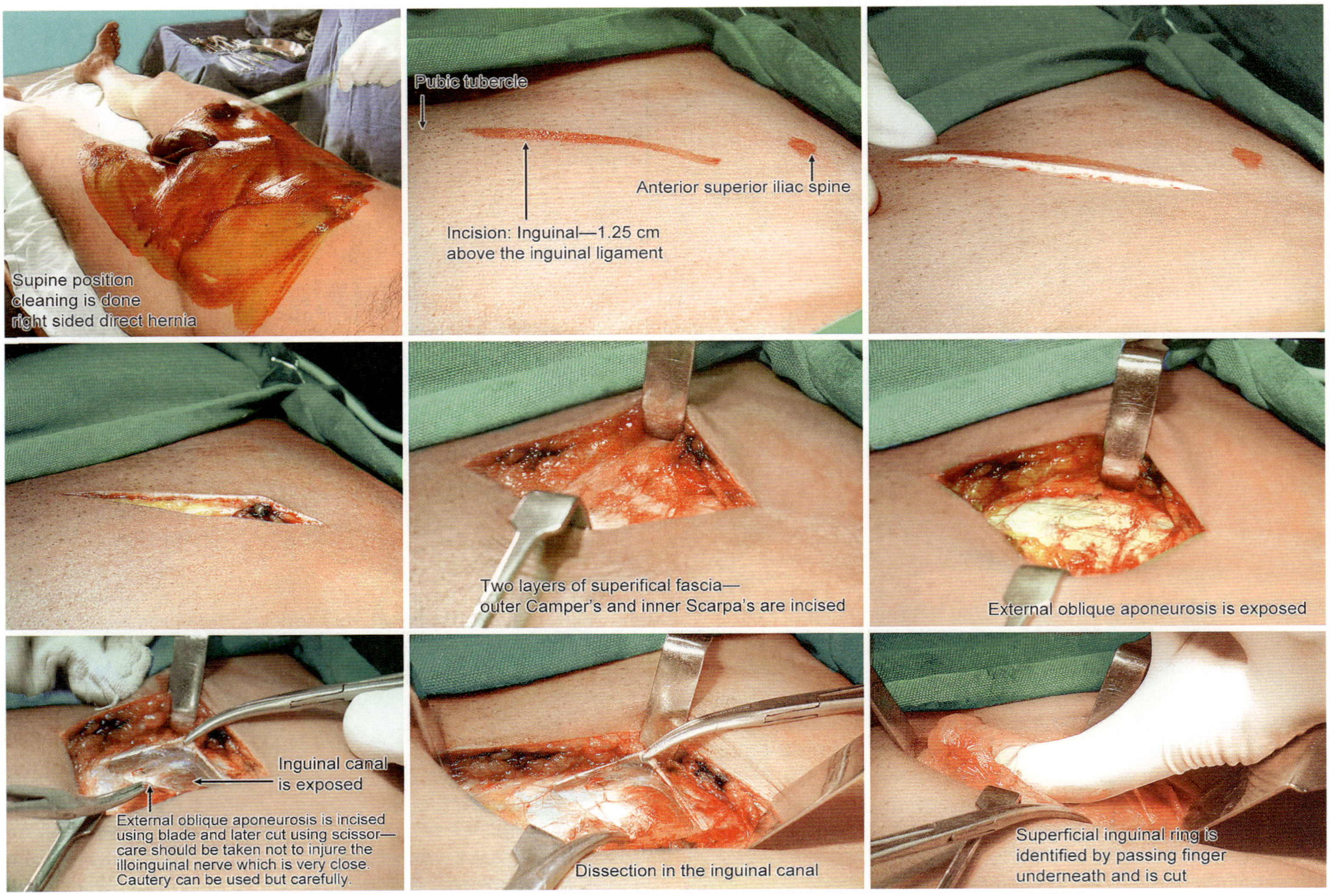

Supine position cleaning is done right sided direct hernia
Pubic tubercle
Anterior superior iliac spine
Incision: Inguinal—1.25 cm above the inguinal ligament
Two layers of superifical fascia—outer Camper's and inner Scarpa's are incised
External oblique aponeurosis is exposed
Inguinal canal is exposed
External oblique aponeurosis is incised using blade and later cut using scissor—care should be taken not to injure the illoinguinal nerve which is very close. Cautery can be used but carefully.
Dissection in the inguinal canal
Superficial inguinal ring is identified by passing finger underneath and is cut

Figs. 19-59(1)

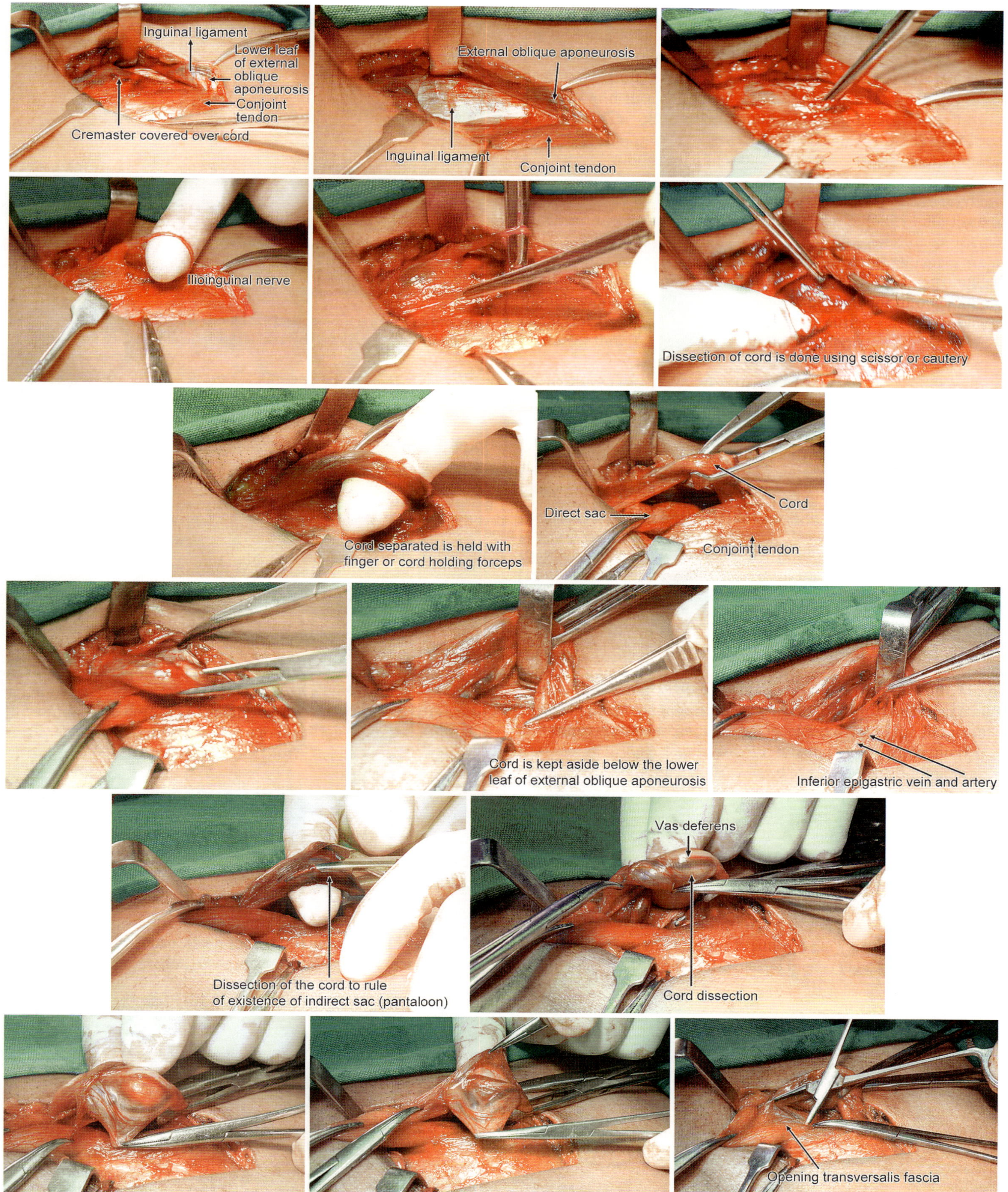
Inguinal ligament
Lower leaf of external oblique aponeurosis
Conjoint tendon
Cremaster covered over cord
External oblique aponeurosis
Inguinal ligament
Conjoint tendon
Ilioinguinal nerve
Dissection of cord is done using scissor or cautery
Cord separated is held with finger or cord holding forceps
Cord
Direct sac
Conjoint tendon
Cord is kept aside below the lower leaf of external oblique aponeurosis
Inferior epigastric vein and artery
Dissection of the cord to rule of existence of indirect sac (pantaloon)
Vas deferens
Cord dissection
Opening transversalis fascia

Figs. 19-59(2)

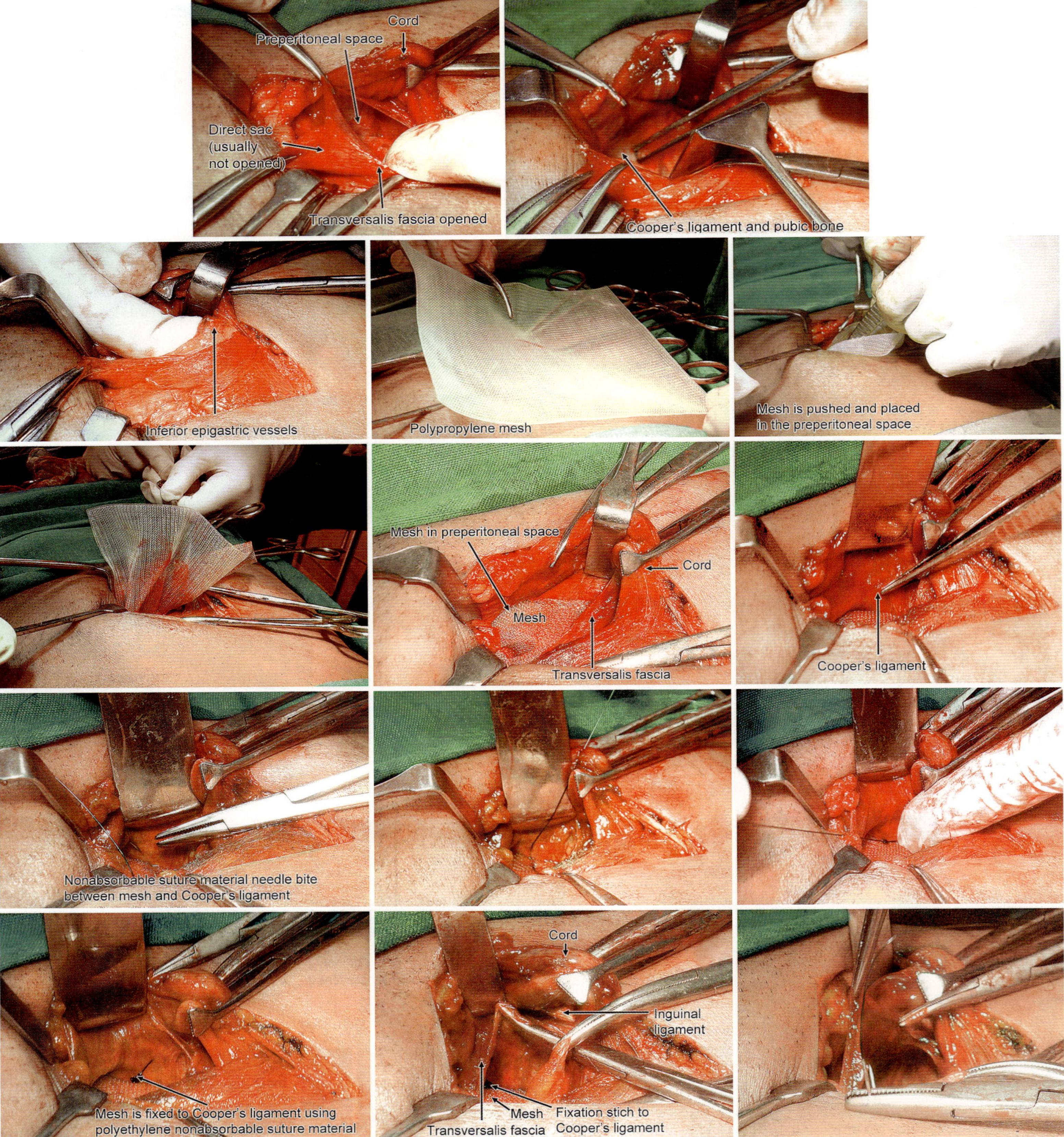
Cord
Preperitoneal space
Direct sac (usually not opened)
Transversalis fascia opened
Cooper's ligament and pubic bone
Inferior epigastric vessels
Polypropylene mesh
Mesh is pushed and placed in the preperitoneal space
Mesh in preperitoneal space
Cord
Mesh
Transversalis fascia
Cooper's ligament
Nonabsorbable suture material needle bite between mesh and Cooper's ligament
Mesh is fixed to Cooper's ligament using polyethylene nonabsorbable suture material
Cord
Inguinal ligament
Mesh
Transversalis fascia
Fixation stich to Cooper's ligament

Figs. 19-59(3)

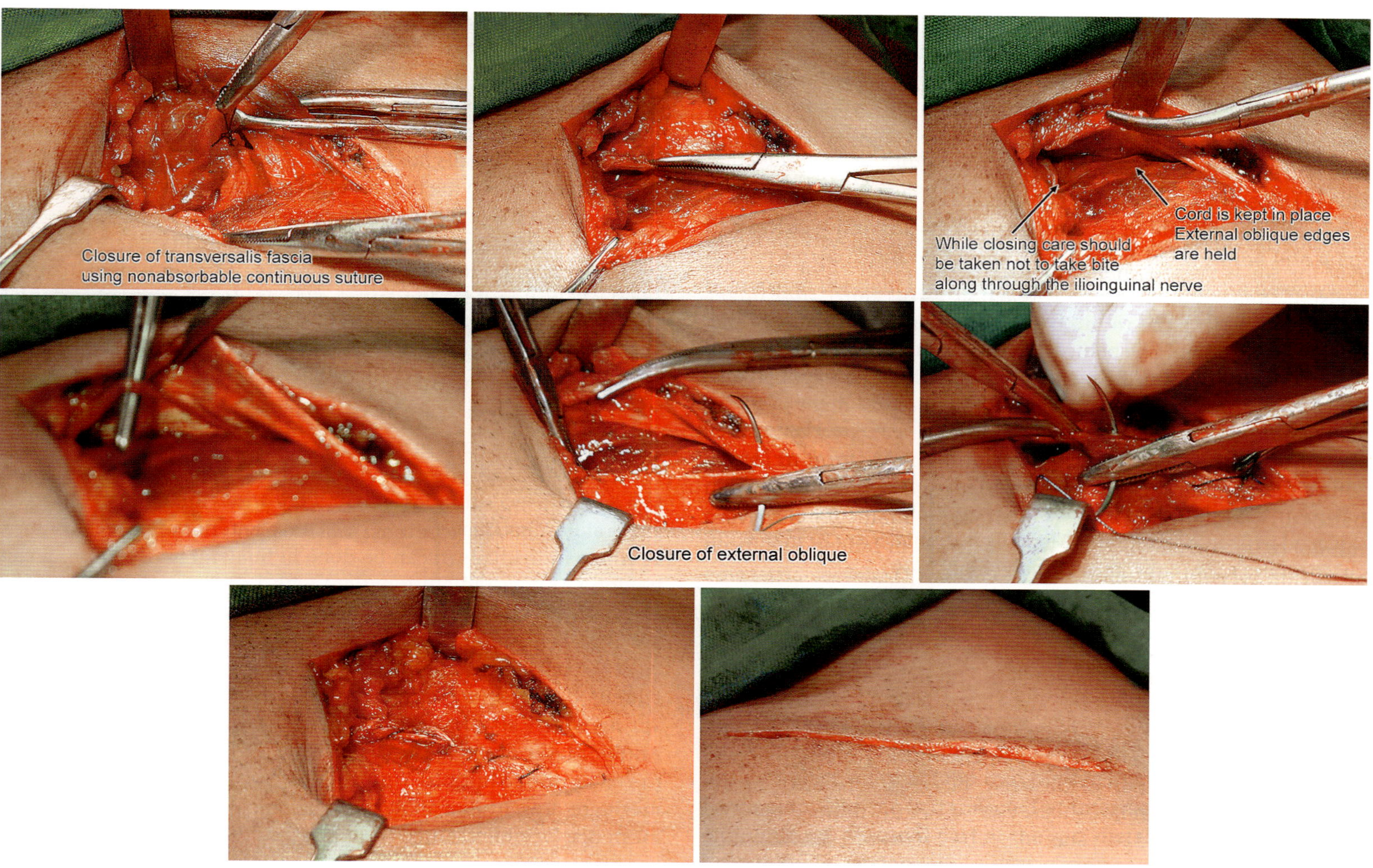

Figs. 19-59(4)

Figs. 19-59(1 to 4): Rives preperitoneal mesh repair—transinguinal approach.

Stoppa's (Rene S Stoppa) giant prosthesis reinforcement of visceral sac (GPRVS—sublay)

It is done in large hernias, hernias in elderly, bilateral hernias, recurrent and re-recurrent hernias, hernia with very lax abdomen, obesity and hernia with collagen diseases like Marfan's syndrome. Horizontal length (size) of the mesh is 2 cm less than distance between two anterior superior iliac spines and vertical length (size) is distance between the umbilicus and pubic symphysis (26 × 15 cm). Dacron polyester mesh is better than polypropylene mesh which is supple, lightly adherent but rapidly fixing. Large mesh is placed between peritoneum and lateral, inferior, anterior abdominal wall which stretches in the lower abdomen and pelvis. It is contraindicated in sepsis, iliac vein thrombosis, when general anaesthesia (GA) or spinal anaesthesia cannot be given to the patient. It is done through lower midline subumbilical incision as a posterior preperitoneal approach across space of Retzius medially and space of Bogros laterally. Procedure is done under GA/spinal/epidural anaesthesia. Local anaesthesia is not used. Patient is placed in supine head down position. Subumbilical midline incision is placed across skin, subcutaneous fascia rectus sheath. Peritoneum is not opened. Space of Retzius in front of the bladder is dissected using finger and peanut swab. Dissection is continued towards *opposite side* of the surgeon first along the space of Bogros. Hernial sac/sacs whether indirect/direct or femoral sac are dissected off from their place. Indirect sac when large can be cut and proximal part is ligated and distal end is left open. Dissection is done further using finger along external iliac vessels, iliopsoas muscle. Funicular elements of sac along the vas deferens and testicular vessels are released so as to make complete parietalisation of the cord. Usual size of the mesh is 26 × 15 cm. Polyester mesh is preferred. Prosthesis mesh is made chevron shaped. It is placed and spread along the myopectineal orifice, on lateral part and towards midline. Mesh should be placed unfolded. Surgeon changes his position by moving on to opposite side to carry on with similar dissection on side where he was standing earlier. Usually such large mesh is placed without any anchorage. Often one vicryl stitch is placed between upper medial end of mesh and lower margin of midline of *umbilical fascia (Richet's)*. Suction drains are placed. Mesh envelops the endoabdominal fascia widely preventing the recurrence below at groin or at lower midline wound. Drains are removed in 2 days. *In Rignault's modification*, procedure is done through Pfannensteil incision (nerve injury and bleeding chances are high in this incision). Unilateral half cut GPRVS is called as *Wantz procedure,* done under local anaesthesia. Migration of mesh into the bladder is the only rare but serious complication which may occur.

Gilbert mesh repair (patch and plug)

After herniotomy, internal ring is plugged by cone shaped (umbrella plug) piece of prolene mesh. Later onlay/inlay mesh repair of posterior wall of the inguinal canal is done.

Gilbert's PHS (Prolene Hernia System) repair (onlay and sublay)

It is an open *transinguinal approach* to place a specially devised mesh in both preperitoneal as inlay and in front as onlay mesh repair. This mesh has got a rounded deeper part which is placed in preperitoneal space and a modified quadrangular part which is placed as onlay. Both parts are connected through a connecting stiff rounded part in between which steadies the mesh in place preventing the displacement. Procedure is usually done under local anaesthesia. Direct sac when present is opened. Transversalis fascia over the sac is cut circumferentially and extra part of the fascia is excised. Preperitoneal space is reached using gauze and finger dissection to place the round part of the mesh; lower part of this rounded mesh should be below and deep to the pubic bone to cover entire myopectineal orifice. Outer part is folded perpendicularly using a sponge holding/flat forceps to visualise the inner part and gently pushed into the preperitoneal space using finger. Using index finger it is spread gently in the preperitoneal space. On either side of connector of the mesh, transversalis fascia is sutured using one each polypropylene sutures to fix the connector. Outer quadrangular part is placed in front horizontally. Medially it should cover 2 cm beyond pubic tubercle like onlay mesh repair **(Fig. 19-60)**.

Using polypropylene interrupted suture below it is sutured to inguinal ligament, above to conjoined tendon by one suture, medially to soft tissue adjacent to pubic tubercle. Cord structure with ilioinguinal nerve is passed through the mesh by making a vertical cut on the wide portion of the anterior part of the mesh near its upper margin adjacent to internal ring and once cord is encircled, mesh is secured around the cord by single suture with crossing over of the leaves of the cut part of the mesh. Slit can also be made on the lateral margin to accommodate the cord structure. Connecting cord (connector) or rounded part should not be cut or cord should not be passed through this. In indirect sac preperitoneal space can also be created through posterior wall of the inguinal canal like in direct sac or through the internal ring space is created by blunt dissection by passing index finger. Pulsation of iliac artery can be felt lateral to the index finger. This dissection can be achieved using a sponge held in an instrument or by index finger. Dissection is between preperitoneal space and transversalis fascia. Inferior epigastric vessels are usually left in place between the two lamina of fascia transversalis but can be securely ligated if difficulty arises. Space of 6 cm radius is created all around centering deep ring. Connector is made to remain either on internal ring or on the direct defect of the posterior wall of inguinal canal. Wound is closed in layers. Skin is closed with subcuticular absorbable suture or N butyl cyanacrylate bond. Patient can be discharged within 24 hours. Wound inspection is done in 7 days. Mild discolouration and oedema may last as long as for 6 weeks. Complications are haematoma, swelling, seroma, infection.

Kugel (Rober D Kugel) groin hernia mesh repair (sublay)

It is done through *posterior preperitoneal* approach with tension free less invasive sutureless repair. *Indications* are indirect, direct or femoral hernias; recurrent hernias after anterior approach (onlay); in young individuals. It can be done in bilateral hernias also. It can be done in post-radiation patient with hernia or recurrence after TEP or TAPP. Kugel patch contains two overlapping layers of knitted polypropylene mesh which are attached to each other ultrasonically. Near the outer edge of the mesh it has got a polyester spring which stiffens the mesh to unfold. 1 cm of mesh extends outer to the spring which also has radial slits to have easy manoeuvrability. Anterior layer of the mesh has got single transverse slit to facilitate the insertion. Multiple 3 mm holes through both layers of the mesh are present that allow tissue contact in better way to prevent mesh displacement. Small V shaped triangular cuts on the anterior layer adjacent to these multiple holes act as sutureless anchors.

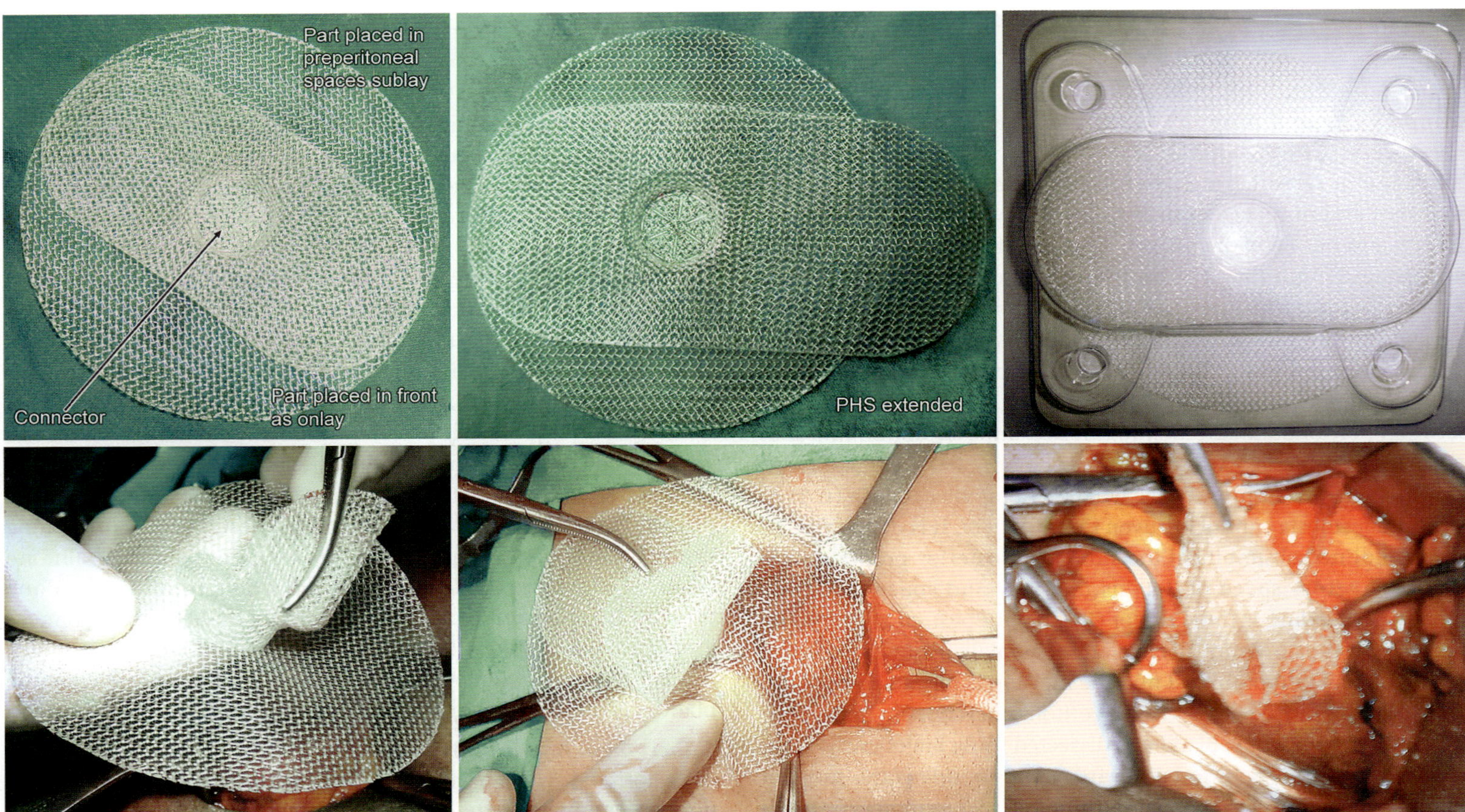

Figs. 19-60(1)

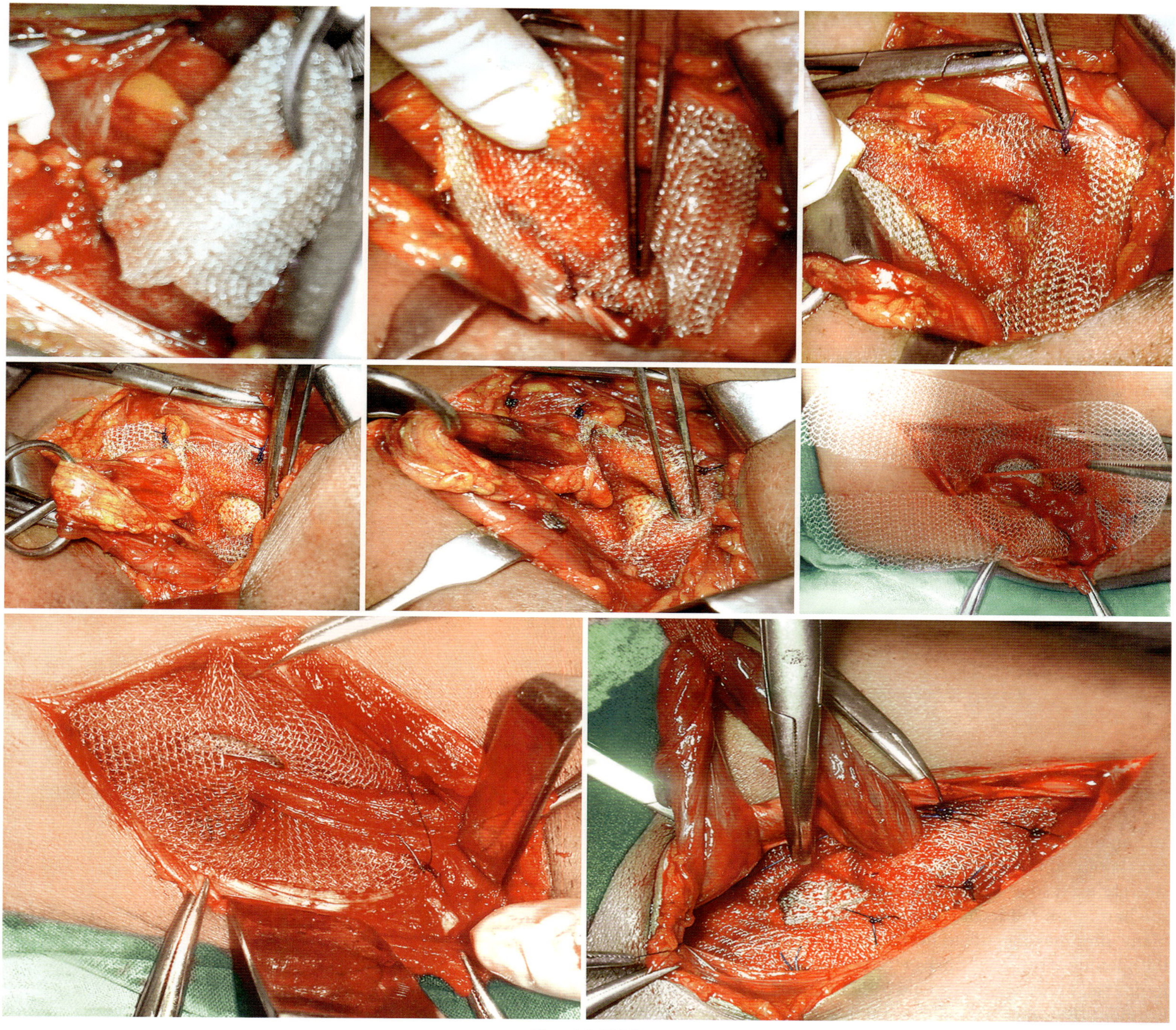

Figs. 19-60(2)

Figs. 19-60(1 and 2): Prolene hernia system (PHS)—surgical technique.

Small 8 × 12 cm and large 11 × 14 cm sizes are available, former is used in indirect sac, latter in direct sac. Incision is above the deep ring and lateral to inferior epigastric vessels. Midpoint of the inguinal ligament is marked. *Oblique incision* line just superior to this point; with 1/3rd lateral and 2/3rd medial to this point is made **(Figs. 19-61A and B)**.

Skin, subcutaneous tissue, external oblique aponeurosis is cut; internal oblique and transversus abdominis muscles are split to reach deeper space. Ilioinguinal and iliohypogastric nerves will not come into the field. Transversalis fascia often which is two layered is split vertically to avoid injury to inferior epigastric vessels. Inferior epigastric vessels are retracted medially. Preperitoneal space is created first superiorly then laterally. Indirect sac is dissected off the deep ring from above; if dissection is difficult, sac can be cut with distal part left open and proximal part being ligated using absorbable 3-zero vicryl. Direct sac is dissected off the defect without opening; its pseudosac which is modified transversalis fascia is dissected off entirely from the peritoneum behind. Often it is needed to make a small incision on the pseudosac to prevent seroma formation as this cut allows dissipation of fluid or blood into the tissue in the inguinal canal in front. As approach is small, proper malleable retractors are necessary. Dissection is carried out down under the pubic bone across Cooper's ligament. Care should be taken not to injure vessels at this place either small veins or aberrant obturator artery. Kugel's mesh patch is placed properly without allowing any tissue bands folding it. Transversalis fascia is sutured with one absorbable suture. Transversus abdominis and internal oblique muscles are not sutured. External oblique aponeurosis is sutured; then subcutaneous tissue and skin. Bilateral hernias are dealt with two separate incisions.

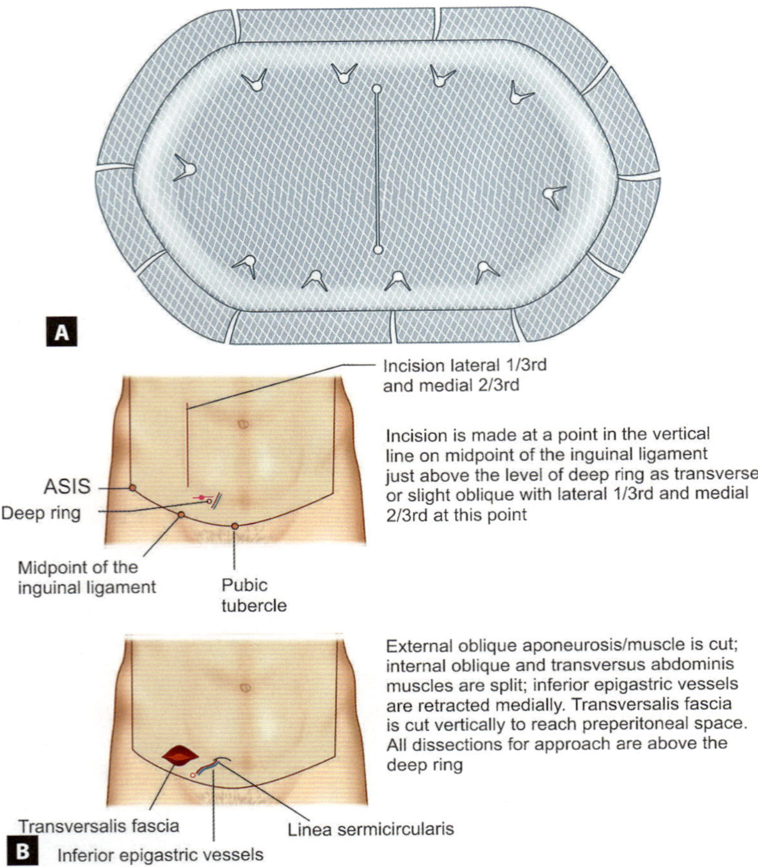

Figs. 19-61A and B: Kugel's procedure for inguinal hernia. It is suprainguinal posterior approach.

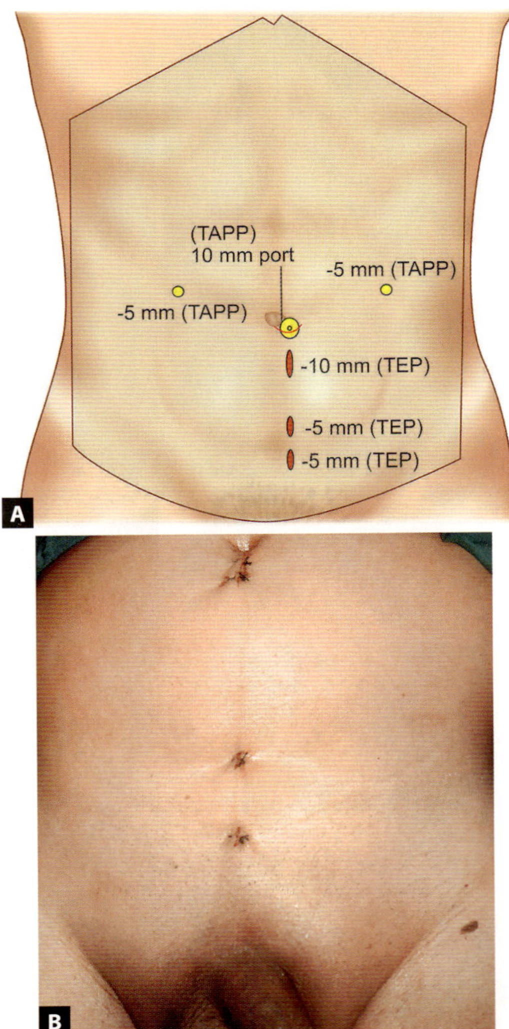

Figs. 19-62A and B: Ports used for TEP (red colour) and for TAPP (yellow colour).

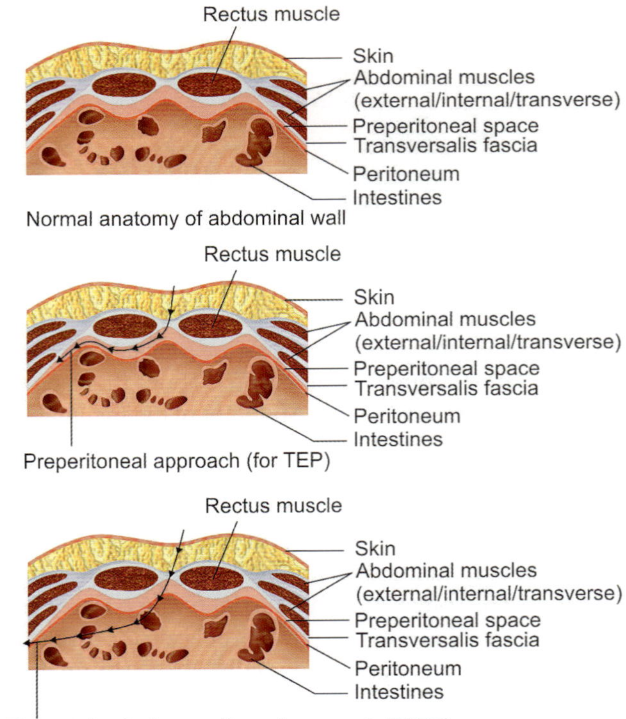

Fig. 19-63: Diagrammatic representations of TEP and TAPP.

Transabdominal preperitoneal mesh repair (TAPP—sublay) using laparoscope (Arregui, 1991)

This is used in large indirect hernia or irreducible inguinal hernia. 10 mm umbilical port is used for laparoscope. 5 mm ports on pararectal point at the or above the level of the umbilicus one on each side are used so as to achieve adequate triangulation. Contents of the hernia are reduced. Hernial sac is dissected in preperitoneal plane after making curved horizontal incision at the upper part of the opening of sac. Incision over the peritoneum is made from lateral to medial. From a point around 3–4 cm lateral to lateral umbilical ligament (inferior epigastric vessels) horizontal incision is made across internal ring on its upper part medially up to medial umbilical ligament. Preperitoneal space is dissected to identify pubic bone, Cooper's ligament, vas, gonadal vessels, and inferior epigastric vessels. Once sac is dissected and excised, a prolene/vipro/ultrapro mesh of 15 × 10 cm size is placed in preperitoneal pace. It is fixed to pubic bone/Cooper's ligament using tacks. Peritoneum is closed with continuous prolene sutures from lateral to medial. It is mainly used in irreducible and large hernias. Thus reperitonealisation should be done properly. TAPP without reperitonealisation **(TAPPWR)** can be done if dual mesh with ePTFE on inner visceral side can be placed after complete dissection in retroperitoneal space without suturing/apposing the peritoneum. ePTFE prevents viscera from getting adherent and eroded by mesh. Neoperitoneum develops on the ePTFE mesh in 10 days. Complications of TAPP are similar to TEP. Additional problems of bowel injury by trocars, problems of pneumoperitoneum can occur. Advantage of TAPP is larger working space **(Figs. 19-62 to 19-65)**.

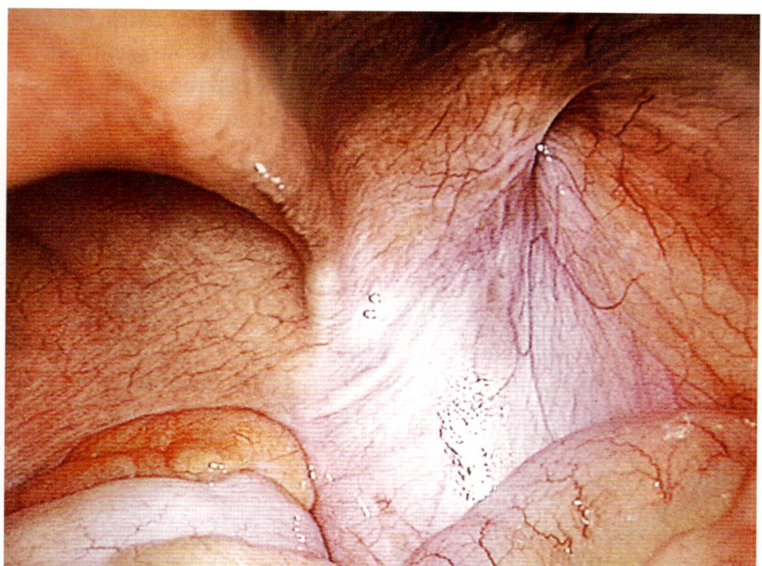

Fig. 19-64: Indirect hernia sac as seen in TAPP.

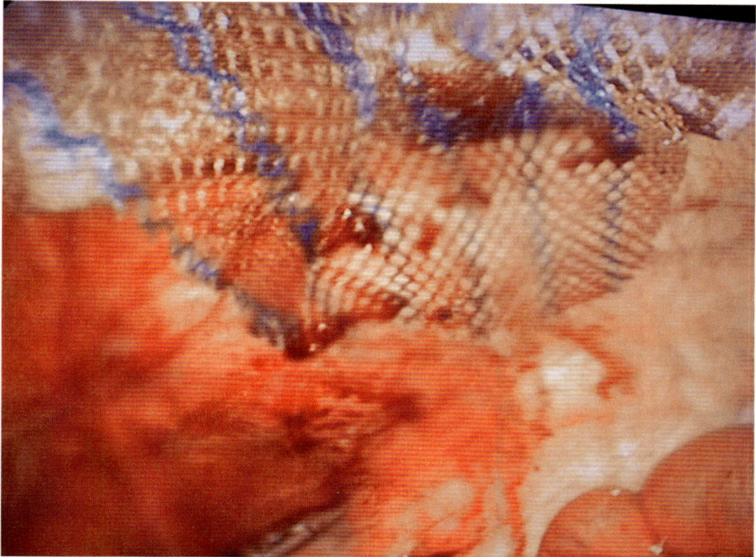

Fig. 19-65: Mesh placement in TAPP procedure.

Cobweb space is avascular and easily identifiable. It is better to use zero degree telescope initially to reach the pubic bone. Touching of the telescope over the hard pubic bone can be felt during dissection. Further dissection allows visualisation of the bone as *light house sign*. Immediate laterally Cooper's ligament can be identified. After CO_2 insufflation, another 5 mm port is inserted 4 cm below the first port in the midline. It is often better to put a hypodermic needle (needle of a syringe) into the space from midline to identify the site of the further ports. Third 5 mm port is inserted in the same line 4 cm below or in the right iliac fossa. Dissection is carried out downwards carefully, then medially up to the pubic tubercle, iliopectineal ligament, laterally to iliac vessels, and inferior epigastric vessels. At this stage 30° telescope is used. Direct sac when present is immediately visualised. It is dissected proximally by traction and countertraction over the white pseudosac (attenuated transversalis fascia) in front. After complete separation many practice to pull this pseudosac proximally to fix it to anterior abdominal wall to prevent the formation of seroma. Entire sac should be dissected down and behind to visualise wide direct defect medial to inferior epigastric vessels. One should remember that inferior epigastric vessels are properly seen only after dissection of the sac in case of direct one. Whereas in indirect sac, first inferior epigastric vessels are seen; then peritoneal sac is seen lateral to it running upwards, medially and proximally in the anterior abdominal wall. Hernial sac descends downwards into the internal ring. Sac is dissected from the deep ring. Usually entire sac can be dissected proximally. It is usual to place an endoloop into the sac but not always necessary. Large complete sac is transected at internal ring with placing an endoloop on proximal part of the sac; distal part of cut sac is left open without ligation.

Triangle of doom should be identified and care should be taken while dissecting in this area. Laterally dissection is done up to anterior superior iliac spine adequately along the iliopsoas to create needed space to place large mesh. *Triangle of pain* should be kept in mind as not to injure lateral femoral cutaneous nerve and femoral branch of genitofemoral nerve **(Fig. 19-66)**.

One should avoid opening peritoneum as it reduces the extraperitoneal space to undertake further part of the procedure.

Totally Extraperitoneal Repair (TEP Repair) Using Laparoscope (First done by McKernon, EH Phillips and Laws 1990, 1993)

This technique is gaining more popularity than TAPP. It does not breach the peritoneal cavity. It is useful for bilateral and recurrent hernias. It is contraindicated in previous midline surgical scar, previous caesarean, previous pelvic surgery or pelvic radiation.

Patient is ideally *catheterised*. Surgeon should stand opposite to the side of the hernia. Camera man stands on the same side proximal to the surgeon. Scrub nurse stands on the opposite side. Monitor is kept near the foot end side on the side of the hernia. Through sub-umbilical vertical/horizontal incision (10 mm) extraperitoneal space is reached. Often special type of balloon is used to create the same.

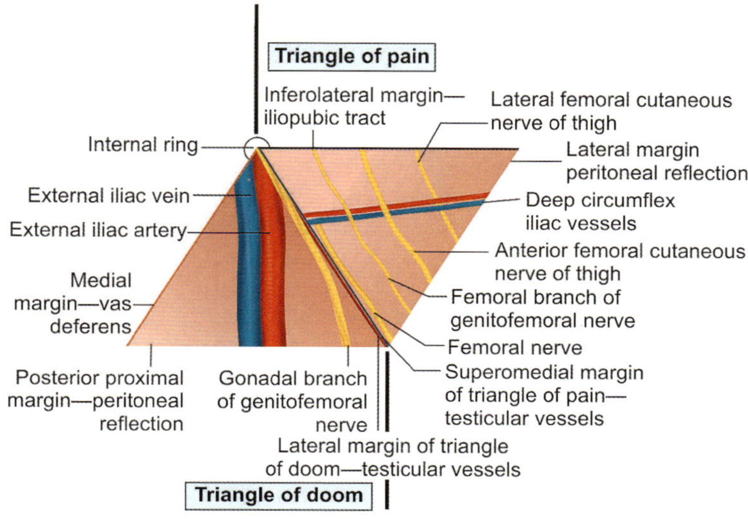

Fig. 19-66: Triangle of doom and triangle of pain.

If it happens, then it is better to place a Verres needle into the peritoneal cavity to deflate it and to increase the CO_2 flow rate. If bleeding occurs through injury of inferior epigastric vessels, it is tackled by placing clips or using bipolar cautery. Iliac vessels injury is catastrophic which needs immediate conversion to open procedure for proper vascular repair.

Mesh is passed through 10 mm port using a reducer after removing the telescope. If difficulty arises in passing mesh then port knob is removed and mesh is directly pushed into the space through the port. Once adequate space is dissected 15 × 15 cm sized mesh is placed and spread. Care should be taken not to have any folding in the mesh. Mesh may be sutured to iliopectineal ligament. Tackers should not be placed laterally and adjacent to vessels. Displacement of mesh is not common. Other side also can be done together. Deflation of gas is done at the end to keep the mesh in place. Port sites are sutured. 10 mm port site needs deeper vicryl suture **(Fig. 19-67)**.

Different port approaches and port placements are used for TEP

1. *Duluq approach:* Veress needle is passed just above the midline across the linea alba into the *space of Retzius* in preperitoneal area. CO_2 is insufflated into the preperitoneal space at a rate of 1 litre/minute with needle tip manipulating at various directions to inflate preperitoneal space adequately. Through a vertical

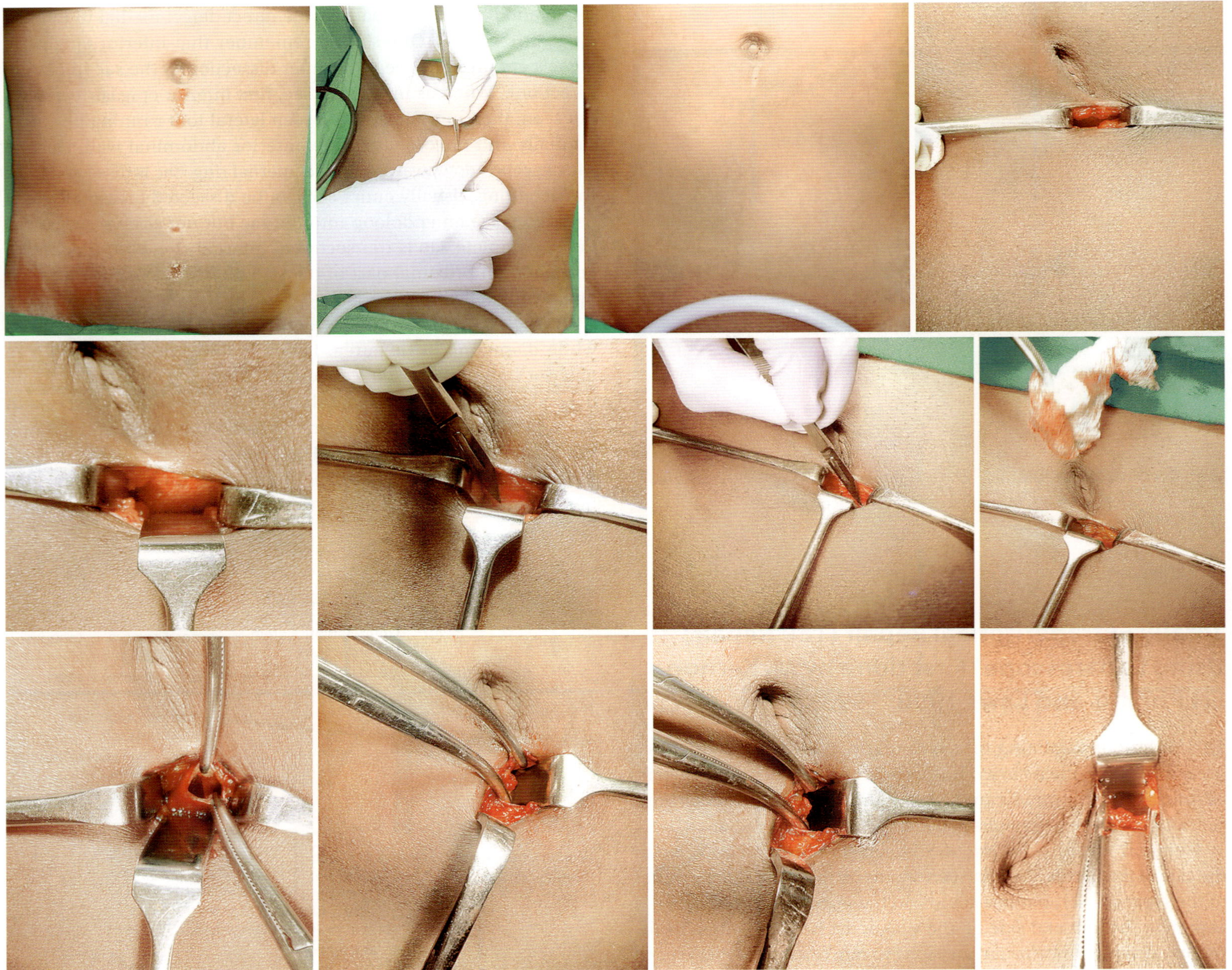

Figs. 19-67(1)

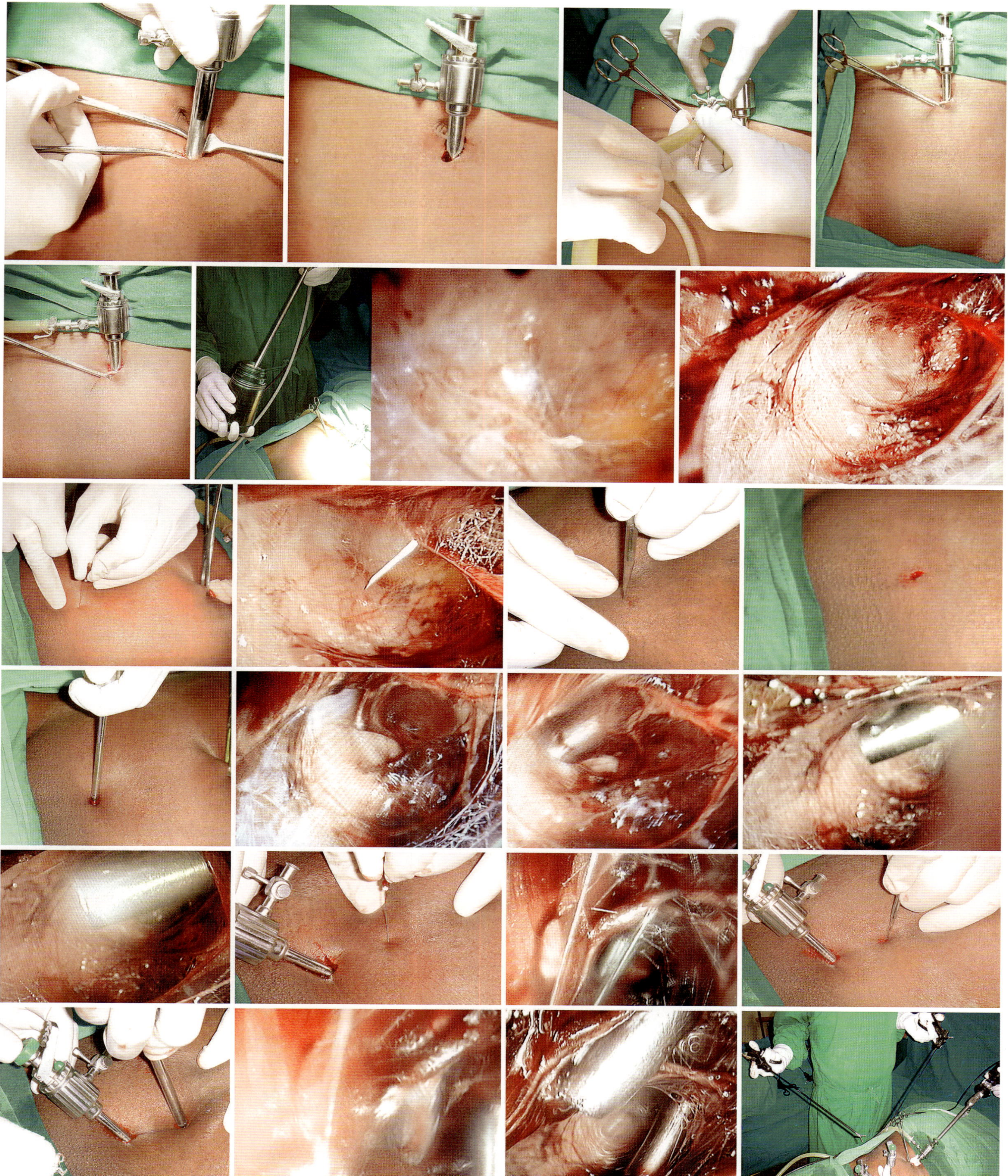

Figs. 19-67(2)

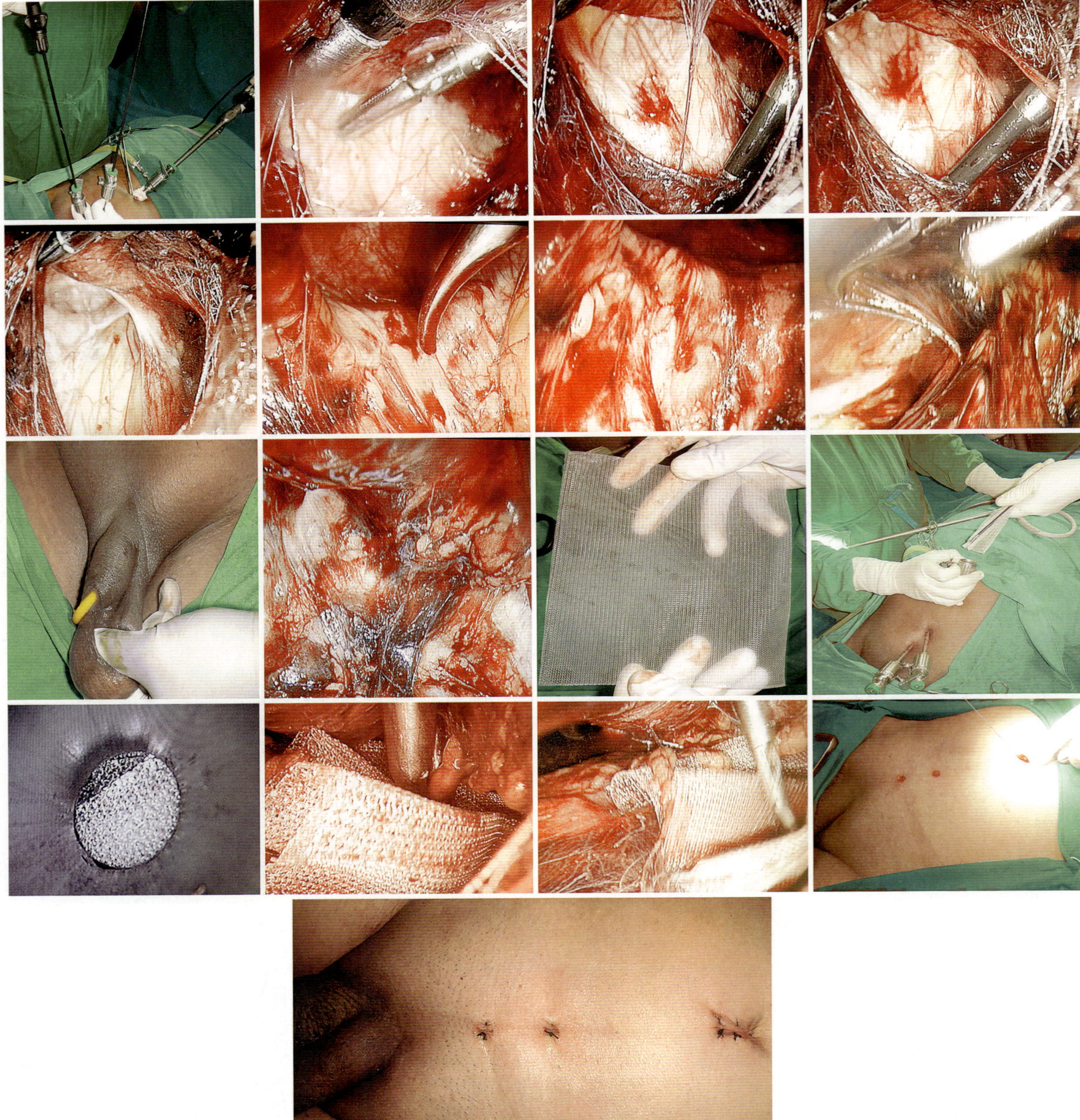

Figs. 19-67(3)

Figs. 19-67(1 to 3): Technical aspects of TEP.

subumbilical incision, 10 mm trocar is passed into the space directed obliquely towards the pubis initially, later at 60° angle. Zero degree telescope is passed to visualise the space and for further dissection using telescope along the cobweb areolar tissue. Further 5 mm trocars are passed as usual.

2. *McKernan's method:* Anterior rectus sheath is exposed through infraumbilical 2 cm vertical incision which is incised vertically to expose the rectus muscle; rectus muscle is retracted laterally to reach posterior rectus sheath; through this route Hassan's cannula is passed to proceed with creation of space and further two 5 mm ports below midline are inserted. 12.5 × 7.5 cm mesh with slit for passage of cord is used.
3. *Phillips TEP using initial peritoneoscopy:* After creating pneumoperitoneum through subumbilical 1 cm incision 10 mm trocars and port is passed into the peritoneal cavity. Under laparoscopic vision additional two 10 mm ports are passed on either side after making skin incision into the preperitoneal space without entering the peritoneal cavity along the lateral borders of the both rectus muscles. Laparoscope with the trocars is slowly withdrawn until preperitoneal space is reached where it is advanced into the preperitoneal space to proceed with the further dissection as usual.

Anatomical Considerations

Preperitoneal space is a potential space in front of the peritoneum, behind the transversalis fascia and anterior rectus muscle. Below in front of the urinary bladder, it is called as *space of Retzius* (medially), laterally it is called as *space of Bogros*. Median umbilical fold is formed by urachus in the midline. Medial umbilical ligament is formed by obliterated umbilical arteries, lateral umbilical fold by inferior epigastric vessels. Three fossae are lying in relation to these folds—supravesical and medial fossae are medial to lateral umbilical fold which are sites of direct hernia whereas lateral fossa is lateral to lateral umbilical fold and is site of indirect hernia.

In 1956 Fruchaud described his myopectineal orifice bounded medially by the lateral border of rectus abdominis, laterally by iliopsoas, superiorly by conjoined tendon and inferiorly by pectin pubis. This area is the site of groin hernia which should be covered by mesh of adequate size to strengthen the defect and to prevent the recurrence. Iliopubic tract is analogue of the inguinal ligament, extends from Cooper's ligament to anterior superior iliac spine which divides endoscopic view of preperitoneal space into superior compartment (contains inferior epigastric artery, Hesselbach's triangle, cord structures and is site of inguinal hernia) and inferior compartment (contains femoral canal, iliac vessels (vein medially; artery laterally), iliopsoas muscle, genitofemoral nerve, lateral femoral cutaneous nerve). External iliac vessels lie in a triangle formed by gonadal vessels laterally, vas deferens medially and peritoneal reflection inferiorly (triangle of doom).

Aberrant obturator artery which is an occasional branch of inferior epigastric artery replacing its pubic branch travels across Cooper's ligament, which during fixation of mesh can cause torrential haemorrhage—*circle of death. Triangle of pain* is formed by gonadal vessels medially, iliopubic tract laterally and peritoneal reflection below. Genitofemoral nerve and lateral cutaneous nerve of thigh traverse this triangle. Injury to these nerves either by dissection or by tacks cause postoperative pain. Tacks/staplers should not be placed in this triangle **(Figs. 19-68 to 19-73)**.

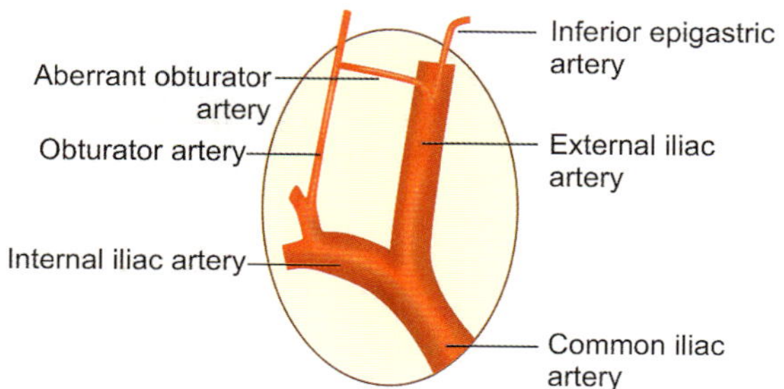

Fig. 19-68: Circle of death.

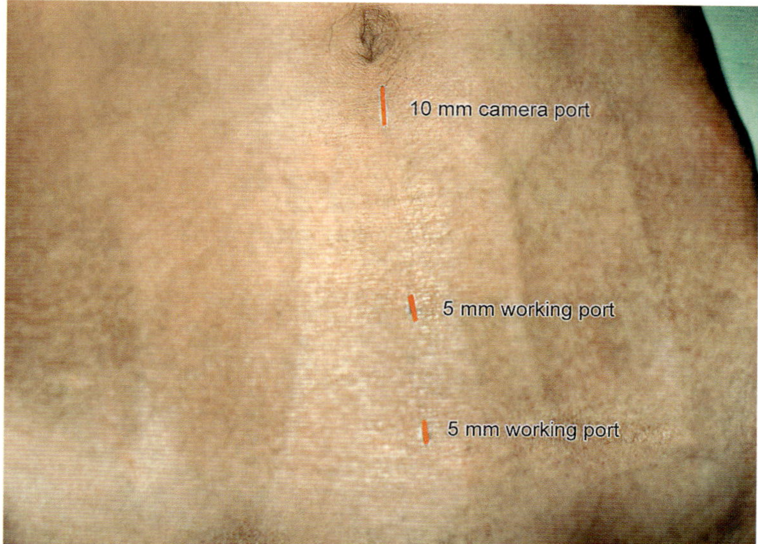

Fig. 19-69: Port incisions in TEP.

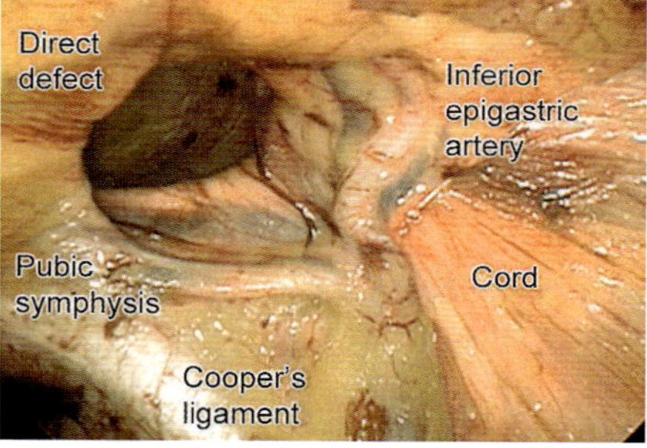

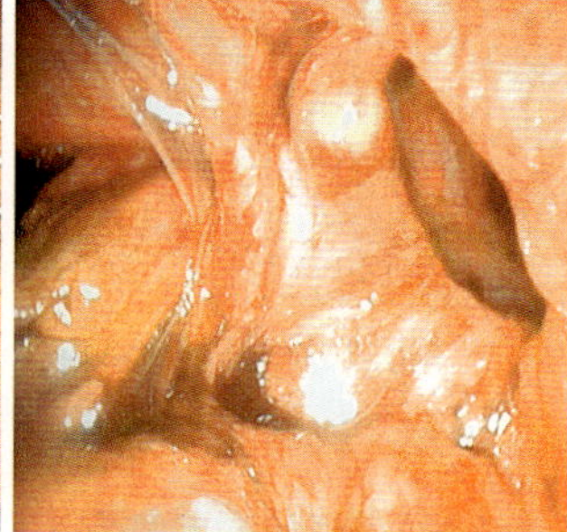

Fig. 19-70: TEP after dissection prior to placement of mesh. Direct defect, inferior epigastric artery, pubic symphysis and Cooper's ligament are clearly seen.

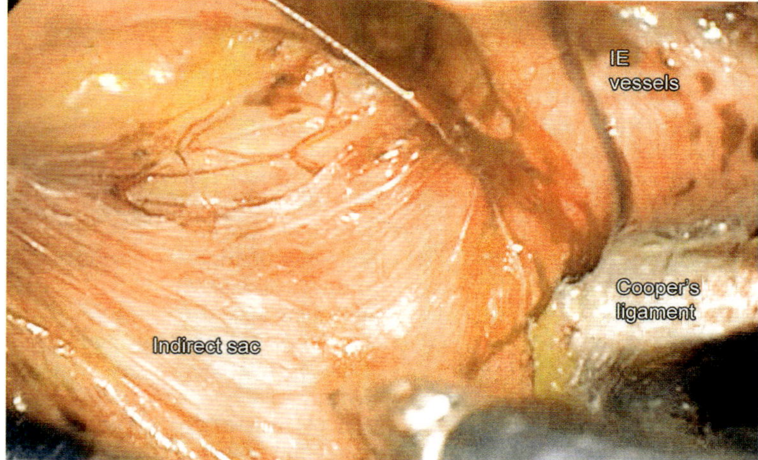

Fig. 19-71: TEP after dissection showing indirect sac, inferior epigastric vessels, Cooper's ligament.

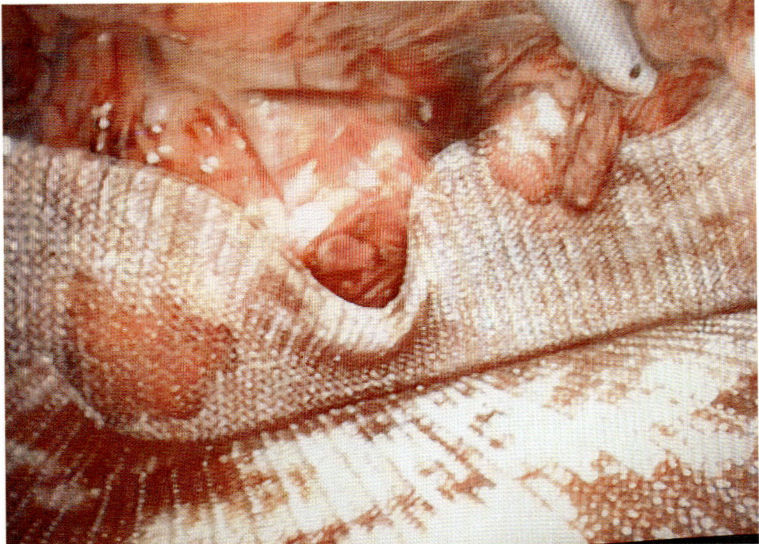

Fig. 19-72: TEP mesh placement in preperitoneal space.

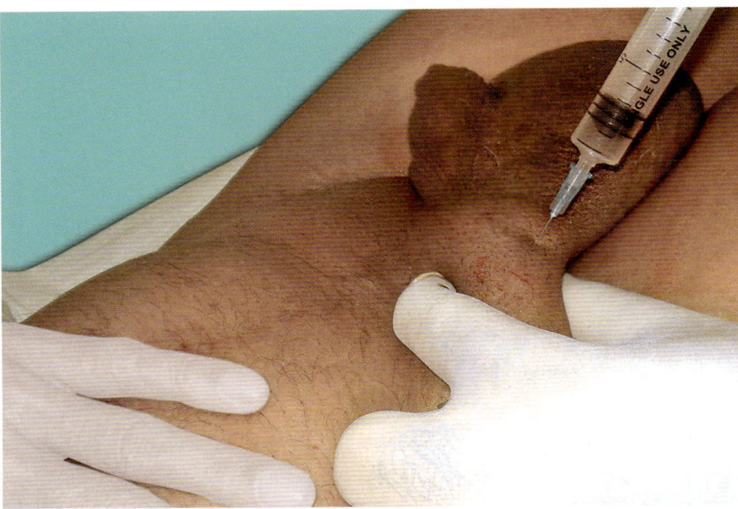

Fig. 19-73: Seroma in groin is common after TEP which can be aspirated safely.

Indications for TEP	*Contraindications for TEP*
♦ Recurrent hernia ♦ Bilateral hernia ♦ Indirect/direct/femoral hernia	♦ Obstructed/strangulated inguinal hernias ♦ Ascites ♦ Bleeding disorders
Landmarks to be identified in TEP	*Principles in TEP*
♦ Pubic bone midline ♦ Inferior epigastric artery ♦ Cooper's ligament ♦ Iliopubic tract ♦ Cord and vas deferens ♦ Psoas muscle and nerves in relation	♦ Supine or head-down supine position ♦ Surgeon standing opposite side of hernia ♦ Camera person placed on opposite side of hernia ♦ Monitor at foot end ♦ Catheterise/empty the bladder properly prior to TEP ♦ Adequate wide space creation ♦ Careful dissection of cord and sac ♦ Ligate indirect sac ♦ Mesh should not be fixed laterally ♦ Size of mesh is 15 × 15 cm ♦ Two point fixation—one at pubic bone other at Cooper's ligament by tacks/staplers

Difficulties and complications in TEP repair

- Difficulty in dissecting indirect sac. Cord/vas injury.
- Inadvertent opening of the sac/peritoneum and creation of pneumoperitoneum.
- Injuries to major structures like iliac vessels: 0.5–1.0%.
- Displacement of mesh or erosion into the structures like urinary bladder—rarely may occur.
- Nerve injury: Lateral cutaneous nerve of thigh and femoral branch of genitofemoral nerve.
- Formation of seroma/haematoma.
- Infection.
- Recurrence.
- Prolapsed of the mesh into the direct hernial defect.

Advantages of TEP repair

- Approach is totally extraperitoneal.
- Small incision.
- Proper placement of mesh in right space that is preperitoneal space.
- Peritoneal cavity is intact and not opened.

STRANGULATED INGUINAL HERNIA

Irreducibility, obstruction and strangulation are the complications of the inguinal hernia. First irreducibility occurs which leads into obstruction and strangulation **(Figs. 19-74 to 19-79)**.

Features of strangulated hernia	*Causes of strangulation*
♦ Tense, tender, irreducible ♦ No impulse on coughing ♦ Shock, toxicity ♦ Features of obstruction when there is enterocele ♦ Abdominal distension, vomiting ♦ Rebound tenderness	♦ Narrow neck ♦ Adhesions ♦ Irreducibility ♦ Long-time, large hernia with adhesions

Patient with strangulated inguinal hernia presents with irreducibility, pain and tenderness, distension of abdomen, vomiting, and toxic features. Initial resuscitation is done with nasogastric aspiration, fluid and electrolyte therapy, antibiotics, urinary catheterisation. Erect X-ray abdomen may show multiple air fluid levels. *Emergency surgery* is needed under general anaesthesia. Inguinal incision extending into the groin is placed. Incision is deepened to reach the external oblique aponeurosis which is cut across the superficial inguinal ring **(Fig. 19-80)**.

Incision is extended and deepened downwards along the root of the scrotum. Sac is identified and held. One should also hold the contents in the sac so has to prevent contents getting reduced and also toxic fluid spilling into the peritoneal cavity. Sac is opened carefully; all toxic fluid in the sac is sucked out thoroughly. Content, either bowel or omentum is held with Babcock's forceps. Viability of the bowel is checked by its colour, texture, peristalsis, mesenteric pulsation or when in doubt by giving 100% oxygen to the patient or after covering the bowel wall using hot mops. If bowel is not viable resection and anastomosis is done. For this, incision may be adequately extended laterally along the lateral abdominal wall. Closing this wound and separate laparotomy incision is not mandatory. Anastomosis is done using interrupted single layer silk or vicryl sutures. *Strangulated omentum* is not uncommon which is treated by omentectomy. *Drains* are placed into the peritoneal cavity as well as into the inguinal wound **(Fig. 19-81)**.

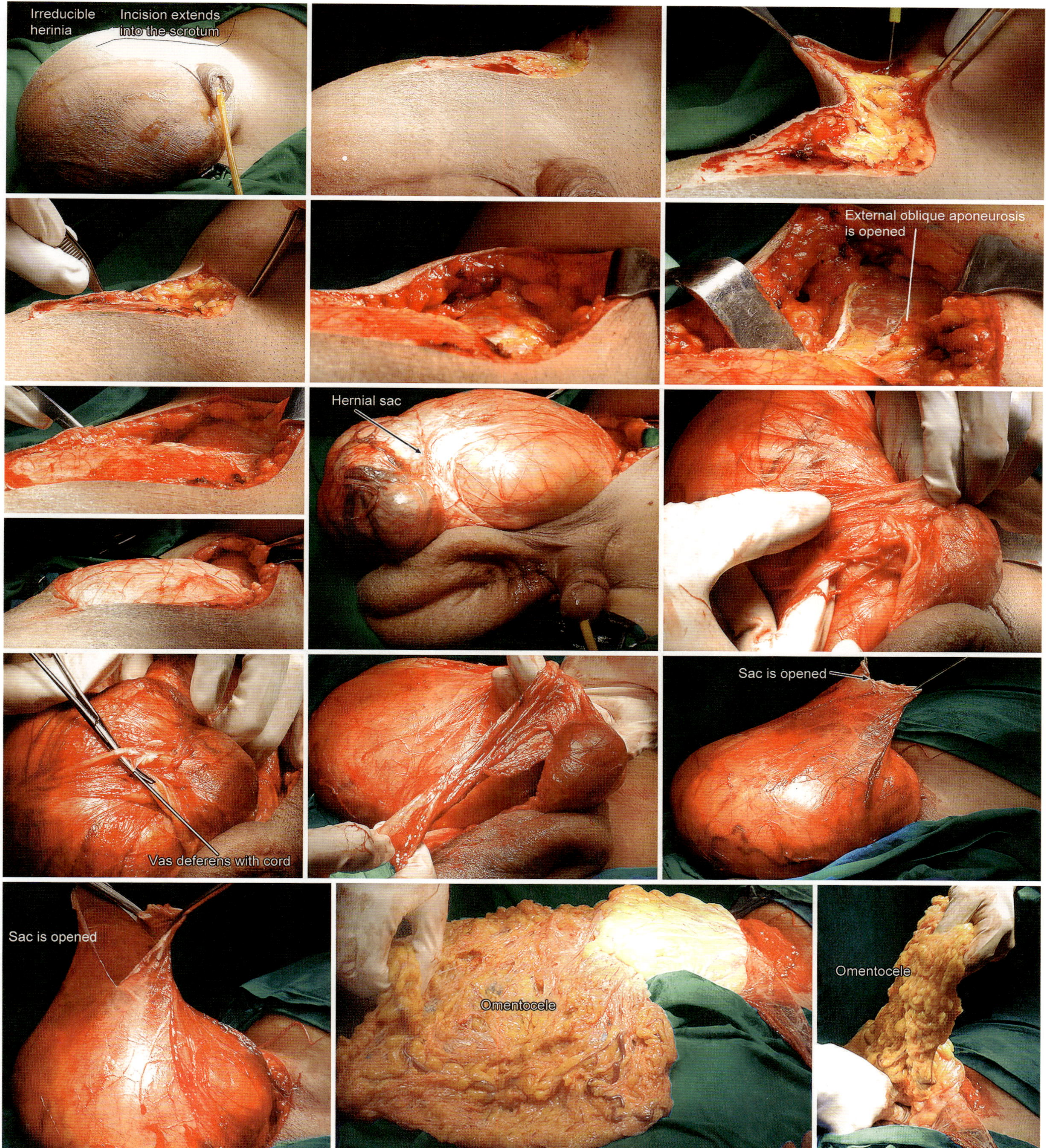
Irreducible herinia
Incision extends into the scrotum
External oblique aponeurosis is opened
Hernial sac
Vas deferens with cord
Sac is opened
Sac is opened
Omentocele
Omentocele

Figs. 19-74(1)

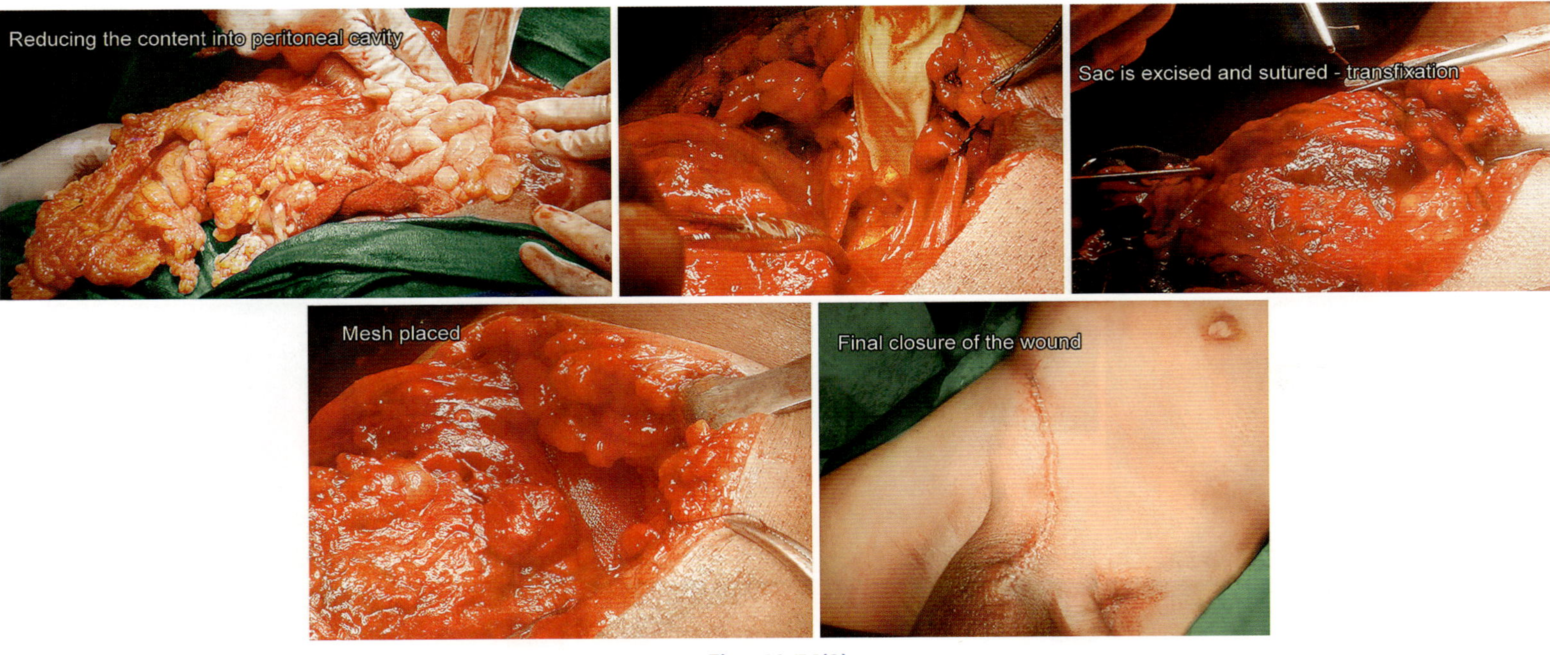

Figs. 19-74(2)

Figs. 19-74(1 and 2): Large irreducible omentocele in a hernia.

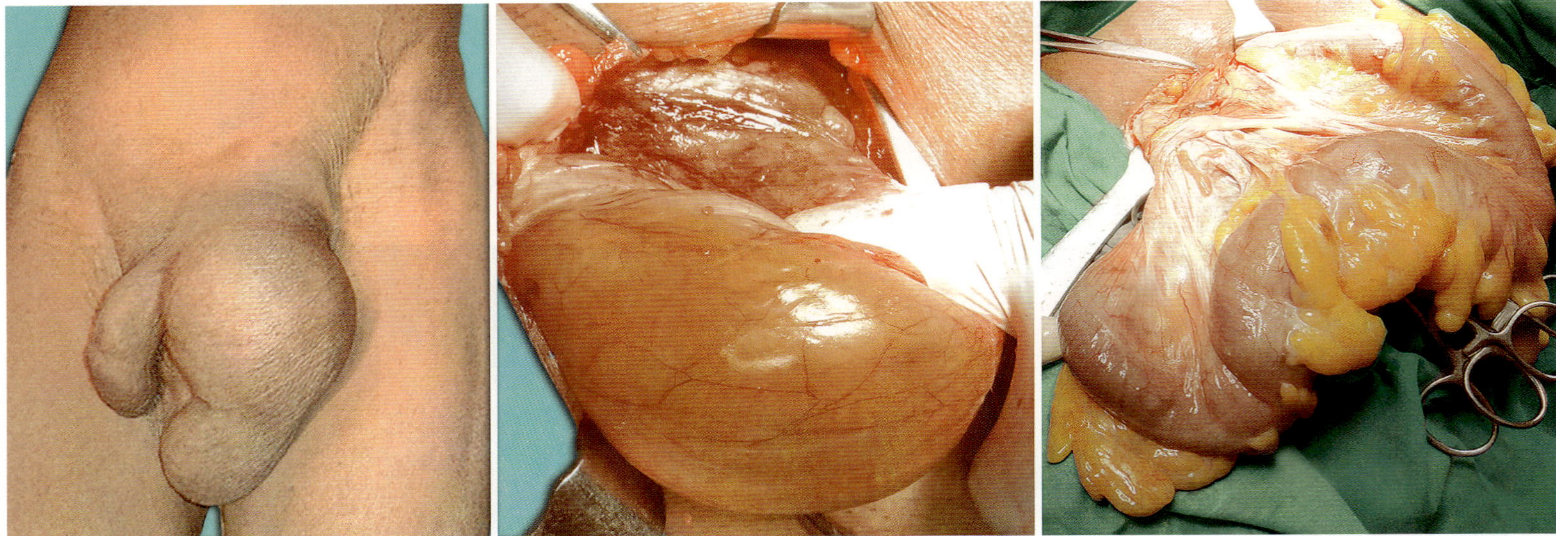

Fig. 19-75: Irreducible hernia—typical look.

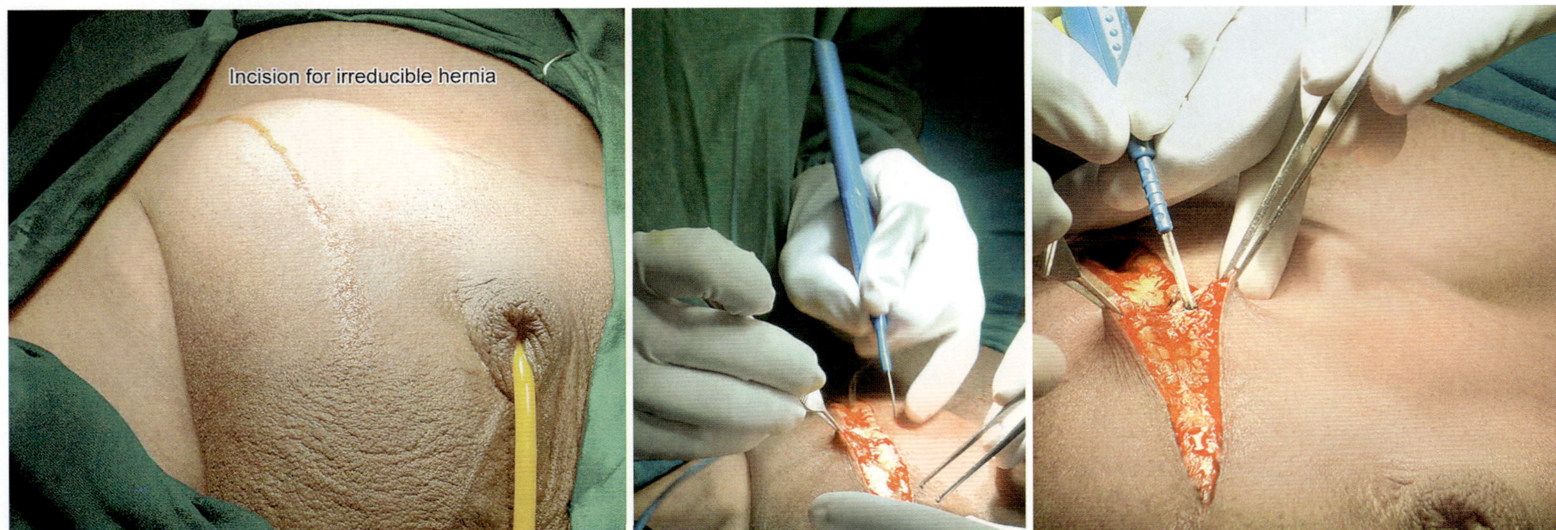

Figs. 19-76(1)

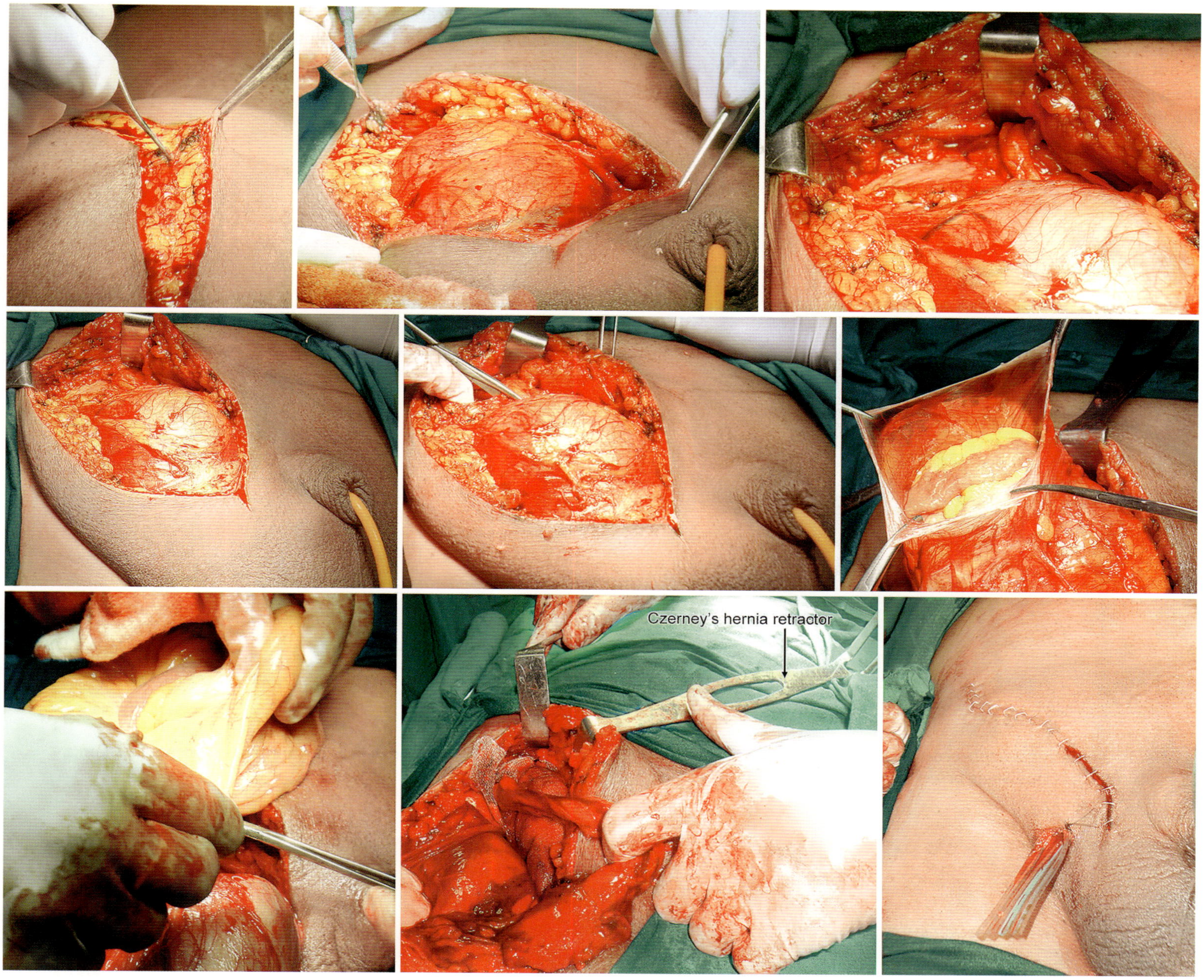

Czerney's hernia retractor

Figs. 19-76(2)

Figs. 19-76(1 and 2): Irreducible enterocele.

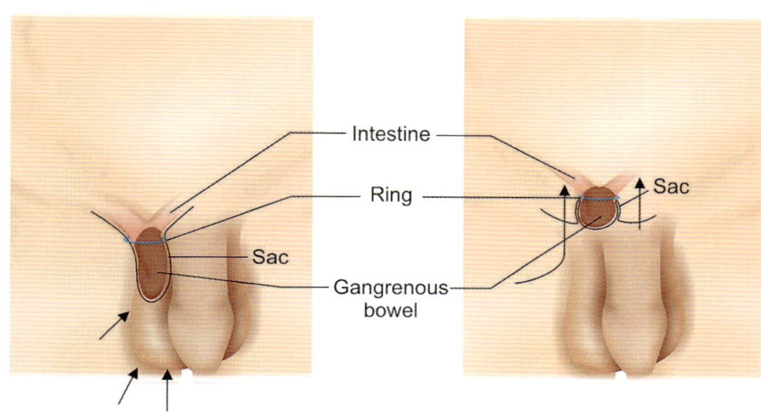

Fig. 19-77: Forced reduction of inguinal hernia will get reduced with the sac with persistent obstruction and strangulation within the peritoneal cavity.

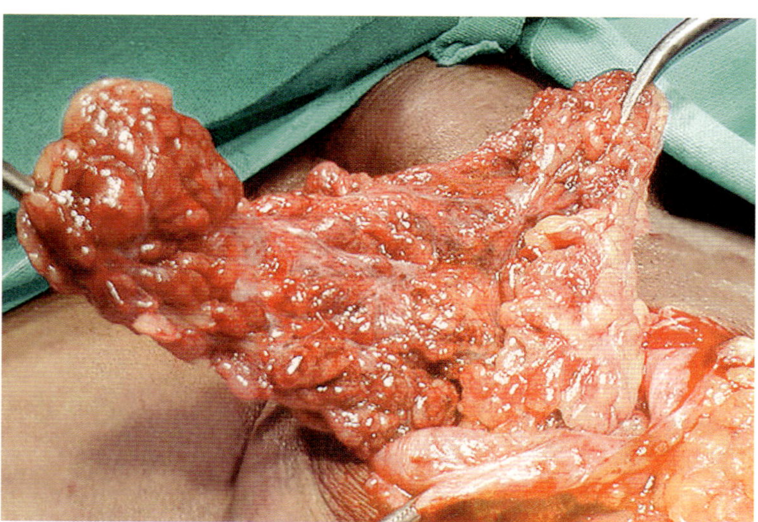

Fig. 19-78: Gangrenous omentum.

Inguinal canal is strengthened by *modified Bassini's repair* using interrupted monofilament polypropylene sutures. Prosthetic mesh is not used as field is contaminated. In later period if hernia recurs then prosthetic mesh is used for repair. Biological mesh can be used during the surgery for strangulated hernia **(Fig. 19-82)**.

Problems in strangulated hernia are—sepsis, leak and fistula formation, ileus, wound infection, peritonitis, intra-abdominal abscess formation like pelvic or subphrenic, electrolyte imbalance, respiratory complications like pneumonia and acute respiratory distress syndrome (ARDS), disseminated intravascular coagulation (DIC).

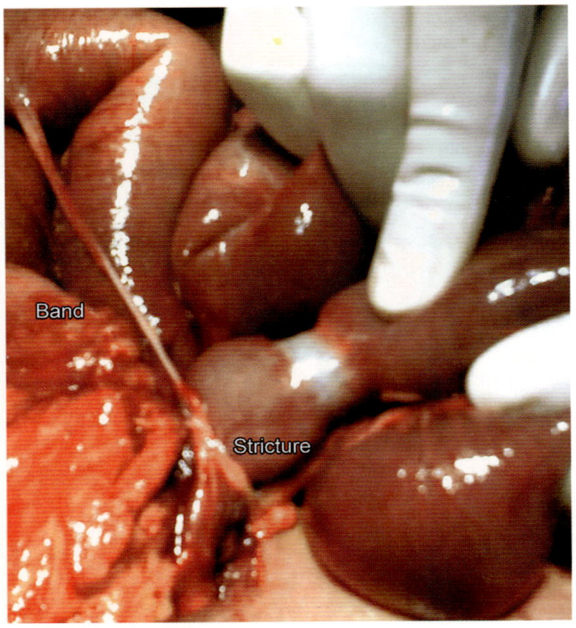

Fig. 19-79: Garry's stricture occurs in long standing obstructed hernia. Stricture develops where bowel developed obstruction at the ring.

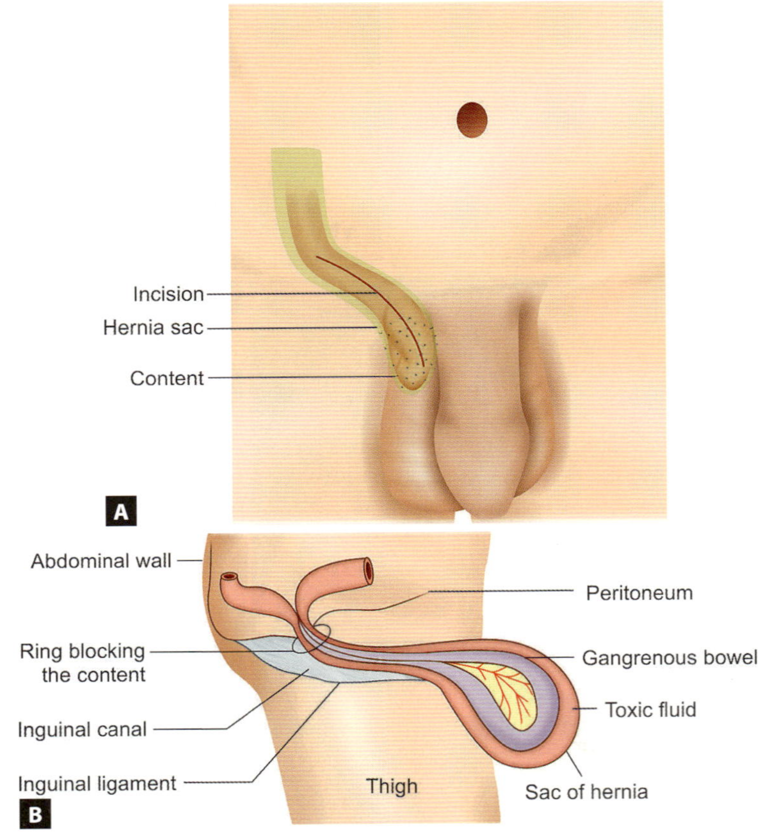

Figs. 19-80A and B: Incision for strangulated inguinal hernia.

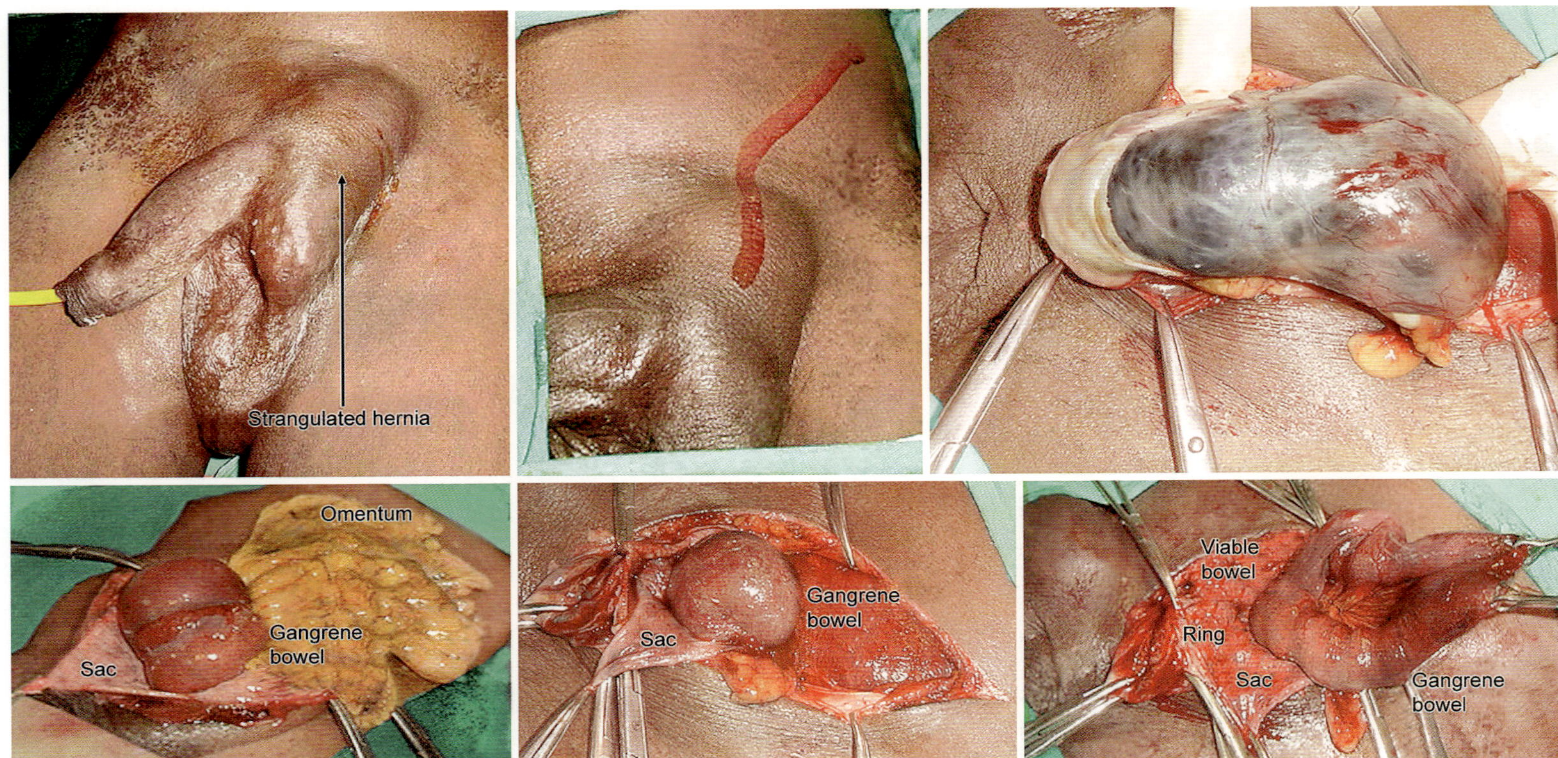

Fig. 19-81: Strangulated hernia—approach. Note the incision placed for strangulated hernia. Only tissue repair is done Modified Bassini's. Mesh is not used.

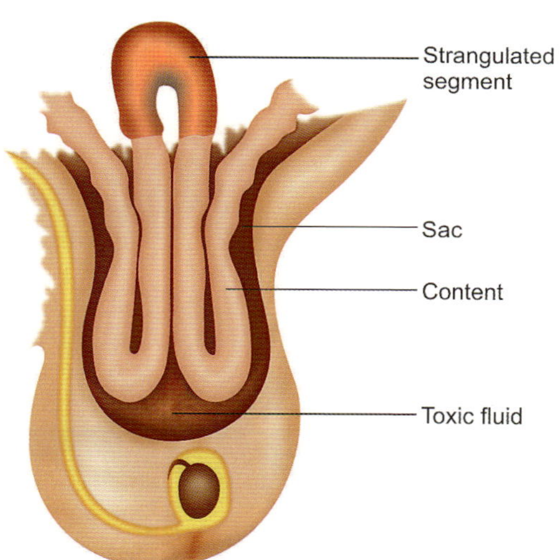

Fig. 19-82: Strangulated hernia with 'W' type bowel content (Maydl's hernia). Inner loop gets strangulated.

INGUINAL HERNIA IN FEMALES

Commonest groin hernia in females is inguinal hernia. Often it may contain Fallopian tube or ovary. Round ligament is attached to labia. Sac is in close relation with round ligament. Sac is adherent and is often difficult to dissect. It is invariably indirect sac. Direct hernia is rare in females. Surgery is the treatment. Laparoscopic or open approach can be used. Round ligament is excised and inguinal canal is entirely closed. Mesh is placed in preperitoneal plane. That also prevents the development of femoral hernia. Incision and technique are same. Bilateral inguinal hernia can be treated surgically in same sitting **(Fig. 19-83)**.

VENTRAL HERNIA

Any protrusion through abdominal wall with the exception of hernia through the inguinofemoral region is defined as *ventral hernia*. Incisional hernia (80%) and primary defects in abdominal fascia which can cause umbilical hernia, epigastric hernia, paraumbilical hernia or Spigelian hernia are grouped under ventral hernia. *Ventral hernia can be*—reducible, irreducible, obstructed, strangulated, single, multiple small defects (*Swiss cheese hernia*) **(Figs. 19-84 to 19-91)**.

Factors responsible for development of incisional hernia

- Vertical incision has got higher chances of incisional hernia than horizontal incision.
- Layered closure of the abdomen has got higher chance than single layer.
- Continuous closure has got higher chances than interrupted closure.
- Using absorbable suture material has got higher chances of hernia than non-absorbable sutures.
- Emergency surgical wound has higher chances than elective surgical wound.
- Laparotomy for peritonitis, acute abdomen, and trauma can commonly cause incisional hernia.
- Drainage through the main laparotomy wound may precipitate formation of incisional hernia.
- Chronic cough, smoking, obstructive uropathy, constipation can precipitate incisional hernia.
- Diabetes, old age, malnutrition, malignancy, anaemia, hypoproteinaemia, jaundice, ascites, liver disease, uraemia, steroid therapy, immunosuppressive diseases are other precipitating factors.

Type of defects in incisional hernia

- Small defect.
- Large and wide defect.
- Very large defect.
- Massive/diffuse.
- Multiple defects.

Incisional hernia may be vertical midline above or below the umbilicus; vertical midline including umbilicus; vertical paramedian; transverse above or below the umbilicus; transverse which crosses the midline; oblique above or below the umbilicus or combined.

It may be less than 5 cm defect; between 5–10 cm; more than 10 cm.

Note:
Size of the defect is important to decide the type of surgical closure in incisional hernia.

Preoperative Preparations for Incisional Hernia Surgery

- Reduction in weight and control of obesity; nutrition, control of anaemia; treatment for diabetes, hypertension, cardiac diseases, respiratory problems; treating the precipitating causes; chest X-ray, ultrasound abdomen to be done. Cessation of smoking, respiratory physiotherapy is important.
- Massive incisional hernia after reduction may cause inferior vena cava (IVC) compression, paralytic ileus and diaphragmatic elevation with respiratory embarrassment (*abdominal compartment syndrome*). It is prevented by prior increasing the capacity of peritoneal cavity by creating pneumoperitoneum using CO_2 so as to increase the intraperitoneal pressure by 12–15 cm of H_2O, daily for 3–6 weeks. Later definitive surgery is done.

Treatment Strategy for Incisional Hernia

It can be non-prosthetic tissue repair or prosthetic repair. *Non-prosthetic repair has become a surgical legacy*. ***Prosthetic repair is the present standard***.

Non-prosthetic Repair

Non-prosthetic repair has got only historical value as recurrence rate is very high (as high as 55%).

Cattell's operation: When the defect is less than 3 cm, and if the patient is having adequate abdominal muscle tone, *layer-by-layer anatomical repair* is done using monofilament non-absorbable suture material like *polypropylene/polyethylene,* ideally with interrupted sutures. Sac should be dissected, ligated and excised prior to repair. Peritoneum and posterior rectus sheath is apposed as first layer and anterior rectus sheath as second layer.

Double breasting of the rectus sheath using interrupted non-absorbable sutures using monofilament suture material. It is overlapping the rectus sheath in two layers with two rows of sutures.

Keel operation is done in large defect. Scar is excised and sac is dissected beyond the margin of the defect. Sac is never opened unless there is obstruction of the content. Sac in inverted using continuous/ interrupted inverting non-absorbable sutures, layer by layer until the defect margins are apposed together which is then again sutured with interrupted sutures (*Keel is inverted beam of the ship running along its bottom*).

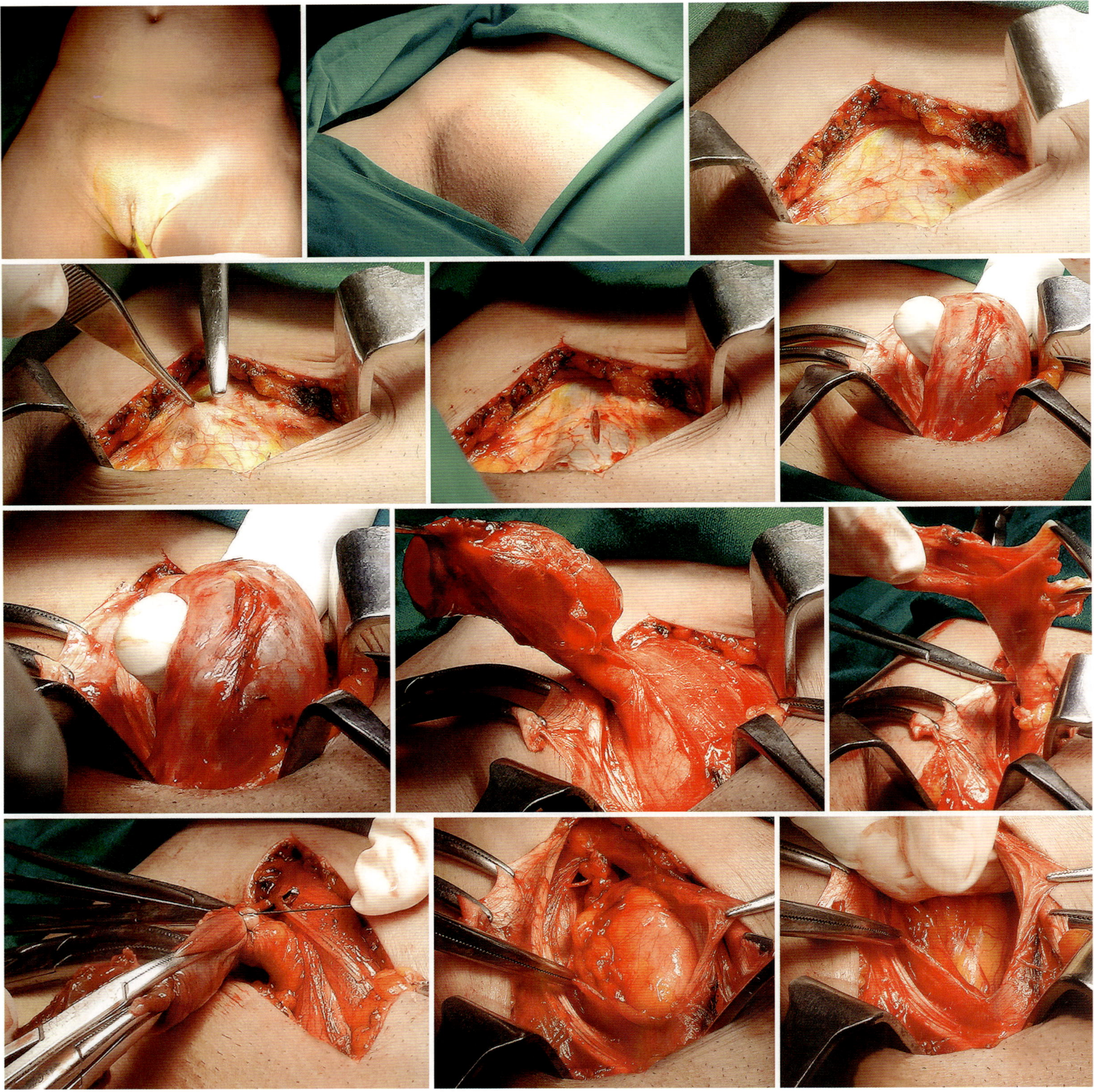

Figs. 19-83(1)

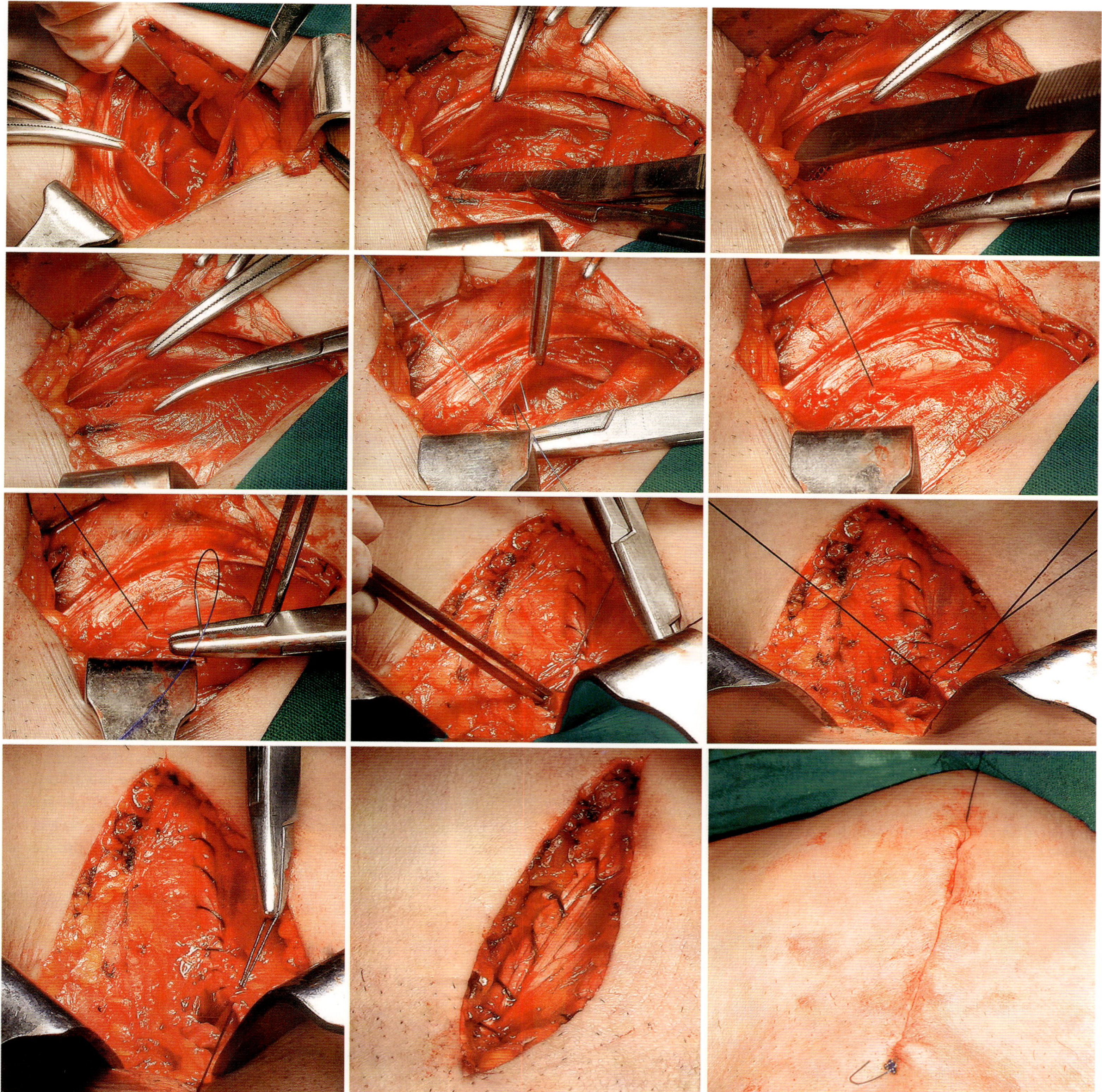

Figs. 19-83(2)

Figs. 19-83(1 and 2): Inguinal hernia repair in female.

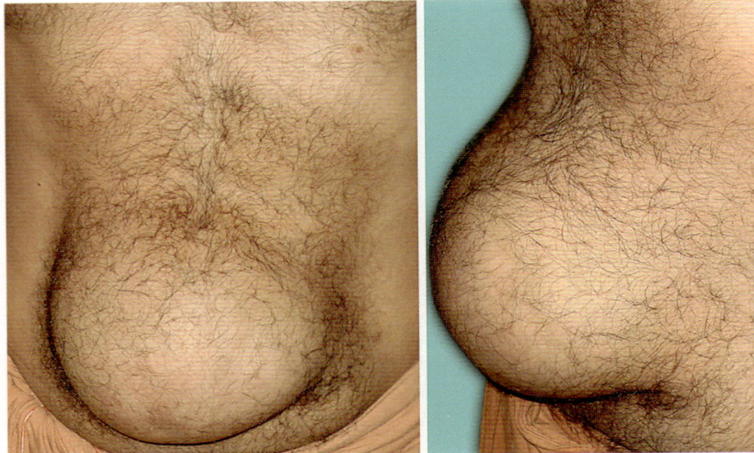

Fig. 19-84: Large ventral hernias. It needs proper mesh repair. Causes—congenital defect, obesity, smoking, chronic cough.

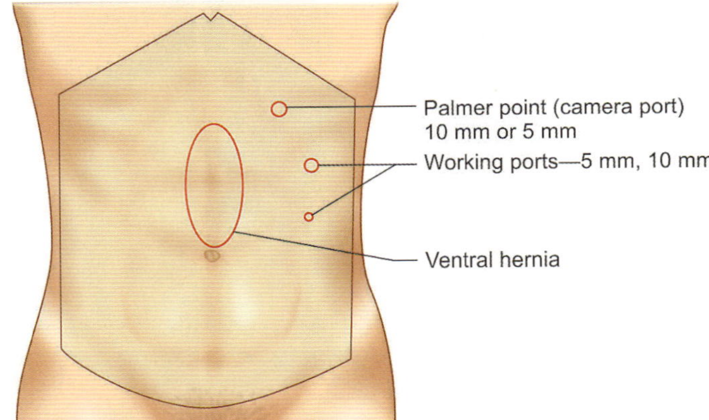

Fig. 19-85: Port placement for laparoscopic ventral hernia repair. Left subcostal point is palmer point.

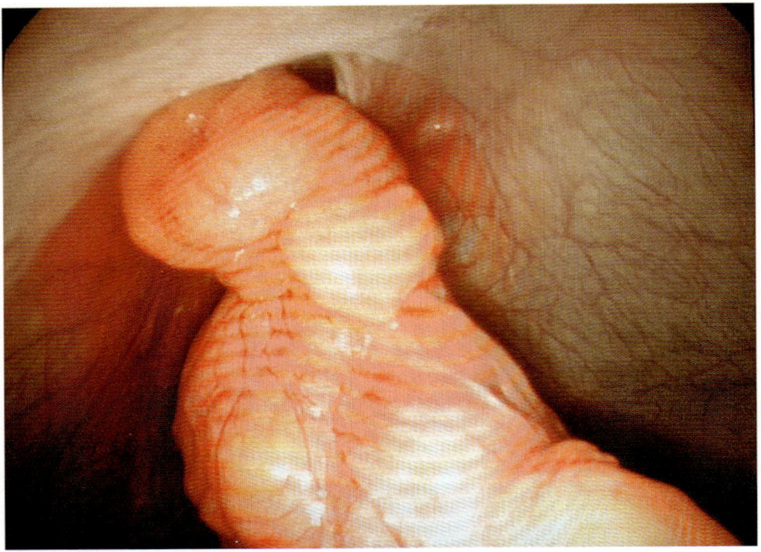

Fig. 19-86: Laparoscopic view of ventral hernia with omentum as irreducible content. Content is released and dual or four-layered mesh is fixed with tackers or sutures.

Nuttall's operation is done for lower midline incisional hernia. Recti attachments are detached from the pubic bones and are crossed over to fix to opposite pubic bones so as to create a firm abdominal wall support by crossed recti muscles **(Figs. 19-92A and B)**.

Prosthetic Repair of Incisional Hernia

It is the Present Standard

It is now universally accepted that prosthetic repair is gold standard for all incisional hernia. Prosthesis used are polypropylene mesh, e-PTFE, Dacron, dual intraperitoneal mesh, biologic grafts.

Open Mesh Repair of the Incisional Hernia

It is always better and ideal with less chances of recurrence. Adequate sized mesh is placed at different planes onlay/overlay or inlay or retrorectus or preperitoneal. Mesh onlay is placing mesh in front of the defect and muscle layer usually after doing simple repair. It has got high recurrence rate (25%) with wound infection. So it is not practiced commonly. Inlay is bridging the defect using prosthetic

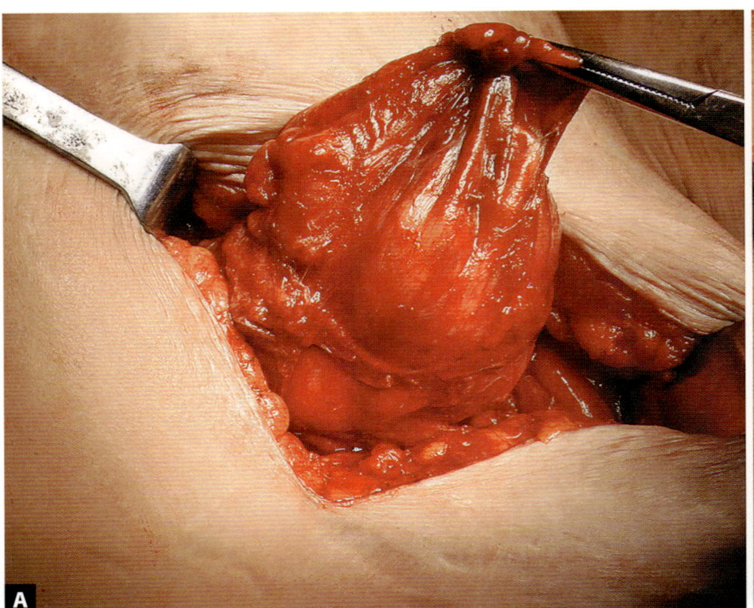

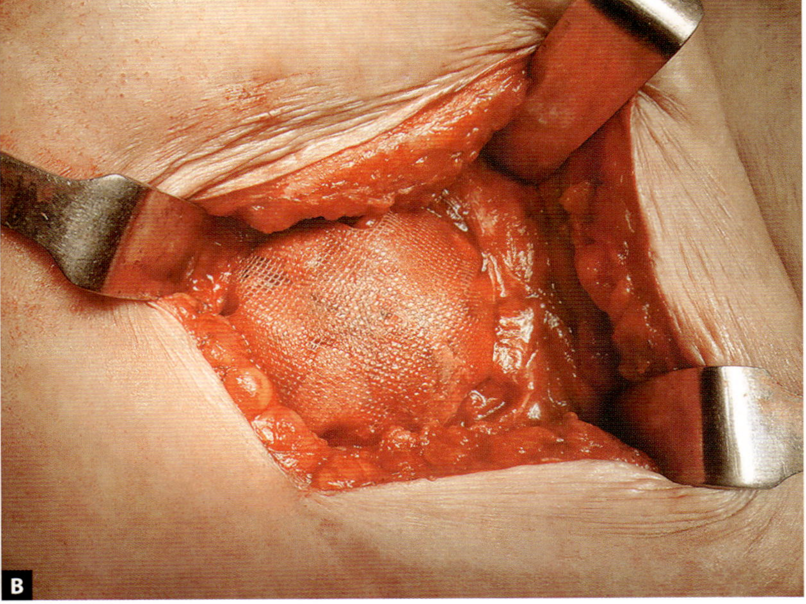

Figs. 19-87A and B: On table look of ventral hernia sac and its mesh repair (in retrorectus plane).

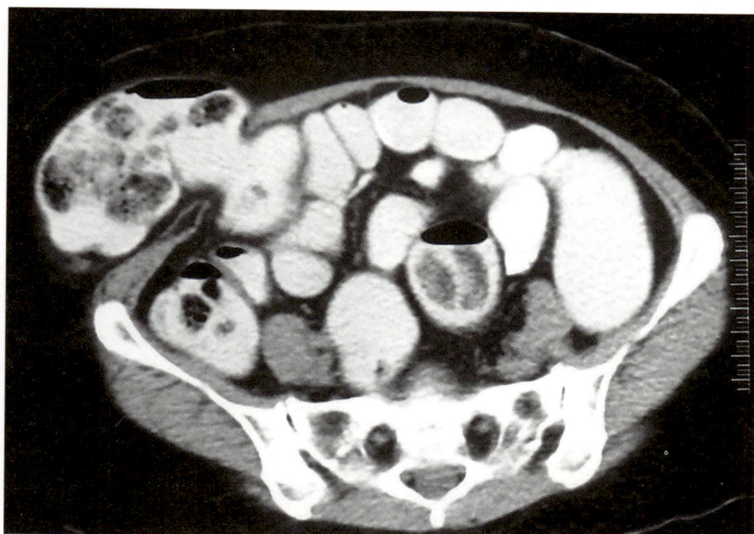

Fig. 19-88: CT scan finding of the ventral hernia.

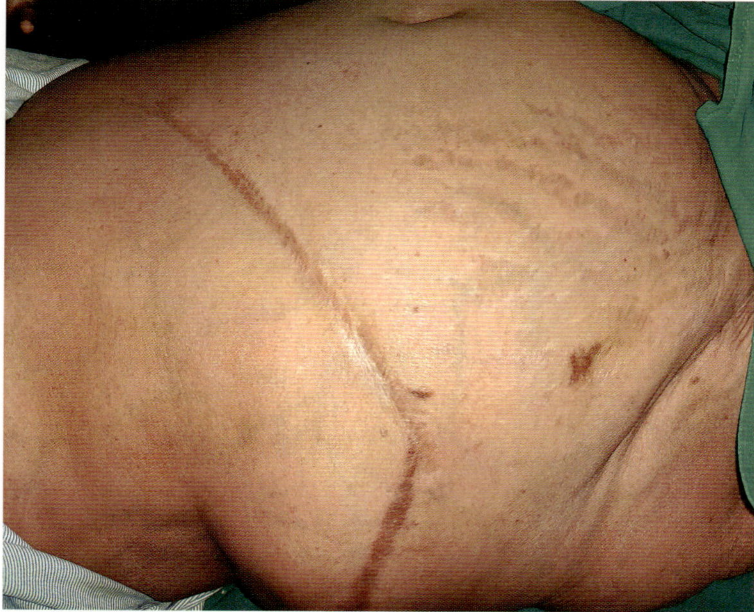

Fig. 19-89: Incisional hernia through right subcostal incision scar.

mesh by suturing mesh to the surrounding myoaponeurotic defect. Repeated contractions of abdominal wall muscles, mesh shrinkage, separation forces of recti leads to the high recurrence rate (20%). So again it is not commonly accepted method. *Rive's Stoppa's mesh placement* for incisional hernia is placing mesh between posterior rectus sheath and rectus muscle. It is *sublay retrorectus mesh* placement. Midline or transverse incision is done. If needed panniculectomy incision may also be used. Hernial sac is dissected using fine scissor and cautery. Bowel may be adherent to sac and so care should be taken not to injure the bowel. Usually peritoneal sac is opened; all adhesions are released. Retrorectal plane is entered by incising the posterior rectus sheath; 5 cm area beyond the defect is dissected. Usually it will be within the rectus muscle area; if dissection is needed beyond that then it is done through intermuscular plane between internal oblique and transverse abdominis or through preperitoneal plane up to the plane of psoas major muscle. Dissection is done using blunt, sharp scissor and cautery. Peritoneum, posterior rectus sheath and transversalis fascia are sutured. Polyester or lightweight polypropylene mesh is ideal **(Fig. 19-93)**.

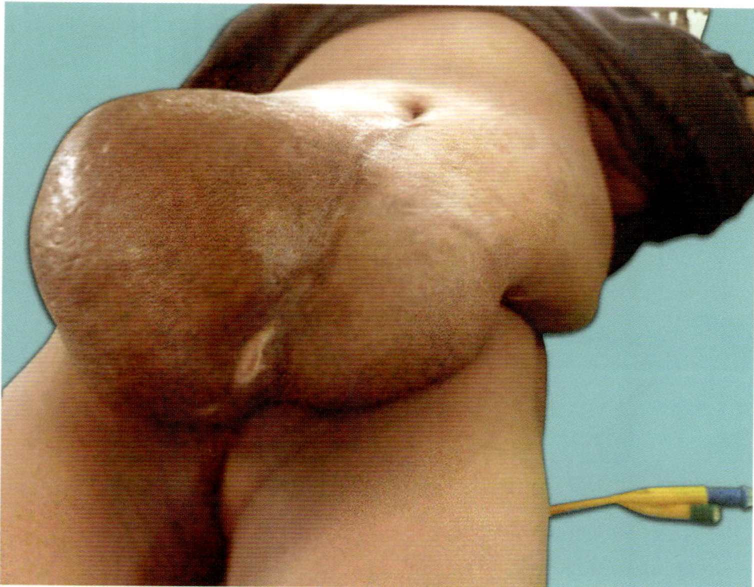

Fig. 19-90: Incisional hernia—large.

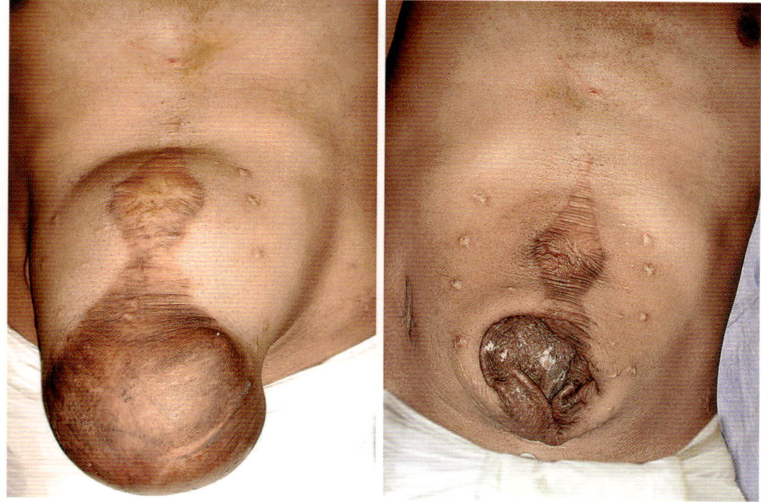

Fig. 19-91: Incisional hernia while coughing; while relaxing it is getting reduced showing thin lax skin.

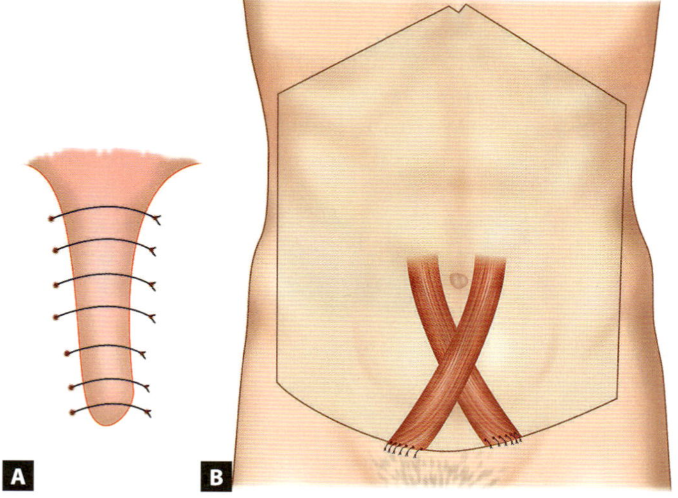

Figs. 19-92A and B: (A) Keel and (B) Nuttall's operation for incisional hernia. It is not used nowadays.

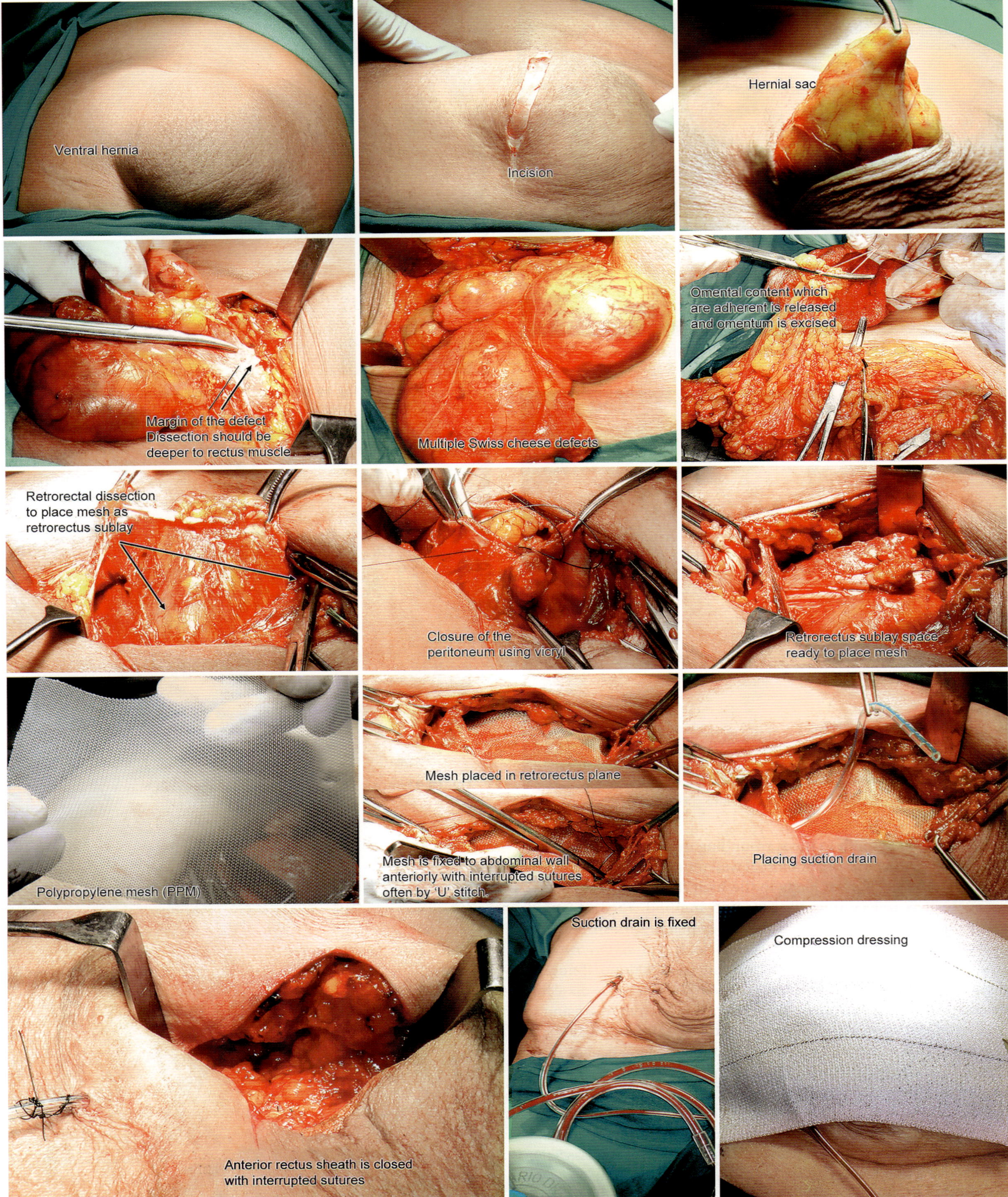

Fig. 19-93: Technique of open ventral hernia repair by placing mesh in retrorectus plane.

Mesh is fixed using polypropylene interrupted sutures to the abdominal wall muscles in its full thickness. 'U' stitches are placed using Reverdin needle. Sutures are placed on one side of the wound from mesh to abdominal wall; once all sutures are placed on one side of the wound, they are tied. Then mesh is fixed similarly on the other side of the wound. Usually around 10 sutures are needed on one side. Absorbable sutures may be used to reduce the chances of chronic abdominal pain. Sutures keep the mesh in place and prevent bulging of the mesh. Often these sutures are brought out through separate stab incisions in the abdominal wall and knots are tied which are buried in the subcutaneous plane. Deeper blind bites on to the peritoneum should not be taken. Linea alba or anterior rectus sheath should be closed to keep the abdominal contour and function normal and also to prevent infection. Commonly polypropylene mesh is used. Other materials used are polyester, Dacron, polytetrafluroethylene (PTFE) mesh, polyglycolic acid mesh (vicryl mesh) or combined polypropylene and polyglycolic acid mesh (vypro mesh). Suction drain should be placed in front of the mesh and in subcutaneous plane as well. Subcutaneous tissue and skin are closed with interrupted sutures. When subcutaneous drain is placed, suturing of subcutaneous fat is not done as strangulation/necrosis of fat can occur by suturing. Mesh repair is ideal approach for incisional hernia. Prevention of infection/haemostasis and drainage are important. Recurrence rate in this type is less than 5% **(Fig. 19-94)**.

Open Intraperitoneal Mesh Repair for Incisional Hernia

It is done whenever peritoneum is not enough to close. Dissection is done similarly. ePTFE mesh is used to place the mesh directly outer to viscera intraperitoneally. Mesh is first fixed to abdominal wall at 12 and 6 o'clock positions to prevent displacement. Continuous mesh fixation suture is placed from 12 o'clock position to 6 o'clock position; later from 6 o'clock to 12 o'clock position. Rectus sheath is sutured in front after placing a suction drain.

Component Separation Technique with Mesh Placement (Autologenous Repair by Vascularised Innervated Muscle Flaps) (Ramirez, 1990)

It is release of the external oblique aponeurosis and separation of the lateral abdominal wall muscles to achieve advancement of the abdominal wall to cause medialisation of the rectus muscle up to 10 cm to achieve reformation of dynamic abdominal wall with midline linea alba closure. Originally it was designed as a non-prosthetic repair but eventually it became popular with additional mesh placement in retrorectus or intraperitoneal area. Vertical incision is made along the hernial sac usually in midline. Sac is identified, dissected, opened and ligated. Flap in front of anterior rectus sheath is raised to identify the external oblique aponeurosis 2–5 cm lateral to the lateral margin of the rectus sheath. Longitudinal incision is made in the external oblique aponeurosis below and beyond the hernial defect usually up to the inguinal ligament; above up to 5 cm above the costal margin. External oblique muscle is then dissected off from the internal oblique in an avascular plane between these two muscles up to posterior axillary line to medialise the rectus muscle along its full length. Additional 4 cm of medialisation can be achieved if needed by incising the posterior rectus sheath longitudinally on its medial aspect. Large prosthetic mesh is now placed after creating plane in retrorectus area or intraperitoneal dual mesh can also be placed. Biologic graft can be used in infected contaminated area. Drain is placed over the mesh. Linea alba is closed. Multiple drains are placed in subcutaneous plane. By this separation technique rectus is advanced for 5 cm in upper abdomen; 7–10 cm in middle and 3 cm in lower abdomen.

It is often of practice that skin fat is first dissected off the anterior rectus sheath for 5 cm beyond the rectus; incision is made in posterior rectus sheath and muscle is separated from the posterior rectus sheath; lastly aponeurosis is incised to separate external oblique from internal oblique to achieve adequate medialisation to close the defect and linea alba.

Separation of component can also be achieved *endoscopically*. 10 mm incision is made adjacent to the tip of 11th rib. External oblique aponeurosis is identified and incised along the line of incision 1 cm to reach an avascular plane between external oblique aponeurosis and internal oblique muscle. Inguinal hernia balloon dissector is placed, directed towards pubic tubercle and is inflated to create adequate space to place a 10 mm port to achieve up to 12 mm Hg pressure with CO_2 insufflation. One 5 mm port is placed in posterior axillary line through which aponeurosis is cut caudally using scissor or cautery. Another 5 mm port is placed medially through which cranial part of the aponeurosis is cut. *Complications of component separation technique are*—seroma/haematoma formation; lateral bulging of the muscle if internal oblique muscle is cut; mesh related complications; paralytic ileus; wound infection; abdominal wall nerve injury and its consequences. Recurrence rate is less than 5%.

Laparoscopic Mesh Repair for Incisional/ Ventral Hernia (1992—LeBlanch and Booth)

It is placing a mesh under the defect laparoscopically in intraperitoneal plane. The only problem of this underlay placement is chances of adhesion and GI fistula formation but it is found to be safer. Laparoscopic preperitoneal mesh placement is also done for smaller defects. Now dual mesh (PTFE) or four layered mesh are available. Presently only these meshes are recommended for use. Here mesh is placed under the peritoneum deep to the defect after reducing the contents. Mesh is fixed with sutures and tacks. In four layer mesh, deepest 1st layer is absorbable cellulose which allows new peritoneum to creep underneath. 2nd layer is PDS/PTFE mesh 3rd layer is polypropylene mesh last 4th layer is again PDS/PTFE mesh. It is ideal but costly.

Exact defect is marked using skin marking pen after cleaning and draping under general anaesthesia. Catheterisation is always better done especially in lower abdominal hernias. After creating pneumoperitoneum ports are placed. Table can be tilted accordingly depending on location of the hernial site. Procedure is done in supine position. Surgeon and cameraman are standing on left side of the patient. Monitor is placed on right side towards leg end. Left Palmer point below the left subcostal margin is used for 10 mm port for 10 mm end or side viewing telescope. 5 mm port with 5 mm telescope can be used if available. Usually open method is used. Hasson cannula is better in this situation. Visiport usage makes creation of this first port site better. Further two 5 mm ports are placed also in the left side along the anterior axillary line. If needed additional port may be used on the opposite side. Hernial contents are reduced with careful dissection. Dissection is done either with bipolar cautery or ideally sharp scissor. Adhesiolysis is done by keeping scissor close to abdominal wall to reduce the chances of bowel perforation. Entire abdominal contents are inspected. Hernial defect is assessed

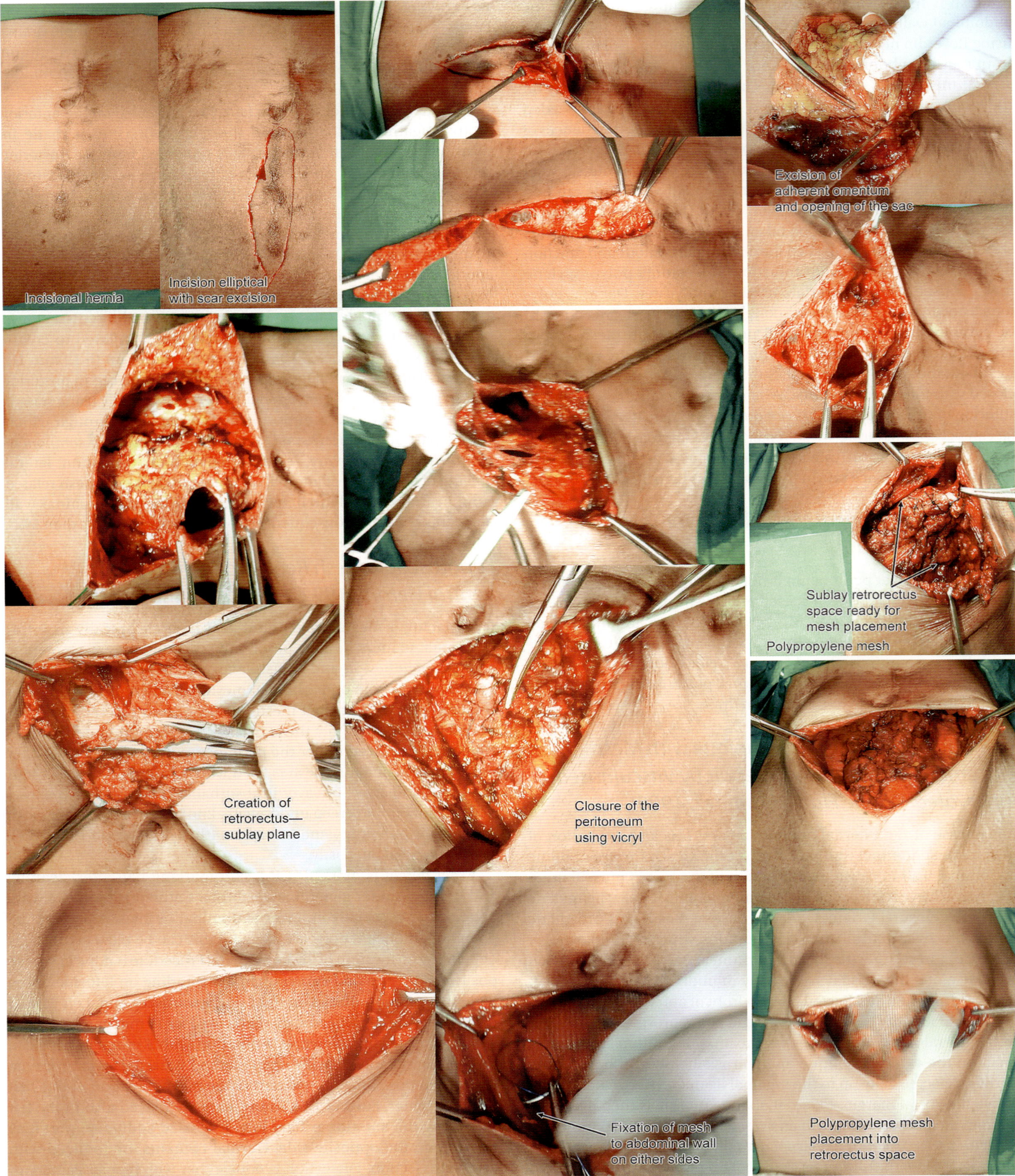
Incisional hernia
Incision elliptical with scar excision
Excision of adherent omentum and opening of the sac
Sublay retrorectus space ready for mesh placement
Polypropylene mesh
Creation of retrorectus—sublay plane
Closure of the peritoneum using vicryl
Fixation of mesh to abdominal wall on either sides
Polypropylene mesh placement into retrorectus space

Figs. 19-94(1)

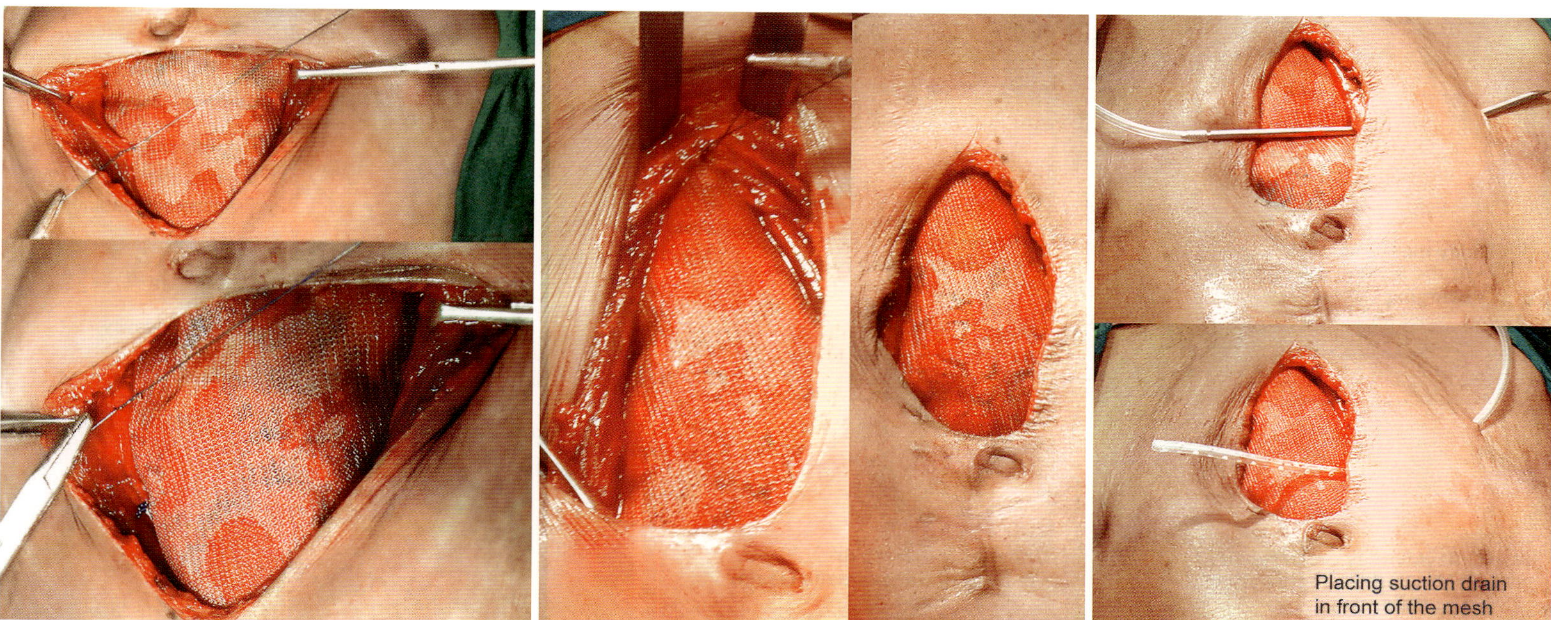

Figs. 19-94(2)

Figs. 19-94(1 and 2): Incisional hernia repair and retrorectus mesh placement. This is the standard technique in open repair. Suction drain should be placed always.

by placing a flexible ruler intra-abdominally through a port under standard insufflation pressure of 12 mm Hg. Dual or four layer mesh with non-adhesive surface facing towards abdominal contents is placed. It is folded carefully and passed inside through 10 mm port. All four corners are sutured using transfascial fixation sutures. It is fixed properly using tackers (helical tacks) or sutures. It is better to place sutures using specialised needle or by intracorporeal suturing and knotting technique. Helical tacks are placed all round at every 5 mm gap. Patient is discharged in 24 hours with abdominal binder for 6 weeks advicing not to lift weight for 6 weeks. *Advantages of laparoscopic ventral hernia repair* are—proper visualisation of entire abdomen; avoidance of unnecessary dissection; identification of multiple/Swiss cheese defects; less recurrence rate; short hospital stay; less morbid surgery; faster recovery; better in obese patients. *Disadvantages, problems and complications* are—seroma formation (20%), cautery or dissection injury to bowel (5%), costly mesh, need for general anaesthesia, mesh folding, displacement, bowel interposition between mesh and peritoneum if mesh is not properly placed, mesh infection, wound infection, recurrence, port site bleeding, port site hernia, inadvertent fall of tackers into the peritoneal cavity and its possible complications like erosion into major vessels and vital structures, paralytic ileus, retention of urine postoperatively after removal of the catheter, abdominal wall neuralgia due to injury to abdominal wall nerves by sutures or tackers, conversion into open method. Complications are classified as intraoperative, early, late.

Different Types of Mesh Repair for Incisional Hernia

- *Rive's Stoppa's method* of placing mesh between posterior rectus sheath and rectus muscle widely—retrorectus approach is better.
- *Under the peritoneum, directly over the content (intraperitoneal):* Now it is accepted but there are chances of adhesions/fistula formation. It is used in laparoscopic repair. Dual mesh/four layered mesh is used.
- *Overlay* mesh placed outer to musculoaponeurotic layer *is not ideal* due to high recurrence rate.
- *Combined inlay and overlay* with two layers of mesh—practiced in few centres.
- *Bridging at myoaponeurotic level outer to peritoneum (inlay):* Adequate sized mesh is placed in the defect level bridging the gap to cover preperitoneum. It is better by principle but still shows high recurrence **(Fig. 19-95)**.

Postoperative Care

Postoperative management is crucial in these patients. Prevention of sepsis, DVT, ileus, mobilisation are important. Heparin should be started to prevent DVT. Early ambulation, fluid and electrolyte management, catheterisation, care of drain (drain should be kept until drainage becomes minimal), abdominal binder is used to support abdominal wall during recovery period.

Additional Problems in Large Incisional Hernia

- While reducing the bulky contents like bowel and omentum, inadequate intra-abdominal capacity leads to increased intra-abdominal pressure causing IVC compression, mesenteric oedema following stasis of splanchnic bed, paralytic ileus, diaphragmatic elevation and respiratory distress (*abdominal compartment syndrome*), urinary and bowel disturbances. Abdominal capacity can be raised by creating regular pneumoperitoneum over the period of 3–6 weeks.
- Lordosis and back pain may be presenting feature.
- Sac and contents may get adherent to the thin skin over the summit of the hernia leading to skin ulceration and occasionally fistula formation.
- Often might need resection of the adherent bowel segment. In such a situation only biologic grafts may be possible. Otherwise primary tissue repair has to be done which has got high recurrence rate.
- Large mesh placement is required.
- Additional lipectomy (panniculectomy) may be done in case of pendulous abdomen.

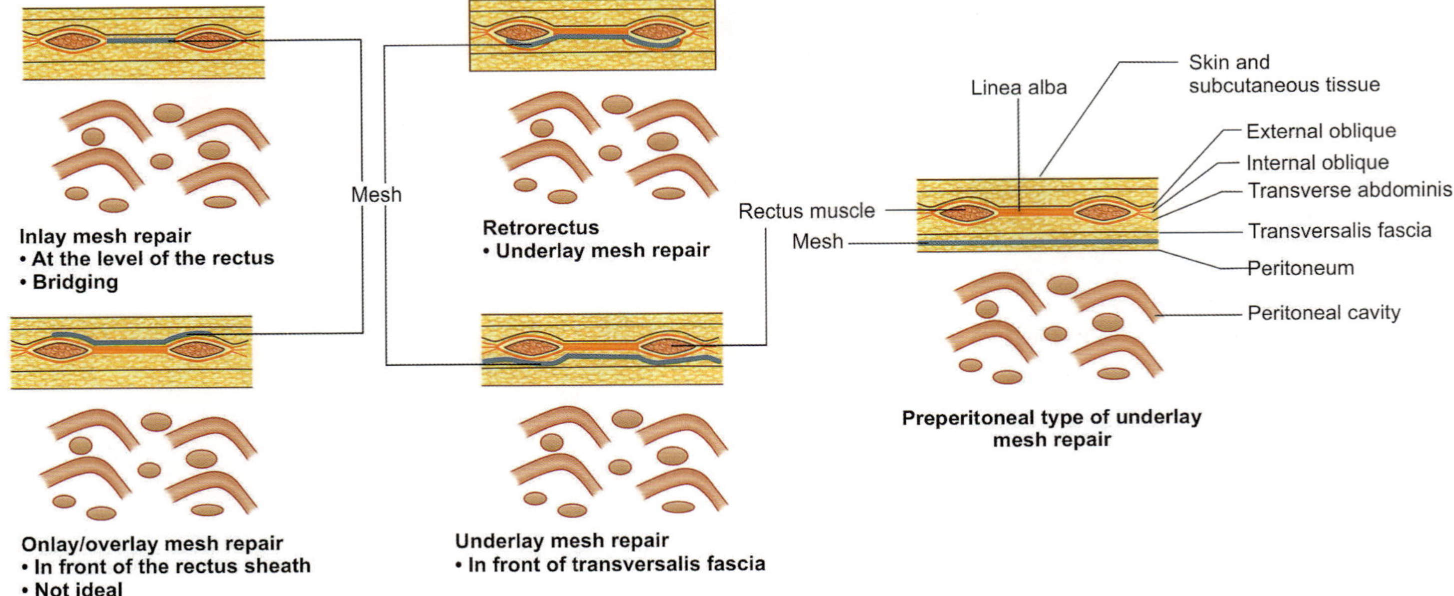

Fig. 19-95: Different levels where mesh can be placed in ventral/incisional hernia—sublay/retrorectus is ideal anatomical plane.

NEWER CONCEPTS IN VENTRAL HERNIA

Current definition of incisional hernia is by Korenkov et al. as "Any abdominal wall gap with or without a bulge in the area of a postoperative scar perceptible or palpable by clinical examination or imaging".

Abdominal wall dynamics are based on Pascal's law of pressure and Laplace's law of wall tension. Abdominopelvic cavity is enveloped by muscles, tendons and bones. If intra-abdominal pressure is more than the abdominal wall pressure then wall ruptures at weakest point causing herniation. Once hernia develops it will continue to enlarge due to increased wall tension. It can develop due to excessive intra-abdominal pressure (cough, urinary strain, constipation. etc.), age, pregnancy, weakness of abdominal wall due to developmental failure, muscle atrophy, genetic weakness of collagen, trauma, previous surgery, ascites, obesity, metabolic diseases, diabetes mellitus, liver cell dysfunction, chronic kidney disease.

Hernia can be—occult; reducible; irreducible; obstructed; strangulated; incarcerated. Hernia can be—ventral wall hernia (epigastric, umbilical, paraumbilical, incisional, spigelian, parastomal); groin hernia (inguinal, femoral); flank hernia (superior and inferior lumbar); pelvic hernia (sciatic, obturator, perineal). Newer classifications have come like EHS (European Hernia Society). Primary ventral hernia has different aetiology which is non-incisional hernia. Incisional ventral hernia is due to failure of previous incision closure and healing process.

It is classified as (EHS)—Midline (M) and Lateral (L). In midline—subxiphoidal; epigastric; umbilical; infraumbilical; suprapubic; (M1; M2; M3; M4; M5). Lateral as subcostal; flank; iliac; lumbar (L1; L2; L3; L4). Recurrence is classified as R0; R1; R3; --- depending on number of recurrence. Multiple defects from same incisional hernia are considered as one with maximum length and outermost widths are taken for measurement for "Grid format". Defect is classified as—small (2 cm); medium (2–4 cm); large (>4 cm).

Incisional hernia grading—Grade/Stage I: Low recurrence, less SSO (surgical site occurrence), <10 cm, clean; Stage II: Moderate recurrence, moderate SSO, <10 cm contaminated OR 10–20 cm clean; Stage III: High recurrence, high SSO, >10 cm contaminated OR any more than 20 cm **(Fig. 19-96)**.

Chevrel and Rath (2000) classification of ventral hernia

Site:
Medial incisional hernias are coded as M, with 4 subgroups:
M1 - supraumbilical incisional hernias
M2 - juxtaumbilical incisional hernias
M3 - subumbilical incisional hernias
M4 - xipho-pubic incisional hernias

Lateral incisional hernias are coded as L, with 4 subgroups:
L1 - subcostal incisional hernias
L2 - transverse incisional hernias
L3 - iliac incisional hernias
L4 - lumber incisional hernias

Width (preoperative measurement) is classified by 5 cm increments:
W1 - <5 cm
W2 - 5 to 10 cm
W3 - 10 to 15 cm
W4 - >15 cm

Recurrence is defined by its number:
No recurrence: R0
First recurrence: R1
Second recurrence: R2, etc.

Giant ventral (incisional hernia): It is important to understand giant abdominal hernia as "loss of domain" and "hernia volume" are major two factors decides the definition and outcome. Loss of domain is defined as hernia contents with adhesions are not reducible to abdominal cavity. Hernia volume >25% of abdominal volume is difficult to manage. So, giant ventral hernia is defined as large ventral hernia (probably >10 cm) with loss of domain and hernia volume >20–25%. Here assessment with CECT abdomen, functional respiratory volume and cardiac status is mandatory. Abdominal volumetry is often used assess the volume ratio. *Problems with giant ventral hernia are*—respiratory failure; recurrence; compartment syndrome; impossible to reduce the content; infection. Proper preoperative preparation is a must with respiratory physiotherapy, reduction in weight, diet, non-invasive ventilation, methods to improve intra-abdominal volume, etc. planning the surgery type, mesh usage also important. Botulinum toxin injection, preoperative

EHS Primary abdominal wall hernia Classification		Diameter cm	Small <2 cm	Medium ≥2–4 cm	Large ≥4 cm
Midline	Epigastric				
	Umbilical				
Lateral	Spigelian				
	Lumbar				

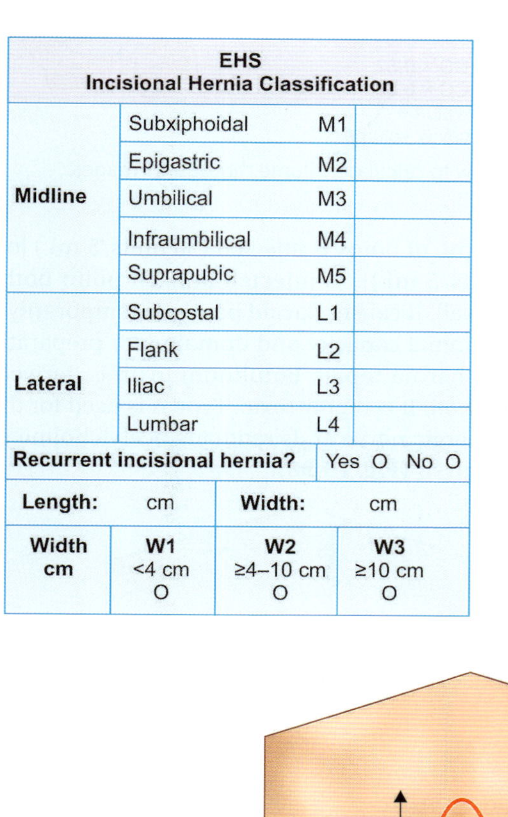

EHS Incisional Hernia Classification			
Midline	Subxiphoidal	M1	
	Epigastric	M2	
	Umbilical	M3	
	Infraumbilical	M4	
	Suprapubic	M5	
Lateral	Subcostal	L1	
	Flank	L2	
	Iliac	L3	
	Lumbar	L4	
Recurrent incisional hernia?		Yes O No O	
Length: cm		Width: cm	
Width cm	W1 <4 cm O	W2 ≥4–10 cm O	W3 ≥10 cm O

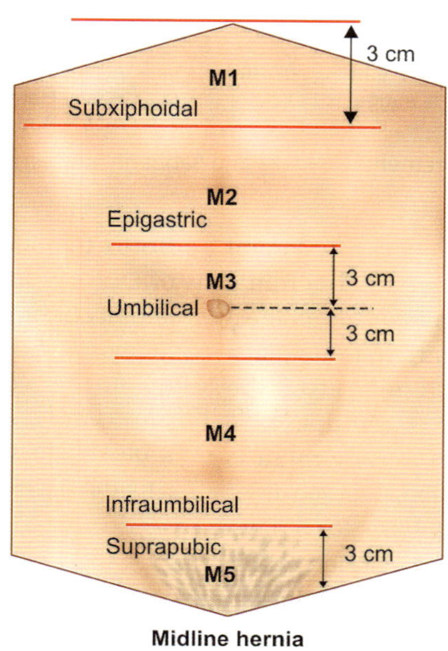

Midline hernia

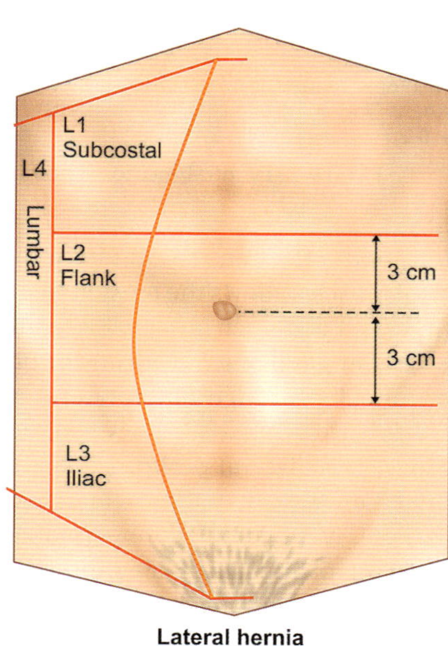

Lateral hernia

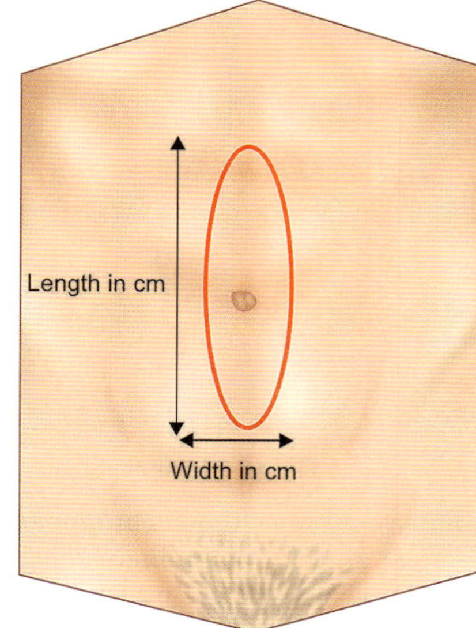

Single defect

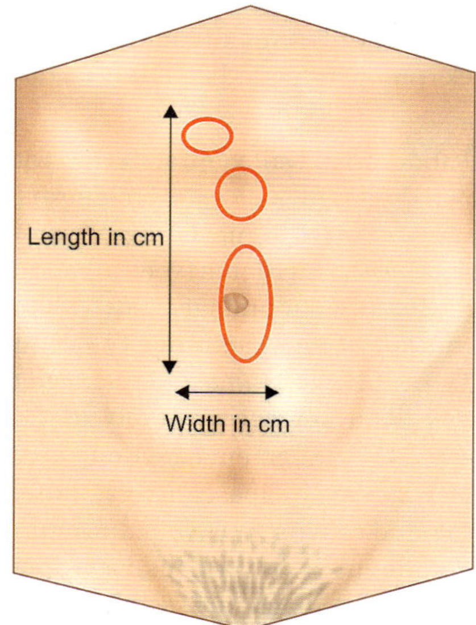

Multiple defects

Fig. 19-96: European Hernia Society (EHS) ventral/incisional hernia classification.

progressive pneumoperitoneum to improve volume of abdomen should be considered. Botulinum toxin A (BTX A) is injected 4 weeks prior to surgery; around 200–500 IU dose (total dose) is used under ultrasound guidance; it is injected over muscular planes of abdominal wall both sides; 3–5 sites each side is selected depending on different regimes; subcostal/anterior axillary line/mid-axillary line/into the muscular planes. BTX A injection lengthens the muscle about 4 cm and brings down the defect size significantly so that closure of the rectus becomes optimum to achieve dynamic closure often with addition of component closure (CST) with or without transversus abdominis release (TR).

Progressive preoperative pneumoperitoneum (PPP) (Goni Moreno's): It is used to gradually inflate the abdomen to prepare for ventral hernia repair like in large ventral, incisional, parastomal hernias and giant hernias with loss of domain (LOD). It is intermittent insufflation of the peritoneal cavity to elongate the contracted oblique muscles which gradually increasing the capacity of abdominal cavity allowing the viscera into the abdominal cavity into the right domain.

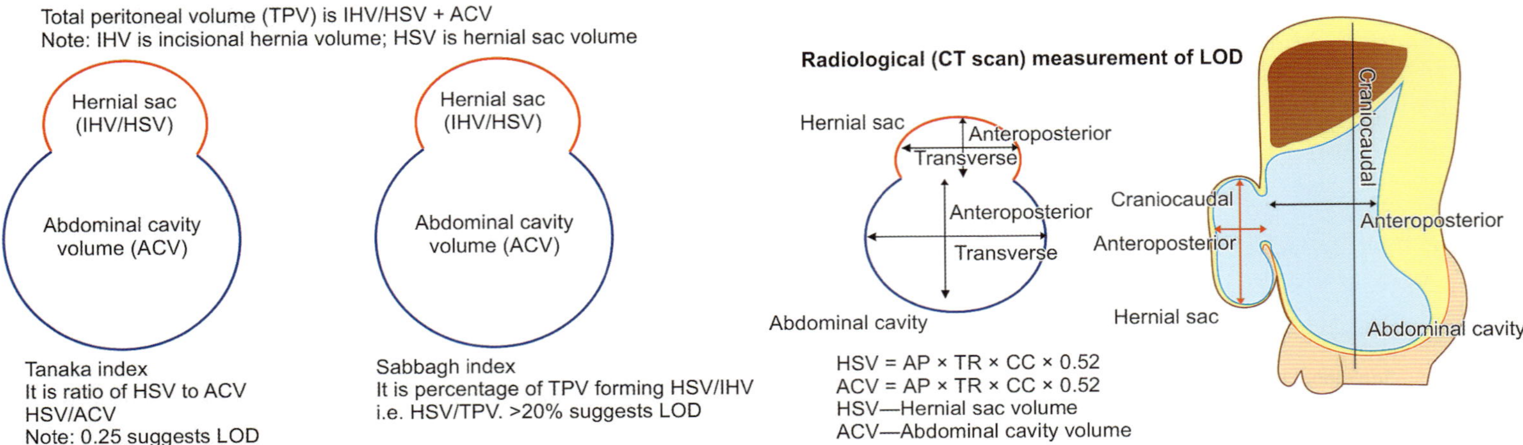

Fig. 19-97: Ventral/incisional hernia measurements—Tanaka and Sabbagh indices; and how to calculate volume through CT mages.

This along with injection of Botulinum toxin A injection to lateral abdominal muscles allows the tension free closure of the abdominal defect. Initial CT abdomen is done; PPP catheter (8 Fr pigtail catheter) is placed under guidance (CT ideally or ultrasound) in a safe place intraperitoneally through anterolateral approach away from the scar or hernia site. (Initially 22 G spinal needle is passed under CT guidance into the lateral peritoneal space; 300 mL of room air is insufflated; later 8 Fr pigtail catheter is passed into the area under CT guidance). Insufflation is done gradually daily basis for 5 days. 800 to 1000 mL of air is insufflated through three way catheter daily (patient tolerance and dyspnoea are good parameters). CT abdomen repeated to confirm the increased abdominal wall capacity. Daily enoxaparin should be injected as DVT prophylaxis. CT scans were done to measure the abdominal wall length from the lateral edge of the quadrates lumborum to medial edge of rectus abdominis muscle. Botox injection is done 2–3 weeks preoperatively; PPP is done 5 days preoperatively.

Loss of domain (LOD): Large abdominal wall ventral hernia with significant bowel content herniated through a defect which forms a second abdominal cavity; usually defect is >10 cm. LOD is measured with preoperative CT volumetric analysis. Incisional (ventral) hernia volume (IHV/HSV [hernia sac volume]), abdominal cavity volume (ACV [excluding IHV]) and total peritoneal volumes (TPV) are assessed. IHV/TPV gives the LOD. In *Tanaka index* percentage of IHV to ACV is taken; in *Sabbagh index* percentage of IHV to total peritoneal cavity (TPV) is assessed. Measurements are done using radiological imaging (CT). *Effects of LOD:* Increased lateral muscle traction; thickened mesentery; altered venous and lymphatic return; dilated oedematous bowel; cutaneous hypoxia causing trophic ulcers; secondary bacterial or/and fungal infection; fistula formation **(Fig. 19-97)**.

Management concept: (1) Recover anatomy; (2) Recover function: (3) Adequate tissue cover; (4) Dynamic closure of midline; (5) Prevent recurrence. ***Preoperative optimisation is crucial***—To stop smoking; make albumin >3.5 gram%; HbA1c <7%; respiratory physiotherapy; weight loss; progressive preoperative pneumoperitoneum (PPP); botox injection to paralyse muscle temporarily to increase the domain. *Procedures are*—Laparoscopic mesh repair (IPOM); component separation (anterior [ACS] or posterior [PCs is better]); transversus abdominis release (TAR); Albanese triple incision; tissue expanders; Hybrid procedures (open dissection from front then laparoscopically placing intraperitoneal underlay mesh).

Botox injection: 3 mL of Botox is injected (30 units/5 mL) [or 5 mL of Dysport (50 units/5 mL)]) is injected at each point both sides lateral abdominal wall. It causes flaccid paralysis temporarily which increases the abdominal capacity and domain as a preparation for the further ventral hernia repair. Botulinum toxin is derived from *Clostridium botulinum*. It is highly toxic. Type A is used for therapy. it blocks the cholinergic nerve ends reducing acetylcholine release causing flaccid paralysis **(Fig. 19-98)**.

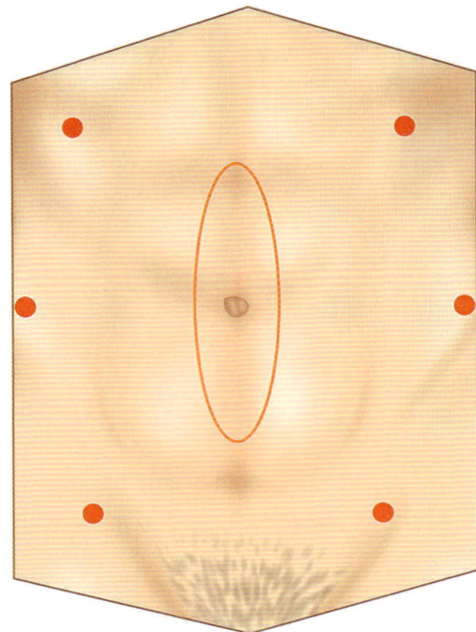

Fig. 19-98: Botulinum toxin A injection sites.

Component separation technique (CST): Albanese first published the open anterior component separation technique; later it was popularised by Ramirez. In a very large primary or incisional hernia, suturing technique or mesh placement leads into difficulty in maintain the dynamic closure of the rectus sheath and also carry high recurrence rate. Relaxing incision in the lateral musculofascial system leads into optimum domain and easy closure of the rectus sheath to maintain the dynamic apposition. Fascial closure restores the crucial structural and functional closure of the anatomical composite structures.

Different types of CST are—(1) Open CST; Laparoscopic CST; (2) CST with mesh augmentation (current standard); (3) Anterior CST wherein external oblique component is incised along the anterior rectus sheath to create plane between external oblique and internal oblique so that adequate medialisation and mesh placement is achieved; (4) Posterior CST wherein posterior rectus sheath in incised vertically to reach transversus abdominis muscle plane to allow medialisation and mesh placement; (5) Posterior CST with transversus abdominis release (TAR) with mesh placement; (6) Posterior CST with TAR with Perforator preserving CST.

Posterior CST with TAR with perforator sparing is ideal. Proper assessment preoperatively is a must. Patient optimisation with weight control, respiratory exercise, control of diabetes, hypertension is important. Injection Botulinum toxin A and progressive preoperative pneumoperitoneum (PPP) if needed should be undertaken. Perioperative antibiotics should be given. General anaesthesia with epidural support is ideal. After cleaning and draping, lengthy midline incision is placed. Hernia sac is dealt with. All adhesions are released. Care should be taken not to open the bowel to avoid contamination. Rectus sheath is opened medially with vertical incision from subcostal region to linea semilunaris. Rectus muscle id identified and reflected laterally and in front. Perforating vessels and nerves entering through the lateral part of the posterior rectus sheath is noticed. Perforators should not be injured. Posterior rectus sheath is opened vertically just medial to the line of perforators from subcostal region to linea semilunaris. It can be achieved from above downwards or from below upwards using 15 number blade or monopolar cautery. While using cautery care should be taken not to fulgurate the perforator vessels and nerve. Once this sheath is incised plane is created behind it between transversalis fascia and internal oblique to visualise the transversus abdominis muscle. TA muscle is vertically released so that adequate lateral plane is created up to midaxillary line and above up to diaphragm, below towards pubic symphysis and Cooper's ligament. 4 cm below the pubic symphysis in front of the bladder and 3 cm below the Cooper's ligament plane should be dissected using finger and cautery. Iliac vessels should be taken care off. Haemostasis should be achieved. Similar dissection should be carried out on opposite side. This causes medialisation of rectus sheath adequately up to 10 cm achieving the dynamic midline closure of peritoneum with posterior rectus sheath. Large mesh 30 × 30 sized is placed in the created plane. Fixation is not necessary but can be done by placing few interrupted polypropylene sutures in front. Suction drain should be placed in front of the mesh. Anterior rectus sheath is also closed with non-absorbable suture material. Postoperatively respiratory physiotherapy, deep vein thrombosis (DVT) prophylaxis with enoxaparin should be done. Antibiotics coverage is done for 72 hours. Drain is removed once drain fluid is less than 25 mL per day. Abdominal binder should be worn by the patient for 6–12 weeks.

Subcutaneous onlay laparoscopic approach for ventral hernia (primary) [SCOLA] with diastasis of rectus abdominis muscle is used in some centres. Diastasis of rectus abdominis muscle is defined as distancing from rectus muscular borders more than 2.2 cm from midline. SCOLA is endo/laparoscopic procedure wherein after placing ports into the subcutaneous plane, dissection is carried out extensively in front of the rectus sheath above up to the subcostal area, below 3 cm below the umbilicus and laterally up to midaxillary line. Hernial sac is identified and dissected. Sac is sutured through intracorporeal suturing. Rectus sheath also sutured with continuous sutures. Adequate sized mesh is placed in the plane and fixed using tackers.

Hybrid procedure: It is done in large incisional hernia with adhesions. Laparoscopy is done by placing camera port at left subcostal point (*Palmer point*). Peritoneal cavity is assessed. Midline incision is placed; hernia sac is dealt with release of all adhesions; care should be taken not to perforate bowel. IPOM dual mesh of adequate size is pushed into the peritoneal cavity through the midline incision wound prior to its closure. Sac is closed; defect is sutured using non-absorbable sutures. Pneumoperitoneum is created; further ports are placed; dual mesh is fixed to the abdominal wall using absorbable spiral tackers achieving sublay intraperitoneal mesh placement. Port sites are closed with their sheaths (if port is 10 cm or more). *Double crown technique* of mesh fixation to abdominal wall by two rows of tackers is ideal.

Extended totally extraperitoneal repair (eTEP) for ventral hernia: it is creation of space in retrorectus plane through a left subcostal 15 mm camera port with further additional ports of 5 mm at left midclavicular line above the linea semilunaris with 5 cm gap between each. Additional 10 mm port is needed at right subcostal region also for camera placement as and when needed. Adequate dissection is done. If needed eTEP Rives Stoppa (eTEP RS) can be achieved in lower abdomen ventral hernia wherein proper dissection should be done under pubic symphysis and Cooper's ligament. Hernia sac is dealt accordingly. If required posterior component separation (eTEP PCST) or with transverses abdominis release (eTEP TAR) can be achieved). Standard polypropylene mesh is placed of proper size which can be fixed using tackers or sutures. Suction drain should be placed.

UMBILICAL HERNIA REPAIR

Anatomy of Umbilical Region

Umbilical ring is a complex structure which is related to linea alba, falciform ligament, obliterated urachus (median umbilical ligament) and umbilical fascia (*Richet's fascia*). It is located at the level of L4 and L5 vertebral disc. It is lower in position in infants. It is water shed area for venous and lymphatic drainage—above umbilicus it drains to axillary vein or lymphatics; below to inguinal area. Umbilical skin is supplied by T10 spinal cord. It is the meeting point of four folds of embryonic plate and three systems—gastrointestinal (vitellointestinal), urinary (urachus), and vascular (umbilical vessels). Umbilical hernia develops due to either absence of umbilical fascia or incomplete closure of umbilical defect. Weakest part in the umbilical cicatrix is the upper part where hernia begins **(Figs. 19-99A and B)**.

Primary Closure of the Defect

An infraumbilical incision is made encircling its lower half. Sac is dissected circumferentially and is released off from the umbilicus and subcutaneous tissue. Sac is opened; contents are reduced; excess part

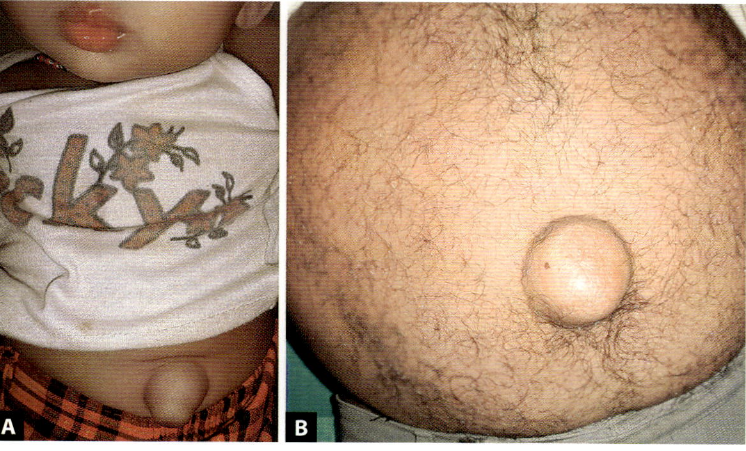

Figs. 19-99A and B: Umbilical hernia in a child and in an adult. Both need surgical intervention. In children primary repair or Mayo's repair is done; in adult mesh repair is done placing mesh retrorectus plane.

is excised up to the umbilical ring. Defect is closed with interrupted non-absorbable polypropylene sutures. Often layer by layer closure of the peritoneum is also advocated. Anterior rectus sheath can be sutured either horizontally (ideally) or vertically. Umbilicoplasty is done by creating umbilical dimpling. Centre of the umbilical flap is inverted by using finger or instrument; from the summit of the inverted umbilical skin absorbable vicryl—3-zero suture bite is taken which is sutured firmly to the sutured rectus sheath defect. Skin is closed often with a suction drain underneath **(Fig. 19-100)**.

Mayo's Operation

Here horizontally opened rectus sheath is approximated as double breasting with upper flap overlapping lower flap in front. Interrupted non-absorbable polypropylene 2-zero sutures are used. Suture bite begins from outer surface of upper flap about 2 cm from cut margin; passes deeper to upper flap reaches the outer surface of the lower flap about 1 cm from the cut margin of the lower flap where the horizontal bite of 5–8 mm width is taken; again bite comes out of the outer surface of the lower flap which later pierces upper flap from deeper aspect to outer aspect to complete the suture. Similar sutures are taken at 5 mm distance. All suture ends are held using small haemostats which are tied together after completion of taking all suture bites. Cut margin of the upper flap which is overhanging on to the lower surface of the lower flap is sutured to the lower flap with continuous or interrupted sutures using polypropylene. It is ideal to place a suction drain underneath the main suture line before tying all knots. Skin is closed using interrupted sutures. Pressure dressing is placed. Procedure is also done for paraumbilical hernia. It is *'vest over pant'* autogenous repair **(Fig. 19-101)**.

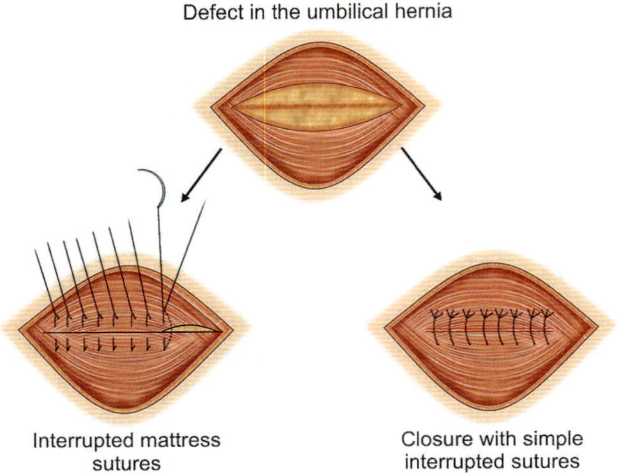

Fig. 19-100: Primary closure of umbilical hernia is done when defect is small. Mayo's repair or mesh repair is better.

Sublay Mesh Repair

In a large umbilical hernia with a degenerated skin on its surface it is often difficult to retain the umbilicus. When umbilicus is tried to be saved, infraumbilical incision should extend laterally about 2 cm on each side at 3 and 9 o'clock positions. Sac is dissected similarly. Sac is excised after excision of redundant sac. Presently it is standard to use polypropylene mesh as sublay or in retrorectus position and then rectus sheath is closed. Mesh placement is better to prevent recurrence in large umbilical hernia. Keeping a suction drain is the usual practice. Umbilical dimpling can be created by placing single vicryl/polypropylene interrupted suture under the centre of skin flap to sutured rectus defect. Skin is closed ideally with interrupted sutures even though many practice absorbable subcuticular suture **(Fig. 19-102)**.

Umbilectomy

Unhealthy thin skin over the large umbilical hernia is a real problem. It is better to do umbilectomy in these patients (excision of umbilical cicatrix). A horizontal elliptical incision is made to encircle the umbilicus. Undermining of skin should not be done. Incision is deepened up to aponeurosis. Umbilical margin is dissected using

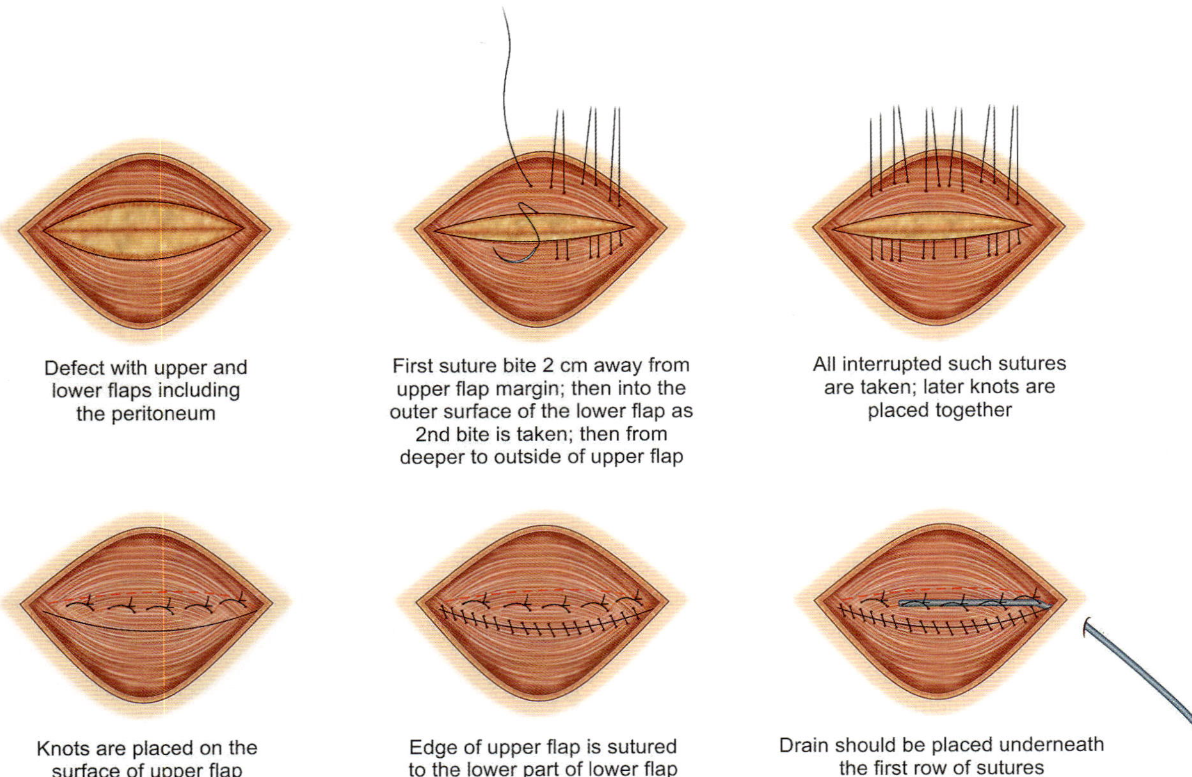

Fig. 19-101: Mayo repair (vest over pant) for umbilical hernia—steps.

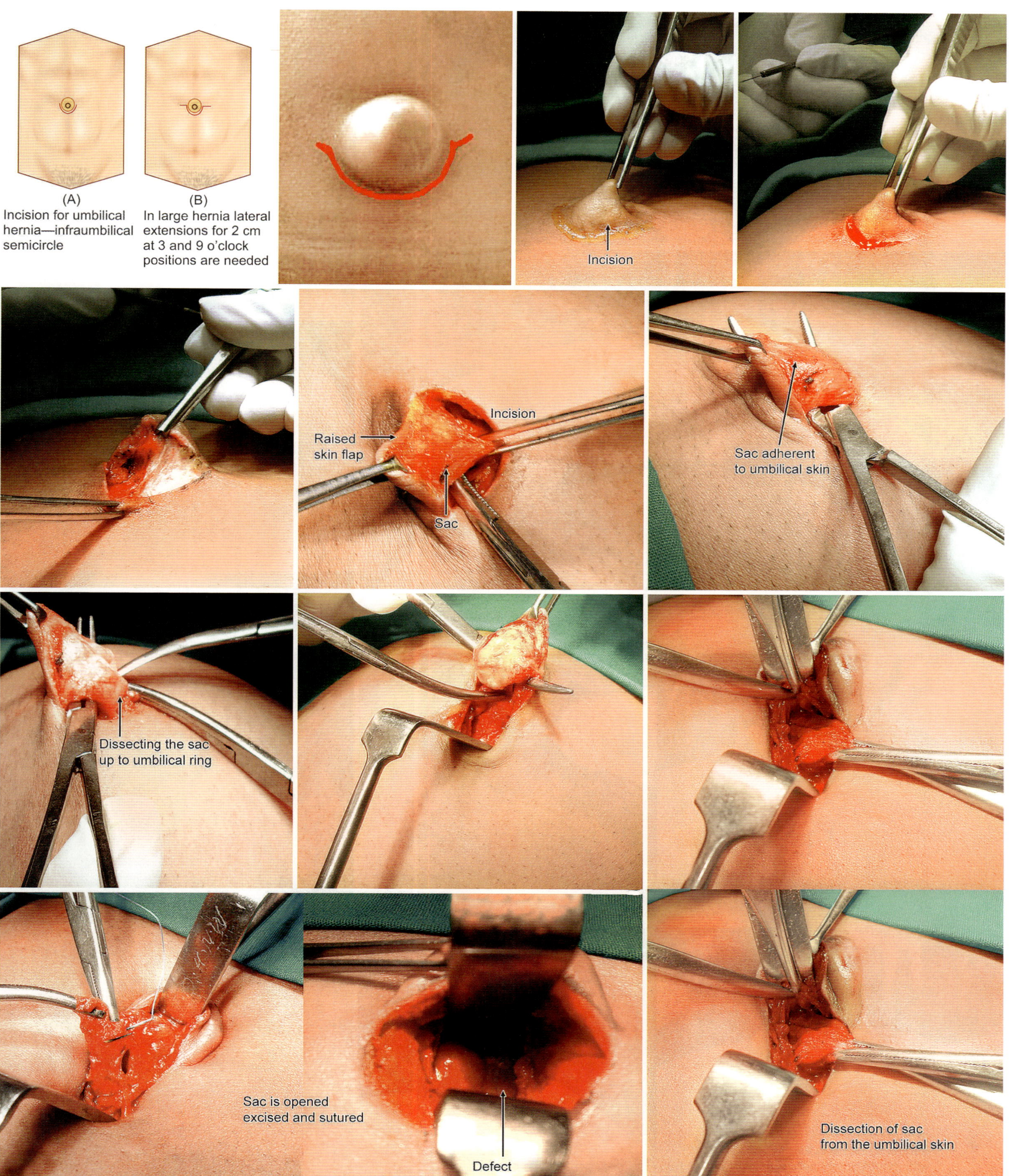
(A)
Incision for umbilical hernia—infraumbilical semicircle
(B)
In large hernia lateral extensions for 2 cm at 3 and 9 o'clock positions are needed
Incision
Incision
Raised skin flap
Sac
Sac adherent to umbilical skin
Dissecting the sac up to umbilical ring
Sac is opened excised and sutured
Defect
Dissection of sac from the umbilical skin

Figs. 19-102(1)

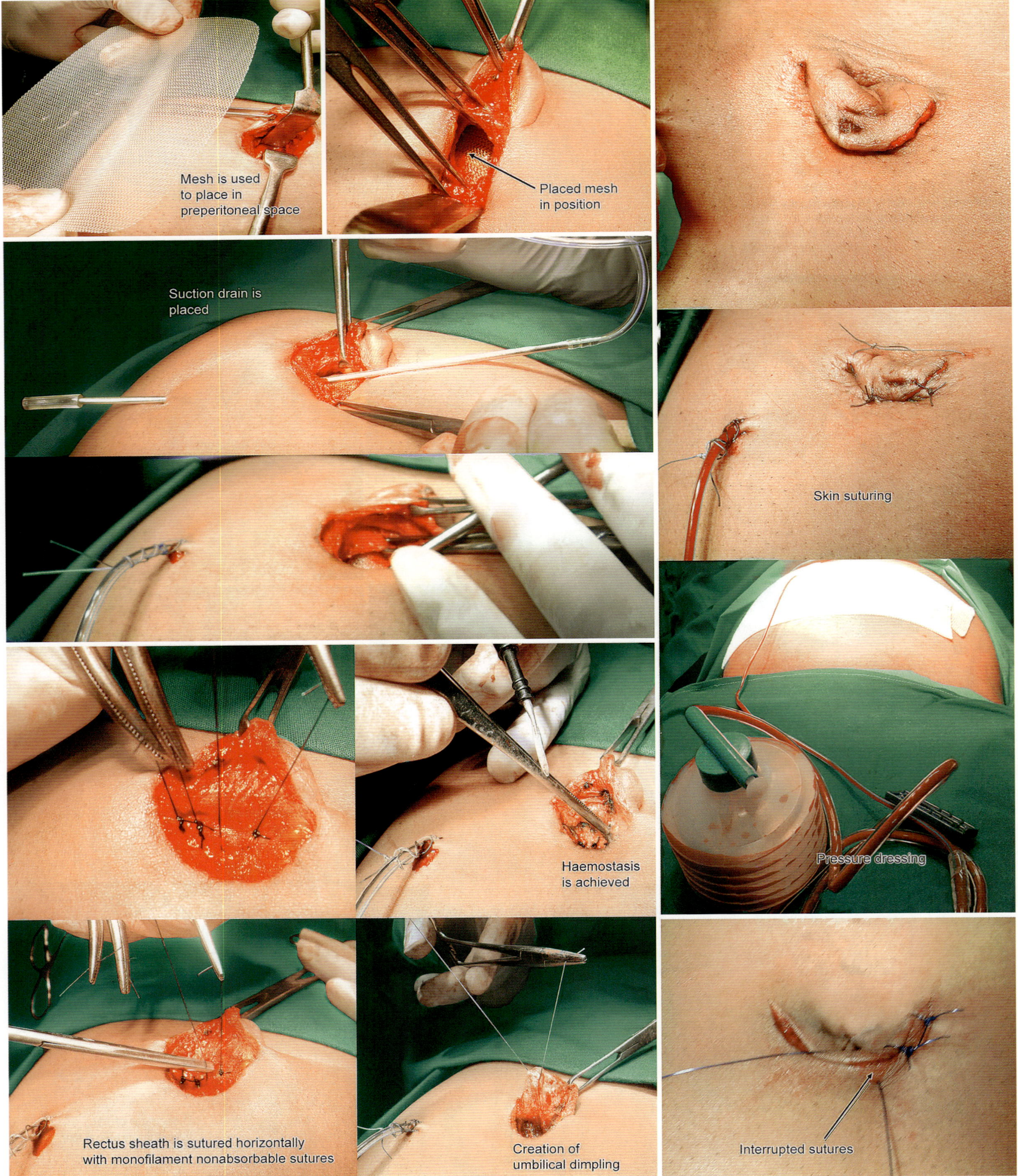

Figs. 19-102(2)

Figs. 19-102(1 and 2): Technique of umbilical hernia repair with sublay mesh placement.

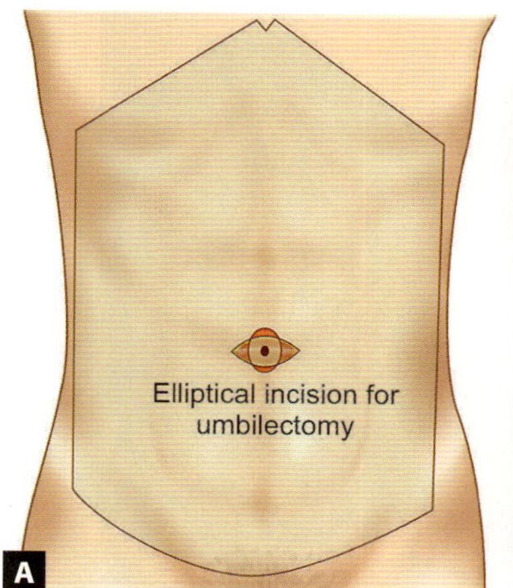

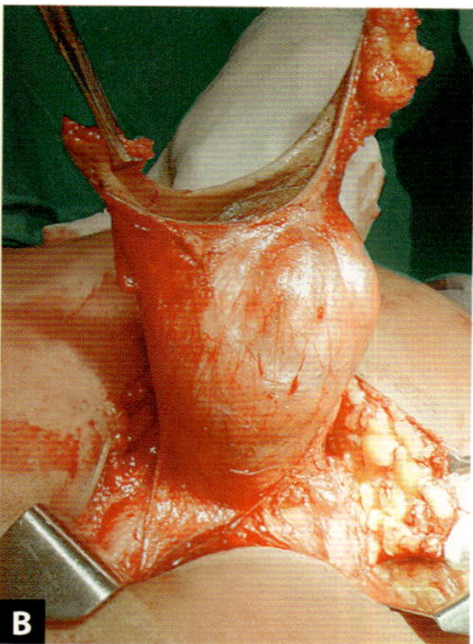

Figs. 19-103A and B: Umbilectomy is needed for large hernia through elliptical incision.

cautery or scissor; sac is opened and excised. Often content is adherent to sac. Sac is carefully dissected off the contents. Adherent omentum needs omentectomy. Often defect may require to be widened to replace the content into the peritoneal cavity. It is achieved by incising the defect laterally (horizontally). Falciform ligament attached to umbilicus is ligated and divided to complete the excision of the umbilicus. Sac is closed using vicryl. Preperitoneal space is created deep to rectus muscle. A polypropylene mesh of adequate size is placed in preperitoneal/retrorectus plane. It is sutured to the margin at different places to abdominal wall in front. It should never be sutured to peritoneum posteriorly. Suction drain is placed in front of the mesh. Rectus sheath is closed using interrupted polypropylene sutures. Subcutaneous drain is often helpful. Skin is closed with interrupted sutures **(Figs. 19-103A and B)**.

Open dual PTFE and polypropylene mesh placement: Umbilical hernia is dissected similarly through subumbilical incision. Redundant sac is excised. Peritoneum is not closed. A special composite mesh containing wider PTFE on the inner side with little smaller polypropylene mesh on the outer aspect is used. It has also got two additional straps attached to the outer part of the main composite mesh which are used to hold and later fix into the defect anteriorly. 4.3 cm and 6.4 cm diameter sized meshes are available. Holding straps folded mesh with PTFE part facing the visceral surface is placed intraperitoneally abutting into the peritoneal surface. Care should be taken to avoid interposition of the bowel between mesh and peritoneal surface. Outer polypropylene part of the mesh is fixed to anterior myoaponeurosis 4 cm away from the margin of the defect using 'U' stitch with knot on the outer surface. First at 3 and 9 o'clock positions sutures are placed; then straps are tugged under the defect in front of the round polypropylene part of the mesh and these straps are fixed using similar 'U' stitches at 6 and 12 o'clock positions. Anterior rectus sheath is approximated horizontally using interrupted sutures. Skin is closed with interrupted sutures after absolute haemostasis. This has got excellent results with low recurrence rate.

Laparoscopic umbilical hernia repair: It is similar like any ventral hernia repair through laparoscopy which is done under general anaesthesia **(Figs. 19-104A and B)**.

Complications

Infection, haematoma/seroma formation, ileus, recurrence. Recurrence rate with primary repairs is very high—40% if defect is more than 1 cm. So mesh repair is ideal in adult umbilical hernia repair.

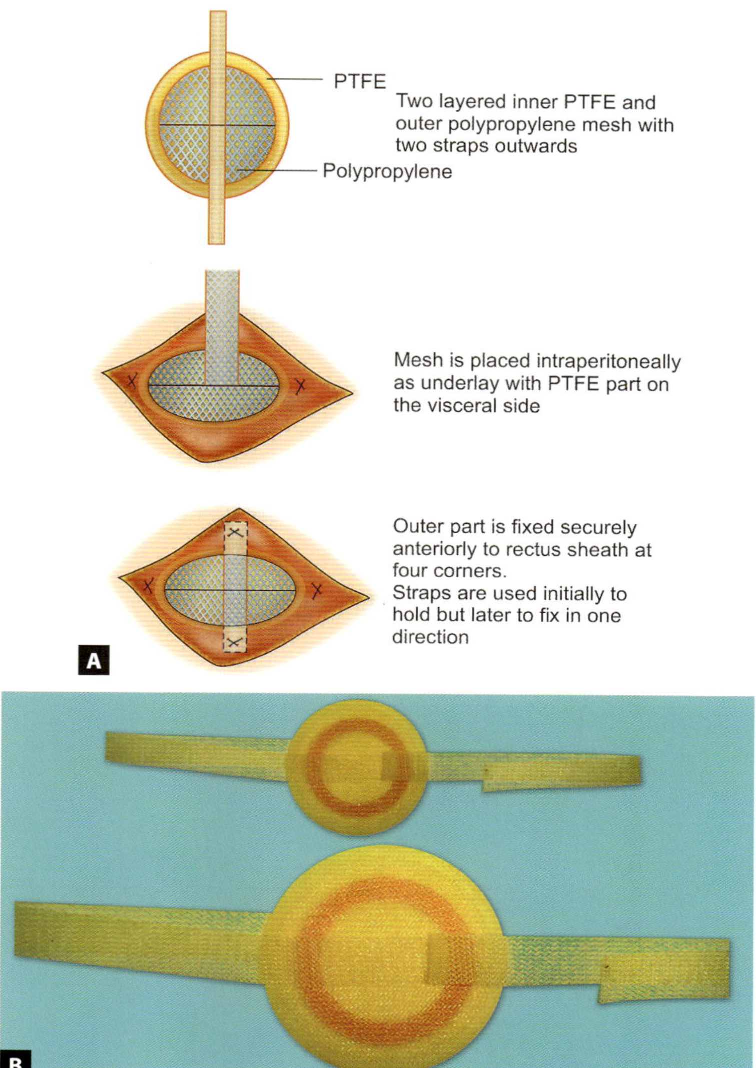

Figs. 19-104A and B: Umbilical hernia repair using open dual polytetrafluoroethylene (PTFE) and polypropylene mesh placement.

EPIGASTRIC HERNIA (FATTY HERNIA OF LINEA ALBA)

It is common (10%); common in males; 20% of epigastric hernias are multiple—Swiss *cheese like*. It occurs usually through a defect in the decussation of the fibres of linea alba, anywhere between xiphoid process and umbilicus. Extraperitoneal fat protrudes through the defect as fatty hernia of the linea alba presenting like a swelling in the upper midline with an impulse on coughing. *It is sacless hernia.* Later protrusion enlarges and drags a pouch of peritoneum, presenting as a *true epigastric hernia*. If the defect is less than 1.5 cm, lateral margin of the defect is formed by only anterior and posterior lamina of the rectus sheath; if the defect is >1.5 cm, then lateral margin is also formed by rectus muscle. Content of true epigastric hernia is usually omentum, sometimes it may be small bowel. It is common in muscular men; manual labourers **(Figs. 19-105 to 19-107)**.

Treatment

Through a vertical incision, sac is dealt with. Defect is closed with non-absorbable interrupted sutures. Large defect is supported with preperitoneal mesh—ideal and better. Complete reconstruction of linea alba is needed from xiphisternum to umbilicus especially in *Swiss cheese* type using different methods like—interrupted primary

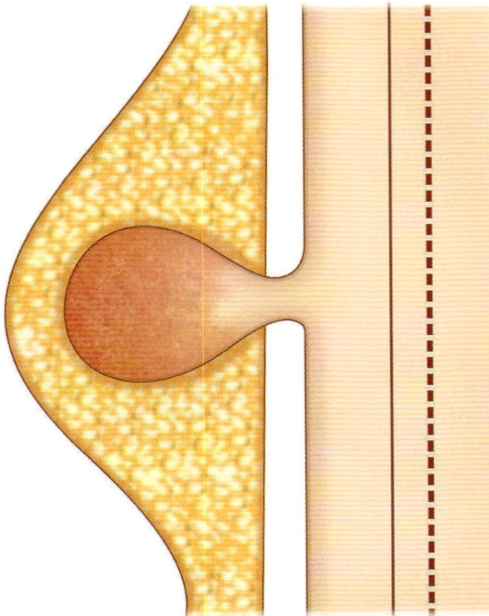

Fig. 19-105: Epigastric hernia.

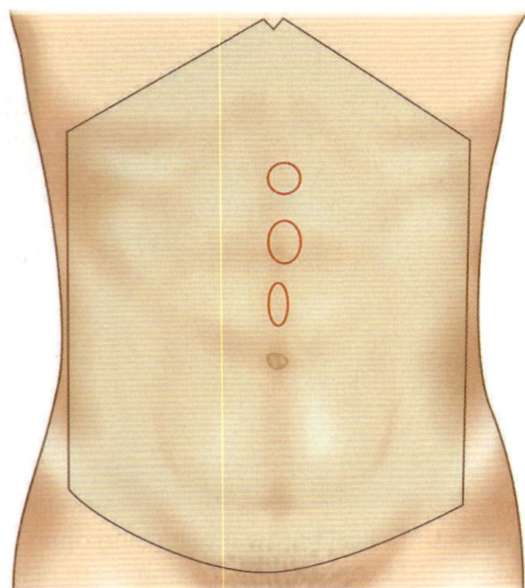

Fig. 19-106: Epigastric hernia with Swiss cheese defects.

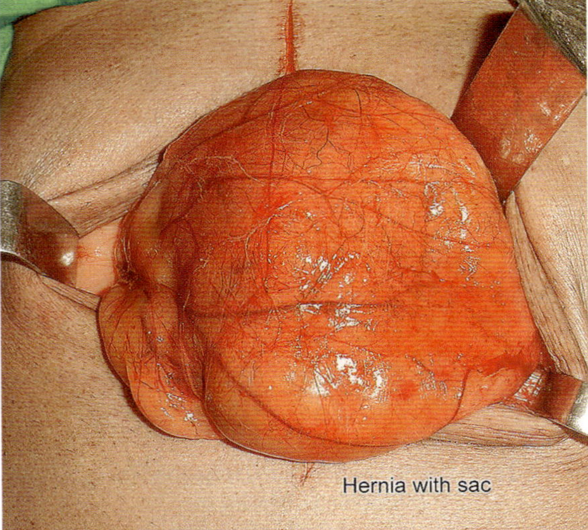

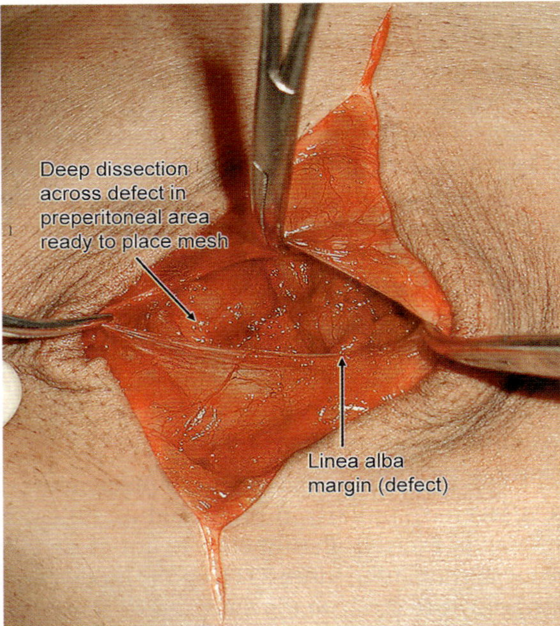

Fig. 19-107: Epigastric hernia on table look.

closure using polypropylene sutures; *modified shoelace technique* is used after removing strip of medial margins of the linea alba; double breasting of the linea alba **(Figs. 19-108 and 19-109)**.

FEMORAL HERNIA REPAIR

Surgical Anatomy of Femoral Canal (Figs. 19-110 and 19-111)

It is the medial most compartment of the femoral sheath which extends from femoral ring above to saphenous opening below. It contains fat, lymphatics, lymph node of Cloquet. It is 1.25 cm long and 1.25 cm wide at the base. Below it is closed by cribriform fascia.

Femoral ring is bounded anteriorly by inguinal ligament and iliopubic tract; posteriorly by iliopectineal ligament of Cooper, pubic bone and pectineal fascia covering the pectineus muscle; medially by concave, sharp lacunar (Gimbernat's) ligament; laterally by a thin septum separating from femoral vein **(Figs. 19-112 and 19-113)**.

Pathology in Femoral Hernia

Through femoral canal, hernial sac descends down vertically up to saphenous opening and then escapes out into the loose areolar tissue to expand out like a ***retort***. Because of its irregular pathway and narrow neck, it is more prone for obstruction and strangulation. During surgery, precaution should be taken about the femoral vein and pubic branch of obturator artery (or abnormal obturator artery) which often may get injured leading to torrential haemorrhage.

Hydrocele of femoral hernia occurs when adherent omentum is the content which secretes fluid into the sac. *Herniation* through a gap in the lacunar ligament (medial) is always strangulated and is called as *Laugier's femoral hernia*. In congenital dislocation of hip, femoral hernia occurs *behind* the femoral vessels—*Narath's femoral hernia*. If sac lies under the pectineal fascia, it is called as *Cloquet's hernia. Strangulation and Richter's hernia are common in femoral hernia.* Often on medial side, a portion of bladder forms the wall of the femoral hernial sac—*sliding femoral hernia*.

Surgical Approaches (Fig. 19-114)

Lockwood (London)—Low Operation

Here sac is approached below the inguinal ligament through groin crease incision so that fundus of sac is dissected by direct vision and repair is done from below. Incision is made 1 cm below the inguinal ligament on its medial portion. Skin and subcutaneous tissue is incised to visualise the swelling with sac. Blunt dissection will reveal the margin of the sac. Commonly sac content is irreducible. Sac is opened; fluid invariably present in the sac is collected for culture and sucked out. Bowel/omentum are held using Babcock's forceps. Viability of bowel or omentum is checked by colour, peristalsis, and blood supply. If content is viable, it is pushed into the peritoneal cavity. If reduction of the content is difficult then constriction at femoral ring should be released. It is done by cutting the inguinal ligament in front. One should not cut the lacunar ligament to release the ring while approaching from below as superior invisible part of the lacunar ligament may be closely related to aberrant obturator artery or pubic branch of obturator artery which communicates with pubic branch of inferior epigastric artery. If this artery is cut both

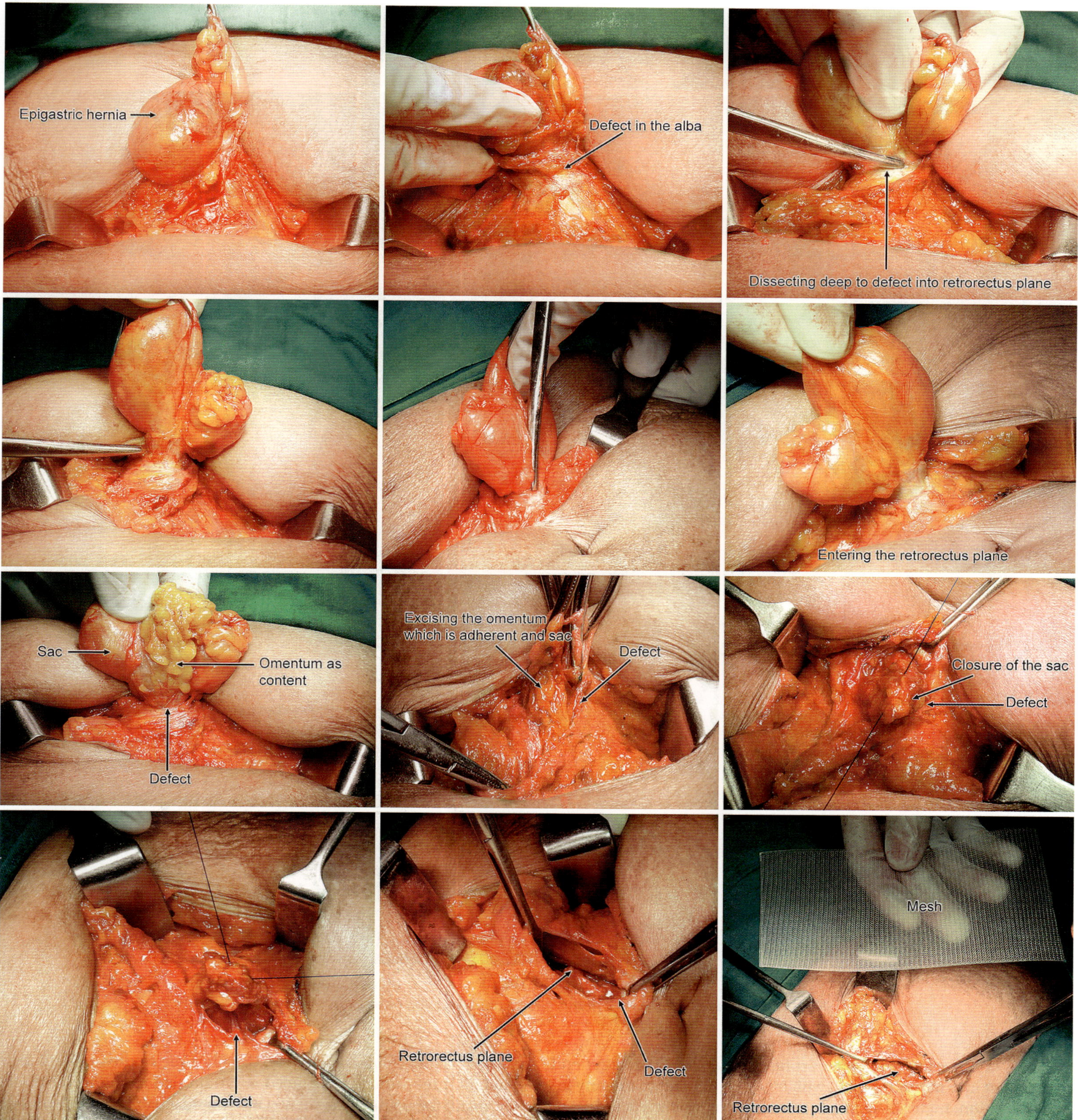

Figs. 19-108(1)

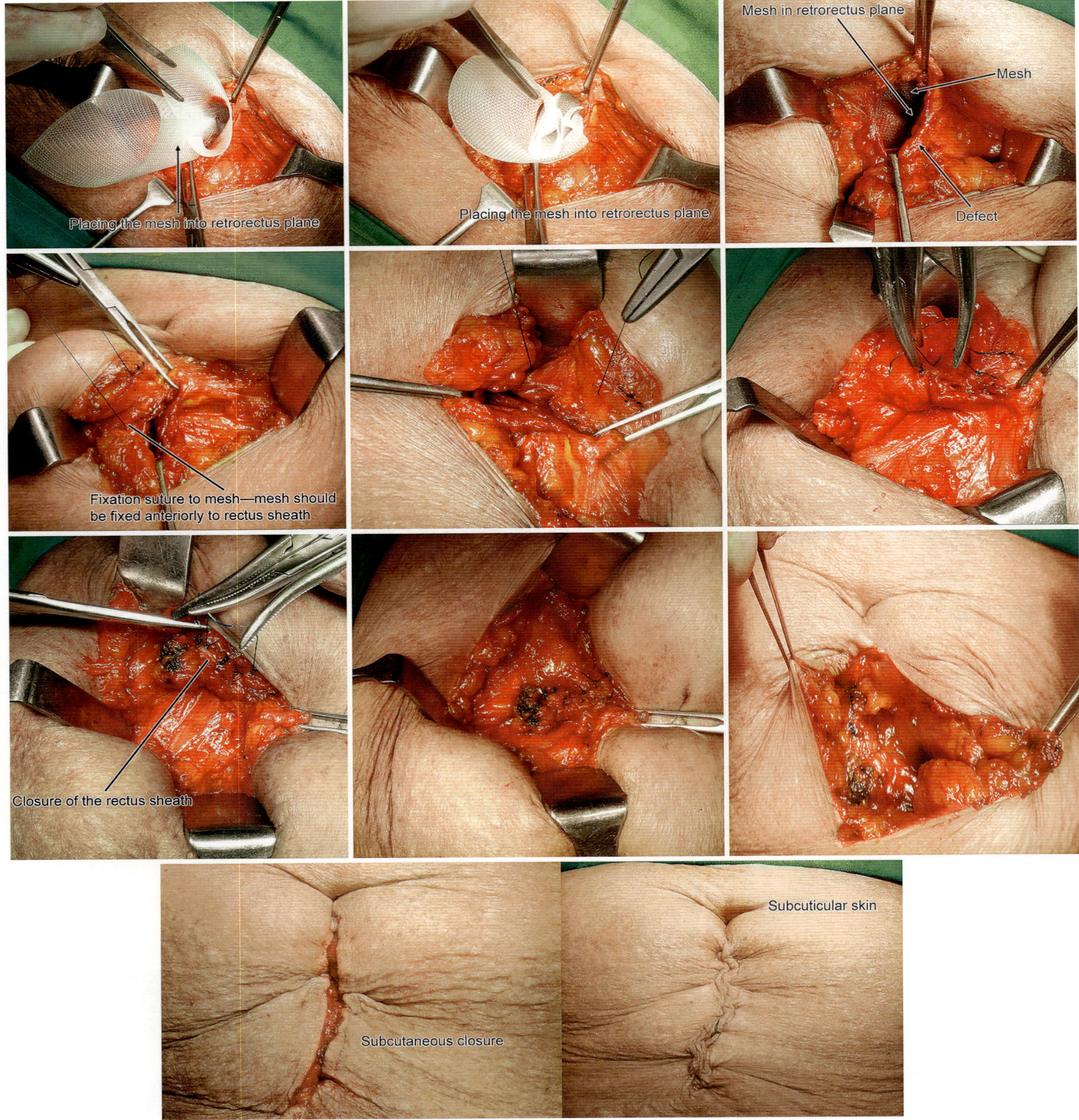

Figs. 19-108(2)

Figs. 19-108(1 and 2): Epigastric hernia dissection, defect and retrorectus mesh repair.

cut ends of the artery will bleed profusely and also medial cut end may retract into obturator fossa which will be difficult to identify for secure ligation. Inguinal ligament is sutured to Cooper's ligament or pectineal fascia using interrupted polypropylene sutures. Femoral vein that is located laterally should be guarded using finger to prevent taking of inadvertent bite. Usually three sutures are sufficient. First all three sutures are placed and then tied together to prevent tearing of the inguinal ligament. One should ensure that constriction of the femoral vein will not occur. J shaped needle if available should be ideal to take suture bites.

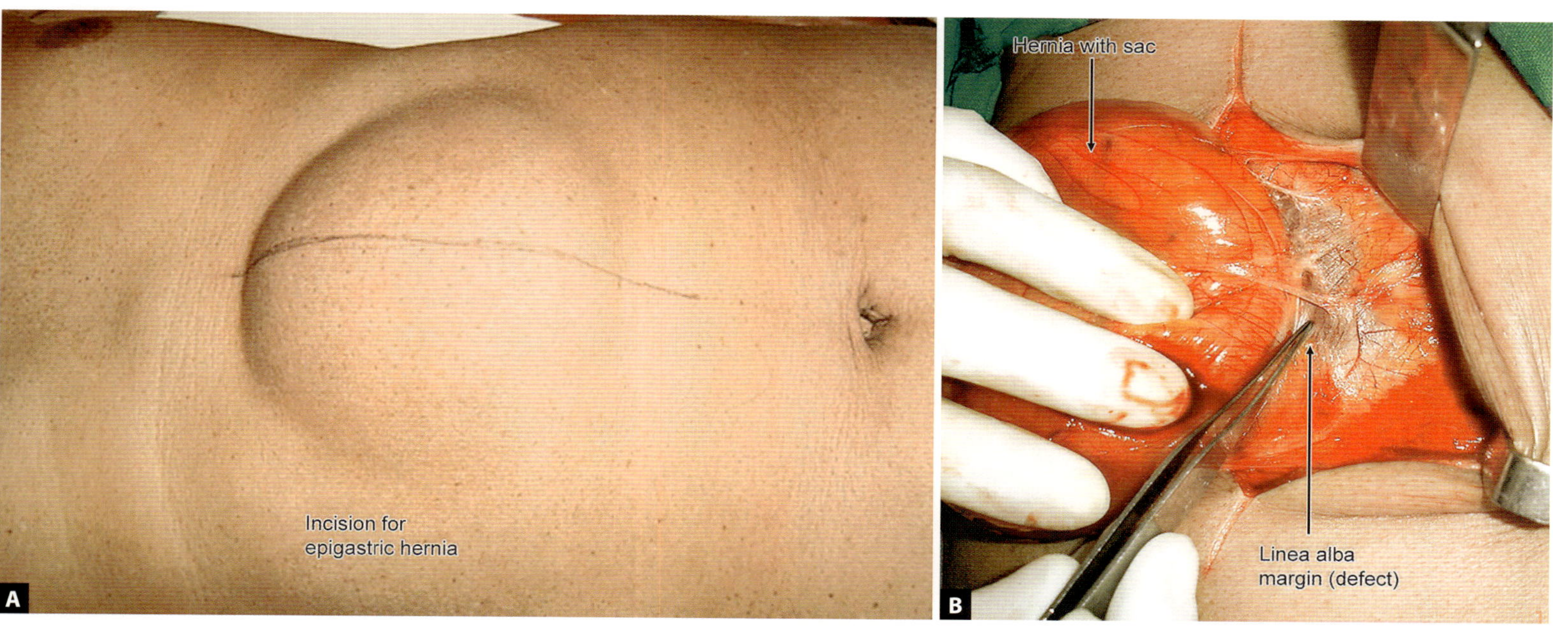

Figs. 19-109A and B: Surgical treatment of epigastric hernia and plane of placing the mesh.

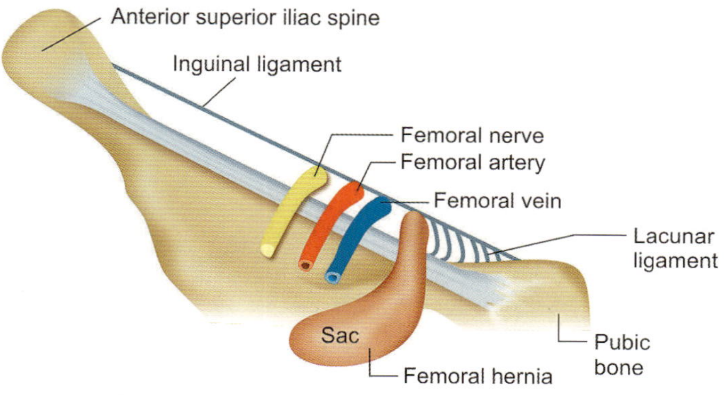

Fig. 19-110: Femoral hernia—surgical anatomy.

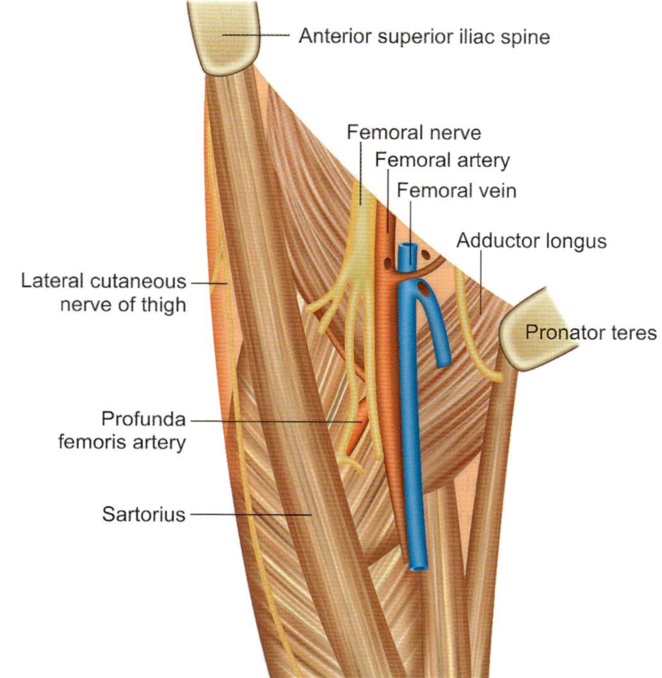

Fig. 19-111: Femoral triangle and its boundaries.

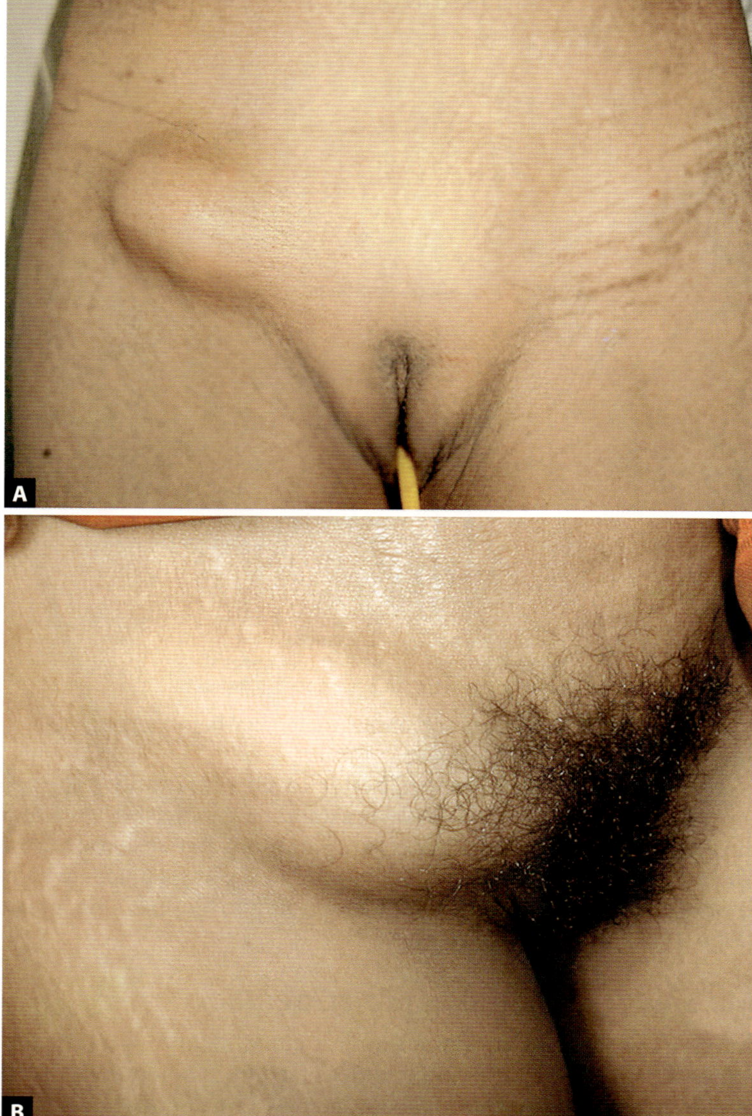

Figs. 19-112A and B: Femoral hernia is common in females.

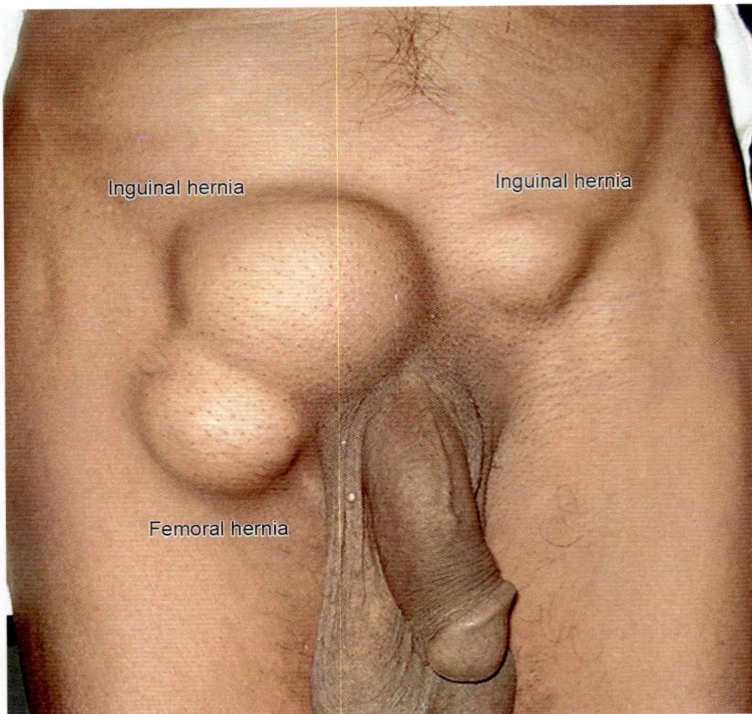

Fig. 19-113: Femoral and direct inguinal hernia in a male patient.

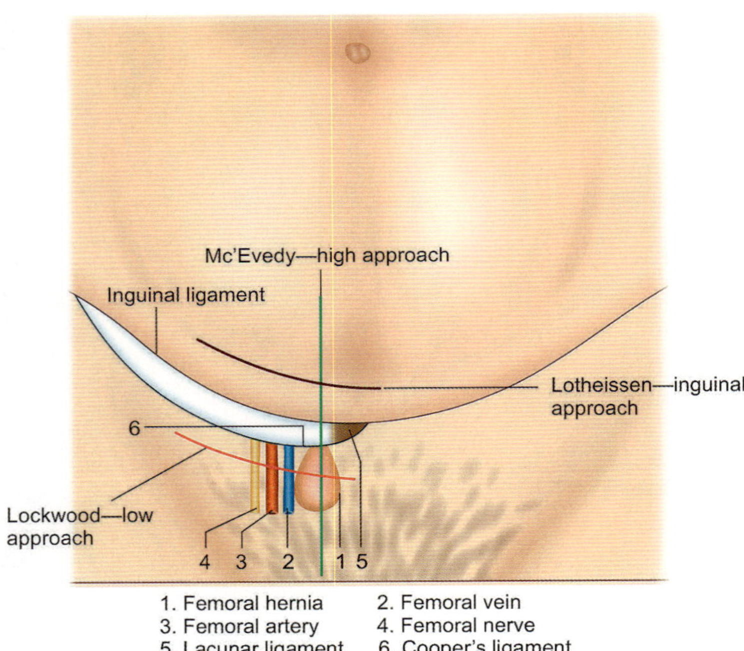

Fig. 19-114: Surgical approaches for femoral hernia repair.

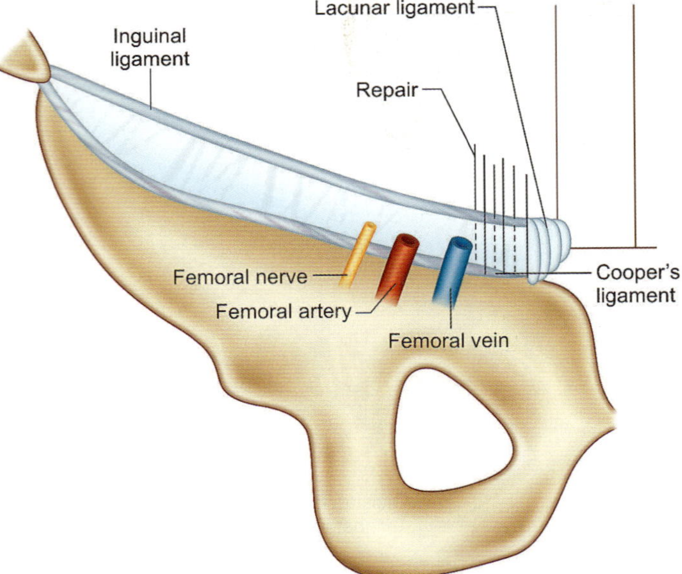

Fig. 19-115: Repair of femoral hernia.

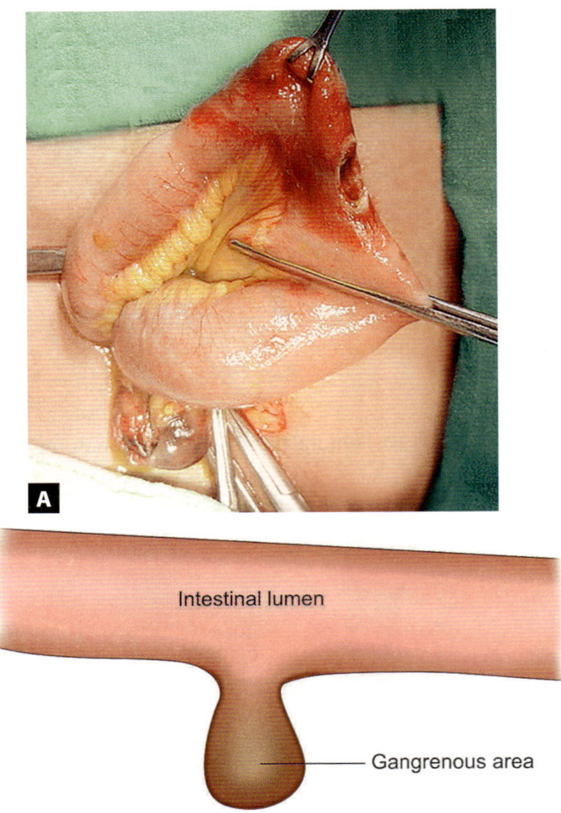

Figs. 19-116A and B: Femoral hernia Richter's type—perforated. Only part of circumference of the bowel is involved (gangrene or ischaemia) in Richter's hernia.

If bowel is gangrenous it is better to do resection by formal laparotomy incision. Other option is extending the incision vertically across into the lower abdomen to complete the resection and anastomosis. In uncontaminated hernia mesh plug is placed which is often sutured into the inguinal ligament and Cooper's ligament **(Figs. 19-115 and 19-116)**.

Mc'Evedy (Manchester) High Operation

An incision is made over the femoral canal extending vertically above the inguinal ligament. Sac is dissected from below, neck from above and repair is done from above. It gives a very good exposure of neck, fundus of sac and repair is also easier. It is done in strangulated femoral hernia.

Lotheissen's (Vienna) Operation

It is through inguinal canal approach (like for inguinal hernia). Transversalis fascia is opened and neck of the sac is identified in the femoral ring. Sac is dissected from above, neck is ligated and repair is done. If release of constriction ring is necessary then cut can be given to lacunar ligament under direct visualisation; one should not injure vessels which is (abnormal obturator artery or pubic branch of inferior epigastric artery) in close proximity to it. If difficulty arises then it is better to cut medial most part of the inguinal ligament to release the neck of the sac **(Fig. 19-117)**.

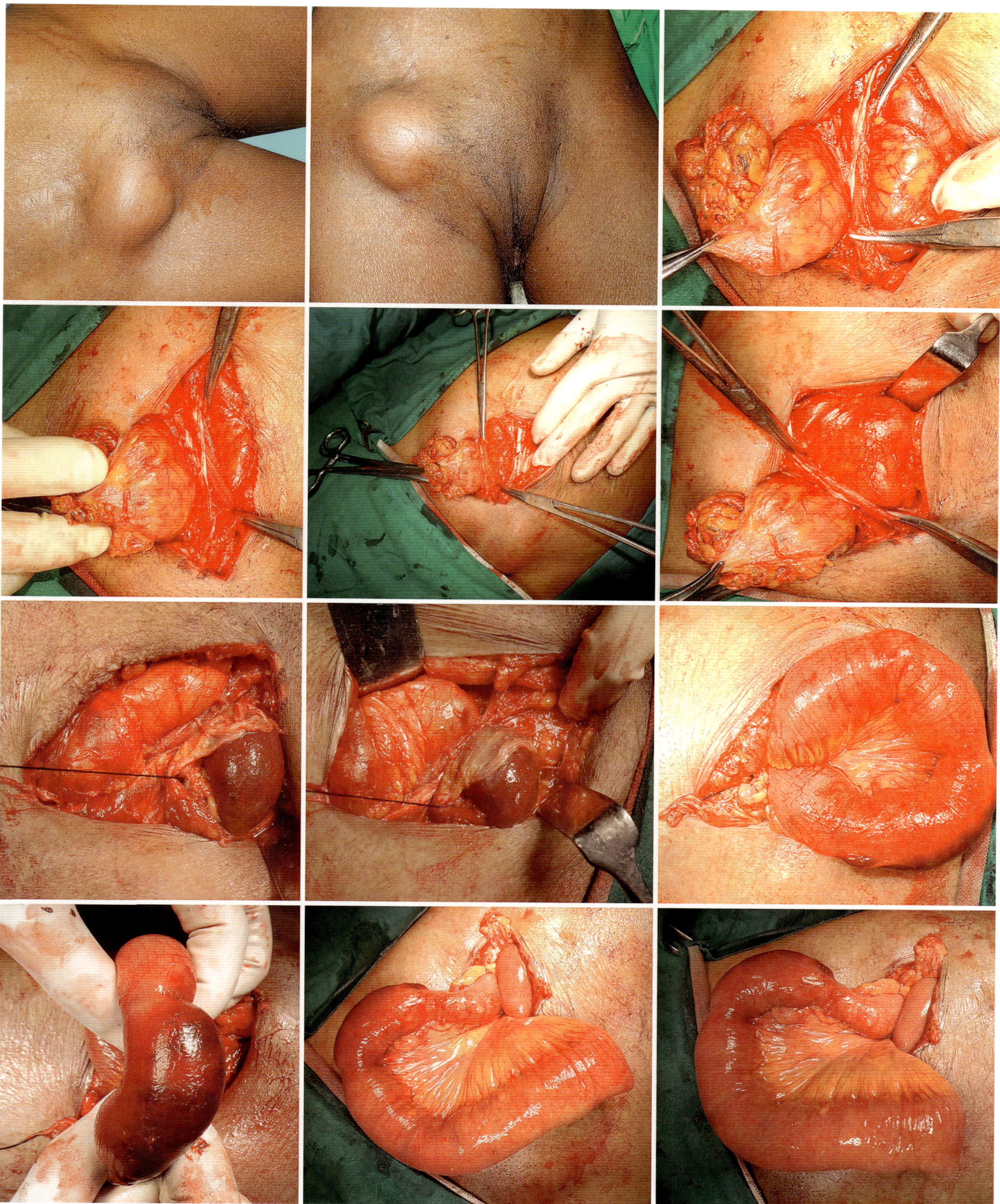

Figs. 19-117(1)

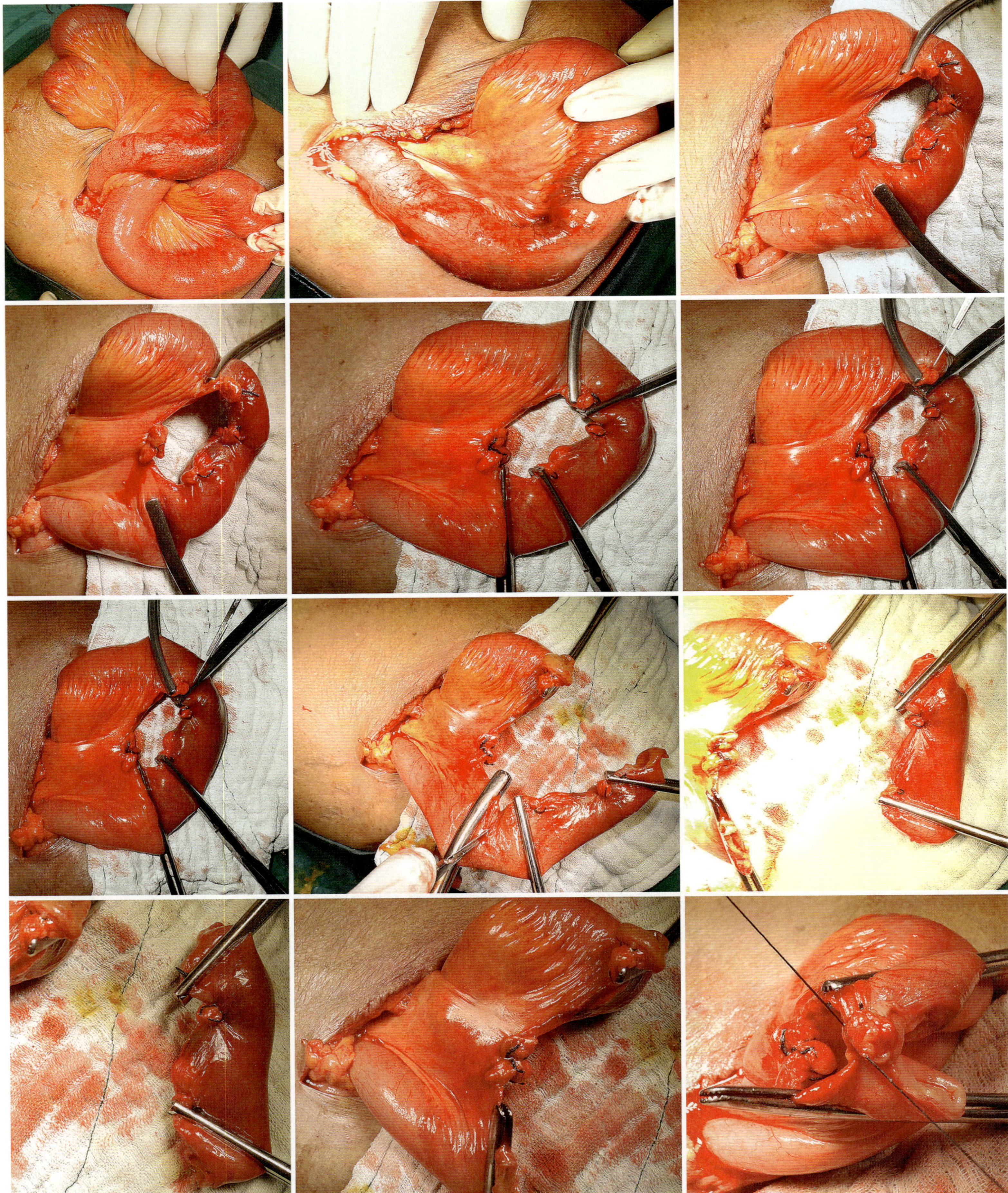

Figs. 19-117(2)

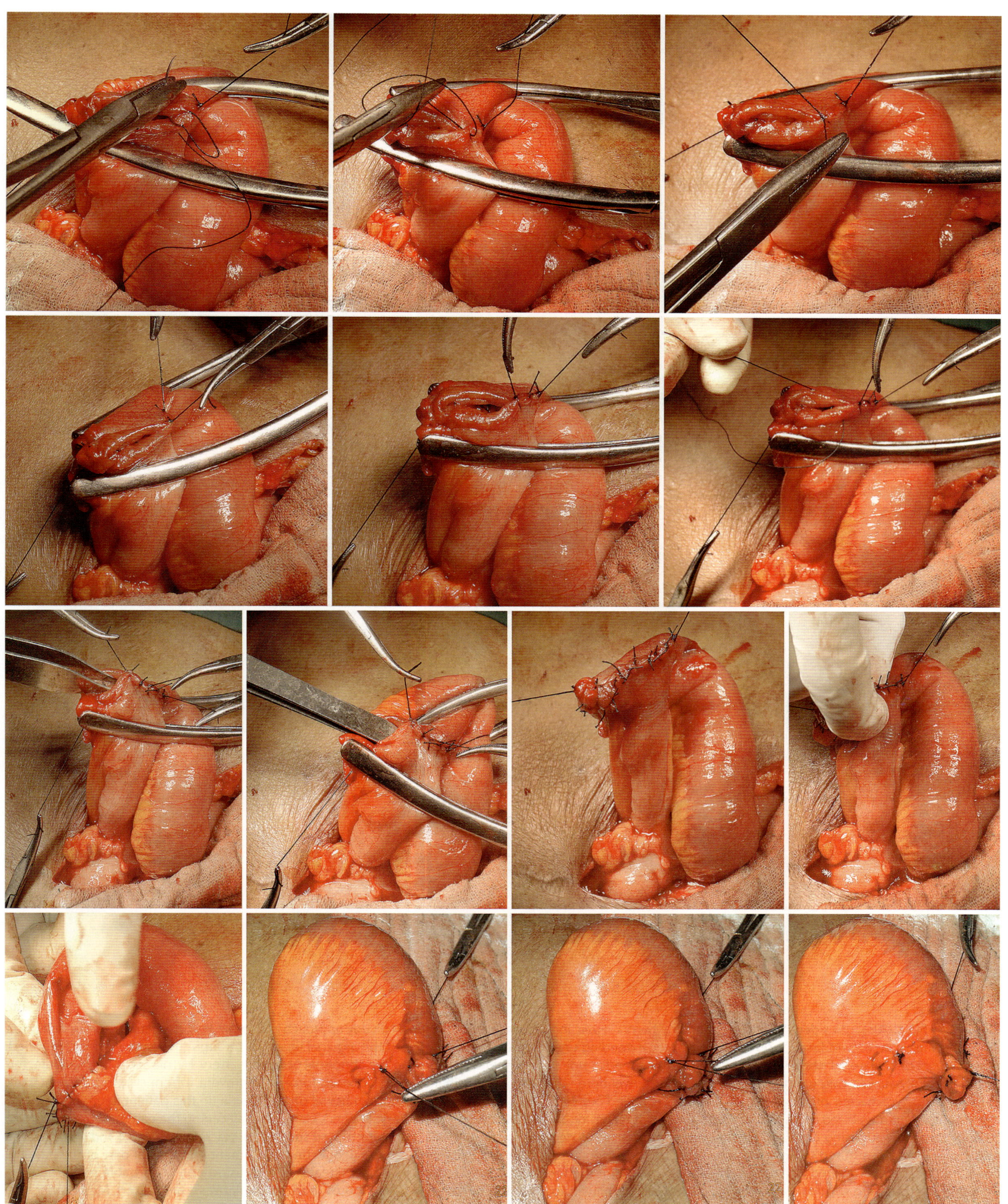

Figs. 19-117(3)

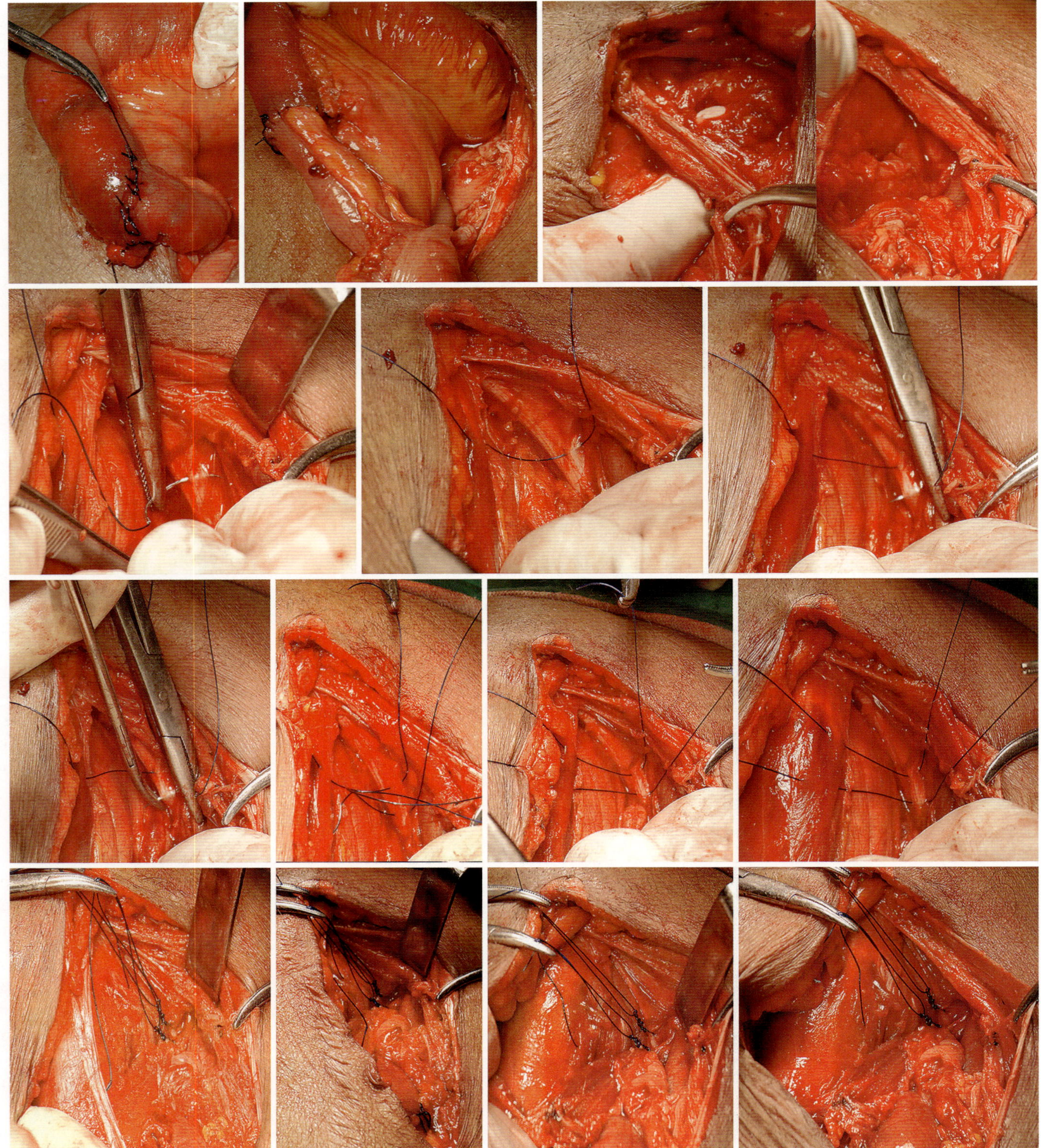

Figs. 19-117(4)

Figs. 19-117(1 to 4): Right sided strangulated femoral hernia repair. Inguinal incision is placed; McEvedy approach is also can be considered. After opening the inguinal canal, transversalis fascia is opened; hernial sac extending underneath the medial side of the inguinal ligament through the femoral ring is identified; tense sac can be released if needed by giving a cut on the medial side so as to avoid the injury to the abnormal obturator artery. Hernia sac is opened; infected fluid is carefully sucked out; gangrenous bowel (small bowel here—Richter's type) is held using Babcock's forceps to prevent it from slipping back into the peritoneal cavity; adjacent proximal and distal bowel is pulled out sufficiently to get adequate normal bowel on either side (in this patient ileum is involved). Occlusion clamps are placed to resect the ileal segment after ligating the corresponding mesentery; Kocher's clamps are placed on the gangrenous sides of the bowel; segment is cut using no. 15 blade; bowel is anastomosed as decided by the surgeon (here interrupted sutures are placed using vicryl and silk—2-zero). Mesenteric defect is sutured using interrupted silk sutures. Femoral hernia defect between Cooper's (iliopectineal) ligament and medial part of the inguinal ligament (lacunar) is repaired by Lotheissen's repair—conjoint tendon is approximated to the iliopectineal ligament using non-absorbable monofilament (polypropylene) 2-zero sutures. 2-zero or 3-zero sutures are placed to close the defect. Here box sutures (horizontal mattress) are placed. Mesh cannot be placed as it is strangulated. If femoral hernia is not obstructed or not strangulated mesh repair is the standard. Laparoscopic mesh repair is also good alternative approach in femoral hernia which is not strangulated.

Lotheissen's repair: After herniotomy, conjoined tendon is sutured to iliopectineal line (ligament) by interrupted sutures (2 or 3), using non-absorbable monofilament sutures. Care should be taken to avoid injury to femoral vein, pubic branch of obturator artery, bladder.

AK Henry's approach: Repair of bilateral femoral hernia through lower midline abdominal incision with extraperitoneal approach.

Laparoscopic approach: It is similar to inguinal hernia either through totally extraperitoneal (TEP) or transabdominal preperitoneal (TAPP) or with placement of mesh to cover the Fruchaud's myopectineal orifice.

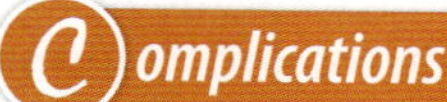

Complications

Bleeding; haematoma, abscess formation.

SPIGELIAN HERNIA

It was first described by Flemish anatomist Adriaan van den Spiegel. It is lateral ventral hernia through *Spigelian fascia* at any point along its line. *Semilunar line of Spiegel* is a line from pubic tubercle to tip of 9th costal cartilage. It marks the lateral margin of the rectus sheath. Semicircular arcuate line (fold) of Douglas is lower end of posterior lamina of rectus sheath below the umbilicus and above the pubis. Spigelian fascia is area between lateral border of the rectus muscle and external and internal oblique and transversus abdominis muscle. Spigelian hernia belt extends from line of Monro (interspinous line) for 6 cm above where spigelian hernia is very common **(Figs. 19-118 and 19-119)**.

Spigelian hernia can occur above (10%) or below (90%) the umbilicus. Below the umbilicus it occurs at the junction of the linea semilunaris and linea semicircularis. In spigelian hernia, defect is formed by internal oblique and transversus abdominis muscle. External oblique is outer to the hernial sac. A vertical or transverse incision is made. External oblique is cut vertically or transversely. Sac can be visualised deep to it. Ring often requires a release by cutting the rectus muscle medially. Sac is opened; contents are reduced; sac is ligated using 3-zero vicryl. In earlier days, defect containing internal oblique and transversus abdominis was closed with interrupted monofilament polypropylene sutures. Now retrorectus mesh placement is done prior to closing the defect.

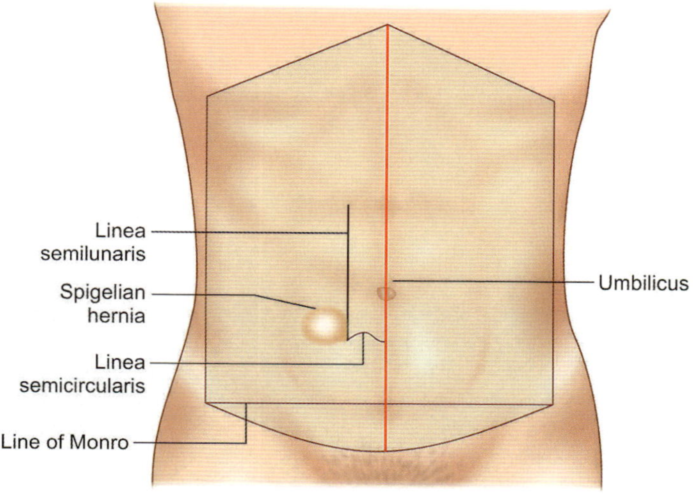

Fig. 19-118: Surgical anatomy of spigelian hernia.

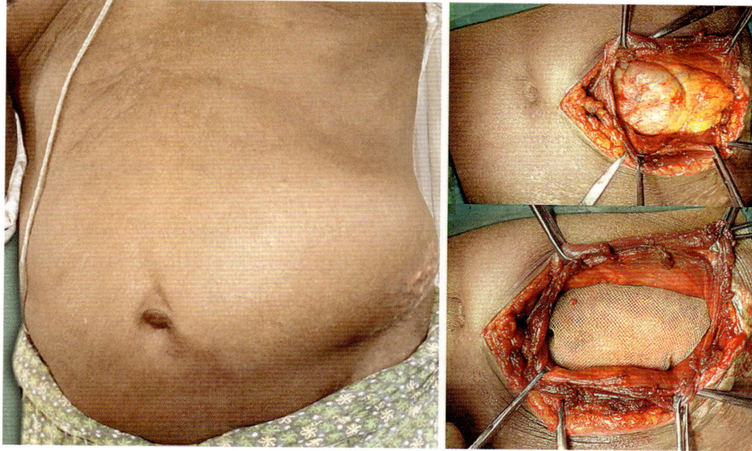

Fig. 19-119: Spigelian hernia and placing mesh after dissection.

BIOMATERIALS USED IN SURGERIES OF HERNIA

There are many biomaterials used in hernia and vascular surgeries. Its efficacy is based on its tissue response.

Response to Prosthetic Material

Inflammatory response occurs in 4 phases. They are: (1) Acute inflammation that occurs within 2–3 days and climaxes after 14 to 21 days. (2) Chronic inflammatory response seals the foreign body. (3) Foreign body reaction with mediators like PDGF, TGF-β, ILGF, EGF recruiting more inflammatory cells, fibroblasts and smooth muscle cells to promote tissue ingrowths. (4) Fibrosis—collagen rich scar tissue forms and builds a three-dimensional frame work around and through the mesh.

Prosthesis

Bursting and ultimate effective strength of the prosthetic material depends on: (1) Pore size, (2) Structural configuration and (3) Filament properties—diameter, type of polymer, monofilament or multifilament.

Classification of pore size—Type I: Pore size >75 μm, e.g. prolene lighter mesh which allows macrophages, fibroblasts, blood vessels and collagen to adhere significantly to the material thereby increases its tensile strength. Type II: Pore size less than 10 μm, e.g. ePTFE attract more histiocytes than fibroblasts, causes formation of immature, loose granulation tissue around the mesh. Type III: Macroporous material with multifilamentous or microporous component, e.g. PTFE mesh, Dacron mesh, braided polypropylene mesh. Type IV: Submicronic pore size e.g. silastic sheeting.

Maximum tensile strength required to maintain abdominal closure is 16 N/cm with normal intra-abdominal pressure being 20 kPa. Conventional prosthetic materials have greater than 32 N/cm, e.g. prolene may rupture at 131 kPa. So, true failure of prosthesis is rare. Recurrence, usually at suture line is due to weakness of prosthesis—tissue interface. Mesh of small pore size causes rigid non-elastic scar plate in tissue. Mesh of large pore size causes elastic flexible soft scar mesh which is always better.

Earlier in olden days of surgical practice, prosthetic materials made of stainless steel and tantalums were used. Usher in 1958 first used inert strong polyethylene Marlex mesh; but it was difficult to sterilise. In 1962 polypropylene which can be sterilised by autoclave was introduced. Presently meshes made of—polypropylene, polyester and polytetrafluoroethylene (PTFE) with combinations of these as composite mesh are available. All these meshes are designed to bear 4 times more than the bursting pressure of the abdominal wall.

Meshes can be *heavyweight (80 g/m²), medium weight or lightweight (<30 g/m²)*. In all these different weight mesh groups, compliance of abdominal wall (abdominal wall movement) was studied using stereography technique to prove that restriction of movement of the abdominal wall is highest in heavyweight mesh and is less with lightweight mesh. Compliance, pain and abdominal wall discomfort depends on the formation of strong scar around the mesh with shrinkage of mesh, stiffness and discomfort. Heavyweight mesh shows shrinkage up to 40%. Lightweight mesh or combination of lightweight mesh with an absorbable component [vypro (LWM with vicryl), ultrapro (LWM with monocryl)] showed less shrinkage. These meshes cannot be placed over viscera directly as it may cause bowel ingrowth into the mesh and fistula formation. Interceed antiadhesive barrier dual mesh is used to place the mesh intraperitoneally. There is theoretical possibility of carcinogenicity of heavyweight mesh which is not identified in humans until now even though it is observed in experimental studies in rats.

Meshes can be: (1) *Non-absorbable* like polypropylene or polyester or ePTFE; (2) *Absorbable* like polyglactin (vicryl); (3) *Composite* absorbable and non-absorbable like vypro with polypropylene and vicryl, ultrapro with polypropylene and absorbable poliglecaprone 25 (glycolide + e-caprolactone). ePTFE (1972) is a common material used as vascular graft. It is now used as intraperitoneal prosthesis as visceral ingrowth into the mesh is not seen. Dual Goretex ePTFE mesh is also used. Polyester meshes (mersilene by Ethicon, Dacron by Bard) are commonly used for Rives and Stoppa procedures. Polyester is softer and supple and does not stiffen and harden as much as heavyweight polypropylene. Only absorbable vicryl mesh is used in splenic and renal trauma which has got 0.5 mm pore size with 0.17 mm thickness. It is inert, non-antigenic which supports well for 60 days. It is placed over the organs using sutures. Absorbable mesh cannot be used for hernia repair **(Fig. 19-120)**.

Lightweight mesh was started by professor Schumpelick, Germany to have strength enough to bear the abdominal wall pressure and stress but flexible and elastic to move with abdominal wall and also being thin with less mass to handle easily. Composite absorbable and non-absorbable mesh is widely used now. *Vypro mesh* contains equal parts of absorbable polyglactin and non-absorbable polypropylene components. Filaments of both are twisted together and knitted to form vypro mesh to make it more elastic with stretching capacity in all directions. Polyglactin component of the mesh loses its tensile strength gradually by hydrolysis in 70–90 days. Due to large pore size of 5 mm tissue ingrowth is better thus preventing non-elastic rigid scar plate formation but to form an *elastic flexible stretchable* (30% stretchable as compared to only 8% stretch of polypropylene mesh) strong biophysical anatomical reinforcement of the defect and abdominal wall with less abdominal wall discomfort. It forms less foreign body mass. It cannot be used in contaminated field. A modified version of vypro mesh with rhombically placed violet polyglactin and polypropylene thread is often used for inguinal hernia repair. Rhomboid part keeps the mesh rigid making intraoperative manipulation easier. Similarly *Ultrapro mesh* contains equal parts of polypropylene and poliglecaprone 25 which like vypro mesh achieves flexible stable scar tissue. It is ideal for tension free repair, TAPP and TEP. Ultrapro mesh contains dyed and undyed parts **(Fig. 19-121)**.

Multilayered mesh has been developed to be placed intraperitoneally to prevent adhesion of bowel/viscera with fistula formation. Sterile multilayered thin flexible mesh contains oxidised regenerated cellulose (ORC) as 1st and innermost layer; polydioxanone (PDS) 2nd deeper layer; soft non-absorbable polypropylene mesh as 3rd deeper layer; again a layer of PDS as deepest 4th layer. First ORC layer prevents adhesions and peritoneum develops on it in 4 weeks. PDS is non-antigenic and gets absorbed in 6 months. This mesh is easier to handle, unroll, less infective, stays intact, creates flexible scar, and incorporates strongly to tissues and abdominal wall. This mesh is used in intraperitoneal placement in all incisional and ventral hernias either through open or laparoscopic methods. It is contraindicated in contaminated areas. *Dual mesh* of different types with cellulose or ePTFE as inner layer and polypropylene part as outer layer is also available for same use. These meshes should be fixed properly to abdominal wall using sutures at regular intervals of 1 cm to prevent gap between mesh and abdominal wall which may be a site of dangerous visceral interposition. Sutures are ideal although tacks are practiced by many.

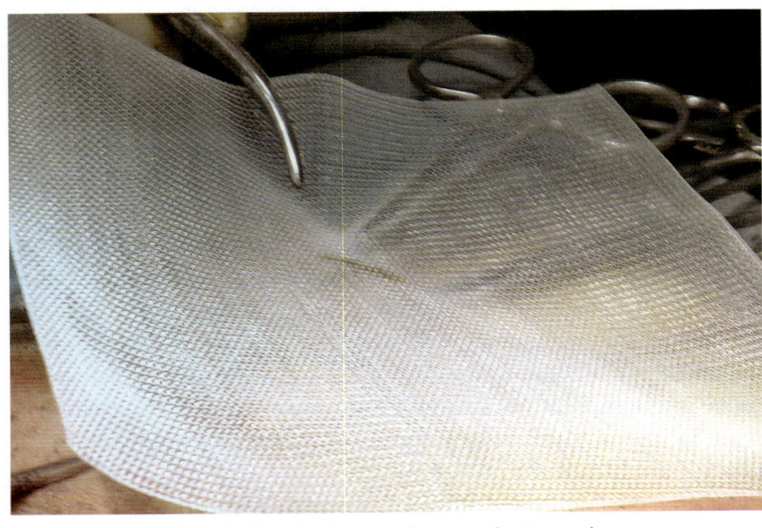

Fig. 19-120: Poylopropylene synthetic mesh.

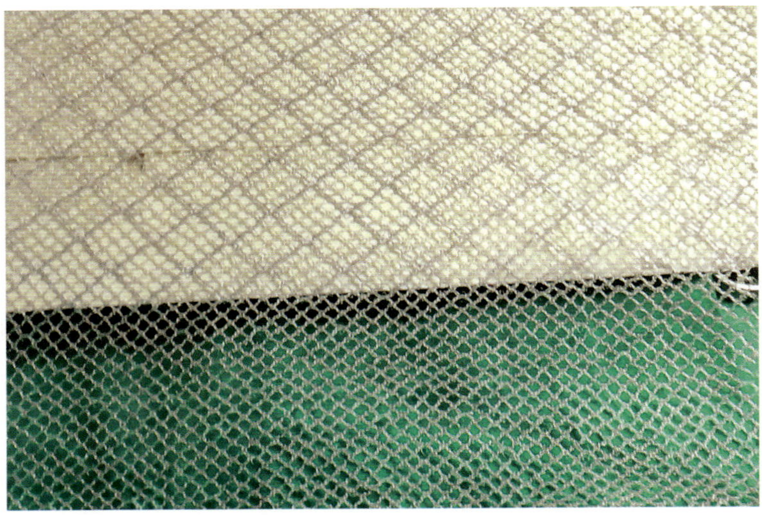

Fig. 19-121: Light weight mesh used in laparoscopic hernia surgery.

Biological meshes are available for use in contaminated fields. Cellular parts of the human or animal (porcine or bovine) tissue are removed to prevent allergic reactions and protein structure is stabilised to act like a collagen implant to scaffold the tissues by allowing natural fibroblast to proliferate. They act as extracellular matrix for ingrowth of new vessels and collagen to create bioscaffolding which controls the bacteria by presence of macrophages and antibiotics when needed in these tissues adequately. Many materials used are—porcine gut submucosa (*surgisis*), cadaver dermis, porcine dermis, bovine pericardium, fetal bovine pericardium. These disappear over the time from the host completely replacing natural collagen tissue.

Surgical technique of placing mesh are: Onlay on the myoaponeurotic fascia (like in Lichtenstein in inguinal hernia; not used in ventral hernia); Inlay is bridging of the myoaponeurotic fascia; Sublay/underlay is either preperitoneal (preferred placement) or intraperitoneal (only dual or similar mesh) placement of the mesh. Mesh should be fixed with permanent sutures preferably of the same material. It should be overlapped for 4–6 cm with normal fascia in order to obtain a solid prosthesis tissue interphase and also taking into account the shrinkage of tissue which occurs, e.g. prolene mesh can shrink up to 40% in the body.

Complications of mesh are: Infection, reaction, extrusion, nerve entrapment, abdominal wall discomfort, visceral erosion and fistula formation, inguinodynia in inguinal hernia repair, seroma formation (5–16%) may be due to potential space, lymphatic disruption, reaction to mesh.

COMPLICATIONS OF HERNIA SURGERY

Complications of hernia surgery are important as often complications may become more problematic than hernia itself. 20 years back where tissue repair was popular recurrence was the most worried complication. Now since recurrence rates have come down due to standard usage of mesh, mesh-related complications have become more common than recurrence. Inguinodynia, mesh extrusion, mesh infection, mesh erosion are the worried problems **(Fig. 19-122)**.

♦ Complications of open hernia surgery ♦ Complications of TEP/TAPP ♦ Complications of other hernia surgery—ventral/femoral	♦ Early ♦ Delayed ♦ Late ♦ Life threatening

Complications of open hernia surgery	*Complications of TEP/TAPP*
♦ Infection ♦ Neural: Groin pain, ostetitis pubis ♦ Ischaemic orchitis—due thrombosis of pampiniform venous plexus (0.5%) ♦ Injury to vas ♦ Injury to viscera ♦ Recurrence ♦ Hydrocele formation ♦ Seroma, haematoma ♦ Inguinodynia ♦ Dysejaculation: Painful, burning sensation just before/during/after ejaculation due to cremaster dysfunction or vas stricture (0.25%)	♦ Subcutaneous emphysema ♦ Pneumothorax, hypercarbia ♦ Vascular ♦ Neural ♦ Visceral ♦ Infection, ileus ♦ Conversion ♦ Recurrence

Immediate	*Late/delayed*
♦ Vascular: Injury to iliac vessels/IE vessels ♦ Visceral injury—bowel/bladder ♦ Vas injury ♦ Anaesthetic complications	♦ Seroma/haematoma ♦ Neural complications ♦ Intestinal obstruction ♦ Bowel adhesion/fistula ♦ Testicular atrophy ♦ Mesh related complications ♦ Recurrence

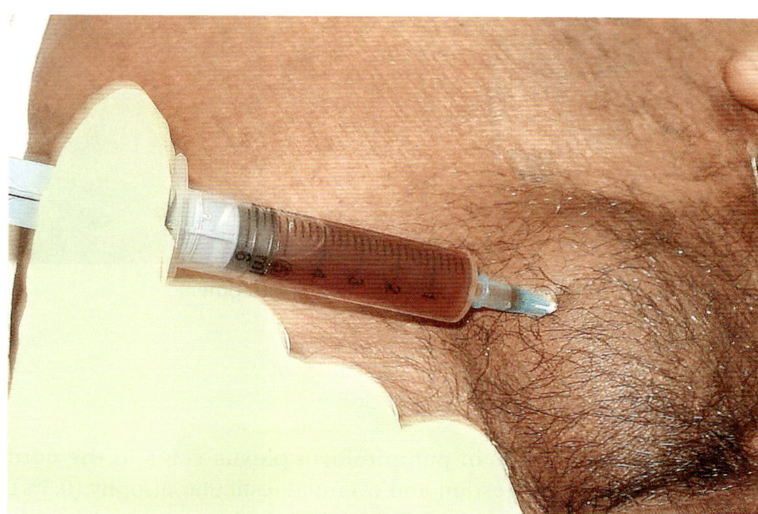

Fig. 19-122: TEP causing haematoma in the groin which is aspirated.

Inguinodynia

It is chronic inguinal pain seen in post-hernia surgery patients (30%)—whether tissue or mesh repair. *Causes are*—traction, cautery, transection, entrapment. Even though it can occur in both tissue and mesh repair, it is more observed in mesh repair especially in onlay mesh repair. It is due to entrapment of nerve in the suture or in the mesh itself or nerve gets adherent to the mesh during fibrosis (perineural fibrosis) (*Mesh inguinodynia*). It may be transient or persistent. Nerves involved are—iliohypogastric, ilioinguinal, genital branch of genitofemoral nerve, paravasal nerves. *Features are*—distressing pain in the groin which often radiates to thigh, scrotum and loin. Arch and twist mobility of pelvis reproduce the pain. Bupivacaine injection relieves the pain. Imaging/nerve conduction studies are of no use. Open method has higher (32–38%) incidence of inguinodynia than TAPP/TEP. In open hernia surgery inguinodynia has replaced recurrence as a primary complication. It is distressing discomfort to both patient and surgeon. Incidence is less in posterior or laparoscopic approach.

It is treated with analgesics/nerve block (injection of steroid, local anaesthetic agents, phenol, and alcohol)/transcutaneous stimulation/cryotherapy/radiofrequency therapy/neurectomy. Neurectomy is done via groin or suprainguinal or laparoscopic or laparotomy approach. Commonly groin approach is used. Ilioinguinal, iliohypogastric and genitofemoral nerves are carefully dissected. Nerve which is causing the problem is transected at a point where it comes out of the internal oblique muscle and proximal end should be ligated, otherwise end neuroma may form to cause recurrence of the pain. This ligated stump is buried in the internal oblique muscle. Just neurolysis may be sufficient but chances of readhesion are higher with recurrence of symptoms. In difficult cases nerve may be transected through laparotomy/laparoscopy approach **(Fig. 19-123)**.

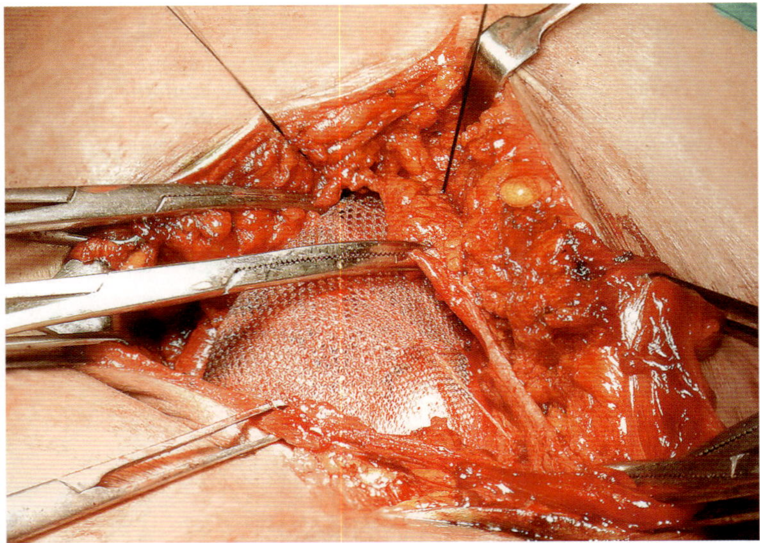

Fig. 19-123: Ilioinguinal nerve entrapment.

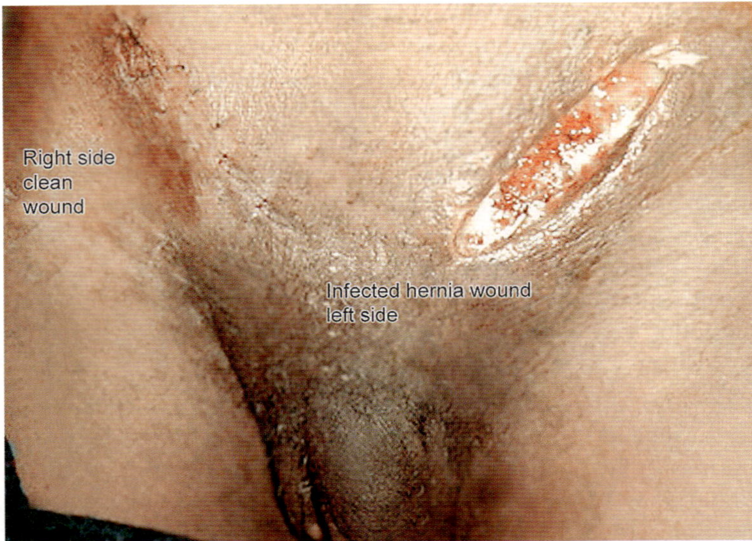

Fig. 19-124: Infection of the hernia surgery wound may increase the chance of recurrence.

Ischaemic Orchitis

It is due to thrombosis of pampiniform plexus veins in the cord leading to venous congestion and eventual testicular atrophy (0.5%). It is commonly observed while managing the recurrent hernia through anterior approach. In such situation it is advisable to use posterior approach. It can occur in laparoscopic hernia repair also.

Wound Infection

It may be surface infection of skin or subcutaneous tissue. It may be deeper infection involving the mesh. Surface infection is controlled by using specific antibiotics. There is risk of mesh extrusion in deeper infection and may require surgical removal of the mesh. Parenteral antibiotics are needed. Prophylactic antibiotic is given at perioperative period 30 minutes prior to skin incision. Focus of infection especially in the skin should be identified prior to surgery and treated properly **(Fig. 19-124)**.

Recurrence

Recurrence after hernia surgery is reduced significantly in last 15 years. It is different for different procedures. Now overall incidence is 1-3%. Bassini's repair—10%; Shouldice repair—1%; hernioplasty—1-3%; other methods—1-5%.

Tissue repair has got higher recurrence than prosthetic repair. *Causes* may be—persisting precipitating aetiologies, smoking, more tension in the wound, infection, mesh displacement, missed indirect sac, patulous internal ring **(Figs. 19-125 to 19-127)**.

Recurrence may be *medial or lateral* recurrence. Medial recurrence is common and is due to the fact that greatest tension in hernia repair occurs adjacent to the pubic tubercle.

Recurrence also often may be classified as *true or false* recurrences. If hernia occurs in inguinal region after inguinal hernia repair it is called as true recurrence. If other groin hernia occurs after inguinal hernia repair like femoral hernia or obturator or other rare types, it is called as false recurrence. But presently hernia is classified grossly as groin hernias and so all recurrences are true recurrences.

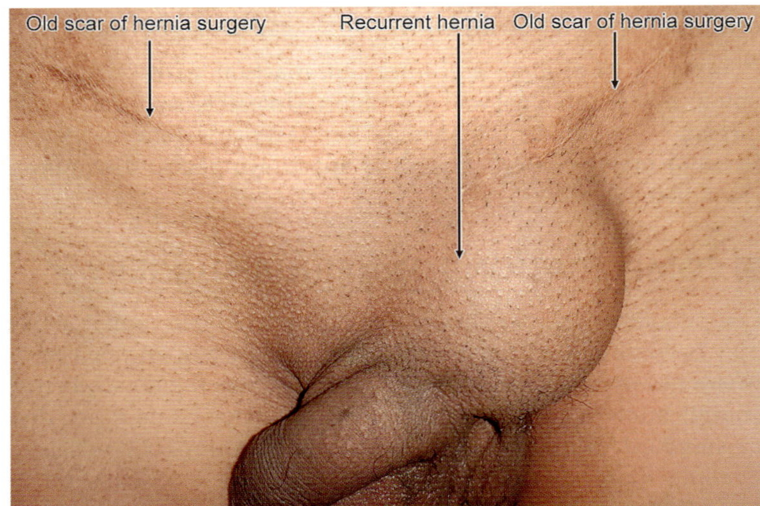

Fig. 19-125: Left sided recurrent hernia.

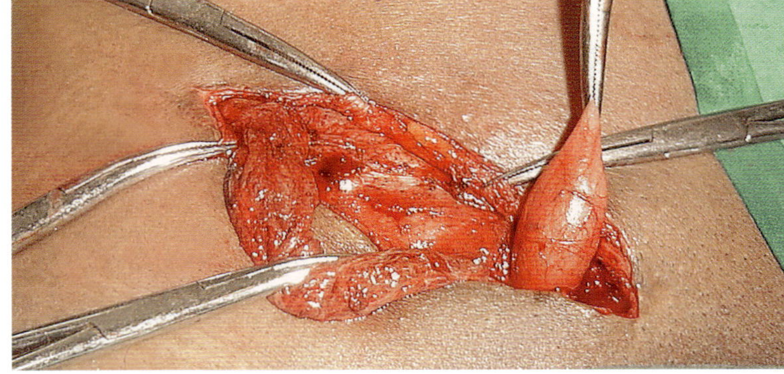

Fig. 19-126: Sac in a recurrent hernia.

Dysejaculation (0.25%)

It is burning or painful sensation just before, during or after ejaculation. It may be due to obstruction to the ejaculate flow caused by stricture in vas deferens or due to cremaster dysfunction.

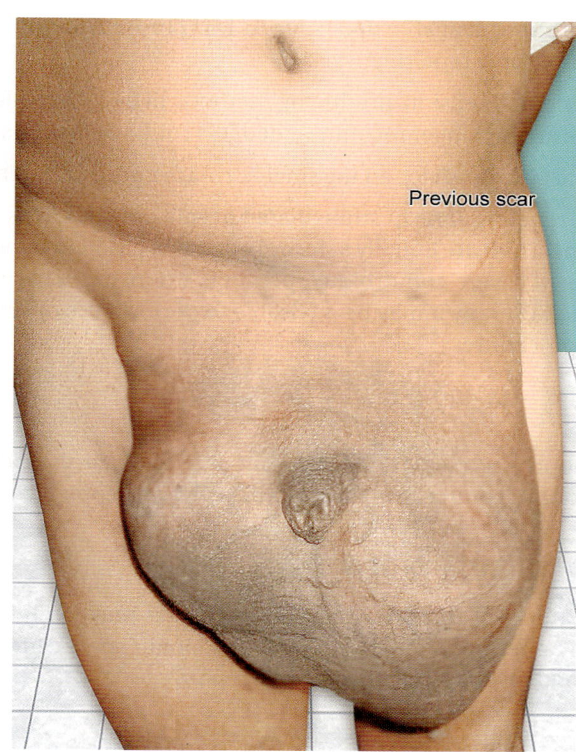

Fig. 19-127: Large recurrent hernia.

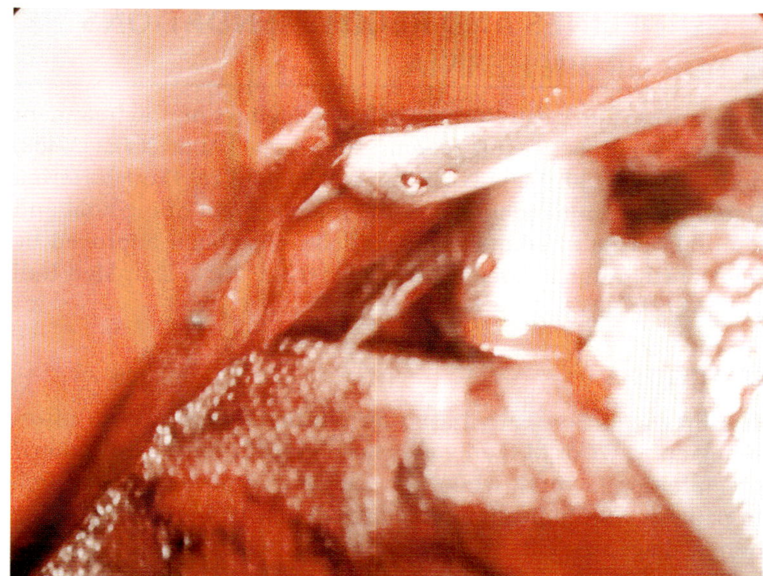

Fig. 19-128: Port site bleeding is a cumbersome problem in TEP surgery. It should be carefully controlled using bipolar cautery. If inferior epigastric vessel is the cause then it may require clipping after changing one of the 5 mm ports into 10 mm.

Hydrocele

Post-herniorrhaphy hydrocele occasionally can occur due to lymphatic obstruction. Deep and superficial rings should not be constrictive while suturing.

Haematoma or Seroma Formation

It is common. It often requires needle aspiration. Open evacuation is usually not required unless haematoma is significantly large. Often haematocele can occur. In TEP bleeding can occur from small vessels, inferior epigastric vessels, or port site. It is dealt with bipolar cautery, clipping or ligaseal **(Fig. 19-128)**.

Infection

Minor infection on the subcutaneous tissue subsides with dressing and antibiotics. Deeper infection may trouble the mesh by infecting it. Infected mesh may get extruded or may form a sinus. Such mesh has to be removed under general anaesthesia. Defect may get fibrosed or later may require a repair **(Figs. 19-129 and 19-130)**.

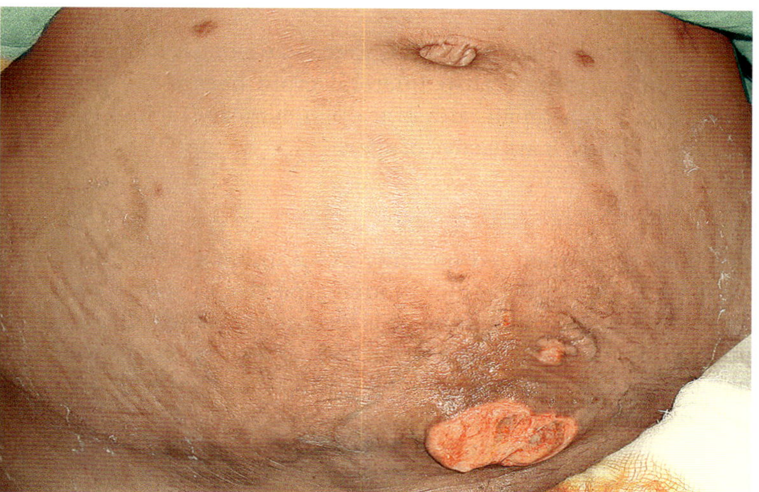

Fig. 19-129: Mesh infection forming fistula after laparoscopic ventral hernia repair.

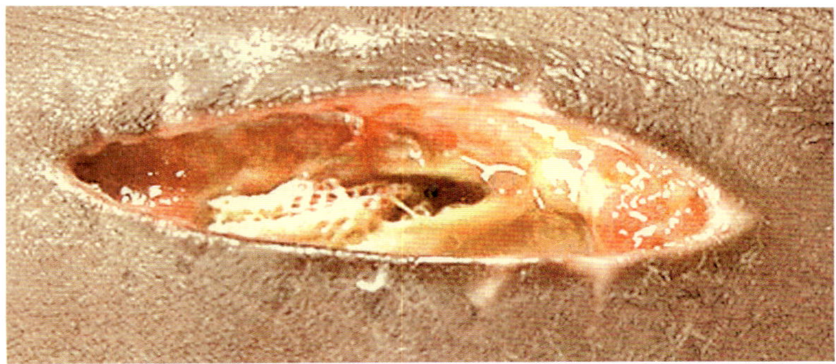

Fig. 19-130: Infection of the mesh after open inguinal hernia surgery.

Major Complications

Injury to iliac vessels, inferior epigastric vessels, pubic branch of inferior epigastric artery or abnormal obturator artery can cause severe torrential haemorrhage. It needs surgical exploration and corrective procedures like repair of injured iliac vessel or ligation of inferior epigastric vessels. Bowel or urinary bladder injury can cause fistula formation. Bowel fistula needs proper evaluation with CT fistulogram and later surgical exploration and resection of the involved segment. Injury to urinary bladder causing urinary fistula can be treated by catheterisation for 3–6 weeks. Once fistula subsides catheter can be removed safely without any problem later. If fistula persists then bladder exploration and excision of fistula tract with suturing and repair of bladder wall is done. Anaesthetic complications like pneumonia, ARDS can be occasionally life threatening.

GUIDELINES AND RECOMMENDATIONS FOR GROIN HERNIA

References: European Hernia Society guidelines on the treatment of inguinal hernia in adult patients. Hernia 2009 Aug;13(4):343-403. doi: 10.1007/s10029-009-0529-7. Epub 2009 Jul 28. Danish Hernia Database recommendations for the management of inguinal and femoral hernia in adults—This guideline has been approved by the Danish Surgical Society December 12th, 2010. Dan Med Bull 2011;58:(2):C4243.

Diagnosis

The diagnosis is mainly based on **clinical examination;** ultrasonography, CT or MRI are rarely needed (with some associations/precipitating factors), while herniography is not recommended. In patients with indicative symptoms of hernia, but no detectable hernia, diagnostic laparoscopy may be an option.

Indication

Hernia repair is recommended in the presence of symptoms affecting daily life.

In Male Patients

With minimal or absent symptoms watchful waiting is recommended; with primary unilateral or bilateral groin hernia the preferred method is mesh repair, either at open surgery (Lichtenstein) or laparoscopically, irrespective of age.

In Females

Repair is recommended not only in symptomatic but also in all asymptomatic patients (due to increased risk of strangulation in females). Laparoscopic approach is recommended whether inguinal or femoral; unilateral or bilateral. Risk of recurrence in women is higher when performing an open repair compared with a laparoscopic repair for a primary hernia.

Due to excellent exposure of the myopectineal orifice including the femoral canal during the laparoscopic dissection it is recommended that all women with a groin hernia (inguinal or femoral) should be offered a laparoscopic repair.

In Young Age

Since young age may be a risk factor for chronic pain, after inguinal hernia repair the use of mesh repair in young male patients (e.g. 18–30 years) is controversial but so far data does not support any disadvantages but rather the contrary. The use of a mesh is, therefore, recommended in all adult patients (>18 years) with indication of inguinal hernia repair.

In Recurrent Hernia

In patients with recurrent hernia with a previous open repair laparoscopic repair is preferred. Patients with recurrence after laparoscopic repair should undergo open mesh repair.

Type of Surgery

Compared to the Lichtenstein operation, laparoscopic repair is associated with less acute pain and faster recovery.

Furthermore, available data suggest less chronic long-term pain after laparoscopic repair.

Conventional tension-producing methods like Bassini, McVay or Shouldice are no longer recommended in a routine elective setting.

Use of a plug mesh for an inguinal hernia is not recommended.

Tissue repair is done in strangulated hernia or with sepsis.

TEP and TAPP are equally safe and effective in skilled hands.

In case of severe comorbidity, previous extensive pelvic surgery or radiation therapy it may be advisable to perform the operation as an open procedure.

In Bilateral Groin Hernia

Laparoscopic approach is preferred but different data show different conclusions in comparison to open versus laparoscopic.

Large Inguinoscrotal Hernia

Large inguinoscrotal or incarcerated hernia may preferably be treated by open repair, although international expert centres have shown good results after laparoscopic repair.

In Direct Hernia

Asymptomatic small direct hernias can be left to be watched carefully; large and symptomatic direct hernia should be operated. Laparoscopic or open Lichtenstein repair is used.

Both sides are operated in single sitting in open method.

Design of Mesh Used

Mesh in Open Repair

14 × 7 cm mesh with 2 cm medial overlap—Lichtenstein repair is used; below continuous sutures non-absorbable; above always interrupted sutures; folding of the mesh should be avoided; three nerves should be safeguarded.

Mesh in Laparoscopic Repair

Minimum 15 × 10 cm sized mesh should be used; larger hernia defects (direct >4 cm; indirect >4 cm)—17 × 12 cm sized mesh may be a need.

Type of Mesh

Recent data suggest that light weight meshes may be followed by less complaint after surgery although the risk of recurrence may be slightly elevated. Slitting the mesh for the passage of cord can be used in open method.

However, it is generally recommended *not to cut a slit* in the mesh in laparoscopic inguinal hernia repair.

Fixation of Mesh

It has been agreed in the database at different national meetings to use non-absorbable monofilament suture material for mesh fixation.

Fixation in Laparoscopy

Mesh fixation in laparoscopic inguinal hernia repair is controversial.

Current evidence suggests that fixation of the mesh with tacks may be followed by increased risk of acute and chronic pain and recent reports have suggested that laparoscopic repair can be performed without fixation or with glue fixation without increased risk of recurrence.

However, because of the limited amount of data, the recommendation is mesh fixation during laparoscopic repair, and this can be performed by *non-absorbable tacks*, absorbable tacks or by glue fixation. There is not yet sufficient data to support one method for another.

Anaesthesia in Hernia Surgery

Elective surgery for groin hernia should be performed in an outpatient setting, using cost-effective local anaesthesia for open mesh repair. General anaesthesia can also be used for open.

General anaesthesia is used and recommended for laparoscopic repair.

Note: Spinal anaesthesia is not recommended.

Antibiotic Need in Hernia Surgery

Routine prophylactic antibiotics are not indicated.
In patients with increased risk of infections antibiotics may be indicated, although the evidence for this is lacking.

Antithrombotic Prophylaxis in Groin Hernia Surgery

In open hernia repair
There are no guidelines available for open inguinal hernia repair, and for this operation, routine prophylaxis is not recommended.

In laparoscopic hernia repair
LMWH is recommended if >2 of following criteria is present—Duration of surgery >1 hour; History of venous thromboembolism, congestive heart failure; Age >40 years; Previous myocardial infarction, immobility, HRT, varicose veins, OCP use, multiparity, peripartum; Cancer, chronic renal failure, inflammatory bowel disease; obesity.

Regime: Single perioperative dose of LMWH.

Hospital Stay

Inguinal hernia surgery as day surgery is as safe and effective as inpatient treatment and more cost effective. This applies for all patients including selected elderly and ASA-III-patients, but may depend on local factors such as social backup, etc. It is therefore recommended that inguinal hernia repair is performed in an outpatient setting unless argued otherwise from specific factors.

Convalescence and Restrictions

It depends on postoperative pain and operative approach—open/laparoscopic. There is no evidence supporting prolonged convalescence periods to avoid recurrence, and patients can therefore be active immediately after surgery when pain is not a hindrance.

Treatment of Chronic Pain (3 Months After Repair)

Surgical treatment is recommended only after 12 months. Neurectomy or mesh removal may be the need.